BNF for children

2009

The essential resource for clinical use of medicines in children

bnfc.org

Published by
BMJ Group
Tavistock Square, London WC1H 9JP, UK

RPS Publishing
RPS Publishing is the wholly-owned publishing organisation of the Royal Pharmaceutical Society of Great Britain
1 Lambeth High Street, London, SE1 7JN, UK

RCPCH Publications Ltd
5–11 Theobalds Road, London WC1X 8SH, UK

Copyright © BMJ Group, RPS Publishing, RCPCH Publications Ltd 2009

ISBN: 978 0 85369 847 0

ISSN: 1747-5503

Printed by GGP Media GmbH, Pössneck, Germany

A catalogue record for this book is available from the British Library.

Paper copies may be obtained through any bookseller or direct from:

RPS Publishing
c/o Macmillan Distribution
Stratton Business Park
Brunel Rd
Houndmills
Basingstoke
RG21 6XS
UK
Tel: +44 (0) 1256 302 692
Fax: +44 (0) 1256 812 558
E-mail: orders@macmillan.co.uk
www.pharmpress.com

RPS Publishing also supplies *BNF for Children* in digital formats suitable for standalone use and for use on a personal digital assistant (PDA).

Distribution of BNFCs
The UK health departments distribute BNFCs to NHS hospitals, doctors, dental surgeons, and community pharmacies. In England BNFCs are mailed individually to NHS general practitioners and community pharmacies; contact the DH Publication Orderline for extra copies or changes relating to mailed BNFCs
Tel: 08701 555 455
In **Wales** telephone the Business Services Centre
Tel: 01495 332 000
For further information on the supply of copies of the BNFC to NHS organisations, see http://tinyurl.com/2uebpp

The *BNF for Children* is for use by health professionals engaged in prescribing, dispensing, and administering medicines to children. It has been prepared under the guidance of the Paediatric Formulary Committee.

BNF for Children has been constructed using robust procedures for gathering, assessing and assimilating information on paediatric drug treatment. It is, however, expected that the reader will be relying on appropriate professional knowledge and expertise to interpret the contents in the context of the circumstances of the individual child. *BNF for Children* should be used in conjunction with other appropriate and up-to-date literature and, where necessary, supplemented by expert advice. *Special care is required in managing childhood conditions with unlicensed medicines or with licensed medicines for unlicensed uses.*

Responsibility for the appropriate use of medicines lies solely with the individual health professional.

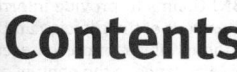

Contents

Preface iv
Acknowledgements v
Editorial Staff vi
Paediatric Formulary Committee 2008–2009 vi
How *BNF for Children* is constructed viii
How to use *BNF for Children* xi
Changes for this edition xiv
Name changes xvii
General guidance 1
Prescription writing 5
Supply of medicines 7
Emergency supply of medicines 9
Drug treatment in children 11
Prescribing in hepatic impairment 12
Prescribing in renal impairment 13
Prescribing in pregnancy 15
Prescribing in breast-feeding 16
Prescribing Controlled Drugs 17
Adverse reactions to drugs 21
Prescribing in palliative care 24
Prescribing in dental practice 31
Drugs and sport 32
Emergency treatment of poisoning 33

Notes on drugs and Preparations
  1: Gastro-intestinal system 49
  2: Cardiovascular system 96
  3: Respiratory system 167
  4: Central nervous system 211
  5: Infections 295
  6: Endocrine system 417
  7: Obstetrics, gynaecology, and urinary-tract disorders 472
  8: Malignant disease and immunosuppression 496
  9: Nutrition and blood 528
  10: Musculoskeletal and joint diseases 599
  11: Eye 620
  12: Ear, nose, and oropharynx 642
  13: Skin 663
  14: Immunological products and vaccines 725
  15: Anaesthesia 761

Appendixes and indices
Appendix 1: Interactions 793
Appendix 2: Borderline substances 878
Appendix 3: Cautionary and advisory labels for dispensed medicines 918
Appendix 4: Intravenous infusions for neonatal intensive care 921

Dental Practitioners' Formulary 924
Nurse Prescribers' Formulary 925
Non-medical prescribing 928
Index of manufacturers 929
Index 945
Medical emergencies in the community .... Inside back cover

Preface

BNF for Children aims to provide prescribers, pharmacists and other healthcare professionals with sound up-to-date information on the use of medicines for treating children.

A joint publication of the British Medical Association, the Royal Pharmaceutical Society of Great Britain, the Royal College of Paediatrics and Child Health, and the Neonatal and Paediatric Pharmacists Group, *BNF for Children* ('BNFC') is published under the authority of a Paediatric Formulary Committee.

Many areas of paediatric practice have suffered from inadequate information on effective medicines. BNFC addresses this significant knowledge gap by providing practical information on the use of medicines in children of all ages from birth to adolescence. *Medicines for Children* (RCPCH Publications Ltd) and the *British National Formulary* itself form the basis for BNFC. Information in BNFC has been validated against emerging evidence, best-practice guidelines, and crucially, advice from a network of clinical experts.

Drawing information from manufacturers' literature where appropriate, BNFC also includes a great deal of advice that goes beyond marketing authorisations (product licences). This is necessary because licensed indications frequently do not cover the clinical needs of children; in some cases, products for use in children need to be specially manufactured or imported. Careful consideration has been given to establishing the clinical need for unlicensed interventions with respect to the evidence and experience of their safety and efficacy; local paediatric formularies, clinical literature and national information resources have been invaluable in this process.

BNFC has been designed for rapid reference and the information presented has been carefully selected to aid decisions on prescribing, dispensing and administration of medicines. Less detail is given on areas such as malignant disease and the very specialist use of medicines generally undertaken in tertiary centres. BNFC should be interpreted in the light of professional knowledge and it should be supplemented as necessary by specialised publications. Information is also available from medicines information services (see inside front cover).

The website (bnfc.org) includes additional information of relevance to healthcare professionals. BNFC is also available on other digital platforms.

BNFC aims to provide information suited to the needs of the clinician and recognises that, although this edition represents a considerable advance in the content and presentation of information on the paediatric use of medicines, further changes will be necessary. Comments from healthcare professionals are therefore very welcome and should be sent to:

British National Formulary Publications, Royal Pharmaceutical Society of Great Britain, 1 Lambeth High Street, London SE1 7JN. bnfc@bnf.org

Acknowledgements

The Paediatric Formulary Committee is grateful to individuals and organisations that have provided advice and information to the *BNF for Children*.

The principal contributors for this edition were:
I. H. Ahmed-Jushuf, M. N. Badminton, S. Bailey, T. G. Barrett, D. N. Bateman, G. D. L. Bates, H. Bedford, R. M. Bingham, I. W. Booth, L. Brook, K. G. Brownlee, R. J. Buckley, M. Burch, I. F. Burgess, R. Carr, T.D. Cheetham, A.J. Cotgrove, J. B. S. Coulter, B. G. Craig, S. M. Creighton, J. H. Cross, A. Dhawan, P. N. Durrington, A. Durward, A.B. Edgar, J.A. Edge, D. A. C. Elliman, N.D. Embleton, J. Gray, J. W. Gregory, P.Gringras, J. Guillebaud, J. P. Harcourt, P. J. Helms, R. F. Howard, R. G. Hull, H. R. Jenkins, B.A. Judd, C. J. H. Kelnar, P. T. Khaw, P. J. Lee, T.H. Lee, S. Lewis-Jones, E. G. H. Lyall, A. MacDonald, D. J. Macrae, P. S. Malone, S.D. Marks, A. G. Marson, A. Y. Manzur, P.J. McKiernan, E. Miller, C. Moss, P. Mulholland, J. M. Neuberger, K. K. Nischal, C. Y. Ng, L. P. Omerod, J. Y. Paton, G. A. Pearson, M.M. Ramsay, J. M. Rennie, I. A. G. Roberts, J. Rogers, K. E. Rogstad, P. C. Rubin, J. W. Sander, N. J. Scolding, M. R. Sharland, N. J. Shaw, G. J. Shortland, O. F. W. Stumper, A. G. Sutcliffe, A. Sutherland, C.J. Taylor, E.A. Taylor, M. A. Thomson, J. A. Vale, J. O. Warner, D.A. Warrell, N. J. A. Webb, A.D. Weeks, R. Welbury, W.P. Whitehouse, C. E. Willoughby, C. Wren, A. Wright, M. M. Yaqoob and S. M. Zuberi.

M.J. Kendall, senior medical adviser for BNF Publications has also provided valuable assistance.

Members of the British Association of Dermatologists Therapy Guidelines Subcommittee, H.K. Bell, L. C. Fuller, J. Hughes, S. Lawton, J. Lear, N.J. Levell, A.J. McDonagh, M.J. Tidman, P.D. Yesudian, and M. F. M. Mustapa (Secretariat) have provided valuable advice.

Members of the Advisory Committee on Malaria Prevention, B. A. Bannister, R. H. Behrens, P. L. Chiodini, F. Genasi, L. Goodyer, D. Hill, R. Jecock, G. Kassianos, D. G. Lalloo, G. Lea, G. Pasvol, M. Powell, D. V. Shingadia, D. A. Warrell, C. J. M. Whitty, and C. Lucas (Secretariat) have also provided valuable advice.

R. Suvarna and colleagues at the MHRA have provided valuable assistance.

Correspondents in the pharmaceutical industry have provided information on new products and commented on products in the *BNF for Children*. NHS Prescription Services have supplied the prices of products in the *BNF for Children*.

Numerous doctors, pharmacists, nurses and others have sent comments and suggestions.

The *BNF for Children* has valuable access to the *Martindale* data banks by courtesy of S. Sweetman and staff.

J. E. Macintyre and staff provided valuable technical assistance

C. Adetola, N. Bansal, A. Breewood, L.M. Britton, I.M. Chiwele, M. Davis, C. Fischetti, S. Foad, E.H. Glover, D.T.H. Griffiths, T. Hamp, J. Humphreys, J.M. James, L.K. Kearney, E. Laughton, A. McLaughlin, A. Melen, H.M.N. Neill, A. Ohene-Djan, O. Ojeleye, A. Parkin, R. Sooriakumaran, R. G. Taljaard, and E.J. Tong provided considerable assistance during the production of this edition of *BNF for Children*.

Xpage have provided technical assistance with the editorial database and typesetting software.

Editorial Staff

Managing Editor: Knowledge Creation
John Martin *BPharm, PhD, MRPharmS*

Assistant Editors

Leigh-Anne Claase *BSc, PhD, MRPharmS*

Bryony Jordan *BSc, DipPharmPract, MRPharmS*

Colin R. Macfarlane *BPharm, MSc, MRPharmS*

Allison F. Patterson *BPharm, MRPharmS*

Rachel S. M. Ryan *BPharm, MRPharmS*

Shama M. S. Wagle *BPharm, DipPharmPract, MRPharmS*

Staff Editors

Onatefe Akporobaro-Iwudibia *MPharm, MRPharmS*

Sejal Amin *BPharm, MSc, MRPharmS*

Angela K. Bennett *MPharm, DipPharmPract, MRPharmS*

Susan E. Clarke *BPharm, DipClinPharm, MRPharmS*

Julia A. Dickin *MPharm, MRPharmS*

Belén Granell Villen *BSc, PGDipClinPharm, MRPharmS*

Manjula Halai *BScChem, MPharm, MRPharmS*

Emma E. Harris *MPharm, DipPharmPract, MRPharmS*

Amy E. Harvey *MPharm, PGDipCommPharm, MRPharmS*

Paul S. Maycock *MPharm, DipPharmPract, MRPharmS*

Elizabeth Nix *DipPharm(NZ), MRPharmS*

Rupal M. Patel *BSc, MRPharmS*

Claire L. Preston *BPharm, MRPharmS*

Shaistah J. Qureshi *MPharm, MRPharmS*

Vinaya K. Sharma *BPharm, MSc, PGDipPIM, MRPharmS*

Editorial Assistant
Jennifer L. Palmer *RegPharmTech*

Senior BNF Administrator
Heidi Homar *BA*

Administrative Assistant
Cristina Lopez-Bueno *BA*

Managing Editor: Digital Development and Delivery
Cornelia Schnelle *MPhil*

Knowledge Systems
Robert C. Buckingham *BSc*
Digital Development Assistant
Philip D. Lee *BSc, PhD*
Digital Development Editor

Sarah Peck *BSc*
Terminologist
Zephyr M. Wastell
Digital Development Assistant

Head of Publishing Services
John Wilson

BNF Publishing Director
Duncan S.T. Enright *MA, PGCE, MInstP, FIDM*

Managing Director, RPS Publishing
Robert Bolick *BA, MA*

Paediatric Formulary Committee 2008–2009

Chair
George W. Rylance
MB, FRCPCH

Committee Members
Jeffrey K. Aronson
MA, MBChB, DPhil, FRCP, FBPharmacolS, FFPM

Judith H. Cope
BPharm, MSc, MRPharmS

Ian Costello
BPharm, MSc, MRPharmS

Simon Keady
BSc, MRPharmS, SP

Martin J. Kendall
MB, ChB, MD, FRCP, FFPM (Chair, Formulary Development Committee)

Neena Modi
MB, ChB, MD, FRCP, FRCPCH

Matthew J. Thatcher
MBBS, FRCS, DRCOG, DMRD

William G. van't Hoff
BSc, MB, MD, FRCPCH, FRCP

David W. Wall
MB, ChB, PGCE, MMEd, PhD, FRCP, FRCGP

Edward R. Wozniak
BSc, MB, BS, FRCP, FRCPCH, DCH

Observers
Jane Houghton
RGN, RSCN, DNCert, MSc

Anita MacDonald
PhD, BSc, RD

Executive Secretary
Heidi Homar
BA

Dental Advisory Group 2008–2009

Chair
David Wray
MD, BDS, MB ChB, FDSRCPS, FDSRCS Ed, F MedSci

Committee Members
Christine Arnold
BDS, DDPHRCS, MCDH

Barry Cockcroft
BDS, FFDS (Eng)

Duncan S.T. Enright *MA, PGCE, MInstP, FIDM*

Martin J. Kendall
OBE, MD, FRCP, FFPM

Lesley P. Longman
BSc, BDS, FDSRCS Ed, PhD

John Martin
BPharm, PhD, MRPharmS

Michelle Moffat
BDS, MFDS RCS Ed, M Paed Dent RPCS, FDS (Paed Dent) RSC Ed

Richard J. Oliver
BDS, BSc, PhD, FDSRCPS, FDS (OS) RCPS

Rachel S.M. Ryan
BPharm, MRPharmS

Secretary
Arianne J. Matlin
MA, MSc, PhD

Executive Secretary
Heidi Homar
BA

> Advice on dental practice
> The **British Dental Association** has contributed to the advice on medicines for dental practice through its representatives on the Dental Advisory Group.

Nurse Prescribers' Advisory Group 2008–2009

Chair
Nicky A. Cullen
PhD, RGN

Committee Members
Una J. Adderley
MSc, BA, RGN, DN

Rebecca F. Cheatle
BSc, RGN

Michele L. Cossey
BPharm, MSc, MRPharmS

Molly Courtenay
PhD, MSc, Cert Ed, BSc, RGN

Duncan S.T. Enright
MA, PGCE, MInstP, FIDM

Penny M. Franklin
RN, RCN, RSCPHN(HV), MA, PGCE

Margaret F. Helliwell
MB, BS, BSc, MFPHM

Bryony Jordan
BSc, DipPharmPract, MRPharmS

Martin J. Kendall
OBE, MD, FRCP, FFPM

Fiona Lynch
BSc, MSc, RGN, RSCN

John Martin
BPharm, PhD, MRPharmS

Paul S. Maycock
MPharm, DipPharmPract, MRPharmS

Maureen P. Morgan
RN, RHV, MBA

Elizabeth J. Plastow
RMN, RGN, RSCPHN(HV), MSc, PGDipEd

Paul G.H. Robinson

Gul Root
BSc, MRPharmS, DMS

Jill M. Shearer
BSc, RGN, RM

Rabina Tindale
RN, RSCN, BSc, DipAEN, PGCE

Vicky Vidler
MA, RGN, RSCN

Executive Secretary
Heidi Homar
BA

How *BNF for Children* is constructed

BNF for Children (BNFC) is unique in bringing together authoritative, independent guidance on best practice with clinically validated drug information, enabling healthcare professionals to select safe and effective medicines for individual children.

Information in BNFC has been validated against emerging evidence, best-practice guidelines, and advice from a network of clinical experts. BNFC includes a great deal of advice that goes beyond marketing authorisations (product licences or summaries of product characteristics). This is necessary because licensed indications frequently do not cover the clinical needs of children; in some cases, products for use in children need to be specially manufactured or imported. Careful consideration has been given to establishing the clinical need for unlicensed interventions with respect to the evidence and experience of their safety and efficacy.

Hundreds of changes are made between editions, and the most clinically significant changes are listed at the front of each edition (p. xiv).

Paediatric Formulary Committee

The Paediatric Formulary Committee (PFC) is responsible for the content of BNFC. The PFC includes a neonatologist and paediatricians appointed by the Royal College of Paediatrics and Child Health, paediatric pharmacists appointed by the Royal Pharmaceutical Society of Great Britain and the Neonatal and Paediatric Pharmacists Group, doctors appointed by the BMJ Publishing Group, a GP appointed by the Royal College of General Practitioners, and representatives from the Medicines and Healthcare products Regulatory Agency (MHRA) and the UK health departments. The PFC decides on matters of policy and reviews amendments to BNFC in the light of new evidence and expert advice. The Committee meets every 6 months and each member also receives proofs of all BNFC chapters for review before publication.

Dental Advisory Group

The Dental Advisory Group oversees the preparation of advice on the drug management of dental and oral conditions; the group includes representatives from the British Dental Association.

Editorial team

BNFC staff editors are pharmacists with a sound understanding of how drugs are used in clinical practice, including paediatrics. Each staff editor is responsible for editing, maintaining, and updating specific chapters of BNFC. During the publication cycle the staff editors review information in BNFC against a variety of sources (see below).

Amendments to the text are drafted when the editors are satisfied that any new information is reliable and relevant. The draft amendments are passed to expert advisers for comment and then presented to the Paediatric Formulary Committee for consideration. Additionally, for each edition, sections are chosen from every chapter for thorough review. These planned reviews aim to verify all the information in the selected sections and to draft any amendments to reflect current best practice.

Staff editors prepare the text for publication and undertake a number of checks on the knowledge at various stages of the production.

Expert advisers

BNFC uses about 80 expert clinical advisers (including doctors, pharmacists, nurses, and dentists) throughout the UK to help with the production of each edition. The role of these expert advisers is to review existing text and to comment on amendments drafted by the staff editors. These clinical experts help to ensure that BNFC remains reliable by:

- commenting on the relevance of the text in the context of best clinical practice in the UK;

- checking draft amendments for appropriate interpretation of any new evidence;
- providing expert opinion in areas of controversy or when reliable evidence is lacking;
- advising on areas where BNFC diverges from summaries of product characteristics;
- advising on the use of unlicensed medicines or of licensed medicines for unlicensed uses ('off-label' use);
- providing independent advice on drug interactions, prescribing in hepatic impairment, renal impairment, pregnancy, breast-feeding, neonatal care, palliative care, and the emergency treatment of poisoning.

In addition to consulting with regular advisers, BNFC calls on other clinical specialists for specific developments when particular expertise is required.

BNFC also works closely with a number of expert bodies that produce clinical guidelines. Drafts or pre-publication copies of guidelines are routinely received for comment and for assimilation into BNFC.

Sources of BNFC information

BNFC uses a variety of sources for its information; the main ones are shown below.

Summaries of product characteristics   BNFC receives summaries of product characteristics (SPCs) of all new products as well as revised SPCs for existing products. The SPCs are a key source of product information and are carefully processed, despite the ever-increasing volume of information being issued by the pharmaceutical industry. Such processing involves:

- verifying the approved names of all relevant ingredients including 'non-active' ingredients (BNFC is committed to using approved names and descriptions as laid down by the Medicines Act);
- comparing the indications, cautions, contra-indications, and side-effects with similar existing drugs. Where these are different from the expected pattern, justification is sought for their inclusion or exclusion;
- seeking independent data on the use of drugs in pregnancy and breast-feeding;
- incorporating the information into BNFC using established criteria for the presentation and inclusion of the data;
- checking interpretation of the information by two staff editors before submitting to a senior editor; changes relating to doses receive an extra check;
- identifying potential clinical problems or omissions and seeking further information from manufacturers or from expert advisers;
- careful validation of any areas of divergence of BNFC from the SPC before discussion by the Committee (in the light of supporting evidence);
- constructing, with the help of expert advisers, a comment on the role of the drug in the context of similar drugs.

Much of this processing is applicable to the following sources as well.

Expert advisers   The role of expert clinical advisers in providing the appropriate clinical context for all BNFC information is discussed above.

Literature   Staff editors monitor core medical, paediatric, and pharmaceutical journals. Research papers and reviews relating to drug therapy are carefully processed. When a difference between the advice in BNFC and the paper is noted, the new information is assessed for reliability and relevance to UK clinical practice. If necessary, new text is drafted and discussed with expert advisers and the Paediatric Formulary Committee. BNFC enjoys a close working relationship with a number of national information providers.

Systematic reviews   BNFC has access to various databases of systematic reviews (including the Cochrane Library and various web-based resources). These are used for answering specific queries, for reviewing existing text and for constructing new text. Staff editors receive training in critical appraisal, literature evaluation, and search strategies. Reviews published in Clinical Evidence are used to validate BNFC advice.

Consensus guidelines The advice in BNFC is checked against consensus guidelines produced by expert bodies. A number of bodies make drafts or pre-publication copies of the guidelines available to BNFC; it is therefore possible to ensure that a consistent message is disseminated. BNFC routinely processes guidelines from the National Institute for Health and Clinical Excellence (NICE), the Scottish Medicines Consortium (SMC), and the Scottish Intercollegiate Guidelines Network (SIGN).

Reference sources Paediatric formularies and reference sources are used to provide background information for the review of existing text or for the construction of new text. The BNFC team works closely with the editorial team that produces *Martindale: The Complete Drug Reference*. BNFC has access to *Martindale* information resources and each team keeps the other informed of significant developments and shifts in the trends of drug usage.

Statutory information BNFC routinely processes relevant information from various Government bodies including Statutory Instruments and regulations affecting the Prescription only Medicines Order. Official compendia such as the British Pharmacopoeia and its addenda are processed routinely to ensure that BNFC complies with the relevant sections of the Medicines Act.

BNFC maintains close links with the Home Office (in relation to controlled drug regulations) and the Medicines and Healthcare products Regulatory Agency (including the British Pharmacopoeia Commission). Safety warnings issued by the Commission on Human Medicines (CHM) and guidelines on drug use issued by the UK health departments are processed as a matter of routine.

Relevant professional statements issued by the Royal Pharmaceutical Society of Great Britain are included in BNFC as are guidelines from bodies such as the Royal College of Paediatrics and Child Health.

BNFC reflects information from the Drug Tariff, the Scottish Drug Tariff, and the Northern Ireland Drug Tariff.

Pricing information NHS Prescription Services provide information on prices of medicinal products and appliances in BNFC. BNFC also receives and processes price lists from product suppliers.

Comments from readers Readers of BNFC are invited to send in comments. Numerous letters and emails are received during the preparation of each edition. Such feedback helps to ensure that BNFC provides practical and clinically relevant information. Many changes in the presentation and scope of BNFC have resulted from comments sent in by users.

Comments from industry Each manufacturer is provided with a complimentary copy of BNFC and invited to comment on it. Close scrutiny of BNFC by the manufacturers provides an additional check and allows them an opportunity to raise issues about BNFC's presentation of the role of various drugs; this is yet another check on the balance of BNFC advice. All comments are looked at with care and, where necessary, additional information and expert advice are sought.

Virtual user groups BNFC has set up virtual user groups across various healthcare professions (e.g. doctors, pharmacists, nurses). The aim of these groups will be to provide feedback to the editors and publishers to ensure that BNF publications continue to serve the needs of its users.

Market research Market research is conducted at regular intervals to gather feedback on specific areas of development, such as drug interactions or changes to the way information is presented in digital formats.

BNFC is an independent professional publication that is kept up-to-date and addresses the day-to-day prescribing information needs of healthcare professionals treating children. Use of this resource throughout the health service helps to ensure that medicines are used safely, effectively, and appropriately in children.

How to use *BNF for Children*

The *BNF for Children* provides information on the use of medicines in children ranging from neonates (including preterm neonates) to adolescents. The terms infant, child, and adolescent are not used consistently in the literature; to avoid ambiguity actual ages are used in the dose statements in *BNF for Children*. The term neonate is used to describe a newborn infant aged 0–28 days. The terms child or children are used generically to describe the entire range from infant to adolescent in *BNF for Children*.

BNF for Children is divided into the following broad areas.

General Guidance

The section on general guidance includes general advice on the use of medicines for managing childhood conditions. It also includes information on prescribing controlled drugs and the management of palliative care. Advice is given on the reporting of adverse reactions. General principles on the use of medicines in hepatic impairment, renal impairment, pregnancy, and breast-feeding are also included in this section.

Notes on conditions, drugs and preparations

The main text consists of classified notes on clinical conditions, drugs and preparations. These notes are divided into 15 chapters, each of which is related

DRUG NAME ◄

Cautions details of precautions required and also any monitoring required

 Hepatic impairment advice for use of drug in these circumstances

 Renal impairment

 Pregnancy

 Breast-feeding

 Counselling Verbal explanation to the patient of specific details of the drug treatment (e.g. posture when taking a medicine)

Contra-indications details of any contra-indications to use of drug

Side-effects details of common and more serious side-effects

Licensed use licensing status where this is of clinical relevance

Indication and dose

 Details of uses and indications

 • By route

  Child dose and frequency of administration (max. dose) for specific age group

 • By alternative route

  Child dose and frequency

[1]**Approved Name** (Non-proprietary) PoM ◄

 Pharmaceutical form colour, coating, active ingredient and amount in dosage form, net price, pack size = basic NHS price. Label: (as in Appendix 3)

1. Exceptions to the prescribing status are indicated by a note or footnote.

Proprietary Name (Manufacturer) PoM NHS

 Pharmaceutical form sugar-free, active ingredient mg/mL, net price, pack size = basic NHS price. Label: (as in Appendix 3)

 Excipients include clinically important excipients or electrolytes

 Note Specific notes about the product e.g. handling

In the case of compound preparations the indications, cautions, contra-indications, side-effects, and interactions of all constituents should be taken into account for prescribing.

When no suitable licensed preparation is available details of preparations that may be imported or formulations available as manufactured specials or extemporaneous preparations are included.

Drugs

The symbol ◢ is used to denote those preparations considered to be less suitable for prescribing. Although such preparations may not be considered as drugs of first choice, their use may be justifiable in certain circumstances.

Prescription-only medicines PoM

This symbol PoM has been placed against preparations that are available only on a prescription from an appropriate practitioner.

The symbol CD indicates that the preparation is subject to the prescription requirements of the Misuse of Drugs Act. For advice on prescribing such preparations see Prescribing Controlled Drugs.

Preparations not available for NHS prescription NHS

This symbol NHS has been placed against preparations that are not prescribable under the NHS. Those prescribable only for specific disorders have a footnote specifying the condition(s) for which the preparation remains available. Some preparations which are not *prescribable* by brand name under the NHS may nevertheless be *dispensed* using the brand name provided that the prescription shows an appropriate non-proprietary name.

Prices

Prices have been calculated from the basic cost used in pricing NHS prescriptions. The price for an extemporaneously prepared preparation has been omitted where the net cost of the ingredients used to make it would give a misleadingly low impression of the final price. Since the prices shown in the *BNF for Children* do not include professional fees and overhead allowances, they are not suitable for quoting to patients seeking private prescriptions or contemplating over-the-counter purchase.

Preparations

Preparations usually follow immediately after the drug which is their main ingredient.

Preparations are included under a non-proprietary title, if they are marketed under such a title, if they are not otherwise prescribable under the NHS, or if they may be prepared extemporaneously.

If proprietary preparations are of a distinctive colour this is stated.

to a particular system of the body or to an aspect of neonatal and paediatric medical care. Each chapter is then divided into sections which begin with *notes* on the selection and use of medicines. Guidance on dental and oral conditions is identified by means of a relevant heading (e.g. Dental and Orofacial pain) in the appropriate sections. The notes are followed by details of relevant drugs and preparations.

Drug entries

Drugs appear under pharmacopoeial or other non-proprietary titles. When there is an *appropriate current monograph* (Medicines Act 1968, Section 65) preference is given to a name at the head of that monograph; otherwise a British Approved Name (BAN), if available, is used. Information on the properties of each drug is organised as shown in the illustration below; the information on cautions, contra-indications, side-effects, dose and indications reflects, as far as possible, the manufacturer's summary of product characteristics.

Side-effects are generally listed in order of frequency and arranged broadly by body systems. Occasionally a rare side-effect might be listed first if it is considered to be particularly important because of its seriousness.

For the majority of drugs, *doses* are expressed in terms of body-weight (i.e. standardised by weight). To calculate the dose for a given child the weight-standardised dose is multiplied by the child's weight (or occasionally by the child's ideal body-weight). The calculated dose should not normally exceed the maximum recommended dose for an adult. For example if the dose is 8 mg/kg (max. 300 mg) a child of 10 kg body-weight should receive 80 mg but a child of 40 kg body-weight should receive 300 mg (rather than 320 mg).

> Doses are expressed for specific age ranges; neonatal doses are preceded by the word Neonate, all other doses are preceded by the word Child. Age ranges in the BNF for Children are described as follows:
>
> Child 1 month–4 years refers to a child from 1 month old up to their 4th birthday;
>
> Child 4–10 years refers to a child from the day of their 4th birthday up to their 10th birthday.
>
> However, a pragmatic approach should be applied to these cut-off points depending on the child's physiological development, condition, and if weight is appropriate for the child's age.

Emergency treatment of poisoning

This chapter provides information on the management of acute poisoning when first seen, although aspects of hospital-based treatment are mentioned.

Appendixes and indexes

The appendixes include information on interactions, borderline substances, and cautionary and advisory labels for dispensed medicines. They are designed for use in association with the main body of the text.

The Dental Practitioners' List and the Nurse Prescribers' List are also included in this section. The indexes consist of the Index of Manufacturers and the Main Index.

Patient Packs

Directive 92/27/EEC specifies the requirements for the labelling of medicines and outlines the format and content of patient information leaflets to be supplied with every medicine; the directive also requires the use of Recommended International Non-proprietary Names for drugs (see p. xvii).

All medicines have approved labelling and patient information leaflets; anyone who supplies a medicine is responsible for providing the relevant information to the patient (see also Appendix 3).

Many medicines are available in manufacturers' original packs complete with patient information leaflets. Where patient packs are available, the *BNF for Children* shows the number of dose units in the packs. In particular clinical circumstances, where patient packs need to be split or medicines are provided in bulk dispensing packs, manufacturers will provide additional supplies of patient information leaflets on request.

During the revision of each edition of this publication careful note is taken of the information that appears on the patient information leaflets. Where it is considered appropriate to alert a prescriber to some specific limitation appearing on the patient information leaflet (for example, in relation to pregnancy) this advice now appears in the *BNF for Children*, see also General guidance, patient information leaflets.

The patient information leaflet also includes details of all inactive ingredients in the medicine. A list of common E numbers and the inactive ingredients to which they correspond is now therefore included in the *BNF for Children* (see inside back cover).

PACT and SPA

PACT (Prescribing Analyses and Cost) and SPA (Scottish Prescribing Analysis) provide prescribers with information about their prescribing.

The *PACT Standard Report*, or in Scotland SPA *Level 1 Report*, is sent to all general practitioners on a quarterly basis. The PACT Standard Report contains an analysis of the practitioner's prescribing and the practice prescribing over the last 3 months, and gives comparisons with the local Primary Care Trust equivalent practice and with a national equivalent. The report also contains details of the practice prescribing for a specific topic; a different topic is chosen each quarter.

The *PACT Catalogue*, or in Scotland SPA *Level 2 Report*, provides a full inventory of the prescriptions issued by a prescriber. The PACT catalogue is available on request for periods between 1 and 24 months. To allow the prescriber to target specific areas of prescribing, a Catalogue may be requested to cover individual preparations, BNF sections, or combinations of BNF chapters.

PACT is also available electronically (www.nhsbsa.nhs.uk). This system gives users on-line access through NHSnet to the 3 years' prescribing data held on the NHS Prescription Services' database; tools for analysing the data are also provided.

Prices in the *BNF for Children*

Basic **net prices** are given in the *BNF for Children* to provide an indication of relative cost. Where there is a choice of suitable preparations for a particular disease or condition the relative cost may be used in making a selection. Cost-effective prescribing must, however, take into account other factors (such as dose frequency and duration of treatment) that affect the total cost. The use of more expensive drugs is justified if it will result in better treatment of the patient or a reduction of the length of an illness or the time spent in hospital.

Prices have generally been calculated from the net cost used in pricing NHS prescriptions dispensed in November 2008; unless an original pack is available these prices are based on the largest pack size of the preparation in use in community pharmacies. The price for an extemporaneously prepared preparation has been omitted where the net cost of the ingredients used to make it would give a misleadingly low impression of the final price.

The unit of 20 is still sometimes used as a basis for comparison, but where suitable original packs or patient packs are available these are priced instead.

Gross prices vary as follows:

1. Costs to the NHS are greater than the net prices quoted and include professional fees and overhead allowances;
2. Private prescription charges are calculated on a separate basis;
3. Over-the-counter sales are at retail price, as opposed to basic net price, and include VAT.

BNF for Children prices are not, therefore, suitable for quoting to patients seeking private prescriptions or contemplating over-the-counter purchases.

A fuller explanation of costs to the NHS may be obtained from the Drug Tariff.

It should be noted that separate Drug Tariffs are applicable to England and Wales, Scotland, and Northern Ireland. Prices in the different tariffs may vary.

Changes for this edition

Significant changes

The *BNF for Children* is revised yearly and numerous changes are made between issues. All copies of *BNF for Children 2008* should therefore be withdrawn and replaced by *BNF for Children 2009*. Significant changes have been made in the following sections for *BNF for Children 2009*:

Adjustment of drug dosages in renal impairment [updated advice and terminology], Prescribing in renal impairment

Salicylate poisoning, Emergency treatment of poisoning

Paracetamol poisoning, Emergency treatment of poisoning

Cyanide poisoning, Emergency treatment of poisoning

Ethylene glycol and methanol poisoning, Emergency treatment of poisoning

Heavy metal poisoning, Emergency treatment of poisoning

Alginate raft-forming oral suspensions, section 1.1.2

Infliximab for subacute manifestations of ulcerative colitis [NICE guidance], section 1.5

Fistulating Crohn's disease, section 1.5

Irritable Bowel Syndrome, section 1.5

Aminosalicylates [monitoring of renal function], section 1.5.1

Management of acute asthma, section 3.1

Beclomethasone dipropionate CFC-free metered dose inhalers [MHRA/CHM advice], section 3.2

Oxygen, section 3.6

Over-the-counter cough and cold medicines [MHRA/CHM advice], section 3.9.1

Melatonin, section 4.1.1

Attention deficit hyperactivity disorder [updated advice], section 4.4

Fentanyl [risk of severe respiratory depression with transdermal patch], section 4.7.2

Pethidine [restricted indications], section 4.7.2

Clostridium difficile infection, section 5.1, Table 1

Hospital-acquired pneumonia, section 5.1, Table 1

Throat infections, sinusitis, and otitis media, section 5.1, Table 1

Tendon damage with quinolones [updated advice], section 5.1.12

Oseltamivir, zanamivir, and amantadine for the prophylaxis and treatment of influenza [updated NICE guidance], section 5.3.4

Oseltamivir [prophylaxis and treatment of influenza in child under 1 year of age], section 5.3.4

Ascaricides (common round worm infections) [updated advice], section 5.5.2

Continuous subcutaneous insulin infusion [NICE guidance], section 6.1.1

Use of oral hypoglycaemic drugs for type 2 diabetes during pregnancy and breast-feeding, section 6.1.2

Use of metformin in renal impairment and risk of lactic acidosis, section 6.1.2.2

Diabetic ketoacidosis [updated advice], section 6.1.3

Treatment of hypoglycaemia [updated advice on glucose-containing liquids], section 6.1.4

Combined hormonal contraceptives and risk factors for venous thromboembolism [addition of smoking], section 7.3.1

Nocturnal enuresis [updated advice], section 7.4.2

Administration of vinca alkaloids [NPSA advice], section 8.1.4

Tacrolimus [MHRA/CHM advice], section 8.2.2

Management of hyperkalaemia, section 9.2.1.1

Drugs unsafe for use in acute porphyria, section 9.8.2

Over-the-counter cough and cold medicines [MHRA/CHM advice], section 12.2.2

Topical oral pain relief products containing salicylates [CHM advice], section 12.3.1

Topical corticosteriods [counselling, application, and labelling requirements], section 13.4

Sunscreen preparations [updated advice on Sun Protection Factor], section 13.8.1

Active immunity [reorganised and updated], section 14.1

Immunisation schedule [table], section 14.1

Vaccines and antisera [reformatted and updated], section 14.4

Risk of neurological and haematological toxic effects with nitrous oxide, section 15.1.2

Enteral feeds and nutritional supplements [new tables], Borderline Substances, Appendix 2

Intravenous infusions for neonatal intensive care, Appendix 4

Dose changes

Changes in dose statements introduced into *BNF for Children 2009*:

Aciclovir [chickenpox and herpes zoster infection], p. 386

Alpha tocopheryl acetate [malabsorption in cystic fibrosis], p. 582

Alprostadil, p. 166

Atomoxetine, p. 234

Atracurium, p. 780

Atropine sulphate [control of muscarinic side-effects of neostigmine in reversal of competitive neuromuscular block], p. 770

Betaine, p. 594

Binocrit®, p. 537

Caffeine, p. 202

Carglumic acid, p. 592

Caspofungin, p. 365

Chlorphenamine [by intramuscular or intravenous injection], p. 194

Chloroquine [treatment of benign malaria], p. 396 and [prophylaxis of malaria], p. 402

Ciprofloxacin, p. 358

Concerta® *XL*, p. 236

Dantrolene, p. 786

Diamorphine [intranasal], p. 252

Diazepam [status epilepticus], p. 284

Digoxin [maintenance doses for 10–18 years], p. 97

Dobutamine, p. 143

Doxycycline [late latent syphilis], p. 330

Epipen®, p. 201

Eprex®, p. 538

Equasym XL®, p. 236

Erythromycin [gastro-intestinal stasis], p. 58

Etanercept, p. 612

European viper venom antiserum [text], p. 47

Folic acid [megaloblastic anaemia], p. 535

Fentanyl [use in anaesthesia], p. 777

Fluconazole [vaginal candidiasis and candidal balanitis], p. 366

Gabapentin [epilepsy], p. 270

Ganciclovir [congenital cytomegalovirus infection of the CNS], p. 388

Glycopyrronnium [control of upper airways secretion and hypersalivation], p. 770

Halothane, p. 767

Hydrocortisone [acute hypersensitivity reactions], p. 451

Hydroxycarbamide, p. 539

Hydroxyzine hydrochloride, p. 195

Ipratropium bromide [by inhalation of nebulised solution], p. 169

Lenograstim [mobilisation of peripheral blood progenitor cells following adjunctive myelosuppressive chemotherapy (to improve yield)], p. 545

Levetiracetam, p. 273

Levothyroxine, p. 438

Lisinopril, p. 133

Medikinet XL®, p. 236

Methotrexate [severe Crohn's disease], p. 75

Methylphenidate, p. 235

Midazolam [intravenous injection for sedation], p. 774

Midazolam [status epilepticus], p. 286

Naloxone, p. 40

Normacol Plus®, p. 79

Pancuronium, p. 781

Pentasa® granules, p. 70

Pholcodine, p. 209

Pralidoxime chloride, p. 47

Propofol [induction of anaesthesia], p. 765

Pseudoephedrine, p. 210

Pulmicort® aerosol inhalation, p. 187

Pyridostigmine, p. 615

Rufinamide, p. 276

Salbutamol [by continuous intravenous infusion], p. 174

Salbutamol [by inhalation of aerosol or nebulised solution], p. 169

Salofalk® granules, p. 70

Sevoflurane [induction of anesthesia], p. 768

Sodium bicarbonate, p. 550

Streptomycin, p. 355

Sucralfate, p. 62

Thiamine [metabolic disorders], p. 576

Timentin®, p. 318

Uniphyllin Continus®, p. 180

Varilrix®, p. 753

Varivax®, p. 754

Vecuronium, p. 782

Vitamin D, p. 578

Warfarin, p. 153

Zanamivir [prevention of influenza], p. 392

Classification changes

Classification changes have been made in the following sections of *BNF for Children 2009*:

Section 1.5.1 Aminosalicylates [new sub-section]

Section 1.5.2 Corticosteroids [new sub-section]

Section 1.5.3 Drugs affecting the immune response [new sub-section]

Section 1.5.4 Food allergy [new sub-section]

Section 5.1.2 Cephalosporins, carbapenems, and other beta-lactams [title change]

Section 5.1.2.1 Cephalosporins [new sub-section]

Section 5.1.2.2 Carbapenems [new sub-section]

Section 5.1.2.3 Other beta-lactam antibiotics [new sub-section]

Section 6.1.2.3 Other antidiabetic drugs [title change]

Section 6.1.6 Oral glucose tolerance test [sub-section title change]

Section 11.8.2 Ocular diagnostic and perioperative preparations [title change]

Deleted preparations

Preparations listed below have been discontinued during the compilation of *BNF for Children 2009*, or are still available but are not considered suitable for inclusion by the Paediatric Formulary Committee (see footnote):

AeroBec® preparations
Agenerase®
Aquasept®
Ascalix®
Benzatropine
Cardilate MR®
Cary'lderm®
Cimetidine[1]
Claforan®
Daclizumab
Daonil®
Efcortelan®
Euglucon®
Flagyl® intravenous infusion
Fletchers'® Enemas

Graneodin®
Halycitrol®
Hydrocortone®
Icthaband®
Idrolax®
Intal® Spincaps
Kloref®
Liquid paraffin[1]
Locoid C®
Navoban®
Neo-Cortef®
Nifopress® Retard
Nystan® cream and ointment
Paraldehyde injection
Phentolamine mesilate[1]

Pulmicort LS®
Rapolyte®
Senokot® granules
Ster-Zac Bath Concentrate®
Tri-Adcortyl® preparations
Tropisetron
Vaseline Dermacare®
Vepesid® infusion
Vibramycin® capsules
Vioform-Hydrocortisone®
Viracept® powder
Viraferon®
Volmax®
Zenapax®

New preparations included in this edition

Preparations included in the relevant sections of *BNF for Children 2009*:

Advagraf®, p. 524
Apidra®, p. 424
Aptivus®, p. 382
Atripla®, p. 378
Avamys®, p. 650
Bumetanide oral liquid, p. 104
Bridion®, p. 784
Cardioxane®, p. 499
Celsentri®, p. 384
Clasteon®, p. 470
Clinitas®, p. 639
Diacomit®, p. 277
Epilim Chronosphere®, p. 280
Ferinject®, p. 532
Ferriprox®, p. 541
Flexbumin®, p. 557
Geloplasma®, p. 557

Grazax®, p. 197
Humira®, p. 612
Intal® CFC-free inhaler, p. 190
Intelence®, p. 383
Isentress®, p. 385
Isoplex®, p. 557
Kuvan®, p. 562
Laxido®, p. 83
LMX 4®, p. 789
Maxitram SR®, p. 260
MucoClear®, p. 208
Mycamine®, p. 370
Myozyme®, p. 591
Nicorette® Invisi patches, p. 293
NuvaRing®, p. 481
Ocusan®, p. 639
Optive®, p. 637

Oxyal®, p. 639
Prezista®, p. 379
Ratiograstim®, p. 545
Rebetol®, p. 394
Retacrit®, p. 538
Rosiced®, p. 710
Sandocal®+D 600, p. 582
Siklos®, p. 539
Tetraspan®, p. 558
Thymoglobuline®, p. 521
Tramquel SR®, p. 260
Vimpat®, p. 271
Vismed®, p. 639
Vismed® Multi, p. 639
Volulyte®, p. 558
Zavesca®, p. 595

---

1. Not considered suitable for inclusion by the Paediatric Formulary Committee

Name changes

European Law requires use of the Recommended International Non-proprietary Name (rINN) for medicinal substances. In most cases the British Approved Name (BAN) and rINN were identical. Where the two differed, the BAN was modified to accord with the rINN.

The following list shows those substances for which the former BAN has been modified to accord with the rINN. Former BANs have been retained as synonyms in *BNF for Children*.

Adrenaline and noradrenaline Adrenaline and noradrenaline are the terms used in the titles of monographs in the European Pharmacopoeia and are thus the official names in the member states. For these substances, BP 2008 shows the European Pharmacopoeia names and the rINNs at the head of the monographs; *BNF for Children* has adopted a similar style.

Former BAN	New BAN
adrenaline	*see above*
amethocaine	tetracaine
aminacrine	aminoacridine
amoxycillin	amoxicillin
amphetamine	amfetamine
amylobarbitone sodium	amobarbital sodium
beclomethasone	beclometasone
bendrofluazide	bendroflumethiazide
benzhexol	trihexyphenidyl
benzphetamine	benzfetamine
busulphan	busulfan
butobarbitone	butobarbital
carticaine	articaine
cephalexin	cefalexin
cephradine	cefradine
chloral betaine	cloral betaine
chlorbutol	chlorobutanol
chlormethiazole	clomethiazole
chlorpheniramine	chlorphenamine
chlorthalidone	chlortalidone
cholecalciferol	colecalciferol
cholestyramine	colestyramine
clomiphene	clomifene
colistin sulphomethate sodium	colistimethate sodium
corticotrophin	corticotropin
cyclosporin	ciclosporin
cysteamine	mercaptamine
danthron	dantron
dexamphetamine	dexamfetamine
dibromopropamidine	dibrompropamidine
dicyclomine	dicycloverine
dienoestrol	dienestrol
dimethicone(s)	dimeticone
dimethyl sulphoxide	dimethyl sulfoxide
dothiepin	dosulepin
doxycycline hydrochloride (hemihydrate hemiethanolate)	doxycycline hyclate
eformoterol	formoterol
ethamsylate	etamsylate
ethinyloestradiol	ethinylestradiol
ethynodiol	etynodiol

Former BAN	New BAN
flumethasone	flumetasone
flupenthixol	flupentixol
flurandrenolone	fludroxycortide
frusemide	furosemide
guaiphenesin	guaifenesin
hexachlorophane	hexachlorophene
hexamine hippurate	methenamine hippurate
hydroxyurea	hydroxycarbamide
indomethacin	indometacin
lignocaine	lidocaine
methotrimeprazine	levomepromazine
methyl cysteine	mecysteine
methylene blue	methylthioninium chloride
methicillin	meticillin
mitozantrone	mitoxantrone
nicoumalone	acenocoumarol
noradrenaline	*see above*
oestradiol	estradiol
oestriol	estriol
oestrone	estrone
oxpentifylline	pentoxifylline
phenobarbitone	phenobarbital
pipothiazine	pipotiazine
polyhexanide	polihexanide
pramoxine	pramocaine
procaine penicillin	procaine benzylpenicillin
prothionamide	protionamide
quinalbarbitone	secobarbital
riboflavine	riboflavin
salcatonin	calcitonin (salmon)
sodium calciumedetate	sodium calcium edetate
sodium cromoglycate	sodium cromoglicate
sodium ironedetate	sodium feredetate
sodium picosulphate	sodium picosulfate
sorbitan monostearate	sorbitan stearate
stibocaptate	sodium stibocaptate
stilboestrol	diethylstilbestrol
sulphacetamide	sulfacetamide
sulphadiazine	sulfadiazine
sulphamethoxazole	sulfamethoxazole
sulphapyridine	sulfapyridine
sulphasalazine	sulfasalazine
sulphathiazole	sulfathiazole
sulphinpyrazone	sulfinpyrazone
tetracosactrin	tetracosactide
thiabendazole	tiabendazole
thioguanine	tioguanine
thiopentone	thiopental
thymoxamine	moxisylyte
thyroxine sodium	levothyroxine sodium
tribavirin	ribavirin
trimeprazine	alimemazine
urofollitrophin	urofollitropin

General guidance

Medicines should be given to children only when they are necessary, and in all cases the potential benefit of administering the medicine should be considered in relation to the risk involved. This is particularly important during pregnancy, when the risk to both mother and fetus must be considered (for further details see Prescribing in Pregnancy).

It is important to discuss treatment options carefully with the child and the child's carer (see also Taking Medicines to Best Effect, below). In particular, the child and the child's carer should be helped to distinguish the adverse effects of prescribed drugs from the effects of the medical disorder. When the beneficial effects of the medicine are likely to be delayed, this should be highlighted.

Taking medicines to best effect   Difficulties in adherence to drug treatment occur regardless of age. Factors that contribute to poor compliance with prescribed medicines include:

- difficulty in taking the medicine (e.g. inability to swallow the medicine);
- unattractive formulation (e.g. unpleasant taste);
- prescription not collected or not dispensed;
- purpose of medicine not clear;
- perceived lack of efficacy;
- real or perceived side-effects;
- carers' or child's perception of the risk and severity of side-effects may differ from that of the prescriber;
- ambiguous instructions for administration.

The prescriber, the child's carer, and the child (if appropriate) should agree on the health outcomes desired and on the strategy for achieving them ('concordance'). The prescriber should be sensitive to religious, cultural, and personal beliefs of the child's family that can affect acceptance of medicines.

Taking the time to explain to the child (and carers) the rationale and the potential adverse effects of treatment may improve compliance. Reinforcement and elaboration of the physician's instructions by the pharmacist and other members of the healthcare team can be important. Giving advice on the management of adverse effects and the possibility of alternative treatments may encourage carers and children to seek advice rather than merely abandon unacceptable treatment.

Simplifying the drug regimen may help; the need for frequent administration may reduce compliance, although there appears to be little difference in compliance between once-daily and twice-daily administration.

Administration of medicines to children   Children should be involved in decisions about taking medicines and encouraged to take responsibility for using them correctly. The degree of such involvement will depend on the child's age, understanding, and personal circumstances.

Occasionally a medicine or its taste has to be disguised or masked with small quantities of food. However, unless specifically permitted (e.g. some formulations of pancreatin), a medicine should **not** be mixed with large quantities of food because the full dose might not be taken and the child might develop an aversion to food if the medicine imparts an unpleasant taste. Medicines should **not** be mixed or administered in a baby's feeding bottle.

Children under 5 years (and some older children) find a liquid formulation more acceptable than tablets or capsules. However, for long-term treatment it may be possible for a child to be taught to take tablets or capsules.

An oral syringe (see below) should be used for accurate measurement and controlled administration of an oral liquid medicine. The unpleasant taste of an oral liquid can be disguised by flavouring it or by giving a favourite food or drink immediately afterwards, but the potential for food-drug interactions should be considered.

Advice should be given on dental hygiene to those receiving medicines containing cariogenic sugars for long-term treatment; sugar-free medicines should be provided whenever possible.

Children with nasal feeding tubes in place for prolonged periods should be encouraged to take medicines by mouth if possible; enteric feeding should generally be interrupted before the medicine is given (particularly if enteral feeds reduce the absorption of a particular drug). Oral liquids can be given through the tube provided that precautions are taken to guard against blockage; the dose should be washed down with warm water. When a medicine is given through a nasogastric tube to a neonate, **sterile water** must be used to accompany the medicine or to wash it down.

The intravenous route is generally chosen when a medicine cannot be given by mouth; reliable access, often a central vein, should be used for children whose treatment involves irritant or inotropic drugs or who need to receive the medicine over a long period or for home therapy. The subcutaneous route is used most commonly for insulin administration. Intramuscular injections should preferably be **avoided** in children, particularly neonates, infants, and young children. However, the intramuscular route may be advantageous for administration of single doses of medicines when intravenous cannulation would be more problematic or painful to the child. Certain drugs, e.g. some vaccines, are only administered intramuscularly.

The intrathecal, epidural and intraosseous routes should be used **only** by staff specially trained to administer medicines by these routes. Local protocols for the management of intrathecal injections must be in place (section 8.1).

Managing medicines in school   Administration of a medicine during schooltime should be avoided if possible; medicines should be prescribed for once or twice-daily administration whenever practicable. If the medicine needs to be taken in school, this should be discussed with parents or carers and the necessary arrangements made in advance; where appropriate, involvement of a school nurse should be sought. *Managing Medicines in Schools and Early Years Settings* produced by the Department of Health provides guidance on using medicines in schools (www.dh.gov.uk).

Patient information leaflets   Manufacturers' patient information leaflets that accompany a medicine cover only the licensed use of the medicine (see *BNF for Children* and Marketing Authorisation, below). Therefore, when a medicine is used outside its licence, it may be appropriate to advise the child and the child's parent or carer that some of the information in the leaflet might not apply to the child's treatment. Where necessary, inappropriate advice in the patient information leaflet should be identified and reassurance provided about the correct use in the context of the child's condition.

Biosimilar medicines   A biosimilar medicine is a new biological product that is similar to a medicine that has already been authorised to be marketed (the biological reference medicine) in the European Union. The active substance of a biosimilar medicine is similar, but not identical, to the biological reference medicine. Biological products are different from standard chemical products in terms of their complexity and although theoretically there should be no important differences between the biosimilar and biological reference medicine in terms of safety or efficacy, when prescribing biological products, it is good practice to use the brand name. This will ensure that substitution of a biosimilar medicine does not occur when the medicine is dispensed.

Biosimilar medicines have black triangle status (▼) at the time of initial marketing. It is important to report suspected adverse reactions to biosimilar medicines using the Yellow Card Scheme (p. 21). For biosimilar medicines, adverse reaction reports should clearly state the brand name of the suspected medicine.

Complementary and alternative medicine   An increasing amount of information on complementary and alternative medicine is becoming available. Where appropriate, the child and the child's carers should be asked about the use of their medicines, including dietary supplements and topical products. The scope of *BNF* *for Children* is restricted to the discussion of conventional medicines but reference is made to complementary treatments if they affect conventional therapy (e.g. interactions with St John's wort—see Appendix 1). Further information on herbal medicines is available at www.mhra.gov.uk.

BNF for Children and marketing authorisation   Where appropriate the *doses, indications, cautions, contra-indications,* and *side-effects* in *BNF for Children* reflect those in the manufacturers' Summaries of Product Characteristics (SPCs) which, in turn, reflect those in the corresponding marketing authorisations (formerly known as Product Licences). *BNF for Children* does not generally include proprietary medicines that are not supported by a valid Summary of Product Characteristics or when the marketing authorisation holder has not been able to supply essential information. When a preparation is available from more than one manufacturer, *BNF for Children* reflects advice that is the most clinically relevant regardless of any variation in the marketing authorisation. Unlicensed products can be obtained from 'special-order' manufacturers or specialist importing companies, see p. 943.

As far as possible, medicines should be prescribed within the terms of the marketing authorisation. However, many children require medicines not specifically licensed for paediatric use. Although medicines cannot be promoted outside the limits of the licence, the Medicines Act does not prohibit the use of unlicensed medicines.

BNF for Children includes advice involving the use of unlicensed medicines or of licensed medicines for unlicensed uses ('off-label' use). Such advice reflects careful consideration of the options available to manage a given condition and the weight of evidence and experience of the unlicensed intervention (see also Unlicensed Medicines, p. 7). Where the advice falls outside a drug's marketing authorisation, *BNF for Children* shows the licensing status in the drug monograph. However, limitations of the marketing authorisation should not preclude unlicensed use where clinically appropriate.

> Prescribing unlicensed medicines or medicines outside the recommendations of their marketing authorisation alters (and probably increases) the prescriber's professional responsibility and potential liability. The prescriber should be able to justify and feel competent in using such medicines.

Drugs and skilled tasks   Prescribers should advise children and their carers if treatment is likely to affect their ability to perform skilled tasks. This applies especially to drugs with sedative effects; patients should be warned that these effects are increased by alcohol.

Oral syringes   An **oral syringe** is supplied when oral liquid medicines are prescribed in doses other than multiples of 5 mL. The oral syringe is marked in 0.5-mL divisions from 1 to 5 mL to measure doses of less than 5 mL. It is provided with an adaptor and an instruction leaflet. The *5-mL spoon* is used for doses of 5 mL (or multiples thereof). Different sizes of oral syringe are available for the accurate measurement of smaller volumes, although these can not be prescribed.

Excipients   Branded oral liquid preparations that do not contain *fructose, glucose,* or *sucrose* are described as 'sugar-free' in *BNF for Children*. Preparations containing hydrogenated glucose syrup, mannitol, maltitol, sorbitol, or xylitol are also marked 'sugar-free' since they do not cause dental caries. Children receiving medicines containing cariogenic sugars, or their carers, should be advised of dental hygiene measures to prevent caries. Sugar-free preparations should be used whenever possible, particularly if treatment is required for a long period.

Where information on the presence of *alcohol, aspartame, gluten, sulphites, tartrazine, arachis (peanut) oil* or *sesame oil* is available, this is indicated in *BNF for Children* against the relevant preparation.

Information is provided on *selected excipients* in skin preparations (section 13.1.3), in vaccines (section 14.1), and on *selected preservatives* and *excipients* in eye drops and injections. Pressurised metered aerosols containing *chlorofluorocarbons* (CFCs) have also been identified.

The presence of *benzyl alcohol* and *polyoxyl castor oil* (polyethoxylated castor oil) in injections is indicated in *BNF for Children*. Benzyl alcohol has been associated with a fatal toxic syndrome in preterm neonates, and therefore, parenteral preparations containing the preservative should not be used in neonates. Polyoxyl castor oils, used as vehicles in intravenous injections, have been associated with severe anaphylactoid reactions.

The presence of *propylene glycol* in oral or parenteral medicines is indicated in *BNF for Children*; it can cause adverse effects if its elimination is impaired, e.g. in renal failure, in neonates and young children, and in slow metabolisers of the substance. It may interact with metronidazole.

> In the absence of information on excipients in *BNF for Children* and in the product literature, contact the manufacturer (see Index of Manufacturers) if it is essential to check details.

Health and safety   When handling chemical or biological materials particular attention should be given to the possibility of allergy, fire, explosion, radiation, or poisoning. Care is required to avoid sources of heat (including hair dryers) when flammable substances are used on the skin or hair. Substances, such as corticosteroids, some antimicrobials, phenothiazines, and many cytotoxics, are irritant or very potent and should be handled with caution; contact with the skin and inhalation of dust should be avoided. Healthcare professionals and carers should guard against exposure to sensitising, toxic or irritant substances if it is necessary to crush tablets or open capsules.

Security of prescriptions   The Councils of the British Medical Association and the Royal Pharmaceutical Society have issued a joint statement on the security and validity of prescriptions.

In particular, prescription forms should:

- not be left unattended at reception desks;
- not be left in a car where they may be visible; and
- when not in use, be kept in a locked drawer within the surgery and at home.

Patient group direction (PGD)   In most cases, the most appropriate clinical care will be provided on an individual basis by a prescriber to a specific child. However, a Patient Group Direction for supply and administration of medicines by other healthcare professionals can be used where it would benefit the child's care without compromising safety.

A Patient Group Direction is a written direction relating to the supply and administration (or administration only) of a licensed prescription-only medicine by certain classes of healthcare professionals; the Direction is signed by a doctor (or dentist) and by a pharmacist. Further information on Patient Group Directions is available in Health Service Circular HSC 2000/026 (England), HDL (2001) 7 (Scotland), and WHC (2000) 116 (Wales).

NICE and Scottish Medicines Consortium   Advice issued by the National Institute for Health and Clinical Excellence (NICE) and by the Scottish Medicines Consortium (SMC) is included in *BNF for Children* when relevant. If advice within a NICE Single Technology Appraisal differs from SMC advice, the Scottish Executive expects NHS Boards within NHS Scotland to comply with the SMC advice. Details of the advice together with updates can be obtained from www.nice.org.uk and from www.scottishmedicines.org.

Prescription writing

> **Shared care**
> In its guidelines on responsibility for prescribing (circular EL (91) 127) between hospitals and general practitioners, the Department of Health has advised that legal responsibility for prescribing lies with the doctor who signs the prescription.

Prescriptions[1] should be written legibly in ink or otherwise so as to be indelible[2], should be dated, should state the full name and address of the patient, and should be signed in ink by the prescriber[3]. The age and the date of birth of the child should preferably be stated, and it is a legal requirement in the case of prescription-only medicines to state the age for children under 12 years.

Wherever appropriate the prescriber should state the current weight of the child to enable the dose prescribed to be checked. Consideration should also be given to including the dose per unit mass e.g. mg/kg or the dose per m^2 body-surface area e.g. mg/m^2 where this would reduce error.

The following should be noted:

(a) The unnecessary use of decimal points should be avoided, e.g. 3 mg, not 3.0 mg.

Quantities of 1 gram or more should be written as 1 g, etc.

Quantities less than 1 gram should be written in milligrams, e.g. 500 mg, not 0.5 g.

Quantities less than 1 mg should be written in micrograms, e.g. 100 micrograms, not 0.1 mg.

When decimals are unavoidable a zero should be written in front of the decimal point where there is no other figure, e.g. 0.5 mL, not .5 mL.

Use of the decimal point is acceptable to express a range, e.g. 0.5 to 1 g.

(b) 'Micrograms' and 'nanograms' should **not** be abbreviated. Similarly 'units' should **not** be abbreviated.

(c) The term 'millilitre' (ml or mL)[4] is used in medicine and pharmacy, and cubic centimetre, c.c., or cm^3 should not be used.

(d) Dose and dose frequency should be stated; in the case of preparations to be taken 'as required' a **minimum dose interval** should be specified.

Care should be taken to ensure the child receives the correct dose of the active drug. Therefore, the dose should normally be stated in terms of the mass of the active drug (e.g. '125 mg 3 times daily'); terms such as '5 mL' or '1 tablet' should be avoided except for compound preparations.

When doses other than multiples of 5 mL are prescribed for *oral liquid preparations* the dose-volume will be provided by means of an **oral syringe**, see p. 3 (except for preparations intended to be measured with a pipette).

(e) The names of drugs and preparations should be written clearly and **not** abbreviated, using approved titles **only** (see also advice in box on p. 6 to **avoid** creating generic titles for modified-release preparations).

(f) The quantity to be supplied may be stated by indicating the number of days of treatment required in the box provided on NHS forms. In most cases the exact amount will be supplied. This does not apply to items directed to be used as required—if the dose and frequency are not given then the quantity to be supplied needs to be stated.

When several items are ordered on one form the box can be marked with the number of days of treatment provided the quantity is added for any item for which the amount cannot be calculated.

(g) Although directions should preferably be in **English without abbreviation**, it is recognised that some Latin abbreviations are used (for details see Inside Back Cover).

General guidance

---

1. These recommendations are acceptable for **prescription-only medicines** (PoM). For items marked CD see also Prescribing Controlled Drugs, p. 17.
2. It is permissible to issue carbon copies of NHS prescriptions as long as they are signed in ink.
3. Computer-generated facsimile signatures do not meet the legal requirement.
4. The use of capital 'L' in mL is a printing convention throughout *BNF for Children*; both 'mL' and 'ml' are recognised SI abbreviations.

General guidance

Abbreviation of titles   In general, titles of drugs and preparations should be written *in full*. Unofficial abbreviations should **not** be used as they may be misinterpreted.

Non-proprietary titles   Where non-proprietary ('generic') titles are given, they should be used for prescribing. This will enable any suitable product to be dispensed, thereby saving delay to the patient and sometimes expense to the health service. The only exception is where there is a demonstrable difference in clinical effect between different manufacturer's versions of the formulation, making it important that the child should always receive the same brand; in such cases, the brand name or the manufacturer should be stated.

> Non-proprietary names of **compound preparations** e.g. co-codamol that appear in *BNF for Children* are those that have been introduced by the British Pharmacopoeia Commission or another recognised body; whenever possible they reflect the names of the active ingredients.
>
> Prescribers should avoid creating their own compound names for the purposes of generic prescribing; such names do not have an approved definition and can be misinterpreted.
>
> Special care should be taken to avoid errors when prescribing compound preparations; in particular the hyphen in the prefix 'co-' should be retained.
>
> Special care should also be taken to avoid creating generic names for **modified-release** preparations where the use of these names could lead to confusion between formulations with different duration of action.

Strengths and quantities   The strength or quantity to be contained in capsules, lozenges, tablets, etc. should be stated by the prescriber. In particular, strengths of liquid preparations should be clearly stated (e.g. 125 mg/5 mL).

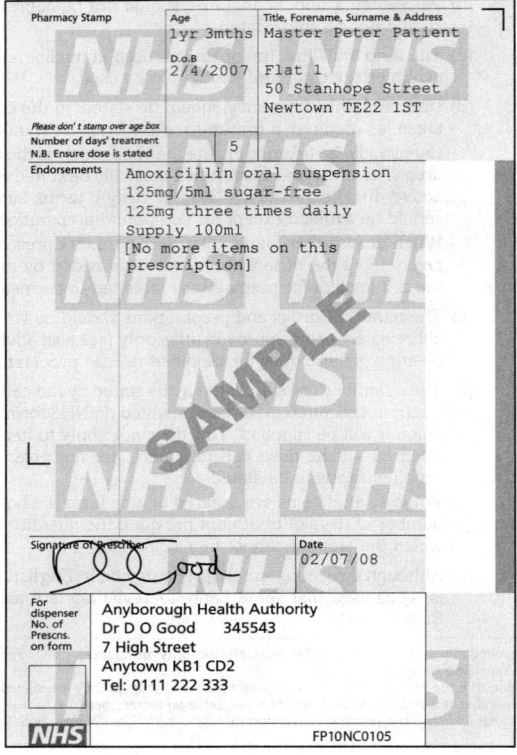

Supply of medicines

When supplying a medicine for a child, the pharmacist should ensure that the child and the child's carer understand the nature and identity of the medicine and how it should be used. The child and the carer should be provided with appropriate information (e.g. how long the medicine should be taken for and what to do if a dose is missed or the child vomits soon after the dose is given).

Safety in the home   Carers and relatives of children must be warned to keep all medicines out of the reach and sight of children. Tablets, capsules and oral and external liquid preparations must be dispensed in a reclosable *child-resistant container* unless:

- the medicine is in an original pack or patient pack such as to make this inadvisable;
- the child's carer will have difficulty in opening a child-resistant container;
- a specific request is made that the product shall not be dispensed in a child-resistant container;
- no suitable child-resistant container exists for a particular liquid preparation.

All patients should be advised to dispose of *unwanted medicines* by returning them to a pharmacy for destruction.

Validity of prescriptions   Where there is any doubt about the authenticity of a prescription, the pharmacist should contact the prescriber. If this is done by telephone, the number should be obtained from the directory rather than relying on the information on the prescription form, which may be false.

Strength and quantities   If a pharmacist receives an incomplete prescription for a systemically administered preparation[1] and considers it would not be appropriate for the patient to return to the prescriber, the following procedures will apply:

(a) an attempt must always be made to contact the prescriber to ascertain the intention;

(b) if the attempt is successful the pharmacist must, where practicable, subsequently arrange for details of quantity, strength where applicable, and dosage to be inserted by the prescriber on the incomplete form;

(c) where, although the prescriber has been contacted, it has not proved possible to obtain the written intention regarding an incomplete prescription, the pharmacist may endorse the form 'p.c.' (prescriber contacted) and add details of the quantity and strength where applicable of the preparation supplied, and of the dose indicated. The endorsement should be initialled and dated by the pharmacist;

(d) where the prescriber cannot be contacted and the pharmacist has sufficient information to make a professional judgement the preparation may be dispensed. If the quantity is missing the pharmacist may supply sufficient to complete up to 5 days' treatment; except that where a combination pack (i.e. a proprietary pack containing more than one medicinal product) or oral contraceptive is prescribed by name only, the smallest pack shall be dispensed. In all cases the prescription must be endorsed 'p.n.c.' (prescriber not contacted), the quantity, the dose, and the strength (where applicable) of the preparation supplied must be indicated, and the endorsement must be initialled and dated;

(e) if the pharmacist has any doubt about exercising discretion, an incomplete prescription must be referred back to the prescriber.

Unlicensed medicines   A drug or formulation that is not covered by a marketing authorisation (see also *BNF for Children* and Marketing Authorisation) may be obtained from a pharmaceutical company, imported by a specialist importer, manufactured by a commercial or hospital licensed manufacturing unit, or prepared extemporaneously (see below) against a prescription.

---

1. With the exception of temazepam, an incomplete prescription is **not** acceptable for controlled drugs in schedules 2 and 3 of the Misuse of Drugs Regulations 2001.

The safeguards that apply to products with marketing authorisation should be extended, as far as possible, to the use of unlicensed medicines. The safety, efficacy, and quality (including labelling) of unlicensed medicines should be assured by means of clear policies on their prescribing, purchase, supply, and administration. Extra care is required with unlicensed medicines because less information may be available on the drug and any formulation of the drug.

The following should be agreed with the supplier when ordering an unlicensed or extemporaneously prepared medicine:

- the specification of the formulation;
- documentation confirming the specification and quality of the product supplied (e.g. a certificate of conformity or of analysis);
- for imported preparations product and licensing information should be supplied in English.

Extemporaneous preparations   A product should be dispensed extemporaneously only when no product with a marketing authorisation is available. Every effort should be made to ensure that an extemporaneously prepared product is stable and that it delivers the requisite dose reliably; the child should be provided with a consistent formulation regardless of where the medicine is supplied to minimise variations in quality. Where there is doubt about the formulation, advice should be sought from a medicines information centre, the pharmacy at a children's hospital, a hospital production unit, a hospital quality control department, or the manufacturer.

In many cases it is preferable to give a licensed product by an unlicensed route (e.g. an injection solution given by mouth) than to prepare a special formulation. When tablets or capsules are cut, dispersed, or used for preparing liquids immediately before administration, it is important to confirm uniform dispersal of the active ingredient, especially if only a portion of the solid content (e.g. a tablet segment) is used or if only an aliquot of the liquid is to be administered.

In some cases the child's clinical condition may require a dose to be administered in the absence of full information on the method of administration. It is important to ensure that the appropriate supporting information is available at the earliest opportunity.

Preparation of products that produce harmful dust (e.g. cytotoxic drugs, hormones, or potentially sensitising drugs such as neomycin) should be **avoided** or undertaken with appropriate precautions to protect staff and carers (see also Safety in the Home, above).

The BP direction that a preparation must be *freshly prepared* indicates that it must be made not more than 24 hours before it is issued for use. The direction that a preparation should be *recently prepared* indicates that deterioration is likely if the preparation is stored for longer than about 4 weeks at 15–25° C.

The term **water** used without qualification means either potable water freshly drawn direct from the public supply and suitable for drinking or freshly boiled and cooled purified water. The latter should be used if the public supply is from a local storage tank or if the potable water is unsuitable for a particular preparation (Water for injections, section 9.2.2).

Labelling medicines   The *name* of the medicine should appear on the label unless the prescriber indicates otherwise; the name shown on the label should be that written on the prescription. The *strength* should also be stated on the label in the case of preparations that are available in different strengths.

Labels should indicate the *total quantity* of the product dispensed in the container to which the label refers. This requirement applies equally to solid, liquid, internal, and external preparations. If a product is dispensed in more than one container, the reference should be to the amount in each container.

Emergency supply of medicines

Emergency supply requested by member of the public

Pharmacists are sometimes called upon by members of the public to make an emergency supply of medicines. The Prescription Only Medicines (Human Use) Order 1997 allows exemptions from the Prescription Only requirements for emergency supply to be made by a person lawfully conducting a retail pharmacy business provided:

(a) that the pharmacist has interviewed the person requesting the prescription-only medicine and is satisfied:

  (i) that there is immediate need for the prescription-only medicine and that it is impracticable in the circumstances to obtain a prescription without undue delay;

  (ii) that treatment with the prescription-only medicine has on a previous occasion been prescribed by a doctor, a dentist, a supplementary prescriber, a community practitioner nurse prescriber (formerly a district nurse or health visitor prescriber), a nurse independent prescriber, or a pharmacist independent prescriber, for the person requesting it;

  (iii) as to the dose that it would be appropriate for the person to take;

(b) that no greater quantity shall be supplied than will provide 5 days' treatment except when the prescription-only medicine is:

  (i) insulin, an ointment or cream, or a preparation for the relief of asthma in an aerosol dispenser when the smallest pack can be supplied;

  (ii) an oral contraceptive when a full cycle may be supplied;

  (iii) an antibiotic in liquid form for oral administration when the smallest quantity that will provide a full course of treatment can be supplied;

(c) that an entry shall be made by the pharmacist in the prescription book stating:

  (i) the date of supply;

  (ii) the name, quantity, and, where appropriate, the pharmaceutical form and strength;

  (iii) the name and address of the patient;

  (iv) the nature of the emergency;

(d) that the container or package must be labelled to show:

  (i) the date of supply;

  (ii) the name, quantity, and, where appropriate, the pharmaceutical form and strength;

  (iii) the name of the patient;

  (iv) the name and address of the pharmacy;

  (v) the words 'Emergency supply';

  (vi) the words 'Keep out of the reach of children' (or similar warning);

(e) that the prescription-only medicine is not a substance specifically excluded from the emergency supply provision, and does not contain a Controlled Drug specified in Schedules 1, 2, or 3 to the Misuse of Drugs Regulations 2001 except for phenobarbital or phenobarbital sodium for the treatment of epilepsy: for details see *Medicines, Ethics and Practice*, No. 32, London, Pharmaceutical Press, 2008 (and subsequent editions as available).

General guidance

Emergency supply requested by prescriber

Emergency supply of a prescription-only medicine may also be made at the request of a doctor, a dentist, a supplementary prescriber, a community practitioner nurse prescriber (formerly a district nurse or health visitor prescriber), a nurse independent prescriber, or a pharmacist independent prescriber, provided:

(a) that the pharmacist is satisfied that the prescriber by reason of some emergency is unable to furnish a prescription immediately;

(b) that the prescriber has undertaken to furnish a prescription within 72 hours;

(c) that the medicine is supplied in accordance with the directions of the prescriber requesting it;

(d) that the medicine is not a substance specifically excluded from the emergency supply provision, and does not contain a Controlled Drug specified in Schedules 1, 2, or 3 to the Misuse of Drugs Regulations 2001 except for phenobarbital or phenobarbital sodium for the treatment of epilepsy: for details see *Medicines, Ethics and Practice*, No. 32, London, Pharmaceutical Press, 2008 (and subsequent editions as available);

(e) that an entry shall be made in the prescription book stating:

    (i) the date of supply;

    (ii) the name, quantity, and, where appropriate, the pharmaceutical form and strength;

    (iii) the name and address of the practitioner requesting the emergency supply;

    (iv) the name and address of the patient;

    (v) the date on the prescription;

    (vi) when the prescription is received the entry should be amended to include the date on which it is received.

Royal Pharmaceutical Society's Guidelines

1. The pharmacist should consider the medical consequences of *not* supplying a medicine in an emergency.
2. If the pharmacist is unable to make an emergency supply of a medicine the pharmacist should advise the patient how to obtain essential medical care.

For conditions that apply to supplies made at the request of a patient, see *Medicines, Ethics and Practice*, No. 32, London Pharmaceutical Press, 2008 (and subsequent editions).

General guidance

Drug treatment in children

Children, and particularly neonates, differ from adults in their response to drugs. Special care is needed in the neonatal period (first 28 days of life) and doses should always be calculated with care; the risk of toxicity is increased by a reduced rate of drug clearance and differing target organ sensitivity.

Many children's doses in *BNF for Children* are standardised by **weight** (and therefore require multiplying by the body-weight in kilograms to determine the child's dose); occasionally, the doses have been standardised by **body surface area** (in m²) (see also How to Use *BNF for Children*, p. xi). These methods should be used rather than attempting to calculate a child's dose on the basis of doses used in adults. If a dose is not stated, prescribers should seek advice from a medicines information centre.

For most drugs the adult maximum dose should not be exceeded. For example if the dose is 8 mg/kg (max. 300 mg) a child of 10 kg body-weight should receive 80 mg but a child of 40 kg body-weight should receive 300 mg (rather than 320 mg). For certain drugs, young children may require a higher dose per kilogram than adults because of their higher metabolic rates. Calculation by body-weight in the overweight child may result in much higher doses being administered than necessary; in such cases, the dose should be calculated from an ideal weight, related to height and age.

Body surface area (BSA) estimates are often preferable to body-weight for calculating paediatric doses since many physiological phenomena correlate better with body surface area.

Body surface area can be estimated from weight; see inside back cover.

Where the dose for children is not stated, prescribers should seek advice from a medicines information centre.

Dose frequency   Most drugs can be administered at slightly irregular intervals during the day. Some drugs, e.g. antimicrobials, are best given at regular intervals. Some flexibility should be allowed in children to avoid waking them during the night. For example, the night-time dose may be given at the child's bedtime.

General guidance

Prescribing in hepatic impairment

Children have a large reserve of hepatic metabolic capacity and modification of the choice and dosage of drugs is usually unnecessary even in apparently severe liver disease. However, special consideration is required in the following situations:

- liver failure characterised by severe derangement of liver enzymes and profound jaundice; the use of sedative drugs, opioids, and drugs such as diuretics and amphotericin which produce hypokalaemia may precipitate hepatic encephalopathy;

- impaired coagulation, which can affect response to oral anticoagulants;

- in cholestatic jaundice elimination may be impaired of drugs such as fusidic acid and rifampicin which are excreted in the bile;

- in hypoproteinaemia, the effect of highly protein-bound drugs such as phenytoin, prednisolone, warfarin, and benzodiazepines may be increased;

- use of hepatotoxic drugs is more likely to cause toxicity in children with liver disease; such drugs should be avoided if possible;

- in neonates, particularly preterm neonates, and also in infants metabolic pathways may differ from older children and adults because liver enzyme pathways may be immature.

Where care is needed in hepatic impairment, this is indicated under the relevant drug in *BNF for Children*.

Prescribing in renal impairment

The use of drugs in children with reduced renal function can give rise to problems for several reasons:

- reduced renal excretion of a drug or its metabolites may produce toxicity;
- sensitivity to some drugs is increased even if elimination is unimpaired;
- many side-effects are tolerated poorly by children with renal impairment;
- some drugs are not effective when renal function is reduced;
- neonates, particularly preterm, may have immature renal function.

Many of these problems can be avoided by reducing the dose or by using alternative drugs.

Principles of dose adjustment in renal impairment

The level of renal function below which the dose of a drug must be reduced depends on the proportion of the drug eliminated by renal excretion and its toxicity.

For many drugs with only minor or no dose-related side-effects, very precise modification of the dose regimen is unnecessary and a simple scheme for dose reduction is sufficient

For more toxic drugs with a small safety margin dose regimens based on glomerular filtration rate should be used. When both efficacy and toxicity are closely related to plasma-drug concentration, recommended regimens should be regarded only as a guide to initial treatment; subsequent doses must be adjusted according to clinical response and plasma-drug concentration.

The total daily maintenance dose of a drug can be reduced either by reducing the size of the individual doses or by increasing the interval between doses. For some drugs, although the size of the maintenance dose is reduced it is important to give a loading dose if an immediate effect is required. This is because it takes about five times the half-life of the drug to achieve steady-state plasma concentration. Because the plasma half-life of drugs excreted by the kidney is prolonged in renal impairment, it can take many doses at the reduced dosage to achieve a therapeutic plasma concentration. The loading dose should usually be the same as the initial dose for a child with normal renal function.

Nephrotoxic drugs should, if possible, be avoided in children with renal disease because the consequences of nephrotoxicity are likely to be more serious when the renal reserve is already reduced.

Glomerular filtration rate is low at birth and increases rapidly during the first 6 months. Thereafter, glomerular filtration rate increases gradually to reach adult levels by 1–2 years of age, when standardised to a typical adult body surface area ($1.73 \, m^2$). In the first weeks after birth, serum creatinine falls; a single measure of serum creatinine provides only a crude estimate of renal function and observing the change over days is of more use. In the neonate, a sustained rise in serum creatinine or a lack of the expected postnatal decline, is indicative of a reduced glomerular filtration rate.

Dose recommendations are based on the severity of renal impairment. This is expressed in terms of **glomerular filtration rate** ($mL/minute/1.73 \, m^2$).

The following equations provide a guide to glomerular filtration rate.

Child over 1 year:
Estimated glomerular filtration rate ($mL/minute/1.73 \, m^2$)$= 40^1 \times$ height (cm)/ serum creatinine (micromol/litre)

Neonate:
Estimated glomerular filtration rate ($mL/minute/1.73 \, m^2$)$= 30^1 \times$ height (cm)/ serum creatinine (micromol/litre)

The serum-creatinine concentration is sometimes used as a measure of renal function but is only a **rough guide** even when corrected for age, weight, and sex.

General guidance

---

1. The values used in these formulas may differ according to locality or laboratory.

General guidance

> **Important**
> The information on dose adjustment in *BNF for Children* is expressed in terms of estimated glomerular filtration rate.
> Renal function in adults is increasingly being reported as estimated glomerular filtration rate (eGFR) normalised to a body surface area of $1.73\,\text{m}^2$; however, eGFR is derived from the MDRD (Modification of Diet in Renal Disease) formula which is not validated for use in children. eGFR derived from the MDRD formula should **not** be used to adjust drug doses in children with renal impairment.

In *BNF for Children*, values for measures of renal function are included where possible. However, where such values are not available, the *BNF for Children* reflects the terms used in the published information.

*Chronic kidney disease in **adults**: UK guidelines for identification, management and referral* (March 2006) defines renal function as follows:

Degree of impairment	eGFR[1] mL/minute/$1.73\,\text{m}^2$
Normal: Stage 1	More than 90 (with other evidence of kidney damage)
Mild: Stage 2	60–89 (with other evidence of kidney damage)
Moderate[2]: Stage 3	30–59
Severe: Stage 4	15–29
Established renal failure: Stage 5	Less than 15

1. Estimated glomerular filtration rate (eGFR) derived from the Modification of Diet in Renal Disease (MDRD) formula for use in patients over 18 years
2. NICE clinical guideline 73 (September 2008)—Chronic kidney disease: Stage 3A eGFR = 45–59, Stage 3B eGFR = 30–44

> **Dialysis**
> For prescribing in children on renal replacement therapy consult specialist literature.

Drug prescribing should be kept to the minimum in all children with severe renal disease.

If even mild renal impairment is considered likely on clinical grounds, renal function should be checked before prescribing **any** drug which requires dose modification.

Where care is needed in renal impairment, this is indicated under the relevant drug entry in *BNF for Children*.

Prescribing in pregnancy

Drugs can have harmful effects on the fetus at any time during pregnancy. It is important to bear this in mind when prescribing for a female of *childbearing age* or for men *trying to father* a child.

During the *first trimester* drugs may produce congenital malformations (teratogenesis), and the period of greatest risk is from the third to the eleventh week of pregnancy.

During the *second* and *third trimesters* drugs may affect the growth and functional development of the fetus or have toxic effects on fetal tissues; and drugs given shortly before term or during labour may have adverse effects on labour or on the neonate after delivery.

BNF for Children identifies drugs which:

● may have harmful effects in pregnancy and indicates the trimester of risk;

● are not known to be harmful in pregnancy.

The information is based on human data but information on *animal* studies has been included for some drugs when its omission might be misleading. Maternal drug doses may require adjustment during pregnancy due to changes in maternal physiology but this is beyond the scope of *BNF for Children*.

Drugs should be prescribed in pregnancy only if the expected benefit to the mother is thought to be greater than the risk to the fetus, and all drugs should be avoided if possible during the first trimester. Drugs which have been extensively used in pregnancy and appear to be usually safe should be prescribed in preference to new or untried drugs; and the smallest effective dose should be used.

Few drugs have been shown conclusively to be teratogenic in humans but no drug is safe beyond all doubt in early pregnancy. Screening procedures are available where there is a known risk of certain defects.

Absence of a drug from the list does not imply safety. It should be noted that *BNF for Children* provides independent advice and may not always agree with the product literature.

Information on drugs and pregnancy is also available from the National Teratology Information Service Telephone:

Tel: (0191) 232 1525

Tel: (0191) 223 1307 (out of hours emergency only)
www.nyrdtc.nhs.uk/Services/teratology/teratology.html

General guidance

Prescribing in breast-feeding

Breast-feeding is beneficial; the immunological and nutritional value of breast milk to the infant is greater than that of formula feeds.

Although there is concern that drugs taken by the mother might affect the infant, there is very little information on this. In the absence of evidence of an effect, the potential for harm to the infant can be inferred from:

- the amount of drug or active metabolite of the drug delivered to the infant (dependent on the pharmacokinetic characteristics of the drug in the mother);
- the efficiency of absorption, distribution and elimination of the drug by the infant (infant pharmacokinetics);
- the nature of the effect of the drug on the infant (pharmacodynamic properties of the drug in the infant).

Most medicines given to a mother cause no harm to breast-fed infants and there are few contra-indications to breast-feeding when maternal medicines are necessary. However, administration of some drugs to nursing mothers can harm the infant. In the first week of life, some such as preterm or jaundiced infants are at a slightly higher risk of toxicity.

Toxicity to the infant can occur if the drug enters the milk in pharmacologically significant quantities. The concentration in milk of some drugs (e.g. fluvastatin) may exceed the concentration in maternal plasma so that therapeutic doses in the mother can cause toxicity to the infant. Some drugs inhibit the infant's sucking reflex (e.g. phenobarbital) while others can affect lactation (e.g. bromocriptine). Drugs in breast milk may, at least theoretically, cause hypersensitivity in the infant even when concentration is too low for a pharmacological effect. *BNF for Children* identifies drugs:

- which should be used with caution or which are contra-indicated in breast-feeding for the reasons given above;
- which, on present evidence, may be given to the mother during breast-feeding, because they appear in milk in amounts which are too small to be harmful to the infant;
- which are not known to be harmful to the infant although they are present in milk in significant amounts.

For many drugs insufficient evidence is available to provide guidance and it is advisable to administer only essential drugs to a mother during breast-feeding. Because of the inadequacy of information on drugs in breast milk information in *BNF for Children* should be used only as a guide; absence of information does not imply safety.

General guidance

Prescribing Controlled Drugs

The Misuse of Drugs Act, 1971 prohibits certain activities in relation to 'Controlled Drugs', in particular their manufacture, supply, and possession. The penalties applicable to offences involving the different drugs are graded broadly according to the *harmfulness attributable to a drug when it is misused* and for this purpose the drugs are defined in the following three classes:

Class A includes: alfentanil, cocaine, diamorphine (heroin), dipipanone, lysergide (LSD), methadone, methylenedioxymethamfetamine (MDMA, 'ecstasy'), morphine, opium, pethidine, phencyclidine, remifentanil, and class B substances when prepared for injection

Class B includes: oral amphetamines, barbiturates, cannabis, cannabis resin, codeine, ethylmorphine, glutethimide, pentazocine, phenmetrazine, and pholcodine

Class C includes: certain drugs related to the amphetamines such as benzfetamine and chlorphentermine, buprenorphine, diethylpropion, mazindol, meprobamate, pemoline, pipradrol, most benzodiazepines, zolpidem, androgenic and anabolic steroids, clenbuterol, chorionic gonadotrophin (HCG), non-human chorionic gonadotrophin, somatotropin, somatrem, and somatropin

The Misuse of Drugs Regulations 2001 define the classes of person who are authorised to supply and possess controlled drugs while acting in their professional capacities and lay down the conditions under which these activities may be carried out. In the regulations drugs are divided into five schedules each specifying the requirements governing such activities as import, export, production, supply, possession, prescribing, and record keeping which apply to them.

Schedule 1 includes drugs such as cannabis and lysergide which are not used medicinally. Possession and supply are prohibited except in accordance with Home Office authority.

Schedule 2 includes drugs such as diamorphine (heroin), morphine, remifentanil, pethidine, secobarbital, glutethimide, amfetamine, and cocaine and are subject to the full controlled drug requirements relating to prescriptions, safe custody (except for secobarbital), the need to keep registers, etc. (unless exempted in Schedule 5).

Schedule 3 includes the barbiturates (except secobarbital, now Schedule 2), buprenorphine, diethylpropion, mazindol, meprobamate, midazolam, pentazocine, phentermine, and temazepam. They are subject to the special prescription requirements (except for temazepam) but not to the safe custody requirements (except for buprenorphine and temazepam) nor to the need to keep registers (although there are requirements for the retention of invoices for 2 years).

Schedule 4 includes in Part I benzodiazepines (except temazepam and midazolam which are in Schedule 3) and zolpidem, which are subject to minimal control. Part II includes androgenic and anabolic steroids, clenbuterol, chorionic gonadotrophin (HCG), non-human chorionic gonadotrophin, somatotropin, somatrem, and somatropin. Controlled Drug prescription requirements do not apply (but see Department of Health Guidance, p. 18) and Schedule 4 Controlled Drugs are not subject to safe custody requirements.

Schedule 5 includes those preparations which, because of their strength, are exempt from virtually all Controlled Drug requirements other than retention of invoices for two years.

Prescriptions   Preparations in Schedules 2 and 3 of the Misuse of Drugs Regulations 2001 (and subsequent amendments) are identified throughout *BNF for Children* by the symbol ⌐CD⌐ (Controlled Drug). The principal legal requirements relating to medical prescriptions are listed below (see also Department of Health Guidance, p. 18).

General guidance

General guidance

> **Prescription requirements**
> Prescriptions for Controlled Drugs that are subject to prescription requirements[1] must be indelible[2] and must be *signed* by the prescriber, *be dated*, and specify the prescriber's *address*. The prescription must always state:
> - The name and address of the patient;
> - In the case of a preparation, the form[3] and where appropriate the strength[4] of the preparation;
> - either the total quantity (in both words and figures) of the preparation[5], or the number (in both words and figures) of dosage units, as appropriate, to be supplied; in any other case, the total quantity (in both words and figures) of the Controlled Drug to be supplied;
> - The dose[6];
> - The words 'for dental treatment only' if issued by a dentist.

A pharmacist is **not** allowed to dispense a Controlled Drug unless all the information required by law is given on the prescription. In the case of a prescription for a Controlled Drug in Schedule 2 or 3, a pharmacist can amend the prescription if it specifies the total quantity only in words or in figures or if it contains minor typographical errors, provided that such amendments are indelible and clearly attributable to the pharmacist[7]. Failure to comply with the regulations concerning the writing of prescriptions will result in inconvenience to patients and carers and delay in supply of the necessary medicine. A prescription for a Controlled Drug in Schedules 2, 3, or 4 is valid for 28 days from the date stated thereon[8].

Instalments and 'repeats' A prescription may order a Controlled Drug to be dispensed by instalments; the amount of instalments and the intervals to be observed must be specified.[9] Prescriptions ordering 'repeats' on the same form are **not** permitted for Controlled Drugs in Schedules 2 or 3.

For a sample prescription, see p. 19

Private prescriptions Private prescriptions for Controlled Drugs in Schedules 2 and 3 must be written on specially designated forms provided by Primary Care Trusts in England, Health Boards in Scotland, Local Health Boards in Wales or the Northern Ireland Central Services Agency; in addition, prescriptions must specify the *prescriber's identification number*. Prescriptions to be supplied by a pharmacist in hospital are exempt from the requirement for private prescriptions.

Department of Health guidance Guidance (June 2006) issued by the Department of Health in England on prescribing and dispensing of Controlled Drugs requires:

- in general, prescriptions for Controlled Drugs in Schedules 2, 3, and 4 to be limited to a supply of up to 30 days' treatment; exceptionally, to cover a justifiable clinical need and after consideration of any risk, a prescription can be issued for a longer period, but the reasons for the decision should be recorded on the patient's notes;
- the patient's identifier to be shown on NHS and private prescriptions for Controlled Drugs in Schedules 2 and 3.

Further information is available at www.dh.gov.uk.

Dependence and misuse The most serious drugs of addiction are **cocaine**, **diamorphine** (heroin), **morphine**, and the **synthetic opioids**.

---

1. All preparations in Schedules 2 and 3, except temazepam.
2. A machine-written prescription is acceptable. The prescriber's signature must be handwritten.
3. The dosage form (e.g. tablets) must be included on a Controlled Drugs prescription irrespective of whether it is implicit in the proprietary name (e.g. *MST Continus*) or whether only one form is available.
4. When more than one strength of a preparation exists the strength required must be specified.
5. The Home Office has advised that quantities of liquid preparations such as methadone mixture should be written in millilitres.
6. The instruction 'one as directed' constitutes a dose but 'as directed' does not.
7. Implementation date for *N. Ireland* not confirmed.
8. The prescriber may forward-date the prescription; the start date may also be specified in the body of the prescription.
9. A total of 14 days' treatment by instalment of any drug listed in Schedule 2 of the Misuse of Drugs Regulations, buprenorphine and diazepam may be prescribed in England. In *England*, forms FP10(MDA) (blue) and FP10H(MDA) (blue) should be used. In *Scotland*, forms GP10 (peach), HBP (blue), or HBPA (pink) should be used. In *Wales* a total of 14 days' treatment by instalment of any drug listed in Schedules 2–5 of the Misuse of Drugs Regulations may be prescribed. In Wales, form WP10(MDA) or form WP10HP(AD) should be used.

Despite marked reduction in the prescribing of **amphetamines** the abuse of illicit amfetamine and related compounds is widespread.

The benzodiazepine **temazepam** has commonly been associated with misuse. The misuse of **barbiturates** is now less common, in line with declining prescription numbers.

Cannabis (Indian hemp) has no approved medicinal use and cannot be prescribed by doctors. Its use is illegal but has become widespread. Cannabis is a mild hallucinogen seldom accompanied by a desire to increase the dose; withdrawal symptoms are unusual. **Lysergide** (lysergic acid diethylamide, LSD) is a much more potent hallucinogen; its use can lead to severe psychotic states which can be life-threatening.

Prescribing drugs likely to cause dependence or misuse   The prescriber has three main responsibilities:

- to avoid creating dependence by introducing drugs to patients without sufficient reason. In this context, the proper use of the morphine-like drugs is well understood. The dangers of other Controlled Drugs are less clear because recognition of dependence is not easy and its effects, and those of withdrawal, are less obvious;

- to see that the patient does not gradually increase the dose of a drug, given for good medical reasons, to the point where dependence becomes more likely. The prescriber should keep a close eye on the amount prescribed to prevent patients or their carers from accumulating stocks. A minimal amount should be prescribed in the first instance, or when seeing a new patient for the first time;

- to avoid being used as an unwitting source of supply for addicts and being vigilant to methods for obtaining medicines which include visiting more than one doctor, fabricating stories, and forging prescriptions.

General guidance

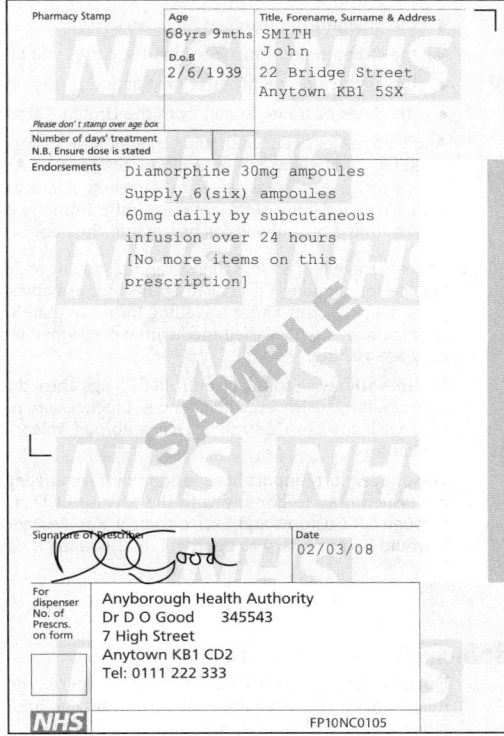

General guidance

Patients under temporary care should be given only small supplies of drugs unless they present an unequivocal letter from their own doctor. It is sensible to reduce dosages steadily or to issue weekly or even daily prescriptions for small amounts if dependence is suspected.

The stealing and misuse of prescription forms could be minimised by the following precautions:

(a) do not leave unattended if called away from the consulting room or at reception desks; do not leave in a car where they may be visible; when not in use, keep in a locked drawer within the surgery and at home;

(b) draw a diagonal line across the blank part of the form under the prescription;

(c) the quantity should be shown in words and figures when prescribing drugs prone to abuse; this is obligatory for controlled drugs (see Prescriptions, above);

(d) alterations are best avoided but if any are made they should be clear and unambiguous; add initials against altered items;

(e) if prescriptions are left for collection they should be left in a safe place in a sealed envelope.

Travelling abroad   Prescribed drugs listed in Schedule 4 Part II (CD Anab) and Schedule 5 of the Misuse of Drugs Regulations 2001 are not subject to export or import licensing. However, patients intending to travel abroad for more than 3 months carrying any amount of drugs listed in Schedules 2, 3, or 4 Part I (CD Benz) will require a personal export/import licence. Further details can be obtained at www.drugs.homeoffice.gov.uk/drugs-laws/licensing/personal, or from the Home Office by contacting (020) 7035 0484 or licensing_enquiry.aadu@homeoffice.gsi.gov.uk.

Applications must be supported by a covering letter from the prescriber and should give details of:

• the patient's name and current address;

• the quantities of drugs to be carried;

• the strength and form in which the drugs will be dispensed;

• the country or countries of destination;

• the dates of travel to and from the United Kingdom.

Applications for licences should be sent to the Home Office, Drugs Licensing, Peel Building, 2 Marsham Street, London, SW1P 4DF. Alternatively, completed application forms can be emailed to licensing_enquiry.aadu@homeoffice.gsi.gov.uk with a scanned copy of the covering letter from the prescriber. A minimum of two weeks should be allowed for processing the application.

Patients travelling for less than 3 months do not require a personal export/import licence for carrying Controlled Drugs, but are advised to carry a letter from the prescribing doctor. Those travelling for more than 3 months are advised to make arrangements to have their medication prescribed by a practitioner in the country they are visiting.

Doctors who wish to take Controlled Drugs abroad while accompanying patients may similarly be issued with licences. Licences are not normally issued to doctors who wish to take Controlled Drugs abroad solely in case a family emergency should arise.

Personal export/import licences do not have any legal status outside the UK and are issued only to comply with the Misuse of Drugs Act and facilitate passage through UK Customs and Excise control. For clearance in the country to be visited it would be necessary to approach that country's consulate in the UK.

Notification of drug misusers

Doctors should report cases of drug misuse to their regional or national drug misuse database or centre—for further advice and contact telephone numbers consult the BNF.

Adverse reactions to drugs

Any drug may produce unwanted or unexpected adverse reactions. Rapid detection and recording of adverse reactions is of vital importance so that unrecognised hazards are identified promptly and appropriate regulatory action is taken to ensure that medicines are used safely. Doctors, dentists, coroners, pharmacists, and nurses (see also self-reporting, below) are urged to report suspected adverse reactions directly to the Medicines and Healthcare products Regulatory Agency (MHRA) through the Yellow Card Scheme using the electronic form at www.yellowcard.gov.uk. Alternatively, prepaid Yellow Cards for reporting are available from the address below and are also bound in this book (inside back cover).

Medicines and Healthcare products Regulatory Agency
CHM
Freepost
London, SW8 5BR.
Tel: (0800 731 6789)

The reporting of **all** suspected adverse drug reactions in children, including those relating to unlicensed or off-label use of medicines, is **strongly encouraged** through the Yellow Card Scheme even if the intensive monitoring symbol (▼) has been removed, because experience in children may still be limited.

The identification and reporting of adverse reactions to drugs in children is particularly important because:

- the action of the drug and its pharmacokinetics in children (especially in the very young) may be different from that in adults;
- drugs may not be extensively tested in children;
- children may be more susceptible to developmental disorders or they may have delayed adverse reactions which do not occur in adults;
- many drugs are not specifically licensed for use in children and are used 'off-label';
- suitable formulations may not be available to allow precise dosing in children;
- the nature and course of illnesses and adverse drug reactions may differ between adults and children.

Suspected adverse reactions to *any* therapeutic agent should be reported, including drugs *(self-medication* as well as those *prescribed)*, blood products, vaccines, radiographic contrast media, complementary and herbal products.

Spontaneous reporting is particularly valuable for recognising possible new hazards rapidly. An adverse reaction should be reported even if it is not certain that the drug has caused it, or if the reaction is well recognised, or if other drugs have been given at the same time. Reports of overdoses (deliberate or accidental) can complicate the assessment of adverse drug reactions, but provide important information on the potential toxicity of drugs.

A 24-hour Freefone service is available to all parts of the UK for advice and information on suspected adverse drug reactions; contact the National Yellow Card Information Service at the MHRA on 0800 731 6789. Outside office hours a telephone-answering machine will take messages.

The following Yellow Card Centres may *follow up* reports:

Yellow Card Centre, North West
70 Pembroke Place
Liverpool, L69 3GF.
Tel: (0151) 794 8206

Yellow Card Centre, Wales
Freepost
Cardiff, CF4 1ZZ.
Tel: (029) 2074 4181 (direct line)

Yellow Card Centre, Northern & Yorkshire
Wolfson Unit
Claremont Place
Newcastle upon Tyne, NE2 4HH.
Tel: (0191) 260 6181 (direct line)

General guidance

Yellow Card Centre, West Midlands
Freepost SW2991
Birmingham, B18 7BR.
Tel: (0121) 507 5672

Yellow Card Centre, Scotland
CARDS, Royal Infirmary of Edinburgh
Freepost RRAR-RUXE-GJGX
Edinburgh, EH16 4SA.
Tel: (0131) 242 2919

The MHRA's database facilitates the monitoring of adverse drug reactions.

More detailed information on reporting and a list of products currently under intensive monitoring can be found on the MHRA website: www.mhra.gov.uk.

Drug Safety Update is a monthly newsletter from the MHRA and the Commission on Human Medicines (CHM); it is available at www.mhra.gov.uk/mhra/drugsafetyupdate.

Self-reporting   Patients, parents, and carers can also report suspected adverse reactions to the MHRA. Reports can be submitted directly to the MHRA through the Yellow Card Scheme using the electronic form at www.yellowcard.gov.uk or by telephone on 0808 100 3352. Alternatively, patient Yellow Cards are available from pharmacies or can be downloaded from www.mhra.gov.uk, where more detailed information on patient reporting is available.

Adverse reactions to medical devices   Suspected adverse reactions to medical devices including dental or surgical materials, intra-uterine devices, and contact lens fluids should be reported. Information on reporting these can be found at: www.mhra.gov.uk.

Prescription-event monitoring   In addition to the MHRA's Yellow Card Scheme, an independent scheme monitors the safety of new medicines using a different approach. The Drug Safety Research Unit identifies patients who have been prescribed selected new medicines and collects data on clinical events in these patients. The data are submitted on a voluntary basis by general practitioners on green forms. More information about the scheme and the Unit's educational material is available from www.dsru.org.

Side-effects in the *BNF for Children*   The *BNF for Children* includes clinically relevant side-effects for most drugs; an exhaustive list is not included for drugs that are used by specialists (e.g. cytotoxic drugs and drugs used in anaesthesia). Where causality has not been established, side-effects in the manufacturers' literature may be omitted from the *BNF for Children*.

In the product literature the frequency of side-effects is generally described as follows:

Very common	greater than 1 in 10
Common	1 in 100 to 1 in 10
Uncommon ['less commonly' in *BNF for Children*]	1 in 1000 to 1 in 100
Rare	1 in 10 000 to 1 in 1000
Very rare	less than 1 in 10 000

Special problems

Symptoms   Children may be poor at expressing the symptoms of an adverse drug reaction and parental opinion may be required.

Delayed drug effects   Some reactions (e.g. cancers, and effects on development) may become manifest months or years after exposure. Any suspicion of such an association should be reported directly to the MHRA through the Yellow Card Scheme.

Congenital abnormalities   When an infant is born with a congenital abnormality or there is a malformed aborted fetus doctors are asked to consider whether this might be an adverse reaction to a drug and to report all drugs (including self-medication) taken during pregnancy.

General guidance

Prevention of adverse reactions

Adverse reactions may be prevented as follows:

- never use any drug unless there is a good indication. If the patient is pregnant do not use a drug unless the need for it is imperative;

- allergy and idiosyncrasy are important causes of adverse drug reactions. Ask if the child has had previous reactions to the drug or formulation;

- prescribe as few drugs as possible and give very clear instructions to the child, parent, or carer;

- whenever possible use a familiar drug; with a new drug be particularly alert for adverse reactions or unexpected events;

- consider if excipients (e.g. colouring agents) may be contributing to the adverse reaction. If the reaction is minor, a trial of an alternative formulation of the same drug may be considered before abandoning the drug;

- obtain a full drug history including asking if the child is already taking other drugs *including over-the-counter medicines*; interactions may occur;

- age and hepatic or renal disease may alter the metabolism or excretion of drugs, particularly in neonates, which can affect the potential for adverse effects. Genetic factors may also be responsible for variations in metabolism, and therefore for the adverse effects of the drug;

- warn the child, parent, or carer if serious adverse reactions are liable to occur.

Defective medicines

During the manufacture or distribution of a medicine an error or accident may occur whereby the finished product does not conform to its specification. While such a defect may impair the therapeutic effect of the product and could adversely affect the health of a patient, it should **not** be confused with an Adverse Drug Reaction where the product conforms to its specification.

The Defective Medicines Report Centre assists with the investigation of problems arising from licensed medicinal products thought to be defective and co-ordinates any necessary protective action. Reports on suspect defective medicinal products should include the brand or the non-proprietary name, the name of the manufacturer or supplier, the strength and dosage form of the product, the product licence number, the batch number or numbers of the product, the nature of the defect, and an account of any action already taken in consequence. The Centre can be contacted at:

The Defective Medicines Report Centre

Medicines and Healthcare products Regulatory Agency

17–157 Market Towers

1 Nine Elms Lane

London SW8 5NQ

(020) 7084 2574 (weekdays 9.00 am–5.00 pm)

or (020) 7210 3000 (urgent calls any other time)

info@mhra.gsi.gov.uk

General guidance

Prescribing in palliative care

Palliative care is the active total care of children and young adults who have incurable, life-limiting conditions and are not expected to survive beyond young adulthood.

The child may be cared for in a hospice or at home according to the needs of the child and the child's family. In all cases, children should receive total care of their physical, emotional, social, and spiritual needs, and their families should be supported throughout. In particular, specialist palliative care is essential for end-of-life care of the child and for supporting the family through death and bereavement.

Drug treatment The number of drugs should be as few as possible. Oral medication is usually appropriate unless there is severe nausea and vomiting, dysphagia, weakness, or coma, when parenteral medication may be necessary.

Pain

Analgesics are more effective in preventing pain than in the relief of established pain; it is important that they are given regularly.

Paracetamol (p. 247) or a **NSAID** (section 10.1.1) given regularly will often make the use of opioid analgesics unnecessary. A NSAID may also control the pain of *bone secondaries*. Radiotherapy and bisphosphonates (section 6.6.2) may also be useful for pain due to bone metastases.

An opioid analgesic (section 4.7.2) such as **codeine** (p. 252), alone or in combination with a non-opioid analgesic at adequate dosage, may be helpful in the control of moderate pain if non-opioid analgesics alone are not sufficient. If these preparations do not control the pain, **morphine** (p. 255) is the most useful opioid analgesic. Alternatives to morphine, including transdermal **fentanyl** (see below and p. 253), are best initiated by those with experience in palliative care. Initiation of an opioid analgesic should not be delayed by concern over a theoretical likelihood of psychological or physical dependence (addiction).

Equivalent single doses of opioid analgesics	
These equivalences are intended **only** as an approximate guide; patients should be carefully monitored after **any** change in medication and dose titration may be required	
Analgesic	Dose
Morphine salts (oral)	10 mg
Diamorphine hydrochloride (subcutaneous)	3 mg
Hydromorphone hydrochloride	1.3 mg
Oxycodone (oral)	5 mg

Oral route Morphine (p. 255) is given *by mouth* as an oral solution or as standard ('immediate release') tablets regularly every 4 hours, the initial dose depending largely on the patient's previous treatment. If the first dose of morphine is no more effective than the previous analgesic, the next dose should be increased by 30–50%, the aim being to choose the lowest dose that prevents pain. The dose should be adjusted with careful assessment of the pain, and the use of adjuvant analgesics (such as NSAIDs) should also be considered. Although low doses of morphine are usually adequate there should be no hesitation in increasing the dose stepwise according to response if necessary.

If pain occurs between regular doses of morphine ('breakthrough pain'), an additional dose ('rescue dose') should be given. An additional dose should also be given 30 minutes before an activity that causes pain (e.g. wound dressing).

When the pain is controlled and the patient's 24-hour morphine requirement is established, the daily dose can be given as a single dose or in 2 divided doses as a *modified-release preparation*. The first dose of the modified-release preparation is given within 4 hours of the last dose of the oral solution.[1]

---

1. Studies have indicated that administration of the last dose of the *oral solution* with the first dose of the *modified-release tablets* is not necessary.

MST Continus® tablets or suspension (p. 257) are designed for twice daily administration; *MXL*® capsules (p. 257) allow administration of the total daily morphine requirement as a single dose.

Alternatively, a *modified-release preparation* may be commenced immediately and the dose adjusted according to pain control. The starting dose of modified-release preparations designed for twice daily administration is usually 200–800 micrograms/kg every 12 hours if no other analgesic (or only paracetamol) has been taken previously, but to replace a weaker opioid analgesic (such as codeine) the starting dose is usually higher. Increments should be made to the dose, not to the frequency of administration, which should remain at every 12 hours.

Morphine, as oral solution or standard formulation tablets, should be prescribed for breakthrough pain; the dose should be about one-sixth of the total daily dose of oral morphine repeated every 4 hours if necessary (review pain management if analgesic required more frequently). Children often require a higher dose of morphine in proportion to their body-weight compared to adults. Children are more susceptible to certain adverse effects of opioids such as urinary retention (which can be eased by carbachol or bethanechol), and opioid-induced pruritus.

Oxycodone (p. 257) is used in a child who requires an opioid but cannot tolerate morphine. If the child is already receiving an opioid, oxycodone should be started at a dose equivalent to the current analgesic.

Parenteral route   Diamorphine (p. 252) is preferred for injection because, being more soluble, it can be given in a smaller volume. The equivalent subcutaneous dose is approximately a third of the oral dose of morphine. *Subcutaneous infusion* of diamorphine via a continuous infusion device can be useful (for details, see p. 28).

If the child can resume taking medicines by mouth, then oral morphine may be substituted for subcutaneous infusion of diamorphine. See table of approximate equivalent doses of morphine and diamorphine, p. 29.

Rectal route   Morphine (p. 257) is also available for *rectal administration* as suppositories.

Transdermal route   Transdermal preparations of fentanyl (p. 254) are available; they are not suitable for acute pain or in those children whose analgesic requirements are changing rapidly because the long time to steady state prevents rapid titration of the dose. Prescribers should ensure that they are familiar with the correct use of transdermal preparations (see under fentanyl, p. 253) because prescribing errors have caused fatalities.

The following 24-hour doses of morphine **by mouth** are considered to be approximately equivalent to the fentanyl patches shown:

Morphine salt 45 mg daily ≡ fentanyl '12' patch

Morphine salt 90 mg daily ≡ fentanyl '25' patch

Morphine salt 180 mg daily ≡ fentanyl '50' patch

Morphine salt 270 mg daily ≡ fentanyl '75' patch

Morphine salt 360 mg daily ≡ fentanyl '100' patch

Morphine (as oral solution or standard formulation tablets) is given for breakthrough pain.

Gastro-intestinal pain   The pain of *bowel colic* may be reduced by loperamide (p. 65). Hyoscine hydrobromide (p. 245) may also be helpful in reducing the frequency of spasms; it is given sublingually at a dose of 10 micrograms/kg (max. 300 micrograms) 3 times daily as *Kwells*® tablets. For the dose by subcutaneous infusion using a continuous infusion device, see p. 28).

Gastric distension pain due to pressure on the stomach may be helped by a preparation incorporating an antacid with an antiflatulent (p. 51) and a prokinetic such as domperidone (p. 58) before meals.

Muscle spasm   The pain of muscle spasm can be helped by a muscle relaxant such as diazepam (p. 618) or baclofen (p. 616).

Neuropathic pain   Patients with neuropathic pain (p. 261) may benefit from a trial of a tricyclic antidepressant, most commonly amitriptyline (p. 229), for

General guidance

several weeks. An anticonvulsant, most commonly carbamazepine (p. 267), may be added or substituted if pain persists; gabapentin is licensed for neuropathic pain in adults.

Pain due to nerve compression may be reduced by a corticosteroid such as dexamethasone, which reduces oedema around the tumour, thus reducing compression.

Nerve blocks can be considered when pain is localised to a specific area. **Transcutaneous electrical nerve stimulation** (TENS) may also help.

Miscellaneous conditions

> Unlicensed indications or routes
> Several recommendations in this section involve unlicensed indications or routes.

Anorexia   Anorexia may be helped by prednisolone or dexamethasone.

Anxiety   Anxiety can be treated with a long-acting benzodiazepine such as diazepam, or by continuous infusion of the short-acting benzodiazepine midazolam. Interventions for more acute episodes of anxiety (such as panic attacks) include short-acting benzodiazepines such as lorazepam given sublingually or midazolam given subcutaneously. Temazepam provides useful night-time sedation in some children.

Capillary bleeding   Capillary bleeding can be treated with tranexamic acid (p. 158) by mouth; treatment is usually continued for one week after the bleeding has stopped but it can be continued at a reduced dose if bleeding persists. Alternatively, gauze soaked in tranexamic acid 100 mg/mL or adrenaline (epinephrine) solution 1 mg/mL (1 in 1000) can be applied to the affected area. Vitamin K may be useful in bleeding associated with liver dysfunction.

Constipation   Constipation is a very common cause of distress and is almost invariable after administration of an opioid analgesic. It should be prevented if possible by the regular administration of laxatives. Suitable laxatives include osmotic laxatives (p. 83) (such as lactulose or macrogols), stimulant laxatives (p. 79) (such as co-danthramer and senna) or the combination of lactulose and a senna preparation. Naloxone given by mouth may help relieve opioid-induced constipation; it is poorly absorbed and there is little risk of it reversing opioid analgesia.

Convulsions   Intractable seizures are relatively common in children dying from non-malignant conditions. Phenobarbital by mouth or as a continuous subcutaneous infusion may be beneficial; continuous infusion of midazolam is an alternative. Both cause drowsiness, but this is rarely a concern in the context of intractable seizures. For breakthrough convulsions diazepam (p. 284) given rectally (as a solution), buccal midazolam (p. 286), or paraldehyde (p. 286) as an enema may be appropriate.

For the use of midazolam by subcutaneous infusion using a continuous infusion device, see p. 28.

Dry mouth   Dry mouth may be caused by certain medications including opioid analgesics, antimuscarinic drugs (e.g. hyoscine), antidepressants and some antiemetics; if possible, an alternative preparation should be considered. Dry mouth may be relieved by good mouth care and measures such as sucking ice or pineapple chunks, chewing gum, or the use of artificial saliva (p. 661); dry mouth associated with candidiasis can be treated by oral preparations of nystatin (p. 658) or miconazole (p. 658); alternatively, fluconazole (p. 366) can be given by mouth.

Dysphagia   A corticosteroid such as dexamethasone may help, temporarily, if there is an obstruction due to tumour. See also Dry Mouth, above.

Dyspnoea   Breathlessness at rest may be relieved by regular oral morphine in carefully titrated doses. Diazepam may be helpful for dyspnoea associated with anxiety. Sublingual lorazepam or subcutaneous or buccal midazolam are alternatives. A nebulised short-acting beta$_2$ agonist (section 3.1.1.1) or a corticosteroid (section 3.2), such as dexamethasone or prednisolone, may also be helpful for bronchospasm or partial obstruction.

General guidance

Excessive respiratory secretion   Excessive respiratory secretion (death rattle) may be reduced by hyoscine hydrobromide patches (p. 245) or by subcutaneous or intravenous injection of hyoscine hydrobromide 10 micrograms/kg (max. 600 micrograms) every 4 to 8 hours; however, care must be taken to avoid the discomfort of dry mouth. Alternatively, glycopyrronium (p. 770) may be given. Benzodiazepines such as rectal diazepam or subcutaneous midazolam may be helpful in the final stages.

Fungating tumours   Fungating tumours can be treated by regular dressing and antibacterial drugs; systemic treatment with metronidazole (p. 356) is often required, but topical metronidazole (p. 709) is also used.

Hiccup   Hiccup due to gastric distension may be helped by a preparation incorporating an antacid with an antiflatulent (p. 52).

Hypercalcaemia   See section 9.5.1.2.

Insomnia   Children with advanced cancer may not sleep because of discomfort, cramps, night sweats, joint stiffness, or fear. There should be appropriate treatment of these problems before hypnotics (p. 212) are used. Benzodiazepines, such as temazepam, may be useful.

Intractable cough   Intractable cough may be relieved by moist inhalations or by regular administration of oral morphine every 4 hours. Methadone linctus should be avoided because it has a long duration of action and tends to accumulate.

Mucosal bleeding   Mucosal bleeding from the mouth and nose occurs commonly in the terminal phase, particularly in a child suffering from haemopoeitic malignancy. Bleeding from the nose caused by a single bleeding point can be arrested by cauterisation or by dressing it. Tranexamic acid (p. 158) may be effective applied topically or given systemically.

Nausea and vomiting   Nausea and vomiting are common in children with advanced cancer. Ideally, the cause should be determined before treatment with an antiemetic (section 4.6) is started.

Nausea and vomiting with opioid therapy are less common in children than in adults but may occur particularly in the initial stages and can be prevented by giving an antiemetic. An antiemetic is usually necessary only for the first 4 or 5 days and therefore combined preparations containing an opioid with an antiemetic are not recommended because they lead to unnecessary antiemetic therapy (and associated side-effects when used long-term).

Metoclopramide has a prokinetic action and is used by mouth for nausea and vomiting associated with gastritis, gastric stasis, and functional bowel obstruction. Drugs with antimuscarinic effects antagonise prokinetic drugs and, if possible, should not therefore be used concurrently.

Haloperidol (p. 219) is used by mouth for most metabolic causes of vomiting (e.g. hypercalcaemia, renal failure).

Cyclizine (p. 239) is used for nausea and vomiting due to mechanical bowel obstruction, raised intracranial pressure, and motion sickness.

Ondansetron (p. 244) is most effective when the vomiting is due to damaged or irritated gut mucosa (e.g. after chemotherapy or radiotherapy).

Antiemetic therapy should be reviewed every 24 hours; it may be necessary to substitute the antiemetic or to add another one.

Levomepromazine (methotrimeprazine) (p. 219) can be used if first-line antiemetics are inadequate. Dexamethasone by mouth can be used as an adjunct.

For the administration of antiemetics by subcutaneous infusion using a syringe driver, see below.

For the treatment of nausea and vomiting associated with cancer chemotherapy, see section 8.1.

Pruritus   Pruritus, even when associated with obstructive jaundice, often responds to simple measures such as application of emollients (p. 666). Ondansetron may be effective in some children. Where opioid analgesics cause pruritus

General guidance

it may be appropriate to review the dose or to switch to an alternative opioid analgesic. In the case of obstructive jaundice, further measures include administration of colestyramine (p. 93).

Raised intracranial pressure   Headache due to raised intracranial pressure often responds to a high dose of a corticosteroid, such as dexamethasone, for 4 to 5 days, subsequently reduced if possible; dexamethasone should be given before 6 p.m. to reduce the risk of insomnia. Treatment of headache and of associated nausea and vomiting should also be considered.

Restlessness and confusion   Restlessness and confusion may require treatment with haloperidol (p. 219) 10–20 micrograms/kg by mouth every 8–12 hours. Levomepromazine (methotrimeprazine) (p. 219) is also used occasionally for restlessness.

Continuous infusion devices

Although drugs can usually be administered *by mouth* to control symptoms in palliative care, the parenteral route may sometimes be necessary. Repeated administration of *intramuscular injections* should be avoided in children, particularly if cachectic. This has led to the use of portable continuous infusion devices such as syringe drivers to give a *continuous subcutaneous infusion*, which can provide good control of symptoms with little discomfort or inconvenience to the patient.

> Syringe driver rate settings
> Staff using syringe drivers should be **adequately trained** and different rate settings should be **clearly identified** and **differentiated**; incorrect use of syringe drivers is a common cause of medication errors.

Indications for the **parenteral route** are:

- inability to take medicines by mouth owing to *nausea and vomiting, dysphagia, severe weakness,* or *coma;*
- *malignant bowel obstruction* for which surgery is inappropriate (avoiding the need for an intravenous infusion or for insertion of a nasogastric tube);
- refusal by the child to take regular medication by mouth.

Bowel colic and excessive respiratory secretions   Hyoscine hydrobromide (p. 245) effectively reduces respiratory secretions and is sedative (but occasionally causes paradoxical agitation); it is given in a *subcutaneous* or *intravenous infusion dose* of 40–60 micrograms/kg/24 hours. Glycopyrronium (p. 770) may also be used.

Hyoscine butylbromide (p. 55) is effective in bowel colic, is less sedative than hyoscine hydrobromide, but is not always adequate for the control of respiratory secretions; it is given by *subcutaneous infusion* (**important:** *hyoscine butylbromide* must not be confused with *hyoscine hydrobromide*, above).

Convulsions   If a child has previously been receiving an antiepileptic drug *or* has a primary or secondary cerebral tumour *or* is at risk of convulsion (e.g. owing to uraemia) antiepileptic medication should not be stopped. Midazolam (p. 286) is the benzodiazepine antiepileptic of choice for *continuous subcutaneous infusion*.

Nausea and vomiting   Levomepromazine (methotrimeprazine) (p. 219) causes sedation in about 50% of patients. Haloperidol (p. 219) has little sedative effect.

Cyclizine (p. 239) is particularly likely to precipitate if mixed with diamorphine or other drugs (see under Mixing and Compatibility); it is given by *subcutaneous infusion*.

Pain control   Diamorphine (p. 252) is the preferred opioid since its high solubility permits a large dose to be given in a small volume (see under Mixing and Compatibility). The table on p. 29 shows approximate equivalent doses of morphine and diamorphine.

Restlessness and confusion   Haloperidol has little sedative effect. Levomepromazine (methotrimeprazine) (p. 219) has a sedative effect. Midazolam is a sedative and an antiepileptic that may be suitable for a very restless patient.

Mixing and compatibility   The general principle that injections should be given into separate sites (and should not be mixed) does not apply to the use of syringe drivers in palliative care. Provided that there is evidence of compatibility, selected injections can be mixed in syringe drivers. Not all types of medication can be used in a subcutaneous infusion. In particular, chlorpromazine, prochlorperazine, and diazepam are **contra-indicated** as they cause skin reactions at the injection site; to a lesser extent cyclizine and levomepromazine (methotrimeprazine) also sometimes cause local irritation.

In theory injections dissolved in water for injections are more likely to be associated with pain (possibly owing to their hypotonicity). The use of physiological saline (sodium chloride 0.9%) however increases the likelihood of precipitation when more than one drug is used; moreover subcutaneous infusion rates are so slow (0.1–0.3 mL/hour) that pain is not usually a problem when water is used as a diluent.

Diamorphine can be given by subcutaneous infusion in a strength of up to 250 mg/mL; up to a strength of 40 mg/mL either *water for injections* or *physiological saline* (sodium chloride 0.9%) is a suitable diluent—above that strength only *water for injections* is used (to avoid precipitation).

The following can be mixed with *diamorphine*:

Cyclizine[1]	Hyoscine hydrobromide
Dexamethasone[2]	Levomepromazine
Haloperidol[3]	Metoclopramide[4]
Hyoscine butylbromide	Midazolam

Subcutaneous infusion solution should be monitored regularly both to check for precipitation (and discoloration) and to ensure that the infusion is running at the correct rate.

Equivalent doses of morphine sulphate and diamorphine hydrochloride

These equivalences are *approximate only* and may need to be adjusted according to response

MORPHINE		PARENTERAL DIAMORPHINE
Morphine sulphate by mouth (oral solution or standard tablets)	Morphine sulphate by subcutaneous infusion	Diamorphine hydrochloride by subcutaneous infusion
every 4 hours	**every 24 hours**	**every 24 hours**
5 mg	15 mg	10 mg
10 mg	30 mg	20 mg
15 mg	45 mg	30 mg
20 mg	60 mg	40 mg
30 mg	90 mg	60 mg
40 mg	120 mg	80 mg
60 mg	180 mg	120 mg
80 mg	240 mg	160 mg
100 mg	300 mg	200 mg
130 mg	390 mg	260 mg
160 mg	480 mg	320 mg
200 mg	600 mg	400 mg

If breakthrough pain occurs give a subcutaneous injection equivalent to one-sixth of the total 24-hour subcutaneous infusion dose. With an intermittent subcutaneous injection absorption is smoother so that the risk of adverse effects at peak absorption is avoided (an even better method is to use a subcutaneous butterfly needle).
To minimise the risk of infection no subcutaneous infusion solution should be used for longer than 24 hours.

---

1. Cyclizine may precipitate at concentrations above 10 mg/mL *or* in the presence of sodium chloride 0.9% *or* as the concentration of diamorphine relative to cyclizine increases; mixtures of diamorphine and cyclizine are also likely to precipitate after 24 hours.
2. Special care is needed to avoid precipitation of dexamethasone when preparing it.
3. Mixtures of haloperidol and diamorphine are likely to precipitate after 24 hours if haloperidol concentration is above 2 mg/mL.
4. Under some conditions, infusions containing metoclopramide become discoloured; such solutions should be discarded.

General guidance

Problems encountered with syringe drivers   The following are problems that may be encountered with syringe drivers and the action that should be taken:

- if the subcutaneous infusion runs *too quickly* check the rate setting and the calculation;

- if the subcutaneous infusion runs *too slowly* check the start button, the battery, the syringe driver, the cannula, and make sure that the injection site is not inflamed;

- if there is an *injection site reaction* make sure that the site does not need to be changed—firmness or swelling at the site of injection is not in itself an indication for change, but pain or obvious inflammation is.

Prescribing in dental practice

> Advice on the drug management of dental and oral conditions is covered in the main text. For ease of access, guidance on such conditions is usually identified by means of a relevant heading (e.g. Dental and Orofacial Pain) in the appropriate sections.

The following is a list of topics of particular relevance to dental surgeons.

General guidance

Prescribing by dental surgeons, see BNF

Oral side-effects of drugs, see BNF

Medical emergencies in dental practice, see BNF

Medical problems in dental practice, see BNF

Drug management of dental and oral conditions

Dental and orofacial pain, p. 246

Neuropathic pain, p. 261

Non-opioid analgesics, p. 246

Opioid analgesics, p. 251

Non-steroidal anti-inflammatory drugs, p. 600

Oral infections

Bacterial infections, p. 297

Phenoxymethylpenicillin, p. 309

Broad-spectrum penicillins (amoxicillin and ampicillin), p. 313

Cephalosporins (cefalexin and cefradine), p. 319

Tetracyclines, p. 329

Macrolides (erythromycin and azithromycin) , p. 336

Clindamycin, p. 339

Metronidazole, p. 355

Fusidic acid p. 709

Fungal infections, p. 657

Local treatment, p. 657

Systemic treatment, p. 361

Viral infections, p. 657

Herpetic gingivostomatitis, local treatment, p. 657

Herpetic gingivostomatitis, systemic treatment, p. 385 and p. 657

Herpes labialis, p. 715

Anaesthetics, anxiolytics and hypnotics

Anaesthesia, sedation, and resuscitation in dental practice, p. 762

Hypnotics, p. 212

Peri-operative anxiolytics, p. 772

Local anaesthesia, p. 787

Oral ulceration and inflammation, p. 654

Mouthwashes and gargles, p. 659

Dry mouth, p. 661

Minerals

Fluorides, p. 571

Aromatic inhalations, p. 208

Nasal decongestants, p. 652

Dental Practitioners' Formulary, p. 924

General guidance

Drugs and sport

UK Sport advises that athletes are personally responsible should a prohibited substance be detected in their body. Information and advice, including the status of specific drugs in sport, can be obtained from UK Sport's Drug Information Database at www.didglobal.com. Alternatively, an advice card listing examples of permitted and prohibited substances is available from:

Drug-Free Sport
UK Sport
40 Bernard Street
London, WC1N 1ST.
Tel: 0800 528 0004
drug-free@uksport.gov.uk
www.uksport.gov.uk

A similar card detailing classes of drugs and doping methods prohibited in football is available from the Football Association.

> **General Medical Council's advice**
> Doctors who prescribe or collude in the provision of drugs or treatment with the intention of improperly enhancing an individual's performance in sport contravene the GMC's guidance, and such actions would usually raise a question of a doctor's continued registration. This does not preclude the provision of any care or treatment where the doctor's intention is to protect or improve the patient's health.

Emergency treatment of poisoning

These notes provide only an overview of the treatment of poisoning and it is strongly recommended that either **TOXBASE** or the **UK National Poisons Information Service** (see below) be consulted when there is doubt about the degree of risk or about appropriate management.

Most childhood poisoning is accidental. Other causes include intentional overdose, drug abuse, iatrogenic and deliberate poisoning. The drugs most commonly involved in childhood poisoning are paracetamol, ibuprofen, orally ingested creams, aspirin, iron preparations, cough medicines, and the contraceptive pill.

Hospital admission   Children who have features of poisoning should generally be admitted to hospital. Children who have taken poisons with delayed actions should also be admitted, even if they appear well. Delayed-action poisons include aspirin, iron, paracetamol, tricyclic antidepressants, and co-phenotrope (diphenoxylate with atropine, *Lomotil*®); the effects of modified-release preparations are also delayed. A note of all relevant information, including what treatment has been given, should accompany the patient to hospital.

Further information and advice

TOXBASE, the primary clinical toxicology database of the National Poisons Information Service, is available on the Internet to registered users at www.toxbase.org. It provides information about routine diagnosis, treatment, and management of patients exposed to drugs, household products, and industrial and agricultural chemicals.

Specialist information and advice on the treatment of poisoning is available day and night from the **UK National Poisons Information Service** on the following number:
Tel: 0844 892 0111

Advice on laboratory analytical services can be obtained from TOXBASE or from the National Poisons Information Service.

Help with identifying capsules or tablets may be available from a regional medicines information centre (see inside front cover).

General care

It is often impossible to establish with certainty the identity of the poison and the size of the dose. Fortunately this is not usually important because only a few poisons (such as opioids, paracetamol, and iron) have specific antidotes; few children require active removal of the poison. In most children, treatment is directed at managing symptoms as they arise. Nevertheless, knowledge of the type and timing of poisoning can help in anticipating the course of events. All relevant information should be sought from the poisoned child and from their carers. However, such information should be interpreted with care because it may not be complete or entirely reliable. Sometimes symptoms arise from other illnesses, and children should be assessed carefully. Accidents may involve a number of domestic and industrial products (the contents of which are not generally known). The **National Poisons Information Service** should be consulted when there is doubt about any aspect of suspected poisoning.

Respiration

Respiration is often impaired in unconscious children. An obstructed airway requires immediate attention. In the absence of trauma, the airway should be opened with simple measures such as chin lift or jaw thrust. An oropharyngeal or nasopharyngeal airway may be useful in children with reduced consciousness to prevent obstruction, provided ventilation is adequate. Intubation and ventilation should be considered in children whose airway cannot be protected or who have respiratory acidosis because of inadequate ventilation; such children should be monitored in a critical care area.

Most poisons that impair consciousness also depress respiration. Assisted ventilation (either mouth-to-mouth or using a bag-valve-mask device) may be needed. Oxygen is not a substitute for adequate ventilation, although it should be given in the highest concentration possible in poisoning with carbon monoxide and irritant gases.

Respiratory stimulants do not help and should be **avoided**.

The potential for pulmonary aspiration of gastric contents should be considered.

Blood pressure

Hypotension is common in severe poisoning with central nervous system depressants; if severe this may lead to irreversible brain damage or renal tubular necrosis. Hypotension should be corrected initially by tilting down the head of the bed and administration of either sodium chloride intravenous infusion or a colloidal infusion. Vasoconstrictor sympathomimetics (section 2.7.2) are rarely required and their use may be discussed with the National Poisons Information Service.

Fluid depletion without hypotension is common after prolonged coma and after aspirin poisoning due to vomiting, sweating, and hyperpnoea.

Hypertension, often transient, occurs less frequently than hypotension in poisoning; it may be associated with sympathomimetic drugs such as amphetamines, phencyclidine, and cocaine.

Heart

Cardiac conduction defects and arrhythmias can occur in acute poisoning, notably with tricyclic antidepressants, some antipsychotics, and some antihistamines. Arrhythmias often respond to correction of underlying hypoxia, acidosis, or other biochemical abnormalities. Ventricular arrhythmias that cause serious hypotension may require treatment. If the QT interval is prolonged, specialist advice should be sought because the use of some anti-arrhythmic drugs may be inappropriate. Supraventricular arrhythmias are seldom life-threatening and drug treatment is best withheld until the child reaches hospital.

Body temperature

Hypothermia may develop in patients of any age who have been deeply unconscious for some hours, particularly following overdose with barbiturates or phenothiazines. It may be missed unless core temperature is measured using a low-reading rectal thermometer or by some other means. Hypothermia is best treated by wrapping the patient (e.g. in a 'space blanket') to conserve body heat.

Hyperthermia can develop in children taking CNS stimulants; children are also at risk when taking therapeutic doses of drugs with antimuscarinic properties. Hyperthermia is initially managed by removing all unnecessary clothing and using a fan. Sponging with tepid water will promote evaporation; iced water should **not** be used. Advice should be sought from the National Poisons Information Service on the management of severe hyperthermia resulting from conditions such as the serotonin syndrome.

Both hypothermia and hyperthermia require **urgent** hospitalisation for assessment and supportive treatment.

Convulsions

Single short-lived convulsions do not require treatment. If convulsions are protracted or recur frequently, lorazepam 100 micrograms/kg (max. 4 mg) or diazepam (preferably as emulsion) 300–400 micrograms/kg (max. 20 mg) should be given by slow intravenous injection into a large vein. Benzodiazepines should not be given by the intramuscular route for convulsions. If the intravenous route is not readily available, diazepam can be administered as a rectal solution or midazolam [unlicensed use] can be given by the buccal route (section 4.8.2).

> The **National Poisons Information Service** (Tel: 0844 892 0111) will provide specialist advice on all aspects of poisoning day and night

Removal and elimination

Prevention of absorption Given by mouth, **activated charcoal** can adsorb many poisons in the gastro-intestinal system, thereby *reducing their absorption*. The **sooner** it is given the **more effective** it is, but it may still be effective up to 1 hour after ingestion of the poison—longer in the case of modified-release preparations or of drugs with antimuscarinic (anticholinergic) properties. It is relatively safe and is particularly useful for the prevention of absorption of poisons that are toxic in small amounts such as antidepressants.

A second dose may occasionally be required when blood-drug concentration continues to rise suggesting delayed drug release or delayed gastric emptying.

For the use of charcoal in active elimination techniques, see below.

Active elimination techniques Repeated doses of **activated charcoal** by mouth may *enhance the elimination* of some drugs after they have been absorbed; repeated doses are given after overdosage with:

Carbamazepine	Quinine
Dapsone	Theophylline
Phenobarbital	

Vomiting should be treated (e.g. with an antiemetic drug) since it may reduce the efficacy of charcoal treatment. In cases of intolerance, the dose may be reduced and the frequency increased but this may compromise efficacy.

Other techniques intended to enhance the elimination of poisons after absorption are only practicable in hospital and are only suitable for a small number of severely poisoned patients. Moreover, they only apply to a limited number of poisons. Examples include:

- haemodialysis for salicylates, phenobarbital, methyl alcohol (methanol), ethylene glycol, and lithium
- alkalinisation of the urine for salicylates.

Removal from the gastro-intestinal tract Gastric lavage is rarely required as benefit rarely outweighs risk; advice should be sought from the National Poisons Information Service if a significant quantity of iron or lithium has been ingested within the previous hour.

Whole bowel irrigation (by means of a bowel cleansing solution) has been used in poisoning with certain modified-release or enteric-coated formulations, in severe poisoning with lithium salts, and if illicit drugs are carried in the gastro-intestinal tract ('body-packing'). However, it is not clear that the procedure improves outcome and advice should be sought from a poisons information centre.

The administration of **laxatives** alone has no role in the management of the poisoned child and is not a recommended method of gut decontamination. The routine use of a laxative in combination with activated charcoal has mostly been abandoned. Laxatives should not be administered to young children because of the likelihood of fluid and electrolyte imbalance.

CHARCOAL, ACTIVATED

Cautions drowsy or comatose child (risk of aspiration); reduced gastro-intestinal motility (risk of obstruction); **not** for poisoning with petroleum distillates, corrosive substances, alcohols, malathion, and metal salts including iron and lithium salts

Contra-indications unprotected airway; gastro-intestinal tract not intact

Side-effects black stools

Indication and dose

Reduction of absorption of poisons
- **By mouth**

  Neonate 1 g/kg

  Child 1 month–12 years 1 g/kg (max. 50 g)

  Child 12–18 years 50 g

Emergency treatment of poisoning

◻ **CHARCOAL, ACTIVATED** *(continued)*

Active elimination of poisons
• **By mouth**

Neonate 1 g/kg every 4 hours

Child 1 month–12 years 1 g/kg (max. 50 g) every 4 hours

Child 12–18 years 50 g every 4 hours

Administration suspension or reconstituted powder may be mixed with soft drinks (e.g. caffeine-free diet cola) or fruit juices to mask the taste

Actidose-Aqua® Advance (Cambridge)
Oral suspension, activated charcoal 1.04 g/5 mL, net price 50-g pack (240 mL) = £8.69

Carbomix® (Beacon)
Powder, activated charcoal, net price 25-g pack = £8.50, 50-g pack = £11.90

Charcodote® (PLIVA)
Oral suspension, activated charcoal 1 g/5 mL, net price 50-g pack = £11.88

Specific drugs

Alcohol

Acute intoxication with alcohol (ethanol) is common in adults but also occurs in children. The features include ataxia, dysarthria, nystagmus, and drowsiness, which may progress to coma, with hypotension and acidosis. Aspiration of vomit is a special hazard and hypoglycaemia may occur in children and some adults. Patients are managed supportively, with particular attention to maintaining a clear airway and measures to reduce the risk of aspiration of gastric contents. The blood glucose is measured and glucose given if indicated.

Analgesics (non-opioid)

Aspirin   The main features of salicylate poisoning are hyperventilation, tinnitus, deafness, vasodilatation, and sweating. Coma is uncommon but indicates very severe poisoning. The associated acid-base disturbances are complex.

Treatment must be in hospital, where plasma salicylate, pH, and electrolytes (particularly potassium) can be measured; absorption of aspirin may be slow and the plasma-salicylate concentration may continue to rise for several hours, requiring repeated measurement. Plasma-salicylate concentration may not correlate with clinical severity in children, and clinical and biochemical assessment is necessary. Generally, the clinical severity of poisoning is low below a plasma-salicylate concentration of 500 mg/litre (3.6 mmol/litre) unless there is evidence of metabolic acidosis. Activated charcoal should be given within 1 hour of ingesting more than 125 mg/kg aspirin. Fluid losses should be replaced and intravenous sodium bicarbonate may be given (ensuring plasma-potassium concentration is maintained within the reference range) to enhance urinary salicylate excretion (optimum urinary pH 7.5–8.5); treatment should be given in a high dependency unit.

Plasma-potassium concentration should be corrected before giving sodium bicarbonate as hypokalaemia may complicate alkalinisation of the urine.

Haemodialysis is the treatment of choice for severe salicylate poisoning and should be considered when the plasma-salicylate concentration exceeds 700 mg/litre (5.1 mmol/litre) or in the presence of severe metabolic acidosis, convulsions, renal failure, pulmonary oedema or persistently high plasma-salicylate concentrations unresponsive to urinary alkalinisation.

NSAIDs   Mefenamic acid has important consequences in overdosage because it can cause convulsions, which if prolonged or recurrent, require treatment with intravenous lorazepam or diazepam.

Overdosage with ibuprofen may cause nausea, vomiting, epigastric pain, and tinnitus, but more serious toxicity is very uncommon. Activated charcoal followed by symptomatic measures are indicated if more than 400 mg/kg has been ingested within the preceding hour.

Paracetamol   Single or repeated doses totalling as little as 150 mg/kg of para-cetamol taken within 24 hours may cause severe hepatocellular necrosis and, much less frequently, renal tubular necrosis. Children at *high-risk* of liver damage, including those taking enzyme-inducing drugs or who are malnourished (see below), may develop liver toxicity with as little as 75 mg/kg of paracetamol taken within 24 hours. Nausea and vomiting, the only early features of poisoning, usually settle within 24 hours. Persistence beyond this time, often associated with the onset of right subcostal pain and tenderness, usually indicates development of hepatic necrosis. Liver damage is maximal 3–4 days after ingestion and may lead to encephalopathy, haemorrhage, hypoglycaemia, cerebral oedema, and death.

Therefore, despite a lack of significant early symptoms, patients who have taken an overdose of paracetamol should be transferred to hospital **urgently**.

Administration of activated charcoal should be considered if paracetamol in excess of 150 mg/kg (or in excess of 75 mg/kg for those considered to be at *high-risk*, see below) is thought to have been ingested within the previous hour.

Acetylcysteine protects the liver if infused within 24 hours of ingesting para-cetamol. It is most effective if given within 8 hours of ingestion, after which effectiveness declines sharply; if more than 24 hours have elapsed advice should be sought either from the National Poisons Information Service or from a liver unit on the management of serious liver damage. In remote areas, **methionine** by mouth is an alternative only if acetylcysteine cannot be given promptly. Once the child reaches hospital the need to continue treatment with the antidote will be assessed from the plasma-paracetamol concentration (related to the time from ingestion).

Children at risk of liver damage and therefore requiring treatment can be identified from a single measurement of the plasma-paracetamol concentration, related to the time from ingestion, provided this time interval is not less than 4 hours; earlier samples may be misleading. The concentration is plotted on a paracetamol treatment graph, with a reference line ('normal treatment line') joining plots of 200 mg/litre (1.32 mmol/litre) at 4 hours and 6.25 mg/litre (0.04 mmol/litre) at 24 hours (see p. 38). Those whose plasma-paracetamol concentration is above the *normal treatment line* are treated with acetylcysteine by intravenous infusion (or, if acetylcysteine is not available, with methionine by mouth, provided the overdose has been taken **within 10–12 hours** *and* the child is not vomiting).

Children at *high-risk* of liver damage include those:

- taking liver enzyme-inducing drugs (e.g. carbamazepine, phenobarbital, phenytoin, primidone, rifampicin, alcohol, St John's wort);
- who are malnourished (e.g. in anorexia, cystic fibrosis, in underweight children with 'failure to thrive', in alcoholism, or those who are HIV-positive);
- who have a febrile illness;
- who have not eaten for a few days.

These children may develop toxicity at **lower** plasma-paracetamol concentra-tions and should be treated if the concentration is above the *high-risk treatment line* (which joins plots that are at 50% of the plasma-paracetamol concentrations of the normal treatment line).The prognostic accuracy of plasma-paracetamol con-centration taken after 15 hours is uncertain, but a concentration above the relevant treatment line should be regarded as carrying a serious risk of liver damage.

The plasma-paracetamol concentration may be difficult to interpret when para-cetamol has been ingested over several hours (staggered overdose). If there is doubt about timing or the need for treatment then the child should be treated with acetylcysteine.

See also Co-proxamol, under Analgesics (opioid).

Emergency treatment of poisoning

The **National Poisons Information Service** (Tel: 0844 892 0111) will provide specialist advice on all aspects of poisoning day and night

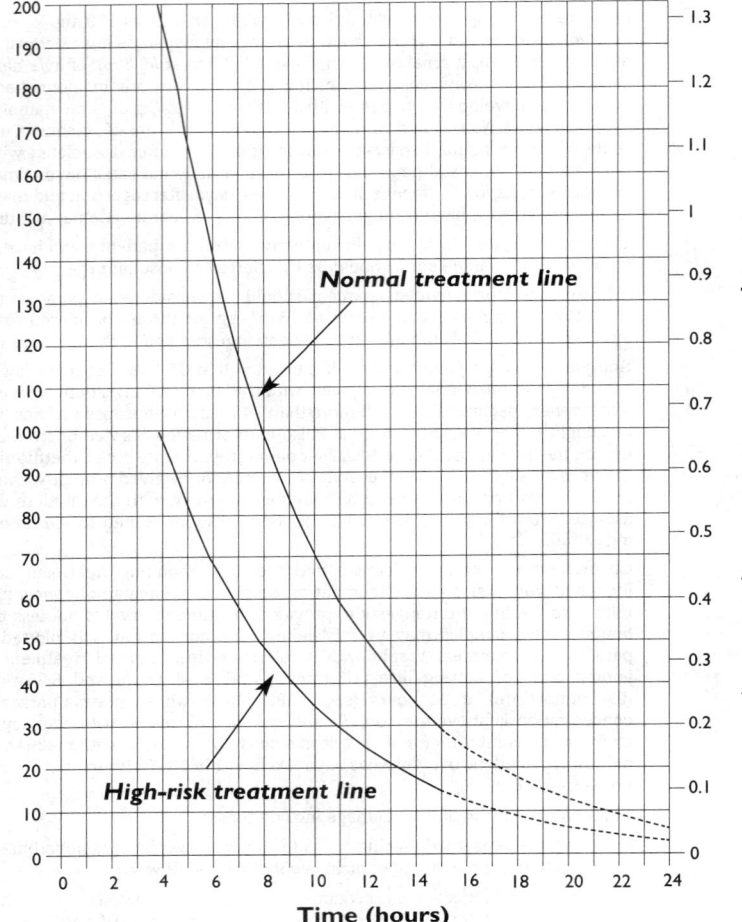

Patients whose plasma-paracetamol concentrations are above the **normal treatment line** should be treated with acetylcysteine by intravenous infusion (or, if acetylcysteine cannot be used, with methionine by mouth, provided the overdose has been taken **within 10–12 hours** and the patient is not vomiting).

Children at *high-risk* of liver damage include those:

- taking liver enzyme-inducing drugs (e.g. carbamazepine, phenobarbital, phenytoin, primidone, rifampicin, alcohol, St John's wort);
- who are malnourished (e.g. in anorexia, cystic fibrosis, in underweight children with failure to thrive, in alcoholism, or those who are HIV-positive);
- who have a febrile illness;
- who have not eaten for a few days.

These children should be treated if their plasma-paracetamol concentration is above the **high-risk treatment line**.

The prognostic accuracy after 15 hours is uncertain but a plasma-paracetamol concentration above the relevant treatment line should be regarded as carrying a serious risk of liver damage.

Graph reproduced courtesy of University of Wales College of Medicine Therapeutics and Toxicology Centre

---

ACETYLCYSTEINE

Cautions asthma (see side-effects below, but do not delay acetylcysteine treatment)

Side-effects hypersensitivity-like reactions managed by reducing infusion rate or suspending until reaction settled—contact the National Poisons Information Service if reaction severe (rash also managed by giving antihistamine; acute asthma by giving nebulised short-acting beta$_2$ agonist)

◁ **ACETYLCYSTEINE** (*continued*)

Indication and dose

Paracetamol overdosage see notes above

• **By intravenous infusion**

Neonate initially 150 mg/kg in 3 mL/kg Glucose 5% and given over 15 minutes, followed by 50 mg/kg in 7 mL/kg Glucose 5% and given over 4 hours, then 100 mg/kg in 14 mL/kg Glucose 5% and given over 16 hours

Child 1 month–5 years (or body-weight under 20 kg) initially 150 mg/kg in 3 mL/kg Glucose 5% and given over 15 minutes, followed by 50 mg/kg in 7 mL/kg Glucose 5% and given over 4 hours, then 100 mg/kg in 14 mL/kg Glucose 5% and given over 16 hours

Child 5–12 years (or body-weight over 20 kg) initially 150 mg/kg in 100 mL Glucose 5% and given over 15 minutes, followed by 50 mg/kg in 250 mL Glucose 5% and given over 4 hours,

then 100 mg/kg in 500 mL Glucose 5% and given over 16 hours

Child 12–18 years initially 150 mg/kg (max. 16.5 g) in 200 mL Glucose 5% and given over 15 minutes, followed by 50 mg/kg (max. 5.5 g) in 500 mL Glucose 5% and given over 4 hours, then 100 mg/kg (max.11 g) in 1 litre Glucose 5% and given over 16 hours

Note Manufacturer also recommends other infusion fluids, but Glucose 5% is preferable

Acetylcysteine (Non-proprietary) ℞
Injection, acetylcysteine 200 mg/mL, net price 10-mL amp = £2.50

Parvolex® (UCB Pharma) ℞
Injection, acetylcysteine 200 mg/mL, net price 10-mL amp = £2.50

▲ METHIONINE

Cautions

Hepatic impairment May precipitate coma in hepatic impairment

Side-effects nausea, vomiting, drowsiness, irritability

Indication and dose

Paracetamol overdosage see notes above

• **By mouth**

Child under 6 years 1 g every 4 hours for a total of 4 doses

Child 6–18 years 2.5 g every 4 hours for a total of 4 doses

Methionine (Pharma Nord)
Tablets, f/c, methionine 500 mg, net price 20-tab pack = £9.95

Methionine (UCB Pharma)
Tablets, DL-methionine 250 mg, net price 200-tab pack = £87.76

Analgesics (opioid)

Opioids (narcotic analgesics) cause varying degrees of coma, respiratory depression, and pinpoint pupils. The specific antidote **naloxone** is indicated if there is coma or bradypnoea. Since naloxone has a shorter duration of action than many opioids, close monitoring and repeated injections are necessary according to the respiratory rate and depth of coma. When repeated administration of naloxone is required, it can be given by continuous intravenous infusion instead and the rate of infusion adjusted according to vital signs. All children should be observed for at least 6 hours after the last dose of naloxone. The effects of some opioids, such as buprenorphine, are only partially reversed by naloxone. Dextropropoxyphene and methadone have very long durations of action; patients may need to be monitored for long periods following large overdoses.

Co-proxamol A combination of dextropropoxyphene and paracetamol (co-proxamol) taken in overdosage is much more likely to cause death than a combination of other opioids and paracetamol. The initial features are those of acute opioid overdosage with coma, respiratory depression, and pinpoint pupils. Patients may die of acute cardiovascular collapse before reaching hospital (particularly if alcohol has also been consumed) unless adequately resuscitated.

Naloxone reverses the opioid effects of dextropropoxyphene; the long duration of action of dextropropoxyphene calls for prolonged monitoring and further doses of naloxone may be required. Norpropoxyphene, a metabolite of dextropropoxyphene, also has cardiotoxic effects which may require treatment with **sodium bicarbonate**, or **magnesium sulphate**, or both; arrhythmias may occur for up to 12 hours. Paracetamol hepatotoxicity may develop later and should be anticipated and treated as indicated above.

The **National Poisons Information Service** (Tel: 0844 892 0111) will provide specialist advice on all aspects of poisoning day and night

Emergency treatment of poisoning

◢ NALOXONE HYDROCHLORIDE

Cautions physical dependence on opioids; cardiac irritability; naloxone is short-acting, see notes above

Indication and dose

> Safe Practice Doses used in acute opioid overdosage may not be appropriate for the management of opioid-induced respiratory depression and sedation in those receiving palliative care and in chronic opioid use; see also section 15.1.7 for management of postoperative respiratory depression

Overdosage with opioids
• **By intravenous injection**

Neonate 10 micrograms/kg; if no response give subsequent dose of 100 micrograms/kg (then review diagnosis); further doses may be required if respiratory function deteriorates

Child 1 month–12 years 10 micrograms/kg; if no response give subsequent dose of 100 micrograms/kg (then review diagnosis); further doses may be required if respiratory function deteriorates

Child 12–18 years 0.4–2 mg; if no response repeat at intervals of 2–3 minutes to a max. of 10 mg (then review diagnosis); further doses may be required if respiratory function deteriorates

• **By subcutaneous or intramuscular injection**
As intravenous injection but only if intravenous route not feasible (onset of action slower)

• **By continuous intravenous infusion using an infusion pump**

Neonate 5–20 micrograms/kg/hour, adjusted according to response

Child 1 month–12 years 5–20 micrograms/kg/hour, adjusted according to response

Child 12–18 years initially 0.24–1.2 mg infused over 1 hour, then using a solution of 4 micrograms/mL infuse at a rate adjusted according to response

Reversal of postoperative respiratory depression, reversal of respiratory and CNS depression in neonate following maternal opioid use during labour section 15.1.7

Administration for *continuous intravenous infusion*, dilute to a concentration of 4 micrograms/mL with Glucose 5% *or* Sodium Chloride 0.9% infusion

Naloxone (Non-proprietary) ℗ℴ𝓂
Injection, naloxone hydrochloride 400 micrograms/mL, net price 1-mL amp = £4.10; 1 mg/mL, 2-mL prefilled syringe = £6.61

Minijet® Naloxone (UCB Pharma) ℗ℴ𝓂
Injection, naloxone hydrochloride 400 micrograms/mL, net price 1-mL disposable syringe = £9.00, 2-mL disposable syringe = £11.78, 5-mL disposable syringe = £11.53

◢ Antidepressants

Tricyclic and related antidepressants Tricyclic and related antidepressants cause dry mouth, coma of varying degree, hypotension, hypothermia, hyperreflexia, extensor plantar responses, convulsions, respiratory failure, cardiac conduction defects, and arrhythmias. Dilated pupils and urinary retention also occur. Metabolic acidosis may complicate severe poisoning; delirium with confusion, agitation, and visual and auditory hallucinations, are common during recovery.

Assessment in hospital is strongly advised in case of poisoning by *tricyclic and related antidepressants* but symptomatic treatment can be given before transfer. Supportive measures to ensure a clear airway and adequate ventilation during transfer are mandatory. Intravenous lorazepam or diazepam (preferably in emulsion form) may be required to treat convulsions. Activated charcoal given within 1 hour of the overdose reduces absorption of the drug. Although arrhythmias are worrying, some will respond to correction of hypoxia and acidosis. The use of anti-arrhythmic drugs is best avoided, but intravenous infusion of sodium bicarbonate can arrest arrhythmias or prevent them in those with an extended QRS duration. Diazepam given by mouth is usually adequate to sedate delirious children but large doses may be required.

Selective serotonin re-uptake inhibitors (SSRIs) Symptoms of poisoning by selective serotonin re-uptake inhibitors include nausea, vomiting, agitation, tremor, nystagmus, drowsiness, and sinus tachycardia; convulsions may occur. Rarely, severe poisoning results in the serotonin syndrome, with marked neuropsychiatric effects, neuromuscular hyperactivity, and autonomic instability; hyperthermia, rhabdomyolysis, renal failure, and coagulopathies may develop.

Management of SSRI poisoning is supportive. Activated charcoal given within 1 hour of the overdose reduces absorption of the drug. Convulsions can be treated with lorazepam, diazepam, or buccal midazolam [unlicensed use] (see p. 34). Contact the National Poisons Information Service for the management of hyperthermia or the serotonin syndrome.

Antimalarials

Overdosage with quinine, chloroquine, or hydroxychloroquine is extremely hazardous and difficult to treat. Urgent advice from the National Poisons Information Service is essential. Life-threatening features include arrhythmias (which can have a very rapid onset) and convulsions (which can be intractable).

Beta-blockers

Therapeutic overdosages with beta-blockers may cause lightheadedness, dizziness, and possibly syncope as a result of bradycardia and hypotension; heart failure may be precipitated or exacerbated. These complications are most likely in children with conduction system disorders or impaired myocardial function. Bradycardia is the most common arrhythmia caused by beta-blockers, but sotalol may induce ventricular tachyarrhythmias (sometimes of the torsade de pointes type). The effects of massive overdosage can vary from one beta-blocker to another; propranolol overdosage in particular may cause coma and convulsions.

Acute massive overdosage must be managed in hospital and expert advice should be obtained. Maintenance of a clear airway and adequate ventilation is mandatory. An intravenous injection of atropine is required to treat bradycardia and hypotension (40 micrograms/kg, max. 3 mg). Cardiogenic shock unresponsive to atropine is probably best treated with an intravenous injection of glucagon (50–150 micrograms/kg, max. 10 mg) [unlicensed indication and dose] in glucose 5% (with precautions to protect the airway in case of vomiting) followed by an intravenous infusion of 50 micrograms/kg/hour. If glucagon is not available, intravenous isoprenaline (available from 'special-order' manufacturers or specialist importing companies, see p. 943) is an alternative. A cardiac pacemaker can be used to increase the heart rate.

> The **National Poisons Information Service** (Tel: 0844 892 0111) will provide specialist advice on all aspects of poisoning day and night

Calcium-channel blockers

Features of calcium-channel blocker poisoning include nausea, vomiting, dizziness, agitation, confusion, and coma in severe poisoning. Metabolic acidosis and hyperglycaemia may occur. Verapamil and diltiazem have a profound cardiac depressant effect causing hypotension and arrhythmias, including complete heart block and asystole. The dihydropyridine calcium-channel blockers cause severe hypotension secondary to profound peripheral vasodilatation.

Activated charcoal should be considered if the child presents within 1 hour of overdosage with a calcium-channel blocker; repeated doses of activated charcoal are considered if a modified-release preparation is involved (although activated charcoal may be effective beyond 1 hour with modified-release preparations). In children with significant features of poisoning, calcium chloride or calcium gluconate (section 9.5.1.1) is given by injection; atropine is given to correct symptomatic bradycardia. For the management of hypotension, the choice of inotropic sympathomimetic depends on whether hypotension is secondary to vasodilatation or to myocardial depression and advice should be sought from the National Poisons Information Service.

Hypnotics and anxiolytics

Benzodiazepines   Benzodiazepines taken alone cause drowsiness, ataxia, dysarthria, and occasionally minor and short-lived depression of consciousness. They potentiate the effects of other central nervous system depressants taken concomitantly. Activated charcoal can be given within 1 hour of ingesting a significant quantity of benzodiazepine, provided the child is awake and the airway is protected. Use of the benzodiazepine antagonist flumazenil can be hazardous, particularly in mixed overdoses involving tricyclic antidepressants or in benzo-diazepine-dependent patients. Flumazenil should be used on **expert advice** only.

Iron salts

Iron poisoning in childhood is usually accidental. The symptoms are nausea, vomiting, abdominal pain, diarrhoea, haematemesis, and rectal bleeding. Hypotension, coma and hepatocellular necrosis can occur later. Coma and shock indicate severe poisoning.

Advice should be sought from the National Poisons Information Service if a significant quantity of iron has been ingested within the previous hour.

Mortality is reduced by intensive and specific therapy with **desferrioxamine**, which chelates iron. The serum-iron concentration is measured as an emergency and intravenous desferrioxamine given to chelate absorbed iron in excess of the expected iron binding capacity. In **severe toxicity** intravenous desferrioxamine should be given *immediately* without waiting for the result of the serum-iron measurement.

DESFERRIOXAMINE MESILATE
(Deferoxamine Mesilate)

Cautions section 9.1.3

Side-effects section 9.1.3

Licensed use licensed for use in children (age range not specified by manufacturer)

Indication and dose

Iron poisoning
* **By continuous intravenous infusion**

> Neonate up to 15 mg/kg/hour, reduced after 4–6 hours; max. 80 mg/kg in 24 hours (in severe cases, higher doses on advice from the National Poisons Information Service)

> Child 1 month–18 years up to 15 mg/kg/hour, reduced after 4–6 hours; max. 80 mg/kg in 24 hours (in severe cases, higher doses on advice from the National Poisons Information Service)

Chronic iron overload section 9.1.3

◢Preparations
Section 9.1.3

Lithium

Most cases of lithium intoxication occur as a complication of long-term therapy and are caused by reduced excretion of the drug due to a variety of factors including dehydration, deterioration of renal function, infections, and co-administration of diuretics or NSAIDs (or other drugs that interact). Acute deliberate overdoses may also occur with delayed onset of symptoms (12 hours or more) due to slow entry of lithium into the tissues and continuing absorption from modified-release formulations.

The early clinical features are non-specific and may include apathy and restlessness which could be confused with mental changes due to the child's depressive illness. Vomiting, diarrhoea, ataxia, weakness, dysarthria, muscle twitching, and tremor may follow. Severe poisoning is associated with convulsions, coma, renal failure, electrolyte imbalance, dehydration, and hypotension.

Therapeutic lithium concentrations are within the range of 0.4–1.0 mmol/litre; concentrations in excess of 2.0 mmol/litre are usually associated with serious toxicity and such cases may need treatment with haemodialysis if neurological symptoms or renal failure are present. In acute overdosage, much higher serum-lithium concentrations may be present without features of toxicity and all that is usually necessary is to take measures to increase urine output (e.g. by increasing fluid intake, but avoiding diuretics). Otherwise, treatment is supportive with special regard to electrolyte balance, renal function, and control of convulsions. Whole-bowel irrigation should be considered for significant ingestion, but advice should be sought from the National Poisons Information Service, p. 33.

> The **National Poisons Information Service** (Tel: 0844 892 0111) will provide specialist advice on all aspects of poisoning day and night

Phenothiazines and related drugs

Phenothiazines cause less depression of consciousness and respiration than other sedatives. Hypotension, hypothermia, sinus tachycardia, and arrhythmias may complicate poisoning. Dystonic reactions can occur with therapeutic doses (particularly with prochlorperazine and trifluoperazine), and convulsions may occur in severe cases. Arrhythmias may respond to correction of hypoxia, acidosis, and other biochemical abnormalities, but specialist advice should be sought if arrhythmias result from a prolonged QT interval; the use of some anti-arrhythmic drugs can worsen such arrhythmias. Dystonic reactions are rapidly abolished by injection of drugs such as procyclidine (section 4.9.2) or diazepam (section 4.8.2, emulsion preferred).

Atypical antipsychotic drugs

Features of poisoning by atypical antipsychotic drugs (section 4.2.1) include drowsiness, convulsions, extrapyramidal symptoms, hypotension, and ECG abnormalities (including prolongation of the QT interval). Management is supportive. Activated charcoal can be given within 1 hour of ingesting a significant quantity of an atypical antipsychotic drug.

Stimulants

Amphetamines   These cause wakefulness, excessive activity, paranoia, hallucinations, and hypertension followed by exhaustion, convulsions, hyperthermia, and coma. The early stages can be controlled by diazepam or lorazepam; advice should be sought from the National Poisons Information Service (p. 33) on the management of hypertension. Later, tepid sponging, anticonvulsants, and artificial respiration may be needed.

Cocaine   Cocaine stimulates the central nervous system, causing agitation, dilated pupils, tachycardia, hypertension, hallucinations, hyperthermia, hypertonia, and hyperreflexia; cardiac effects include chest pain, myocardial infarction, and arrhythmias.

Initial treatment of cocaine poisoning involves intravenous administration of diazepam to control agitation and cooling measures for hyperthermia (see p. 34); hypertension and cardiac effects require specific treatment and expert advice should be sought.

Ecstasy   Ecstasy (methylenedioxymethamphetamine, MDMA) may cause severe reactions, even at doses that were previously tolerated. The most serious effects are delirium, coma, convulsions, ventricular arrhythmias, hyperthermia, rhabdomyolysis, acute renal failure, acute hepatitis, disseminated intravascular coagulation, adult respiratory distress syndrome, hyperreflexia, hypotension and intracerebral haemorrhage; hyponatraemia has also been associated with ecstasy use and syndrome of inappropriate antidiuretic hormone secretion (SIADH) can occur.

Treatment of methylenedioxymethamphetamine poisoning is supportive, with diazepam to control severe agitation or persistent convulsions and close monitoring including ECG. Self-induced water intoxication should be considered in patients with ecstasy poisoning.

'Liquid ecstasy' is a term used for sodium oxybate (gamma-hydroxybutyrate, GHB), which is a sedative.

Theophylline

Theophylline and related drugs are often prescribed as modified-release formulations and toxicity can therefore be delayed. They cause vomiting (which may be severe and intractable), agitation, restlessness, dilated pupils, sinus tachycardia, and hyperglycaemia. More serious effects are haematemesis, convulsions, and supraventricular and ventricular arrhythmias. Severe hypokalaemia may develop rapidly.

Repeated doses of activated charcoal can be used to eliminate theophylline even if more than 1 hour has elapsed after ingestion and especially if a modified-release preparation has been taken (see also under Active Elimination Techniques). Ondansetron (section 4.6) may be effective for severe vomiting that is resistant to other antiemetics. Hypokalaemia is corrected by intravenous infusion of potassium chloride in 0.9% sodium chloride and may be so severe as to require high doses under ECG monitoring. Convulsions should be controlled by intravenous administration of diazepam (emulsion preferred). Sedation with lorazepam or diazepam (emulsion preferred) may be necessary in agitated children.

Provided the child does **not** suffer from asthma, a short-acting beta-blocker (section 2.4) can be administered intravenously to reverse severe tachycardia, hypokalaemia, and hyperglycaemia.

Other poisons

Consult either the National Poisons Information Service day and night or TOXBASE, see p. 33.

> The **National Poisons Information Service** (Tel: 0844 892 0111) will provide specialist advice on all aspects of poisoning day and night

Cyanides

Oxygen should be administered to children with cyanide poisoning. The choice of antidote depends on the severity of poisoning, certainty of diagnosis, and the cause. Dicobalt edetate is the antidote of choice when there is a strong clinical suspicion of severe cyanide poisoning. Dicobalt edetate itself is toxic, associated with anaphylactic reactions, and is potentially fatal if administered in the absence of cyanide poisoning. A regimen of sodium nitrite followed by sodium thiosulphate is an alternative if dicobalt edetate is not available.

Hydroxocobalamin can be considered for victims of smoke inhalation who show signs of significant cyanide poisoning. The usual dose is 70 mg/kg (max. 5 g) by intravenous infusion (given once or twice according to severity). *Cyanokit®* provides hydroxocobalamin 2.5 g/bottle (no other preparation of hydroxocobalamin is suitable)—contact the National Poisons Information Service for advice.

DICOBALT EDETATE

Cautions owing to toxicity to be used only for definite cyanide poisoning when patient tending to lose, or has lost, consciousness; **not** to be used as a precautionary measure

Side-effects hypotension, tachycardia, and vomiting; anaphylactic reactions including facial and laryngeal oedema and cardiac abnormalities

Indication and dose

Severe poisoning with cyanides
- **By intravenous injection**
  Consult the National Poisons Information Service

¹**Dicobalt Edetate** (Cambridge) [PoM]
Injection, dicobalt edetate 15 mg/mL, net price 20-mL (300-mg) amp = £13.75
1. [PoM] restriction does not apply where administration is for saving life in emergency

SODIUM NITRITE

Side-effects flushing and headache due to vasodilatation

Indication and dose

Poisoning with cyanides (used in conjunction with sodium thiosulphate)
  See under preparation

¹**Sodium Nitrite** [PoM]
Injection, sodium nitrite 3% (30 mg/mL) in water for injections
Dose
- **By intravenous injection over 5–20 minutes**
  Child 1 month–18 years 4–10 mg/kg max. 300 mg (0.13–0.33 mL/kg, max. 10 mL, of 3% solution) followed by sodium thiosulphate injection 400 mg/kg, max. 12.5 g (0.8 mL/kg, max. 25 mL, of 50% solution) over 10 minutes

Available from 'special-order' manufacturers or specialist importing companies, see p. 943
1. [PoM] restriction does not apply where administration is for saving life in emergency

◣ SODIUM THIOSULPHATE

Indication and dose

Poisoning with cyanides (used in conjunction with sodium nitrite)

  See above under Sodium Nitrite

[1] **Sodium Thiosulphate** (PoM)

Injection, sodium thiosulphate 50% (500 mg/mL) in water for injections

Available from 'special-order' manufacturers or specialist importing companies, see p. 943

1. (PoM) restriction does not apply where administration is for saving life in emergency

Ethylene glycol and methanol

Fomepizole (available from 'special-order' manufacturers or specialist importing companies, see p. 943) is the treatment of choice for ethylene glycol and methanol (methyl alcohol) poisoning. If necessary, ethanol (by mouth or by intravenous infusion) can be used with caution in children. Advice on the treatment of ethylene glycol and methanol poisoning should be obtained from the National Poisons Information Service. It is important to start antidote treatment promptly in cases of suspected poisoning with these agents.

Heavy metals

Heavy metal antidotes include dimercaprol and sodium calcium edetate. Other antidotes include succimer (DMSA) and unithiol (DMPS) [both unlicensed]; they may be useful in certain cases of heavy metal poisoning but the advice of the National Poisons Information Service should be sought.

◣ DIMERCAPROL

(BAL)

Cautions hypertension, pregnancy and breast-feeding; **interactions:** Appendix 1 (dimercaprol)

Renal impairment discontinue or use with extreme caution if impairment develops during treatment

Contra-indications not indicated for iron, cadmium, or selenium poisoning; severe hepatic impairment (unless due to arsenic poisoning)

Side-effects hypertension, tachycardia, malaise, nausea, vomiting, salivation, lacrimation, sweating, burning sensation (mouth, throat, and eyes), feeling of constriction of throat and chest, headache, muscle spasm, abdominal pain, tingling of extremities; pyrexia; local pain and abscess at injection site

Licensed use licensed for use in children (age range not specified by manufacturer)

Indication and dose

Poisoning by antimony, arsenic, bismuth, gold, mercury

● **By intramuscular injection**

  Child 1 month–18 years 2.5–3 mg/kg every 4 hours for 2 days, 2–4 times on the third day, then 1–2 times daily for 10 days or until recovery

Dimercaprol (Sovereign) (PoM)

Injection, dimercaprol 50 mg/mL. Net price 2-mL amp = £42.73

Note Contains arachis (peanut) oil as solvent

◣ SODIUM CALCIUM EDETATE

(Sodium Calciumedetate)

Cautions renal impairment

Side-effects nausea, diarrhoea, abdominal pain, pain at site of injection, thrombophlebitis if given too rapidly, renal damage particularly in overdosage; hypotension, lacrimation, myalgia, nasal congestion, sneezing, malaise, thirst, fever, chills, headache and zinc depletion also reported

Licensed use licensed for use in children (age range not specified by manufacturer)

Indication and dose

Lead poisoning

● **By intravenous infusion**

  Child 1 month–18 years 40 mg/kg twice daily for up to 5 days; if necessary a second course

can be given at least 7 days after the first course, and a third course can be given at least 7 days after the second course

Administration for *intravenous infusion*, dilute to a concentration of not more 30 mg/mL with Glucose 5% *or* Sodium Chloride 0.9%; give over at least 1 hour

Ledclair® (Durbin) (PoM)

Injection, sodium calcium edetate 200 mg/mL, net price 5-mL amp = £7.29

Noxious gases

Carbon monoxide   Carbon monoxide poisoning is usually due to inhalation of smoke, car exhaust, or fumes caused by blocked flues or incomplete combustion of fuel gases in confined spaces.

Immediate treatment of carbon monoxide poisoning is essential. The child should be moved to fresh air, the airway cleared, and high-flow **oxygen** 100% administered as soon as available. Artificial respiration should be given as necessary and continued until adequate spontaneous breathing starts, or stopped only after persistent and efficient treatment of cardiac arrest has failed. The child should be admitted to hospital because complications may arise after a delay of hours or days. Cerebral oedema may occur in severe poisoning and is treated with an intravenous infusion of mannitol (section 2.2.5). Referral for hyperbaric oxygen treatment should be discussed with the National Poisons Information Service if the patient is or has been unconscious, or has psychiatric or neurological features other than a headache or has myocardial ischaemia or an arrhythmia, or has a blood carboxyhaemoglobin concentration of more than 20%, or is pregnant.

Sulphur dioxide, chlorine, phosgene, ammonia   All of these gases can cause upper respiratory tract and conjunctival irritation. Pulmonary oedema, with severe breathlessness and cyanosis may develop suddenly up to 36 hours after exposure. Death may occur. Children are kept under observation and those who develop pulmonary oedema are given oxygen. Assisted ventilation may be necessary in the most serious cases.

CS Spray

CS spray, which is used for riot control, irritates the eyes (hence 'tear gas') and the respiratory tract; symptoms normally settle spontaneously within 15 minutes. If symptoms persist, the patient should be removed to a well-ventilated area, and the exposed skin washed with soap and water after removal of contaminated clothing. Contact lenses should be removed and rigid ones washed (soft ones should be discarded). Eye symptoms should be treated by irrigating the eyes with physiological saline (or water if saline is not available) and advice sought from an ophthalmologist. Patients with features of severe poisoning, particularly respiratory complications, should be admitted to hospital for symptomatic treatment.

Nerve agents

Treatment of nerve agent poisoning is similar to organophosphorus insecticide poisoning (see below), but advice must be sought from the National Poisons Information Service. The risk of cross-contamination is significant; adequate decontamination and protective clothing for healthcare personnel are essential. In emergencies involving the release of nerve agents, kits ('NAAS pods') containing **pralidoxime** can be obtained through the Ambulance Service from the National Blood Service (or the Welsh Blood Service in South Wales or designated hospital pharmacies in Northern Ireland and Scotland—see TOXBASE for list of designated centres).

The **National Poisons Information Service** (Tel: 0844 892 0111) will provide specialist advice on all aspects of poisoning day and night

Pesticides

Organophosphorus insecticides   Organophosphorus insecticides are usually supplied as powders or dissolved in organic solvents. All are absorbed through the bronchi and intact skin as well as through the gut and inhibit cholinesterase activity, thereby prolonging and intensifying the effects of acetylcholine. Toxicity between different compounds varies considerably, and onset may be delayed after skin exposure.

Anxiety, restlessness, dizziness, headache, miosis, nausea, hypersalivation, vomiting, abdominal colic, diarrhoea, bradycardia, and sweating are common features of organophosphorus poisoning. Muscle weakness and fasciculation may develop and progress to generalised flaccid paralysis, including the ocular and respiratory muscles. Convulsions, coma, pulmonary oedema with copious bronchial secretions, hypoxia, and arrhythmias occur in severe cases. Hyperglycaemia and glycosuria without ketonuria may also be present.

Further absorption of the organophosphorus insecticide should be prevented by moving the child to fresh air, removing soiled clothing, and washing contaminated skin. In severe poisoning it is vital to ensure a clear airway, frequent removal of bronchial secretions, and adequate ventilation and oxygenation; gastric lavage may be considered provided that the airway is protected. **Atropine** will reverse the muscarinic effects of acetylcholine and is given intravenously in a dose of 20 micrograms/kg (max. 2 mg) as atropine sulphate every 5 to 10 minutes (according to the severity of poisoning) until the skin becomes flushed and dry, the pupils dilate, and bradycardia is abolished.

Pralidoxime chloride, a cholinesterase reactivator, is used as an adjunct to atropine in moderate or severe poisoning. It improves muscle tone within 30 minutes of administration. Pralidoxime chloride is continued until the patient has not required atropine for 12 hours. Pralidoxime chloride can be obtained from designated centres, the names of which are held by the National Poisons Information Service (see p. 33).

◣ PRALIDOXIME CHLORIDE

Cautions renal impairment, myasthenia gravis

Contra-indications poisoning with carbamates or organophosphorus compounds without anticholinesterase activity

Side-effects drowsiness, dizziness, disturbances of vision, nausea, tachycardia, headache, hyperventilation, and muscular weakness

Licensed use licensed for use in children (age range not specified by manufacturer)

Indication and dose

Adjunct to atropine in the treatment of poisoning by organophosphorus insecticide or nerve agent

• **By intravenous infusion over 20 minutes**

  Child under 18 years initially 30 mg/kg, followed by 8 mg/kg/hour; usual max. 12 g in 24 hours

  Note The loading dose may be administered **by intravenous injection** (diluted to a concentration of 50 mg/mL with water for injections) over at least 5 minutes if pulmonary oedema is present or if it is not practical to administer an intravenous infusion; pralidoxime chloride doses may differ from those in product literature

[1] **Pralidoxime chloride** ⓅⓄⓂ

  Injection, powder for reconstitution pralidoxime chloride 1 g/vial

  Available as *Protopam*® (from designated centres for organophosphorus insecticide poisoning or from the National Blood Service (or Welsh Ambulance Services for Mid West and South East Wales) — see TOXBASE for list of designated centres)

  1. ⓅⓄⓂ restriction does not apply where administration is for saving life in emergency

▰▰▰▰▰ Snake bites and animal stings

Snake bites　Envenoming from snake bite is uncommon in the UK. Many exotic snakes are kept, some illegally, but the only indigenous venomous snake is the adder (*Vipera berus*). The bite may cause local and systemic effects. Local effects include pain, swelling, bruising, and tender enlargement of regional lymph nodes. Systemic effects include early anaphylactic symptoms (transient hypotension with syncope, angioedema, urticaria, abdominal colic, diarrhoea, and vomiting), with later persistent or recurrent hypotension, ECG abnormalities, spontaneous systemic bleeding, coagulopathy, adult respiratory distress syndrome, and acute renal failure. Fatal envenoming is rare but the potential for severe envenoming must not be underestimated.

Early anaphylactic symptoms should be treated with **adrenaline (epinephrine)** (section 3.4.3). Indications for antivenom treatment include systemic envenoming, especially hypotension (see above), ECG abnormalities, vomiting, haemostatic abnormalities, and marked local envenoming such that after bites on the hand or foot, swelling extends beyond the wrist or ankle within 4 hours of the bite. The contents of one vial (10 mL) of **European viper venom antiserum** (available from Movianto) is given *by intravenous injection* over 10–15 minutes or *by intravenous infusion* over 30 minutes after diluting in sodium chloride intravenous infusion 0.9% (use 5 mL diluent/kg body-weight). The **same dose** should be used for **adults** and **children**. The dose can be repeated in 1–2 hours if symptoms of **systemic envenoming** persist. For children who present with clinical features of severe envenoming (e.g. shock, ECG abnormalities, and rapidly advancing local swelling), an initial dose of 2 vials (20 mL) of the antiserum is recommended. Adrenaline (epinephrine) injection must be immediately to hand for treatment of anaphylactic reactions to the antivenom (for the management of anaphylaxis see section 3.4.3).

Antivenom is available for bites by certain foreign snakes and spiders, stings by scorpions and fish. For information on identification, management, and for supply in an emergency, telephone the National Poisons Information Service (Tel: 0844 892 0111).

Insect stings   Stings from ants, wasps, hornets, and bees cause local pain and swelling but seldom cause severe direct toxicity unless many stings are inflicted at the same time. If the sting is in the mouth or on the tongue local swelling may threaten the upper airway. The stings from these insects are usually treated by cleaning the area with a topical antiseptic. Bee stings should be removed as quickly as possible. Anaphylactic reactions require immediate treatment with intramuscular **adrenaline** (**epinephrine**); self-administered (or administered by a carer) intramuscular adrenaline (e.g. *EpiPen®*) is the best first-aid treatment for children with severe hypersensitivity. An inhaled bronchodilator should be used for asthmatic reactions. For the management of anaphylaxis, see section 3.4.3. A short course of an **oral antihistamine** or a **topical corticosteroid** may help to reduce inflammation and relieve itching. A vaccine containing extracts of bee and wasp venom can be used to reduce the risk of severe anaphylaxis and systemic reactions in children with systemic hypersensitivity to bee or wasp stings (section 3.4.2).

Marine stings   The severe pain of weeverfish (*Trachinus vipera*) and Portuguese man-o'-war stings can be relieved by immersing the stung area immediately in uncomfortably hot, but not scalding, water (not more than $45°$ C). Children stung by jellyfish and Portuguese man-o'-war around the UK coast should be removed from the sea as soon as possible. Adherent tentacles should be lifted off carefully (wearing gloves or using tweezers) or washed off with seawater. Alcoholic solutions, including suntan lotions, should **not** be applied because they can cause further discharge of stinging hairs. Ice packs will reduce pain and a slurry of baking soda (sodium bicarbonate), but not vinegar, may be useful for treating stings from UK species.

> The **National Poisons Information Service** (Tel: 0844 892 0111) will provide specialist advice on all aspects of poisoning day and night

1 Gastro-intestinal system

1.1 Dyspepsia and gastro-oesophageal reflux disease................................. **50**
1.1.1 Antacids and simeticone.. 51
1.1.2 Compound alginate preparations... 53

1.2 Antispasmodics and other drugs altering gut motility **54**

1.3 Antisecretory drugs and mucosal protectants............................. **58**
1.3.1 H$_2$-receptor antagonists 60
1.3.2 Selective antimuscarinics 62
1.3.3 Chelates and complexes 62
1.3.4 Prostaglandin analogues 62
1.3.5 Proton pump inhibitors 62

1.4 Acute diarrhoea **64**
1.4.1 Adsorbents and bulk-forming drugs 65
1.4.2 Antimotility drugs 65

1.5 Chronic bowel disorders **66**
1.5.1 Aminosalicylates 68
1.5.2 Corticosteroids 72
1.5.3 Drugs affecting the immune response 74
1.5.4 Food allergy 76

1.6 Laxatives **77**
1.6.1 Bulk-forming laxatives 78
1.6.2 Stimulant laxatives 79
1.6.3 Faecal softeners 82
1.6.4 Osmotic laxatives 83
1.6.5 Bowel cleansing solutions 85
1.6.6 Peripheral opioid-receptor antagonists.. 87

1.7 Local preparations for anal and rectal disorders **87**
1.7.1 Soothing anal and rectal preparations 88
1.7.2 Compound anal and rectal preparations with corticosteroids 88
1.7.3 Rectal sclerosants 89
1.7.4 Management of anal fissures.. 89

1.8 Stoma and enteral feeding tubes **90**

1.9 Drugs affecting intestinal secretions **91**
1.9.1 Drugs affecting biliary composition and flow 91
1.9.2 Bile acid sequestrants 92
1.9.3 Aprotinin 93
1.9.4 Pancreatin... 93

This chapter includes advice on the drug management of the following:
Clostridium difficile infection, p. 68
constipation, p. 77
Crohn's disease, p. 66
food allergy, p. 76
Helicobacter pylori infection, p. 59
irritable bowel syndrome, p. 68
malabsorption syndromes, p. 68
NSAID-associated ulcers, p. 60
ulcerative colitis, p. 66

1.1 Dyspepsia and gastro-oesophageal reflux disease

1.1.1 Antacids and simeticone
1.1.2 Compound alginate preparations

Dyspepsia

Dyspepsia covers pain, fullness, early satiety, bloating, and nausea. It can occur with gastric and duodenal ulceration (section 1.3), gastro-oesophageal reflux disease, gastritis, and upper gastro-intestinal motility disorders, but most commonly it is of uncertain origin.

Children with dyspepsia should be advised about lifestyle changes (see Gastro-oesophageal reflux disease, below). Some medications may cause dyspepsia—these should be stopped, if possible.

A compound alginate preparation (section 1.1.2) may provide relief from dyspepsia; persistent dyspepsia requires investigation. Treatment with a H_2-receptor antagonist (section 1.3.1) or a proton pump inhibitor (section 1.3.5) should be initiated only on the advice of a hospital specialist.

Helicobacter pylori may be present in children with dyspepsia. *H. pylori* eradication therapy (section 1.3) should be considered for persistent dyspepsia if it is ulcer-like. However, most children with functional (investigated, non-ulcer) dyspepsia do not benefit symptomatically from *H. pylori* eradication.

Gastro-oesophageal reflux disease

Gastro-oesophageal reflux disease includes non-erosive gastro-oesophageal reflux and erosive oesophagitis. Uncomplicated gastro-oesophageal reflux is common in infancy and most symptoms, such as intermittent vomiting or repeated, effortless regurgitation, resolve without treatment between 12 and 18 months of age. Older children with gastro-oesophageal reflux disease may have heartburn, acid regurgitation and dysphagia. Oesophageal inflammation (oesophagitis), ulceration or stricture formation may develop in early childhood; gastro-oesophageal reflux disease may also be associated with chronic respiratory disorders including asthma.

Parents and carers of *neonates* and *infants* should be reassured that most symptoms of uncomplicated gastro-oesophageal reflux resolve without treatment. An increase in the frequency and a decrease in the volume of feeds may reduce symptoms. A feed thickener or pre-thickened formula feed (Appendix 2) can be used on the advice of a dietician. If necessary, a suitable alginate-containing preparation (section 1.1.2) can be used instead of thickened feeds.

Older children should be advised about life-style changes such as weight reduction if overweight, and the avoidance of alcohol and smoking. An alginate-containing antacid (section 1.1.2) can be used to relieve symptoms.

Children who do not respond to these measures or who have problems such as respiratory disorders or suspected oesophagitis need to be referred to hospital. On the advice of a paediatrician, a **histamine H_2-receptor antagonist** (section 1.3.1) can be used to relieve symptoms of gastro-oesophageal reflux disease, promote mucosal healing and permit reduction in antacid consumption. A **proton pump inhibitor** (section 1.3.5) can be used for the treatment of moderate, non-erosive oesophagitis that is unresponsive to an H_2-receptor antagonist. Endoscopically confirmed *erosive*, *ulcerative*, or *stricturing* disease in children is usually treated with a proton pump inhibitor. Reassessment is necessary if symptoms persist despite 4–6 weeks of treatment; long-term use of an H_2-receptor antagonist or proton pump inhibitor should not be undertaken without full assessment of the underlying condition. For endoscopically confirmed *erosive*, *ulcerative*, or *stricturing* disease, the proton pump inhibitor usually needs to be maintained at the minimum effective dose.

Motility stimulants (section 1.2), such as domperidone or erythromycin may improve gastro-oesophageal sphincter contraction and accelerate gastric emptying. Evidence for the long-term efficacy of motility stimulants in the management of gastro-oesophageal reflux in children is unconvincing.

For advice on specialised formula feeds, see section 9.4.2.

1.1.1 Antacids and simeticone

Antacids (usually containing aluminium or magnesium compounds) can be used for short-term relief of intermittent symptoms of *ulcer dyspepsia* and *non-erosive gastro-oesophageal reflux* (see section 1.1) in children; they are also used in functional (non-ulcer) dyspepsia, but the evidence of benefit is uncertain.

Aluminium- and **magnesium-containing** antacids, being relatively insoluble in water, are long-acting if retained in the stomach. Magnesium-containing antacids tend to be laxative whereas aluminium-containing antacids may be constipating; antacids containing both magnesium and aluminium may reduce these colonic side-effects. Aluminium-containing antacids should not be used in children with renal impairment, or in neonates and infants because accumulation may lead to increased plasma-aluminium concentrations.

Complexes such as **hydrotalcite** confer no special advantage.

Calcium-containing antacids can induce rebound acid secretion; with modest doses the clinical significance of this is doubtful, but prolonged high doses also cause hypercalcaemia and alkalosis.

Simeticone (activated dimeticone) is used to treat infantile colic, but the evidence of benefit is uncertain. Simeticone is added to an antacid as an antifoaming agent to relieve flatulence; such preparations may also be useful for the relief of hiccup in palliative care (see Prescribing in Palliative Care, p. 27).

Alginates act as mucosal protectants in gastro-oesophageal reflux disease (section 1.1.2). The amount of additional ingredient or antacid in individual preparations varies widely, as does their sodium content, so that preparations may not be freely interchangeable.

Interactions   Antacids should preferably not be taken at the same time as other drugs since they may impair absorption. Antacids may also damage enteric coatings designed to prevent dissolution in the stomach. See also **Appendix 1** (antacids, calcium salts).

> **Low Na^+**
> The words 'low Na^+' added after some preparations indicate a sodium content of less than 1 mmol per tablet or 10-mL dose.

Aluminium- and magnesium-containing antacids

ALUMINIUM HYDROXIDE

Cautions see notes above; **interactions:** Appendix 1 (antacids)

Renal impairment risk of aluminium accumulation and aluminium toxicity. Absorption of aluminium from aluminium salts is increased by citrates, which are contained in many effervescent preparations

Pregnancy use with caution especially in first trimester

Contra-indications hypophosphataemia; neonates and infants

Gastro-intestinal system **1**

◌ **ALUMINIUM HYDROXIDE (continued)**

Side-effects see notes above

Indication and dose

Dyspepsia for dose see preparations

Hyperphosphataemia section 9.5.2.2

◀Co-magaldrox
Co-magaldrox is a mixture of aluminium hydroxide and
magnesium hydroxide; the proportions are expressed in
the form x/y where x and y are the strengths in milligrams
per unit dose of magnesium hydroxide and aluminium
hydroxide respectively

Maalox® (Sanofi-Aventis)
Suspension, sugar-free, co-magaldrox 195/220
(magnesium hydroxide 195 mg, dried aluminium

hydroxide 220 mg/5 mL (low Na$^+$)). Net price
500 mL = £2.79

Dose
• **By mouth**
   Child 14–18 years 10–20 mL 20–60 minutes after
   meals and at bedtime, or when required

Mucogel® (Chemidex)
Suspension, sugar-free, co-magaldrox 195/220
(magnesium hydroxide 195 mg, dried aluminium
hydroxide 220 mg/5 mL (low Na$^+$)). Net price
500 mL = £1.71

Dose
• **By mouth**
   Child 12–18 years 10–20 mL 3 times daily, 20–60
   minutes after meals and at bedtime, or when required

MAGNESIUM TRISILICATE

Cautions heart failure, hypertension; metabolic or
respiratory alkalosis, hypermagnesaemia; **interactions:** Appendix 1 (antacids)

Renal impairment increased risk of toxicity—
avoid or reduce dose. Magnesium trisilicate mixture has a high sodium content

Pregnancy use with caution especially in first
trimester; avoid antacid preparations containing
high sodium content

Contra-indications severe renal failure; hypophosphataemia

Side-effects see notes above; silica-based renal
stones reported on long-term treatment

Indication and dose

Dyspepsia for dose see under preparation

**Magnesium Trisilicate Mixture, BP
(Magnesium Trisilicate Oral Suspension)**
Oral suspension, 5% each of magnesium trisilicate,
light magnesium carbonate, and sodium bicarbonate in a suitable vehicle with a peppermint flavour. Contains about 6 mmol Na$^+$/10 mL

Dose
• **By mouth**
   Child 5–12 years 5–10 mL with water 3 times daily or
   as required
   Child 12–18 years 10–20 mL with water 3 times daily
   or as required

Aluminium-magnesium complexes

HYDROTALCITE
**Aluminium magnesium carbonate hydroxide
hydrate**

Cautions see notes above; **interactions:** Appendix 1 (antacids)

Side-effects see notes above

Indication and dose

Dyspepsia for dose see under preparation

Hydrotalcite (Peckforton)
Suspension, hydrotalcite 500 mg/5 mL (low Na$^+$).
Net price 500-mL pack = £1.96

Note The brand name *Altacite®* 𝖭𝖧𝖲 is used for hydrotalcite
suspension; for *Altacite Plus®* suspension, see below

Dose
• **By mouth**
   Child 6–12 years 5 mL 4 times daily (between meals
   and at bedtime)
   Child 12–18 years 10 mL 4 times daily (between
   meals and at bedtime)

Antacid preparations containing simeticone

Altacite Plus® (Peckforton)
Suspension, sugar-free, co-simalcite 125/500
(simeticone 125 mg, hydrotalcite 500 mg)/5 mL
(low Na$^+$). Net price 500 mL = £1.96

Dose
• **By mouth**
   Child 8–12 years 5 mL 4 times daily (between meals
   and at bedtime) when required

   Child 12–18 years 10 mL 4 times daily (between
   meals and at bedtime) when required

Gastro-intestinal system

1

Asilone® (Thornton & Ross)

Suspension, sugar-free, dried aluminium hydroxide 420 mg, simeticone 135 mg, light magnesium oxide 70 mg/5 mL (low Na$^+$). Net price 500 mL = £1.95

Dose

- **By mouth**

  Child 12–18 years 5–10 mL after meals and at bedtime or when required up to 4 times daily

Maalox Plus® (Sanofi-Aventis)

Suspension, sugar-free, dried aluminium hydroxide 220 mg, simeticone 25 mg, magnesium hydroxide 195 mg/5 mL (low Na$^+$). Net price 500 mL = £2.79

Dose

- **By mouth**

  Child 2–5 years 5 mL 3 times daily

  Child 5–12 years 5–10 mL 3–4 times daily

  Child 12–18 years 5–10 mL 4 times daily (after meals and at bedtime) or when required

Simeticone alone

◢ SIMETICONE

Activated dimeticone

Indication and dose

Colic or wind pain for dose see under individual preparations

Dentinox® (DDD) ◢

Colic drops (= emulsion), simeticone 21 mg/2.5-mL dose. Net price 100 mL = £1.73

Dose

- **By mouth**

  Neonate 2.5 mL with or after each feed (max. 6 doses in 24 hours); may be added to bottle feed

Child 1 month–2 years 2.5 mL with or after each feed (max. 6 doses in 24 hours); may be added to bottle feed

Note The brand name *Dentinox®* is also used for other preparations including teething gel

Infacol® (Forest) ◢

Liquid, sugar-free, simeticone 40 mg/mL (low Na$^+$). Net price 50 mL = £2.26. Counselling, use of dropper

Dose

- **By mouth**

  Neonate 0.5–1 mL before feeds

  Child 1 month–2 years 0.5–1 mL before feeds

1.1.2   Compound alginate preparations

Alginate taken in combination with an antacid increases the viscosity of stomach contents and can protect the oesophageal mucosa from acid reflux. Some alginate-containing preparations form a viscous gel ('raft') that floats on the surface of the stomach contents, thereby reducing symptoms of reflux. Alginate-containing preparations are used in the management of mild symptoms of dyspepsia and gastro-oesophageal reflux disease (see section 1.1). Antacids may damage enteric coatings designed to prevent dissolution in the stomach. For **interactions**, see Appendix 1 (antacids, calcium salts).

Preparations containing aluminium should not be used in children with renal impairment, or in neonates and infants.

Alginate raft-forming oral suspensions

The following preparations contain sodium alginate, sodium bicarbonate, and calcium carbonate in a suitable flavoured vehicle, and conform to the specification for Alginate Raft-forming Oral Suspension, BP.

Acidex® (Pinewood)

Liquid, sugar-free, sodium alginate 250 mg, sodium bicarbonate 133.5 mg, calcium carbonate 80 mg/5 mL. Contains about 3 mmol Na$^+$/5 mL, net price 500 mL (aniseed- or peppermint-flavour) = £1.70

Dose

- **By mouth**

  Child 6–12 years 5–10 mL after meals and at bedtime

  Child 12–18 years 10–20 mL after meals and at bedtime

Peptac® (IVAX)

Suspension, sugar-free, sodium bicarbonate 133.5 mg, sodium alginate 250 mg, calcium carbonate 80 mg/5 mL. Contains 3.1 mmol Na$^+$/5mL. Net price 500 mL (aniseed- or peppermint-flavoured) = £2.16

Dose

  Child 6–12 years 5–10 mL after meals and at bedtime

  Child 12–18 years 10–20 mL after meals and at bedtime

Gastro-intestinal system

1

Other compound alginate preparations

Gastrocote® (Actavis)

Tablets, alginic acid 200 mg, dried aluminium hydroxide 80 mg, magnesium trisilicate 40 mg, sodium bicarbonate 70 mg. Contains about 1 mmol Na⁺/tablet. Net price 100-tab pack = £3.51

Cautions diabetes mellitus (high sugar content)

Dose
• **By mouth**
  Child 6–18 years 1–2 tablets chewed 4 times daily (after meals and at bedtime)

Liquid, sugar-free, peach-coloured, dried aluminium hydroxide 80 mg, magnesium trisilicate 40 mg, sodium alginate 220 mg, sodium bicarbonate 70 mg/5 mL. Contains 2.13 mmol Na⁺/5 mL. Net price 500 mL = £2.67

Dose
• **By mouth**
  Child 6–18 years 5–15 mL 4 times daily (after meals and at bedtime)

Gaviscon® Advance (R&C)

Tablets, sugar-free, sodium alginate 500 mg, potassium bicarbonate 100 mg. Contains 2.25mmol Na⁺, 1 mmol K⁺/tablet. Net price 60–tab pack (peppermint-flavour) = £3.24
Excipients include aspartame (section 9.4.1)

Dose
• **By mouth**
  Child 6–12 years 1 tablet to be chewed after meals and at bedtime (under medical advice only)
  Child 12–18 years 1–2 tablets to be chewed after meals and at bedtime

Suspension, sugar-free, aniseed- or peppermint-flavour, sodium alginate 500 mg, potassium bicarbonate 100 mg/5 mL. Contains 2.3 mmol Na⁺, 1 mmol K⁺/5 mL, net price 250 mL = £2.70, 500 mL = £5.40

Dose
• **By mouth**
  Child 2–12 years 2.5–5 mL after meals and at bedtime (under medical advice only)
  Child 12–18 years 5–10 mL after meals and at bedtime

Gaviscon® Infant (R&C)

Oral powder, sugar-free, sodium alginate 225 mg, magnesium alginate 87.5 mg, with colloidal silica and mannitol/dose (half dual-sachet). Contains 0.92 mmol Na⁺/dose. Net price 15 dual-sachets (30 doses) = £2.46

Dose
• **By mouth**
  Neonate body-weight under 4.5 kg 1 'dose' (half dual-sachet) mixed with feeds (or water, for breast-fed infants) when required (max. 6 times in 24 hours)
  Neonate body-weight over 4.5 kg 2 'doses' (1 dual-sachet) mixed with feeds (or water, for breast-fed infants) when required (max. 6 times in 24 hours)

  Child 1 month–2 years
  Body-weight under 4.5 kg dose as for neonate
  Body-weight over 4.5 kg 2 'doses' (1 dual-sachet) mixed with feeds (or water, for breast-fed infants) when required (max. 6 times in 24 hours)

Note Not to be used in preterm neonates, or where excessive water loss likely (e.g. fever, diarrhoea, vomiting, high room temperature), or if intestinal obstruction. Not to be used with other preparations containing thickening agents

> Safe Practice Each half of the dual-sachet is identified as 'one dose'. To avoid errors prescribe as 'dual-sachet' with directions in terms of 'dose'

Rennie® Duo (Roche Consumer Health)

Suspension, sugar-free, calcium carbonate 600 mg, magnesium carbonate 70 mg, sodium alginate 150 mg/5 mL. Contains 2.6 mmol Na⁺/5 mL. Net price 500 mL (mint flavour) = £2.67

Dose
• **By mouth**
  Child 12–18 years 10 mL after meals and at bedtime; an additional 10 mL may be taken between doses for heartburn if necessary, max. 80 mL daily

Excipients include propylene glycol

Topal® (Fabre)

Tablets, alginic acid 200 mg, dried aluminium hydroxide 30 mg, light magnesium carbonate 40 mg with lactose 220 mg, sucrose 880 mg, sodium bicarbonate 40 mg (low Na⁺). Net price 42-tab pack = £1.67

Cautions diabetes mellitus (high sugar content)

Dose
• **By mouth**
  Child 12–18 years 1–3 tablets chewed 4 times daily (after meals and at bedtime)

1.2 Antispasmodics and other drugs altering gut motility

Drugs in this section include antimuscarinic compounds and drugs believed to be direct relaxants of intestinal smooth muscle. The smooth muscle relaxant properties of antimuscarinic and other antispasmodic drugs may be useful in *irritable bowel syndrome*.

The dopamine-receptor antagonist **domperidone** stimulates transit in the gut.

Antimuscarinics

Antimuscarinics (formerly termed 'anticholinergics') reduce intestinal motility. They are occasionally used for the management of *irritable bowel syndrome* but the evidence of their value has not been established and response varies. Other indications for antimuscarinic drugs include asthma and airways disease (section 3.1.2), motion sickness (section 4.6), urinary frequency and enuresis (section 7.4.2), mydriasis and cycloplegia (section 11.5), premedication (section 15.1.3), palliative care (p. 26), and as an antidote to organophosphorus poisoning (p. 47).

Antimuscarinics that are used for gastro-intestinal smooth muscle spasm include the tertiary amine **dicycloverine hydrochloride** (dicyclomine hydrochloride) and the quaternary ammonium compounds **propantheline bromide** and **hyoscine butylbromide**. The quaternary ammonium compounds are less lipid soluble than atropine and so are less likely to cross the blood-brain barrier; they are also less well absorbed from the gastro-intestinal tract.

Dicycloverine hydrochloride may also have some direct action on smooth muscle. Hyoscine butylbromide is advocated as a gastro-intestinal antispasmodic, but it is poorly absorbed; the injection may be useful in endoscopy and radiology.

Cautions   Antimuscarinics should be used with caution in children (especially children with Down's syndrome) due to increased risk of side-effects; they should also be used with caution in hypertension, conditions characterised by tachycardia (including hyperthyroidism, cardiac insufficiency, cardiac surgery), pyrexia, pregnancy, and in children susceptible to angle-closure glaucoma. Antimuscarinics are not used in children with gastro-oesophageal reflux disease, diarrhoea or ulcerative colitis. **Interactions:** Appendix 1 (antimuscarinics).

Contra-indications   Antimuscarinics are contra-indicated in myasthenia gravis (but may be used to decrease muscarinic side-effects of anticholinesterases—section 10.2.1), paralytic ileus, and pyloric stenosis.

Side-effects   Side-effects of antimuscarinics include constipation, transient bradycardia (followed by tachycardia, palpitation and arrhythmias), reduced bronchial secretions, urinary urgency and retention, dilatation of the pupils with loss of accommodation, photophobia, dry mouth, flushing and dryness of the skin. Side-effects that occur occasionally include nausea, vomiting, and giddiness.

1 Gastro-intestinal system

DICYCLOVERINE HYDROCHLORIDE
(Dicyclomine hydrochloride)

Cautions   see notes above

Contra-indications   see notes above; child under 6 months

Breast-feeding   avoid—present in milk; apnoea reported in infant

Side-effects   see notes above

Indication and dose

Symptomatic relief of gastro-intestinal disorders characterised by smooth muscle spasm
• By mouth

Child 6 months–2 years 5–10 mg 3–4 times daily 15 minutes before feeds

Child 2–12 years 10 mg 3 times daily

Child 12–18 years 10–20 mg 3 times daily

Merbentyl® (Sanofi-Aventis) (PoM)
Tablets, dicycloverine hydrochloride 10 mg, net price 20 = £1.01; 20 mg (*Merbentyl 20®*), 84-tab pack = £8.47

Syrup, dicycloverine hydrochloride 10 mg/5 mL, net price 120 mL = £1.84

Note Dicycloverine hydrochloride can be sold to the public provided that max. single dose is 10 mg and max. daily dose is 60 mg

◀Compound preparations
Kolanticon® (Peckforton)
Gel, sugar-free, dicycloverine hydrochloride 2.5 mg, dried aluminium hydroxide 200 mg, light magnesium oxide 100 mg, simeticone 20 mg/5 mL, net price 200 mL = £2.21, 500 mL = £2.79

Dose
Child 12–18 years 10–20 mL every 4 hours when required

HYOSCINE BUTYLBROMIDE

Cautions   see notes above; also intestinal and urinary outlet obstruction

Pregnancy   manufacturer advises use only if potential benefit outweighs risk

Breast-feeding   amount too small to be harmful

Contra-indications   see notes above

Side-effects   see notes above

Licensed use   *tablets* not licensed for use in children under 6 years; *injection* not licensed for use in children (age range not specified by manufacturer)

◁ **HYOSCINE BUTYLBROMIDE (continued)**

Indication and dose

Symptomatic relief of gastro-intestinal or gen-ito-urinary disorders characterised by smooth muscle spasm
• **By mouth**
  Child 6–12 years 10 mg 3 times daily
  Child 12–18 years 20 mg 4 times daily

Excessive respiratory secretions and bowel colic in palliative care (see also p. 28)
• **By mouth**
  Child 1 month–2 years 300–500 micrograms/kg (max. 5 mg) 3–4 times daily
  Child 2–5 years 5 mg 3–4 times daily
  Child 5–12 years 10 mg 3–4 times daily
  Child 12–18 years 10–20 mg 3–4 times daily

• **By intramuscular or intravenous injection**
  Child 1 month–4 years 300–500 micrograms/kg (max. 5 mg) 3–4 times daily
  Child 5–12 years 5–10 mg 3–4 times daily
  Child 12–18 years 10–20 mg 3–4 times daily

Acute spasm, spasm in diagnostic procedures
• **By intramuscular or intravenous injection**
  Child 2–6 years 5 mg repeated after 30 minutes if necessary (may be repeated more frequently in endoscopy), max. 15 mg daily
  Child 6–12 years 5–10 mg repeated after 30 minutes if necessary (may be repeated more frequently in endoscopy), max. 30 mg daily
  Child 12–18 years 20 mg repeated after 30 minutes if necessary (may be repeated more frequently in endoscopy), max. 80 mg daily

Administration for *intravenous injection*, may be diluted with Glucose 5% or Sodium Chloride 0.9%; give over at least 1 minute.

For administration *by mouth*, injection solution may be used; content of ampoule may be stored in a refrigerator for up to 24 hours after opening

Buscopan® (Boehringer Ingelheim) [PoM]
Tablets, coated, hyoscine butylbromide 10 mg, net price 56-tab pack = £2.59
Note Hyoscine butylbromide tablets can be sold to the public provided single dose does not exceed 20 mg, daily dose does not exceed 80 mg, and pack does not contain a total of more than 240 mg

Injection, hyoscine butylbromide 20 mg/mL. Net price 1-mL amp = 20p

---

◢ PROPANTHELINE BROMIDE

Cautions see notes above
  Hepatic impairment manufacturer advises caution
  Renal impairment manufacturer advises caution
  Pregnancy manufacturer advises avoid
  Breast-feeding may suppress lactation
Contra-indications see notes above
Side-effects see notes above
Licensed use *tablets* not licensed for use in children under 12 years

Indication and dose

Symptomatic relief of gastro-intestinal disorders characterised by smooth muscle spasm
• **By mouth**
  Child 1 month–12 years 300 micrograms/kg (max. 15 mg) 3–4 times daily at least one hour before food
  Child 12–18 years 15 mg 3 times daily at least one hour before meals and 30 mg at night (max. 120 mg daily)

Pro-Banthine® (Concord) [PoM]
Tablets, pink, s/c, propantheline bromide 15 mg, net price 112-tab pack = £15.32. Label: 23

◢ Extemporaneous formulations available see Extemporaneous Preparations, p. 8

◢ Other antispasmodics

Alverine, **mebeverine**, and **peppermint oil** are believed to be direct relaxants of intestinal smooth muscle and may relieve pain in *irritable bowel syndrome* and primary dysmenorrhoea. They have no serious adverse effects; peppermint oil occasionally causes heartburn.

◢ ALVERINE CITRATE

Cautions
  Pregnancy caution
  Breast-feeding little information available—manufacturer advises avoid
Contra-indications paralytic ileus

Side-effects nausea; headache, dizziness; pruritus, rash; hepatitis also reported

◁ **ALVERINE CITRATE (continued)**

Indication and dose

Adjunct in gastro-intestinal disorders characterised by smooth muscle spasm, dysmenorrhoea
• By mouth
   Child 12–18 years 60–120 mg 1–3 times daily

Spasmonal® (Norgine)
Capsules, alverine citrate 60 mg (blue/grey), net
price 100-cap pack = £11.95; 120 mg (*Spasmonal®
Forte*, blue/grey), 60-cap pack = £13.80

■ MEBEVERINE HYDROCHLORIDE

Cautions avoid in acute porphyria (section 9.8.2)
   Pregnancy not known to be harmful—manufacturers advise caution

Contra-indications paralytic ileus

Side-effects *rarely* allergic reactions (including
rash, urticaria, angioedema)

Licensed use *tablets and liquid* not licensed for
use in children under 10 years; *granules* not
licensed for use in children under 12 years; *modified-release capsules* not licensed for use in children under 18 years

Indication and dose

Adjunct in gastro-intestinal disorders characterised by smooth muscle spasm
• By mouth
   Child 3–4 years 25 mg 3 times daily, preferably
   20 minutes before meals

   Child 4–8 years 50 mg 3 times daily, preferably
   20 minutes before meals

   Child 8–10 years 100 mg 3 times daily, preferably 20 minutes before meals

   Child 10–18 years 135–150 mg 3 times daily,
   preferably 20 minutes before meals

¹**Mebeverine Hydrochloride** (Non-proprietary) [PoM]
Tablets, mebeverine hydrochloride 135 mg, net
price 20 = £2.21

Oral suspension, mebeverine hydrochloride (as
mebeverine embonate) 50 mg/5 mL. Contains Na⁺
0.87 mmol/5 mL. Net price 300 mL = £107.00
1. Mebeverine hydrochloride can be sold to the public for
children over 10 years, for symptomatic relief of
irritable bowel syndrome, provided that max. single
dose is 135 mg and max. daily dose is 405 mg

Colofac® (Solvay) [PoM]
Tablets, s/c, mebeverine hydrochloride 135 mg.
Net price 20 = £1.50

◢ **Modified release**
Colofac® MR (Solvay) [PoM]
Capsules, m/r, mebeverine hydrochloride 200 mg,
net price 60-cap pack = £6.67. Label: 25
Dose
Irritable bowel syndrome
• By mouth
   Child 12–18 years 1 capsule twice daily preferably 20
   minutes before food

◢ **Compound preparations**
¹**Fybogel® Mebeverine** (R&C) [PoM]
Granules, buff, effervescent, ispaghula husk 3.5 g,
mebeverine hydrochloride 135 mg/sachet. Contains 2.5 mmol K⁺/sachet, net price 10 sachets =
£2.50. Label: 13, 22, counselling, see below
Excipients include aspartame (section 9.4.1)
Dose
Irritable bowel syndrome
• By mouth
   Child 12–18 years 1 sachet in water, morning and
   evening 30 minutes before food; an additional sachet
   may also be taken before the midday meal if necessary

Counselling Preparations that swell in contact with liquid
should always be carefully swallowed with water and
should not be taken immediately before going to bed
1. 10-sachet pack can be sold to the public for use in
children over 12 years

■ PEPPERMINT OIL

Cautions sensitivity to menthol
   Breast-feeding significant levels of menthol in
   breast milk unlikely

Side-effects heartburn, perianal irritation; *rarely*,
allergic reactions (including rash, headache,
bradycardia, muscle tremor, ataxia)
Local irritation Capsules should not be broken or chewed
because peppermint oil may irritate mouth or oesophagus

Indication and dose

Relief of abdominal colic and distension, particularly in irritable bowel syndrome
• By mouth
   Child 15–18 years 1–2 capsules, swallowed
   whole with water, 3 times daily for up to 3
   months if necessary

Colpermin® (McNeil)
Capsules, e/c, light blue/dark blue, blue band,
peppermint oil 0.2 mL. Net price 100-cap pack =
£12.05. Label: 5, 25
Excipients include arachis (peanut) oil

1

Gastro-intestinal system

Gastro-intestinal system · 1

Motility stimulants

Domperidone and **metoclopramide** (section 4.6) are dopamine receptor antagonists which stimulate gastric emptying and small intestinal transit, and enhance the strength of oesophageal sphincter contraction. Metoclopramide and occasionally domperidone can cause acute dystonic reactions—for further details of this and other side-effects, see section 4.6.

A low dose of **erythromycin** stimulates gastro-intestinal motility and may be used on the advice of a paediatric gastroenterologist to promote tolerance of enteral feeds; erythromycin may be less effective as a prokinetic drug in preterm neonates than in older children.

DOMPERIDONE

Cautions see under Domperidone (section 4.6)

Side-effects see under Domperidone (section 4.6); also QT-interval prolongation reported

Licensed use not licensed for use in gastro-intestinal stasis; not licensed for use in children for gastro-oesophageal reflux disease

Indication and dose

Gastro-oesophageal reflux disease (but efficacy not proven, see section 1.1), gastro-intestinal stasis
• By mouth

 Neonate 100–300 micrograms/kg 4–6 times daily before feeds

 Child 1 month–12 years 200–400 micrograms/kg (max. 20 mg) 3–4 times daily before food

 Child 12–18 years 10–20 mg, 3–4 times daily before food

Nausea and vomiting section 4.6

◀Preparations
Section 4.6

ERYTHROMYCIN

Cautions see section 5.1.5; **interactions:** Appendix 1 (macrolides)

Side-effects see section 5.1.5

Licensed use not licensed for use in gastro-intestinal stasis

Indication and dose

Gastro-intestinal stasis
• By mouth

 Neonate 3 mg/kg 4 times daily

 Child 1 month–18 years 3 mg/kg 4 times daily

• By intravenous infusion

 Neonate 3 mg/kg 4 times daily

 Child 1 month–1 year 3 mg/kg 4 times daily

◀Preparations
Section 5.1.5

1.3 Antisecretory drugs and mucosal protectants

1.3.1 H₂-receptor antagonists
1.3.2 Selective antimuscarinics
1.3.3 Chelates and complexes
1.3.4 Prostaglandin analogues
1.3.5 Proton pump inhibitors

Peptic ulceration commonly involves the stomach, duodenum, and lower oesophagus; after gastric surgery it involves the gastro-enterostomy stoma.

Healing can be promoted by general measures, stopping smoking and taking antacids and by antisecretory drug treatment, but relapse is common when treatment ceases. Nearly all duodenal ulcers and most gastric ulcers not associated with NSAIDs are caused by *Helicobacter pylori*.

The management of *H. pylori* infection and of NSAID-associated ulcers is discussed below.

Helicobacter pylori infection

Eradication of *Helicobacter pylori* reduces the recurrence of gastric and duodenal ulcers and the risk of rebleeding. The presence of *H. pylori* should be confirmed before starting eradication treatment. If possible, the antibacterial sensitivity of the organism should be established at the time of endoscopy and biopsy. Acid inhibition combined with antibacterial treatment is highly effective in the eradication of *H. pylori*; reinfection is rare. Antibiotic-associated colitis is an uncommon risk.

Treatment to eradicate *H. pylori* infection in children should be initiated under specialist supervision. One-week triple-therapy regimens that comprise omeprazole, amoxicillin, and either clarithromycin or metronidazole are recommended. Resistance to clarithromycin or to metronidazole is much more common than to amoxicillin and can develop during treatment. A regimen containing amoxicillin and clarithromycin is therefore recommended for initial therapy and one containing amoxicillin and metronidazole for eradication failure. There is usually no need to continue antisecretory treatment (with a proton pump inhibitor or H_2-receptor antagonist), however, if the ulcer is large, or complicated by haemorrhage or perforation then antisecretory treatment is continued for a further 3 weeks. Lansoprazole may be considered if omeprazole is unsuitable. Treatment failure usually indicates antibacterial resistance, poor compliance, or familial reinfection.

Two-week triple-therapy regimens offer the possibility of higher eradication rates compared to one-week regimens, but adverse effects are common and poor compliance is likely to offset any possible gain.

Two-week dual-therapy regimens using a proton pump inhibitor and a single antibacterial produce low rates of *H. pylori* eradication and are **not** recommended.

For the role of *H. pylori* eradication therapy in children starting or taking NSAIDs, see NSAID-associated ulcers, below.

Recommended regimens for *Helicobacter pylori* eradication

Eradication therapy	Age range	Oral dose (to be used in combination with omeprazole, section 1.3.5)
Amoxicillin	1–6 years	250 mg twice daily (with clarithromycin)
		125 mg 3 times daily (with metronidazole)
	6–12 years	500 mg twice daily (with clarithromycin)
		250 mg 3 times daily (with metronidazole)
	12–18 years	1 g twice daily (with clarithromycin)
		500 mg 3 times daily (with metronidazole)
Clarithromycin	1–12 years	7.5 mg/kg (max. 500 mg) twice daily (with metronidazole or amoxicillin)
	12–18 years	500 mg twice daily (with metronidazole or amoxicillin)
Metronidazole	1–6 years	100 mg twice daily (with clarithromycin)
		100 mg 3 times daily (with amoxicillin)
	6–12 years	200 mg twice daily (with clarithromycin)
		200 mg 3 times daily (with amoxicillin)
	12–18 years	400 mg twice daily (with clarithromycin)
		400 mg 3 times daily (with amoxicillin)

Gastro-intestinal system

1

Gastro-intestinal system   **1**

Test for *Helicobacter pylori*

^{13}C-Urea breath test kits are available for confirming the presence of gastro-duodenal infection with *Helicobacter pylori*. The test involves collection of breath samples before and after ingestion of an oral solution of ^{13}C-urea; the samples are sent for analysis by an appropriate laboratory. The test should not be performed within 4 weeks of treatment with an antibacterial or within 2 weeks of treatment with an antisecretory drug. A specific ^{13}C-Urea breath test kit for children is available (*Helicobacter Test INFAI for children of the age 3–11*®). However the appropriateness of testing for *H. pylori* infection in children has not been established. Breath, saliva, faecal, and urine tests for *H. pylori* are frequently unreliable in children; the most accurate method of diagnosis is endoscopy with biopsy.

Helicobacter Test INFAI for children of the age 3-11® (Infai) [PoM]
Oral powder, ^{13}C-urea 45 mg, net price 1 kit (including 4 breath sample containers, straws) = £19.20 (spectrometric analysis included)

Helicobacter Test INFAI® (Infai) [PoM]
Oral powder, ^{13}C-urea 75 mg, net price 1 kit (including 4 breath-sample containers, straws) = £19.20 (spectrometric analysis included); 1 kit (including 2 breath bags) = £14.20 (spectroscopic analysis not included); 50-test set = £855.00 (spectrometric analysis included)

NSAID-associated ulcers

Gastro-intestinal bleeding and ulceration can occur with NSAID use (section 10.1.1). In adults, the risk of serious upper gastro-intestinal side-effects varies between individual NSAIDs (see Gastro-intestinal side-effects, p. 602). Whenever possible, NSAIDs should be **withdrawn** if an ulcer occurs.

Children at high risk of developing gastro-intestinal complications include those with a history of peptic ulcer disease or serious upper gastro-intestinal complication, those taking other medicines that increase the risk of upper gastro-intestinal side-effects, or those with serious co-morbidity. In children at risk of ulceration, a proton pump inhibitor (section 1.3.5) or an H$_2$-receptor antagonist, such as ranitidine, may be considered for protection against gastric and duodenal ulcers associated with non-selective NSAIDs.

NSAID use and *H. pylori* infection are independent risk factors for gastro-intestinal bleeding and ulceration. In children already taking a NSAID, eradication of *H. pylori* is unlikely to reduce the risk of NSAID-induced bleeding or ulceration. However, in children about to start long-term NSAID treatment who are *H. pylori* positive and have dyspepsia or a history of gastric or duodenal ulcer, eradication of *H. pylori* may reduce the overall risk of ulceration.

If the *NSAID can be discontinued* in a child who has developed an ulcer, a proton pump inhibitor usually produces the most rapid healing, alternatively the ulcer can be treated with an H$_2$-receptor antagonist.

If *NSAID treatment needs to continue*, the ulcer is treated with a proton pump inhibitor (section 1.3.5).

1.3.1   H$_2$-receptor antagonists

Histamine H$_2$-receptor antagonists heal *gastric* and *duodenal ulcers* by reducing gastric acid output as a result of histamine H$_2$-receptor blockade; they are also used to relieve symptoms of *dyspepsia* and *gastro-oesophageal reflux disease* (section 1.1). H$_2$-receptor antagonists should not normally be used for *Zollinger–Ellison syndrome* because proton pump inhibitors (section 1.3.5) are more effective.

Maintenance treatment with low doses has largely been replaced in *Helicobacter pylori* positive children by eradication regimens (section 1.3).

H$_2$-receptor antagonist therapy can promote healing of *NSAID-associated ulcers* (section 1.3).

Treatment with a H$_2$-receptor antagonist has not been shown to be beneficial in haematemesis and melaena, but prophylactic use reduces the frequency of bleeding from *gastroduodenal erosions in hepatic coma*, and possibly in other conditions requiring intensive care. Treatment also reduces the risk of *acid aspiration* in obstetric patients at delivery (Mendelson's syndrome).

H$_2$-receptor antagonists are also used to reduce the degradation of pancreatic enzyme supplements (section 1.9.4) in children with cystic fibrosis.

Side-effects   Side-effects of the H$_2$-receptor antagonists include diarrhoea and other gastro-intestinal disturbances, altered liver function tests (rarely liver damage), headache, dizziness, rash, and tiredness. Rare side-effects include acute pancreatitis, bradycardia, AV block, confusion, depression, and hallucinations particularly in the very ill, hypersensitivity reactions (including fever, arthralgia, myalgia, anaphylaxis), blood disorders (including agranulocytosis, leucopenia, pancytopenia, thrombocytopenia), and skin reactions (including erythema multiforme and toxic epidermal necrolysis). There have been occasional reports of gynaecomastia and impotence.

◤ RANITIDINE

Cautions   acute porphyria; **interactions:** Appendix 1 (histamine H$_2$-antagonists)

Renal impairment   use half normal dose if estimated glomerular filtration rate less than 50 mL/minute/1.73 m^2

Pregnancy   manufacturer advises avoid unless essential, but not known to be harmful

Breast-feeding   significant amount present in milk, but not known to be harmful

Side-effects   see notes above; also *rarely* tachycardia, agitation, visual disturbances, alopecia; *very rarely* interstitial nephritis

Licensed use   *oral* preparations not licensed for use in children under 3 years; *injection* not licensed for use in children under 6 months

Indication and dose

Reflux oesophagitis, benign gastric and duodenal ulceration, prophylaxis of stress ulceration, other conditions where gastric acid reduction is beneficial (see notes above and section 1.9.4)

● **By mouth**

Neonate 2 mg/kg 3 times daily but absorption unreliable; max. 3 mg/kg 3 times daily

Child 1–6 months 1 mg/kg 3 times daily; max. 3 mg/kg 3 times daily

Child 6 months–3 years 2–4 mg/kg twice daily

Child 3–12 years 2–4 mg/kg (max. 150 mg) twice daily; increased up to 5 mg/kg (max. 300 mg) twice daily in severe gastro-oesophageal reflux disease

Child 12–18 years 150 mg twice daily *or* 300 mg at night; increased if necessary, to 300 mg twice daily *or* 150 mg 4 times daily for up to 12 weeks in moderate to severe gastro-oesophageal reflux disease

Note In fat malabsorption syndrome, give 1–2 hours before food to enhance effects of pancreatic enzyme replacement

● **By slow intravenous injection**

Neonate 0.5–1 mg/kg every 6–8 hours

Child 1 month–18 years 1 mg/kg (max. 50 mg) every 6–8 hours (may be given as an intermittent infusion at a rate of 25 mg/hour)

Zollinger–Ellison syndrome (but see notes above)

● **By mouth**

Child 12–18 years 150 mg 3 times daily (doses up to 6 g daily in divided doses have been used)

Administration   For *slow intravenous injection* dilute to a concentration of 2.5 mg/mL with Glucose 5%, Sodium Chloride 0.9%, *or* Compound Sodium Lactate. Give over at least 3 minutes

[1]**Ranitidine** (Non-proprietary) ℗⊙ℳ
Tablets, ranitidine (as hydrochloride) 150 mg, net price 60-tab pack = £1.27; 300 mg, 30-tab pack = £1.32
Brands include *Ranitic*®

Effervescent tablets, ranitidine (as hydrochloride) 150 mg, net price 60-tab pack = £10.74; 300 mg, 30-tab pack = £11.25. Label: 13
Excipients may include sodium (check with supplier)

Oral solution, ranitidine (as hydrochloride) 75 mg/5 mL, 100 mL = £7.44, 300 mL = £21.43
Excipients may include alcohol (check with supplier)
1. Ranitidine can be sold to the public for children over 16 years (provided packs do not contain more than 2 weeks' supply) for the short-term symptomatic relief of heartburn, dyspepsia, and hyperacidity, and for the prevention of these symptoms when associated with consumption of food or drink (max. single dose 75 mg, max. daily dose 300 mg)

Zantac® (GSK) ℗⊙ℳ
Tablets, f/c, ranitidine (as hydrochloride) 150 mg, net price 60-tab pack = £1.30; 300 mg, 30-tab pack = £1.30

Effervescent tablets, pale yellow, ranitidine (as hydrochloride) 150 mg (contains 14.3 mmol Na$^+$/tablet), net price 60-tab pack = £25.94; 300 mg (contains 20.8 mmol Na$^+$/tablet), 30-tab pack = £25.51. Label: 13
Excipients include aspartame (section 9.4.1)

Syrup, sugar-free, ranitidine (as hydrochloride) 75 mg/5 mL. Net price 300 mL = £20.76
Excipients include alcohol 8%

Injection, ranitidine (as hydrochloride) 25 mg/mL. Net price 2-mL amp = 60p

1.3.2 **Selective antimuscarinics**

Classification not used in *BNF for Children*.

1.3.3 **Chelates and complexes**

Sucralfate is a complex of aluminium hydroxide and sulphated sucrose that appears to act by protecting the mucosa from acid-pepsin attack; it has minimal antacid properties. Sucralfate can be used to prevent stress ulceration in children receiving intensive care. It should be used with caution in this situation (**important**: reports of bezoar formation, see CSM advice below).

SUCRALFATE

Cautions administration of sucralfate and enteral feeds should be separated by 1 hour; **interactions**: Appendix 1 (sucralfate)

Renal impairment use with caution; aluminium is absorbed and may accumulate

Breast-feeding amount probably too small to be harmful

Bezoar formation Following reports of bezoar formation associated with sucralfate, the **CSM** has advised caution in seriously ill patients, especially those receiving concomitant enteral feeds or those with predisposing conditions such as delayed gastric emptying

Side-effects constipation; *less frequently* diarrhoea, nausea, indigestion, flatulence, gastric discomfort, back pain, dizziness, headache, drowsiness, bezoar formation (see above), dry mouth, and rash

Licensed use not licensed for use in children under 15 years; tablets not licensed for prophylaxis of stress ulceration

Indication and dose

Prophylaxis of stress ulceration in child under intensive care
* By mouth
  Child 1 month–2 years 250 mg 4–6 times daily
  Child 2–12 years 500 mg 4–6 times daily

Child 12–15 years 1 g 4–6 times daily
Child 15–18 years 1 g 6 times daily; max. 8 g daily

Benign gastric and duodenal ulceration
* By mouth
  Child 1 month–2 years 250 mg 4–6 times daily
  Child 2–12 years 500 mg 4–6 times daily
  Child 12–15 years 1 g 4–6 times daily
  Child 15–18 years 2 g twice daily (on rising and at bedtime) *or* 1 g 4 times daily (1 hour before meals and at bedtime) taken for 4–6 weeks, or in resistant cases up to 12 weeks; max. 8 g daily

Administration for administration *by mouth*, sucralfate should be given 1 hour before meals, see also Cautions, above; *oral suspension* blocks fine-bore feeding tubes; crushed *tablets* may be dispersed in water.

Antepsin® (Chugai) (PoM)
Tablets, scored, sucralfate 1 g, net price 50-tab pack = £4.81. Label: 5

Suspension, sucralfate, 1 g/5 mL, net price 250 mL (aniseed- and caramel-flavoured) = £4.81. Label: 5

1.3.4 **Prostaglandin analogues**

Classification not used in *BNF for Children*.

1.3.5 **Proton pump inhibitors**

The proton pump inhibitors **omeprazole** and **lansoprazole** inhibit gastric acid secretion by blocking the hydrogen-potassium adenosine triphosphatase enzyme system (the 'proton pump') of the gastric parietal cell. Omeprazole is currently only licensed in children for the treatment of *gastro-oesophageal reflux disease* with severe symptoms. Lansoprazole is not licensed for use in children, but may be considered when the available formulations of omeprazole are unsuitable. Proton pump inhibitors are effective short-term treatments for *gastric* and *duodenal ulcers*; they are also used in combination with antibacterials for the eradication of *Helicobacter pylori* (see p. 59 for specific regimens). An initial short course of a proton pump inhibitor is the treatment of choice in *gastro-oesophageal reflux disease* with severe symptoms; children with endoscopically confirmed *erosive*, *ulcerative*, or *stricturing oesophagitis* usually need to be maintained on a proton pump inhibitor.

Proton pump inhibitors are also used for the prevention and treatment of NSAID-associated ulcers (see p. 60). In the child who need to continue NSAID treatment after an ulcer has healed, the dose of proton pump inhibitor should not normally be reduced because asymptomatic ulcer deterioration may occur.

Proton pump inhibitors are effective in the treatment of the *Zollinger-Ellison syndrome* (including cases resistant to other treatment). They are also used to reduce the degradation of pancreatic enzyme supplements (section 1.9.4) in children with cystic fibrosis.

Side-effects   Side-effects of the proton pump inhibitors include gastro-intestinal disturbances (including nausea, vomiting, abdominal pain, flatulence, diarrhoea, constipation), and headache. Less frequent side-effects include dry mouth, peripheral oedema, dizziness, sleep disturbances, fatigue, paraesthesia, arthralgia, myalgia, rash, and pruritus. Other side-effects reported *rarely* or *very rarely* include taste disturbance, stomatitis, hepatitis, jaundice, hypersensitivity reactions (including anaphylaxis, bronchospasm), fever, depression, hallucinations, confusion, gynaecomastia, interstitial nephritis, hyponatraemia, blood disorders (including leucopenia, leucocytosis, pancytopenia, thrombocytopenia), visual disturbances, sweating, photosensitivity, alopecia, Stevens-Johnson syndrome, and toxic epidermal necrolysis. By decreasing gastric acidity, proton pump inhibitors may increase the risk of gastro-intestinal infections (including *Clostridium difficile* infection).

▮ LANSOPRAZOLE

Cautions interactions: Appendix 1 (proton pump inhibitors)

Hepatic impairment   may accumulate in severe impairment

Pregnancy   manufacturer advises avoid

Breast-feeding   present in milk in *animal* studies—manufacturer advises avoid

Side-effects   see notes above; also glossitis, pancreatitis, anorexia, restlessness, tremor, impotence, petechiae, and purpura; *very rarely* colitis, raised serum cholesterol or triglycerides

Licensed use   not licensed for use in children

Indication and dose

Gastro-oesophageal reflux disease, acid-related dyspepsia, treatment of duodenal and benign gastric ulcer including those complicating NSAID therapy, fat malabsorption despite pancreatic enzyme replacement therapy in cystic fibrosis
- By mouth

  Child body-weight under 30 kg 0.5–1 mg/kg (max. 15 mg) once daily in the morning

  Child body-weight over 30 kg 15–30 mg once daily in the morning

Administration   for administration by a *nasogastric tube* or an *oral syringe, Zoton FasTab®* can be dispersed in a small amount of water

Zoton® (Wyeth) ⒫ⓄⓂ

FasTab® (= orodispersible tablet), lansoprazole 15 mg, net price 28-tab pack = £5.97; 30 mg, 14-tab pack = £5.47, 28-tab pack = £11.00. Label: 5, 22, counselling, administration
Excipients include aspartame (section 9.4.1)

Counselling Tablets should be placed on the tongue, allowed to disperse and swallowed, or may be swallowed whole with a glass of water.

▮ OMEPRAZOLE

Cautions interactions: Appendix 1 (proton pump inhibitors)

Hepatic impairment   no more than 700 micrograms/kg (max. 20 mg) once daily

Pregnancy   not known to be harmful

Breast-feeding   present in milk but not known to be harmful

Side-effects   see notes above; also agitation and impotence

Licensed use   *capsules* and *tablets* not licensed for use in children except for severe ulcerating reflux oesophagitis in children over 1 year; *injection* not licensed for use in children under 12 years

Indication and dose

Gastro-oesophageal reflux disease, acid-related dyspepsia, treatment of duodenal and benign gastric ulcers including those complicating NSAID therapy, prophylaxis of acid aspiration, Zollinger-Ellison syndrome, fat malabsorption despite pancreatic enzyme replacement therapy in cystic fibrosis
- By mouth

  Neonate 700 micrograms/kg once daily, increased if necessary after 7–14 days to 1.4 mg/kg; some neonates may require up to 2.8 mg/kg once daily

  Child 1 month–2 years 700 micrograms/kg once daily, increased if necessary to 3 mg/kg (max. 20 mg) once daily

  Child body-weight 10–20 kg 10 mg once daily increased if necessary to 20 mg once daily (in severe ulcerating reflux oesophagitis, max. 12 weeks at higher dose)

1   Gastro-intestinal system

⌐ **OMEPRAZOLE (continued)**

Child body-weight over 20 kg 20 mg once daily increased if necessary to 40 mg once daily (in severe ulcerating reflux oesophagitis, max. 12 weeks at higher dose)

• **By intravenous injection over 5 minutes *or* by intravenous infusion**

Child 1 month–12 years initially 500 micrograms/kg (max. 20 mg) once daily, increased to 2 mg/kg (max. 40 mg) once daily if necessary

Child 12–18 years 40 mg once daily

Helicobacter pylori eradication (in combination with antibacterials see p. 59)

• **By mouth**

Child 1–12 years 1–2 mg/kg (max. 40 mg) once daily

Child 12–18 years 40 mg once daily

Administration for administration *by mouth*, swallow whole, *or* disperse *Losec MUPS®* tablets in water, *or* mix capsule contents *or Losec MUPS®* tablets with fruit juice or yoghurt. Preparations consisting of an e/c tablet within a capsule should **not** be opened.

For administration through an *enteral feeding tube*, use *Losec MUPS®* or the contents of a capsule containing omeprazole dispersed in a large volume of water, or in 10 mL Sodium Bicarbonate 8.4% (1 mmol Na^+/mL) (allow to stand for 10 minutes before administration).

For *intermittent intravenous infusion*, dilute reconstituted solution to a concentration of 400 micrograms/mL with Glucose 5% *or* Sodium Chloride 0.9%; give over 20–30 minutes

Omeprazole (Non-proprietary) ⒫ⓞⓜ

Capsules, enclosing e/c granules, omeprazole 10 mg, net price 28-cap pack = £1.87; 20 mg, 28-cap pack = £1.75; 40 mg, 7-cap pack = £2.04, 28-cap pack = £58.00. Counselling, administration

Note Some preparations consist of an e/c tablet within a capsule; brands include *Mepradec®*
Dental prescribing on NHS Gastro-resistant omeprazole capsules may be prescribed

Tablets, e/c, omeprazole 10 mg, net price 28-tab pack = £6.13; 20 mg, 28-tab pack = £5.37; 40 mg, 7-tab pack = £5.08. Label: 25

Intravenous infusion, powder for reconstitution, omeprazole (as sodium salt), net price 40-mg vial = £5.21

Losec® (AstraZeneca) ⒫ⓞⓜ

MUPS® (multiple-unit pellet system = dispersible tablets), f/c, omeprazole 10 mg (light pink), net price 28-tab pack = £19.34; 20 mg (pink), 28-tab pack = £29.22; 40 mg (red-brown), 7-tab pack = £14.61. Counselling, administration

Capsules, enclosing e/c granules, omeprazole 10 mg (pink), net price 28-cap pack = £19.34; 20 mg (pink/brown), 28-cap pack = £29.22; 40 mg (brown), 7-cap pack = £14.61. Counselling, administration

Intravenous infusion, powder for reconstitution, omeprazole (as sodium salt), net price 40-mg vial = £5.41

Injection, powder for reconstitution, omeprazole (as sodium salt), net price 40-mg vial (with solvent) = £5.41

1.4 Acute diarrhoea

1.4.1 Adsorbents and bulk-forming drugs
1.4.2 Antimotility drugs

The priority in acute diarrhoea, as in gastro-enteritis, is the prevention or reversal of fluid and electrolyte depletion—this is particularly important in infants. For details of **oral rehydration preparations**, see section 9.2.1.2. Severe dehydration requires immediate admission to hospital and urgent replacement of fluid and electrolytes.

Antimotility drugs (section 1.4.2) relieve symptoms of diarrhoea. They are used in the management of uncomplicated acute diarrhoea in adults, but are **not** recommended for use in children under 12 years. Fluid and electrolyte replacement (section 9.2.1.2) are of prime importance in the treatment of acute diarrhoea.

Antispasmodics (section 1.2) are occasionally of value in treating abdominal cramp associated with diarrhoea but they should **not** be used for primary treatment. Antispasmodics and antiemetics should be **avoided** in young children with gastro-enteritis since they are rarely effective and have troublesome side-effects.

Antibacterial drugs are generally unnecessary in simple gastro-enteritis because the complaint usually resolves quickly without such treatment, and infective diarrhoeas in the UK often have a viral cause. Systemic bacterial infection does, however, need appropriate systemic treatment; for drugs used in campylobacter enteritis, shigellosis, and salmonellosis, see p. 298

Colestyramine (cholestyramine, section 1.9.2) binds unabsorbed bile salts and provides symptomatic relief of diarrhoea following ileal disease or resection.

Gastro-intestinal system

1

1.4.1 Adsorbents and bulk-forming drugs

Adsorbents such as kaolin are **not** recommended for *acute diarrhoeas*. Bulk-forming drugs, such as ispaghula, methylcellulose, and sterculia (section 1.6.1) are rarely effective in controlling faecal consistency in ileostomy and colostomy.

1.4.2 Antimotility drugs

Antimotility drugs have a role in the management of uncomplicated *acute diarrhoea* in adults but not in children under 12 years; see also section 1.4. However, in the case of dehydration, fluid and electrolyte replacement (section 9.2.1.2) are of primary importance.

For comments on their role in *chronic bowel disorders* see section 1.5. Antimotility drugs are also used in children with *stoma* (section 1.8).

CODEINE PHOSPHATE

Cautions see section 4.7.2; tolerance and dependence may occur with prolonged use; **interactions:** Appendix 1 (opioid analgesics)

Contra-indications see section 4.7.2; also conditions where inhibition of peristalsis should be avoided, where abdominal distension develops, or in acute diarrhoeal conditions such as acute ulcerative colitis or antibiotic-associated colitis

Side-effects see section 4.7.2

Indication and dose

Diarrhoea (but see notes above)
• By mouth
   Child 12–18 years 30 mg (range 15–60 mg) 3–4 times daily

Pain section 4.7.2

Codeine Phosphate (Non-proprietary) (PoM)
Tablets, codeine phosphate 15 mg, net price 28 = £1.08; 30 mg, 28 = £1.24; 60 mg, 28 = £1.73. Label: 2
Note As for schedule 2 controlled drugs, travellers needing to take codeine phosphate tablets abroad may require a doctor's letter explaining why codeine is necessary.

CO-PHENOTROPE

A mixture of diphenoxylate hydrochloride and atropine sulphate in the mass proportions 100 parts to 1 part respectively

Cautions see under Codeine Phosphate (section 4.7.2); also young children are particularly susceptible to **overdosage** and symptoms may be delayed and observation is needed for at least 48 hours after ingestion; presence of subclinical doses of atropine may give rise to atropine side-effects in susceptible individuals or in overdosage (section 1.2); **interactions:** Appendix 1 (antimuscarinics, opioid analgesics)

Pregnancy may depress neonatal respiration; withdrawal effects in neonates of dependent mothers; gastric stasis and risk of inhalation pneumonia in mother during labour

Breast-feeding may be present in milk

Contra-indications see under Antimuscarinics (section 1.2) and Codeine Phosphate (section 4.7.2); also jaundice

Side-effects see under Antimuscarinics (section 1.2) and Codeine Phosphate (section 4.7.2); also fever

Licensed use not licensed for use in children under 4 years

Indication and dose

See preparations

Administration for administration *by mouth* tablets may be crushed

Co-phenotrope (Non-proprietary) (PoM)
Tablets, co-phenotrope 2.5/0.025 (diphenoxylate hydrochloride 2.5 mg, atropine sulphate 25 micrograms), net price 20 = £1.79
Brands include *Lomotil*®

Dose

Control of faecal consistency after colostomy or ileostomy, adjunct to rehydration in acute diarrhoea (but see notes above)
• By mouth
   Child 2–4 years half tablet 3 times daily
   Child 4–9 years 1 tablet 3 times daily
   Child 9–12 years 1 tablet 4 times daily
   Child 12–16 years 2 tablets 3 times daily
   Child 16–18 years initially 4 tablets then 2 tablets 4 times daily

Note Co-phenotrope 2.5/0.025 can be sold to the public for children over 16 years (provided packs do not contain more than 20 tablets) as an adjunct to rehydration in acute diarrhoea (max. daily dose 10 tablets)

LOPERAMIDE HYDROCHLORIDE

Cautions see notes above; **interactions:** Appendix 1 (loperamide)
   Hepatic impairment risk of accumulation—manufacturer advises avoid

Pregnancy manufacturer advises avoid—no information available

Breast-feeding amount probably too small to be harmful

1
Gastro-intestinal system

◁ **LOPERAMIDE HYDROCHLORIDE** (*continued*)

Contra-indications   conditions where inhibition of peristalsis should be avoided, where abdominal distension develops, or in conditions such as active ulcerative colitis or antibiotic-associated colitis

Side-effects   abdominal cramps, dizziness, drowsiness, and skin reactions including urticaria; paralytic ileus and abdominal bloating also reported

Licensed use   *capsules* not licensed for use in children under 8 years; *syrup* not licensed for use in children under 4 years; not licensed for use in children for chronic diarrhoea

Indication and dose

Chronic diarrhoea
● **By mouth**

Child 1 month–1 year 100–200 micrograms/kg twice daily, 30 minutes before feeds; up to 2 mg/kg daily in divided doses occasionally required

Child 1–12 years 100–200 micrograms/kg (max. 2mg) 3–4 times daily; up to 1.25 mg/kg daily in divided doses may be required (max. 16 mg daily)

Child 12–18 years 2–4 mg 2–4 times daily (max. 16 mg daily)

Acute diarrhoea (but see notes above)
● **By mouth**

Child 4–8 years 1 mg 3–4 times daily for *up to 3 days only*

Child 8–12 years 2 mg 4 times daily for up to 5 days

Child 12–18 years initially 4 mg, then 2 mg after each loose stool for up to 5 days (usual dose 6–8 mg daily; max. 16 mg daily)

Loperamide (Non-proprietary) ℞
Capsules, loperamide hydrochloride 2 mg, net price 30-cap pack = £1.07

Tablets, loperamide hydrochloride 2 mg, net price 30-tab pack = £2.15
Brands include *Norimode®*
Note Loperamide can be sold to the public, for use in children over 12 years, provided it is licensed and labelled for the treatment of acute diarrhoea

Imodium® (Janssen-Cilag) ℞
Capsules, green/grey, loperamide hydrochloride 2 mg. Net price 30-cap pack = £1.13

Syrup, sugar-free, red, loperamide hydrochloride 1 mg/5 mL. Net price 100 mL = 98p

◢ Compound preparations
Imodium® Plus (McNeil)
Caplets (= tablets), loperamide hydrochloride 2 mg, simeticone 125 mg, net price 6-tab pack = £2.14, 12-tab pack = £3.40
Dose
Acute diarrhoea with abdominal colic
Child 12–18 years initially 1 caplet, then 1 caplet after each loose stool; max. 4 caplets daily for up to 2 days

1.5 Chronic bowel disorders

Individual symptoms of chronic bowel disorders need specific treatment including dietary manipulation as well as drug treatment and the maintenance of a liberal fluid intake.

Inflammatory bowel disease

Chronic inflammatory bowel diseases include *ulcerative colitis* and *Crohn's disease*. The treatment of inflammatory bowel disease in children should be initiated and supervised by a paediatric gastroenterologist. Effective management requires drug therapy, attention to nutrition, and in severe or chronic active disease, surgery.

Aminosalicylates (balsalazide, mesalazine, olsalazine, and sulfasalazine), and **corticosteroids** (hydrocortisone, budesonide, and prednisolone) form the basis of drug treatment.

Treatment of acute ulcerative colitis and Crohn's disease   Acute mild to moderate disease affecting the rectum (proctitis) or the recto-sigmoid (distal colitis) is treated initially with local application of an aminosalicylate (section 1.5.1); alternatively a local corticosteroid (section 1.5.2) can be used but it is less effective. Foam preparations and suppositories are useful for children who have difficulty retaining liquid enemas.

Diffuse inflammatory bowel disease or disease that does not respond to local therapy requires oral treatment. Mild disease affecting the upper colon can be treated with an oral aminosalicylate alone; a combination of a local and an oral aminosalicylate can be used in distal colitis. Refractory or moderate inflammatory bowel disease usually requires adjunctive use of an oral corticosteroid such as **prednisolone** (section 1.5.2) for 4–8 weeks. Modified-release **budesonide** is used for children with Crohn's disease affecting the ileum and the ascending colon; it causes fewer systemic side-effects than oral prednisolone but may be less effective.

Active Crohn's disease affecting the small intestine may be treated with **enteral nutrition** (Appendix 2) for 6–8 weeks. Alternatively, an oral corticosteroid may be used but at the expense of side-effects; the dose of the corticosteroid is reduced gradually over 8–10 weeks.

Severe inflammatory bowel disease calls for hospital admission and treatment with an intravenous corticosteroid such as **hydrocortisone** (p. 451) or **methyl-prednisolone** (p. 452); other therapy may include intravenous fluid and electro-lyte replacement, and possibly parenteral nutrition. Children with ulcerative colitis that fails to respond adequately to these measures may benefit from a short course of ciclosporin. Children with unresponsive or chronically active Crohn's disease may benefit from azathioprine, mercaptopurine, or once-weekly methotrexate.

Infliximab (section 1.5.3) is used in specialist centres for children with severe active Crohn's disease whose condition has not responded adequately to treatment with a corticosteroid and a conventional immunosuppressant or who are intolerant of them. Infliximab has also been used for the treatment of severe, refractory ulcerative colitis. There are concerns about the long-term safety of infliximab in children; hepatosplenic T-cell lymphoma has been reported.

Crohn's disease of the mouth or of the perineum is more common in children than in adults and it is difficult to treat; elimination diets and the use of a topical corticosteroid (section 13.4) may be beneficial, but a systemic corticosteroid (section 6.3.2) and occasionally azathioprine may be required in severe cases.

NICE guidance

Infliximab for Crohn's disease (April 2002)
Infliximab is recommended for the treatment of severe active Crohn's disease (with or without fistulae) when treatment with immunomodulating drugs and corticosteroids has failed or is not tolerated and when surgery is inappropri-ate. Treatment may be repeated if the condition responded to the initial course but relapsed subsequently. Infliximab should be prescribed only by a gastroenterologist.

NICE guidance

Infliximab for subacute manifestations of ulcerative colitis (April 2008)
Infliximab is **not** recommended for the treatment of subacute manifestations of moderate to severe active ulcerative colitis that would normally be man-aged in an outpatient setting.

Maintenance of remission of acute ulcerative colitis and Crohn's disease
Smoking cessation (section 4.10) may reduce the risk of relapse in Crohn's disease and should be encouraged. **Aminosalicylates** are of great value in the main-tenance of remission of ulcerative colitis. They are of less value in the main-tenance of remission of Crohn's disease; an oral formulation of mesalazine is available for the long-term management of ileal disease. Corticosteroids are **not** suitable for maintenance treatment because of their side-effects. In resistant or frequently relapsing cases either **azathioprine** (section 1.5.3) or **mercaptopurine** (section 1.5.3) may be helpful. **Methotrexate** (section 1.5.3) is used in Crohn's disease when azathioprine or mercaptopurine are ineffective or not tolerated. **Infliximab** (p. 75) can be used for maintenance therapy in Crohn's disease or ulcerative colitis in children who respond to the initial induction course of this drug. There are concerns about the long-term safety of infliximab in children.

Fistulating Crohn's disease   Treatment may not be necessary for simple, asymptomatic perianal fistulas. **Metronidazole** (section 5.1.11) or **ciprofloxacin** (section 5.1.12) may be beneficial for the treatment of fistulating Crohn's disease [both unlicensed for this indication]. Metronidazole by mouth is usually used at a dose of 7.5 mg/kg 3 times daily for 1 month but no longer than 3 months because of concerns about developing peripheral neuropathy. Ciprofloxacin by mouth is given at a dose of 5 mg/kg twice daily. Other antibacterials should be given if specifically indicated (e.g. sepsis associated with fistulas and perianal disease) and for managing bacterial overgrowth in the small bowel. Fistulas may also require surgical exploration and local drainage.

Either **azathioprine** or **mercaptopurine** is used as a second-line treatment for fistulating Crohn's disease and continued for maintenance. **Infliximab** is used for fistulating Crohn's disease refractory to conventional treatments and it can be continued as maintenance therapy.

Adjunctive treatment of inflammatory bowel disease   Due attention should be paid to diet; high-fibre or low-residue diets should be used as appropriate.

Antimotility drugs such as codeine phosphate and loperamide, and antispasmodic drugs may precipitate paralytic ileus and megacolon in active ulcerative colitis; treatment of the inflammation is more logical. Laxatives may be required in proctitis. Diarrhoea resulting from the loss of bile-salt absorption (e.g. in terminal ileal disease or bowel resection) may improve with **colestyramine** (section 1.9.2), which binds bile salts.

Irritable bowel syndrome

Irritable bowel syndrome can present with pain, constipation, or diarrhoea. Some children have important psychological aggravating factors which respond to reassurance. The **fibre** intake of children with irritable bowel syndrome should be reviewed. If an increase in dietary fibre is required, soluble fibre (e.g. oats, ispaghula husk, or sterculia) is recommended; insoluble fibre (e.g. bran) should be avoided. A **laxative** (section 1.6) can be used to treat constipation. An osmotic laxative, such as a macrogol, is preferred; lactulose may cause bloating. **Loperamide** (section 1.4.2) may relieve diarrhoea and antispasmodic drugs (section 1.2) may relieve pain. Opioids with a central action, such as codeine, are better avoided because of the risk of dependence.

Clostridium difficile infection

Antibiotic-associated colitis is caused by colonisation of the colon with *Clostridium difficile* which may follow antibacterial therapy. It is usually of acute onset, but may run a chronic course; it is a particular hazard of clindamycin but few antibacterials are free of this side-effect. Oral **metronidazole** (section 5.1.11) or oral **vancomycin** (section 5.1.7) are used as specific treatment; vancomycin may be preferred for very sick patients. Metronidazole can be given by intravenous infusion if oral treatment is inappropriate.

Malabsorption syndromes

Individual conditions need specific management and also general nutritional consideration. Coeliac disease (gluten enteropathy) usually needs a gluten-free diet (Appendix 2) and pancreatic insufficiency needs pancreatin supplements (section 1.9.4).

For further information on foods for special diets (ACBS), see Appendix 2.

1.5.1 Aminosalicylates

Sulfasalazine is a combination of 5-aminosalicylic acid ('5-ASA') and sulfapyridine; sulfapyridine acts only as a carrier to the colonic site of action but still causes side-effects. In the newer aminosalicylates, **mesalazine** (5-aminosalicylic acid), **balsalazide** (a prodrug of 5-aminosalicylic acid) and **olsalazine** (a dimer of 5-aminosalicylic acid which cleaves in the lower bowel), the sulphonamide-related side-effects of sulfasalazine are avoided, but 5-aminosalicylic acid alone can still cause side-effects including blood disorders (see recommendation below) and lupus-like syndrome also seen with sulfasalazine.

Cautions   Renal function should be monitored before starting an oral aminosalicylate, at 3 months of treatment, and then annually during treatment (more frequently in renal impairment). Blood disorders can occur with aminosalicylates (see recommendation below).

Gastro-intestinal system

1

> **Blood disorders**
>
> Children receiving aminosalicylates and their carers should be advised to report any unexplained bleeding, bruising, purpura, sore throat, fever or malaise that occurs during treatment. A blood count should be performed and the drug stopped immediately if there is suspicion of a blood dyscrasia.

Contra-indications Aminosalicylates should be avoided in salicylate hypersensitivity.

Side-effects Side-effects of the aminosalicylates include diarrhoea, nausea, vomiting, abdominal pain, exacerbation of symptoms of colitis, headache, hypersensitivity reactions (including rash and urticaria); side-effects that occur rarely include acute pancreatitis, hepatitis, myocarditis, pericarditis, lung disorders (including eosinophilia and fibrosing alveolitis), peripheral neuropathy, blood disorders (including agranulocytosis, aplastic anaemia, leucopenia, methaemoglobinaemia, neutropenia, and thrombocytopenia—see also recommendation above), renal dysfunction (interstitial nephritis, nephrotic syndrome), myalgia, arthralgia, skin reactions (including lupus erythematosus-like syndrome, Stevens-Johnson syndrome), alopecia.

◢ BALSALAZIDE SODIUM

Cautions see notes above; also history of asthma; **interactions:** Appendix 1 (aminosalicylates)
Blood disorders see recommendation above

Renal impairment manufacturer advises avoid in moderate to severe impairment

Pregnancy manufacturer advises avoid

Breast-feeding manufacturer advises avoid

Contra-indications see notes above

Hepatic impairment avoid in severe impairment

Side-effects see notes above; also cholelithiasis

Licensed use not licensed for use in children under 18 years

Indication and dose

Treatment of mild to moderate ulcerative colitis and maintenance of remission

* By mouth

    Child 12–18 years acute attack, 2.25 g 3 times daily until remission occurs or for up to max. 12 weeks; maintenance, 1.5 g twice daily, adjusted according to response (max. 3 g twice daily)

Colazide® (Shire) ℗ℴℳ
Capsules, beige, balsalazide sodium 750 mg. Net price 130-cap pack = £39.00. Label: 21, 25, counselling, blood disorder symptoms (see recommendation above)

◢ MESALAZINE

Cautions see notes above; **interactions:** Appendix 1 (aminosalicylates)
Blood disorders see recommendation above

Renal impairment use with caution; avoid if estimated glomerular filtration rate less than $20 \, mL/minute/1.73 \, m^2$

Pregnancy negligible quantity crosses placenta

Breast-feeding diarrhoea reported but manufacturers advise negligible amounts detected in breast milk

Contra-indications see notes above; blood clotting abnormalities

Hepatic impairment avoid in severe impairment

Side-effects see notes above

Licensed use *Asacol®* (all preparations), *Ipocol®*, *Salofalk®* rectal enema, not licensed for use in children under 18 years; *Pentasa®* tablets and suppositories, *Salofalk®* tablets and suppositories, not licensed for use in children under 15 years; *Mesren MR®, Pentasa®* granules, *Salofalk®* rectal foam, not licensed for use in children under 12 years; *Salofalk®* granules not licensed for use in children under 6 years; *Pentasa®* retention enema, no dose recommendation for children (age range not specified by manufacturer)

Indication and dose

Treatment of mild to moderate ulcerative colitis and maintenance of remission for dose see under preparations below

Note The delivery characteristics of oral mesalazine preparations may vary; these preparations should not be considered interchangeable

Asacol® (Procter & Gamble Pharm.) ℗ℴℳ
Foam enema, mesalazine 1 g/metered application, net price 14-application canister with disposable applicators and plastic bags = £28.37. Counselling, blood disorder symptoms (see recommendation above)
Excipients include disodium edetate, hydroxybenzoates (parabens), polysorbate 20, sodium metabisulphite

Dose

Acute attack affecting the rectosigmoid region
* By rectum

    Child 12–18 years 1 metered application (mesalazine 1 g) into the rectum daily for 4–6 weeks

Acute attack affecting the descending colon
* By rectum

    Child 12–18 years 2 metered applications (mesalazine 2 g) once daily for 4–6 weeks

1

Gastro-intestinal system

◁ **MESALAZINE (continued)**

Suppositories, mesalazine 250 mg, net price 20-suppos pack = £5.12; 500 mg, 10-suppos pack = £5.12. Counselling, blood disorder symptoms (see recommendation above)

Dose

Treatment and maintenance of remission of ulcerative colitis affecting the rectosigmoid region
• By rectum
   Child 12–18 years 250–500 mg 3 times daily, with last dose at bedtime

Asacol® MR (Procter & Gamble Pharm.) [PoM]

Tablets, red, e/c, mesalazine 400 mg, net price 90-tab pack = £31.22, 120-tab pack = £41.62. Label: 5, 25, counselling, blood disorder symptoms (see recommendation above)

Dose

Acute attack
• By mouth
   Child 12–18 years 800 mg 3 times daily

Maintenance of remission of ulcerative colitis and Crohn's ileo-colitis
• By mouth
   Child 12–18 years 400–800 mg 2–3 times daily

Note Preparations that lower stool pH (e.g. lactulose) may prevent release of mesalazine

Ipocol® (Sandoz) [PoM]

Tablets, e/c, mesalazine 400 mg, net price 120-tab pack = £41.62. Label: 5, 25, counselling, blood disorder symptoms (see recommendation above)

Dose

Acute attack
• By mouth
   Child 12–18 years 800 mg 3 times daily

Maintenance of remission
• By mouth
   Child 12–18 years 400–800 mg 3 times daily

Mesren MR® (IVAX) [PoM]

Tablets, red-brown, e/c, mesalazine 400 mg, net price 90-tab pack = £20.29, 120-tab pack = £27.05. Label: 5, 25, counselling, blood disorder symptoms (see recommendation above)

Dose

Acute attack
• By mouth
   Child 12–18 years 800 mg 3 times daily

Maintenance of remission
• By mouth
   Child 12–18 years 400–800 mg 3 times daily

Pentasa® (Ferring) [PoM]

Tablets, m/r, scored, mesalazine 500 mg (grey), net price 100-tab pack = £25.48. Counselling, administration (see dose), blood disorder symptoms (see recommendation above)

Dose

Acute attack
• By mouth
   Child 5–15 years 15–20 mg/kg (max. 1 g) 3 times daily
   Child 15–18 years 1–2 g twice daily; total daily dose may alternatively be given in 3 divided doses

Maintenance of remission
• By mouth
   Child 5–15 years 10 mg/kg (max. 500 mg) 2–3 times daily
   Child 15–18 years 500 mg 3 times daily; total daily dose may alternatively be given in 2 divided doses

Administration tablets may be halved, quartered, or dispersed in water, but should not be chewed

Granules, m/r, pale brown, mesalazine 1 g/sachet, net price 50-sachet pack = £30.02; 2 g/sachet, 60-sachet pack = £72.05. Counselling, administration (see dose), blood disorder symptoms (see recommendation above)

Dose

Acute attack
• By mouth
   Child 5–12 years 15–20 mg/kg (max. 1 g) 3 times daily
   Child 12–18 years 1–2 g twice daily; total daily dose may alternatively be given in 3–4 divided doses

Maintenance of remission
• By mouth
   Child 5–12 years 10 mg/kg (max. 500 mg) 2–3 times daily
   Child 12–18 years 2 g once daily

Administration contents of one sachet should be weighed and divided immediately before use; discard any remaining granules. Granules should be placed on tongue and washed down with water or orange juice without chewing

Retention enema, mesalazine 1 g in 100-mL pack. Net price 7 enemas = £18.09. Counselling, blood disorder symptoms (see recommendation above)

Dose

Acute attack affecting the rectosigmoid region
• By rectum
   Child 12–18 years 1 g at bedtime

Suppositories, mesalazine 1 g. Net price 28-suppos pack = £41.55. Counselling, blood disorder symptoms (see recommendation above)

Dose

Acute attack, ulcerative proctitis
• By rectum
   Child 12–18 years 1 g daily for 2–4 weeks

Maintenance, ulcerative proctitis
• By rectum
   Child 12–18 years 1 g daily

Salofalk® (Dr Falk) [PoM]

Tablets, e/c, yellow, mesalazine 250 mg. Net price 100-tab pack = £17.40. Label: 5, 25, counselling, blood disorder symptoms (see recommendation above)

Dose

Acute attack
• By mouth
   Child 12–18 years 500 mg 3 times daily

Maintenance of remission
• By mouth
   Child 12–18 years 250–500 mg 2–3 times daily

⌐ MESALAZINE (*continued*)

Granules, m/r, grey, e/c, vanilla-flavoured, mesalazine 500 mg/sachet, net price 100-sachet pack = £29.30; 1 g/sachet, 50-sachet pack = £29.30; 1.5 g/sachet, 60-sachet pack = £49.80. Counselling, administration (see dose), blood disorder symptoms (see recommendation above)
Excipients include aspartame (section 9.4.1)

Dose

Acute attack
- By mouth
  Child 6–15 years and body-weight under 40 kg 10–15 mg/kg 3 times daily
  Child 6–15 years and body-weight over 40 kg 1.5–3 g once daily (preferably in the morning) *or* 0.5–1 g 3 times daily
  Child 15–18 years 1.5–3 g once daily (preferably in the morning) *or* 0.5–1 g 3 times daily

Maintenance of remission
- By mouth
  Child 6–15 years and body-weight under 40 kg 7.5–15 mg/kg twice daily *or* 250 mg 3 times daily
  Child 6–15 years and body-weight over 40 kg 500 mg 3 times daily
  Child 15–18 years 500 mg 3 times daily

Administration Granules should be placed on tongue and washed down with water without chewing
Note Preparations that lower stool pH (e.g. lactulose) may prevent release of mesalazine

Suppositories, mesalazine 500 mg. Net price 30-suppos pack = £15.90. Counselling, blood disorder symptoms (see recommendation above)

Dose

Acute attack
- By rectum
  Child 12–18 years 0.5–1 g 2–3 times daily adjusted according to response

Enema, mesalazine 2 g in 59-mL pack. Net price 7 enemas = £31.20. Counselling, blood disorder symptoms (see recommendation above)

Dose

Acute attack *or* maintenance
- By rectum
  Child 12–18 years 2 g once daily at bedtime

Rectal foam, mesalazine 1 g/metered application, net price 14-application canister with disposable applicators and plastic bags = £31.10. Counselling, blood disorder symptoms (see recommendation above)
Excipients include cetostearyl alcohol, disodium edetate, polysorbate 60, propylene glycol, sodium metabisulphite

Dose

Mild ulcerative colitis affecting sigmoid colon and rectum
- By rectum
  Child 12–18 years 2 metered applications (mesalazine 2 g) into the rectum at bedtime increased if necessary to 2 metered applications (mesalazine 2 g) twice daily

---

◢ OLSALAZINE SODIUM

Cautions see notes above; **interactions:** Appendix 1 (aminosalicylates)
Blood disorders see recommendation above

Renal impairment use with caution; manufacturer advises avoid in significant impairment

Pregnancy manufacturer advises avoid unless potential benefit outweighs risk

Breast-feeding manufacturer advises avoid unless potential benefit outweighs risk—may cause diarrhoea in infant

Contra-indications see notes above

Side-effects see notes above; watery diarrhoea common; also reported, tachycardia, palpitation, pyrexia, blurred vision, and photosensitivity

Licensed use not licensed for use in children under 12 years

Indication and dose

Treatment of acute attack of mild ulcerative colitis
- By mouth
  Child 2–18 years 500 mg twice daily after food increased if necessary over 1 week to max. 1 g 3 times daily

Maintenance of remission of mild ulcerative colitis
- By mouth
  Child 2–18 years 250–500 mg twice daily after food

Administration Capsules can be opened and contents sprinkled on food

Dipentum® (UCB Pharma) ⟨PoM⟩
Capsules, brown, olsalazine sodium 250 mg. Net price 112-cap pack = £20.57. Label: 21, counselling, blood disorder symptoms (see recommendation above)

Tablets, yellow, scored, olsalazine sodium 500 mg. Net price 60-tab pack = £22.04. Label: 21, counselling, blood disorder symptoms (see recommendation above)

◢ SULFASALAZINE
(Sulphasalazine)

Cautions see notes above; also history of allergy; hepatic impairment; G6PD deficiency (section 9.1.5); slow acetylator status; risk of haematological and hepatic toxicity (differential white cell, red cell, and platelet counts initially and at

monthly intervals for first 3 months; liver function tests at monthly intervals for first 3 months); upper gastro-intestinal side-effects common with doses over 4 g daily; acute porphyria (section

1 Gastro-intestinal system

◁ **SULFASALAZINE** (*continued*)

9.8.2); **interactions:** Appendix 1 (aminosalicylates)

Blood disorders see recommendation above

Renal impairment risk of toxicity including crystalluria—ensure high fluid intake; avoid in severe impairment

Pregnancy theoretical risk of neonatal haemolysis in third trimester; adequate folate supplements should be given to mother

Breast-feeding small amount in milk (1 report of bloody diarrhoea and rashes); theoretical risk of neonatal haemolysis especially in G6PD-deficient infants

Contra-indications see notes above; also sulphonamide hypersensitivity; child under 2 years of age

Side-effects see notes above; also loss of appetite; fever; blood disorders (including Heinz body anaemia, megaloblastic anaemia); hypersensitivity reactions (including exfoliative dermatitis, epidermal necrolysis, pruritus, photosensitisation, anaphylaxis, serum sickness); ocular complications (including periorbital oedema); stomatitis, parotitis; ataxia, aseptic meningitis, vertigo, tinnitus, insomnia, depression, hallucinations; kidney reactions (including proteinuria, crystalluria, haematuria); oligospermia; urine may be coloured orange; some soft contact lenses may be stained

Indication and dose

Treatment of acute attack of mild to moderate and severe ulcerative colitis, active Crohn's disease

• **By mouth**

  Child 2–12 years 10–15 mg/kg (max. 1 g) 4–6 times daily until remission occurs; increased to max. 60 mg/kg daily in divided doses, if necessary

  Child 12–18 years 1–2 g 4 times daily until remission occurs

Maintenance of remission of mild to moderate and severe ulcerative colitis

• **By mouth**

  Child 2–12 years 5–7.5 mg/kg (max. 500 mg) 4 times daily

  Child 12–18 years 500 mg 4 times daily

Treatment of mild to moderate or severe ulcerative colitis and maintenance of remission, active Crohn's disease

• **By rectum as suppositories**

  Child 5–8 years 500 mg twice daily

  Child 8–12 years 500 mg in the morning and 1 g at night

  Child 12–18 years 0.5–1 g twice daily

Juvenile idiopathic arthritis section 10.1.3

Sulfasalazine (Non-proprietary) [PoM]
Tablets, sulfasalazine 500 mg. Net price 112 = £9.21. Label: 14, counselling, blood disorder symptoms (see recommendation above), contact lenses may be stained

Tablets, e/c, sulfasalazine 500 mg. Net price 112-tab pack = £21.52. Label: 5, 14, 25, counselling, blood disorder symptoms (see recommendation above), contact lenses may be stained
Brands include *Sulazine EC*®

Salazopyrin® (Pharmacia) [PoM]
Tablets, yellow, scored, sulfasalazine 500 mg. Net price 112-tab pack = £6.97. Label: 14, counselling, blood disorder symptoms (see recommendation above), contact lenses may be stained

EN-Tabs® (= tablets e/c), yellow, f/c, sulfasalazine 500 mg. Net price 112-tab pack = £8.43. Label: 5, 14, 25, counselling, blood disorder symptoms (see recommendation above), contact lenses may be stained

Suspension, yellow, sulfasalazine 250 mg/5 mL. Net price 500 mL = £18.84. Label: 14, counselling, blood disorder symptoms (see recommendation above), contact lenses may be stained

Suppositories, yellow, sulfasalazine 500 mg. Net price 10 = £3.30. Label: 14, counselling, blood disorder symptoms (see recommendation above), contact lenses may be stained

1.5.2 **Corticosteroids**

For the role of corticosteroids in acute ulcerative colitis and Crohn's disease, see Inflammatory Bowel Disease, p. 66.

BUDESONIDE

Cautions section 6.3.2; **interactions:** Appendix 1 (corticosteroids)

  Hepatic impairment plasma-budesonide concentration may increase

Contra-indications section 6.3.2

Side-effects section 6.3.2

Licensed use not licensed for use in children

Indication and dose

See preparations

Administration Capsules can be opened and the contents mixed with apple or orange juice

◻ BUDESONIDE (*continued*)

Budenofalk® (Dr Falk) PoM

Capsules, pink, enclosing e/c pellets, budesonide 3 mg, net price 100-cap pack = £76.70. Label: 5, 10, steroid card, 22, 25

Dose

> Mild to moderate Crohn's disease affecting ileum or ascending colon, chronic diarrhoea due to collagenous colitis
> • **By mouth**
>> **Child 12–18 years** 3 mg 3 times daily for up to 8 weeks; reduce dose for the last 2 weeks of treatment. See also section 6.3.2

Entocort® (AstraZeneca) PoM

CR Capsules, grey/pink, enclosing e/c, m/r granules, budesonide 3 mg, net price 100-cap pack = £99.00. Label: 5, 10, steroid card, 22, 25

Note Dispense in original container (contains desiccant)

Dose

> Mild to moderate Crohn's disease affecting the ileum or ascending colon
> • **By mouth**
>> **Child 12–18 years** 9 mg once daily in the morning before breakfast for up to 8 weeks; reduce dose for the last 2–4 weeks of treatment. See also section 6.3.2

Enema, budesonide 2 mg/100 mL when dispersible tablet reconstituted in isotonic saline vehicle, net price pack of 7 dispersible tablets and bottles of vehicle = £33.00

Dose

> Ulcerative colitis involving rectal and recto-sigmoid disease
> • **By rectum**
>> **Child 12–18 years** 1 enema at bedtime for 4 weeks

◼ HYDROCORTISONE

Cautions section 6.3.2; systemic absorption may occur; prolonged use should be avoided

Contra-indications intestinal obstruction, bowel perforation, recent intestinal anastomoses, extensive fistulas; untreated infection

Side-effects section 6.3.2; also local irritation

Indication and dose

> Inflammatory bowel disease
> • **By intravenous administration**
> See p. 451
>
> • **By rectum**
> See preparations

Colifoam® (Meda) PoM

Foam in aerosol pack, hydrocortisone acetate 10%, net price 14-application cannister with applicator = £8.21

Excipients include cetyl alcohol, hydroxybenzoates (parabens), propylene glycol

Dose

> Ulcerative colitis, proctitis, proctosigmoiditis
> • **By rectum**
>> **Child 2–18 years** initially 1 metered application (125 mg hydrocortisone acetate) inserted into the rectum once or twice daily for 2–3 weeks, then once on alternate days

---

◼ PREDNISOLONE

Cautions section 6.3.2; systemic absorption may occur; prolonged use should be avoided

Contra-indications section 6.3.2; intestinal obstruction, bowel perforation, recent intestinal anastomoses, extensive fistulas; untreated infection

Side-effects section 6.3.2

Licensed use *Predfoam®*, *Predsol®* retention enema not licensed for use in children (age range not specified by manufacturer)

Indication and dose

> Ulcerative colitis, Crohn's disease see also under preparations, below
> • **By mouth**
>> **Child 2–18 years** 2 mg/kg (max. 60 mg) once daily until remission occurs, followed by reducing doses
>
> • **By rectum**
> See under preparations

Other indications section 6.3.2

◢ Oral preparations
Section 6.3.2

◢ Rectal preparations

Predenema® (Forest) PoM

Retention enema, prednisolone 20 mg (as sodium metasulphobenzoate) in 100-mL single-dose disposable pack. Net price 1 (standard tube) = 71p, 1 (long tube) = £1.21

Dose

> Ulcerative colitis
> • **By rectum**
>> **Child 12–18 years** initially 20 mg at bedtime for 2–4 weeks, continued if good response

1

Gastro-intestinal system

◁ **PREDNISOLONE (continued)**

Predfoam® (Forest) [PoM]
Foam in aerosol pack, prednisolone 20 mg (as metasulphobenzoate sodium)/metered application, net price 14-application cannister with disposable applicators = £6.32
Excipients include cetostearyl alcohol, disodium edetate, polysorbate 20, sorbic acid

Dose
Proctitis and distal ulcerative colitis
• By rectum
Child 12–18 years 1 metered application (20 mg prednisolone) inserted into the rectum once or twice daily for 2 weeks, continued for further 2 weeks if good response

Predsol® (UCB Pharma) [PoM]
Suppositories, prednisolone 5 mg (as sodium phosphate). Net price 10 = £1.40

Dose
Proctitis and rectal complications of Crohn's disease
• By rectum
Child 2–18 years 5 mg inserted night and morning after a bowel movement

1.5.3 Drugs affecting the immune response

Azathioprine, **mercaptopurine**, or once weekly **methotrexate** are used to induce remission in unresponsive or chronically active Crohn's disease. Azathioprine or mercaptopurine may also be helpful for retaining remission in frequently relapsing inflammatory bowel disease; once weekly methotrexate is used in Crohn's disease when azathioprine or mercaptopurine are ineffective or not tolerated. Response to azathioprine or mercaptopurine may not become apparent for several months. Folic acid (section 9.1.2) should be given to reduce the possibility of methotrexate toxicity. Folic acid can be given at a dose of 5 mg weekly; alternative regimens may be used in some settings.

Ciclosporin (cyclosporin) is a potent immunosuppressant and is markedly nephrotoxic. In children with severe ulcerative colitis unresponsive to other treatment, ciclosporin may reduce the need for urgent colorectal surgery.

AZATHIOPRINE

Cautions see section 8.2.1; **interactions:** Appendix 1 (azathioprine)
Contra-indications see section 8.2.1
Side-effects see section 8.2.1
Licensed use not licensed for use in ulcerative colitis or Crohn's disease

Indication and dose
Severe ulcerative colitis and Crohn's disease
• By mouth
Child 2–18 years initially 2 mg/kg (if necessary up to 3 mg/kg) once daily, then reduced according to response to lowest effective dose; total daily dose may alternatively be given in 2 divided doses

Transplantation rejection section 8.2.1

Rheumatic diseases section 10.1.3

◀Preparations
Section 8.2.1

CICLOSPORIN

Cautions see section 8.2.2; **interactions:** Appendix 1 (ciclosporin)
Contra-indications see section 8.2.2
Side-effects see section 8.2.2
Licensed use not licensed for use in ulcerative colitis

Indication and dose
Refractory ulcerative colitis
• By mouth
Child 2–18 years initially 2 mg/kg twice daily, dose adjusted according to blood-ciclosporin concentration and response; max. 5 mg/kg twice daily
Important For advice on counselling and conversion between preparations, see section 8.2.2

• By intravenous infusion
Child 3–18 years initially 0.5–1 mg/kg twice daily, dose adjusted according to blood-ciclosporin concentration and response

Nephrotic syndrome section 8.2.2

Transplantation rejection and auto-immune conditions section 8.2.2

Atopic dermatitis and psoriasis section 13.5.3

Administration for *intermittent intravenous infusion*, dilute to a concentration of 0.5–2.5 mg/mL with Glucose 5% *or* Sodium Chloride 0.9% and give over 2–6 hours; not to be used with PVC equipment; observe for at least 30 minutes after starting infusion and at frequent intervals thereafter

◀Preparations
Section 8.2.2

▲ MERCAPTOPURINE

Cautions see section 8.1.3; see also Azathioprine, section 8.2.1

Contra-indications see section 8.1.3

Side-effects see section 8.1.3

Licensed use not licensed for use in severe ulcerative colitis and Crohn's disease; for other indications, see section 8.1.3

Indication and dose

Severe ulcerative colitis and Crohn's disease
• By mouth
   Child 2–18 years 1–1.5 mg/kg once daily (initial max. 50 mg; may be increased to 75 mg once daily)

Acute leukaemias section 8.1.3

◀Preparations
Section 8.1.3

▲ METHOTREXATE

Cautions section 10.1.3

Contra-indications section 10.1.3

Side-effects section 10.1.3

Licensed use not licensed for use in children for non-malignant conditions

Indication and dose

Severe acute Crohn's disease
• By subcutaneous or intramuscular injection
   Child 7–18 years 15 mg/m^2 (max. 25 mg) once weekly

Maintenance of remission of severe Crohn's disease
• By mouth or by subcutaneous or intramuscular injection
   Child 7–18 years 15 mg/m^2 (max. 25 mg) once weekly; dose reduced according to response to lowest effective dose

Safe Practice Note that the above dose is a **weekly** dose. To avoid error with low-dose methotrexate, it is recommended that:
• the child or their carer is carefully advised of the **dose** and **frequency** and the reason for taking methotrexate and any other prescribed medicine (e.g. folic acid);
• only one strength of methotrexate tablet (usually 2.5 mg) is prescribed and dispensed;
• the prescription and the dispensing label clearly show the dose and frequency of methotrexate administration;
• the child or their carer is warned to report immediately the onset of any feature of blood disorders (e.g. sore throat, bruising, and mouth ulcers), liver toxicity (e.g. nausea, vomiting, abdominal discomfort, and dark urine), and respiratory effects (e.g. shortness of breath).

Malignant disease section 8.1.3

Rheumatic disease section 10.1.3

Psoriasis section 13.5.3

◀Preparations
Section 10.1.3

Cytokine modulators

Infliximab is a monoclonal antibody which inhibits the pro-inflammatory cytokine, tumour necrosis factor alpha. It should be administered under specialist supervision where adequate resuscitation facilities are available and is used in the treatment of severe refractory or fistulating Crohn's disease in children. Infliximab should be used only when treatment with other immunomodulating drugs has failed or is not tolerated and for children in whom surgery is inappropriate.

▲ INFLIXIMAB

Cautions hepatic impairment; renal impairment; monitor for infections before, during, and for 6 months after treatment (see also Tuberculosis below); heart failure (discontinue if symptoms develop or worsen; avoid in moderate or severe heart failure); demyelinating CNS disorders (risk of exacerbation); history of malignancy (consider discontinuing treatment if malignancy develops); history of prolonged immunosuppressant or PUVA treatment in patients with psoriasis; **interactions:** Appendix 1 (infliximab)
Tuberculosis Children should be evaluated for tuberculosis before treatment. Active tuberculosis should be treated with standard treatment (section 5.1.9) for at least 2 months before starting infliximab. Children who have previously received adequate treatment for tuberculosis can start infliximab but should be monitored every 3 months for possible recurrence. In those without active tuberculosis but who were previously not treated adequately, chemoprophylaxis should ideally be completed before starting infliximab. Children and their carers should be advised to seek medical attention if symptoms suggestive of tuberculosis (e.g. persistent cough, weight loss, and fever) develop
Hypersensitivity reactions Hypersensitivity reactions (including fever, chest pain, hypotension, hypertension, dyspnoea, pruritus, urticaria, serum sickness-like reactions, angioedema, anaphylaxis) reported during or within 1–2 hours after infusion (risk greatest during first or

1
Gastro-intestinal system

◻ **INFLIXIMAB** (*continued*)

second infusion or in children who discontinue other immunosuppressants). All children should be observed carefully for 1–2 hours after infusion and resuscitation equipment should be available for immediate use. Prophylactic antipyretics, antihistamines, or hydrocortisone may be administered. Readministration not recommended after infliximab-free interval of more than 16 weeks—risk of delayed hypersensitivity reactions. Children and carers should be advised to keep Alert card with them at all times and seek medical advice if symptoms of delayed hypersensitivity develop

Contra-indications severe infections (see also under cautions)

Pregnancy avoid; manufacturer advises adequate contraception during and for at least 6 months after last dose

Breast-feeding avoid; manufacturer advises avoid for at least 6 months after last dose

Side-effects see under Cytokine Modulators (section 10.1.3) and Cautions above; also diarrhoea, dyspepsia; flushing, chest pain; dyspnoea; dizziness, fatigue; sinusitis; rash, increased sweating, dry skin; *less commonly* constipation, gastro-oesophageal reflux, cholecystitis, palpitation, arrhythmia, hypertension, hypotension, vasospasm, cyanosis, bradycardia, syncope, oedema, thrombophlebitis, epistaxis, pleurisy, confusion, agitation, nervousness, amnesia, sleep disturbances, vaginitis, demyelinating disorders, antibody formation, pyelonephritis, myalgia, arthralgia, eye disorders, abnormal skin pigmentation, ecchymosis, cheilitis, and alopecia; *rarely* hepatitis, intestinal stenosis, intestinal perforation, gastro-intestinal haemorrhage, pancreatitis, hepatosplenic T-cell lymphoma, circulatory failure, meningitis, seizure, neuropathy, paraesthesia, and lymphoma; *very rarely* pericardial effusion, and skin reactions (including Stevens-Johnson syndrome and toxic epidermal necrolysis); also

reported interstitial lung disease and transverse myelitis

Licensed use not licensed for fistulating Crohn's disease in children

Indication and dose

Severe active Crohn's disease
● **By intravenous infusion**
   Child 6–18 years initially 5 mg/kg, then 5 mg/kg 2 weeks and 6 weeks after initial dose, then 5 mg/kg every 8 weeks; interval between maintenance doses adjusted according to response; discontinue if no response within 10 weeks of initial dose

Fistulating Crohn's disease
● **By intravenous infusion**
   Child 6–18 years initially 5 mg/kg, then 5 mg/kg 2 weeks and 6 weeks after initial dose, then if condition has responded, consult literature for guidance on further doses

Administration for *intravenous infusion* reconstitute each 100-mg vial of powder with 10 mL Water for Injections; to dissolve, gently swirl vial without shaking; allow to stand for 5 minutes; dilute required dose with Sodium Chloride 0.9% to a final volume of 250 mL and give through a low protein-binding filter (1.2 micron or less) over at least 2 hours; start infusion within 3 hours of reconstitution

Remicade® (Schering-Plough) ▼ PoM
Intravenous infusion, powder for reconstitution, infliximab, net price 100-mg vial = £419.62.
Label: 10, alert card, counselling, tuberculosis and hypersensitivity reactions

1.5.4 Food allergy

Allergy with classical symptoms of vomiting, colic and diarrhoea caused by specific foods such as cow's milk should be managed by strict avoidance. The condition should be distinguished from symptoms of occasional food intolerance in children with irritable bowel syndrome. **Sodium cromoglicate** (sodium cromoglycate) may be helpful as an adjunct to dietary avoidance.

SODIUM CROMOGLICATE
(Sodium cromoglycate)

Side-effects occasional nausea, rashes, and joint pain

Indication and dose

Food allergy (in conjunction with dietary restriction)
● **By mouth**
   Child 2–14 years 100 mg 4 times daily before meals, dose may be increased after 2–3 weeks to a max. 40 mg/kg daily and then reduced according to response
   Child 14–18 years 200 mg 4 times daily before meals, dose may be increased after 2–3 weeks to max. 40 mg/kg daily and then reduced according to response

Asthma section 3.3

Allergic conjunctivitis section 11.4.2

Allergic rhinitis section 12.2.1

Administration capsules may be swallowed whole or the contents dissolved in hot water and diluted with cold water before taking

Nalcrom® (Sanofi-Aventis) PoM
Capsules, sodium cromoglicate 100 mg. Net price 100-cap pack = £62.17. Label: 22, counselling, administration

1.6 Laxatives

1.6.1 Bulk-forming laxatives
1.6.2 Stimulant laxatives
1.6.3 Faecal softeners
1.6.4 Osmotic laxatives
1.6.5 Bowel cleansing solutions
1.6.6 Peripheral opioid-receptor antagonists

Before prescribing laxatives it is important to be sure that the child *is* constipated and that the constipation is *not* secondary to an underlying undiagnosed complaint.

Laxatives should be prescribed by a healthcare professional experienced in the management of constipation in children. Delays of greater than 3 days between stools may increase the likelihood of pain on passing hard stools leading to anal fissure, anal spasm and eventually to a learned response to avoid defaecation.

In infants, increased intake of fluids, particularly fruit juice containing sorbitol (e.g. prune, pear, or apple), may be sufficient to soften the stool. In infants under 1 year with mild constipation, **lactulose** (section 1.6.4) can be used to soften the stool; glycerol suppositories may be used to clear faecal impaction. The infant should be referred to a hospital paediatric specialist if these measures fail.

In children over 1 year with infrequent bowel motion or hard stools, if increased fluid and fibre intake is insufficient, an osmotic laxative containing **macrogols** or **lactulose** (section 1.6.4) can be used. If there is evidence of minor faecal retention, the addition of a **stimulant laxative** (section 1.6.2) may overcome withholding but may lead to colic or, in the presence of faecal impaction in the rectum, an increase of faecal overflow.

In children with faecal impaction, an oral preparation containing **macrogols** (section 1.6.4) is used to clear faecal mass and to establish and maintain soft well-formed stools. Rectal administration of laxatives may be effective but this route is frequently distressing for the child and may lead to a persistence of withholding. If the impacted mass is not expelled following treatment with macrogols, referral to hospital may be necessary. Enemas may be administered under heavy sedation in hospital or alternatively, a **bowel cleansing solution** (section 1.6.5) may be tried. In severe cases or where the child is afraid, manual evacuation under anaesthetic may be appropriate.

Long-term regular use of laxatives is essential to maintain well-formed stools and prevent recurrence of faecal impaction; intermittent use may provoke relapses.

> For children with chronic constipation, it may be necessary to exceed the licensed doses of some laxatives. Parents and carers of children should be advised to adjust the dose of laxative in order to establish a regular pattern of bowel movements in which stools are soft, well-formed, and passed without discomfort.

Pregnancy If dietary and lifestyle changes fail to control constipation in pregnancy, moderate doses of poorly absorbed laxatives may be used. A bulk-forming laxative should be tried first. An osmotic laxative, such as lactulose, can also be used. Bisacodyl or senna may be suitable, if a stimulant effect is necessary.

Laxatives are also of value in *drug-induced constipation* (see Prescribing in Palliative Care, p. 26), in *distal intestinal obstruction syndrome* in children with cystic fibrosis, for the expulsion of *parasites* after anthelmintic treatment, and to clear the alimentary tract before *surgery and radiological procedures* (section 1.6.5).

> The laxatives that follow have been divided into 5 main groups (sections 1.6.1–1.6.5). This simple classification disguises the fact that some laxatives have a complex action.

1 Gastro-intestinal system

Gastro-intestinal system

1

1.6.1 Bulk-forming laxatives

Bulk-forming laxatives are of value if the diet is deficient in fibre. They relieve constipation by increasing faecal mass which stimulates peristalsis; children and their carers should be advised that the full effect may take some days to develop.

During treatment with bulk-forming laxatives, adequate fluid intake must be maintained to avoid intestinal obstruction. Proprietary preparations containing a bulking agent such as ispaghula husk are often difficult to administer to children; unprocessed wheat **bran**, taken with food or fruit juice, is a most effective bulk-forming preparation. Finely ground bran, though more palatable, has poorer water-retaining properties, but can be taken as bran bread or biscuits in appropriately increased quantities. Oat bran is also used.

Bulk-forming laxatives may be used in the management of children with *haemorrhoids, anal fissure,* and *irritable bowel syndrome.*

ISPAGHULA HUSK

Cautions adequate fluid intake should be maintained to avoid intestinal obstruction

Contra-indications difficulty in swallowing, intestinal obstruction, colonic atony, faecal impaction

Side-effects flatulence and abdominal distension (especially during the first few days of treatment), gastro-intestinal obstruction or impaction; hypersensitivity reported

Licensed use *Regulan®* not licensed for use in children under 6 years; *Fybogel®* and *Ispagel Orange®* not licensed for use in children under 6 years (unless on specialist practitioner's advice); *Isogel®* licensed for use in children (age range not specified by manufacturer)

Indication and dose

See under preparations

Counselling Preparations that swell in contact with liquid should always be carefully swallowed with water and should not be taken immediately before going to bed

Fibrelief® (Manx)
Granules, sugar- and gluten-free, ispaghula husk 3.5 g/sachet (natural or orange flavour), net price 10 sachets = £1.23, 30 sachets = £2.07. Label: 13, counselling, see above
Excipients include aspartame (section 9.4.1)

Dose
Constipation
• By mouth
  Child 12–18 years 1–6 sachets daily in water in 1–3 divided doses

Fybogel® (R&C)
Granules, buff, effervescent, sugar- and gluten-free, ispaghula husk 3.5 g/sachet (low Na⁺), net price 30 sachets (plain, lemon, or orange flavour) = £3.84. Label: 13, counselling, see above
Excipients include aspartame 16 mg/sachet (see section 9.4.1)

Dose
Constipation
• By mouth
  Child 2–12 years ½–1 level 5-mL spoonful in water twice daily preferably after meals

  Child 12–18 years 1 sachet *or* 2 level 5-mL spoonfuls in water twice daily preferably after meals

Isogel® (Potters)
Granules, brown, sugar- and gluten-free, ispaghula husk 90%. Net price 200 g = £2.67. Label: 13, counselling, see above

Dose
Constipation
• By mouth
  Child 2–12 years 1 level 5-mL spoonful in water once or twice daily, preferably at mealtimes

  Child 2–12 years 2 level 5-mL spoonfuls in water once or twice daily, preferably at mealtimes

Note May be difficult to obtain

Ispagel Orange® (LPC)
Granules, beige, effervescent, sugar- and gluten-free, ispaghula husk 3.5 g/sachet, net price 30 sachets = £2.10. Label: 13, counselling, see above
Excipients include aspartame (section 9.4.1)

Dose
Constipation
• By mouth
  Child 2–12 years ½–1 level 5-mL spoonful in water twice daily preferably after meals

  Child 12–18 years 1 sachet (or 2 level 5-mL spoonfuls) in water 1–3 times daily preferably after meals

Regulan® (Procter & Gamble)
Powder, beige, sugar- and gluten-free, ispaghula husk 3.4 g/5.85-g sachet (orange or lemon/lime flavour). Net price 30 sachets = £2.54. Label: 13, counselling, see above
Excipients include aspartame (section 9.4.1)

Dose
Constipation
• By mouth
  Child 2–12 years ½–1 level 5-mL spoonful in water 1–3 times daily

  Child 12–18 years 1 sachet in 150 mL water 1–3 times daily

METHYLCELLULOSE

Cautions see under Ispaghula Husk

Contra-indications see under Ispaghula Husk; also infective bowel disease

◁ **METHYLCELLULOSE (continued)**

Side-effects   see under Ispaghula Husk

Licensed use   no age limit specified by manufacturer

Indication and dose

See under preparation below

Counselling Preparations that swell in contact with liquid should always be carefully swallowed with water and should not be taken immediately before going to bed

Celevac® (Amdipharm)

Tablets, pink, scored, methylcellulose '450' 500 mg. Net price 112-tab pack = £2.69.Counselling, see above and dose

Dose

Constipation, diarrhoea (see notes above)
* **By mouth**

    Child 7–12 years 2 tablets twice daily

    Child 12–18 years 3–6 tablets twice daily.

Administration In constipation the dose should be taken with at least 300 mL liquid. In diarrhoea, ileostomy, and colostomy control, minimise liquid intake for 30 minutes before and after dose

◢Extemporaneous formulations available see Extemporaneous Preparations, p. 8

■ **STERCULIA**

Cautions   see under Ispaghula Husk

Contra-indications   see under Ispaghula Husk

Side-effects   see under Ispaghula Husk

Indication and dose

Constipation for dose see under preparation

Counselling Preparations that swell in contact with liquid should always be carefully swallowed with water and should not be taken immediately before going to bed

Normacol® (Norgine)

Granules, coated, gluten-free, sterculia 62%. Net price 500 g = £6.18; 60 × 7-g sachets = £5.19. Label: 25, 27, counselling, see above

Dose

* **By mouth**

    Child 6–12 years ½–1 heaped 5-mL spoonful or the contents of ½–1 sachet, washed down without chewing with plenty of liquid once or twice daily after meals

    Child 12–18 years 1–2 heaped 5-mL spoonfuls or the contents of 1–2 sachets, washed down without chewing with plenty of liquid once or twice daily after meals

Administration May be mixed with soft food (e.g. yoghurt) before swallowing, followed by plenty of liquid.

Normacol Plus® (Norgine)

Granules, brown, coated, gluten-free, sterculia 62%, frangula (standardised) 8%. Net price 500 g = £6.60; 60 × 7 g sachets = £5.56. Label: 25, 27, Counselling, see above

Dose

* **By mouth**

    Child 6–12 years ½-1 heaped 5-mL spoonful or the contents of ½-1 sachet, washed down without chewing with plenty of liquid, once or twice daily after meals

    Child 12–18 years 1–2 heaped 5-mL spoonfuls or the contents of 1–2 sachets, washed down without chewing with plenty of liquid, once or twice daily after meals

---

■ **1.6.2** **Stimulant laxatives**

Stimulant laxatives include **bisacodyl**, **sodium picosulphate**, and members of the **anthraquinone** group, **senna** and **dantron** (danthron). The indications for dantron are limited (see below) by its potential carcinogenicity (based on *rodent* carcinogenicity studies) and evidence of genotoxicity. Powerful stimulants such as **cascara** (an anthraquinone) and **castor oil** are obsolete. **Docusate sodium** probably acts both as a stimulant and as a softening agent.

Stimulant laxatives increase intestinal motility and often cause abdominal cramp; they should be avoided in intestinal obstruction. Stools should be softened by increasing dietary fibre and liquid or with an osmotic laxative (section 1.6.4) before giving a stimulant laxative. In chronic constipation, especially where withholding of stool occurs, additional doses of a stimulant laxative may be required. Long-term use of stimulant laxatives is sometimes necessary (see section 1.6), but excessive use can cause diarrhoea and related effects such as hypokalaemia.

Glycerol suppositories act as a lubricant and as a rectal stimulant by virtue of the mildly irritant action of glycerol.

■ **BISACODYL**

Cautions   prolonged use (risk of electrolyte imbalance)

Pregnancy   see p. 77

Contra-indications   ileus, intestinal obstruction, acute abdominal conditions, acute inflammatory bowel disease, severe dehydration

Side-effects   see notes above; nausea and vomiting; colitis also reported; *suppositories* local irritation

80 1.6.2 Stimulant laxatives

◁ **BISACODYL** (*continued*)

Indication and dose

Constipation (tablets act in 10–12 hours; suppositories act in 20–60 minutes)

● **By mouth**

Child 4–10 years 5 mg at night

Child 10–18 years 5–10 mg at night; increased if necessary (max. 20 mg)

● **By rectum (suppository)**

Child 2–10 years 5 mg in the morning

Child 10–18 years 10 mg in the morning

Bowel clearance before radiological procedures and surgery

● **By mouth and by rectum**

Child 4–10 years *by mouth*, 5 mg at bedtime for 2 days before procedure and, if necessary, *by rectum*, 5 mg suppository 1 hour before procedure

Child 10–18 years *by mouth*, 10 mg at bedtime for 2 days before procedure and, if necessary, *by rectum*, 10 mg suppository 1 hour before procedure

Bisacodyl (Non-proprietary)

Tablets, e/c, bisacodyl 5 mg. Net price 20 = 65p. Label: 5, 25

Suppositories, bisacodyl 10 mg. Net price 12 = 89p

Paediatric suppositories, bisacodyl 5 mg. Net price 5 = 94p

Note The brand name *Dulcolax®* ⓈⒽ (Boehringer Ingelheim) is used for bisacodyl tablets, net price 10-tab pack = 74p; suppositories (10 mg), 10 = £1.57; paediatric suppositories (5 mg), 5 = 94p
The brand names *Dulcolax® Liquid* and *Dulcolax® Perles* are used for sodium picosulfate preparations

---

▌**DANTRON**
(Danthron)

Cautions avoid prolonged contact with skin (as in incontinent patients or infants wearing nappies)—risk of irritation and excoriation; *rodent* studies indicate potential carcinogenic risk

Pregnancy manufacturer advises avoid—no information available

Breast-feeding manufacturer advises avoid—limited information available

Contra-indications see Bisacodyl above

Side-effects see notes above; also urine may be coloured red

Indication and dose

Constipation in terminally ill children for dose see under preparations

◀**With poloxamer '188'** (as co-danthramer)
Note Co-danthramer suspension 5 mL = one co-danthramer capsule, **but** strong co-danthramer suspension 5 mL = two strong co-danthramer capsules

Co-danthramer (Non-proprietary) ⓅⓄⓜ

Capsules, co-danthramer 25/200 (dantron 25 mg, poloxamer '188' 200 mg). Net price 60-cap pack = £12.86. Label: 14, (urine red)

Dose

● **By mouth**

Child 6–12 years 1 capsule at night (restricted indications, see notes above)

Child 12–18 years 1–2 capsules at night (restricted indications, see notes above)

Strong capsules, co-danthramer 37.5/500 (dantron 37.5 mg, poloxamer '188' 500 mg). Net price 60-cap pack = £15.55. Label: 14, (urine red)

Dose

● **By mouth**

Child 12–18 years 1–2 capsules at night (restricted indications, see notes above)

Suspension, co-danthramer 25/200 in 5 mL (dantron 25 mg, poloxamer '188' 200 mg/5 mL). Net price 300 mL = £11.27, 1 litre = £37.57. Label: 14, (urine red)
Brands include *Codalax®* ⓈⒽ, *Danlax®*

Dose

● **By mouth**

Child 2–12 years 2.5–5 mL at night (restricted indications, see notes above)

Child 12–18 years 5–10 mL at night (restricted indications, see notes above)

Strong suspension, co-danthramer 75/1000 in 5 mL (dantron 75 mg, poloxamer '188' 1 g/5 mL). Net price 300 mL = £30.13. Label: 14, (urine red)
Brands include *Codalax Forte®* ⓈⒽ

Dose

● **By mouth**

Child 12–18 years 5 mL at night (restricted indications, see notes above)

◀**With docusate sodium** (as co-danthrusate)
Co-danthrusate (Non-proprietary) ⓅⓄⓜ

Capsules, co-danthrusate 50/60 (dantron 50 mg, docusate sodium 60 mg). Net price 63-cap pack = £14.50. Label: 14, (urine red)
Brands include *Normax®* ⓈⒽ

Dose

● **By mouth**

Child 6–12 years 1 capsule at night (restricted indications, see notes above)

Child 12–18 years 1–3 capsules at night (restricted indications, see notes above)

Suspension, yellow, co-danthrusate 50/60 (dantron 50 mg, docusate sodium 60 mg/5 mL). Net price 200 mL = £8.75. Label: 14, (urine red)
Brands include *Normax®*

Dose

● **By mouth**

Child 6–12 years 5 mL at night (restricted indications, see notes above)

Child 12–18 years 5–15 mL at night (restricted indications, see notes above)

◢ DOCUSATE SODIUM
(Dioctyl sodium sulphosuccinate)

Cautions see notes above; do not give with liquid paraffin

Pregnancy not known to be harmful—manufacturer advises caution

Breast-feeding present in milk following oral administration—manufacturer advises caution

Contra-indications see notes above; also for *rectal preparations*, haemorrhoids or anal fissure

Side-effects see notes above

Licensed use *adult oral solution and capsules* not licensed for use in children under 12 years

Indication and dose

Constipation
• By mouth

Child 6 months–2 years 12.5 mg 3 times daily (use paediatric oral solution)

Child 2–12 years 12.5–25 mg 3 times daily (use paediatric oral solution)

Child 12–18 years up to 500 mg daily in divided doses

Note Oral preparations act within 1–2 days; response to rectal administration usually occurs within 20 minutes; recommended doses may be exceeded on specialist advice

Adjunct in abdominal radiological procedures
• By mouth

Child 12–18 years 400 mg with barium meal

Administration for administration *by mouth*, solution may be mixed with milk or squash

Dioctyl® (UCB Pharma)
Capsules, yellow/white, docusate sodium 100 mg, net price 30-cap pack = £2.40, 100-cap pack = £8.00

Docusol® (Typharm)
Adult oral solution, sugar-free, docusate sodium 50 mg/5 mL, net price 300 mL = £2.48

Paediatric oral solution, sugar-free, docusate sodium 12.5 mg/5 mL, net price 300 mL = £1.63

◢ Rectal preparations
Norgalax Micro-enema® (Norgine)
Enema, docusate sodium 120 mg in 10-g single-dose disposable packs. Net price 10-g unit = 60p
Dose
• By rectum
Child 12–18 years 1 enema as a single dose

◢ GLYCEROL
(Glycerin)

Indication and dose

Constipation
• By rectum

Child 1 month–1 year 1-g suppository as required

Child 1–12 years 2-g suppository as required

Child 12–18 years 4-g suppository as required

Glycerol Suppositories, BP
(Glycerin Suppositories)
Suppositories, gelatin 140 mg, glycerol 700 mg, purified water to 1 g. Net price 12 = £1.07 (infant, 1-g mould), £1.03 (child, 2-g mould), £1.54 (adult, 4-g mould)

Administration Moisten with water before insertion

◢ SENNA

Cautions see notes above

Pregnancy see p. 77

Breast-feeding not known to be harmful

Contra-indications see notes above

Side-effects see notes above

Licensed use *syrup* not licensed for use in children under 2 years

Indication and dose

Constipation for dose see under preparations

Note Onset of action 8–12 hours; initial dose should be low; recommended doses may be exceeded on specialist advice

Senna (Non-proprietary)
Tablets, total sennosides (calculated as sennoside B) 7.5 mg. Net price 60 = £1.70
Brands include *Senokot®* [NHS]
Dose
• By mouth
Child 6–12 years 1–2 tablets at night (or in the morning if preferred)
Child 12–18 years 2–4 tablets at night (or in the morning if preferred)

1 Gastro-intestinal system

Gastro-intestinal system

1

◻ **SENNA (*continued*)**

Manevac® (Galen)
Granules, coated, senna fruit 12.4%, ispaghula 54.2%, net price 400 g = £7.45. Label: 25, 27, counselling, see below

Dose
• **By mouth**
  Child 5–12 years 1 level 5-mL spoonful once daily
  Child 12–18 years 1–2 level 5-mL spoonfuls after evening meal and, if necessary, before breakfast or every 6 hours in resistant cases for 1–3 days

  Administration granules can be taken mixed with a cold or warm drink *or* be sprinkled on food
  Counselling Preparations that swell in contact with liquid should always be carefully swallowed with water and should not be taken immediately before going to bed

Senokot® (R&C)
Tablets ▣▣, see above

Syrup, sugar-free, brown, total sennosides (calculated as sennoside B) 7.5 mg/5 mL. Net price 500 mL = £2.69

Dose
• **By mouth**
  Child 1 month–2 years 0.5 mL/kg (max. 2.5 mL) once daily
  Child 2–6 years 2.5–5 mL once daily in the morning
  Child 6–12 years 5–10 mL at night *or* in the morning
  Child 12–18 years 10–20 mL once daily, usually at bedtime

SODIUM PICOSULFATE
(Sodium picosulphate)

Cautions see notes above; active inflammatory bowel disease (avoid if fulminant)

Pregnancy see p. 77

Breast-feeding not known to be present in milk but manufacturer advises avoid unless potential benefit outweighs risk

Contra-indications see notes above; severe dehydration

Side-effects see notes above

Licensed use *elixir*, licensed for use in children (age range not specified by manufacturer; *Perles®* not licensed for use in children under 4 years

Indication and dose
  Constipation
  • **By mouth**
    Child 1 month–4 years 250 micrograms/kg (max. 5 mg) at night
    Child 4–10 years 2.5–5 mg at night
    Child 10–18 years 5–10 mg at night
    Note onset of action 6–12 hours; recommended doses may be exceeded on specialist advice

Bowel evacuation before abdominal radiological and endoscopic procedures on the colon, and surgery section 1.6.5

Sodium Picosulfate (Non-proprietary)
Elixir, sodium picosulfate 5 mg/5 mL, net price 100 mL = £1.85
Note The brand name *Dulcolax® Liquid* (Boehringer Ingelheim) is used for sodium picosulfate elixir 5 mg/5 mL

Dulcolax® (Boehringer Ingelheim)
Perles® (= capsules), sodium picosulfate 2.5 mg, net price 20-cap pack = £1.93, 50-cap pack = £2.73
Note The brand name *Dulcolax®* is also used for bisacodyl tablets and suppositories

◀Bowel cleansing solutions
Section 1.6.5

1.6.3 Faecal softeners

Enemas containing **arachis oil** (ground-nut oil, peanut oil) lubricate and soften impacted faeces and promote a bowel movement.

Bulk laxatives (section 1.6.1) and non-ionic surfactant 'wetting' agents e.g. docusate sodium (section 1.6.2) also have softening properties. Such drugs are useful for oral administration in the management of anal fissure; glycerol suppositories (section 1.6.2) are useful for rectal use.

ARACHIS OIL

Cautions intestinal obstruction; hypersensitivity to soya

Contra-indications inflammatory bowel disease, hypersensitivity to arachis oil or peanuts

Licensed use licensed for use in children (age range not specified by manufacturer

Indication and dose
  Impacted faeces
  • **By rectum**
    Child 3–7 years 45–65 mL as required

    Child 7–12 years 65–100 mL as required
    Child 12–18 years 100–130 mL as required

Administration warm enema in warm water before use

Arachis Oil Enema (Non-proprietary)
Enema, arachis (peanut) oil in 130-mL single-dose disposable packs. Net price 130 mL = £7.98

1.6.4 Osmotic laxatives

Osmotic laxatives increase the amount of water in the large bowel, either by drawing fluid from the body into the bowel or by retaining the fluid they were administered with.

Lactulose is a semi-synthetic disaccharide which is not absorbed from the gastro-intestinal tract. It produces an osmotic diarrhoea of low faecal pH, and discourages the proliferation of ammonia-producing organisms. It is therefore useful in the treatment of *hepatic encephalopathy*.

Macrogols are inert polymers of ethylene glycol which sequester fluid in the bowel; giving fluid with macrogols may reduce the dehydrating effect sometimes seen with osmotic laxatives. Macrogols are an effective non-traumatic means of evacuation in children with faecal impaction and can be used in the long-term management of chronic constipation.

Saline purgatives such as **magnesium hydroxide** are commonly abused but are satisfactory for occasional use; adequate fluid intake should be maintained. **Magnesium salts** are useful where rapid bowel evacuation is required. **Sodium salts** should be avoided as they may give rise to sodium and water retention in susceptible individuals. **Phosphate enemas** are useful in bowel clearance before radiology, endoscopy, and surgery. Enemas containing **phosphate** or **sodium citrate**, and oral **bowel cleansing solutions** (section 1.6.5) should only be used on the advice of a specialist practitioner.

LACTULOSE

Cautions lactose intolerance; **interactions:** Appendix 1 (lactulose)

Contra-indications galactosaemia, intestinal obstruction

Side-effects flatulence, cramps, and abdominal discomfort

Licensed use not licensed for use in children for hepatic encephalopathy

Indication and dose

Constipation (may take up to 48 hours to act)
- **By mouth**
   Child 1 month–1 year 2.5 mL twice daily, adjusted according to response
   Child 1–5 years 5 mL twice daily, adjusted according to response

   Child 5–10 years 10 mL twice daily, adjusted according to response
   Child 10–18 years initially 15 mL twice daily, adjusted according to response

Hepatic encephalopathy
- **By mouth**
   Child 12–18 years 30–50 mL 3 times daily; adjust dose to produce 2–3 soft stools per day

Lactulose (Non-proprietary)
Solution, lactulose 3.1–3.7 g/5 mL with other ketoses. Net price 300-mL pack = £2.51, 500-mL pack = £2.90
Brands include *Duphalac*® ⟨NHS⟩, *Lactugal*®, *Regulose*®

MACROGOLS
(Polyethylene glycols)

Cautions discontinue if symptoms of fluid and electrolyte disturbance; see also preparations below

Pregnancy manufacturer advises use only if essential—no information available

Breast-feeding no information available, but absorption from gastro-intestinal tract negligible

Contra-indications intestinal perforation or obstruction, paralytic ileus, severe inflammatory conditions of the intestinal tract (such as Crohn's disease, ulcerative colitis, and toxic megacolon); see also preparations below

Side-effects abdominal distension and pain, nausea

Licensed use *Movicol*® *Paediatric Plain* not licensed for use in faecal impaction in children under 5 years, or for chronic constipation in children under 2 years

Indication and dose
See under preparations below

Laxido® (Galen)
Oral powder, orange-flavoured, macrogol '3350' (polyethylene glycol '3350') 13.125 g, sodium bicarbonate 178.5 mg, sodium chloride 350.7 mg, potassium chloride 46.6 mg/sachet, net price 20-sachet pack = £3.56, 30-sachet pack = £5.34. Label: 13

Note Also available in natural flavour (sugar-free)

Cautions patients with cardiovascular impairment should not take more than 2 sachets in any 1 hour

Dose
Chronic constipation
- **By mouth**
   Child 12–18 years 1–3 sachets daily in divided doses usually for up to 2 weeks; maintenance, 1–2 sachets daily
   Administration Mix contents of each sachet in half a glass (approx. 125 mL) of water

1

Gastro-intestinal system

◁ **MACROGOLS (continued)**

Faecal impaction
• By mouth

Child 12–18 years 8 sachets daily, usually for max. 3 days

Administration Mix contents of 8 sachets in 1 litre of water. After reconstitution the solution should be kept in a refrigerator and discarded if unused after 6 hours

Movicol® (Norgine)

Oral powder, macrogol '3350' (polyethylene glycol '3350') 13.125 g, sodium bicarbonate 178.5 mg, sodium chloride 350.7 mg, potassium chloride 46.6 mg/sachet, net price 20-sachet pack (lime- and lemon- flavoured) = £4.63, 30-sachet pack (lime- and lemon- or chocolate- or plain- flavoured) = £6.95, 50-sachet pack (lime- and lemon- or plain-flavoured) = £11.58. Label: 13

Note Amount of potassium chloride varies according to flavour of *Movicol®* as follows: plain-flavour = 50.2 mg/sachet; lime and lemon flavour = 46.6 mg/sachet; chocolate flavour = 31.7 mg/sachet. 1 sachet when reconstituted with 125 mL water provides K⁺ 5.4 mmol/litre

Cautions patients with cardiovascular impairment should not take more than 2 sachets in any 1 hour

Dose

Chronic constipation
• By mouth

Child 12–18 years 1–3 sachets daily in divided doses usually for up to 2 weeks; maintenance, 1–2 sachets daily

Administration Mix contents of each sachet in half a glass (approx. 125 mL) of water

Faecal impaction
• By mouth

Child 12–18 years 8 sachets daily, usually for max. 3 days

Administration Mix contents of 8 sachets in 1 litre of water. After reconstitution the solution should be kept in a refrigerator and discarded if unused after 6 hours

Movicol®-Half (Norgine)

Oral powder, macrogol '3350' (polyethylene glycol '3350') 6.563 g, sodium bicarbonate 89.3 mg, sodium chloride 175.4 mg, potassium chloride 23.3 mg/sachet, net price 20-sachet pack (lime and

lemon flavour) = £2.78, 30-sachet pack = £4.17. Label: 13

Cautions patients with impaired cardiovascular function should not take more than 4 sachets in any 1 hour

Dose

Chronic constipation
• By mouth

Child 12–18 years 2–6 sachets daily in divided doses usually for up to 2 weeks; maintenance, 2–4 sachets daily

Administration Mix content of each sachet dissolved in quarter of a glass (approx. 60–65 mL) of water

Faecal impaction
• By mouth

Child 12–18 years 16 sachets daily, usually for max. 3 days

Administration Mix contents of 16 sachets in 1 litre of water. After reconstitution the solution should be kept in a refrigerator and discarded if unused after 6 hours

Movicol® Paediatric Plain (Norgine) PoM

Oral powder, macrogol '3350' (polyethylene glycol '3350') 6.563 g, sodium bicarbonate 89.3 mg, sodium chloride 175.4 mg, potassium chloride 25.1 mg/sachet, net price 30-sachet pack = £4.63. Label: 13

Cautions *with high doses,* impaired gag reflex, reflux oesophagitis, impaired consciousness

Contra-indications cardiovascular impairment, renal impairment——no information available

Dose

Chronic constipation, prevention of faecal impaction
• By mouth

Child 1–6 years 1 sachet daily; adjust dose to produce regular soft stools (max. 4 sachets daily)

Child 6–12 years 2 sachets daily; adjust dose to produce regular soft stools (max. 4 sachets daily)

Administration Mix content of each sachet in quarter of a glass (approx. 60–65 mL) of water

Faecal impaction
• By mouth

Child 1–5 years (treat until impaction resolves or for max. 7 days) 2 sachets on first day, then 4 sachets daily for 2 days, then 6 sachets daily for 2 days, then 8 sachets daily for 2 days

Child 5–12 years (treat until impaction resolves or for max. 7 days) 4 sachets on first day, then increased in steps of 2 sachets daily to max. 12 sachets daily

Administration Mix each sachet in quarter of a glass (approx. 60–65 mL) of water; total daily dose to be taken over a 12-hour period

---

▮ **MAGNESIUM SALTS**

Cautions see also notes above; **interactions:** Appendix 1 (antacids)

Hepatic impairment avoid in hepatic coma if risk of renal impairment

Renal impairment avoid or reduce dose; increased risk of toxicity

Contra-indications acute gastro-intestinal conditions

Side-effects colic

Indication and dose

Constipation see under preparations below

◁Magnesium hydroxide
Magnesium Hydroxide Mixture, BP

Aqueous suspension containing about 8% hydrated magnesium oxide. Do not store in cold place

Dose
• By mouth

Child 3–12 years 5–10 mL with water at bedtime when required

Child 12–18 years 30–45 mL with water at bedtime when required

◁Bowel cleansing solutions
Section 1.6.5

■ PHOSPHATES (RECTAL)

Cautions see also notes above; *with enema*, electrolyte disturbances, renal impairment, congestive heart failure, ascites, uncontrolled hypertension, maintain adequate hydration

Contra-indications acute gastro-intestinal conditions (including gastro-intestinal obstruction, inflammatory bowel disease, and conditions associated with increased colonic absorption)

Side-effects local irritation; *with enema*, electrolyte disturbances

Indication and dose

Constipation, bowel evacuation before abdominal radiological procedures, endoscopy, and surgery

    For dose see preparations

Carbalax® (Forest)
Suppositories, sodium acid phosphate (anhydrous) 1.3 g, sodium bicarbonate 1.08 g, net price 12 = £2.01

Dose
- **By rectum**
    Child 12–18 years 1 suppository, inserted 30 minutes before evacuation required; moisten with water before use

Fleet® Ready-to-use Enema (De Witt)
Enema, sodium acid phosphate 21.4 g, sodium phosphate 9.4 g/118 mL, net price 133-mL pack (delivers 118 mL dose) with standard tube = 57p

- **By rectum**
    Child 3–7 years 40–60 mL once daily
    Child 7–12 years 60–90 mL once daily
    Child 12–18 years 90–118 mL once daily

Phosphates Enema BP Formula B
Enema, sodium dihydrogen phosphate dihydrate 12.8 g, disodium phosphate dodecahydrate 10.24 g, purified water, freshly boiled and cooled, to 128 mL. Net price 128 mL with standard tube = £2.98, with long rectal tube = £3.98

Dose
- **By rectum**
    Child 3–7 years 45–65 mL once daily
    Child 7–12 years 65–100 mL once daily
    Child 12–18 years 100–128 mL once daily

■ SODIUM CITRATE (RECTAL)

Cautions see notes above

Contra-indications acute gastro-intestinal conditions

Indication and dose

Constipation for dose see under preparations

Micolette Micro-enema® (Pinewood)
Enema, sodium citrate 450 mg, sodium lauryl sulphoacetate 45 mg, glycerol 625 mg, together with citric acid, potassium sorbate, and sorbitol in a viscous solution, in 5-mL single-dose disposable packs with nozzle. Net price 5 mL = 31p

Dose
- **By rectum**
    Child 3–18 years 5–10 mL as a single dose

Micralax Micro-enema® (UCB Pharma)
Enema, sodium citrate 450 mg, sodium alkylsulphoacetate 45 mg, sorbic acid 5 mg, together with

glycerol and sorbitol in a viscous solution in 5-mL single-dose disposable packs with nozzle. Net price 5 mL = 41p

Dose
- **By rectum**
    Child 3–18 years 5 mL as a single dose

Relaxit Micro-enema® (Crawford)
Enema, sodium citrate 450 mg, sodium lauryl sulphate 75 mg, sorbic acid 5 mg, together with glycerol and sorbitol in a viscous solution in 5-mL single-dose disposable packs with nozzle. Net price 5 mL = 32p

Dose
- **By rectum**
    Child 1 month–18 years 5 mL as a single dose (insert only half nozzle length in child under 3 years)

1.6.5 Bowel cleansing solutions

Bowel cleansing solutions are used before colonic surgery, colonoscopy, or radiological examination to ensure the bowel is free of solid contents. They are **not** treatments for constipation.

Gastrografin® is an **amidotrizoate** radiological contrast medium with high osmolality; it is used in the treatment of meconium ileus in neonates and in the management of distal intestinal obstruction syndrome in children with cystic fibrosis.

■ BOWEL CLEANSING SOLUTIONS

Cautions recent gastro-intestinal surgery; heart disease; inflammatory bowel disease; reflux oesophagitis; impaired gag reflex; administer

solution via nasogastric tube in semi-conscious or unconscious patients

Renal impairment avoid *Citramag®* and *Picolax®* if estimated glomerular filtration rate less than

Gastro-intestinal system

1

Gastro-intestinal system

1

△ **BOWEL CLEANSING SOLUTIONS (continued)**

30 mL/minute/1.73 m² (risk of hypermagnesaemia); manufacturer of *Fleet Phospho-soda®* advises avoid in significant renal impairment

Pregnancy no evidence of harm in *animal* studies; manufacturer advises caution especially in first trimester

Breast-feeding not excreted in breast milk

Contra-indications gastro-intestinal obstruction, gastric retention, gastro-intestinal ulceration, perforated bowel, congestive cardiac failure; toxic colitis, toxic megacolon or ileus

Side-effects nausea, vomiting, abdominal pain (usually transient—reduced by taking more slowly), abdominal distension, anal discomfort; *less frequently* headache, rash, and electrolyte disturbances

Licensed use *Klean-Prep®* not licensed for use in children

Indication and dose

Clearance of bowel prior to radiological examination, colonoscopy, or surgery

For dose see under preparations

Citramag® (Sanochemia)
Oral powder, sugar-free, effervescent, magnesium carbonate 11.57 g, anhydrous citric acid 17.79 g/sachet, net price 10-sachet pack (lemon and lime flavour) = £14.90. Label: 10, patient information leaflet, 13, counselling, see below

Dose
- **By mouth**

  Child 5–10 years on day before procedure, one-third of a sachet at 8 a.m. and one-third of a sachet between 2 and 4 p.m.

  Child 10–18 years on day before procedure, ½–1 sachet at 8 a.m. and ½–1 sachet between 2 and 4 p.m.

Counselling The patient information leaflet advises that hot water (200 mL) is needed to make the solution and provides guidance on the timing and procedure for reconstitution; it also mentions need for high fluid, low residue diet beforehand (according to hospital advice), and explains that only clear fluids can be taken after *Citramag®* until procedure completed

Fleet Phospho-soda® (De Witt)
Oral solution, sugar-free, sodium dihydrogen phosphate dihydrate 24.4 g, disodium phosphate dodecahydrate 10.8 g/45 mL. Contains about 217 mmol Na⁺/45 mL. Net price 2 × 45-mL bottles = £4.79. Label: 10, patient information leaflet, counselling

Dose
- **By mouth**

  Child 15–18 years 45 mL diluted with half a glass (120 mL) of cold water, followed by one full glass (240 mL) of cold water

  Timing of doses is dependent on the time of the procedure

  For morning procedure, first dose should be taken at 7 a.m. and second at 7 p.m. on day before the procedure

  For afternoon procedure, first dose should be taken at 7 p.m. on day before and second dose at 7 a.m. on day of the procedure

  Solid food must not be taken during dosing period; clear liquids or water should be substituted for meals

  Acts within half to 6 hours of first dose

Klean-Prep® (Norgine)
Oral powder, sugar-free, macrogol '3350' (polyethylene glycol '3350') 59 g, anhydrous sodium sulphate 5.685 g, sodium bicarbonate 1.685 g, sodium chloride 1.465 g, potassium chloride 743 mg/sachet, net price 4 sachets = £8.56. Label: 10, patient information leaflet, counselling
Excipients include aspartame (section 9.4.1)

Note Allergic reactions reported. 1 sachet when reconstituted with 1 litre water provides Na⁺ 125 mmol, K⁺ 10 mmol

Dose

Clearance of bowel prior to radiological examination, colonoscopy or surgery
- **By mouth**

  Child 12–18 years a glass (approx. 250 mL) of reconstituted solution every 10–15 minutes, or by nasogastric tube 20–30 mL/minute, until 4 litres have been consumed or watery stools are free of solid matter. The solution from all 4 sachets should be drunk within 4–6 hours (250 mL drunk rapidly every 10–15 minutes)

  Alternatively total volume for administration given in 2 divided doses, first dose taken on the evening before examination and second dose on the morning of the examination

Distal intestinal obstruction syndrome
- **By mouth, nasogastric or gastrostomy tube**

  Child 1–18 years 10 mL/kg/hour for 30 minutes, then 20 mL/kg/hour for 30 minutes, then increase to 25 mL/kg/hour if tolerated; max. 100 mL/kg (or 4 litres) over 4 hours; repeat 4-hour treatment if necessary

Administration Each sachet should be made up to 1 litre with water; flavouring such as clear fruit cordials may be added if required; to facilitate gastric emptying domperidone (section 1.2) may be given 30 minutes before starting. After reconstitution the solution should be kept in a refrigerator and discarded if unused after 24 hours.

Picolax® (Ferring)
Oral powder, sugar-free, sodium picosulfate 10 mg/sachet, with magnesium citrate. Contains 87 mmol Mg²⁺ and 5 mmol K⁺/sachet. Net price 2-sachet pack = £3.53. Label: 10, patient information leaflet, 13, counselling, see below

Dose

Bowel evacuation on day before radiological procedure, endoscopy, or surgery
- **By mouth**

  Child 1–2 years ¼ sachet before 8 a.m. then ¼ sachet 6–8 hours later

  Child 2–4 years ½ sachet before 8 a.m. then ½ sachet 6–8 hours later

  Child 4–9 years 1 sachet before 8 a.m. then ½ sachet 6–8 hours later

  Child 9–18 years 1 sachet before 8 a.m. then 1 sachet 6–8 hours later

Note Acts within 3 hours of first dose. Low residue diet recommended on the day before procedure and copious intake of water or other clear fluids recommended during treatment

Counselling. One sachet should be reconstituted with 150 mL (approx. half a glass) of cold water; children and carers should be warned that heat is generated during reconstitution and that the solution should be allowed to cool before drinking

▲ AMIDOTRIZOATES
Diatrizoates

Cautions asthma or history of allergy, latent hyperthyroidism, dehydration and electrolyte disturbance (correct first); in children with oesophageal fistulae (aspiration may lead to pulmonary oedema); benign nodular goitre; enteritis; risk of anaphylactoid reactions increased by concomitant administration of beta-blockers

Pregnancy manufacturer advises caution

Contra-indications hypersensitivity to iodine, hyperthyroidism

Side-effects diarrhoea, nausea, vomiting; also reported, abdominal pain, intestinal perforation, bowel necrosis, oral mucosal blistering, hypersensitivity reactions, pyrexia, headache, dizziness, disturbances in consciousness, hyperthyroidism, electrolyte disturbances, and skin reactions (including toxic epidermal necrolysis)

Licensed use not licensed for use in distal intestinal obstruction syndrome

Indication and dose

Uncomplicated meconium ileus
- **By rectum**

  Neonate 15–30 mL as a single dose

Distal intestinal obstruction syndrome
- **By mouth or by rectum**

  Child 1 month–2 years 15–30 mL as a single dose

  Child body-weight 15–25 kg 50 mL as a single dose

  Child body-weight over 25 kg 100 mL as a single dose

Administration Intravenous prehydration is essential in neonates and infants. Fluid intake should be encouraged for 3 hours after administration. *By mouth*, for child bodyweight under 25 kg, dilute *Gastrografin®* with 3 times its volume of water or fruit juice; for child bodyweight over 25 kg, dilute *Gastrografin®* with twice its volume of water or fruit juice. *By rectum*, administration must be carried out slowly under radiological supervision to ensure required site is reached. For child under 5 years, dilute *Gastrografin®* with 5 times its volume of water; for child over 5 years dilute *Gastrografin®* with 4 times its volume of water. Administer using a large syringe and soft rubber catheter (No.8 French); the buttocks may be taped tightly together to minimise leakage, but a balloon catheter should not be used.

Radiological investigations dose to be recommended by radiologist

Gastrografin® (Bayer)
Solution, sodium amidotrizoate 100 mg, meglumine amidotrizoate 660 mg/mL, net price 100-mL bottle = £15.58
Excipients include disodium edetate

1.6.6 Peripheral opioid-receptor antagonists
Classification not used in *BNF for Children*.

1.7 Local preparations for anal and rectal disorders

1.7.1 Soothing anal and rectal preparations
1.7.2 Compound anal and rectal preparations with corticosteroids
1.7.3 Rectal sclerosants
1.7.4 Management of anal fissures

In children with perianal soreness or pruritus ani, good toilet hygiene is essential; the use of alcohol-free 'wet-wipes' after each bowel motion, regular bathing and the avoidance of local irritants such as bath additives is recommended. Excoriated skin is best treated with a protective barrier emollient (section 13.2.2); in children over 1 month, **hydrocortisone** ointment or cream (section 13.4) or a compound rectal preparation (section 1.7.2) may be used for a short period of time, up to a maximum of 7 days.

Pruritus ani caused by threadworm infection requires treatment with an anthelmintic (section 5.5.1). Topical application of **white soft paraffin** or other bland emollient (section 13.2.1) may reduce anal irritation caused by threadworms.

Perianal erythema caused by streptococcal infection should be treated initially with an oral antibacterial such as **phenoxymethylpenicillin** (section 5.1.1.1) or **erythromycin** (section 5.1.5), while awaiting results of culture and sensitivity testing.

Perianal candidiasis (thrush) requires treatment with a topical antifungal preparation (section 13.10.2). For treatment of vulvovaginal candidiasis, see section 7.2.2.

Proctitis associated with inflammatory bowel disease in children is treated with corticosteroids and aminosalicylates (section 1.5).

For the management of anal fissures, see section section 1.7.4.

1
Gastro-intestinal system

1.7.1 Soothing anal and rectal preparations

Haemorrhoids in children are rare, but may occur in infants with portal hypertension. Soothing rectal preparations containing mild astringents such as bismuth subgallate, zinc oxide, and hammamelis may provide symptomatic relief, but proprietary preparations which also contain lubricants, vasoconstrictors, or mild antiseptics may cause further perianal irritation.

Local anaesthetics may be used to relieve pain in children with anal fissures or pruritus ani, but local anaesthetics are absorbed through the rectal mucosa and may cause sensitisation of the anal skin. Excessive use of local anaesthetics may result in systemic effects, see section 15.2. Preparations containing local anaesthetics should be used for no longer than 2–3 days.

Lidocaine (lignocaine) ointment (section 15.2) may be applied before defaecation to relieve pain associated with anal fissure, but local anaesthetics can cause stinging initially and this may aggravate the child's fear of pain.

Other local anaesthetics such as tetracaine (amethocaine), cinchocaine (dibucaine), and pramocaine (pramoxine) may be included in rectal preparations, but these are more irritant than lidocaine.

Corticosteroids are often combined with local anaesthetics and soothing agents in topical preparations for haemorrhoids and proctitis. Topical preparations containing corticosteroids (section 1.7.2) should not be used long-term or if infection (such as herpes simplex) is present. For further information on the use of topical corticosteroids, see section 13.4.

1.7.2 Compound anal and rectal preparations with corticosteroids

Anugesic-HC® (Pfizer) [PoM]
Cream, benzyl benzoate 1.2%, bismuth oxide 0.875%, hydrocortisone acetate 0.5%, Peru balsam 1.85%, pramocaine hydrochloride 1%, zinc oxide 12.35%. Net price 30 g (with rectal nozzle) = £3.71

Dose
Haemorrhoids, pruritus ani
• By rectum
   Child 12–18 years apply night and morning and after a bowel movement; do not use for longer than 7 days

Suppositories, buff, benzyl benzoate 33 mg, bismuth oxide 24 mg, bismuth subgallate 59 mg, hydrocortisone acetate 5 mg, Peru balsam 49 mg, pramocaine hydrochloride 27 mg, zinc oxide 296 mg, net price 12 = £2.69

Dose
Haemorrhoids, pruritus ani
• By rectum
   Child 12–18 years insert 1 suppository night and morning and after a bowel movement; do not use for longer than 7 days

Anusol-HC® (McNeil) [PoM]
Ointment, benzyl benzoate 1.25%, bismuth oxide 0.875%, bismuth subgallate 2.25%, hydrocortisone acetate 0.25%, Peru balsam 1.875%, zinc oxide 10.75%. Net price 30 g (with rectal nozzle) = £3.50

Dose
Haemorrhoids, pruritus ani
• By rectum
   Child 12–18 years apply night and morning and after a bowel movement; do not use for longer than 7 days

Suppositories, benzyl benzoate 33 mg, bismuth oxide 24 mg, bismuth subgallate 59 mg, hydro-

cortisone acetate 10 mg, Peru balsam 49 mg, zinc oxide 296 mg. Net price 12 = £2.46

Dose
Haemorrhoids, pruritus ani
• By rectum
   Child 12–18 years insert 1 suppository night and morning and after a bowel movement; do not use for longer than 7 days

Perinal® (Dermal)
Spray application, hydrocortisone 0.2%, lidocaine hydrochloride 1%. Net price 30-mL pack = £6.39

Dose
Haemorrhoids, pruritus ani
• By rectum
   Child 2–18 years spray once over the affected area up to 3 times daily; do not use for longer than 7 days without medical advice (child under 14 years, on medical advice only)

Proctofoam HC® (Meda) [PoM]
Foam in aerosol pack, hydrocortisone acetate 1%, pramocaine hydrochloride 1%. Net price 21.2-g pack (approx. 40 applications) with applicator = £5.06

Dose
Pain and irritation associated with local, non-infected anal or perianal conditions
• By rectum
   Child 12–18 years 1 applicatorful (4–6 mg hydrocortisone acetate, 4–6 mg pramocaine hydrochloride) by rectum 2–3 times daily and after a bowel movement (max. 4 times daily); do not use for longer than 7 days

Proctosedyl® (Aventis Pharma) [PoM]
Ointment, cinchocaine (dibucaine) hydrochloride 0.5%, hydrocortisone 0.5%. Net price 30 g = £9.40 (with cannula)

Dose

Haemorrhoids, pruritus ani
- By rectum
  Child 1 month–18 years apply morning and night and after a bowel movement, externally or by rectum; do not use for longer than 7 days

Suppositories, cinchocaine (dibucaine) hydrochloride 5 mg, hydrocortisone 5 mg. Net price 12 = £4.24

Dose

Haemorrhoids, pruritus ani
- By rectum
  Child 12–18 years insert 1 suppository night and morning and after a bowel movement; do not use for longer than 7 days

Scheriproct® (Valeant) [PoM]
Ointment, cinchocaine (dibucaine) hydrochloride 0.5%, prednisolone hexanoate 0.19%. Net price 30 g = £3.00

Dose

Haemorrhoids, pruritus ani
- By rectum
  Child 1 month–18 years apply twice daily for 5–7 days (3–4 times daily on 1st day if necessary), then once daily for a few days after symptoms have cleared

Suppositories, cinchocaine (dibucaine) hydrochloride 1 mg, prednisolone hexanoate 1.3 mg. Net price 12 = £1.41

Dose

Haemorrhoids, pruritus ani
- By rectum
  Child 12–18 years insert 1 suppository daily after a bowel movement, for 5–7 days (in severe cases initially 2–3 times daily)

Ultraproct® (Meadow) [PoM]
Ointment, cinchocaine (dibucaine) hydrochloride 0.5%, fluocortolone caproate 0.095%, fluocortolone pivalate 0.092%, net price 30 g (with rectal nozzle) = £4.57

Dose

Haemorrhoids, pruritus ani
  Child 1 month–18 years apply twice daily for 5–7 days (3–4 times daily on 1st day if necessary), then once daily for a few days after symptoms have cleared

Suppositories, cinchocaine (dibucaine) hydrochloride 1 mg, fluocortolone caproate 630 micrograms, fluocortolone pivalate 610 micrograms, net price 12 = £2.15

Dose

Haemorrhoids, pruritus ani
- By rectum
  Child 12–18 years insert 1 suppository daily after a bowel movement, for 5–7 days (in severe cases initially 2–3 times daily) then 1 suppository every other day for 1 week

Uniroid-HC® (Chemidex) [PoM]
Ointment, cinchocaine (dibucaine) hydrochloride 0.5%, hydrocortisone 0.5%. Net price 30 g (with applicator) = £4.23

Dose

Haemorrhoids, pruritus ani
- By rectum
  Child 1 month–18 years apply twice daily and after a bowel movement, externally or by rectum; do not use for longer than 7 days (child under 12 years, on medical advice only)

Suppositories, cinchocaine (dibucaine) hydrochloride 5 mg, hydrocortisone 5 mg. Net price 12 = £1.91

Dose

Haemorrhoids, pruritus ani
- By rectum
  Child 12–18 years insert 1 suppository twice daily and after a bowel movement; do not use for longer than 7 days

Xyloproct® (AstraZeneca) [PoM]
Ointment (water-miscible), aluminium acetate 3.5%, hydrocortisone acetate 0.275%, lidocaine 5%, zinc oxide 18%, net price 20 g (with applicator) = £2.26

Dose

Haemorrhoids, pruritus ani
- By rectum
  Child 1 month–18 years apply several times daily; short-term use only

1.7.3 Rectal sclerosants

Classification not used in *BNF for Children*.

1.7.4 Management of anal fissures

The management of anal fissures includes stool softening (section 1.6) and the short-term use of a topical preparation containing a local anaesthetic (section 1.7.1). If these measures are inadequate, children with chronic anal fissures should be referred for specialist treatment in hospital. Topical **glyceryl trinitrate**, 0.05% or 0.1% ointment, may be used in children to relax the anal sphincter, relieve pain and aid healing of anal fissures. Excessive application of topical nitrates causes side-effects such as headache, flushing, dizziness, and postural hypotension.

Before considering surgery, **diltiazem** 2% ointment may be used in children with chronic anal fissures resistant to topical nitrates.

Ointments containing glyceryl trinitrate in a range of strengths or diltiazem 2% are available as manufactured specials (see Special-order Manufacturers, p. 943).

1.8 Stoma and enteral feeding tubes

Stoma

Prescribing for children with stoma calls for special care. The following is a brief account of some of the main points to be borne in mind.

When a solid-dose formulation such as a capsule or a tablet is given the contents of the ostomy bag should be checked for any remnants; response to treatment should be carefully monitored because of the possibility of incomplete absorption. *Enteric-coated* and *modified-release* preparations are **unsuitable**, particularly in children with an ileostomy, as there may not be sufficient release of the active ingredient.

Laxatives   Enemas and washouts should be used in children with stoma only under specialist supervision; they should **not** be prescribed for those with an ileostomy as they may cause rapid and severe loss of water and electrolytes.

Children with colostomy may suffer from constipation and whenever possible it should be treated by increasing fluid intake or dietary fibre. If a laxative (section 1.6) is required, it should generally be used for short periods only.

Antidiarrhoeals   Loperamide, **codeine phosphate,** and **co-phenotrope** (section 1.4.2) are effective for controlling excessive stool losses. Bulk-forming drugs (section 1.6.1) may be tried but it is often difficult to adjust the dose appropriately.

Antibacterials should **not** be given for an episode of acute diarrhoea.

Antacids   The tendency to diarrhoea from magnesium salts or constipation from aluminium salts may be increased in children with stoma.

Diuretics   Diuretics should be used with caution in children with an ileostomy because they may become excessively dehydrated and potassium depletion may easily occur. It is usually advisable to use a **potassium-sparing** diuretic (section 2.2.3).

Digoxin   Children with stoma are particularly susceptible to hypokalaemia. This predisposes children on digoxin to digoxin toxicity; potassium supplements (section 9.2.1.1) or a potassium-sparing diuretic (section 2.2.3) may be advisable.

Analgesics   Opioid analgesics (section 4.7.2) may cause troublesome constipation in children with colostomy. When a non-opioid analgesic is required **paracetamol** is usually suitable; anti-inflammatory analgesics may cause gastric irritation and bleeding.

Iron preparations   Iron supplements may cause loose stools and sore skin at the stoma site. If this is troublesome and if iron is definitely indicated a parenteral iron preparation (section 9.1.1.2) should be used. Modified-release iron preparations should be **avoided**.

Care of stoma   Children and carers are usually given advice about the use of *cleansing agents, protective creams, lotions, deodorants,* or *sealants* whilst in hospital, either by the surgeon or by a stoma-care nurse. Voluntary organisations offer help and support to patients with stoma.

Enteral feeding tubes

Care is required in choosing an appropriate formulation of a drug for administration through a nasogastric narrow-bore feeding tube or through a percutaneous endoscopic gastrostomy (PEG) or jejunostomy tube. Liquid preparations (or soluble tablets) are preferred; injection solutions may also be suitable for administration through an enteral tube.

If a solid formulation of a medicine needs to be given, it should be given as a suspension of particles fine enough to pass through the tube. It is possible to crush many immediate-release tablets but enteric-coated or modified-release preparations should **not** be crushed.

Enteral feeds may affect the absorption of drugs and it is therefore important to consider the timing of drug administration in relation to feeds. If more than one drug needs to be given, they should be given separately and the tube should be flushed with water after each drug has been given.

Clearing blockages   Carbonated (sugar-free) drinks may be marginally more effective than water in unblocking feeding tubes, but mildly acidic liquids (such as pineapple juice or cola-based drinks) can coagulate protein in feeds, causing further blockage. If these measures fail to clear the enteral feeding tube, an alkaline solution containing pancreatic enzymes may be introduced into the tube (followed after at least 5 minutes by water). Specific products designed to break up blockages caused by formula feeds are also available.

1.9 Drugs affecting intestinal secretions

1.9.1   Drugs affecting biliary composition and flow
1.9.2   Bile acid sequestrants
1.9.3   Aprotinin
1.9.4   Pancreatin

1.9.1 Drugs affecting biliary composition and flow

Bile acids (**ursodeoxycholic** and **chenodeoxycholic acid**) may be used as dietary supplements in children with inborn errors of bile acid synthesis. Ursodeoxycholic acid is used to improve the flow of bile in children with cholestatic conditions such as familial intrahepatic cholestasis, biliary atresia in infants, cystic-fibrosis-related liver disease, and cholestasis caused by total parenteral nutrition or following liver transplantation. Ursodeoxycholic acid may also relieve the severe itching associated with cholestasis.

In sclerosing cholangitis, ursodeoxycholic acid is used to lower liver enzyme and serum-bilirubin concentrations.

Ursodeoxycholic acid is also used in the treatment of intrahepatic cholestasis in pregnancy.

Smith-Lemli-Opitz syndrome   Chenodeoxycholic and ursodeoxycholic acid have been used with cholesterol in children with Smith-Lemli-Opitz syndrome. Chenodeoxycholic acid is also used in combination with cholic acid to treat bile acid synthesis defects but cholic acid is difficult to obtain. Chenodeoxycholic acid and cholesterol are available from 'special-order' manufacturers or specialist importing companies, see p. 943.

1

Gastro-intestinal system

▌ URSODEOXYCHOLIC ACID

Cautions interactions: Appendix 1 (ursodeoxycholic acid)

Hepatic impairment avoid in chronic liver disease (but used in primary biliary cirrhosis)

Pregnancy no evidence of harm but manufacturer advises avoid

Breast-feeding not known to be harmful but manufacturer advises avoid

Contra-indications radio-opaque stones; non-functioning gall bladder (in patients with radiolucent gallstones)

Side-effects *rarely*, diarrhoea

Licensed use not licensed for use in children for indications shown below

Indication and dose

Cholestasis
• By mouth
> **Neonate** 5 mg/kg 3 times daily, adjust dose and frequency according to response, max. 10 mg/kg 3 times daily

> **Child 1 month–2 years** 5 mg/kg 3 times daily, adjust dose and frequency according to response, max. 10 mg/kg 3 times daily

Improvement of hepatic metabolism of essential fatty acids and bile flow, in children with cystic fibrosis
• By mouth
> **Child 1 month–18 years** 10–15 mg/kg twice daily; total daily dose may alternatively be given in 3 divided doses

Cholestasis associated with total parenteral nutrition
• By mouth
> **Neonate** 10 mg/kg 3 times daily

> **Child 1 month–18 years** 10 mg/kg 3 times daily

◺ URSODEOXYCHOLIC ACID *(continued)*

Sclerosing cholangitis
- **By mouth**

  Child 1 month–18 years 5–10 mg/kg 2–3 times daily, adjusted according to response, max. 15 mg/kg 3 times daily

Ursodeoxycholic Acid (Non-proprietary) ℗ℴℳ
Tablets, ursodeoxycholic acid 150 mg, net price 60-tab pack = £18.51. Label: 21

Capsules, ursodeoxycholic acid 250 mg, net price 60-cap pack = £35.11. Label: 21

Destolit® (Norgine) ℗ℴℳ
Tablets, scored, ursodeoxycholic acid 150 mg, net price 60-tab pack = £18.39. Label: 21

Urdox® (CP) ℗ℴℳ
Tablets, f/c, ursodeoxycholic acid 300 mg, net price 60-tab pack = £26.50. Label: 21

Ursofalk® (Dr Falk) ℗ℴℳ
Capsules, ursodeoxycholic acid 250 mg, net price 60-cap pack = £31.10, 100-cap pack = £32.85. Label: 21

Suspension, sugar-free, ursodeoxycholic acid 250 mg/5 mL, net price 250 mL = £28.50. Label: 21

Ursogal® (Galen) ℗ℴℳ
Tablets, scored, ursodeoxycholic acid 150 mg, net price 60-tab pack = £17.05. Label: 21

Capsules, ursodeoxycholic acid 250 mg, net price 60-cap pack = £30.50. Label: 21

Other preparations for bile synthesis defects

◤ CHENODEOXYCHOLIC ACID

Cautions see under Ursodeoxycholic Acid
  Pregnancy avoid—fetotoxicity reported in *animal* studies

Contra-indications see under Ursodeoxycholic Acid

Side-effects see under Ursodeoxycholic Acid

Licensed use not licensed

Indication and dose

  Cerebrotendinous xanthomatosis
  - **By mouth**

    Neonate 5 mg/kg 3 times daily

    Child 1 month–18 years 5 mg/kg 3 times daily

  Defective synthesis of bile acid
  - **By mouth**

    Neonate initially 5 mg/kg 3 times daily, reduced to 2.5 mg/kg 3 times daily

    Child 1 month–18 years initially 5 mg/kg 3 times daily, reduced to 2.5 mg/kg 3 times daily

  Smith-Lemli-Opitz syndrome see notes above
  - **By mouth**

    Neonate 7 mg/kg once daily or in divided doses

    Child 1 month–18 years 7 mg/kg once daily or in divided doses

Administration for administration *by mouth*, add the contents of a 250-mg capsule to 25 mL of sodium bicarbonate solution 8.4% (1 mmol/mL) to produce a suspension containing cheno-deoxycholic acid 10 mg/mL; use immediately after preparation, discard any remaining suspension

Chenofalk (Non-proprietary) ℗ℴℳ
Capsules, chenodeoxycholic acid 250mg
Available from 'special-order' manufacturers or specialist importing companies, see p. 943

◤ CHOLESTEROL

Cautions consult product literature

Contra-indications consult product literature

Licensed use not licensed

Indication and dose

  Smith-Lemli-Opitz syndrome
  - **By mouth**

    Neonate 5–10 mg/kg 3–4 times daily

    Child 1 month–18 years 5–10 mg/kg 3–4 times daily (doses up to 15 mg/kg 4 times daily have been used)

Administration cholesterol powder can be mixed with a vegetable oil before administration

Cholesterol Powder (Non-proprietary)
Available from 'special-order' manufacturers or specialist importing companies, see p. 943

1.9.2 Bile acid sequestrants

Colestyramine (cholestyramine) is an anion-exchange resin that forms an insoluble complex with bile acids in the gastro-intestinal tract; it is used to relieve diarrhoea associated with surgical procedures such as ileal resection, or following radiation therapy. Colestyramine is also used in the treatment of familial hypercholesterolaemia (see section 2.12), and to relieve pruritus in children with partial biliary obstruction, (for treatment of pruritus, see section 3.4.1). Colestyramine is

(Left margin: Gastro-intestinal system 1)

not absorbed from the gastro-intestinal tract, but will interfere with the absorption of a number of drugs, so timing of administration is important.

◤ COLESTYRAMINE
(Cholestyramine)

Cautions see section 2.12

Contra-indications see section 2.12

Side-effects see section 2.12

Licensed use not licensed for use in children under 6 years

Indication and dose

Pruritus associated with partial biliary obstruction and primary biliary cirrhosis, diarrhoea associated with Crohn's disease, ileal resection, vagotomy, diabetic vagal neuropathy, and radiation

• By mouth

Child 1 month–1 year 1 g once daily in a suitable liquid, adjusted according to response; total daily dose may alternatively be given in 2–4 divided doses (max. 9 g daily)

Child 1–6 years 2 g once daily in a suitable liquid, adjusted according to response; total daily dose may alternatively be given in 2–4 divided doses (max. 18 g daily)

Child 6–12 years 4 g once daily in a suitable liquid, adjusted according to response; total daily dose may alternatively be given in 2–4 divided doses (max. 24 g daily)

Child 12–18 years 4–8 g once daily in a suitable liquid, adjusted according to response; total daily dose may alternatively be given in 2–4 divided doses (max. 36 g daily)

Counselling Other drugs should be taken at least 1 hour before or 4–6 hours after colestyramine to reduce possible interference with absorption

Note For treatment of diarrhoea induced by bile acid malabsorption, if no response within 3 days an alternative therapy should be initiated

Hypercholesterolaemia section 2.12

Administration The contents of one sachet should be mixed with at least 150 mL of water or other suitable liquid such as fruit juice, skimmed milk, thin soups, or pulpy fruits with a high moisture content

◤ Preparations
Section 2.12

1.9.3 Aprotinin

Classification not used in *BNF for Children*.

1.9.4 Pancreatin

Pancreatin containing a mixture of protease, lipase and amylase in varying proportions aids the digestion of starch, fat, and protein. Supplements of pancreatin are given by mouth to compensate for reduced or absent exocrine secretion in cystic fibrosis, and following pancreatectomy, total gastrectomy, or chronic pancreatitis.

The dose of pancreatin is adjusted according to size, number, and consistency of stools, and the nutritional status of the child; extra allowance will be needed if snacks are taken between meals. Daily dose should not exceed 10 000 lipase units per kg body-weight per day, (**important**: see CSM advice on Higher-strength preparations below).

Pancreatin preparations			
Preparation	Protease units	Amylase units	Lipase units
Creon® 10 000 capsule, e/c granules	600	8000	10 000
Creon® Micro e/c granules (per 100 mg)	200	3600	5000
Nutrizym 10® capsule, e/c minitablets	500	9000	10 000
Pancrex® granules (per gram)	300	4000	5000
Pancrex V® capsule, powder	430	9000	8000
Pancrex V '125'® capsule, powder	160	3300	2950
Pancrex V® e/c tablet	110	1700	1900
Pancrex V® Forte e/c tablet	330	5000	5600
Pancrex V® powder (per gram)	1400	30 000	25 000

Higher-strength pancreatin preparations *Pancrease HL*® and *Nutrizym 22*® have been associated with the development of large bowel strictures (fibrosing colonopathy) in children with cystic fibrosis aged between 2 and 13 years. The **CSM** (1995) has recommended the following:

- *Pancrease HL®*, *Nutrizym 22®* should not be used in children under 16 years with cystic fibrosis;

- the total dose of pancreatic enzyme supplements used in patients with cystic fibrosis should not usually exceed 10 000 units of lipase per kg body-weight daily;

- if a patient on any pancreatin preparation develops new abdominal symptoms (or any change in existing abdominal symptoms) the patient should be reviewed to exclude the possibility of colonic damage.

Possible risk factors are gender (boys at greater risk than girls), more severe cystic fibrosis, and concomitant use of laxatives. The peak age for developing fibrosing colonopathy is between 2 and 8 years.

Higher-strength pancreatin preparations			
Preparation	Protease units	Amylase units	Lipase units
Creon® 25 000 capsule, e/c pellets	1000	18 000	25 000
Creon® 40 000 capsule, e/c granules	1600	25 000	40 000
Nutrizym 22® capsule, e/c minitablets	1100	19 800	22 000
Pancrease HL® capsule, e/c minitablets	1250	22 500	25 000

Pancreatin is inactivated by gastric acid therefore pancreatin preparations are best taken with food (or immediately before or after food). In children with cystic fibrosis with persistent fat malabsorption despite optimal use of enzyme replacement, an **H$_2$-receptor antagonist** (section 1.3.1), or a **proton pump inhibitor** (section 1.3.5) may improve fat digestion and absorption. Enteric-coated preparations are designed to deliver a higher enzyme concentration in the duodenum (provided the capsule contents are swallowed whole without chewing). If the capsules are opened the enteric-coated granules should be mixed with milk, slightly acidic soft food or liquid such as apple juice, and then swallowed immediately without chewing. Any left-over food or liquid containing pancreatin should be discarded. Since pancreatin is also inactivated by heat, excessive heat should be avoided if preparations are mixed with liquids or food.

Pancreatin can irritate the perioral skin and buccal mucosa if retained in the mouth, and excessive doses can cause perianal irritation. Hypersensitivity reactions may occur particularly if the powder is handled.

PANCREATIN

Cautions see CSM advice above; hyperuricaemia and hyperuricosuria have been associated with very high doses; **interactions:** Appendix 1 (pancreatin)

Side-effects nausea, vomiting, abdominal discomfort; skin and mucosal irritation (see notes above)

Indication and dose

Pancreatic insufficiency for dose see individual preparations, below

Creon® 10 000 (Solvay)

Capsules, brown/clear, enclosing buff-coloured e/c granules of pancreatin (pork), providing: protease 600 units, lipase 10 000 units, amylase 8000 units. Net price 100-cap pack = £16.66. Counselling, see dose

Dose
- By mouth

  Child 1 month–18 years initially 1–2 capsules with each meal either taken whole or contents mixed with fluid or soft food (then swallowed immediately without chewing), see notes above

Creon® Micro (Solvay)

Gastro-resistant granules, brown, pancreatin (pork), providing: protease 200 units, lipase 5000 units, amylase 3600 units per 100 mg, net price 20 g = £31.50. Counselling, see dose

Dose
- By mouth

  Neonate initially 100 mg before each feed; granules can be mixed with a small amount of breast milk or formula feed and administered immediately (manufacturer recommends mixing with a small amount of apple juice before administration)

  Child 1 month–18 years initially 100 mg before each feed or meal; granules can be mixed with a small amount of milk or soft food and administered immediately (manufacturer recommends mixing with acidic liquid or pureed fruit before administration); see notes above

  Note 100 mg granules = one measured scoopful (scoop supplied with product). Granules should not be chewed before swallowing.

◻ **PANCREATIN** (*continued*)

Nutrizym 10® (Merck)

Capsules, red/yellow, enclosing e/c minitablets of pancreatin (pork) providing minimum of: protease 500 units, lipase 10 000 units, amylase 9000 units. Net price 100 = £14.47. Counselling, see dose

Dose

• **By mouth**

Child 1 month–18 years 1–2 capsules with meals and 1 capsule with snacks, swallowed whole or contents taken with water or mixed with soft food (then swallowed immediately without chewing, see notes above); higher doses may be required according to response

Pancrex® (Paines & Byrne)

Granules, pancreatin (pork), providing minimum of: protease 300 units, lipase 5000 units, amylase 4000 units/g. Net price 300 g = £20.39. Label: 25, counselling, see dose
Excipients include lactose (7 g per 10 g dose)

Dose

• **By mouth**

Child 2–18 years 5–10 g just before meals washed down or mixed with milk or water

Pancrex V® (Paines & Byrne)

Capsules, pancreatin (pork), providing minimum of: protease 430 units, lipase 8000 units, amylase 9000 units. Net price 300-cap pack = £15.80. Counselling, see dose

Dose

• **By mouth**

Child 1 month–1 year contents of 1–2 capsules mixed with feeds

Child 1–18 years 2–6 capsules with meals, swallowed whole or sprinkled on food

Capsules '125', pancreatin (pork), providing minimum of: protease 160 units, lipase 2950 units, amylase 3300 units. Net price 300-cap pack = £9.72. Counselling, see dose

Dose

• **By mouth**

Neonate contents of 1–2 capsules in each feed (or mix with feed and give by spoon)

Tablets, e/c, pancreatin (pork), providing minimum of: protease 110 units, lipase 1900 units, amylase 1700 units. Net price 300-tab pack = £4.51. Label: 5, 25, counselling, see dose

Dose

• **By mouth**

Child 2–18 years 5–15 tablets before meals

Tablets forte, e/c, pancreatin (pork), providing minimum of: protease 330 units, lipase 5600 units, amylase 5000 units. Net price 300-tab pack = £13.74. Label: 5, 25, counselling, see dose

Dose

• **By mouth**

Child 2–18 years 6–10 tablets before meals

Powder, pancreatin (pork), providing minimum of: protease 1400 units, lipase 25 000 units, amylase

30 000 units/g. Net price 300 g = £24.28. Counselling, see dose

Dose

• **By mouth**

Neonate 250–500 mg with each feed

Child 1 month–18 years 0.5–2 g with meals, washed down or mixed with milk or water

◢ **Higher-strength preparations**

See **CSM** warning above

Counselling It is important to ensure adequate hydration at all times in children receiving higher-strength pancreatin preparations.

Creon® 25 000 (Solvay) ⒫ⓞⓜ

Capsules, orange/clear, enclosing brown-coloured e/c pellets of pancreatin (pork), providing: protease (total) 1000 units, lipase 25 000 units, amylase 18 000 units, net price 100-cap pack = £30.03. Counselling, see above and under dose

Dose

• **By mouth**

Child 2–18 years initially 1 capsule with meals either taken whole or contents mixed with fluid or soft food (then swallowed immediately without chewing), see notes above

Creon® 40 000 (Solvay) ⒫ⓞⓜ

Capsules, brown/clear, enclosing brown-coloured e/c granules of pancreatin (pork), providing: protease (total) 1600 units, lipase 40 000 units, amylase 25 000 units, net price 100-cap pack = £60.00. Counselling, see above and under dose

Dose

• **By mouth**

Child 2–18 years initially 1–2 capsules with meals either taken whole or contents mixed with fluid or soft food (then swallowed immediately without chewing), see notes above

Nutrizym 22® (Merck) ⒫ⓞⓜ

Capsules, red/yellow, enclosing e/c minitablets of pancreatin (pork), providing minimum of: protease 1100 units, lipase 22 000 units, amylase 19 800 units. Net price 100-cap pack = £33.33. Counselling, see above and under dose

Dose

• **By mouth**

Child 15–18 years 1–2 capsules with meals and 1 capsule with snacks, swallowed whole or contents taken with water or mixed with soft food (then swallowed immediately without chewing), see notes above

Pancrease HL® (Janssen-Cilag) ⒫ⓞⓜ

Capsules, enclosing light brown e/c minitablets of pancreatin (pork), providing minimum of: protease 1250 units, lipase 25 000 units, amylase 22 500 units. Net price 100 = £33.65. Counselling, see above and under dose

Dose

• **By mouth**

Child 15–18 years 1–2 capsules during each meal and 1 capsule with snacks swallowed whole or contents mixed with slightly acidic liquid or soft food (then swallowed immediately without chewing), see notes above

1

Gastro-intestinal system

2 Cardiovascular system

2.1 **Positive inotropic drugs**...**97**
2.1.1 Cardiac glycosides 97
2.1.2 Phosphodiesterase inhibitors 99

2.2 **Diuretics**..**100**
2.2.1 Thiazides and related diuretics 101
2.2.2 Loop diuretics 103
2.2.3 Potassium-sparing diuretics and aldosterone antagonists................ 104
2.2.4 Potassium-sparing diuretics with other diuretics 106
2.2.5 Osmotic diuretics 107
2.2.6 Mercurial diuretics 107
2.2.7 Carbonic anhydrase inhibitors 107
2.2.8 Diuretics with potassium 107

2.3 **Anti-arrhythmic drugs**..**107**
2.3.1 Management of arrhythmias 107
2.3.2 Drugs for arrhythmias 108

2.4 **Beta-adrenoceptor blocking drugs** **113**

2.5 **Hypertension** **119**
2.5.1 Vasodilator antihypertensive drugs and pulmonary hypertension 121
2.5.2 Centrally acting antihypertensive drugs 127
2.5.3 Adrenergic neurone blocking drugs 128
2.5.4 Alpha-adrenoceptor blocking drugs 128
2.5.5 Drugs affecting the renin-angiotensin system 130

2.6 **Nitrates, calcium-channel blockers, and other antianginal drugs**................**135**
2.6.1 Nitrates 135
2.6.2 Calcium-channel blockers 136
2.6.3 Other antianginal drugs 141
2.6.4 Peripheral vasodilators and related drugs...................................... 141

2.7 **Sympathomimetics** **142**
2.7.1 Inotropic sympathomimetics 142
2.7.2 Vasoconstrictor sympathomimetics 144
2.7.3 Cardiopulmonary resuscitation 146

2.8 **Anticoagulants and protamine** **147**
2.8.1 Parenteral anticoagulants 147
2.8.2 Oral anticoagulants.. 151
2.8.3 Protamine sulphate 153

2.9 **Antiplatelet drugs**...**154**

2.10 **Myocardial infarction and fibrinolysis**..**156**
2.10.1 Management of myocardial infarction 156
2.10.2 Fibrinolytic drugs 156

2.11 **Antifibrinolytic drugs and haemostatics** **158**

2.12 **Lipid-regulating drugs** **159**

2.13 **Local sclerosants**..**164**

2.14 **Drugs affecting the ductus arteriosus**..**164**

This chapter also includes advice on the drug management of the following:
> arrhythmias, p. 107
> heart failure, p. 100
> hypertension, p. 119
> pulmonary hypertension, p. 123

2.1 Positive inotropic drugs

2.1.1 Cardiac glycosides
2.1.2 Phosphodiesterase inhibitors

Positive inotropic drugs increase the force of contraction of the myocardium. Drugs which produce inotropic effects include cardiac glycosides, phosphodiesterase inhibitors, and some sympathomimetics (section 2.7.1).

2.1.1 Cardiac glycosides

The cardiac glycoside digoxin increases the force of myocardial contraction and reduces conductivity within the atrioventricular (AV) node.

Digoxin is most useful in the treatment of supraventricular tachycardias, especially for controlling ventricular response in persistent atrial fibrillation (section 2.3.1). Digoxin has a limited role in children with chronic heart failure; for reference to the role of digoxin in heart failure, see section 2.2.

For the management of atrial fibrillation, the maintenance dose of digoxin is determined on the basis of the ventricular rate at rest, which should not be allowed to fall below an acceptable level for the child.

Digoxin is now rarely used for rapid control of heart rate (see section 2.3.2), even with intravenous administration, response may take many hours; persistence of tachycardia is therefore not an indication for exceeding the recommended dose. The intramuscular route is **not** recommended.

Unwanted effects depend both on the concentration of digoxin in the plasma and on the sensitivity of the conducting system or of the myocardium, which is often increased in heart disease. It can sometimes be difficult to distinguish between toxic effects and clinical deterioration because the symptoms of both are similar. Also, the plasma-digoxin concentration alone cannot indicate toxicity reliably but the likelihood of toxicity increases progressively through the range 1.5 to 3 micrograms/litre for digoxin. Renal function is very important in determining digoxin dosage.

Hypokalaemia predisposes the child to digitalis toxicity and should be avoided; it is managed by giving a potassium-sparing diuretic or, if necessary, potassium supplements (or foods rich in potassium).

Toxicity can often be managed by discontinuing digoxin and correcting hypokalaemia if appropriate; serious manifestations require urgent specialist management. **Digoxin-specific antibody fragments** are available for reversal of life-threatening overdosage (see below).

▲ DIGOXIN

Cautions sick sinus syndrome; thyroid disease; hypoxia; severe respiratory disease; avoid hypokalaemia, hypomagnesaemia, hypercalcaemia, and hypoxia (risk of digitalis toxicity); monitor serum electrolytes and renal function; avoid rapid intravenous administration (risk of hypertension and reduced coronary flow); **interactions:** Appendix 1 (cardiac glycosides)

Renal impairment reduce dose; toxicity increased by electrolyte disturbances, adjust dose according to plasma-digoxin concentration

Pregnancy may need dosage adjustment

Breast-feeding amount too small to be harmful

Contra-indications intermittent complete heart block, second degree AV block; supraventricular arrhythmias associated with accessory conducting pathways e.g. Wolff-Parkinson-White syndrome (although can be used in infancy); ventricular tachycardia or fibrillation; hypertrophic cardiomyopathy (unless concomitant atrial fibrillation and heart failure—but with caution); myocarditis; constrictive pericarditis (unless to control atrial fibrillation or improve systolic dysfunction—but use with caution)

Side-effects see notes above; also nausea, vomiting, diarrhoea; arrhythmias, conduction disturbances; dizziness; blurred or yellow vision; rash,

◁ DIGOXIN (*continued*)

eosinophilia; *less commonly* depression; *very rarely* anorexia, intestinal ischaemia and necrosis, psychosis, apathy, confusion, headache, fatigue, weakness, gynaecomastia on long-term use, and thrombocytopenia

Pharmacokinetics For plasma-digoxin concentration assay, blood should ideally be taken at least 6 hours after a dose; plasma-digoxin concentration should be maintained in the range 0.8–2 micrograms/litre (see also notes above)

Licensed use heart failure, supraventricular arrhythmias

Indication and dose

Supraventricular arrhythmias and chronic heart failure (see also notes above) consult product literature for details

• **By mouth**

Neonate under 1.5 kg initially 25 micrograms/kg in 3 divided doses for 24 hours then 4–6 micrograms/kg daily in 1–2 divided doses

Neonate 1.5–2.5 kg initially 30 micrograms/kg in 3 divided doses for 24 hours then 4–6 micrograms/kg daily in 1–2 divided doses

Neonate over 2.5 kg initially 45 micrograms/kg in 3 divided doses for 24 hours then 10 micrograms/kg daily in 1–2 divided doses

Child 1 month–2 years initially 45 micrograms/kg in 3 divided doses for 24 hours then 10 micrograms/kg daily in 1–2 divided doses

Child 2–5 years initially 35 micrograms/kg in 3 divided doses for 24 hours then 10 micrograms/kg daily in 1–2 divided doses

Child 5–10 years initially 25 micrograms/kg (max. 750 micrograms) in 3 divided doses for 24 hours then 6 micrograms/kg daily (max. 250 micrograms daily) in 1–2 divided doses

Child 10–18 years initially 0.75–1.5 mg in 3 divided doses for 24 hours then 62.5–250 micrograms daily in 1–2 divided doses (higher doses may be necessary)

• **By intravenous infusion (but rarely necessary)**

Neonate under 1.5 kg initially 20 micrograms/kg in 3 divided doses for 24 hours then 4–6 micrograms/kg daily in 1–2 divided doses

Neonate 1.5–2.5 kg initially 30 micrograms/kg in 3 divided doses for 24 hours then 4–6 micrograms/kg daily in 1–2 divided doses

Neonate over 2.5 kg initially 35 micrograms/kg in 3 divided doses for 24 hours then 10 micrograms/kg daily in 1–2 divided doses

Child 1 month–2 years initially 35 micrograms/kg in 3 divided doses for 24 hours then 10 micrograms/kg daily in 1–2 divided doses

Child 2–5 years initially 35 micrograms/kg in 3 divided doses for 24 hours then 10 micrograms/kg daily in 1–2 divided doses

Child 5–10 years initially 25 micrograms/kg (max. 500 micrograms) in 3 divided doses for 24 hours then 6 micrograms/kg daily (max. 250 micrograms daily) in 1–2 divided doses

Child 10–18 years initially 0.5–1 mg in 3 divided doses for 24 hours then 62.5–250 micrograms daily in 1–2 divided doses (higher doses may be necessary)

Less urgent digitalisation

• **By mouth**

Rapid digitalisation may not always be required.

Child 10–18 years 250–500 micrograms daily (higher dose may be divided) for 5–7 days followed by maintenance dose

Note The above doses may need to be reduced if digoxin (or another cardiac glycoside) has been given in the preceding 2 weeks. When switching from intravenous to oral route may need to increase dose by 20–30% to maintain the same plasma digoxin concentration. Plasma monitoring may be required when changing formulation to take account of varying bioavailabilities. For plasma concentration monitoring, blood should ideally be taken at least 6 hours after a dose

Administration For *intravenous infusion*, dilute with sodium chloride 0.9% intravenous infusion *or* glucose 5% to a max. concentration of 62.5 micrograms/mL; loading doses should be given over 30–60 minutes and maintenance dose over 10–20 minutes. Protect from light.

For *oral* administration, oral solution must **not** be diluted

Digoxin (Non-proprietary) ⟨PoM⟩
Tablets, digoxin 62.5 micrograms, net price 28 = £1.66; 125 micrograms, 28 = £1.34; 250 micrograms, 28 = £1.37

Injection, digoxin 250 micrograms/mL, net price 2-mL amp = 70p
Excipients include alcohol, propylene glycol (see excipients)
Available from Antigen

Paediatric injection, digoxin 100 micrograms/mL
Available from 'special-order' manufacturers or specialist importing companies, see p. 943

Lanoxin® (GSK) ⟨PoM⟩
Tablets, digoxin 125 micrograms, net price 20 = 32p; 250 micrograms (scored), 20 = 32p

Injection, digoxin 250 micrograms/mL, net price 2-mL amp = 66p

Lanoxin-PG® (GSK) ⟨PoM⟩
Tablets, blue, digoxin 62.5 micrograms. Net price 20 = 32p

Elixir, yellow, digoxin 50 micrograms/mL. Do not dilute, measure with pipette. Net price 60 mL = £5.35. Counselling, use of pipette

Digoxin-specific antibody

Digoxin-specific antibody fragments are indicated for the treatment of known or strongly suspected digoxin or digitoxin overdosage, in situations where mea-

see p. 943

sures beyond the withdrawal of the cardiac glycoside and correction of any electrolyte abnormalities are felt to be necessary (see also notes above).

Digibind® (GSK) (PoM)
Injection, powder for preparation of infusion, digoxin-specific antibody fragments (F(ab)) 38 mg. Net price per vial = £93.97 (hosp. and poisons centres only)

Dose
Consult product literature or Poisons Information Centre

2.1.2 Phosphodiesterase inhibitors

Enoximone and **milrinone** are selective phosphodiesterase inhibitors which exert most of their effect on the myocardium. They possess positive inotropic and vasodilator activity and are useful in infants and children with low cardiac output especially after cardiac surgery. Phosphodiesterase inhibitors should be limited to short-term use because long-term oral administration has been associated with increased mortality in adults with congestive heart failure.

ENOXIMONE

Cautions heart failure associated with hypertrophic cardiomyopathy, stenotic or obstructive valvular disease or other outlet obstruction; monitor blood pressure, heart rate, ECG, central venous pressure, fluid and electrolyte status, renal function, platelet count, hepatic enzymes; avoid extravasation; **interactions**: Appendix 1 (phosphodiesterase inhibitors)

Hepatic impairment dose reduction may be required

Renal impairment consider dose reduction

Pregnancy manufacturer advises use only if potential benefit outweighs risk

Breast-feeding manufacturer advises caution—no information available

Side-effects ectopic beats; less frequently ventricular tachycardia or supraventricular arrhythmias (more likely in children with pre-existing arrhythmias); hypotension; also headache, insomnia, nausea and vomiting, diarrhoea; occasionally, chills, oliguria, fever, urinary retention; upper and lower limb pain

Licensed use not licensed for use in children

Indication and dose

Congestive heart failure, low cardiac output following cardiac surgery
• **By intravenous injection and continuous intravenous infusion**

Neonate initial loading dose of 500 micrograms/kg *by slow intravenous injection*, followed by 5–20 micrograms/kg/minute *by continuous intravenous infusion* over 24 hours adjusted according to response; max 24 mg/kg over 24 hours

Child 1 month–18 years initial loading dose of 500 micrograms/kg *by slow intravenous injection*, followed by 5–20 micrograms/kg/minute *by continuous intravenous infusion* over 24 hours adjusted according to response; max. 24 mg/kg over 24 hours

Administration for *intravenous* administration dilute to concentration of 2.5 mg/mL with sodium chloride 0.9% intravenous infusion *or* water for injections; the initial loading dose should be given by slow intravenous injection over at least 15 minutes. Use plastic apparatus—crystal formation if glass used

Perfan® (INCA-Pharm) (PoM)
Injection, enoximone 5 mg/mL. For dilution before use. Net price 20-mL amp = £15.02
Excipients include alcohol, propylene glycol

MILRINONE

Cautions see under Enoximone; also correct hypokalaemia; monitor renal function; **interactions**: Appendix 1 (phosphodiesterase inhibitors)

Renal impairment reduce dose and monitor response

Pregnancy manufacturer advises use only if potential benefit outweighs risk

Breast-feeding manufacturer advises caution—no information available

Side-effects ectopic beats, ventricular tachycardia, supraventricular arrhythmias (more likely in children with pre-existing arrhythmias), hypotension; headache; *less commonly* ventricular fibrillation, chest pain, tremor, hypokalaemia,

thrombocytopenia; *very rarely* bronchospasm, anaphylaxis, and rash

Licensed use not licensed for use in children under 18 years

Indication and dose

Congestive heart failure, low cardiac output following cardiac surgery, shock
• **By intravenous infusion**

Neonate initially 50–75 micrograms/kg over 30–60 minutes (reduce or omit initial dose if at risk of hypotension) then 30–45 micrograms/kg/hour by *continuous intravenous infusion* for 2–3 days (usually for 12 hours after cardiac surgery)

◁ **MILRINONE (continued)**

Child 1 month–18 years initially 50–75 micrograms/kg over 30–60 minutes (reduce or omit initial dose if at risk of hypotension) then 30–45 micrograms/kg/hour by *continuous intravenous infusion* for 2–3 days (usually for 12 hours after cardiac surgery)

Administration for *intravenous infusion* dilute with glucose 5% *or* sodium chloride 0.9% *or* sodium chloride and glucose intravenous infusion to a concentration of 200 micrograms/mL (higher concentrations of 400 micrograms/mL have been used); loading dose may be given undiluted if fluid-restricted

Primacor® (Sanofi-Aventis) ⒫ⓄⓂ
Injection, milrinone (as lactate) 1 mg/mL, net price 10-mL amp = £16.61

2.2 Diuretics

Diuretics are used for a variety of conditions in children including pulmonary oedema (caused by conditions such as respiratory distress syndrome and bronchopulmonary dysplasia), congestive heart failure, and hypertension. Hypertension in children is often resistant to therapy and may require the use of several drugs in combination (see section 2.5). Maintenance of fluid and electrolyte balance can be difficult in children on diuretics, particularly neonates whose renal function may be immature.

Loop diuretics (section 2.2.2) are used for pulmonary oedema, congestive heart failure, and in renal disease.

Thiazides (section 2.2.1) are used less commonly than loop diuretics but are often used in combination with loop diuretics or spironolactone in the management of pulmonary oedema and, in lower doses, for hypertension associated with cardiac disease.

Aminophylline infusion has been used with intravenous furosemide to relieve fluid overload in critically ill children.

Heart failure   Heart failure is less common in children than in adults; it can occur as a result of congenital heart disease (e.g. septal defects), dilated cardiomyopathy, myocarditis, or cardiac surgery. Drug treatment of heart failure due to left ventricular systolic dysfunction is covered below; optimal management of heart failure with preserved left ventricular function is not established.

Acute heart failure can occur after cardiac surgery or as a complication in severe acute infections with or without myocarditis. Therapy consists of volume loading, vasodilator or inotropic drugs.

Chronic heart failure is initially treated with a **loop diuretic** (section 2.2.2), usually furosemide supplemented with spironolactone, amiloride, or potassium.

If diuresis with furosemide is insufficient, the addition of metolazone or a thiazide diuretic (section 2.2.1) can be considered. With metolazone, the resulting diuresis can be profound and care is needed to avoid potentially dangerous electrolyte disturbance.

If diuretics are insufficient an ACE inhibitor, titrated to the maximum tolerated dose, can be used. **ACE inhibitors** (section 2.5.5.1) are used for the treatment of all grades of heart failure in adults and can also be useful for children with heart failure. Addition of digoxin can be considered in children who remain symptomatic despite treatment with a diuretic and an ACE inhibitor.

Some beta-blockers improve outcome in adults with heart failure, but data on beta-blockers in children are limited. **Carvedilol** (section 2.4) has vasodilatory properties and therefore (like ACE inhibitors) also lowers afterload.

In children receiving specialist cardiology care, the selective phosphodiesterase inhibitor **enoximone** is sometimes used by mouth for its inotropic and vasodilator effects. **Spironolactone** (section 2.2.3) is usually used as a potassium-sparing drug with a loop diuretic; in adults low doses of spironolactone are effective in the treatment of heart failure. Careful monitoring of serum potassium is necessary if spironolactone is used in combination with an ACE inhibitor.

Potassium loss   Hypokalaemia can occur with both thiazide and loop diuretics. The risk of hypokalaemia depends on the duration of action as well as the potency and is thus greater with thiazides than with an equipotent dose of a loop diuretic.

Hypokalaemia is particularly dangerous in children being treated with cardiac glycosides. In hepatic failure hypokalaemia caused by diuretics can precipitate encephalopathy.

The use of potassium-sparing diuretics (section 2.2.3) avoids the need to take potassium supplements.

2.2.1 Thiazides and related diuretics

Thiazides and related compounds are moderately potent diuretics; they inhibit sodium reabsorption at the beginning of the distal convoluted tubule. They are usually administered early in the day so that the diuresis does not interfere with sleep.

In the management of *hypertension* a low dose of a thiazide produces a maximal or near-maximal blood pressure lowering effect, with very little biochemical disturbance. Higher doses cause more marked changes in plasma potassium, sodium, uric acid, glucose, and lipids, with little advantage in blood pressure control. For reference to the use of thiazides in chronic heart failure see section 2.2.

Bendroflumethiazide is licensed for use in children; **chlorothiazide** is also used.

Chlortalidone (chlorthalidone), a thiazide-related compound, has a longer duration of action than the thiazides and may be given on alternate days in younger children.

Metolazone is particularly effective when combined with a loop diuretic (even in renal failure) and is most effective when given 30–60 minutes before furosemide; profound diuresis can occur and the child should therefore be monitored carefully.

Cautions See also section 2.2. Thiazides and related diuretics can exacerbate diabetes, gout, and systemic lupus erythematosus. Electrolytes should be monitored particularly with high doses, long-term use, or in renal impairment. Thiazides and related diuretics should also be used with caution in nephrotic syndrome, hyperaldosteronism, malnourishment, hepatic impairment (avoid if severe), renal impairment, pregnancy, and breast-feeding; **interactions:** Appendix 1 (diuretics).

Contra-indications Thiazides and related diuretics should be avoided in refractory hypokalaemia, hyponatraemia, and hypercalcaemia, symptomatic hyperuricaemia, and Addison's disease.

Side-effects Side-effects of thiazides and related diuretics include mild gastrointestinal disturbances, postural hypotension, altered plasma-lipid concentrations, metabolic and electrolyte disturbances including hypokalaemia (see also notes above), hyponatraemia, hypomagnesaemia, hypercalcaemia, hyperglycaemia, hypochloraemic alkalosis, and hyperuricaemia, and gout. Less common side-effects include blood disorders including agranulocytosis, leucopenia and thrombocytopenia, and impotence. Pancreatitis, intrahepatic cholestasis, cardiac arrhythmias, headache, dizziness, paraesthesia, visual disturbances, and hypersensitivity reactions (including pneumonitis, pulmonary oedema, photosensitivity, and severe skin reactions) have also been reported.

BENDROFLUMETHIAZIDE
(Bendrofluazide)

Cautions see notes above

Hepatic impairment use with caution in mild to moderate impairment; avoid in severe impairment; hypokalaemia may precipitate coma (potassium-sparing diuretics can prevent)

Renal impairment use with caution; avoid if estimated glomerular filtration rate less than 30 mL/minute/1.73 m^2—ineffective

Pregnancy not used to treat gestational hypertension; may cause neonatal thrombocytopenia, bone marrow suppression, jaundice, electrolyte disturbances, and hypoglycaemia; placental perfusion may be reduced; stimulation of labour, uterine inertia, and meconium staining also reported

Breast-feeding amount too small to be harmful; large doses may suppress lactation

Contra-indications see notes above

Side-effects see notes above

Indication and dose

Oedema and hypertension
- By mouth

  Child 1 month–2 years 50–100 micrograms/kg daily adjusted according to response

  Child 2–12 years initially 50–400 micrograms/kg daily (max. 10 mg daily) then 50–100 micrograms/kg daily adjusted according to response

  Child 12–18 years initially 5–10 mg daily or on alternate days (2.5 mg in hypertension) as a single morning dose, adjusted according to response

2

Cardiovascular system

◁ **BENDROFLUMETHIAZIDE** (*continued*)

Bendroflumethiazide (Non-proprietary) PoM
Tablets, bendroflumethiazide 2.5 mg, net price 28 = 83p; 5 mg, 28 = 86p
Brands include *Aprinox®*, *Neo-NaClex®*

◀Extemporaneous formulations available see Extemporaneous Preparations, p. 8

◢ CHLOROTHIAZIDE

Cautions see notes above; also neonate (theoretical risk of kernicterus if very jaundiced)

Hepatic impairment use with caution in mild to moderate impairment; avoid in severe impairment; hypokalaemia may precipitate coma (potassium-sparing diuretics can prevent)

Renal impairment use with caution; avoid if estimated glomerular filtration rate less than 30 mL/minute/1.73m²—ineffective

Pregnancy not used to treat gestational hypertension; may cause neonatal thrombocytopenia, bone marrow suppression, jaundice, electrolyte disturbances, and hypoglycaemia; placental perfusion may be reduced; stimulation of labour, uterine inertia, and meconium staining also reported

Breast-feeding amount too small to be harmful; large doses may suppress lactation

Contra-indications see notes above

Side-effects see notes above

Licensed use not licensed

Indication and dose

Heart failure, hypertension, ascites
• By mouth

Neonate 10–20 mg/kg twice daily

Child 1–6 months 10–20 mg/kg twice daily

Child 6 months–12 years 10 mg/kg twice daily (max. 1 g daily)

Child 12–18 years 0.25–1 g once daily or 125–500 mg twice daily

Chronic hypoglycaemia section 6.1.4

Diabetes insipidus section 6.5.2

◀Preparations
Chlorothiazide oral suspension 250 mg/5 mL is available from 'special-order' manufacturers or specialist importing companies, see p. 943

◢ CHLORTALIDONE

(Chlorthalidone)

Cautions see notes above

Hepatic impairment use with caution in mild to moderate impairment; avoid in severe impairment; hypokalaemia may precipitate coma (potassium-sparing diuretics can prevent)

Renal impairment avoid if estimated glomerular filtration rate less than 30 mL/minute/1.73 m²—ineffective

Pregnancy not used to treat gestational hypertension; may cause neonatal thrombocytopenia, bone marrow suppression, jaundice, electrolyte disturbances, and hypoglycaemia; placental perfusion may be reduced; stimulation of labour, uterine inertia, and meconium staining also reported

Breast-feeding amount too small to be harmful; large doses may suppress lactation

Contra-indications see notes above

Side-effects see notes above; also *rarely* jaundice

Indication and dose

Hypertension
• By mouth

Child 5–12 years 0.5–1 mg/kg in the morning every 48 hours; max. 1.7 mg/kg every 48 hours

Child 12–18 years 25 mg daily in the morning, increased to 50 mg daily if necessary (but see notes above)

Stable heart failure
• By mouth

Child 5–12 years 0.5–1 mg/kg in the morning every 48 hours; max. 1.7 mg/kg every 48 hours

Child 12–18 years 25–50 mg daily in the morning, increased if necessary to 100–200 mg daily (reduce to lowest effective dose for maintenance)

Ascites, oedema in nephrotic syndrome
• By mouth

Child 5–12 years 0.5–1 mg/kg in the morning every 48 hours; max. 1.7 mg/kg every 48 hours

Child 12–18 years up to 50 mg daily

Hygroton® (Alliance) PoM
Tablets, yellow, scored, chlortalidone 50 mg, net price 28-tab pack = £1.64

◢ METOLAZONE

Cautions see notes above; also acute porphyria (section 9.8.2)

Hepatic impairment use with caution in mild to moderate impairment; avoid in severe impairment; hypokalaemia may precipitate coma (potassium-sparing diuretics can prevent)

Renal impairment remains effective in moderate impairment but risk of excessive diuresis

Pregnancy not used to treat gestational hypertension; may cause neonatal thrombocytopenia, bone marrow suppression, jaundice, electrolyte disturbances, and hypoglycaemia; placental perfu-

2 Cardiovascular system

◻ **METOLAZONE** (*continued*)

sion may be reduced; stimulation of labour, uterine inertia, and meconium staining also reported

Breast-feeding amount too small to be harmful; large doses may suppress lactation

Contra-indications see notes above

Side-effects see notes above; also chills, chest pain

Licensed use not licensed for use in children

Indication and dose

> Oedema resistant to loop diuretics; adjunct to loop diuretics to induce diuresis
> • **By mouth**
>> **Child 1 month–12 years** 100–200 micrograms/kg once or twice daily

> **Child 12–18 years** 5–10 mg once daily in the morning, increased to 5–10 mg twice daily in resistant oedema

Administration Tablets may be crushed and mixed with water immediately before use

Metenix 5® (Sanofi-Aventis) [PoM]
Tablets, blue, metolazone 5 mg, net price 100-tab pack = £18.94

◢Extemporaneous formulations available see Extemporaneous Preparations, p. 8

2.2.2 Loop diuretics

Loop diuretics inhibit reabsorption of sodium, potassium, and chloride from the ascending limb of the loop of Henlé in the renal tubule and are powerful diuretics. Hypokalaemia may develop, and care is needed to avoid hypotension.

Furosemide (frusemide) and **bumetanide** are similar in activity; they produce dose-related diuresis. In children with impaired renal function very large doses may occasionally be needed; in such doses both drugs can cause deafness and bumetanide can cause myalgia. Furosemide is used extensively in children. It can be used for pulmonary oedema (e.g. in respiratory distress syndrome and bronchopulmonary dysplasia), congestive heart failure, and in renal disease. Furosemide may occasionally cause ototoxicity but the risk can be reduced by giving large oral doses in 2 or more divided doses. Long-term use of furosemide in neonates can lead to nephrocalcinosis because it increases urinary calcium excretion; a thiazide diuretic may be an alternative in this case.

◢ **FUROSEMIDE**

(Frusemide)

Cautions see section 2.2; also monitor electrolytes; hypotension; correct hypovolaemia before using in oliguria; comatose and precomatose states associated with liver cirrhosis; impaired micturition; gout; hepatorenal syndrome; some liquid preparations contain alcohol, caution especially in neonates; **interactions:** Appendix 1 (diuretics)

Hepatic impairment hypokalaemia may precipitate coma (use potassium-sparing diuretic to prevent this)

Renal impairment may need high doses; deafness and tinnitus may follow rapid intravenous injection

Pregnancy not to be used to treat hypertension in pregnancy

Breast-feeding amount too small to be harmful; may inhibit lactation

Contra-indications hypovolaemia, dehydration, severe hypokalaemia, severe hyponatraemia; renal failure due to nephrotoxic or hepatotoxic drugs, anuria

Side-effects mild gastro-intestinal disturbances; hypotension; hyperglycaemia (less common than with thiazides), hyperuricaemia and gout; electrolyte disturbances including hyponatraemia, hypokalaemia (see also section 2.2), increased calcium excretion (nephrocalcinosis and nephrolithiasis reported in preterm infants), and hypomagnesaemia, metabolic alkalosis; *rarely* paraesthesia, blood disorders (including thrombocytopenia, leucopenia, agranulocytosis, aplastic anaemia, haemolytic anaemia), bone marrow depression (withdraw treatment), tinnitus and deafness (usually with large parenteral doses and rapid administration, in renal impairment, or in hypoproteinaemia), and hypersensitivity reactions (including rashes, photosensitivity, eosinophilia, exfoliative dermatitis, purpura, and anaphylaxis), pancreatitis, intrahepatic cholestasis

Indication and dose

> Oedema
> • **By mouth**
>> **Neonate** 0.5–2 mg/kg every 12–24 hours (every 24 hours if postmenstrual age under 31 weeks)

>> **Child 1 month–12 years** 0.5–2 mg/kg 2–3 times daily (every 24 hours if postmenstrual age under 31 weeks); higher doses may be required in resistant oedema; max. 12 mg/kg daily, not to exceed 80 mg daily

>> **Child 12–18 years** 20–40 mg daily, increased in resistant oedema to 80–120 mg daily

> • **By slow intravenous injection**
>> **Neonate** 0.5–1 mg/kg every 12–24 hours (every 24 hours if post-menstrual age under 31 weeks)

>> **Child 1 month–12 years** 0.5–1 mg/kg (max. 4 mg/kg) repeated every 8 hours as necessary

2 Cardiovascular system

◁ **FUROSEMIDE** *(continued)*

Child 12–18 years 20–40 mg repeated every 8 hours as necessary; higher doses may be required in resistant cases

● **By continuous intravenous infusion**

Child 1 month–18 years 0.1–2 mg/kg/hour (following cardiac surgery, initially 100 micrograms/kg/hour, doubled every 2 hours until urine output exceeds 1 mL/kg/hour)

Oliguria
● **By mouth**

Child 12–18 years initially 250 mg daily; if necessary, dose increased in steps of 250 mg given every 4–6 hours; max. single dose 2 g (rarely used)

● **By intravenous infusion**

Child 1 month–12 years 2–5 mg/kg up to 4 times daily (max. 1 g daily)

Child 12–18 years initially 250 mg over 1 hour (rate not exceeding 4 mg/minute), increase to 500 mg over 2 hours if satisfactory urine output not obtained, then give a further 1 g over 4 hours if no satisfactory response within subsequent hour, if no response obtained dialysis probably required; effective dose (up to 1 g) can be repeated every 24 hours

Administration For administration *by mouth* tablets may be crushed and mixed with water *or* injection solution diluted and given by mouth; for *intravenous injection* give over 5–10 minutes at a usual rate of 100 micrograms/kg/minute (not exceeding 500 micrograms/kg/minute), max. 4 mg/minute; for *intravenous infusion* dilute with sodium chloride 0.9% intravenous infusion to a concentration of 1–2 mg/mL—glucose solutions unsuitable (infusion pH must be above 5.5)

Furosemide (Non-proprietary) ᴾᵒᴹ
Tablets, furosemide 20 mg, net price 28 = 81p; 40 mg, 28-tab pack = 86p; 500 mg, 28 = £4.37
Brands include *Froop®*, *Rusyde®*

Oral solution, sugar-free, furosemide, net price 20 mg/5 mL, 150 mL = £12.68; 40 mg/5 mL, 150 mL = £16.31; 50 mg/5 mL, 150 mL = £17.68
Brands include *Frusol®* (contains alcohol 10%)

Injection, furosemide 10 mg/mL, net price 2-mL amp = 55p; 5-mL amp = 66p; 25-mL amp = £2.50

Lasix® (Sanofi-Aventis) ᴾᵒᴹ
Injection, furosemide 10 mg/mL, net price 2-mL amp = 78p

Note Large-volume furosemide injections also available; brands include *Minijet®*

▌ **BUMETANIDE**

Cautions see under Furosemide
Hepatic impairment hypokalaemia may precipitate coma (use potassium-sparing diuretic to prevent this)
Renal impairment may need high doses
Pregnancy not to be used for treating hypertension in pregnancy
Breast-feeding manufacturer advises avoid if possible—no information available
Contra-indications see under Furosemide
Side-effects see under Furosemide; also headache, dizziness, fatigue, gynaecomastia, myalgia
Licensed use not licensed for use in children under 12 years

Indication and dose
Oedema
● **By mouth**

Child 1 month–12 years 15–50 micrograms/kg 1–4 times daily (max. single dose 2 mg); do not exceed 5 mg daily

Child 12–18 years 1 mg in the morning, repeated after 6–8 hours if necessary; severe cases up to 5 mg daily

● **By intravenous injection**

Child 12–18 years 1–2 mg, repeated after 20 minutes if necessary

● **By intravenous infusion over 30–60 minutes**

Child 1 month–12 years 25–50 micrograms/kg
Child 12–18 years 1–5 mg

Administration For *intravenous infusion*, dilute with glucose 5% intravenous infusion *or* sodium chloride 0.9% intravenous infusion to a concentration of 24 micrograms/mL

Bumetanide (Non-proprietary) ᴾᵒᴹ
Tablets, bumetanide 1 mg, net price 28-tab pack = £1.22; 5 mg, 28-tab pack = £2.53

Oral liquid, bumetanide 1 mg/5 mL, net price 150 mL = £128.00

Injection, bumetanide 500 micrograms/mL, net price 4-mL amp = £1.79

Burinex® (LEO) ᴾᵒᴹ
Tablets, scored, bumetanide 1 mg, net price 28-tab pack = £1.52; 5 mg, 28-tab pack = £9.67

◢Extemporaneous formulations available see Extemporaneous Preparations, p. 8

2.2.3 **Potassium-sparing diuretics and aldosterone antagonists**

Spironolactone is the most commonly used potassium-sparing diuretic in children; it is an aldosterone antagonist and enhances potassium retention and sodium excretion in the distal tubule. Spironolactone is combined with other diuretics to reduce urinary potassium loss. It is also used in the long-term management of Bartter's syndrome and high doses can help to control ascites

(vertical left margin) **2** Cardiovascular system

in babies with chronic neonatal hepatitis. The clinical value of spironolactone in the management of pulmonary oedema in preterm neonates with chronic lung disease is uncertain.

Potassium canrenoate, given intravenously, is an alternative aldosterone antagonist that may be useful if a potassium-sparing diuretic is required and the child is unable to take oral medication. It is metabolised to canrenone, which is also a metabolite of spironolactone.

Amiloride on its own is a weak diuretic. It causes retention of potassium and is therefore given with thiazide or loop diuretics as an alternative to giving potassium supplements (see section 2.2.4 for compound preparations with thiazides or loop diuretics).

A potassium-sparing diuretic such as spironolactone or amiloride may also be used in the management of amphotericin-induced hypokalaemia.

Potassium supplements must **not** be given with potassium-sparing diuretics. Administration of a potassium-sparing diuretic to a child receiving an ACE inhibitor or an angiotensin-II receptor antagonist (section 2.5.5) can also cause severe hyperkalaemia.

◢ AMILORIDE HYDROCHLORIDE

Cautions monitor electrolytes; diabetes mellitus; **interactions:** Appendix 1 (diuretics)

Renal impairment monitor plasma-potassium concentration (high risk of hyperkalaemia in renal impairment); manufacturers advise avoid in severe impairment

Pregnancy not to be used for treating hypertension in pregnancy

Breast-feeding manufacturer advises avoid—no information available

Contra-indications hyperkalaemia; anuria; Addison's disease

Side-effects include gastro-intestinal disturbances, dry mouth, rashes, confusion, postural hypotension, hyperkalaemia, hyponatraemia

Licensed use Not licensed for use in children

Indication and dose

> Adjunct to thiazide or loop diuretics in oedema or congestive heart failure (where potassium conservation desirable)
> • By mouth
>
> > Neonate 100–200 micrograms/kg twice daily

> Child 1 month–12 years 100–200 micrograms/kg twice daily; max. 20 mg daily
>
> Child 12–18 years 5–10 mg twice daily

Amiloride (Non-proprietary) PoM
Tablets, amiloride hydrochloride 5 mg, net price 28-tab pack = £1.03p

Oral solution, sugar-free, amiloride hydrochloride 5 mg/5 mL, net price 150 mL = £39.73
Brands include *Amilamont®* (*excipients include* propylene glycol, see Excipients p. 3)

◢ Compound preparations with thiazide or loop diuretics
See section 2.2.4

◢ Aldosterone antagonists

◢ SPIRONOLACTONE

Cautions potential metabolic products carcinogenic in *rodents*; monitor electrolytes (discontinue if hyperkalaemia); acute porphyria (section 9.8.2); **interactions:** Appendix 1 (diuretics)

Renal impairment monitor plasma-potassium concentration; high risk of hyperkalaemia in renal impairment; manufacturer advises avoid if rapidly deteriorating or severe impairment

Pregnancy feminisation of male fetus in *animal* studies

Breast-feeding metabolites present in milk but unlikely to be harmful; manufacturer advises avoid

Contra-indications hyperkalaemia, hyponatraemia; Addison's disease

Side-effects gastro-intestinal disturbances; impotence, gynaecomastia; menstrual irregularities; lethargy, headache, confusion; rashes; hyperkalaemia (discontinue); hyponatraemia; hepatotoxicity, osteomalacia, and blood disorders reported

Licensed use Not licensed for reduction of hypokalaemia induced by diuretics or amphotericin

Indication and dose

> Diuresis in congestive heart failure, ascites and oedema, reduction of hypokalaemia induced by diuretics or amphotericin
> • By mouth
>
> > Neonate 1–2 mg/kg daily in 1–2 divided doses; up to 7 mg/kg daily in resistant ascites

2
Cardiovascular system

◁ **SPIRONOLACTONE** (*continued*)

> **Child 1 month–12 years** 1–3 mg/kg daily in 1–2 divided doses; up to 9 mg/kg daily in resistant ascites
>
> **Child 12–18 years** 50–100 mg daily in 1–2 divided doses; up to 9 mg/kg daily (max. 400 mg daily) in resistant ascites

Spironolactone (Non-proprietary) [PoM]
Tablets, spironolactone 25 mg, net price 28 = £1.76; 50 mg, 28 = £2.53; 100 mg, 28 = £3.55. Label: 21

Oral suspensions, spironolactone 5 mg/5 mL, 10 mg/5 mL, 25 mg/5 mL, 50 mg/5 mL, and 100 mg/5 mL
Available from 'special-order' manufacturers or specialist importing companies, see p. 943

Aldactone® (Pharmacia) [PoM]
Tablets, f/c, spironolactone 25 mg (buff), net price 100-tab pack = £8.89; 50 mg (off-white), 100-tab pack = £17.78; 100 mg (buff), 28-tab pack = £9.96. Label: 21

■ POTASSIUM CANRENOATE

Cautions potential metabolic products carcinogenic in *rodents*; monitor electrolytes (discontinue if hyperkalaemia); hypotension; acute porphyria (section 9.8.2); **interactions**: Appendix 1 (diuretics)

Renal impairment use with caution and monitor plasma-potassium concentration if estimated glomerular filtration rate 30–60 mL/minute/1.73 m²; avoid if estimated glomerular filtration rate less than 30 mL/minute/1.73 m²

Contra-indications hyperkalaemia; hyponatraemia

Pregnancy crosses placenta; feminisation and undescended testes in male fetus in *animal* studies—manufacturer advises avoid

Breast-feeding present in breast milk—manufacturer advises avoid

Side-effects drowsiness, headache, ataxia; menstrual irregularities; hyperuricaemia; pain at injection site on rapid administration; *less commonly* thrombocytopenia, eosinophilia, and hyperkalaemia; *rarely* hepatotoxicity, agranulocytosis, osteomalacia, hoarseness and deepening of voice, hypersensitivity reactions (including urticaria and erythema), and alopecia; also gas-

tro-intestinal disturbances, hypotension, transient confusion with high doses, hyponatraemia, hypochloraemic acidosis, mastalgia, gynaecomastia, and hirsutism

Licensed use not licensed for use in the UK

Indication and dose

> Short-term diuresis in congestive heart failure, oedema, and ascites
>
> • **By intravenous injection over at least 3 minutes or intravenous infusion**
>
> **Neonate** 1–2 mg/kg twice daily
>
> **Child 1 month–12 years** 1–2 mg/kg twice daily
>
> **Child 12–18 years** 1–2 mg/kg (max. 200 mg) twice daily

Note To convert to equivalent oral spironolactone dose, multiply potassium canrenoate dose by 0.7

Administration consult product literature

◢ **Preparations**

Potassium canrenoate injection is available from 'special-order' manufacturers or specialist importing companies, see p. 943

2.2.4 Potassium-sparing diuretics with other diuretics

Although it is preferable to prescribe diuretics separately in children, the use of fixed combinations may be justified in older children if compliance is a problem. The most commonly used preparations are listed below (but they may not be licensed for use in children—consult product literature), for other preparations see the BNF. For **interactions**, see Appendix 1 (diuretics).

◢ **Amiloride with thiazides**

Co-amilozide (Non-proprietary) [PoM]
Tablets, co-amilozide 2.5/25 (amiloride hydrochloride 2.5 mg, hydrochlorothiazide 25 mg), net price 28-tab pack = £2.57
Brands include *Moduret 25*®

◢ **Amiloride with loop diuretics**

Co-amilofruse (Non-proprietary) [PoM]
Tablets, co-amilofruse 2.5/20 (amiloride hydrochloride 2.5 mg, furosemide 20 mg). Net price 28-tab pack = £1.19, 56-tab pack = £1.63
Brands include *Frumil LS*®

Tablets, co-amilofruse 5/40 (amiloride hydrochloride 5 mg, furosemide 40 mg). Net price 28-tab pack = £1.24, 56-tab pack = £1.61
Brands include *Frumil*®

Tablets, co-amilofruse 10/80 (amiloride hydrochloride 10 mg, furosemide 80 mg), net price 28-tab pack = £9.33

2.2.5 Osmotic diuretics

Mannitol is used to treat cerebral oedema, raised intra-ocular pressure, peripheral oedema, and ascites.

MANNITOL

Cautions extravasation causes inflammation and thrombophlebitis; monitor fluid and electrolyte balance, serum osmolality, and pulmonary and renal function; assess cardiac function before and during treatment; **interactions:** Appendix 1 (mannitol)

Renal impairment caution in severe impairment

Pregnancy manufacturer advises avoid unless essential—no information available

Breast-feeding manufacturer advises avoid unless essential—no information available

Contra-indications severe heart failure; severe pulmonary oedema; intracranial bleeding (except during craniotomy); anuria; severe dehydration

Side-effects *less commonly* hypotension, thrombophlebitis, fluid and electrolyte imbalance; *rarely* dry mouth, thirst, nausea, vomiting, oedema, raised intracranial pressure, arrhythmia, hypertension, pulmonary oedema, chest pain, headache, convulsions, dizziness, chills, fever, urinary retention, focal osmotic nephrosis, dehydration, cramp, blurred vision, rhinitis, skin necrosis, and hypersensitivity reactions (including urticaria and anaphylaxis); *very rarely* congestive heart failure and acute renal failure

Licensed use not licensed for use in children under 12 years

Indication and dose

Cerebral oedema, raised intra-ocular pressure
- **By intravenous infusion over 30–60 minutes**
  Child 1 month–12 years 0.25–1.5 g/kg repeated if necessary 1–2 times after 4–8 hours
  Child 12–18 years 0.25–2 g/kg repeated if necessary 1–2 times after 4–8 hours

Peripheral oedema and ascites
- **By intravenous infusion over 2–6 hours**
  Child 1 month–18 years 1–2 g/kg

Administration examine infusion for crystals; if crystals present, dissolve by warming infusion fluid (allow to cool to body temperature before administration); for mannitol 20%, an in-line filter is recommended (15-micron filters have been used)

Mannitol (Baxter) [PoM]
Intravenous infusion, mannitol 10%, net price 500-mL *Viaflex*® bag = £1.87, 500-mL *Viaflo*® bag = £2.15; 20%, 250-mL *Viaflex*® bag = £2.70, 250-mL *Viaflo*® bag = £3.10, 500-mL *Viaflex*® bag = £2.72, 500-mL *Viaflo*® bag = £3.12

2.2.6 Mercurial diuretics

Classification not used in *BNF for Children*.

2.2.7 Carbonic anhydrase inhibitors

The carbonic anhydrase inhibitor **acetazolamide** is a weak diuretic although it is little used for its diuretic effect. Acetazolamide and eye drops of dorzolamide and brinzolamide inhibit the formation of aqueous humour and are used in glaucoma (section 11.6). In children, acetazolamide is also used in the treatment of epilepsy (section 4.8.1), and raised intracranial pressure (section 11.6).

2.2.8 Diuretics with potassium

Diuretics and potassium supplements should be prescribed separately for children.

2.3 Anti-arrhythmic drugs

2.3.1 Management of arrhythmias
2.3.2 Drugs for arrhythmias

2.3.1 Management of arrhythmias

Management of an arrhythmia requires precise diagnosis of the type of arrhythmia; electrocardiography and referral to a paediatric cardiologist is essential; underlying causes such as heart failure require appropriate treatment.

2 Cardiovascular system

Arrhythmias may be broadly divided into bradycardias, supraventricular tachycardias, and ventricular arrhythmias.

Bradycardia   Adrenaline (epinephrine) is useful in the treatment of symptomatic bradycardia in an infant or child.

Supraventricular tachycardias

In supraventricular tachycardia adenosine is given by rapid intravenous injection. If adenosine is ineffective, intravenous amiodarone, flecainide, or a beta-blocker (such as esmolol, see section 2.4) can be tried; verapamil can also be considered in children over 1 year. Atenolol, sotalol (section 2.4), and flecainide are used for the prophylaxis of paroxysmal supraventricular tachycardias.

The use of d.c. shock and vagal stimulation also have a role in the treatment of supraventricular tachycardia.

Syndromes associated with accessory conducting pathways   Amiodarone, flecainide, or a beta-blocker is used to prevent recurrence of supraventricular tachycardia in infants and young children with these syndromes (e.g. Wolff-Parkinson-White syndrome).

Atrial flutter   In atrial flutter without structural heart defects, sinus rhythm is restored with d.c. shock or cardiac pacing; drug treatment is usually not necessary. Amiodarone is used in atrial flutter when structural heart defects are present or after heart surgery. Sotalol (section 2.4) may also be considered.

Atrial fibrillation   Atrial fibrillation is very rare in children. To restore sinus rhythm d.c. shock is used; beta-blockers, alone or together with digoxin, may be useful for ventricular rate control.

Ectopic tachycardia   Intravenous amiodarone is used in conjunction with body cooling and synchronised pacing in *postoperative* junctional ectopic tachycardia. Oral amiodarone or flecainide are used in *congenital* junctional ectopic tachycardia.

Amiodarone, flecainide, or a beta-blocker are used in atrial ectopic tachycardia; amiodarone is preferred in those with poor ventricular function.

Ventricular tachycardia and ventricular fibrillation

Pulseless ventricular tachycardia or ventricular fibrillation require resuscitation, see Paediatric Advanced Life Support algorithm (inside back cover). Amiodarone is used in resuscitation for pulseless ventricular tachycardia or ventricular fibrillation unresponsive to d.c. shock; lidocaine can be used as an alternative only if amiodarone is not available.

Amiodarone is also used in a haemodynamically stable child where drug treatment is required; lidocaine can be used as an alternative only if amiodarone is not available.

Torsade de pointes   Torsade de pointes is a form of ventricular tachycardia associated with long QT syndrome, which may be congenital or drug induced. Episodes may be self-limiting, but are frequently recurrent and can cause impairment or loss of consciousness. If not controlled, the arrhythmia can progress to ventricular fibrillation and sometimes death. Intravenous magnesium sulphate (section 9.5.1.3) can be used to treat torsade de pointes (dose recommendations vary—consult local guidelines). Anti-arrhythmics can further prolong the QT interval, thus worsening the condition.

2.3.2 Drugs for arrhythmias

Anti-arrhythmic drugs can be classified clinically as those acting on supraventricular arrhythmias (adenosine, digoxin, and verapamil), those acting on both supraventricular and ventricular arrhythmias (amiodarone, beta-blockers, flecainide and procainamide), and those acting on ventricular arrhythmias (lidocaine (lignocaine)). For the treatment of bradycardia, see section 2.3.1.

2 Cardiovascular system

Anti-arrhythmic drugs can also be classified according to their effects on the electrical behaviour of myocardial cells during activity (the Vaughan Williams classification) although this classification is of less clinical significance:

Class I: membrane stabilising drugs (e.g. lidocaine, flecainide)

Class II: beta-blockers

Class III: amiodarone and sotalol (also Class II)

Class IV: calcium-channel blockers (includes verapamil but not dihydropyridines)

Cautions   The negative inotropic effects of anti-arrhythmic drugs tend to be additive. Therefore special care should be taken if two or more are used, especially if myocardial function is impaired. Most or all drugs that are effective in countering arrhythmias can also provoke them in some circumstances; moreover, hypokalaemia enhances the arrhythmogenic (pro-arrhythmic) effect of many drugs.

Adenosine is the treatment of choice for terminating supraventricular tachycardias, including those associated with accessory conducting pathways (e.g. Wolff-Parkinson-White syndrome). It is also used in the diagnosis of supraventricular arrhythmias. It is not negatively inotropic and does not cause significant hypotension; it can be used safely in children with impaired cardiac function or postoperative arrhythmias. The injection should be administered by rapid intravenous injection into a central or large peripheral vein.

Amiodarone is useful in the management of both supraventricular and ventricular tachyarrhythmias. It may be given by intravenous infusion and by mouth and causes little or no myocardial depression. Unlike oral amiodarone, intravenous amiodarone acts relatively rapidly. Intravenous amiodarone is also used in cardiopulmonary resuscitation for ventricular fibrillation or pulseless ventricular tachycardia unresponsive to d.c. shock (see algorithm, inside back cover).

Amiodarone has a very long half-life (extending to several weeks) and only needs to be given once daily (but high doses may cause nausea unless divided). Many weeks or months may be required to achieve steady-state plasma-amiodarone concentration; this is particularly important when drug interactions are likely (see also Appendix 1).

Most patients taking amiodarone develop corneal microdeposits (reversible on withdrawal of treatment); these rarely interfere with vision, but drivers may be dazzled by headlights at night. However, if vision is impaired or if optic neuritis or optic neuropathy occur, amiodarone must be stopped to prevent blindness and expert advice sought. Because of the possibility of phototoxic reactions, children and carers should be advised to shield the child's skin from light during treatment and for several months after discontinuing amiodarone; a wide-spectrum sunscreen (section 13.8.1) should be used to protect against both long-wave ultraviolet and visible light.

Amiodarone contains iodine and can cause disorders of thyroid function; both hypothyroidism and hyperthyroidism can occur. Clinical assessment alone is unreliable, and laboratory tests should be performed before treatment and every 6 months. Thyroxine (T4) may be raised in the absence of hyperthyroidism; therefore tri-iodothyronine (T3), T4, and thyroid-stimulating hormone (thyrotrophin, TSH) should all be measured. A raised T3 and T4 with a very low or undetectable TSH concentration suggests the development of thyrotoxicosis. The thyrotoxicosis may be very refractory, and amiodarone should usually be withdrawn at least temporarily to help achieve control; treatment with carbimazole may be required. Hypothyroidism can be treated with replacement therapy without withdrawing amiodarone if it is essential; careful supervision is required.

Pneumonitis should always be suspected if new or progressive shortness of breath or cough develops in a patient taking amiodarone. Fresh neurological symptoms should raise the possibility of peripheral neuropathy. Amiodarone is also associated with hepatotoxicity (see under amiodarone, below).

Beta-blockers act as anti-arrhythmic drugs principally by attenuating the effects of the sympathetic system on automaticity and conductivity within the heart, for details see section 2.4. For special reference to the role of **sotalol** in ventricular arrhythmias, see section 2.4.

2

Cardiovascular system

Oral administration of **digoxin** (section 2.1.1) slows the ventricular rate in atrial fibrillation and in atrial flutter. However, intravenous infusion of digoxin is rarely effective for rapid control of ventricular rate.

Flecainide is useful for the treatment of resistant re-entry supraventricular tachycardia, ventricular tachycardia, ventricular ectopic beats, arrhythmias associated with accessory conducting pathways (e.g. Wolff-Parkinson-White syndrome), and paroxysmal atrial fibrillation. Flecainide crosses the placenta and can be used to control fetal supraventricular arrhythmias.

Lidocaine (lignocaine) can be used in cardiopulmonary resuscitation in children with ventricular fibrillation or pulseless ventricular tachycardia unresponsive to d.c. shock, but only if amiodarone is not available. Doses may need to be reduced in children with persistently poor cardiac output and hepatic or renal failure (see under lidocaine, below).

Verapamil (section 2.6.2) can cause severe haemodynamic compromise (refractory hypotension and cardiac arrest) when used for the acute treatment of arrhythmias in neonates and infants; it is contra-indicated in children under 1 year. It is also contra-indicated in those with congestive heart failure, syndromes associated with accessory conducting pathways (e.g. Wolff-Parkinson-White syndrome) and in most receiving concomitant beta-blockers. It can be useful in older children with supraventricular tachycardia.

ADENOSINE

Cautions atrial fibrillation or flutter with accessory pathway (conduction down anomalous pathway may increase); asthma; ECG monitoring should be carried out and resuscitation facilities should be available during administration; **interactions**: Appendix 1 (adenosine)

Pregnancy no evidence of harm

Breast-feeding no information available—unlikely to be present in milk owing to short half-life

Contra-indications second- or third-degree AV block and sick sinus syndrome (unless pacemaker fitted)

Side-effects include transient facial flush, chest pain, dyspnoea, bronchospasm, choking sensation, nausea, light-headedness; severe bradycardia reported (requiring temporary pacing); ECG may show transient rhythm disturbances

Licensed use not licensed for use in children

Indication and dose

Arrhythmias (see also section 2.3.1), diagnosis of arrhythmias
• **By intravenous injection**

Neonates 150 micrograms/kg; if necessary repeat injection every 1–2 minutes increasing dose by 50–100 micrograms/kg until tachycardia terminated or max. single dose of 300 micrograms/kg given

Child 1 month–1 year 150 micrograms/kg; if necessary repeat injection every 1–2 minutes increasing the dose by 50–100 micr-

ograms/kg until tachycardia terminated or max. single dose of 500 micrograms/kg given

Child 1–12 years 100 micrograms/kg; if necessary repeat injection every 1–2 minutes increasing dose by 50–100 micrograms/kg until tachycardia terminated or max. single dose of 500 micrograms/kg given

Child 12–18 years initially 3 mg; if necessary followed by 6 mg after 1–2 minutes, and then by 12 mg after a further 1–2 minutes
Note In some children over 12 years 3-mg dose ineffective (e.g. if a small peripheral vein is used for administration) and higher initial dose sometimes used; however, those with *heart transplant* are **very sensitive** to the effects of adenosine, and should **not** receive higher initial doses. In children receiving dipyridamole reduce dose to a quarter of usual dose of adenosine

Administration by *rapid intravenous injection* over 2 seconds into central or large peripheral vein followed by rapid Sodium Chloride 0.9% flush; Injection solution may be diluted with Sodium Chloride 0.9% if required

Adenocor® (Sanofi-Synthelabo) [PoM]
Injection, adenosine 3 mg/mL in physiological saline, net price 2-mL vial = £4.45 (hosp. only)
Note Intravenous infusion of adenosine (*Adenoscan®*, Sanofi Winthrop) may be used in conjunction with radionuclide myocardial perfusion imaging in patients who cannot exercise adequately or for whom exercise is inappropriate—consult product literature

AMIODARONE HYDROCHLORIDE

Cautions liver-function and thyroid-function tests required before treatment and then every 6 months (see notes above for tests of thyroid function); hypokalaemia (measure serum-potassium concentration before treatment); pulmonary function tests and chest x-ray required before treatment; heart failure; severe bradycardia and

conduction disturbances in excessive dosage; intravenous use may cause moderate and transient fall in blood pressure (circulatory collapse precipitated by rapid administration or overdosage) or severe hepato-cellular toxicity (monitor transaminases closely); ECG monitoring and resuscitation facilities must be available during

◁ **AMIODARONE HYDROCHLORIDE** (*continued*)

intravenous use; acute porphyria (section 9.8.2); avoid benzyl alcohol containing injections in neonates (see Excipients, p. 3); **interactions:** Appendix 1 (amiodarone)

Contra-indications (except in cardiac arrest) sinus bradycardia, sino-atrial heart block; unless pacemaker fitted avoid in severe conduction disturbances or sinus node disease; thyroid dysfunction; iodine sensitivity; avoid *intravenous use* in severe respiratory failure, circulatory collapse, or severe arterial hypotension; avoid bolus injection in congestive heart failure or cardiomyopathy

Pregnancy possible risk of neonatal goitre if amiodarone used in second or third trimester; use only if no alternative

Breast-feeding avoid; significant amount present in milk—theoretical risk of neonatal thyroid dysfunction

Side-effects nausea, vomiting, taste disturbances, raised serum transaminases (may require dose reduction or withdrawal if accompanied by acute liver disorders), jaundice; bradycardia (see Cautions); pulmonary toxicity (including pneumonitis and fibrosis); tremor, sleep disorders; hypothyroidism, hyperthyroidism; reversible corneal microdeposits (sometimes with night glare); phototoxicity, persistent slate-grey skin discoloration (see also notes above); *less commonly* onset or worsening of arrhythmia, conduction disturbances (see Cautions), peripheral neuropathy and myopathy (usually reversible on withdrawal); *very rarely* chronic liver disease including cirrhosis, sinus arrest, bronchospasm (in patients with severe respiratory failure), ataxia, benign intracranial hypertension, headache, vertigo, epididymo-orchitis, impotence, haemolytic or aplastic anaemia, thrombocytopenia, rash (including exfoliative dermatitis), hypersensitivity including vasculitis, alopecia, impaired vision due to optic neuritis or optic neuropathy (including blindness), anaphylaxis on rapid injection, also hypotension, respiratory distress syndrome, sweating, and hot flushes

Licensed use Not licensed for use in children under 3 years

Indication and dose

Supraventricular and ventricular arrhythmias see notes above (initiated in hospital or under specialist supervision)

• **By mouth**

Neonate initially 5–10 mg/kg twice daily for 7–10 days, then reduced to maintenance dose of 5–10 mg/kg once daily

Child 1 month–12 years initially 5–10 mg/kg (max. 200 mg) twice daily for 7–10 days, then reduced to maintenance dose of 5–10 mg/kg once daily (max. 200 mg daily)

Child 12–18 years 200 mg 3 times daily for 1 week then 200 mg twice daily for 1 week then usually 200 mg daily adjusted according to response

• **By intravenous infusion**

Neonate initially 5 mg/kg over 30 minutes then 5 mg/kg over 30 minutes every 12–24 hours

Child 1 month–18 years initially 5–10 mg/kg over 20 minutes–2 hours then *by continuous infusion* 300 micrograms/kg/hour, increased according to response to max. 1.5 mg/kg/hour; do not exceed 1.2 g in 24 hours

Ventricular fibrillation or pulseless ventricular tachycardia refractory to defibrillation (see also section 2.3.1)

• **By intravenous injection**

Neonate 5 mg/kg over at least 3 minutes

Child 1 month–18 years 5 mg/kg (max. 300 mg) over at least 3 minutes

Administration Intravenous administration via central venous catheter preferred. For *intravenous infusion* dilute with Glucose 5% to a concentration of not less than 600 micrograms/mL; incompatible with Sodium Chloride infusion; avoid equipment containing the plasticizer di-2-ethyl-hexphthalate (DEHP).

For administration *by mouth*, tablets may be crushed and dispersed in water; injection solution should **not** be given orally (irritant)

Amiodarone (Non-proprietary) PoM
Tablets, amiodarone hydrochloride 100 mg, net price 28-tab pack = £1.39; 200 mg, 28-tab pack = £1.42. Label: 11
Brands include *Amyben*®

Injection, amiodarone hydrochloride 30 mg/mL, net price 10-mL prefilled syringe = £10.25
Excipients may include benzyl alcohol (avoid in neonates unless no safer alternative available, see Excipients, p. 3)

Sterile concentrate, amiodarone hydrochloride 50 mg/mL, net price 3-mL amp = £1.33, 6-mL amp = £2.86. For dilution and use as an infusion
Excipients may include benzyl alcohol (avoid in neonates unless no safer alternative available, see Excipients, p. 3)

◢Extemporaneous formulations available see Extemporaneous Preparations, p. 8

Cordarone X® (Sanofi-Aventis) PoM
Tablets, scored, amiodarone hydrochloride 100 mg, net price 28-tab pack = £4.45; 200 mg, 28-tab pack = £7.27. Label: 11

Sterile concentrate, amiodarone hydrochloride 50 mg/mL, net price 3-mL amp = £1.33. For dilution and use as an infusion
Excipients include benzyl alcohol (avoid in neonates unless no safer alternative available, see Excipients, p. 3)

▲ **FLECAINIDE ACETATE**

Cautions children with pacemakers (especially those who may be pacemaker dependent because stimulation threshold may rise appreciably); atrial fibrillation following heart surgery; monitor ECG

2

Cardiovascular system

◁ **FLECAINIDE ACETATE** (*continued*)

and have resuscitation facilities available during intravenous use; **interactions**: Appendix 1 (flecainide)

Hepatic impairment avoid or reduce dose in severe impairment; monitor plasma concentration (see pharmacokinetics below)

Renal impairment reduce dose by 25–50% if estimated glomerular filtration rate less than 35 mL/minute/1.73 m^2 and monitor plasma-flecainide concentration

Pregnancy used in pregnancy to treat maternal and fetal arrhythmias in specialist centres; toxicity reported in *animal* studies; infant hyperbilirubinaemia also reported

Breast-feeding significant amount present in milk but not known to be harmful

Contra-indications heart failure; abnormal left ventricular function; long-standing atrial fibrillation where conversion to sinus rhythm not attempted; haemodynamically significant valvular heart disease; avoid in sinus node dysfunction, atrial conduction defects, second-degree or greater AV block, bundle branch block or distal block unless pacing rescue available

Side-effects oedema, pro-arrhythmic effects; dyspnoea; dizziness, asthenia, fatigue, fever; visual disturbances; *rarely* pneumonitis, hallucinations, depression, confusion, amnesia, dyskinesia, convulsions, peripheral neuropathy; *also reported* gastro-intestinal disturbances, anorexia, hepatic dysfunction, flushing, syncope, drowsiness, tremor, vertigo, headache, anxiety, insomnia, ataxia, paraesthesia, hypoaesthesia, anaemia, leucopenia, thrombocytopenia, corneal deposits, tinnitus, increased antinuclear antibodies, hypersensitivity reactions (including rash, urticaria, and photosensitivity), increased sweating

Pharmacokinetics plasma-flecainide concentration for optimal response 200–800 micrograms/litre; blood sample should be taken immediately before next dose

Licensed use Not licensed for use in children under 12 years

Indication and dose

Resistant re-entry supraventricular tachycardia, ventricular ectopic beats or ventricular tachycardia, arrhythmias associated with accessory conduction pathways (e.g. Wolff-Parkinson-White syndrome), paroxysmal atrial fibrillation
• By mouth

Neonate 2 mg/kg 2–3 times daily adjusted according to response and plasma-flecainide concentration

Child 1 month–12 years 2 mg/kg 2–3 times daily adjusted according to response and plasma-flecainide concentration (max. 8 mg/kg/day or 300 mg daily)

Child 12–18 years initially 50–100 mg twice daily; max. 300 mg daily (max. 400 mg daily for ventricular arrhythmias in heavily built children)

• By slow intravenous injection or intravenous infusion

Neonate 1–2 mg/kg over 10–30 minutes; if necessary followed by continuous infusion at a rate of 100–250 micrograms/kg/hour until arrhythmia controlled; transfer to *oral* treatment as above

Child 1 month–12 years 2 mg/kg over 10–30 minutes; if necessary followed by continuous infusion at a rate of 100–250 micrograms/kg/hour until arrhythmia controlled (max. cumulative dose 600 mg in 24 hours); transfer to *oral* treatment as above

Child 12–18 years 2 mg/kg (max. 150 mg) over 10–30 minutes; if necessary followed by continuous infusion at a rate of 1.5 mg/kg/hour for 1 hour, then reduced to 100–250 micrograms/kg/hour until arrhythmia controlled (max. cumulative dose 600 mg in first 24 hours); transfer to *oral* treatment as above

Administration for administration *by mouth*, milk, infant formula, and dairy products may reduce absorption of flecainide—separate doses from feeds. Liquid has a local anaesthetic effect and should be given at least 30 minutes before or after food. Do not store liquid in refrigerator as precipitation occurs.

For *intravenous administration*, give initial dose over 30 minutes in children with sustained ventricular tachycardia or cardiac failure.

Dilute injection using Glucose 5%; concentrations of more than 300 micrograms/mL are unstable in chloride containing solutions

Flecainide (Non-proprietary) ℞PoM
Tablets, flecainide acetate 50 mg, net price 60-tab pack = £9.81; 100 mg, 60-tab pack = £15.04

Liquid, available from 'special-order' manufacturers or specialist importing companies, see p. 943

Tambocor® (3M) ℞PoM
Tablets, flecainide acetate 50 mg, net price 60-tab pack = £14.46; 100 mg (scored), 60-tab pack = £20.66

Injection, flecainide acetate 10 mg/mL, net price 15-mL amp = £4.40

◢Modified release
Tambocor® XL (Meda) ℞PoM
Capsules, m/r, grey/pink, flecainide acetate 200 mg, net price 30-cap pack = £14.77. Label: 25
Dose
Supraventricular arrhythmias
• By mouth
Child 12–18 years 200 mg once daily
Note Not to be used to control arrhythmias in acute situations; children stabilised on 200 mg daily of immediate-release flecainide may be transferred to *Tambocor® XL*

◢ LIDOCAINE HYDROCHLORIDE
(Lignocaine hydrochloride)

Cautions lower doses in congestive heart failure and following cardiac surgery; monitor ECG; resuscitation facilities should be available; **interactions:** Appendix 1 (lidocaine)

Hepatic impairment manufacturer advises caution—increased risk of side-effects

Renal impairment possible accumulation of lidocaine and active metabolite; manufacturers advise caution in severe impairment

Pregnancy crosses the placenta but not known to be harmful in *animal* studies—use if benefit outweighs risk

Breast-feeding present in milk but amount too small to be harmful

Contra-indications sino-atrial disorders, all grades of atrioventricular block, severe myocardial depression; acute porphyria (section 9.8.2)

Side-effects dizziness, paraesthesia, or drowsiness (particularly if injection too rapid); other CNS effects include confusion, respiratory depression and convulsions; hypotension and bradycardia (may lead to cardiac arrest); *rarely* hypersensitivity reactions including anaphylaxis

Licensed use not licensed for use in children under 1 year

Indication and dose

Ventricular arrhythmias, pulseless ventricular tachycardia or ventricular fibrillation

• **By intravenous or intraosseous injection, and intravenous infusion**

Neonate 0.5–1 mg/kg by injection followed by infusion of 0.6–3 mg/kg/hour; if infusion not immediately available following initial injection, injection of 0.5–1 mg/kg may be repeated at intervals of not less than 5 minutes (to max. total dose 3 mg/kg)

Child 1 month–12 years 0.5–1 mg/kg by injection followed by infusion of 0.6–3 mg/kg/hour; if infusion not immediately available following initial injection, injection of 0.5–1 mg/kg may be repeated at intervals of not less than 5 minutes (to max. total dose 3 mg/kg)

Child 12–18 years 50–100 mg by injection followed by infusion of 120 mg over 30 minutes *then* 240 mg over 2 hours *then* 60 mg/hour; reduce dose further if infusion continued beyond 24 hours; if infusion not immediately available following initial injection, injection of 50–100 mg may be repeated at intervals of not less than 5 minutes (to max. 300 mg in 1 hour)

Administration For *intravenous infusion* dilute with glucose 5% intravenous infusion or sodium chloride 0.9%

For use as a local anaesthetic see section 15.2

Lidocaine (Non-proprietary) ▣ⁿᵒᵐ̲
Injection 2%, lidocaine hydrochloride 20 mg/mL, net price 2-mL amp = 28p; 5-mL amp = 26p; 10-mL amp = 60p; 20-mL amp = 61p
Available from Braun

Infusion, lidocaine hydrochloride 0.1% (1 mg/mL) and 0.2% (2 mg/mL) in glucose intravenous infusion 5%. 500-mL containers
Available from Baxter

Minijet® Lignocaine (UCB Pharma) ▣ⁿᵒᵐ̲
Injection, lidocaine hydrochloride 1% (10 mg/mL), net price 10-mL disposable syringe = £4.85; 2% (20 mg/mL), 5-mL disposable syringe = £4.73

▣ 2.4 Beta-adrenoceptor blocking drugs

Beta-adrenoceptor blocking drugs (beta-blockers) block the beta-adrenoceptors in the heart, peripheral vasculature, bronchi, pancreas, and liver.

Many beta-blockers are available but experience in children is limited to the use of only a few.

Differences between beta-blockers may affect choice. The water-soluble beta-blockers, atenolol and sotalol, are less likely to enter the brain and may therefore cause less sleep disturbance and nightmares. Water-soluble beta-blockers are excreted by the kidneys and dosage reduction is often necessary in renal impairment.

Some beta-blockers, such as atenolol, have an intrinsically longer duration of action and need to be given only once daily. Carvedilol and labetalol are beta-blockers which have, in addition, an arteriolar vasodilating action and thus lower peripheral resistance. Although carvedilol and labetalol possess both alpha- and beta-blocking properties, these drugs have no important advantages over other beta-blockers in the treatment of hypertension.

Beta-blockers slow the heart and can depress the myocardium; they are contra-indicated in children with second- or third-degree heart block. Sotalol may prolong the QT interval, and it occasionally causes life-threatening ventricular arrhythmias (**important:** particular care is required to avoid hypokalaemia in children taking sotalol).

Beta-blockers can precipitate asthma and they should be **avoided** in children with a history of asthma or bronchospasm; if there is no alternative, a cardioselective beta-blocker can be used with extreme caution under specialist supervision. Atenolol and metoprolol have less effect on the beta$_2$ (bronchial) receptors and are, therefore, relatively *cardioselective*, but they are **not** *cardiospecific*. They have a lesser effect on airways resistance but are **not** free of this side-effect.

Beta-blockers are also associated with fatigue, coldness of the extremities, and sleep disturbances with nightmares (may be less common with the water-soluble beta-blockers, see above).

Beta-blockers are not contra-indicated in diabetes; however, they can lead to a small deterioration of glucose tolerance and interfere with metabolic and autonomic responses to hypoglycaemia. The cardioselective beta-blockers (e.g. atenolol and metoprolol) may be preferable in diabetes but beta-blockers should be avoided altogether in those with frequent episodes of hypoglycaemia.

Hypertension　Beta-blockers are effective for reducing blood pressure (section 2.5), but their mode of action is not understood; they reduce cardiac output, alter baroceptor reflex sensitivity, and block peripheral adrenoceptors. Some beta-blockers depress plasma renin secretion. It is possible that a central effect may also partly explain their mode of action. Blood pressure can usually be controlled with relatively few side-effects. In general the dose of beta-blocker does not have to be high.

Labetalol may be given intravenously for *hypertensive emergencies* in children (section 2.5); however, care is needed to avoid dangerous hypotension or beta-blockade, particularly in neonates. **Esmolol** is also used intravenously for the treatment of hypertension particularly in the peri-operative period.

Beta-blockers can be used to control the pulse rate in children with *phaeochromocytoma* (section 2.5.4). However, they should never be used alone as beta-blockade without concurrent alpha-blockade may lead to a hypertensive crisis; phenoxybenzamine should always be used together with the beta-blocker.

Arrhythmias　In arrhythmias (section 2.3), beta-blockers act principally by attenuating the effects of the sympathetic system on automaticity and conductivity within the heart. They can be used alone or in conjunction with digoxin to control the ventricular rate in *atrial fibrillation*. Beta-blockers are also useful in the management of *supraventricular tachycardias* and *ventricular tachycardias* particularly to prevent recurrence of the tachycardia.

Esmolol is a relatively cardioselective beta-blocker with a very short duration of action, used intravenously for the short-term treatment of supraventricular arrhythmias and sinus tachycardia, particularly in the peri-operative period.

Sotalol is a non-cardioselective beta-blocker with additional class III anti-arrhythmic activity. Atenolol and sotalol suppress ventricular ectopic beats and non-sustained ventricular tachycardia (section 2.3.1). However, the pro-arrhythmic effects of sotalol, particularly in children with sick sinus syndrome, may prolong the QT interval and induce torsade de pointes.

Heart failure　Beta-blockers may produce benefit in heart failure by blocking sympathetic activity and the addition of a beta-blocker such as **carvedilol** to other treatment for heart failure may be beneficial. Treatment should be initiated by those experienced in the management of heart failure (see section 2.2 for details on heart failure).

Thyrotoxicosis　Beta-blockers are used in the management of *thyrotoxicosis* including neonatal thyrotoxicosis; **propranolol** can reverse clinical symptoms within 4 days. Beta-blockers are also used for the pre-operative preparation for thyroidectomy; the thyroid gland is rendered less vascular, thus facilitating surgery (section 6.2.2).

Other uses　In tetralogy of Fallot, esmolol or propranolol may be given intravenously in the initial management of *cyanotic spells*; propranolol is given by mouth for preventing cyanotic spells. If a severe cyanotic spell in a child with congenital heart disease persists despite optimal use of 100% oxygen, propranolol is given by intravenous infusion (for dose, see below). If cyanosis is still present after 10 minutes, sodium bicarbonate intravenous infusion is given in a dose of 1 mmol/kg to correct acidosis (or dose calculated according to arterial blood gas results); sodium bicarbonate 4.2% intravenous infusion is appropriate for a child under 1 year and sodium bicarbonate 8.4% intravenous infusion in children over 1 year. If blood-glucose concentration is less than 3 mmol/litre, glucose 10% intravenous infusion is given in a dose of 2 mL/kg (glucose 200 mg/kg) over 10 minutes, followed by morphine in a dose of 100 micrograms/kg by intravenous or intramuscular injection.

Beta-blockers are also used in the *prophylaxis of migraine* (section 4.7.4.2). Betaxolol, carteolol, levobunolol, and timolol are used topically in *glaucoma* (section 11.6).

◢ PROPRANOLOL HYDROCHLORIDE

Cautions see notes above; also avoid abrupt withdrawal; first-degree AV block; portal hypertension (risk of deterioration in liver function); diabetes (see also notes above); history of obstructive airways disease (introduce cautiously and monitor lung function—see also Bronchospasm below); myasthenia gravis; symptoms of thyrotoxicosis may be masked (see also notes above); psoriasis; history of hypersensitivity—may increase sensitivity to allergens and result in more serious hypersensitivity response, also may reduce response to adrenaline (epinephrine); **interactions**: Appendix 1 (beta-blockers), **important**: verapamil interaction, see also p. 140

Hepatic impairment reduce oral dose in liver disease

Renal impairment manufacturer advises caution—dose reduction may be required

Pregnancy may cause intra-uterine growth restriction, neonatal hypoglycaemia, and bradycardia; risk greater in severe hypertension

Breast-feeding present in milk but amount probably too small to be harmful; monitor infant for symptoms of beta-blockade

Contra-indications asthma (**important**: see Bronchospasm below), uncontrolled heart failure, marked bradycardia, hypotension, sick sinus syndrome, second- or third- degree AV block, cardiogenic shock, metabolic acidosis, severe peripheral arterial disease; phaeochromocytoma (apart from specific use with alpha-blockers, see also notes above)
Bronchospasm The CSM has advised that beta-blockers, including those considered to be cardioselective, should not be given to patients with a history of asthma or bronchospasm. However, in rare situations where there is no alternative a cardioselective beta-blocker is given to these patients with extreme caution and under specialist supervision

Side-effects see notes above; also gastro-intestinal disturbances; bradycardia, heart failure, hypotension, conduction disorders, peripheral vasoconstriction (including exacerbation of intermittent claudication and Raynaud's phenomenon); bronchospasm (see above), dyspnoea; headache, fatigue, sleep disturbances, paraesthesia, dizziness, psychoses; sexual dysfunction; purpura, thrombocytopenia; visual disturbances; exacerbation of psoriasis, alopecia; *rarely* rashes and dry eyes (reversible on withdrawal); **overdosage**: see Emergency Treatment of Poisoning, p. 41

Licensed use not licensed for treatment of hypertension in children under 12 years

Indication and dose

Arrhythmias
● **By mouth**

> **Neonate** 250–500 micrograms/kg 3 times daily, adjusted according to response

> **Child 1 month–18 years** 250–500 micrograms/kg 3–4 times daily, adjusted according to response; max. 1 mg/kg 4 times daily, total daily dose not to exceed 160 mg daily

● **By slow intravenous injection, with ECG monitoring**

> **Neonate** 20–50 micrograms/kg repeated if necessary every 6–8 hours

> **Child 1 month–18 years** 25–50 micrograms/kg repeated every 6–8 hours if necessary

Hypertension
● **By mouth**

> **Neonate** initially, 250 micrograms/kg 3 times daily, increased if necessary to max. 2 mg/kg 3 times daily

> **Child 1 month–12 years** 0.25–1 mg/kg 3 times daily, increased at weekly intervals to max. 5 mg/kg daily

> **Child 12–18 years** initially 80 mg twice daily; increased at weekly intervals as required; maintenance 160–320 mg daily; slow-release preparations may be used for once daily administration

Tetralogy of Fallot
● **By mouth**

> **Neonate** 0.25–1 mg/kg 2–3 times daily, max. 2 mg/kg 3 times daily

> **Child 1 month–12 years** 0.25–1 mg/kg 3–4 times daily, max. 5 mg/kg daily

● **By slow intravenous injection with ECG monitoring**

> **Neonate** initially 15–20 micrograms/kg (max. 100 micrograms/kg), repeated every 12 hours if necessary

> **Child 1 month–12 years** initially 15–20 micrograms/kg (max. 100 micrograms/kg), repeated every 6–8 hours if necessary; higher doses rarely necessary

2

Cardiovascular system

◁ **PROPRANOLOL HYDROCHLORIDE (continued)**

Migraine prophylaxis
• **By mouth**

Child 2–12 years 200–500 micrograms/kg 3 times daily; max. 4 mg/kg daily, usual dose 10–20 mg 2–3 times daily

Child 12–18 years 20–40 mg 2–3 times daily; maintenance 80–160 mg daily

Administration Give by slow intravenous injection over at least 3–5 minutes. Rate of administration should not exceed 1 mg/minute. May be diluted with Sodium Chloride 0.9% or Glucose 5%. Incompatible with bicarbonate.
Note Excessive bradycardia can be countered with intravenous injection of atropine sulphate; for **overdosage** see Emergency Treatment of Poisoning, p. 41

Propranolol (Non-proprietary) [PoM]
Tablets, propranolol hydrochloride 10 mg, net price 28 = 91p; 40 mg, 28 = 97p; 80 mg, 56 = £1.68; 160 mg, 56 = £3.29. Label: 8
Brands include *Angilol*®

Oral solution, propranolol hydrochloride 5 mg/5 mL, net price 150 mL = £12.50; 10 mg/5 mL, 150 mL = £16.45; 50 mg/5 mL, 150 mL = £19.98. Label: 8
Brands include *Syprol*®

Inderal® (AstraZeneca) [PoM]
Injection, propranolol hydrochloride 1 mg/mL, net price 1-mL amp = 21p

◢ **Modified release**
Note Modified-release preparations for once daily administration; use in older children only

Half-Inderal LA® (AstraZeneca) [PoM]
Capsules, m/r, lavender/pink, propranolol hydrochloride 80 mg. Net price 28-cap pack = £5.40. Label: 8, 25
Note Modified-release capsules containing propranolol hydrochloride 80 mg also available; brands include *Bedranol SR*®, *Half Beta Prograne*®

Inderal-LA (AstraZeneca) [PoM]
Capsules, m/r, lavender/pink, propranolol hydrochloride 160 mg. Net price 28-cap pack = £6.67. Label: 8, 25
Note Modified-release capsules containing propranolol hydrochloride 160 mg also available; brands include *Bedranol SR*®, *Beta-Prograne*®, *Slo-Pro*®

◢ ATENOLOL

Cautions see under Propranolol Hydrochloride

Renal impairment initially use 50% of usual dose if estimated glomerular filtration rate 10–35 mL/minute/1.73 m^2; initially use 30–50% of usual dose if estimated glomerular filtration rate less than 10 mL/minute/1.73 m^2

Pregnancy may cause intra-uterine growth restriction, neonatal hypoglycaemia, and bradycardia; risk greater in severe hypertension

Breast-feeding present in milk in greater amounts than some other beta-blockers; possible toxicity due to beta-blockade—monitor infant and use with caution

Contra-indications see under Propranolol Hydrochloride

Side-effects see under Propranolol Hydrochloride

Licensed use not licensed for use in children under 12 years

Indication and dose

Hypertension
• **By mouth**

Neonate 0.5–2 mg/kg once daily; may be given in 2 divided doses

Child 1 month–12 years 0.5–2 mg/kg once daily (doses higher than 50 mg daily rarely necessary); may be given in 2 divided doses

Child 12–18 years 25–50 mg once daily (higher doses rarely necessary); may be given in 2 divided doses

Arrhythmias
• **By mouth**

Neonate 0.5–2 mg/kg once daily; may be given in 2 divided doses

Child 1 month–12 years 0.5–2 mg/kg once daily (max. 100 mg daily); may be given in 2 divided doses

Child 12–18 years 50–100 mg once daily; may be given in 2 divided doses

Atenolol (Non-proprietary) [PoM]
Tablets, atenolol 25 mg, net price 28-tab pack = 81p; 50 mg, 28-tab pack = 85p; 100 mg, 28-tab pack = 86p. Label: 8
Brands include *Atenix*®

Tenormin® (AstraZeneca) [PoM]
'25' tablets, f/c, atenolol 25 mg, net price 28-tab pack = £4.41. Label: 8

LS tablets, orange, f/c, scored, atenolol 50 mg, net price 28-tab pack = £5.11. Label: 8

Tablets, orange, f/c, scored, atenolol 100 mg, net price 28-tab pack = £6.50. Label: 8

Syrup, sugar-free, atenolol 25 mg/5 mL, net price 300 mL = £8.55. Label: 8

▇ CARVEDILOL

Cautions see under Propranolol Hydrochloride; monitor renal function during dose titration in children with heart failure who also have low blood pressure, renal impairment, ischaemic heart disease, or diffuse vascular disease

Pregnancy see under Propranolol Hydrochloride; also lack of experience in human pregnancy limits any assessment of fetal risk

Breast-feeding present in milk in *animal* studies but amount probably too small to be harmful; monitor infant for symptoms of alpha- and beta-blockade

Contra-indications see under Propranolol Hydrochloride; acute or decompensated heart failure requiring intravenous inotropes

Hepatic impairment avoid

Side-effects postural hypotension, dizziness, headache, fatigue, gastro-intestinal disturbances, bradycardia; occasionally diminished peripheral circulation, peripheral oedema and painful extremities, dry mouth, dry eyes, eye irritation or disturbed vision, impotence, disturbances of micturition, influenza-like symptoms; rarely angina, AV block, exacerbation of intermittent claudication or Raynaud's phenomenon; allergic skin reactions, exacerbation of psoriasis, nasal stuffiness, wheezing, depressed mood, sleep dis-

turbances, paraesthesia, heart failure, changes in liver enzymes, thrombocytopenia, leucopenia also reported

Licensed use not licensed for use in children under 18 years

Indication and dose

Adjunct in heart failure (limited information available)

● **By mouth**

Child 2–18 years initially 50 micrograms/kg (max. 3.125 mg) twice daily, double dose at intervals of at least 2 weeks up to 350 micrograms/kg (max. 25 mg) twice daily

Carvedilol (Non-proprietary) ℙℴ𝕄

Tablets, carvedilol 3.125 mg, net price 28-tab pack = £5.73; 6.25 mg, 28-tab pack = £6.09; 12.5 mg, 28-tab pack = £1.54; 25 mg, 28-tab pack = £2.14. Label: 8

Eucardic® (Roche) ℙℴ𝕄

Tablets, scored, carvedilol 3.125 mg (pink), net price 28-tab pack = £7.57; 6.25 mg (yellow), 28-tab pack = £8.41; 12.5 mg (peach), 28-tab pack = £9.35; 25 mg (peach), 28-tab pack = £11.68. Label: 8

▇ ESMOLOL HYDROCHLORIDE

Cautions see under Propranolol Hydrochloride

Renal impairment manufacturer advises caution

Contra-indications see under Propranolol Hydrochloride

Side-effects see under Propranolol Hydrochloride; infusion causes venous irritation and thrombophlebitis

Licensed use not licensed for use in children

Indication and dose

Arrhythmias, hypertensive emergencies (see also notes above and section 2.5)

● **By intravenous administration**

Child 1 month–18 years initially by *intravenous injection* over 1 minute 500 micrograms/kg then by *intravenous infusion* 50 micrograms/kg/minute for 4 minutes (rate reduced if low blood pressure or low heart rate); if inadequate response, repeat loading dose and increase maintenance infusion by 50 micrograms/kg/minute increments; repeat until effective or

max. infusion of 200 micrograms/kg/minute reached; doses over 300 micrograms/kg/minute not recommended

Tetralogy of Fallot

● **By intravenous administration**

Neonate initially by *intravenous injection* over 1–2 minutes 600 micrograms/kg then if necessary by *intravenous infusion* 300–900 micrograms/kg/minute

Administration Dilute injection solution (with Glucose 5% *or* Sodium Chloride 0.9%) to a concentration of 10 mg/mL (20 mg/mL if fluid restricted) and give through central venous catheter; incompatible with bicarbonate

Brevibloc® (Baxter) ℙℴ𝕄

Injection, esmolol hydrochloride 10 mg/mL, net price 10-mL vial = £7.79, 250-mL infusion bag = £89.69

▇ LABETALOL HYDROCHLORIDE

Cautions see under Propranolol Hydrochloride; interferes with laboratory tests for catecholamines; liver damage (see below)

Liver damage Severe hepatocellular damage reported after both short-term and long-term treatment. Appropriate laboratory testing needed at first symptom of liver dysfunction and if laboratory evidence of damage (or if jaundice) labetalol should be stopped and not restarted

Renal impairment dose reduction may be required

Pregnancy use in treatment of maternal hypertension does not pose risk, except possibly in first trimester, monitor neonate for signs of alpha- and beta-blockade

Breast-feeding present in milk but amount probably too small to be harmful—monitor infant for possible symptoms of alpha- and beta-blockade

Contra-indications see under Propranolol Hydrochloride

2

Cardiovascular system

◁ LABETALOL HYDROCHLORIDE (continued)

Side-effects postural hypotension (avoid upright position during and for 3 hours after intravenous administration), tiredness, weakness, headache, rashes, scalp tingling, difficulty in micturition, epigastric pain, nausea, vomiting; liver damage (see above); rarely lichenoid rash

Licensed use not licensed for use in children

Indication and dose

Hypertensive emergencies see also section 2.5
- **By intravenous infusion**

  Neonate 500 micrograms/kg/hour adjusted at intervals of at least 15 minutes according to response; max. 4 mg/kg/hour

  Child 1 month–12 years initially 0.5–1 mg/kg/hour adjusted at intervals of at least 15 minutes according to response; max. 3 mg/kg/hour

  Child 12–18 years 30–120 mg/hour adjusted at intervals of at least 15 minutes according to response
  Note Consult local guidelines. In hypertensive encephalopathy reduce blood pressure to normotensive level over 24–48 hours (more rapid reduction may lead to cerebral infarction, blindness, and death). If child fitting, reduce blood pressure rapidly, but not to normal levels

Hypertension
- **By mouth**

  Child 1 month–12 years 1–2 mg/kg 3–4 times a day

  Child 12–18 years initially 50–100 mg twice daily increased if required at intervals of 3–14 days to usual dose of 200–400 mg twice daily (3–4 divided doses if higher); max. 2.4 g daily
  Administration Injection may be given orally with squash or juice

- **By intravenous injection**

  Child 1 month–12 years 250–500 micrograms/kg as a single dose; max. 20 mg

  Child 12–18 years 50 mg over at least 1 minute, repeated after 5 minutes if necessary; max. total dose 200 mg

  Note Excessive bradycardia can be countered with intravenous injection of atropine sulphate; for **overdosage** see p. 41

Administration for *intravenous infusion*, dilute to a concentration of 1 mg/mL in Glucose 5% or Sodium Chloride and Glucose 5%; if fluid restricted may be given undiluted, preferably through a central venous catheter

Labetalol Hydrochloride (Non-proprietary) ⟨PoM⟩
Tablets, f/c, labetalol hydrochloride 100 mg, net price 56 = £7.80; 200 mg, 56 = £11.83; 400 mg, 56 = £17.73. Label: 8, 21

Trandate® (UCB Pharma) ⟨PoM⟩
Tablets, all orange, f/c, labetalol hydrochloride 50 mg, net price 56-tab pack = £3.79; 100 mg, 56-tab pack = £4.17; 200 mg, 56-tab pack = £6.77; 400 mg, 56-tab pack = £9.42. Label: 8, 21

Injection, labetalol hydrochloride 5 mg/mL, net price 20-mL amp = £2.12

◣ Extemporaneous formulations available see Extemporaneous Preparations, p. 8

METOPROLOL TARTRATE

Cautions see under Propranolol Hydrochloride
  Hepatic impairment reduce dose in severe impairment

  Pregnancy see under Propranolol Hydrochloride
  Breast-feeding present in milk but amount probably too small to be harmful—monitor infant for possible symptoms of beta-blockade

Contra-indications see under Propranolol Hydrochloride

Side-effects see under Propranolol Hydrochloride

Licensed use not licensed for use in children

Indication and dose

Hypertension
- **By mouth**

  Child 1 month–12 years initially 1 mg/kg twice daily, increased if necessary to max. 8 mg/kg daily in 2–4 divided doses

  Child 12–18 years initially 50–100 mg daily increased if necessary to 200 mg daily in 1–2 divided doses; max. 400 mg daily (but high doses rarely necessary)

Arrhythmias
- **By mouth**

  Child 12–18 years usually 50 mg 2–3 times daily; up to 300 mg daily in divided doses if necessary

Metoprolol Tartrate (Non-proprietary) ⟨PoM⟩
Tablets, metoprolol tartrate 50 mg, net price 28 = £1.39, 56 = £1.54; 100 mg, 28 = £1.88, 56 = £2.24. Label: 8

Lopresor® (Novartis) ⟨PoM⟩
Tablets, f/c, scored, metoprolol tartrate 50 mg (pink), net price 56-tab pack = £2.57; 100 mg (blue), 56-tab pack = £6.68. Label: 8

◣ Extemporaneous formulations available see Extemporaneous Preparations, p. 8

SOTALOL HYDROCHLORIDE

Cautions see under Propranolol Hydrochloride; correct hypokalaemia, hypomagnesaemia, or other electrolyte disturbances; severe or prolonged diarrhoea; reduce dose or discontinue if corrected QT interval exceeds 550 msec; **inter-**

⌐ **SOTALOL HYDROCHLORIDE** (*continued*)

actions: Appendix 1 (beta-blockers), **important:** verapamil interaction see also p. 140

Renal impairment halve normal dose if estimated glomerular filtration rate 30–60 mL/minute/1.73 m^2; use one-quarter normal dose if estimated glomerular filtration rate 10–30 mL/minute/1.73 m^2; avoid if estimated glomerular filtration rate less than 10 mL/minute/1.73 m^2

Pregnancy see under Propranolol Hydrochloride

Breast-feeding present in milk; possible toxicity due to beta-blockade—monitor infant

CSM advice The use of sotalol should be limited to the treatment of ventricular arrhythmias or prophylaxis of supraventricular arrhythmias (see above). It should no longer be used for angina, hypertension, thyrotoxicosis or for secondary prevention after myocardial infarction; when stopping sotalol for these indications, the dose should be reduced gradually

Contra-indications see under Propranolol Hydrochloride; congenital or acquired long QT syndrome; torsade de pointes

Side-effects see under Propranolol Hydrochloride; arrhythmogenic (pro-arrhythmic) effect (torsade de pointes—increased risk in females)

Licensed use not licensed for use in children under 12 years

Indication and dose

Ventricular arrhythmias, life-threatening ventricular tachyarrhythmia and supraventricular arrhythmias initiated under specialist supervision and ECG monitoring and measurement of corrected QT interval

• **By mouth**

Neonate initially 1 mg/kg twice daily, increased as necessary every 3–4 days to max. 4 mg/kg twice daily

Atrial flutter, ventricular arrhythmias, life-threatening ventricular tachyarrhythmia and supraventricular arrhythmias initiated under specialist supervision and ECG monitoring and measurement of corrected QT interval

• **By mouth**

Child 1 month–12 years initially 1 mg/kg twice daily, increased as necessary every 2–3 days to max. 4 mg/kg twice daily (max. 80 mg twice daily)

Child 12–18 years initially 80 mg once daily *or* 40 mg twice daily, increased gradually at intervals of 2–3 days to usual dose 80–160 mg twice daily; higher doses of 480–640 mg daily for life-threatening ventricular arrhythmias under specialist supervision

Administration tablets may be crushed and dispersed in water

Note Excessive bradycardia can be countered with intravenous injection of atropine sulphate; for **overdosage** see Emergency Treatment of Poisoning, p. 41

Sotalol (Non-proprietary) ⟨PoM⟩
Tablets, sotalol hydrochloride 40 mg, net price 56 = £1.34; 80 mg, 56-tab pack = £1.99; 160 mg, 28-tab pack = £2.21. Label: 8

Beta-Cardone® (UCB Pharma) ⟨PoM⟩
Tablets, scored, sotalol hydrochloride 40 mg (green), net price 56-tab pack = £1.34; 80 mg (pink), 56-tab pack = £1.99; 200 mg, 28-tab pack = £2.50. Label: 8

Sotacor® (Bristol-Myers Squibb) ⟨PoM⟩
Tablets, scored, sotalol hydrochloride 80 mg, net price 28-tab pack = £3.25; 160 mg, 28-tab pack = £6.41. Label: 8

Injection, sotalol hydrochloride 10 mg/mL, net price 4-mL amp = £1.76

◀ Extemporaneous formulations available see Extemporaneous Preparations, p. 8

2 Cardiovascular system

2.5 Hypertension

2.5.1 Vasodilator antihypertensive drugs and pulmonary hypertension
2.5.2 Centrally acting antihypertensive drugs
2.5.3 Adrenergic neurone blocking drugs
2.5.4 Alpha-adrenoceptor blocking drugs
2.5.5 Drugs affecting the renin-angiotensin system

Hypertension in children and adolescents can have a substantial effect on long-term health. Possible causes of hypertension (e.g. congenital heart disease, renal disease and endocrine disorders) and the presence of any complications (e.g. left ventricular hypertrophy) should be established. Treatment should take account of contributory factors and any factors that increase the risk of cardiovascular complications.

Serious hypertension is rare in *neonates* but it can present with signs of congestive heart failure; the cause is often renal and can follow embolic arterial damage.

Children (or their parents or carers) should be given advice on lifestyle changes to reduce blood pressure or cardiovascular risk; these include weight reduction (in obese children), reduction of dietary salt, reduction of total and saturated fat, increasing exercise, increasing fruit and vegetable intake, and smoking cessation (in children who smoke).

Indications for antihypertensive therapy in children include symptomatic hypertension, secondary hypertension, hypertensive target-organ damage, diabetes mellitus, persistent hypertension despite lifestyle measures (see above), and pulmonary hypertension (section 2.5.1.2). The effect of antihypertensive treatment on growth and development is not known; treatment should be started only if benefits are clear.

Antihypertensive therapy should be initiated with a single drug at the lowest recommended dose; the dose can be increased until the target blood pressure is achieved. Once the highest recommended dose is reached, or sooner if the patient begins to experience side-effects, a second drug may be added if blood pressure is not controlled. If more than one drug is required, these should be given as separate products because there is little paediatric experience in using fixed-dose combination products.

Acceptable drug classes for use in children with hypertension include **ACE inhibitors** (section 2.5.5.1), **alpha-blockers** (section 2.5.4), **beta-blockers** (section 2.4), **calcium-channel blockers** (section 2.6.2), and **thiazide diuretics** (section 2.2.1). There is limited information on the use of **angiotensin-II receptor antagonists** (section 2.5.5.2) in children. Diuretics and beta-blockers have a long history of safety and efficacy in children. The newer classes of antihypertensive drugs, including ACE inhibitors and calcium-channel blockers have been shown to be safe and effective in short-term studies in children. Refractory hypertension may require additional treatment with agents such as **minoxidil** (section 2.5.1.1) or **clonidine** (section 2.5.2).

Other measures to reduce cardiovascular risk   **Aspirin** (section 2.9) may be used to reduce the risk of cardiovascular events; however, concerns about an increased risk of bleeding and Reye's syndrome need to be considered.

A **statin** can be of benefit in older children who have a high risk of cardiovascular disease and have hypercholesterolaemia (see section 2.12).

Hypertension in diabetes   Hypertension can occur in type 2 diabetes and treatment prevents both macrovascular and microvascular complications. ACE inhibitors (section 2.5.5.1) may be considered in children with diabetes and microalbuminaemia or proteinuric renal disease (see also section 6.1.5). Beta-blockers are best avoided in children with, or at a high risk of developing, diabetes, especially when combined with a thiazide diuretic.

Hypertension in renal disease   ACE inhibitors may be considered in children with micro-albuminuria or proteinuric renal disease (see also section 6.1.5). High doses of loop diuretics may be required. Specific cautions apply to the use of ACE inhibitors in renal impairment, see section 2.5.5.1, but ACE inhibitors may be effective. Dihydropyridine calcium-channel blockers may be added.

Hypertension in pregnancy   High blood pressure in pregnancy may usually be due to pre-existing essential hypertension or to pre-eclampsia. **Methyldopa** (section 2.5.2) is safe in pregnancy. Beta-blockers are effective and safe in the third trimester. Modified-release preparations of **nifedipine** [unlicensed] are also used for hypertension in pregnancy. Intravenous administration of **labetalol** (section 2.4) can be used to control hypertensive crises; alternatively **hydralazine** (section 2.5.1.1) may be used by the intravenous route.

Hypertensive emergencies   Hypertensive emergencies in children may be accompanied by signs of hypertensive encephalopathy, including seizures. Controlled reduction in blood pressure over 72–96 hours is essential; rapid reduction can reduce perfusion leading to organ damage. It may be necessary to infuse fluids particularly during the first 12 hours to expand plasma volume should the blood pressure drop too rapidly. Once blood pressure is controlled oral therapy should be started.

Controlled reduction of blood pressure is achieved by **sodium nitroprusside** (section 2.5.1.1). **Esmolol** (section 2.4) is useful for short-term use and has a short duration of action. **Nicardipine** (section 2.6.2) may be administered as a continuous intravenous infusion but it is not licensed for this use. In less severe cases, nifedipine capsules (section 2.6.2) can be used.

In resistant cases, **diazoxide** (section 2.5.1.1) is given intravenously, but it can cause sudden hypotension. Other antihypertensive drugs which may be given intravenously include hydralazine (section 2.5.1.1) and **clonidine** (section 2.5.2).

Hypertension in acute nephritis occurs as a result of sodium and water retention; it should be treated with sodium and fluid restriction, and with furosemide (section 2.2.2); antihypertensive drugs may be added if necessary.

For advice on short-term management of hypertensive episodes in phaeochromocytoma, see under Phaeochromocytoma, section 2.5.4.

2.5.1 Vasodilator antihypertensive drugs and pulmonary hypertension

2.5.1.1 Vasodilator antihypertensives

Vasodilators have a potent hypotensive effect, especially when used in combination with a beta-blocker and a thiazide. **Important:** for a warning on the hazards of a very rapid fall in blood pressure, see Hypertensive Emergencies, p. 120.

Sodium nitroprusside is given by intravenous infusion to control severe hypertensive crisis when parenteral treatment is necessary. At low doses it reduces systemic vascular resistance and increases cardiac output; at high doses it can produce profound systemic hypotension—continuous blood pressure monitoring is therefore essential. Sodium nitroprusside may also be used to control paradoxical hypertension after surgery for coarctation of the aorta.

Diazoxide has also been used by intravenous injection in hypertensive emergencies; however it is not first-line therapy.

Hydralazine is given by mouth as an adjunct to other antihypertensives for the treatment of resistant hypertension but is rarely used; when used alone it causes tachycardia and fluid retention. The incidence of side-effects is lower if the dose is kept low, but systemic lupus erythematosus should be suspected if there is unexplained weight loss, arthritis, or any other unexplained ill health.

Minoxidil should be reserved for the treatment of severe hypertension resistant to other drugs. Vasodilatation is accompanied by increased cardiac output and tachycardia and children develop fluid retention. For this reason the addition of a beta-blocker and a diuretic (usually furosemide, in high dosage) are mandatory. Hypertrichosis is troublesome and renders this drug unsuitable for females.

Prazosin and doxazosin (section 2.5.4) have alpha-blocking and vasodilator properties.

DIAZOXIDE

Cautions during prolonged use monitor white cell and platelet count, and regularly assess growth, bone, and psychological development; **interactions:** Appendix 1 (diazoxide)

Renal impairment dose reduction may be required

Contra-indications

Pregnancy prolonged use may produce alopecia, hypertrichosis, and impaired glucose tolerance in neonate; inhibits uterine activity during labour

Breast-feeding manufacturer advises avoid—no information available

Side-effects tachycardia, hypotension, hyperglycaemia, sodium and water retention; *rarely* cardiomegaly, hyperosmolar non-ketotic coma, leucopenia, thrombocytopenia, and hirsuitism

Licensed use intractable hypoglycaemia (section 6.1.4)

Indication and dose

Hypertensive emergencies initiated on specialist advice
- **By intravenous injection**

    Child 1 month–18 years 1–3 mg/kg (max. 150 mg) as a single dose, repeat dose after 5–15 minutes until blood pressure controlled; max. 4 doses in 24 hours

Administration intravenous injection over 30 seconds. Do not dilute

Resistant hypertension
- **By mouth**

    Neonate initially 1.7 mg/kg 3 times daily, adjusted according to response; usual max. 15 mg/kg daily

    Child 1 month–18 years initially 1.7 mg/kg 3 times daily, adjusted according to response; usual max. 15 mg/kg daily

Intractable hypoglycaemia section 6.1.4

◁ DIAZOXIDE (*continued*)

Eudemine® (Goldshield) [PoM] ◢
Injection, diazoxide 15 mg/mL, net price 20-mL amp = £30.00

Tablets, section 6.1.4

◢ Extemporaneous formulations available see Extemporaneous Preparations, p. 8

HYDRALAZINE HYDROCHLORIDE

Cautions cerebrovascular disease; occasionally blood pressure reduction too rapid even with low parenteral doses; manufacturer advises test for antinuclear factor and for proteinuria every 6 months and check acetylator status before increasing dose, but evidence of clinical value unsatisfactory; **interactions:** Appendix 1 (hydralazine)

Hepatic impairment reduce dose

Renal impairment reduce dose if estimated glomerular filtration rate less than 30 mL/minute/1.73 m²

Pregnancy manufacturer advises avoid before third trimester; no reports of serious harm following use in third trimester

Breast-feeding present in milk but not known to be harmful; monitor infant

Contra-indications idiopathic systemic lupus erythematosus, severe tachycardia, high output heart failure, myocardial insufficiency due to mechanical obstruction, cor pulmonale; acute porphyria (section 9.8.2)

Side-effects tachycardia, palpitation, flushing, hypotension, fluid retention, gastro-intestinal disturbances; headache, dizziness; systemic lupus erythematosus-like syndrome after long-term therapy (especially in slow acetylator individuals); rarely rashes, fever, peripheral neuritis, polyneuritis, paraesthesia, arthralgia, myalgia, increased lacrimation, nasal congestion, dyspnoea, agitation, anxiety, anorexia; blood disorders (including leucopenia, thrombocytopenia, haemolytic anaemia), abnormal liver function, jaundice, raised plasma creatinine, proteinuria and haematuria reported

Licensed use not licensed for use in children

Indication and dose

Hypertension
• By mouth

Neonate 250–500 micrograms/kg every 8–12 hours increased as necessary to max. 2–3 mg/kg every 8 hours

Child 1 month–12 years 250–500 micrograms/kg every 8–12 hours increased as necessary to max. 7.5 mg/kg daily (not exceeding 200 mg daily)

Child 12–18 years 25 mg twice daily, increased to usual max. 50–100 mg twice daily

• By slow intravenous injection

Neonate 100–500 micrograms/kg repeated every 4–6 hours as necessary; max 3 mg/kg daily

Child 1 month–12 years 100–500 micrograms/kg repeated every 4–6 hours as necessary; max 3 mg/kg daily (not exceeding 60 mg daily)

Child 12–18 years 5–10 mg repeated every 4–6 hours as necessary

• By continuous intravenous infusion (preferred route in cardiac patients)

Neonate 12.5–50 micrograms/kg/hour

Child 1 month–12 years 12.5–50 micrograms/kg/hour; max. 3 mg/kg daily

Child 12–18 years initially 3–9 mg/hour; max. 3 mg/kg daily

Administration For *intravenous injection* initially reconstitute 20 mg with 1 mL water for injections, then dilute to a concentration of 0.5–1 mg/mL with sodium chloride 0.9% intravenous infusion and administer over 5–20 minutes. For administration *by mouth* diluted injection may be given orally. For *continuous intravenous infusion* initially reconstitute 20 mg with 1 mL water for injections, then dilute with sodium chloride 0.9% or Ringer's solution. Incompatible with glucose intravenous infusion

Hydralazine (Non-proprietary) [PoM]
Tablets, hydralazine hydrochloride 25 mg, net price 56 = £11.79; 50 mg, 56 = £18.54

Apresoline® (Amdipharm) [PoM]
Tablets, yellow, s/c, hydralazine hydrochloride 25 mg, net price 84-tab pack = £2.82
Excipients include gluten

Injection, powder for reconstitution, hydralazine hydrochloride, net price 20-mg amp = £1.84

◢ Extemporaneous formulations available see Extemporaneous Preparations, p. 8

MINOXIDIL

Cautions see notes above; acute porphyria (section 9.8.2); **interactions:** Appendix 1 (vasodilator antihypertensives)

Renal impairment use with caution in significant impairment

Pregnancy neonatal hirsutism reported

Breast-feeding present in milk but not known to be harmful

Contra-indications phaeochromocytoma

Side-effects sodium and water retention; weight gain, peripheral oedema, tachycardia, hypertrichosis; reversible rise in creatinine and blood

2 Cardiovascular system

◿ **MINOXIDIL (continued)**

urea nitrogen; occasionally, gastro-intestinal disturbances, breast tenderness, rashes

Indication and dose

Severe hypertension
* **By mouth**

Child 1 month–12 years initially 200 micrograms/kg daily in 1–2 divided doses, increased in steps of 100–200 micrograms/kg daily at intervals of at least 3 days; max. 1 mg/kg daily

Child 12–18 years initially 5 mg daily in 1–2 divided doses increased in steps of 5–10 mg at

intervals of at least 3 days; max. 100 mg daily (seldom necessary to exceed 50 mg daily)

Loniten® (Pharmacia) ℞
Tablets, scored, minoxidil 2.5 mg, net price 60-tab pack = £8.88; 5 mg, 60-tab pack = £15.83; 10 mg, 60-tab pack = £30.68

◢ Extemporaneous formulations available see Extemporaneous Preparations, p. 8

■ SODIUM NITROPRUSSIDE

Cautions hypothyroidism, hyponatraemia, impaired cerebral circulation, hypothermia; monitor blood pressure and blood-cyanide concentration, and if treatment exceeds 3 days also blood-thiocyanate concentration; avoid sudden withdrawal—terminate infusion over 15–30 minutes; **interactions:** Appendix 1 (nitroprusside)

Hepatic impairment avoid in severe liver impairment

Renal impairment cyanide or thiocyanate metabolites may accumulate—avoid prolonged use

Pregnancy potential for accumulation of cyanide in fetus—avoid prolonged use

Breast-feeding no information available; caution advised due to thiocyanate metabolite

Contra-indications severe vitamin B_{12} deficiency; Leber's optic atrophy; compensatory hypertension

Side-effects associated with over rapid reduction in blood pressure (reduce infusion rate): headache, dizziness, nausea, retching, abdominal pain, perspiration, palpitation, anxiety, retrosternal discomfort; occasionally reduced platelet count, acute transient phlebitis
Cyanide Side-effects caused by excessive plasma concentration of the cyanide metabolite include tachycardia,

sweating, hyperventilation, arrhythmias, marked metabolic acidosis (discontinue and give antidote, see p. 44)

Licensed use not licensed for use in the UK

Indication and dose

Hypertensive emergencies
* **By continuous infusion**

Neonate 500 nanograms/kg/minute then increased in steps of 200 nanograms/kg/minute as necessary to max. 8 micrograms/kg/minute (max. 4 micrograms/kg/minute if used for longer than 24 hours)

Child 1 month–18 years 500 nanograms/kg/minute then increased in steps of 200 nanograms/kg/minute as necessary to max. 8 micrograms/kg/minute (max. 4 micrograms/kg/minute if used for longer than 24 hours)

Administration For *continuous intravenous infusion* in glucose 5%, infuse *via* infusion device to allow precise control; protect infusion from light. For further details, consult product literature

Sodium Nitroprusside (Non-proprietary) ℞
Intravenous infusion, powder for reconstitution, sodium nitroprusside 10 mg/mL. For dilution and use as an infusion. Available from 'special-order' manufacturers or specialist importing companies, see p. 943

2.5.1.2 Pulmonary hypertension

Only pulmonary *arterial* hypertension is currently suitable for drug treatment. Pulmonary arterial hypertension includes persistent pulmonary hypertension of the newborn, idiopathic pulmonary arterial hypertension in children, and pulmonary hypertension related to congenital heart disease and cardiac surgery.

Some types of pulmonary hypertension are treated with vasodilator antihypertensive therapy and oxygen. Diuretics (section 2.2) may also have a role in children with right-sided heart failure.

Initial treatment of *persistent pulmonary hypertension of the newborn* involves the administration of **nitric oxide**; **epoprostenol** can be used until nitric oxide is available. Oral sildenafil may be helpful in less severe cases. Epoprostenol and sildenafil can cause profound systemic hypotension. In rare circumstances either **tolazoline** or **magnesium sulphate** can be given by intravenous infusion when nitric oxide and epoprostenol have failed.

Treatment of *idiopathic pulmonary arterial hypertension* is determined by acute vasodilator testing; drugs used for treatment include calcium-channel blockers (usually **nifedipine**, section 2.6.2), long-term intravenous **epoprostenol**, nebulised **iloprost**, **bosentan**, or **sildenafil**. Anticoagulation (usually with warfarin) may also be required to prevent secondary thrombosis.

2 Cardiovascular system

Inhaled nitric oxide is a potent and selective pulmonary vasodilator. It acts on cyclic gaunosine monophosphate (cGMP) resulting in smooth muscle relaxation. Inhaled nitric oxide is used in the treatment of persistent pulmonary hypertension of the newborn, and may also be useful in other forms of arterial pulmonary hypertension. Dependency can occur with high doses and prolonged use; to avoid rebound pulmonary hypertension the drug should be withdrawn gradually, often with the aid of sildenafil.

Excess nitric oxide can cause methaemoglobinaemia; therefore, methaemoglobin concentration should be measured regularly, particularly in neonates.

Nitric oxide increases the risk of haemorrhage by inhibiting platelet aggregation, but it does not usually cause bleeding.

Epoprostenol (prostacyclin) is a prostaglandin and a potent vasodilator. It is used in the treatment of persistent pulmonary hypertension of the newborn, idiopathic pulmonary arterial hypertension, and in the acute phase following cardiac surgery. It is given by continuous 24-hour intravenous infusion.

Epoprostenol is a powerful inhibitor of platelet aggregation and there is a possible risk of haemorrhage. It is sometimes used as an antiplatelet in renal dialysis either alone or with heparin (see section 2.8.1). It can also cause serious systemic hypotension and, if withdrawn suddenly, can cause pulmonary hypertensive crisis.

Children on prolonged treatment can become tolerant to epoprostenol, and therefore require an increase in dose.

Iloprost is a synthetic analogue of epoprostenol and is efficacious when nebulised in adults with pulmonary arterial hypertension, but experience in children is limited. It is more stable than epoprostenol and has a longer half-life.

Bosentan is a dual endothelin receptor antagonist used orally in the treatment of idiopathic pulmonary arterial hypertension. The concentration of endothelin, a potent vasoconstrictor, is raised in sustained pulmonary hypertension.

Sildenafil, a vasodilator developed for the treatment of erectile dysfunction, is also used for pulmonary arterial hypertension. It is used either alone or as an adjunct to other drugs and has relatively few side-effects.

Sildenafil is a selective phosphodiesterase type-5 inhibitor. Inhibition of this enzyme in the lungs enhances the vasodilatory effects of nitric oxide and promotes relaxation of vascular smooth muscle.

Sildenafil has also been used in pulmonary hypertension for weaning children off inhaled nitric oxide following cardiac surgery, and less successfully in idiopathic pulmonary arterial hypertension.

Tolazoline is now rarely used to correct pulmonary artery vasospasm in pulmonary hypertension of the newborn as better alternatives are available (see above). Tolazoline is an alpha-blocker and produces both pulmonary and systemic vasodilation.

BOSENTAN

Cautions not to be initiated if systemic systolic blood pressure is below 85 mmHg; monitor liver function before and at monthly intervals during treatment, and 2 weeks after dose increase (reduce dose or suspend treatment if liver enzymes raised significantly) — discontinue if symptoms of liver impairment (see Contra-indications below); monitor haemoglobin before and during treatment (monthly for first 4 months, then 3-monthly thereafter), withdraw treatment gradually; **interactions:** Appendix 1 (bosentan)

Contra-indications acute porphyria (section 9.8.2)

Hepatic impairment avoid in moderate and severe hepatic impairment

Pregnancy avoid (teratogenic in *animal* studies); effective contraception required during and for at least 3 months after administration (hormonal contraception not considered effective); monthly pregnancy tests advised

Breast-feeding manufacturer advises avoid—no information available

Side-effects gastro-intestinal disturbances, dry mouth, rectal haemorrhage, hepatic impairment (see Cautions, above); flushing, hypotension, palpitation, oedema, chest pain; dyspnoea; headache, dizziness, fatigue; back pain and pain in extremities; anaemia; hypersensitivity reactions (including rash, pruritus, and anaphylaxis)

Licensed use not licensed for use in children under 12 years

◻ **BOSENTAN** (*continued*)

Indication and dose

Idiopathic pulmonary arterial hypertension
* By mouth

     Child 3–18 years and body-weight 10–20 kg
     initially 31.25 mg once daily increased after 4
     weeks to 31.25 mg twice daily

     Child 3–18 years and body-weight 20–40 kg
     initially 31.25 mg twice daily increased after 4
     weeks to 62.5 mg twice daily

     Child 12–18 years and body-weight over 40 kg
     initially 62.5 mg twice daily increased after 4

weeks to 125 mg twice daily; max. 250 mg twice
daily

Administration Tablets may be cut, or suspended
in water or non-acidic liquid. Suspension is stable
at room-temperature (max. 25°C) for 24 hours

Tracleer® (Actelion) ▼ (PoM)
     Tablets, f/c, orange, bosentan (as monohydrate)
     62.5 mg, net price 56-tab pack = £1541.00; 125 mg,
     56-tab pack = £1541.00

▰ EPOPROSTENOL

Cautions anticoagulant monitoring required when
given with heparin; haemorrhagic diathesis; avoid
abrupt withdrawal (see notes above); monitor
blood pressure; concomitant use of drugs that
increase risk of bleeding

     Pregnancy manufacturer advises use with cau-
     tion—no information available

Contra-indications severe left ventricular dysfunction; pulmonary veno-occlusive disease

Side-effects see notes above; gastro-intestinal
disturbances, hypotension, bradycardia, tachycardia, pallor, flushing, sweating with higher
doses; headache; lassitude, anxiety, agitation; dry
mouth, jaw pain, chest pain; also reported,
hyperglycaemia and injection-site reactions

Licensed use not licensed for use in children

Indication and dose

Persistent pulmonary hypertension of the
newborn
* By continuous intravenous infusion

     Neonate initially 2 nanograms/kg/minute
     adjusted according to response; usual max.
     20 nanograms/kg/minute (rarely up to 40 nan-
     ograms/kg/minute)

Idiopathic pulmonary arterial hypertension
* By continuous intravenous infusion

     Child 1 month–18 years initially 2 nanograms/
     kg/minute increased as necessary to 40 nan-
     ograms/kg/minute

Administration consult product literature

Flolan® (GSK) (PoM)
     Infusion, powder for reconstitution, epoprostenol
     (as sodium salt), net price 500-microgram vial (with
     diluent) = £64.57; 1.5-mg vial (▼) (with diluent) =
     £130.07

▰ ILOPROST

Cautions unstable pulmonary hypertension with
advanced right heart failure; hypotension (do not
initiate if systolic blood pressure below
85 mmHg); acute pulmonary infection; severe
asthma; **interactions:** Appendix 1 (iloprost)

     Hepatic impairment dose may need to be halved
     in liver cirrhosis—initially 2.5 micrograms at inter-
     vals of at least 3 hours (max. 6 times daily),
     adjusted according to response

Contra-indications decompensated cardiac failure (unless under medical supervision); severe
coronary heart disease; severe arrhythmias;
congenital or acquired valvular defects of the
myocardium; pulmonary veno-occlusive disease;
conditions which increase risk of haemorrhage

     Pregnancy manufacturer advises avoid (toxicity
     in *animal* studies); effective contraception must be
     used during treatment

     Breast-feeding manufacturer advises avoid—no
     information available

Side-effects vasodilatation, hypotension, syncope, cough, headache, throat or jaw pain;
nausea, vomiting, diarrhoea, chest pain, dys-

pnoea, bronchospasm, and wheezing also
reported

Licensed use not licensed for use in children
under 18 years

Indication and dose

Idiopathic or familial pulmonary arterial
hypertension
* By inhalation of nebulised solution

     Child 8–18 years initial dose 2.5 micrograms
     increased to 5 micrograms for second dose, if
     tolerated maintain at 5 micrograms 6–9 times
     daily according to response; reduce to
     2.5 micrograms 6–9 times daily if higher dose
     not tolerated

Raynaud's syndrome section 2.6.4.1

Ventavis® (Schering Health) ▼ (PoM)
     Nebuliser solution, iloprost (as trometamol)
     10 micrograms/mL, net price 30 × 1-mL (10 micr-
     ogram) unit-dose vials = £425.00, 168 × 1-mL =
     £2377.20. For use with *Prodose®* (NHS) or *Venta-Neb®*
     (NHS) nebuliser

2 Cardiovascular system

MAGNESIUM SULPHATE

Cautions see section 9.5.1.3

Side-effects see section 9.5.1.3

Licensed use see section 9.5.1.3

Indication and dose

Persistent pulmonary hypertension of the newborn
- By intravenous infusion

  Neonate initially 200 mg/kg over 20–30 minutes; if response occurs, then by continuous intravenous infusion of 20–75 mg/kg/hour to maintain plasma-magnesium concentration between 3.5–5.5 mmol/litre), given for up to 5 days

Neonatal hypocalcaemia see section 9.5.1.3

Hypomagnesaemia see section 9.5.1.3

Administration For *intravenous infusion* dilute with glucose 5% *or* sodium chloride 0.9% intravenous infusion to a max. concentration of 100 mg/mL (200 mg/mL if fluid restricted)

Magnesium Sulphate (Non-proprietary) PoM
Injection, magnesium sulphate 50% (Mg^{2+} approx. 2 mmol/mL), net price 2-mL (1-g) amp= £3.80, 5-mL (2.5-g) amp = £3.00, 10-mL (5-g) amp = £3.35; prefilled 10-mL (5-g) syringe = £4.95

SILDENAFIL

Cautions hypotension (avoid if severe); intravascular volume depletion; left ventricular outflow obstruction; autonomic dysfunction; avoid abrupt withdrawal; other cardiovascular disease; pulmonary veno-occlusive disease; predisposition to priapism; anatomical deformation of the penis; bleeding disorders or active peptic ulceration; ocular disorders; initiate cautiously if child also on epoprostenol, iloprost, bosentan or nitric oxide; **interactions**: Appendix 1 (sildenafil)

Hepatic impairment reduce dose if not tolerated in mild to moderate impairment; manufacturer advises avoid in severe impairment

Renal impairment reduce dose if not tolerated

Contra-indications recent history of stroke; history of non-arteritic anterior ischaemic optic neuropathy; hereditary degenerative retinal disorders; avoid concomitant use of nitrates

Side-effects gastro-intestinal disturbances, dry mouth; flushing, oedema; bronchitis, cough; headache, migraine, night sweats, paraesthesia, insomnia, anxiety, tremor, vertigo; fever, influenza-like symptoms; anaemia; back and limb pain, myalgia; visual disturbances, retinal haemorrhage, photophobia, painful red eyes; nasal congestion, epistaxis; cellulitis, alopecia; *less commonly* gynaecomastia, priapism; *also reported* rash, retinal vascular occlusion, non-arteritic anterior ischaemic optic neuropathy (discontinue if sudden visual impairment occurs), and sudden hearing loss (advise patient to seek medical help)

Licensed use not licensed for use in children under 18 years

Indication and dose

Pulmonary hypertension after cardiac surgery, weaning from nitric oxide, idiopathic pulmonary arterial hypertension, persistent pulmonary hypertension of the newborn
- By mouth

  Neonate initially 250–500 micrograms/kg every 4–8 hours, adjusted according to response; max. 2 mg/kg every 4 hours; start with lower dose and frequency especially if used with other vasodilators (see Cautions above); withdraw gradually

  Child 1 month– 18 years initially 250–500 micrograms/kg every 4–8 hours, adjusted according to response; max. 2 mg/kg every 4 hours; start with lower dose and frequency especially if used with other vasodilators (see Cautions above)

Administration tablet may be dissolved in water or blackcurrant drink and given by mouth or through a nasogastric tube

Viagra® (Pfizer) PoM NHS
Tablets, all blue, f/c, sildenafil (as citrate), 25 mg, net price 4-tab pack = £16.59, 8-tab pack = £33.19; 50 mg, 4-tab pack = £19.34, 8-tab pack = £38.67; 100 mg, 4-tab pack = £23.50, 8-tab pack = £46.99

Revatio® (Pfizer) ▼ PoM
Tablets, f/c, sildenafil (as citrate), 20 mg, net price 90-tab pack = £373.50

◢Extemporaneous formulations available see Extemporaneous Preparations, p. 8

TOLAZOLINE

Cautions mitral stenosis; cardiotoxic accumulation may occur with continuous infusion, particularly in renal impairment—monitor blood pressure regularly for sustained systemic hypotension; **interactions**: Appendix 1 (alpha-blockers)

Renal impairment accumulates in renal impairment; risk of cardiotoxicity; lower doses may be necessary

Contra-indications peptic ulcer disease

Side-effects nausea, vomiting, diarrhoea, epigastric pain; flushing, tachycardia, cardiac arrhythmias; headache, shivering, sweating; oliguria, metabolic alkalosis, haematuria, blood dyscrasias (including thrombocytopenia); blotchy skin; at high doses severe hypotension, marked hypertension, renal failure, and haemorrhage reported

Licensed use not licensed for use in children

◁ **TOLAZOLINE** (*continued*)

Indication and dose

Correction of pulmonary vasospasm in neonates
• **By intravenous injection and continuous intravenous infusion (maintenance)**

Neonate initially 1 mg/kg *by intravenous injection* over 2–5 minutes, followed if necessary *by continuous intravenous infusion* of 200 micrograms/kg/hour with careful blood pressure monitoring; doses above 300 micrograms/kg/hour associated with cardiotoxicity and renal failure

• **By endotracheal administration**

Neonate 200 micrograms/kg

Administration For *continuous intravenous infusion* dilute with glucose 5% *or* sodium chloride 0.9% intravenous infusion. Prepare a fresh solution every 24 hours.

For *endotracheal administration* dilute with 0.5–1 mL of sodium chloride 0.9% solution for injection

Tolazoline (Non-proprietary)
Injection, tolazoline 25 mg/mL
Available from 'special-order' manufacturers or specialist importing companies, see p. 943

2.5.2 Centrally acting antihypertensive drugs

Methyldopa, a centrally acting antihypertensive, is of little value in the management of refractory sustained hypertension in infants and children. On prolonged use it is associated with fluid retention (which may be alleviated by concomitant use of diuretics).

Methyldopa is effective for the management of hypertension in pregnancy.

Clonidine is also a centrally acting antihypertensive but has the disadvantage that sudden withdrawal may cause a hypertensive crisis. Clonidine is also used under specialist supervision for pain management, sedation, and opioid withdrawal, attention deficit hyperactivity disorder, and Tourette syndrome.

2 Cardiovascular system

◾ CLONIDINE HYDROCHLORIDE ◿

Cautions must be withdrawn gradually to avoid hypertensive crisis; Raynaud's syndrome or other occlusive peripheral vascular disease; history of depression; avoid in acute porphyria (section 9.8.2); **interactions:** Appendix 1 (clonidine)
Skilled tasks Drowsiness may affect performance of skilled tasks (e.g. driving); effects of alcohol may be enhanced

Pregnancy may lower fetal heart rate, but risk to fetus should be balanced against risk of uncontrolled maternal hypertension; avoid intravenous injection

Breast-feeding present in milk—manufacturer advises avoid

Side-effects dry mouth, sedation, depression, fluid retention, bradycardia, Raynaud's phenomenon, headache, dizziness, euphoria, nocturnal unrest, rash, nausea, constipation, rarely impotence

Licensed use not licensed for use in children

Indication and dose

Severe hypertension
• **By mouth**

Child 2–18 years initially 0.5–1 microgram/kg 3 times daily, increased gradually if necessary; max. 25 micrograms/kg daily in divided doses (not exceeding 1.2 mg daily)

• **By slow intravenous injection**

Child 2–18 years 2–6 micrograms/kg (max. 300 micrograms) as a single dose

Administration For *intravenous injection* give over 10–15 minutes; compatible with sodium chloride 0.9% *or* glucose 5% intravenous infusion.

For administration *by mouth* tablets may be crushed and dissolved in water

Catapres® (Boehringer Ingelheim) ℞ ◿
Tablets, scored, clonidine hydrochloride 100 micrograms, net price 100-tab pack = £5.60; 300 micrograms, 100-tab pack = £13.04. Label: 3, 8

Injection, clonidine hydrochloride 150 micrograms/mL, net price 1-mL amp = 29p

◿Extemporaneous formulations available see Extemporaneous Preparations, p. 8

◾ METHYLDOPA

Cautions withdraw treatment gradually; monitor blood counts and liver-function before treatment and at intervals during first 6–12 weeks *or* if

unexplained fever occurs; history of depression; positive direct Coombs' test in up to 20% of patients (may affect blood cross-matching); inter-

◁ **METHYLDOPA** (*continued*)

ference with laboratory tests; **interactions:**
Appendix 1 (methyldopa)
Skilled tasks Drowsiness may affect performance of
skilled tasks (e.g. driving); effects of alcohol may be
enhanced

Hepatic impairment manufacturer advises caution in history of liver disease; avoid in active liver disease

Renal impairment start with small dose; increased sensitivity to hypotensive and sedative effect

Pregnancy not known to be harmful

Breast-feeding amount too small to be harmful

Contra-indications depression, active liver disease, phaeochromocytoma; acute porphyria (section 9.8.2)

Side-effects gastro-intestinal disturbances, dry mouth, stomatitis, sialadenitis; bradycardia, postural hypotension, oedema; sedation, headache, dizziness, asthenia, myalgia, arthralgia, paraesthesia, nightmares, mild psychosis, depression, impaired mental acuity, parkinsonism, Bell's palsy; hepatitis, jaundice; pancreatitis; haemolytic anaemia; bone-marrow depression, leucopenia, thrombocytopenia, eosinophilia; hypersensitivity reactions including lupus erythematosus-like syndrome, drug fever, myocarditis, pericarditis; rashes (including toxic epi-

dermal necrolysis); nasal congestion, failure of ejaculation, impotence, decreased libido, gynaecomastia, hyperprolactinaemia, amenorrhoea

Indication and dose

Refractory hypertension (but see notes above)

• **By mouth**

Child 1 month–12 years initially 2.5 mg/kg 3 times daily, increased as necessary at intervals of at least 2 days to max. 65 mg/kg daily (not exceeding 3 g daily)

Child 12–18 years initially 250 mg 2–3 times daily increased as necessary at intervals of at least 2 days to max. 3 g daily

Methyldopa (Non-proprietary) ⒫ⓄⓂ
Tablets, coated, methyldopa (anhydrous) 125 mg, net price 56 tab pack = £13.60; 250 mg, 56 tab pack = £8.36; 500 mg, 56 tab pack = £12.78. Label: 3, 8

Aldomet® (MSD) ⒫ⓄⓂ
Tablets, yellow, f/c, methyldopa (anhydrous) 250 mg, net price 60 = £1.88; 500 mg, 30 = £1.90. Label: 3, 8

◢Extemporaneous formulations available see Extemporaneous Preparations, p. 8

2.5.3 Adrenergic neurone blocking drugs

Adrenergic neurone blocking drugs prevent the release of noradrenaline from postganglionic adrenergic neurones. These drugs do not control supine blood pressure and may cause postural hypotension. For this reason they have largely fallen from use in adults and are rarely used in children.

2.5.4 Alpha-adrenoceptor blocking drugs

Doxazosin and **prazosin** have post-synaptic alpha-blocking and vasodilator properties and rarely cause tachycardia. They can, however, reduce blood pressure rapidly after the first dose and should be introduced with caution.

Alpha-blockers can be used with other antihypertensive drugs in the treatment of resistant hypertension.

◢ DOXAZOSIN

Cautions care with initial dose (postural hypotension); cataract surgery (risk of intra-operative floppy iris syndrome); susceptibility to heart failure; **interactions:** Appendix 1 (alpha-blockers)
Driving May affect performance of skilled tasks e.g. driving

Hepatic impairment no information available—manufacturer advises caution

Pregnancy no evidence of teratogenicity, manufacturer advises use only when potential benefit outweighs risk

Breast-feeding accumulates in milk in *animal* studies—manufacturer advises avoid

Side-effects gastro-intestinal disturbances; oedema, hypotension, postural hypotension; dyspnoea, rhinitis, coughing; asthenia, fatigue, vertigo, dizziness, headache, paraesthesia, sleep disturbance, anxiety, depression; respiratory-tract infection, urinary-tract infection, influenza-like symptoms; back pain, myalgia; *less commonly* weight changes, flushing, hypoaesthesia, syn-

cope, tremor, agitation, micturition disturbances, impotence, epistaxis, arthralgia, tinnitus, hypersensitivity reactions (including pruritus, purpura, rash), alopecia; *very rarely* cholestasis, hepatitis, jaundice, bronchospasm, gynaecomastia, priapism, abnormal ejaculation, leucopenia, thrombocytopenia, blurred vision

Licensed use not licensed for use in children

Indication and dose

Hypertension (see notes above)

• **By mouth**

Child 6–12 years 500 micrograms once daily, increased at 1-week intervals to 2–4 mg daily

Child 12–18 years 1 mg daily, increased after 1–2 weeks to 2 mg once daily, and thereafter to 4 mg once daily if necessary; usual max. 4 mg daily (rarely up to 16 mg daily may be required)

Dysfunctional voiding section 7.4.1

2 Cardiovascular system

◻ **DOXAZOSIN** (*continued*)

Doxazosin (Non-proprietary) `PoM`
Tablets, doxazosin (as mesilate) 1 mg, net price 28-tab pack = 93p; 2 mg, 28-tab pack = 97p; 4 mg, 28-tab pack = £1.42. Counselling, driving
Brands include *Doxadura*®

Cardura® (Pfizer) `PoM`
Tablets, doxazosin (as mesilate) 1 mg, net price 28-tab pack = £10.56; 2 mg, 28-tab pack = £14.08. Counselling, driving

◢ Extemporaneous formulations available see Extemporaneous Preparations, p. 8

◢ **Modified-release**
Note Children stabilised on immediate-release doxazosin can be transferred to the equivalent dose of modified-release doxazosin

Doxazosin (Non-proprietary) `PoM`
Tablets, m/r, doxazosin (as mesilate) 4 mg, net price 28-tab pack = £6.33. Label: 25, counselling, driving
Brands include *Doxadura*® XL, *Slocinx*® XL

Cardura® **XL** (Pfizer) `PoM`
Tablets, m/r, doxazosin (as mesilate) 4 mg, net price 28-tab pack = £6.33; 8 mg, 28-tab pack = £12.67. Label: 25, counselling, driving

---

◢ **PRAZOSIN**

Cautions first dose may cause collapse due to hypotension (therefore should be taken on retiring to bed); **interactions:** Appendix 1 (alpha-blockers)

Hepatic impairment start with low doses and adjust according to response

Renal impairment start with low doses in moderate to severe impairment; increase with caution

Pregnancy no evidence of teratogenicity; manufacturer advises use only when potential benefit outweighs risk

Breast-feeding present in milk; manufacturer advises use with caution

Contra-indications not recommended for congestive heart failure due to mechanical obstruction (e.g. aortic stenosis)

Side-effects gastro-intestinal disturbances; postural hypotension, oedema, palpitation; dyspnoea, nasal congestion; drowsiness, headache, depression, nervousness, vertigo; urinary frequency; weakness; blurred vision; *less commonly* tachycardia, insomnia, paraesthesia, sweating, impotence, arthralgia, eye disorders, tinnitus, epistaxis, allergic reactions including rash, pruritus, and urticaria; *rarely* pancreatitis, flushing, vasculitis, bradycardia, hallucinations, worsening of narcolepsy, gynaecomastia, priapism, urinary incontinence, and alopecia

Licensed use not licensed for use in children under 12 years

Indication and dose

Hypertension (see notes above)
• **By mouth**
Child 1 month–12 years 10–15 micrograms/kg 2–4 times daily (initial dose at bedtime) increa-sed gradually to max. 500 micrograms/kg daily in divided doses (not exceeding 20 mg daily)

Child 12–18 years 500 micrograms 2–3 times daily (initial dose at bedtime), increased after 3–7 days to 1 mg 2–3 times daily for a further 3–7 days; further increased gradually if necessary to max. 20 mg daily in divided doses

Congestive heart failure (but rarely used, see section 2.2)
• **By mouth**
Child 1 month–12 years 5 micrograms/kg twice daily (initial dose at bedtime), increased gradually to max. 100 micrograms/kg daily in divided doses

Child 12–18 years 500 micrograms 2–4 times daily (initial dose at bedtime), increasing to 4 mg daily in divided doses; maintenance 4–20 mg daily in divided doses

Administration For *oral* administration tablets may be dispersed in water

Prazosin (Non-proprietary) `PoM`
Tablets, prazosin (as hydrochloride) 500 micrograms, net price 56-tab pack = £2.51; 1 mg, 56-tab pack = £3.23; 2 mg, 56-tab pack = £4.39; 5 mg, 56-tab pack = £8.75. Label: 3, counselling, initial dose

Hypovase® (Pfizer) `PoM`
Tablets, prazosin (as hydrochloride) 500 micrograms, net price 60-tab pack = £2.69; 1 mg, scored, 60-tab pack = £3.46. Label: 3, counselling, initial dose

2

Cardiovascular system

Phaeochromocytoma

Long-term management of phaeochromocytoma involves surgery. However, surgery should not take place until there is adequate blockade of both alpha- and beta-adrenoceptors. Alpha-blockers are used in the short-term management of hypertensive episodes in phaeochromocytoma. Once alpha blockade is established, tachycardia can be controlled by the cautious addition of a beta-blocker (section 2.4); a cardioselective beta-blocker is preferred. There is no nationwide consensus on the optimal drug regimen or doses used for the management of phaeochromocytoma.

Phenoxybenzamine, a powerful alpha-blocker, is effective in the management of phaeochromocytoma but it has many side-effects. Phenoxybenzamine has also been used to treat severe shock in the presence of adequate circulating blood volume, and to lower systemic vascular resistance after cardiac surgery.

PHENOXYBENZAMINE HYDROCHLORIDE

Cautions congestive heart failure; severe heart disease (see also Contra-indications); cerebrovascular disease (avoid if history of cerebrovascular accident); carcinogenic in *animals*; avoid in acute porphyria (section 9.8.2); avoid infusion in hypovolaemia; avoid extravasation (irritant to tissues); avoid contact with skin (risk of contact sensitisation)

Renal impairment use with caution

Pregnancy hypotension in newborn may occur—use with caution

Breast-feeding may be present in milk

Contra-indications history of cerebrovascular accident

Side-effects postural hypotension with dizziness and marked compensatory tachycardia, lassitude, nasal congestion, miosis, inhibition of ejaculation; rarely gastro-intestinal disturbances; decreased sweating and dry mouth after intravenous infusion; idiosyncratic profound hypotension within few minutes of starting infusion

Licensed use not licensed for use in children

Indication and dose

Hypertension in phaeochromocytoma
• By mouth
  Child 1 month–18 years 0.5–1 mg/kg twice daily adjusted according to response

• By intravenous infusion
  Child 1 month–18 years 0.5–1 mg/kg daily adjusted according to response; occasionally up to 2 mg/kg daily may be required; do not repeat dose within 24 hours

Severe shock following cardiac surgery
• By intravenous infusion
  Child 1 month–18 years initially 1 mg/kg then if necessary 500 micrograms/kg every 8–12 hours adjusted according to response

Administration for administration *by mouth*, capsules may be opened; for *intravenous infusion*, dilute with Sodium Chloride 0.9% and give over at least 2 hours; max. 4 hours between dilution and completion of infusion

Phenoxybenzamine (Goldshield) [PoM]
Injection concentrate, phenoxybenzamine hydrochloride 50 mg/mL. To be diluted before use. Net price 2-mL amp = £57.14 (hosp. only)

Dibenyline® (Goldshield) [PoM]
Capsules, red/white, phenoxybenzamine hydrochloride 10 mg. Net price 30-cap pack = £10.84
Note May be difficult to obtain

2.5.5 Drugs affecting the renin-angiotensin system

2.5.5.1 Angiotensin-converting enzyme inhibitors
2.5.5.2 Angiotensin-II receptor antagonists

2.5.5.1 Angiotensin-converting enzyme inhibitors

Angiotensin-converting enzyme inhibitors (ACE inhibitors) inhibit the conversion of angiotensin I to angiotensin II. The main indications of ACE inhibitors in children are shown below. In infants and young children, captopril is often considered first.

Initiation under specialist supervision Treatment with ACE inhibitors should be initiated under specialist supervision and with careful clinical monitoring in children.

Heart failure ACE inhibitors have a valuable role in all grades of heart failure, usually combined with a loop diuretic (section 2.2). Potassium supplements and potassium-sparing diuretics should be discontinued before introducing an ACE inhibitor because of the risk of hyperkalaemia. In adults, a low dose of spironolactone may be beneficial in severe heart failure and can be used with an ACE inhibitor provided serum potassium is monitored carefully. Profound first-dose hypotension can occur when ACE inhibitors are introduced to children with heart failure who are already taking a high dose of a loop diuretic (see Cautions below). Temporary withdrawal of the loop diuretic reduces the risk, but can cause severe rebound pulmonary oedema.

Hypertension   ACE inhibitors may be considered for hypertension when thiazides and beta-blockers are contra-indicated, not tolerated, or fail to control blood pressure; they may be considered for hypertension in children with type 1 diabetes with nephropathy (see also section 6.1.5). ACE inhibitors can reduce blood pressure very rapidly in some patients particularly in those receiving diuretic therapy (see Cautions, below); the first dose should preferably be given at bedtime.

Diabetic nephropathy   For comment on the role of ACE inhibitors in the management of diabetic nephropathy, see section 6.1.5.

Renal effects   Renal function and electrolytes should be checked before starting ACE inhibitors (or increasing the dose) and monitored during treatment (more frequently if features mentioned below are present). Hyperkalaemia and other side-effects of ACE inhibitors are more common in children with impaired renal function and the dose may need to be reduced (see under individual drugs).

Concomitant treatment with NSAIDs increases the risk of renal damage, and potassium-sparing diuretics (or potassium-containing salt substitutes) increase the risk of hyperkalaemia.

In children with severe bilateral renal artery stenosis (or severe stenosis of the artery supplying a single functioning kidney), ACE inhibitors reduce or abolish glomerular filtration and are likely to cause severe and progressive renal failure. They are therefore contra-indicated in children known to have these forms of critical renovascular disease.

ACE inhibitor treatment is unlikely to have an adverse effect on overall renal function in children with severe unilateral renal artery stenosis and a normal contralateral kidney, but glomerular filtration is likely to be reduced (or even abolished) in the affected kidney and the long-term consequences are unknown.

ACE inhibitors are therefore best avoided in those with known or suspected renovascular disease, unless the blood pressure cannot be controlled by other drugs. If they are used in these circumstances renal function needs to be monitored.

ACE inhibitors should also be used with particular caution in children who have undiagnosed and clinically silent renovascular disease. ACE inhibitors are useful for the management of hypertension and proteinuria in children with nephritis. They are thought to have a beneficial effect by reducing intra-glomerular hypertension and protecting the glomerular capillaries and membrane.

Cautions   ACE inhibitors need to be initiated with care in children receiving diuretics (**important**: see Concomitant diuretics, below); first doses can cause hypotension especially in children taking high doses of diuretics, on a low-sodium diet, on dialysis, dehydrated or with heart failure (see above). Discontinue if marked elevation of hepatic enzymes or jaundice (risk of hepatic necrosis). Renal function should be monitored before and during treatment, and the dose reduced in renal impairment (see also above and under individual drugs). For use in known renovascular disease, see Renal Effects above. The risk of agranulocytosis is possibly increased in collagen vascular disease (blood counts recommended). ACE inhibitors should be used with care in children with severe or symptomatic aortic stenosis (risk of hypotension) and in hypertrophic cardiomyopathy. They should be used with care (or avoided) in those with a history of idiopathic or hereditary angioedema. Children with primary aldosteronism and Afro-Caribbean children may respond less well to ACE inhibitors. **Interactions**: Appendix 1 (ACE inhibitors).

Anaphylactoid reactions To prevent anaphylactoid reactions, ACE inhibitors should be avoided during dialysis with high-flux polyacrylonitrile membranes and during low-density lipoprotein apheresis with dextran sulphate; they should also be withheld before desensitisation with wasp or bee venom

Concomitant diuretics   ACE inhibitors can cause a very rapid fall in blood pressure in volume-depleted children; treatment should therefore be initiated with very low doses. In some children the diuretic dose may need to be reduced or the diuretic discontinued at least 24 hours beforehand (may not be possible in heart failure—risk of pulmonary oedema). If high-dose diuretic therapy cannot be stopped, close observation is recommended after administration of the first dose of ACE inhibitor, for at least 2 hours or until the blood pressure has stabilised.

Contra-indications   ACE inhibitors are contra-indicated in children with hyper-sensitivity to ACE inhibitors (including angioedema) and in bilateral renovascular disease (see also above). ACE inhibitors should not be used in pregnancy unless essential—they may adversely affect fetal and neonatal blood pressure control and renal function, and possibly cause skull defects and oligohydramnios; toxicity in *animal* studies has been reported.

Side-effects   ACE inhibitors can cause profound hypotension (see Cautions), renal impairment (see Renal effects above), and a persistent dry cough. They can also cause angioedema (onset may be delayed; higher incidence reported in Afro-Caribbean patients), rash (which may be associated with pruritus and urticaria), pancreatitis, and upper respiratory-tract symptoms such as sinusitis, rhinitis, and sore throat. Gastro-intestinal effects reported with ACE inhibitors include nausea, vomiting, dyspepsia, diarrhoea, constipation, and abdominal pain. Altered liver function tests, cholestatic jaundice, hepatitis, fulminant hepatic necrosis, and hepatic failure have been reported—discontinue if marked elevation of hepatic enzymes or jaundice. Hyperkalaemia, hypoglycaemia and blood disorders including thrombocytopenia, leucopenia, neutropenia, and haemolytic anaemia have also been reported. Other reported side-effects include headache, dizziness, fatigue, malaise, taste disturbance, paraesthesia, bronchospasm, fever, serositis, vasculitis, myalgia, arthralgia, positive antinuclear antibody, raised erythrocyte sedimentation rate, eosinophilia, leucocytosis, and photosensitivity.

Neonates   The neonatal response to treatment with ACE inhibitors is very variable, and some neonates develop profound hypotension with even small doses; a test-dose should be used initially and increased cautiously. Adverse effects such as apnoea, seizures, renal failure, and severe unpredictable hypotension are very common in the first month of life and it is therefore recommended that ACE inhibitors are avoided whenever possible, particularly in preterm neonates.

◢ CAPTOPRIL

Cautions see notes above; acute porphyria (section 9.8.2)

Renal impairment see notes above; start with low dose and adjust according to response

Breast-feeding avoid in first few weeks after delivery—risk of profound neonatal hypotension; can be used in older infant if essential but monitor infant's blood pressure

Contra-indications see notes above

Pregnancy avoid unless essential (see notes above)

Side-effects see notes above; tachycardia, serum sickness, weight loss, stomatitis, maculopapular rash, photosensitivity, flushing and acidosis

Licensed use not licensed for use in children under 18 years

Indication and dose

Hypertension, heart failure, proteinuria in nephritis (under specialist supervision)
- **By mouth**

  Neonate (caution, see neonatal information above) test dose, 10–50 micrograms/kg (10 micrograms/kg in neonate less than 37 weeks post-menstrual age), monitor blood pressure carefully for 1–2 hours; if tolerated give 10–50 micrograms/kg 2–3 times daily increased as necessary to max. 2 mg/kg daily in divided doses (max. 300 micrograms/kg daily in divided doses in neonate less than 37 weeks post-menstrual age)

  Child 1 month–12 years test dose, 100 micrograms/kg (max. 6.25 mg), monitor blood pressure carefully for 1–2 hours; if tolerated give 100–300 micrograms/kg 2–3 times a day, increased as necessary to max. 6 mg/kg daily in divided doses (max. 4 mg/kg daily in divided doses for child 1 month–1 year)

  Child 12–18 years test dose, 100 micrograms/kg or 6.25 mg, monitor blood pressure carefully for 1–2 hours; if tolerated give 12.5–25 mg 2–3 times a day, increased as necessary to max. 150 mg daily in divided doses

Diabetic nephropathy (under specialist supervision)
- **By mouth**

  Child 12–18 years test dose, 100 micrograms/kg or 6.25 mg, monitor blood pressure carefully for 1–2 hours; if tolerated, give 12.5–25 mg 2–3 times a day, increased as necessary to max. 150 mg daily in divided doses

Administration Administer under close supervision, see notes above. Give test dose whilst child supine. Tablets can be dispersed in water

Captopril (Non-proprietary) ℗⚪ℳ
Tablets, captopril 12.5 mg, net price 56-tab pack = £1.59; 25 mg, 56-tab pack = £1.70; 50 mg, 56-tab pack = £2.22
Brands include *Ecopace®*, *Kaplon®*, *Tensopril®*

Liquid, various strengths available from 'special-order' manufacturers or specialist importing companies, see p. 943

◁ **CAPTOPRIL** *(continued)*

Capoten® (Squibb) PoM
Tablets, captopril 12.5 mg (scored), net price 56-tab pack = £9.82; 25 mg, 56-tab pack = £11.19, 50 mg (scored), 56-tab pack = £19.07 (also available as *Acepril®*)

◢ Extemporaneous formulations available see Extemporaneous Preparations, p. 8

ENALAPRIL MALEATE

Cautions see notes above

Hepatic impairment monitor closely

Renal impairment see notes above; start with low dose and adjust according to response

Breast-feeding avoid in first few weeks after delivery—risk of profound neonatal hypotension; can be used in older infant if essential but monitor infant's blood pressure

Contra-indications see notes above

Pregnancy avoid unless essential (see notes above)

Side-effects see notes above; also dyspnoea; depression, asthenia; blurred vision; *less commonly* dry mouth, peptic ulcer, anorexia, ileus; arrhythmias, palpitation, flushing; confusion, nervousness, drowsiness, insomnia, vertigo; impotence; muscle cramps; tinnitus; alopecia, sweating; hyponatraemia; *rarely* stomatitis, glossitis, Raynaud's syndrome, pulmonary infiltrates, allergic alveolitis, abnormal dreams, gynaecomastia, Stevens-Johnson syndrome, toxic epidermal necrolysis, exfoliative dermatitis, pemphigus; *very rarely* gastro-intestinal angio-edema

Licensed use not licensed for use in children for congestive heart failure, proteinuria in nephritis or diabetic nephropathy; not licensed for use in children less than 20 kg for hypertension

Indication and dose

Hypertension, congestive heart failure, proteinuria in nephritis (under specialist supervision)
• **By mouth**

Neonate (limited information) initially 10 micrograms/kg once daily, monitor blood pressure carefully for 1–2 hours, increased as necessary up to 500 micrograms/kg daily in 1–3 divided doses

Child 1 month–12 years initially 100 micrograms/kg once daily, monitor blood pressure carefully for 1–2 hours, increased as necessary up to max. 1 mg/kg daily in 1–2 divided doses

Child 12–18 years initially 2.5 mg once daily, monitor blood pressure carefully for 1–2 hours, usual maintenance dose 10–20 mg daily in 1–2 divided doses; max. 40 mg daily in 1–2 divided doses if body-weight over 50 kg

Diabetic nephropathy (under specialist supervision)
• **By mouth**

Child 12–18 years initially 2.5 mg once daily, monitor blood pressure carefully for 1–2 hours, usual maintenance dose 10–20 mg daily in 1–2 divided doses; max. 40 mg daily in 1–2 divided doses if body-weight over 50 kg

Administration Tablets may be crushed and suspended in water immediately before use

Enalapril Maleate (Non-proprietary) PoM
Tablets, enalapril maleate 2.5 mg, net price 28-tab pack = £1.31; 5 mg, 28-tab pack = £1.10; 10 mg, 28-tab pack = £1.12; 20 mg, 28-tab pack = £1.22
Brands include *Ednyt®*

Liquid, various strengths available from 'special-order' manufacturers or specialist importing companies, see p. 943

Innovace® (MSD) PoM
Tablets, enalapril maleate 2.5 mg, net price 28-tab pack = £5.35; 5 mg (scored), 28-tab pack = £7.51; 10 mg (red), 28-tab pack = £10.53; 20 mg (peach), 28-tab pack = £12.51

LISINOPRIL

Cautions see notes above

Renal impairment see notes above; start with low dose and adjust according to response

Breast-feeding avoid—no information available

Contra-indications see notes above

Pregnancy avoid unless essential (see notes above)

Side-effects see notes above; also *less commonly* tachycardia, palpitation, cerebrovascular accident, Raynaud's syndrome, confusion, mood changes, vertigo, sleep disturbances, asthenia, impotence; *rarely* dry mouth, gynaecomastia, alopecia, psoriasis; *very rarely* allergic alveolitis, pulmonary infiltrates, profuse sweating, pemphi-gus, Stevens-Johnson syndrome, and toxic epidermal necrolysis

Licensed use not licensed for use in children

Indication and dose

Hypertension (under specialist supervision)

Child 6–12 years initially 70 micrograms/kg (max. 5 mg) once daily, increased in intervals of 1–2 weeks to max. 600 micrograms/kg (*or* 40 mg) once daily

Child 12–18 years initially 2.5 mg once daily; usual maintenance dose 10–20 mg once daily; max. 80 mg once daily

2

Cardiovascular system

◁ **LISINOPRIL** (*continued*)

Heart failure (adjunct) (under specialist supervision)

Child 12–18 years initially 2.5 mg once daily; increased in steps no greater than 10 mg at intervals of at least 2 weeks up to max. 35 mg once daily if tolerated

Lisinopril (Non-proprietary) ℞
Tablets, lisinopril (as dihydrate) 2.5 mg, net price 28-tab pack = 91p; 5 mg, 28-tab pack = £1.02; 10 mg, 28-tab pack = £1.10; 20 mg, 28-tab pack = £1.37

Liquid, various strengths available from 'special-order' manufacturers or specialist importing companies, see p. 943

Carace® (Bristol-Myers Squibb) ℞
Tablets, lisinopril 5 mg (scored), net price 28-tab pack = £8.51; 10 mg (yellow, scored), 28-tab pack = £10.51; 20 mg (orange, scored), 28-tab pack = £11.89

Zestril® (AstraZeneca) ℞
Tablets, lisinopril (as dihydrate) 2.5 mg, net price 28-tab pack = £6.26; 5 mg (pink), 28-tab pack = £7.86; 10 mg (pink), 28-tab pack = £9.70; 20 mg (pink), 28-tab pack = £10.97

◢ Extemporaneous formulations available see Extemporaneous Preparations, p. 8

2.5.5.2 Angiotensin-II receptor antagonists

Losartan is a specific angiotensin-II receptor antagonist with many properties similar to those of the ACE inhibitors. However, unlike ACE inhibitors, losartan does not inhibit the breakdown of bradykinin and other kinins, and therefore does not appear to cause the persistent dry cough which commonly complicates ACE inhibitor therapy. It is therefore an alternative for children who have to discontinue an ACE inhibitor because of persistent cough.

Losartan can be used as an alternative to an ACE inhibitor in the management of hypertension; however, evidence for its use in children is very limited.

◢ LOSARTAN POTASSIUM

Cautions renal artery stenosis (see also Renal Effects under ACE inhibitors, section 2.5.5.1); monitor plasma-potassium concentration (particularly in children with renal impairment); aortic or mitral valve stenosis; hypertrophic cardiomyopathy; children with primary aldosteronism and Afro-Caribbean children, particularly those with left ventricular hypertrophy, may not benefit from losartan; **interactions**: Appendix 1 (angiotensin-II receptor antagonists)

Hepatic impairment manufacturer advises avoid in children 6–16 years—no information available; child 17–18 years consider dose reduction in mild to moderate impairment, avoid in severe impairment (no information available)

Renal impairment manufacturer advises avoid in children 6–16 years with estimated glomerular filtration rate less than 30 mL/minute/1.73m²—no information available

Contra-indications

Pregnancy avoid unless essential—may adversely affect fetal and neonatal blood pressure control and renal function; also possible skull defects and oligohydramnios; toxicity in *animal* studies

Breast-feeding avoid—no information available

Side-effects diarrhoea, symptomatic hypotension including dizziness (particularly in children with intravascular volume depletion e.g. those taking high-dose diuretics); cough, asthenia, vertigo, migraine, hyperkalaemia; arthralgia, myalgia; urticaria, pruritus, rash; *rarely* hepatitis, anaemia (in severe renal disease or following renal transplant), thrombocytopenia, vasculitis (including Henoch-Schönlein purpura), anaphylaxis, and angioedema

Licensed use not licensed for use in children

Indication and dose

Hypertension (under specialist supervision)
● **By mouth**

Child 6–16 years
Body-weight 20–50 kg initially 25 mg once daily; adjusted according to response to max. 50 mg once daily

Body-weight 50 kg and over initially 50 mg once daily adjusted according to response to max. 100 mg once daily

Child 16–18 years initially 50 mg once daily (intravascular volume depletion, initially 25 mg once daily); if necessary increased after several weeks to 100 mg once daily

Cozaar® (MSD) ℞
Tablets, f/c, losartan potassium 25 mg, net price 28-tab pack = £16.18; 50 mg (scored), 28-tab pack = £12.80; 100 mg, 28-tab pack = £16.18

2.6 Nitrates, calcium-channel blockers, and other antianginal drugs

2.6.1 Nitrates
2.6.2 Calcium-channel blockers
2.6.3 Other antianginal drugs
2.6.4 Peripheral vasodilators and related drugs

Nitrates and calcium-channel blockers have a vasodilating and, consequently, blood-pressure lowering effect. Vasodilators can act in heart failure by arteriolar dilatation, which reduces both peripheral vascular resistance and left ventricular pressure during systole resulting in improved cardiac output. They can also cause venous dilatation, which results in dilatation of capacitance vessels, increase of venous pooling, and diminution of venous return to the heart (decreasing left ventricular end-diastolic pressure).

2.6.1 Nitrates

Nitrates are potent coronary vasodilators, but their principal benefit follows from a reduction in venous return which reduces left ventricular work. Unwanted effects such as flushing, headache, and postural hypotension may limit therapy, especially if the child is unusually sensitive to the effects of nitrates or is hypovolaemic.

For the use of glyceryl trinitrate in extravasation, see section 10.3.

Children receiving nitrates continuously throughout the day can develop tolerance (with reduced therapeutic effects). Reduction of blood-nitrate concentrations to low levels for 4 to 8 hours each day usually maintains effectiveness in such patients.

GLYCERYL TRINITRATE

Cautions hypothyroidism, malnutrition, hypothermia; head trauma, cerebral haemorrhage; hypoxaemia or other ventilation and perfusion abnormalities; metal-containing transdermal systems should be removed before cardioversion or diathermy; avoid abrupt withdrawal; tolerance (see notes above); **interactions**: Appendix 1 (nitrates)

Hepatic impairment caution in severe hepatic impairment

Renal impairment use with caution in severe impairment

Pregnancy not known to be harmful but most manufacturers advise avoid unless potential benefit outweighs risk

Breast-feeding no information available—manufacturers advise use only if potential benefit outweighs risk

Contra-indications hypersensitivity to nitrates; hypotensive conditions and hypovolaemia; hypertrophic cardiomyopathy, aortic stenosis, cardiac tamponade, constrictive pericarditis, mitral stenosis; marked anaemia, closed-angle glaucoma

Side-effects postural hypotension, tachycardia (but paradoxical bradycardia also reported); throbbing headache, dizziness, *less commonly* nausea, vomiting, heartburn; flushing
Injection Specific side-effects following injection (particularly if given too rapidly) include severe hypotension, diaphoresis, apprehension, restlessness, muscle twitching, retrosternal discomfort, palpitation, abdominal pain, syncope; prolonged administration has been associated with methaemoglobinaemia

Licensed use not licensed for use in children

Indication and dose

Hypertension during and after cardiac surgery, cardiac failure after cardiac surgery, coronary vasoconstriction in myocardial ischaemia, vasoconstriction in shock

- **By continuous intravenous infusion**

  Neonate 0.2–0.5 micrograms/kg/minute, dose adjusted according to response; usual dose 1–3 micrograms/kg/minute; max. 10 micrograms/kg/minute

  Child 1 month–18 years initially 0.2–0.5 micrograms/kg/minute, dose adjusted according to response, usual dose 1–3 micrograms/kg/minute; max. 10 micrograms/kg/minute (do not exceed 200 micrograms/minute)

Administration for *continuous intravenous infusion* dilute to max. concentration of 400 micrograms/mL (but concentration of 1 mg/mL has been used via a central venous catheter) with Glucose 5% or Sodium Chloride 0.9%.

Glass or polyethylene apparatus is preferable; loss of potency will occur if PVC is used.

Neonatal intensive care, dilute 3 mg/kg bodyweight to a final volume of 50 mL with infusion fluid; an intravenous infusion rate of 1 mL/hour provides a dose of 1 microgram/kg/minute

Glyceryl Trinitrate (Non-proprietary) [PoM]
Injection, glyceryl trinitrate 5 mg/mL. To be diluted before use. Net price 5-mL amp = £6.49; 10-mL amp = £12.98
Excipients include ethanol, propylene glycol

2

Cardiovascular system

◁ **GLYCERYL TRINITRATE (continued)**

Nitrocine® (UCB Pharma) PoM
Injection, glyceryl trinitrate 1 mg/mL. To be diluted before use or given undiluted with syringe pump. Net price 10-mL amp = £7.34; 50-mL bottle = £17.21
Excipients include propylene glycol

Nitronal® (Merck) PoM
Injection, glyceryl trinitrate 1 mg/mL. To be diluted before use or given undiluted with syringe pump. Net price 5-mL vial = £1.92; 50-mL vial = £15.67

2.6.2 Calcium-channel blockers

Calcium-channel blockers (less correctly called 'calcium-antagonists') interfere with the inward displacement of calcium ions through the slow channels of active cell membranes. They influence the myocardial cells, the cells within the specialised conducting system of the heart, and the cells of vascular smooth muscle. Thus, myocardial contractility may be reduced, the formation and propagation of electrical impulses within the heart may be depressed, and coronary or systemic vascular tone may be diminished.

Calcium-channel blockers differ in their predilection for the various possible sites of action and, therefore, their therapeutic effects are disparate, with much greater variation than those of beta-blockers. There are important differences between verapamil, diltiazem, and the dihydropyridine calcium-channel blockers (amlodipine, nicardipine, nifedipine, and nimodipine). Verapamil and diltiazem should usually be **avoided** in heart failure because they may further depress cardiac function and cause clinically significant deterioration.

Verapamil is used for the treatment of hypertension (section 2.5) and arrhythmias (section 2.3.2). However, it is no longer first-line treatment for arrhythmias in children because it has been associated with fatal collapse especially in infants under 1 year; adenosine is now recommended for first-line use.

Verapamil is a highly negatively inotropic calcium channel-blocker and it reduces cardiac output, slows the heart rate, and may impair atrioventricular conduction. It may precipitate heart failure, exacerbate conduction disorders, and cause hypotension at high doses and should **not** be used with beta-blockers (see p. 140). Constipation is the most common side-effect.

Nifedipine relaxes vascular smooth muscle and dilates coronary and peripheral arteries. It has more influence on vessels and less on the myocardium than does verapamil, and unlike verapamil has no anti-arrhythmic activity. It rarely precipitates heart failure because any negative inotropic effect is offset by a reduction in left ventricular work. Short-acting formulations of nifedipine are not recommended for long-term management of hypertension; their use may be associated with large variations in blood pressure and reflex tachycardia. However, they may be used if a modified-release preparation delivering the appropriate dose is not available or if a child is unable to swallow (a liquid preparation may be prepared using capsules). Nifedipine may also be used for the management of angina due to coronary artery disease in Kawasaki disease or progeria and in the management of Raynaud's syndrome.

Nicardipine has similar effects to those of nifedipine and may produce less reduction of myocardial contractility; it is used to treat hypertensive crisis.

Amlodipine also resembles nifedipine and nicardipine in its effects and does not reduce myocardial contractility or produce clinical deterioration in heart failure. It has a longer duration of action and can be given once daily. Nifedipine and amlodipine are used for the treatment of hypertension. Side-effects associated with vasodilatation such as flushing and headache (which become less obtrusive after a few days), and ankle swelling (which may respond only partially to diuretics) are common.

Nimodipine is related to nifedipine but the smooth muscle relaxant effect preferentially acts on cerebral arteries. Its use is confined to prevention and treatment of vascular spasm following aneurysmal subarachnoid haemorrhage.

Diltiazem is a peripheral vasodilator and also has mild depressor effects on the myocardium. It is used in the treatment of Raynaud's syndrome.

Withdrawal There is some evidence that sudden withdrawal of calcium-channel blockers may be associated with an exacerbation of myocardial ischaemia.

▲ AMLODIPINE

Cautions interactions: Appendix 1 (calcium-channel blockers)

Hepatic impairment half-life prolonged—may need dose reduction

Pregnancy no information available—manufacturer advises avoid, but risk to fetus should be balanced against risk of uncontrolled maternal hypertension

Breast-feeding no information available—manufacturer advises avoid

Contra-indications cardiogenic shock, significant aortic stenosis, acute porphyria (section 9.8.2)

Side-effects abdominal pain, nausea; palpitation, flushing, oedema; headache, dizziness, sleep disturbances, fatigue; *less commonly* gastro-intestinal disturbances, dry mouth, taste disturbances, hypotension, syncope, chest pain, dyspnoea, rhinitis, mood changes, asthenia, tremor, paraesthesia, urinary disturbances, impotence, gynaecomastia, weight changes, myalgia, muscle cramps, back pain, arthralgia, visual disturbances, tinnitus, pruritus, rashes (including isolated reports of erythema multiforme), sweating, alopecia, purpura, and skin discolouration; *very rarely* gastritis, pancreatitis, hepatitis, jaundice, cholestasis, gingival hyperplasia, myocardial infarction, arrhythmias, tachycardia, vasculitis, coughing, peripheral neuropathy, hyperglycaemia, thrombocytopenia, angioedema, and urticaria

Licensed use not licensed for use in children

Indication and dose

Hypertension
• By mouth

Child 1 month–12 years initially 100–200 micrograms/kg once daily; if necessary increase at intervals of 1–2 weeks up to 400 micrograms/kg once daily; max. 10 mg once daily

Child 12–18 years initially 5 mg once daily; if necessary increase at intervals of 1–2 weeks to max. 10 mg once daily

Administration Tablets may be dispersed in water

Note Tablets from various suppliers may contain different salts (e.g. amlodipine besilate, amlodipine maleate, and amlodipine mesilate) but the strength is expressed in terms of amlodipine (base); tablets containing different salts are considered interchangeable

Amlodipine (Non-proprietary) ℗ⓞ𝐌

Tablets, amlodipine (as maleate or as mesilate) 5 mg, net price 28-tab pack = £1.12; 10 mg, 28-tab pack = £1.29

Brands include Amlostin®

Istin® (Pfizer) ℗ⓞ𝐌

Tablets, amlodipine (as besilate) 5 mg, net price 28-tab pack = £13.04; 10 mg, 28-tab pack = £19.47

◢ Extemporaneous formulations available see Extemporaneous Preparations, p. 8

▲ DILTIAZEM HYDROCHLORIDE

Cautions heart failure or significantly impaired left ventricular function, bradycardia (avoid if severe), first degree AV block, or prolonged PR interval; **interactions:** Appendix 1 (calcium-channel blockers)

Hepatic impairment reduce dose

Renal impairment start with smaller dose

Breast-feeding significant amount present in milk—no evidence of harm but avoid unless no safer alternative

Contra-indications severe bradycardia, left ventricular failure with pulmonary congestion, second- or third-degree AV block (unless pacemaker fitted), sick sinus syndrome, acute porphyria (but see section 9.8.2)

Pregnancy avoid

Side-effects bradycardia, sino-atrial block, AV block, palpitation, dizziness, hypotension, malaise, asthenia, headache, hot flushes, gastro-intestinal disturbances, oedema (notably of ankles); rarely rashes (including erythema multiforme and exfoliative dermatitis), photosensitivity; hepatitis, gynaecomastia, gum hyperplasia, extrapyramidal symptoms, depression reported

Licensed use not licensed for use in children

Indication and dose

Raynaud's syndrome
• By mouth

Child 12–18 years 30–60 mg 2–3 times daily

◢ Standard formulations

Note These formulations are licensed as generics and there is no requirement for brand name dispensing. Although their means of formulation has called for the strict designation 'modified-release' their duration of action corresponds to that of tablets requiring administration more frequently

Diltiazem (Non-proprietary) ℗ⓞ𝐌

Tablets, m/r (but see note above), diltiazem hydrochloride 60 mg, net price 84 = £3.34. Label: 25

Brands include *Optil®*

Tildiem® (Sanofi-Synthelabo) ℗ⓞ𝐌

Tablets, m/r (but see note above), off-white, diltiazem hydrochloride 60 mg, net price 90-tab pack = £8.28. Label: 25

▲ NICARDIPINE HYDROCHLORIDE

Cautions congestive heart failure or significantly impaired left ventricular function; avoid grapefruit juice (may affect metabolism); **interactions:** Appendix 1 (calcium-channel blockers)

Hepatic impairment reduce dose

Renal impairment start with smaller dose

Pregnancy may inhibit labour; toxicity in *animal* studies; manufacturer advises avoid, but risk to

2

Cardiovascular system

◁ NICARDIPINE HYDROCHLORIDE (*continued*)

fetus should be balanced against risk of uncontrolled maternal hypertension

Contra-indications cardiogenic shock; advanced aortic stenosis; acute porphyria (section 9.8.2)

Breast-feeding no information available—manufacturer advises avoid

Side-effects dizziness, headache, peripheral oedema, flushing, palpitation, nausea; also gastro-intestinal disturbances, drowsiness, insomnia, tinnitus, hypotension, rashes, dyspnoea, paraesthesia, frequency of micturition; thrombocytopenia, depression and impotence reported

Licensed use not licensed for use in children

Indication and dose

Hypertensive crisis
• By continuous intravenous infusion

Neonate initially 500 nanograms/kg/minute, adjusted according to response; usual maintenance of 1–4 micrograms/kg/minute

Child 1 month–18 years initially 500 nanograms/kg/minute, adjusted according to response; usual maintenance of 1–4 micrograms/kg/minute (max. 250 micrograms/minute)

Administration for *intravenous infusion*, dilute to a concentration of 100 micrograms/mL with Glucose 5% *or* Sodium Chloride 0.9%; to minimise peripheral venous irritation, change site of infusion every 12 hours

Cardene IV® PoM

Injection, nicardipine 2.5 mg/mL (10-mL ampoule)
Available from 'special-order' manufacturers or specialist importing companies, see p. 943

■ NIFEDIPINE

Cautions see notes above; also poor cardiac reserve; heart failure or significantly impaired left ventricular function (heart failure deterioration observed); severe hypotension; diabetes mellitus; avoid grapefruit juice (may affect metabolism); **interactions:** Appendix 1 (calcium-channel blockers)

Hepatic impairment dose reduction may be required in severe liver disease

Pregnancy may inhibit labour; manufacturer advises avoid before week 20, but risk to fetus should be balanced against risk of uncontrolled maternal hypertension; use only if other treatment options are not indicated or have failed

Breast-feeding amount too small to be harmful but manufacturer advises avoid

Contra-indications cardiogenic shock; advanced aortic stenosis; acute porphyria (section 9.8.2)

Side-effects gastro-intestinal disturbance; hypotension, oedema, vasodilatation, palpitation; headache, dizziness, lethargy, asthenia; *less commonly* tachycardia, hypotension, syncope, chills, nasal congestion, dyspnoea, anxiety, sleep disturbance, vertigo, migraine, paraesthesia, tremor, polyuria, dysuria, nocturia, erectile dysfunction, epistaxis, myalgia, joint swelling, visual disturbance, sweating, and hypersensitivity reactions (including angioedema, jaundice, pruritus, urticaria, and rash); *rarely* anorexia, gum hyperplasia, mood disturbances, hyperglycaemia, male infertility, purpura, and photosensitivity reactions; also reported dysphagia, intestinal obstruction, intestinal ulcer, bezoar formation, gynaecomastia, agranulocytosis, and anaphylaxis

Licensed use not licensed for use in children

Indication and dose

Hypertensive crisis, acute angina in Kawasaki disease or progeria
• By mouth (see Administration, below)

Child 1 month–18 years 250–500 micrograms/kg as a single dose

Hypertension, angina in Kawasaki disease or progeria
• By mouth

Child 1 month–12 years 200–300 micrograms/kg 3 times daily; max. 3 mg/kg daily *or* 90 mg daily

Child 12–18 years 5–20 mg 3 times daily; max. 90 mg daily
Note Dose frequency depends on preparation used

Raynaud's syndrome
• By mouth

Child 2–18 years 2.5–10 mg 2–4 times daily; start with low doses at night and increase gradually to avoid postural hypotension
Note Dose frequency depends on preparation used

Persistent hyperinsulinaemic hypoglycaemia
see also section 6.1.4
• By mouth

Neonates 100–200 micrograms/kg (max. 600 micrograms/kg) 4 times daily

Administration for rapid effect in hypertensive crisis or acute angina, use capsules or use liquid if 5- or 10-mg dose inappropriate; if liquid unavailable, extract contents of capsule via a syringe and use immediately—cover syringe with foil to protect contents from light; capsule contents may be diluted with water if necessary

Modified-release tablets may be crushed—this may alter the release profile; crushed tablets should be administered within 30–60 seconds to avoid significant loss of potency of drug

Nifedipine (Non-proprietary) PoM

Capsules, nifedipine 5 mg, net price 84-cap pack = £2.84; 10 mg, 84-cap pack = £3.94
Dose
Give 3 times daily

◻ **NIFEDIPINE** *(continued)*

Oral liquid, available from 'special-order' manufacturers or specialist importing companies, see p. 943

Adalat® (Bayer) (PoM)
Capsules, orange, nifedipine 5 mg, net price 90-cap pack = £6.08; 10 mg, 90-cap pack = £7.74
Dose
    Give 3 times daily

◀ **Modified release**
Note Different versions of modified-release preparations may not have the same clinical effect. To avoid confusion between these different formulations of nifedipine, prescribers should specify the brand to be dispensed. Modified-release formulations may not be suitable for dose titration in hepatic disease

Adalat® LA (Bayer) (PoM)
LA 20 tablets, m/r, f/c, pink, nifedipine 20 mg, net price 28-tab pack = £5.27. Label: 25
LA 30 tablets, m/r, f/c, pink, nifedipine 30 mg, net price 28-tab pack = £7.59. Label: 25
LA 60 tablets, m/r, f/c, pink, nifedipine 60 mg, net price 28-tab pack = £9.69. Label: 25
Counselling Tablet membrane may pass through gastro-intestinal tract unchanged, but being porous has no effect on efficacy
Cautions dose form not appropriate for use in hepatic impairment or where there is a history of oesophageal or gastro-intestinal obstruction, decreased lumen diameter of the gastro-intestinal tract, or inflammatory bowel disease (including Crohn's disease)
Dose
    Give once daily

Adalat® Retard (Bayer) (PoM)
Retard 10 tablets, m/r, f/c, grey-pink, nifedipine 10 mg, net price 56-tab pack = £8.50. Label: 25
Retard 20 tablets, m/r, f/c, grey-pink, nifedipine 20 mg, net price 56-tab pack = £10.20. Label: 25
Dose
    Give twice daily

Adipine® MR (Chiesi) (PoM)
Tablets, m/r, nifedipine 10 mg (apricot), net price 56-tab pack = £5.96; 20 mg (pink), 56-tab pack = £7.43. Label: 21, 25
Dose
    Give twice daily

Adipine® XL (Chiesi) (PoM)
Tablets, m/r, red, nifedipine 30 mg, net price 28-tab pack = £5.89. Label: 25
Dose
    Give once daily

Coracten SR® (UCB Pharma) (PoM)
Capsules, m/r, nifedipine 10 mg (grey/pink, enclosing yellow pellets), net price 60-cap pack = £4.70; 20 mg (pink/brown, enclosing yellow pellets), 60-cap pack = £6.52. Label: 25
Dose
    Give twice daily

Coracten XL® (UCB Pharma) (PoM)
Capsules, m/r, nifedipine 30 mg (brown), net price 28-cap pack = £5.89; 60 mg (orange), 28-cap pack = £8.84. Label: 25
Dose
    Give once daily

Fortipine LA 40® (Goldshield) (PoM)
Tablets, m/r, nifedipine 40 mg, net price 30-tab pack = £9.60. Label: 21, 25
Dose
    Give 1–2 times daily

Hypolar® Retard 20 (Sandoz) (PoM)
Tablets, m/r, red, f/c, nifedipine 20 mg, net price 56-tab pack = £5.75. Label: 25
Dose
    Give twice daily

Nifedipress® MR (Dexcel) (PoM)
Tablets, m/r, pink, nifedipine 10 mg, net price 56-tab pack = £9.23; 20 mg, 56–tab pack = £10.06. Label: 25
Dose
    Give twice daily
Note Also available as *Calchan®* MR

Tensipine MR® (Genus) (PoM)
Tablets, m/r, pink-grey, nifedipine 10 mg, net price 56-tab pack = £4.30; 20 mg, 56-tab pack = £5.49. Label: 21, 25
Dose
    Give twice daily

Valni XL® (Winthrop) (PoM)
Tablets, m/r, red, nifedipine 30 mg, net price 28-tab pack = £9.89; 60 mg, 28-tab pack = £14.71. Label: 25
Cautions dose form not appropriate for use in hepatic impairment, or where there is a history of oesophageal or gastro-intestinal obstruction, decreased lumen diameter of the gastro-intestinal tract, inflammatory bowel disease, or ileostomy after proctocolectomy
Dose
    Give once daily

2

Cardiovascular system

NIMODIPINE

Cautions cerebral oedema or severely raised intracranial pressure; hypotension; avoid concomitant administration of nimodipine tablets and infusion, other calcium-channel blockers, or beta-blockers; concomitant nephrotoxic drugs; avoid grapefruit juice (may affect metabolism); **interactions**: Appendix 1 (calcium-channel blockers, alcohol (infusion only))

Hepatic impairment elimination reduced in cirrhosis—monitor blood pressure; reduce oral dose by 50% in children with severe cirrhosis

Renal impairment manufacturer advises monitor renal function closely

Pregnancy manufacturer advises use only if potential benefit outweighs risks

Contra-indications acute porphyria (section 9.8.2)

Side-effects hypotension, variation in heart-rate, flushing, headache, gastro-intestinal disorders, nausea, sweating and feeling of warmth; thrombocytopenia and ileus reported

Licensed use not licensed for use in children

Indication and dose

Treatment of vasospasm following subarachnoid haemorrhage under specialist advice only

• By intravenous infusion

Child 1 month–12 years initially 15 micrograms/kg/hour (max. 500 micrograms/hour) or initially 7.5 micrograms/kg/hour if blood pressure unstable; increase after 2 hours to 30 micrograms/kg/hour (max. 2 mg/hour) if no severe decrease in blood pressure; continue for at least 5 days (max. 14 days)

Child 12–18 years initially 500 micrograms/hour (up to 1 mg/hour if body-weight over 70 kg and blood pressure stable), increase after 2 hours to 1–2 mg/hour if no severe fall in blood pressure; continue for at least 5 days (max. 14 days)

Prevention of vasospasm following subarachnoid haemorrhage

• By mouth

Child 1 month–18 years 0.9–1.2 mg/kg (max. 60 mg) 6 times daily, starting within 4 days of haemorrhage and continued for 21 days

Administration for *continuous intravenous infusion*, administer undiluted *via* a Y-piece on a central venous catheter connected to a running infusion of Glucose 5%, Sodium Chloride 0.9%, *or* Compound Sodium Lactate; not to be added to an infusion container; incompatible with polyvinyl chloride giving sets or containers; protect infusion from light.

For administration *by mouth*, tablets may be crushed or halved but are light sensitive—administer immediately

Nimotop® (Bayer) [PoM]
Tablets, yellow, f/c, nimodipine 30 mg, net price 100-tab pack = £38.85

Intravenous infusion, nimodipine 200 micrograms/mL; also contains ethanol 20% and macrogol '400' 17%. Net price 50-mL vial (with polyethylene infusion catheter) = £13.24

Note Polyethylene, polypropylene, or glass apparatus should be used; PVC should be avoided

VERAPAMIL HYDROCHLORIDE

Cautions first-degree AV block; patients taking beta-blockers (**important**: see below); avoid grapefruit juice (may affect metabolism); **interactions**: Appendix 1 (calcium-channel blockers)
Verapamil and beta-blockers Verapamil injection should not be given to patients recently treated with beta-blockers because of the risk of hypotension and asystole. The suggestion that when verapamil injection has been given first, an interval of 30 minutes before giving a beta-blocker is sufficient has not been confirmed.
It may also be hazardous to give verapamil and a beta-blocker together by mouth (should only be contemplated if myocardial function well preserved).

Hepatic impairment oral dose may need to be reduced

Pregnancy may reduce uterine blood flow with fetal hypoxia; manufacturer advises avoid during first trimester unless absolutely necessary; may inhibit labour

Breast-feeding amount too small to be harmful

Contra-indications hypotension, bradycardia, second- and third-degree AV block, sick sinus syndrome, cardiogenic shock, sino-atrial block; history of heart failure or significantly impaired left ventricular function, even if controlled by therapy; atrial flutter or fibrillation complicating syndromes associated with accessory conducting pathways (e.g. Wolff-Parkinson-White syndrome); acute porphyria (section 9.8.2)

Side-effects constipation; *less commonly* nausea, vomiting, flushing, headache, dizziness, fatigue, ankle oedema; *rarely* allergic reactions (erythema, pruritus, urticaria, angioedema, Stevens-Johnson syndrome); myalgia, arthralgia, paraesthesia, erythromelalgia; increased prolactin concentration; gynaecomastia and gingival hyperplasia after long-term treatment; after intravenous administration or high doses, hypotension, heart failure, bradycardia, heart block, and asystole; hypersensitivity reactions involving reversibly raised liver function tests

Licensed use Modified release preparation not licensed for use in children

Indication and dose

Hypertension, prophylaxis of supraventricular arrhythmias under specialist advice only

• By mouth

Child 1–2 years 20 mg 2–3 times daily

Child 2–18 years 40–120 mg 2–3 times daily

◁ **VERAPAMIL HYDROCHLORIDE** (*continued*)

Treatment of supraventricular arrhythmias

• **By intravenous injection over 2–3 minutes (with ECG and blood-pressure monitoring and under specialist advice)**

Child 1–18 years 100–300 micrograms/kg (max. 5 mg) as a single dose, repeated after 30 minutes if necessary

Administration for *intravenous injection*, may be diluted with Glucose 5% *or* Sodium Chloride 0.9%; incompatible with solutions of pH greater than 6

Verapamil (Non-proprietary) PoM

Tablets, coated, verapamil hydrochloride 40 mg, net price 84-tab pack = £1.54; 80 mg, 84-tab pack = £1.68; 120 mg, 28-tab pack = £1.41; 160 mg, 56-tab pack = £20.23

Oral solution, verapamil hydrochloride 40 mg/5 mL, net price 150 mL = £36.90
Brands include *Zolvera*®

Cordilox® (Dexcel) PoM

Tablets, yellow, f/c, verapamil hydrochloride 40 mg, net price 84-tab pack = £1.50; 80 mg, 84-tab pack = £2.05; 120 mg, 28-tab pack = £1.15; 160 mg, 56-tab pack = £2.80

Injection, verapamil hydrochloride 2.5 mg/mL, net price 2-mL amp = £1.11

Securon® (Abbott) PoM

Injection, verapamil hydrochloride 2.5 mg/mL, net price 2-mL amp = £1.08

◀ Extemporaneous formulations available see Extemporaneous Preparations, p. 8

◀ **Modified release**

Half Securon SR® (Abbott) PoM

Tablets, m/r, f/c, verapamil hydrochloride 120 mg, net price 28-tab pack = £7.50. Label: 25

Dose

Give once daily (doses above 240 mg daily, give 2–3 times daily)

Securon SR® (Abbott) PoM

Tablets, m/r, pale green, f/c, scored, verapamil hydrochloride 240 mg, net price 28-tab pack = £6.29. Label: 25

Dose

Give once daily (doses above 240 mg daily, give 2–3 times daily)

Univer® (Cephalon) PoM

Capsules, m/r, verapamil hydrochloride 120 mg (yellow/dark blue), net price 28-cap pack = £7.51; 180 mg (yellow), 56-cap pack = £18.15; 240 mg (yellow/dark blue), 28-cap pack = £12.24. Label: 25

Dose

Give once daily

Verapress MR® (Dexcel) PoM

Tablets, m/r, pale green, f/c, verapamil hydrochloride 240 mg, net price 28-tab pack = £9.90. Label: 25

Dose

Give 1–2 times daily

Note Also available as *Cordilox*® *MR*

Vertab® **SR 240** (Chiesi) PoM

Tablets, m/r, pale green, f/c, scored, verapamil hydrochloride 240 mg, net price 28-tab pack = £8.63. Label: 25

Dose

Give 1–2 times daily

2.6.3 **Other antianginal drugs**

Classification not used in *BNF for Children*.

2.6.4 **Peripheral vasodilators and related drugs**

Raynaud's syndrome consists of recurrent, long-lasting, and episodic vasospasm of the fingers and toes often associated with exposure to cold. Management includes avoidance of exposure to cold and stopping smoking (if appropriate). More severe symptoms may require vasodilator treatment, which is most often successful in primary Raynaud's syndrome. **Nifedipine** and **diltiazem** (section 2.6.2) are useful for reducing the frequency and severity of vasospastic attacks. In very severe cases, where digital infarction is likely, intravenous infusion of the prostacyclin analogue **iloprost** may be helpful.

Vasodilator therapy is not established as being effective for *chilblains* (section 13.13).

▇ **ILOPROST**

Cautions see section 2.5.1.2
Contra-indications see section 2.5.1.2
Side-effects see section 2.5.1.2
Licensed use not licensed for use in children

Indication and dose

Pulmonary hypertension section 2.5.1.2

Raynaud's syndrome see notes above

• **By intravenous infusion**

Child 12–18 years initially 30 nanograms/kg/hour, increased gradually to 60–120 nanograms/kg/hour given over 6 hours daily for 3–5 days

2 Cardiovascular system

◿ **ILOPROST** (*continued*)

Administration For intravenous infusion dilute with Glucose 5% or Sodium Chloride 0.9% to a concentration of 200 nanograms/mL; alternatively, may be diluted to a concentration of 2 micrograms/mL and given via syringe driver

Iloprost (Non-proprietary)
Concentrate for infusion, iloprost 100 micrograms/mL (as iloprost trometamol).
For dilution and use as an intravenous infusion
Note available on a named patient basis from Bayer in 0.5 mL and 1 mL ampoules

2.7 Sympathomimetics

2.7.1 Inotropic sympathomimetics
2.7.2 Vasoconstrictor sympathomimetics
2.7.3 Cardiopulmonary resuscitation

The properties of sympathomimetics vary according to whether they act on alpha or on beta adrenergic receptors. Response to sympathomimetics can also vary considerably in children, particularly neonates. It is important to titrate the dose to the desired effect and to monitor the child closely.

2.7.1 Inotropic sympathomimetics

The cardiac stimulants **dobutamine** and **dopamine** act on beta$_1$ receptors in cardiac muscle and increase contractility with little effect on rate.

Dopamine has a variable, unpredictable, and dose dependent impact on vascular tone. Low dose infusion (2 micrograms/kg/minute) normally causes vasodilatation, but there is little evidence that this is clinically beneficial; moderate doses increase myocardial contractility and cardiac output in older children, but in neonates moderate doses may cause a reduction in cardiac output. High doses cause vasoconstriction and increase vascular resistance, and should therefore be used with caution following cardiac surgery, or where there is co-existing neonatal pulmonary hypertension.

In neonates the response to inotropic sympathomimetics varies considerably, particularly in those born prematurely; careful dose titration and monitoring are necessary.

Isoprenaline injection is available from 'special-order' manufacturers or specialist importing companies, see p. 943.

Shock   Shock is a medical emergency associated with a high mortality. The underlying causes of shock such as haemorrhage, sepsis or myocardial insufficiency should be corrected. Additional treatment is dependent on the type of shock.

Septic shock is associated with severe hypovolaemia (due to vasodilation and capillary leak) which should be corrected with crystalloids or colloids (section 9.2.2). If hypotension persists despite volume replacement, **dopamine** should be started. For shock refractory to treatment with dopamine, if cardiac output is high and peripheral vascular resistance is low (warm shock), **noradrenaline** (norepinephrine) (section 2.7.2) should be added *or* if cardiac output is low and peripheral vascular resistance is high (cold shock), **adrenaline** (epinephrine) (section 2.7.2) should be added. Additionally, in cold shock, a vasodilator such as **milrinone** (section 2.1.2), **glyceryl trinitrate** (section 2.6.1), or **sodium nitroprusside** (on specialist advice only) (section 2.5.1.1) can be used to reduce vascular resistance.

If the shock is resistant to volume expansion and catecholamines, and there is suspected or proven adrenal insufficiency, low dose **hydrocortisone** (section 6.3.2) can be used. ACTH-stimulated plasma-cortisol concentration should be measured; however, hydrocortisone can be started without such information.

Alternatively, if the child is resistant to catecholamines, and vascular resistance is low, **vasopressin** (section 6.5.2) can be added.

Neonatal septic shock can be complicated by the transition from fetal to neonatal circulation. Treatment to reverse right ventricular failure, by decreasing pulmonary artery pressures, is commonly needed in neonates with fluid-refractory shock and persistent pulmonary hypertension of the newborn (section 2.5.1.2). Rapid administration of fluid in neonates with patent ductus arteriosus may cause left-to-right shunting and congestive heart failure induced by ventricular overload.

In *cardiogenic shock*, the aim is to improve cardiac output and to reduce the afterload on the heart. If central venous pressure is low, cautious volume expansion with a colloid or crystalloid can be used. An inotrope such as **adrenaline** (epinephrine) (section 2.7.2) or **dopamine** should be given to increase cardiac output. **Dobutamine** is a peripheral vasodilator and is an alternative if hypotension is not significant.

Milrinone (section 2.1.2) has both inotropic and vasodilatory effects and can be used when vascular resistance is high. Alternatively, **glyceryl trinitrate** (2.6.1) or **sodium nitroprusside** (on specialist advice only) (section 2.5.1.1) can be used to reduce vasoconstriction.

Hypovolaemic shock should be treated with a crystalloid or colloid solution (or whole or reconstituted blood if source of hypovolaemia is haemorrhage) and further steps to improve cardiac output and decrease vascular resistance can be taken, as in cardiogenic shock.

The use of sympathomimetic inotropes and vasoconstrictors should preferably be confined to the intensive care setting and undertaken with invasive haemodynamic monitoring.

For advice on the management of anaphylactic shock, see section 3.4.3.

DOBUTAMINE

Cautions hyperthyroidism; **interactions**: Appendix 1 (sympathomimetics)

Pregnancy no information available

Contra-indications marked obstruction of cardiac ejection, such as idiopathic hypertrophic subaortic stenosis

Side-effects tachycardia and marked increase in systolic blood pressure indicate overdosage; phlebitis; *rarely* thrombocytopenia

Licensed use not licensed for use in children

Indication and dose

Inotropic support in low cardiac output states, after cardiac surgery, cardiomyopathies, shock
• By continuous intravenous infusion

Neonate initially 5 micrograms/kg/minute, adjusted according to response to 2–15 micrograms/kg/minute; max. 20 micrograms/kg/minute

Child 1 month–18 years initially 5 micrograms/kg/minute adjusted according to response to 2–20 micrograms/kg/minute

Administration for *continuous intravenous infusion*, using infusion pump, dilute to a concentration of 0.5–1 mg/mL (max. 5 mg/mL if fluid restricted) with Glucose 5% or Sodium Chloride 0.9%; infuse higher concentration solutions through central venous catheter only. Incompatible with bicarbonate and other strong alkaline solutions.
Neonatal intensive care, dilute 30 mg/kg bodyweight to a final volume of 50 mL with infusion fluid; an intravenous infusion rate of 0.5 mL/hour provides a dose of 5 micrograms/kg/minute

Dobutamine (Non-proprietary) [PoM]
Strong sterile solution, dobutamine (as hydrochloride) 12.5 mg/mL. For dilution and use as an intravenous infusion. Net price 20-mL amp = £5.20

DOPAMINE HYDROCHLORIDE

Cautions correct hypovolaemia; hyperthyroidism; **interactions**: Appendix 1 (sympathomimetics)

Pregnancy manufacturer advises use only if potential benefit outweighs risk

Contra-indications tachyarrhythmia, phaeochromocytoma

Side-effects nausea and vomiting, peripheral vasoconstriction, hypotension, hypertension, tachycardia

Licensed use not licensed for use in children under 12 years

Indication and dose

To correct the haemodynamic imbalance due to acute hypotension, shock, cardiac failure, adjunct following cardiac surgery
• By continuous intravenous infusion

Neonate initially 3 micrograms/kg/minute, adjusted according to response (max. 20 micrograms/kg/minute)

Child 1 month–18 years initially 5 micrograms/kg/minute adjusted according to response (max. 20 micrograms/kg/minute)

Administration for *continuous intravenous infusion*, dilute to a max. concentration of 3.2 mg/mL with Glucose 5% *or* Sodium Chloride 0.9%. Infuse higher concentrations through central venous catheter using a syringe pump to avoid extrava-

2

Cardiovascular system

◁ **DOPAMINE HYDROCHLORIDE (continued)**

sation and fluid overload. Incompatible with bicarbonate and other alkaline solutions.
Neonatal intensive care, dilute 30 mg/kg body-weight to a final volume of 50 mL with infusion fluid; an intravenous infusion rate of 0.3 mL/hour provides a dose of 3 micrograms/kg/minute

Dopamine (Non-proprietary) PoM
Sterile concentrate, dopamine hydrochloride 40 mg/mL, net price 5-mL amp = £3.88; 160 mg/mL, net price 5-mL amp = £14.75. For dilution and use as an intravenous infusion

Intravenous infusion, dopamine hydrochloride 1.6 mg/mL in glucose 5% intravenous infusion, net price 250-mL container (400 mg) = £11.69; 3.2 mg/mL, 250-mL container (800 mg) = £22.93 (both hosp. only)

Select-A-Jet® Dopamine (UCB Pharma) PoM
Strong sterile solution, dopamine hydrochloride 40 mg/mL. For dilution and use as an intravenous infusion. Net price 5-mL vial = £5.01; 10-mL vial = £8.05

2.7.2 Vasoconstrictor sympathomimetics

Vasoconstrictor sympathomimetics raise blood pressure transiently by acting on alpha-adrenergic receptors to constrict peripheral vessels. They are sometimes used as an emergency method of elevating blood pressure where other measures have failed (see also section 2.7.1).

The danger of vasoconstrictors is that although they raise blood pressure they also reduce perfusion of vital organs such as the kidney.

Ephedrine is used to reverse hypotension caused by spinal and epidural anaesthesia.

Metaraminol is used as a vasopressor during cardiopulmonary bypass.

Phenylephrine causes peripheral vasoconstriction and increases arterial pressure.

Ephedrine, metaraminol and phenylephrine are rarely needed in children and should be used under specialist supervision.

Noradrenaline (norepinephrine) is reserved for children with low systemic vascular resistance that is unresponsive to fluid resuscitation following septic shock, spinal shock, and anaphylaxis.

Adrenaline (epinephrine) is mainly used for its inotropic action. Low doses (acting on beta receptors) cause systemic and pulmonary vasodilation, with some increase in heart rate and stroke volume and also an increase in contractility; high doses act predominantly on alpha receptors causing intense systemic vasoconstriction.

EPHEDRINE HYDROCHLORIDE

Cautions hyperthyroidism, diabetes mellitus, hypertension, susceptibility to angle-closure glaucoma, **interactions**: Appendix 1 (sympathomimetics)

Renal impairment use with caution

Pregnancy increased fetal heart rate reported

Contra-indications

Breast-feeding irritability and disturbed sleep reported in breast-fed infants

Side-effects nausea, vomiting, anorexia; tachycardia (sometimes bradycardia) arrhythmias, anginal pain, vasoconstriction with hypertension, vasodilation with hypotension, dizziness and flushing; dyspnoea; headache, anxiety, restlessness, confusion, psychoses, insomnia, tremor; difficulty in micturition, urine retention; sweating, hypersalivation; changes in blood-glucose concentration

Indication and dose

Reversal of hypotension from epidural and spinal anaesthesia

• **By slow intravenous injection of a solution containing ephedrine hydrochloride 3 mg/mL**

Child 1–12 years 500–750 micrograms/kg *or* 17–25 mg/m² every 3–4 minutes according to response; max. 30 mg during episode

Child 12–18 years 3–7.5 mg (max. 9 mg) repeated every 3–4 minutes according to response, max. 30 mg during episode

Nasal congestion section 12.2.2

Administration By slow intravenous injection, via central line.

Ephedrine Hydrochloride (Non-proprietary) PoM
Injection, ephedrine hydrochloride 3 mg/mL, net price 10-mL amp = £2.83; 30 mg/mL, net price 1-mL amp = £1.70

METARAMINOL

Cautions see under Noradrenaline; longer duration of action than noradrenaline (norepinephrine), see below; cirrhosis; **interactions:** Appendix 1 (sympathomimetics)
Hypertensive response Metaraminol has a longer duration of action than noradrenaline, and an excessive vasopressor response may cause a prolonged rise in blood pressure

Breast-feeding manufacturer advises caution—no information available

Contra-indications see under Noradrenaline

Pregnancy may reduce placental prefusion—manufacturer advises use only if potential benefit outweighs risk

Side-effects see under Noradrenaline; tachycardia; fatal ventricular arrhythmia reported in Laennec's cirrhosis

Licensed use Not licensed for use in children

Indication and dose

Acute hypotension
* **By intravenous infusion**

    Child 12–18 years 15–100 mg adjusted according to response

Emergency treatment of acute hypotension
* **By intravenous administration**

    Child 12–18 years initially by intravenous injection 0.5–5 mg, then by intravenous infusion 15–100 mg adjusted according to response

Administration for *intravenous infusion* dilute to a concentration of 30–200 micrograms/mL with Glucose 5% *or* Sodium Chloride 0.9% and give through a central venous catheter

Metaraminol (Non-proprietary) ⃞PoM
Injection, metaraminol 10 mg (as tartrate)/mL.
Available from 'special-order' manufacturers or specialist importing companies, see p. 943

NORADRENALINE/NOREPINEPHRINE

Cautions coronary, mesenteric, or peripheral vascular thrombosis; Prinzmetal's variant angina, hyperthyroidism, diabetes mellitus; hypoxia or hypercapnia; uncorrected hypovolaemia; extravasation at injection site may cause necrosis; **interactions:** Appendix 1 (sympathomimetics)

Contra-indications hypertension (monitor blood pressure and rate of flow frequently)

Pregnancy avoid—may reduce placental perfusion

Side-effects hypertension, headache, bradycardia, arrhythmias, peripheral ischaemia

Licensed use not licensed for use in children

Indication and dose

Acute hypotension (septic shock) or shock secondary to excessive vasodilation (as noradrenaline)
* **By continuous intravenous infusion**

    Neonate 20–100 nanograms(base)/kg/minute adjusted according to response; max. 1 microgram(base)/kg/minute

    Child 1 month–18 years 20–100 nanograms(base)/kg/minute adjusted according to response; max. 1 microgram(base)/kg/minute

Note 1 mg of noradrenaline acid tartrate is equivalent to 500 micrograms of the base. Dose expressed as the base

Administration for *continuous intravenous infusion*, dilute to a max. concentration of noradrenaline (base) 40 micrograms/mL (higher concentrations can be used if fluid-restricted) with Glucose 5% *or* Sodium Chloride and Glucose. Infuse through central venous catheter; discard if discoloured. Incompatible with bicarbonate or alkaline solutions.

Neonatal intensive care, dilute 600 micrograms (base)/kg body-weight to a final volume of 50 mL with infusion fluid; an intravenous infusion rate of 0.1 mL/hour provides a dose of 20 nanograms (base)/kg/minute

Noradrenaline/Norepinephrine (Non-proprietary) ⃞PoM
Injection, noradrenaline acid tartrate 2 mg/mL (equivalent to noradrenaline base 1 mg/mL). For dilution before use. Net price 2-mL amp = £1.01, 4-mL amp = £1.50, 20-mL amp = £6.35
Excipients may include sodium metabisulphite

PHENYLEPHRINE HYDROCHLORIDE

Cautions see under Noradrenaline; longer duration of action than noradrenaline (norepinephrine), see below; coronary disease
Hypertensive response Phenylephrine has a longer duration of action than noradrenaline, and an excessive vasopressor response may cause a prolonged rise in blood pressure

Contra-indications see under Noradrenaline; severe hyperthyroidism

Pregnancy avoid if possible; malformations reported following use in first trimester; fetal hypoxia and bradycardia reported in late pregnancy and labour

Side-effects see under Noradrenaline; tachycardia or reflex bradycardia

Licensed use not licensed for use in children by intravenous infusion or injection

Indication and dose

Acute hypotension
* **By subcutaneous or intramuscular injection (but intravenous injection preferred, see below)**

    Child 1–12 years 100 micrograms/kg every 1–2 hours as needed (max. 5 mg)

2

Cardiovascular system

◁ **PHENYLEPHRINE HYDROCHLORIDE (*continued*)**

Child 12–18 years 2–5 mg, followed if necessary by further doses of 1–10 mg (max. initial dose 5 mg)

- **By slow intravenous injection**

Child 1–12 years 5–20 micrograms/kg (max. 500 micrograms) repeated as necessary after at least 15 minutes

Child 12–18 years 100–500 micrograms repeated as necessary after at least 15 minutes

- **By intravenous infusion**

Child 1–16 years 100–500 nanograms/kg/minute, adjusted according to response

Child 16–18 years initially up to 180 micrograms/minute reduced to 30–60 micrograms/minute according to response

Administration for *intravenous injection* dilute to a concentration of 1 mg/mL with Water for Injections and administer slowly.

For *intravenous infusion* dilute to a concentration of 20 micrograms/mL with Glucose 5% *or* Sodium Chloride 0.9% and administer as a continuous infusion via a central venous catheter using a controlled infusion device

Phenylephrine (Sovereign) [PoM]
Injection, phenylephrine hydrochloride 10 mg/mL (1%), net price 1-mL amp = £5.50

ADRENALINE/EPINEPHRINE

Cautions diabetes mellitus, hyperthyroidism, hypertension, arrhythmias, cerebrovascular disease, avoid extravasation, monitor urine output, limb perfusion (especially at higher doses), central venous pressures and ECG; **interactions:** Appendix 1 (sympathomimetics)

Side-effects nausea, vomiting, sweating, tachycardia, dyspnoea, anxiety, tremor, headache, weakness, dizziness and hyperglycaemia , cold extremities; in overdosage hypertension, arrhythmias, cerebral haemorrhage, pulmonary oedema

Indication and dose

Acute hypotension

- **By continuous intravenous infusion**

Neonate initially 100 nanograms/kg/minute adjusted according to response; higher doses up to 1.5 micrograms/kg/minute have been used in acute hypotension

Child 1 month–18 years initially 100 nanograms/kg/minute adjusted according to

response; higher doses up to 1.5 micrograms/kg/minute have been used in acute hypotension

Anaphylaxis section 3.4.3

Administration for *continuous intravenous infusion* dilute with Glucose 5% *or* Sodium Chloride 0.9% and give through a central venous catheter. Incompatible with bicarbonate and alkaline solutions.

Neonatal intensive care, dilute 3 mg/kg body-weight to a final volume of 50 mL with infusion fluid; an intravenous infusion rate of 0.1 mL/hour provides a dose of 100 nanograms/kg/minute
Note These infusions are usually made up with adrenaline 1 in 1000 (1 mg/mL) solution; this concentration of adrenaline is not licensed for intravenous administration

◀Preparations
Section 3.4.3

2.7.3 Cardiopulmonary resuscitation

The algorithms for cardiopulmonary resuscitation (see inside back cover) reflect the recommendations of the Resuscitation Council (UK); they cover paediatric basic life support, paediatric advanced life support, and newborn life support. The guidelines are available at www.resus.org.uk.

Paediatric advanced life support   Cardiopulmonary (cardiac) arrest in children is rare and frequently represents the terminal event of progressive shock or respiratory failure.

During cardiopulmonary arrest in children without intravenous access, the intraosseous route is chosen because it provides rapid and effective response; if circulatory access cannot be gained, the endotracheal tube can be used. When the endotracheal route is used ten times the intravenous dose should be used; the drug should be injected quickly down a narrow bore suction catheter beyond the tracheal end of the tube and then flushed in with 1 or 2 mL of sodium chloride 0.9%. The endotracheal route is useful for lipid-soluble drugs, including lidocaine, adrenaline, atropine, and naloxone. Drugs that are not lipid-soluble (e.g. sodium bicarbonate and calcium chloride) should **not** be administered by this route because they will injure the airways.

For the management of acute anaphylaxis see section 3.4.3.

2.8 Anticoagulants and protamine

2.8.1 Parenteral anticoagulants
2.8.2 Oral anticoagulants
2.8.3 Protamine sulphate

Although thrombotic episodes are uncommon in childhood, anticoagulants may be required in children with congenital heart disease; in children undergoing haemodialysis; for preventing thrombosis in children requiring chemotherapy and following surgery; and for systemic venous thromboembolism secondary to inherited thrombophilias, systemic lupus erythematosus, or indwelling central venous catheters.

2.8.1 Parenteral anticoagulants

Heparin

Heparin initiates anticoagulation rapidly but has a short duration of action. It is now often referred to as being **standard** or **unfractionated heparin** to distinguish it from the **low molecular weight heparins** (see p. 149), which have a longer duration of action. For children at high risk of bleeding, heparin is more suitable than low molecular weight heparin because its effect can be terminated rapidly by stopping the infusion.

Heparin is used in both the treatment and prophylaxis of thromboembolic disease; however, it is mainly used to prevent further clotting rather than to lyse existing clots—surgery or a thrombolytic drug may be necessary if a thrombus obstructs major vessels.

Treatment   For the initial treatment of thrombotic episodes heparin is given as an intravenous loading dose, followed by continuous intravenous infusion (using an infusion pump) or by intermittent subcutaneous injection; the use of intermittent intravenous injection is no longer recommended. Alternatively, a low molecular weight heparin may be given for initial treatment. An oral anticoagulant (usually warfarin, section 2.8.2) is started at the same time as the heparin (the heparin needs to be continued for at least 5 days and until the INR has been in the therapeutic range for 2 consecutive days). Laboratory monitoring of coagulation activity, preferably on a daily basis, involves determination of the activated partial thromboplastin time (APTT) or of the anti-Factor Xa concentration. Local guidelines on recommended APTT for neonates and children should be followed.

Prophylaxis   Low-dose heparin by subcutaneous injection is used to prevent thrombotic episodes in 'high-risk' patients; laboratory monitoring of APTT or anti-Factor Xa concentration is also required in prophylactic regimens in children. **Aspirin** (section 2.9) and **warfarin** (section 2.8.2) can also be used for prophylaxis.

Pregnancy   Heparins are used for the management of thromboembolic disease in pregnancy because they do not cross the placenta. Low molecular weight heparins are preferred because they have a lower risk of osteoporosis and of heparin-induced thrombocytopenia. Low molecular weight heparins are eliminated more rapidly in pregnancy, requiring alteration of the dosage regimen for drugs such as dalteparin, enoxaparin, and tinzaparin. Treatment should be stopped at the onset of labour and advice sought from a specialist on continuing therapy after birth.

Extracorporeal circuits   Heparin is also used in the maintenance of extracorporeal circuits in cardiopulmonary bypass and haemodialysis.

Haemorrhage   If haemorrhage occurs it is usually sufficient to withdraw heparin, but if rapid reversal of the effects of heparin is required, protamine sulphate (section 2.8.3) is a specific antidote (but only partially reverses the effects of low molecular weight heparins).

2   Cardiovascular system

▲ HEPARIN

Cautions see notes above; concomitant use of drugs that increase risk of bleeding; **interactions:** Appendix 1 (heparin)

Heparin-induced thrombocytopenia Clinically important heparin-induced thrombocytopenia is immune-mediated and does not usually develop until after 5–10 days; it can be complicated by thrombosis. Platelet counts should be measured just before treatment with heparin or low molecular weight heparins, and regular monitoring of platelet counts is recommended if given for longer than 4 days. Signs of heparin-induced thrombocytopenia include a 50% reduction of platelet count, thrombosis, or skin allergy. If heparin-induced thrombocytopenia is strongly suspected or confirmed, heparin should be **stopped** and an alternative anticoagulant, such as danaparoid, should be given. Ensure platelet counts return to normal range in those who require warfarin

Hyperkalaemia Inhibition of aldosterone secretion by heparin (including low molecular weight heparins) can result in hyperkalaemia; patients with diabetes mellitus, chronic renal failure, acidosis, raised plasma potassium, or those taking potassium-sparing drugs seem to be more susceptible. The risk appears to increase with duration of therapy and the CSM has recommended that plasma-potassium concentration should be measured in children at risk of hyperkalaemia before starting heparin and monitored regularly thereafter, particularly if heparin is to be continued for longer than 7 days

Hepatic impairment risk of bleeding increased—possibly reduce dose in severe impairment

Renal impairment risk of bleeding increased in severe impairment—dose may need to be reduced

Pregnancy does not cross the placenta; maternal osteoporosis reported after prolonged use; multi-dose vials may contain benzyl alcohol—some manufacturers advise avoid

Breast-feeding not excreted in milk due to high molecular weight

Contra-indications haemophilia and other haemorrhagic disorders, thrombocytopenia (including history of heparin-induced thrombocytopenia), recent cerebral haemorrhage, severe hypertension; severe liver disease (including oesophageal varices), peptic ulcer; after major trauma or recent surgery to eye or nervous system; acute bacterial endocarditis; spinal or epidural anaesthesia with treatment doses of heparin; hypersensitivity to heparin or low molecular weight heparins

Side-effects haemorrhage (see notes above), thrombocytopenia (see Cautions), rarely rebound hyperlipidaemia following heparin withdrawal, priapism, hyperkalaemia (see Cautions), osteoporosis (risk lower with low molecular weight heparins), alopecia on prolonged use, injection-site reactions, skin necrosis, and hypersensitivity reactions (including urticaria, angioedema, and anaphylaxis)

Licensed use Some preparations licensed for use in children

Indication and dose

Maintenance of neonatal umbilical arterial catheter
• **By intravenous infusion**
  Neonate 0.5 units/hour

Treatment of thrombotic episodes
• **By intravenous administration**
  Neonate initially 75 units/kg (50 units/kg if under 35 weeks post-menstrual age) *by intravenous injection*, then *by continuous intravenous infusion* 25 units/kg/hour, adjusted according to APTT

  Child 1 month–1 year initially 75 units/kg *by intravenous injection*, then *by continuous intravenous infusion* 25 units/kg/hour, adjusted according to APTT

  Child 1–18 years initially 75 units/kg *by intravenous injection*, then *by continuous intravenous infusion* 20 units/kg/hour, adjusted according to APTT

• **By subcutaneous injection**
  Child 1 month–18 years 250 units/kg twice daily, adjusted according to APTT

Prophylaxis of thrombotic episodes
• **By subcutaneous injection**
  Child 1 month–18 years 100 units/kg (max. 5000 units) twice daily, adjusted according to APTT

Prevention of clotting in extracorporeal circuits
consult product literature

Administration for *continuous intravenous infusion*, dilute with Glucose 5% *or* Sodium Chloride 0.9%. *Maintenance of neonatal umbilical arterial catheter*, dilute 50 units to a final volume of 50 mL with Sodium Chloride 0.45% *or* use ready-made bag containing 500 units in 500 mL Sodium Chloride 0.9%; infuse at 0.5 mL/hour

Neonatal intensive care (treatment of thrombosis), dilute 1250 units/kg body-weight to a final volume of 50 mL with infusion fluid; an intravenous infusion rate of 1 mL/hour provides a dose of 25 units/kg/hour

Heparin Sodium (Non-proprietary) ⓅⓄⓂ
Injection, heparin sodium 1000 units/mL, net price 1-mL amp = 37p, 5-mL amp = 93p, 5-mL vial = 92p, 10-mL amp = £1.60, 20-mL amp = £2.63; 5000 units/mL, 1-mL amp = 72p, 5-mL amp = £1.87, 5-mL vial = £2.09; 25 000 units/mL, 0.2-mL amp = 92p, 1-mL amp = £1.90, 5-mL vial = £3.68
Excipients may include benzyl alcohol (avoid in neonates, see Excipients, p. 3)

Heparin Calcium (Non-proprietary) ⓅⓄⓂ
Injection, heparin calcium 25 000 units/mL, net price 0.2-mL amp = 73p

Low molecular weight heparins

Dalteparin, **enoxaparin**, and **tinzaparin** are low molecular weight heparins used for treatment and prophylaxis of thrombotic episodes in children. Their duration of action is longer than that of unfractionated heparin and in adults and older children *once-daily subcutaneous* dosage is sometimes possible; however, younger children require relatively higher doses (possibly due to larger volume of distribution, altered heparin pharmacokinetics, or lower plasma concentrations of antithrombin) and twice daily dosage is sometimes necessary. Low molecular weight heparins are convenient to use, especially in children with poor venous access. Routine monitoring of anti-Factor Xa activity is not usually required except in neonates; monitoring may also be necessary in severely ill children and those with renal or hepatic impairment.

Haemorrhage   See under Heparin.

Hepatic impairment   Reduce dose in severe hepatic impairment—risk of bleeding may be increased.

Renal impairment   See under individual drug.

Pregnancy   Not known to be harmful, low molecular weight heparins do not cross the placenta.

Breast-feeding   Due to the relatively high molecular weight of these drugs and inactivation in the gastro-intestinal tract, passage into breast-milk and absorption by the nursing infant are likely to be negligible; however manufacturers advise avoid.

◢ DALTEPARIN SODIUM

Cautions   see under Heparin and notes above

Hepatic impairment   see notes above

Renal impairment   risk of bleeding may be increased—dose reduction and monitoring of anti-factor Xa may be required; use of unfractionated heparin may be preferable

Pregnancy   see notes above

Breast-feeding   see notes above

Contra-indications   see under Heparin

Side-effects   see under Heparin

Licensed use   not licensed for use in children

Indication and dose

> Treatment of thrombotic episodes
> • By subcutaneous injection
>
> Neonate 100 units/kg twice daily
>
> Child 1 month–12 years 100 units/kg twice daily
>
> Child 12–18 years 200 units/kg (max. 18 000 units) once daily, if increased risk of bleeding reduced to 100 units/kg twice daily

> Treatment of venous thromboembolism in pregnancy
> • By subcutaneous injection
>
> Child 12–18 years early pregnancy body-weight under 50 kg, 5000 units twice daily; body-weight 50–70 kg, 6000 units twice daily;

> body-weight 70–90 kg, 8000 units twice daily; body-weight over 90 kg, 10 000 units twice daily

> Prophylaxis of thrombotic episodes
> • By subcutaneous injection
>
> Neonate 100 units/kg once daily
>
> Child 1 month–12 years 100 units/kg once daily
>
> Child 12–18 years 2500–5000 units once daily

Fragmin® (Pharmacia) ⒫ₒ̅ₘ̅

Injection (single-dose syringe), dalteparin sodium 12 500 units/mL, net price 2500-unit (0.2-mL) syringe = £1.86; 25 000 units/mL, 5000-unit (0.2-mL) syringe = £2.82, 7500-unit (0.3-mL) syringe = £4.23, 10 000-unit (0.4-mL) syringe = £5.65, 12 500-unit (0.5-mL) syringe = £7.06, 15 000-unit (0.6-mL) syringe = £8.47, 18 000-unit (0.72-mL) syringe = £10.16

Injection, dalteparin sodium 2500 units/mL (for subcutaneous or intravenous use), net price 4-mL (10 000-unit) amp = £5.12; 10 000-units/mL (for subcutaneous or intravenous use), 1-mL (10 000-unit) amp = £5.12; 25 000 units/mL (for subcutaneous use only), 4-mL (100 000-unit) vial = £48.66

Injection (graduated syringe), dalteparin sodium 10 000 units/mL, net price 1-mL (10 000-unit) syringe = £5.65

◢ ENOXAPARIN SODIUM

Cautions   see under Heparin and notes above

Hepatic impairment   see notes above

Renal impairment   risk of bleeding may be increased; reduce dose if estimated glomerular filtration rate less than 30 mL/minute/1.73 m²; mon-

2

Cardiovascular system

◻ **ENOXAPARIN SODIUM** (*continued*)

itoring of anti-factor Xa may be required; use of unfractionated heparin may be preferable

Pregnancy see notes above

Breast-feeding see notes above

Contra-indications see under Heparin

Side-effects see under Heparin

Licensed use not licensed for use in children

Indication and dose

Treatment of thrombotic episodes
• By subcutaneous injection

Neonate 1.5–2 mg/kg twice daily

Child 1–2 months 1.5 mg/kg twice daily

Child 2 months–18 years 1 mg/kg twice daily

Treatment of venous thromboembolism in pregnancy
• By subcutaneous injection

Child 12–18 years early pregnancy body-weight under 50 kg, 40 mg (4000 units) twice daily; body-weight 50–70 kg, 60 mg (6000 units) twice daily; body-weight 70–90 kg, 80 mg (8000 units) twice daily; body-weight over 90 kg, 100 mg (10 000 units) twice daily

Prophylaxis of thrombotic episodes
• By subcutaneous injection

Neonate 750 micrograms/kg twice daily

Child 1–2 months 750 micrograms/kg twice daily

Child 2 months–18 years 500 micrograms/kg twice daily; max. 40 mg daily

Clexane® (Rhône-Poulenc Rorer) PoM
Injection, enoxaparin sodium 100 mg/mL, net price 20-mg (0.2-mL, 2000-units) syringe = £3.15, 40-mg (0.4-mL, 4000-units) syringe = £4.20, 60-mg (0.6-mL, 6000-units) syringe = £4.75, 80-mg (0.8-mL, 8000-units) syringe = £5.40, 100-mg (1-mL, 10 000-units) syringe = £6.69, 300-mg (3-mL, 30 000-units) vial (*Clexane® Multi-Dose*) = £22.20; 150 mg/mL (*Clexane® Forte*), 120-mg (0.8-mL, 12 000-units) syringe = £9.77, 150-mg (1-mL, 15 000-units) syringe = £11.10

TINZAPARIN SODIUM

Cautions see under Heparin and notes above

Hepatic impairment see notes above

Renal impairment risk of bleeding may be increased—dose reduction and monitoring of anti-factor Xa may be required; unfractionated heparin may be preferable

Pregnancy see notes above; also vials contain benzyl alcohol—manufacturer advises avoid

Breast-feeding see notes above

Contra-indications see under Heparin

Side-effects see under Heparin

Licensed use not licensed for use in children

Indication and dose

Treatment of thrombotic episodes
• By subcutaneous injection

Child 1–2 months 275 units/kg once daily

Child 2 months–1 year 250 units/kg once daily

Child 1–5 years 240 units/kg once daily

Child 5–10 years 200 units/kg once daily

Child 10–18 years 175 units/kg once daily

Treatment of venous thromboembolism in pregnancy
• By subcutaneous injection

Child 12–18 years 175 units/kg once daily (based on early pregnancy body-weight)

Prophylaxis of thrombotic episodes
• By subcutaneous injection

Child 1 month–18 years 50 units/kg once daily

Innohep® (LEO) PoM
Injection, tinzaparin sodium 10 000 units/mL, net price 2500-unit (0.25-mL) syringe = £1.98, 3500-unit (0.35-mL) syringe = £2.77, 4500-unit (0.45-mL) syringe = £3.56, 20 000-unit (2-mL) vial = £10.56

Injection, tinzaparin sodium 20 000 units/mL, net price 0.5-mL (10 000-unit) syringe = £8.98, 0.7-mL (14 000-unit) syringe = £12.57, 0.9-mL (18 000-unit) syringe = £16.16, 2-mL (40 000-unit) vial = £34.20
Excipients include benzyl alcohol (in vials) (avoid in neonates, see Excipients, p. 3), sulphites (in 20 000 units/mL vial and syringe)

Heparinoids

Danaparoid is a heparinoid that has a role in children who develop thrombocytopenia in association with heparin, providing they have no evidence of cross-reactivity.

DANAPAROID SODIUM

Cautions recent bleeding or risk of bleeding; concomitant use of drugs that increase risk of bleeding; antibodies to heparins (risk of antibody-induced thrombocytopenia)

Hepatic impairment use with caution in moderate impairment (increased risk of bleeding); avoid in severe impairment unless no alternative

Renal impairment use with caution in moderate impairment; increased risk of bleeding (monitor

◁ **DANAPAROID SODIUM** (*continued*)

anti-Factor Xa activity); avoid in severe impairment unless child has heparin-induced thrombocytopenia and no alternative available

Pregnancy limited information available but not known to be harmful—manufacturer advises avoid

Breast-feeding amount probably too small to be harmful but manufacturer advises avoid

Contra-indications haemophilia and other haemorrhagic disorders, thrombocytopenia (unless patient has heparin-induced thrombocytopenia), recent cerebral haemorrhage, severe hypertension, active peptic ulcer (unless this is the reason for operation), diabetic retinopathy, acute bacterial endocarditis, spinal or epidural anaesthesia with treatment doses of danaparoid

Side-effects haemorrhage; hypersensitivity reactions (including rash)

Licensed use not licensed for use in children

Indication and dose

Thromboembolic disease in children with history of heparin-induced thrombocytopenia
• By intravenous administration

Neonate initially 30 units/kg *by intravenous injection* then *by continuous intravenous infusion* 1.2–2 units/kg/hour adjusted according to coagulation activity

Child 1 month–16 years initially 30 units/kg (max. 1250 units if bodyweight under 55 kg, 2500 units if over 55 kg) *by intravenous injection* then *by continuous intravenous infusion* 1.2–2 units/kg/hour adjusted according to coagulation activity

Child 16–18 years initially 2500 units (1250 units if bodyweight under 55 kg, 3750 units if over 90 kg) *by intravenous injection* then *by continuous intravenous infusion* 400 units/hour for 2 hours, *then* 300 units/hour for 2 hours, *then* 200 units/hour for 5 days adjusted according to coagulation activity

Administration for *intravenous infusion*, dilute with Glucose 5% *or* Sodium Chloride 0.9%

Organan® (Organon) [PoM]
Injection, danaparoid sodium 1250 units/mL, net price 0.6-mL amp (750 units) = £29.80

Heparin flushes

The use of heparin flushes should be kept to a minimum. For maintaining patency of peripheral venous catheters, sodium chloride 0.9% injection is as effective as heparin flushes. The role of heparin flushes in maintaining patency of arterial and central venous catheters is unclear.

Heparin Sodium (Non-proprietary) [PoM]
Solution, heparin sodium 10 units/mL, net price 5-mL amp = 25p; 100 units/mL, 2-mL amp = 28p
Excipients may include benzyl alcohol (avoid in neonates, see Excipients, p. 3)

Epoprostenol

Epoprostenol (prostacyclin) can be given to inhibit platelet aggregation during renal dialysis either alone or with heparin. For its use in pulmonary hypertension, see section 2.5.1.2. It is a potent vasodilator and therefore its side-effects include flushing, headache, and hypotension.

2.8.2 Oral anticoagulants

Oral anticoagulants antagonise the effects of vitamin K and take at least 48 to 72 hours for the anticoagulant effect to develop fully; if an immediate effect is required, heparin must be given concomitantly.

Uses Warfarin is the drug of choice for the treatment of systemic thromboembolism in children (not neonates) after initial heparinisation. It may also be used occasionally for the treatment of intravascular or intracardiac thrombi. Warfarin is used prophylactically in those with chronic atrial fibrillation, dilated cardiomyopathy, certain forms of reconstructive heart surgery, mechanical prosthetic heart valves, and some forms of hereditary thrombophilia (e.g. homozygous protein C deficiency).

Heparin or a low molecular weight heparin (section 2.8.1) is usually preferred for the prophylaxis of venous thromboembolism in children undergoing surgery; alternatively warfarin can be continued in selected children currently taking warfarin and who are at a high risk of thromboembolism (seek expert advice).

2 Cardiovascular system

Dose Whenever possible, the base-line prothrombin time should be determined but the initial dose should not be delayed whilst awaiting the result.

An induction dose is usually given over 4 days (see under Warfarin Sodium below). The subsequent maintenance dose depends on the prothrombin time, reported as INR (international normalised ratio) and should be taken at the same time each day. The following indications and target INRs[1] for **adults** take into account recommendations of the British Society for Haematology[2];

- INR 2.5 for treatment of deep-vein thrombosis and pulmonary embolism (including those associated with antiphospholipid syndrome or for recurrence in patients no longer receiving warfarin), for atrial fibrillation, cardioversion (higher target values, such as an INR of 3, can be used for up to 4 weeks before the procedure to avoid cancellations due to low INR), dilated cardiomyopathy, mural thrombus, symptomatic inherited thrombophilia, coronary artery thrombosis (if anticoagulated), and paroxysmal nocturnal haemoglobinuria;

- INR 3.5 for recurrent deep-vein thrombosis and pulmonary embolism (in patients currently receiving warfarin with INR above 2);

- For mechanical prosthetic heart valves, the recommended target INR depends on the type and location of the valve. Generally, a target INR of 3 is recommended for mechanical aortic valves, and 3.5 for mechanical mitral valves.

Monitoring It is essential that the INR be determined daily or on alternate days in early days of treatment, *then* at longer intervals (depending on response[3]) *then* up to every 12 weeks.

Haemorrhage The main adverse effect of all oral anticoagulants is haemorrhage. Checking the INR and omitting doses when appropriate is essential; if the anticoagulant is stopped but not reversed, the INR should be measured 2–3 days later to ensure that it is falling. The following recommendations are based on the result of the INR and whether there is major or minor bleeding; the recommendations (which take into account the recommendations of the British Society for Haematology) apply to **adults** taking warfarin:

- Major bleeding—stop warfarin; give phytomenadione (vitamin K_1) 5–10 mg by slow intravenous injection; give prothrombin complex concentrate (factors II, VII, IX, and X) 30–50 units/kg *or* (if no concentrate available) fresh frozen plasma 15 mL/kg

- INR > 8.0, no bleeding or minor bleeding—stop warfarin, restart when INR < 5.0; if there are other risk factors for bleeding give phytomenadione (vitamin K_1) 500 micrograms by slow intravenous injection or 5 mg by mouth (for partial reversal of anticoagulation give smaller oral doses of phytomenadione e.g. 0.5–2.5 mg using the intravenous preparation orally); repeat dose of phytomenadione if INR still too high after 24 hours

- INR 6.0–8.0, no bleeding or minor bleeding—stop warfarin, restart when INR < 5.0

- INR < 6.0 but more than 0.5 units above target value—reduce dose or stop warfarin, restart when INR < 5.0

- Unexpected bleeding at therapeutic levels—always investigate possibility of underlying cause e.g. unsuspected renal or gastro-intestinal tract pathology

Pregnancy Oral anticoagulants are teratogenic and should not be given in the first trimester of pregnancy. Adolescents at risk of pregnancy should be warned of this danger since stopping warfarin before the sixth week of gestation largely avoids the risk of fetal abnormality. Oral anticoagulants cross the placenta with risk of placental or fetal haemorrhage, especially during the last few weeks of pregnancy and at delivery. Therefore, if at all possible, oral anticoagulants should be avoided in pregnancy, especially in the first and third trimesters. Difficult decisions may have to be made, particularly in those with prosthetic heart valves

1. An INR which is within 0.5 units of the target value is generally satisfactory; larger deviations require dosage adjustment. Target values (rather than ranges) are now recommended.
2. Guidelines on Oral Anticoagulation (warfarin): third edition—2005 update. *Br J Haematol* 2005; **132**: 277–285.
3. Change in child's clinical condition, particularly associated with liver disease, intercurrent illness, or drug administration, necessitates more frequent testing. See also **interactions**, Appendix 1 (warfarin). Major changes in diet (especially involving salads and vegetables) and in alcohol consumption may also affect warfarin control.

or with a history of recurrent venous thrombosis, pulmonary embolism, or atrial fibrillation.

Babies of mothers taking warfarin at the time of delivery need to be offered immediate prophylaxis with at least 100 micrograms/kg of intramuscular phytomenadione (vitamin K$_1$), see section 9.6.6.

Dietary differences   Infant formula is supplemented with vitamin K, which makes formula-fed infants resistant to warfarin; they may therefore need higher doses. In contrast breast milk contains low concentrations of vitamin K making breast-fed infants more sensitive to warfarin.

Treatment booklets   Anticoagulant treatment booklets should be issued to children or their carers, and are available for distribution to local healthcare professionals from Health Authorities and from:
3M Security Printing and Systems Limited
Gorse Street
Chadderton
Oldham, OL9 9QH.
Tel: 0845 610 1112
nhsforms@spsl.uk.com

These booklets include advice for children or their carers on anticoagulant treatment, an alert card to be carried by the patient at all times, and a section for recording of INR results and dosage information. Electronic copies are also available at www.npsa.nhs.uk/nrls/alerts-and-directives/alerts/anticoagulant.

WARFARIN SODIUM

Cautions   see notes above; also recent surgery; concomitant use of drugs that increase risk of bleeding; bacterial endocarditis (increased risk of bleeding; use only if warfarin otherwise indicated); **interactions**: Appendix 1 (warfarin)

Hepatic impairment   avoid in severe impairment, especially if prothrombin time already prolonged

Renal impairment   use with caution (avoid in severe impairment)

Breast-feeding   not excreted in breast milk; no evidence of harm

Contra-indications   peptic ulcer, severe hypertension

Pregnancy   see notes above

Side-effects   haemorrhage—see notes above; other side-effects reported include hypersensitivity, rash, alopecia, diarrhoea, unexplained drop in haematocrit, 'purple toes', skin necrosis, jaundice, hepatic dysfunction; also nausea, vomiting, and pancreatitis

Licensed use   not licensed for use in children

Indication and dose

Treatment and prophylaxis of thrombotic episodes
• By mouth

Neonate (under specialist advice) 200 micrograms/kg as a single dose on first day, reduced to 100 micrograms/kg once daily for following 3 days (but if INR still below 1.4 use 200 micrograms/kg once daily, or if INR above 3 use 50 micrograms/kg once daily, if INR above 3.5 omit dose); then adjusted according to INR, usual maintenance 100–300 micrograms/kg once daily (may need up to 400 micrograms/kg once daily especially if bottle fed—see notes above)

Child 1 month–18 years 200 micrograms/kg (max. 10 mg) as a single dose on first day, reduced to 100 micrograms/kg (max. 5 mg) once daily for following 3 days (but if INR still below 1.4 use 200 micrograms/kg (max. 10 mg) once daily, or if INR above 3 use 50 micrograms/kg (max. 2.5 mg) once daily, or if INR above 3.5 omit dose); then adjusted according to INR, usual maintenance 100–300 micrograms/kg once daily (may need up to 400 micrograms/kg once daily especially if bottle fed—see notes above)

Note Induction dose may need to be altered according to condition (e.g. abnormal liver function tests, cardiac failure), concomitant interacting drugs, and if baseline INR above 1.3

Warfarin (Non-proprietary) [PoM]
Tablets, warfarin sodium 500 micrograms (white), net price 28-tab pack = 93p; 1 mg (brown), 28 = £1.03; 3 mg (blue), 28 = £1.14; 5 mg (pink), 28 = £1.24. Label: 10, anticoagulant card
Brands include *Marevan*®

◢ Extemporaneous formulations available see Extemporaneous Preparations, p. 8

2.8.3 Protamine sulphate

Protamine sulphate is used to treat overdosage of heparin and low molecular weight heparins. The long half-life of low molecular weight heparins should be taken into consideration when determining the dose of protamine sulphate; the effects of low molecular weight heparins can persist for up to 24 hours after administration. Excessive doses of protamine sulphate can have an anticoagulant effect.

Cardiovascular system

<table>
<tr><td>

■ **PROTAMINE SULPHATE**
(Protamine Sulfate)

Cautions see above; also monitor activated partial thromboplastin time or other appropriate blood clotting parameters; if increased risk of allergic reaction to protamine (includes previous treatment with protamine or protamine insulin, allergy to fish, and adolescent males who are infertile)

Side-effects nausea, vomiting, lassitude, flushing, hypotension, hypertension, bradycardia, dyspnoea, rebound bleeding, back pain; hypersensitivity reactions (including angioedema, anaphylaxis) and pulmonary oedema reported

Indication and dose

Overdosage with intravenous injection or intravenous infusion of heparin

• **By intravenous injection (rate not exceeding 5 mg/minute)**

   Child 1 month–18 years *to neutralise each 100 units of unfractionated heparin*, 1 mg if less than 30 minutes lapsed since overdose, 500–750 micrograms if 30–60 minutes lapsed, 375–500 micrograms if 60–120 minutes lapsed, 250–375 micrograms if over 120 minutes lapsed; max. 50 mg

</td><td>

Overdosage with subcutaneous injection of heparin

• **By intravenous injection and intravenous infusion**

   Child 1 month–18 years 1 mg neutralises approx. 100 units of unfractionated heparin; give 50–100% of the total dose by *intravenous injection* (rate not exceeding 5 mg/minute), then give any remainder of dose by *intravenous infusion* over 8–16 hours; max. total dose 50 mg

Overdosage with subcutaneous injection of low molecular weight heparin

• **By intermittent intravenous injection (rate not exceeding 5 mg/minute) or by continuous intravenous infusion**

   Child 1 month–18 years 1 mg neutralises approx. 100 units low molecular weight heparin (consult product literature of low molecular weight heparin for details); max. 50 mg

Administration may be diluted if necessary with Sodium Chloride 0.9%

Protamine Sulphate (Non-proprietary) ᴾᵒᴹ
   Injection, protamine sulphate 10 mg/mL, net price 5-mL amp = £1.14, 10-mL amp = £4.15

Prosulf® (CP) ᴾᵒᴹ
   Injection, protamine sulphate 10 mg/mL, net price 5-mL amp = 96p (glass), £1.20 (polypropylene)

</td></tr>
</table>

2.9 Antiplatelet drugs

Antiplatelet drugs decrease platelet aggregation and may inhibit thrombus formation in the arterial circulation, where anticoagulants have little effect.

Aspirin has limited use in children because it has been associated with Reye's syndrome. The CSM has advised that aspirin-containing preparations should not be given to children and adolescents under 16 years, unless specifically indicated, such as for Kawasaki syndrome (see below), for prophylaxis of clot formation after cardiac surgery, or for prophylaxis of stroke in children at high risk.

If aspirin causes dyspepsia, or if the child is at a high risk of gastro-intestinal bleeding, a proton pump inhibitor (section 1.3.5) or a H₂-receptor antagonist (section 1.3.1) can be added.

Dipyridamole is also used as an antiplatelet drug to prevent clot formation after cardiac surgery and may be used with specialist advice for treatment of persistent coronary artery aneurysms in Kawasaki syndrome.

Kawasaki syndrome   Initial treatment is with high-dose aspirin and a single dose of intravenous normal immunoglobulin (p. 757); this combination has an additive anti-inflammatory effect resulting in faster resolution of fever and a decreased incidence of coronary artery complications. After the acute phase, when the patient is afebrile, aspirin is continued at a lower dose to prevent coronary artery abnormalities.

■ **ASPIRIN (antiplatelet)**
(Acetylsalicylic Acid)

Cautions asthma; uncontrolled hypertension; previous peptic ulceration (but manufacturers may advise avoidance of low-dose aspirin in history of peptic ulceration); concomitant use of drugs that increase risk of bleeding; G6PD deficiency (section 9.1.5); **interactions**: Appendix 1 (aspirin)

Hepatic impairment avoid in severe impairment—increased risk of gastro-intestinal bleeding

Renal impairment use with caution (avoid in severe impairment); sodium and water retention; deterioration in renal function; increased risk of gastro-intestinal bleeding

Pregnancy use with caution during third trimester; impaired platelet function and risk of

2 Cardiovascular system (side margin)

◁ **ASPIRIN (antiplatelet) (*continued*)**

haemorrhage; delayed onset and increased duration of labour with increased blood loss; avoid analgesic doses if possible in last few weeks (low doses probably not harmful); with high doses, closure of fetal ductus arteriosus *in utero* and possibly persistent pulmonary hypertension of newborn; kernicterus in jaundiced neonates

Contra-indications children under 16 years (risk of Reye's syndrome) unless for indications below; active peptic ulceration; haemophilia and other bleeding disorders

Hypersensitivity Aspirin and other NSAIDs are **contra-indicated** in history of hypersensitivity to aspirin or any other NSAID—which includes those in whom attacks of asthma, angioedema, urticaria, or rhinitis have been precipitated by aspirin or any other NSAID

Breast-feeding avoid—possible risk of Reye's syndrome; regular use of high doses could impair platelet function and produce hypoprothrombinaemia in infant if neonatal vitamin K stores low

Side-effects bronchospasm; gastro-intestinal haemorrhage (occasionally major), also other haemorrhage (e.g. subconjunctival)

Licensed use Not licensed for use in children under 16 years

Indication and dose

Kawasaki syndrome
• By mouth

Neonate initially 8 mg/kg 4 times daily for 2 weeks *or* until afebrile, followed by 5 mg/kg once daily for 6–8 weeks; if no evidence of coronary lesions after 8 weeks, discontinue treatment or seek expert advice

Child 1 month–12 years initially 7.5–12.5 mg/kg 4 times daily for 2 weeks or until afebrile, then 2–5 mg/kg once daily for 6–8 weeks; if no evidence of coronary lesions after 8 weeks, discontinue treatment or seek expert advice

Antiplatelet, prevention of thrombus formation after cardiac surgery
• By mouth

Neonate 1–5 mg/kg once daily

Child 1 month–12 years 1–5 mg/kg (usual max. 75 mg) once daily

Child 12–18 years 75 mg once daily

Aspirin (Non-proprietary) [PoM]
Dispersible tablets, aspirin 75 mg, net price 28 = 83p; 300 mg, 100-tab pack = £4.93 Label: 13, 21, 32

Tablets, e/c, aspirin 75 mg, net price 28-tab pack = 83p; 56-tab pack = £1.08; 300 mg, 100-tab pack = £4.74. Label: 5, 25, 32
Brands include *Micropirin*®

Suppositories, available from 'special-order' manufacturers or specialist importing companies, see p. 943

Angettes 75® (Bristol-Myers Squibb)
Tablets, aspirin 75 mg, net price 28-tab pack = 94p. Label: 32

Caprin® (Pinewood) [PoM]
Tablets, e/c, pink, aspirin 75 mg, net price 28-tab pack = £1.55, 56-tab pack = £3.08, 100-tab pack = £5.24; 300 mg, 100-tab pack = £4.89. Label: 5, 25, 32

Nu-Seals® Aspirin (Alliance) [PoM]
Tablets, e/c, aspirin 75 mg, net price 56-tab pack = £2.60; 300 mg, 100-tab pack = £3.46. Label: 5, 25, 32

▊ **DIPYRIDAMOLE**

Cautions aortic stenosis, left ventricular outflow obstruction, heart failure; may exacerbate migraine; hypotension; myasthenia gravis (risk of exacerbation); concomitant use of drugs that increase risk of bleeding; coagulation disorders; **interactions**: Appendix 1 (dipyridamole)

Pregnancy not known to be harmful

Breast-feeding small amount present in milk—manufacturer advises caution

Side-effects gastro-intestinal effects, dizziness, myalgia, throbbing headache, hypotension, hot flushes and tachycardia; hypersensitivity reactions such as rash, urticaria, severe bronchospasm and angioedema; increased bleeding during or after surgery; thrombocytopenia reported

Licensed use Not licensed for use in children

Indication and dose

Kawasaki syndrome
• By mouth
Child 1 month–12 years 1 mg/kg 3 times daily

Prevention of thrombus formation after cardiac surgery
• By mouth

Child 1 month–12 years 2.5 mg/kg twice daily

Child 12–18 years 100–200 mg 3 times daily

Administration Injection solution can be given orally

Dipyridamole (Non-proprietary) [PoM]
Tablets, coated, dipyridamole 25 mg, net price 84 = £4.28; 100 mg, 84 = £3.19. Label: 22

Oral suspension, dipyridamole 50 mg/5 ml, net price 150 mL = £37.00

Persantin® (Boehringer Ingelheim) [PoM]
Tablets, both s/c, dipyridamole 25 mg (orange), net price 84-tab pack = £1.57; 100 mg, 84-tab pack = £4.38. Label: 22

Injection, dipyridamole 5 mg/mL, net price 2-mL amp = 11p

2

Cardiovascular system

2.10 Myocardial infarction and fibrinolysis

2.10.1 Management of myocardial infarction
2.10.2 Fibrinolytic drugs

2.10.1 Management of myocardial infarction

Classification not used in *BNF for Children*.

2.10.2 Fibrinolytic drugs

Fibrinolytic drugs act as thrombolytics by activating plasminogen to form plasmin, which degrades fibrin and so breaks up thrombi.

Alteplase, **streptokinase**, and **urokinase** are used in children to dissolve intravascular thrombi and unblock occluded arteriovenous shunts, catheters, and indwelling central lines blocked with fibrin clots. Treatment should be started as soon as possible after a clot has formed and discontinued once a pulse in the affected limb is detected, or the shunt or catheter unblocked.

The safety and efficacy of treatment remains uncertain, especially in neonates. A fibrinolytic drug is probably only appropriate where arterial occlusion threatens ischaemic damage; an anticoagulant may stop the clot getting bigger. Alteplase is the preferred fibrinolytic in children and neonates; there is less risk of adverse effects including allergic reactions.

Cautions   Thrombolytic drugs should be used with caution if there is a risk of bleeding including that from venepuncture or invasive procedures. They should also be used with caution in external chest compression, pregnancy (see individual drugs), hypertension, other conditions in which thrombolysis might give rise to embolic complications such as enlarged left atrium with atrial fibrillation (risk of dissolution of clot and subsequent embolisation), and recent or concurrent use of drugs that increase the risk of bleeding.

Contra-indications   Thrombolytic drugs are contra-indicated in recent haemorrhage, trauma, or surgery (including dental extraction), coagulation defects, bleeding diatheses, aortic dissection, aneurysm, coma, history of cerebrovascular disease especially recent events or with any residual disability, recent symptoms of possible peptic ulceration, heavy vaginal bleeding, severe hypertension, active pulmonary disease with cavitation, acute pancreatitis, pericarditis, bacterial endocarditis, severe liver disease, and oesophageal varices; also in the case of streptokinase, previous allergic reactions to streptokinase.

Prolonged persistence of antibodies to streptokinase can reduce the effectiveness of subsequent treatment; therefore, streptokinase should not be used again beyond 4 days of first administration. Streptokinase should also be avoided in children who have had streptococcal infection in the last 12 months.

Side-effects   Side-effects of thrombolytics are mainly bleeding, nausea, and vomiting. Reperfusion can cause cerebral and pulmonary oedema. Hypotension can also occur and can usually be controlled by elevating the patient's legs, or by reducing the rate of infusion or stopping it temporarily. Back pain, fever, and convulsions have been reported. Bleeding is usually limited to the site of injection, but intracerebral haemorrhage or bleeding from other sites can occur. Serious bleeding calls for discontinuation of the thrombolytic and may require administration of coagulation factors and antifibrinolytic drugs (e.g. tranexamic acid). Thrombolytics can cause allergic reactions (including rash, flushing and uveitis) and anaphylaxis has been reported (for details of management see Allergic Emergencies, section 3.4.3). Guillain-Barré syndrome has been reported rarely after streptokinase treatment.

◢ ALTEPLASE
(rt-PA, tissue-type plasminogen activator)
Cautions   see notes above; in children who have had *acute stroke*, monitor for intracranial haemorrhage and monitor blood pressure

Hepatic impairment   avoid in severe impairment—increased risk of bleeding

Pregnancy   no evidence of teratogenicity; possibility of premature separation of placenta in first 18 weeks; risk of maternal haemorrhage throughout pregnancy and during post-partum use; theoretical risk of fetal haemorrhage throughout pregnancy

◻ **ALTEPLASE** (*continued*)

Contra-indications see notes above; in children who have had an *acute stroke*, convulsion accompanying stroke, severe stroke, history of stroke in children with diabetes, stroke in last 3 months, hypoglycaemia, hyperglycaemia

Side-effects see notes above; also risk of cerebral bleeding increased in acute stroke

Licensed use Not licensed for use in children

Indication and dose

Intravascular thrombosis doses may vary—consult local guidelines

- **By intravenous infusion**

  Neonate 100–500 micrograms/kg/hour for 3–6 hours; use ultrasound assessment to monitor effect before considering a second course of treatment

  Child 1 month–18 years 100–500 micrograms/kg/hour for 3–6 hours; max. 100 mg total daily dose; use ultrasound assessment to monitor effect before considering a second course of treatment

Administration dissolve in Water for Injections to a concentration of 1 mg/mL or 2 mg/mL and infuse intravenously; alternatively dilute further in Sodium Chloride 0.9% to a concentration of not less than 200 micrograms/mL; not to be diluted in Glucose

Occluded arteriovenous shunts, catheters, and indwelling central lines
- **By injection direct into catheter or central line**

  Child 1 month–18 years using 1 mg/mL solution, instill up to 2 mL according to dead-space of catheter or central line; aspirate lysate after 4 hours; flush with sodium chloride 0.9% injection

Actilyse® (Boehringer Ingelheim) (PoM)
Injection, powder for reconstitution, alteplase 10 mg (5.8 million units)/vial, net price per vial (with diluent) = £135.00; 20 mg (11.6 million units)/vial (with diluent and transfer device) = £180.00; 50 mg (29 million units)/vial (with diluent, transfer device, and infusion bag) = £300.00

STREPTOKINASE

Cautions see notes above

Hepatic impairment avoid in severe hepatic impairment—increased risk of bleeding

Pregnancy possibility of premature separation of placenta in first 18 weeks; risk of maternal haemorrhage throughout pregnancy and during post-partum use; theoretical risk of fetal haemorrhage throughout pregnancy

Contra-indications see notes above

Side-effects see notes above

Licensed use Licensed for use in children for intravascular dissolution of thrombi and emboli

Indication and dose

Intravascular thrombosis
- **By intravenous infusion**

  Child 1 month–12 years initially 2500–4000 units/kg over 30 minutes, followed

by *continuous intravenous infusion* of 500–1000 units/kg/hour for up to 3 days until reperfusion occurs

  Child 12–18 years initially 250 000 units over 30 minutes, followed by *continuous intravenous infusion* of 100 000 units/hour for up to 3 days until reperfusion occurs

Administration May be diluted with Glucose 5% or Sodium Chloride 0.9% after reconstitution. Monitor fibrinogen concentration closely; if fibrinogen concentration less than 1g/litre, stop streptokinase infusion and start heparin; restart streptokinase once fibrinogen concentration reaches 1g/litre

Streptase® (CSL Behring) (PoM)
Injection, powder for reconstitution, streptokinase, net price 250 000-unit vial = £15.91; 750 000-unit vial = £41.72; 1.5 million-unit vial = £83.44 (hosp. only)

UROKINASE

Cautions see notes above

Hepatic impairment avoid in severe hepatic impairment—increased risk of bleeding

Pregnancy possibility of premature separation of placenta; risk of maternal haemorrhage throughout pregnancy and during post-partum use; theoretical risk of fetal haemorrhage throughout pregnancy

Contra-indications see notes above

Side-effects see notes above

Licensed use not licensed for use in children

Indication and dose

Intravascular thrombosis
- **By intravenous injection and infusion**

  Neonate 4400 units/kg as a single dose *by intravenous injection* in 15 mL diluent, followed

by 4400 units/kg/hour *by intravenous infusion* for 6–12 hours, adjusted according to response

  Child 1 month–18 years 4400 units/kg as a single dose *by intravenous injection* in 15 mL diluent, followed by 4400 units/kg/hour *by intravenous infusion* for 6–12 hours, adjusted according to response

Administration May be diluted, after reconstitution, with Sodium Chloride 0.9%

Occluded arteriovenous shunts, catheters, and indwelling central lines
- **By injection directly into catheter or central line**

  Neonate 5000–10 000 units in sodium chloride 0.9% to fill catheter dead-space **only**; leave for 2–4 hours then aspirate the lysate; flush with heparinised saline

◁ **UROKINASE** *(continued)*

Child 1 month–18 years 5000–10 000 units in sodium chloride 0.9% to fill catheter dead-space **only**; leave for 2–4 hours then aspirate the lysate; flush with heparinised saline

Syner-KINASE® (Syner-Med) [PoM]
Injection, powder for reconstitution, urokinase, net price 25 000-unit vial = £45.95; 100 000-unit vial = £112.95
Note 10 000-unit vial, 50 000-unit vial, and 250 000-unit vial also available from 'special-order' manufacturers or specialist importing companies, see p. 943

2.11 Antifibrinolytic drugs and haemostatics

Fibrin dissolution can be impaired by the administration of **tranexamic acid**, which inhibits fibrinolysis. It can be used to prevent bleeding or treat bleeding associated with excessive fibrinolysis (e.g. in prostatectomy, bladder surgery, in dental extraction in children with haemophilia, and in traumatic hyphaema) and in the management of menorrhagia. Tranexamic acid may also be used in hereditary angioedema, epistaxis, and thrombolytic overdose.

Desmopressin (section 6.5.2) is used in the management of mild to moderate haemophilia and von Willebrands' disease. It is also used for testing fibrinolytic response.

TRANEXAMIC ACID

Cautions massive haematuria (avoid if risk of ureteric obstruction); not for use in disseminated intravascular coagulation; irregular menstrual bleeding (establish cause before initiating therapy); regular liver function tests in long-term treatment of hereditary angioedema
Renal impairment manufacturer advises reduce dose in mild to moderate renal impairment; avoid in severe renal impairment
Pregnancy no evidence of teratogenicity in *animal* studies; manufacturer advises use only if potential benefit outweighs risk—crosses the placenta
Breast-feeding small amount present in milk—antifibrinolytic effect in infant unlikely
Contra-indications thromboembolic disease
Side-effects nausea, vomiting, diarrhoea (reduce dose); *rarely* disturbances in colour vision (discontinue), thromboembolic events, allergic skin reactions; giddiness and hypotension on *rapid intravenous injection*
Licensed use Licensed for inhibition of fibrinolysis

Indication and dose

Inhibition of fibrinolysis, hereditary angio-edema (section 3.4.3)
• **By mouth**
Child 1 month–18 years 15–25 mg/kg (max. 1.5 g) 2–3 times daily
• **By intravenous injection over at least 10 minutes**
Child 1 month–18 years 10 mg/kg (max. 1 g) 2–3 times daily
• **By continuous intravenous infusion**
Child 1 month–18 years 45 mg/kg over 24 hours

Prevention of excessive bleeding after dental procedures (e.g. in haemophilia)
• **By intravenous injection (pre-operatively) and by mouth (post-operatively)**
Child 6–18 years 10 mg/kg (max. 1.5 g) *by intravenous injection* pre-operatively, followed by 15–25 mg/kg (max. 1.5 g) 2–3 times daily *by mouth* for up to 8 days
• **Mouthwash 5% solution (specialist use only)**
Child 6–18 years rinse mouth with 5–10 mL 4 times daily for 2 days; not to be swallowed
Note Mouthwash available only as extemporaneously prepared preparation, see Extemporaneous Preparations, p. 8

Menorrhagia
• **By mouth**
Child 12–18 years 1 g 3–4 times daily for up to 4 days; max. 4 g daily (initiate when menstruation has started)

Administration For *intravenous administration*, dilute with Glucose 5% *or* Sodium Chloride 0.9%

Tranexamic acid (Non-proprietary) [PoM]
Tablets, tranexamic acid 500 mg, net price 60-tab pack = £7.80

Cyklokapron® (Meda) [PoM]
Tablets, f/c, scored, tranexamic acid 500 mg, net price 60-tab pack = £14.30

Cyklokapron® (Pfizer) [PoM]
Injection, tranexamic acid 100 mg/mL, net price 5-mL amp = £1.55

Blood products
Classification not used in *BNF for Children*.

2.12 Lipid-regulating drugs

Atherosclerosis begins in childhood and raised serum-cholesterol in children is associated with cardiovascular disease in adulthood. Lowering the cholesterol, without hindering growth and development in children and adolescents, should reduce the risk of cardiovascular disease in later life.

The risk factors for developing cardiovascular disease include raised serum cholesterol concentration, smoking, hypertension, impaired glucose tolerance, male sex, ethnicity, obesity, triglyceride concentration, chronic kidney disease, and a family history of cardiovascular disease. In children with heterozygous familial hypercholesterolaemia, the family history of cardiovascular disease is most important when considering initiation of a lipid-regulating drug. Homozygous familial hypercholesterolaemia is rare and requires specialist management.

Secondary causes of hypercholesterolaemia should be addressed, these include diet, diabetes mellitus, hypothyroidism (see below), nephrotic syndrome, obstructive biliary disease, glycogen storage disease, and drugs such as corticosteroids.

Treatment   Dietary intervention is the mainstay of treatment of hypercholesterolaemia in children. The aim is to reduce the risk of atherosclerosis whilst ensuring adequate growth and development. Advice should also be given on lifestyle measures (e.g. increased exercise, and if appropriate, stopping smoking). Blood pressure should also be reduced if required (section 2.5).

When 6–12 months of dietary intervention alone has failed, drug therapy is indicated in children 10 years and over (rarely necessary in younger children) who are at a high risk of developing cardiovascular disease. Dietary therapy and lifestyle measures should continue even if lipid-regulating drugs have been introduced.

Lipid-regulating drugs are considered if dietary intervention fails to reduce total serum-cholesterol adequately; experience of their use in children is limited and they should be initiated on specialist advice.

Statins (**atorvastatin**, **pravastatin**, and **simvastatin**) are generally well tolerated; atorvastatin and simvastatin are considered to be the drugs of first choice. **Bile acid sequestrants** are also available but tolerability of and compliance with these drugs is poor, and their use is declining.

Evidence for the use of a **fibrate** (**bezafibrate** or **fenofibrate**) in children is limited; fibrates should be considered only if dietary intervention and treatment with a statin and a bile acid sequestrant is unsuccessful or contra-indicated.

In hypertriglyceridaemia which cannot be controlled by very strict diet, omega-3 fatty acid compounds can be considered.

Hypothyroidism   Children with hypothyroidism should receive adequate thyroid replacement therapy before their requirement for lipid-regulating treatment is assessed because correction of hypothyroidism itself may resolve the lipid abnormality. Untreated hypothyroidism increases the risk of myositis with lipid-regulating drugs.

> CSM advice (muscle effects)
> The CSM has advised that rhabdomyolysis associated with lipid-regulating drugs such as the fibrates and statins appears to be rare (approx. 1 case in every 100 000 treatment years) but may be increased in those with renal impairment and possibly in those with hypothyroidism (see also notes above). Concomitant treatment with drugs that increase plasma-statin concentration increase the risk of muscle toxicity; concomitant treatment with a fibrate and a statin may also be associated with an increased risk of serious muscle toxicity.

Statins

The statins (**atorvastatin**, **pravastatin**, and **simvastatin**) competitively inhibit 3-hydroxy-3-methylglutaryl coenzyme A (HMG CoA) reductase, an enzyme involved in cholesterol synthesis, especially in the liver. They are more effective

2 Cardiovascular system

than other classes of drugs in lowering LDL-cholesterol but less effective than the fibrates in reducing triglycerides. Statins also increase concentrations of HDL-cholesterol.

Statins reduce cardiovascular disease events and total mortality in adults, irrespective of the initial cholesterol concentration.

Cautions Statins should be used with caution in those with a history of liver disease or with a high alcohol intake (use should be avoided in active liver disease). Hypothyroidism should be managed adequately before starting treatment with a statin (see p. 159). Liver-function tests should be carried out before and within 1–3 months of starting treatment and thereafter at intervals of 6 months for 1 year, unless indicated sooner by signs or symptoms suggestive of hepatotoxicity. Treatment should be discontinued if serum transaminase concentration rises to, and persists at, 3 times the upper limit of the reference range. Statins should be used with caution in those with risk factors for myopathy or rhabdomyolysis; children or their carers should be advised to report unexplained muscle pain (see Muscle Effects below). Statins should be avoided in acute porphyria (section 9.8.2). **Interactions**: Appendix 1 (statins)

Contra-indications Statins are contra-indicated in active liver disease (or persistently abnormal liver function tests), in pregnancy (adequate contraception required during treatment and for 1 month afterwards), and during breast-feeding.

Side-effects Statins can cause various muscular side-effects, including myositis, which can lead to rhabdomyolysis. Muscular effects are rare but often significant (see below and CSM advice (Muscle effects), p. 159). Statins can cause gastro-intestinal disturbances, and very rarely pancreatitis. They can also cause altered liver function tests, and rarely hepatitis and jaundice; hepatic failure has been reported very rarely. Other side-effects include sleep disturbance, headache, dizziness, depression, paraesthesia, hypoaesthesia, asthenia, peripheral neuropathy, amnesia, fatigue, sexual dysfunction, thrombocytopenia, arthralgia, visual disturbance, alopecia, and hypersensitivity reactions (including rash, pruritus, urticaria, and very rarely lupus erythematosus-like reactions). In very rare cases statins can cause interstitial lung disease; if patients develop symptoms such as dyspnoea, cough, and weight loss, they should seek medical attention.

Muscle effects Myalgia, myositis, and myopathy have been reported with the statins; if myopathy is suspected and creatine kinase is markedly elevated (more than 5 times upper limit of normal), treatment should be discontinued; in children at high risk of muscle effects, a statin should not be started if creatine kinase is elevated. Children at high risk of myopathy include those with a personal or family history of muscular disorders, previous history of muscular toxicity or liver disease (see also CSM advice, p. 159). There is also an increased incidence of myopathy if the statins are given with a fibrate, with lipid-lowering doses of nicotinic acid, or with immunosuppressants such as ciclosporin; close monitoring of liver function and, if symptomatic, of creatine kinase is required in patients receiving these drugs. Rhabdomyolysis with acute renal impairment secondary to myoglobinuria has also been reported.

Counselling Advise children or their carers to report promptly unexplained muscle pain, tenderness, or weakness.

◢ ATORVASTATIN

Cautions see notes above; also haemorrhagic stroke

Hepatic impairment avoid in active liver disease or unexplained persistent elevations in serum transaminases

Contra-indications see notes above

Pregnancy avoid—congenital anomalies reported; decreased synthesis of cholesterol possibly affects fetal development

Breast-feeding manufacturer advises avoid—no information available

Side-effects see notes above; also chest pain; back pain; pruritus; *less commonly* anorexia, malaise, weight gain, hypoglycaemia, hyperglycaemia, and tinnitus; *rarely* cholestatic jaundice and peripheral oedema; *very rarely* taste disturbances, gynaecomastia, hearing loss, Stevens-Johnson syndrome, and toxic epidermal necrolysis

Indication and dose

Hyperlipidaemia including familial hypercholesterolaemia
• **By mouth**

Child 10–17 years initially 10 mg once daily, increased if necessary, at intervals of at least 4 weeks to usual max. 20 mg once daily

Child 17–18 years initially 10 mg once daily, increased if necessary, at intervals of at least 4 weeks to max. 80 mg once daily

Note Reduced dose required with concomitant ciclosporin, clarithromycin, or itraconazole—seek specialist advice

ATORVASTATIN (*continued*)

Lipitor® (Pfizer) PoM
Tablets, all f/c, atorvastatin (as calcium trihydrate) 10 mg, net price 28-tab pack = £18.03; 20 mg, 28-tab pack = £24.64; 40 mg, 28-tab pack = £28.21; 80 mg, 28-tab pack = £28.21. Counselling, muscle effects, see notes above

PRAVASTATIN SODIUM

Cautions see notes above

Hepatic impairment avoid in active liver disease or unexplained persistent elevations in serum transaminases

Renal impairment start with lower doses in moderate to severe impairment

Contra-indications see notes above

Pregnancy avoid—congenital anomalies reported; decreased synthesis of cholesterol possibly affects fetal development

Breast-feeding small amounts present in breast milk—manufacturer advises avoid

Side-effects see notes above; *less commonly* abnormal urination (including dysuria, nocturia, and frequency); *very rarely* fulminant hepatic necrosis

Licensed use licensed in children over 8 years for familial hypercholesterolaemia

Indication and dose

Hyperlipidaemia including familial hypercholesterolaemia
- By mouth

Child 8–14 years 10 mg once daily at night, adjusted at intervals of at least 4 weeks to max. 20 mg once daily at night

Child 14–18 years 10 mg once daily at night, adjusted at intervals of at least 4 weeks to max. 40 mg once daily at night

Pravastatin (Non-proprietary) PoM
Tablets, pravastatin sodium 10 mg, net price 28-tab pack = £1.73; 20 mg, 28-tab pack = £2.22; 40 mg, 28-tab pack = £2.77
Counselling muscle effects, see notes above

Lipostat® (Squibb) PoM
Tablets, all yellow, pravastatin sodium 10 mg, net price 28-tab pack = £15.05; 20 mg, 28-tab pack = £27.61; 40 mg, 28-tab pack = £27.61. Counselling, muscle effects, see notes above

SIMVASTATIN

Cautions see notes above

Hepatic impairment avoid in active liver disease or unexplained persistent elevations in serum transaminases

Renal impairment doses above 5 mg daily (10 mg daily in children over 10 years) should be used with caution if estimated glomerular filtration rate less than 30 mL/minute/1.73 m^2

Contra-indications see notes above

Pregnancy avoid—congenital anomalies reported; decreased synthesis of cholesterol possibly affects fetal development

Breast-feeding manufacturer advises avoid—no information available

Side-effects see notes above; also *rarely* anaemia

Licensed use not licensed for use in children

Indication and dose

Hyperlipidaemia including familial hypercholesterolaemia
- By mouth

Child 5–10 years initially 5 mg at night increased, if necessary, at intervals of at least 4 weeks to max. 20 mg at night

Child 10–18 years initially 10 mg at night increased, if necessary, at intervals of at least 4 weeks to max. 40 mg at night

Note Reduced dose required with concomitant ciclosporin, danazol, fibrates, amiodarone, diltiazem, or verapamil—seek specialist advice

Simvastatin (Non-proprietary) PoM
Tablets, simvastatin 10 mg, net price 28-tab pack = 85p; 20 mg, 28-tab pack = 95p; 40 mg, 28-tab pack = £1.37; 80 mg, 28-tab pack = £2.94. Counselling, muscle effects, see notes above
Brands include *Simvador®*

Zocor® (MSD) PoM
Tablets, all f/c, simvastatin 10 mg (peach), net price 28-tab pack = £18.03; 20 mg (tan), 28-tab pack = £29.69; 40 mg (red), 28-tab pack = £29.69; 80 mg (red), 28-tab pack = £29.69. Counselling, muscle effects, see notes above

Bile acid sequestrants

Colestyramine (cholestyramine) and **colestipol** are bile acid sequestrants used in the management of hypercholesterolaemia. They act by binding bile acids, preventing their reabsorption; this promotes hepatic conversion of cholesterol into bile acids; the resultant increased LDL-receptor activity of liver cells increases the clearance of LDL-cholesterol from the plasma. Thus both compounds effectively reduce LDL-cholesterol but can aggravate hypertriglyceridaemia. Bile acid sequestrants are not well tolerated and compliance with treatment is poor, therefore they are rarely used in children.

Cautions Bile acid sequestrants interfere with the absorption of fat-soluble vitamins; supplements of vitamins A, D and K may be required when treatment is prolonged and the child's growth and development should be monitored. **Interactions:** Appendix 1 (bile acid sequestrants).

Side-effects As bile acid sequestrants are not absorbed, gastro-intestinal side-effects predominate. Constipation is common, but diarrhoea has occurred, as have nausea, vomiting, and gastro-intestinal discomfort. Hypertriglyceridaemia may be aggravated. An increased bleeding tendency has been reported due to hypoprothrombinaemia associated with vitamin K deficiency.

Counselling Other drugs should be taken at least 1 hour before or 4–6 hours after bile acid sequestrants to reduce possible interference with absorption.

COLESTYRAMINE
(Cholestyramine)

Cautions see notes above

Hepatic impairment interferes with absorption of fat-soluble vitamins and may aggravate malabsorption in primary biliary cirrhosis; likely to be ineffective in complete biliary obstruction

Pregnancy use with caution—drug not absorbed but may cause fat soluble vitamin deficiency on prolonged use

Breast-feeding use with caution—drug not absorbed but may cause fat soluble vitamin deficiency on prolonged use

Contra-indications complete biliary obstruction (not likely to be effective)

Side-effects see notes above; intestinal obstruction reported rarely and hyperchloraemic acidosis reported on prolonged use

Licensed use licensed in children over 6 years to reduce cholesterol; see also section 1.9.2

Indication and dose

Familial hypercholesterolaemia
• By mouth

Child 6–12 years initially 4 g once daily increased to 4 g up to 3 times daily according to response

Child 12–18 years initially 4 g once daily increased by 4 g at weekly intervals to 12–24 g daily in 1–4 divided doses, then adjusted according to response; max. 36 g daily

Cholestatic pruritus section 1.9.2

Diarrhoea section 1.9.2

Administration The contents of each sachet should be mixed with at least 150 mL of water or other suitable liquid such as fruit juice, skimmed milk, thin soups, and pulpy fruits with a high moisture content; total daily dose may be given as a single dose if tolerated

Colestyramine (Non-proprietary) ℗ₒ𝖬
Powder, sugar-free, colestyramine (anhydrous) 4 g/sachet, net price 50-sachet pack = £18.20.
Label: 13, counselling, avoid other drugs at same time (see notes above)
Excipients may include aspartame (section 9.4.1)

Questran® (Bristol-Myers Squibb) ℗ₒ𝖬
Powder, colestyramine (anhydrous) 4 g/sachet, net price 50-sachet pack = £11.42. Label: 13, counselling, avoid other drugs at same time (see notes above)
Excipients include sucrose 3.79g/sachet

Questran Light® (Bristol-Myers Squibb) ℗ₒ𝖬
Powder, sugar-free, colestyramine (anhydrous) 4 g/sachet, net price 50-sachet pack = £16.99.
Label: 13, counselling, avoid other drugs at same time (see notes above)
Excipients include aspartame (section 9.4.1)

COLESTIPOL HYDROCHLORIDE

Cautions see notes above

Pregnancy use with caution—drug not absorbed but may cause fat soluble vitamin deficiency on prolonged use

Breast-feeding use with caution—drug not absorbed but may cause fat soluble vitamin deficiency on prolonged use

Side-effects see notes above

Licensed use not licensed for use in children

Indication and dose

Familial hypercholesterolaemia
• By mouth

Child 12–18 years initially 5 g 1–2 times daily increased if necessary in 5-g increments at intervals of 1 month to max. of 30 g daily in 1–2 divided doses

Administration The contents of each sachet should be mixed with at least 100 mL of water or other suitable liquid such as fruit juice, skimmed milk, thin soups, cereals, yoghurt, and pulpy fruits with a high moisture content; total daily dose may be given as a single dose if tolerated

◿ **COLESTIPOL HYDROCHLORIDE** (*continued*)

Colestid® (Pharmacia) PoM
Granules, yellow, colestipol hydrochloride 5 g/
sachet, net price 30 sachets = £15.05. Label: 13,
counselling, avoid other drugs at same time (see
notes above)

Colestid Orange, granules, yellow/orange, colestipol hydrochloride 5 g/sachet, with aspartame, net
price 30 sachets = £15.05. Label: 13, counselling,
avoid other drugs at same time (see notes above)

Ezetimibe

Ezetimibe inhibits the intestinal absorption of cholesterol. It is given in combination with a statin or alone if a statin is inappropriate. If ezetimibe is used in
combination with a statin, there is an increased risk of rhabdomyolysis (see also
CSM advice on p. 159).

EZETIMIBE

Cautions interactions: Appendix 1 (ezetimibe)

Hepatic impairment avoid in moderate and
severe impairment—may accumulate

Pregnancy manufacturer advises use only if
potential benefit outweighs risk—no information
available

Contra-indications

Breast-feeding present in milk in *animal* studies—manufacturer advises avoid

Side-effects gastro-intestinal disturbances; headache, fatigue; myalgia; *rarely* arthralgia, hypersensitivity reactions (including rash, angioedema,
and anaphylaxis), hepatitis; *very rarely* pancreatitis, cholelithiasis, cholecystitis, thrombocytopenia, raised creatine kinase, myopathy, and rhabdomyolysis

Indication and dose

Adjunct to dietary measures and statin treatment in primary hypercholesterolaemia and
homozygous familial hypercholesterolaemia
(ezetimibe alone in primary hypercholesterolaemia if statin inappropriate or not tolerated)
adjunct to dietary measures in homozygous
sitosterolaemia

Child 10–18 years 10 mg once daily

Ezetrol® (MSD, Schering-Plough) ▼ PoM
Tablets, ezetimibe 10 mg, net price 28-tab pack =
£26.31

Fibrates

Bezafibrate and **fenofibrate** act mainly by decreasing serum triglycerides; they
have variable effects on LDL-cholesterol. Fibrates may reduce the risk of coronary heart disease in those with low HDL-cholesterol or with raised triglycerides.

Fibrates can cause a myositis-like syndrome, especially in children with impaired
renal function. Also, combination of a fibrate with a statin increases the risk of
muscle effects (especially rhabdomyolysis) and should be used with caution (see
CSM advice, p. 159).

There is limited evidence to support their use in children and they should only be
considered if treatment with a statin and a bile acid sequestrant is unsuccessful or
contra-indicated.

BEZAFIBRATE

Cautions correct hypothyroidism before initiating
treatment (see Lipid-regulating Drugs, p. 159);
see under Myotoxicity below; **interactions:**
Appendix 1 (fibrates)

Myotoxicity Special care needed in patients with renal
disease, as progressive increases in serum creatinine
concentration or failure to follow dosage guidelines may
result in myotoxicity (rhabdomyolysis); discontinue if
myotoxicity suspected or creatine kinase concentration
increases significantly

Hepatic impairment avoid in severe impairment

Renal impairment reduce dose if estimated
glomerular filtration rate 15–60 mL/minute/
1.73 m²; avoid if estimated glomerular filtration rate
less than 15 mL/minute/1.73 m²; see also Myotoxicity above

Contra-indications hypoalbuminaemia, primary
biliary cirrhosis, gall bladder disease, nephrotic
syndrome

Pregnancy embryotoxicity in *animal* studies—
manufacturers advise avoid

Breast-feeding manufacturer advises avoid—no
information available

Side-effects gastro-intestinal disturbances, anorexia; *less commonly* cholestasis, weight gain,
dizziness, headache, fatigue, drowsiness, renal
impairment, raised serum creatinine (unrelated
to renal impairment), erectile dysfunction, myotoxicity (with myasthenia or myalgia)—particular
risk in renal impairment (see Cautions), urticaria,
pruritus, photosensitivity reactions; *very rarely*
gallstones, hypoglycaemia, anaemia, leucopenia,

2

Cardiovascular system

◁ **BEZAFIBRATE** (*continued*)

thrombocytopenia, increased platelet count, alopecia, Stevens-Johnson syndrome, and toxic epidermal necrolysis

Licensed use not licensed for use in children

Indication and dose

Hyperlipidaemia including familial hypercholesterolaemia (on specialist advice only)

• **By mouth**

Child 10–18 years 200 mg once daily adjusted according to response to max. 200 mg 3 times daily

Bezafibrate (Non-proprietary) [PoM]
Tablets, bezafibrate 200 mg, net price 100-tab pack = £11.23. Label: 21

Bezalip® (Roche) [PoM]
Tablets, f/c, bezafibrate 200 mg, net price 100-tab pack = £9.15. Label: 21

◢ **FENOFIBRATE**

Cautions see under Bezafibrate; liver function tests recommended every 3 months for first year (discontinue treatment if significantly raised)

Hepatic impairment avoid in severe impairment

Renal impairment reduce dose if estimated glomerular filtration rate less than 60 mL/minute/1.73 m²; avoid if estimated glomerular filtration rate less than 15 mL/minute/1.73 m²

Contra-indications gall bladder disease; photosensitivity to ketoprofen

Pregnancy embryotoxicity in animal studies—manufacturer advises avoid

Breast-feeding manufacturer advises avoid—no information available

Side-effects see under Bezafibrate; also *very rarely* hepatitis, pancreatitis, and interstitial pneumopathies

Licensed use *Lipantil® Micro 67* is licensed for use in children with hypercholesterolaemia

Indication and dose

Hyperlipidaemias including familial hypercholesterolaemia (on specialist advice only)

• **By mouth**

Child 4–15 years 1 capsule/20 kg body-weight daily

Child 15–18 years initially 3 capsules daily in divided doses; usual range 2-4 capsules daily

Lipantil® (Solvay) [PoM]
Lipantil® Micro 67 capsules, yellow, fenofibrate (micronised) 67 mg, net price 90-cap pack = £23.30. Label: 21

2.13 Local sclerosants

Classification not used in *BNF for Children*.

2.14 Drugs affecting the ductus arteriosus

Closure of the ductus arteriosus

Patent ductus arteriosus is a frequent problem in premature neonates with respiratory distress syndrome. Substantial left-to-right shunting through the ductus arteriosus may increase the risk of intraventricular haemorrhage, necrotising enterocolitis, bronchopulmonary dysplasia, and possibly death.

Indometacin or ibuprofen can be used to close the ductus arteriosus. **Indometacin** has been used for many years and is effective but it reduces cerebral blood flow, and causes a transient fall in renal and gastro-intestinal blood flow. **Ibuprofen** may also be used; it has little effect on renal function (there may be a small reduction in sodium excretion) when used in doses for closure of the ductus arteriosus; gastro-intestinal problems are uncommon.

If drug treatment fails to close the ductus arteriosus, surgery may be indicated.

◢ **IBUPROFEN**

Cautions may mask symptoms of infection; monitor for bleeding; monitor gastro-intestinal function; allergic disorders; **interactions:** Appendix 1 (NSAIDs)

Hepatic impairment avoid in severe liver disease

Renal impairment use lowest effective dose and monitor renal function; sodium and water retention; deterioration in renal function possibly lead-

---

2 Cardiovascular system

⌒ **IBUPROFEN** (*continued*)

ing to renal failure; avoid if possible in severe impairment

Contra-indications life-threatening infection; active bleeding especially intracranial or gastro-intestinal; thrombocytopenia or coagulation defects; marked unconjugated hyperbilirubinaemia; known or suspected necrotising enterocolitis; pulmonary hypertension

Side-effects intestinal perforation; intraventricular haemorrhage; ischaemic brain injury; bronchopulmonary dysplasia, pulmonary haemorrhage; thrombocytopenia, neutropenia, oliguria, haematuria, fluid retention, hyponatraemia; *less commonly* gastro-intestinal haemorrhage; hypoxaemia

Licensed use Orphan licence for the injection for closure of ductus arteriosus in premature neonates less than 34 weeks gestational age

Indication and dose

Closure of ductus arteriosus
• By slow intravenous injection

> Neonate initially 10 mg/kg as a single dose followed at 24-hour intervals by 2 doses of 5 mg/kg; course may be repeated after 48 hours if necessary

Mild to moderate pain, pain and inflammation of soft tissue injuries and rheumatic disease, pyrexia section 10.1.1

Administration By slow intravenous injection over 15 minutes, preferably undiluted. May be diluted, with Glucose 5% *or* Sodium Chloride 0.9%

Pedea® (Orphan Europe) [PoM]
Intravenous solution, ibuprofen 5 mg/mL, net price 4 × 2-mL vials = £263.00

◢ INDOMETACIN

Cautions see notes above; also may mask symptoms of infection; may reduce urine output by 50% or more (monitor carefully—see also under Anuria or Oliguria, below) and precipitate renal impairment especially if extracellular volume depleted, heart failure, sepsis, or concomitant use of nephrotoxic drugs; may induce hyponatraemia; inhibition of platelet aggregation (monitor for bleeding); **interactions:** Appendix 1 (NSAIDs)

Anuria or oliguria If anuria or marked oliguria (urinary output less than 0.6 mL/kg/hour), delay further doses until renal function returns to normal

Hepatic impairment can cause fluid retention; avoid in severe hepatic impairment

Renal impairment use lowest effective dose and monitor renal function; sodium and water retention; deterioration in renal function possibly leading to renal failure; avoid if possible in severe impairment

Contra-indications untreated infection, bleeding (especially with active intracranial haemorrhage or gastro-intestinal bleeding); thrombocytopenia, coagulation defects, necrotising enterocolitis

Side-effects haemorrhagic, renal, gastro-intestinal, metabolic, and coagulation disorders; pulmonary hypertension, intracranial bleeding, fluid retention, and exacerbation of infection

Indication and dose

Closure of ductus arteriosus
• By intravenous infusion over 20–30 minutes

> Neonate under 48 hours initially 200 micrograms/kg as a single dose followed by (if urine output adequate) 2 doses of 100 micrograms/kg at intervals of 12–24 hours; course may be repeated after 48 hours if necessary
>
> Neonate 2–7 days initially 200 micrograms/kg as a single dose followed by (if urine output adequate) 2 doses of 200 micrograms/kg at intervals of 12–24 hours; course may be repeated after 48 hours if necessary
>
> Neonate over 7 days initially 200 micrograms/kg as a single dose followed by (if urine output adequate) 2 doses of 250 micrograms/kg at intervals of 12–24 hours; course may be repeated after 48 hours if necessary
> Note In some units *by intravenous infusion* initially 100 micrograms/kg (200 micrograms/kg if symptomatic) then 100 micrograms/kg every 24 hours for 5 further doses

Pain and inflammation in rheumatic disease section 10.1.1

Administration For *intravenous infusion* dilute each vial with 1–2 mL Sodium Chloride 0.9% *or* Water for Injections

Indocid PDA® (IDIS) [PoM]
Injection, powder for reconstitution, indometacin (as sodium trihydrate), net price 3 × 1-mg vials = £43.50 (hosp. only)

2 Cardiovascular system

◢ Maintenance of patency

In the newborn with duct-dependent congenital heart disease it is often necessary to maintain the patency of the ductus arteriosus whilst awaiting surgery.

Alprostadil (prostaglandin E1) and **dinoprostone** (prostaglandin E2) are potent vasodilators that are effective for maintaining the patency of the ductus arteriosus. They are usually given by continuous intravenous infusion, but oral dosing of dinoprostone is still used in some centres.

During the infusion of a prostaglandin, the newborn requires careful monitoring of heart rate, blood pressure, respiratory rate, and core body temperature. In the event of complications such as apnoea, profound bradycardia, or severe hypotension, the infusion should be temporarily stopped and the complication dealt with; the infusion should be restarted at a lower dose. Recurrent or prolonged apnoea may require ventilatory support in order for the prostaglandin infusion to continue.

ALPROSTADIL

Cautions see notes above; also history of haemorrhage; avoid in hyaline membrane disease; monitor arterial pressure, respiratory rate, heart rate, temperature, and venous blood pressure in arm and leg; facilities for intubation and ventilation must be immediately available; **interactions**: Appendix 1 (alprostadil)

Side-effects apnoea (particularly in neonates under 2 kg), flushing, bradycardia, hypotension, tachycardia, cardiac arrest, oedema, diarrhoea, fever, convulsions, disseminated intravascular coagulation, hypokalaemia; cortical proliferation of long bones; weakening of the wall of the ductus arteriosus and pulmonary artery may follow prolonged use; gastric-outlet obstruction reported

Indication and dose

Maintaining patency of the ductus arteriosus
• By continuous intravenous infusion

Neonate initially 5–10 nanograms/kg/minute, adjusted according to response in steps of 5–10 nanograms/kg/minute; max. 100 nanograms/kg/minute (but associated with increased side-effects)

Note Alprostadil doses in BNFC may differ from those in product literature

Administration dilute 150 micrograms/kg bodyweight to a final volume of 50 mL with Glucose 5% or Sodium Chloride 0.9%; an intravenous infusion rate of 0.1 mL/hour provides a dose of 5 nanograms/kg/minute. Undiluted solution must not come into contact with the barrel of the plastic syringe; add the required volume of alprostadil to a volume of infusion fluid in the syringe and then make up to final volume

Prostin VR® (Pharmacia) [PoM]
Intravenous solution, alprostadil 500 micrograms/mL in alcohol. For dilution and use as an infusion. Net price 1–mL amp = £75.19 (hosp.only)

DINOPROSTONE

Cautions see notes above; also history of haemorrhage; avoid in hyaline membrane disease; monitor arterial oxygenation, heart rate, temperature, and blood pressure in arm and leg; facilities for intubation and ventilation must be immediately available; **interactions**: Appendix 1 (prostaglandins)

Contra-indications

Hepatic impairment manufacturer advises avoid in hepatic impairment

Renal impairment manufacturer advises avoid in renal impairment

Side-effects nausea, vomiting, diarrhoea; flushing, bradycardia, hypotension, cardiac arrest; respiratory depression and apnoea, particularly with high doses and in low birth-weight neonates; bronchospasm; pyrexia and raised white blood cell count, shivering; local reactions, erythema; if used for longer than 5 days, gastric outlet obstruction; cortical hyperostosis (prolonged use)

Licensed use not licensed for use in children

Indication and dose

Maintaining patency of the ductus arteriosus
• By continuous intravenous infusion

Neonate initially 5–10 nanograms/kg/minute, increased as necessary in 5 nanogram/kg/minute increments to 20 nanograms/kg/minute
Note Doses up to 100 nanograms/kg/minute have been used but are associated with increased side-effects

• By mouth

Neonate 20–25 micrograms/kg every 1–2 hours doubled if necessary; if treatment continues for more than 1 week gradually reduce the dose

Administration for continuous intravenous infusion, dilute to a concentration of 1 microgram/mL with Glucose 5% or Sodium Chloride 0.9%.
For administration by mouth, injection solution can be given orally; dilute with water

Prostin® E2 (Pharmacia) [PoM]
Intravenous solution, for dilution and use as an infusion, dinoprostone 1 mg/mL, net price 0.75-mL amp = £8.52; 10 mg/mL, 0.5-mL amp = £18.40 (both hosp. only)

◄Extemporaneous formulations available see Extemporaneous Preparations, p. 8

2 Cardiovascular system

3 Respiratory system

3.1 Bronchodilators **168**
3.1.1 Adrenoceptor agonists 172
3.1.2 Antimuscarinic bronchodilators 178
3.1.3 Theophylline 178
3.1.4 Compound bronchodilator preparations 180
3.1.5 Peak flow meters, inhaler devices, and nebulisers 181

3.2 Corticosteroids **184**

3.3 Cromoglicate and related therapy and leukotriene receptor antagonists **189**
3.3.1 Cromoglicate and related therapy 189
3.3.2 Leukotriene receptor antagonists 190

3.4 Antihistamines, immunotherapy, and allergic emergencies **191**
3.4.1 Antihistamines 191
3.4.2 Allergen immunotherapy 196
3.4.3 Allergic emergencies 198

3.5 Respiratory stimulants and pulmonary surfactants **202**
3.5.1 Respiratory stimulants 202
3.5.2 Pulmonary surfactants 203

3.6 Oxygen **204**

3.7 Mucolytics **206**

3.8 Aromatic inhalations **208**

3.9 Cough preparations **208**
3.9.1 Cough suppressants 208
3.9.2 Expectorant and demulcent cough preparations 209

3.10 Systemic nasal decongestants **210**

3

Respiratory system

This chapter includes advice on the drug management of the following:

acute asthma, p. 168

anaphylaxis, p. 198

angioedema, p. 201

chronic asthma, p. 170

croup, p. 169

3.1 Bronchodilators

3.1.1 Adrenoceptor agonists

3.1.2 Antimuscarinic bronchodilators

3.1.3 Theophylline

3.1.4 Compound bronchodilator preparations

3.1.5 Peak flow meters, inhaler devices, and nebulisers

Asthma

Drugs used in the management of asthma include beta$_2$ agonists (section 3.1.1), antimuscarinic bronchodilators (section 3.1.2), theophylline (section 3.1.3), corticosteroids (section 3.2), cromoglicate and nedocromil (section 3.3.1), and leukotriene receptor antagonists (section 3.3.2).

For tables outlining the management of chronic asthma and management of acute asthma, see p. 170 and p. 171.

Administration of drugs for asthma

Inhalation   This route delivers the drug directly to the airways; the dose required is smaller than when given by mouth and side-effects are reduced. See Inhaler devices, section 3.1.5.

Solutions for nebulisation for use in acute severe asthma are administered over 5–10 minutes from a nebuliser, usually driven by oxygen in hospital. See Nebulisers, section 3.1.5.

Oral   Systemic side-effects occur more frequently when a drug is given orally rather than by inhalation. Oral corticosteroids, theophylline, and leukotriene receptor antagonists are sometimes required for the management of asthma. Oral administration of a beta$_2$ agonist is generally not recommended for children, but may be necessary in infants and young children unable to use an inhaler device.

Parenteral   Drugs such as beta$_2$ agonists, corticosteroids, and aminophylline can be given by injection in acute severe asthma when drug administration by nebulisation is inadequate or inappropriate; in these circumstances the child should generally be treated in a high-dependency or intensive care unit.

Pregnancy and breast-feeding

Women with asthma should be closely monitored during pregnancy. Well-controlled asthma has no important effects on pregnancy, labour, or the fetus. Drugs for asthma should preferably be administered by inhalation to minimise fetal drug exposure. Women planning to become pregnant should be counselled about the importance of taking their asthma medication regularly to maintain good control.

Severe exacerbations of asthma can have an adverse effect on pregnancy and should be treated promptly with conventional therapy, including oral or parenteral administration of a corticosteroid and nebulisation of a beta$_2$ agonist; prednisolone is the preferred corticosteroid for oral administration since very little of the drug reaches the fetus. Oxygen should be given immediately to maintain an arterial oxygen saturation of 94–98% and prevent maternal and fetal hypoxia.

Inhaled drugs, theophylline, and prednisolone can be taken as normal during pregnancy and breast-feeding.

Management of acute asthma[1]

> **Important**
> Regard each emergency consultation as being for **severe acute asthma** until shown otherwise.
>
> Failure to respond adequately **at any time** requires immediate transfer to hospital.

1. Advice on the management of acute asthma is based on the recommendations of the British Thoracic Society and Scottish Intercollegiate Guidelines Network (updated May 2008); updates available at www.brit-thoracic.org.uk

Severe acute asthma can be fatal and must be treated promptly and energetically. Treatment of severe acute asthma is safer in hospital where resuscitation facilities are immediately available. Treatment should **never** be delayed for investigations, children should **never** be sedated, and the possibility of a pneumothorax should be considered. If the child's condition deteriorates despite pharmacological treatment, urgent transfer to a paediatric intensive care unit should be arranged. For a table outlining the management of severe acute asthma, see Management of acute asthma p. 171.

Mild to moderate acute asthma   Administer a **short-acting beta₂ agonist** using a pressurised metered-dose inhaler with a spacer device; for a child under 3 years use a close-fitting facemask. Give 1 puff every 15–30 seconds up to a maximum of 10 puffs; repeat dose after 10–20 minutes if necessary.

Give **prednisolone** by mouth, child under 12 years 1–2 mg/kg (max. 40 mg) once daily for 3–5 days; if the child has been taking an oral corticosteroid for more than a few days, give prednisolone 2 mg/kg (max. 60 mg) once daily. For children 12–18 years, give prednisolone 40–50 mg daily for at least 5 days.

If response is poor or if a relapse occurs within 3–4 hours, transfer child **immediately** to hospital for assessment and further treatment.

Children under 18 months often respond poorly to bronchodilators; nebulised beta₂ agonists have been associated with mild (but occasionally severe) paradoxical bronchospasm and transient worsening of oxygen saturation; response to prednisolone may also be poor in this age group.

Severe or life-threatening acute asthma   Transfer **immediately** to hospital. Administer high-flow **oxygen** (section 3.6) using a close-fitting face mask or nasal prongs.

Treat severe or life-threatening acute exacerbations of asthma with an inhaled **short-acting beta₂ agonist** (as above). Treatment of life-threatening asthma should be initiated with nebulised salbutamol 2.5 mg or terbutaline 5 mg (via an oxygen-driven nebuliser if available); nebulised doses may be doubled for children over 5 years. Repeat the dose every 10–20 minutes or as necessary, then reduce the frequency on improvement.

If response is poor, add nebulised **ipratropium bromide** 250 micrograms every 20–30 minutes over the first 2 hours, then reduce the frequency on improvement.

Give **prednisolone** by mouth, child under 12 years 1–2 mg/kg (max. 40 mg) once daily for 3–5 days; if the child has been taking an oral corticosteroid for more than a few days, give prednisolone 2 mg/kg (max. 60 mg) once daily. For children 12–18 years, give prednisolone 40–50 mg daily for at least 5 days. If oral administration is not possible, use intravenous **hydrocortisone** (preferably as sodium succinate) 4 mg/kg (child under 2 years max. 25 mg, 2–5 years 50 mg, 5–18 years 100 mg) 3–4 times daily.

If the condition does not respond or is life-threatening, transfer the child to an intensive care unit and treat with a parenteral **short-acting beta₂ agonist** (e.g. salbutamol) (section 3.1.1.1) or parenteral **aminophylline** (section 3.1.3). Children over 2 years with severe asthma may be helped by intravenous infusion of **magnesium sulphate** 40 mg/kg (max. 2 g) over 20 minutes (section 9.5.1.3), but evidence of benefit is limited.

Croup

Mild croup is largely self-limiting, but treatment with a single dose of a corticosteroid (e.g. **dexamethasone** 150 micrograms/kg) by mouth is of benefit.

Severe croup (or mild croup that might cause complications) calls for hospital admission—a single dose of either dexamethasone 150 micrograms/kg or prednisolone 1–2 mg/kg, can be administered by mouth before transfer to hospital. In hospital, dexamethasone 150 micrograms/kg (by mouth or by injection) or budesonide 2 mg by nebulisation (section 3.2) will often reduce symptoms; the dose may be repeated after 12 hours if necessary.

For severe croup not effectively controlled with corticosteroid treatment, nebulised **adrenaline** (section 3.4.3) solution 1 in 1000 (1 mg/mL) can be given with close clinical monitoring in a dose of 400 micrograms/kg (max. 5 mg) repeated after 30 minutes if necessary (the dose may be diluted with sterile sodium chloride 0.9% solution). The effects of nebulised adrenaline last 2–3 hours; the child needs to be carefully monitored for recurrence of the obstruction.

Management of chronic asthma

Start at **step most appropriate** to initial severity; before initiating a new drug consider whether diagnosis is correct, check compliance and inhaler technique, and eliminate trigger factors for acute exacerbations

Child 5–18 years

Step 1: occasional relief bronchodilator

Inhaled short-acting beta$_2$ agonist as required (up to once daily)

Note Move to step 2 if needed more than twice a week, or if night-time symptoms more than once a week, or if exacerbation in the last 2 years

Step 2: regular inhaled preventer therapy

Inhaled short-acting beta$_2$ agonist as required

plus

Regular standard-dose[1] inhaled corticosteroid (alternatives[2] are considerably less effective)

Step 3: inhaled corticosteroid + inhaled long-acting beta$_2$ agonist

Inhaled short-acting beta$_2$ agonist as required

plus

Regular standard-dose[1] inhaled corticosteroid

plus

Regular inhaled long-acting beta$_2$ agonist (salmeterol *or* formoterol)

If asthma not controlled

Increase dose of inhaled corticosteroid to upper end of standard dose range[1]

and

Either stop long-acting beta$_2$ agonist if of no benefit

Or continue long-acting beta$_2$ agonist if of some benefit

If asthma still not controlled and long-acting beta$_2$ agonist stopped, add one of

> Leukotriene receptor antagonist
> Modified-release oral theophylline
> Modified-release oral beta$_2$ agonist

Step 4: high-dose inhaled corticosteroid + regular bronchodilators

Inhaled short-acting beta$_2$ agonist as required

with

Regular high-dose[3] inhaled corticosteroid

plus

Inhaled long-acting beta$_2$ agonist (if of benefit)

plus

A 6-week sequential therapeutic trial of one or more of

> Leukotriene receptor antagonist
> Modified-release oral theophylline
> Modified-release oral beta$_2$ agonist

Step 5: regular corticosteroid tablets

Refer to respiratory paediatrician

Inhaled short-acting beta$_2$ agonist as required

with

Regular high-dose[3] inhaled corticosteroid

and

One or more long-acting bronchodilators (see step 4)

plus

Regular prednisolone tablets (as single daily dose)

Note In addition to regular prednisolone, continue high-dose inhaled corticosteroid (in exceptional cases may exceed licensed doses)

Stepping down

Review treatment every 3 months; if control achieved stepwise reduction may be possible; reduce dose of *inhaled* corticosteroid slowly (consider reduction every 3 months, decreasing dose by up to 50% each time) to the lowest dose which controls asthma

Child under 5 years[4]

Step 1: occasional relief bronchodilator

Short-acting beta$_2$ agonist as required (not more than once daily)

Note Preferably by inhalation (less effective and more side-effects when given as tablets or syrup)

Move to step 2 if needed more than twice a week, or if night-time symptoms more than once a week, or if exacerbation in last 2 years

Step 2: regular preventer therapy

Inhaled short-acting beta$_2$ agonist as required

plus

Regular standard-dose[1] inhaled corticosteroid

Or leukotriene receptor antagonist if inhaled corticosteroid cannot be used

Step 3: add-on therapy

Child under 2 years:

Refer to respiratory paediatrician

Child 2–5 years:

Inhaled short-acting beta$_2$ agonist as required

plus

Regular standard-dose[1] inhaled corticosteroid

plus

Leukotriene receptor antagonist

Step 4: persistent poor control

Refer to respiratory paediatrician

Stepping down

Regularly review need for treatment

1. **Standard doses** of inhaled corticosteroids (metered-dose inhaler used with large-volume spacer)
   Beclometasone dipropionate or **budesonide**:
   Child under 12 years 100–200 micrograms twice daily;
   Child 12–18 years 100–400 micrograms twice daily.
   Fluticasone propionate:
   Child 4–12 years 50–100 micrograms twice daily;
   Child 12–18 years 50–200 micrograms twice daily.
   Mometasone furoate (given through dry powder inhaler):
   Child 12–18 years 200 micrograms twice daily

2. Alternatives to inhaled corticosteroid are leukotriene receptor antagonists, theophylline, inhaled nedocromil, or inhaled cromoglicate

3. **High doses** of inhaled corticosteroids (metered-dose inhaler used with large-volume spacer)
   Beclometasone dipropionate or **budesonide**:
   Child 5–12 years 200–400 micrograms twice daily;
   Child 12–18 years 0.4–1 mg twice daily.
   Fluticasone propionate:
   Child 5–12 years 100–200 micrograms twice daily;
   Child 12–18 years 200–500 micrograms twice daily.
   Mometasone furoate (given through dry powder inhaler):
   Child 12–18 years up to 400 micrograms twice daily.
   Note. Failure to achieve control with these doses is unusual, see also Side-effects of Inhaled Corticosteroids, section 3.2

4. Lung-function measurements cannot be used to guide management in those under 5 years

Advice on the management of chronic asthma is based on the recommendations of the British Thoracic Society and Scottish Intercollegiate Guidelines Network (updated May 2008); updates available at www.brit-thoracic.org.uk

Management of acute asthma

Important The assessment of acute asthma in early childhood can be difficult. Children with severe or life-threatening acute asthma may not be distressed and may not have all of these abnormalities; the presence of any should alert the doctor. Regard each emergency consultation as being for **severe acute asthma** until shown otherwise		

Moderate acute asthma	Severe acute asthma	Life-threatening acute asthma
• Respiration Child 2–5 years ≤ 50 breaths/minute, 5–12 years ≤ 30 breaths/minute, 12–18 years < 25 breaths/minute • Pulse Child 2–5 years ≤ 130 beats/minute, 5–12 years ≤ 120 beats/minute, 12–18 years < 110 beats/minute • Arterial oxygen saturation ≥ 92% • Peak flow Child 5–12 years ≥ 50% of predicted or best, 12–18 years > 50% of predicted or best *Treat at home or in surgery and assess response to treatment*	• Child under 12 years too breathless to talk or feed, 12–18 years cannot complete sentences in one breath • Use of accessory breathing muscles • Respiration Child 2–5 years > 50 breaths/minute, 5–12 years > 30 breaths/minute, 12–18 years ≥ 25 breaths/minute • Pulse Child 2–5 years > 130 beats/minute, 5–12 years >120 beats/minute, 12–18 years ≥ 110 beats/minute • Arterial oxygen saturation < 92% • Peak flow Child 5–12 years < 50% of predicted or best, 12–18 years 33-50% of predicted or best *Send immediately to hospital*	Arterial oxygen saturation < 92% plus any of the following: • Silent chest • Poor respiratory effort • Cyanosis • Reduced level of consciousness • Peak flow < 33% of predicted or best *Send immediately to hospital; consult with senior medical staff and refer to paediatric intensive care*
Treatment • Inhaled **short-acting beta₂ agonist** via a large-volume spacer (and a close-fitting face mask if child under 3 years) or oxygen-driven nebuliser (if available); give 4–10 puffs of **salbutamol** 100 micrograms/metered inhalation each inhaled separately, and repeat at 10–20 minute intervals if necessary *or* give nebulised **salbutamol**, Child under 5 years 2.5 mg, 5–12 years 2.5–5 mg, 12–18 years 5 mg *or* terbutaline Child under 5 years 5 mg, 5–12 years 5–10 mg, 12–18 years 10 mg, and repeat at 10–20 minute intervals if necessary • **Prednisolone** by mouth Child under 12 years 1–2 mg/kg (max. 40 mg) daily for 3–5 days; if the child has been taking an oral corticosteroid for more than a few days, give prednisolone 2 mg/kg (max. 60 mg); Child 12–18 years 40–50 mg daily for at least 5 days *Monitor response for 15–30 minutes* *If response is poor or a relapse occurs in 3–4 hours, send immediately to hospital for assessment and further treatment*	**Treatment** • High-flow **oxygen** (if available) • Inhaled **short-acting beta₂ agonist** via a large-volume spacer (and a close-fitting face mask if child under 3 years) or oxygen-driven nebuliser (if available); give 4–10 puffs of **salbutamol** 100 micrograms/metered inhalation each inhaled separately, and repeat at 10–20 minute intervals or as necessary *or* give nebulised **salbutamol**, Ch ld under 5 years 2.5 mg, 5–12 years 2.5–5 mg, 12–18 years 5 mg *or* **terbutaline** Child under 5 years 5 mg, 5–12 years 5–10 mg, 12–18 years 10 mg, and repeat at 10–20 minute intervals or as necessary • **Prednisolone** by mouth as for moderate acute asthma *or* intravenous **hydrocortisone** (preferably as sodium succinate) 4 mg/kg (Child under 2 years max. 25 mg, 2–5 years 50 mg, 5–18 years 100 mg) 3–4 times daily until conversion to oral prednisolone is possible *Monitor response for 15–30 minutes* *If response is poor:* • Inhaled **ipratropium bromide** via oxygen-driven nebuliser (if available), Child under 12 years, 250 micrograms, 12–18 years, 500 micrograms and repeat at 20–30 minute intervals if necessary *Refer those who fail to respond and require ventilatory support to a paediatric intensive care or high-dependency unit* • Consider intravenous **beta₂ agonists, aminophylline**, or **magnesium sulphate** [unlicensed indication] only after consultation with senior medical staff *If symptoms improve, follow up as for moderate acute asthma*	**Treatment** • High-flow **oxygen** (if available) • Inhaled **short-acting beta₂ agonist** via oxygen-driven nebuliser (if available); give **salbutamol**, Child under 5 years 2.5 mg, 5–12 years 2.5–5 mg, 12–18 years 5 mg, or **terbutaline**, Child under 5 years 5 mg, 5–12 years 5–10 mg, 12–18 years 10 mg, and repeat as necessary; reserve **intravenous beta₂ agonists** for those in whom inhaled therapy cannot be used reliably or there is no current effect • **Prednisolone** by mouth as for moderate acute asthma *or* intravenous **hydrocortisone** (preferably as sodium succinate) 4 mg/kg (Child under 2 years, max. 25 mg, 2–5 years 50 mg, 5–18 years 100 mg) 3–4 times daily until conversion to oral prednisolone is possible • Inhaled **ipratropium bromide** via oxygen-driven nebuliser (if available), Child under 12 years 250 micrograms, 12–18 years 500 micrograms and repeat at 20–30 minute intervals if necessary *Monitor response for 15–30 minutes* • Consider intravenous **beta₂ agonists, aminophylline**, or **magnesium sulphate** [unlicensed indication] only after consultation with senior medical staff *If symptoms improve, follow up as for moderate acute asthma*
Follow up in all cases Monitor symptoms and peak flow Set up asthma action plan and check inhaler technique with child and carer Review by general practitioner within 48 hours; modify treatment according to the Management of Chronic Asthma table, p. 170		

Advice on the management of acute asthma is based on the recommendations of the British Thoracic Society and Scottish Intercollegiate Guidelines Network (updated May 2008); updates available at www.brit-thoracic.org.uk

3 Respiratory system

3.1.1 Adrenoceptor agonists
(Sympathomimetics)

3.1.1.1 Selective beta$_2$ agonists
3.1.1.2 Other adrenoceptor agonists

The selective beta$_2$ agonists (selective beta$_2$-adrenoceptor agonists, selective beta$_2$ stimulants) such as salbutamol or terbutaline are the safest and most effective short-acting beta$_2$ agonists for the treatment of asthma. Less selective beta$_2$ agonists, such as orciprenaline, are no longer recommended for the treatment of asthma.

Adrenaline (epinephrine), which has both alpha- and beta-adrenoceptor agonist properties, is used in the emergency management of allergic and anaphylactic reactions (section 3.4.3); it is also used as a nebuliser solution to treat severe croup.

3.1.1.1 Selective beta$_2$ agonists

Selective beta$_2$ agonists produce bronchodilation. A short-acting beta$_2$ agonist is used for immediate relief of asthma symptoms while a long-acting beta$_2$ agonist is used in addition to an inhaled corticosteroid in children requiring prophylactic treatment.

Short-acting beta$_2$ agonists Mild to moderate symptoms of asthma respond rapidly to the inhalation of a selective short-acting beta$_2$ agonist such as **salbutamol** or **terbutaline**. If beta$_2$ agonist inhalation is needed more often than once daily, prophylactic treatment should be considered, using a stepped approach as outlined in the Management of Chronic Asthma, p. 170. Regular treatment with an inhaled short-acting beta$_2$ agonist is less effective than 'as required' inhalation and is not appropriate prophylactic treatment.

A short-acting beta$_2$ agonist inhaled immediately before exertion reduces *exercise-induced asthma*; however, frequent exercise-induced asthma probably reflects poor overall control and calls for reassessment of asthma treatment.

Long-acting beta$_2$ agonists **Formoterol** (eformoterol) and **salmeterol** are longer-acting beta$_2$ agonists which are administered by inhalation. Added to regular inhaled corticosteroid treatment, they have a role in the long-term control of chronic asthma (see Management of Chronic Asthma, p. 170) and they can be useful in nocturnal asthma. Salmeterol should not be used for the relief of an asthma attack; it has a slower onset of action than salbutamol or terbutaline. Formoterol is licensed for short-term symptom relief and for the prevention of exercise-induced bronchospasm; its speed of onset of action is similar to that of salbutamol.

> CHM advice
> To ensure safe use, the CHM has advised that for the management of chronic asthma, long-acting beta$_2$ agonists (formoterol and salmeterol) should:
> - be added only if regular use of standard-dose inhaled corticosteroids has failed to control asthma adequately;
> - not be initiated in patients with rapidly deteriorating asthma;
> - be introduced at a low dose and the effect monitored before considering dose increase;
> - be discontinued in the absence of benefit;
> - be reviewed as clinically appropriate: stepping down therapy should be considered when good long-term asthma control has been achieved.
>
> Children and their carers should be advised to report any deterioration in symptoms following initiation of treatment with a long-acting beta$_2$ agonist, see Management of Chronic Asthma, p. 170.

Management of Chronic Asthma, see p. 170
Management of Acute Asthma, see p. 168
For guidance on the use of inhalers and spacer devices, see section 3.1.5

Inhalation   A *pressurised metered-dose inhaler* is an effective method of drug administration in mild to moderate chronic asthma; to deliver the drug effectively particularly in children under 12 years, a spacer device should be used (see also NICE guidance, section 3.1.5). When a pressurised metered-dose inhaler with a spacer is unsuitable or inconvenient, a *dry-powder inhaler* or *breath-actuated inhaler* may be used instead if the child is able to use the device effectively. At recommended inhaled doses the duration of action of salbutamol and terbutaline is about 3 to 5 hours and for salmeterol and formoterol is about 12 hours. The **dose**, the frequency, and the maximum number of inhalations in 24 hours of the beta$_2$ agonist should be **stated explicitly** to the child and the child's carer. High doses of beta$_2$ agonists can be dangerous in some children (see Cautions, below). Excessive use is usually an indication of **inadequately controlled** asthma and should be managed with a prophylactic drug such as an inhaled corticosteroid. The child and the child's carer should be advised to seek medical advice when the prescribed dose of beta$_2$ agonist fails to provide the usual degree of symptomatic relief because this usually indicates a worsening of the asthma and the child may require alternative medication (see Management of Chronic Asthma, p. 170).

Children and their carers should be advised to follow manufacturers' instructions on the care and cleansing of inhaler devices.

CFC-free inhalers   Chlorofluorocarbon (CFC) propellants in pressurised metered-dose inhalers are being replaced by hydrofluoroalkane (HFA) propellants. Children receiving CFC-free inhalers and their carers should be reassured about the efficacy of the new inhalers and counselled that the aerosol may feel and taste different to their previous CFC-based inhaler; any difficulty with the new inhaler should be discussed with the doctor or pharmacist.

Nebuliser (or respirator) solutions of salbutamol and terbutaline are used for the treatment of severe acute asthma both in hospital and in general practice. Children with a severe attack of asthma should have oxygen if possible during nebulisation since beta$_2$ agonists can increase arterial hypoxaemia, see also section 3.1.5.

Oral   Oral preparations of beta$_2$ agonists may be used for children if an inhaler device cannot be used but inhaled beta$_2$ agonists are more effective and have fewer side-effects. A modified-release formulation of salbutamol may be of value in nocturnal asthma as an alternative to modified-release theophylline preparations (section 3.1.3), but an inhaled long-acting beta$_2$ agonist is preferable.

Parenteral   Beta$_2$ agonists can be given intravenously in children with severe or life-threatening acute asthma. Chronic asthma unresponsive to stepwise treatment (see Management of Chronic Asthma, p. 170) may benefit from continuous subcutaneous infusion of a beta$_2$ agonist but this should be used only under the supervision of a respiratory specialist; the evidence of benefit is uncertain and it may be difficult to withdraw such treatment once started.

Cautions   Beta$_2$ agonists should be used with caution in diabetes—monitor blood glucose (risk of ketoacidosis, especially when a beta$_2$ agonist is given intravenously). Beta$_2$ agonists should also be used with caution in hyperthyroidism, cardiovascular disease, arrhythmias, susceptibility to QT-interval prolongation, and hypertension. If high doses of beta$_2$ agonists are needed during pregnancy they should be given by inhalation because a parenteral beta$_2$ agonist can affect the myometrium and possibly cause cardiac problems; see also Pregnancy and Breast-feeding, section 3.1. **Interactions:** Appendix 1 (sympathomimetics, beta$_2$).

Hypokalaemia   The CSM has advised that potentially serious hypokalaemia may result from beta$_2$ agonist therapy. Particular caution is required in severe asthma, because this effect may be potentiated by concomitant treatment with theophylline and its derivatives, corticosteroids, and diuretics, and by hypoxia. Plasma-potassium concentration should therefore be monitored in severe asthma.

Side-effects   Side-effects of the beta$_2$ agonists include fine tremor (particularly in the hands), nervous tension, headache, peripheral dilatation and palpitation. Other side-effects include tachycardia, arrhythmias, peripheral vasodilation, myocardial ischaemia, and disturbances of sleep and behaviour. Muscle cramps and

3

Respiratory system

hypersensitivity reactions including paradoxical bronchospasm (occasionally severe), urticaria, angioedema, hypotension, and collapse have also been reported. High doses of beta$_2$ agonists are associated with hypokalaemia (for CSM advice, see Hypokalaemia, p. 173).

FORMOTEROL FUMARATE
(Eformoterol fumarate)

Cautions see notes above

Hepatic impairment metabolism possibly reduced in severe cirrhosis

Pregnancy see section 3.1 (manufacturers advise use only if potential benefit outweighs risk)

Breast-feeding amount in milk probably too small to be harmful but manufacturers advise avoid

Side-effects see notes above; nausea, dizziness, rash, taste disturbances, and pruritus also reported

Indication and dose

Reversible airways obstruction (including nocturnal asthma and prevention of exercise-induced bronchospasm) in patients requiring long-term regular bronchodilator therapy see also Management of Chronic Asthma, p. 170; for dose see preparations below

Counselling Advise children and carers not to exceed prescribed dose, and to follow manufacturer's directions; if a previously effective dose of inhaled formoterol fails to provide adequate relief, a doctor's advice should be obtained as soon as possible

Formoterol (Non-proprietary) PoM

Dry powder for inhalation, formoterol fumarate 12 micrograms/metered inhalation, net price 120-dose unit = £24.80. Counselling, dose

Brands include *Easyhaler® Formoterol*

Dose

Chronic asthma
- **By inhalation of powder**

Child 6–18 years 12 micrograms twice daily, increased to 24 micrograms twice daily in more severe airways obstruction

Atimos Modulite® (Chiesi) ▼ PoM

Aerosol inhalation, formoterol fumarate 12 micrograms/metered inhalation, net price 100-dose unit = £31.28. Counselling, dose

Dose

Chronic Asthma
- **By aerosol inhalation**

Child 12–18 years 12 micrograms twice daily, increased to max. 24 micrograms twice daily in more severe airways obstruction

Foradil® (Novartis) PoM

Dry powder for inhalation, formoterol fumarate 12 micrograms/capsule, net price 60-cap pack (with inhaler device) = £29.23. Counselling, dose

Dose

Chronic asthma
- **By inhalation of powder**

Child 5–18 years 12 micrograms twice daily, increased to 24 micrograms twice daily in more severe airways obstruction

Oxis® (AstraZeneca) PoM

Turbohaler®(= dry powder inhaler), formoterol fumarate 6 micrograms/inhalation, net price 60-dose unit = £24.80; 12 micrograms/inhalation, 60-dose unit = £24.80. Counselling, dose

Dose

Chronic asthma
- **By inhalation of powder**

Child 6–18 years 6–12 micrograms 1–2 times daily; occasionally up to 48 micrograms daily may be needed (max. single dose 12 micrograms); reassess treatment if additional doses required on more than 2 days a week

Relief of bronchospasm
- **By inhalation of powder**

Child 6–18 years 6–12 micrograms

Prevention of exercise-induced bronchospasm
- **By inhalation of powder**

Child 6–18 years 6–12 micrograms before exercise

Compound preparations

For **compound preparations** containing formoterol, see section 3.2

SALBUTAMOL
(Albuterol)

Cautions see notes above

Side-effects see notes above

Licensed use not licensed for use in hyperkalaemia; syrup not licensed for use in children under 2 years; modified-release tablets not licensed for use in children under 3 years; injection not licensed for use in children; *Pulvinal® Salbutamol* not licensed for use in children under 6 years

Indication and dose

Acute asthma
- **By aerosol or nebulised solution inhalation**
See Management of Acute Asthma, p. 168

- **By intravenous injection over 5 minutes (see also Management of Acute Asthma, p. 168)**

Child 1 month–2 years 5 micrograms/kg as a single dose

Child 2–18 years 15 micrograms/kg (max. 250 micrograms) as a single dose

◻ **SALBUTAMOL** (*continued*)

• **By continuous intravenous infusion**

    Child 1 month–18 years 1–2 micrograms/kg/ minute, adjusted according to response and heart rate up to 5 micrograms/kg/minute; doses above 2 micrograms/kg/minute should be given in an intensive care setting

Exacerbations of reversible airways obstruction (including nocturnal asthma) and prevention of allergen- or exercise-induced bronchospasm, see also Management of Chronic Asthma, p. 170

• **By aerosol inhalation**

    Child 1 month–18 years 100–200 micrograms (1–2 puffs); for persistent symptoms up to 4 times daily

• **By inhalation of powder**

    (for *Asmasal Clickhaler®*, *Salbulin Novolizer®*, and *Ventolin Accuhaler®* doses, see under preparations)

    Child 5–12 years 200 micrograms; for persistent symptoms up to 4 times daily

    Child 12–18 years 200–400 micrograms; for persistent symptoms up to 4 times daily

• **By mouth (but use by inhalation preferred)**

    Child 1 month–2 years 100 micrograms/kg (max. 2 mg) 3–4 times daily

    Child 2–6 years 1–2 mg 3–4 times daily

    Child 6–12 years 2 mg 3–4 times daily

    Child 12–18 years 4 mg (sensitive patients initially 2 mg) 3–4 times daily; max. single dose 8 mg (but unlikely to provide extra benefit or to be tolerated)

Severe hyperkalaemia (section 9.2.1.1)

• **By intravenous injection over 5 minutes**

    Neonate 4 micrograms/kg as a single dose; repeat if necessary

    Child 1 month–18 years 4 micrograms/kg as a single dose; repeat if necessary

• **By inhalation of nebulised solution (but intravenous injection preferred)**

    Neonate 2.5–5 mg as a single dose; repeat if necessary

    Child 1 month–18 years 2.5–5 mg as a single dose; repeat if necessary

Administration for *continuous intravenous infusion*, dilute to a concentration of 200 micrograms/mL with Glucose 5%, Sodium Chloride 0.9%, *or* Water for injections; if fluid-restricted, can be given undiluted through central venous catheter. For *intravenous injection*, dilute to a concentration of 50 micrograms/mL with Glucose 5%, Sodium Chloride 0.9%, *or* Water for injections

For *nebulisation*, dilute nebuliser solution with a suitable volume of sterile Sodium Chloride 0.9% solution according to nebuliser type and duration of administration; salbutamol and ipratropium bromide solutions are compatible and can be mixed for nebulisation.

◀Oral
Salbutamol (Non-proprietary) ⓅⓄⓂ

    Tablets, salbutamol (as sulphate) 2 mg, net price 28-tab pack = £12.71; 4 mg, 28-tab pack = £12.20

    Oral solution, salbutamol (as sulphate) 2 mg/5 mL, net price 150 mL = £1.27
    Brands include *Salapin®* (sugar-free)

Ventmax® SR (Chiesi) ⓅⓄⓂ

    Capsules, m/r, salbutamol (as sulphate) 4 mg (green/grey), net price 56-cap pack = £8.57; 8 mg (white), 56-cap pack = £10.28. Label: 25
Dose
    Chronic asthma (but see notes above)
    • **By mouth**
        Child 3–12 years 4 mg twice daily
        Child 12–18 years 8 mg twice daily

Ventolin® (A&H) ⓅⓄⓂ

    Syrup, sugar-free, salbutamol (as sulphate) 2 mg/ 5 mL, net price 150 mL = 60p

◀Parenteral
Ventolin® (A&H) ⓅⓄⓂ

    Injection, salbutamol (as sulphate) 500 micrograms/mL, net price 1-mL amp = 40p

    Solution for intravenous infusion, salbutamol (as sulphate) 1 mg/mL. Dilute before use. Net price 5-mL amp = £2.58

◀Inhalation
    Counselling Advise children and carers not to exceed prescribed dose and to follow manufacturer's directions; if a previously effective dose of inhaled salbutamol fails to provide at least 3 hours relief, a doctor's advice should be obtained as soon as possible.
    Patients receiving CFC-free inhalers should be reassured about their efficacy and counselled that aerosol may feel and taste different (see notes above)

Salbutamol (Non-proprietary) ⓅⓄⓂ

    Aerosol inhalation, salbutamol 100 micrograms/ metered inhalation, net price 200-dose unit = £2.88. Counselling, dose
    Excipients include CFC propellants

    Aerosol inhalation, salbutamol (as sulphate) 100 micrograms/metered inhalation, net price 200-dose unit = £2.99. Counselling, dose, change to CFC-free inhaler
    Excipients include HFA-134a (a non-CFC propellant)
    Brands include *Salamol®*
    Note Can be supplied against a generic prescription but if CFC-free not specified will be reimbursed at price for CFC-containing inhaler

    Dry powder for inhalation, salbutamol 100 micrograms/metered inhalation, net price 200-dose unit = £3.46; 200 micrograms/metered inhalation, 100-dose unit = £5.05, 200-dose unit = £6.92. Counselling, dose
    Brands include *Easyhaler® Salbutamol*, *Pulvinal® Salbutamol*

    Inhalation powder, *hard capsule* (for use with *Cyclohaler®* device), salbutamol 200 micrograms, net price 120-cap pack = £8.99; 400 micrograms, 120-cap pack = £12.99. Counselling, dose
    Brands include *Salbutamol Cyclocaps®*

3

Respiratory system

◁ **SALBUTAMOL** (*continued*)

Nebuliser solution, salbutamol (as sulphate) 1 mg/
mL, net price 20 × 2.5 mL (2.5 mg) = £1.99; 2 mg/
mL, 20 × 2.5 mL (5 mg) = £3.98. May be diluted
with sterile sodium chloride 0.9%
Brands include *Salamol Steri-Neb®*

Airomir® (IVAX) [PoM]

Aerosol inhalation, salbutamol (as sulphate)
100 micrograms/metered inhalation, net price 200-
dose unit = £1.97. Counselling, dose, change to
CFC-free inhaler
Excipients include HFA-134a (a non-CFC propellant)

Note Can be supplied against a generic prescription but if
'CFC-free' not specified will be reimbursed at price for
CFC-containing inhaler

Autohaler (breath-actuated aerosol inhalation),
salbutamol (as sulphate) 100 micrograms/metered
inhalation, net price 200-dose unit = £6.02. Counselling, dose, change to CFC-free inhaler
Excipients include HFA-134a (a non-CFC propellant),

Asmasal Clickhaler® (UCB Pharma) [PoM]

Dry powder for inhalation, salbutamol (as sulphate)
95 micrograms/metered inhalation, net price 200-
dose unit = £5.88. Counselling, dose

Dose

Acute bronchospasm
• **By inhalation of powder**
Child 5–18 years 1–2 puffs; for persistent symptoms
up to 4 times daily (but see also Management of
Chronic Asthma, p. 170)

Prophylaxis of allergen- or exercise-induced bron-
chospasm
• **By inhalation of powder**
Child 5–18 years 1–2 puffs

Salamol Easi-Breathe® (IVAX) [PoM]

Aerosol inhalation , salbutamol 100 micrograms/
metered inhalation, net price 200-dose breath-
actuated unit = £6.30. Counselling, dose
Excipients include HFA-134a (a non-CFC propellant)

Salbulin Novolizer® (Meda) [PoM]

Dry powder for inhalation, salbutamol (as sulphate)
100 micrograms/metered inhalation, net price
refillable 200-dose unit = £4.95; 200-dose refill =
£2.75. Counselling, dose

Dose

Acute bronchospasm
• **By inhalation of powder**
Child 6–12 years 100-200 micrograms; for persistent
symptoms up to 400 micrograms daily (but see also
Management of Chronic Asthma, p. 170)

Child 12–18 years 100-200 micrograms; for persistent
symptoms up to 800 micrograms daily (but see also
Management of Chronic Asthma, p. 170)

Prophylaxis of allergen- or exercise-induced bron-
chospasm
• **By inhalation of powder**
Child 6–12 years 100–200 micrograms
Child 12–18 years 200 micrograms

Ventolin® (A&H) [PoM]

Accuhaler® (dry powder for inhalation), disk containing 60 blisters of salbutamol (as sulphate)
200 micrograms/blister with *Accuhaler®* device, net
price = £5.12. Counselling, dose

Dose

Acute bronchospasm
• **By inhalation of powder**
Child 5–18 years 200 micrograms; for persistent
symptoms up to 4 times daily but see also Management of Chronic Asthma, p. 170

Prophylaxis of allergen- or exercise-induced bron-
chospasm
• **By inhalation of powder**
Child 5–18 years 200 micrograms

Evohaler® *aerosol inhalation*, salbutamol (as sulphate) 100 micrograms/metered inhalation, net
price 200-dose unit = £1.50. Counselling, dose,
change to CFC-free inhaler
Excipients include HFA-134a (a non-CFC propellant)

Note Can be supplied against a generic prescription but if
CFC-free not specified will be reimbursed at price for
CFC-containing inhaler

Nebules® (for use with nebuliser), salbutamol (as
sulphate) 1 mg/mL, net price 20 × 2.5 mL (2.5 mg)
= £1.75; 2 mg/mL, 20 × 2.5 mL (5 mg) = £2.95. May
be diluted with sterile sodium chloride 0.9%

Respirator solution (for use with a nebuliser or
ventilator), salbutamol (as sulphate) 5 mg/mL. Net
price 20 mL = £2.27 (hosp. only). May be diluted
with sterile sodium chloride 0.9%

◢ SALMETEROL

Note Not for immediate relief of acute attacks; existing
corticosteroid therapy should not be reduced or withdrawn

Cautions see notes above

Side-effects see notes above; nausea, dizziness,
arthralgia, and rash also reported

Indication and dose

Reversible airways obstruction (including
nocturnal asthma and prevention of exercise-
induced bronchospasm) in patients requiring
long-term regular bronchodilator therapy see
also Management of Chronic Asthma, p. 170

• **By inhalation**
Child 5–12 years 50 micrograms (2 puffs or 1
blister) twice daily

◻ **SALMETEROL** (*continued*)

Child 12–18 years 50 micrograms (2 puffs or 1 blister) twice daily; up to 100 micrograms (4 puffs or 2 blisters) twice daily in more severe airways obstruction

Counselling Advise children and carers that salmeterol should **not** be used for relief of acute attacks, not to exceed prescribed dose, and to follow manufacturer's directions; if a previously effective dose of inhaled salmeterol fails to provide adequate relief, a doctor's advice should be obtained as soon as possible

Serevent® (A&H) ⒫ₒₘ

Accuhaler® (dry powder for inhalation), disk containing 60 blisters of salmeterol (as xinafoate) 50 micrograms/blister with *Accuhaler®* device, net price = £29.26. Counselling, dose

Evohaler® aerosol inhalation, salmeterol (as xinafoate) 25 micrograms/metered inhalation, net price 120-dose unit = £29.26. Counselling, dose, change to CFC-free inhaler

Excipients include HFA-13Ha (a non-CFC propellant)

Diskhaler® (dry powder for inhalation), disks containing 4 blisters of salmeterol (as xinafoate) 50 micrograms/blister, net price 15 disks with *Diskhaler®* device = £35.79, 15-disk refill = £35.15. Counselling, dose, change to CFC-free inhaler

◀Compound preparations

For **compound preparations** containing salmeterol, see section 3.2

🔳 **TERBUTALINE SULPHATE**

Cautions see notes above
Side-effects see notes above
Licensed use tablets not licensed for use in children under 7 years; injection not licensed for use in children under 2 years

Indication and dose

Acute asthma

• **By inhalation of nebulised solution**
see Management of Acute Asthma, p. 168

• **By subcutaneous or slow intravenous injection**
Child 2–15 years 10 micrograms/kg (max. 300 micrograms) up to 4 times daily
Child 15–18 years 250–500 micrograms up to 4 times daily

• **By continuous intravenous infusion**
Child 1 month–18 years initially 2–4 micrograms/kg as a loading dose, then 1–10 micrograms/kg/hour according to response and heart rate (doses above 10 micrograms/kg/hour with close monitoring)

Exacerbations of reversible airways obstruction (including nocturnal asthma) and prevention of exercise-induced bronchospasm see Management of Chronic Asthma, p. 170

• **By inhalation of powder**
Child 5–18 years 500 micrograms (1 inhalation) up to 4 times daily (for occasional use only)

• **By mouth (but not recommended)**
Child 1 month–7 years 75 micrograms/kg (max. 2.5 mg) 3 times daily
Child 7–15 years 2.5 mg 2–3 times daily
Child 15–18 years initially 2.5 mg 3 times daily, increased if necessary to 5 mg 3 times daily

Administration For *continuous intravenous infusion*, dilute to a concentration of 5 micrograms/mL with Glucose 5% *or* Sodium Chloride 0.9%; if fluid-restricted, dilute to a concentration of 100 micrograms/mL

For *nebulisation*, dilute nebuliser solution with sterile Sodium Chloride 0.9% solution according to nebuliser type and duration of administration; terbutaline and ipratropium bromide solutions are compatible and may be mixed for nebulisation.

◀Oral and parenteral

Bricanyl® (AstraZeneca) ⒫ₒₘ
Tablets, scored, terbutaline sulphate 5 mg, net price 20 = 82p

Syrup, sugar-free, terbutaline sulphate 1.5 mg/5 mL, net price 100 mL = £2.00

Injection, terbutaline sulphate 500 micrograms/mL, net price 1-mL amp = 30p; 5-mL amp = £1.40

◀Inhalation

Counselling Advise children and carers not to exceed prescribed dose and to follow manufacturer's directions; if a previously effective dose of inhaled terbutaline fails to provide at least 3 hours relief, a doctor's advice should be obtained as soon as possible

Bricanyl® (AstraZeneca) ⒫ₒₘ
Turbohaler® (= dry powder inhaler), terbutaline sulphate 500 micrograms/metered inhalation, net price 100-dose unit = £6.92. Counselling, dose

Respules® (= single-dose units for nebulisation), terbutaline sulphate 2.5 mg/mL, net price 20 × 2-mL units (5-mg) = £4.04

3.1.1.2 **Other adrenoceptor agonists**

Adrenaline (epinephrine) injection (1 in 1000) is used in the emergency treatment of acute allergic and anaphylactic reactions (section 3.4.3), in angioedema (section 3.4.3), and in cardiopulmonary resuscitation (section 2.7.3). Adrenaline solution (1 in 1000) is used by nebulisation in the management of severe croup (section 3.1).

3 Respiratory system

3.1.2 Antimuscarinic bronchodilators

Ipratropium by nebulisation can be added to other standard treatment in life-threatening acute asthma or if acute asthma fails to improve with standard therapy (see Management of Acute Asthma, p. 168). Ipratropium can be used to provide short-term relief in chronic asthma, but short-acting beta$_2$ agonists act more quickly and are preferred.

The aerosol inhalation of ipratropium has a maximum effect 30–60 minutes after use; its duration of action is 3 to 6 hours.

IPRATROPIUM BROMIDE

Cautions risk of glaucoma (see below), bladder outflow obstruction; **interactions**: Appendix 1 (antimuscarinics)

Glaucoma *Acute angle-closure glaucoma* reported with nebulised ipratropium, particularly when given with nebulised salbutamol (and possibly other beta$_2$ agonists); care needed to protect the child's eyes from nebulised drug or from drug powder

Side-effects dry mouth; *less commonly* nausea and headache; *rarely* constipation, tachycardia, palpitation, paradoxical bronchospasm, urinary retention, blurred vision, angle-closure glaucoma, and hypersensitivity reactions including rash, urticaria, and angioedema

Indication and dose

Acute asthma
• **By inhalation of nebulised solution**
  See Management of Acute Asthma, section 3.1

Reversible airways obstruction see notes above
• **By aerosol inhalation**
  Child 1 month–6 years 20 micrograms 3 times daily
  Child 6–12 years 20–40 micrograms 3 times daily
  Child 12–18 years 20–40 micrograms 3–4 times daily

• **By inhalation of powder**
  Child 12–18 years 40 micrograms 3–4 times daily (dose may be doubled in less responsive condition)

Counselling Advise child and carer not to exceed prescribed dose and to follow manufacturer's directions

Rhinitis section 12.2.2

Ipratropium Bromide (Non-proprietary) [PoM]
Nebuliser solution, ipratropium bromide 250 micrograms/mL, net price 20 × 1-mL (250-microgram) unit-dose vials = £6.75, 60 × 1-mL = £21.78; 20 × 2-mL (500-microgram) = £7.43, 60 × 2-mL = £26.97

Atrovent® (Boehringer Ingelheim) [PoM]
Aerocaps® (dry powder for inhalation; for use with *Atrovent Aerohaler®*), green, ipratropium bromide 40 micrograms, net price pack of 100 caps with *Aerohaler®* = £14.53; 100 caps = £10.53. Counselling, dose
Note One *Atrovent Aerocap®* is equivalent to 2 puffs of *Atrovent®* metered aerosol inhalation

Aerosol inhalation ▼, ipratropium bromide 20 micrograms/metered inhalation, net price 200-dose unit = £4.21. Counselling, dose, change to CFC-free inhaler
Excipients include HFA-134a (a non-CFC propellant)

Nebuliser solution, isotonic, ipratropium bromide 250 micrograms/mL, net price 20 × 1-mL unit-dose vials = £5.18, 60 × 1-mL vials = £15.55; 20 × 2-mL vials = £6.08, 60 × 2-mL vials = £18.24

Ipratropium Steri-Neb® (IVAX) [PoM]
Nebuliser solution, isotonic, ipratropium bromide 250 micrograms/mL, net price 20 × 1-mL (250-microgram) unit-dose vials = £8.72; 20 × 2-mL (500-microgram) = £9.94

Respontin® (A&H) [PoM]
Nebuliser solution, isotonic, ipratropium bromide 250 micrograms/mL, net price 20 × 1-mL (250-microgram) unit-dose vials = £5.07; 20 × 2-mL (500-microgram) = £5.95

3.1.3 Theophylline

Theophylline is a bronchodilator used for asthma, see Management of Chronic Asthma p. 170. It may have an additive effect when used in conjunction with small doses of beta$_2$ agonists; the combination may increase the risk of side-effects, including hypokalaemia (see p. 173).

Theophylline is given by injection as **aminophylline**, a mixture of theophylline with ethylenediamine, which is 20 times more soluble than theophylline alone. Aminophylline injection is rarely needed for severe attacks of asthma (see Management of Acute Asthma, section 3.1). It must be given by **very slow** intravenous injection (over at least 20 minutes) or by intravenous infusion; it is too irritant for intramuscular use. Intravenous aminophylline may be used as a respiratory stimulant in neonates with apnoea, but **caffeine** (section 3.5.1) is usually preferred. Measurement of plasma-theophylline concentration may be helpful and is **essential** if a loading dose of aminophylline is to be given to children who are taking theophylline, because serious side-effects such as convulsions and arrhythmias can occasionally precede other symptoms of toxicity.

Theophylline is metabolised in the liver. Plasma-theophylline concentration is *increased* in heart failure, cirrhosis, viral infections, and by drugs that inhibit its metabolism. The plasma-theophylline concentration is *decreased* in smokers and by drugs that induce liver metabolism. Particular care is required when introducing or withdrawing drugs that interact with theophylline. For other interactions of theophylline see Appendix 1.

Plasma-theophylline concentration In most individuals a plasma-theophylline concentration of 10–20 mg/litre (55–110 micromol/litre) is required for satisfactory bronchodilation, but a lower concentration of 5–15 mg/litre may be effective. Adverse effects can occur within the range 10–20 mg/litre and both the frequency and severity increase if the concentration exceeds 20 mg/litre. In neonates, toxic symptoms sometimes occur when the plasma-theophylline concentration exceeds 14 mg/litre (78 micromol/litre). If theophylline is used in the treatment of *neonatal apnoea*, the usual target range is 8–12 mg/litre (44–66 micromol/litre).

Plasma-theophylline concentration is measured 5 days after starting oral treatment and at least 3 days after any dose adjustment. A blood sample should be taken 1–2 hours after an oral dose (after 4–6 hours in the case of a modified-release preparation). If aminophylline is given intravenously, a blood sample should be taken 4–6 hours after starting treatment; in a child already taking theophylline, plasma-theophylline concentration should be determined before giving the intravenous dose.

◢ THEOPHYLLINE

Cautions cardiac disease, hypertension, hyperthyroidism; peptic ulcer; epilepsy; fever; **CSM** advice on hypokalaemia risk, p. 173; avoid in acute porphyria (section 9.8.2); monitor plasma-theophylline concentration (see notes above); **interactions:** Appendix 1 (theophylline) and notes above

Hepatic impairment reduce dose

Pregnancy neonatal irritability and apnoea reported

Breast-feeding present in milk—irritability in infant reported; modified-release preparations preferable

Side-effects tachycardia, palpitation, nausea and other gastro-intestinal disturbances, headache, CNS stimulation, insomnia, arrhythmias, and convulsions especially if given rapidly by intravenous injection; **overdosage:** see Emergency Treatment of Poisoning, p. 43

Licensed use *Slo-Phyllin®* capsules not licensed for use in children under 2 years

Indication and dose

Chronic asthma

see under preparations below and Management of Chronic Asthma p. 170
Note Plasma-theophylline concentration for optimum response 10–20 mg/litre (55–110 micromol/litre); narrow margin between therapeutic and toxic dose, see also notes above

◢ Modified release

Note The rate of absorption from modified-release preparations can vary between different brands. The Council of the Royal Pharmaceutical Society of Great Britain advises pharmacists that if a general practitioner prescribes a modified-release oral theophylline preparation without specifying a brand name, the pharmacist should contact the prescriber and agree the brand to be dispensed. Additionally, it is essential that a child discharged from hospital should be maintained on the brand on which that child was stabilised as an in-patient.

Nuelin SA® (3M)
SA tablets, m/r, theophylline 175 mg. Net price 60-tab pack = £3.19. Label: 21, 25
Dose
Chronic asthma
• By mouth
Child 6–12 years 175 mg every 12 hours
Child 12–18 years 175–350 mg every 12 hours

SA 250 tablets, m/r, scored, theophylline 250 mg. Net price 60-tab pack = £4.46. Label: 21, 25
Dose
Chronic asthma
• By mouth
Child 6–12 years 125–250 mg every 12 hours
Child 12–18 years 250–500 mg every 12 hours

Slo-Phyllin® (Merck)
Capsules, m/r, theophylline 60 mg (white/clear, enclosing white pellets), net price 56-cap pack = £2.76; 125 mg (brown/clear, enclosing white pellets), 56-cap pack = £3.48; 250 mg (blue/clear, enclosing white pellets), 56-cap pack = £4.34. Label: 25, or counselling, see below
Dose
Chronic asthma
• By mouth
Child 6 months–2 years (body-weight under 10 kg) 12 mg/kg every 12 hours
Child 2–6 years (body-weight over 10 kg) 60–120 mg every 12 hours
Child 6–12 years 125–250 mg every 12 hours
Child 12–18 years 250–500 mg every 12 hours
Administration Contents of the capsule (enteric-coated granules) may be sprinkled on to a spoonful of soft food (e.g. yoghurt) and swallowed without chewing

3 Respiratory system

◻ THEOPHYLLINE (*continued*)

Uniphyllin Continus® (Napp)
Tablets, m/r, scored, theophylline 200 mg, net price
56-tab pack = £3.13; 300 mg, 56-tab pack = £4.77;
400 mg, 56-tab pack = £5.65. Label: 25

Dose
Chronic asthma
• By mouth
   Child 2–12 years 9 mg/kg (up to 200 mg) every 12
   hours; some children with chronic asthma may require
   10–16 mg/kg (max. 400 mg) every 12 hours

Child 12–18 years 200 mg every 12 hours, increased
according to response to 400 mg every 12 hours
Note May be appropriate to give larger evening or
morning dose to achieve optimum therapeutic effect
when symptoms most severe; in children whose night
or daytime symptoms persist despite other therapy,
who are not currently receiving theophylline, total
daily requirement may be added as a single evening or
morning dose

◤ AMINOPHYLLINE

Note Aminophylline is a stable mixture or combination of
theophylline and ethylenediamine; the ethylenediamine
confers greater solubility in water

Cautions see under Theophylline; also rapid
intravenous injection can cause arrhythmias

Side-effects see under Theophylline; also allergy
to ethylenediamine can cause urticaria, erythema, and exfoliative dermatitis

Licensed use *Minijet® Aminophylline* not licensed
for use in children under 6 months

Indication and dose
   Note To avoid excessive dosage in obese children,
   dose should be calculated on the basis of ideal weight
   for height

Chronic asthma (see also Management of
Chronic Asthma, p. 170)
• By mouth
   See under preparations below

Severe acute asthma not previously treated
with theophylline (with close monitoring; see
also Management of Acute Asthma, section 3.1)
• By intravenous injection over at least 20 minutes
   Child 1 month–18 years 5 mg/kg (max. 500 mg)
   then by intravenous infusion

Severe acute asthma (with close monitoring; see
also Management of Acute Asthma, section 3.1)
• By intravenous infusion
   Child 1 month–9 years 1 mg/kg/hour adjusted
   according to plasma-theophylline concentration
   Child 9–16 years 800 micrograms/kg/hour
   adjusted according to plasma-theophylline
   concentration
   Child 16–18 years 500 micrograms/kg/hour
   adjusted according to plasma-theophylline
   concentration

Note Plasma-theophylline concentration for optimum
response in asthma 10–20 mg/litre (55–110 micromol/
litre); narrow margin between therapeutic and toxic dose,

see also notes above on plasma-theophylline concentration; children taking oral theophylline or aminophylline
should not normally receive intravenous aminophylline
unless plasma-theophylline concentration is available to
guide dosage

Neonatal apnoea (but see notes above)
• By intravenous injection over 20 minutes
   Neonate initially 6 mg/kg, then 2.5 mg/kg every
   12 hours (increased if necessary to 3.5 mg/kg
   every 12 hours)

Note Plasma-theophylline concentration for optimum
response in neonatal apnoea 8–12 mg/litre (44–
66 micromol/litre), see also notes above

Administration For *intravenous infusion*, dilute to a
concentration of 1 mg/mL with Glucose 5% *or*
Sodium Chloride 0.9%

Aminophylline (Non-proprietary) PoM
Injection, aminophylline 25 mg/mL, net price 10-
mL amp = 72p
Brands include *Minijet® Aminophylline*

Injection, aminophylline 2 mg/mL, 20-mL amp;
5 mg/mL, 20-mL amp
Available from 'special-order' manufacturers or specialist
importing companies, see p. 943

◢Modified release
Note Advice about modified-release theophylline preparations on p. 179 also applies to modified-release aminophylline preparations

Phyllocontin Continus® (Napp)
Tablets, m/r, yellow, f/c, aminophylline hydrate
225 mg, net price 56-tab pack = £2.54. Label: 25
Dose
Chronic asthma (see also Management of Chronic
Asthma, p. 170)
• By mouth
   Child body-weight over 40 kg initially 1 tablet twice
   daily, increased after 1 week to 2 tablets twice daily
   according to plasma-theophylline concentration

Note Brands of modified-release tablets containing
aminophylline 225 mg include *Norphyllin® SR*

3.1.4 Compound bronchodilator preparations

In general, children are best treated with single-ingredient preparations, such as a
selective beta₂ agonist (section 3.1.1.1) or ipratropium bromide (section 3.1.2), so
that the dose of each drug can be adjusted. This flexibility is lost with compound
bronchodilator preparations.

3.1.5 Peak flow meters, inhaler devices, and nebulisers

Peak flow meters

Peak flow meters may be used to assess lung function in children over 5 years with asthma, but symptom monitoring is the most reliable assessment of asthma control. They are best used for short periods to assess the severity of asthma and to monitor response to treatment; continuous use of peak flow meters may detract from compliance with inhalers.

Standard Range Peak Flow Meter

Conforms to standard EN 13826

MicroPeak®, range 60–800 litres/minute, net price = £6.50, replacement mouthpiece = 38p (Micro Medical)

Mini-Wright®, range 60–800 litres/minute, net price = £6.86, replacement mouthpiece = 38p (Clement Clarke)

Piko-1®, range 15–999 litres/minute, net price = £9.50, replacement mouthpiece = 38p (nSPIRE Health)

Pocketpeak®, range 60–800 litres/minute, net price = £6.53, replacement mouthpiece = 38p (nSPIRE Health)

Vitalograph®, range 50–800 litres/minute, net price = £4.50 (a child's peak flow meter is also available), replacement mouthpiece = 40p (Vitalograph)

Note Readings from new peak flow meters are often lower than those obtained from old Wright-scale peak flow meters and the correct recording chart should be used

Low Range Peak Flow Meter

Compliant to standard EN 13826 except for scale range

Mini-Wright®, range 30–400 litres/minute, net price = £6.90, replacement mouthpiece = 38p (Clement Clarke)

Pocketpeak®, range 50–400 litres/minute, net price = £6.53, replacement mouthpiece = 38p (nSPIRE Health)

Note Readings from new peak flow meters are often lower than those obtained from old Wright-scale peak flow meters and the correct recording chart should be used

Drug delivery devices

Inhaler devices   A *pressurised metered-dose inhaler* is an effective method of drug administration in mild to moderate chronic asthma; to deliver the drug effectively, a spacer device should also be used (see also NICE guidance, below). By the age of 3 years, a child can usually be taught to use the spacer device without a mask. As soon as a child is able to use the mouthpiece, then this is the preferred delivery system.

Dry powder inhalers may be useful in children over 5 years, who are unwilling or unable to use a pressurised metered-dose inhaler with a spacer device; breath-actuated inhalers may be useful in older children if they are able to use the device effectively. The child or child's carer should be instructed carefully on the use of the inhaler. It is important to check that the inhaler is being used correctly; poor inhalation technique may be mistaken for a lack of response to the drug.

On changing from a pressurised metered-dose inhaler to a dry powder inhaler, the child may notice a lack of sensation in the mouth and throat previously associated with each actuation; coughing may occur more frequently following use of a dry-powder inhaler.

CFC-free metered-dose inhalers should be cleaned **weekly** according to the manufacturer's instructions.

> **NICE guidance**
>
> Inhaler devices for children with chronic asthma (children under 5 years, August 2000; children 5–15 years, March 2002)
>
> A child's needs, ability to develop and maintain effective technique, and likelihood of good compliance should govern the choice of inhaler and spacer device; only then should cost be considered.
>
> For children aged under 5 years:
>
> - corticosteroid and bronchodilator therapy should be delivered by pressurised metered-dose inhaler **and** spacer device, with a facemask if necessary;
> - if this is not effective, and depending on the child's condition, nebulised therapy may be considered and, in children over 3 years, a dry powder inhaler may also be considered [but see notes above].
>
> For children aged 5–15 years:
>
> - corticosteroid therapy should be routinely delivered by a pressurised metered-dose inhaler **and** spacer device;
> - children and their carers should be trained in the use of the chosen device; suitability of the device should be reviewed at least annually. Inhaler technique and compliance should be monitored.

3 Respiratory system

Spacer devices Spacer devices are particularly useful for infants, for children with poor inhalation technique, or for nocturnal asthma, because the device reduces the need for co-ordination between actuation of a pressurised metered-dose inhaler and inhalation. The spacer device reduces the velocity of the aerosol and subsequent impaction on the oropharynx and allows more time for evaporation of the propellant so that a larger proportion of the particles can be inhaled and deposited in the lungs. Smaller-volume spacers may be more manageable for pre-school children and infants. The spacer device used must be compatible with the prescribed metered-dose inhaler.

Use and care of spacer devices The suitability of the spacer device should be carefully assessed; opening the one-way valve is dependent on the child's inspiratory flow. Some devices can be tipped to 45° to open the valve during inhaler actuation and inspiration to assist the child.

Inhalation from the spacer device should follow the actuation as soon as possible because the drug aerosol is very short-lived. The total dose (which may be more than a single puff) should be administered as single actuations (tidal breathing for 10–20 seconds or 5–6 breaths between each actuation) for children with good inspiratory flow. Larger doses may be necessary for a child with acute broncho-spasm; for guidance on the Management of Acute Asthma, see section 3.1.

The device should be cleansed once a month by washing in mild detergent and then allowed to dry in air; the mouthpiece should be wiped clean of detergent before use. More frequent cleaning should be avoided since any electrostatic charge may affect drug delivery. Spacer devices should be replaced every 6–12 months.

Able Spacer® (Clement Clarke)
Spacer device, small-volume device. For use with all pressurised (aerosol) inhalers, net price standard device = £4.20; with infant, child or adult mask = £6.86

AeroChamber® Plus (GSK)
Spacer device, medium-volume device. For use with all pressurised (aerosol) inhalers, net price standard device (blue) = £4.43, with mask (blue) = £7.40; infant device (orange) with mask = £7.40; child device (yellow) with mask = £7.40

Babyhaler® (A&H)
Spacer device, paediatric use with *Flixotide®*, *Seretide®*, *Serevent®*, and *Ventolin®* inhalers, net price = £11.34

Haleraid® (A&H)
Inhalation aid, device to place over pressurised (aerosol) inhalers to aid when strength in hands is impaired (e.g. arthritis). For use with *Flixotide®*, *Seretide®*, *Serevent®*, *Ventolin®* inhalers. Available as *Haleraid®-120* for 120-dose inhalers and *Haleraid®-200* for 200-dose inhalers, net price = 80p

NebuChamber® (AstraZeneca)
Spacer device, for use with *Pulmicort®* aerosol inhalers, net price = £8.56.

Nebuhaler® (AstraZeneca)
Spacer device, large-volume device. For use with *Pulmicort®* inhalers, net price with paediatric mask = £4.28

Optichamber® (Respironics)
Spacer device, for use with all pressurised (aerosol) inhalers, net price = £4.28; with small or medium mask = £7.40

PARI Vortex Spacer® (Pari)
Spacer device, medium-volume device. For use with all pressurised (aerosol) inhalers, net price with mouthpiece = £6.07; with mask for infant or child = £7.91; with adult mask = £9.97

Pocket Chamber® (nSPIRE Health)
Spacer device, small-volume device. For use with all pressurised (aerosol) inhalers, net price = £4.18; with infant, small, medium, or large mask = £9.75

Volumatic® (A&H)
Spacer inhaler, large-volume device. For use with *Clenil Modulite®*, *Flixotide®*, *Seretide®*, *Serevent®*, and *Ventolin®* inhalers, net price = £2.75; with paediatric mask = £2.75

Nebulisers

In England and Wales nebulisers and compressors are not available on the NHS (but they are free of VAT); some nebulisers (but not compressors) are available on form GP10A in Scotland (for details consult Scottish Drug Tariff).
For details of jet nebulisers, home compressors with nebulisers, and compressors, see current BNF.

A nebuliser converts a solution of a drug into an aerosol for inhalation. It is used to deliver higher doses of drug to the airways than is usual with standard inhalers. The main indications for use of a nebuliser are:

- to deliver a beta$_2$ agonist or ipratropium to a child with an *acute exacerbation* of asthma or of airways obstruction;
- to deliver *prophylactic medication* to a child unable to use other conventional devices;

- to deliver an antibacterial (such as colistin or tobramycin) to a child with chronic purulent infection (as in cystic fibrosis or bronchiectasis);
- to deliver budesonide to a child with severe croup;
- to deliver pentamidine for the prophylaxis and treatment of pneumocystis pneumonia to a child with AIDS.

The proportion of a nebuliser solution that reaches the lungs depends on the type of nebuliser and although it can be as high as 30% it is more frequently close to 10% and sometimes below 10%. The remaining solution is left in the nebuliser as residual volume or it is deposited in the mouthpiece and tubing. The extent to which the nebulised solution is deposited in the airways or alveoli depends on particle size. Particles with a median diameter of 1–5 microns are deposited in the airways and are therefore appropriate for asthma whereas a particle size of 1–2 microns is needed for alveolar deposition of pentamidine to combat pneumocystis infection. The type of nebuliser is therefore chosen according to the deposition required and according to the viscosity of the solution (antibacterial solutions usually being more viscous).

Some jet nebulisers are able to increase drug output during inspiration and hence increase efficiency.

Nebulised bronchodilators are appropriate for children with chronic persistent asthma or those with severe acute asthma. In chronic asthma, nebulised bronchodilators should only be used to relieve persistent daily wheeze (see Management of Chronic Asthma table, p. 170). The use of nebulisers in chronic persistent asthma should be considered only:

- after a review of the diagnosis and use of current inhaler devices;
- if the airflow obstruction is significantly reversible by bronchodilators without unacceptable side-effects;
- if the child does not benefit from use of conventional inhaler device, such as pressurised metered-dose inhaler plus spacer;
- if the child is complying with the prescribed dose and frequency of anti-inflammatory treatment including regular use of high-dose inhaled corticosteroid.

When a nebuliser is prescribed, the child or child's carer must:

- have clear instructions from doctor, specialist nurse or pharmacist on the use of the nebuliser (and on peak-flow monitoring—see notes above);
- be instructed not to treat acute attacks without also seeking medical help;
- have regular follow up with doctor or specialist nurse.

Jet nebulisers are more widely used than ultrasonic nebulisers. Most jet nebulisers require an optimum flow rate of 6–8 litres/minute and in hospital can be driven by piped air or oxygen; in acute asthma the nebuliser should always be driven by oxygen. Domiciliary oxygen cylinders do not provide an adequate flow rate therefore an electrical compressor is required for domiciliary use.

> **Safe practice**
> The Department of Health has reminded users of the need to use the correct grade of tubing when connecting a nebuliser to a medical gas supply or compressor.

For a list of available devices see BNF (section 3.1.5).

Nebuliser diluent

Nebulisation may be carried out using an undiluted nebuliser solution or it may require dilution beforehand. The usual diluent is sterile sodium chloride 0.9% (physiological saline).

Sodium Chloride (Non-proprietary) PoM
Nebuliser solution, sodium chloride 0.9%, net price
20 × 2.5 mL = £5.49
Brands include *Saline Steripoule®*, *Saline Steri-Neb®*

3
Respiratory system

3.2 Corticosteroids

Corticosteroids are effective in the management of *asthma*; they reduce airway inflammation.

An inhaled corticosteroid is used regularly for prophylaxis of asthma when a child requires a beta$_2$ agonist more than twice a week, or if symptoms disturb sleep more than once a week, or if the child has suffered exacerbations in the last 2 years requiring a systemic corticosteroid or a nebulised bronchodilator (see Management of Chronic Asthma, p. 170).

In adults, current or previous smoking reduces the effectiveness of inhaled corticosteroids and higher doses may be necessary.

Corticosteroid inhalers must be used regularly for maximum benefit; alleviation of symptoms usually occurs 3 to 7 days after initiation but may take longer. **Beclometasone dipropionate** (beclomethasone dipropionate), **budesonide**, **fluticasone propionate,** and **mometasone furoate** appear to be equally effective. A spacer device should be used for administering inhaled corticosteroids in children under 15 years (see NICE guidance, section 3.1.5); a spacer device is also useful in children over 15 years, particularly if high doses are required.

High doses of inhaled corticosteroids can be prescribed for children who respond only partially to standard doses of an inhaled corticosteroid and a long-acting beta$_2$ agonist or to other long-acting bronchodilators (see Management of Chronic Asthma, p. 170). High doses should be continued only if there is clear benefit over the lower dose. The recommended maximum dose of an inhaled corticosteroid should not generally be exceeded; however, if a higher dose is required it should be initiated and supervised by a respiratory paediatrician. The use of high doses of an inhaled corticosteroid can minimise the requirement for an oral corticosteroid.

Cautions of inhaled corticosteroids   Systemic therapy may be required during periods of stress, such as during severe infections, or when airways obstruction or mucus prevent drug access to smaller airways. An inhaled corticosteroid may be used during pregnancy and breast-feeding, see p. 168; **interactions**: Appendix 1 (corticosteroids).

Paradoxical bronchospasm   The potential for paradoxical bronchospasm (calling for discontinuation and alternative therapy) should be borne in mind—mild bronchospasm may be prevented by inhalation of a short-acting beta$_2$ agonist beforehand (or by transfer from an aerosol inhalation to a dry powder inhalation if suitable).

CFC-free inhalers   Chlorofluorocarbon (CFC) propellants in pressurised aerosol inhalers are being replaced by hydrofluoroalkane (HFA) propellants. Carers of children and children receiving CFC-free pressurised inhalers should be reassured about the efficacy of the new inhalers and counselled that the aerosol may feel and taste different; any difficulty with the new inhaler should be discussed with the doctor, asthma nurse specialist, or pharmacist.

Doses for CFC-free corticosteroid inhalers may be different from those that contain CFCs, see also MHRA/CHM advice below.

> MHRA/CHM advice (July 2008)
> Beclometasone dipropionate CFC-free pressurised metered-dose inhalers (*Qvar®* and *Clenil Modulite®*) are **not** interchangeable and should be prescribed by brand name; *Qvar®* has extra-fine particles, is more potent than traditional beclometasone dipropionate CFC-containing inhalers, and is approximately twice as potent as *Clenil Modulite®*.

Side-effects of inhaled corticosteroids   Inhaled corticosteroids have considerably fewer systemic effects than oral corticosteroids, but adverse effects have been reported.

High doses of inhaled corticosteroids (see Management of Chronic Asthma, p. 170) used for prolonged periods can induce adrenal suppression. Inhaled corticosteroids have occasionally been associated with adrenal crisis and coma in children; excessive doses should be **avoided**. Children using high doses of inhaled corticosteroids should be under the supervision of a paediatrician for the duration of the treatment; they should be given a 'steroid card' (section 6.3.2) and

Respiratory system

3

specific written advice to consider corticosteroid replacement during an episode of stress, such as a severe intercurrent illness or an operation.

In adults, bone mineral density is sometimes reduced following long-term inhalation of higher doses of corticosteroids, predisposing patients to osteoporosis (section 6.6). It is, therefore, sensible to ensure that the dose of an inhaled corticosteroid is no higher than necessary to keep a child's asthma under good control.

Growth restriction associated with systemic corticosteroid therapy does not seem to occur with recommended doses of inhaled corticosteroids; although initial growth velocity may be reduced, there appears to be no effect on achieving normal adult height. However, the CSM has recommended that the height of children receiving prolonged treatment with inhaled corticosteroid is monitored; if growth is slowed, referral to a paediatrician should be considered.

Hoarseness and candidiasis of the mouth or throat have been reported, usually only with high doses (see also below). Hypersensitivity reactions (including rash and angioedema) have been reported rarely. Other side-effects that have very rarely been reported include paradoxical bronchospasm, anxiety, depression, sleep disturbances, and behavioural changes including hyperactivity and irritability.

Candidiasis The risk of oral candidiasis can be reduced by using a spacer device with the corticosteroid inhaler; rinsing the mouth with water (or cleaning the child's teeth) after inhalation of a dose may also be helpful. Antifungal oral suspension or lozenges (section 12.3.2) can be used to treat oral candidiasis while continuing corticosteroid therapy.

Oral   An acute attack of asthma should be treated with a short course (3–5 days) of oral corticosteroid, see Management of Acute Asthma, p. 168. The dose can usually be stopped abruptly in a mild exacerbation of asthma (see also Withdrawal of Corticosteroids, section 6.3.2) but it should be reduced gradually in children with poorer asthma control, to reduce the possibility of serious relapse.

In chronic continuing asthma, when the response to other drugs has been inadequate, longer term administration of an oral corticosteroid may be necessary; in such cases high doses of an inhaled corticosteroid should be continued to minimise oral corticosteroid requirements.

An oral corticosteroid should normally be taken as a single dose in the morning to reduce the disturbance to circadian cortisol secretion. Dosage should always be titrated to the lowest dose that controls symptoms.

Parenteral   For the use of hydrocortisone injection in the emergency treatment of acute severe asthma, see Management of Acute Asthma, p. 168.

3

Respiratory system

▲ BECLOMETASONE DIPROPIONATE
(Beclomethasone Dipropionate)

Cautions see notes above

Side-effects see notes above

Licensed use *Becodisk®-400, Clenil Modulate®*-200 and -250, and *Qvar®* are not licensed for use in children under 12 years

Indication and dose

Prophylaxis of asthma

see Management of Chronic Asthma, p. 170
Important for *Asmabec Clickhaler®*, *Becodisks®*, and *Qvar®* doses see under preparations below

Beclometasone (Non-proprietary) PoM
Aerosol inhalation, beclometasone dipropionate 50 micrograms/metered inhalation, net price 200-dose unit = £5.69; 100 micrograms/metered inhalation, 200-dose unit = £9.91; 200 micrograms/metered inhalation, 200-dose unit = £17.25; 250 micrograms/metered inhalation, 200-dose unit

= £22.88. Label: 8, counselling, dose; also 10 and steroid card with high doses
Excipients include CFC propellants
Brands include *Beclazone®*

Dry powder for inhalation, beclometasone dipropionate 100 micrograms/metered inhalation, net price 100-dose unit = £5.58; 200 micrograms/metered inhalation, 100-dose unit = £10.29, 200-dose unit = £15.60; 400 micrograms/metered inhalation, 100-dose unit = £20.41. Label: 8, counselling, dose; also 10 and steroid card with high doses
Brands include *Pulvinal® Beclometasone Dipropionate*, *Easyhaler® Beclometasone Dipropionate*

Inhalation powder, hard capsule (for use with *Cyclohaler®* device), beclometasone dipropionate 100 micrograms, net price 120-cap pack = £15.99; 200 micrograms, 120-cap pack = £25.00; 400 micrograms, 120-cap pack = £32.25. Label: 8, counselling, dose; also 10 and steroid card with high doses
Brands include *Beclometasone Cyclocaps®*

◁ **BECLOMETASONE DIPROPIONATE** (*continued*)

Asmabec Clickhaler® (UCB Pharma) PoM
Dry powder for inhalation, beclometasone dipropionate 50 micrograms/metered inhalation, net price 200-dose unit = £6.68; 100 micrograms/metered inhalation, 200-dose unit = £9.81; 250 micrograms/metered inhalation, 100-dose unit = £12.31. Label: 8, counselling, dose; also 10 and steroid card with high doses

Dose

Prophylaxis of asthma
• **By inhalation of powder**
  Child 6–12 years 50–200 micrograms twice daily, adjusted as necessary
  Child 12–18 years 100–400 micrograms twice daily, adjusted as necessary; max. 1 mg twice daily

Beclazone Easi-Breathe® (IVAX) PoM
Aerosol inhalation (breath-actuated), beclometasone dipropionate 50 micrograms/metered inhalation, net price 200-dose unit = £3.26; 100 micrograms/metered inhalation, 200-dose unit = £10.30; 250 micrograms/metered inhalation, 200-dose unit = £20.25. Label: 8, counselling, dose; also 10 and steroid card with high doses
Excipients include CFC propellants

Becodisks® (A&H) PoM
Dry powder for inhalation, disks containing 8 blisters of beclometasone dipropionate 100 micrograms/blister, net price 15 disks with *Diskhaler®* device = £12.00, 15-disk refill = £11.42; 200 micrograms/blister, 15 disks with *Diskhaler®* device = £22.87, 15-disk refill = £22.28; 400 micrograms/blister, 15 disks with *Diskhaler®* device = £45.14, 15-disk refill = £44.57. Label: 8, counselling, dose; also 10 and steroid card with high doses

Dose

Prophylaxis of asthma
• **By inhalation of powder**
  Child 5–12 years 100–200 micrograms twice daily, adjusted as necessary
  Child 12–18 years 400–800 micrograms twice daily, adjusted as necessary

Clenil Modulite® (Chiesi) ▼ PoM
Aerosol inhalation, beclometasone dipropionate 50 micrograms/metered inhalation, net price 200-dose unit = £3.85; 100 micrograms/metered inhalation = £7.72; 200 micrograms/metered inhalation = £16.83; 250 micrograms/metered inhalation = £16.95. Label: 8, counselling, dose; also 10 and steroid card with high doses
Excipients include HFA-134a (a non-CFC propellant)

Dose

Prophylaxis of asthma
• **By aerosol inhalation**
  Child 2–12 years 100–200 micrograms twice daily

Child 12–18 years 200–400 micrograms twice daily adjusted as necessary up to 1 mg twice daily

Note *Clenil Modulite®* is not interchangeable with other CFC-free beclometasone dipropionate inhalers; the MHRA has advised (August 2006 and July 2008) that CFC-free beclometasone dipropionate inhalers should be prescribed by brand name
Dental prescribing on NHS *Clenil Modulite®* 50 micrograms/metered inhalation may be prescribed

Qvar® (IVAX) PoM
Aerosol inhalation, beclometasone dipropionate 50 micrograms/metered inhalation, net price 200-dose unit = £7.87; 100 micrograms/metered inhalation, 200-dose unit = £17.21. Label: 8, counselling, dose; also 10 and steroid card with high doses
Excipients include HFA-134a (a non-CFC propellant)

Autohaler® (breath-actuated aerosol inhalation), beclometasone dipropionate 50 micrograms/metered inhalation, net price 200-dose unit = £7.87; 100 micrograms/metered inhalation, 200-dose unit = £17.21. Label: 8, counselling, dose; also 10 and steroid card with high doses
Excipients include HFA-134a (a non-CFC propellant)

Easi-Breathe® (breath-actuated aerosol inhalation), beclometasone dipropionate 50 micrograms/metered inhalation, net price 200-dose = £7.74; 100 micrograms/metered inhalation, 200-dose = £16.95. Label: 8, counselling, dose; also 10 and steroid card with high doses
Excipients include HFA-134a (a non-CFC propellant)

Dose

Prophylaxis of asthma
• **By aerosol inhalation**
  Child 12–18 years 50–200 micrograms twice daily, increased if necessary to max. 400 micrograms twice daily

Important When switching a child with well-controlled asthma from another corticosteroid inhaler, initially a 100-microgram metered dose of *Qvar®* should be prescribed for:
• 200–250 micrograms of beclometasone dipropionate or budesonide
• 100 micrograms of fluticasone propionate

When switching a child with poorly controlled asthma from another corticosteroid inhaler, initially a 100-microgram metered dose of *Qvar®* should be prescribed for 100 micrograms of beclometasone dipropionate, budesonide, or fluticasone propionate; the dose of *Qvar®* should be adjusted according to response
Note The MHRA has advised (August 2006 and July 2008) that beclometasone dipropionate CFC-free inhalers should be prescribed by brand name

---

BUDESONIDE

Cautions see notes above
Side-effects see notes above
Licensed use *Pulmicort®* nebuliser solution not licensed for use in children under 3 months; not licensed for use in bronchopulmonary dysplasia

Indication and dose

Prophylaxis of asthma see Management of Chronic Asthma, p. 170, and preparations below

Croup
• **By inhalation of nebuliser suspension**
  Child over 1 month 2 mg as single dose or in 2 divided doses separated by 30 minutes; dose may be repeated after 12 hours if necessary

◁ **BUDESONIDE** (*continued*)

Bronchopulmonary dysplasia with assisted ventilation

• **By aerosol inhalation**

Neonate 400 micrograms twice daily

Child 1–4 months 400 micrograms twice daily

Bronchopulmonary dysplasia with spontaneous respiration

• **By inhalation of nebuliser suspension**

Neonate 500 micrograms twice daily

Child 1–4 months 500 micrograms twice daily; for severe symptoms in child body-weight 2.5 kg or over, 1 mg twice daily

Administration For *aerosol inhalation* in ventilated babies with bronchopulmonary dysplasia, use medium-volume spacer (section 3.1.5) attached directly to endotracheal tube; hand-ventilate through spacer, using a bag system; inflate chest 10 times between activations of inhaler

Budesonide (Non-proprietary) PoM

Dry powder for inhalation, budesonide 100 micrograms/metered inhalation, net price 200-dose unit = £9.25; 200 micrograms/metered inhalation 200-dose unit = £18.50; 400 micrograms/metered inhalation 100-dose unit = £18.50. Label: 8, counselling, dose; also 10 and steroid card with high doses
Brands include *Easyhaler® Budesonide*

Inhalation powder, hard capsule (for use with *Cyclohaler®* device), budesonide 200 micrograms, net price 100-cap pack = £15.48; 400 micrograms, 50-cap pack = £15.48. Label: 8, counselling, dose; also 10 and steroid card with high doses
Brands include *Budesonide Cyclocaps®*

Dose

Prophylaxis of asthma

• **By inhalation of powder**

Child 6–12 years 100-400 micrograms twice daily, adjusted as necessary; alternatively, in mild to moderate asthma, 200–400 micrograms as a single dose each evening if stabilised on daily dose given in 2 divided doses

Child 12–18 years 100–800 micrograms twice daily, adjusted as necessary; alternatively, in mild to moderate asthma, 200–400 micrograms as a single dose each evening if stabilised on daily dose given in 2 divided doses (max. 800 micrograms)

Novolizer® (Viatris) ▼ PoM

Dry powder for inhalation, budesonide 200 micrograms, net price refillable inhaler device and 100-dose cartridge = £14.86; 100-dose refill cartridge = £9.59. Label: 8, counselling, dose; also 10 and steroid card with high doses

Dose

Prophylaxis of asthma

• **By inhalation of powder**

Child 6–12 years 200-400 micrograms twice daily, adjusted as necessary; alternatively, in mild to moderate asthma, 200–400 micrograms as a single dose each evening if stabilised on daily dose given in 2 divided doses

Child 12–18 years 200–800 micrograms twice daily, adjusted as necessary; alternatively, in mild to moderate asthma, 200–400 micrograms as a single dose each evening if stabilised on daily dose given in 2 divided doses (max. 800 micrograms)

Pulmicort® (AstraZeneca) PoM

Aerosol inhalation ▼, budesonide 100 micrograms/metered inhalation, net price 120-dose unit = £9.60; 200 micrograms/metered inhalation, net price 120-dose unit = £13.20. Label: 8, counselling, dose, change to CFC-free inhaler; also 10 and steroid card with high doses
Excipients include HFA–134a (a non-CFC propellant)

Dose

Prophylaxis of asthma

• **By aerosol inhalation**

Child 2–12 years 100–400 micrograms twice daily, adjusted as necessary

Child 12–18 years 100–400 micrograms twice daily, adjusted as necessary; max. 800 micrograms twice daily

Turbohaler® (= dry powder inhaler), budesonide 100 micrograms/metered inhalation, net price 200-dose unit = £18.50; 200 micrograms/metered inhalation, 100-dose unit = £18.50; 400 micrograms/metered inhalation, 50-dose unit = £18.50. Label: 8, counselling, dose; also 10 and steroid card with high doses

Dose

Prophylaxis of asthma

• **By inhalation of powder**

Child 6–12 years 100-400 micrograms twice daily, adjusted as necessary; alternatively, in mild to moderate asthma, 200–400 micrograms as a single dose each evening if stabilised on daily dose given in 2 divided doses

Child 12–18 years 100–800 micrograms twice daily, adjusted as necessary; alternatively, in mild to moderate asthma, 200–400 micrograms as a single dose each evening if stabilised on daily dose given in 2 divided doses (max. 800 micrograms)

Respules® (= single-dose units for nebulisation), budesonide 250 micrograms/mL, net price 20 × 2-mL (500-microgram) unit = £32.00; 500 micrograms/mL, 20 × 2-mL (1-mg) unit = £44.64. May be diluted with sterile sodium chloride 0.9%. Label: 8, counselling, dose, 10, steroid card

Dose

Prophylaxis of asthma

• **By inhalation of nebuliser suspension**

Child 3 months–12 years initially 0.5–1 mg twice daily, reduced to 250–500 micrograms twice daily

Child 12–18 years initially 1–2 mg twice daily, reduced to 0.5–1 mg twice daily

◣ **Compound preparations**

Symbicort® (AstraZeneca) PoM

Symbicort 100/6 Turbohaler® (= dry powder inhaler), budesonide 100 micrograms, formoterol fumarate 6 micrograms/metered inhalation, net price 120-dose unit = £33.00. Label: 8, counselling, dose

Dose

Prophylaxis of asthma

• **By inhalation of powder**

Child 6–12 years 2 puffs twice daily reduced to 1 puff once daily if control maintained

Child 12–18 years 1–2 puffs twice daily reduced to 1 puff once daily if control maintained

3

Respiratory system

◁ **BUDESONIDE (continued)**

Symbicort 200/6 Turbohaler® (= dry powder inhaler), budesonide 200 micrograms, formoterol fumarate 6 micrograms/metered inhalation, net price 120-dose unit = £38.00. Label: 8, counselling, dose; also 10 and steroid card with high doses

Dose

Prophylaxis of asthma
• By inhalation of powder
   Child 12–18 years 1–2 puffs twice daily reduced in well-controlled asthma to 1 puff once daily

Symbicort 400/12 Turbohaler® (= dry powder inhaler), budesonide 400 micrograms, formoterol fumarate 12 micrograms/metered inhalation, net price 60-dose unit = £38.00. Label: 8, counselling, dose; also 10 and steroid card with high doses

Dose

Prophylaxis of asthma
• By inhalation of powder
   Child 12–18 years 1 puff twice daily; may be reduced in well-controlled asthma to 1 puff once daily

◼ CICLESONIDE

Cautions see notes above

Side-effects see notes above

Indication and dose

Prophylaxis of asthma
• By aerosol inhalation
   Child 12–18 years 160 micrograms daily as a single dose reduced to 80 micrograms daily if control maintained

Alvesco® (Nycomed) ▼ PoM
Aerosol inhalation, ciclesonide 80 micrograms/metered inhalation, net price 120-dose unit = £28.56; 160 micrograms/metered inhalation, 60-dose unit = £16.80, 120-dose unit = £33.60. Label: 8, counselling, dose
Excipients include HFA-134a (a non-CFC propellant)

◼ FLUTICASONE PROPIONATE

Cautions see notes above

Side-effects see notes above; also *very rarely* dyspepsia, hyperglycaemia, and arthralgia

Indication and dose

Prophylaxis of asthma see Management of Chronic Asthma, p. 170, and preparations below

Flixotide® (A&H) PoM
Accuhaler® (dry powder for inhalation), disk containing 60 blisters of *fluticasone propionate* 50 micrograms/blister with *Accuhaler®* device, net price = £6.38; 100 micrograms/blister with *Accuhaler®* device = £8.93; 250 micrograms/blister with *Accuhaler®* device = £21.26; 500 micrograms/blister with *Accuhaler®* device = £36.14. Label: 8, counselling, dose; also 10 and steroid card with high doses

Dose

Prophylaxis of asthma
• By inhalation of powder
   Child 5–16 years 50–100 micrograms twice daily adjusted as necessary; max. 200 micrograms twice daily
   Child 16–18 years 100–500 micrograms twice daily, adjusted as necessary; max. 1 mg twice daily

Diskhaler® (dry powder for inhalation), fluticasone propionate 100 micrograms/blister, net price 15 disks of 4 blisters with *Diskhaler®* device = £12.71, 15-disk refill = £12.18; 250 micrograms/blister, 15 disks of 4 blisters with *Diskhaler®* device = £24.11, 15-disk refill = £23.58; 500 micrograms/blister, 15 disks of 4 blisters with *Diskhaler®* device = £40.05, 15-disk refill = £39.52. Label: 8, counselling, dose; also 10 and steroid card with high doses

Dose

Prophylaxis of asthma
• By inhalation of powder
   Child 5–16 years 100–200 micrograms twice daily
   Child 16–18 years 100–500 micrograms twice daily adjusted as necessary; max. 1 mg twice daily

Evohaler® *aerosol inhalation*, fluticasone propionate 50 micrograms/metered inhalation, net price 120-dose unit = £5.44; 125 micrograms/metered inhalation, 120-dose unit = £21.26; 250 micrograms/metered inhalation, 120-dose unit = £36.14. Label: 8, counselling, dose, change to CFC-free inhaler; also 10 and steroid card with high doses
Excipients include HFA-134a (a non-CFC propellant)

Dose

Prophylaxis of asthma
• By aerosol inhalation
   Child 4–16 years 50–100 micrograms twice daily adjusted as necessary; max. 200 micrograms twice daily
   Child 16–18 years 100–500 micrograms twice daily adjusted as necessary; max. 1 mg twice daily

Nebules® (= single-dose units for nebulisation) fluticasone propionate 250 micrograms/mL, net price 10 × 2-mL (500-microgram) unit = £9.34; 1 mg/mL, 10 × 2-mL (2-mg) unit = £37.35. May be diluted with sterile sodium chloride 0.9%. Label: 8, counselling, dose, 10, steroid card

Dose

Prophylaxis of asthma
• By inhalation of nebuliser suspension
   Child 4–16 years 1 mg twice daily
   Child 16–18 years 0.5–2 mg twice daily

◀Compound preparations
Seretide® (A&H) PoM
Seretide 100 Accuhaler® (dry powder for inhalation), disk containing 60 blisters of fluticasone propionate 100 micrograms, salmeterol (as xinafoate) 50 micrograms/blister with *Accuhaler®* device, net price = £31.19. Label: 8, counselling, dose

Dose

Prophylaxis of asthma
• By inhalation of powder
   Child 5–18 years 1 blister twice daily, reduced to 1 blister once daily if control maintained

◁ **FLUTICASONE PROPIONATE** (*continued*)

Seretide 250 Accuhaler® (dry powder for inhalation), disk containing 60 blisters of fluticasone propionate 250 micrograms, salmeterol (as xinafoate) 50 micrograms/blister with *Accuhaler®* device, net price = £36.65. Label: 8, counselling, dose, 10, steroid card

Dose
Prophylaxis of asthma
- **By inhalation of powder**
  Child 12–18 years 1 blister twice daily

Seretide 500 Accuhaler® (dry powder for inhalation), disk containing 60 blisters of fluticasone propionate 500 micrograms, salmeterol (as xinafoate) 50 micrograms/blister with *Accuhaler®* device, net price = £40.92. Label: 8, counselling, dose, 10, steroid card

Dose
Prophylaxis of asthma
- **By inhalation of powder**
  Child 12–18 years 1 blister twice daily

Seretide 50 Evohaler® (aerosol inhalation), fluticasone propionate 50 micrograms, salmeterol (as xinafoate) 25 micrograms/metered inhalation, net price 120-dose unit = £18.14. Label: 8, counselling, dose, change to CFC-free inhaler
Excipients include HFA-134a (a non-CFC propellant)

Dose
Prophylaxis of asthma
- **By aerosol inhalation**
  Child 5–18 years 2 puffs twice daily, reduced to 2 puffs once daily if control maintained

Seretide 125 Evohaler® (aerosol inhalation), fluticasone propionate 125 micrograms, salmeterol (as xinafoate) 25 micrograms/metered inhalation, net price 120-dose unit = £36.65. Label: 8, counselling, dose, change to CFC-free inhaler, 10, steroid card
Excipients include HFA-134a (a non-CFC propellant)

Dose
Prophylaxis of asthma
- **By aerosol inhalation**
  Child 12–18 years 2 puffs twice daily

Seretide 250 Evohaler® (aerosol inhalation), fluticasone propionate 250 micrograms, salmeterol (as xinafoate) 25 micrograms/metered inhalation, net price 120-dose unit = £62.29. Label: 8, counselling, dose, change to CFC-free inhaler, 10, steroid card
Excipients include HFA-134a (a non-CFC propellant)

Dose
Prophylaxis of asthma
- **By aerosol inhalation**
  Child 12–18 years 2 puffs twice daily

MOMETASONE FUROATE

Cautions see notes above

Side-effects see notes above; also pharyngitis, headache; *less commonly* palpitation

Indication and dose
Prophylaxis of asthma see also Management of Chronic Asthma, p. 170
- **By inhalation of powder**
  Child 12–18 years 200–400 micrograms as a single dose in the evening or in 2 divided doses; dose increased to 400 micrograms twice daily if necessary

Asmanex® (Schering-Plough) ▼ PoM
Twisthaler (= dry powder inhaler), mometasone furoate 200 micrograms/metered inhalation, net price 30-dose unit = £16.00, 60-dose unit = £24.00; 400 micrograms/metered inhalation, 30-dose unit = £22.20, 60-dose unit = £36.75. Label: 8, counselling, dose, 10, steroid card
Note The *Scottish Medicines Consortium* has advised (November 2003) that *Asmanex®* is restricted for use following failure of first-line inhaled corticosteroids

---

3.3 Cromoglicate and related therapy and leukotriene receptor antagonists

3.3.1 Cromoglicate and related therapy
3.3.2 Leukotriene receptor antagonists

3.3.1 Cromoglicate and related therapy

The mode of action of **sodium cromoglicate** and **nedocromil** is not completely understood; they may be of value as *prophylaxis* in asthma with an allergic basis, but the evidence for benefit of sodium cromoglicate in children is contentious. Prophylaxis with cromoglicate or nedocromil is less effective than with inhaled corticosteroids (see Management of Chronic Asthma, p. 170).

Nedocromil may be of some benefit in the prophylaxis of exercise-induced asthma.

3 Respiratory system

For the use of sodium cromoglicate and nedocromil in allergic conjunctivitis see section 11.4.2; sodium cromoglicate is used also in allergic rhinitis (section 12.2.1) and allergy-related diarrhoea (section 1.5.4).

SODIUM CROMOGLICATE
(Sodium Cromoglycate)

Cautions discontinue if eosinophilic pneumonia occurs

Side-effects coughing, transient bronchospasm, and throat irritation; *very rarely* hypersensitivity reactions (including angioedema); rhinitis and headache also reported

Indication and dose

Prophylaxis of asthma (see also Management of Chronic Asthma, p. 170)

• **By aerosol inhalation**

Child 5–18 years 10 mg (2 puffs) 4 times daily, increased if necessary to 6–8 times daily; an additional dose may also be taken before exercise; maintenance, 5 mg (1 puff) 4 times daily

> **Food allergy** section 1.5.4

> **Allergic conjunctivitis** section 11.4.2

> **Allergic rhinitis** section 12.2.1

Intal® CFC-free inhaler (Sanofi-Aventis) PoM
Aerosol inhalation, sodium cromoglicate 5 mg/metered inhalation, net price 112-dose unit = £15.44. Label: 8, Counselling, change to CFC-free inhaler
Excipients include HFA-227 (a non-CFC propellant)

NEDOCROMIL SODIUM

Side-effects see under Sodium Cromoglicate; also headache, nausea, vomiting, dyspepsia and abdominal pain; bitter taste (masked by mint flavour)

Licensed use not licensed for use in children under 6 years

Indication and dose

Prophylaxis of asthma (but see notes above)

Counselling Regular use is necessary

• **By aerosol inhalation**

Child 5–18 years 4 mg (2 puffs) 4 times daily, when control achieved may be possible to reduce to twice daily

> **Allergic conjunctivitis** section 11.4.2

Tilade CFC-free inhaler® (Sanofi-Aventis) ▼ PoM
Aerosol inhalation, mint-flavoured, nedocromil sodium 2 mg/metered inhalation. Net price 112-dose unit = £39.94. Label: 8, counselling, change to CFC-free inhaler
Excipients include HFA-227 (a non-CFC propellant)

3.3.2 Leukotriene receptor antagonists

The leukotriene receptor antagonists, **montelukast** and **zafirlukast**, block the effects of cysteinyl leukotrienes in the airways; they can be used with an inhaled corticosteroid (see Management of Chronic Asthma, p. 170) but adequate control is not always achieved. Montelukast has not been shown to be more effective than a standard dose of inhaled corticosteroid but the two drugs appear to have an additive effect. The leukotriene receptor antagonists may be of benefit in exercise-induced asthma and in those with concomitant rhinitis but they are less effective in children with severe asthma who are also receiving high doses of other drugs.

Churg-Strauss syndrome Churg-Strauss syndrome has occurred very rarely in association with the use of leukotriene receptor antagonists; in many of the reported cases the reaction followed the reduction or withdrawal of oral corticosteroid therapy. The CSM has advised that prescribers should be alert to the development of eosinophilia, vasculitic rash, worsening pulmonary symptoms, cardiac complications, or peripheral neuropathy.

MONTELUKAST

Cautions interactions: Appendix 1 (leukotriene receptor antagonists)

Pregnancy manufacturer advises avoid unless essential

Breast-feeding manufacturer advises avoid unless essential

Side-effects abdominal pain, thirst; hyperkinesia (in young children), headache; *very rarely* Churg-Strauss syndrome (see notes above); dry mouth, diarrhoea, dyspepsia, nausea, vomiting, hepatic disorders, palpitation, oedema, increased bleeding, hypersensitivity reactions (including anaphylaxis and skin reactions), depression, tre-

◁ **MONTELUKAST** (*continued*)

mor, asthenia, dizziness, hallucinations, suicidal thoughts and behaviour, paraesthesia, hypoaesthesia, sleep disturbances, abnormal dreams, agitation, aggression, seizures, arthralgia, and myalgia also reported

Indication and dose

Prophylaxis of asthma see notes above and Management of Chronic Asthma, p. 170

• **By mouth**

Child 6 months–6 years 4 mg once daily in the evening

Child 6–15 years 5 mg once daily in the evening

Child 15–18 years 10 mg once daily in the evening

Symptomatic relief of seasonal allergic rhinitis in children with asthma

• **By mouth**

Child 15–18 years 10 mg once daily in the evening

Singulair® (MSD) [PoM]
Chewable tablets, pink, cherry-flavoured, montelukast (as sodium salt) 4 mg, net price 28-tab pack = £25.69; 5 mg, 28-tab pack = £25.69. Label: 24
Excipients include aspartame equivalent to phenylalanine 674 micrograms/4-mg tablet and 842 micrograms/5-mg tablet (section 9.4.1)

Granules, montelukast (as sodium salt) 4 mg, net price 28-sachet pack = £25.69. Counselling, administration
Counselling Granules may be swallowed whole or mixed with cold food (but not fluid) and taken immediately

Tablets, beige, f/c, montelukast (as sodium salt) 10 mg, net price 28-tab pack = £26.97
Note The *Scottish Medicines Consortium* has advised (June 2007) that *Singulair®* chewable tablets and granules are restricted for use as an alternative to low-dose inhaled corticosteroids for children 2–14 years with mild persistent asthma who have not recently had serious asthma attacks that required oral corticosteroid use, and who are not capable of using inhaled corticosteroids; *Singulair®* chewable tablets and granules should be initiated by a specialist in paediatric asthma

▌ ZAFIRLUKAST

Cautions interactions: Appendix 1 (leukotriene receptor antagonists)
Hepatic disorders Children or their carers should be told how to recognise development of liver disorder and advised to seek medical attention if symptoms or signs such as persistent nausea, vomiting, malaise or jaundice develop

Renal impairment manufacturer advises caution in moderate to severe impairment

Pregnancy manufacturer advises use only if potential benefit outweighs risk

Contra-indications hepatic impairment

Breast-feeding present in milk—manufacturer advises avoid

Side-effects gastro-intestinal disturbances; headache; *rarely* bleeding disorders, hypersensitivity

reactions including angioedema and skin reactions, arthralgia, myalgia, hepatitis, hyperbilirubinaemia, thrombocytopenia; *very rarely* Churg-Strauss syndrome (see notes above), agranulocytosis

Indication and dose

Prophylaxis of asthma see notes above and Management of Chronic Asthma, p. 170

• **By mouth**

Child 12–18 years 20 mg twice daily

Accolate® (AstraZeneca) [PoM]
Tablets, f/c, zafirlukast 20 mg, net price 56-tab pack = £28.26. Label: 23

3   **Respiratory system**

3.4 Antihistamines, immunotherapy, and allergic emergencies

3.4.1 Antihistamines
3.4.2 Allergen immunotherapy
3.4.3 Allergic emergencies

3.4.1 Antihistamines

Antihistamines (histamine H_1-receptor antagonists) are classified as *sedating* or *non-sedating*, according to their relative potential for CNS depression. Antihistamines differ in their duration of action, incidence of drowsiness, and antimuscarinic effects; the response to an antihistamine may vary from child to child (see Side-effects, p. 192). Either a sedating or a non-sedating antihistamine may be used to treat an acute allergic reaction; for conditions with more persistent symptoms, a non-sedating antihistamine should be used regularly.

Oral antihistamines are used in the treatment of nasal allergies, particularly seasonal allergic rhinitis (hay fever), and may be of some value in vasomotor rhinitis; rhinorrhoea and sneezing is reduced, but antihistamines are usually less effective for nasal congestion. Antihistamines are used topically to treat allergic reactions in the eye (section 11.4.2) and in the nose (section 12.2.1). Topical application of antihistamines to the skin is not recommended (section 13.3).

An oral antihistamine may be used to prevent urticaria, and for the treatment of acute urticarial rashes, pruritus, insect bites, and stings. Antihistamines are also used in the management of nausea and vomiting (section 4.6), of migraine (section 4.7.4.1), and the adjunctive management of anaphylaxis and angioedema (section 3.4.3).

Sedating antihistamines are occasionally useful when insomnia is associated with urticaria and pruritus (section 4.1.1). Most of the sedating antihistamines are relatively short acting, but promethazine may be effective for up to 12 hours. **Alimemazine** (trimeprazine) and **promethazine** have a more sedative effect than **chlorphenamine** (chlorpheniramine) and **cyclizine** (section 4.6). Chlorphenamine is used as an adjunct to adrenaline (epinephrine) in the emergency treatment of anaphylaxis and angioedema (section 3.4.3).

The *non-sedating* antihistamine **cetirizine** is safe and effective in children; it causes less sedation and psychomotor impairment than the sedating antihistamines. Other non-sedating antihistamines that are used in children include **desloratadine** (an active metabolite of loratadine), **fexofenadine** (an active metabolite of terfenadine), **levocetirizine** (an isomer of cetirizine), **loratadine**, and **mizolastine**. Most non-sedating antihistamines are long-acting (usually 12–24 hours). There is little evidence that desloratadine or levocetirizine confer any additional benefit—they should be reserved for children who cannot tolerate other therapies.

Cautions and contra-indications   Antihistamines should be used with caution in hepatic impairment (see below) and in children with epilepsy. Most antihistamines should be avoided in acute porphyria, but some are thought to be safe (see section 9.8.2). Sedating antihistamines should not be given to children under 2 years, except on specialist advice, because the safety of such use has not been established. Sedating antihistamines have significant antimuscarinic activity—they should **not** be used in neonates and should be used with caution in children with urinary retention, glaucoma, or pyloroduodenal obstruction. **Interactions:** see Appendix 1 (antihistamines).

Hepatic impairment   Sedating antihistamines should be avoided in children with severe liver disease—increased risk of coma.

Pregnancy and breast-feeding   There is no evidence of teratogenicity associated with the use of antihistamines, except for hydroxyzine and loratadine where embryotoxicity has been reported with high doses in *animal* studies. However, manufacturers of some antihistamines advise avoiding use during pregnancy. The use of sedating antihistamines in the latter part of the third trimester may cause adverse effects in neonates such as irritability, paradoxical excitability, and tremor. Significant amounts of some antihistamines are present in breast milk; although not known to be harmful, manufacturers advise avoiding use in mothers who are breast-feeding.

Side-effects   Drowsiness is a significant side-effect with most of the older antihistamines although paradoxical stimulation may occur rarely in children, especially with high doses. Drowsiness may diminish after a few days of treatment and is considerably less of a problem with the newer antihistamines (see also notes above). Side-effects that are more common with the older antihistamines include headache, psychomotor impairment, and antimuscarinic effects such as urinary retention, dry mouth, blurred vision, and gastro-intestinal disturbances. Other rare side-effects of antihistamines include hypotension, palpitation, arrhythmias, extrapyramidal effects, dizziness, confusion, depression, sleep disturbances, tremor, convulsions, hypersensitivity reactions (including bronchospasm, angioedema, anaphylaxis, rashes, and photosensitivity reactions), blood disorders, and liver dysfunction.

Non-sedating antihistamines

Skilled tasks   Although drowsiness is rare, children and their carers should be advised that it can occur and may affect performance of skilled tasks (e.g. cycling or driving); alcohol should be avoided.

◢ CETIRIZINE HYDROCHLORIDE

Cautions see notes above

Renal impairment use half normal dose if estimated glomerular filtration rate less than 30 mL/minute/1.73 m²

Contra-indications see notes above

Side-effects see notes above

Licensed use not licensed for use in children under 6 years except for use in children 2–6 years for treatment of seasonal allergic rhinitis

Indication and dose

Symptomatic relief of allergy such as hay fever, chronic idiopathic urticaria, atopic dermatitis
- **By mouth**
  Child 1–2 years 250 micrograms/kg twice daily

Child 2–6 years 5 mg once daily *or* 2.5 mg twice daily

Child 6–18 years 10 mg once daily *or* 5 mg twice daily

Cetirizine (Non-proprietary)
Tablets, cetirizine hydrochloride 10 mg, net price 30-tab pack = 97p. Counselling, skilled tasks
Dental prescribing on NHS Cetirizine 10 mg tablets may be prescribed

Oral solution, cetirizine hydrochloride 5 mg/5 mL, net price 200 mL = £2.43. Counselling, skilled tasks

◢ DESLORATADINE

Note Desloratadine is a metabolite of loratadine

Cautions see notes above

Contra-indications see notes above; also hypersensitivity to loratadine

Side-effects see notes above; *rarely* myalgia; *very rarely* hallucinations

Indication and dose

Symptomatic relief of allergy such as hay fever, chronic idiopathic urticaria
- **By mouth**
  Child 1–6 years 1.25 mg once daily

Child 6–12 years 2.5 mg once daily

Child 12–18 years 5 mg once daily

Neoclarityn® (Schering-Plough) ⒫ⓄⓂ
Tablets, blue, f/c, desloratadine 5 mg, net price 30-tab pack = £7.04. Counselling, skilled tasks

Syrup, desloratadine 2.5 mg/5 mL, net price 100 mL (bubblegum-flavour) = £7.04. Counselling, skilled tasks

◢ FEXOFENADINE HYDROCHLORIDE

Note Fexofenadine is a metabolite of terfenadine

Cautions see notes above

Contra-indications see notes above

Side-effects see notes above

Indication and dose

Symptomatic relief of seasonal allergic rhinitis
- **By mouth**
  Child 6–12 years 30 mg twice daily
  Child 12–18 years 120 mg once daily

Symptomatic relief of chronic idiopathic urticaria
- **By mouth**
  Child 12–18 years 180 mg once daily

Fexofenadine (Non-proprietary) ⒫ⓄⓂ
Tablets, f/c, fexofenadine hydrochloride 120 mg, net price 30-tab pack = £5.92; 180 mg, 30-tab pack = £7.49. Label: 5, counselling, skilled tasks

Telfast® (Aventis Pharma) ⒫ⓄⓂ
Tablets, f/c, peach, fexofenadine hydrochloride 30 mg, net price 60-tab pack = £5.68; 120 mg, 30-tab pack = £6.23; 180 mg, 30-tab pack = £7.89. Label: 5, counselling, skilled tasks

◢ LEVOCETIRIZINE HYDROCHLORIDE

Note Levocetirizine is an isomer of cetirizine

Cautions see notes above

Renal impairment estimated glomerular filtration rate 30–50 mL/minute/1.73 m², reduce dose frequency to alternate days; estimated glomerular filtration rate 10–30 mL/minute/1.73 m², reduce dose frequency to every 3 days; estimated glomerular filtration rate less than 10 mL/minute/1.73 m², avoid

Contra-indications see notes above

Side-effects see notes above; *very rarely* weight gain

Licensed use tablets not licensed for use in children under 6 years

Indication and dose

Symptomatic relief of allergy such as hay fever, urticaria
- **By mouth**
  Child 2–6 years 1.25 mg twice daily
  Child 6–18 years 5 mg once daily

3

Respiratory system

◁ **LEVOCETIRIZINE HYDROCHLORIDE (*continued*)**

Xyzal® (UCB Pharma) [PoM]
Tablets, f/c, levocetirizine hydrochloride 5 mg, net price 30-tab pack = £5.20. Counselling, skilled tasks

Oral solution, levocetirizine hydrochloride 2.5 mg/ 5 mL, net price 200 mL = £6.00. Counselling, skilled tasks

LORATADINE

Cautions see notes above

Contra-indications see notes above

Side-effects see notes above

Indication and dose

Symptomatic relief of allergy such as hay fever, chronic idiopathic urticaria
• By mouth
  Child 2–6 years 5 mg once daily
  Child 6–18 years 10 mg once daily

Loratadine (Non-proprietary)
Tablets, loratadine 10 mg, net price 30-tab pack = £1.24. Counselling, skilled tasks

Dental prescribing on NHS Loratadine 10 mg tablets may be prescribed

Syrup, loratadine 5 mg/5 mL, net price 100 mL = £5.16. Counselling, skilled tasks

MIZOLASTINE

Cautions see notes above

Contra-indications see notes above; also susceptibility to QT-interval prolongation (including cardiac disease and hypokalaemia)

Hepatic impairment manufacturer recommends avoid in significant hepatic impairment

Side-effects see notes above; weight gain; anxiety, asthenia; *less commonly* arthralgia and myalgia

Indication and dose

Symptomatic relief of allergy such as hay fever, urticaria
• By mouth
  Child 12–18 years 10 mg once daily

Mizollen® (Sanofi-Aventis) [PoM]
Tablets, m/r, f/c, scored, mizolastine 10 mg, net price 30-tab pack = £5.77. Label: 25, counselling, skilled tasks

Sedating antihistamines

Skilled tasks Drowsiness may affect performance of skilled tasks (e.g. cycling or driving); sedating effects enhanced by alcohol.

ALIMEMAZINE TARTRATE
(Trimeprazine tartrate)

Cautions see notes above

Contra-indications see notes above

Renal impairment avoid

Side-effects see notes above

Licensed use not licensed for use in children under 2 years

Indication and dose

Urticaria, pruritus
• By mouth
  Child 6 months–2 years 250 micrograms/kg (max. 2.5 mg) 3–4 times daily—specialist use only
  Child 2–5 years 2.5 mg 3–4 times daily
  Child 5–12 years 5 mg 3–4 times daily

Child 12–18 years 10 mg 2–3 times daily, in severe cases up to max. 100 mg daily

Premedication section 15.1.4
• By mouth
  Child 2–7 years up to max. 2 mg/kg 1–2 hours before operation

Vallergan® (Sanofi-Aventis) [PoM]
Tablets, blue, f/c, alimemazine tartrate 10 mg, net price 28-tab pack = £3.89. Label: 2

Syrup, straw-coloured, alimemazine tartrate 7.5 mg/5 mL, net price 100 mL = £4.44. Label: 2

Syrup forte, alimemazine tartrate 30 mg/5 mL, net price 100 mL = £6.86. Label: 2

CHLORPHENAMINE MALEATE
(Chlorpheniramine maleate)

Cautions see notes above

Contra-indications see notes above

Side-effects see notes above; also exfoliative dermatitis and tinnitus reported; injections may cause transient hypotension or CNS stimulation and may be irritant

Respiratory system

3

◁ **CHLORPHENAMINE MALEATE (continued)**

Licensed use *syrup* not licensed for use in children under 1 year; *tablets* not licensed for use in children under 6 years; *injection* not licensed for use in neonates

Indication and dose

Symptomatic relief of allergy such as hay fever, urticaria

• **By mouth**

Child 1 month–2 years 1 mg twice daily

Child 2–6 years 1 mg every 4–6 hours, max. 6 mg daily

Child 6–12 years 2 mg every 4–6 hours, max. 12 mg daily

Child 12–18 years 4 mg every 4–6 hours, max. 24 mg daily

Emergency treatment of anaphylactic reactions, symptomatic relief of allergy

• **By intramuscular or intravenous injection**

Child under 6 months 250 micrograms/kg (max. 2.5 mg), repeated if required up to 4 times in 24 hours

Child 6 months–6 years 2.5 mg, repeated if required up to 4 times in 24 hours

Child 6–12 years 5 mg, repeated if required up to 4 times in 24 hours

Child 12–18 years 10 mg, repeated if required up to 4 times in 24 hours

Administration for *intravenous injection*, give over 1 minute; if small dose required, dilute with Sodium Chloride 0.9%

Chlorphenamine (Non-proprietary)

Tablets, chlorphenamine maleate 4 mg, net price 28 = £1.12. Label: 2

Dental prescribing on NHS Chlorphenamine tablets may be prescribed

Oral solution, chlorphenamine maleate 2 mg/5 mL, net price 150 mL = £2.25. Label: 2

Dental prescribing on NHS Chlorphenamine oral solution may be prescribed

Injection PoM[1], chlorphenamine maleate 10 mg/mL, net price 1-mL amp = £1.62

1. PoM restriction does not apply where administration is for saving life in emergency

Piriton® (GSK Consumer Healthcare)

Tablets, yellow, scored, chlorphenamine maleate 4 mg, net price 28 = £1.62. Label: 2

Syrup, chlorphenamine maleate 2 mg/5 mL, net price 150 mL = £2.39. Label: 2

HYDROXYZINE HYDROCHLORIDE

Cautions see notes above

Renal impairment use half normal dose

Contra-indications see notes above

Side-effects see notes above

Licensed use *Ucerax®* syrup not licensed for use in children under 1 year

Indication and dose

Pruritus

• **By mouth**

Child 6 months–6 years initially 5–15 mg at night, increased if necessary to 50 mg daily in 3–4 divided doses

Child 6–12 years initially 15–25 mg at night, increased if necessary to 50–100 mg daily in 3–4 divided doses

Child 12–18 years initially 25 mg at night, increased if necessary to 100 mg in 3–4 divided doses

Atarax® (Alliance) PoM

Tablets, both s/c, hydroxyzine hydrochloride 10 mg (orange), net price 84-tab pack = £1.82; 25 mg (green), 28-tab pack = £1.22. Label: 2

Ucerax® (UCB Pharma) PoM

Tablets JHS, f/c, scored, hydroxyzine hydrochloride 25 mg, net price 25-tab pack = £1.22. Label: 2

Syrup, hydroxyzine hydrochloride 10 mg/5 mL. Net price 200-mL pack = £1.78. Label: 2

KETOTIFEN

Cautions see notes above

Contra-indications see notes above

Side-effects see notes above; also irritability, nervousness; *less commonly* cystitis; *rarely* weight gain; *very rarely* Stevens-Johnson syndrome

Indication and dose

Symptomatic relief of allergy such as allergic rhinitis

• **By mouth**

Child 3–18 years 1 mg twice daily

Zaditen® (Novartis) PoM

Tablets, scored, ketotifen (as hydrogen fumarate) 1 mg, net price 60-tab pack = £10.75. Label: 2, 21

Elixir, ketotifen (as hydrogen fumarate), 1 mg/5 mL, net price 300 mL (strawberry-flavoured) = £12.73. Label: 2, 21

3 Respiratory system

PROMETHAZINE HYDROCHLORIDE

Cautions see notes above

Contra-indications see notes above; severe coronary artery disease

Side-effects see notes above; also restlessness

Indication and dose

Symptomatic relief of allergy such as hay fever, insomnia associated with urticaria and pruritus
• By mouth
  Child 2–5 years 5 mg twice daily *or* 5–15 mg at night
  Child 5–10 years 5–10 mg twice daily *or* 10–25 mg at night
  Child 10–18 years 10–20 mg 2–3 times daily *or* 25 mg at night increased to 25 mg twice daily if necessary

Sedation section 4.1.1

Nausea and vomiting section 4.6

Phenergan® (Sanofi-Aventis)
Tablets, both blue, f/c, promethazine hydrochloride 10 mg, net price 56-tab pack = £2.05; 25 mg, 56-tab pack = £3.06. Label: 2
Dental prescribing on NHS May be prescribed as Promethazine Hydrochloride Tablets 10 mg or 25 mg

Elixir, golden, promethazine hydrochloride 5 mg/5 mL. Net price 100 mL = £1.93. Label: 2
Dental prescribing on NHS May be prescribed as Promethazine Hydrochloride Oral Solution 5 mg/5 mL

3.4.2 Allergen immunotherapy

Immunotherapy using allergen vaccines containing house dust mite, animal dander (cat or dog), or extracts of grass and tree pollen can improve symptoms of asthma and allergic rhino-conjunctivitis in children. A vaccine containing extracts of wasp and bee venom is used to reduce the risk of severe anaphylaxis and systemic reactions in children with hypersensitivity to wasp and bee stings. Children requiring immunotherapy must be referred to a hospital specialist for accurate allergy diagnosis, assessment, and treatment.

> In view of concerns about the safety of desensitising vaccines, it is recommended that they are used by specialists and only for the following indications:
>
> • seasonal allergic hay fever (caused by pollen) that has not responded to anti-allergic drugs;
>
> • hypersensitivity to wasp and bee venoms.
>
> Desensitising vaccines should generally be avoided or used with particular care in children with asthma.

Desensitising vaccines should be avoided in pregnant women, in children under 5 years, and in those taking beta-blockers (adrenaline will be ineffective if a hypersensitivity reaction occurs), or ACE inhibitors (risk of severe anaphylactoid reactions).

Hypersensitivity reactions to immunotherapy (especially to wasp and bee venom extracts) can be life-threatening; bronchospasm usually develops within 1 hour and anaphylaxis within 30 minutes of injection. Therefore the child needs to be monitored for at least 1 hour after injection. If symptoms or signs of hypersensitivity develop (e.g. rash, urticaria, bronchospasm, faintness), **even when mild**, the child should be observed until these have **resolved completely**.

For details of the management of anaphylactic shock, see section 3.4.3.

Each set of allergen extracts usually contains vials for the administration of graded amounts of allergen. Maintenance sets containing vials at the highest strength are also available. Product literature must be consulted for details of allergens, vial strengths, and administration.

BEE AND WASP ALLERGEN EXTRACTS

Cautions see notes above and consult product literature
CSM advice The CSM has advised that facilities for cardiopulmonary resuscitation must be immediately available and children monitored closely for 1 hour after each injection

Contra-indications see notes above and consult product literature

Side-effects consult product literature

Indication and dose

Hypersensitivity to wasp or bee venom (see notes above)
• By subcutaneous injection
  Consult product literature

◁ **BEE AND WASP ALLERGEN EXTRACTS (***continued***)**

Pharmalgen® (ALK-Abelló) P̲o̲M̲
Bee venom extract (*Apis mellifera*) or wasp venom extract (*Vespula* spp.). Net price initial treatment set = £59.77 (bee), £73.28 (wasp); maintenance treatment set = £69.54 (bee), £89.45 (wasp)

■ GRASS AND TREE POLLEN EXTRACTS

Cautions see notes above and consult product literature
  CSM advice The CSM has advised that facilities for cardiopulmonary resuscitation must be immediately available and children must be monitored closely for 1 hour after each injection

Contra-indications see notes above and consult product literature

Side-effects consult product literature

Indication and dose

  Treatment of seasonal allergic hay fever due to grass or tree pollen (see notes above)

    See under preparations, below

Pollinex® (Allergy) P̲o̲M̲
Grasses and rye or tree pollen extract, net price initial treatment set (3 vials) and extension course treatment (1 vial) = £320.00
Dose
  • **By subcutaneous injection**
    Consult product literature

◀ Grass pollen extract
Grazax® (ALK-Abelló) ▼ P̲o̲M̲
Oral lyophilisates (= freeze-dried tablets), grass pollen extract 75 000 units, net price 30-tab pack = £67.50. Counselling, administration

Dose
  • **By mouth**
    Child 5–18 years 1 tablet daily; start treatment at least 4 months before start of pollen season and continue for up to 3 years

  Counselling Tablets should be placed under the tongue and allowed to disperse

---

Omalizumab

Omalizumab is a monoclonal antibody that binds to immunoglobulin E (IgE). It is licensed for use as additional therapy in children over 12 years with proven IgE-mediated sensitivity to inhaled allergens, whose severe persistent allergic asthma cannot be controlled adequately with high-dose inhaled corticosteroid together with a long-acting beta$_2$ agonist. Omalizumab should be initiated by physicians experienced in the treatment of severe persistent asthma.

Churg-Strauss syndrome has occurred rarely in patients given omalizumab; the reaction is usually associated with the reduction or withdrawal of oral corticosteroid therapy. Churg-Strauss syndrome can present as eosinophilia, vasculitic rash, cardiac complications, worsening pulmonary symptoms, or peripheral neuropathy. Hypersensitivity reactions can also occur immediately following treatment with omalizumab or sometimes more than 24 hours after the first injection.

For details on the management of anaphylactic shock, see section 3.4.3.

NICE guidance
Omalizumab for severe persistent allergic asthma (November 2007)
Omalizumab is recommended as additional therapy for the prophylaxis of severe persistent allergic asthma in children over 12 years, who cannot be controlled adequately with high-dose inhaled corticosteroids and long-acting beta$_2$ agonists in addition to leukotriene receptor antagonists, theophylline, oral corticosteroids, oral beta$_2$ agonists, and smoking cessation where clinically appropriate. The following conditions apply:

  • confirmation of IgE-mediated allergy to a perennial allergen by clinical history and allergy skin testing;

  • either 2 or more severe exacerbations of asthma requiring hospital admission within the previous year, or 3 or more severe exacerbations of asthma within the previous year, at least one of which required hospital admission, and a further 2 which required treatment or monitoring in excess of the patient's usual regimen, in an accident and emergency unit.

Omalizumab should be initiated and monitored by a physician experienced in both allergy and respiratory medicine in a specialist centre, and discontinued at 16 weeks in patients who have not shown an adequate response to therapy.

3

Respiratory system

▲ OMALIZUMAB

Cautions autoimmune disease; susceptibility to helminth infections—discontinue if infection does not respond to anthelmintic

Hepatic impairment manufacturer advises caution—no information available

Renal impairment manufacturer advises caution—no information available

Pregnancy manufacturer advises avoid unless essential; no evidence of teratogenicity in *animal* studies

Contra-indications

Breast-feeding manufacturer advises avoid—present in milk in *animal* studies

Side-effects headache; injection-site reactions; *less commonly* nausea, diarrhoea, dyspepsia, flushing, fatigue, dizziness, drowsiness, paraesthesia, weight gain, influenza-like symptoms, photosensitivity, hypersensitivity reactions

(including hypotension, bronchospasm, laryngoedema, rash, pruritus, serum sickness, and anaphylaxis); Churg-Strauss syndrome (see notes above), thrombocytopenia, arthralgia, myalgia, and alopecia also reported

Indication and dose

Prophylaxis of severe persistent allergic asthma (see notes above)

• By subcutaneous injection

Child 12–18 years according to immunoglobulin E concentration and body-weight, consult product literature

Xolair® (Novartis) ▼ [PoM]
Injection, powder for reconstitution, omalizumab, net price 150-mg vial = £256.15 (with solvent)
Excipients include sucrose 108 mg/vial

3.4.3 Allergic emergencies

Adrenaline (**epinephrine**) provides physiological reversal of the immediate symptoms (such as laryngeal oedema, bronchospasm, and hypotension) associated with hypersensitivity reactions such as *anaphylaxis* and *angioedema*.

Anaphylaxis

Anaphylactic shock requires prompt treatment of *laryngeal oedema, bronchospasm,* and *hypotension*. Atopic individuals are particularly susceptible. Insect stings are a recognised risk (in particular wasp and bee stings). Latex and certain foods, including eggs, fish, cow's milk protein, peanuts, and tree nuts may also precipitate anaphylaxis. Medicinal products particularly associated with anaphylaxis include blood products, vaccines, allergen immunotherapy preparations, antibacterials, aspirin and other NSAIDs, heparin, and neuromuscular blocking drugs. In the case of drugs, anaphylaxis is more likely after parenteral administration; resuscitation facilities must always be available when giving injections associated with special risk. Refined arachis (peanut) oil, which may be present in some medicinal products, is unlikely to cause an allergic reaction—nevertheless it is wise to check the full formula of preparations which may contain allergenic fats or oils.

Treatment of anaphylaxis
First-line treatment includes:

• securing the airway, restoration of blood pressure (laying the child flat and raising the legs, or in the recovery position if unconscious or nauseous and at risk of vomiting);

• administering **adrenaline** (epinephrine) by **intramuscular** injection (for doses see Intramuscular Adrenaline, p. 199); the dose should be repeated if necessary at 5-minute intervals according to blood pressure, pulse, and respiratory function [**important**: possible need for *intravenous route using dilute solution* (Adrenaline 1 in 10 000), see Intravenous Adrenaline p. 199];

• administering high-flow **oxygen** (section 3.6) and **intravenous fluids** (section 9.2.2);

• administering an antihistamine, such as **chlorphenamine** (chlorpheniramine), by slow intravenous injection or intramuscular injection (section 3.4.1) as adjunctive treatment given after adrenaline injection and the antihistamine continued orally for 24 to 48 hours according to clinical response to prevent relapse.

Continuing respiratory deterioration requires further treatment with **bronchodilators** including inhaled or intravenous salbutamol (see p. 174), inhaled ipratropium (see p. 178), intravenous aminophylline (see p. 180), or intravenous magnesium sulphate [unlicensed indication] (see Management of Acute Asthma,

p. 168). In addition to oxygen, assisted respiration and possibly emergency tracheotomy may be necessary.

An intravenous corticosteroid (section 6.3.2) such as **hydrocortisone** (as sodium succinate) is of secondary value in the initial management of anaphylactic shock because the onset of action is delayed for several hours, but should be given to prevent further deterioration in severely affected children and continued for 24–48 hours according to clinical response.

When a child is so ill that there is doubt as to the adequacy of the circulation, the initial injection of adrenaline may need to be given as a *dilute solution by the intravenous route*, or by the intraosseous route if venous access is difficult—for details of cautions, dose and strength, see under Intravenous Adrenaline (Epinephrine), below.

Some children with severe allergy to insect stings or foods are encouraged to carry prefilled adrenaline syringes for *self-administration* during periods of risk.

Children who are suspected of having had an anaphylactic reaction should be referred to a specialist for specific allergy diagnosis; avoidance of the allergen is the principal treatment.

Intramuscular adrenaline (epinephrine)

The *intramuscular route* is the *first choice route* for the administration of adrenaline in the management of anaphylactic shock. Adrenaline has a rapid onset of action after intramuscular administration and in the shocked patient its absorption from the intramuscular site is faster and more reliable than from the subcutaneous site. The intravenous route should be reserved for extreme emergency when there is doubt about the adequacy of the circulation; for details of cautions, dose and strength see Intravenous Adrenaline (Epinephrine), below.

Carers of children or the child with severe allergy should ideally be instructed in the self-administration of adrenaline by intramuscular injection (for details see Self-administration of Adrenaline (Epinephrine), p. 200).

Prompt injection of adrenaline is of paramount importance. The following adrenaline doses are based on the revised recommendations of the Working Group of the Resuscitation Council (UK).

Dose of *intramuscular* injection of adrenaline (epinephrine) for anaphylactic shock		
Age range	Dose	Volume of adrenaline **1 in 1000** (1 mg/mL)
Under 6 years	150 micrograms	0.15 mL[1]
6–12 years	300 micrograms	0.3 mL
12–18 years	500 micrograms	0.5 mL[2]
These doses may be repeated several times if necessary at 5-minute intervals according to blood pressure, pulse and respiratory function.		

1. Use suitable syringe for measuring small volume
2. 300 micrograms (0.3 mL) if child is small or prepubertal

Intravenous adrenaline (epinephrine)

Intravenous adrenaline should be given only by those experienced in its use, in a setting where patients can be carefully monitored; it should be given to children only when intravenous access is already available.

Where the child is severely ill and there is real doubt about adequacy of the circulation and absorption from the intramuscular injection site, adrenaline may be given by **slow** *intravenous injection*. Children may respond to as little as 1 microgram/kg (0.01 mL/kg) of the dilute 1 in 10 000 adrenaline injection by **slow** *intravenous injection* over several minutes, repeated according to response. A single dose of adrenaline by intravenous injection should not exceed 50 micrograms; if multiple doses are required consider giving adrenaline by slow intravenous *infusion*. Great vigilance is needed to ensure that the *correct strength* of

3

Respiratory system

adrenaline injection is used; anaphylactic shock kits need to make a *very clear distinction* between the 1 in 10 000 strength and the 1 in 1000 strength. It is also important that, where intramuscular injection might still succeed, time should not be wasted seeking intravenous access.

For reference to the use of the intravenous route for *acute hypotension*, see section 2.7.2.

Self-administration of adrenaline (epinephrine)

Children at considerable risk of anaphylaxis need to carry (or have available) adrenaline at all times and the child, or child's carers, need to be *instructed in advance* how to inject it. Packs for self-administration need to be **clearly labelled with instructions** on how to administer adrenaline (intramuscularly, preferably at the midpoint of the outer thigh, through light clothing if necessary). It is important to ensure that an adequate supply is provided to treat symptoms until medical assistance is available.

Adrenaline for administration by intramuscular injection is available in 'auto-injectors', pre-assembled syringes (e.g. *Anapen®* or *EpiPen®*) fitted with a needle suitable for very rapid administration (if necessary by a bystander or a healthcare provider if it is the only preparation available). A syringe delivering 300 micrograms of adrenaline is recommended for a child over 30 kg. A syringe delivering 150 micrograms of adrenaline is recommended for a child 15–30 kg, but on the basis of a dose of 10 micrograms/kg, 300 micrograms may be more appropriate for some children.

ADRENALINE/EPINEPHRINE

Cautions heart disease, hypertension, arrhythmias, cerebrovascular disease, phaeochromocytoma; diabetes mellitus, hyperthyroidism; susceptibility to angle-closure glaucoma
Interactions Severe anaphylaxis in children on non-cardioselective beta-blockers may not respond to adrenaline injection calling for intravenous injection of salbutamol (see section 3.1.1.1); furthermore, adrenaline may cause severe hypertension and bradycardia in those receiving non-cardioselective beta-blockers. Other **interactions**, see Appendix 1 (sympathomimetics).

Side-effects nausea, vomiting; tachycardia, arrhythmias, palpitation, cold extremities, hypertension (risk of cerebral haemorrhage); dyspnoea, pulmonary oedema (on excessive dosage or extreme sensitivity); anxiety, tremor, restlessness, headache, weakness, dizziness; hyperglycaemia; urinary retention; sweating; tissue necrosis at injection site

Indication and dose

Emergency treatment of acute anaphylaxis, angioedema
• By intramuscular injection (preferably midpoint in anterolateral thigh) of 1 in 1000 (1 mg/mL) solution
See notes and table above

Acute anaphylaxis when there is doubt as to the adequacy of the circulation
• By slow intravenous injection of 1 in 10 000 (100 micrograms/mL) solution (extreme caution—specialist use only)
See notes above

Safe Practice Intravenous route should be used with **extreme care** by specialists only, see notes above

Croup (section 3.1)
• By inhalation of nebulised solution of adrenaline 1 in 1000 (1 mg/mL)
Child 1 month–12 years 400 micrograms/kg (max. 5 mg), repeated after 30 minutes if necessary
Administration For nebulisation, dilute adrenaline 1 in 1000 solution with sterile sodium chloride 0.9% solution

Acute hypotension, low cardiac output section 2.7.2

Cardiopulmonary resuscitation section 2.7.3

◢Intramuscular or subcutaneous
[1]**Adrenaline/Epinephrine 1 in 1000** (Non-proprietary) PoM
Injection, adrenaline (as acid tartrate) 1 mg/mL, net price 0.5-mL amp = 49p; 1-mL amp = 56p
Excipients include sulphites

[1]**Minijet® Adrenaline 1 in 1000** (UCB Pharma) PoM
Injection, adrenaline (as hydrochloride) 1 in 1000 (1 mg/mL). Net price 1 mL (with 25 gauge × 0.25 inch needle for subcutaneous injection) = £9.81, 1 mL (with 21 gauge × 1.5 inch needle for intramuscular injection) = £5.78 (both disposable syringes)
Excipients include sulphites

---

1. PoM restriction does not apply to adrenaline injection 1 mg/mL where administration is for saving life in emergency

◻ **ADRENALINE/EPINEPHRINE** (*continued*)

◢ Intravenous
Extreme caution, see notes above

Adrenaline/Epinephrine 1 in 10 000, Dilute (Non-proprietary) [PoM]
Injection, adrenaline (as acid tartrate) 100 micrograms/mL, 10-mL amp, 1-mL and 10-mL prefilled syringe
Excipients include sulphites

Minijet® Adrenaline 1 in 10 000 (UCB Pharma) [PoM]
Injection, adrenaline (as hydrochloride) 1 in 10 000 (100 micrograms/mL), net price 3-mL prefilled syringe = £5.70; 10-mL prefilled syringe = £5.30
Excipients include sulphites

◢ Intramuscular injection for self-administration
Anapen® (Lincoln Medical) [PoM]
[1]Anapen® 0.3 mg solution for injection (delivering a single dose of adrenaline 300 micrograms), adrenaline 1 mg/mL (1 in 1000), net price 1.05-mL auto-injector device = £30.67
Excipients include sulphites
Note 0.75 mL of the solution remains in the auto-injector device after use

Dose
Acute anaphylaxis
● By intramuscular injection
  Child over 30 kg 300 micrograms repeated after 10–15 minutes as necessary

Anapen® Junior 0.15 mg solution for injection (delivering a single dose of adrenaline 150 micrograms), adrenaline 500 micrograms/mL (1 in 2000), net price 1.05-mL auto-injector device = £30.67
Excipients include sulphites
Note 0.75 mL of the solution remains in the auto-injector device after use

Dose
Acute anaphylaxis
● By intramuscular injection
  Child 15–30 kg 150 micrograms (but on the basis of a dose of 10 micrograms/kg, 300 micrograms may be more appropriate for some children) repeated after 10–15 minutes as necessary

EpiPen® (ALK-Abelló) [PoM]
[1]EpiPen® Auto-injector 0.3 mg (delivering a single dose of adrenaline 300 micrograms), adrenaline 1 mg/mL (1 in 1000), net price 2-mL auto-injector = £28.05
Excipients include sulphites
Note 1.7 mL of the solution remains in the *Auto-injector* after use

Dose
Acute anaphylaxis
● By intramuscular injection
  Child over 30 kg 300 micrograms repeated after 5–15 minutes as necessary

Epipen® Jr Auto-injector 0.15 mg (delivering a single dose of adrenaline 150 micrograms), adrenaline 500 micrograms/mL (1 in 2000), net price 2-mL auto-injector = £28.05
Excipients include sulphites
Note 1.7 mL of the solution remains in the *Auto-injector* after use

Dose
Acute anaphylaxis
● By intramuscular injection
  Child 15–30 kg 150 micrograms (but on the basis of a dose of 10 micrograms/kg, 300 micrograms may be more appropriate for some children) repeated after 5–15 minutes as necessary

Angioedema

Angioedema is dangerous if *laryngeal oedema* is present. In this circumstance adrenaline (epinephrine) injection and oxygen should be given as described under Anaphylaxis (see above); antihistamines and corticosteroids should also be given (see again above). Tracheal intubation may be necessary. In some children with laryngeal oedema, adrenaline 1 in 1000 (1 mg/mL) solution may be given by nebuliser. However, nebulised adrenaline cannot be relied upon for a systemic effect—intramuscular adrenaline should be used.

Hereditary angioedema The administration of C_1 esterase inhibitor (in fresh frozen plasma or in partially purified form) may terminate acute attacks of *hereditary angioedema*, but is not practical for long-term prophylaxis. **Tranexamic acid** (section 2.11) is used for short-term or long-term prophylaxis of hereditary angioedema; short-term prophylaxis is started several days before planned procedures which may trigger an acute attack of hereditary angioedema (e.g. dental work) and continued for 2–5 days afterwards. **Danazol** [unlicensed indication, see BNF section 6.7.2] is best avoided in children because of its androgenic effects but it can be used for short-term prophylaxis of hereditary angioedema.

1. [PoM] restriction does not apply to adrenaline injection 1 mg/mL where administration is for saving life in emergency

3

Respiratory system

3.5 Respiratory stimulants and pulmonary surfactants

3.5.1 Respiratory stimulants
3.5.2 Pulmonary surfactants

3.5.1 Respiratory stimulants

Respiratory stimulants (analeptic drugs), such as caffeine and doxapram, should only be given under **expert supervision** in hospital; it is important to rule out any underlying disorder, such as seizures, hypoglycaemia, or infection, causing respiratory exhaustion before starting treatment with a respiratory stimulant.

Caffeine (as caffeine base) is licensed for the treatment of idiopathic apnoea in preterm neonates; it is used in preference to theophylline. Caffeine can also be used to improve trigger ventilation, or assist extubation in ventilated infants. Caffeine has fewer adverse effects and a longer half-life than theophylline in neonates. It is well absorbed when given orally; intravenous treatment is rarely necessary. Plasma-caffeine concentration should be measured if the child has previously been treated with theophylline. The therapeutic range for plasma-caffeine concentration is usually 10–20 mg/litre (50–100 micromol/litre), but a concentration of 25–35 mg/litre (130–180 micromol/litre) may be required.

Doxapram may be given by continuous intravenous infusion or by mouth for preterm neonates and infants who continue to have troublesome apnoea despite treatment with caffeine. When given by continuous intravenous infusion, blood pressure monitoring and frequent measurement of arterial blood gas and pH are necessary to ensure correct dosage.

CAFFEINE

Cautions gastro-oesophageal reflux; cardiovascular disease; monitor plasma-caffeine concentration (see notes above); monitor closely for 1 week after stopping treatment

Side-effects hypertension, tachycardia; irritability, restlessness; hypoglycaemia, hyperglycaemia; fluid and electrolyte imbalance

Licensed use not licensed for use as an adjunct to extubation in pre-term neonates

Indication and dose

Neonatal apnoea, adjunct to extubation in pre-term neonates
• By mouth

Neonate initially 10 mg/kg, then 2.5–5 mg/kg once daily starting 24 hours after initial dose (some neonates may require 10 mg/kg/day)

• By intravenous infusion

Neonate initially 10 mg/kg over 30 minutes, then 2.5–5 mg/kg over 10 minutes once daily starting 24 hours after initial dose (some neonates may require 10 mg/kg/day)

Note Dose expressed as caffeine base

Safe practice When prescribing, always state dose in terms of caffeine base
Caffeine base 1 mg = caffeine *citrate* 2 mg

Caffeine (Non-proprietary) (PoM)
Injection, caffeine 5 mg/mL, net price 1-mL amp = £4.44
Electrolytes Na$^+$ < 0.5 mmol/amp

◀Caffeine citrate preparations
Caffeine citrate oral liquid available from 'special-order' manufacturers or specialist importing companies, see p. 943

DOXAPRAM HYDROCHLORIDE

Cautions impaired cardiac reserve; risk of QT interval prolongation; **interactions:** Appendix 1 (doxapram)

Contra-indications severe hypertension, thyrotoxicosis, epilepsy, physical obstruction of respiratory tract

Side-effects perineal warmth, dizziness, sweating, moderate increase in blood pressure and heart rate; hyperexcitability; high doses may cause convulsions; oral dose may cause slowed gastric emptying

Licensed use not licensed for use in children

Indication and dose

Neonatal apnoea (see notes above)
• By intravenous infusion

Neonate initially 2.5 mg/kg over 5–10 minutes, then by *continuous intravenous infusion* 300 microgram/kg/hour adjusted according to response, up to max. 1.5 mg/kg/hour

• By mouth (after initial intravenous dose)

Neonate 6 mg/kg 4 times daily

◁ **DOXAPRAM HYDROCHLORIDE** (*continued*)

Administration for *intravenous infusion*, dilute injection solution (20 mg/mL) to a concentration of 1 mg/mL with Glucose 5% *or* Sodium Chloride 0.9%

For administration *by mouth*, dilute doxapram injection solution with Glucose 5% if necessary

Dopram® (Anpharm) [PoM]
Injection, doxapram hydrochloride 20 mg/mL. Net price 5-mL amp = £3.00

Intravenous infusion, doxapram hydrochloride 2 mg/mL in glucose 5%. Net price 500-mL bottle = £21.33

3.5.2 Pulmonary surfactants

Pulmonary surfactants derived from animal lungs, **beractant** and **poractant alfa** are used to prevent and treat respiratory distress syndrome (hyaline membrane disease) in preterm neonates. Prophylactic use of a pulmonary surfactant may reduce the need for mechanical ventilation and is more effective than 'rescue treatment' in preterm neonates of 29 weeks or less post-menstrual age.

Pulmonary surfactants may also be of benefit in neonates with meconium aspiration syndrome or intrapartum streptococcal infection.

Pulmonary immaturity with surfactant deficit is the commonest reason for respiratory failure in the neonate, especially in those of less than 30 weeks postmenstrual age. Betamethasone (section 6.3.2) given to the mother (at least 12 hours but preferably 48 hours) before delivery substantially enhances pulmonary maturity in the neonate.

Cautions   Continuous monitoring is required to avoid hyperoxaemia caused by rapid improvement in arterial oxygen concentration.

Side-effects   Pulmonary haemorrhage has been rarely associated with pulmonary surfactants, especially in more preterm neonates. Obstruction of the endotracheal tube by mucous secretions has also been reported.

3
Respiratory system

BERACTANT

Cautions see notes above

Side-effects see notes above

Licensed use licensed for use in respiratory distress syndrome in newborn premature infants, birth-weight over 700 g, and as prophylaxis in neonates less than 32 weeks post-menstrual age

Indication and dose

Treatment of respiratory distress syndrome in preterm neonate; prophylaxis of respiratory distress syndrome in preterm neonate
• By endotracheal tube

Neonate phospholipid 100 mg/kg equivalent to a volume of 4 mL/kg, preferably within 8 hours of birth; may be repeated within 48 hours at intervals of at least 6 hours for up to 4 doses

Survanta® (Abbott) [PoM]
Suspension, beractant (bovine lung extract) providing phospholipid 25 mg/mL, with lipids and proteins, net price 8-mL vial = £306.43

PORACTANT ALFA

Cautions   see notes above

Side-effects   see notes above

Licensed use licensed for use in respiratory distress syndrome in newborn premature infants, birth-weight over 700 g, and as prophylaxis in neonates 24–32 weeks post-menstrual age

Indication and dose

Treatment of respiratory distress syndrome or hyaline membrane disease in preterm neonate; prophylaxis of respiratory distress syndrome in preterm neonate
• By endotracheal tube

Neonate *treatment*, 100–200 mg/kg; further doses of 100 mg/kg may be repeated 12 hours later and after further 12 hours if still intubated; max. total dose 300–400 mg/kg; *prophylaxis*, 100–200 mg/kg soon after birth (preferably within 15 minutes); further doses of 100 mg/kg may be repeated 6–12 hours later and after further 12 hours if still intubated; max. total dose 300–400 mg/kg

Curosurf® (Chiesi) [PoM]
Suspension, poractant alfa (porcine lung phospholipid fraction) 80 mg/mL, net price 1.5-mL vial = £298.74; 3-mL vial = £580.64

3.6 Oxygen

Oxygen should be regarded as a drug. It is prescribed for hypoxaemic patients to increase alveolar oxygen tension and decrease the work of breathing. The concentration of oxygen required depends on the condition being treated; administration of an inappropriate concentration of oxygen may have serious or even fatal consequences. High concentrations of oxygen can cause pulmonary epithelial damage (bronchopulmonary dysplasia), convulsions, and retinal damage, especially in preterm neonates.

Oxygen is probably the most common drug used in medical emergencies. It should be prescribed initially to achieve a normal or near-normal oxygen saturation. In most acutely ill children with an expected or known normal or low arterial carbon dioxide (P_aCO_2), oxygen saturation should be maintained above 92%; some clinicians may aim for a target of 94–98%. In some clinical situations, such as carbon monoxide poisoning, (see also Emergency Treatment of Poisoning, p. 46), it is more appropriate to aim for the highest possible oxygen saturation until the child is stable. Hypercapnic respiratory failure is rare in children; in those children at risk, a lower oxygen saturation target of 88-92% is indicated, see below.

High concentration oxygen therapy, with concentrations of up to 60%, is safe in uncomplicated cases of conditions such as pneumonia, pulmonary embolism, pulmonary fibrosis, shock, severe trauma, sepsis, or anaphylaxis. In such conditions, low arterial oxygen (P_aO_2) is usually associated with low or normal arterial carbon dioxide (P_aCO_2) and there is little risk of hypoventilation and carbon dioxide retention.

In severe acute asthma, the arterial carbon dioxide (P_aCO_2) is usually subnormal but as asthma deteriorates it may rise steeply. These patients usually require a high concentration (40–60%) of oxygen and if the arterial carbon dioxide (P_aCO_2) remains high despite treatment, intermittent positive pressure ventilation needs to be considered urgently. Where facilities for blood gas measurements are not immediately available, for example while transferring the patient to hospital, 35% to 50% oxygen delivered through a conventional mask is recommended.

For neonates and infants with breathing difficulties, *high concentration oxygen therapy* is usually given in an incubator or by nasal cannula if the concentration of oxygen required is less than 50%; a humidified headbox must be used for concentration of oxygen greater than 60%.

Low concentration oxygen therapy (controlled oxygen therapy) is reserved for children at risk of hypercapnic respiratory failure, which is more likely in children with:

- advanced cystic fibrosis;
- advanced non-cystic fibrosis bronchiectasis;
- severe kyphoscoliosis or severe ankylosing spondylitis;
- severe lung scarring caused by tuberculosis;
- musculoskeletal disorders with respiratory weakness, especially if on home ventilation;
- an overdose of opioids, benzodiazepines, or other drugs causing respiratory depression.

Until blood gases can be measured, initial oxygen should be given using a controlled concentration of 28% or less, titrated towards a target concentration of 88-92%. The aim is to provide the child with enough oxygen to achieve an acceptable arterial oxygen tension without worsening carbon dioxide retention and respiratory acidosis.

Domiciliary oxygen   Oxygen should only be prescribed for use in the home after careful evaluation in hospital by a respiratory care specialist. Children and their carers should be advised of the risks of continuing to smoke when receiving oxygen, including the risk of fire. Smoking cessation therapy (section 4.10) should be tried before home oxygen prescription.

Long-term oxygen therapy

The aim of long-term oxygen therapy is to maintain oxygen saturation of at least 92%. Children (especially those with chronic neonatal lung disease) often require supplemental oxygen, either for 24-hours a day or during periods of sleep; many children are eventually weaned off long-term oxygen therapy as their condition improves.

Long-term oxygen therapy should be considered for children with conditions such as:

- bronchopulmonary dysplasia (chronic neonatal lung disease);
- congenital heart disease with pulmonary hypertension;
- pulmonary hypertension secondary to pulmonary disease;
- interstitial lung disease and obliterative bronchiolitis;
- cystic fibrosis;
- obstructive sleep apnoea syndrome;
- neuromuscular or skeletal disease requiring non-invasive ventilation;
- pulmonary malignancy or other terminal disease with disabling dyspnoea.

Increased respiratory depression is seldom a problem in children with stable respiratory failure treated with low concentrations of oxygen although it may occur during exacerbations; children and their carers should be warned to call for medical help if drowsiness or confusion occurs.

Short-burst oxygen therapy

Oxygen is occasionally prescribed for short-burst (intermittent) use for episodes of breathlessness.

Ambulatory oxygen therapy

Ambulatory oxygen is prescribed for children on long-term oxygen therapy who need to be away from home on a regular basis.

Oxygen therapy equipment

Under the NHS oxygen may be supplied as **oxygen cylinders**. Oxygen flow can be adjusted by means of an oxygen flow meter. Oxygen delivered from a cylinder should be passed through a humidifier if used for long periods.

Oxygen concentrators are more economical for children who require oxygen for long periods, and in England and Wales can be ordered on the NHS on a regional tendering basis (see below). A concentrator is recommended for a child who requires oxygen for more than 8 hours a day (or 21 cylinders per month). Exceptionally, if a higher concentration of oxygen is required the output of 2 oxygen concentrators can be combined using a 'Y' connection.

A nasal cannula is usually preferred to a face mask for long-term oxygen therapy from an oxygen concentrator. Nasal cannulas can, however, cause dermatitis and mucosal drying in sensitive individuals.

Giving oxygen by nasal cannula allows the child to talk, eat, and drink, but the concentration is not controlled and the method may not be appropriate for acute respiratory failure. When oxygen is given through a nasal cannula at a rate of 1–2 litres/minute the inspiratory oxygen concentration is usually low, but it varies with ventilation and can be high if the child is underventilating.

Arrangements for supplying oxygen

The following services may be ordered in England and Wales:

- emergency oxygen;
- short-burst (intermittent) oxygen therapy;
- long-term oxygen therapy;
- ambulatory oxygen.

The type of oxygen service (or combination of services) should be ordered on a Home Oxygen Order Form (HOOF); the amount of oxygen required (hours per day) and flow rate should be specified. The supplier will determine the appropriate equipment to be provided. Special needs or preferences should be specified on the HOOF.

3

Respiratory system

The clinician should obtain the patient's consent to pass on the patient's details to the supplier and the fire brigade. The supplier will contact the patient to make arrangements for delivery, installation, and maintenance of the equipment. The supplier will also train the patient to use the equipment.

The clinician should send order forms to the supplier by facsimile (see below); a copy of the HOOF should be sent to the Primary Care Trust or Local Health Board. The supplier will continue to provide the service until a revised order is received, or until notified that the patient no longer requires the home oxygen service.

HOOF and further instructions are available at www.bprs.co.uk/oxygen.html.

Eastern England South West	BOC Medical *to order:* Tel: 0800 136 603 Fax: 0800 169 9989
North East South East London Kent, Surrey, and Sussex South West London Thames Valley, Hampshire, and Isle of Wight	Air Liquide *to order:* Tel: 0500 823 773 Fax: 0800 781 4610
North West Yorkshire and Humberside East Midlands West Midlands North London Wales	Air Products *to order:* Tel: 0800 373 580 Fax: 0800 214 709

In **Scotland**, refer the child for assessment by a paediatric respiratory consultant. If the need for a concentrator is confirmed the consultant will arrange for the provision of a concentrator through the Common Services Agency. In **Northern Ireland** oxygen concentrators and cylinders should be prescribed on form HS21; oxygen concentrators are supplied by a local contractor. In **Scotland** and **Northern Ireland**, prescriptions for oxygen cylinders and accessories can be dispensed by pharmacies contracted to provide domiciliary oxygen services.

3.7 Mucolytics

Mucolytics, such as **carbocisteine** and **mecysteine**, are used to facilitate mucociliary clearance and expectoration by reducing sputum viscosity but evidence of efficacy is limited.

Dornase alfa is a genetically engineered version of a naturally occurring human enzyme which cleaves extracellular deoxyribonucleic acid (DNA); it is used to reduce sputum viscosity in children with cystic fibrosis. Dornase alfa is administered by inhalation using a jet nebuliser (section 3.1.5), usually once daily at least 1 hour before physiotherapy; however, alternate-day therapy may be as effective as daily treatment. Not all children benefit from treatment with dornase alfa; improvement occurs within 2 weeks, but in more severely affected children a trial of 6–12 weeks may be required.

Nebulised **hypertonic sodium chloride** solution may improve mucociliary clearance in children with cystic fibrosis.

Mesna (*Mistabron®*, available from 'special-order' manufacturers or specialist importing companies, see p. 943) is used in some children with cystic fibrosis when other mucolytics have failed to reduce sputum viscosity; 3–6 mL of a 20% solution is nebulised twice daily.

Acetylcysteine has been used to treat meconium ileus in neonates and distal intestinal obstruction syndrome in children with cystic fibrosis, but evidence of efficacy is lacking. *Gastrografin®* (section 1.6.5), or a bowel cleansing preparation containing macrogols (section 1.6.5), is usually more effective. Acetylcysteine may be used as a mucolytic to prevent further obstruction.

Respiratory system

3

ACETYLCYSTEINE

Cautions history of peptic ulceration; asthma

Side-effects hypersensitivity-like reactions including rashes and anaphylaxis

Licensed use not licensed for use in meconium ileus or for distal intestinal obstructive syndrome in children with cystic fibrosis

Indication and dose

Meconium ileus (but see notes above)
- By mouth

    NEONATE 200–400 mg up to 3 times daily if necessary

Treatment of distal intestinal obstructive syndrome (but see notes above)
- By mouth

    Child 1 month–2 years 0.4–3 g as a single dose

    Child 2–7 years 2–3 g as a single dose

    Child 7–18 years 4–6 g as a single dose

Prevention of distal intestinal obstruction syndrome
- By mouth

    Child 1 month–2 years 100–200 mg 3 times daily

    Child 2–12 years 200 mg 3 times daily

    Child 12–18 years 200–400 mg 3 times daily

Administration For *oral* administration, use oral granules, *or* dilute injection solution (200 mg/mL) to a concentration of 50 mg/mL; orange or blackcurrant juice or cola drink may be used as a diluent to mask the bitter taste

Acetylcysteine (Non-proprietary) [PoM]
Oral granules, acetylcysteine 100 mg/sachet; 200 mg/sachet. Label: 13
Available from 'special-order' manufacturers or specialist importing companies, see p. 943

◢ Injection
See Emergency treatment of poisoning, p. 38

CARBOCISTEINE

Cautions history of peptic ulceration

Pregnancy manufacturer advises avoid in first trimester

Contra-indications active peptic ulceration

Side-effects *rarely* gastro-intestinal bleeding; hypersensitivity reactions (including rash and anaphylaxis) also reported

Indication and dose

Reduction of sputum viscosity
- By mouth

    Child 2–5 years 62.5–125 mg 4 times daily

    Child 5–12 years 250 mg 3 times daily

    Child 12–18 years initially 2.25 g daily in divided doses, then 1.5 g daily in divided doses as condition improves

Carbocisteine (Sanofi-Aventis) [PoM]
Capsules, carbocisteine 375 mg, net price 120-cap pack = £16.68
Brands include *Mucodyne®*

Oral liquid, carbocisteine 125 mg/5 mL, net price 300 mL = £4.57; 250 mg/5 mL, 300 mL = £5.84
Brands include *Mucodyne® Paediatric* 125 mg/5 mL (cherry- and raspberry-flavoured) and *Mucodyne®* 250 mg/5 mL (cinnamon- and rum-flavoured)

DORNASE ALFA

Phosphorylated glycosylated recombinant human deoxyribonuclease 1 (rhDNase)

Cautions

Pregnancy no evidence of teratogenicity; manufacturer advises use only if potential benefit outweighs risk

Breast-feeding amount probably too small to be harmful—manufacturer advises caution

Side-effects pharyngitis, voice changes, chest pain; occasionally laryngitis, rashes, urticaria, conjunctivitis

Indication and dose

Management of cystic fibrosis patients with a forced vital capacity (FVC) of greater than 40% of predicted to improve pulmonary function
- By inhalation of nebulised solution (by jet nebuliser)

    Child 5–18 years 2500 units (2.5 mg) once daily

Pulmozyme® (Roche) [PoM]
Nebuliser solution, dornase alfa 1000 units (1 mg)/mL. Net price 2.5-mL (2500 units) vial = £17.57
Note For use undiluted with jet nebulisers only; ultrasonic nebulisers are unsuitable

MECYSTEINE HYDROCHLORIDE

(Methyl Cysteine Hydrochloride)

Cautions history of peptic ulceration

Contra-indications

Pregnancy manufacturer advises avoid

Breast-feeding manufacturer advises avoid

Indication and dose

Reduction of sputum viscosity
- By mouth

    Child 5–12 years 100 mg 3 times daily

3

Respiratory system

◻ **MECYSTEINE HYDROCHLORIDE (*continued*)**

Child 12–18 years 200 mg 4 times daily for 2 days, then 200 mg 3 times daily for 6 weeks, then 200 mg twice daily

Visclair® (Ranbaxy)
Tablets, yellow, s/c, e/c, mecysteine hydrochloride 100 mg, net price 100= £17.65. Label: 5, 22, 25

Hypertonic sodium chloride

Nebulised hypertonic sodium chloride solution (3–7 %) is used to mobilise lower respiratory tract secretions in mucous consolidation (e.g. cystic fibrosis).

MucoClear® (Pari)
Nebuliser solution, sodium chloride 6%, net price 20 × 4 ml = £12.98; 60 × 4 ml = £29.98

Dose
• By inhalation of nebulised solution
  Child 4 mL twice daily

3.8 Aromatic inhalations

Inhalations containing volatile substances such as eucalyptus oil are traditionally used to relieve congestion and ease breathing. Although the vapour may contain little of the additive it encourages deliberate inspiration of warm moist air which is often comforting. Boiling water should not be used for inhalations owing to the risk of scalding.

Strong aromatic decongestants (applied as rubs or to pillows) are not recommended for infants under the age of 3 months. **Sodium chloride 0.9%** solution given as nasal drops can be used to liquefy mucous secretions and relieve nasal congestion in infants and young children.

Benzoin Tincture, Compound, BP
(Friars' Balsam)
Tincture, balsamic acids approx. 4.5%. Label: 15
Dose
Nasal congestion
• By inhalation
  Add one teaspoonful to a pint of hot, **not** boiling, water and inhale the vapour

Menthol and Eucalyptus Inhalation, BP 1980
Inhalation, racementhol or levomenthol 2 g, eucalyptus oil 10 mL, light magnesium carbonate 7 g, water to 100 mL
Dose
Nasal congestion
• By inhalation
  Add one teaspoonful to a pint of hot, **not** boiling, water and inhale the vapour

Dental prescribing on the NHS May be prescribed as Menthol and Eucalyptus Inhalation BP, 1980

Karvol® (Crookes) 〔NHS〕
Inhalation capsules, levomenthol 35.55 mg, with chlorobutanol, pine oils, terpineol, and thymol, net price 10-cap pack = £2.25; 20-cap pack = £4.06
Inhalation solution, levomenthol 7.9%, with chlorobutanol, pine oils, terpineol, and thymol, net price 12-mL dropper bottle = £1.90
Dose
Nasal congestion
• By inhalation
  Express into handkerchief or add to a pint of hot, **not** boiling, water the contents of 1 capsule or 6 drops of solution; avoid in infants under 3 months

---

3.9 Cough preparations

3.9.1 Cough suppressants
3.9.2 Expectorant and demulcent cough preparations

3.9.1 Cough suppressants

Cough may be a symptom of an underlying disorder such as asthma (section 3.1), gastro-oesophageal reflux disease (section 1.1), or rhinitis (section 12.2.1), which should be addressed before prescribing cough suppressants. Cough may be associated with smoking or environmental pollutants. Cough can also result from bronchiectasis including that associated with cystic fibrosis; cough can also have a significant habit component. There is little evidence of any significant benefit from the use of cough suppressants in children with acute cough in ambulatory settings. Cough suppressants may cause sputum retention and this can be harmful in children with bronchiectasis.

The use of cough suppressants containing **pholcodine** or similar opioid analgesics is not generally recommended in children and should be avoided altogether in children under 6 years, see MHRA/CHM advice below.

Sedating antihistamines (section 3.4.1) are used as the cough suppressant component of many compound cough preparations on sale to the public; all tend to cause drowsiness which may reflect their main mode of action.

MHRA/CHM advice (March 2008 and February 2009)
Children under 6 years should not be given over-the-counter cough and cold medicines containing the following ingredients:

- brompheniramine, chlorphenamine, diphenhydramine, doxylamine, promethazine, or triprolidine (antihistamines);
- dextromethorphan or pholcodine (cough suppressants);
- guaifenesin or ipecacuanha (expectorants);
- phenylephrine, pseudoephedrine, ephedrine, oxymetazoline, or xylometazoline (decongestants).

Over-the-counter cough and cold medicines can be considered for children aged 6–12 years after basic principles of best care have been tried. Children should not be given more than 1 cough or cold preparation at a time because different brands may contain the same active ingredient; care should be taken to give the correct dose.

PHOLCODINE

Cautions may cause sputum retention

Contra-indications

Hepatic impairment avoid or reduce dose—may precipitate coma

Pregnancy avoid in third trimester, respiratory depression and withdrawal effects in neonate

Side-effects nausea, sputum retention, constipation

Indication and dose

Dry or painful cough (but not generally recommended for children, see notes above)

- By mouth

  Child 6–12 years 2–5 mg 3–4 times daily

  Child 12–18 years 5–10 mg 3–4 times daily

Pholcodine Linctus, BP
Linctus (= oral solution), pholcodine 5 mg/5 mL in a suitable flavoured vehicle, containing citric acid monohydrate 1%. Net price 100 mL = 43p
Brands include *Pavacol-D*® (sugar-free), *Galenphol*® (sugar-free)

Pholcodine Linctus, Strong, BP
Linctus (= oral solution), pholcodine 10 mg/5 mL in a suitable flavoured vehicle, containing citric acid monohydrate 2%. Net price 100 mL = 35p
Brands include *Galenphol*®

Galenphol® (Thornton & Ross)
Paediatric linctus (= oral solution), orange, sugar-free, pholcodine 2 mg/5 mL. Net price 90-mL pack = £1.11

3.9.2 Expectorant and demulcent cough preparations

Simple linctus and other demulcent cough preparations containing soothing substances, such as syrup or glycerol, may temporarily relieve a dry irritating cough. These preparations have the advantage of being harmless and inexpensive and sugar-free versions are available.

Expectorants are claimed to promote expulsion of bronchial secretions but there is no evidence that any drug can specifically facilitate expectoration.

Compound cough preparations for children are on sale to the public but should not be used in children under 6 years; the rationale for some is dubious. Care should be taken to give the correct dose and to not use more than one preparation at a time, see MHRA/CHM advice above.

Simple Linctus, Paediatric, BP
Linctus (= oral solution), citric acid monohydrate 0.625% in a suitable vehicle with an anise flavour. Net price 100 mL = 72p
A sugar-free version is also available

Dose
Cough
- By mouth
  Child 1 month–12 years 5–10 mL 3–4 times daily

3

Respiratory system

Simple Linctus, BP

Linctus (= oral solution), citric acid monohydrate 2.5% in a suitable vehicle with an anise flavour. Net price 100 mL = 42p

A sugar-free version is also available

Dose

Cough
• **By mouth**
Child 12–18 years 5 mL 3–4 times daily

3.10 Systemic nasal decongestants

Nasal congestion in children due to allergic or vasomotor rhinitis should be treated with oral antihistamines (section 3.4.1), topical nasal preparations containing corticosteroids (section 12.2.1), or topical decongestants (section 12.2.2).

There is little evidence to support the use of systemic decongestants in children.

Pseudoephedrine has few sympathomimetic effects, and is commonly combined with other ingredients (including antihistamines) in preparations intended for the relief of cough and cold symptoms but it should not be used in children under 6 years, see MHRA/CHM advice, p. 209.

PSEUDOEPHEDRINE HYDROCHLORIDE

Cautions hypertension, heart disease, diabetes, hyperthyroidism, raised intra-ocular pressure; **interactions:** Appendix 1 (sympathomimetics)

Hepatic impairment caution in severe hepatic impairment

Renal impairment manufacturer advises caution in moderate to severe renal impairment

Pregnancy defective closure of the abdominal wall (gastrochisis) reported very rarely in newborns after first trimester exposure

Breast-feeding amount too small to be harmful

Contra-indications treatment with MAOI within previous 2 weeks

Side-effects tachycardia, anxiety, restlessness, insomnia; *rarely* hallucinations, rash; urinary retention also reported

Indication and dose

Congestion of mucous membranes of upper respiratory tract
• **By mouth**
Child 6–12 years 30 mg 3–4 times daily
Child 12–18 years 60 mg 3–4 times daily

[1]**Galpseud®** (Thornton & Ross) ⌧
Tablets, pseudoephedrine hydrochloride 60 mg, net price 20 = £1.06

Linctus, sugar-free, pseudoephedrine hydrochloride 30 mg/5 mL, net price 100 mL = 69p

[1]**Sudafed®** (McNeil) ⌧
Tablets, red, f/c, pseudoephedrine hydrochloride 60 mg, net price 24 = £2.12

Elixir, red, pseudoephedrine hydrochloride 30 mg/ 5 mL, net price 100 mL = £1.48

---

1. Can be sold to the public provided no more than 720 mg of pseudoephedrine salts are supplied, and ephedrine base (or salts) are not supplied at the same time; for details see *Medicines, Ethics and Practice*, No. 32, London, Pharmaceutical Press, 2008 (and subsequent editions as available)

4 Central nervous system

4.1 Hypnotics and anxiolytics 211
4.1.1 Hypnotics 212
4.1.2 Anxiolytics 214
4.1.3 Barbiturates 215

4.2 Drugs used in psychoses and related disorders 215
4.2.1 Antipsychotic drugs 215
4.2.2 Antipsychotic depot injections 225
4.2.3 Antimanic drugs 225

4.3 Antidepressant drugs 228
4.3.1 Tricyclic antidepressant drugs 229
4.3.2 Monoamine-oxidase inhibitors 231
4.3.3 Selective serotonin re-uptake inhibitors 231
4.3.4 Other antidepressant drugs 234

4.4 CNS stimulants and other drugs for attention deficit hyperactivity disorder 234

4.5 Drugs used in the treatment of obesity 237

4.6 Drugs used in nausea and vertigo 237

4.7 Analgesics 245
4.7.1 Non-opioid analgesics 246
4.7.2 Opioid analgesics 249
4.7.3 Neuropathic pain 261
4.7.4 Antimigraine drugs 261

4.8 Antiepileptics 264
4.8.1 Control of epilepsy 264
4.8.2 Drugs used in status epilepticus 283
4.8.3 Febrile convulsions 287

4.9 Drugs used in dystonias and related disorders 288
4.9.1 Dopaminergic drugs used in dystonias 288
4.9.2 Antimuscarinic drugs used in dystonias 289
4.9.3 Drugs used in essential tremor, chorea, tics, and related disorders 290

4.10 Drugs used in substance dependence 291
4.11 Drugs for dementia 294

4.1 Hypnotics and anxiolytics

4.1.1 Hypnotics
4.1.2 Anxiolytics
4.1.3 Barbiturates

Most anxiolytics ('sedatives') will induce sleep when given at night and most hypnotics will sedate when given during the day. Hypnotics and anxiolytics should be reserved for short courses to alleviate acute conditions after causal factors have been established.

The role of drug therapy in the management of anxiety disorders in children and adolescents is uncertain; drug therapy should be initiated only by specialists after psychosocial interventions have failed. Benzodiazepines and tricyclic antidepressants have been used but adverse effects may be problematic.

Central nervous system

4

Skilled tasks Hypnotics and anxiolytics may impair judgement and increase reaction time, and so affect ability to drive or perform skilled tasks; they increase the effects of alcohol. Moreover the hangover effects of a night dose may impair performance on the following day.

CSM advice
1. Benzodiazepines are indicated for the short-term relief (two to four weeks only) of anxiety that is severe, disabling or subjecting the individual to unacceptable distress, occurring alone or in association with insomnia or short-term psychosomatic, organic, or psychotic illness.
2. The use of benzodiazepines to treat short-term 'mild' anxiety is inappropriate and unsuitable.
3. Benzodiazepines should be used to treat insomnia only when it is severe, disabling, or subjecting the individual to extreme distress.

4.1.1 Hypnotics

The prescribing of hypnotics to children, except for occasional use such as for sedation for procedures (section 15.1.4), is not justified. There is a risk of habituation with prolonged use. Problems settling children at night should be managed with behavioural therapy.

Dental procedures Some anxious children may benefit from the use of a hypnotic for 1 to 3 nights before the dental appointment. Hypnotics do not relieve pain, and if pain interferes with sleep an appropriate analgesic should be given.

Chloral and derivatives

Chloral hydrate and derivatives were formerly popular hypnotics for children. **Triclofos** causes fewer gastro-intestinal disturbances than chloral hydrate.

Chloral hydrate and triclofos are now mainly used for sedation during diagnostic procedures (section 15.1.4) and in intensive care units. These drugs accumulate on prolonged use.

CHLORAL HYDRATE

Cautions reduce dose in debilitated; avoid prolonged use (and abrupt withdrawal thereafter); avoid contact with skin and mucous membranes; **interactions:** Appendix 1 (anxiolytics and hypnotics)

Hepatic impairment can precipitate coma; reduce dose in mild to moderate hepatic impairment; avoid in severe impairment
Skilled tasks Drowsiness may persist the next day and affect performance of skilled tasks (e.g. driving); effects of alcohol enhanced

Contra-indications severe cardiac disease, gastritis, acute porphyria (section 9.8.2)

Renal impairment manufacturer advises avoid in severe impairment

Pregnancy avoid

Breast-feeding sedation in infant—manufacturer advises avoid

Side-effects gastric irritation (nausea and vomiting reported), abdominal distention, flatulence, headache, tolerance, dependence, excitement, delirium (especially on abrupt withdrawal), ketonuria, and rash

Licensed use not licensed for sedation for painless procedures

Indication and dose
Insomnia (but not recommended)
* **By mouth or by rectum (if oral route not available)**

Neonate 30–50 mg/kg at bedtime

Child 1 month–12 years 30–50 mg/kg (max. 1 g) at night

Child 12–18 years 0.5–1 g (max. 2 g) at night

Sedation for painless procedures
* **By mouth or by rectum (if oral route not available)**

Neonate 30–50 mg/kg 45–60 minutes before procedure; doses up to 100 mg/kg may be used with respiratory monitoring

Child 1 month–12 years 30–50 mg/kg (max. 1 g) 45–60 minutes before procedure; higher doses up to 100 mg/kg (max. 2 g) may be used

Child 12–18 years 1–2 g 45–60 minutes before procedure

Administration for administration *by mouth* dilute liquid with plenty of water or juice to mask unpleasant taste.

◁ **CHLORAL HYDRATE** (*continued*)

Chloral Mixture, BP 2000 PoM
(Chloral Oral Solution)
Mixture, chloral hydrate 500 mg/5 mL in a suitable vehicle. Available from 'special-order' manufacturers or specialist importing companies, see p. 943

Chloral Elixir, Paediatric, BP 2000 PoM
(Chloral Oral Solution, Paediatric)
Elixir, chloral hydrate 200 mg/5mL (4%) in a suitable vehicle with a black currant flavour. Available from 'special-order' manufacturers or specialist importing companies, see p. 943

Chloral Hydrate (Non-proprietary) PoM
Suppositories, chloral hydrate 25 mg, 50 mg, 60 mg, 100 mg, 200 mg, 500 mg. Available from 'special-order' manufacturers or specialist importing companies, see p. 943

◀Cloral betaine

Welldorm® (Alphashow) PoM
Tablets, blue-purple, f/c, cloral betaine 707 mg (≡ chloral hydrate 414 mg). Net price 30-tab pack = £7.90. Label: 19, 27

Dose

Short-term treatment of insomnia
• By mouth
> Child 12–18 years 1–2 tablets with water or milk at bedtime, max. 5 tablets (chloral hydrate 2 g) daily

Elixir, red, chloral hydrate 143.3 mg/5 mL. Net price 150-mL pack = £6.67. Label: 19, 27

Dose

Short-term treatment of insomnia
• By mouth
> Neonate 1–1.75 mL/kg (chloral hydrate 30–50 mg/kg) with water or milk at bedtime
>
> Child 1 month–12 years 1–1.75 mL/kg (chloral hydrate 30–50 mg/kg) with water or milk at bedtime; max. 35 mL (chloral hydrate 1 g) daily
>
> Child 12–18 years 15–45 mL (chloral hydrate 0.4–1.3 g) with water or milk at bedtime; max. 70 mL (chloral hydrate 2 g) daily

---

▌ TRICLOFOS SODIUM

Cautions avoid prolonged use (and abrupt withdrawal thereafter); **interactions:** Appendix 1 (anxiolytics and hypnotics)

Hepatic impairment can precipitate coma

Renal impairment start with small doses in severe impairment, increased cerebral sensitivity
Skilled tasks Drowsiness may persist the next day and affect performance of skilled tasks (e.g. driving); effects of alcohol enhanced

Contra-indications cardiac disease; gastritis; acute porphyria (section 9.8.2); pregnancy; breast-feeding

Side-effects abdominal distension, flatulence, gastric irritation including nausea and vomiting, dependence, malaise, ataxia, drowsiness, headache, lightheadedness, vertigo, confusion, paranoia, excitement, nightmares, delirium (especially on abrupt withdrawal), ketonuria, blood disorders, skin reactions, and urticaria

Licensed use not licensed for sedation for painless procedures

Indication and dose

Insomnia (but not recommended)
• By mouth
> Neonate 25–30 mg/kg at night

> Child 1 month–1 year 25–30 mg/kg at night
>
> Child 1–5 years 250–500 mg at night
>
> Child 6–12 years 0.5–1 g at night
>
> Child 12–18 years 1–2 g at night

Sedation for painless procedures
• By mouth
> Neonate 25–30 mg/kg 45–60 minutes before procedure
>
> Child 1 month–18 years 30–50 mg/kg (max. 2 g) 45–60 minutes before procedure; higher doses up to 100 mg/kg (max. 2 g) may be used but respiratory monitoring is required

Triclofos Oral Solution, BP PoM
(Triclofos Elixir)
Oral solution, triclofos sodium 500 mg/5 mL. Net price 300 mL = £28.23. Label: 19

4
Central nervous system

▌ Antihistamines

Some **antihistamines** (section 3.4.1) such as promethazine are used for occasional insomnia in adults; their prolonged duration of action can often cause drowsiness the following day. The sedative effect of antihistamines may diminish after a few days of continued treatment; antihistamines are associated with headache, psychomotor impairment and antimuscarinic effects.

The use of antihistamines as hypnotics in children is not usually justified.

PROMETHAZINE HYDROCHLORIDE

Cautions section 3.4.1

Contra-indications section 3.4.1

Side-effects section 3.4.1

Licensed use not licensed for use in children under 2 years

Indication and dose

Sedation (short-term use)
- **By mouth**

  Child 2–5 years 15–20 mg

  Child 5–10 years 20–25 mg

  Child 10–18 years 25–50 mg

Sedation in intensive care
- **By mouth or by slow intravenous injection or by deep intramuscular injection**

  Child 1 month–12 years 0.5–1 mg/kg (max. 25 mg) 4 times daily, adjusted according to response

Child 12–18 years 25–50 mg 4 times daily, adjusted according to response

Allergy and urticaria section 3.4.1

Nausea and vomiting section 4.6

Phenergan® (Rhône-Poulenc Rorer)
Injection [PoM] [1], promethazine hydrochloride 25 mg/ mL, net price 1-mL amp = 70p
1. [PoM] restriction does not apply where administration is for saving life in emergency

◢ Oral preparations
Section 3.4.1

Melatonin

Melatonin is a pineal hormone which may affect sleep pattern. Clinical experience suggests that it may be of value for treating sleep onset insomnia and delayed sleep phase syndrome in children with conditions such as visual impairment, cerebral palsy, attention deficit hyperactivity disorder, autism, and learning difficulties. It is also sometimes used before magnetic resonance imaging (MRI), computed tomography (CT), or EEG investigations. Little is known about its long-term effects in children, but there is a theoretical basis for an effect on sexual development. Treatment with melatonin should be initiated and supervised by a specialist, but may be continued by general practitioners under a shared-care arrangement. The need for continuing melatonin therapy should be reviewed every 6 months.

MELATONIN

Cautions interactions: Appendix 1 (melatonin)

Renal impairment no information available— manufacturer advises caution

Contra-indications autoimmune disease

Hepatic impairment manufacturer advises avoid

Pregnancy no information available—manufacturer advises avoid

Breast-feeding present in milk—manufacturer advises avoid

Side-effects abdominal pain, constipation, dry mouth, weight gain, drowsiness, dizziness, migraine, asthenia, sleep disorders, restlessness, nervousness, irritability, and sweating; *rarely* flatulence, halitosis, hypersalivation, vomiting, hypertriglyceridaemia, aggression, agitation, fatigue, impaired memory, mood changes, hot flushes, priapism, increased libido, leucopenia,

thrombocytopenia, muscle cramp, lacrimation, visual disturbances, and skin reactions

Licensed use not licensed for use in children

Indication and dose

Sleep onset insomnia and delayed sleep phase syndrome (see notes above)
- **By mouth**

  Child 1 month–18 years initially 2–3 mg increased if necessary after 1–2 weeks to 4– 6 mg; max. 10 mg

Circadin® (Lundbeck) ▼ [PoM]
Tablets, m/r, melatonin 2 mg, net price 21-tab pack = £10.77. Label: 2, 21, 25
Note Other formulations of melatonin are available from 'special-order' manufacturers or specialist importing companies, see p. 943

4.1.2 Anxiolytics

Anxiolytic treatment should be used in children only to relieve acute anxiety (and related insomnia) caused by fear (e.g. before surgery, section 15.1.4.1).

Anxiolytic treatment should be limited to the lowest possible dose for the shortest possible time (see CSM advice, section 4.1).

Buspirone

Buspirone is thought to act at specific serotonin ($5HT_{1A}$) receptors; safety and efficacy in children have yet to be determined.

4.1.3 Barbiturates

Classification not used in *BNF for Children*.

4.2 Drugs used in psychoses and related disorders

4.2.1 Antipsychotic drugs
4.2.2 Antipsychotic depot injections
4.2.3 Antimanic drugs

Advice on doses above *BNF for Children* upper limit

1. Consider alternative approaches including adjuvant therapy.
2. Bear in mind risk factors, including obesity.
3. Consider potential for drug interactions—see **interactions**: Appendix 1 (antipsychotics).
4. Carry out ECG to exclude untoward abnormalities such as prolonged QT interval; repeat ECG periodically and reduce dose if prolonged QT interval or other adverse abnormality develops.
5. Increase dose slowly and not more often than once weekly.
6. Carry out regular pulse, blood pressure, and temperature checks; ensure that patient maintains adequate fluid intake.
7. Consider high-dose therapy to be for limited period and review regularly; abandon if no improvement after 3 months (return to standard dosage).

Important When prescribing an antipsychotic for administration on an emergency basis, the intramuscular dose should be **lower** than the corresponding oral dose (owing to absence of first-pass effect), particularly if the child is very active (increased blood flow to muscle considerably increases the rate of absorption). The prescription should specify the dose for **each route** and should **not** imply that the same dose can be given by mouth or by intramuscular injection. The dose of antipsychotic for emergency use should be reviewed at least **daily**.

4.2.1 Antipsychotic drugs

There is little information on the efficacy and safety of antipsychotic drugs in children and adolescents and much of the information available has been extrapolated from adult data; in particular, little is known about the long-term effects of antipsychotic drugs on the developing nervous system. Antipsychotic drugs should be initiated and managed under the close supervision of an appropriate specialist.

Antipsychotic drugs are also known as 'neuroleptics' and (misleadingly) as 'major tranquillisers'. Antipsychotic drugs generally tranquillise without impairing consciousness and without causing paradoxical excitement but they should not be regarded merely as tranquillisers. For conditions such as schizophrenia the tranquillising effect is of secondary importance.

In the short term they are used to calm disturbed children whatever the underlying psychopathology, which may be schizophrenia, brain damage, mania, toxic delirium, or agitated depression. Antipsychotic drugs are used to alleviate severe anxiety but this too should be a short-term measure.

Schizophrenia   Antipsychotic drugs relieve florid psychotic symptoms such as thought disorder, hallucinations, and delusions, and prevent relapse. Although they are usually less effective in apathetic withdrawn children, they sometimes appear to have an activating influence. Children with acute schizophrenia generally respond better than those with chronic symptoms.

Long-term treatment of a child with a definite diagnosis of schizophrenia may be necessary even after the first episode of illness in order to prevent the manifest illness from becoming chronic. Withdrawal of drug treatment requires careful surveillance because children who appear well on medication may suffer a disastrous relapse if treatment is withdrawn inappropriately. In addition the need for continuation of treatment may not become immediately evident because relapse is often delayed for several weeks after cessation of treatment.

Antipsychotic drugs are considered to act by interfering with dopaminergic transmission in the brain by blocking dopamine D_2 receptors, which may give rise to the extrapyramidal effects described below, and also to hyperprolactinaemia. Antipsychotic drugs may also affect cholinergic, alpha-adrenergic, histaminergic, and serotonergic receptors.

Choice of drug is influenced by the potential for side-effects and is often guided by individual circumstances e.g. the psychological effects of potential weight gain. The drugs most commonly used in children are haloperidol, risperidone, and olanzapine.

Cautions and contra-indications   Antipsychotic drugs should be used with **caution** in children with hepatic impairment (can precipitate coma), renal impairment (start with small dose; increased cerebral sensitivity), cardiovascular disease, epilepsy (and conditions predisposing to epilepsy), depression, myasthenia gravis, or a personal or family history of angle-closure glaucoma (avoid chlorpromazine, pericyazine and prochlorperazine in these conditions). Caution is also required in severe respiratory disease and in children with a history of jaundice or who have blood dyscrasias (perform blood counts if unexplained infection or fever develops). As photosensitisation may occur with higher dosages, children should avoid direct sunlight.

Antipsychotic drugs may be **contra-indicated** in comatose states, CNS depression, and phaeochromocytoma. Most antipsychotic drugs are best avoided during pregnancy unless essential; extrapyramidal effects may occur in neonates. Although the amount present in breast milk is probably too small to be harmful, *animal* studies indicate possible adverse effects of these drugs on developing nervous system and therefore it is advisable to discontinue breast-feeding during treatment; **interactions:** Appendix 1 (antipsychotics).

Skilled tasks   Drowsiness may affect performance of skilled tasks (e.g. driving or operating machinery), especially at start of treatment; effects of alcohol are enhanced.

Withdrawal   Withdrawal of antipsychotic drugs after long-term therapy should always be gradual and closely monitored to avoid the risk of acute withdrawal syndromes or rapid relapse.

Side-effects   Extrapyramidal symptoms are the most troublesome. They occur most frequently with the piperazine phenothiazines (such as perphenazine, prochlorperazine, and trifluoperazine), the butyrophenones (such as haloperidol), and the depot preparations. They are easy to recognise but cannot be predicted accurately because they depend on the dose, the type of drug, and on individual susceptibility.

Extrapyramidal symptoms consist of:

- *parkinsonian symptoms* (including tremor), which may appear gradually (but less commonly than in adults);

- *dystonia* (abnormal face and body movements) and *dyskinesia*, which appear after only a few doses;

- *akathisia* (restlessness), which characteristically occurs after large initial doses and may resemble an exacerbation of the condition being treated; and

- *tardive dyskinesia* (rhythmic, involuntary movements of tongue, face, and jaw), which usually develops on long-term therapy or with high dosage, but it may develop on short-term treatment with low doses—short-lived tardive dyskinesia may occur after withdrawal of the drug.

Parkinsonian symptoms remit if the drug is withdrawn and may be suppressed by the administration of **antimuscarinic** drugs (section 4.9.2). However, routine administration of such drugs is not justified because not all children are affected and because they may unmask or worsen tardive dyskinesia.

Tardive dyskinesia is of particular concern because it may be irreversible on withdrawing therapy and treatment is usually ineffective. However, some manufacturers suggest that drug withdrawal at the earliest signs of tardive dyskinesia (fine vermicular movements of the tongue) may halt its full development. Tardive dyskinesia may occur and treatment must be carefully and regularly reviewed.

Hypotension and interference with temperature regulation are dose-related side-effects.

Neuroleptic malignant syndrome (hyperthermia, fluctuating level of consciousness, muscle rigidity, and autonomic dysfunction with pallor, tachycardia, labile blood pressure, sweating, and urinary incontinence) is a rare but potentially fatal side-effect of some antipsychotic drugs. Discontinuation of the antipsychotic is essential because there is no proven effective treatment, but cooling, bromocriptine, and dantrolene have been used. The syndrome, which usually lasts for 5–7 days after drug discontinuation, may be unduly prolonged if depot preparations have been used.

Other side-effects include: drowsiness; apathy; agitation, excitement and insomnia; convulsions; dizziness; headache; confusion; gastro-intestinal disturbances; nasal congestion; antimuscarinic symptoms (such as dry mouth, constipation, difficulty with micturition, and blurred vision); cardiovascular symptoms (such as hypotension, tachycardia, and arrhythmias); ECG changes (cases of sudden death have occurred); endocrine effects such as menstrual disturbances, galactorrhoea, gynaecomastia, impotence, and weight gain; blood dyscrasias (such as agranulocytosis and leucopenia), photosensitisation, contact sensitisation and rashes, and jaundice (including cholestatic); corneal and lens opacities, and purplish pigmentation of the skin, cornea, conjunctiva, and retina.

Overdosage: for poisoning with phenothiazines and related compounds, see Emergency Treatment of Poisoning, p. 43.

Classification of antipsychotics   The **phenothiazine** derivatives can be divided into 3 main groups.

> *Group 1*: chlorpromazine, levomepromazine (methotrimeprazine), and promazine, generally characterised by pronounced sedative effects and moderate antimuscarinic and extrapyramidal side-effects.

> *Group 2*: pericyazine and pipotiazine, generally characterised by moderate sedative effects, marked antimuscarinic effects, but fewer extrapyramidal side-effects than groups 1 or 3.

> *Group 3*: perphenazine, prochlorperazine, and trifluoperazine, generally characterised by fewer sedative effects, fewer antimuscarinic effects, but more pronounced extrapyramidal side-effects than groups 1 and 2.

Drugs of other chemical groups resemble the phenothiazines of *group 3* in their clinical properties. They include the **butyrophenones** (e.g. haloperidol); **diphenylbutylpiperidines** (e.g. pimozide); **thioxanthenes** (flupentixol and zuclopenthixol); and the **substituted benzamides** (e.g. sulpiride).

For details of the newer antipsychotic drugs amisulpride, clozapine, olanzapine, quetiapine, and risperidone, see under Atypical Antipsychotics, p. 221.

Choice   As indicated above, the various drugs differ somewhat in predominant actions and side-effects. Selection is influenced by the degree of sedation required and the child's susceptibility to extrapyramidal side-effects. However, the differences between antipsychotic drugs are less important than the great variability in response; moreover, tolerance to secondary effects such as sedation usually develops. The atypical antipsychotic drugs may be appropriate if extrapyramidal side-effects are a particular concern (see under Atypical Antipsychotics, p. 221). **Clozapine** is used for schizophrenia when other antipsychotic drugs are ineffective or not tolerated.

Prescribing of more than one antipsychotic drug at the same time is **not** recommended; it may constitute a hazard and there is no significant evidence that side-effects are minimised.

Chlorpromazine is still widely used despite the wide range of adverse effects associated with it. It has a marked sedating effect and is useful for treating violent children without causing stupor.

Pimozide (see CSM warning, p. 220) is less sedating than chlorpromazine.

Sulpiride in high doses controls florid positive symptoms, but in lower doses it has an alerting effect on children with apathetic withdrawn schizophrenia.

4 Central nervous system

Haloperidol and **trifluoperazine** are also of value but their use is limited by the high incidence of extrapyramidal symptoms. Haloperidol may be preferred for the rapid control of hyperactive psychotic states; it causes less hypotension than chlorpromazine.

Other uses Nausea and vomiting (section 4.6), choreas, motor tics, and intractable hiccup.

Equivalent doses of oral antipsychotic drugs

These equivalences are intended **only** as an approximate guide; individual dosage instructions should **also** be checked; children should be carefully monitored after **any** change in medication

Antipsychotic drug	Daily dose
Chlorpromazine	100 mg
Clozapine	50 mg
Haloperidol	2–3 mg
Pimozide	2 mg
Risperidone	0.5–1 mg
Sulpiride	200 mg
Trifluoperazine	5 mg

Important These equivalences must **not** be extrapolated beyond the max. dose for the drug. Higher doses require careful titration in specialist units and the equivalences shown here may not be appropriate

Dosage

After an initial period of stabilisation, the total daily oral dose can be given as a single dose in most children. For the advice of The Royal College of Psychiatrists on doses above the *BNF for Children* upper limit, see p. 215.

CHLORPROMAZINE HYDROCHLORIDE

Warning Owing to the risk of contact sensitisation, pharmacists, nurses, and other health workers should avoid direct contact with chlorpromazine; tablets should not be crushed and solutions should be handled with care

Cautions see notes above; also children should remain supine and the blood pressure monitored for 30 minutes after intramuscular injection

Contra-indications see notes above

Side-effects see notes above; also intramuscular injection may be painful, cause hypotension and tachycardia, and give rise to nodule formation

Indication and dose

Childhood schizophrenia and other psychoses (under specialist supervision)
- By mouth

Child 1–6 years 500 micrograms/kg every 4–6 hours adjusted according to response (max. 40 mg daily)

Child 6–12 years 10 mg 3 times daily, adjusted according to response (max. 75 mg daily)

Child 12–18 years 25 mg 3 times daily (*or* 75 mg at night), adjusted according to response, to usual maintenance dose of 75–300 mg daily (but up to 1 g daily may be required)

Relief of acute symptoms of psychoses (under specialist supervision) but see also Cautions and Side-effects
- By deep intramuscular injection

Child 1–6 years 500 micrograms/kg every 6–8 hours (max. 40 mg daily)

Child 6–12 years 500 micrograms/kg every 6–8 hours (max. 75 mg daily)

Child 12–18 years 25–50 mg every 6–8 hours

Induction of hypothermia (to prevent shivering) (under specialist supervision)
- By deep intramuscular injection

Child 1–12 years initially 0.5–1 mg/kg, followed by maintenance 500 micrograms/kg every 4–6 hours

Child 12–18 years 25–50 mg every 6–8 hours

Chlorpromazine (Non-proprietary) PoM
Tablets, coated, chlorpromazine hydrochloride 25 mg, 28-tab pack = £3.35; 50 mg, 28-tab pack = £3.40; 100 mg, 28-tab pack = £3.57. Label: 2, 11
Brands include *Chloractil®*

Oral solution, chlorpromazine hydrochloride 25 mg/5 mL, net price 150 mL = £1.47, 100 mg/5 mL, 150 mL = £3.57. Label: 2, 11

Injection, chlorpromazine hydrochloride 25 mg/mL, net price 1-mL amp = 60p; 2-mL amp = 63p

Largactil® (Sanofi-Aventis) PoM
Injection, chlorpromazine hydrochloride 25 mg/mL. Net price 2-mL amp = 63p

■ HALOPERIDOL

Cautions see notes above; also subarachnoid haemorrhage and metabolic disturbances such as hypokalaemia, hypocalcaemia, or hypomagnesaemia

Contra-indications see notes above

Side-effects see notes above, but less sedating and fewer antimuscarinic or hypotensive symptoms; pigmentation and photosensitivity reactions rare; extrapyramidal symptoms, particularly dystonic reactions and akathisia especially in thyrotoxic patients; *rarely* weight loss; hypoglycaemia; inappropriate antidiuretic hormone secretion

Licensed use not licensed for use in children for nausea and vomiting in palliative care

Indication and dose

Schizophrenia and other psychoses, mania, short-term adjunctive management of psychomotor agitation, excitement and violent or dangerously impulsive behaviour (under specialist supervision)

• By mouth

Child 12–18 years initially 0.5–3 mg 2–3 times daily *or* 3–5 mg 2–3 times daily in severely affected or resistant disease; in resistant schizophrenia up to 30 mg daily may be needed; adjusted according to response to lowest effective maintenance dose (as low as 5–10 mg daily)

Motor tics (including Tourette syndrome) (under specialist supervision)

• By mouth

Child 5–12 years 12.5–25 micrograms/kg twice daily, adjusted according to response up to 10 mg daily

Child 12–18 years 1.5 mg 3 times daily, adjusted according to response up to 10 mg daily

Nausea and vomiting in palliative care

• By mouth

Child 12–18 years 1.5 mg once daily at night, increased to 1.5 mg twice daily if necessary; max. 5 mg twice daily

• By continuous intravenous or subcutaneous infusion

Child 1 month–12 years 25–85 micrograms/kg over 24 hours

Child 12–18 years 1.5–5 mg over 24 hours

Haloperidol (Non-proprietary) ℞
Tablets, haloperidol 500 micrograms, net price 28-tab pack = 91p; 1.5 mg, 28-tab pack = £1.62; 5 mg, 28-tab pack = £3.93; 10 mg, 28-tab pack = £4.27; 20 mg, 28-tab pack = £11.17. Label: 2

Dozic® (Rosemont) ℞
Oral liquid, sugar-free, haloperidol 1 mg/mL, net price 100-mL pack = £6.86. Label: 2

Haldol® (Janssen-Cilag) ℞
Tablets, both scored, haloperidol 5 mg (blue), net price 100-tab pack = £7.35; 10 mg (yellow), 100-tab pack = £14.37. Label: 2

Oral liquid, sugar-free, haloperidol 2 mg/mL, net price 100-mL pack (with pipette) = £4.72. Label: 2

Injection, haloperidol 5 mg/mL, net price 1-mL amp = 30p

Serenace® (IVAX) ℞
Capsules, green, haloperidol 500 micrograms, net price 30-cap pack = 98p. Label: 2

Tablets, haloperidol 1.5 mg, net price 30-tab pack = £1.73; 5 mg (pink), 30-tab pack = £4.90; 10 mg (pale pink), 30-tab pack = £8.81. Label: 2

Oral liquid, sugar-free, haloperidol 2 mg/mL, net price 500-mL pack = £43.83. Label: 2

■ LEVOMEPROMAZINE
(Methotrimeprazine)

Cautions see notes above; children receiving large initial doses should remain supine

Contra-indications see notes above

Side-effects see notes above; occasionally raised erythrocyte sedimentation rate occurs

Indication and dose

Restlessness and confusion in palliative care

• By continuous subcutaneous infusion

Child 1–12 years 0.35–3 mg/kg over 24 hours

Child 12–18 years 12.5–200 mg over 24 hours

Nausea and vomiting in palliative care

• By continuous intravenous or subcutaneous infusion

Child 1 month–12 years 100–400 micrograms/kg over 24 hours

Child 12–18 years 5–25 mg over 24 hours

Administration for administration by *subcutaneous infusion* dilute with a suitable volume of Sodium Chloride 0.9%

Nozinan® (Link) ℞
Tablets, scored, levomepromazine maleate 25 mg, net price 84-tab pack = £20.26. Label: 2

Injection, levomepromazine hydrochloride 25 mg/mL, net price 1-mL amp = £2.01

■ PERICYAZINE
(Periciazine)
Cautions see notes above

Contra-indications see notes above

Side-effects see notes above; more sedating; hypotension common when treatment initiated; respiratory depression

4 Central nervous system

◻ **PERICYAZINE (continued)**

Licensed use tablets not licensed for use in children

Indication and dose

> Schizophrenia, psychoses (severe mental or behavioural disorders only) (under specialist supervision)
>
> • By mouth
>
>> **Child 1–12 years** initially 500 micrograms daily for 10-kg child, increased by 1 mg for each additional 5 kg to max. total daily dose of 10 mg; dose may be gradually increased according to response but maintenance should not exceed twice initial dose
>
>> **Child 12–18 years** initially 25 mg 3 times daily increased at weekly intervals by steps of 25 mg according to response; usual max. 100 mg 3 times daily; total daily dose may alternatively be given in 2 divided doses

Neulactil® (Sanofi-Aventis) ⟨PoM⟩

Tablets, yellow, scored, pericyazine 2.5 mg, net price 84-tab pack = £9.23; 10 mg, 84-tab pack = £24.95. Label: 2

Syrup forte, brown, pericyazine 10 mg/5 mL. Net price 100-mL pack = £12.08. Label: 2

PERPHENAZINE

Cautions see notes above

Contra-indications see notes above

Side-effects see notes above; less sedating; extrapyramidal symptoms, especially dystonia, more frequent, particularly at high dosage; *rarely* systemic lupus erythematosus

Indication and dose

> Schizophrenia and other psychoses, mania, short-term adjunctive management of anxiety, severe psychomotor agitation, excitement, violent or dangerously impulsive behaviour (under specialist supervision)
>
> • By mouth
>
>> **Child 14–18 years** initially 4 mg 3 times daily adjusted according to the response; max. 24 mg daily

Fentazin® (Goldshield) ⟨PoM⟩

Tablets, both s/c, perphenazine 2 mg, net price 100-tab pack = £22.38; 4 mg, 100-tab pack = £26.34. Label: 2

PIMOZIDE

Cautions see notes above

CSM warning Following reports of sudden unexplained death, the CSM recommends ECG before treatment. The CSM also recommends that patients on pimozide should have an annual ECG (if the QT interval is prolonged, treatment should be reviewed and either withdrawn or dose reduced under close supervision) and that pimozide should **not** be given with other antipsychotic drugs (including depot preparations), tricyclic antidepressants or other drugs which prolong the QT interval, such as certain antimalarials, anti-arrhythmic drugs and certain antihistamines and should **not** be given with drugs which cause electrolyte disturbances (especially diuretics)

Contra-indications see notes above; history of arrhythmias or congenital QT prolongation

Side-effects see notes above; less sedating; serious arrhythmias reported; glycosuria and, *rarely*, hyponatraemia reported

Licensed use not licensed for use in Tourette syndrome

Indication and dose

> Schizophrenia (under specialist supervision)
>
> • By mouth
>
>> **Child 12–18 years** initially 1 mg daily, increased according to response in steps of 2–4 mg at intervals of not less than 1 week; usual dose range 2–20 mg daily

> Tourette syndrome (under specialist supervision)
>
> • By mouth
>
>> **Child 2–12 years** 1–4 mg daily
>
>> **Child 12–18 years** 2–10 mg daily

Orap® (Janssen-Cilag) ⟨PoM⟩

Tablets, scored, green, pimozide 4 mg, net price 100-tab pack = £27.41. Label: 2

SULPIRIDE

Cautions see notes above; also excited, agitated, or aggressive children (even low doses may aggravate symptoms)

Pregnancy limited experience in humans but no evidence of harm in *animal* studies

Contra-indications see notes above; also acute porphyria (section 9.8.2)

Side-effects see notes above; also hepatitis

Licensed use not licensed for use in Tourette syndrome

Indication and dose

> Schizophrenia (under specialist supervision)
>
> • By mouth
>
>> **Child 14–18 years** 200–400 mg twice daily; max. 800 mg daily in predominantly negative

Central nervous system **4**

◁ **SULPIRIDE** (*continued*)

symptoms, dose increased to max. 2.4 g daily in mainly positive symptoms

Tourette syndrome (under specialist supervision)
● **By mouth**
Child 2–12 years 50–400 mg twice daily
Child 12–18 years 100–400 mg twice daily

Sulpiride (Non-proprietary) [PoM]
Tablets, sulpiride 200 mg, net price 30-tab pack = £6.92; 56-tab pack = £6.46; 400 mg, 30-tab pack = £12.87. Label: 2

Dolmatil® (Sanofi-Synthelabo) [PoM]
Tablets, both scored, sulpiride 200 mg, net price 100-tab pack = £13.85; 400 mg (f/c), 100-tab pack = £36.29. Label: 2

Sulpor® (Rosemont) [PoM]
Oral solution, sugar-free, lemon- and aniseed-flavoured, sulpiride 200 mg/5 mL, net price 150 mL = £25.38. Label: 2

▰ TRIFLUOPERAZINE

Cautions see notes above

Contra-indications see notes above

Side-effects see notes above; extrapyramidal symptoms more frequent, especially at doses exceeding 6 mg daily; pancytopenia; thrombocytopenia; hyperthermia; anorexia

Indication and dose

Schizophrenia and other psychoses, short-term adjunctive management of psychomotor agitation, excitement and violent or dangerously impulsive behaviour (under specialist supervision)
● **By mouth**
Child 12–18 years initially 5 mg twice daily, increased by 5 mg daily after 1 week, then at intervals of 3 days, according to response

Short-term adjunctive management of severe anxiety (under specialist supervision)
● **By mouth**
Child 3–6 years up to 500 micrograms twice daily

Child 6–12 years up to 2 mg twice daily

Child 12–18 years 1–2 mg twice daily, increased if necessary to 3 mg twice daily

Antiemetic section 4.6

Trifluoperazine (Non-proprietary) [PoM]
Tablets, coated, trifluoperazine (as hydrochloride) 1 mg, net price 100-tab pack = £6.10; 5 mg, 100-tab pack = £5.32. Label: 2

Oral solution, trifluoperazine (as hydrochloride) 5 mg/5 mL, net price 150-mL pack = £9.33. Label: 2

Stelazine® (Goldshield) [PoM]
Tablets, blue, f/c, trifluoperazine (as hydrochloride) 1 mg, net price 112-tab pack = £3.43; 5 mg, 112-tab pack = £4.89. Label: 2

Syrup, sugar-free, yellow, trifluoperazine (as hydrochloride) 1 mg/5 mL, net price 200-mL pack = £2.95. Label: 2

▰ Atypical antipsychotics

The 'atypical antipsychotic' drugs **amisulpride**, **clozapine**, **olanzapine**, **quetiapine**, and **risperidone** may be better tolerated than other antipsychotic drugs; extrapyramidal symptoms may be less frequent than with older antipsychotic drugs.

Clozapine, olanzapine, and quetiapine cause little or no elevation of prolactin concentration; when changing from other antipsychotic drugs, a reduction in prolactin may increase fertility.

Clozapine is used for the treatment of schizophrenia only in children unresponsive to, or intolerant of, conventional antipsychotic drugs. It can cause agranulocytosis and its use is restricted to patients registered with a clozapine Patient Monitoring Service (see under Clozapine).

Cautions and contra-indications While atypical antipsychotic drugs have not generally been associated with clinically significant prolongation of the QT interval, they should be used with care if prescribed with other drugs that increase the QT interval. Atypical antipsychotic drugs should be used with caution in children with cardiovascular disease, or a history of epilepsy; **interactions**: Appendix 1 (antipsychotics).

Skilled tasks Atypical antipsychotic drugs may affect performance of skilled tasks (e.g. driving); effects of alcohol are enhanced.

Withdrawal Withdrawal of antipsychotic drugs after long-term therapy should always be gradual and closely monitored to avoid the risk of acute withdrawal syndromes or rapid relapse.

Side-effects Side-effects of the atypical antipsychotic drugs include weight gain, dizziness, postural hypotension (especially during initial dose titration) which may be associated with syncope or reflex tachycardia in some children, extrapyramidal symptoms (usually mild and transient and which respond to dose reduction or to an antimuscarinic drug), and occasionally tardive dyskinesia on long-term administration (discontinue drug on appearance of early signs). Hyperglycaemia and sometimes diabetes can occur, particularly with clozapine, olanzapine and risperidone; monitoring weight and plasma glucose may identify the development of hyperglycaemia. Neuroleptic malignant syndrome has been reported rarely. Hypersalivation associated with clozapine therapy can be treated with hyoscine hydrobromide (p. 245) provided that patients are not at particular risk from the additive antimuscarinic side-effects of hyoscine and clozapine.

AMISULPRIDE

Cautions see notes above

Renal impairment halve dose if estimated glomerular filtration rate 30–60 mL/minute/1.73 m²; use one-third dose if estimated glomerular filtration rate 10–30 mL/minute/1.73 m²; no information available if estimated glomerular filtration rate less than 10 mL/minute/1.73 m²

Contra-indications see notes above; phaeochromocytoma, prolactin-dependent tumours

Pregnancy avoid

Breast-feeding avoid

Side-effects see notes above; also insomnia, anxiety, agitation, drowsiness, gastro-intestinal disorders such as constipation, nausea, vomiting, and dry mouth; hyperprolactinaemia; *occasionally* bradycardia; *rarely* seizures

Indication and dose

Acute psychotic episode (under specialist supervision)
- By mouth
  Child 15–18 years 200–400 mg twice daily adjusted according to response; max. 1.2 g daily

Predominantly negative symptoms (under specialist supervision)
- By mouth
  Child 15–18 years 50–300 mg daily

Amisulpride (Non-proprietary) ℗oM
Tablets, amisulpride 50 mg, net price 60-tab pack = £19.00; 100 mg, 60-tab pack = £33.73; 200 mg, 60-tab pack = £56.47; 400 mg, 60-tab pack = £112.45. Label: 2

Solian® (Sanofi-Synthelabo) ℗oM
Tablets, scored, amisulpride 50 mg, net price 60-tab pack = £23.69; 100 mg, 60-tab pack = £36.72; 200 mg, 60-tab pack = £61.38, 400 mg, 60-tab pack = £122.76. Label: 2

Solution, 100 mg/mL, net price 60 mL (caramel flavour) = £30.69. Label: 2

CLOZAPINE

Cautions see notes above; monitor leucocyte and differential blood counts (see Agranulocytosis, below); susceptibility to angle-closure glaucoma; taper off other antipsychotics before starting; close medical supervision during initiation (risk of collapse because of hypotension)

Hepatic impairment monitor hepatic function regularly; avoid in symptomatic, or progressive liver disease or hepatic failure

Pregnancy manufacturers advise caution
Withdrawal On planned withdrawal reduce dose over 1–2 weeks to avoid risk of rebound psychosis. If abrupt withdrawal necessary observe child carefully
Agranulocytosis Neutropenia and potentially fatal agranulocytosis reported. Leucocyte and differential blood counts must be normal before starting; monitor counts every week for 18 weeks then at least every 2 weeks and if clozapine continued and blood count stable after 1 year at least every 4 weeks (and 4 weeks after discontinuation); if leucocyte count below 3000/mm³ or if absolute neutrophil count below 1500/mm³ discontinue permanently and refer to haematologist. Avoid drugs which depress leucopoiesis; children (or carers) should

report immediately symptoms of infection, especially influenza-like illness
Myocarditis and cardiomyopathy Fatal myocarditis (most commonly in first 2 months) and cardiomyopathy reported. The CSM has advised:
- physical examination and medical history before starting clozapine;
- specialist examination if cardiac abnormalities or history of heart disease found—clozapine initiated only in absence of severe heart disease and if benefit outweighs risk;
- persistent tachycardia especially in first 2 months should prompt observation for other indicators for myocarditis or cardiomyopathy;
- if myocarditis or cardiomyopathy suspected clozapine should be stopped and child evaluated urgently by cardiologist;
- discontinue permanently in clozapine-induced myocarditis or cardiomyopathy

Gastro-intestinal obstruction Reactions resembling gastro-intestinal obstruction reported. Clozapine should be used cautiously with drugs which cause constipation (e.g. antimuscarinic drugs) or in children with history of colo-

◁ **CLOZAPINE (continued)**

nic disease or bowel surgery. Monitor for constipation and prescribe laxative if required

Contra-indications severe cardiac disorders (e.g. myocarditis; see Cautions); history of neutropenia or agranulocytosis (see Cautions); bone-marrow disorders; paralytic ileus (see Cautions); alcoholic and toxic psychoses; history of circulatory collapse; drug intoxication; coma or severe CNS depression; uncontrolled epilepsy

Renal impairment manufacturer advises avoid in severe renal impairment

Breast-feeding avoid

Side-effects see notes above; also constipation (see Cautions), hypersalivation, dry mouth, nausea, vomiting, anorexia; tachycardia, ECG changes, hypertension; drowsiness, headache, tremor, seizures, fatigue, impaired temperature regulation; urinary incontinence and retention; leucopenia, eosinophilia, leucocytosis; blurred vision; sweating; *less commonly* agranulocytosis (**important**: see Cautions); *rarely* dysphagia, hepatitis, cholestatic jaundice, pancreatitis, circulatory collapse, arrhythmia, myocarditis (**important**: see Cautions), pericarditis, thromboembolism, agitation, confusion, delirium, anaemia; *very rarely* parotid gland enlargement, intestinal obstruction (see Cautions), cardiomyopathy, myocardial infarction, respiratory depression, priapism, interstitial nephritis, thrombocytopenia, thrombocythaemia, hyperlipidaemia, fulminant hepatic necrosis, and skin reactions

Licensed use not licensed for use in children under 16 years

Indication and dose

Schizophrenia in children unresponsive to, or intolerant of, conventional antipsychotic drugs (under specialist supervision)

• **By mouth**

Child 12–18 years 12.5 mg once or twice on first day then 25–50 mg on second day then

increased gradually (if well tolerated) in steps of 25–50 mg daily over 14–21 days up to 300 mg daily in divided doses (larger dose at night, up to 200 mg daily may be taken as a single dose at bedtime; if necessary may be further increased in steps of 50–100 mg once (preferably) or twice weekly; usual dose 200–450 mg daily (max. 900 mg daily)

Note *Restarting* after *interval of more than 2 days*, 12.5 mg once or twice on first day (but may be feasible to increase more quickly than on initiation)—extreme caution if previous respiratory or cardiac arrest with initial dosing

Clozaril® (Novartis) PoM

Tablets, yellow, clozapine 25 mg (scored), net price 28-tab pack = £6.17, 84-tab pack (hosp. only) = £18.49; 100 mg, 28-tab pack = £24.64, 84-tab pack (hosp. only) = £73.92. Label: 2, 10, patient information leaflet

Note Child, prescriber, and supplying pharmacist must be registered with the Clozaril Patient Monitoring Service—takes several days to do this

Denzapine® (Merz) PoM

Tablets, yellow, scored, clozapine 25 mg, net price 28-tab pack = £6.17, 84-tab pack = £18.49; 100 mg, 28-tab pack = £24.64, 84-tab pack = £73.92. Label: 2, 10, patient information leaflet

Note Child, prescriber, and supplying pharmacist must be registered with the Denzapine Patient Monitoring Service—takes several days to do this

Zaponex® (IVAX) PoM

Tablets, yellow, scored, clozapine 25 mg, net price 84-tab pack = £22.17; 100 mg, 84-tab pack = £50.00. Label: 2, 10, patient information leaflet

Note Child, prescriber, and supplying pharmacist must be registered with the Zaponex Treatment Access System—takes several days to do this

OLANZAPINE

Cautions see notes above; also susceptibility to angle-closure glaucoma, paralytic ileus, diabetes mellitus (risk of exacerbation or ketoacidosis), low leucocyte or neutrophil count, bone-marrow depression, hyper-eosinophilic disorders, myeloproliferative disease

Hepatic impairment initial dose 5mg daily, increased slowly

Renal impairment initial dose 5mg daily, increased slowly

Pregnancy manufacturer advises use only if potential benefit outweighs risk; neonatal lethargy, tremor and hypertonia reported when used in third trimester

Contra-indications

Breast-feeding manufacturer advises avoid—present in milk

Side-effects see notes above; also mild, transient antimuscarinic effects; drowsiness, speech difficulty, abnormal gait, hallucinations, akathisia, asthenia, increased appetite, increased body

temperature, raised triglyceride concentration, oedema, hyperprolactinaemia (but clinical manifestations rare); urinary incontinence; eosinophilia; *less commonly* hypotension, bradycardia, QT interval prolongation, photosensitivity; *rarely* seizures, leucopenia, rash; *very rarely* thromboembolism, hypercholesterolaemia, hypothermia, urinary retention, priapism, thrombocytopenia, neutropenia, rhabdomyolysis, hepatitis, pancreatitis; *with injection*, injection-site reactions, sinus pause, hypoventilation

Licensed use not licensed for use in children

Indication and dose

Schizophrenia, combination therapy for mania (under specialist supervision)

• **By mouth**

Child 12–18 years initially 5–10 mg daily adjusted to usual range of 5–20 mg daily; doses greater than 10 mg daily only after reassessment; max. 20 mg daily

4 Central nervous system

◻ **OLANZAPINE** *(continued)*

Monotherapy for mania (under specialist supervision)
- **By mouth**

  Child 12–18 years 15 mg daily adjusted to usual range of 5–20 mg daily; doses greater than 15 mg only after reassessment; max. 20 mg daily

Note When one or more factors present that might result in slower metabolism (e.g. female gender, non-smoker) consider lower initial dose and more gradual dose increase

Zyprexa® (Lilly) [PoM]
Tablets, f/c, olanzapine 2.5 mg, net price 28-tab pack = £33.29; 5 mg, 28-tab pack = £48.78; 7.5 mg,

56-tab pack = £146.34; 10 mg, 28-tab pack = £79.45, 15 mg (blue), 28-tab pack = £119.18; 20 mg (pink), 28-tab pack = £158.90. Label: 2

Orodispersible tablet (*Velotab®*), yellow, olanzapine 5 mg, net price 28-tab pack = £48.78; 10 mg, 28-tab pack = £79.45; 15 mg, 28-tab pack = £119.18; 20 mg, 28-tab pack = £158.90. Label: 2, counselling, administration
Excipients include aspartame (section 9.4.1)

Counselling *Velotab®* may be placed on the tongue and allowed to dissolve or dispersed in water, orange juice, apple juice, milk, or coffee

▌QUETIAPINE

Cautions see notes above; cerebrovascular disease

Hepatic impairment manufacturer advises initial dose of 25 mg daily

Renal impairment manufacturer advises initial dose of 25 mg daily

Pregnancy manufacturer advises use only if potential benefit outweighs risk

Contra-indications

Breast-feeding avoid

Side-effects see notes above; also drowsiness, dyspepsia, constipation, dry mouth, mild asthenia, rhinitis, tachycardia; leucopenia, neutropenia and occasionally eosinophilia reported; elevated plasma-triglyceride and cholesterol concentrations, reduced plasma-thyroid hormone concentrations; possible QT interval prolongation; rest-

less leg syndrome; *rarely* oedema; *very rarely* priapism

Licensed use not licensed for use in children

Indication and dose

Schizophrenia (under specialist supervision)
- **By mouth**

  Child 12–18 years initially 25 mg twice daily adjusted in steps of 25–50 mg according to response; max. 750 mg daily

Seroquel® (AstraZeneca) [PoM]
Tablets, f/c, quetiapine (as fumarate) 25 mg (peach), net price 60-tab pack = £33.83; 100 mg (yellow), 60-tab pack = £113.10; 150 mg (pale yellow), 60-tab pack = £113.10; 200 mg (white), 60-tab pack = £113.10; 300 mg (white), 60-tab pack = £170.00. Label: 2

▌RISPERIDONE

Cautions see notes above; monitor height, body-weight, bowel habit, pulse, blood pressure, and developmental status including sexual maturation; assess for movement disorders before starting and monitor neurological parameters during treatment; family history of sudden cardiac death (perform ECG)

Hepatic impairment initially 500 micrograms twice daily increased in steps of 500 micrograms twice daily to 1-2 mg twice daily

Renal impairment initially 500 micrograms twice daily increased in steps of 500 micrograms twice daily to 1-2 mg twice daily

Pregnancy manufacturer advises use only if potential benefit outweighs risk; extrapyramidal effects reported in neonate when taken in third trimester

Contra-indications breast-feeding

Side-effects see notes above; also sleep disturbances, agitation, anxiety, and headache; *less commonly* constipation, nausea and vomiting, dyspepsia, abdominal pain, hypertension, impaired concentration, dizziness, fatigue, hyperprolactinaemia, sexual dysfunction, urinary incontinence, abnormal vision, and rash; *rarely* seizures, hyponatraemia, abnormal temperature

regulation, and epistaxis; oedema and blood disorders also reported

Licensed use not licensed for use in children under 15 years for psychoses; not licensed for use in autism

Indication and dose

Acute and chronic psychoses (under specialist supervision)
- **By mouth**

  Child 12–18 years 2 mg in 1–2 divided doses on first day *then* 4 mg in 1–2 divided doses on second day (slower titration appropriate in some children); usual dose range 4–6 mg daily; doses above 10 mg daily only if benefit considered to outweigh risk (max. 16 mg daily)

Short-term treatment (up to 6 weeks) of persistent aggression in conduct disorder (under specialist supervision)
- **By mouth**

  Child 5–18 years and body-weight under 50 kg initially 250 micrograms once daily increased according to response in steps of 250 micrograms on alternate days; usual dose 500 micrograms daily (up to 750 micrograms once daily has been required)

◁ **RISPERIDONE** (*continued*)

Child 5–18 years and body-weight over 50 kg initially 500 micrograms once daily increased according to response in steps of 500 micrograms on alternate days; usual dose 1 mg daily (up to 1.5 mg once daily has been required)

Short-term treatment of severe aggression in autism (under specialist supervision)
● **By mouth**
Child over 5 years and 15–20 kg 250 micrograms daily increased if necessary after 3 days to 500 micrograms daily; thereafter increased by 250 micrograms daily at 2-week intervals to max. 1.5 mg daily

Child over 20 kg up to 12 years 250 micrograms daily increased if necessary after 3 days to 750 micrograms daily; thereafter increased by 500 micrograms daily at 2-week intervals; max. daily dose 2.5 mg if under 45 kg; max. daily dose 3.5 mg if over 45 kg

Risperidone (Non-proprietary) ▼ PoM
Tablets, risperidone 500 micrograms, net price 20-tab pack = £4.34; 1 mg, 20-tab pack = £7.62, 60-tab pack = £17.93; 2 mg, 60-tab pack = £41.80; 3 mg, 60-tab pack = £60.69; 4 mg, 60-tab pack = £81.15; 6 mg, 28-tab pack = £57.87. Label: 2

Orodispersible tablets, risperidone 1 mg, net price 28-tab pack = £18.39; 2 mg 28-tab pack = £33.31. Label: 2, counselling, administration
Counselling Tablets should be placed on the tongue, allowed to dissolve and swallowed

Liquid, risperidone 1 mg/mL, net price 100-mL pack = £55.25. Label: 2, counselling, use of dose syringe
Note Liquid may be diluted with mineral water, orange juice or black coffee (should be taken immediately)

Risperdal® (Janssen-Cilag) ▼ PoM
Tablets, f/c, scored, risperidone 500 micrograms (brown-red), net price 20-tab pack = £7.06; 1 mg (white), 20-tab pack = £11.61, 60-tab pack = £34.84; 2 mg (orange), 60-tab pack = £68.69; 3 mg (yellow), 60-tab pack = £101.01; 4 mg (green), 60-tab pack = £133.34; 6 mg (yellow), 28-tab pack = £94.28. Label: 2

Orodispersible tablets (*Quicklet®*), pink, risperidone 500 micrograms, net price 28-tab pack = £11.43; 1 mg, 28-tab pack = £18.39; 2 mg, 28-tab pack = £34.66; 3 mg, 28-tab pack = £50.34; 4 mg, 28-tab pack = £64.84. Label: 2, counselling, administration
Excipients include aspartame (section 9.4.1)

Counselling Tablets should be placed on the tongue, allowed to dissolve and swallowed

Liquid, risperidone 1 mg/mL, net price 100-mL pack = £56.12. Label: 2, counselling, use of dose syringe
Note Liquid may be diluted with mineral water, orange juice or black coffee (should be taken immediately)

4.2.2 Antipsychotic depot injections

There is limited information on the use of antipsychotic depot injections in children and use should be restricted to specialist centres.

4.2.3 Antimanic drugs

Drugs are used in mania to control acute attacks and to prevent their recurrence.

Benzodiazepines

Use of benzodiazepines (section 4.1) may be helpful in the initial stages of treatment until lithium achieves its full effect; they should not be used for long periods because of the risk of dependence.

Antipsychotic drugs

In an acute attack of mania, treatment with an antipsychotic drug (section 4.2.1) is usually required because it may take a few days for lithium to exert its antimanic effect. Lithium may be given concurrently with the antipsychotic drug, and treatment with the antipsychotic gradually tailed off as lithium becomes effective. Alternatively, lithium therapy may be commenced once the child's mood has been stabilised with the antipsychotic. The adjunctive use of atypical antipsychotics such as olanzapine (section 4.2.1) and risperidone with either lithium or valproic acid may also be of benefit.

High doses of haloperidol may be hazardous when used with lithium; irreversible toxic encephalopathy has been reported.

Carbamazepine

Carbamazepine (section 4.8.1) may be used for the prophylaxis of bipolar disorder (manic-depressive disorder) in children unresponsive to lithium; it seems to be

4 Central nervous system

particularly effective in those with rapid-cycling manic-depressive illness (4 or more affective episodes per year).

Valproic acid

Valproic acid (as the semisodium salt) is licensed in adults for the treatment of manic episodes associated with bipolar disorder. It may be useful in children unresponsive to lithium. Sodium valproate (section 4.8.1) has also been used.

Lithium

Lithium salts are used in the prophylaxis and treatment of mania, in the prophylaxis of bipolar disorder (manic-depressive disorder) and in the prophylaxis of recurrent depression (unipolar illness or unipolar depression). Lithium should be used in children only on the advice of a specialist.

The decision to give prophylactic lithium must be based on careful consideration of the likelihood of recurrence in the individual child, and the benefit weighed against the risks. In long-term use lithium has been associated with thyroid disorders and mild cognitive and memory impairment. Long-term treatment should therefore be undertaken only with careful assessment of risk and benefit, and with regular monitoring of thyroid function. The need for continued therapy should be assessed regularly and children should be maintained on lithium after 3–5 years only if benefit persists.

Serum concentrations   Lithium salts have a narrow therapeutic/toxic ratio and should not be prescribed unless facilities for monitoring serum-lithium concentrations are available. There seem few if any reasons for preferring one or other of the salts of lithium available. Doses are adjusted to achieve serum-lithium concentration of 0.4–1 mmol/litre on samples taken 12 hours after the preceding dose. It is important to determine the optimum range for each individual child.

Overdosage, usually with serum-lithium concentration of over 1.5 mmol/litre, may be fatal and toxic effects include tremor, ataxia, dysarthria, nystagmus, renal impairment, and convulsions. If these potentially hazardous signs occur, treatment should be stopped, serum-lithium concentrations redetermined, and steps taken to reverse lithium toxicity. In mild cases withdrawal of lithium and administration of generous amounts of sodium and fluid will reverse the toxicity. Serum-lithium concentration in excess of 2 mmol/litre require urgent treatment as indicated under Emergency Treatment of Poisoning, p. 42.

Interactions   Lithium toxicity is made worse by sodium depletion, therefore concurrent use of diuretics (particularly thiazides) is hazardous and should be avoided. For other **interactions** with lithium, see Appendix 1 (lithium).

Withdrawal   While there is no clear evidence of withdrawal or rebound psychosis, abrupt discontinuation of lithium increases the risk of relapse. If lithium is to be discontinued, the dose should be reduced gradually over a period of a few weeks and children and carers should be warned of possible relapse if it is discontinued abruptly.

> **Lithium cards**
> A lithium treatment card available from pharmacies tells children and carers how to take lithium preparations, what to do if a dose is missed, and what side-effects to expect. It also explains why regular blood tests are important and warns that some medicines and illnesses can change serum-lithium concentration.
> Cards may be purchased from the National Pharmacy Association.
> Tel: (01727) 858 687 sales@npa.co.uk

LITHIUM CARBONATE

Cautions measure serum-lithium concentration regularly (every 3 months on stabilised regimens), measure renal function and thyroid function every 6–12 months on stabilised regimens and advise children and carers to seek attention if symptoms of hypothyroidism develop (females are at greater risk) e.g. lethargy, feeling cold; maintain adequate sodium and fluid intake; test renal function before initiating and if evidence of toxicity, avoid in cardiac disease, and conditions with sodium imbalance such as Addison's disease; reduce dose or discontinue in diarrhoea,

◻ **LITHIUM CARBONATE** (*continued*)

vomiting and intercurrent infection (especially if sweating profusely); psoriasis (risk of exacerbation); diuretic treatment, myasthenia gravis; surgery (section 15.1); if possible avoid abrupt withdrawal (see notes above); **interactions:** Appendix 1 (lithium)

Counselling Children should maintain adequate fluid intake and avoid dietary changes which reduce or increase sodium intake; lithium treatment cards are available from pharmacies (see above)

Renal impairment avoid if possible or reduce dose and monitor serum-lithium concentration carefully

Pregnancy avoid if possible in first trimester (risk of teratogenicity, including cardiac abnormalities); dose requirements increased in second and third trimesters (but return to normal abruptly on delivery); close monitoring of serum-lithium concentration advised (risk of toxicity in neonate)

Breast-feeding present in milk and risk of toxicity in infant—manufacturer advises avoid

Side-effects gastro-intestinal disturbances, fine tremor, renal impairment (particularly impaired urinary concentration and polyuria), polydipsia, leucocytosis; also weight gain and oedema (may respond to dose reduction); hyperparathyroidism and hypercalcaemia reported; signs of intoxication are blurred vision, increasing gastro-intestinal disturbances (anorexia, vomiting, diarrhoea), muscle weakness, increased CNS disturbances (mild drowsiness and sluggishness increasing to giddiness with ataxia, coarse tremor, lack of co-ordination, dysarthria), and require withdrawal of treatment; with severe **overdosage** (serum-lithium concentration above 2 mmol/litre) hyperreflexia and hyperextension of limbs, convulsions, toxic psychoses, syncope, renal failure, circulatory failure, coma, and occasionally, death; goitre, raised antidiuretic hormone concentration, hypothyroidism, hypokalaemia, ECG changes, and kidney changes may also occur; see also Emergency Treatment of Poisoning, p. 42

Indication and dose

Treatment and prophylaxis of mania, bipolar disorder, recurrent depression (see also notes above), aggressive or self-mutilating behaviour

• **By mouth**

See under preparations below, adjusted to achieve a serum-lithium concentration of 0.4–1 mmol/litre 12 hours after a dose on days 4–7 of treatment, then every week until dosage has

remained constant for 4 weeks and every 3 months thereafter; doses are initially divided throughout the day, but once daily administration is preferred when serum-lithium concentration stabilised

Note **Preparations vary widely in bioavailability**; changing the preparation requires the same precautions as initiation of treatment

Note Lithium carbonate 200 mg ≡ lithium citrate 509 mg

Camcolit® (Norgine) [PoM]

Camcolit 250® tablets, f/c, scored, lithium carbonate 250 mg (Li⁺ 6.8 mmol), net price 100-tab pack = £3.09 Label: 10, lithium card, counselling, see above

Camcolit 400® tablets, m/r, f/c, scored, lithium carbonate 400 mg (Li⁺ 10.8 mmol), net price 100-tab pack = £4.13. Label: 10, lithium card, 25, counselling, see above

Dose

Treatment

• **By mouth**

(see above for advice on bioavailability and serum-lithium monitoring)

Child 12–18 years initially 1–1.5 g daily

Prophylaxis

• **By mouth**

(see above for advice on bioavailability and serum-lithium monitoring)

Child 12–18 years initially 300–400 mg daily

Liskonum® (GSK) [PoM]

Tablets, m/r, f/c, scored, lithium carbonate 450 mg (Li⁺ 12.2 mmol), net price 60-tab pack = £2.88. Label: 10, lithium card, 25, counselling, see above

Dose

Treatment

• **By mouth**

(see above for advice on bioavailability and serum-lithium monitoring)

Child 12–18 years initially 225–675 mg twice daily

Prophylaxis

• **By mouth**

(see above for advice on bioavailability and serum-lithium monitoring)

Child 12–18 years initially 225–450 mg twice daily

▊ **LITHIUM CITRATE**

Cautions see under Lithium Carbonate and notes above

Counselling Patients should maintain an adequate fluid intake and should avoid dietary changes which might reduce or increase sodium intake; lithium treatment cards are available from pharmacies (see above)

Side-effects see under Lithium Carbonate and notes above

Licensed use not licensed for use in children

Indication and dose

See under Lithium Carbonate and notes above

• **By mouth**

Adjust to achieve serum-lithium concentration of 0.4–1 mmol/litre as described under Lithium Carbonate above

Note **Preparations vary widely in bioavailability**; changing the preparation requires the same precautions as initiation of treatment

Note Lithium carbonate 200 mg ≡ lithium citrate 509 mg

4 Central nervous system

◁ **LITHIUM CITRATE** (*continued*)

Li-Liquid® (Rosemont) [PoM]
  Oral solution, lithium citrate 509 mg/5 mL (Li⁺
  5.4 mmol/5 mL), yellow, net price 150-mL pack =
  £5.79; 1.018 g/5 mL (Li⁺ 10.8 mmol/5 mL), orange,
  150-mL pack = £11.58. Label: 10, lithium card,
  counselling, see above

Priadel® (Sanofi-Synthelabo) [PoM]
  Liquid, sugar-free, lithium citrate 520 mg/5 mL
  (approx. Li⁺ 5.4 mmol/5 mL), net price 150-mL
  pack = £5.84. Label: 10, lithium card, counselling,
  see above

4.3 Antidepressant drugs

4.3.1 Tricyclic antidepressant drugs
4.3.2 Monoamine-oxidase inhibitors
4.3.3 Selective serotonin re-uptake inhibitors
4.3.4 Other antidepressant drugs

> Depression in children should be managed by an appropriate specialist and
> treatment should involve psychological therapy.

The major classes of antidepressant drugs include the tricyclics and related
antidepressant drugs, the selective serotonin re-uptake inhibitors (SSRIs), and
the monoamine oxidase inhibitors (MAOIs).

Choice of antidepressant drug should be based on the individual child's requirements, including the presence of concomitant disease, existing therapy, suicide
risk, and previous response to antidepressant therapy.

When drug treatment of depression is considered necessary in children, the SSRIs
should be considered first-line treatment; following a safety and efficacy review,
fluoxetine is licensed to treat depression in children.

Tricyclic antidepressant drugs should generally be avoided for the treatment of
depression in children.

St John's wort (*Hypericum perforatum*) is a popular unlicensed herbal remedy for
treating mild depression in adults. In the absence of adequate evidence of safety
or efficacy in children, St John's wort should not be used for the treatment of
depression in children. It interacts with a number of conventional drugs, see
Appendix 1 (St John's wort).

> Hyponatraemia and antidepressant therapy
> Hyponatraemia (possibly due to inappropriate secretion of antidiuretic
> hormone) has been associated with all types of antidepressants; however, it
> has been reported more frequently with SSRIs than with other antidepressant
> drugs. The CSM has advised that hyponatraemia should be considered in all
> children who develop drowsiness, confusion, or convulsions while taking an
> antidepressant drug.

> Suicidal behaviour and antidepressant therapy
> The use of antidepressant drugs has been linked with suicidal thoughts and
> behaviour. Where necessary, children should be monitored for suicidal
> behaviour, self-harm, and hostility, particularly at the beginning of treatment
> or if the dose is changed.

Withdrawal   Gastro-intestinal symptoms of nausea, vomiting, and anorexia,
accompanied by headache, giddiness, 'chills', and insomnia, and sometimes by
hypomania, panic-anxiety, and extreme motor restlessness may occur if an antidepressant is stopped suddenly after regular administration for 8 weeks or more.
The dose should preferably be reduced gradually over about 4 weeks, or longer if
withdrawal symptoms emerge (6 months in children who have been on long-term
maintenance treatment). SSRIs have been associated with a specific withdrawal
syndrome (section 4.3.3).

Anxiety   Management of *acute anxiety* in children with drug treatment is contentious (section 4.1.2). For *chronic anxiety* (of longer than 4 weeks' duration), it
may be appropriate to use an antidepressant drug before a benzodiazepine.

4.3.1 Tricyclic antidepressant drugs

> The safety and efficacy of tricyclic antidepressant drugs in the treatment of depression in children has not been established. Treatment should be managed by an appropriate specialist and should involve psychological therapy.

For reference to the role of some tricyclic antidepressant drugs in some forms of *neuralgia*, see section 4.7.3, and in *nocturnal enuresis* in children, see section 7.4.2.

Dosage It is important to use doses that are sufficiently high for effective treatment but not so high as to cause toxic effects. Low doses should be used for initial treatment.

In most children the long half-life of tricyclic antidepressant drugs allows **once-daily** administration, usually at night; the use of modified-release preparations is therefore unnecessary.

Choice Tricyclic antidepressant drugs should generally be avoided for the treatment of depression in children (see above). Tricyclic and related antidepressant drugs block the re-uptake of both serotonin and noradrenaline, although to different extents. For example, clomipramine is more selective for serotonergic transmission, and imipramine is more selective for noradrenergic transmission. Tricyclic antidepressant drugs can be roughly divided into those with additional sedative properties and those without. Those with **sedative** properties include amitriptyline and doxepin. Those with **less sedative** properties include imipramine and nortriptyline.

Amitriptyline and **imipramine** have more marked antimuscarinic and cardiac side-effects than some other tricyclic or related antidepressant drugs, such as **doxepin**; this may be important in some children.

Side-effects *Arrhythmias* and *heart block* occasionally follow the use of tricyclic antidepressant drugs, particularly amitriptyline, and may be a factor in the sudden death of children with cardiac disease. They are also sometimes associated with *convulsions* (and should be prescribed with special caution in epilepsy as they lower the convulsive threshold).

Other side-effects of tricyclic antidepressant drugs include *drowsiness, dry mouth, blurred vision, constipation,* and *urinary retention* (all attributed to antimuscarinic activity), and sweating. The child should be encouraged to persist with treatment as some tolerance to these side-effects seems to develop. They are reduced if low doses are given initially and then gradually increased, but this must be balanced against the need to obtain a full therapeutic effect as soon as possible.

Neuroleptic malignant syndrome (section 4.2.1) may, *very rarely*, arise in the course of antidepressant drug treatment.

Suicidal behaviour has been linked with antidepressant drugs (see p. 228).

Overdosage Limited quantities of tricyclic antidepressant drugs should be prescribed at any one time because their cardiovascular effects are dangerous in overdosage. In particular, overdosage with **amitriptyline** is associated with a relatively high rate of fatality. For advice on overdosage see Emergency Treatment of Poisoning, p. 40.

Withdrawal If possible tricyclic antidepressant drugs should be withdrawn slowly (see also section 4.3.1).

AMITRIPTYLINE HYDROCHLORIDE

Cautions cardiac disease (particularly with arrhythmias, see Contra-indications below), history of epilepsy, thyroid disease, phaeochromocytoma, history of mania, psychoses (may aggravate psychotic symptoms), susceptibility to angle-closure glaucoma, history of urinary retention, concurrent electroconvulsive therapy; if possible avoid abrupt withdrawal; anaesthesia (increased risk of arrhythmias and hypotension, see surgery section 15.1); acute porphyria (section 9.8.2); see section 7.4.2 for additional nocturnal enuresis

warnings; **interactions**: Appendix 1 (antidepressants, tricyclic)

Skilled tasks Drowsiness may affect performance of skilled tasks (e.g. driving); effects of alcohol enhanced

Hepatic impairment sedative effects increased; avoid in severe hepatic impairment

Pregnancy manufacturer advises use only if potential benefit outweighs risk

Breast-feeding amount too small to be harmful but manufacturer advises avoid

4 Central nervous system

⌐ **AMITRIPTYLINE HYDROCHLORIDE (continued)**

Contra-indications arrhythmias (particularly heart block), not indicated in manic phase, severe liver disease

Side-effects dry mouth, sedation, blurred vision (disturbance of accommodation, increased intra-ocular pressure), constipation, nausea, difficulty with micturition; cardiovascular side-effects (such as ECG changes, arrhythmias, postural hypotension, tachycardia, syncope, particularly with high doses); sweating, tremor, rashes and hypersensitivity reactions (including urticaria, photosensitivity); behavioural disturbances, hypomania or mania, confusion or delirium, headache, interference with sexual function, blood—glucose changes; increased appetite and weight gain (occasionally weight loss); endocrine side-effects such as testicular enlargement, gynaecomastia, galactorrhoea; also convulsions (see also Cautions), movement disorders and dyskinesias, dysarthria, paraesthesia, taste disturbances, tinnitus, fever, agranulocytosis, leucopenia, eosinophilia, purpura, thrombocytopenia, hyponatraemia (see Hyponatraemia and Antidepressant Therapy, p. 228), abnormal liver function tests (jaundice); for a general outline of side-effects see also notes above; **overdosage:** see Emergency Treatment of Poisoning, p. 40 (high rate of fatality—see Overdosage, p. 229)

Licensed use not licensed for use in neuropathic pain

Indication and dose

> Depression (but see notes above)
> - By mouth
>> Child 16–18 years 10–25 mg 3 times daily (total daily dose may alternatively be given as a single dose at bedtime) increased gradually as necessary to 150–200 mg daily

> Nocturnal enuresis
> - By mouth
>> Child 6–11 years 10–20 mg at night
>> Child 11–16 years 25–50 mg at night
>> Note Max. period of treatment (including gradual withdrawal) 3 months—full physical examination before further course, see also section 7.4.2

> Neuropathic pain in palliative care
> - By mouth
>> Child 2–12 years initially 200–500 micrograms/kg (max. 25 mg) once daily at night, increased if necessary; max. 1 mg/kg twice daily on specialist advice
>> Child 12–18 years initially 10–25 mg once daily at night, increased gradually if necessary to usual dose 75 mg at night; higher doses on specialist advice

Amitriptyline (Non-proprietary) ℗ℴℳ
Tablets, coated, amitriptyline hydrochloride 10 mg, net price 28 = 97p; 25 mg, 28 = 97p; 50 mg, 28 = £1.12. Label: 2

Oral solution, amitriptyline hydrochloride 25 mg/5 mL, net price 150 mL = £13.30; 50 mg/5 mL, 150 mL = £14.48. Label: 2

▞ DOXEPIN

Cautions see under Amitriptyline Hydrochloride
Contra-indications see under Amitriptyline Hydrochloride

Breast-feeding manufacturer advises avoid—accumulation of doxepin metabolite may cause sedation and respiratory depression

Side-effects see under Amitriptyline Hydrochloride

Indication and dose

> Depressive illness, particularly where sedation is required (but see notes above)
> - By mouth
>> Child 12–18 years initially 75 mg daily in divided doses or as a single dose at bedtime, adjusted according to response; usual maintenance 30–300 mg daily (doses above 100 mg given in 3 divided doses)

Sinepin® (Marlborough) ℗ℴℳ
Capsules, doxepin (as hydrochloride) 25 mg, net price 28-cap pack = £3.77; 50 mg, 28-cap pack = £5.71. Label: 2

▞ IMIPRAMINE HYDROCHLORIDE

Cautions see under Amitriptyline Hydrochloride
Pregnancy tachycardia, irritability, and muscle spasms reported in neonates when used in third trimester

Contra-indications see under Amitriptyline Hydrochloride

Side-effects see under Amitriptyline Hydrochloride, but less sedating
Licensed use not licensed for use for attention deficit hyperactivity disorder

◁ **IMIPRAMINE HYDROCHLORIDE** (*continued*)

Indication and dose

Nocturnal enuresis
- **By mouth**

  Child 6–8 years 25 mg at bedtime

  Child 8–11 years 25–50 mg at bedtime

  Child 11–18 years 50–75 mg at bedtime
  Note Max. period of treatment (including gradual withdrawal) 3 months—full physical examination before further course, see also section 7.4.2

Attention deficit hyperactivity disorder (under specialist supervision)
- **By mouth**

  Child 6–18 years 10–30 mg twice daily

Imipramine (Non-proprietary) ℗ℴℳ
Tablets, coated, imipramine hydrochloride 10 mg, net price 28-tab pack = £1.20; 25 mg, 28-tab pack = £1.17. Label: 2

NORTRIPTYLINE

Cautions see under Amitriptyline Hydrochloride; manufacturer advises plasma-nortriptyline concentration monitoring if dose above 100 mg daily, but evidence of practical value uncertain

Contra-indications see under Amitriptyline Hydrochloride

Side-effects see under Amitriptyline Hydrochloride, but less sedating

Indication and dose

Depression (but see notes above)
- **By mouth**

  Child 12–18 years low dose initially increased as necessary to 30–50 mg daily in divided doses *or* as a single dose (max. 150 mg daily)

Nocturnal enuresis
- **By mouth**

  Child 6–8 years 10 mg at night

  Child 8–11 years 10–20 mg at night

  Child 11–18 years 25–35 mg at night
  Note Max. period of treatment (including gradual withdrawal) 3 months—full physical examination and ECG before further course, see also section 7.4.2

Allegron® (King) ℗ℴℳ
Tablets, nortriptyline (as hydrochloride) 10 mg, net price 100-tab pack = £12.06; 25 mg (orange, scored), 100-tab pack = £24.02. Label: 2

4.3.2 Monoamine-oxidase inhibitors (MAOIs)

Classification not used in *BNF for Children*.

4.3.3 Selective serotonin re-uptake inhibitors

Citalopram, **escitalopram**, **fluoxetine**, **fluvoxamine**, **paroxetine**, and **sertraline** selectively inhibit the re-uptake of serotonin (5-hydroxytryptamine, 5-HT); they are termed selective serotonin re-uptake inhibitors (SSRIs).

CSM advice (depressive illness in children and adolescents)
The CSM has advised that the balance of risks and benefits for the treatment of depressive illness in individuals under 18 years is considered unfavourable for the SSRIs **citalopram**, **escitalopram**, **paroxetine**, and **sertraline**, and for **mirtazapine** and **venlafaxine**. Clinical trials have failed to show efficacy and have shown an increase in harmful outcomes. However, it is recognised that specialists may sometimes decide to use these drugs in response to individual clinical need; children and adolescents should be monitored carefully for suicidal behaviour, self-harm or hostility, particularly at the beginning of treatment. Only **fluoxetine** has been shown in clinical trials to be effective for treating depressive illness in children and adolescents. However, it is possible that, in common with the other SSRIs, it is associated with a small risk of self-harm and suicidal thoughts. Overall, the balance of risks and benefits for fluoxetine in the treatment of depressive illness in individuals under 18 years is considered favourable, but children and adolescents must be carefully monitored as above.

Cautions SSRIs should be used with caution in children with epilepsy (avoid if poorly controlled, discontinue if convulsions develop), cardiac disease, diabetes mellitus, susceptibility to angle-closure glaucoma, a history of mania or bleeding disorders (especially gastro-intestinal bleeding), and if used together with other drugs that increase the risk of bleeding. They should also be used with caution in those receiving concurrent electroconvulsive therapy (prolonged seizures reported with fluoxetine). SSRIs may also impair performance of skilled tasks (e.g. driving). **Interactions:** Appendix 1 (antidepressants, SSRI).

Withdrawal Gastro-intestinal disturbances, headache, anxiety, dizziness, paraesthesia, sleep disturbances, fatigue, influenza-like symptoms, and sweating are the most common features of abrupt withdrawal of an SSRI or marked reduction of the dose; the dose should be tapered over a few weeks to avoid these effects.

Contra-indications SSRIs should not be used if the child enters a manic phase.

Side-effects SSRIs are less sedating and have fewer antimuscarinic and cardiotoxic effects than tricyclic antidepressant drugs (section 4.3.1). Side-effects of the SSRIs include gastro-intestinal effects (dose-related and fairly common—include nausea, vomiting, dyspepsia, abdominal pain, diarrhoea, constipation), anorexia with weight loss (increased appetite and weight gain also reported) and hypersensitivity reactions including rash (consider discontinuation—may be sign of impending serious systemic reaction, possibly associated with vasculitis), urticaria, angioedema, anaphylaxis, arthralgia, myalgia and photosensitivity; other side-effects include dry mouth, nervousness, anxiety, headache, insomnia, tremor, dizziness, asthenia, hallucinations, drowsiness, convulsions (see Cautions above), galactorrhoea, sexual dysfunction, urinary retention, sweating, hypomania or mania (see Cautions above), movement disorders and dyskinesias, visual disturbances, hyponatraemia (see Hyponatraemia and Antidepressant Therapy, p. 228), and bleeding disorders including ecchymoses and purpura. Suicidal behaviour has been linked with antidepressants, see p. 228.

CITALOPRAM

Cautions see notes above

Hepatic impairment use doses at lower end of range

Renal impairment no information available for estimated glomerular filtration rate less than $20 \, mL/minute/1.73 \, m^2$

Pregnancy manufacturers advise use only if potential benefit outweighs risk; risk of neonatal withdrawal

Breast-feeding present in milk—manufacturer advises avoid

Contra-indications see notes above

Side-effects see notes above; also palpitation, tachycardia, postural hypotension, coughing, yawning, confusion, impaired concentration, malaise, amnesia, migraine, paraesthesia, abnormal dreams, taste disturbance, increased salivation, rhinitis, tinnitus, polyuria, micturition disorders, euphoria

Licensed use not licensed for use in children

Indication and dose

Major depression (but see CSM advice, above)
- **By mouth as tablets**

  Child 12–18 years initially 10 mg once daily, increased if necessary to 20 mg once daily over 2–4 weeks; max. 60 mg once daily

- **By mouth as oral drops**

  Child 12–18 years initially 8 mg once daily increased if necessary to 16 mg once daily over 2–4 weeks; max. 48 mg once daily

Citalopram (Non-proprietary) [PoM]
Tablets, citalopram (as hydrobromide) 10 mg, net price 28-tab pack = £1.08; 20 mg, 28-tab pack = £1.25; 40 mg, 28-tab pack = £1.46. Counselling, driving

Oral drops, citalopram (as hydrochloride) 40 mg/mL, net price 15-mL pack = £19.66. Counselling, driving, administration

Note 4 drops (8 mg) can be considered equivalent in therapeutic effect to 10-mg tablet
Mix with water, orange juice, or apple juice before taking

Cipramil® (Lundbeck) [PoM]
Tablets, f/c, citalopram (as hydrobromide) 10 mg, net price 28-tab pack = £8.97; 20 mg (scored), 28-tab pack = £14.91; 40 mg, 28-tab pack = £25.20. Counselling, driving

Oral drops, sugar-free, citalopram (as hydrochloride) 40 mg/mL, net price 15-mL pack = £20.16. Counselling, driving, administration

Note 4 drops (8 mg) can be considered equivalent in therapeutic effect to 10-mg tablet
Mix with water, orange juice, or apple juice before taking

FLUOXETINE

Cautions see notes above

Hepatic impairment reduce dose; avoid in severe hepatic impairment

Pregnancy manufacturer advises use only if potential benefit outweighs risk (no evidence of teratogenicity)

Breast-feeding present in breast milk, manufacturer advises avoid

Contra-indications see notes above

Side-effects see notes above; also vasodilatation, postural hypotension, pharyngitis, dyspnoea, chills, taste disturbances, sleep disturbances,

◻ **FLUOXETINE** (*continued*)

euphoria, confusion, yawning, impaired concentration, changes in blood sugar, alopecia, urinary frequency; *rarely* pulmonary inflammation and fibrosis; *very rarely* hepatitis, toxic epidermal necrolysis, and neuroleptic malignant syndrome-like event

Indication and dose

Major depression

• **By mouth**

Child 8–18 years 10 mg once daily increased after 1–2 weeks if necessary, max. 20 mg once daily

Long duration of action Consider the long half-life of fluoxetine when adjusting dosage (or in overdosage)

Fluoxetine (Non-proprietary) ᴾᵒᴹ

Capsules, fluoxetine (as hydrochloride) 20 mg, net price 30-cap pack = £1.02; 60 mg, 30-cap pack = £55.76. Counselling, driving
Brands include *Oxactin*®

Liquid, fluoxetine (as hydrochloride) 20 mg/5 mL, net price 70 mL = £7.41. Counselling, driving
Brands include *Prozep*®

Prozac® (Lilly) ᴾᵒᴹ

Capsules, fluoxetine (as hydrochloride) 20 mg (green/yellow), net price 30-cap pack = £14.21. Counselling, driving

Liquid, fluoxetine (as hydrochloride) 20 mg/5 mL, net price 70 mL = £13.26. Counselling, driving

---

▉ FLUVOXAMINE MALEATE

Cautions see notes above

Hepatic impairment reduce dose

Renal impairment start with smaller dose

Pregnancy manufacturers advise use only if potential benefit outweighs risk; risk of neonatal withdrawal

Breast-feeding present in milk—manufacturer advises avoid

CSM advice The CSM has advised that concomitant use of fluvoxamine and theophylline or aminophylline should usually be avoided; see also **interactions**: Appendix 1 (antidepressants, SSRIs)

Contra-indications see notes above

Side-effects see notes above; palpitation, tachycardia (may also cause bradycardia); *rarely* postural hypotension, confusion, ataxia, paraesthesia, malaise, taste disturbance, neuroleptic malignant syndrome-like event, abnormal liver function tests, usually symptomatic (discontinue treatment)

Indication and dose

Obsessive-compulsive disorder

• **By mouth**

Child 8–18 years initially 25 mg daily increased if necessary in steps of 25 mg every 4–7 days according to response (total daily doses above 50 mg in 2 divided doses); max. 100 mg twice daily

Note If no improvement in obsessive-compulsive disorder within 10 weeks, treatment should be reconsidered

Fluvoxamine (Non-proprietary) ᴾᵒᴹ

Tablets, fluvoxamine maleate 50 mg, net price 60-tab pack = £6.80; 100 mg, 30-tab pack = £8.34. Counselling, driving

Faverin® (Solvay) ᴾᵒᴹ

Tablets, f/c, scored, fluvoxamine maleate 50 mg, net price 60-tab pack = £17.10; 100 mg, 30-tab pack = £17.10. Counselling, driving

---

▉ SERTRALINE

Cautions see notes above; renal impairment

Hepatic impairment reduce dose in mild or moderate hepatic impairment; avoid in severe impairment

Pregnancy manufacturers advise use only if potential benefit outweighs risk; risk of neonatal withdrawal

Breast-feeding present in milk but not known to be harmful in short-term use

Contra-indications see notes above

Side-effects see notes above; pancreatitis, hepatitis, jaundice, liver failure, tachycardia, postural hypotension, amnesia, paraesthesia, aggression, urinary incontinence, and menstrual irregularities also reported

Licensed use not licensed for use in children for depression

Indication and dose

Obsessive-compulsive disorder

• **By mouth**

Child 6–12 years initially 25 mg daily increased to 50 mg daily after 1 week, further increased if necessary in steps of 50 mg at intervals of at least 1 week; max. 200 mg daily

Child 12–18 years initially 50 mg daily increased if necessary in steps of 50 mg over several weeks; usual range 50–200 mg daily

Major depression (but see CSM advice, above)

• **By mouth**

Child 12–18 years initially 50 mg once daily increased if necessary in steps of 50 mg daily at intervals of at least a week; max. 200 mg once daily

Sertraline (Non-proprietary) ᴾᵒᴹ

Tablets, sertraline (as hydrochloride) 50 mg, net price 28-tab pack = £1.37; 100 mg, 28-tab pack = £1.80. Counselling, driving

Lustral® (Pfizer) ᴾᵒᴹ

Tablets, both f/c, sertraline (as hydrochloride) 50 mg (scored), net price 28-tab pack = £17.82; 100 mg, 28-tab pack = £29.16. Counselling, driving

4 Central nervous system

4.3.4 **Other antidepressant drugs**

Classification not used in *BNF for Children*.

4.4 **CNS stimulants and other drugs for attention deficit hyperactivity disorder**

CNS stimulants should only be prescribed for children with severe and persistent symptoms of *attention deficit hyperactivity disorder* (ADHD), when the diagnosis has been confirmed by a specialist; treatment may be continued by general practitioners under a shared-care arrangement. Treatment often needs to be continued into adolescence, and may need to be continued into adulthood.

Drug treatment of ADHD should be part of a comprehensive treatment programme. The choice of drug should take into consideration co-morbid conditions (such as tic disorders, Tourette syndrome, and epilepsy), different adverse effects of the drugs, potential for drug misuse, and preferences of the child and carers. **Methylphenidate** and **atomoxetine** are used for the management of ADHD; **dexamfetamine** (dexamphetamine) is an alternative in children who do not respond to these drugs. Growth is not generally affected by treatment with CNS stimulants but it is advisable to monitor growth during treatment.

A tricyclic antidepressant such as **imipramine** (section 4.3.1) is sometimes used in the treatment of ADHD; it should not be prescribed concomitantly with a CNS stimulant.

Modafinil is used for the treatment of daytime sleepiness associated with narcolepsy; dependence with long-term use cannot be excluded and it should therefore be used with caution.

Dexamfetamine and methylphenidate [both unlicensed] are also used to treat narcolepsy.

ATOMOXETINE

Cautions cardiovascular disease including hypertension and tachycardia; monitor growth; QT-interval prolongation (avoid concomitant administration of drugs that prolong QT-interval); history of seizures; susceptibility to angle-closure glaucoma; **interactions**: Appendix 1 (atomoxetine)

Hepatic disorders Following rare reports of hepatic disorders, the CSM has advised that children and carers should be advised of the risk and be told how to recognise symptoms; prompt medical attention should be sought in case of abdominal pain, unexplained nausea, malaise, darkening of the urine or jaundice

Suicidal ideation Following reports of suicidal thoughts and behaviour, CSM has advised that children and carers should be informed about the risk and told to report clinical worsening, suicidal thoughts or behaviour, irritability, agitation, or depression

Hepatic impairment see hepatic disorders above; also halve dose in moderate liver disease; quarter dose in severe liver disease

Pregnancy no information available; manufacturer advises avoid unless potential benefit outweighs risk

Breast-feeding manufacturer advises avoid—present in milk in *animal* studies

Side-effects anorexia, dry mouth, nausea, vomiting, abdominal pain, constipation, dyspepsia, flatulence; palpitation, tachycardia, increased blood pressure, postural hypotension, hot flushes; sleep disturbance, dizziness, headache, fatigue, lethargy, depression, anxiety, irritability, tremor, rigors; urinary retention, prostatitis, sexual dysfunction, menstrual disturbances; mydriasis, conjunctivitis; dermatitis, pruritus, rash, sweating; *less commonly* suicidal ideation

(see Suicidal Ideation, above), cold extremities; *very rarely* hepatic disorders (see Hepatic Disorders, above), seizures, Raynaud's phenomenon, and angle-closure glaucoma

Indication and dose

Attention deficit hyperactivity disorder initiated by specialist

• By mouth

Child over 6 years (body-weight under 70 kg) initially 500 micrograms/kg daily for 7 days then increased according to response to usual maintenance dose 1.2 mg/kg daily; usual max. 100 mg daily, but may be increased to 1.8 mg/kg (max. 120 mg) daily under the direction of a specialist

Child (body-weight over 70 kg) initially 40 mg daily for 7 days then increased according to response to usual maintenance dose 80 mg daily; usual max. 100 mg daily, but may be increased to max. 120 mg daily under the direction of a specialist

Note Total daily dose may be given *either* as a single dose in the morning *or* in 2 divided doses with last dose no later than early evening

Strattera® (Lilly) ▼ PoM

Capsules, atomoxetine (as hydrochloride) 10 mg (white), net price 7-cap pack = £15.02, 28-cap pack = £60.06; 18 mg (gold/white), 7-cap pack = £15.02, 28-cap pack = £60.06; 25 mg (blue/white), 7-cap pack = £15.02, 28-cap pack = £60.06; 40 mg (blue), 7-cap pack = £15.02, 28-cap pack = £60.06; 60 mg (blue/gold), 28-cap pack = £60.06. Label: 3

■ DEXAMFETAMINE SULPHATE
(Dexamphetamine sulphate)

Cautions mild hypertension (contra-indicated if moderate or severe)—monitor blood pressure; history of epilepsy (discontinue if convulsions occur); tics and Tourette syndrome (use with caution)—discontinue if tics occur; monitor growth (see below); avoid abrupt withdrawal; data on safety and efficacy of long-term use not complete; acute porphyria (see section 9.8.2); **interactions:** Appendix 1 (sympathomimetics)
Growth restriction Monitor height and weight as growth restriction may occur during prolonged therapy (drug-free periods may allow catch-up in growth but withdraw slowly to avoid inducing depression or renewed hyperactivity).

Contra-indications cardiovascular disease including moderate to severe hypertension, hyperexcitability or agitated states, hyperthyroidism, history of drug or alcohol abuse, glaucoma
Skilled tasks May affect performance of skilled tasks (e.g. driving); effects of alcohol unpredictable

Pregnancy manufacturer advises avoid (retrospective evidence of uncertain significance suggesting possible embryotoxicity)

Breast-feeding significant amount in milk—avoid

Side-effects insomnia, restlessness, irritability and excitability, nervousness, night terrors, euphoria, tremor, dizziness, headache; convulsions (see also Cautions); dependence and tolerance, sometimes psychosis; anorexia, gastro-intestinal symptoms, growth restriction (see also under Cautions); dry mouth, sweating, tachycardia (and anginal pain), palpitation, increased blood pressure; visual disturbances; cardiomyopathy reported with chronic use; central stimulants have provoked choreoathetoid movements, tics and Tourette syndrome in predisposed individuals (see also Cautions above); **overdosage:** see Emergency Treatment of Poisoning, p. 43

Indication and dose

Refractory attention deficit hyperactivity disorder initiated by specialist
• By mouth

Child 4–6 years initially 2.5 mg once daily, increased if necessary by 2.5 mg at intervals of 1 week; usual max. 20 mg daily; maintenance dose given in 2–3 divided doses

Child 6–18 years initially 5–10 mg once daily, increased if necessary by 5 mg at intervals of 1 week; usual max. 20 mg daily (older children have received max. 40 mg); maintenance dose given in 2–3 divided doses

Administration tablets can be halved

Dexedrine® (UCB Pharma) ⃞CD⃞
Tablets, scored, dexamfetamine sulphate 5 mg. Net price 28-tab pack = £3.00. Counselling, driving

■ METHYLPHENIDATE HYDROCHLORIDE

Cautions monitor growth (if prolonged treatment), blood pressure and full blood count; anxiety or agitation; tics or a family history of Tourette syndrome; epilepsy (discontinue if increased seizure frequency); avoid abrupt withdrawal; **interactions:** Appendix 1 (sympathomimetics)

Pregnancy limited experience—manufacturer advises avoid unless potential benefit outweighs risk; toxicity in *animals*

Contra-indications severe depression, suicidal ideation; drug or alcohol dependence, psychosis; hyperthyroidism; cardiovascular disease

Breast-feeding no information available—manufacturer advises avoid

Side-effects abdominal pain, nausea, vomiting, dyspepsia, dry mouth; anorexia, reduced weight gain; tachycardia, palpitation, arrhythmias, changes in blood pressure; tics (*very rarely* Tourette syndrome), insomnia, nervousness, asthenia, depression, irritability, aggression, headache, drowsiness, dizziness, movement disorders; fever, arthralgia; rash, pruritus, alopecia; *less commonly* diarrhoea, abnormal dreams, confusion, suicidal ideation, urinary frequency, haematuria, muscle cramps, epistaxis; *rarely* growth restriction, visual disturbances; *very rarely* hepatic dysfunction, cerebral arteritis, psychosis, seizures, neuroleptic malignant syndrome, tolerance and dependence, blood disorders including leucopenia and thrombocytopenia, exfoliative dermatitis, and erythema multiforme

Licensed use not licensed for use in children under 6 years

Indication and dose

Attention deficit hyperactivity disorder initiated by specialist
• By mouth

Child 4–6 years 2.5 mg twice daily increased if necessary at weekly intervals by 2.5 mg daily to max. 1.4 mg/kg daily in divided doses; discontinue if no response after 1 month, suspend treatment every 1–2 years to assess condition

Child 6–18 years initially 5 mg 1–2 times daily, increased if necessary at weekly intervals by 5–10 mg daily; usual max. 60 mg daily in divided doses but may be increased to 2.1 mg/kg daily (max. 90 mg daily) under the direction of a specialist; discontinue if no response after 1 month, suspend treatment every 1–2 years to assess condition
Evening dose If effect wears off in evening (with rebound hyperactivity) a dose at bedtime may be appropriate (establish need with trial bedtime dose)
Note Treatment may be started using a modified-release preparation

Administration *Equasym®* and *Ritalin®* tablets may be halved; contents of *Equasym XL®* capsules can be sprinkled on a tablespoon of apple sauce, then swallowed immediately without chewing

◁ **METHYLPHENIDATE HYDROCHLORIDE (continued)**

Methylphenidate Hydrochloride (Non-proprietary) (CD)
Tablets, methylphenidate hydrochloride 5 mg, net
price 30-tab pack = £2.78; 10 mg, 30-tab pack =
£5.80; 20 mg, 30-tab pack = £9.98
Brands include *Equasym*®, *Medikinet*®

Ritalin® (Novartis) (CD)
Tablets, scored, methylphenidate hydrochloride
10 mg, net price 30-tab pack = £5.57

▲Modified release

Concerta® **XL** (Janssen-Cilag) (CD)
Tablets, m/r, methylphenidate hydrochloride
18 mg (yellow), net price 30-tab pack = £29.70;
27 mg (grey), 30-tab pack = £35.06; 36 mg (white),
30-tab pack = £40.43. Label: 25

Counselling Tablet membrane may pass through gastro-
intestinal tract unchanged
Cautions dose form not appropriate for use in dysphagia
or if gastro-intestinal lumen restricted

Dose
• **By mouth**
  Child 6–18 years initially 18 mg once daily (in the
  morning), increased if necessary in weekly steps of
  18 mg according to response; usual max. 54 mg
  daily, but may be increased to 2.1 mg/kg daily (max.
  108 mg daily) under the direction of a specialist; discontinue if no response after 1 month; suspend treatment every 1–2 years to assess condition
  Note Total daily dose of 15 mg of standard-release
  formulation is considered equivalent to *Concerta*® *XL*
  18 mg once daily

Equasym XL® (UCB Pharma) (CD)
Capsules, m/r, methylphenidate hydrochloride
10 mg (white/green), net price 30-cap pack =
£25.00; 20 mg (white/blue), 30-cap pack = £30.00;
30 mg (white/brown), 30-cap pack = £35.00.
Label: 25

Dose
• **By mouth**
  Child 6–18 years initially 10 mg once daily in the
  morning before breakfast, increased gradually if
  necessary; usual max. 60 mg daily, but may be
  increased to 2.1 mg/kg daily (max. 90 mg daily) under
  the direction of a specialist; discontinue if no response
  after 1 month; suspend treatment every 1–2 years to
  assess condition

Medikinet XL® (Flynn) (CD)
Capsules, m/r, methylphenidate hydrochloride
10 mg (lilac/white), net price 28-cap pack = £21.00;
20 mg (lilac), 28-cap pack = £28.00; 30 mg (purple/
light grey), 28-cap pack = £33.72; 40 mg (purple/
grey), 28-cap pack = £44.95. Label: 25

Dose
• **By mouth**
  Child 6–18 years 10 mg once daily in the morning
  with breakfast, adjusted according to response; usual
  max. 60 mg daily, but may be increased to 2.1 mg/kg
  daily (max. 90 mg daily) under the direction of a
  specialist; discontinue if no response after 1 month;
  suspend treatment every 1–2 years to assess condition
  Note Contents of capsule can be sprinkled on a tablespoon of apple sauce (then swallowed immediately without chewing)

▮ **MODAFINIL**

Cautions monitor blood pressure and heart rate in
hypertension (see Contra-indications); possibility
of dependence; **interactions**: Appendix 1 (modafinil)

Hepatic impairment halve dose in severe liver
disease

Renal impairment manufacturer advises use half
normal dose in severe impairment

Contra-indications moderate to severe uncontrolled hypertension, arrhythmia; history of left
ventricular hypertrophy, of cor pulmonale, or of
clinically significant stimulant-induced mitral-
valve prolapse (including ischaemic ECG
changes, chest pain and arrhythmias)

Pregnancy manufacturer advises avoid

Breast-feeding manufacturer advises avoid—no
information available

Side-effects dry mouth, appetite changes, gastro-
intestinal disturbances (including nausea, diarrhoea, constipation, and dyspepsia), abdominal
pain; tachycardia, vasodilation, chest pain, palpitation; headache (uncommonly migraine),
anxiety, sleep disturbances, dizziness, depression,
confusion, paraesthesia, asthenia; visual disturbances; *less commonly* mouth ulcers, glossitis,
pharyngitis, dysphagia, taste disturbance,
increased thirst, hypertension, hypotension,
bradycardia, arrhythmia, peripheral oedema,
hypercholesterolaemia, rhinitis, dyspnoea, agita-

tion, dyskinesia, amnesia, emotional lability,
abnormal dreams, tremor, decreased libido,
weight changes, hyperglycaemia, urinary frequency, menstrual disturbances, eosinophilia,
leucopenia, myasthenia, muscle cramps, dry eye,
sinusitis, epistaxis, myalgia, arthralgia, acne,
sweating, rash, and pruritus; *very rarely* psychosis,
mania, Stevens-Johnson syndrome, and toxic
epidermal necrolysis

Licensed use not licensed for use in children
under 12 years

Indication and dose

Narcolepsy
• **By mouth**
  Child 5–12 years initially 100 mg daily in the
  morning, dose adjusted according to response
  to 100–400 mg daily *either* in 2 divided doses
  morning and at noon *or* as a single dose in the
  morning

  Child 12–18 years 200 mg daily, *either* in 2
  divided doses morning and at noon *or* as a single
  dose in the morning, dose adjusted according to
  response to 200–400 mg daily in 2 divided doses
  or as a single dose

Provigil® (Cephalon) ▼ (PoM)
Tablets, modafinil 100 mg, net price 30-tab pack =
£55.80; 200 mg, 30-tab pack = £111.60

4.5 Drugs used in the treatment of obesity

Obesity is associated with many health problems including cardiovascular disease, diabetes mellitus, gallstones, and osteoarthritis. Factors that aggravate obesity may include depression, other psychosocial problems, and some drugs.

The main treatment of the obese individual is a suitable diet, carefully explained to the individual or carer, with appropriate support and encouragement; increased physical activity should also be encouraged. If appropriate, smoking cessation (while maintaining body weight) may be worthwhile before attempting supervised weight loss, since cigarette smoking may be more harmful than obesity.

Obesity should be managed in an appropriate setting by staff who have been trained in the management of obesity in children; the individual or carer should receive advice on diet and lifestyle modification and should be monitored for changes in weight as well as in blood pressure, blood lipids, and other associated conditions.

NICE has recommended (December 2006) that drug treatment should only be considered for obese children after dietary, exercise, and behavioural approaches have been started, and who have associated conditions such as orthopaedic problems or sleep apnoea; treatment is intended both to facilitate weight loss and to maintain reduced weight. Initial treatment should involve a 6–12 month trial of orlistat or sibutramine, with regular reviews of effectiveness, tolerance, and adherence.

Choice   **Orlistat**, a lipase inhibitor, reduces the absorption of dietary fat. Some weight loss in those taking orlistat probably results from a reduction in fat intake to avoid severe gastro-intestinal effects including steatorrhoea. Vitamin supplementation (especially of vitamin D) may be considered if there is concern about deficiency of fat-soluble vitamins.

Sibutramine is a centrally acting appetite suppressant that inhibits the re-uptake of noradrenaline and serotonin.

There is little evidence to guide selection between orlistat and sibutramine, but it may be appropriate to choose orlistat for those who have a high intake of fat whereas sibutramine may be chosen for those who cannot control their eating; the cautions, contra-indications and side-effects of the two drugs should also be considered. On stopping treatment with orlistat or sibutramine there may be a gradual reversal of weight loss.

Combination therapy involving more than one anti-obesity drug should not be used until further information about efficacy and long-term safety is available.

Thyroid hormones have no place in the treatment of obesity except in biochemically proven hypothyroid children. The use of diuretics, chorionic gonadotrophin, or amphetamines is not appropriate for weight reduction.

4.6 Drugs used in nausea and vertigo

Antiemetics should be prescribed only when the cause of vomiting is known because otherwise they may delay diagnosis. Antiemetics are unnecessary and sometimes harmful when the cause can be treated, such as in diabetic ketoacidosis, or in digoxin or antiepileptic overdose.

If antiemetic drug treatment is indicated, the drug is chosen according to the aetiology of vomiting.

Antihistamines are effective against nausea and vomiting resulting from many underlying conditions. There is no evidence that any one antihistamine is superior to another but their duration of action and incidence of adverse effects (drowsiness and antimuscarinic effects) differ.

The **phenothiazines** are dopamine antagonists and act centrally by blocking the chemoreceptor trigger zone. They may be considered for the prophylaxis and treatment of nausea and vomiting associated with diffuse neoplastic disease, radiation sickness, and the emesis caused by drugs such as opioids, general anaesthetics, and cytotoxics. **Prochlorperazine**, **perphenazine**, and **trifluoperazine** are less sedating than **chlorpromazine**; severe dystonic reactions sometimes occur with phenothiazines (see below). Other antipsychotic drugs including

haloperidol and **levomepromazine** (methotrimeprazine) (section 4.2.1) are also used for the relief of nausea in palliative care (see p. 27 and p. 28). Some phenothiazines are available as rectal suppositories, which can be useful in children with persistent vomiting or with severe nausea; for children over 12 years prochlorperazine can also be administered as a buccal tablet which is placed between the upper lip and the gum.

Metoclopramide is an effective antiemetic and its activity closely resembles that of the phenothiazines. Metoclopramide also acts directly on the gastro-intestinal tract and it may be superior to the phenothiazines for emesis associated with gastroduodenal, hepatic, and biliary disease. In postoperative nausea and vomiting, metoclopramide has limited efficacy. For the role of metoclopramide in cytotoxic-induced nausea and vomiting see section 8.1.

> Acute dystonic reactions
> Phenothiazines and metoclopramide can all induce acute dystonic reactions such as facial and skeletal muscle spasms and oculogyric crises; children (especially girls, young women, and those under 10 kg) are particularly susceptible. With metoclopramide, dystonic effects usually occur shortly after starting treatment and subside within 24 hours of stopping it. An antimuscarinic drug such as procyclidine (section 4.9.2) is used to abort dystonic attacks.

Domperidone acts at the chemoreceptor trigger zone; it has the advantage over metoclopramide and the phenothiazines of being less likely to cause central effects such as sedation and dystonic reactions because it does not readily cross the blood-brain barrier. For the role of domperidone in cytotoxic-induced nausea and vomiting see section 8.1. Domperidone is also used to treat vomiting due to emergency hormonal contraception (section 7.3.5).

Granisetron and **ondansetron** are specific $5HT_3$ antagonists which block $5HT_3$ receptors in the gastro-intestinal tract and in the CNS. They are of value in the management of nausea and vomiting in children receiving cytotoxics and in postoperative nausea and vomiting.

Nabilone is a synthetic cannabinoid with antiemetic properties. It may be used for nausea and vomiting caused by cytotoxic chemotherapy that is unresponsive to conventional antiemetics. Side-effects such as drowsiness and dizziness occur frequently with standard doses.

Dexamethasone (section 6.3.2) has antiemetic effects. For the role of dexamethasone in cytotoxic-induced nausea and vomiting see section 8.1.

Vomiting during pregnancy

Nausea in the first trimester of pregnancy is generally mild and does not require drug therapy. On rare occasions if vomiting is severe, short-term treatment with an antihistamine, such as **promethazine**, may be required. **Prochlorperazine** or **metoclopramide** may be considered as second-line treatments. If symptoms do not settle in 24 to 48 hours then specialist opinion should be sought. Hyperemesis gravidarum is a more serious condition, which requires intravenous fluid and electrolyte replacement and sometimes nutritional support. Supplementation with thiamine must be considered in order to reduce the risk of Wernicke's encephalopathy.

Postoperative nausea and vomiting

The incidence of postoperative nausea and vomiting depends on many factors including the anaesthetic used, and the type and duration of surgery. The aim is to prevent postoperative nausea and vomiting from occurring. Drugs used include some **phenothiazines** (e.g. prochlorperazine), **metoclopramide**, **$5HT_3$ antagonists**, **antihistamines** (such as cyclizine), and **dexamethasone**. A combination of two antiemetic drugs acting at different sites may be needed in resistant postoperative nausea and vomiting.

Opioid-induced nausea and vomiting

Cyclizine, ondansetron, and prochlorperazine are used to relieve opioid-induced nausea and vomiting; ondansetron has the advantage of not producing sedation.

Central nervous system

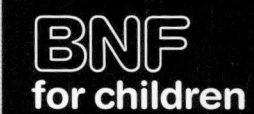

Dear BNFC user

Welcome to *BNF for Children* 2009. We have highlighted below some of the key changes you will find in this new edition.

New sections

Intravenous infusions for neonatal intensive care
A new appendix on intravenous infusions for neonatal intensive care has been added to this edition (Appendix 4, p. 921). As well as providing practical information on preparing intravenous infusions in this setting, it includes a table of detailed administration instructions for key drugs. Drug-specific information can also be found in the Administration section of the monographs.

How BNFC is constructed
This new section (p. viii) provides valuable insight into how the national prescribing resource is constructed.

Updated advice

Caffeine
Caffeine (as caffeine base) is now licensed for the treatment of apnoea of prematurity. For safety reasons, the caffeine monograph in BNFC (p. 202) recommends that the dose should be expressed in terms of caffeine base and *not* caffeine citrate.

Hospital-acquired pneumonia
Guidance on the treatment of hospital-acquired pneumonia has been revised in Table 1, section 5.1 (p. 300). Children with early-onset infection can be treated in a similar way to children with severe community-acquired pneumonia of unknown aetiology. More broad-spectrum antibacterials are recommended for children with late-onset infection that occurs more than 5 days after admission to hospital, for life-threatening infection, or if resistant organisms are suspected.

Otitis media
Most uncomplicated cases of acute otitis media resolve without antibacterial treatment. In children without systemic features, antibacterial treatment may be started after 72 hours if there is no improvement. Guidance on earlier antibacterial treatment of otitis media has been updated in BNFC (p. 303 and p. 646) to take into account the

recommendations of the NICE guidance: *Prescribing of antibiotics for self-limiting respiratory tract infections in adults and children in primary care (July 2008)*. Earlier treatment can be considered if the condition deteriorates, if the child is systemically unwell, if the child is at high risk of serious complications (e.g. in immunosuppression, cystic fibrosis), if mastoiditis is present, or in children under 2 years of age with bilateral otitis media. Perforation of the tympanic membrane in children with acute otitis media usually resolves spontaneously without treatment, but a systemic antibacterial can be given if there is no improvement.

Influenza
Safety data on the use of oseltamivir in children under 1 year of age is limited and it is not licensed for use in this age group. Furthermore, oseltamivir may be ineffective in neonates and very young infants because they may not be able to metabolise oseltamivir to its active form. BNFC recommends that in exceptional circumstances, oseltamivir can be used under specialist supervision for the treatment or post-exposure prophylaxis of influenza in children under 1 year of age (p. 390). The Department of Health has advised (May 2009) that, during a pandemic, treatment of children under 1 year with oseltamivir can be overseen by healthcare professionals experienced in assessing children.

BNFC also includes a summary of the latest NICE guidance on the prevention and treatment of influenza (p. 391).

New safety information

Inadvertent switching between tacrolimus proprietary products
There have been reports to the MHRA of serious medication errors occurring when patients were switched between different preparations of tacrolimus. *Prograf* ® is an immediate-release preparation taken twice daily, and *Advagraf* ® is a prolonged-release preparation taken once daily. Substitution between *Prograf* ® and *Advagraf* ® should be made only under the close supervision of a transplant specialist. *Advagraf* ® is not licensed for use in children, but BNFC has included the MHRA/CHM advice (December 2008) in section 8.2.2 (p. 524) so that healthcare professionals are alerted to the danger of switching between tacrolimus proprietary products.

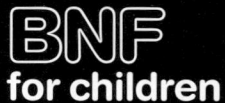
BNF for children

Reorganised sections in BNFC 2009

Chapter 14: Immunological products and vaccines
The chapter on immunological products and vaccines has been updated and reformatted as follows:

- section 14.1 now includes information that is common to all vaccines, including cautions, contra-indications, and side-effects, as well as other advice, such as administration of vaccines to those who are immunocompromised because of drugs or disease (e.g. HIV infection), and in pregnancy and during breast-feeding;
- the immunisation schedule has been moved into a table for ease of use;
- section 14.4 has been restructured to follow the same style as the rest of BNFC, i.e. notes for prescribers followed by a monograph and preparation entries.

Appendix 2: Borderline substances
The appendix on borderline substances (Appendix 2) has been revised. Tables of ACBS-approved enteral feeds and nutritional supplements have been created, based on their energy and protein content. There are separate tables for feeds and supplements suitable for use in children and infants. Additional nutritional information is included for standard dilutions of powder formulations throughout the appendix.

Guidance notes at the beginning of Appendix 2, and in Chapter 9 (p. 562), have also been updated to provide more information on the use of enteral feeds and nutritional supplements in children, and the use of special feeds for infants with specific food intolerance.

e-newsletter

The e-newsletter is 1 year old and thriving! If you have not registered, we recommend that you visit the e-newsletter archive at http://bnfc.org/bnfc/bnfcextra/current/450066.htm to find out what you are missing. Newsletters are free, and alert you to significant changes in the clinical content of the BNF and BNFC and to the way that this information is delivered. Newsletters also review clinical case studies to help put this therapeutic advice into practice and provide tips on using the publications effectively. If you would like to be kept informed of the latest changes that are influencing clinical practice, please sign up at http://bnf.org/newsletter.

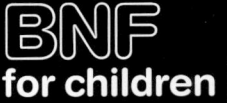
BNF
for children

Digital developments

Index added to online versions of BNFC

BNFC online is now available with a browseable index. This has been developed in response to feedback from users and is intended to give access to the content via an additional route that will be familiar to the many readers who have traditionally used print versions of BNFC. In addition, users who are unsure of the precise spelling of a particular drug name or condition may feel more comfortable browsing the index, rather than relying on the misspelling algorithm that is part of the BNFC search function.

The index complements the existing search functionality by providing links to entries in the main body of BNFC text and to information in Appendixes 2 and 4 (Borderline Substances and Intravenous infusions for Neonatal Intensive Care). Advice in Appendix 1 (Interactions) is not indexed, but this section can be easily accessed by browsing the main hierarchy or by using the interactions search engine.

Distribution of BNFCs

The UK health departments distribute BNFCs to NHS hospitals, doctors, and community pharmacies. For information on the supply of copies of the BNFC to NHS organisations, see the DH website http://tinyurl.com/2uebpp. Alternatively, copies may be obtained through any bookseller or direct from www.pharmpress.com.

Pharmaid

Numerous requests have been received from developing countries for BNFCs. The Pharmaid scheme of the Commonwealth Pharmacists Association will dispatch old BNFCs to Commonwealth countries. BNFCs will be collected from certain community pharmacies in November. For further details check the health press or contact:

Betty Falconbridge
Tel: 020 7572 2364
Email: admin@commonwealthpharmacy.org

Feedback

We welcome feedback from you. If you have any comments or suggestions please let us know at bnfc@bnf.org.

Motion sickness

Antiemetics should be given to prevent motion sickness rather than after nausea or vomiting develop. The most effective drug for the prevention of motion sickness is **hyoscine hydrobromide**. For children over 10 years old, a transdermal hyoscine patch provides prolonged activity but it needs to be applied several hours before travelling. The sedating antihistamines are slightly less effective against motion sickness, but are generally better tolerated than hyoscine. If a sedative effect is desired **promethazine** is useful, but generally a slightly less sedating antihistamine such as **cyclizine** or **cinnarizine** is preferred. The 5HT$_3$ antagonists, domperidone, metoclopramide, and the phenothiazines (except the antihistamine phenothiazine promethazine) are **ineffective** in motion sickness.

Other vestibular disorders

Management of vestibular diseases is aimed at treating the underlying cause as well as treating symptoms of the balance disturbance and associated nausea and vomiting.

Antihistamines (such as cinnarizine), and **phenothiazines** (such as prochlorperazine) are effective for prophylaxis and treatment of nausea and vertigo resulting from vestibular disorders; however, when nausea and vertigo are associated with middle ear surgery, treatment can be difficult.

Cytotoxic chemotherapy

For the management of nausea and vomiting induced by cytotoxic chemotherapy, see section 8.1.

Palliative care

For the management of nausea and vomiting in palliative care, see p. 27 and p. 28.

Migraine

For the management of nausea and vomiting associated with migraine, see p. 263.

Antihistamines

CINNARIZINE

Cautions see section 3.4.1

Hepatic impairment sedation inappropriate in severe liver disease—avoid

Pregnancy manufacturer advises avoid

Breast-feeding although not known to be harmful, manufacturer advises avoid

Contra-indications see section 3.4.1

Side-effects see section 3.4.1; also *rarely* weight gain, sweating, lichen planus, and lupus-like skin reactions

Indication and dose

Relief of symptoms of vestibular disorders
• By mouth
Child 5–12 years 15 mg 3 times daily
Child 12–18 years 30 mg 3 times daily

Motion sickness
• By mouth
Child 5–12 years 15 mg 2 hours before travel then 7.5 mg every 8 hours during journey if necessary
Child 12–18 years 30 mg 2 hours before travel then 15 mg every 8 hours during journey if necessary

Cinnarizine (Non-proprietary)
Tablets, cinnarizine 15 mg, net price 84-tab pack = £15.91. Label: 2

Stugeron® (Janssen-Cilag)
Tablets, scored, cinnarizine 15 mg, net price 15-tab pack = £1.48, 100-tab pack = £3.49. Label: 2

CYCLIZINE

Cautions see section 3.4.1; severe heart failure; may counteract haemodynamic benefits of opioids; **interactions**: Appendix 1 (antihistamines)

Hepatic impairment sedation inappropriate in severe liver disease—avoid
Skilled tasks Drowsiness may affect performance of skilled tasks (e.g. driving); effects of alcohol enhanced

Contra-indications see section 3.4.1

Side-effects see section 3.4.1

Licensed use tablets not licensed for use in children under 6 years; injection not licensed for use in children

◁ **CYCLIZINE** (*continued*)

Indication and dose

Nausea and vomiting of known cause; nausea and vomiting associated with vestibular disorders and palliative care

* **By mouth or by intravenous injection over 3–5 minutes**

  Child 1 month–6 years 0.5–1 mg/kg up to 3 times daily; max. single dose 25 mg

  Child 6–12 years 25 mg up to 3 times daily

  Child 12–18 years 50 mg up to 3 times daily

* **By rectum**

  Child 2–6 years 12.5 mg up to 3 times daily

  Child 6–12 years 25 mg up to 3 times daily

  Child 12–18 years 50 mg up to 3 times daily

* **By continuous intravenous or subcutaneous infusion**

  Child 1 month–2 years 3 mg/kg over 24 hours

  Child 2–5 years 50 mg over 24 hours

  Child 6–12 years 75 mg over 24 hours

  Child 12–18 years 150 mg over 24 hours

Administration for administration *by mouth*, tablets may be crushed

Valoid® (Amdipharm)

Tablets, scored, cyclizine hydrochloride 50 mg. Net price 100 = £7.41. Label: 2

Injection (PoM), cyclizine lactate 50 mg/mL. Net price 1-mL amp = 49p

Cyclizine (Non-proprietary)

Suppositories, 12.5 mg, 25 mg, 50 mg, 100 mg. Available from 'special-order' manufacturers or specialist importing companies, see p. 943

PROMETHAZINE HYDROCHLORIDE

Cautions see section 3.4.1

Contra-indications see section 3.4.1

Side-effects see section 3.4.1 but more sedating

Indication and dose

Nausea and vomiting

* **By mouth**

  Child 2–5 years 5 mg at bedtime on night before travel, repeat following morning if necessary

  Child 5–10 years 10 mg at bedtime on night before travel, repeat following morning if necessary

  Child 10–18 years 20–25 mg at bedtime on night before travel, repeat following morning if necessary

Allergy and urticaria section 3.4.1

Sedation section 4.1.1

◀ Preparations
Section 3.4.1

PROMETHAZINE TEOCLATE

Cautions see section 3.4.1

Contra-indications see section 3.4.1

Side-effects see section 3.4.1

Licensed use not licensed to treat vomiting of pregnancy

Indication and dose

Nausea, vomiting, labyrinthine disorders

* **By mouth**

  Child 5–10 years 12.5–37.5 mg daily

  Child 10–18 years 25–75 mg daily (max. 100 mg)

Motion sickness prevention

* **By mouth**

  Child 5–10 years 12.5 mg at bedtime on night before travel *or* 12.5 mg 1–2 hours before travel

  Child 10–18 years 25 mg at bedtime on night before travel *or* 25 mg 1–2 hours before travel

Severe vomiting during pregnancy

* **By mouth**

  25 mg at bedtime increased if necessary to max. 100 mg daily (but see also Vomiting During Pregnancy, p. 238)

Avomine® (Manx)

Tablets, scored, promethazine teoclate 25 mg. Net price 10-tab pack = £1.13; 28-tab pack = £3.13. Label: 2

Phenothiazines and related drugs

CHLORPROMAZINE HYDROCHLORIDE

Cautions see Chlorpromazine Hydrochloride, section 4.2.1

Contra-indications see Chlorpromazine Hydrochloride, section 4.2.1

Side-effects see Chlorpromazine Hydrochloride, section 4.2.1

Indication and dose

Nausea and vomiting of terminal illness (where other drugs are unsuitable)

• By mouth

Child 1–6 years 500 micrograms/kg every 4–6 hours; max. 40 mg daily

Child 6–12 years 500 micrograms/kg every 4–6 hours; max. 75 mg daily

Child 12–18 years 10–25 mg every 4–6 hours

• By deep intramuscular injection

Child 1–6 years 500 micrograms/kg every 6–8 hours; max. 40 mg daily

Child 6–12 years 500 micrograms/kg every 6–8 hours; max. 75 mg daily

Child 12–18 years initially 25 mg then 25–50 mg every 3–4 hours until vomiting stops

◢Preparations
Section 4.2.1

PERPHENAZINE

Cautions see Perphenazine, section 4.2.1

Contra-indications see Perphenazine, section 4.2.1

Side-effects see Perphenazine, section 4.2.1; extrapyramidal symptoms

Indication and dose

Severe nausea and vomiting unresponsive to other antiemetics

• By mouth

Child 14–18 years 4 mg 3 times daily, adjusted according to response, max. 24 mg daily

◢Preparations
Section 4.2.1

PROCHLORPERAZINE

Cautions see Prochlorperazine, section 4.2.1; hypotension more likely after intramuscular injection

Contra-indications see Prochlorperazine, section 4.2.1

Side-effects see Prochlorperazine, section 4.2.1; extrapyramidal symptoms, particularly dystonias, more frequent; respiratory depression may occur in susceptible children

Licensed use injection not licensed for use in children

Indication and dose

Prevention and treatment of nausea and vomiting

• By mouth

Child 1–12 years and over 10 kg 250 micrograms/kg 2–3 times daily

Child 12–18 years 5–10 mg, repeated if necessary up to 3 times daily

• By intramuscular injection

Child 2–5 years, 1.25–2.5 mg, repeated if necessary up to 3 times daily

Child 5–12 years 5–6.25 mg, repeated if necessary up to 3 times daily

Child 12–18 years 12.5 mg, repeated if necessary up to 3 times daily

Note Doses are expressed as prochlorperazine maleate or mesilate; 1 mg prochlorperazine maleate ≡ 1 mg prochlorperazine mesilate

Prochlorperazine (Non-proprietary) ℗ₒₘ
Tablets, prochlorperazine maleate 5 mg, net price 28 = £2.09, 84 = £4.14. Label: 2

Stemetil® (Castlemead) ℗ₒₘ
Tablets, prochlorperazine maleate 5 mg (off-white), net price 84-tab pack = £6.18. Label: 2

Syrup, straw-coloured, prochlorperazine mesilate 5 mg/5 mL. Net price 100-mL pack = £3.48. Label: 2

Injection, prochlorperazine mesilate 12.5 mg/mL. Net price 1-mL amp = 54p

◢Buccal preparation
Buccastem® (R&C) ℗ₒₘ
Tablets (buccal), pale yellow, prochlorperazine maleate 3 mg. Net price 5 × 10-tab pack = £5.75. Label: 2, counselling, administration, see under Dose below

Dose
• By mouth
Child 12–18 years 1–2 tablets twice daily; tablets are placed high between upper lip and gum and left to dissolve

▲ TRIFLUOPERAZINE

Cautions see Trifluoperazine section 4.2.1

Contra-indications see Trifluoperazine section 4.2.1

Side-effects see Trifluoperazine section 4.2.1; extrapyramidal symptoms

Indication and dose

> Severe nausea and vomiting unresponsive to other antiemetics
> • **By mouth**
> > **Child 3–5 years** up to 500 micrograms twice daily

> **Child 6–12 years** up to 2 mg twice daily

> **Child 12–18 years** 1–2 mg twice daily; max. 3 mg twice daily

◀Preparations
Section 4.2.1

Domperidone and metoclopramide

▲ DOMPERIDONE

Cautions children; **interactions**: Appendix 1 (domperidone)

> **Renal impairment** manufacturer advises reduce dose in renal impairment

> **Breast-feeding** amount probably too small to be harmful

Contra-indications prolactinaemia; where increased gastro-intestinal motility harmful

> **Hepatic impairment** avoid

> **Pregnancy** manufacturer advises avoid

Side-effects *rarely* gastro-intestinal disturbances (including cramps), and hyperprolactinaemia; *very rarely* extrapyramidal effects and rashes

Indication and dose

> Nausea and vomiting
> • **By mouth**
> > **Child over 1 month and body-weight up to 35 kg** 250–500 micrograms/kg 3–4 times daily; max. 2.4 mg/kg in 24 hours
> > **Body-weight 35 kg and over** 10–20 mg 3–4 times daily, max. 80 mg daily

> • **By rectum**
> > **Body-weight 15–35 kg** 30 mg twice daily
> > **Body-weight over 35 kg** 60 mg twice daily

> Gastro-intestinal stasis section 1.2

Domperidone (Non-proprietary) [PoM]
Tablets, 10 mg (as maleate), net price 30-tab pack = £1.37; 100-tab pack = £2.55

Suspension, domperidone 5 mg/mL, net price 200-mL pack = £7.00

Motilium® (Winthrop) [PoM]
Tablets, f/c, domperidone 10 mg (as maleate), net price 30-tab pack = £2.82; 100-tab pack = £9.41

Suspension, sugar-free, domperidone 5 mg/5 mL, net price 200-mL pack = £2.16

Suppositories, domperidone 30 mg, net price 10 = £3.18

▲ METOCLOPRAMIDE HYDROCHLORIDE

Cautions atopic allergy (including asthma); may mask underlying disorders such as cerebral irritation; epilepsy; acute porphyria (section 9.8.2); **interactions**: Appendix 1 (metoclopramide)

> **Hepatic impairment** reduce dose

> **Renal impairment** avoid or use small dose; increased risk of extrapyramidal reactions in severe impairment

> **Pregnancy** not known to be harmful but manufacturer advises use only when compelling reasons

Contra-indications gastro-intestinal obstruction, perforation or haemorrhage; 3–4 days after gastro-intestinal surgery; phaeochromocytoma

> **Breast-feeding** small amount present in milk; manufacturer advises avoid large single doses

Side-effects extrapyramidal effects (see p. 238), hyperprolactinaemia, occasionally tardive dyskinesia on prolonged administration; also reported, anxiety, confusion, drowsiness, restlessness, diarrhoea, depression, neuroleptic malignant syndrome, rashes, pruritus, oedema; cardiac conduction abnormalities reported following intravenous administration; *rarely* methaemoglobinaemia (more severe in G6PD deficiency)

Licensed use not licensed for use in neonates as a prokinetic

Indication and dose

> Severe intractable vomiting of known cause, vomiting associated with radiotherapy and cytotoxics, aid to gastro-intestinal intubation, as a prokinetic in neonates
> • **By mouth, or by intramuscular injection or by intravenous injection over 1–2 minutes**
> > **Neonate** 100 micrograms/kg every 6–8 hours (by mouth or by intravenous injection only)

> > **Child 1 month–1 year and body-weight up to 10 kg** 100 micrograms/kg (max. 1 mg) twice daily

◁ **METOCLOPRAMIDE HYDROCHLORIDE (*continued*)**

Child 1–3 years and body-weight 10–14 kg
1 mg 2–3 times daily

Child 3–5 years and body-weight 15–19 kg
2 mg 2–3 times daily

Child 5–9 years and body-weight 20–29 kg
2.5 mg 3 times daily

Child 9–18 years and body-weight 30–60 kg
5 mg 3 times daily

Child 15–18 years and body-weight over 60 kg
10 mg 3 times daily
Note Daily dose of metoclopramide should not normally exceed 500 micrograms/kg

Premedication in diagnostic procedures
• **By mouth as a single dose 5–10 minutes before examination**

Child 1 month–3 years and body-weight up to 14 kg 100 micrograms/kg, max. 1 mg

Child 3–5 years and body-weight 15–19 kg
2 mg

Child 5–9 years and body-weight 20–29 kg
2.5 mg

Child 9–15 years and body-weight 30–60 kg
5 mg

Child 15–18 years and body-weight over 60 kg
10 mg

Metoclopramide (Non-proprietary) PoM
Tablets, metoclopramide hydrochloride 10 mg, net price 28-tab pack = 90p

Oral solution, metoclopramide hydrochloride 5 mg/5 mL, net price 100-mL pack = £3.83. Counselling, use of pipette

Note Sugar-free versions are available and can be ordered by specifying 'sugar-free' on the prescription

Injection, metoclopramide hydrochloride 5 mg/mL, net price 2-mL amp = 26p

Maxolon® (Amdipharm) PoM
Tablets, scored, metoclopramide hydrochloride 10 mg, net price 84-tab pack = £5.25

Syrup, sugar-free, metoclopramide hydrochloride 5 mg/5 mL. Net price 200-mL pack = £3.83

Paediatric liquid, sugar-free, metoclopramide hydrochloride 1 mg/mL. Net price 15-mL pack with pipette = £1.51. Counselling, use of pipette

Injection, metoclopramide hydrochloride 5 mg/mL. Net price 2-mL amp = 27p

◀Compound preparations (for migraine)
Section 4.7.4.1

5HT₃ antagonists

GRANISETRON

Cautions
Pregnancy manufacturer advises use only when compelling reasons—no information available
Breast-feeding manufacturer advises avoid—no information available
Side-effects constipation, headache, rash; hypersensitivity reactions reported; *rarely* movement disorders
Licensed use sterile solution not licensed for use in children under 2 years

Indication and dose
Treatment and prevention of nausea and vomiting induced by cytotoxic chemotherapy or radiotherapy
• **By mouth**

Child 12–18 years 1–2 mg within 1 hour before start of treatment, then 1 mg twice daily during treatment (total daily dose may alternatively be given as a single dose); when intravenous infusion also used, max. combined total 9 mg in 24 hours

• **By intravenous infusion**

Child 1 month–12 years prevention, 40 micrograms/kg (max. 3 mg) before start of cytotoxic therapy; treatment, 40 micrograms/kg (max. 3 mg) repeated within 24 hours if necessary (not less than 10 minutes after initial dose)

• **By intravenous injection or by intravenous infusion**

Child 12–18 years prevention, 3 mg before start of cytotoxic therapy (up to 2 additional 3-mg doses may be given within 24 hours); treatment, 3 mg repeated if necessary (doses must not be given less than 10 minutes apart), max. 9 mg in 24 hours

Administration for *intravenous infusion*, dilute 3 mL in 10–30 mL Glucose 5% *or* Sodium Chloride 0.9%, *or* Compound Sodium Lactate; give over 5 minutes

Kytril® (Roche) PoM
Tablets, f/c, granisetron (as hydrochloride) 1 mg, net price 10-tab pack = £65.49; 2 mg, 5-tab pack = £65.49

Sterile solution, granisetron (as hydrochloride) 1 mg/mL, for dilution and use as injection or infusion, net price 1-mL amp = £8.60, 3-mL amp = £25.79

4

Central nervous system

▲ ONDANSETRON

Cautions QT interval prolongation (avoid concomitant administration of drugs that prolong QT interval)

Hepatic impairment reduce dose in moderate or severe hepatic impairment

Pregnancy no information available; manufacturer advises avoid unless potential benefit outweighs risk

Breast-feeding manufacturer advises avoid—no information available

Side-effects constipation; headache; flushing; injection-site reactions; *less commonly* hiccups, hypotension, bradycardia, chest pain, arrhythmias, movement disorders, seizures; *on intravenous administration, rarely* dizziness, transient visual disturbances (*very rarely* transient blindness)

Licensed use oral and parenteral preparations not licensed for use in children under 2 years

Indication and dose

Prevention and treatment of chemotherapy- and radiotherapy-induced nausea and vomiting

• By slow intravenous injection or by intravenous infusion

Child 1–12 years 5 mg/m² immediately before chemotherapy (max. single dose 8 mg), then **either** repeat every 8–12 hours during chemotherapy and for at least 24 hours afterwards **or** give by mouth

Child 12–18 years 8 mg immediately before chemotherapy, then **either** repeated every 8–12 hours during chemotherapy and for at least 24 hours afterwards **or** give by mouth

• By mouth following intravenous administration

Child 1–12 years 4 mg every 8–12 hours for up to 5 days

Child 12–18 years 8 mg every 8–12 hours for up to 5 days

Treatment and prevention of postoperative nausea and vomiting

• By slow intravenous injection

Child 2–12 years 100 micrograms/kg (max. 4 mg), as a single dose before, during, or after induction of anaesthesia

Child 12–18 years 4 mg, as a single dose at induction of anaesthesia

Administration for *slow intravenous injection*, give over 2–5 minutes

For *intravenous infusion*, dilute to a concentration of 320–640 micrograms/mL with Glucose 5% *or* Sodium Chloride 0.9% *or* Ringer's Solution; give over at least 15 minutes

Ondansetron (Non-proprietary) ℞

Tablets, ondansetron (as hydrochloride) 4 mg, net price 30-tab pack = £89.69; 8 mg, 10-tab pack = £59.71
Brands include *Ondemet*®

Injection, ondansetron (as hydrochloride) 2 mg/mL, net price 2-mL amp = £5.39, 4-mL amp = £10.79
Brands include *Ondemet*®

Zofran® (GSK) ℞

Tablets, yellow, f/c, ondansetron (as hydrochloride) 4 mg, net price 30-tab pack = £107.91; 8 mg, 10-tab pack = £71.94

Oral lyophilisates (*Zofran Melt*®), ondansetron 4 mg, net price 10-tab pack = £35.97; 8 mg, 10-tab pack = £71.94. Counselling, administration
Excipients include aspartame (section 9.4.1)

Counselling Tablets should be placed on the tongue, allowed to disperse and swallowed

Syrup, sugar-free, strawberry-flavoured, ondansetron (as hydrochloride) 4 mg/5 mL, net price 50-mL pack = £35.97

Injection, ondansetron (as hydrochloride) 2 mg/mL, net price 2-mL amp = £5.99; 4-mL amp = £11.99

Cannabinoid

▲ NABILONE

Cautions history of psychiatric disorder; hypertension; heart disease; adverse effects on mental state can persist for 48–72 hours after stopping; **interactions:** Appendix 1 (nabilone)
Skilled tasks Drowsiness may affect performance of skilled tasks (e.g. driving); effects of alcohol enhanced

Contra-indications

Hepatic impairment avoid in severe hepatic impairment

Pregnancy manufacturer advises avoid unless essential

Breast-feeding no information available—manufacturer advises avoid

Side-effects drowsiness, vertigo, euphoria, dry mouth, ataxia, visual disturbance, concentration difficulties, sleep disturbance, dysphoria, hypotension, headache and nausea; also confusion, disorientation, hallucinations, psychosis, depression, decreased coordination, tremors, tachycardia, decreased appetite, and abdominal pain
Behavioural effects Children and carers should be made aware of possible changes of mood and other adverse behavioural effects

Licensed use not licensed for use in children

Indication and dose

Nausea and vomiting caused by cytotoxic chemotherapy, unresponsive to conventional antiemetics (under close observation, preferably in hospital setting)

• By mouth

Consult local treatment protocol for details

Nabilone (Valeant) ℞

Capsules, blue/white, nabilone 1 mg. Net price 20-cap pack = £125.84. Label: 2, counselling, behavioural effects

Hyoscine

HYOSCINE HYDROBROMIDE
(Scopolamine Hydrobromide)

Cautions urinary retention, cardiovascular disease, gastro-intestinal obstruction; **interactions:** Appendix 1 (antimuscarinics)

Skilled tasks Drowsiness may affect performance of skilled tasks (e.g. driving) and may persist for up to 24 hours or longer after removal of patch; effects of alcohol enhanced

Hepatic impairment manufacturer advises caution

Renal impairment manufacturer advises caution

Pregnancy manufacturer advises use only if potential benefit outweighs risk; injection may depress neonatal respiration

Breast-feeding amount too small to be harmful

Contra-indications closed-angle glaucoma

Side-effects drowsiness, dry mouth, dizziness, blurred vision, difficulty with micturition

Licensed use not licensed for use in excessive respiratory secretions or hypersalivation associated with clozapine therapy

Indication and dose

Motion sickness
- **By mouth**

    Child 4–10 years 75–150 micrograms 30 minutes before start of journey, repeated every 6 hours if required; max. 3 doses in 24 hours

    Child 10–18 years 150–300 micrograms 30 minutes before start of journey, repeated every 6 hours if required; max. 3 doses in 24 hours

- **By topical application**

    Child 10–18 years apply 1 patch (1 mg) to hairless area of skin behind ear 5–6 hours before journey; replace if necessary after 72 hours, siting replacement patch behind the other ear

Excessive respiratory secretions
- **By mouth or by sublingual administration**

    Child 2–12 years 10 micrograms/kg, max. 300 micrograms 4 times daily

    Child 12–18 years 300 micrograms 4 times daily

- **By transdermal route**

    Child 1 month–3 years 250 micrograms every 72 hours (quarter of a patch)

Child 3–10 years 500 micrograms every 72 hours (half a patch)

Child 10–18 years 1 mg every 72 hours (one patch)

- **By subcutaneous injection, intravenous injection, intravenous infusion, or subcutaneous infusion**

    See Prescribing in Palliative Care, p. 26 and p. 28

Hypersalivation associated with clozapine therapy
- **By mouth**

    Child 12–18 years 300 micrograms up to 3 times daily; max. 900 micrograms daily

Premedication section 15.1.3

Administration *patch* applied to hairless area of skin behind ear; if less than whole patch required **either** cut with scissors along full thickness ensuring membrane is not peeled away **or** cover portion to prevent contact with skin

For administration *by mouth*, injection solution may be given orally

Joy-Rides® (GSK Consumer Healthcare)
Chewable tablets, hyoscine hydrobromide 150 micrograms, net price 12-tab pack = £1.49. Label: 2, 24

Kwells® (Bayer Consumer Care)
Chewable tablets, hyoscine hydrobromide 150 micrograms (*Kwells® Kids*), net price 12-tab pack = £1.52; 300 micrograms, 12-tab pack = £1.52. Label: 2

Scopoderm TTS® (Novartis Consumer Health) [PoM]
Patch, self-adhesive, pink, releasing hyoscine approx. 1 mg/72 hours when in contact with skin. Net price 2 = £4.30. Label: 19, counselling, see below

Counselling Explain accompanying instructions to child and carer, in particular emphasise advice to wash hands after handling and to wash application site after removing, and to use one patch at a time

---

4.7 Analgesics

4.7.1 Non-opioid analgesics
4.7.2 Opioid analgesics
4.7.3 Neuropathic pain
4.7.4 Antimigraine drugs

The non-opioid drugs (section 4.7.1), paracetamol and ibuprofen (and other NSAIDs), are particularly suitable for pain in musculoskeletal conditions, whereas the opioid analgesics (section 4.7.2) are more suitable for moderate to severe pain, particularly of visceral origin.

4

Central nervous system

Pain in palliative care   For advice on pain relief in palliative care, see p. 24.

Pain in sickle-cell disease   The pain of mild sickle-cell crises is managed with paracetamol, an NSAID, codeine, or dihydrocodeine. Severe crises may require the use of morphine or diamorphine; concomitant use of an NSAID (section 10.1.1) may potentiate analgesia and allow lower doses of the opioid to be used. A mixture of nitrous oxide and oxygen (*Entonox*®, *Equanox*®) may also be used.

Dental and orofacial pain   Analgesics should be used judiciously in dental care as a **temporary** measure until the cause of the pain has been dealt with.

Dental pain of inflammatory origin, such as that associated with pulpitis, apical infection, localised osteitis (dry socket) or pericoronitis is usually best managed by treating the infection, providing drainage, restorative procedures, and other local measures. Analgesics provide temporary relief of pain (usually for about 1 to 7 days) until the causative factors have been brought under control. In the case of pulpitis, intra-osseous infection or abscess, reliance on analgesics alone is usually inappropriate.

Similarly the pain and discomfort associated with acute problems of the oral mucosa (e.g. acute herpetic gingivostomatitis, erythema multiforme) may be relieved by **benzydamine** (p. 655) or topical anaesthetics until the cause of the mucosal disorder has been dealt with. However, where a child is febrile, the antipyretic action of **paracetamol** (p. 247) or **ibuprofen** (p. 604) is often helpful.

The *choice* of an analgesic for dental purposes should be based on its suitability for the child. Most dental pain is relieved effectively by non-steroidal anti-inflammatory drugs (NSAIDs) e.g. ibuprofen (section 10.1.1). **Paracetamol** has analgesic and antipyretic effects but no anti-inflammatory effect.

Opioid analgesics (section 4.7.2) such as **dihydrocodeine** act on the central nervous system and are traditionally used for *moderate to severe pain*. However, opioid analgesics are relatively ineffective in dental pain and their side-effects can be unpleasant.

Combining a non-opioid with an opioid analgesic can provide greater relief of pain than either analgesic given alone. However, this applies only when an adequate dose of each analgesic is used. Most combination analgesic preparations have not been shown to provide greater relief of pain than an adequate dose of the non-opioid component given alone. Moreover, combination preparations have the disadvantage of an increased number of side-effects.

Any analgesic given before a dental procedure should have a low risk of increasing postoperative bleeding. In the case of pain after the dental procedure, taking an analgesic before the effect of the local anaesthetic has worn off can improve control. Postoperative analgesia with ibuprofen is usually continued for about 24 to 72 hours.

Dysmenorrhoea   Paracetamol or a NSAID (section 10.1.1) will generally provide adequate relief of pain from dysmenorrhoea. Alternatively use of a combined hormonal contraceptive in adolescent girls may prevent the pain.

4.7.1 Non-opioid analgesics

Paracetamol has analgesic and antipyretic properties but no demonstrable anti-inflammatory activity; unlike opioid analgesics, it does not cause respiratory depression and is less irritant to the stomach than the NSAIDs. **Overdosage** with paracetamol is particularly dangerous as it may cause hepatic damage which is sometimes not apparent for 4 to 6 days (see Emergency Treatment of Poisoning, p. 37).

Non-steroidal anti-inflammatory analgesics (NSAIDs, section 10.1.1) are particularly useful for the treatment of children with chronic disease accompanied by pain and inflammation. Some of them are also used in the short-term treatment of mild to moderate pain including transient musculoskeletal pain but paracetamol is now often preferred. They are also suitable for the relief of pain in *dysmenorrhoea* and to treat pain caused by *secondary bone tumours*, many of which produce lysis of bone and release prostaglandins (see Prescribing in Palliative Care, p. 24). Due to an association with Reye's syndrome (section 2.9), **aspirin** should be avoided in children under 16 years except in Kawasaki syndrome or for its antiplatelet action (section 2.9). NSAIDs are also used for peri-operative analgesia (section 15.1.4.2).

Dental and orofacial pain   Most dental pain is relieved effectively by NSAIDs (section 10.1.1).

Paracetamol is less irritant to the stomach than NSAIDs. Paracetamol is a suitable analgesic for children; sugar-free versions can be requested by specifying 'sugar-free' on the prescription.

For further information on the management of dental and orofacial pain, see notes above, p. 246.

Compound analgesic preparations

Compound analgesic preparations that contain a simple analgesic (such as aspirin or paracetamol) with an opioid component reduce the scope for effective titration of the individual components in the management of pain of varying intensity.

Compound analgesic preparations containing paracetamol or aspirin with a *low dose* of an opioid analgesic (e.g. 8 mg of codeine phosphate per compound tablet) may be used in older children but the advantages have not been substantiated. The low dose of the opioid may be enough to cause opioid side-effects (in particular, constipation) and can complicate the treatment of **overdosage** (see p. 39) yet may not provide significant additional relief of pain.

A *full dose* of the opioid component (e.g. 60 mg codeine phosphate) in compound analgesic preparations effectively augments the analgesic activity but is associated with the full range of opioid side-effects (including nausea, vomiting, severe constipation, drowsiness, respiratory depression, and risk of dependence on long-term administration). For details of the **side-effects** of opioid analgesics, see p. 249.

PARACETAMOL
(Acetaminophen)

Cautions   alcohol dependence; **interactions**: Appendix 1 (paracetamol)

Hepatic impairment   dose-related toxicity—avoid large doses

Renal impairment   increase *infusion* dose interval to every 6 hours if estimated glomerular filtration rate less than 30 mL/minute/1.73m^2

Pregnancy   not known to be harmful

Breast-feeding   amount too small to be harmful

Side-effects   side-effects rare, but rashes, blood disorders (including thrombocytopenia, leucopenia, neutropenia) reported; hypotension also reported on infusion; **important**: liver damage (and less frequently renal damage) following **overdosage**, see Emergency Treatment of Poisoning, p. 37

Licensed use   not licensed for use in children under 2 months by mouth; doses for severe symptoms not licensed

Indication and dose

Pain; pyrexia with discomfort
• By mouth

> **Neonate 28–32 weeks postmenstrual age**
> 20 mg/kg as a single dose then 10–15 mg/kg every 8–12 hours as necessary; max. 30 mg/kg daily in divided doses

> **Neonate over 32 weeks postmenstrual age**
> 20 mg/kg as a single dose then 10–15 mg/kg every 6–8 hours as necessary; max. 60 mg/kg daily in divided doses

> **Child 1–3 months** 30–60 mg every 8 hours as necessary; *for severe symptoms* 20 mg/kg as a single dose then 15–20 mg/kg every 6–8 hours; max. 60 mg/kg daily in divided doses

> **Child 3–12 months** 60–120 mg every 4–6 hours (max. 4 doses in 24 hours); *for severe symptoms* 20 mg/kg every 6 hours (max. 90 mg/kg daily in divided doses) for 48 hours (or longer if necessary and if adverse effects ruled out) then 15 mg/kg every 6 hours

> **Child 1–5 years** 120–250 mg every 4–6 hours (max. 4 doses in 24 hours); *for severe symptoms* 20 mg/kg every 6 hours (max. 90 mg/kg daily in divided doses) for 48 hours (or longer if necessary and if adverse effects ruled out) then 15 mg/kg every 6 hours

> **Child 6–12 years** 250–500 mg every 4–6 hours (max. 4 doses in 24 hours); *for severe symptoms* 20 mg/kg (max. 1 g) every 6 hours (max. 90 mg/kg daily in divided doses, not to exceed 4 g) for 48 hours (or longer if necessary and if adverse effects ruled out) then 15 mg/kg every 6 hours; max. 4 g daily

> **Child 12–18 years** 500 mg every 4–6 hours; *for severe symptoms* 1 g every 4–6 hours (max. 4 doses in 24 hours)

• By rectum

> **Neonate 28–32 weeks postmenstrual age**
> 20 mg/kg as a single dose then 15 mg/kg every 12 hours as necessary; max. 30 mg/kg daily in divided doses

> **Neonate over 32 weeks postmenstrual age**
> 30 mg/kg as a single dose then 20 mg/kg every 8 hours as necessary; max. 60 mg/kg daily in divided doses

> **Child 1–3 months** 30–60 mg every 8 hours as necessary; *for severe symptoms* 30 mg/kg as a single dose then 20 mg/kg every 8 hours; max. 60 mg/kg daily in divided doses

4 Central nervous system

◁ **PARACETAMOL** (*continued*)

Child 3–12 months 60–125 mg every 4–6 hours as necessary (max. 4 doses in 24 hours); *for severe symptoms* 40 mg/kg as a single dose then 20 mg/kg every 4–6 hours (max. 90 mg/kg daily in divided doses) for 48 hours (or longer if necessary and if adverse effects ruled out) then 15 mg/kg every 6 hours

Child 1–5 years 125–250 mg every 4–6 hours as necessary (max. 4 doses in 24 hours); *for severe symptoms* 40 mg/kg as a single dose then 20 mg/kg every 4–6 hours (max. 90 mg/kg daily in divided doses) for 48 hours (or longer if necessary and if adverse effects ruled out) then 15 mg/kg every 6 hours

Child 5–12 years 250–500 mg every 4–6 hours as necessary (max. 4 doses in 24 hours); *for severe symptoms* 40 mg/kg (max. 1 g) as a single dose then 20 mg/kg every 6 hours (max. 90 mg/kg daily in divided doses) for 48 hours (or longer if necessary and if adverse effects ruled out) then 15 mg/kg every 6 hours

Child 12–18 years 500 mg every 4–6 hours; *for severe symptoms* 1 g every 4–6 hours; max. 4 g daily in divided doses

• **By intravenous infusion over 15 minutes**

Neonate 7.5 mg/kg every 4–6 hours; max. 30 mg/kg daily

Child body-weight under 10 kg 7.5 mg/kg every 4–6 hours; max. 30 mg/kg daily

Child body-weight 10–50 kg 15 mg/kg every 4–6 hours; max. 60 mg/kg daily

Child body-weight over 50 kg 1 g every 4–6 hours; max. 4 g daily

Post-immunisation pyrexia in infants (see also p. 727)

• **By mouth**

Child 2–3 months 60 mg as a single dose repeated once after 6 hours if necessary

Paracetamol (Non-proprietary)
Tablets and caplets [PoM] [1], paracetamol 500 mg. Net price 16 = 17p, 32 = £1.14, 100 = £1.56. Label: 29, 30
Brands include *Panadol®* [JHS]

Capsules [PoM] [1], paracetamol 500 mg, net price 32-cap pack = £1.05. Label: 29, 30
Brands include *Panadol Capsules®* [JHS]

Soluble tablets (= Dispersible tablets) [PoM] [2], paracetamol 500 mg. Net price 60-tab pack = £4.03. Label: 13, 29, 30
Brands include *Panadol Soluble®* [JHS] (contains Na⁺ 18.6 mmol/tablet)

Paediatric soluble tablets (= Paediatric dispersible tablets), paracetamol 120 mg. Net price 16-tab pack = 89p. Label: 13, 30
Brands include *Disprol® Soluble Paracetamol* [JHS]

Oral suspension 120 mg/5 mL (= Paediatric Mixture), paracetamol 120 mg/5 mL. Net price 100 mL = 42p. Label: 30

Note BP directs that when Paediatric Paracetamol Oral Suspension or Paediatric Paracetamol Mixture is prescribed Paracetamol Oral Suspension 120 mg/5 mL should be dispensed; sugar-free versions can be ordered by specifying 'sugar-free' on the prescription
Brands include *Calpol® Paediatric, Calpol® Paediatric sugar-free, Disprol® Paediatric, Medinol® Paediatric sugar-free, Paldesic®, Panadol®* sugar-free

Oral suspension 250 mg/5 mL (= Mixture), paracetamol 250 mg/5 mL. Net price 100 mL = 66p. Label: 30
Brands include *Calpol® 6 Plus* [JHS]*, Medinol® Over 6* [JHS]*, Paldesic®*

Suppositories, paracetamol 60 mg, net price 10 = £9.96; 125 mg, 10 = £11.50; 250 mg, 10 = £23.00; 500 mg, 10 = £10.36. Label: 30
Brands include *Alvedon®*
Note other strengths available from 'special-order' manufacturers or specialist importing companies, see p. 943
Dental prescribing on NHS Paracetamol Tablets, Paracetamol Soluble Tablets 500 mg, and Paracetamol Oral Suspension may be prescribed

Perfalgan® (Bristol-Myers Squibb) ▼ [PoM]
Intravenous infusion, paracetamol 10 mg/mL, net price 50-mL vial = £1.80, 100-mL vial = £1.98
Administration give undiluted or dilute to a concentration of 1 mg/mL in Glucose 5% *or* Sodium Chloride 0.9%; use within 1 hour of dilution

◀ Co-codamol 8/500
When co-codamol tablets, dispersible (or effervescent) tablets, or capsules are prescribed and **no strength is stated**, tablets, dispersible (or effervescent) tablets, or capsules, respectively, containing codeine phosphate **8 mg** and paracetamol **500 mg** should be dispensed.

[2] **Co-codamol 8/500** (Non-proprietary) [PoM] ◀
Tablets, co-codamol 8/500 (codeine phosphate 8 mg, paracetamol 500 mg) Net price 30-tab pack = £1.05. Label: 29, 30
Brands include *Panadeine®* [JHS]

Dose
Pain, pyrexia
• **By mouth**
Child 6–12 years ½–1 tablet every 4–6 hours; max. 4 tablets daily
Child 12–18 years 1–2 tablets every 4–6 hours; max. 8 tablets daily

Effervescent *or* dispersible tablets, co-codamol 8/500 (codeine phosphate 8 mg, paracetamol

---

1. Can be sold to the public provided packs contain no more than 32 capsules or tablets; pharmacists can sell multiple packs up to a total quantity of 100 capsules or tablets in justifiable circumstances; for details see *Medicines, Ethics and Practice*, No. 32, London, Pharmaceutical Press, 2008 (and subsequent editions as available)
2. Can be sold to the public under certain circumstances; for exemptions see *Medicines, Ethics and Practice*, No. 32, London, Pharmaceutical Press, 2008 (and subsequent editions as available)

◻ **PARACETAMOL** *(continued)*

500 mg), net price 100-tab pack = £4.53. Label: 13, 29, 30

Brands include *Paracodol®* ⟨JHS⟩

Note The Drug Tariff allows tablets of co-codamol labelled 'dispersible' to be dispensed against an order for 'effervescent' and *vice versa*

Dose

Pain, pyrexia
• **By mouth**

Child 6–12 years ½–1 tablet in water every 4–6 hours; max. 4 tablets daily

Child 12–18 years 1–2 tablets in water every 4–6 hours; max. 8 tablets daily

Capsules, co-codamol 8/500 (codeine phosphate 8 mg, paracetamol 500 mg). Net price 10-cap pack = £1.10, 20-cap pack = £1.66. Label: 29, 30

Brands include *Paracodol®* ⟨JHS⟩

Dose

Pain, pyrexia
• **By mouth**

Child 12–18 years 1–2 capsules every 4 hours; max. 8 capsules daily

4.7.2 Opioid analgesics

Opioid analgesics are usually used to relieve moderate to severe pain particularly of visceral origin. Repeated administration may cause tolerance, but this is no deterrent in the control of pain in terminal illness, for guidelines see Prescribing in Palliative Care, p. 24. Regular use of a potent opioid may be appropriate for certain cases of chronic non-malignant pain; treatment should be supervised by a specialist and the child should be assessed at regular intervals.

Cautions Opioids should be used with caution in children with impaired respiratory function and asthma (avoid during an acute attack), hypotension, shock, obstructive or inflammatory bowel disorders, diseases of the biliary tract, and convulsive disorders. A reduced dose is recommended in hypothyroidism or adrenocortical insufficiency. Repeated use of opioid analgesics is associated with the development of psychological and physical dependence; although this is rarely a problem with therapeutic use, caution is advised if prescribing for patients with a history of drug dependence. Avoid abrupt withdrawal after long-term treatment. Transdermal preparations (fentanyl or buprenorphine patches) are not suitable for acute pain or in those children whose analgesic requirements are changing rapidly, because the long time to steady state prevents rapid titration of the dose.

Palliative care In the control of pain in terminal illness, the cautions listed above should not necessarily be a deterrent to the use of opioid analgesics.

Contra-indications Opioid analgesics should be avoided in children with acute respiratory depression, and when there is a risk of paralytic ileus. They are also contra-indicated in conditions associated with raised intracranial pressure, and in head injury (opioid analgesics interfere with pupillary responses vital for neurological assessment). Comatose children should not be treated with opioid analgesics.

Side-effects Opioid analgesics share many side-effects, although qualitative and quantitative differences exist. The most common side-effects include nausea and vomiting (particularly in initial stages), constipation, dry mouth and biliary spasm; larger doses produce muscle rigidity, hypotension and respiratory depression (for reversal of opioid-induced respiratory depression, see section 15.1.7); neonates, particularly if preterm, may be more susceptible. Other common side-effects of opioid analgesics include bradycardia, tachycardia, palpitation, oedema, postural hypotension, hallucinations, vertigo, euphoria, dysphoria, mood changes, dependence, dizziness, confusion, drowsiness, sleep disturbances, headache, sexual dysfunction, difficulty with micturition, urinary retention, ureteric spasm, miosis, visual disturbances, sweating, flushing, rash, urticaria, and pruritus. **Overdosage:** see Emergency Treatment of Poisoning, p. 39.

Interactions See Appendix 1 (opioid analgesics) (**important:** special hazard with *pethidine and possibly other opioids* and MAOIs).

Skilled tasks Drowsiness may affect performance of skilled tasks (e.g. driving); effects of alcohol enhanced.

4 Central nervous system

Choice   **Morphine** remains the most valuable opioid analgesic for severe pain although it frequently causes nausea and vomiting. It is the standard against which other opioid analgesics are compared. In addition to relief of pain, morphine also confers a state of euphoria and mental detachment.

Morphine is the opioid of choice for the oral treatment of *severe pain in palliative care*. It is given regularly every 4 hours (or every 12 or 24 hours as modified-release preparations). For guidelines on dosage adjustment in palliative care, see p. 24 .

Buprenorphine has both opioid agonist and antagonist properties and may precipitate withdrawal symptoms, including pain, in children dependent on other opioids. It has abuse potential and may itself cause dependence. It has a much longer duration of action than morphine and sublingually is an effective analgesic for 6 to 8 hours. Unlike most opioid analgesics, the effects of buprenorphine are only partially reversed by naloxone. It is used rarely in children.

Codeine is used for the relief of mild to moderate pain but is too constipating for long-term use.

Diamorphine (heroin) is a powerful opioid analgesic. It may cause less nausea and hypotension than morphine. In *palliative care* the greater solubility of diamorphine allows effective doses to be injected in smaller volumes and this is important in the emaciated child.

Diamorphine is sometimes given by the intranasal route to treat acute pain in children, for example, in accident and emergency units; however, as yet, there is limited safety and efficacy data to support this practice.

Dihydrocodeine has an analgesic efficacy similar to that of codeine; doses may be given every 4 hours.

Alfentanil, fentanyl and **remifentanil** are used by injection for intra-operative analgesia (section 15.1.4.3). Fentanyl is available in a transdermal drug delivery system as a self-adhesive patch which is changed every 72 hours.

Methadone is less sedating than morphine and acts for longer periods. In prolonged use, methadone should not be administered more often than twice daily to avoid the risk of accumulation and opioid overdosage. Methadone may be used instead of morphine when excitation (or exacerbation of pain) occurs with morphine. Methadone may also be used to treat children with neonatal abstinence syndrome (section 4.10).

Papaveretum should not be used in children; morphine is easier to prescribe and less prone to error with regard to the strength and dose.

Pethidine produces prompt but short-lasting analgesia; it is less constipating than morphine, but even in high doses is a less potent analgesic. Its use in children is not recommended. Pethidine is used for analgesia in labour; however, other opioids, such as morphine or diamorphine, are often preferred for obstetric pain.

Tramadol is used in older children and produces analgesia by two mechanisms: an opioid effect and an enhancement of serotonergic and adrenergic pathways. It has fewer of the typical opioid side-effects (notably, less respiratory depression, less constipation and less addiction potential); psychiatric reactions have been reported.

Dose   Doses of opioids may need to be **adjusted individually** according to the degree of analgesia and side-effects; response to opioids varies widely, particularly in the neonatal period. Opioid overdosage can have serious consequences and the dose should be calculated and **checked with care**.

Postoperative analgesia   A combination of opioid and non-opioid analgesics is used to treat post-operative pain (section 15.1.4.2). The use of intra-operative opioids affects the prescribing of postoperative analgesics and in many cases delays the need for a postoperative analgesic. A postoperative opioid analgesic should be given with care since it may potentiate any residual respiratory depression (for the treatment of opioid-induced respiratory depression, see section 15.1.7).

Morphine is used most widely. **Tramadol** is not as effective in severe pain as other opioid analgesics. **Buprenorphine** may antagonise the analgesic effect of previously administered opioids and is generally not recommended. **Pethidine** is unsuitable for post-operative pain because it is metabolised to norpethidine which may accumulate, particularly in neonates and in renal impairment; norpethidine stimulates the central nervous system and may cause convulsions.

Opioids are also given epidurally [unlicensed route] in the postoperative period but are associated with side-effects such as pruritus, urinary retention, nausea and vomiting; respiratory depression can be delayed, particularly with morphine.

For details of patient-controlled analgesia (PCA) and nurse-controlled analgesia (NCA) to relieve postoperative pain, consult hospital protocols. Formulations specifically designed for PCA are available (*Pharma-Ject® Morphine Sulphate*).

Dental and orofacial pain Opioid analgesics are **relatively ineffective** in dental pain. Like other opioids, **dihydrocodeine** often causes nausea and vomiting which limits its value in dental pain; if taken for more than a few doses it is also liable to cause constipation. Dihydrocodeine is not very effective in post-operative dental pain.

For the management of dental and orofacial pain, see p. 246.

Addicts Although caution is necessary, addicts (and ex-addicts) may be treated with analgesics in the same way as other people when there is a real clinical need. Doctors do not require a special licence to prescribe opioid analgesics for addicts for relief of pain due to organic disease or injury.

Dependence and withdrawal Psychological dependence rarely occurs when opioids are used for pain relief but tolerance can develop during long-term treatment; they should be withdrawn gradually to avoid abstinence symptoms. For information on the treatment of neonatal abstinence syndrome, see section 4.10.

◢ BUPRENORPHINE

Cautions see notes above; also impaired consciousness; effects only partially reversed by naloxone

Hepatic impairment avoid or reduce dose—may precipitate coma

Renal impairment reduce dose or avoid, increased and prolonged effect; increased cerebral sensitivity

Pregnancy depresses neonatal respiration; withdrawal effects in neonates of dependent mothers; gastric stasis and risk of inhalation pneumonia in mother during labour

Breast-feeding amount too small to be harmful; manufacturer advises contra-indicated in the treatment of opioid dependence

Contra-indications see notes above; also myasthenia gravis

Side-effects see notes above; can induce mild withdrawal symptoms in children dependent on opioids; also diarrhoea, abdominal pain, anorexia, dyspepsia; vasodilatation; dyspnoea; paraesthesia, asthenia, fatigue, agitation, anxiety; *less commonly* flatulence, taste disturbance, hypertension, syncope, hypoxia, wheezing, cough, restlessness, depersonalisation, dysarthria, impaired memory, hypoaesthesia, tremor, influenza-like symptoms, pyrexia, rhinitis, rigors, muscle cramp, myalgia, tinnitus, dry eye, and dry skin; *rarely* paralytic ileus, dysphagia, diverticulitis, impaired concentration, and psychosis; *very rarely* retching, hyperventilation, hiccups, and muscle fasciculation

Licensed use sublingual tablets not licensed for use in children under 6 years; injection not licensed for use in children under 6 months

Indication and dose

Moderate to severe pain

* By sublingual administration

  Child body-weight 16–25 kg 100 micrograms every 6–8 hours

  Child body-weight 25–37.5 kg 100–200 micrograms every 6–8 hours

  Child body-weight 37.5–50 kg 200–300 micrograms every 6–8 hours

  Child body-weight over 50 kg 200–400 micrograms every 6–8 hours

* By intramuscular or by slow intravenous injection

  Child 6 months–12 years 3–6 micrograms/kg every 6–8 hours, max. 9 micrograms/kg

  Child 12–18 years 300–600 micrograms every 6–8 hours

Administration for administration *by mouth*, tablets may be halved

Temgesic® (Schering-Plough) [CD]
Tablets (sublingual), buprenorphine (as hydrochloride), 200 micrograms, net price 50-tab pack = £5.33; 400 micrograms, 50-tab pack = £10.66. Label: 2, 26

Injection, buprenorphine (as hydrochloride) 300 micrograms/mL, net price 1-mL amp = 49p

CODEINE PHOSPHATE

Cautions see notes above; also cardiac arrhythmias; myasthenia gravis; acute abdomen; gallstones

Variation in metabolism The capacity to metabolise codeine can vary considerably between individuals and lead to either reduced therapeutic effect or marked increase in side-effects

Hepatic impairment avoid or reduce dose—may precipitate coma

Renal impairment reduce dose or avoid; increased and prolonged effect; increased cerebral sensitivity

Pregnancy depresses neonatal respiration; withdrawal effects in neonates of dependent mothers; gastric stasis and risk of inhalation pneumonia in mother during labour

Breast-feeding amount usually too small to be harmful; however, mothers vary considerably in their capacity to metabolise codeine—risk of morphine overdose in infant

Contra-indications see notes above

Side-effects see notes above; also abdominal pain, anorexia, seizures, malaise, hypothermia, and muscle fasciculation; pancreatitis also reported

Licensed use tablets not licensed for use in children; injection not licensed for use in children under 1 year

Indication and dose

Mild to moderate pain
- By mouth or by rectum or by subcutaneous injection or by intramuscular injection

Neonate 0.5–1 mg/kg every 4–6 hours

Child 1 month–12 years 0.5–1 mg/kg every 4–6 hours, max. 240 mg daily

Child 12–18 years 30–60 mg every 4–6 hours, max. 240 mg daily

Codeine Phosphate (Non-proprietary)
Tablets [PoM], codeine phosphate 15 mg, net price 28 = £1.08; 30 mg, 28 = £1.24; 60 mg, 28 = £1.73. Label: 2

Syrup [PoM], codeine phosphate 25 mg/5 mL. Net price 100 mL = 90p. Label: 2

Injection [CD], codeine phosphate 60 mg/mL. Net price 1-mL amp = £2.44

DIAMORPHINE HYDROCHLORIDE
(Heroin Hydrochloride)

Cautions see notes above; also severe diarrhoea; toxic psychosis, CNS depression; severe cor pulmonale

Hepatic impairment avoid or reduce dose—may precipitate coma

Renal impairment reduce dose or avoid; increased and prolonged effect; increased cerebral sensitivity

Pregnancy depresses neonatal respiration; withdrawal effects in neonates of dependent mothers; gastric stasis and risk of inhalation pneumonia in mother during labour

Breast-feeding therapeutic doses unlikely to affect infant; withdrawal symptoms in infants of dependent mothers; breast-feeding not best method of treating dependence in offspring

Contra-indications see notes above; also delayed gastric emptying; phaeochromocytoma

Side-effects see notes above; also anorexia, taste disturbance; syncope; asthenia; raised intracranial pressure; myocardial infarction also reported

Licensed use intranasal route not licensed

Indication and dose

Acute or chronic pain
- By mouth

Child 1 month–12 years 100–200 micrograms/kg (max. 10 mg) every 4 hours as necessary

Child 12–18 years 5–10 mg every 4 hours as necessary

- By intravenous administration

Neonate (ventilated) initially by intravenous injection over 30 minutes, 50 micrograms/kg then by continuous intravenous infusion, 15 micrograms/kg/hour

Neonate (non-ventilated) by continuous intravenous infusion 2.5–7 micrograms/kg/hour

Child 1 month–12 years by continuous intravenous infusion 12.5–25 micrograms/kg/hour

- By intravenous injection

Child 1–3 months 20 micrograms/kg every 6 hours as necessary

Child 3–6 months 25–50 micrograms/kg every 6 hours as necessary

Child 6–12 months 75 micrograms/kg every 4 hours as necessary

Child 1–12 years 75–100 micrograms/kg every 4 hours as necessary

Child 12–18 years 2.5–5 mg every 4 hours as necessary

- By continuous subcutaneous infusion
See Prescribing in Palliative Care, p. 24

- By subcutaneous or by intramuscular injection
Child 12–18 years 5 mg every 4 hours as necessary

Acute pain in an emergency setting; short painful procedures
- Intranasally (but see p. 250)

Child 3–18 years 100 micrograms/kg, max. 10 mg

Administration for intravenous infusion, dilute in Glucose 5% or Sodium Chloride 0.9%; Glucose 5% is preferable

For intranasal administration, diamorphine powder should be dissolved in sufficient volume of Water for Injections to provide the requisite dose

⌐ **DIAMORPHINE HYDROCHLORIDE** (*continued*)

in 0.2mL of solution; use solution immediately after preparation

Diamorphine (Non-proprietary) CD
Tablets, diamorphine hydrochloride 10 mg. Net price 100-tab pack = £12.92. Label: 2

Injection, powder for reconstitution, diamorphine hydrochloride. Net price 5-mg amp = £2.69, 10-mg amp = £3.37, 30-mg amp = £3.60, 100-mg amp = £9.92, 500-mg amp = £43.44

◄ Extemporaneous formulations available see Extemporaneous Preparations, p. 8

◢ DIHYDROCODEINE TARTRATE

Cautions see notes above; also pancreatitis; severe cor pulmonale

Hepatic impairment avoid or reduce dose—may precipitate coma

Renal impairment reduce dose or avoid; increased and prolonged effect; increased cerebral sensitivity

Pregnancy depresses neonatal respiration—withdrawal effects in neonates of dependent mothers; gastric stasis and risk of inhalation pneumonia in mother during labour

Breast-feeding manufacturer advises use only if potential benefit outweighs risk

Contra-indications see notes above

Side-effects see notes above; also paralytic ileus, abdominal pain, and parasthesia

Licensed use most preparations not licensed for use in children under 4 years

Indication and dose

> Moderate to severe pain
> • **By mouth or by intramuscular injection or by subcutaneous injection**
>> **Child 1–4 years** 500 micrograms/kg every 4–6 hours
>> **Child 4–12 years** 0.5–1 mg/kg (max. 30 mg) every 4–6 hours
>> **Child 12–18 years** 30 mg (max. 50 mg by intramuscular or deep subcutaneous injection) every 4–6 hours

Dihydrocodeine (Non-proprietary)
Tablets PoM, dihydrocodeine tartrate 30 mg. Net price 28 = £1.34. Label: 2, 21
Dental prescribing on NHS Dihydrocodeine Tablets 30 mg may be prescribed

Oral solution PoM, dihydrocodeine tartrate 10 mg/ 5 mL. Net price 150 mL = £3.08. Label: 2, 21

Injection CD, dihydrocodeine tartrate 50 mg/mL. Net price 1-mL amp = £2.29

DF 118 Forte® (Martindale) PoM
Tablets, dihydrocodeine tartrate 40 mg. Net price 100-tab pack = £11.51. Label: 2, 21
Dose
> Severe pain
> • **By mouth**
>> **Child 12–18 years** 40–80 mg 3 times daily; max. 240 mg daily

◄ Modified release
DHC Continus® (Napp) PoM
Tablets, m/r, dihydrocodeine tartrate 60 mg, net price 56-tab pack = £5.50; 90 mg, 56-tab pack = £8.66; 120 mg, 56-tab pack = £11.57. Label: 2, 25
Dose
> Chronic severe pain
> • **By mouth**
>> **Child 12–18 years** 60–120 mg every 12 hours

◢ FENTANYL

Cautions see notes above; also diabetes mellitus, impaired consciousness, cerebral tumour, myasthenia gravis

> **Transdermal fentanyl**
> Fever or external heat Monitor patients using patches for increased side-effects if fever present (increased absorption possible); avoid exposing application site to external heat (may also increase absorption)
> Respiratory depression Risk of fatal respiratory depression, particularly in patients not previously treated with a strong opioid analgesic; manufacturer recommends use only in opioid tolerant patients

Hepatic impairment avoid or reduce dose—may precipitate coma

Renal impairment reduce dose or avoid; increased and prolonged effect; increased cerebral sensitivity

Pregnancy depresses neonatal respiration; withdrawal effects in neonates of dependent mothers;

gastric stasis and risk of inhalation pneumonia in mother during labour

Breast-feeding amount too small to be harmful

Contra-indications see notes above

Side-effects see notes above; also abdominal pain, anorexia, dyspepsia, mouth ulcer, taste disturbance, dry mouth; vasodilatation; apnoea; anxiety; myoclonus; *less commonly* flatulence, diarrhoea, laryngospasm, dyspnoea, hypoventilation, depersonalisation, dysarthria, amnesia, incoordination, paraesthesia, malaise, agitation, tremor, and muscle weakness; *rarely* hiccups and arrhythmia; *very rarely* paralytic ileus, haemoptysis, psychosis, and seizures; shock, asystole, pyrexia, ataxia, and muscle fasciculation also reported; *with patches*, local reactions such as rash, erythema, and itching reported

Licensed use lozenges not licensed for use in children

4

Central nervous system

◻ **FENTANYL** (*continued*)

Indication and dose

Severe chronic pain

● **By transdermal route**

Child 2–16 years currently treated with strong opioid analgesic, initial dose based on previous 24-hour opioid requirement (consult product literature)

Child 16–18 years child **not currently treated** with strong 'opioid analgesic (but see Cautions, p. 249), one '12' or '25 micrograms/hour' patch replaced after 72 hours; child **currently treated** with strong opioid analgesic, initial dose based on previous 24-hour opioid requirement (consult product literature)

Dose adjustment When starting, evaluation of the analgesic effect should **not** be made before the system has been worn for **24 hours** (to allow for the gradual increase in plasma-fentanyl concentration)—previous analgesic therapy should be phased out gradually from time of first patch application; if necessary dose should be adjusted at 72-hour intervals in steps of 12–25 micrograms/hour. More than one patch may be used at a time for doses greater than 100 micrograms/hour (but applied at *same time* to avoid confusion)—consider additional or alternative analgesic therapy if dose required exceeds 300 micrograms/hour (**important**: it may take up to 25 hours for the plasma-fentanyl concentration to decrease by 50%—replacement opioid therapy should be initiated at a low dose and increased gradually).

Long duration of action In view of the long duration of action, children who have had severe side-effects should be monitored for up to 24 hours after patch removal

Breakthrough pain and premedication analgesia, see under preparation below

Peri-operative analgesia section 15.1.4.3

Conversion (from oral morphine to transdermal fentanyl), see Prescribing in Palliative Care, p. 25

Administration For *patches*, apply to dry, non-irritated, non-irradiated, non-hairy skin on torso or upper arm, removing after 72 hours and siting replacement patch on a different area (avoid using the same area for several days).

◢ Lozenges

Actiq® (Cephalon) ⃝CD

Lozenge, (with oromucosal applicator), fentanyl (as citrate) 200 micrograms, net price 3 = £18.58, 30 = £185.80; 400 micrograms, 3 = £18.58, 30 = £185.80; 600 micrograms, 3 = £18.58, 30 = £185.80; 800 micrograms, 3 = £18.58, 30 = £185.80; 1.2 mg,

3 = £18.58, 30 = £185.80; 1.6 mg, 3 = £18.58, 30 = £185.80. Label: 2

Dose

Breakthrough pain

● **By transmucosal application (lozenge with oromucosal applicator)**

Child 2–18 years (over 10 kg body-weight) 15–20 micrograms/kg as a single dose; max. dose 400 micrograms

Note If more than 4 episodes of breakthrough pain each day, adjust dose of background analgesic

Premedication analgesia

● **By transmucosal application (lozenge with oromucosal applicator)**

Child 2–18 years (over 10 kg body-weight) 15–20 micrograms/kg as a single dose; max. 400 micrograms

◢ Patches

Prescriptions Prescriptions for fentanyl patches can be written to show the strength in terms of the release rate and it is acceptable to write '*Fentanyl 25 patches*' to prescribe patches that release fentanyl 25 micrograms per hour. The dosage should be expressed in terms of the interval between applying a patch and replacing it with a new one, e.g. '*one patch to be applied every 72 hours*'. The total quantity of patches should be written in words and figures.

Fentanyl (Non-proprietary) ⃝CD

Patches, self-adhesive, fentanyl, '12' patch (releasing approx. 12 micrograms/hour for 72 hours), net price 5 = £18.85; '25' patch (releasing approx. 25 micrograms/hour for 72 hours), 5 = £26.94; '50' patch (releasing approx. 50 micrograms/hour for 72 hours), 5 = £50.32; '75' patch (releasing approx. 75 micrograms/hour for 72 hours), 5 = £70.15; '100' patch (releasing approx. 100 micrograms/hour for 72 hours), 5 = £86.46. Label: 2, counselling, administration

Brands include *Matrifen*®, *Osmanil*®, *Tilofyl*®, *Victanyl*®

Durogesic DTrans® (Janssen-Cilag) ⃝CD

Patches, self-adhesive, transparent, fentanyl, '12' patch (releasing approx. 12 micrograms/hour for 72 hours), net price 5 = £18.85; '25' patch (releasing approx. 25 micrograms/hour for 72 hours), 5 = £26.94; '50' patch (releasing approx. 50 micrograms/hour for 72 hours), 5 = £50.32; '75' patch (releasing approx. 75 micrograms/hour for 72 hours), 5 = £70.15; '100' patch (releasing approx. 100 micrograms/hour for 72 hours), 5 = £88.32. Label: 2, counselling, administration

---

◤ **HYDROMORPHONE HYDROCHLORIDE**

Cautions see notes above; also pancreatitis; toxic psychosis

Hepatic impairment avoid or reduce dose—may precipitate coma

Renal impairment reduce dose or avoid; increased and prolonged effect; increased cerebral sensitivity

Pregnancy depresses neonatal respiration; withdrawal effects in neonates of dependent mothers;

gastric stasis and risk of inhalation pneumonia in mother during labour

Breast-feeding manufacturer advises avoid—no information available

Contra-indications see notes above; also acute abdomen

Side-effects see notes above; also paralytic ileus, seizures, asthenia, agitation, and myoclonus

◻ **HYDROMORPHONE HYDROCHLORIDE** (*continued*)

Indication and dose

Severe pain in cancer

• **By mouth**

Child 12–18 years 1.3 mg every 4 hours, increased if necessary according to severity of pain

Administration Swallow whole capsule or sprinkle contents on soft food

Palladone® (Napp) ⒸⒹ

Capsules, hydromorphone hydrochloride 1.3 mg (orange/clear), net price 56-cap pack = £8.82; 2.6 mg (red/clear), 56-cap pack = £17.64. Label: 2, counselling, see below

◀**Modified release**

Palladone® SR (Napp) ⒸⒹ

Capsules, m/r, hydromorphone hydrochloride 2 mg (yellow/clear), net price 56-cap pack = £20.98; 4 mg (pale blue/clear), 56-cap pack = £28.75; 8 mg (pink/clear), 56-cap pack = £56.08; 16 mg (brown/clear), 56-cap pack = £106.53; 24 mg (dark blue/clear), 56-cap pack = £159.82. Label: 2, counselling, see below

Dose

Severe pain in cancer

• **By mouth**

Child 12–18 years 4 mg every 12 hours, increased if necessary according to severity of pain

Counselling Swallow whole or open capsule and sprinkle contents on soft food

---

METHADONE HYDROCHLORIDE

Cautions see notes above; also myasthenia gravis; history of cardiac conduction abnormalities, family history of sudden death (ECG monitoring recommended); see also QT Interval Prolongation, below)

Qt interval prolongation The CHM has recommended that children with the following risk factors for QT interval prolongation are carefully monitored while taking methadone: heart or liver disease, electrolyte abnormalities, or concomitant treatment with drugs that can prolong QT interval; children requiring more than 100 mg daily should also be monitored

Hepatic impairment avoid or reduce dose in liver disease—may precipitate coma

Renal impairment reduce dose or avoid; increased and prolonged effect; increased cerebral sensitivity

Pregnancy depresses neonatal respiration; withdrawal effects in neonates of dependent mothers; gastric stasis and risk of inhalation pneumonia in mother during labour

Breast-feeding withdrawal symptoms in infant; breast-feeding permissible during maintenance but dose should be as low as possible and infant monitored to avoid sedation

Contra-indications see notes above; also phaeochromocytoma

Side-effects see notes above; also QT interval prolongation; torsade de pointes, hypothermia, restlessness, raised intracranial pressure, dysmenorrhoea, dry eyes, and hyperprolactinaemia

Licensed use not licensed for use in children

Indication and dose

Neonatal opioid withdrawal dose may vary, consult local guidelines

• **By mouth**

Neonate initially 100 micrograms/kg increased by 50 micrograms/kg every 6 hours until symptoms are controlled; for maintenance, total daily dose that controls symptoms given in 2 divided doses; to withdraw, reduce dose over 7–10 days

Methadone (Non-proprietary) ⒸⒹ

Oral solution 1 mg/mL, methadone hydrochloride 1 mg/mL, net price 30 mL = 60p, 50 mL = £1.03, 100 mL = £1.35, 500 mL = £9.52. Label: 2
Brands include *Eptadone®*,*Metharose®* (sugar-free), *Physeptone* (also as sugar-free)

Safe Practice This preparation is 2½ times the strength of Methadone Linctus; many preparations of this strength are licensed for opioid dependence only but some are also licensed for analgesia in severe pain

---

MORPHINE SALTS

Cautions see notes above; also pancreatitis, myasthenia gravis, cardiac arrhythmias, severe cor pulmonale

Hepatic impairment may precipitate coma in hepatic impairment—avoid or reduce dose (although many such children tolerate morphine well)

Renal impairment reduce dose or avoid, increased and prolonged effect; increased cerebral sensitivity

Pregnancy depresses neonatal respiration; withdrawal effects in neonates of dependent mothers; gastric stasis and risk of inhalation pneumonia in mother during labour

Breast-feeding therapeutic doses unlikely to affect infant; withdrawal symptoms in infants of dependent mothers; breast-feeding not best method of treating dependence in offspring

Contra-indications see notes above; also delayed gastric emptying, acute abdomen; heart failure secondary to chronic lung disease; phaeochromocytoma

Side-effects see notes above; also paralytic ileus, abdominal pain, anorexia, dyspepsia, exacerbation of pancreatitis, taste disturbance; hypertension, hypothermia, syncope, bronchospasm, inhibition of cough reflex; restlessness, seizures, paraesthesia, asthenia, malaise, disorientation, excitation, agitation, delirium, raised intracranial pressure; amenorrhoea, myoclonus, muscle fasciculation, and rhabdomyolysis

4 Central nervous system

◻ **MORPHINE SALTS (continued)**

Licensed use *Oramorph®* solution not licensed for use in children under 1 year; *Oramorph®* unit dose vials not licensed for use in children under 6 years; *Sevredol®* tablets not licensed for use in children under 3 years; *MST Continus®* preparations licensed to treat children with cancer pain (age-range not specified by manufacturer); *MXL®* capsules not licensed for use in children under 1 year

Indication and dose

Pain

• **By subcutaneous injection**

Neonate initially 100 micrograms/kg every 6 hours, adjusted according to response

Child 1–6 months initially 100–200 micrograms/kg every 6 hours, adjusted according to response

Child 6 months–2 years initially 100–200 micrograms/kg every 4 hours, adjusted according to response

Child 2–12 years initially 200 micrograms/kg every 4 hours, adjusted according to response

Child 12–18 years initially 2.5–10 mg every 4 hours, adjusted according to response

• **By intravenous injection over at least 5 minutes**

Neonate initially 50 micrograms/kg every 6 hours, adjusted according to response

Child 1–6 months initially 100 micrograms/kg every 6 hours, adjusted according to response

Child 6 months–12 years initially 100 micrograms/kg every 4 hours, adjusted according to response

Child 12–18 years initially 2.5 mg every 4 hours, adjusted according to response

• **By intravenous injection and infusion**

Neonate initially *by intravenous injection* (over at least 5 minutes) 25–100 micrograms/kg then *by continuous intravenous infusion* 5–40 micrograms/kg/hour adjusted according to response

Child 1–6 months initially *by intravenous injection* (over at least 5 minutes) 100–200 micrograms/kg then *by continuous intravenous infusion* 10–30 micrograms/kg/hour adjusted according to response

Child 6 months–12 years initially *by intravenous injection* (over at least 5 minutes) 100–200 micrograms/kg then *by continuous intravenous infusion* 20–30 micrograms/kg/hour adjusted according to response

Child 12–18 years initially *by intravenous injection* (over at least 5 minutes) 2.5–10 mg then *by continuous intravenous infusion* 20–30 micrograms/kg/hour adjusted according to response

• **By mouth or by rectum**

Child 1–12 months initially 80–200 micrograms/kg every 4 hours, adjusted according to response

Child 1–2 years initially 200–400 micrograms/kg every 4 hours, adjusted according to response

Child 2–12 years initially 200–500 micrograms/kg (max. 20 mg) every 4 hours, adjusted according to response

Child 12–18 years initially 5–20 mg every 4 hours, adjusted according to response

• **By continuous subcutaneous infusion**

Child 1–3 months 10 micrograms/kg/hour

Child 3 months–18 years 20 micrograms/kg/hour

Neonatal opioid withdrawal under specialist supervision

• **By mouth**

Neonate initially 40 micrograms/kg every 4 hours until symptoms controlled, increase dose if necessary; reduce frequency gradually over 6–10 days, and stop when 40 micrograms/kg once daily achieved; dose may vary, consult local guidelines

Administration for *continuous intravenous infusion*, dilute with Glucose 5% or 10% *or* Sodium Chloride 0.9%

Neonatal intensive care, dilute 2.5 mg/kg body-weight to a final volume of 50 mL with infusion fluid; an intravenous infusion rate of 0.1 mL/hour provides a dose of 5 micrograms/kg/hour

◄Oral solutions

Note For advice on transfer from oral solutions of morphine to modified-release preparations of morphine, see Prescribing in Palliative Care, p. 24

Morphine Oral Solutions

[PoM] or [CD]

Oral solutions of morphine can be prescribed by writing the formula:
Morphine hydrochloride 5 mg
Chloroform water to 5 mL

Note The proportion of morphine hydrochloride may be altered when specified by the prescriber; if above 13 mg per 5 mL the solution becomes [CD]. For sample prescription see Controlled Drugs and Drug Dependence, p. 19. It is usual to adjust the strength so that the dose volume is 5 or 10 mL.

Oramorph® (Boehringer Ingelheim)
Oramorph® oral solution [PoM], morphine sulphate 10 mg/5 mL. Net price 100-mL pack = £1.87; 300-mL pack = £5.21; 500-mL pack = £7.86. Label: 2

Oramorph® concentrated oral solution [CD], sugar-free, morphine sulphate 100 mg/5 mL. Net price 30-mL pack = £5.24; 120-mL pack = £19.57 (both with calibrated dropper). Label: 2

△ **MORPHINE SALTS** (*continued*)

◢Tablets

Sevredol® (Napp) ⒸⒹ

Tablets, f/c, scored, morphine sulphate 10 mg (blue), net price 56-tab pack = £5.61; 20 mg (pink), 56-tab pack = £11.21; 50 mg (pale green), 56-tab pack = £28.02. Label: 2

◢Modified-release 12-hourly oral preparations

MST Continus® (Napp) ⒸⒹ

Tablets, m/r, f/c, morphine sulphate 5 mg (white), net price 60-tab pack = £3.29; 10 mg (brown), 60-tab pack = £5.48; 15 mg (green), 60-tab pack = £9.61; 30 mg (purple), 60-tab pack = £13.17; 60 mg (orange), 60-tab pack = £25.69; 100 mg (grey), 60-tab pack = £40.66; 200 mg (green), 60-tab pack = £81.34. Label: 2, 25

Suspension (= sachet of granules to mix with water), m/r, pink, morphine sulphate 20 mg/sachet, net price 30-sachet pack = £24.58; 30 mg/sachet, 30-sachet pack = £25.54; 60 mg/sachet, 30-sachet pack = £51.09; 100 mg/sachet, 30-sachet pack = £85.15; 200 mg/sachet pack, 30-sachet pack = £170.30. Label: 2, 13

Dose

• **By mouth**

Every 12 hours, dose adjusted according to daily morphine requirements; for further advice on determining dose, see Prescribing in Palliative Care, p. 24; dosage requirements should be reviewed if the brand is altered

Note Prescriptions must also specify 'tablets' or 'suspension' (i.e. 'MST Continus tablets' or 'MST Continus suspension')

◢Modified-release 24-hourly oral preparations

MXL® (Napp) ⒸⒹ

Capsules, m/r, morphine sulphate 30 mg (light blue), net price 28-cap pack = £10.91; 60 mg (brown), 28-cap pack = £14.95; 90 mg (pink), 28-cap pack = £22.04; 120 mg (green), 28-cap pack = £29.15; 150 mg (blue), 28-cap pack = £36.43; 200 mg (red-brown), 28-cap pack = £46.15. Label: 2, counselling, see below

Dose

• **By mouth**

Every 24 hours, dose adjusted according to daily morphine requirements; for further advice on determining dose, see Prescribing in Palliative Care, p. 24; dosage requirements should be reviewed if the brand is altered

Counselling Swallow whole or open capsule and sprinkle contents on soft food

Note Prescriptions must also specify 'capsules' (i.e. 'MXL capsules')

◢Suppositories

Morphine (Non-proprietary) ⒸⒹ

Suppositories, morphine hydrochloride or sulphate 10 mg, net price 12 = £8.69; 15 mg, 12 = £7.50; 20 mg, 12 = £33.22; 30 mg, 12 = £10.90. Label: 2

Available from Aurum, Martindale

Note Both the strength of the suppositories and the morphine salt contained in them must be specified by the prescriber

Morphine sulphate 5 mg suppositories available from 'special-order' manufacturers or specialist importing companies, see p. 943

◢Injections

Morphine Sulphate (Non-proprietary) ⒸⒹ

Injection, morphine sulphate 10, 15, 20, and 30 mg/mL, net price 1- and 2-mL amp (all) = 72p–£1.40

Intravenous infusion, morphine sulphate 1 mg/mL, net price 50-mL vial = £5.00; 2 mg/mL, 50-mL vial = £5.89

Minijet® Morphine Sulphate (UCB Pharma) ⒸⒹ

Injection, morphine sulphate 1 mg/mL, net price 10-mL disposable syringe = £7.58

◢Injection with antiemetic

Caution **Not recommended** in palliative care, see Nausea and Vomiting, p. 27

Cyclimorph® (Amdipharm) ⒸⒹ

Cyclimorph-10® Injection, morphine tartrate 10 mg, cyclizine tartrate 50 mg/mL. Net price 1-mL amp = £1.34

Dose

Moderate to severe pain (short-term use only)

• **By subcutaneous, intramuscular, or intravenous injection**

Child 12–18 years 1 mL, repeated not more often than every 4 hours, max. 3 doses in any 24-hour period

Cyclimorph-15® Injection, morphine tartrate 15 mg, cyclizine tartrate 50 mg/mL. Net price 1-mL amp = £1.39

Dose

Moderate to severe pain (short-term use only)

• **By subcutaneous, intramuscular, or intravenous injection**

Child 12–18 years 1 mL, repeated not more often than every 4 hours, max. 3 doses in any 24-hour period

4 Central nervous system

◼ **OXYCODONE HYDROCHLORIDE**

Cautions see notes above; also toxic psychosis; pancreatitis

Contra-indications see notes above; also acute abdomen; delayed gastric emptying; chronic constipation; cor pulmonale; acute porphyria (section 9.8.2)

Hepatic impairment avoid in moderate to severe impairment

Renal impairment reduce dose or avoid, increased and prolonged effect; increased cerebral sensitivity

Pregnancy depresses neonatal respiration; withdrawal effects in neonates of dependent mothers; gastric stasis and risk of inhalation pneumonia in mother during labour

Breast-feeding present in milk—manufacturer advises avoid

Central nervous system 4

◁ **OXYCODONE HYDROCHLORIDE** (*continued*)

Side-effects see notes above; also diarrhoea, abdominal pain, anorexia, dyspepsia; broncho-spasm, dyspnoea, impaired cough reflex; asthenia, anxiety; chills; muscle fasciculation; *less commonly* paralytic ileus, gastritis, flatulence, dysphagia, taste disturbance, belching, hiccups, vasodilatation, supraventricular tachycardia, syncope, amnesia, hypoaesthesia, restlessness, seizures, pyrexia, amenorrhoea, hypotonia, paraesthesia, disorientation, malaise, agitation, speech disorder, tremor, and dry skin

Licensed use not licensed for use in children

Indication and dose

Moderate to severe pain in palliative care (see also Prescribing in Palliative Care, p. 25)

- By mouth

   Child 1 month–12 years initially 200 micrograms/kg (up to 5 mg) every 4–6 hours, dose increased if necessary according to severity of pain

   Child 12–18 years initially 5 mg every 4–6 hours, dose increased if necessary according to severity of pain

Oxynorm® (Napp) ℂ𝔻

Capsules, oxycodone hydrochloride 5 mg (orange/beige), net price 56-cap pack = £12.07; 10 mg (white/beige), 56-cap pack = £24.14; 20 mg (pink/beige), 56-cap pack = £48.27. Label: 2

Liquid (= oral solution), sugar-free, oxycodone hydrochloride 5 mg/5 mL, net price 250 mL = £10.26. Label: 2

Concentrate (= concentrated oral solution), sugar-free, oxycodone hydrochloride 10 mg/mL, net price 120 mL = £49.25. Label: 2

◢ Modified release
OxyContin® (Napp) ℂ𝔻

Tablets, f/c, m/r, oxycodone hydrochloride 5 mg (blue), net price 28-tab pack = £13.23; 10 mg (white), 56-tab pack = £26.45; 20 mg (pink), 56-tab pack = £52.89; 40 mg (yellow), 56-tab pack = £105.80; 80 mg (green), 56-tab pack = £211.61. Label: 2, 25

Dose

Moderate to severe pain in palliative care
- By mouth
   Child 8–12 years initially, 5 mg every 12 hours, increased if necessary according to severity of pain
   Child 12–18 years initially, 10 mg every 12 hours, increased if necessary according to severity of pain

---

PAPAVERETUM

Safe Practice Do **not** confuse with papaverine
A mixture of 253 parts of morphine hydrochloride, 23 parts of papaverine hydrochloride and 20 parts of codeine hydrochloride
The CSM has advised that to avoid confusion the figures of 7.7 mg/mL or 15.4 mg/mL should be used for prescribing purposes

Cautions see notes above; supraventricular tachycardia

Contra-indications see notes above; heart failure secondary to chronic lung disease; phaeochromocytoma

Side-effects see notes above; also hypothermia

Indication and dose

Premedication, postoperative analgesia, severe chronic pain
- By subcutaneous or intramuscular injection
   Neonate 115 micrograms/kg repeated every 4 hours if necessary

   Child 1–12 months 154 micrograms/kg repeated every 4 hours if necessary
   Child 1–6 years 1.93–3.85 mg repeated every 4 hours if necessary
   Child 6–12 years 3.85–7.7 mg repeated every 4 hours if necessary
   Child 12–18 years 7.7–15.4 mg repeated every 4 hours if necessary

- By intravenous injection
   Generally 25–50% of the corresponding subcutaneous or intramuscular dose

Papaveretum (Non-proprietary) ℂ𝔻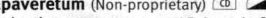
Injection, papaveretum 15.4 mg/mL (providing the equivalent of 10 mg of anhydrous morphine/mL), net price 1-mL amp = £1.64

PETHIDINE HYDROCHLORIDE

Cautions see notes above; not suitable for severe continuing pain; accumulation of metabolites may result in neurotoxicity; myasthenia gravis; cardiac arrhythmias, severe cor pulmonale

Hepatic impairment avoid or reduce dose—may precipitate coma

Renal impairment reduce dose or avoid; increased and prolonged effect; increased cerebral sensitivity

Pregnancy depresses neonatal respiration; withdrawal effects in neonates of dependent mothers;

gastric stasis and risk of inhalation pneumonia in mother during labour

Breast-feeding present in milk but not known to be harmful

Contra-indications see notes above; phaeochromocytoma

Side-effects see notes above; also restlessness and hypothermia; convulsions reported in **overdosage**

◻ **PETHIDINE HYDROCHLORIDE** (*continued*)

Indication and dose

Obstetric analgesia
- By subcutaneous or by intramuscular injection

    Child 12–18 years 50–100 mg, repeated 1–3 hours later if necessary; max. 400 mg in 24 hours

Pethidine (Non-proprietary) CD
Injection, pethidine hydrochloride 50 mg/mL, net price 1-mL amp = 53p, 2-mL amp = 56p; 10 mg/mL, 5-mL amp = £3.17, 10-mL amp = £2.18

▮ TRAMADOL HYDROCHLORIDE

Cautions see notes above; impaired conscious-ness; excessive bronchial secretions; not suitable as substitute in opioid-dependent patients
General anaesthesia Not recommended for analgesia during potentially light planes of general anaesthesia (possibly increased intra-operative recall reported)

Hepatic impairment avoid or reduce dose—may precipitate coma

Renal impairment reduce dose or avoid; increased and prolonged effect; increased cerebral sensitivity

Pregnancy embryotoxic in *animal studies*—manufacturers advise avoid; depresses neonatal respiration; withdrawal effects in neonates of dependent mothers; gastric stasis and risk of inhalation pneumonia in mother during labour

Breast-feeding amount probably too small to be harmful, but manufacturer advises avoid

Contra-indications see notes above; uncontrolled epilepsy; acute porphyria (section 9.8.2)

Side-effects see notes above; also diarrhoea; fatigue; *less commonly* retching, gastritis, and flatulence; *rarely* anorexia, syncope, hypertension, bronchospasm, dyspnoea, wheezing, seizures, paraesthesia, and muscle weakness; blood disorders also reported

Licensed use not licensed for use in children under 12 years

Indication and dose

Moderate to severe pain
- By mouth

    Child 12–18 years 50–100 mg not more often than every 4 hours; total of more than 400 mg daily not usually required

- By intramuscular injection or by intravenous injection (over 2–3 minutes) or by intravenous infusion

    Child 12–18 years 50–100 mg every 4–6 hours

Postoperative pain
- By mouth

    Child 12–18 years 100 mg initially then 50 mg every 10–20 minutes if necessary during first hour to total max. 250 mg (including initial dose) in first hour, *then* 50–100 mg every 4–6 hours; max. 600 mg daily

Administration for *intravenous infusion*, dilute with Glucose 5% *or* Sodium Chloride 0.9% *or* Compound Sodium Lactate *or* Ringer's Solution

Tramadol Hydrochloride (Non-proprietary) PoM
Capsules, tramadol hydrochloride 50 mg. Net price 30-cap pack = £1.39, 100-cap pack = £2.21. Label: 2
Brands include *Tramake*®

Injection, tramadol hydrochloride 50 mg/mL. Net price 2-mL amp = £1.15

Zamadol® (Meda) PoM
Capsules, tramadol hydrochloride 50 mg, net price 100-cap pack = £8.00. Label: 2

Orodispersible tablets (*Zamadol Melt*®), tramadol hydrochloride 50 mg, net price 60-tab pack = £7.12, 100-tab pack = £11.88. Label: 2, counselling, administration
Excipients include aspartame (section 9.4.1)
Counselling *Zamadol Melt*® should be sucked and then swallowed. May also be dispersed in water

Injection, tramadol hydrochloride 50 mg/mL, net price 2-mL amp = £1.10

Zydol® (Grünenthal) PoM
Capsules, green/yellow, tramadol hydrochloride 50 mg, net price 30-cap pack = £3.35, 100-cap pack = £16.91. Label: 2

Soluble tablets, tramadol hydrochloride 50 mg, net price 20-tab pack = £3.95, 100-tab pack = £17.27. Label: 2, 13

Injection, tramadol hydrochloride 50 mg/mL. Net price 2-mL amp = £1.24

◀Modified-release 12-hourly preparations
Dromadol® **SR** (IVAX) PoM
Tablets, m/r, tramadol hydrochloride 100 mg (white), net price 60-tab pack = £12.78; 150 mg (beige), 60-tab pack = £19.17; 200 mg (orange), 60-tab pack = £25.56. Label: 2, 25
Dose

Moderate to severe pain
- By mouth
    Child 12–18 years initially 100 mg twice daily increased if necessary; usual max. 200 mg twice daily

Larapam® **SR** (Sandoz) PoM
Tablets, m/r, tramadol hydrochloride 100 mg, net price 60-tab pack = £18.25; 150 mg, 60-tab pack = £27.35; 200 mg, 60-tab pack = £36.50. Label: 2, 25
Dose

Moderate to severe pain
- By mouth
    Child 12–18 years initially 100 mg twice daily increased if necessary; usual max. 200 mg twice daily

4 Central nervous system

◁ **TRAMADOL HYDROCHLORIDE** (*continued*)

Mabron® (Morningside) [PoM]
Tablets, m/r, tramadol hydrochloride 100 mg, net price 60-tab pack = £18.26; 150 mg, 60-tab pack = £27.39; 200 mg, 60-tab pack = £36.52. Label: 2, 25

Dose
> Moderate to severe pain
> • By mouth
>> **Child 12–18 years** 100 mg twice daily increased if necessary; usual max. 200 mg twice daily

Maxitram SR® (Chiesi) [PoM]
Capsules, m/r, tramadol hydrochloride 50 mg (white), net price 60-cap pack = £4.55; 100 mg (yellow), 60-cap pack = £12.14; 150 mg (yellow), 60-cap pack = £18.21; 200 mg (yellow), 60-cap pack = £24.28. Label: 2, 25

Dose
> Moderate to severe pain
> • By mouth
>> **Child 12–18 years** initially 100 mg twice daily increased if necessary; usual max. 200 mg twice daily

Tramquel SR® (Meda) [PoM]
Capsules, m/r, tramadol hydrochloride 50 mg (dark green), net price 60-cap pack = £7.64; 100 mg (white), 60-cap pack = £15.28; 150 mg (dark green), 60-cap pack = £22.92; 200 mg (yellow), 60-cap pack = £30.55. Label: 2, counselling, administration

Dose
> Moderate to severe pain
> • By mouth
>> **Child 12–18 years** 50–100 mg twice daily increased if necessary; usual max. 200 mg twice daily

> Administration Swallow whole or open capsule and swallow contents immediately without chewing

Zamadol® SR (Meda) [PoM]
Capsules, m/r, tramadol hydrochloride 50 mg (green), net price 60-cap pack = £7.64; 100 mg (yellow), 60-cap pack = £15.28; 150 mg (dark green), 60-cap pack = £22.92; 200 mg (yellow), 60-cap pack = £30.55. Label: 2, counselling, administration

Dose
> Moderate to severe pain
> • By mouth
>> **Child 12–18 years** 50–100 mg twice daily increased if necessary to 150–200 mg twice daily; total of more than 400 mg daily not usually required

> Administration Swallow whole or open capsule and swallow contents immediately without chewing

Zeridame® SR (Actavis) [PoM]
Tablets, m/r, tramadol hydrochloride 100 mg, net price 60-tab pack = £18.26; 150 mg, 60-tab pack = £27.39; 200 mg, 60-tab pack = £36.52. Label: 2, 25

Dose
> Moderate to severe pain
> • By mouth
>> **Child 12–18 years** 100 mg twice daily, increased if necessary; usual max. 200 mg twice daily

Zydol SR® (Grünenthal) [PoM]
Tablets, m/r, f/c, tramadol hydrochloride 100 mg, net price 60-tab pack = £18.26; 150 mg (beige), 60-tab pack = £27.39; 200 mg (orange), 60-tab pack = £36.52. Label: 2, 25

Dose
> Moderate to severe pain
> • By mouth
>> **Child 12–18 years** 100 mg twice daily increased if necessary to 150–200 mg twice daily; total of more than 400 mg daily not usually required

◀ Modified-release 24-hourly preparations
Tradorec XL® (Labopharm) [PoM]
Tablets, m/r, tramadol hydrochloride 100 mg, net price 30-tab pack = £14.10; 200 mg, 30-tab pack = £14.98; 300 mg, 30-tab pack = £22.47. Label: 2, 25

Dose
> Moderate to severe pain
> • By mouth
>> **Child 12–18 years** initially 100 mg once daily, increased if necessary to max. 400 mg once daily

Zamadol® 24hr (Meda) [PoM]
Tablets, f/c, m/r, tramadol hydrochloride 150 mg, net price 28-tab pack = £10.70; 200 mg, 28-tab pack = £14.26; 300 mg, 28-tab pack = £21.39; 400 mg, 28-tab pack = £28.51. Label: 2, 25

Dose
> Moderate to severe pain
> • By mouth
>> **Child 12–18 years** initially 150 mg once daily increased if necessary; max. 400 mg once daily

Zydol XL® (Grünenthal) [PoM]
Tablets, m/r, f/c, tramadol hydrochloride 150 mg, net price 30-tab pack = £15.22; 200 mg, 30-tab pack = £20.29; 300 mg, 30-tab pack = £30.44; 400 mg, 30-tab pack = £40.59. Label: 2, 25

Dose
> Moderate to severe pain
> • By mouth
>> **Child 12–18 years** 150 mg once daily increased if necessary; more than 400 mg once daily not usually required

◀ With paracetamol
Tramacet (Janssen-Cilag) [PoM]
Tablets, f/c, yellow, tramadol hydrochloride 37.5 mg, paracetamol 325 mg, net price 60-tab pack = £10.07. Label: 2, 25, 29, 30

Dose
> Moderate to severe pain
> • By mouth
>> **Child 12–18 years** 2 tablets not more than every 6 hours; max. 8 tablets daily

4.7.3 Neuropathic pain

Neuropathic pain, which occurs as a result of damage to neural tissue, includes *postherpetic neuralgia, phantom limb pain, complex regional pain syndrome* (reflex sympathetic dystrophy, causalgia) *compression neuropathies, peripheral neuropathies* (e.g. due to diabetes, haematological malignancies, rheumatoid arthritis, alcoholism, drug misuse), *trauma, central pain* (e.g. pain following stroke, spinal cord injury and syringomyelia) and *idiopathic neuropathy*. The pain occurs in an area of sensory deficit and may be described as burning, shooting or scalding and is often accompanied by pain that is evoked by a non-noxious stimulus (allodynia).

Neuropathic pain is generally managed with a tricyclic antidepressant such as amitriptyline (p. 229) or antiepileptic drugs such as carbamazepine (p. 267). Neuropathic pain may respond only partially to opioid analgesics. Nerve blocks, transcutaneous electrical nerve stimulation (TENS) and, in selected cases, central electrical stimulation may help. Many children with chronic neuropathic pain require multidisciplinary management, including physiotherapy and psychological support. A corticosteroid may help to relieve pressure in compression neuropathy and thereby reduce pain.

For the management of neuropathic pain in *palliative care*, see p. 25.

Chronic facial pain   Chronic oral and facial pain including persistent idiopathic facial pain (also termed 'atypical facial pain') and temporomandibular dysfunction (previously termed temporomandibular joint pain dysfunction syndrome) may call for prolonged use of analgesics or for other drugs. Tricyclic antidepressants (section 4.3.1) may be useful for facial pain [unlicensed indication], but are not on the Dental Practitioners' List. Disorders of this type require specialist referral and psychological support to accompany drug treatment. Children on long-term therapy need to be monitored both for progress and for side-effects.

4.7.4 Antimigraine drugs

4.7.4.1 Treatment of acute migraine
4.7.4.2 Prophylaxis of migraine
4.7.4.3 Cluster headache

4.7.4.1 Treatment of acute migraine

Treatment of a migraine attack should be guided by response to previous treatment and the severity of the attacks. A **simple analgesic** such as paracetamol (preferably in a soluble or dispersible form) or an NSAID, usually ibuprofen, is often effective; concomitant **antiemetic** treatment may be required. If treatment with an analgesic is inadequate, an attack may be treated with a specific antimigraine compound such as the $5HT_1$ agonist **sumatriptan**. **Ergot alkaloids** are associated with many side-effects and should be avoided.

Excessive use of acute treatments for migraine (opioid and non-opioid analgesics, $5HT_1$ agonists, and ergotamine) is associated with medication-overuse headache (analgesic-induced headache); therefore, increasing consumption of these medicines needs careful management.

Analgesics

ANALGESICS

◢Paracetamol
    Section 4.7.1

◢Non-steroidal anti-inflammatory drugs (NSAIDs)
    Section 10.1.1

◢With antiemetics
Migraleve® (McNeil) ◢
    Tablets, all f/c, *pink tablets*, buclizine hydrochloride 6.25 mg, paracetamol 500 mg, codeine phosphate

8 mg; *yellow tablets*, paracetamol 500 mg, codeine phosphate 8 mg. Net price 48-tab *Migraleve* [PoM] (32 pink + 16 yellow) = £5.10; 48 pink (*Migraleve Pink*) = £5.56. Label: 2, (*Migraleve Pink*), 17, 30

Dose
    Treatment of acute migraine
    • By mouth
        Child under 10 years only under close medical supervision

◁ **ANALGESICS** (*continued*)

Child 10–14 years 1 pink tablet at onset of attack, or if it is imminent then 1 yellow tablet every 4 hours if necessary; max. 1 pink and 3 yellow tablets in 24 hours

Child 14–18 years 2 pink tablets at onset of attack, or if it is imminent, then 2 yellow tablets every 4 hours if necessary; max. in 24 hours 2 pink and 6 yellow

Paramax® (Sanofi-Synthelabo) [PoM]
Tablets, scored, paracetamol 500 mg, metoclopramide hydrochloride 5 mg. Net price 42-tab pack = £8.03. Label: 17, 30

Sachets, effervescent powder, sugar-free, the contents of 1 sachet = 1 tablet; to be dissolved in ¼ tumblerful of liquid before administration. Net price 42-sachet pack = £10.43. Label: 13, 17, 30

Dose

Treatment of acute migraine
• **By mouth**

Child 12–18 years 1 at onset of attack then 1 every 4 hours when necessary to max. of 3 in 24 hours (max. dose of metoclopramide 500 micrograms/kg daily)

Important Metoclopramide can cause **severe extra-pyramidal effects** (for further details, see p. 238 and p. 242)

5HT₁ agonists

5HT₁ agonists are used in the treatment of acute migraine attacks; treatment of children should be initiated by a specialist. The 5HT₁ agonists ('triptans') act on the 5HT (serotonin) 1B/1D receptors and they are therefore sometimes referred to as 5HT$_{1B/1D}$-receptor agonists. A 5HT₁ agonist may be used during the established headache phase of an attack and is the preferred treatment in those who fail to respond to conventional analgesics.

Sumatriptan is used for migraine in children and it may also be of value in cluster headache (section 4.7.4.3).

SUMATRIPTAN

Cautions pre-existing cardiac disease; history of seizures; 5HT₁ agonists are recommended as monotherapy and should not be taken concurrently with other therapies for acute migraine; sensitivity to sulphonamides; **interactions:** Appendix 1 (5HT₁ agonists)
Skilled tasks Drowsiness may affect performance of skilled tasks (e.g. driving)

Hepatic impairment reduce dose of oral therapy; avoid in severe impairment

Renal impairment manufacturer advises caution

Pregnancy limited experience—avoid unless potential benefit outweighs risk

Breast-feeding present in milk but not known to be harmful; withhold breast-feeding for 12 hours

Contra-indications vasospasm; previous cerebrovascular accident or transient ischaemic attack; peripheral vascular disease; moderate and severe hypertension

Side-effects nausea, vomiting; sensations of tingling, heat, heaviness, pressure, or tightness of any part of the body (including throat and chest—discontinue if intense, may be due to coronary vasoconstriction or to anaphylaxis), transient increase in blood pressure, flushing; drowsiness, dizziness, weakness; *very rarely* ischaemic colitis, hypotension, bradycardia or tachycardia, palpitation, arrhythmias, myocardial infarction, Raynaud's syndrome, seizures, tremor, dystonia, nystagmus, and visual disturbances; nasal irritation and epistaxis with nasal spray

Licensed use tablets not licensed for use in children

Indication and dose

Treatment of acute migraine
• **By mouth**

Child 6–10 years 25 mg as a single dose, repeated once after at least 2 hours if migraine recurs

Child 10–12 years 50 mg as a single dose, repeated once after at least 2 hours if migraine recurs

Child 12–18 years 50–100 mg as a single dose, repeated once after at least 2 hours if migraine recurs

• **Intranasally**

Child 12–18 years 10–20 mg as a single dose, repeated once after at least 2 hours if migraine recurs; max. 40 mg in 24 hours

Note Child not responding to initial dose should not take second dose for same attack

¹**Sumatriptan** (Non-proprietary) [PoM]
Tablets, sumatriptan (as succinate) 50 mg, net price 6-tab pack = £9.09; 100 mg, 6-tab pack = £13.77. Label: 3, 10, patient information leaflet
1. Sumatriptan 50 mg tablets can be sold to the public to treat previously diagnosed migraine; max. daily dose 100 mg

Imigran® (GSK) [PoM]
Tablets, sumatriptan (as succinate) 50 mg, net price 6-tab pack = £27.62, 12-tab pack = £52.48; 100 mg, 6-tab pack = £44.64, 12-tab pack = £89.28. Label: 3, 10, patient information leaflet

Nasal spray, sumatriptan 10 mg/0.1-mL actuation, net price 2 unit-dose spray device = £12.28; 20 mg/0.1-mL actuation, 2 unit-dose spray device = £12.28, 6 unit-dose spray device = £36.83. Label: 3, 10, patient information leaflet

◻ **SUMATRIPTAN** (*continued*)

Imgran Radis® (GSK) [PoM]

Tablets, f/c, sumatriptan (as succinate) 50 mg (pink), net price 6-tab pack = £24.87, 12-tab pack =

£49.77; 100 mg (white), 6-tab pack = £44.64, 12-tab pack = £89.28. Label: 3, 10, patient information leaflet

---

Antiemetics

Antiemetics (section 4.6), including **metoclopramide**, **domperidone**, phenothiazines, and antihistamines, relieve the nausea associated with migraine attacks. Antiemetics may be given by intramuscular injection or rectally if vomiting is a problem. Metoclopramide and domperidone have the added advantage of promoting gastric emptying and normal peristalsis; a single dose should be given at the onset of symptoms (**important:** for warnings relating to extrapyramidal effects of metoclopramide see p. 238 and p. 242).

4.7.4.2 Prophylaxis of migraine

Where migraine attacks are frequent, possible provoking factors such as stress should be sought; combined oral contraceptives may also provoke migraine. Preventive treatment should be considered if migraine attacks interfere with school and social life, particularly for children who:

- suffer at least two attacks a month;
- suffer an increasing frequency of headaches;
- suffer significant disability despite suitable treatment for migraine attacks;
- cannot take suitable treatment for migraine attacks.

In children it is often possible to stop prophylaxis after a period of treatment.

Propranolol (section 2.4) may be effective in preventing migraine in children but it is contra-indicated in those with asthma. Side-effects such as depression and postural hypotension can further limit its use.

Pizotifen, an antihistamine and serotonin antagonist, taken at night or twice daily, may also be used but its efficacy in children has not been clearly established. Common side-effects include drowsiness and weight gain.

Topiramate (section 4.8.1) is licensed for migraine prophylaxis. Treatment should be supervised by a specialist.

PIZOTIFEN

Cautions urinary retention; susceptibility to angle-closure glaucoma, renal impairment; **interactions:** Appendix 1 (pizotifen)

Skilled tasks Drowsiness may affect performance of skilled tasks (e.g. driving); effects of alcohol enhanced

Pregnancy manufacturer advises avoid unless potential benefit outweighs risk

Breast-feeding amount probably too small to be harmful but manufacturer advises avoid

Side-effects antimuscarinic effects, drowsiness, increased appetite and weight gain; occasionally nausea, dizziness; *rarely* anxiety, aggression and depression; CNS stimulation may occur

Licensed use *Sanomigran®* elixir and 500-microgram tablets not licensed for use in children under 2 years; 1.5-mg tablets not licensed for use in children

Indication and dose

Prophylaxis of migraine
- **By mouth**

Child 5–10 years initially 500 micrograms at night increased according to response up to 500 micrograms 3 times daily; max. single dose at night 1 mg; max. 1.5 mg in 24 hours

Child 10–12 years initially 1 mg at night increased according to response up to 500 micrograms 3 times daily; max. single dose at night 1 mg; max. 1.5 mg in 24 hours

Child 12–18 years initially 1.5 mg at night increased according to response to 1.5 mg 3 times daily; max. single dose 3 mg; max. 4.5 mg in 24 hours

Pizotifen (Non-proprietary) [PoM]

Tablets, pizotifen (as hydrogen malate), 500 micrograms, net price 28-tab pack = £1.37; 1.5 mg, 28-tab pack = £2.75. Label: 2

Sanomigran® (Novartis) [PoM]

Tablets, both ivory-yellow, s/c, pizotifen (as hydrogen malate), 500 micrograms, net price 60-tab pack = £2.57; 1.5 mg, 28-tab pack = £4.28. Label: 2

Elixir, pizotifen (as hydrogen malate) 250 micrograms/5 mL, net price 300 mL = £4.51. Label: 2

4.7.4.3 Cluster headache

Cluster headache rarely responds to standard analgesics. **Sumatriptan** given by subcutaneous injection is the drug of choice for the *treatment* of cluster headache; treatment should be initiated by a specialist. Alternatively, 100% **oxygen** at a rate of 7–12 litres/minute is useful in aborting an attack.

4.8 Antiepileptics

4.8.1 Control of epilepsy
4.8.2 Drugs used in status epilepticus
4.8.3 Febrile convulsions

4.8.1 Control of epilepsy

The decision about when to start treatment with an antiepileptic drug and the choice of medication depend on frequency of seizures, neurological findings, the identification of an epilepsy syndrome, and the wishes of the child and carers. For the majority of children, epilepsy is controlled with a single antiepileptic drug.

The object of treatment is to prevent the occurrence of seizures by maintaining an effective dose of one or more antiepileptic drugs. Careful adjustment of doses is necessary, starting with low doses and increasing gradually until seizures are controlled or there are significant adverse effects.

When choosing an antiepileptic drug to use, the seizure type, concomitant medication, co-morbidity, age, and sex should be taken into account. For women of child-bearing age, see Pregnancy and Breast-feeding, p. 266.

The frequency of administration is often determined by the plasma half-life, and should be kept as low as possible to encourage better adherence. Most antiepileptics, when used in usual dosage, may be given twice daily. Lamotrigine, phenobarbital and phenytoin, which have long half-lives, can be given as a daily dose at bedtime. However, with large doses, some antiepileptics may need to be given 3 times daily to avoid adverse effects associated with high peak plasma-drug concentrations. Young children metabolise antiepileptics more rapidly than adults and therefore require more frequent doses and a higher amount per kilogram body-weight.

Management When monotherapy with a first-line antiepileptic drug has failed, monotherapy with a second drug should be tried. The changeover from one antiepileptic drug to another should be cautious, slowly withdrawing the first drug only when the new regimen has been established. Combination therapy with 2 or more antiepileptic drugs may be necessary, but the concurrent use of antiepileptic drugs may increase adverse effects and the risk of drug interactions (see below). If combination therapy does not bring about worthwhile benefits, revert to the regimen (monotherapy or combination therapy) that provided the best balance between tolerability and efficacy.

Interactions Interactions between antiepileptics are complex and may increase toxicity without a corresponding increase in antiepileptic effect. Interactions are usually caused by *hepatic enzyme induction* or *hepatic enzyme inhibition*; *displacement from protein binding sites* is not usually a problem. These interactions are highly variable and unpredictable.

Significant interactions that occur **between antiepileptics** themselves are as follows:

> Note Check under each drug for possible interactions when two or more antiepileptic drugs are used

Carbamazepine
often lowers plasma concentration of clobazam, clonazepam, lamotrigine, an active metabolite of oxcarbazepine, and of phenytoin (but may also raise phenytoin concentration), tiagabine, topiramate, and valproate

sometimes lowers plasma concentration of ethosuximide, and primidone (but tendency for corresponding increase in plasma-phenobarbital concentration)

Ethosuximide
sometimes raises plasma concentration of phenytoin

Gabapentin
no interactions with gabapentin reported

Lamotrigine
sometimes raises plasma concentration of an active metabolite of carbamazepine (but evidence is conflicting)

Levetiracetam
no interactions with levetiracetam reported

Oxcarbazepine
sometimes lowers plasma concentration of carbamazepine (but may raise concentration of an active metabolite of carbamazepine)

sometimes raises plasma concentration of phenytoin

often raises plasma concentration of phenobarbital

Phenobarbital *or* Primidone
often lowers plasma concentration of carbamazepine, clonazepam, lamotrigine, an active metabolite of oxcarbazepine, and of phenytoin (but may also raise phenytoin concentration), tiagabine, and valproate

sometimes lowers plasma concentration of ethosuximide

Phenytoin
often lowers plasma concentration of clonazepam, carbamazepine, lamotrigine, an active metabolite of oxcarbazepine, and of tiagabine, topiramate, and valproate

often raises plasma concentration of phenobarbital

sometimes lowers plasma concentration of ethosuximide, and primidone (by increasing conversion to phenobarbital)

Stiripentol
often raises plasma concentration of carbamazepine, clobazam, phenobarbital, and phenytoin

Topiramate
sometimes raises plasma concentration of phenytoin

Valproate
sometimes lowers plasma concentration of an active metabolite of oxcarbazepine

often raises plasma concentration of an active metabolite of carbamazepine, and of lamotrigine, primidone, phenobarbital, and phenytoin (but may also lower)

sometimes raises plasma concentration of ethosuximide, and primidone (and tendency for significant increase in plasma-phenobarbital concentration)

Vigabatrin
often lowers plasma concentration of phenytoin

sometimes lowers plasma concentration of phenobarbital and primidone

For other important interactions see **Appendix 1**; for advice on hormonal contraception and enzyme-inducing drugs (including antiepileptics), see section 7.3.1 and section 7.3.2.

Withdrawal   Antiepileptics should be withdrawn under specialist supervision. Abrupt withdrawal, particularly of the barbiturates and benzodiazepines, should be avoided because this may precipitate severe rebound seizures. Reduction in dosage should be gradual and, in the case of barbiturates, the withdrawal process may take months.

The decision to withdraw antiepileptics from a seizure-free child, and its timing, depends on individual circumstances such as the type of epilepsy and its cause. Even in children who have been seizure-free for several years, there is a significant risk of seizure recurrence on drug withdrawal.

Drugs should be gradually withdrawn over at least 2–3 months by reducing the daily dose by 10–25% at intervals of 1–2 weeks. Benzodiazepines may need to be withdrawn over 6 months or longer.

In children receiving several antiepileptic drugs, only one drug should be withdrawn at a time.

Monitoring   Routine measurement of plasma concentrations of antiepileptic drugs is not usually justified, because the target concentration ranges are arbitrary and often vary between individuals. However, plasma-drug concentrations may be measured in children with worsening seizures, status epilepticus, suspected non-compliance, or suspected toxicity. Similarly, haematological and biochemical monitoring should only be undertaken if clinically indicated.

Driving   Older children suffering from epilepsy may drive a motor vehicle provided that they have been seizure-free for one year or, if subject to attacks only while asleep, have established a 3-year period of asleep attacks without awake attacks. Those affected by drowsiness should not drive or operate machinery.

Guidance issued by the Drivers Medical Unit of the Driver and Vehicle Licensing Agency (DVLA) recommends that patients should be advised not to drive during withdrawal of antiepileptic drugs, or for 6 months afterwards.

Pregnancy and breast-feeding   There is an increased risk of teratogenicity associated with the use of antiepileptic drugs (especially if the child takes two or more antiepileptic drugs). However, the benefit of antiepileptic treatment usually outweighs the potential teratogenic risk, and treatment should not be stopped during pregnancy without discussing with a specialist (see also under individual drugs). In view of the increased risk of neural tube and other defects associated, in particular, with **carbamazepine**, **lamotrigine**, **oxcarbazepine**, **phenytoin**, and **valproate**, women taking antiepileptic drugs who *may become pregnant* should be **informed of the possible consequences**. Those who *wish to become pregnant* should be referred to an appropriate specialist for advice. Young women who become pregnant should be **counselled** and offered **antenatal screening** (including alpha-fetoprotein measurement and a second trimester ultrasound scan).

To counteract the risk of neural tube defects adequate folate supplements are advised for women before and during pregnancy; to prevent recurrence of neural tube defects, women should receive folic acid 5 mg daily (section 9.1.2)—this dose may also be appropriate for women receiving antiepileptic drugs.

The concentration of antiepileptic drugs in the blood can change during pregnancy, particularly in the later stages. The dose of antiepileptic drugs should be monitored carefully during pregnancy and after birth, and adjustments made on a clinical basis.

Routine injection of vitamin K (section 9.6.6) at birth effectively counteracts any antiepileptic-associated risk of neonatal haemorrhage.

Breast-feeding is acceptable with all antiepileptic drugs, taken in normal doses, with the possible exception of the barbiturates, and also some of the more recently introduced ones, see under individual drugs.

Partial seizures with or without secondary generalisation

Carbamazepine, **lamotrigine**, **oxcarbazepine**, and **sodium valproate** are the drugs of choice for partial (focal) seizures; second-line drugs include clobazam, gabapentin, levetiracetam, tiagabine, and topiramate.

Generalised seizures

Tonic-clonic seizures   The drugs of choice for tonic-clonic seizures are **carbamazepine**, **lamotrigine**, **levetiracetam**, and **sodium valproate**. For children who have tonic-clonic seizures as part of the syndrome of primary generalised epilepsy, **sodium valproate** is the drug of choice. Second-line drugs include clobazam, oxcarbazepine, and topiramate.

Absence seizures   **Ethosuximide** and **sodium valproate** are the drugs of choice in typical absence seizures; **lamotrigine** can be used if these are unsuitable. Sodium valproate is also highly effective in treating the generalised tonic-clonic seizures which may co-exist with absence seizures in idiopathic primary generalised epilepsy.

Myoclonic seizures   Myoclonic seizures (myoclonic jerks) occur in a variety of syndromes, and response to treatment varies considerably. **Sodium valproate** is the drug of choice and **clobazam, clonazepam, ethosuximide, lamotrigine, levetiracetam,** or **topiramate** are second-line drugs for treating myoclonic seizures.

Atypical absence, atonic, and tonic seizures   *Atypical absence* and *atonic seizures* may be managed with **sodium valproate, lamotrigine,** or **ethosuximide**. *Tonic seizures* may be treated with **sodium valproate**. Second-line drugs for atypical absence, atonic, and tonic seizures include clobazam, clonazepam, levetiracetam, and topiramate; tonic seizures may rarely be aggravated by benzodiazepines.

Epilepsy syndromes

Infantile spasms   Vigabatrin is the drug of choice for infantile spasms associated with tuberous sclerosis. In spasms of other causes, high doses of corticosteroids such as **prednisolone** (section 6.3.2) or **tetracosactide** (section 6.5.1) may be more effective. Second-line alternatives include clobazam, clonazepam, sodium valproate, and topiramate; nitrazepam is used but it is sedating.

Lennox-Gastaut syndrome   Lamotrigine, sodium valproate, and topiramate are first-line drugs for treating Lennox-Gastaut syndrome. Clobazam, clonazepam, ethosuximide, levetiracetam, and rufinamide are also used.

Landau-Kleffner syndrome   Prednisolone, lamotrigine, and sodium valproate are commonly used to treat Landau-Kleffner syndrome. Alternatives include clobazam, levetiracetam and topiramate.

Neonatal seizures   Seizures can occur before delivery, but they are most common up to 24 hours after birth. Seizures in neonates occur as a result of biochemical disturbances, inborn errors of metabolism, hypoxic ischaemic encephalopathy, drug withdrawal, severe jaundice (kernicterus), meningitis, stroke, or cerebral haemorrhage or malformation.

Seizures caused by biochemical imbalance and those in neonates with inherited abnormal pyridoxine or biotin metabolism should be corrected by treating the underlying cause (section 9.6.2). Seizures caused by drug withdrawal following intra-uterine exposure are treated with a drug withdrawal regimen.

Phenobarbital may be preferred when there is a risk of seizure recurrence in neonates; phenytoin is an alternative. The benzodiazepines (clonazepam, diazepam, lorazepam, and midazolam) and rectal paraldehyde may be useful in the management of seizures which are likely to be brief with little risk of recurrence.

Carbamazepine and oxcarbazepine

Carbamazepine is a drug of choice for simple and complex partial seizures and for tonic-clonic seizures secondary to a focal discharge. It can exacerbate myoclonic and absence seizures. It is essential to initiate carbamazepine therapy at a low dose and build this up slowly in small increments every 3–7 days. Reversible blurring of vision, dizziness, and unsteadiness are dose-related, and may be dose-limiting. These side-effects may be reduced by altering the timing of medication; use of modified-release tablets also significantly lessens the incidence of dose-related side-effects.

Oxcarbazepine may be used for the treatment of partial seizures with or without secondarily generalised tonic-clonic seizures. Oxcarbazepine induces hepatic enzymes to a lesser extent than carbamazepine.

CARBAMAZEPINE

Cautions   cardiac disease (see also Contra-indications); skin reactions (see also Blood, Hepatic or Skin disorders, below and under Side-effects); test for HLA-B*1502 allele in individuals of Han Chinese or Thai origin—risk of Stevens-Johnson syndrome in the presence of HLA-B*1502 allele; history of haematological reactions to other drugs; manufacturer recommends blood counts and hepatic and renal function tests (but evidence of practical value unsatisfactory); may exacerbate absence and myoclonic seizures; susceptibility to angle-closure glaucoma; avoid abrupt with-

4 Central nervous system

◻ **CARBAMAZEPINE** (*continued*)

drawal; **interactions:** see p. 264 and Appendix 1 (carbamazepine)

Hepatic impairment metabolism impaired in advanced liver disease

Renal impairment manufacturer advises caution

Pregnancy see Pregnancy and Breast-feeding, p. 266

Breast-feeding see notes above; amount probably too small to be harmful

Blood, hepatic or skin disorders Children or their carers should be told how to recognise signs of blood, liver, or skin disorders, and advised to seek immediate medical attention if symptoms such as fever, sore throat, rash, mouth ulcers, bruising, or bleeding develop. Leucopenia which is severe, progressive or associated with clinical symptoms requires withdrawal (if necessary under cover of suitable alternative).

Contra-indications AV conduction abnormalities (unless paced); history of bone marrow depression, acute porphyria (section 9.8.2)

Side-effects nausea and vomiting, dizziness, drowsiness, headache, ataxia, confusion and agitation, visual disturbances (especially diplopia and often associated with peak plasma concentrations); constipation or diarrhoea, anorexia; mild transient generalised erythematous rash may occur in a large number of children (withdraw if worsens or is accompanied by other symptoms); leucopenia and other blood disorders (including thrombocytopenia, agranulocytosis and aplastic anaemia); other side-effects include cholestatic jaundice, hepatitis and acute renal failure, Stevens-Johnson syndrome, toxic epidermal necrolysis, alopecia, thromboembolism, arthralgia, fever, proteinuria, lymph node enlargement, cardiac conduction disturbances (sometimes arrhythmias), dyskinesias, paraesthesia, depression, impotence (and impaired fertility), gynaecomastia, galactorrhoea, aggression, activation of psychosis; photosensitivity, pulmonary hypersensitivity (with dyspnoea and pneumonitis), hyponatraemia, oedema, and disturbances of bone metabolism (with osteomalacia) also reported; suicidal ideation; suppositories may cause occasional rectal irritation

Pharmacokinetics plasma concentration for optimum response 4–12 mg/litre (20–50 micromol/litre) measured after 1–2 weeks

Licensed use licensed for use in children with generalised tonic-clonic and partial seizures only

Indication and dose

> Partial and generalised tonic-clonic seizures, neuropathic pain, some movement disorders (e.g. paroxysmal kinesigenic choreoathetosis), mood stabilisation
>
> • **By mouth**
>
> **Child 1 month–12 years** initially 5 mg/kg at night or 2.5 mg/kg twice daily, increased as necessary by 2.5–5 mg/kg every 3–7 days; usual maintenance dose 5 mg/kg 2–3 times daily; doses up to 20 mg/kg daily have been used
>
> **Child 12–18 years** initially 100–200 mg 1–2 times daily, increased slowly to usual maintenance dose 200–400 mg 2–3 times daily; in some cases doses up to 1.8 g daily may be needed

• **By rectum**

> **Child 1 month–18 years** use approx. 25% more than the oral dose (max. 250 mg) up to 4 times daily

Note Different preparations may vary in bioavailability; to avoid reduced effect or excessive side-effects, it may be prudent to avoid changing the formulation (see also notes above on how side-effects may be reduced)

Administration Oral liquid has been used rectally—should be retained for at least 2 hours (but may have laxative effect)

Carbamazepine (Non-proprietary) ⒫ⓞⓜ

Tablets, carbamazepine 100 mg, net price 28 = £5.40; 200 mg, 28 = £4.71; 400 mg, 28 = £6.59. Label: 3, 8, counselling, blood, hepatic or skin disorder symptoms (see above), driving (see notes above)

Brands include *Epimaz*®

Dental prescribing on NHS Carbamazepine Tablets may be prescribed

---

Tegretol® (Novartis) ⒫ⓞⓜ

Tablets, all scored, carbamazepine 100 mg, net price 84-tab pack = £2.43; 200 mg, 84-tab pack = £4.50; 400 mg, 56-tab pack = £5.90. Label: 3, 8, counselling, blood, hepatic or skin disorder symptoms (see above), driving (see notes above)

Chewtabs, orange, carbamazepine 100 mg, net price 56-tab pack = £3.72; 200 mg, 56-tab pack = £6.92. Label: 3, 8, 21, 24, counselling, blood, hepatic or skin disorder symptoms (see above), driving (see notes above)

Liquid, sugar-free, carbamazepine 100 mg/5 mL. Net price 300-mL pack = £7.20. Label: 3, 8, counselling, blood, hepatic or skin disorder symptoms (see above), driving (see notes above)

Suppositories, carbamazepine 125 mg, net price 5 = £9.45; 250 mg, 5 = £12.60. Label: 3, 8, counselling, blood, hepatic or skin disorder symptoms (see above), driving (see notes above)

Dose

> Epilepsy for short-term use (max. 7 days) when oral therapy temporarily not possible

Note Suppositories of 125 mg may be considered to be approximately equivalent in therapeutic effect to tablets of 100 mg but final adjustment should always depend on clinical response (plasma concentration monitoring recommended); max. dose *by rectum* 250 mg 4 times daily

---

◢ Modified release

Carbagen® **SR** (Generics) ⒫ⓞⓜ

Tablets, m/r, f/c, both scored, carbamazepine 200 mg, net price 56-tab pack = £4.88; 400 mg, 56-tab pack = £9.63. Label: 3, 8, 25, counselling, blood, hepatic or skin disorder symptoms (see above), driving (see notes above)

Dose

> **Child 5–18 years** as above; total daily dose given in 1–2 divided doses

◻ **CARBAMAZEPINE** (*continued*)

Tegretol® Retard (Novartis) PoM
Tablets, m/r, both scored, carbamazepine 200 mg (beige-orange), net price 56-tab pack = £5.52; 400 mg (brown-orange), 56-tab pack = £10.86. Label: 3, 8, 25, counselling, blood, hepatic or skin disorder symptoms (see above), driving (see notes above)

Dose

> Child 5–18 years as above; total daily dose given in 2 divided doses

Administration *Tegretol® Retard* tablets can be halved but should not be chewed

◢ OXCARBAZEPINE

Cautions hypersensitivity to carbamazepine; avoid abrupt withdrawal; hyponatraemia (monitor plasma-sodium concentration in patients at risk), heart failure (monitor body-weight), cardiac conduction disorders; avoid in acute porphyria (section 9.8.2); **interactions:** see p. 264 and Appendix 1 (oxcarbazepine)

Hepatic impairment manufacturer advises caution in severe impairment—no information available

Renal impairment use half initial dose if estimated glomerular filtration rate less than 30 mL/minute/1.73 m², increased according to response at intervals of at least 1 week

Pregnancy see Pregnancy and Breast-feeding, p. 266

Breast-feeding present in milk; amount probably too small to be harmful but manufacturer advises avoid

Blood, hepatic or skin disorders Children or their carers should be told how to recognise signs of blood, liver, or skin disorders, and advised to seek immediate medical attention if symptoms such as lethargy, confusion, muscular twitching, fever, sore throat, rash, blistering, mouth ulcers, bruising, or bleeding develop

Side-effects nausea, vomiting, constipation, diarrhoea, abdominal pain, dizziness, headache, drowsiness, agitation, amnesia, asthenia, ataxia, confusion, impaired concentration, depression, tremor, hyponatraemia, acne, alopecia, rash, nystagmus, visual disorders including diplopia; *less commonly* urticaria, leucopenia; *very rarely* hepatitis, pancreatitis, arrhythmias, hypersensitivity reactions, thrombocytopenia, systemic lupus erythematosus, Stevens-Johnson syndrome, and toxic epidermal necrolysis; suicidal ideation

Indication and dose

> Monotherapy and adjunctive therapy of partial seizures with or without secondarily generalised tonic-clonic seizures
>
> • **By mouth**
>
> Child 6–18 years initially 4–5 mg/kg (max. 300 mg) twice daily, increased according to response in steps of up to 5 mg/kg twice daily at weekly intervals (usual maintenance dose for adjunctive therapy 15 mg/kg twice daily); max. 23 mg/kg twice daily

Note In adjunctive therapy the dose of concomitant anti-epileptics may need to be reduced when using high doses of oxcarbazepine

Oxcarbazepine (Non-proprietary) PoM
Tablets, oxcarbazepine 150 mg, net price 50-tab pack = £10.00; 300 mg, 50-tab pack = £19.93; 600 mg, 50-tab pack = £39.48. Label: 3, 8, counselling, blood, hepatic or skin disorders (see above), driving (see notes above)

Trileptal® (Novartis) PoM
Tablets, f/c, scored, oxcarbazepine 150 mg (green), net price 50-tab pack = £10.00; 300 mg (yellow), 50-tab pack = £20.00; 600 mg (pink), 50-tab pack = £40.00. Label: 3, 8, counselling, blood, hepatic or skin disorders (see above), driving (see notes above)

Oral suspension, sugar-free, oxcarbazepine 300 mg/5 mL, net price 250 mL (with oral syringe) = £40.00. Label: 3, 8, counselling, blood, hepatic or skin disorders (see above), driving (see notes above)
Excipients include propylene glycol (see Excipients, p. 3)

Ethosuximide

Ethosuximide is used in typical absence seizures; it may also be used in myoclonic seizures and in atypical absence, atonic, and tonic seizures.

◢ ETHOSUXIMIDE

Cautions avoid abrupt withdrawal; hepatic impairment; renal impairment; avoid in acute porphyria (section 9.8.2); **interactions:** see p. 264 and Appendix 1 (ethosuximide)

Pregnancy may be teratogenic but see Pregnancy and Breast-feeding, p. 266

Breast-feeding present in milk but unlikely to be harmful; manufacturer advises avoid

Blood disorders Children or their carers should be told how to recognise signs of blood disorders, and advised to seek immediate medical attention if symptoms such as fever, sore throat, mouth ulcers, bruising, or bleeding develop

Side-effects gastro-intestinal disturbances (including nausea, vomiting, diarrhoea, abdominal pain, and anorexia), weight loss; *less frequently* headache, fatigue, drowsiness, dizziness, hiccup, ataxia, mild euphoria, irritability, aggression, and impaired concentration; *rarely* tongue swelling, sleep disturbances, night terrors, depression, psychosis, photophobia, dyskinesia, increased libido, vaginal bleeding, myopia, gingival hypertrophy, and rash; also reported, hyperactivity, increase in seizure frequency, blood disorders such as leucopenia, agranulocytosis,

4

Central nervous system

◻ **ETHOSUXIMIDE (continued)**

pancytopenia, and aplastic anaemia (blood counts required if features of infection), systemic lupus erythematosus, and Stevens-Johnson syndrome; suicidal ideation

Indication and dose

Absence seizures, atypical absence, myoclonic seizures

• **By mouth**

Child 1 month–6 years initially 5 mg/kg (max. 125 mg) twice daily, increased gradually over 2–3 weeks up to maintenance dose of 10–20 mg/kg (max. 500 mg) twice daily; total daily dose may rarely be given in 3 divided doses

Child 6–18 years initially 250 mg twice daily, increased by 250 mg at intervals of 4–7 days to usual dose of 500–750 mg twice daily; occasionally up to 1 g twice daily may be needed

Ethosuximide (Non-proprietary) ⒫ⓄⓂ

Capsules, ethosuximide 250 mg, net price 56-cap pack = £38.23. Label: 8, counselling, blood disorders (see above), driving (see notes above)

Emeside® (Chemidex) ⒫ⓄⓂ

Syrup, black currant, ethosuximide 250 mg/5 mL, net price 200-mL pack = £6.60. Label: 8, counselling, blood disorders (see above), driving (see notes above)

Zarontin® (Pfizer) ⒫ⓄⓂ

Syrup, yellow, ethosuximide 250 mg/5 mL, net price 200-mL pack = £4.48. Label: 8, counselling, blood disorders (see above), driving (see notes above)

Gabapentin

Gabapentin is used as adjunctive therapy for the treatment of partial seizures with or without secondary generalisation; it can be used as monotherapy in children over 12 years.

GABAPENTIN

Cautions avoid abrupt withdrawal (may cause anxiety, insomnia, nausea, pain, and sweating—taper off over at least 1 week); diabetes mellitus, false positive readings with some urinary protein tests; **interactions**: Appendix 1 (gabapentin)

Renal impairment reduce dose if estimated glomerular filtration rate less than 80 mL/minute/1.73 m²; consult product literature

Pregnancy see Pregnancy and Breast-feeding, p. 266; toxicity in *animal* studies

Breast-feeding present in milk—manufacturer advises use only if potential benefit outweighs risk

Side-effects diarrhoea, dry mouth, dyspepsia, nausea, vomiting, constipation, abdominal pain, flatulence, appetite changes, gingivitis, weight gain; hypertension, vasodilation, oedema; dyspnoea, cough, rhinitis; confusion, depression, hostility, sleep disturbances, headache; dizziness, anxiety, amnesia, ataxia, dysarthria, nystagmus, tremor, asthenia, paraesthesia, hyperkinesia; influenza-like symptoms; impotence, urinary incontinence; leucopenia; myalgia, arthralgia; diplopia, amblyopia; rash, purpura, pruritus, acne; *rarely* pancreatitis, hepatitis, jaundice, palpitation, hallucinations, movement disorders, thrombocytopenia, blood-glucose fluctuations in patients with diabetes, tinnitus, acute renal failure, Stevens-Johnson syndrome, and alopecia; suicidal ideation

Licensed use not licensed for use in children under 6 years; not licensed at doses over 50 mg/kg daily in children under 12 years

Indication and dose

Adjunctive treatment of partial seizures with or without secondary generalisation

• **By mouth**

Child 2–6 years 10 mg/kg once daily on day 1, then 10 mg/kg twice daily on day 2, then 10 mg/kg 3 times daily on day 3, increased according to response to usual dose of 30–70 mg/kg daily in 3 divided doses

Child 6–12 years 10 mg/kg once daily (max. 300 mg) on day 1, then 10 mg/kg (max. 300 mg) twice daily on day 2, then 10 mg/kg (max. 300 mg) 3 times daily on day 3; usual dose 25–35 mg/kg daily in 3 divided doses; max. 70 mg/kg daily in 3 divided doses

Child 12–18 years 300 mg once daily on day 1, then 300 mg twice daily on day 2, then 300 mg 3 times daily on day 3 or initially 300 mg 3 times daily on day 1; then increased according to response in steps of 300 mg daily (in 3 divided doses) every 2–3 days; usual dose 0.9–3.6 g daily in 3 divided doses

Monotherapy for partial seizures with or without secondary generalisation

• **By mouth**

Child 12–18 years 300 mg once daily on day 1, then 300 mg twice daily on day 2, then 300 mg 3 times daily on day 3 or initially 300 mg 3 times daily on day 1; then increased according to response in steps of 300 mg daily (in 3 divided doses) every 2–3 days; usual dose 0.9–3.6 g daily in 3 divided doses

Note Some children may not tolerate daily increments; longer intervals (up to weekly) may be more appropriate

Administration capsules can be opened but the bitter taste is difficult to mask

◁ **GABAPENTIN** (*continued*)

Gabapentin (Non-proprietary) [PoM]

Capsules, gabapentin 100 mg, net price 100-cap pack = £5.78; 300 mg, 100-cap pack = £8.96; 400 mg, 100-cap pack = £9.24. Label: 3, 5, 8, counselling, driving (see notes above)

Tablets, gabapentin 600 mg, net price 100-tab pack = £106.00; 800 mg, 100-tab pack= £83.38. Label: 3, 5, 8, counselling, driving (see notes above)

Neurontin® (Pfizer) [PoM]

Capsules, gabapentin 100 mg (white), net price 100-cap pack = £22.86; 300 mg (yellow), 100-cap pack = £53.00; 400 mg (orange), 100-cap pack = £61.33. Label: 3, 5, 8, counselling, driving (see notes above)

Tablets, f/c, gabapentin 600 mg, net price 100-tab pack = £106.00; 800 mg, 100-tab pack = £122.66. Label: 3, 5, 8, counselling, driving (see notes above)

Lacosamide

Lacosamide is licensed for adjunctive treatment of partial seizures with or without secondary generalisation.

The *Scottish Medicines Consortium* (p. 4) has advised (January 2009) that lacosamide (*Vimpat®*) is accepted for restricted use within NHS Scotland as adjunctive treatment for partial seizures with or without secondary generalisation in patients from 16 years. It is restricted for specialist use in refractory epilepsy.

LACOSAMIDE

Cautions conduction problems or severe cardiac disease (increased risk of PR-interval prolongation); **interactions:** Appendix 1 (lacosamide)

Hepatic impairment manufacturer advises caution in severe hepatic impairment—no information available

Renal impairment manufacturer advises caution; max. 250 mg daily if estimated glomerular filtration rate is less than 30 mL/minute/1.73 m²

Pregnancy see Pregnancy and Breast-feeding, p. 266; manufacturer advises avoid unless potential benefit outweighs risk

Breast-feeding manufacturer advises avoid—present in milk in *animal* studies

Contra-indications second- or third-degree AV block

Side-effects nausea, vomiting, flatulence, constipation; dizziness, headache, depression, diplopia, nystagmus, impaired coordination, impaired memory, cognitive disorder, drowsiness, tremor, asthenia, fatigue; pruritus; *less commonly* PR-interval prolongation; suicidal ideation

Indication and dose

Adjunctive treatment of partial seizures with or without secondary generalisation

- **By intravenous infusion over 15–60 minutes (for up to 5 days) or by mouth**

  Child 16–18 years initially 50 mg twice daily, increased in steps of 50 mg twice daily every week to max. 200 mg twice daily

Administration for *intravenous infusion*, give undiluted or dilute with Glucose 5% or Sodium Chloride 0.9% or Compound Sodium Lactate solution

Vimpat® (UCB Pharma) ▼ [PoM]

Tablets, f/c, lacosamide 50 mg (pink), net price 14-tab pack = £9.01; 100 mg (yellow), 14-tab pack = £18.02, 56-tab pack = £72.08; 150 mg (salmon), 14-tab pack = £27.03, 56-tab pack £108.12; 200 mg (blue), 56-tab pack = £144.16. Label: 8, counselling, driving (see notes above)

Syrup, lacosamide 15 mg/mL, net price 200 mL = £38.61. Label: 8, counselling, driving (see notes above)

Excipients include aspartame (section 9.4.1)

Intravenous infusion, lacosamide 10 mg/mL net price 200-mg vial = £29.70

Electrolytes Na⁺ 2.6 mmol/200-mg vial

Lamotrigine

Lamotrigine is an antiepileptic for partial seizures and primary and secondarily generalised tonic-clonic seizures. It may be tried for atypical absence, atonic, and tonic seizures particularly in children with Lennox-Gastaut syndrome. Lamotrigine may cause serious skin rash; dose recommendations should be adhered to closely.

Lamotrigine is used either as sole treatment or as an adjunct to treatment with other antiepileptic drugs. Valproate increases plasma-lamotrigine concentration whereas the enzyme inducing antiepileptics reduce it; care is therefore required in choosing the appropriate initial dose and subsequent titration. Where the potential for interaction is not known, treatment should be initiated with lower doses such as those used with valproate.

4 Central nervous system

◢ LAMOTRIGINE

Cautions closely monitor and consider with-drawal if rash, fever, or signs of hypersensitivity syndrome develop; avoid abrupt withdrawal (taper off over 2 weeks or longer) unless serious skin reaction occurs; **interactions:** see p. 264 and Appendix 1 (lamotrigine)

Blood disorders The CSM has advised prescribers to be alert for symptoms and signs suggestive of bone-marrow failure such as anaemia, bruising, or infection. Aplastic anaemia, bone-marrow depression and pancytopenia have been associated rarely with lamotrigine

Hepatic impairment halve dose in moderate impairment; quarter dose in severe impairment

Renal impairment manufacturer advises caution in renal failure; metabolite may accumulate

Pregnancy see Pregnancy and Breast-feeding, p. 266; risk of teratogenesis

Breast-feeding present in milk, but limited data suggest no harmful effect on neonate

Side-effects rash (see Skin Reactions, below); hypersensitivity syndrome (possibly including rash, fever, lymphadenopathy, hepatic dysfunc-tion, blood disorders, disseminated intravascular coagulation and multi-organ dysfunction); nausea, vomiting, diarrhoea, hepatic dysfunction; headache, fatigue, dizziness, sleep disturbances, tremor, movement disorders, agitation, confu-sion, hallucinations, occasional increase in sei-zure frequency; blood disorders (including leucopenia, thrombocytopenia, pancytopenia—see Blood Disorders, above); arthralgia; lupus erythematosus-like effect; photosensitivity; nys-tagmus, diplopia, blurred vision, conjunctivitis; suicidal ideation

Skin reactions Serious skin reactions including Stevens-Johnson syndrome and toxic epidermal necrolysis (rarely with fatalities) have developed especially in children; most rashes occur in the first 8 weeks. Rash is sometimes associated with hypersensitivity syndrome (see Side-effects, above) and is more common in patients with history of allergy or rash from other antiepileptic drugs. Consider withdrawal if rash or signs of hypersensitivity syndrome develop. The CSM has advised that factors associated with increased risk of serious skin reactions include concomitant use of valproate, initial lamotrigine dosing higher than recommended, and more rapid dose escalation than recommended.

Counselling Warn children and their carers to see their doctor immediately if rash or signs or symptoms of hypersensitivity syndrome develop

Indication and dose

Monotherapy and adjunctive treatment of par-tial seizures and primary and secondarily gen-eralised tonic-clonic seizures; seizures asso-ciated with Lennox-Gastaut syndrome

- **By mouth**
  Adjunctive therapy *with valproate*

  Child 2–12 years initially 150 micrograms/kg once daily for 14 days (those weighing under 13 kg may receive 2 mg on alternate days for first 14 days) then 300 micrograms/kg once daily for further 14 days, thereafter increased by max. of 300 micrograms/kg daily every 7–14 days; usual maintenance 1–5 mg/kg daily in 1–2 divided doses (max. single dose 100 mg)

  Child 12–18 years initially 25 mg on alternate days for 14 days then 25 mg daily for further 14 days, thereafter increased by max. 25–50 mg daily every 7–14 days; usual maintenance 100–200 mg daily in 1–2 divided doses

  Adjunctive therapy (with enzyme inducing drugs) *without valproate*

  Child 2–12 years initially 300 micrograms/kg twice daily for 14 days then 600 micrograms/kg twice daily for further 14 days, thereafter increased by max. 1.2 mg/kg daily every 7–14 days; usual maintenance 2.5–7.5 mg/kg (max. single dose 200 mg) twice daily

  Child 12–18 years initially 50 mg daily for 14 days then 50 mg twice daily for further 14 days, thereafter increased by max. 100 mg daily every 7–14 days; usual maintenance 100–200 mg twice daily (up to 700 mg daily has been required)

  Adjunctive therapy *with oxcarbazepine*

  Child 2–12 years initially 300 micrograms/kg daily in 1–2 divided doses for 14 days then 600 micrograms/kg daily in 1–2 divided doses for further 14 days, thereafter increased by max. 600 micrograms/kg daily every 7–14 days; usual maintenance 1–10 mg/kg daily in 1–2 divided doses; max. 200 mg daily

  Child 12–18 years initially 25 mg daily for 14 days, increased to 50 mg daily for further 14 days, then increased by max. 50–100 mg daily every 7–14 days; usual maintenance 100–200 mg daily in 1–2 divided doses

  Monotherapy

  Child 12–18 years initially 25 mg daily for 14 days, increased to 50 mg daily for further 14 days, then increased by max. 50–100 mg daily every 7–14 days; usual maintenance as mono-therapy, 100–200 mg daily in 1–2 divided doses (up to 500 mg daily has been required)

Note Dose titration should be repeated if restarting after interval of more than 5 days

Safe Practice Do not confuse the different combina-tions; see also notes above

Lamotrigine (Non-proprietary) ℞

Tablets, lamotrigine 25 mg, net price 56-tab pack = £3.45; 50 mg, 56-tab pack = £4.13; 100 mg, 56-tab pack = £5.45; 200 mg, 30-tab pack = £27.53, 56-tab pack = £9.36. Label: 8, counselling, driving (see notes above), skin reactions (see above)

Dispersible tablets, lamotrigine 5 mg, net price 28-tab pack = £2.87; 25 mg, 56-tab pack = £3.87; 100 mg, 56-tab pack = £7.70. Label: 8, 13, coun-selling, driving (see notes above), skin reactions (see above)

Lamictal® (GSK) ℞

Tablets, yellow, lamotrigine 25 mg, net price 21-tab pack ('*Valproate Add-on therapy' Starter Pack*) = £7.65, 42-tab pack ('*Monotherapy' Starter Pack*) = £15.30, 56-tab pack = £20.41; 50 mg, 42-tab pack ('*Non-valproate Add-on therapy' Starter Pack*) = £26.02, 56-tab pack = £34.70; 100 mg, 56-tab pack = £59.86; 200 mg, 56-tab pack = £101.76. Label: 8, counselling, driving (see notes above), skin reac-tions (see above)

◻ **LAMOTRIGINE** (*continued*)

Dispersible tablets, chewable, lamotrigine 2 mg, net price 30-tab pack = £ 8.71; 5 mg, 28-tab pack = £8.14; 25 mg, 56-tab pack = £20.41; 100 mg, 56-tab pack = £59.86. Label: 8, 13, counselling, driving (see notes above) , skin reactions (see above)

Levetiracetam

Levetiracetam is used for monotherapy and adjunctive treatment of partial seizures with or without secondary generalisation, and for adjunctive treatment of myoclonic seizures and generalised tonic-clonic seizures.

▲ LEVETIRACETAM

Cautions avoid abrupt withdrawal

Hepatic impairment halve dose in severe hepatic impairment if creatinine clearance less than 70 mL/minute/1.73 m^2

Renal impairment reduce dose if estimated glomerular filtration is less than 80 mL/minute/ 1.73 m^2

Pregnancy see Pregnancy and Breast-feeding, p. 266; manufacturer advises use only if potential benefit outweighs risk—toxicity in *animal* studies

Breast-feeding present in milk—manufacturer advises avoid; see also notes above

Side-effects nausea, vomiting, dyspepsia, diarr-hoea, abdominal pain, anorexia, weight changes; cough; drowsiness, asthenia, amnesia, ataxia, seizures, dizziness, headache, tremor, hyperkine-sia, depression, emotional lability, insomnia, anxiety, impaired balance and attention, aggres-sion, irritability; thrombocytopenia; myalgia; visual disturbances; pruritus, rash; *also reported* pancreatitis, hepatic dysfunction, confusion, psychosis, hallucinations, suicidal ideation, paraesthesia, leucopenia, pancytopenia, and alo-pecia

Indication and dose

Monotherapy of partial seizures with or without secondary generalisation
* **By mouth or by intravenous infusion**

   Child 16–18 years initially 250 mg once daily increased according to response in steps of 250 mg twice daily every 2 weeks; max. 1.5 g twice daily

Adjunctive treatment of partial seizures with or without secondary generalisation; adjunctive treatment of myoclonic seizures; adjunctive treatment of tonic-clonic seizures
* **By mouth or by intravenous infusion**

   Child 4–18 years (12–18 years for myoclonic or tonic-clonic seizures), body-weight under 50 kg initially 10 mg/kg once daily, adjusted in steps not exceeding 10 mg/kg twice daily every 2 weeks; max. 30 mg/kg twice daily

   Child 12–18 years, body-weight over 50 kg initially 250 mg twice daily, adjusted in steps of 500 mg twice daily every 2–4 weeks; max. 1.5 g twice daily

Administration for *intravenous infusion*, dilute requisite dose with at least 100 mL Glucose 5% *or* Sodium Chloride 0.9% *or* Compound Sodium Lactate solution; give over 15 minutes
For administration of *oral solution*, requisite dose may be diluted in a glass of water

Keppra® (UCB Pharma) [PoM]
Tablets, f/c, levetiracetam 250 mg (blue), net price 60-tab pack = £29.70; 500 mg (yellow), 60-tab pack = £52.30; 750 mg (orange), 60-tab pack = £89.10; 1 g (white), 60-tab pack = £101.10. Label: 8

Oral solution, sugar-free, levetiracetam 100 mg/mL, net price 300 mL = £71.00. Label: 8

Concentrate for intravenous infusion, levetirace-tam 100 mg/mL. For dilution before use. Net price 5-mL vial = £13.50
Electrolytes Na$^+$ <0.5 mmol/vial

Phenobarbital and other barbiturates

Phenobarbital (phenobarbitone) is effective for tonic-clonic, partial seizures and neonatal seizures but may cause behavioural disturbances and hyperkinesia. It may be tried for atypical absence, atonic, and tonic seizures. Rebound seizures may be a problem on withdrawal. Monitoring plasma concentrations is less useful than with other drugs because tolerance occurs.

Primidone is largely converted to phenobarbital and this is probably responsible for its antiepileptic action. It is used rarely in children.

▲ PHENOBARBITAL
(Phenobarbitone)

Cautions see also notes above; debilitated; resp-iratory depression (avoid if severe); avoid abrupt

withdrawal (dependence with prolonged use); history of drug and alcohol abuse; avoid in acute

◻ **PHENOBARBITAL** *(continued)*

porphyria (see section 9.8.2); **interactions:** see p. 264 and Appendix 1 (barbiturates)

Hepatic impairment may precipitate coma; avoid in severe impairment

Renal impairment use with caution

Pregnancy see Pregnancy and Breast-feeding, p. 266

Breast-feeding avoid if possible; drowsiness may occur

Side-effects hepatitis, cholestasis; hypotension; respiratory depression; drowsiness, lethargy, depression, ataxia, behavioural disturbances, nystagmus, irritability, hallucinations, impaired memory and cognition, hyperactivity; osteomalacia; megaloblastic anaemia (may be treated with folic acid), agranulocytosis, thrombocytopenia; allergic skin reactions; *very rarely* Stevens-Johnson syndrome and toxic epidermal necrolysis; suicidal ideation; **overdosage:** see Emergency Treatment of Poisoning, p. 35

Pharmacokinetics trough plasma concentration for optimum response 15–40 mg/litre (60–180 micromol/litre)

Indication and dose

All forms of epilepsy except absence seizures
• **By mouth or by intravenous injection**

> **Neonate** initially 20 mg/kg *by slow intravenous injection* then 2.5–5 mg/kg once daily either *by slow intravenous injection* or *by mouth*; dose and frequency adjusted according to response

• **By mouth**

> **Child 1 month–12 years** initially 1–1.5 mg/kg twice daily, increased by 2 mg/kg daily as required; usual maintenance dose 2.5–4 mg/kg once or twice daily

> **Child 12–18 years** 60–180 mg once daily

Status epilepticus section 4.8.2

Note For therapeutic purposes phenobarbital and phenobarbital sodium may be considered equivalent in effect

Administration for administration *by mouth*, tablets may be crushed

For *intravenous injection*, dilute to a concentration of 20 mg/mL with Water for Injections; give over 20 minutes (no faster than 1 mg/kg/minute)

Phenobarbital (Non-proprietary) ⒸⒹ
Tablets, phenobarbital 15 mg, net price 28-tab pack = 88p; 30 mg, 28-tab pack = 59p; 60 mg, 28-tab pack = 69p. Label: 2, 8, counselling, driving (see notes above)

Elixir, phenobarbital 15 mg/5 mL in a suitable flavoured vehicle, containing alcohol 38%, net price 100 mL = 77p. Label: 2, 8, counselling, driving (see notes above)

Note Some hospitals supply **alcohol-free** formulations of varying phenobarbital strengths

Injection, phenobarbital sodium 200 mg/mL in propylene glycol 90% and water for injections 10%, net price 1-mL amp = £2.00

Note Must be diluted before intravenous administration (see Administration)

PRIMIDONE

Cautions see under Phenobarbital; **interactions:** see p. 264 and Appendix 1 (primidone)

Hepatic impairment reduce dose, may precipitate coma

Renal impairment see Phenobarbital

Pregnancy see Phenobarbital

Breast-feeding see Phenobarbital

Side-effects see under Phenobarbital; also nausea and visual disturbances; *less commonly* vomiting, headache, and dizziness; *rarely* arthralgia

Pharmacokinetics monitor plasma concentrations of derived phenobarbital. Optimum range as for phenobarbital

Indication and dose

All forms of epilepsy except absence seizures (but see notes above)
• **By mouth**

> **Child under 2 years** initially 125 mg daily at bedtime, increased by 125 mg every 3 days according to response; usual maintenance, 125–250 mg twice daily

> **Child 2–5 years** initially 125 mg daily at bedtime, increased by 125 mg every 3 days according to response; usual maintenance, 250–375 mg twice daily

> **Child 5–9 years** initially 125 mg daily at bedtime, increased by 125 mg every 3 days according to response; usual maintenance, 375–500 mg twice a day

> **Child 9–18 years** initially 125 mg daily at bedtime, increased by 125 mg every 3 days to 250 mg twice daily, then increased according to response by 250 mg every 3 days to max. 750 mg twice daily

Mysoline® (Acorus) ⓅⓄⓂ
Tablets, scored, primidone 250 mg, net price 100-tab pack = £12.60. Label: 2, 8, counselling, driving (see notes above)

Phenytoin

Phenytoin is effective for tonic-clonic, partial, and neonatal seizures but it may worsen myoclonus. It has a narrow therapeutic index and the relationship between dose and plasma concentration is non-linear; small dosage increases in some children may produce large rises in plasma concentrations with acute toxic side-effects. Monitoring of plasma concentration can assist dosage adjustment. A few missed doses or a small change in drug absorption may result in a marked change in plasma concentration.

Phenytoin may cause coarse facies, acne, hirsutism, and gingival hyperplasia and so may be particularly undesirable in adolescent patients.

When only parenteral administration is possible, **fosphenytoin** (section 4.8.2), a pro-drug of phenytoin, may be convenient to give. Whereas phenytoin can be given intravenously only, fosphenytoin may also be given by intramuscular injection.

PHENYTOIN

Cautions see notes above; avoid abrupt withdrawal; manufacturer recommends blood counts (but evidence of practical value unsatisfactory); avoid in acute porphyria (section 9.8.2); **interactions**: see p. 264 and Appendix 1 (phenytoin)

Hepatic impairment reduce dose

Pregnancy see Pregnancy and Breast-feeding, p. 266; changes in plasma protein binding may make interpretation of plasma-phenytoin concentrations difficult; increased doses may be required in the third trimester

Breast-feeding small amounts present in milk, but not known to be harmful

Blood or skin disorders Children and their carers should be told how to recognise signs of blood or skin disorders, and advised to seek immediate medical attention if symptoms such as fever, sore throat, rash, mouth ulcers, bruising, or bleeding develop. Leucopenia which is severe, progressive, or associated with clinical symptoms requires withdrawal (if necessary under cover of suitable alternative)

Side-effects nausea, vomiting, constipation; insomnia, transient nervousness, tremor, paraesthesia, dizziness, headache, anorexia; gingival hypertrophy and tenderness; rash (discontinue; if mild re-introduce cautiously but discontinue immediately if recurrence), acne, hirsutism, coarse facies; *rarely* hepatoxicity, peripheral neuropathy, dyskinesia, lymphadenopathy, osteomalacia, blood disorders (including megaloblastic anaemia (may be treated with folic acid), leucopenia, thrombocytopenia, and aplastic anaemia), polyarteritis nodosa, lupus erythematosis, Stevens-Johnson syndrome, and toxic epidermal necrolysis; also reported pneumonitis and interstitial nephritis; suicidal ideation; *with excessive dosage* nystagmus, diplopia, slurred speech, ataxia, confusion, and hyperglycaemia

Pharmacokinetics therapeutic plasma-phenytoin concentrations reduced in first 3 months of life because of reduced protein binding

Trough plasma concentration for optimum response:

Neonate–3 months, 6–15 mg/litre (25–60 micromol/litre)

Child 3 months–18 years, 10–20 mg/litre (40–80 micromol/litre)

Licensed use licensed for use in children (age range not specified by manufacturer)

Indication and dose

All forms of epilepsy except absence seizures
• **By intravenous injection (over 20–30 minutes) and by mouth**

Neonate initial loading dose *by slow intravenous injection* (section 4.8.2) 18 mg/kg then *by mouth* 2.5–5 mg/kg twice daily adjusted according to response and plasma-phenytoin concentration (usual max. 7.5 mg/kg twice daily)

• **By mouth**

Child 1 month–12 years initially 1.5–2.5 mg/kg twice daily, then adjusted according to response and plasma-phenytoin concentration to 2.5–5 mg/kg twice daily (usual max. 7.5 mg/kg twice daily *or* 300 mg daily)

Child 12–18 years initially 75–150 mg twice daily then adjusted according to response and plasma-phenytoin concentration to 150–200 mg twice daily (usual max. 300 mg twice daily)

Status epilepticus, acute symptomatic seizures associated with head trauma or neurosurgery section 4.8.2

Administration for administration *by mouth*, interrupt enteral feeds for at least 1–2 hours before and after giving phenytoin; give with water to enhance absorption

For administration by *intravenous injection* and *intravenous infusion*, see p. 287

Phenytoin (Non-proprietary) ℞
Tablets, coated, phenytoin sodium 100 mg, net price 28-tab pack = £30.00. Label: 8, counselling, administration, blood or skin disorder symptoms (see above), driving (see notes above)

Note On the basis of single dose tests there are no clinically relevant differences in bioavailability between available phenytoin sodium tablets and capsules but there may be a pharmacokinetic basis for maintaining the same brand of phenytoin in some patients

Epanutin® (Pfizer) ℞
Capsules, phenytoin sodium 25 mg (white/purple), net price 28-cap pack = 66p; 50 mg (white/pink), 28-cap pack = 67p; 100 mg (white/orange), 84-cap pack = £2.83; 300 mg (white/green), 28-cap pack = £2.83. Label: 8, counselling, administration, blood or skin disorder symptoms (see above), driving (see notes above)

4 Central nervous system

◁ PHENYTOIN (*continued*)

Infatabs® (= chewable tablets), yellow, scored, phenytoin 50 mg, net price 112 = £7.38. Label: 8, 24, counselling, blood or skin disorder symptoms (see above), driving (see notes above)

Note Contain phenytoin 50 mg (as against phenytoin sodium) therefore care is needed on changing to capsules or tablets containing phenytoin sodium

Suspension, red, phenytoin 30 mg/5 mL, net price 500 mL = £4.27. Label: 8, counselling, administration, blood or skin disorder symptoms (see above), driving (see notes above)

Note Suspension of phenytoin 90 mg in 15 mL may be considered to be approximately equivalent in therapeutic effect to capsules or tablets containing phenytoin sodium 100 mg, but nevertheless care is needed in making changes

◢ Parenteral preparations
Section 4.8.2

Rufinamide

Rufinamide is licensed for the adjunctive treatment of seizures in Lennox-Gastaut syndrome.

The *Scottish Medicines Consortium* (p. 4) has advised (October 2008) that rufinamide (*Inovelon®*) is accepted for restricted use within NHS Scotland as adjunctive therapy in the treatment of seizures associated with Lennox-Gastaut syndrome in patients 4 years and above. It is restricted for use when alternative traditional antiepileptic drugs are unsatisfactory.

◢ RUFINAMIDE

Cautions closely monitor and consider withdrawal if rash, fever, or other signs of hypersensitivity syndrome (see Side-effects) develop; avoid abrupt withdrawal; **interactions:** see p. 264 and Appendix 1 (rufinamide)

Hepatic impairment manufacturer advises caution and careful dose titration in mild to moderate hepatic impairment and to avoid in severe impairment

Pregnancy see Pregnancy and Breast-feeding, p. 266; manufacturer advises avoid unless potential benefit outweighs risk—toxicity in *animal* studies; effective contraception must be used during treatment

Contra-indications

Breast-feeding manufacturer advises avoid—no information available

Side-effects nausea, vomiting, constipation, diarrhoea, dyspepsia, abdominal pain; rhinitis, epistaxis; weight loss, anorexia, dizziness, headache, drowsiness, insomnia, anxiety, fatigue, increase in seizure frequency, impaired coordination, hyperactivity, tremor, gait disturbances; influenza-like symptoms; oligomenorrhoea; back pain; nystagmus, diplopia, blurred vision; rash, and acne; hypersensitivity syndrome (possibly including rash, fever, lymphadenopathy, hepatic dysfunction, haematuria, and multi-organ dysfunction) also reported

Hypersensitivity syndrome Serious hypersensitivity syndrome (see above) has developed especially in children and upon initiation of therapy; consider withdrawal if rash or signs or symptoms of hypersensitivity syndrome develop

Counselling Warn children and their carers to seek immediate medical attention if signs or symptoms of hypersensitivity syndrome develop

Indication and dose

Adjunctive treatment of seizures in Lennox-Gastaut syndrome
• **By mouth**

Child 4–18 years body-weight less than 30 kg, initially 100 mg twice daily increased according to response in steps of 100 mg twice daily up to every 2 days; max. 500 mg twice daily (max. 300 mg twice daily if adjunctive therapy *with valproate*)

Child 4–18 years body-weight over 30 kg, initially 200 mg twice daily increased according to response in steps of 200 mg twice daily up to every 2 days; body-weight 30–50 kg max. 900 mg twice daily; body-weight 50–70 kg max. 1.2 g twice daily; body-weight over 70 kg max. 1.6 g twice daily

Administration Tablets may be crushed and given in half a glass of water

Inovelon® (Eisai) ▼ PoM
Tablets, pink, f/c, scored, rufinamide 100 mg, net price 10-tab pack = £8.58; 200 mg, 60-tab pack = £51.48; 400 mg, 60-tab pack = £85.80. Label: 21, counselling, driving (see notes above), hypersensitivity syndrome (see above)

Stiripentol

Stiripentol is licensed for use in combination with clobazam and valproate as adjunctive therapy of refractory generalised tonic-clonic seizures in children with severe myoclonic epilepsy in infancy (Dravet Syndrome). It should be used under specialist supervision.

▲ STIRIPENTOL

Cautions perform full blood count and liver function tests prior to initiating treatment and every 6 months thereafter; monitor growth; **interactions:** Appendix 1 (stiripentol)

Pregnancy see Pregnancy and Breast-feeding, p. 266; manufacturer advises use only if the potential benefit outweighs risk

Breast-feeding present in milk in *animal* studies

Contra-indications history of psychosis

Hepatic impairment manufacturer advises avoid—no information available

Renal impairment manufacturer advises avoid—no information available

Side-effects nausea, vomiting; aggression, anorexia, ataxia, drowsiness, dystonia, hyperexcitability, hyperkinesia, hypotonia, irritability, sleep disorders, weight loss; neutropenia; *less commonly* fatigue, photosensitivity, rash, and urticaria

Indication and dose

Severe myoclonic epilepsy in infancy
- By mouth

 Child 3–18 years initially 10 mg/kg in 2–3 divided doses; titrate dose over minimum of 3 days to max. 50 mg/kg/day in 2–3 divided doses

Diacomit® (Alan Pharmaceuticals) [PoM]
Capsules, stiripentol 250 mg (pink), net price 60-cap pack = £248.00; 500 mg (white), 60-cap pack = £493.00. Label: 1, 8, 21, counselling, administration

Powder, stiripentol 250 mg, net price 60-sachet pack = £284.00; 500 mg, 60-sachet pack = £493.00. Label: 1, 8, 13, 21, counselling, administration
Excipients include aspartame (section 9.4.1)
Counselling Do not take with milk, diary products, carbonated drinks, fruit juice, or with food or drink that contains caffeine

---

Tiagabine

Tiagabine is used as adjunctive treatment for partial seizures, with or without secondary generalisation.

▲ TIAGABINE

Cautions avoid in acute porphyria (section 9.8.2); avoid abrupt withdrawal; **interactions:** Appendix 1 (tiagabine)

Hepatic impairment in mild to moderate impairment, initial maintenance dose is 5–10 mg 1–2 times daily; avoid in severe impairment

Pregnancy see Pregnancy and Breast-feeding, p. 266; no evidence of teratogenicity in *animal* studies, but manufacturer advises use only if potential benefit outweighs risk

Breast-feeding manufacturer advises avoid unless potential benefit outweighs risk
Driving May impair performance of skilled tasks (e.g. driving)

Side-effects diarrhoea; dizziness, tiredness, nervousness, tremor, impaired concentration, emotional lability, speech impairment; *rarely* confusion, depression, drowsiness, psychosis, nonconvulsive status epilepticus, bruising, and visual disturbances; suicidal ideation; leucopenia also reported

Indication and dose

Adjunctive treatment *with enzyme-inducing drugs* for partial seizures with or without secondary generalisation not satisfactorily controlled by other antiepileptics
- By mouth

 Child 12–18 years initially 5 mg twice daily for 1 week then increased at weekly intervals in steps of 5–10 mg daily; usual maintenance dose 30–45 mg daily in 2–3 divided doses (doses above 30 mg daily given in 3 divided doses)

Adjunctive treatment *with non-enzyme-inducing drugs* for partial seizures with or without secondary generalisation not satisfactorily controlled by other antiepileptics
- By mouth

 Child 12–18 years initially 5 mg twice daily for 1 week then increased at weekly intervals in steps of 5–10 mg daily; initial maintenance dose 15–30 mg daily in 2–3 divided doses (doses above 30 mg daily given in 3 divided doses)

Gabitril® (Cephalon) [PoM]
Tablets, f/c, tiagabine (as hydrochloride) 5 mg, net price 100-tab pack = £43.37; 10 mg, 100-tab pack = £86.74; 15 mg, 100-tab pack = £130.11. Label: 21

Topiramate

Topiramate can be given alone or as adjunctive treatment in generalised tonic-clonic seizures or partial seizures with or without secondary generalisation. It can also be used as adjunctive treatment for seizures associated with Lennox-Gastaut syndrome. Topiramate is also licensed for prophylaxis of migraine (section 4.7.4.2).

TOPIRAMATE

Cautions avoid abrupt withdrawal; ensure adequate hydration (especially if predisposition to nephrolithiasis or in strenuous activity or warm environment); avoid in acute porphyria (section 9.8.2); **interactions:** see p. 264 and Appendix 1 (topiramate)

Hepatic impairment use with caution—clearance may be decreased

Renal impairment longer time to steady-state plasma concentration

Pregnancy see Pregnancy and Breast-feeding, p. 266; manufacturer advises avoid unless potential benefit outweighs risk—toxicity in *animal* studies

Breast-feeding manufacturer advises avoid—present in milk

CSM advice Topiramate has been associated with acute myopia with secondary angle-closure glaucoma, typically occurring within 1 month of starting treatment. Choroidal effusions resulting in anterior displacement of the lens and iris have also been reported. The CSM advises that if raised intra-ocular pressure occurs:

*   seek specialist ophthalmological advice;

*   use appropriate measures to reduce intra-ocular pressure;

*   stop topiramate as rapidly as feasible

Side-effects nausea, abdominal pain, dyspepsia, diarrhoea, dry mouth, taste disturbances, weight loss, anorexia; paraesthesia, hypoaesthesia, headache, fatigue, dizziness, speech disorder, drowsiness, insomnia, impaired memory and concentration, anxiety, depression; visual disturbances; *less commonly* suicidal ideation; *rarely* reduced sweating, metabolic acidosis, and alopecia; *very rarely* leucopenia, thrombocytopenia, and serious skin reactions

Indication and dose

Monotherapy of generalised tonic-clonic seizures or partial seizures with or without secondary generalisation

*   By mouth

    Child 6–16 years initially 0.5–1 mg/kg at night for 1 week then increased in steps of 250–500 micrograms/kg twice daily at intervals of 1–2 weeks; usual dose 1.5–3 mg/kg twice daily; max. 7.5 mg/kg twice daily

Child 16–18 years initially 25 mg at night for 1 week then increased in steps of 12.5–25 mg twice daily at intervals of 1–2 weeks; usual dose 50 mg twice daily; max. 200 mg twice daily

Adjunctive treatment of generalised tonic-clonic seizures or partial seizures with or without secondary generalisation, adjunctive treatment of seizures in Lennox-Gastaut syndrome

*   By mouth

    Child 2–16 years initially 25 mg at night for 1 week then increased in steps of 0.5–1.5 mg/kg twice daily at intervals of 1–2 weeks; usual dose 2.5–4.5 mg/kg twice daily; max. 7.5 mg/kg twice daily

    Child 16–18 years initially 25 mg at night for 1 week then increased in steps of 12.5–25 mg twice daily at intervals of 1–2 weeks; usual dose 100–200 mg twice daily; max. 400 mg twice daily

Migraine prophylaxis

*   By mouth

    Child 16–18 years initially 25 mg daily at night for 1 week then increased in steps of 25 mg daily at intervals of 1 week; usual dose 50–100mg daily in 2 divided doses

Note If child cannot tolerate titration regimens recommended above then smaller steps or longer interval between steps may be used

Topamax® (Janssen-Cilag) ▼ PoM
Tablets, f/c, topiramate 25 mg, net price 60-tab pack = £20.48; 50 mg (light yellow), 60-tab pack = £33.64; 100 mg (yellow), 60-tab pack = £60.26; 200 mg (salmon), 60-tab pack = £117.02. Label: 3, 8, counselling, driving (see notes above)

Sprinkle capsules, topiramate 15 mg, net price 60-cap pack = £15.70; 25 mg, 60-cap pack = £23.55; 50 mg, 60-cap pack = £38.69. Label: 3, 8, counselling, administration, driving (see notes above)

Counselling Swallow whole or open capsule and sprinkle contents on soft food

Valproate

Valproate (as either sodium valproate or valproic acid) is effective in controlling tonic-clonic seizures, particularly in primary generalised epilepsy. It is a drug of choice in primary generalised epilepsy, generalised absences and myoclonic seizures, and can be tried in atypical absence, atonic, and tonic seizures. Valproate should generally be avoided in children under 2 years especially if they are on other antiepileptics, but may be required in infants with continuing epileptic tendency. Sodium valproate has widespread metabolic effects, and may have dose-related side-effects.

Valproic acid (as semisodium valproate) (section 4.2.3) is licensed for acute mania associated with bipolar disorder.

SODIUM VALPROATE

Cautions see notes above; monitor liver function before therapy and during first 6 months especially in children most at risk (see also below); measure full blood count and ensure no undue

◻ **SODIUM VALPROATE** (*continued*)

potential for bleeding before starting and before surgery; systemic lupus erythematosus; false-positive urine tests for ketones; avoid sudden withdrawal; **interactions:** see p. 264 and Appendix 1 (valproate)

Hepatic impairment avoid if possible; see also Contra-indications and Liver Toxicity below

Renal impairment reduce dose; adjust dosage according to free serum valproic acid concentration

Pregnancy see Pregnancy and Breast-feeding, p. 266; neonatal bleeding (related to hypofibrinaemia) and neonatal hepatotoxicity also reported

Breast-feeding amount too small to be harmful

Liver toxicity Liver dysfunction (including fatal hepatic failure) has occurred in association with valproate (especially in children under 3 years and in those with metabolic or degenerative disorders, organic brain disease or severe seizure disorders associated with mental retardation) usually in first 6 months and usually involving multiple antiepileptic therapy. Raised liver enzymes during valproate treatment are usually transient but children should be reassessed clinically and liver function (including prothrombin time) monitored until return to normal—discontinue if abnormally prolonged prothrombin time (particularly in association with other relevant abnormalities)

Blood or hepatic disorders Children and their carers should be told how to recognise signs of blood or liver disorders and advised to seek immediate medical attention if symptoms develop

Pancreatitis Children and their carers should be told how to recognise signs and symptoms of pancreatitis and advised to seek immediate medical attention if symptoms such as abdominal pain, nausea and vomiting develop; discontinue if pancreatitis is diagnosed

Contra-indications active liver disease, family history of severe hepatic dysfunction; acute porphyria (section 9.8.2)

Side-effects nausea, gastric irritation, diarrhoea; weight gain; hyperammonaemia, thrombocytopenia; transient hair loss (regrowth may be curly); *less frequently* increased alertness, aggression, hyperactivity, behavioural disturbances, ataxia, tremor, and vasculitis; *rarely* hepatic dysfunction (see under Cautions; withdraw treatment immediately if persistent vomiting and abdominal pain, anorexia, jaundice, oedema, malaise, drowsiness, or loss of seizure control), lethargy, drowsiness, confusion, stupor, hallucinations, menstrual disturbances, anaemia, leucopenia, pancytopenia, hearing loss, and rash; *very rarely* pancreatitis (see under Cautions), peripheral oedema, increase in bleeding time, extrapyramidal symptoms, encephalopathy, coma, gynaecomastia, Fanconi's syndrome, hirsutism, enuresis, hyponatraemia, acne, toxic epidermal necrolysis, and Stevens-Johnson syndrome; suicidal ideation

Indication and dose

All forms of epilepsy
• **By mouth or by rectum**

Neonate initially 20 mg/kg once daily; usual maintenance dose 10 mg/kg twice daily

Child 1 month–12 years initially 5–7.5 mg/kg twice daily; usual maintenance dose 12.5–15 mg/kg twice daily (up to 30 mg/kg twice daily in infantile spasms; monitor clinical

chemistry and haematological parameters if dose exceeds 20 mg/kg twice daily)

Child 12–18 years initially 300 mg twice daily increased in steps of 200 mg daily at 3-day intervals; usual maintenance dose 0.5–1 g twice daily; max. 1.25 g twice daily

Note If switching from oral therapy to intravenous therapy, the intravenous dose should be the same as the established oral dose

• **By intravenous injection over 3–5 minutes**

Neonate 10 mg/kg twice daily

Child 1 month–18 years 10 mg/kg twice daily

• **By continuous intravenous infusion**

Child 1 month–12 years initially 10 mg/kg *by intravenous injection* then *by continuous intravenous infusion* 20–40 mg/kg daily

Child 12–18 years initially 10 mg/kg *by intravenous injection* then up to max. 2.5 g daily *by continuous intravenous infusion*

Administration for *rectal administration*, sodium valproate oral solution may be given rectally and retained for 15 minutes (may require dilution with water to prevent rapid expulsion).

For *intravenous injection*, may be diluted in Glucose 5% *or* Sodium Chloride 0.9%.

For *continuous intravenous infusion*, dilute injection solution with Glucose 5% *or* Sodium Chloride 0.9%

◢Oral

Sodium Valproate (Non-proprietary) ℗ₒ𝗠

Tablets (crushable), scored, sodium valproate 100 mg, net price 100 = £4.67. Label: 8, counselling, pancreatitis, blood or hepatic disorder symptoms (see above), driving (see notes above)

Tablets, e/c, sodium valproate 200 mg, net price 100-tab pack = £5.71; 500 mg, 100-tab pack = £12.15. Label: 5, 8, 25, counselling, pancreatitis, blood or hepatic disorder symptoms (see above), driving (see notes above)
Brands include *Orlept*®

Oral solution, sodium valproate 200 mg/5 mL, net price 300 mL = £6.20. Label: 8, counselling, pancreatitis, blood or hepatic disorder symptoms (see above), driving (see notes above)
Brands include *Orlept*® sugar-free

Epilim® (Sanofi-Synthelabo) ℗ₒ𝗠

Tablets (crushable), scored, sodium valproate 100 mg, net price 100 = £4.67. Label: 8, counselling, pancreatitis, blood or hepatic disorder symptoms (see above), driving (see notes above)

Tablets, both e/c, lilac, sodium valproate 200 mg, net price 100 = £7.70; 500 mg, 100 = £19.25. Label: 5, 8, 25, counselling, pancreatitis, blood or hepatic disorder symptoms (see above), driving (see notes above)

Liquid, red, sugar-free, sodium valproate 200 mg/5 mL, net price 300-mL pack = £7.78. Label: 8, counselling, pancreatitis, blood or hepatic disorder symptoms (see above), driving (see notes above)

4 Central nervous system

Central nervous system

◻ **SODIUM VALPROATE (continued)**

Syrup, red, sodium valproate 200 mg/5 mL, net price 300-mL pack = £7.78. Label: 8, counselling, pancreatitis, blood or hepatic disorder symptoms (see above), driving (see notes above)

◢ Modified release

Epilim Chrono® (Sanofi-Synthelabo) ᴘᴏᴹ
Tablets, m/r, lilac, sodium valproate 200 mg (as sodium valproate and valproic acid), net price 100-tab pack = £9.71; 300 mg, 100-tab pack = £14.56; 500 mg, 100-tab pack = £24.25. Label: 8, 25, counselling, pancreatitis, blood or hepatic disorder symptoms (see above), driving (see notes above)

Dose

Child body-weight over 20 kg as above, total daily dose given in 1–2 divided doses

Epilim Chronosphere® (Sanofi-Aventis) ᴘᴏᴹ
Granules, m/r, sodium valproate 50 mg (as sodium valproate and valproic acid), net price 30-sachet pack = £30.00; 100 mg, 30-sachet pack = £30.00; 250 mg, 30-sachet pack = £30.00; 500 mg, 30-sachet pack = £30.00; 750 mg, 30-sachet pack = £30.00. Label: 8, 25, counselling, administration, pancreatitis, blood or hepatic disorder symptoms (see above), driving (see notes above)

Dose

Child as above, total daily dose given in 1–2 divided doses

Counselling Granules may be mixed with cold food or drink and swallowed immediately without chewing

Episenta® (Beacon) ᴘᴏᴹ
Capsules, m/r, sodium valproate 150 mg, net price 100-cap pack = £5.70; 300 mg, 100-cap pack = £10.90. Label: 8, 25, counselling, administration, pancreatitis, blood or hepatic disorder symptoms (see above), driving (see notes above)

Dose

Child as above, total daily dose given in 1–2 divided doses

Counselling Contents of capsule may be mixed with cold food or drink and swallowed immediately without chewing

Granules, m/r, sodium valproate 500 mg, net price 100-sachet pack = £18.00; 1 g, 100-sachet pack = £35.50. Label: 8, 25, counselling, administration, pancreatitis, blood or hepatic disorder symptoms (see above), driving (see notes above)

Dose

Child as above, total daily dose given in 1–2 divided doses

Counselling Granules may be mixed with cold food or drink and swallowed immediately without chewing

◢ Parenteral

Epilim® Intravenous (Sanofi-Synthelabo) ᴘᴏᴹ
Injection, powder for reconstitution, sodium valproate, net price 400-mg vial (with 4-mL amp water for injections) = £11.58

Episenta® (Beacon) ᴘᴏᴹ
Injection, sodium valproate 100 mg/mL, net price 3-mL amp = £7.00, 10-mL amp = £23.33

◢ Valproic acid

Convulex® (Pharmacia) ᴘᴏᴹ
Capsules, e/c, valproic acid 150 mg, net price 100-cap pack = £3.68; 300 mg, 100-cap pack = £7.35; 500 mg, 100-cap pack = £12.25. Label: 8, 25, counselling, pancreatitis, blood or hepatic disorder symptoms (see above), driving (see notes above)

Dose

Child as for sodium valproate, total daily dose given in 2–4 divided doses

Equivalence to sodium valproate Manufacturer advises that *Convulex®* has a 1:1 dose relationship with products containing sodium valproate, but nevertheless care is needed in making changes

Vigabatrin

For partial epilepsy with or without secondary generalisation, **vigabatrin** is given in combination with other antiepileptic treatment; its use is restricted to children in whom all other combinations are inadequate or are not tolerated. It can be used as sole therapy in the management of infantile spasms.

About one-third of those treated with vigabatrin have suffered visual field defects; counselling and **careful monitoring** for this side-effect are required (see also Visual Field Defects under Cautions below). Vigabatrin has prominent behavioural side-effects in some children.

◼ VIGABATRIN

Cautions closely monitor neurological function; avoid sudden withdrawal (taper off over 2–4 weeks); history of psychosis, depression or behavioural problems; absence seizures (may be exacerbated); **interactions:** see p. 264 and Appendix 1 (vigabatrin)

Renal impairment consider reduced dose or increased dose interval if estimated glomerular filtration rate less than 60 mL/minute/1.73 m²

Pregnancy see Pregnancy and Breast-feeding, p. 266

Breast-feeding see notes above; present in milk—manufacturer advises avoid

Visual field defects Vigabatrin is associated with visual field defects. The CSM has advised that onset of symptoms varies from 1 month to several years after starting. In most cases, visual field defects have persisted despite discontinuation. Product literature advises visual field testing before treatment and at 6-month intervals; a pro-

▢ **VIGABATRIN** (*continued*)

cedure for testing visual fields in those with a developmental age of less than 9 years is available from the manufacturers. Children and their carers should be warned to report any new visual symptoms that develop and those with symptoms should be referred for an urgent ophthalmological opinion. Gradual withdrawal of vigabatrin should be considered.

Contra-indications visual field defects

Side-effects drowsiness (rarely encephalopathic symptoms consisting of marked sedation, stupor, and confusion with non-specific slow wave EEG—reduce dose or withdraw), fatigue, visual field defects (see also under Cautions), dizziness, nervousness, irritability, behavioural effects such as excitation and agitation; depression, abnormal thinking, headache, nystagmus, ataxia, tremor, paraesthesia, impaired concentration; *less commonly* confusion, aggression, psychosis, mania, memory disturbance, visual disturbance (e.g. diplopia); also weight gain, oedema, gastro-intestinal disturbances, alopecia, rash; *less commonly*, urticaria, occasional increase in seizure frequency (especially if myoclonic), decrease in liver enzymes, slight decrease in haemoglobin; photophobia and retinal disorders (e.g. peripheral retinal atrophy); optic neuritis, optic atrophy, hallucinations also reported

Indication and dose

Adjunctive treatment of partial seizures with or without secondary generalisation not satisfactorily controlled with other antiepileptics

• **By mouth**

Neonate initially 15–20 mg/kg twice daily increased over 2–3 weeks to usual maintenance dose 30–40 mg/kg twice daily; max. 75 mg/kg twice daily

Child 1 month–2 years initially 15–20 mg/kg twice daily increased over 2–3 weeks to usual maintenance dose 30–40 mg/kg twice daily; max. 75 mg/kg twice daily

Child 2–12 years initially 15–20 mg/kg (max. 250 mg) twice daily increased over 2–3 weeks to usual maintenance dose 30–40 mg/kg (max. 1.5 g) twice daily

Child 12–18 years initially 250 mg twice daily increased over 2–3 weeks to usual maintenance dose 1–1.5 g twice daily
Administration Tablets may be crushed and dispersed in liquid

• **By rectum**

Child 1 month–18 years dose as for oral therapy, see above
Administration dissolve contents of sachet in small amount of water and administer rectally

Infantile spasms as monotherapy
• **By mouth**

Neonate initially 15–25 mg/kg twice daily adjusted according to response over 7 days to usual maintenance dose 40–50 mg/kg twice daily; max. 75 mg/kg twice daily

Child 1 month–2 years initially 15–25 mg/kg twice daily adjusted according to response over 7 days to usual maintenance dose 40–50 mg/kg twice daily; max. 75 mg/kg twice daily

Sabril® (Aventis Pharma) ℗ℴ𝕄
Tablets, f/c, scored, vigabatrin 500 mg, net price 100-tab pack = £30.84. Label: 3, 8, counselling, driving (see notes above)

Powder, sugar-free, vigabatrin 500 mg/sachet. Net price 50-sachet pack = £17.08. Label: 3, 8, 13, counselling, driving (see notes above)

Note The contents of a sachet should be dissolved in water or a soft drink immediately before taking

---

Benzodiazepines

Clonazepam is occasionally used in tonic-clonic or partial seizures, but its sedative side-effects may be prominent. **Clobazam** may be used as adjunctive therapy in the treatment of epilepsy, but the effectiveness of these and other **benzodiazepines** may wane considerably after weeks or months of continuous therapy.

◢ CLOBAZAM

Cautions see under Diazepam (section 4.8.2)
 Hepatic impairment may precipitate coma
 Renal impairment start with small doses in severe impairment; increased cerebral sensitivity
 Pregnancy avoid regular use (risk of neonatal withdrawal symptoms); use only if clear indication such as seizure control (high doses during late pregnancy or labour may cause neonatal hypothermia, hypotonia and respiratory depression)
 Breast-feeding present in milk—avoid if possible

Contra-indications see under Diazepam (section 4.8.2)

Side-effects see under Diazepam (section 4.8.2)

Licensed use not licensed for use in children under 3 years

Indication and dose

Adjunctive therapy for epilepsy, monotherapy under specialist supervision for catamenial (menstruation) seizures (usually for 7–10 days each month, just before and during menstruation), cluster seizures

• **By mouth**

Child 1 month–12 years initially 125 micrograms/kg twice daily increased every 5 days to usual maintenance dose of 250 micrograms/kg twice daily; max. 500 micrograms/kg twice daily, not exceeding 15 mg twice daily

4 Central nervous system

◁ **CLOBAZAM** (*continued*)

Child 12–18 years initially 10 mg twice daily increased every 5 days to usual maintenance dose of 10–15 mg twice daily; max. 30 mg twice daily

¹**Clobazam** (Non-proprietary) ⟨PoM⟩ ⟨NHS⟩
Tablets, clobazam 10 mg. Net price 30-tab pack = £9.74. Label: 2 or 19, 8, counselling, driving (see notes above)
Brands include *Frisium®* ⟨NHS⟩

Tablets, clobazam 5 mg available on a named patient basis
1. ⟨NHS⟩ except for epilepsy and endorsed 'SLS'

◢Extemporaneous formulations available see Extemporaneous Preparations, p. 8

◼ CLONAZEPAM

Cautions see notes above; respiratory disease; spinal or cerebellar ataxia; myasthenia gravis (avoid if unstable); history of alcohol or drug abuse, depression or suicidal ideation; debilitated; avoid sudden withdrawal; acute porphyria (section 9.8.2); **interactions:** see p. 264 and Appendix 1 (anxiolytics and hypnotics)

Hepatic impairment can precipitate coma; reduce dose in mild to moderate impairment; avoid in severe impairment

Renal impairment start with small doses; increased cerebral sensitivity

Pregnancy avoid regular use (risk of neonatal withdrawal symptoms); use only if clear indication such as seizure control (high doses during late pregnancy or labour may cause neonatal hypothermia, hypotonia and respiratory depression)

Breast-feeding present in milk—avoid if possible
Driving Drowsiness may affect performance of skilled tasks (e.g. driving); effects of alcohol enhanced

Contra-indications respiratory depression; acute pulmonary insufficiency; sleep apnoea syndrome

Side-effects drowsiness, fatigue, dizziness, muscle hypotonia, coordination disturbances; also poor concentration, restlessness, confusion, amnesia, dependence, and withdrawal; salivary or bronchial hypersecretion in infants and small children; *rarely* gastro-intestinal symptoms, respiratory depression, headache, paradoxical effects including aggression and anxiety, sexual dysfunction, urinary incontinence, urticaria, pruritus, reversible hair loss, skin pigmentation changes; dysarthria, and visual disturbances on long-term treatment; blood disorders reported; **overdosage:** see Emergency Treatment of Poisoning, p. 41

Indication and dose

All forms of epilepsy
• **By mouth**

Child 1 month–1 year initially 250 micrograms at night for 4 nights, increased over 2–4 weeks to usual maintenance dose of 0.5–1 mg at night (may be given in 3 divided doses if necessary)

Child 1–5 years initially 250 micrograms at night for 4 nights, increased over 2–4 weeks to usual maintenance of 1–3 mg at night (may be given in 3 divided doses if necessary)

Child 5–12 years initially 500 micrograms at night for 4 nights, increased over 2–4 weeks to usual maintenance dose of 3–6 mg at night (may be given in 3 divided doses if necessary)

Child 12–18 years initially 1 mg at night for 4 nights, increased over 2–4 weeks to usual maintenance dose of 4–8 mg at night (may be given in 3–4 divided doses if necessary)

Note Clonazepam doses in BNFC may differ from those in product literature

Administration for administration *by mouth*, injection solution may be given orally

Rivotril® (Roche) ⟨PoM⟩
Tablets, both scored, clonazepam 500 micrograms (beige), net price 100 = £3.92; 2 mg (white), 100 = £5.23. Label: 2, 8, counselling, driving (see notes above)

Injection, section 4.8.2

Liquid, clonazepam 2.5 mg/mL
Available from 'special-order' manufacturers or specialist importing companies, see p. 943

◢Extemporaneous formulations available see Extemporaneous Preparations, p. 8

◼ NITRAZEPAM

Cautions avoid abrupt withdrawal; respiratory disease; acute porphyria (section 9.8.2); muscle weakness and myasthenia gravis; **interactions:** Appendix 1 (anxiolytics and hypnotics)

Hepatic impairment can precipitate coma; avoid in severe hepatic impairment

Renal impairment start with small doses; increased cerebral sensitivity

Contra-indications respiratory depression, acute pulmonary insufficiency, sleep apnoea syndrome; marked neuromuscular respiratory weakness including myasthenia gravis

Side-effects drowsiness, confusion, ataxia; see also under Diazepam (section 4.8.2); **overdo-**

sage: see Emergency Treatment of Poisoning p. 41

Licensed use not licensed for use in children

Indication and dose

Infantile spasms
• **By mouth**

Child 1 month–2 years initially 125 micrograms/kg twice daily, adjusted according to response over 2–3 weeks to 250 micrograms/kg twice daily; max. 500 micrograms/kg (not exceeding 5 mg) twice daily; total daily dose may alternatively be given in 3 divided doses

◻ **NITRAZEPAM** (*continued*)

Nitrazepam (Non-proprietary) PoM
Oral suspension, nitrazepam 2.5 mg/5 mL, net price 150 mL = £5.30. Label: 1, 8
Brands include *Somnite®* JHS

Other drugs

Acetazolamide (section 11.6), a carbonic anhydrase inhibitor, has a specific role in treating epilepsy associated with menstruation. It can also be used in conjunction with other antiepileptics for tonic-clonic or partial seizures.

Piracetam is used as adjunctive treatment for cortical myoclonus.

4.8.2 Drugs used in status epilepticus

Immediate measures to manage status epilepticus include positioning the child to avoid injury, supporting respiration including the provision of oxygen, maintaining blood pressure, and the correction of any hypoglycaemia. **Pyridoxine** (section 9.6.2) should be administered if the status epilepticus is caused by pyridoxine deficiency.

Convulsive status epilepticus should be treated urgently with intravenous **lorazepam**. Intravenous **diazepam** is effective but it is associated with a high risk of venous thrombophlebitis (reduced by using an emulsion formulation of diazepam injection). **Clonazepam** can also be used as an alternative.

Where facilities for resuscitation are not immediately available, **midazolam** can be given into the buccal cavity, or **diazepam** can be administered as a rectal solution; the buccal route may be more acceptable in children.

> **Important**
> If seizures recur or fail to respond within 30 minutes, phenytoin sodium, fosphenytoin, or phenobarbital sodium should be used.
> If these measures fail to control seizures within 60 minutes, anaesthesia with thiopental (section 15.1.1) or midazolam (section 15.1.4) should be instituted with full intensive care support. Lidocaine infusion has also been used but requires specialist management.

Phenytoin sodium may be given by slow intravenous injection, with ECG monitoring, followed by the maintenance dosage if appropriate. Intramuscular use of phenytoin is not recommended (absorption is slow and erratic).

Alternatively, **fosphenytoin**, a pro-drug of phenytoin, can be given more rapidly and when given intravenously causes fewer injection-site reactions than phenytoin. Intravenous administration requires ECG monitoring. Although it can also be given intramuscularly, absorption is too slow by this route for treatment of status epilepticus. Doses of fosphenytoin should be expressed in terms of phenytoin sodium.

Paraldehyde given rectally causes little respiratory depression and is therefore useful where facilities for resuscitation are poor.

For **neonatal seizures**, see p. 267.

Non-convulsive status epilepticus   The urgency to treat non-convulsive status epilepticus depends upon the severity of the child's condition. If there is incomplete loss of awareness, oral antiepileptic therapy should be restarted or continued. Children who fail to respond to oral antiepileptic therapy or have complete lack of awareness can be treated in the same way as convulsive status epilepticus although anaesthesia is rarely needed.

CLONAZEPAM

Cautions see section 4.8.1; facilities for reversing respiratory depression with mechanical ventilation must be at hand (but see also notes above) Intravenous infusion Intravenous infusion of clonazepam is potentially hazardous (especially if prolonged), calling for close and constant observation and best carried out in specialist centres with intensive care facilities. Prolonged infusion may lead to accumulation and delay recovery

Contra-indications see section 4.8.1; avoid injections containing benzyl alcohol in neonates (see under preparations below)

4   Central nervous system

Central nervous system 4

◻ CLONAZEPAM (continued)

Side-effects see section 4.8.1; hypotension and apnoea

Indication and dose

Status epilepticus

• **By intravenous injection over at least 2 minutes**

Neonate 100 micrograms/kg repeated after 24 hours if necessary (avoid unless there is no safer alternative)

Child 1 month–12 years 50 micrograms/kg (max. 1 mg) repeated if necessary

Child 12–18 years 1 mg repeated if necessary

• **By intravenous infusion**

Child 1 month–12 years initially 50 micrograms/kg (max. 1 mg) by intravenous injection then by intravenous infusion 10 micrograms/kg/hour adjusted according to response; max. 60 micrograms/kg/hour

Child 12–18 years initially 1 mg by intravenous injection then by intravenous infusion 10 micrograms/kg/hour adjusted according to response; max. 60 micrograms/kg/hour

Other forms of epilepsy section 4.8.1

Administration for *intravenous injection*, dilute to a concentration of 500 micrograms/mL with Water for Injections

For *intravenous infusion*, dilute to a concentration of 12 micrograms/mL with Glucose 5% *or* Sodium Chloride 0.9%; incompatible with bicarbonate; adsorbed on PVC—glass infusion apparatus preferred (if PVC apparatus used, complete infusion within 2 hours)

Rivotril® (Roche) (PoM)
Injection, clonazepam 1 mg/mL in solvent, net price 1-mL amp (with 1 mL water for injections) = 63p
Excipients include benzyl alcohol (avoid in neonates unless there is no safer alternative available, see Excipients, p. 3), ethanol, propylene glycol

◢Oral preparations
Section 4.8.1

◢ DIAZEPAM

Cautions respiratory disease, muscle weakness and myasthenia gravis, history of drug or alcohol abuse, marked personality disorder; avoid prolonged use (and abrupt withdrawal thereafter); when given parenterally, close observation required until full recovery from sedation; when given intravenously, facilities for reversing respiratory depression with mechanical ventilation must be at hand (but see also notes above); porphyria (section 9.8.2); **interactions:** Appendix 1 (anxiolytics and hypnotics)

Hepatic impairment reduce dose as may precipitate coma; avoid in severe impairment

Renal impairment start with small doses; increased cerebral sensitivity

Pregnancy avoid regular use (risk of neonatal withdrawal symptoms); use only if clear indication such as seizure control (high doses during late pregnancy or labour may cause neonatal hyperthermia, hypotonia, and respiratory depression)

Breast-feeding avoid if possible—present in milk
Skilled tasks Drowsiness may affect performance of skilled tasks (e.g. driving); effects of alcohol enhanced

Contra-indications respiratory depression; marked neuromuscular respiratory weakness including unstable myasthenia gravis; acute pulmonary insufficiency; sleep apnoea syndrome; not for chronic psychosis; should not be used alone in depression or in anxiety with depression; avoid injections containing benzyl alcohol in neonates (see under preparations below)

Side-effects drowsiness and lightheadedness the next day; confusion and ataxia; amnesia; dependence; paradoxical increase in aggression (see also section 4.1); muscle weakness; *occasionally:* headache, vertigo, hypotension, salivation changes, gastro-intestinal disturbances, visual disturbances, dysarthria, tremor, changes in libido, incontinence, urinary retention; blood disorders and jaundice reported; skin reactions; on intravenous injection, pain, thrombophlebitis, and rarely apnoea; **overdosage:** see Emergency Treatment of Poisoning, p. 41

Licensed use *Diazepam Rectubes®* and *Stesolid Rectal Tubes®* not licensed for use in children under 1 year

Indication and dose

Status epilepticus, febrile convulsions (section 4.8.3), convulsions caused by poisoning

• **By intravenous injection over 3–5 minutes**

Neonate 300–400 micrograms/kg repeated once after 10 minutes if necessary

Child 1 month–12 years 300–400 micrograms/kg repeated once after 10 minutes if necessary

Child 12–18 years 10–20 mg repeated once after 10 minutes if necessary

• **By rectum (as rectal solution)**

Neonate 1.25–2.5 mg repeated once after 10 minutes if necessary

Child 1 month–2 years 5 mg repeated once after 10 minutes if necessary

Child 2–12 years 5–10 mg repeated once after 10 minutes if necessary

Child 12–18 years 10 mg repeated once after 10 minutes if necessary

Muscle spasm section 10.2.2

Peri-operative use section 15.1.4.1

◻ **DIAZEPAM** *(continued)*

Diazepam (Non-proprietary) [PoM]
Injection (solution), diazepam 5 mg/mL. Net price
2-mL amp = 45p
Excipients include benzyl alcohol (avoid in neonates, see
Excipients, p. 3), ethanol, propylene glycol

Injection (emulsion), diazepam 5 mg/mL (0.5%).
Net price 2-mL amp = 84p
Brands include *Diazemuls®*

Rectal tubes (= rectal solution), diazepam 2 mg/
mL, net price 1.25-mL (2.5-mg) tube = 90p, 2.5-mL
(5-mg) tube = £1.27; 4 mg/mL, 2.5-mL (10-mg)
tube = £1.65
Brands include *Diazepam Rectubes®*, *Stesolid®*

◀ Oral preparations
Section 15.1.4.1

▰ FOSPHENYTOIN SODIUM

Note Fosphenytoin is a pro-drug of phenytoin

Cautions see Phenytoin Sodium; resuscitation
facilities must be available; **interactions:** see
p. 264 and Appendix 1 (phenytoin)

Hepatic impairment consider 10–25% reduction
in dose or infusion rate (except initial dose for
status epilepticus)

Renal impairment consider 10–25% reduction in
dose or infusion rate (except initial dose for status
epilepticus)

Pregnancy see Phenytoin (section 4.8.1)

Breast-feeding see Phenytoin (section 4.8.1)

Contra-indications see Phenytoin Sodium

Side-effects see Phenytoin Sodium
CSM advice Intravenous infusion of fosphenytoin has
been associated with severe cardiovascular reactions
including asystole, ventricular fibrillation, and cardiac
arrest. Hypotension, bradycardia, and heart block have
also been reported. The CSM advises:

- monitor heart rate, blood pressure, and respiratory
  function for duration of infusion

- observe patient for at least 30 minutes after infusion

- if hypotension occurs, reduce infusion rate or discontinue

- reduce dose or infusion rate in renal or hepatic
  impairment

Indication and dose

Expressed as **phenytoin sodium equivalent** (PE);
fosphenytoin sodium 1.5 mg ≡ phenytoin sodium
1 mg

Status epilepticus
- **By intravenous infusion (at a rate of 2–
  3 mg(PE)/kg/minute)**
  Child 5–18 years initially 20 mg(PE)/kg, then

(at a rate of 1–2 mg(PE)/kg/minute) 4–
5 mg(PE)/kg; total daily dose may be given in 1–
4 divided doses; adjusted according to response
and trough plasma-phenytoin concentration

Prophylaxis or treatment of seizures associated
with neurosurgery or head injury
- **By intravenous infusion (at a rate of 1–
  2 mg(PE)/kg/minute)**
  Child 5–18 years initially 10–15 mg(PE)/kg
  then 4–5 mg(PE)/kg daily; total daily dose may
  be given in 1–4 divided doses; adjusted
  according to response and trough plasma-
  phenytoin concentration

Temporary substitution for oral phenytoin
- **By intravenous infusion (at a rate of 1–
  2 mg(PE)/kg/minute)**
  Child 5–18 years same dose and dosing frequency as oral phenytoin therapy

Note Fosphenytoin sodium doses in BNFC may differ
from those in product literature

Note Prescriptions for fosphenytoin sodium should
state the dose in terms of phenytoin sodium equivalent (PE)

Administration for *intermittent intravenous infusion*,
dilute to a concentration of 1.5–25 mg (PE)/mL
with Glucose 5% *or* Sodium Chloride 0.9%

Pro-Epanutin® (Pfizer) [PoM]
Injection, fosphenytoin sodium 75 mg/mL
(equivalent to phenytoin sodium 50 mg/mL), net
price 10-mL vial = £40.00
Electrolytes phosphate 3.7 micromol/mg fosphenytoin sodium (phosphate 5.6 micromol/mg phenytoin sodium)

▰ LORAZEPAM

Cautions see under Diazepam; facilities for
reversing respiratory depression with mechanical
ventilation must be at hand

Contra-indications see under Diazepam

Side-effects see under Diazepam; hypotension
and apnoea

Indication and dose
Status epilepticus
- **By slow intravenous injection**

  Neonate 100 micrograms/kg as a single dose,
  repeated once after 10 minutes if necessary

  Child 1 month–12 years 100 micrograms/kg
  (max. 4 mg) as a single dose, repeated once after
  10 minutes if necessary

  Child 12–18 years 4 mg as a single dose,
  repeated once after 10 minutes if necessary

Administration for *intravenous injection*, dilute with
an equal volume of Sodium Chloride 0.9% *or*
Water for Injections (for neonates, dilute injection
solution to a concentration of 100 micrograms/
mL); give slowly into a large vein at a rate not
exceeding 50 micrograms/kg over 3–5 minutes.

◀ Preparations
Section 15.1.4.1

4 Central nervous system

MIDAZOLAM

Cautions section 15.1.4

Contra-indications section 15.1.4

Side-effects section 15.1.4

Licensed use buccal liquid and injection not licensed for use in status epilepticus

Indication and dose

Status epilepticus
* **By buccal administration**

    Neonate 300 micrograms/kg repeated once after 10 minutes if necessary

    Child 1–6 months 300 micrograms/kg (max. 2.5 mg), repeated once after 10 minutes if necessary

    Child 6 months–1 year 2.5 mg, repeated once after 10 minutes if necessary

    Child 1–5 years 5 mg, repeated once after 10 minutes if necessary

    Child 5–10 years 7.5 mg, repeated once after 10 minutes if necessary

    Child 10–18 years 10 mg, repeated once after 10 minutes if necessary

* **By intravenous administration**

    Neonate initially *by intravenous injection* 150–200 micrograms/kg followed *by continuous infusion* of 1 microgram/kg/minute (increased by 1 microgram/kg/minute every 15 minutes until seizure controlled; max. 5 micrograms/kg/minute)

    Child 1 month–18 years initially *by intravenous injection* 150–200 micrograms/kg followed *by continuous intravenous infusion* of 1 microgram/kg/minute (increased by 1 microgram/kg/minute every 15 minutes) until seizure controlled; max. 5 micrograms/kg/minute

Administration for *intravenous injection*, dilute with Glucose 5% or Sodium Chloride 0.9%; rapid intravenous injection (less than 2 minutes) may cause seizure-like myoclonus in preterm neonate
For *buccal administration*, injection solution may be given buccally or by mouth

◢Preparations
Section 15.1.4

PARALDEHYDE

Cautions bronchopulmonary disease, hepatic impairment; **interactions**: Appendix 1 (paraldehyde)

Pregnancy manufacturer advises avoid—crosses placenta

Breast-feeding present in milk—manufacturer advises avoid unless essential

Contra-indications gastric disorders; rectal administration in colitis

Side-effects rashes; rectal irritation after enema

Licensed use not licensed for use in children as an enema

Indication and dose

Status epilepticus
* **By rectum (doses expressed as undiluted paraldehyde)**

    Neonate 0.4 mL/kg (max. 0.5 mL) as a single dose

    Child 1–3 months 0.5 mL as a single dose

    Child 3–6 months 1 mL as a single dose

    Child 6 months–1 year 1.5 mL as a single dose

    Child 1–2 years 2 mL as a single dose

    Child 2–5 years 3–4 mL as a single dose

    Child 5–18 years 5–10 mL as a single dose

Administration for *rectal administration*, do not administer paraldehyde undiluted

Paraldehyde (Non-proprietary) [PoM]
Enema, 8–50%, available from 'special-order' manufacturers or specialist importing companies, see p. 943

PHENOBARBITAL SODIUM
Phenobarbitone sodium

Cautions see under Phenobarbital (section 4.8.1)

Side-effects see under Phenobarbital (section 4.8.1)

Indication and dose

Status epilepticus
* **By slow intravenous injection**

    Neonate initially 20 mg/kg then 2.5–5 mg/kg once or twice daily

    Child 1 month–12 years initially 20 mg/kg then 2.5–5 mg/kg once or twice daily

    Child 12–18 years initially 20 mg/kg (max. 1 g) then 300 mg twice daily

Other forms of epilepsy section 4.8.1

Note For therapeutic purposes phenobarbital and phenobarbital sodium may be considered equivalent in effect

Administration for *intravenous injection*, dilute to a concentration of 20 mg/mL with Water for Injections; give over 20 minutes (no faster than 1 mg/kg/minute)

◁ **PHENOBARBITAL SODIUM** (*continued*)

Phenobarbital (Non-proprietary) ⒸⒹ
Injection, phenobarbital sodium 200 mg/mL, net price 1-mL amp = £2.00
Excipients include propylene glycol 90% (see Excipients, p. 3)
Note Must be diluted before intravenous administration (see Administration)

◀Oral preparations
Section 4.8.1

■ **PHENYTOIN SODIUM**

Cautions hypotension and heart failure; resuscitation facilities must be available; injection solutions alkaline (irritant to tissues); see also p. 274; **interactions**: see p. 264 and Appendix 1 (phenytoin)

Contra-indications sinus bradycardia, sino-atrial block, and second- and third-degree heart block; Stokes-Adams syndrome; acute porphyria (section 9.8.2)

Side-effects intravenous injection may cause cardiovascular and CNS depression (particularly if injection too rapid) with arrhythmias, hypotension, and cardiovascular collapse; alterations in respiratory function (including respiratory arrest); injection-site reactions, see also p. 274

Indication and dose

Status epilepticus, acute symptomatic seizures associated with trauma or neurosurgery
• **By slow intravenous injection or infusion (with blood-pressure and ECG monitoring)**

Neonate initially 18 mg/kg as a loading dose then 2.5–5 mg/kg twice daily

Child 1 month–12 years initially 18 mg/kg as a loading dose then 2.5–5 mg/kg twice daily

Child 12–18 years initially 18 mg/kg as a loading dose then up to 100 mg 3–4 times daily

• **By intramuscular injection**
Not recommended (see notes above)

Other forms of epilepsy section 4.8.1

Note Phenytoin sodium doses in BNFC may differ from those in product literature

Administration before and after administration flush intravenous line with Sodium Chloride 0.9%.
For *intravenous injection*, give at rate not exceeding 1 mg/kg/minute (max. 50 mg/minute).
For *intravenous infusion*, dilute to a concentration not exceeding 10 mg/mL with Sodium Chloride 0.9% and give through an in-line filter (0.22–0.50 micron) at a rate not exceeding 1 mg/kg/minute (max. 50 mg/minute); complete administration within 1 hour of preparation

Phenytoin (Non-proprietary) ⒫ⓄⓂ
Injection, phenytoin sodium 50 mg/mL with propylene glycol 40% and alcohol 10% in water for injections, net price 5-mL amp = £3.40

Epanutin® Ready-Mixed Parenteral (Pfizer) ⒫ⓄⓂ
Injection, phenytoin sodium 50 mg/mL with propylene glycol 40% and alcohol 10% in water for injections. Net price 5-mL amp = £4.88

◀Oral preparations
Section 4.8.1

4 Central nervous system

4.8.3 **Febrile convulsions**

Brief febrile convulsions need no specific treatment; antipyretic medication e.g. **paracetamol** (section 4.7.1) is commonly used to reduce fever and prevent further convulsions but evidence to support this practice is lacking. *Prolonged febrile convulsions* (those lasting 15 minutes or longer), *recurrent convulsions*, or those occurring in a child at known risk must be treated more actively, as there is the possibility of resulting brain damage. **Diazepam** (section 4.8.2) is the drug of choice given either by slow intravenous injection or preferably rectally in solution, repeated if necessary. The rectal solution is generally preferred as satisfactory absorption is achieved within minutes and administration is much easier. Suppositories are not suitable because absorption is too slow.

Intermittent prophylaxis (i.e. the anticonvulsant administered at the onset of fever) is possible in only a small proportion of children; rectal administration of **diazepam** is the treatment of choice.

Long-term anticonvulsant prophylaxis for febrile convulsions is rarely indicated. Anticonvulsant treatment needs to be considered only for children at risk from prolonged or complex febrile convulsions, including those whose first seizure occurred at under 14 months or who have neurological abnormalities or who have had previous prolonged or focal convulsions.

4.9 Drugs used in dystonias and related disorders

4.9.1 Dopaminergic drugs used in dystonias
4.9.2 Antimuscarinic drugs used in dystonias
4.9.3 Drugs used in essential tremor, chorea, tics, and related disorders

Dystonias may result from conditions such as cerebral palsy or may be related to a deficiency of the neurotransmitter dopamine as in Segawa syndrome.

4.9.1 Dopaminergic drugs used in dystonias

Levodopa, the amino-acid precursor of dopamine, acts by replenishing depleted striatal dopamine. It is given with an extracerebral **dopa-decarboxylase inhibitor** that reduces the peripheral conversion of levodopa to dopamine, thereby limiting side-effects such as nausea, vomiting and cardiovascular effects; additionally, effective brain-dopamine concentrations can be achieved with lower doses of levodopa. The extracerebral dopa-decarboxylase inhibitor most commonly used in children is carbidopa (in **co-careldopa**).

Levodopa therapy should be initiated at a low dose and increased in small steps; the final dose should be as low as possible. Intervals between doses should be chosen to suit the needs of the individual child.

In severe dystonias related to cerebral palsy, improvement can be expected within 2 weeks. Children with Segawa syndrome are particularly sensitive to levodopa; they may even become symptom free on small doses. Levodopa also has a role in treating metabolic disorders such as defects in tetrahydrobiopterin synthesis and dihydrobiopterin reductase deficiency. For the use of tetrahydrobiopterin in metabolic disorders see section 9.4.1.

Children may experience nausea within 2 hours of taking a dose; nausea and vomiting with co-careldopa is rarely dose-limiting but domperidone (section 4.6) may be useful in controlling these effects.

In dystonic cerebral palsy treatment with larger doses of levodopa is associated with the development of potentially troublesome motor complications including response fluctuations and dyskinesias. Response fluctuations are characterised by large variations in motor performance, with normal function during the 'on' period, and weakness and restricted mobility during the 'off' period.

Sudden onset of sleep
Excessive daytime sleepiness and sudden onset of sleep can occur with co-careldopa.

Children starting treatment with these drugs, and their carers, should be warned of the possibility of these effects and of the need to exercise caution when performing skilled tasks e.g. driving or operating machinery.

Children who have suffered excessive sedation or sudden onset of sleep should refrain from performing skilled tasks until those effects have stopped recurring.

CO-CARELDOPA

A mixture of carbidopa and levodopa; the proportions are expressed in the form *x/y* where *x* and *y* are the strengths in milligrams of carbidopa and levodopa respectively

Cautions see also notes above; pulmonary disease, peptic ulceration, cardiovascular disease, diabetes mellitus, osteomalacia, open-angle glaucoma, history of skin melanoma (risk of activation), psychiatric illness (avoid if severe); warn children and carers about excessive drowsiness (see notes above); in prolonged therapy, psychiatric, hepatic, haematological, renal, and cardiovascular surveillance is advisable; warn patients to resume normal activities gradually; avoid abrupt withdrawal; **interactions:** Appendix 1 (levodopa)

Contra-indications closed-angle glaucoma

Pregnancy manufacturers advise toxicity in *animal* studies

Breast-feeding may suppress lactation; present in milk—manufacturers advise avoid

Side-effects see also notes above; anorexia, nausea and vomiting, insomnia, agitation, postural hypotension (rarely labile hypertension), dizziness, tachycardia, arrhythmias, reddish discoloration of urine and other body fluids, rarely hypersensitivity; abnormal involuntary movements and psychiatric symptoms which include hypomania and psychosis may be dose-limiting; depression, drowsiness, headache, flushing,

◁ **CO-CARELDOPA** (*continued*)

sweating, gastro-intestinal bleeding, peripheral neuropathy, taste disturbance, pruritus, rash, and liver enzyme changes also reported; syndrome resembling neuroleptic malignant syndrome reported on withdrawal

Licensed use   not licensed for use in children

Indication and dose

Dopamine-sensitive dystonias including Segawa syndrome and dystonias related to cerebral palsy

• **By mouth, expressed as levodopa**

    Child 3 months–18 years initially 250 micrograms/kg 2–3 times daily of a preparation containing 1:4 carbidopa:levodopa, increased according to response every 2–3 days to max. 1 mg/kg three times daily

Treatment of defects in tetrahydrobiopterin synthesis and dihydrobiopterin reductase deficiency

• **By mouth, expressed as levodopa**

    Neonate initially 250–500 micrograms/kg 4 times daily of a preparation containing 1:4 carbidopa:levodopa, increased according to response every 4–5 days to maintenance dose of 2.5–3 mg/kg 4 times daily; at higher doses consider preparation containing 1:10 carbidopa:levodopa; review regularly (every 3–6 months)

Child 1 month–18 years initially 250–500 micrograms/kg 4 times daily of a preparation containing 1:4 carbidopa:levodopa, increased according to response every 4–5 days to maintenance dose of 2.5–3 mg/kg 4 times daily; at higher doses consider preparation containing 1:10 carbidopa:levodopa; review regularly (every 3–6 months in early childhood)

Sinemet® (Bristol-Myers Squibb) [PoM]
Sinemet-62.5® tablets, yellow, scored, co-careldopa 12.5/50 (carbidopa 12.5 mg (as monohydrate), levodopa 50 mg), net price 90-tab pack = £6.54. Label: 14, counselling, driving, see notes above

Note 2 tablets *Sinemet-62.5®* ≡ 1 tablet *Sinemet Plus®*; *Sinemet-62.5®* previously known as *Sinemet LS®*

Sinemet-110® tablets, blue, scored, co-careldopa 10/100 (carbidopa 10 mg (as monohydrate), levodopa 100 mg), net price 90-tab pack = £6.84. Label: 14, counselling, driving, see notes above

Sinemet-Plus® tablets, yellow, scored, co-careldopa 25/100 (carbidopa 25 mg (as monohydrate), levodopa 100 mg), net price 90-tab pack = £10.05. Label: 14, counselling, driving, see notes above

Sinemet-275® tablets, blue, scored, co-careldopa 25/250 (carbidopa 25 mg (as monohydrate), levodopa 250 mg), net price 90-tab pack = £14.28. Label: 14, counselling, driving, see notes above

4.9.2   Antimuscarinic drugs used in dystonias

Antimuscarinic drugs help to control dystonias.

The antimuscarinic drugs **procyclidine** and **trihexyphenidyl** (benzhexol) reduce the symptoms of dystonias, including those induced by antipsychotic drugs; there is no justification for giving them routinely in the absence of dystonic symptoms. Tardive dyskinesia is not improved by antimuscarinic drugs and may be made worse.

No important differences exist between the antimuscarinic drugs, but some children tolerate one better than another.

Cautions   Antimuscarinics should be used with caution in cardiovascular disease, hypertension, psychotic disorders, pyrexia, and in those susceptible to angle-closure glaucoma. Antimuscarinics should not be withdrawn abruptly in children receiving long-term treatment. Antimuscarinics are liable to abuse. They should also be used with caution in hepatic impairment, renal impairment, pregnancy, and breast-feeding. **Interactions**: Appendix 1 (Antimuscarinics).

Driving   May affect performance of skilled tasks (e.g. driving).

Contra-indications   Antimuscarinics should be avoided in gastro-intestinal obstruction and myasthenia gravis.

Side-effects   Side-effects of antimuscarinics include constipation, dry mouth, nausea, vomiting, tachycardia, dizziness, confusion, euphoria, hallucinations, impaired memory, anxiety, restlessness, urinary retention, blurred vision, and rash. Angle-closure glaucoma may occur very rarely.

▌PROCYCLIDINE HYDROCHLORIDE

Cautions   see notes above

    Pregnancy   manufacturers advise use only if potential benefit outweighs risk

Breast-feeding   no information available

Contra-indications   see notes above

Side-effects   see notes above

4   Central nervous system

◿ PROCYCLIDINE HYDROCHLORIDE (*continued*)

Licensed use not licensed for use in children

Indication and dose

Dystonias
● By mouth
Child 7–12 years 1.25 mg 3 times daily
Child 12–18 years 2.5 mg 3 times daily

Acute dystonia
● By intramuscular or intravenous injection
Child under 2 years 0.5–2 mg as a single dose
Child 2–10 years 2–5 mg as a single dose
Child 10–18 years 5–10 mg (occasionally more than 10 mg)
Note Usually effective in 5–10 minutes but may need 30 minutes for relief

Procyclidine (Non-proprietary) ℗ℴ𝕄
Tablets, procyclidine hydrochloride 5 mg, net price 28-tab pack = £3.26. Counselling, driving

Arpicolin® (Rosemont) ℗ℴ𝕄
Syrup, sugar-free, procyclidine hydrochloride 2.5 mg/5 mL, net price 150 mL = £4.22; 5 mg/5 mL, 150 mL pack = £7.54. Counselling, driving

Kemadrin® (GSK) ℗ℴ𝕄
Tablets, scored, procyclidine hydrochloride 5 mg, net price 20 = 94p. Counselling, driving

Kemadrin® (Auden Mckenzie) ℗ℴ𝕄
Injection, procyclidine hydrochloride 5 mg/mL, net price 2-mL amp = £1.49

▌ TRIHEXYPHENIDYL HYDROCHLORIDE
(Benzhexol hydrochloride)

Cautions see notes above
Pregnancy manufacturer advises use only if potential benefit outweighs risk
Breast-feeding manufacturer advises avoid
Contra-indications see notes above
Side-effects see notes above
Licensed use not licensed for use in children

Indication and dose

Dystonia
● By mouth
Child 1 month–18 years 1–2 mg daily in 1–2 divided doses, adjusted according to response

Trihexyphenidyl (Non-proprietary) ℗ℴ𝕄
Tablets, trihexyphenidyl hydrochloride 2 mg, net price 84-tab pack = £24.63; 5 mg, 100-tab pack = £14.63. Counselling, before or after food, driving

Broflex® (Alliance) ℗ℴ𝕄
Syrup, pink, black currant, trihexyphenidyl hydrochloride 5 mg/5 mL, net price 200 mL = £6.20. Counselling, driving

▌ 4.9.3 ▐ Drugs used in essential tremor, chorea, tics, and related disorders

Haloperidol may be useful in improving motor tics and symptoms of Tourette syndrome and related choreas (see section 4.2.1). **Pimozide** (section 4.2.1) and **sulpiride** (section 4.2.1) are also used in Tourette syndrome.

Propranolol or another beta-adrenoceptor blocking drug (section 2.4) may be useful in treating essential tremor or tremor associated with anxiety or thyrotoxicosis.

▌ BOTULINUM TOXIN TYPE A

Cautions neurological disorders; history of dysphagia or aspiration
Pregnancy manufacturers advise avoid unless essential—toxicity in *animal* studies
Breast-feeding manufacturers advise avoid (or avoid unless essential)—no information available
Contra-indications generalised disorders of muscle activity (e.g. myasthenia gravis)
Side-effects increased electrophysiologic jitter in some distant muscles; misplaced injections may paralyse nearby muscle groups and excessive doses may paralyse distant muscles; influenza-like symptoms, *rarely* arrhythmias, myocardial infarction, seizures, hypersensitivity reactions including rash, pruritus and anaphylaxis, antibody formation (substantial deterioration in

response), and injection-site reactions; *very rarely* exaggerated muscle weakness, dysphagia, and aspiration
Specific side-effects in paediatric cerebral palsy Drowsiness, paraesthesia, urinary incontinence, myalgia

Indication and dose

In children over 2 years for dynamic equinus foot deformity caused by spasticity in ambulant paediatric cerebral palsy for dose consult product literature (**important: information specific to each individual preparation and not interchangeable**)

4 Central nervous system

◻ **BOTULINUM TOXIN TYPE A** (*continued*)

Botox® (Allergan) [PoM]
Injection, powder for reconstitution, botulinum A neurotoxin complex, net price 50-unit vial = £72.30; 100-unit vial = £128.93

Dysport® (Ipsen) [PoM]
Injection, powder for reconstitution, botulinum A toxin-haemagglutinin complex, net price 500-unit vial = £164.50

4.10 Drugs used in substance dependence

This section includes drugs used in the treatment of neonatal abstinence syndrome and cigarette smoking.

Treatment of alcohol or opioid dependence in children requires specialist management. The health departments of the UK have produced a report, *Drug Misuse and Dependence* which contains guidelines on clinical management.

Drug Misuse and Dependence, London, The Stationery Office, 1999 can be obtained from:
The Publications Centre
PO Box 276
London, SW8 5DT.
Tel: (087) 0600 5522
Fax: (087) 0600 5533

or from The Stationery Office bookshops and through all good booksellers.

Neonatal abstinence syndrome   Neonatal abstinence syndrome occurs at birth as a result of intra-uterine exposure to opioids or high-dose benzodiazepines.

Treatment is usually initiated if:

- feeding becomes a problem and tube feeding is required;

- there is profuse vomiting or watery diarrhoea;

- the baby remains very unsettled after two consecutive feeds despite gentle swaddling and the use of a pacifier.

Treatment involves weaning the baby from the drug on which it is dependent. **Morphine** or **methadone** (section 4.7.2) can be used in babies of mothers who have been taking opioids. Morphine is widely used because the dose can be easily adjusted, but methadone may provide smoother control of symptoms. Weaning babies from opioids usually takes 7–10 days.

Weaning babies from benzodiazepines that have a long half-life is difficult to manage; **chlorpromazine** (section 4.2.1) may be used in these situations but excessive sedation may occur. For babies who are dependent on barbiturates, phenobarbital (section 4.8.1) may be tried, although it does not control gastro-intestinal symptoms.

Cigarette smoking

Smoking cessation interventions are a cost-effective way of reducing ill health and prolonging life. Smokers should be advised to stop and offered help if interested in doing so, with follow-up where appropriate.

Where possible, smokers should have access to a smoking cessation clinic for behavioural support. **Nicotine replacement therapy** is an effective aid to smoking cessation for those smoking more than 10 cigarettes a day. It is regarded as the pharmacological treatment of choice in the management of smoking cessation.

Cigarette smoking should stop completely before starting a smoking cessation regimen including nicotine replacement therapy. If complete smoking cessation is not possible some nicotine preparations are licensed for use as part of a programme to reduce smoking before stopping completely; the smoking cessation regimen can be followed during a quit attempt.

4 Central nervous system

4 Central nervous system

NICOTINE

Cautions severe or unstable cardiovascular disease (including hospitalisation for severe arrhythmias, recent myocardial infarction, or recent cerebrovascular accident)—initiate under medical supervision; uncontrolled hyperthyroidism; diabetes mellitus (monitor blood-glucose concentration closely when initiating treatment); phaeochromocytoma; *oral preparations*, oesophagitis, gastritis, peptic ulcers; *patches*, exercise may increase absorption and side-effects, skin disorders (patches should not be placed on broken skin)

Hepatic impairment manufacturers advise caution in moderate to severe hepatic impairment

Renal impairment manufacturers advise caution in severe renal impairment

Pregnancy use only if smoking cessation without nicotine replacement therapy fails; intermittent therapy preferred but avoid liquorice-flavoured nicotine products

Breast-feeding present in milk; intermittent therapy preferred

Note Most warnings under Cautions also apply to continuation of cigarette smoking

Side-effects gastro-intestinal disturbances (including nausea, vomiting, dyspepsia); headache, dizziness; influenza-like symptoms; dry mouth; rash; *less frequently* palpitation; *rarely* atrial fibrillation; *with nasal spray*, sneezing, epistaxis, watering eyes, ear sensations; *with lozenges*, thirst, paraesthesia of mouth, taste disturbances; *with patches*, skin reactions (discontinue if severe)—vasculitis also reported, blood pressure changes; *with patches* or *lozenges*, sleep disturbances, nightmares, chest pain; *with gum* or *lozenges*, mouth ulceration, increased salivation; *with gum, lozenge, sublingual tablets,* or *inhalator*, hiccups, throat irritation

Indication and dose

See under preparations, below

Nicorette® (McNeil)

Nicorette Microtab (sublingual), nicotine (as a cyclodextrin complex) 2 mg, net price starter pack of 2 × 15-tablet discs with dispenser = £3.99; refill pack of 7 × 15-tablet discs = £11.12. Label: 26

Dose

Smoking cessation
• **By sublingual administration**

Child 12–18 years individuals smoking *20 cigarettes or less daily*, 2 mg each hour; for patients who fail to stop smoking or have significant withdrawal symptoms, consider increasing to 4 mg each hour; individuals smoking *more than 20 cigarettes daily*, 4 mg each hour. Max. 80 mg daily; treatment continued for up to 8 weeks followed by gradual reduction over 4 weeks; review treatment if abstinence not achieved within 3 months

Nicorette chewing gum, sugar-free, nicotine (as resin) 2 mg, net price pack of 15 = £1.71, pack of 30 = £3.25, pack of 105 = £8.89; 4 mg, net price pack of 15 = £2.11, pack of 30 = £3.99, pack of 105 = £10.83

Note Also available in mint, freshfruit, freshmint, and icy white flavours

Dose

Smoking cessation
• **By mouth**

Child 12–18 years individuals *smoking 20 cigarettes or less daily*, initially chew one 2-mg piece slowly (chew gum until taste becomes strong, then rest gum between cheek and gum, when taste fades start chewing again) for approx. 30 minutes when urge to smoke occurs; individuals smoking *more than 20 cigarettes daily* or needing more than 15 pieces of 2-mg gum daily should use the 4-mg gum; max. 15 pieces of 4-mg gum daily; treatment continued for up to 8 weeks followed by gradual reduction over 4 weeks; review treatment if abstinence not achieved within 3 months

Smoking reduction
• **By mouth**

Child 12–18 years chew one piece when urge to smoke occurs between smoking episodes (chew gum until taste becomes strong, then rest gum between cheek and gum, when taste fades start chewing again); reduce smoking within 6 weeks and attempt smoking cessation within 6 months; review treatment if abstinence not achieved within 9 months

Note Children under 18 years should consult a healthcare professional before starting smoking-reduction regimen

◁ **NICOTINE** (*continued*)

Nicorette patches, self-adhesive, all beige, nicotine, *'5 mg' patch* (releasing approx. 5 mg/16 hours), net price 7 = £9.07; *'10 mg' patch* (releasing approx. 10 mg/16 hours), 7 = £9.07; *'15 mg' patch* (releasing approx. 15 mg/16 hours), 2 = £2.85, 7 = £9.07

Dose

Smoking cessation
• **By transdermal route**

Child 12–18 years apply on waking to dry, non-hairy skin on hip, chest, or upper arm, removing after approx. 16 hours, usually when retiring to bed; site next patch on different area (avoid using same area on consecutive days); initially '15-mg' patch for 16 hours daily for 8 weeks then if abstinence achieved '10-mg' patch for 16 hours daily for 2 weeks then '5-mg' patch for 16 hours daily for 2 weeks; review treatment if abstinence not achieved within 3 months—further courses may be given if considered beneficial

Nicorette Invisi patches, self-adhesive, beige, nicotine, *'10 mg'* patch (releasing approx. 10 mg/16 hours), net price 7 = £14.83; *'15 mg'* patch (releasing approx. 15 mg/16 hours), 7 = £14.83; *'25 mg'* patch (releasing approx. 25 mg/16 hours), 7 = £14.83

Dose

Smoking cessation
• **By transdermal route**

Child 12–18 years apply on waking to dry, non-hairy skin on hip, chest, or upper arm, removing after approx. 16 hours, usually when retiring to bed; site next patch on different area (avoid using same area on consecutive days); individuals smoking *10 or more cigarettes daily*, initially '25-mg' patch for 16 hours daily for 8 weeks then if abstinence achieved '15-mg' patch for 16 hours daily for 2 weeks then '10-mg' patch for 16 hours daily for 2 weeks; individuals smoking *less than 10 cigarettes daily*, initially '15-mg' patch for 16 hours daily for 8 weeks then '10-mg' patch for 16 hours daily for 4 weeks; review treatment if abstinence not achieved within 3 months—further courses may be given if considered beneficial

Note Patients using the '25-mg' patch who experience excessive side-effects that do not resolve within a few days should change to '15-mg' patch for the remainder of the initial 8-week course before switching to the '10-mg' patch for the final 4 weeks

Nicorette nasal spray, nicotine 500 micrograms/metered spray, net price 200-spray unit = £12.26

Dose

Smoking cessation
• **Intranasally**

Child 12–18 years apply 1 spray into each nostril as required to max. twice an hour for 16 hours daily (max. 64 sprays daily) for 8 weeks, then reduce gradually over next 4 weeks (reduce by half at end of first 2 weeks, stop altogether at end of next 2 weeks); review treatment if abstinence not achieved within 3 months

Nicorette inhalator (nicotine-impregnated plug for use in inhalator mouthpiece), nicotine 10 mg/cartridge, net price 6-cartridge (starter) pack = £3.99, 42-cartridge (refill) pack = £12.82

Dose

Smoking cessation
• **By inhalation**

Child 12–18 years inhale when urge to smoke occurs; initially use between 6 and 12 cartridges daily for up to 8 weeks, then reduce gradually over 4 weeks (reduce by half over first 2 weeks, stop altogether at end of next 2 weeks); review treatment if abstinence not achieved within 3 months

Smoking reduction
• **By inhalation**

Child 12–18 years inhale when urge to smoke occurs between smoking episodes; reduce smoking within 6 weeks and attempt smoking cessation within 6 months; review treatment if abstinence not achieved within 9 months

Note Children under 18 years should consult a healthcare professional before starting smoking-reduction regimen

Nicotinell® (Novartis Consumer Health)

Chewing gum, sugar-free, nicotine 2 mg, net price pack of 12 = £1.71, pack of 24 = £3.01, pack of 96 = £8.26; 4 mg, pack of 12 = £1.70, pack of 24 = £3.30, pack of 96 = £10.26

Note Also available in fruit, liquorice, and mint flavours

Dose

Smoking cessation
• **By mouth**

Child 12–18 years individuals smoking *20 cigarettes or less daily*, initially chew one 2-mg piece slowly (chew gum until taste becomes strong, then rest gum between cheek and gum, when taste fades start chewing again) for approx. 30 minutes when urge to smoke occurs; individuals smoking *more than 20 cigarettes daily* should use the 4-mg strength; max. 60 mg daily; withdraw gradually; review treatment if abstinence not achieved within 3 months

Nicotinell mint lozenge, sugar-free, nicotine (as bitartrate) 1 mg, net price pack of 12 = £1.71, pack of 36 = £4.27, pack of 96 = £9.12; 2 mg, net price pack of 12 = £1.99, pack of 36 = £4.95, pack of 96 = £10.60. Label: 24

Excipients include aspartame (section 9.4.1)

Dose

Smoking cessation
• **By mouth**

Child 12–18 years individuals smoking *30 cigarettes or less daily*, initially suck one 1-mg lozenge every 1–2 hours when urge to smoke occurs; individuals smoking *more than 30 cigarettes daily* should use 2-mg strength; max. 30 mg daily; withdraw gradually; review treatment if abstinence not achieved within 3 months

TTS Patches, self-adhesive, all yellowish-ochre, nicotine, *'10' patch* (releasing approx. 7 mg/24 hours), net price 7 = £9.12; *'20' patch* (releasing approx. 14 mg/24 hours), net price 2 = £2.57, 7 = £9.40; *'30' patch* (releasing approx. 21 mg/24 hours), net price 2 = £2.85, 7 = £9.97, 21 = £24.51

Dose

Smoking cessation
• **By transdermal route**

Child 12–18 years apply to dry, non-hairy skin on trunk or upper arm, removing after 24 hours and siting replacement patch on a different area (avoid using the same area for several days); individuals smoking *less than 20 cigarettes daily*, initially '20' patch daily; individuals smoking *20 or more cigarettes daily*, initially '30' patch daily; withdraw gradually, reducing dose every 3–4 weeks; review treatment if abstinence not achieved within 3 months

4

Central nervous system

◁ **NICOTINE (continued)**

NiQuitin® (GSK Consumer Healthcare)

Chewing gum, sugar-free, mint-flavour, nicotine 2 mg (white), net price pack of 12 = £1.71, pack of 24 = £2.85, pack of 96 = £8.55; 4 mg (yellow), pack of 12 = £1.71, pack of 24 = £2.85, pack of 96 = £8.55

Dose

Smoking cessation

• **By mouth**

Child 12–18 years initially chew 1 piece slowly (chew gum until taste becomes strong, then rest gum between cheek and gum, when taste fades start chewing again) for approx. 30 minutes, when urge to smoke occurs; max. 15 pieces daily; withdraw gradually; review treatment if abstinence not achieved within 3 months

Smoking reduction

• **By mouth**

Child 12–18 years chew 1 piece when urge to smoke occurs between smoking episodes (chew gum until taste becomes strong, then rest gum between cheek and gum, when taste fades start chewing again); reduce smoking within 6 weeks and attempt cessation within 6 months; review treatment if abstinence not achieved within 9 months

Note Children under 18 years should consult a healthcare professional before starting smoking-reduction regimen

Temporary abstinence

• **By mouth**

Child 12–18 years chew 1 piece when urge to smoke occurs between smoking episodes; max. 15 pieces daily; review treatment if unable to undertake permanent quit attempt within 6 months

Lozenges, sugar-free, nicotine (as polacrilex) 2 mg, net price pack of 36 = £5.12, pack of 72 = £9.97; 4 mg, pack of 36 = £5.12, pack of 72 = £9.97. Contains 0.65 mmol Na^+/lozenge. Label: 24

Excipients include aspartame (section 9.4.1)

Dose

Smoking cessation

• **By mouth**

Child 12–18 years initially suck 1 lozenge every 1–2 hours when urge to smoke occurs (max. 15 lozenges daily) for 6 weeks, then 1 lozenge every 2–4 hours for 3 weeks, then 1 lozenge every 4–8 hours for 3 weeks; withdrawal gradually; review treatment if abstinence not achieved within 3 months

Smoking reduction

• **By mouth**

Child 12–18 years suck 1 lozenge when urge to smoke occurs between smoking episodes (max. 15 lozenges daily); reduce smoking within 6 weeks and attempt cessation within 6 months; review treatment if abstinence not achieved within 3 months

Note Children under 18 years should consult a healthcare professional before starting a smoking-reduction regimen

Temporary abstinence

• **By mouth**

Child 12–18 years suck 1 lozenge every 1–2 hours when urge to smoke occurs between smoking episodes (max. 15 lozenges daily); review treatment if unable to undertake permanent quit attempt within 6 months

Patches, self-adhesive, pink/beige, nicotine '7 mg' patch (releasing approx. 7 mg/24 hours), net price 7 = £9.97; '14 mg' patch (releasing approx. 14 mg/24 hours), 7 = £9.97; '21 mg' patch (releasing approx. 21 mg/24 hours), 7 = £9.97, 14 = £18.79

Note Also available as a clear patch

Dose

Smoking cessation

• **By transdermal route**

Child 12–18 years apply on waking to dry, non-hairy skin, removing after 24 hours and siting replacement patch on different area (avoid using same area for 7 days); individuals smoking 10 or more cigarettes daily, initially '21-mg' patch daily for 6 weeks then '14-mg' patch daily for 2 weeks then '7-mg' patch daily for 2 weeks. Individuals smoking less than 10 cigarettes daily, initially '14-mg' patch daily for 6 weeks then '7-mg' patch daily for 2 weeks; review treatment if abstinence not achieved within 3 months

Note Patients using the '21-mg' patch who experience excessive side-effects, which do not resolve within a few days, should change to '14-mg' patch for the remainder of the initial 6 weeks before switching to the '7-mg' patch for the final 2 weeks

4.11 Drugs for dementia

Classification not used in *BNF for Children*.

5 Infections

5.1	**Antibacterial drugs**	**296**
5.1.1	Penicillins	308
5.1.2	Cephalosporins, carbapenems, and other beta-lactams	319
5.1.3	Tetracyclines	328
5.1.4	Aminoglycosides	331
5.1.5	Macrolides	335
5.1.6	Clindamycin	339
5.1.7	Some other antibacterials	340
5.1.8	Sulphonamides and trimethoprim	346
5.1.9	Antituberculosis drugs	348
5.1.10	Antileprotic drugs	355
5.1.11	Metronidazole	355
5.1.12	Quinolones	357
5.1.13	Urinary-tract infections	360
5.2	**Antifungal drugs**	**361**
5.3	**Antiviral drugs**	**372**
5.3.1	HIV infection	372
5.3.2	Herpesvirus infections	385
5.3.3	Viral hepatitis	390
5.3.4	Influenza	390
5.3.5	Respiratory syncytial virus	392
5.4	**Antiprotozoal drugs**	**394**
5.4.1	Antimalarials	395
5.4.2	Amoebicides	407
5.4.3	Trichomonacides	408
5.4.4	Antigiardial drugs	408
5.4.5	Leishmaniacides	409
5.4.6	Trypanocides	409
5.4.7	Drugs for toxoplasmosis	409
5.4.8	Drugs for pneumocystis pneumonia	411
5.5	**Anthelmintics**	**413**
5.5.1	Drugs for threadworms	413
5.5.2	Ascaricides	414
5.5.3	Drugs for tapeworm infections	415
5.5.4	Drugs for hookworms	415
5.5.5	Schistosomicides	416
5.5.6	Filaricides	416
5.5.7	Drugs for cutaneous larva migrans	416
5.5.8	Drugs for strongyloidiasis	416

5

Infections

This chapter includes advice on the drug management of the following:

anthrax, p. 357

bacterial infections (summary of treatment and prophylaxis), p. 298–308

Lyme disease, p. 312

MRSA infections, p. 310

oral infections, p. 297 and p. 302

Notifiable diseases

Doctors must notify the Proper Officer of the local authority (usually the consultant in communicable disease control) when attending a patient suspected of suffering from any of the diseases listed below; a form is available from the Proper Officer.

Anthrax	Ophthalmia neonatorum
Cholera	Paratyphoid fever
Diphtheria	Plague
Dysentery (amoebic or bacillary)	Poliomyelitis, acute
Encephalitis, acute	Rabies
Food poisoning	Relapsing fever
Haemorrhagic fever (viral)	Rubella
Hepatitis, viral	Scarlet fever
Leprosy	Smallpox
Leptospirosis	Tetanus
Malaria	Tuberculosis
Measles	Typhoid fever
Meningitis	Typhus
Meningococcal septicaemia (without meningitis)	Whooping cough
Mumps	Yellow fever

Note It is good practice for doctors to also inform the consultant in communicable disease control of instances of other infections (e.g. psittacosis) where there could be a public health risk.

5.1 Antibacterial drugs

5.1.1 Penicillins
5.1.2 Cephalosporins, carbapenems, and other beta-lactams
5.1.3 Tetracyclines
5.1.4 Aminoglycosides
5.1.5 Macrolides
5.1.6 Clindamycin
5.1.7 Some other antibacterials
5.1.8 Sulphonamides and trimethoprim
5.1.9 Antituberculosis drugs
5.1.10 Antileprotic drugs
5.1.11 Metronidazole
5.1.12 Quinolones
5.1.13 Urinary-tract infections

Choice of a suitable drug Before selecting an antibacterial the clinician must first consider two factors—the child and the known or likely causative organism. Factors related to the child which must be considered include history of allergy, renal and hepatic function, susceptibility to infection (i.e. whether immunocompromised), ability to tolerate drugs by mouth, severity of illness, ethnic origin, age and, if an adolescent female, whether pregnant, breast-feeding or taking an oral contraceptive.

The known or likely organism and its antibacterial sensitivity, in association with the above factors, will suggest one or more antibacterials, the final choice depending on the microbiological, pharmacological, and toxicological properties.

The principles involved in selection of an antibacterial must allow for a number of variables including age, changing renal and hepatic function, increasing bacterial resistance, and new information on side-effects. Duration of therapy, dosage, and route of administration depend on site, type and severity of infection and response.

Antibacterial policies Local policies often limit the antibacterials that may be used to achieve reasonable economy consistent with adequate cover, and to reduce the development of resistant organisms. A policy may indicate a range of drugs for general use, and permit other drugs only on the advice of the microbiologist or paediatric infectious diseases specialist.

Before starting therapy   The following principles should be considered before starting:

- Viral infections should not be treated with antibacterials. However, antibacterials are occasionally helpful in controlling secondary bacterial infection (e.g. acute necrotising ulcerative gingivitis secondary to herpes simplex infections);

- Samples should be taken for culture and sensitivity testing whenever possible; **'blind'** antibacterial prescribing for unexplained pyrexia usually leads to further difficulty in establishing the diagnosis;

- Knowledge of **prevalent organisms** and their current **sensitivity** is of great help in choosing an antibacterial before bacteriological confirmation is available. Generally, narrow-spectrum antibacterials are preferred to broad-spectrum antibacterials unless there is a clear clinical indication (e.g. life-threatening sepsis);

- The **dose** of an antibacterial varies according to a number of factors including age, weight, hepatic function, renal function, and severity of infection. The prescribing of the so-called 'standard' dose in serious infections may result in failure of treatment or even death of the patient; therefore it is important to prescribe a dose appropriate to the condition. An inadequate dose may also increase the likelihood of antibacterial resistance. On the other hand, for an antibacterial with a narrow margin between the toxic and therapeutic dose (e.g. an aminoglycoside) it is also important to avoid an excessive dose and the concentration of the drug in the plasma may need to be monitored;

- The **route** of administration of an antibacterial often depends on the severity of the infection. Life-threatening infections often require intravenous therapy. Antibacterials that are well absorbed may be given by mouth even for some serious infections. Parenteral administration is also appropriate when the oral route cannot be used (e.g. because of vomiting) or if absorption is inadequate (e.g. in neonates and young children). Whenever possible painful intramuscular injections should be avoided in children;

- **Duration** of therapy depends on the nature of the infection and the response to treatment. Courses should not be unduly prolonged because they encourage resistance, they may lead to side-effects and they are costly. However, in certain infections such as tuberculosis or chronic osteomyelitis it is necessary to treat for prolonged periods.

Oral bacterial infections   Antibacterial drugs should only be prescribed for the *treatment* of oral infections on the basis of defined need. They may be used in conjunction with (but not as an alternative to) other appropriate measures, such as providing drainage or extracting a tooth.

The 'blind' prescribing of an antibacterial for unexplained pyrexia, cervical lymphadenopathy, or facial swelling can lead to difficulty in establishing the diagnosis. A sample should always be taken for bacteriology in the case of severe oral infection.

Oral infections which may require antibacterial treatment include acute periapical or periodontal abscess, cellulitis, acutely created oral-antral communication (and acute sinusitis), severe pericoronitis, localised osteitis, acute necrotising ulcerative gingivitis, and destructive forms of chronic periodontal disease. Most of these infections are readily resolved by the early establishment of drainage and removal of the cause (typically an infected necrotic pulp). Antibacterials may be indicated if treatment has to be delayed and they are essential in immunocompromised patients or in those with conditions such as diabetes. Certain rarer infections including bacterial sialadenitis, osteomyelitis, actinomycosis, and infections involving fascial spaces such as Ludwig's angina, require antibiotics and specialist hospital care.

Antibacterial drugs may also be useful after dental surgery in some cases of spreading infection. Infection may spread to involve local lymph nodes, to fascial spaces (where it can cause airway obstruction), or into the bloodstream (where it can lead to cavernous sinus thrombosis and other serious complications). Extension of an infection can also lead to maxillary sinusitis; osteomyelitis is a complication, which usually arises when host resistance is reduced.

If the oral infection fails to respond to antibacterial treatment within 48 hours the antibacterial should be changed, preferably on the basis of bacteriological investigation. Failure to respond may also suggest an incorrect diagnosis, lack of essential additional measures (such as drainage), poor host resistance, or poor patient compliance.

Combination of a penicillin (or erythromycin) with metronidazole may sometimes be helpful for the treatment of severe or resistant oral infections.

See also **Penicillins** (section 5.1.1), **Cephalosporins** (section 5.1.2.1), **Tetracyclines** (section 5.1.3), **Macrolides** (section 5.1.5), **Clindamycin** (section 5.1.6), **Metronidazole** (section 5.1.11), **Fusidic acid** (section 13.10.1.2) .

Superinfection   In general, broad-spectrum antibacterial drugs such as the cephalosporins are more likely to be associated with adverse reactions related to the selection of resistant organisms e.g. *fungal infections* or *antibiotic-associated colitis* (pseudomembranous colitis); other problems associated with superinfection include vaginitis and pruritus ani.

Therapy   Suggested treatment is shown in Table 1. When the pathogen has been isolated treatment may be changed to a more appropriate antibacterial if necessary. If no bacterium is cultured the antibacterial can be continued or stopped on clinical grounds. Infections for which prophylaxis is useful are listed in table 2.

Switching from parenteral to oral treatment   The ongoing parenteral administration of an antibacterial should be reviewed regularly. In older children it may be possible to switch to an oral antibacterial; in neonates and infants this should be done more cautiously because of the relatively high incidence of bacteraemia and the possibility of variable oral absorption.

Prophylaxis   Infections for which antibacterial prophylaxis is useful are listed in Table 2. In most situations, only a short course of prophylactic antibacterial is needed. Longer-term antibacterial prophylaxis is appropriate in specific indications such as vesico-ureteric reflux

Table 1. Summary of antibacterial therapy

> If treating a patient suspected of suffering from a notifiable disease, the consultant in communicable disease control should be informed (see p. 296)

Gastro-intestinal system

Gastro-enteritis
Antibacterial not usually indicated
  Frequently self-limiting and may not be bacterial

Campylobacter enteritis
Erythromycin[1] *or* ciprofloxacin
  Frequently self-limiting; treat severe infection

Salmonella
Ciprofloxacin *or* cefotaxime
  Treat invasive or severe infection; treat less severe infection in those at risk of developing invasive infection (e.g. immunocompromised, haemoglobinopathy, or child under 3 months)

Shigellosis
Azithromycin [unlicensed indication] *or* ciprofloxacin
  Antibacterial not indicated for mild cases. Amoxicillin or trimethoprim may be used if organism sensitive

Typhoid fever
Ciprofloxacin *or* cefotaxime *or* ceftriaxone
  Chloramphenicol may be an alternative; infections from Indian subcontinent, Middle-East, and South-East Asia may be multiple-antibacterial-resistant and sensitivity should be tested—azithromycin [unlicensed indication] may be an option in disease caused by multiple-antibacterial-resistant organisms

***Clostridium difficile* infection**
Oral metronidazole *or* oral vancomycin
  Treat for 7–10 days. Use vancomycin for severe infection or in patients intolerant of metronidazole. Give metronidazole by intravenous infusion if oral treatment inappropriate

Necrotising enterocolitis in neonates
Benzylpenicillin + gentamicin + metronidazole *or* amoxicillin[2] + gentamicin + metronidazole *or* amoxicillin[2] + cefotaxime + metronidazole

1. Where erythromycin is suggested another macrolide (e.g. azithromycin or clarithromycin) may be used.
2. Where amoxicillin is suggested ampicillin may be used.

Peritonitis
A cephalosporin (*or* amoxicillin + gentamicin) + metronidazole

Peritoneal dialysis-associated peritonitis
Either vancomycin[1] + ceftazidime added to dialysis fluid *or* vancomycin added to dialysis fluid + ciprofloxacin by mouth
> Treat for 14 days or longer

Cardiovascular system

Endocarditis: initial 'blind' therapy
Flucloxacillin (*or* benzylpenicillin if symptoms less severe) + gentamicin
> Substitute flucloxacillin (or benzylpenicillin) with vancomycin + rifampicin if cardiac prostheses present, or if penicillin-allergic, or if meticillin-resistant *Staphylococcus aureus* suspected

Endocarditis caused by staphylococci
Flucloxacillin (*or* vancomycin + rifampicin if penicillin-allergic or if meticillin-resistant *Staphylococcus aureus*)
> Treat for at least 4 weeks; treat prosthetic valve endocarditis for at least 6 weeks and if using flucloxacillin add rifampicin for at least 2 weeks

Endocarditis caused by streptococci (e.g. viridans streptococci)
Benzylpenicillin (*or* vancomycin[1] if penicillin-allergic or highly penicillin-resistant) + gentamicin
> Treat endocarditis caused by fully sensitive streptococci with benzylpenicillin or vancomycin alone for 4 weeks *or* (if no intra-cardiac abcess or infected emboli) with benzylpenicillin + gentamicin for 2 weeks. Treat more resistant organisms for 4–6 weeks (stopping gentamicin after 2 weeks for organisms moderately sensitive to penicillin); if aminoglycoside cannot be used and if streptococci moderately sensitive to penicillin, treat with benzylpenicillin alone for 4 weeks. Treat prosthetic valve endocarditis for at least 6 weeks (stopping gentamicin after 2 weeks if organisms fully sensitive to penicillin)

Endocarditis caused by enterococci (e.g. *Enterococcus faecalis*)
Amoxicillin[2] (*or* vancomycin[1] if penicillin-allergic or penicillin-resistant) + gentamicin
> Treat for at least 4 weeks (at least 6 weeks for prosthetic valve endocarditis); if gentamicin-resistant, substitute gentamicin with streptomycin

Endocarditis caused by haemophilus, actinobacillus, cardiobacterium, eikenella, and kingella species ('HACEK' organisms)
Amoxicillin[2] (*or* ceftriaxone if amoxicillin-resistant) + gentamicin
> Treat for 4 weeks (6 weeks for prosthetic valve endocarditis); stop gentamicin after 2 weeks

Respiratory system

Haemophilus influenzae epiglottitis
Cefotaxime *or* ceftriaxone *or* chloramphenicol

Uncomplicated community-acquired pneumonia
Neonate and child under 6 months, treat as for severe community acquired pneumonia of unknown aetiology

Child 6 months–5 years, oral amoxicillin[2] or oral erythromycin[3]

Child 5–18 years, oral erythromycin[3] (*or* oral amoxicillin[2] if *Streptococcus pneumoniae* suspected)
> Add flucloxacillin if staphylococci suspected, e.g. in influenza or measles; treat for 7 days (14–21 days for infections caused by staphylococci); pneumococci with decreased penicillin sensitivity being isolated but not yet common in UK; use erythromycin[3] if atypical pathogens suspected (more common in children over 5 years) or if penicillin-allergic

Severe community-acquired pneumonia of unknown aetiology
Neonate, benzylpenicillin + gentamicin

Child 1 month–18 years, cefuroxime *or* co-amoxiclav (or benzylpenicillin if lobar or *Streptococcus pneumoniae* suspected)
> Use erythromycin[3] if atypical pathogens such as mycoplasma (more common in children over 5 years) or chlamydia suspected or if penicillin allergic; in pneumococcal infection add vancomycin to beta-lactam antibacterial if organism highly penicillin- and cephalosporin-resistant; add flucloxacillin if staphylococci suspected; treat for 10 days (14–21 days if staphylococci, legionella, or Gram-negative enteric bacilli suspected)

Pneumonia possibly caused by atypical pathogens
Erythromycin[3]
> Severe Legionella infections may require addition of rifampicin; tetracycline is an alternative for chlamydial and mycoplasma infections in children over 12 years; treat for at least 14 days (14–21 days for legionella)

---

1. Where vancomycin is suggested teicoplanin may be used.
2. Where amoxicillin is suggested ampicillin may be used.
3. Where erythromycin is suggested another macrolide (e.g. azithromycin or clarithromycin) may be used.

5

Infections

Hospital-acquired pneumonia

Early-onset infection (less than 5 days after admission to hospital), treat as for severe community-acquired pneumonia of unknown aetiology; if life-threatening infection or if resistant organisms suspected, treat as for late-onset hospital-acquired pneumonia

Late-onset infection (more than 5 days after admission to hospital), an antipseudomonal penicillin (e.g. piperacillin with tazobactam) *or* a broad-spectrum cephalosporin (e.g. ceftazidime) *or* another antipseudomonal beta-lactam
Treat for 7 days (longer if pseudomonas confirmed); add vancomycin if MRSA suspected; add an aminoglycoside for severe illness caused by *Pseudomonas aeruginosa*

Cystic fibrosis

Staphylococcal lung infection in cystic fibrosis

Flucloxacillin (*or* erythromycin[1] *or* clindamycin if penicillin-allergic)
In severe exacerbation use flucloxacillin or a broad-spectrum cephalosporin (e.g. cefuroxime); substitute with vancomycin[2] if meticillin-resistant *Staphylococcus aureus* suspected, and if necessary, add either rifampicin or sodium fusidate

Haemophilus influenzae lung infection in cystic fibrosis

Amoxicillin *or* a broad-spectrum cephalosporin
In severe exacerbation use a third-generation cephalosporin (e.g. cefotaxime)

Pseudomonal lung infection in cystic fibrosis

Ciprofloxacin + *nebulised* colistin
In severe exacerbation treat with a parenteral aminoglycoside + an antipseudomonal beta-lactam antibacterial, and continue nebulised antibacterial

Central nervous system

Meningitis: Initial empirical therapy

- Transfer patient urgently to hospital.

- If bacterial meningitis and especially if *meningococcal disease* suspected, general practitioners should give benzylpenicillin (see p. 309 for dose) before urgent transfer to hospital; cefotaxime (section 5.1.2) may be an alternative in penicillin allergy; chloramphenicol may be used if history of immediate hypersensitivity reaction to penicillins or to cephalosporins

- Consider adjunctive treatment with dexamethasone (section 6.3.2) starting before or with first dose of antibacterial; avoid dexamethasone in septic shock, suspected meningococcal septicaemia, or if immunocompromised, or in meningitis following surgery

- In hospital, if aetiology unknown:
Neonate and Child 1–3 months, cefotaxime + amoxicillin[3]
Child 3 months–18 years, cefotaxime

Meningitis caused by group B streptococcus

Benzylpenicillin + gentamicin *or* cefotaxime alone
Treat for 14 days

Meningitis caused by meningococci

Benzylpenicillin *or* cefotaxime
Treat for at least 5 days; substitute chloramphenicol if history of anaphylaxis to penicillin or to cephalosporins. To eliminate nasopharyngeal carriage see Table 2, section 5.1.

Meningitis caused by pneumococci

Cefotaxime
Treat for 10–14 days; substitute benzylpenicillin if organism penicillin-sensitive; if organism highly penicillin- and cephalosporin-resistant, add vancomycin and if necessary rifampicin. Consider early adjunctive treatment with dexamethasone (but may reduce penetration of vancomycin into cerebrospinal fluid; section 6.3.2)

Meningitis caused by *Haemophilus influenzae*

Cefotaxime
Treat for at least 10 days; substitute chloramphenicol if history of anaphylaxis to penicillin or to cephalosporins or if organism resistant to cefotaxime. Consider early adjunctive treatment with dexamethasone (section 6.3.2). For *H. influenzae* type b give rifampicin for 4 days before hospital discharge (see Table 2, section 5.1)

Meningitis caused by Listeria

Amoxicillin[3] + gentamicin
Treat for at least 14 days. Consider stopping gentamicin after one week

---

1. Where erythromycin is suggested another macrolide (e.g. azithromycin or clarithromycin) may be used.
2. Where vancomycin is suggested teicoplanin may be used.
3. Where amoxicillin is suggested ampicillin may be used.

Urinary tract

Urinary-tract infection

Child under 3 months of age, i/v amoxicillin[1] + gentamicin *or* i/v cephalosporin alone

Child over 3 months of age with uncomplicated lower urinary-tract infection, trimethoprim *or* nitrofurantoin *or* oral cephalosporin (e.g. cefalexin) *or* amoxicillin[1]
Treat for 3 days. Re-assess child if unwell 24–48 hours after initial assessment. Use amoxicillin only if organism sensitive

Child over 3 months of age with acute pyelonephritis, a cephalosporin or co-amoxiclav
Treat for 7–10 days

Genital system

Syphilis

Neonatal congenital syphilis, benzylpenicillin
Treat for 10 days. Also consider treating neonates with suspected congenital syphilis whose mothers were treated inadequately for syphilis, or whose mothers were treated for syphilis in the 4 weeks before delivery, or whose mothers were treated with non-penicillin antibacterials for syphilis

Other syphilis infections, benzathine benzylpenicillin [unlicensed] *or* doxycycline *or* erythromycin
Doxycycline is an option in children over 12 years. Treat early syphilis (infection of less than 2 years) with benzathine benzylpenicillin as a single dose (repeat dose after 7 days for females in the third trimester of pregnancy) or with doxycycline or erythromycin for 14 days. Treat late latent syphilis (asymptomatic infection of more than 2 years) with doxycycline for 28 days or with benzathine benzylpenicillin once weekly for 2 weeks. Treat asymptomatic contacts of patients with infectious syphilis with doxycycline for 14 days. Contact tracing recommended

Uncomplicated gonorrhoea

Child under 12 years, ceftriaxone

Child 12–18 years, cefixime [unlicensed indication] *or* ciprofloxacin
Single dose treatment in uncomplicated infection. Choice depends on locality where infection acquired. Pharyngeal infection requires treatment with ceftriaxone. Use ciprofloxacin only if organism sensitive. Contact-tracing recommended; remember chlamydia

Uncomplicated genital chlamydial infection, non-gonococcal urethritis and non-specific genital infection

Child under 12 years, erythromycin for 14 days

Child 12–18 years, single dose of azithromycin *or* doxycycline for 7 days
Contact tracing recommended

Pelvic inflammatory disease

Child 12–18 years, doxycycline + metronidazole + i/m ceftriaxone
Treat for at least 14 days (use i/m ceftriaxone as a single dose). In severely ill patients initial treatment with doxycycline + i/v ceftriaxone (as a single dose) + i/v metronidazole, then switch to oral treatment with doxycycline + metronidazole to complete 14 days' treatment. Contact tracing recommended

Blood

Septicaemia: Initial empirical therapy

Neonate less than 48 hours old, benzylpenicillin + gentamicin *or* amoxicillin[1] + cefotaxime

Neonate more than 48 hours old, flucloxacillin + gentamicin *or* amoxicillin[1] + cefotaxime

Child 1 month–18 years, community-acquired septicaemia, aminoglycoside + amoxicillin[1] *or* cefotaxime alone *or* ceftriaxone alone
Use aminoglycoside + broad spectrum antipseudomonal beta-lactam antibacterial if pseudomonas suspected; add metronidazole if anaerobic infection suspected; add flucloxacillin *or* vancomycin[2] if Gram-positive infection suspected

Child 1 month–18 years, hospital-acquired septicaemia, a broad-spectrum antipseudomonal beta-lactam antibacterial (e.g. piperacillin with tazobactam, *Timentin®*, ceftazidime, imipenem (with cilastatin as *Primaxin®*) or meropenem)
Add aminoglycoside if pseudomonas suspected, or if multiple-resistant organisms suspected, or if severe sepsis; add vancomycin[2] if meticillin-resistant *Staphylococcus aureus* suspected; add metronidazole to broad-spectrum cephalosporin if anaerobic infection suspected

1. Where amoxicillin is suggested ampicillin may be used.
2. Where vancomycin is suggested teicoplanin may be used.

5

Infections

Septicaemia related to vascular catheter

Vancomycin[1]
Add a broad-spectrum antipseudomonal beta-lactam if Gram-negative sepsis suspected, especially in the immunocompromised. Consider removing vascular catheter, particularly if infection caused by *Staphylococcus aureus*, pseudomonas, or candida

Meningococcal septicaemia

Benzylpenicillin *or* cefotaxime
If meningococcal disease suspected, general practitioners advised to give a single dose of benzyl-penicillin before urgent transfer to hospital (see under Benzylpenicillin, section 5.1.1.1); cefotaxime (section 5.1.2) may be an alternative in penicillin allergy; chloramphenicol may be used if history of immediate hypersensitivity to penicillin or to cephalosporins. To eliminate nasopharyngeal carriage give rifampicin or ciprofloxacin before hospital discharge (see Table 2, section 5.1)

Musculoskeletal system

Osteomyelitis

Flucloxacillin *or* clindamycin if penicillin-allergic (*or* vancomycin[1] if resistant *Staphylococcus epidermidis* or meticillin-resistant *Staph. aureus*)
Treat acute infection for 4–6 weeks and chronic infection for at least 12 weeks; if child under 5 years of age and not immunised against *Haemophilus influenzae*, add cefotaxime *or* ceftriaxone to flucloxacillin; combine vancomycin[1] with either fusidic acid or rifampicin if prostheses present or if life-threatening condition

Septic arthritis

Flucloxacillin *or* clindamycin if penicillin-allergic (*or* vancomycin[1] if resistant *Staphylococcus epidermidis* or meticillin-resistant *Staph. aureus*)
Treat usually for 6 weeks (longer if infection complicated or if prosthesis is present). If child under 5 years of age and not immunised against *Haemophilus influenzae*, use cefotaxime + flucloxacillin *or* ceftriaxone + flucloxacillin. Combine vancomycin[1] with either fusidic acid or rifampicin if prosthesis present or if life-threatening condition

Eye

Purulent conjunctivitis

Neonate, neomycin eye drops

Child 1 month–18 years, chloramphenicol *or* gentamicin eye-drops

Congenital chlamydial conjunctivitis

Erythromycin (by mouth)
Treat for 14 days

Congenital gonococcal conjunctivitis

Ceftriaxone
Single-dose treatment

Ear, nose, and oropharynx

Pericoronitis

Metronidazole *or* amoxicillin
Antibacterial required only in presence of systemic features of infection or of trismus or persistent swelling despite local treatment; treat for 3 days or until symptoms resolve

Acute necrotising ulcerative gingivitis

Metronidazole *or* amoxicillin
Antibacterial required only if systemic features of infection; treat for 3 days or until symptoms resolve

Periapical or periodontal abscess

Amoxicillin *or* metronidazole
Antibacterial required only in severe disease with cellulitis or if systemic features of infection; treat for 5 days

Periodontitis

Metronidazole *or* doxycycline
Antibacterial required for severe disease or disease unresponsive to local treatment; doxycycline is an option in children over 12 years

Throat infections

Phenoxymethylpenicillin (*or* erythromycin[2] if penicillin-allergic)
Most throat infections are caused by viruses and many do not require antibacterial therapy. Consider antibacterial if history of valvular heart disease, if marked systemic upset, if peritonsillar cellulitis or abscess, or if at increased risk from acute infection (e.g. in immunosuppression, cystic fibrosis); prescribe antibacterial for beta-haemolytic streptococcal pharyngitis; treat for 10 days. **Avoid** amoxicillin if possibility of glandular fever, see section 5.1.1.3. Initial parenteral therapy (in severe infection) with benzylpenicillin, then oral therapy with phenoxymethylpenicillin *or* amoxicillin[3]

---

1. Where vancomycin is suggested teicoplanin may be used.
2. Where erythromycin is suggested another macrolide (e.g. azithromycin or clarithromycin) may be used.
3. Where amoxicillin is suggested ampicillin may be used.

Sinusitis

Amoxicillin[1] *or* erythromycin[2]

Antibacterial should usually be used only for persistent symptoms and purulent discharge lasting at least 7 days or if severe symptoms. Also consider antibacterial for those at high risk of serious complications (e.g. in immunosuppression, cystic fibrosis). Treat for 7 days. Consider oral co-amoxiclav if no improvement after 48 hours. Initial parenteral therapy with co-amoxiclav or cefuroxime may be required in severe infections

Otitis externa

Flucloxacillin (*or* erythromycin[2] if penicillin-allergic)

Consider systemic antibacterial if spreading cellulitis or child systemically unwell. Use ciprofloxacin (or an aminoglycoside) if pseudomonas suspected, see section 12.1.1

Otitis media

Amoxicillin[1] (*or* erythromycin[2] if penicillin-allergic)

Many infections caused by viruses. Most uncomplicated cases resolve without antibacterial treatment. In children without systemic features, antibacterial treatment may be started after 72 hours if no improvement. Consider earlier treatment if deterioration, if systemically unwell, if at high risk of serious complications (e.g. in immunosuppression, cystic fibrosis), if mastoiditis present, or in children under 2 years of age with bilateral otitis media. Treat for 5 days (longer if severely ill); consider co-amoxiclav if no improvement after 48 hours; initial parenteral therapy in severe infection with co-amoxiclav or cefuroxime

Skin

Impetigo

Topical fusidic acid (*or* mupirocin if meticillin-resistant *Staphylococcus aureus*); oral flucloxacillin *or* erythromycin[2] if widespread

Topical treatment for 7 days usually adequate; max. duration of topical treatment 10 days; seek local microbiology advice before using topical treatment in hospital; oral treatment for 7 days; add phenoxymethylpenicillin to flucloxacillin if streptococcal infection suspected

Erysipelas

Phenoxymethylpenicillin (or erythromycin[2] if penicillin-allergic)

Add flucloxacillin to phenoxymethylpenicillin if staphylococcus suspected; substitute benzylpenicillin for phenoxymethylpenicillin if parenteral treatment required

Cellulitis

Benzylpenicillin + flucloxacillin (or erythromycin[2] alone if penicillin-allergic)

Substitute phenoxymethylpenicillin for benzylpenicillin if oral treatment appropriate; discontinue flucloxacillin if streptococcal infection confirmed. Substitute treatment with broad-spectrum antibacterials if patients at risk from anaerobic or Gram-negative infections (e.g. use co-amoxiclav alone for facial infection, orbital infection, or infection caused by animal or human bites. Use ceftazidime + clindamycin in immunocompromised patients)

Animal and human bites

Co-amoxiclav alone (*or* clindamycin if penicillin-allergic)

Cleanse wound thoroughly; for tetanus-prone wound, give human tetanus immunoglobulin (with adsorbed diphtheria [low dose] and tetanus vaccine if necessary, according to immunisation history and risk of infection), see under Tetanus Vaccines, section 14.4; consider rabies prophylaxis (section 14.4) for bites from animals in endemic countries; assess risk of blood-borne viruses

Acne—see section 13.6

Paronychia or 'septic spots' in neonate

Flucloxacillin

Add aminoglycoside if systemically unwell

Surgical wound infection

Flucloxacillin *or* co-amoxiclav

Table 2. Summary of antibacterial prophylaxis

Prevention of recurrence of rheumatic fever

Phenoxymethylpenicillin by mouth

Child 1 month–6 years 125 mg twice daily

Child 6–18 years 250 mg twice daily

or

Erythromycin by mouth

Child 1 month–2 years 125 mg twice daily

Child 2–18 years 250 mg twice daily

1. Where amoxicillin is suggested ampicillin may be used.
2. Where erythromycin is suggested another macrolide (e.g. azithromycin or clarithromycin) may be used.

Prevention of secondary case of invasive group A streptococcal infection[1]

Phenoxymethylpenicillin by mouth

Neonate 12.5 mg/kg (max. 62.5 mg) every 6 hours for 10 days

Child 1 month–1 year 62.5 mg every 6 hours for 10 days

Child 1–6 years 125 mg every 6 hours for 10 days

Child 6–12 years 250 mg every 6 hours for 10 days

Child 12–18 years 250–500 mg every 6 hours for 10 days

If child penicillin allergic,

either erythromycin by mouth

Child 1 month–2 years 125 mg every 6 hours for 10 days

Child 2–8 years 250 mg every 6 hours for 10 days

Child 8–18 years 250–500 mg every 6 hours for 10 days

or azithromycin by mouth [unlicensed indication]

Child 6 months–12 years 12 mg/kg (max. 500 mg) once daily for 5 days

Child 12–18 years 500 mg once daily for 5 days

Prevention of secondary case of meningococcal meningitis[2]

Rifampicin by mouth

Neonate 5 mg/kg every 12 hours for 2 days

Child 1 month–1 year 5 mg/kg every 12 hours for 2 days

Child 1–12 years 10 mg/kg (max. 600 mg) every 12 hours for 2 days

Child 12–18 years 600 mg every 12 hours for 2 days

or

Ciprofloxacin by mouth [unlicensed indication]

Child 2–5 years 125 mg as a single dose

Child 5–12 years 250 mg as a single dose

Child 12–18 years 500 mg as a single dose

or

Ceftriaxone by intramuscular injection [unlicensed indication] (preferred if pregnant)

Child 1 month–12 years 125 mg as a single dose

Child 12–18 years 250 mg as a single dose

Prevention of secondary case of Haemophilus influenzae type b disease[2]

Rifampicin by mouth

Child 1–3 months 10 mg/kg once daily for 4 days

Child 3 months–12 years 20 mg/kg (max. 600 mg) once daily for 4 days

Child 12–18 years 600 mg once daily for 4 days

Prevention of secondary case of diphtheria in non-immune patient

Erythromycin by mouth

Child 1 month–2 years 125 mg every 6 hours for 7 days

Child 2–8 years 250 mg every 6 hours for 7 days

Child 8–18 years 500 mg every 6 hours for 7 days

Treat for further 10 days if nasopharyngeal swabs positive after first 7 days' treatment

1. For details of those who should receive chemoprophylaxis contact a consultant in communicable disease control (or a consultant in infectious diseases or the local Health Protection Agency Laboratory)
2. For details of those who should receive chemoprophylaxis contact a consultant in communicable disease control (or a consultant in infectious diseases or the local Health Protection Agency laboratory). Unless there has been direct exposure of the mouth or nose to infectious droplets from a patient with meningococcal disease who has received less than 24 hours of antibacterial treatment, healthcare workers do not generally require chemoprophylaxis.

Prevention of secondary case of pertussis in non-immune patient or partially immune patient

Erythromycin[1] by mouth

Child 1 month–2 years 125 mg every 6 hours for 7 days

Child 2–8 years 250 mg every 6 hours for 7 days

Child 8–18 years 250–500 mg every 6 hours for 7 days

Note Pertussis vaccine inappropriate for outbreak since 3 injections required for protection

Prevention of pneumococcal infection in asplenia or in patients with sickle cell disease

Phenoxymethylpenicillin by mouth

Child 1 month–6 years 125 mg every 12 hours

Child 6–12 years 250 mg every 12 hours

Child 12–18 years 500 mg every 12 hours

If cover also needed for *H. influenzae* in child give amoxicillin instead

Child 1 month–5 years 125 mg every 12 hours

Child 5–12 years 250 mg every 12 hours

Child 12–18 years 500 mg every 12 hours

Note Antibiotic prophylaxis is not fully reliable; for vaccines in asplenia see p. 727

Prevention of *Staphylococcus aureus* lung infection in cystic fibrosis

Flucloxacillin by mouth

Child 1 month–18 years 12.5–25 mg/kg (max. 1 g) 4 times daily (total daily dose may alternatively be given in 2 divided doses)

Use cefradine (section 5.1.2) if flucloxacillin cannot be used

Prevention of tuberculosis in susceptible close contacts or those who have become tuberculin positive[2]

Isoniazid for 6 months

Neonate 5 mg/kg daily

Child 1 month –12 years 5 mg/kg daily (max. 300 mg daily)

Child 12–18 years 300 mg daily

or isoniazid + rifampicin for 3 months

Child 1 month–12 years isoniazid 5 mg/kg daily (max. 300 mg daily) + rifampicin 10 mg/kg daily (max. 450 mg daily if body-weight less than 50 kg; max. 600 mg daily if body-weight over 50 kg)

Child 12–18 years isoniazid 300 mg daily + rifampicin 600 mg daily (rifampicin 450 mg daily if body-weight less than 50 kg)

or (if isoniazid-resistant tuberculosis) rifampicin for 6 months

Child 1 month–12 years 10 mg/kg daily (max. 450 mg daily if body-weight less than 50 kg; max. 600 mg daily if body-weight over 50 kg)

Child 12–18 years 600 mg daily (450 mg daily if body-weight less than 50 kg)

1. Where erythromycin is suggested another macrolide (e.g. azithromycin or clarithromycin) may be used.
2. For details of those who should receive chemoprophylaxis contact the lead clinician for local tuberculosis services (or a consultant in communicable disease control). See also section 5.1.9, for advice on immunocompromised patients and on prevention of tuberculosis

Prevention of gas-gangrene in high lower-limb amputations or following major trauma

i/v benzylpenicillin

Child 1 month–12 years 25 mg/kg (max. 600mg) every 6 hours for 5 days

Child 12–18 years 300–600 mg every 6 hours for 5 days

or if penicillin-allergic i/v or oral metronidazole

Child 1 month–12 years 7.5mg/kg (max. 500mg) every 8 hours for 5 days

Child 12–18 years 400–500 mg every 8 hours for 5 days

Prevention of infection in gastro-intestinal procedures

Operations on stomach or oesophagus

Single dose[1] of i/v gentamicin *or* i/v cefuroxime

Open biliary surgery

Single dose[1] of i/v cefuroxime + i/v metronidazole[2] *or* i/v gentamicin + i/v metronidazole[2]

Resections of colon and rectum, and resections in inflammatory bowel disease, and appendicectomy

Single dose[1] of i/v gentamicin + i/v metronidazole[2] *or* i/v cefuroxime + i/v metronidazole[2] *or* i/v co-amoxiclav alone

Endoscopic retrograde cholangiopancreatography

Single dose of i/v gentamicin *or* oral or i/v ciprofloxacin
Prophylaxis particularly recommended if bile stasis, pancreatic pseudocyst, previous cholangitis or neutropenia

Prevention of infection in orthopaedic surgery

Management of fractures

Single dose[1] of i/v cefuroxime or i/v flucloxacillin
Substitute i/v vancomycin if history of allergy to penicillins or to cephalosporins or if high risk of meticillin-resistant *Staphylococcus aureus*; use cefuroxime + metronidazole for complex open fractures with extensive soft-tissue damage; prophylaxis continued for 24 hours in open fractures (longer if complex open fractures)

Prevention of infection in obstetric surgery

Termination of pregnancy

Single dose[1] of oral metronidazole
If genital chlamydial infection cannot be ruled out, give doxycycline (section 5.1.3) postoperatively

Prevention of infection in vascular surgery

Reconstructive arterial surgery of abdomen, pelvis or legs

Single dose[1] of i/v cefuroxime
Add i/v metronidazole for patients at risk from anaerobic infections including those with diabetes, gangrene or undergoing amputation; add i/v vancomycin if high risk of meticillin-resistant *Staphylococcus aureus*

1. Additional intra-operative or postoperative doses of antibacterial may be given for prolonged procedures or if there is major blood loss
2. Metronidazole may alternatively be given by suppository but to allow adequate absorption, it should be given 2 hours before surgery

Prevention of endocarditis

NICE Guidance

Antimicrobial prophylaxis against infective endocarditis in children and adults undergoing interventional procedures (March 2008)

Antibacterial prophylaxis and chlorhexidine mouthwash are **not** recommended for the prevention of endocarditis in patients undergoing dental procedures.

Antibacterial prophylaxis is **not** recommended for the prevention of endocarditis in patients undergoing procedures of the:

- upper and lower respiratory tract (including ear, nose, and throat procedures and bronchoscopy);
- genito-urinary tract (including urological, gynaecological, and obstetric procedures);
- upper and lower gastro-intestinal tract.

While these procedures can cause bacteraemia, there is no clear association with the development of infective endocarditis. Prophylaxis may expose patients to the adverse effects of antimicrobials when the evidence of benefit has not been proven.

Any infection in patients at risk of endocarditis[1] should be investigated promptly and treated appropriately to reduce the risk of endocarditis.

If patients at risk of endocarditis[1] are undergoing a gastro-intestinal or genito-urinary tract procedure at a site where infection is suspected, they should receive appropriate antibacterial therapy that includes cover against organisms that cause endocarditis.

Patients at risk of endocarditis[1] should be:

- advised to maintain good oral hygiene;
- told how to recognise signs of infective endocarditis, and advised when to seek expert advice.

Dermatological procedures

Advice of a Working Party of the British Society for Antimicrobial Chemotherapy is that patients who undergo dermatological procedures[2] do not require antibacterial prophylaxis against endocarditis.

Joint prostheses and dental treatment

Joint prostheses and dental treatment

Advice of a Working Party of the British Society for Antimicrobial Chemotherapy is that patients with prosthetic joint implants (including total hip replacements) do not require antibacterial prophylaxis for dental treatment. The Working Party considers that it is unacceptable to expose patients to the adverse effects of antibacterials when there is no evidence that such prophylaxis is of any benefit, but that those who develop any intercurrent infection require prompt treatment with antibacterials to which the infecting organisms are sensitive.

The Working Party has commented that joint infections have rarely been shown to follow dental procedures and are even more rarely caused by oral streptococci.

5

Infections

---

1. Patients at risk of endocarditis include those with valve replacement, acquired valvular heart disease with stenosis or regurgitation, structural congenital heart disease (including surgically corrected or palliated structural conditions, but excluding isolated atrial septal defect, fully repaired ventricular septal defect, fully repaired patent ductus arteriosus, and closure devices considered to be endothelialised), hypertrophic cardiomyopathy, or a previous episode of infective endocarditis.
2. The British Association of Dermatologists Therapy Guidelines and Audit Subcommittee advise that such dermatological procedures include skin biopsies and excision of moles or of malignant lesions

> **Immunosuppression and indwelling intraperitoneal catheters**
> Advice of a Working Party of the British Society for Antimicrobial Che-
> motherapy is that patients who are immunosuppressed (including transplant
> patients) and patients with indwelling intraperitoneal catheters do not require
> antibacterial prophylaxis for dental treatment provided there is no other
> indication for prophylaxis.
>
> The Working Party has commented that there is little evidence that dental
> treatment is followed by infection in immunosuppressed and immunodeficient
> patients nor is there evidence that dental treatment is followed by infection in
> patients with indwelling intraperitoneal catheters.

5.1.1 Penicillins

5.1.1.1 Benzylpenicillin and phenoxymethylpenicillin

5.1.1.2 Penicillinase-resistant penicillins

5.1.1.3 Broad-spectrum penicillins

5.1.1.4 Antipseudomonal penicillins

5.1.1.5 Mecillinams

The penicillins are bactericidal and act by interfering with bacterial cell wall
synthesis. They diffuse well into body tissues and fluids, but penetration into the
cerebrospinal fluid is poor except when the meninges are inflamed. They are
excreted in the urine in therapeutic concentrations.

Hypersensitivity reactions   The most important side-effect of the penicillins is
hypersensitivity which causes rashes and anaphylaxis and can be fatal. Allergic
reactions to penicillins occur in 1–10% of exposed individuals; anaphylactic
reactions occur in fewer than 0.05% of treated patients. Individuals with a history
of anaphylaxis, urticaria, or rash immediately after penicillin administration are at
risk of immediate hypersensitivity to a penicillin; these individuals should not
receive a penicillin. Children who are allergic to one penicillin will be allergic to all
because the hypersensitivity is related to the basic penicillin structure. As patients
with a history of immediate hypersensitivity to penicillins may also react to the
cephalosporins and other beta-lactam antibiotics, they should not receive these
antibiotics; aztreonam may be less likely to cause hypersensitivity in penicillin-
sensitive patients and can be used with caution. If a penicillin (or another beta-
lactam antibiotic) is essential in a child with immediate hypersensitivity to penicillin then specialist advice should be sought on hypersensitivity testing or using a
beta-lactam antibiotic with a different structure to the penicillin that caused the
hypersensitivity (see also p. 319).

Individuals with a history of a minor rash (i.e. non-confluent, non-pruritic rash
restricted to a small area of the body) or a rash that occurs more than 72 hours
after penicillin administration are probably not allergic to penicillin and in these
individuals a penicillin should not be withheld unnecessarily for serious infections;
the possibility of an allergic reaction should, however, be borne in mind. Other
beta-lactam antibiotics (including cephalosporins) can be used in these patients.

A rare but serious toxic effect of the penicillins is encephalopathy due to cerebral
irritation. This may result from excessively high doses or in patients with severe
renal failure. The penicillins should **not** be given by intrathecal injection because
they can cause encephalopathy which may be fatal.

Another problem relating to high doses of penicillin, or normal doses given to
patients with renal failure, is the accumulation of electrolyte since most injectable
penicillins contain either sodium or potassium.

Diarrhoea frequently occurs during oral penicillin therapy. It is most common
with broad-spectrum penicillins, which can also cause antibiotic-associated colitis.

5.1.1.1 Benzylpenicillin and phenoxymethylpenicillin

Benzylpenicillin (Penicillin G) remains an important and useful antibiotic but is
inactivated by bacterial beta-lactamases. It is effective for many streptococcal
(including pneumococcal), gonococcal, and meningococcal infections and also

for anthrax (section 5.1.12), diphtheria, gas-gangrene, leptospirosis, and treatment of Lyme disease (section 5.1.1.3) in children. It is also used in combination with gentamicin for the empirical treatment of sepsis in neonates less than 48 hours old. Pneumococci, meningococci, and gonococci which have decreased sensitivity to penicillin have been isolated; **benzylpenicillin is no longer the drug of first choice for pneumococcal meningitis**. Although benzylpenicillin is effective in the treatment of tetanus, metronidazole (section 5.1.11) is preferred. Benzylpenicillin is inactivated by gastric acid and absorption from the gastro-intestinal tract is low; therefore it must be given by injection.

Benzathine benzylpenicillin (available from 'special-order' manufacturers or specialist importing companies, see p. 943) is used for the treatment of early syphilis and late latent syphilis.

Phenoxymethylpenicillin (Penicillin V) has a similar antibacterial spectrum to benzylpenicillin, but is less active. It is gastric acid-stable, so is suitable for oral administration. It should not be used for serious infections because absorption can be unpredictable and plasma concentrations variable. It is indicated principally for respiratory-tract infections in children, for streptococcal tonsillitis, and for continuing treatment after one or more injections of benzylpenicillin when clinical response has begun. It should not be used for meningococcal or gonococcal infections. Phenoxymethylpenicillin is used for prophylaxis against streptococcal infections following rheumatic fever and against pneumococcal infections following splenectomy or in sickle cell disease.

Oral infections   Phenoxymethylpenicillin is effective for dentoalveolar abscess.

BENZYLPENICILLIN SODIUM
(Penicillin G)

Cautions history of allergy; false-positive urinary glucose (if tested for reducing substances); **interactions:** Appendix 1 (penicillins)

Renal impairment neurotoxicity—high doses may cause convulsions. Estimated glomerular filtration rate 10–50 mL/minute/1.73 m², use normal dose every 8–12 hours; estimated glomerular filtration rate less than 10 mL/minute/1.73 m² use normal dose every 12 hours

Pregnancy not known to be harmful

Breast-feeding trace amounts in breast milk—not known to be harmful but be alert for hypersensitivity in infant

Contra-indications penicillin hypersensitivity

Side-effects hypersensitivity reactions including urticaria, fever, joint pains, rashes, angioedema, anaphylaxis, serum sickness-like reactions; *rarely* CNS toxicity including convulsions (especially with high doses or in severe renal impairment), interstitial nephritis, haemolytic anaemia, leucopenia, thrombocytopenia and coagulation disorders; also reported diarrhoea (including antibiotic-associated colitis)

Indication and dose

Mild to moderate susceptible infections (including throat infections, otitis media, pneumonia, cellulitis, neonatal sepsis, Table 1, section 5.1)

- **By intramuscular injection or by slow intravenous injection or infusion (intravenous route recommended in neonates and infants)**

  Preterm neonate and neonate under 7 days 25 mg/kg every 12 hours; dose doubled in severe infection

  Neonate 7–28 days 25 mg/kg every 8 hours; dose doubled in severe infection

  Child 1 month–18 years 25 mg/kg every 6 hours; increased to 50 mg/kg every 4–6 hours (max. 2.4 g every 4 hours) in severe infection

Endocarditis (combined with another antibacterial if necessary, see Table 1, section 5.1)

- **By slow intravenous injection or infusion**
  Child 1 month–18 years 25 mg/kg every 4 hours, increased if necessary to 50 mg/kg (max. 2.4 g) every 4 hours

Meningitis, meningococcal disease

- **By slow intravenous injection or infusion**

  Preterm neonate and neonate 75 mg/kg every 8 hours

  Child 1 month–18 years 50 mg/kg every 4–6 hours (max. 2.4 g every 4 hours)
  Important. If bacterial meningitis and especially if meningococcal disease is suspected general practitioners are advised to give a single injection of benzylpenicillin by intravenous injection (or by intramuscular injection) before transferring the patient urgently to hospital. Suitable doses are: Infant under 1 year 300 mg; Child 1–9 years 600 mg, 10 years and over 1.2 g. In penicillin allergy, cefotaxime (section 5.1.2) may be an alternative; chloramphenicol may be used if there is a history of anaphylaxis to penicillins

Treatment or prevention of neonatal group B streptococcus infection

- **By slow intravenous injection or infusion**

  Preterm neonate and neonate under 7 days 50 mg/kg every 12 hours

  Neonate 7–28 days 50 mg/kg every 8 hours

Prophylaxis in limb amputation Table 2, section 5.1

5

Infections

◻ **BENZYLPENICILLIN SODIUM (*continued*)**

Administration Intravenous route recommended in neonates and infants. For *intravenous infusion*, dilute with Glucose 5% *or* Sodium Chloride 0.9%; give over 15–30 minutes. Longer administration time is particularly important when using doses of 50 mg/kg (or greater) to avoid CNS toxicity

> Safe practice Intrathecal injection of benzylpenicillin is **not** recommended

Crystapen® (Genus) [PoM]
Injection, powder for reconstitution, benzylpenicillin sodium (unbuffered), net price 600-mg vial = 46p, 2-vial 'GP pack' = £1.90; 1.2-g vial = 92p
Electrolytes Na⁺ 1.68 mmol/600-mg vial; 3.36 mmol/1.2-g vial

PHENOXYMETHYLPENICILLIN
(Penicillin V)

Cautions see under Benzylpenicillin; **interactions:** Appendix 1 (penicillins)

Renal impairment no dose adjustment required

Contra-indications see under Benzylpenicillin

Side-effects see under Benzylpenicillin

Indication and dose

Susceptible infections including oral infections, tonsillitis, otitis media, erysipelas, cellulitis
- **By mouth**
  Child 1 month–1 year 62.5 mg 4 times daily; increased in severe infection to ensure at least 12.5 mg/kg 4 times daily

  Child 1–6 years 125 mg 4 times daily; increased in severe infection to ensure at least 12.5 mg/kg 4 times daily

  Child 6–12 years 250 mg 4 times daily; increased in severe infection to ensure at least 12.5 mg/kg 4 times daily

  Child 12–18 years 500 mg 4 times daily; increased in severe infection up to 1 g 4 times daily

Prevention of pneumococcal infection in asplenia or sickle cell disease, see Table 2, section 5.1

Prevention of recurrence of rheumatic fever, see Table 2, section 5.1

Prevention of group A streptococcal infection, see Table 2, section 5.1

Phenoxymethylpenicillin (Non-proprietary) [PoM]
Tablets, phenoxymethylpenicillin (as potassium salt) 250 mg, net price 28-tab pack = £1.25. Label: 9, 23

Oral solution, phenoxymethylpenicillin (as potassium salt) for reconstitution with water, net price 125 mg/5 mL, 100 mL = £1.90; 250 mg/5 mL, 100 mL = £2.59. Label: 9, 23
Dental prescribing on NHS Phenoxymethylpenicillin Tablets and Oral Solution may be prescribed

---

5.1.1.2 Penicillinase-resistant penicillins

Most staphylococci are now resistant to benzylpenicillin because they produce penicillinases. **Flucloxacillin**, however, is not inactivated by these enzymes and is thus effective in infections caused by penicillin-resistant staphylococci, which is the main indication for its use. Flucloxacillin is acid-stable and can, therefore, be given by mouth as well as by injection.

Flucloxacillin is well absorbed from the gut. For CSM warning on cholestatic jaundice see under Flucloxacillin.

MRSA Infection from *Staphylococcus aureus* strains resistant to meticillin [now discontinued] (meticillin-resistant *Staph. aureus*, MRSA) and to flucloxacillin can be difficult to manage. Treatment is guided by the sensitivity of the infecting strain.

Rifampicin (section 5.1.9) or **sodium fusidate** (section 5.1.7) should **not** be used alone because resistance may develop rapidly. **Clindamycin** alone or a combination of rifampicin and sodium fusidate can be used for *skin and soft-tissue infections* caused by MRSA; a **tetracycline** is an alternative in children over 12 years of age. A **glycopeptide** (e.g. vancomycin, section 5.1.7) can be used for severe skin and soft-tissue infections associated with MRSA. A combination of a glycopeptide and sodium fusidate *or* a glycopeptide and rifampicin can be considered for skin and soft-tissue infections that have failed to respond to a single antibacterial. **Linezolid** (section 5.1.7) or the combination of the streptogramin antibiotics **quinupristin** and **dalfopristin** (section 5.1.7) should be reserved for skin and soft-tissue infections that have not responded to other antibacterials or for children who cannot tolerate other antibacterials.

A **glycopeptide** can be used for *pneumonia* associated with MRSA. **Linezolid** or **quinupristin** and **dalfopristin** should be reserved for hospital-acquired pneumonia that has not responded to other antibacterials or for children who cannot tolerate other antibacterials.

Trimethoprim or **nitrofurantoin** can be used for *urinary-tract infections* caused by MRSA; a **tetracycline** is an alternative in children over 12 years of age. A **glycopeptide** can be used for urinary-tract infections that are severe or resistant to other antibacterials.

A **glycopeptide** can be used for *septicaemia* associated with MRSA.

For the management of endocarditis, osteomyelitis, or septic arthritis associated with MRSA, see Table 1, section 5.1.

Prophylaxis with vancomycin or teicoplanin (alone or in combination with another antibacterial active against other pathogens) is appropriate for patients undergoing surgery if:

- there is a history of MRSA colonisation or infection without documented eradication;
- there is a risk that the patient's MRSA carriage has recurred;
- the patient comes from an area with a high prevalence of MRSA.

It is important that hospitals have infection control guidelines to minimise MRSA transmission, including policies on isolation and treatment of MRSA carriers and on hand hygiene. For eradication of nasal carriage of MRSA, see section 12.2.3.

FLUCLOXACILLIN

Cautions see under Benzylpenicillin (section 5.1.1.1); also hepatic impairment (see CSM advice below)

> CSM advice (hepatic disorders) CSM has advised that very rarely cholestatic jaundice and hepatitis may occur up to several weeks after treatment with flucloxacillin has been stopped. Administration for more than 2 weeks and increasing age are risk factors. CSM has reminded that:
> - flucloxacillin should not be used in patients with a history of hepatic dysfunction associated with flucloxacillin;
> - flucloxacillin should be used with caution in patients with hepatic impairment;
> - careful enquiry should be made about hypersensitivity reactions to beta-lactam antibacterials.

Renal impairment use normal dose every 8 hours if estimated glomerular filtration rate less than 10 mL/minute/1.73 m^2

Pregnancy not known to be harmful

Breast-feeding trace amounts in breast milk—not known to be harmful but be alert for hypersensitivity in infant

Contra-indications see under Benzylpenicillin (section 5.1.1.1)

Side-effects see under Benzylpenicillin (section 5.1.1.1); also gastro-intestinal disturbances; *very rarely* hepatitis and cholestatic jaundice reported (see also CSM advice above)

Indication and dose

Infections due to beta-lactamase-producing staphylococci including otitis externa; adjunct in pneumonia, impetigo, cellulitis
- By mouth

  Neonate under 7 days 25 mg/kg twice daily

  Neonate 7–21 days 25 mg/kg 3 times daily

  Neonate 21–28 days 25 mg/kg 4 times daily

  Child 1 month–2 years 62.5–125 mg 4 times daily

  Child 2–10 years 125–250 mg 4 times daily

  Child 10–18 years 250–500 mg 4 times daily

- By intramuscular injection

  Child 1 month–18 years 12.5–25 mg/kg every 6 hours (max. 500 mg every 6 hours)

- By slow intravenous injection or by intravenous infusion

  Neonate under 7 days 25 mg/kg every 12 hours; may be doubled in severe infection

  Neonate 7–21 days 25 mg/kg every 8 hours; may be doubled in severe infection

  Neonate 21–28 days 25 mg/kg every 6 hours; may be doubled in severe infection

  Child 1 month–18 years 12.5–25 mg/kg every 6 hours (max. 1 g every 6 hours); may be doubled in severe infection

Osteomyelitis (Table 1, section 5.1), cerebral abscess, staphylococcal meningitis
- By slow intravenous injection or by intravenous infusion

  Neonate under 7 days 50–100 mg/kg every 12 hours

  Neonate 7–21 days 50–100 mg/kg every 8 hours

  Neonate 21–28 days 50–100 mg/kg every 6 hours

  Child 1 month–18 years 50 mg/kg (max. 2 g) every 6 hours

◻ **FLUCLOXACILLIN** *(continued)*

Endocarditis (Table 1, section 5.1)
- **By slow intravenous injection or by intravenous infusion**
  Child 1 month–18 years 50 mg/kg (max. 2 g) every 6 hours

Prevention of staphylococcal lung infection in cystic fibrosis
  Table 2, section 5.1

Staphylococcal lung infection in cystic fibrosis
- **By mouth**
  Child 1 month–18 years 12.5–25 mg/kg (max. 1 g) 4 times daily; total daily dose may alternatively be given in 3 divided doses

Administration for *intermittent intravenous infusion*, dilute reconstituted solution in Glucose 5% *or* Sodium Chloride 0.9% and give over 30–60 minutes; alternatively, may be given *via drip tub-*

ing in Glucose 5% *or* Sodium Chloride 0.9% *or* Ringer's Solution *or* Compound Sodium Lactate

Flucloxacillin (Non-proprietary) ᴾᵒᴹ
  Capsules, flucloxacillin (as sodium salt) 250 mg, net price 28 = £2.38; 500 mg, 28 = £4.30. Label: 9, 23
  Brands include *Floxapen®*, *Fluclomix®*, *Ladropen®*

  Oral solution (= elixir or syrup), flucloxacillin (as sodium salt) for reconstitution with water, 125 mg/5 mL, net price 100 mL = £2.97; 250 mg/5 mL, 100 mL = £8.84. Label: 9, 23

  Suspension (= syrup), flucloxacillin (as magnesium salt) for reconstitution with water, 125 mg/5 mL, net price 100 mL = £3.25; 250 mg/5 mL, 100 mL = £6.48. Label: 9, 23
  Brands include *Floxapen®*

  Injection, powder for reconstitution, flucloxacillin (as sodium salt). Net price 250-mg vial = £1.23; 500-mg vial = £2.45; 1-g vial = £4.90

5.1.1.3 Broad-spectrum penicillins

Ampicillin is active against certain Gram-positive and Gram-negative organisms but is inactivated by penicillinases including those produced by *Staphylococcus aureus* and by common Gram-negative bacilli such as *Escherichia coli*. Ampicillin is also active against *Listeria* spp. and enterococci. Almost all staphylococci, approx. 60% of *E. coli* strains and approx. 20% of *Haemophilus influenzae* strains are now resistant. The likelihood of resistance should therefore be considered before using ampicillin for the 'blind' treatment of infections; in particular, it should not be used for hospital patients without checking sensitivity.

Ampicillin can be given by mouth, but less than half the dose is absorbed and absorption is further decreased by the presence of food in the gut. Ampicillin is well excreted in the bile and urine.

Amoxicillin (amoxycillin) is a derivative of ampicillin and has a similar antibacterial spectrum. It is better absorbed than ampicillin when given by mouth, producing higher plasma and tissue concentrations; unlike ampicillin, absorption is not affected by the presence of food in the stomach.

Amoxicillin or ampicillin are principally indicated for the treatment of community-acquired pneumonia and middle ear infections, both of which may be due to *Streptococcus pneumoniae* and *H. influenzae*, and for urinary-tract infections (section 5.1.13). They are also used in the treatment of endocarditis and listerial meningitis. Amoxicillin may also be used for the treatment of Lyme disease [not licensed], see below.

Maculopapular rashes occur commonly with ampicillin (and amoxicillin) but are not usually related to true penicillin allergy. They often occur in children with glandular fever; broad-spectrum penicillins should not therefore be used for 'blind' treatment of a sore throat. Rashes are also common in children with acute or chronic lymphocytic leukaemia or in cytomegalovirus infection.

Co-amoxiclav consists of amoxicillin with the beta-lactamase inhibitor clavulanic acid. Clavulanic acid itself has no significant antibacterial activity but, by inactivating beta-lactamases, it makes the combination active against beta-lactamase-producing bacteria that are resistant to amoxicillin. These include resistant strains of *Staph. aureus*, *E. coli*, and *H. influenzae*, as well as many *Bacteroides* and *Klebsiella* spp. Co-amoxiclav should be reserved for infections likely, or known, to be caused by amoxicillin-resistant beta-lactamase-producing strains; for CSM warning on cholestatic jaundice see under Co-amoxiclav.

A combination of ampicillin with flucloxacillin (as co-fluampicil) is available to treat infections involving either streptococci or staphylococci (e.g. cellulitis).

Lyme disease   Lyme disease should generally be treated by those experienced in its management. **Amoxicillin** [unlicensed indication], **cefuroxime axetil** or **doxycycline** are the antibacterials of choice for *early Lyme disease* or *Lyme arthritis*

but doxycycline should only be used in children over 12 years of age. If these antibacterials are contra-indicated a **macrolide** (e.g. erythromycin) can be used for early Lyme disease. Intravenous administration of **ceftriaxone**, **cefotaxime** (section 5.1.2.1), or **benzylpenicillin** (p. 309) is recommended for Lyme disease associated with cardiac or neurological complications. The duration of treatment is usually 2–4 weeks; Lyme arthritis may require further treatment.

Oral infections   Amoxicillin or ampicillin are as effective as phenoxymethylpenicillin (section 5.1.1.1) but they are better absorbed; however, they may encourage emergence of resistant organisms.

Like phenoxymethylpenicillin, amoxicillin and ampicillin are ineffective against bacteria that produce beta-lactamases.

AMOXICILLIN
(Amoxycillin)

Cautions   see under Ampicillin; maintain adequate hydration with high doses (particularly during parenteral therapy)

Renal impairment   risk of crystalluria with high doses (particularly during parenteral therapy) in mild to moderate impairment; reduce dose in severe impairment; rashes more common and risk of crystalluria

Contra-indications   see under Ampicillin

Side-effects   see under Ampicillin

Indication and dose

> Susceptible infections including urinary-tract infections, sinusitis; *Haemophilus influenzae* infections
> * By mouth
>> **Neonate under 7 days** 30 mg/kg (max. 62.5 mg) twice daily; dose doubled in severe infection
>> **Neonate 7–28 days** 30 mg/kg (max. 62.5 mg) 3 times daily; dose doubled in severe infection
>> **Child 1 month–1 year** 62.5 mg 3 times daily; dose doubled in severe infection
>> **Child 1–5 years** 125 mg 3 times daily; dose doubled in severe infection
>> **Child 5–18 years** 250 mg 3 times daily; dose doubled in severe infection
> * By intramuscular injection
>> **Child 1 month–18 years** 30 mg/kg every 8 hours (max. 500 mg every 8 hours)
> * By intravenous injection or infusion
>> **Neonate under 7 days** 30 mg/kg every 12 hours; dose doubled in severe infection
>> **Neonate 7–28 days** 30 mg/kg every 8 hours; dose doubled in severe infection
>> **Child 1 month–18 years** 20–30 mg/kg (maximum 500 mg) every 8 hours; dose doubled in severe infection (max. 4 g daily)

> Uncomplicated community-acquired pneumonia (Table 1, section 5.1), invasive salmonellosis
> * By mouth
>> **Child 1 month–1 year** 125 mg 3 times daily
>> **Child 1–5 years** 250 mg 3 times daily
>> **Child 5–18 years** 500 mg 3 times daily

> * By slow intravenous injection or by intravenous infusion
>> **Neonate under 7 days** 50 mg/kg every 12 hours
>> **Neonate 7–28 days** 50 mg/kg every 8 hours
>> **Child 1 month–18 years** 30 mg/kg every 8 hours; dose doubled in severe infection (max. 4 g daily)

> Listerial meningitis (in combination with another antibacterial, Table 1, section 5.1), group B streptococcal infection, enterococcal endocarditis (in combination with another antibiotic)
> * By intravenous infusion
>> **Neonate under 7 days** 50 mg/kg every 12 hours; dose may be doubled in meningitis
>> **Neonate 7–28 days** 50 mg/kg every 8 hours; dose may be doubled in meningitis
>> **Child 1 month–18 years** 50 mg/kg every 4–6 hours (max. 2 g every 4 hours)

> Otitis media
> * By mouth
>> **Child 1 month–18 years** 40 mg/kg daily in 3 divided doses (max. 3 g daily in 3 divided doses)

> Cystic fibrosis (treatment of asymptomatic *H. influenzae* carriage or mild exacerbations)
> * By mouth
>> **Child 1 month–1 year** 125 mg 3 times daily
>> **Child 1–7 years** 250 mg 3 times daily
>> **Child 7–18 years** 500 mg 3 times daily

> *Helicobacter pylori* eradication section 1.3

Administration   Displacement value may be significant when reconstituting injection, consult local guidelines. Dilute intravenous injection to a concentration of 50 mg/mL (100 mg/mL for neonates). May be further diluted with Glucose 5% *or* Glucose 10% *or* Sodium chloride 0.9% *or* 0.45% for intravenous infusion. Give intravenous infusion over 30 minutes when using doses over 30 mg/kg

5

Infections

◁ **AMOXICILLIN** *(continued)*

Amoxicillin (Non-proprietary) PoM
Capsules, amoxicillin (as trihydrate) 250 mg, net price 21 = £1.14 ; 500 mg, 21 = £1.56. Label: 9
Brands include *Amix®*, *Amoram®*, *Amoxident®*, *Galenamox®*, *Rimoxallin®*

Oral suspension, amoxicillin (as trihydrate) for reconstitution with water, 125 mg/5 mL, net price 100 mL = £1.37; 250 mg/5 mL, 100 mL = £1.54. Label: 9

Note Sugar-free versions are available and can be ordered by specifying 'sugar-free' on the prescription
Brands include *Amoram®*, *Galenamox®*, *Rimoxallin®*

Sachets, sugar-free, amoxicillin (as trihydrate) 3 g/sachet, net price 2-sachet pack = £5.56, 14-sachet pack = £31.94. Label: 9, 13

Injection, powder for reconstitution, amoxicillin (as sodium salt), net price 250-mg vial = 32p; 500-mg vial = 66p; 1-g vial = £1.16
Dental prescribing on NHS Amoxicillin Capsules and Oral Suspension may be prescribed. Amoxicillin Sachets may be prescribed as Amoxicillin Oral Powder

Amoxil® (GSK) PoM
Capsules, both maroon/gold, amoxicillin (as trihydrate), 250 mg, net price 21-cap pack = £3.59; 500 mg, 21-cap pack = £7.19. Label: 9

Paediatric suspension, amoxicillin 125 mg (as trihydrate)/1.25 mL when reconstituted with water, net price 20 mL (peach- strawberry- and lemon-flavoured) = £3.38. Label: 9, counselling , use of pipette
Excipients include sucrose 600 mg/1.25 mL

Sachets SF, powder, sugar-free, amoxicillin (as trihydrate) 3 g/sachet, 2-sachet pack (peach- strawberry- and lemon-flavoured) = £2.99. Label: 9, 13

Injection, powder for reconstitution, amoxicillin (as sodium salt), net price 500-mg vial = 58p; 1-g vial = £1.16
Electrolytes Na⁺ 3.3 mmol/g

◤ AMPICILLIN

Cautions history of allergy; erythematous rashes common in glandular fever, cytomegalovirus infection, and acute or chronic lymphocytic leukaemia (see notes above); **interactions:** Appendix 1 (penicillins)

Renal impairment if estimated glomerular filtration rate less than 10 mL/minute/1.73 m² reduce dose or frequency—rashes more common

Pregnancy not known to be harmful

Breast-feeding trace amounts in breast milk—not known to be harmful but be alert for hypersensitivity in infant

Contra-indications penicillin hypersensitivity

Side-effects nausea, vomiting, diarrhoea; rashes (discontinue treatment); rarely, antibiotic-associated colitis; see also under Benzylpenicillin (section 5.1.1.1)

Indication and dose

Susceptible infections including urinary-tract infections, otitis media, sinusitis, oral infections (Table 1, section 5.1), *Haemophilus influenzae* infections, invasive salmonellosis
• **By mouth**

Neonate under 7 days 30 mg/kg (max. 62.5 mg) twice daily; dose doubled in severe infection

Neonate 7–21 days 30 mg/kg (max. 62.5 mg) 3 times daily; dose doubled in severe infection

Neonate 21–28 days 30 mg/kg (max. 62.5 mg) 4 times daily; dose doubled in severe infection

Child 1 month–1 year 62.5 mg 4 times daily; dose doubled in severe infection

Child 1–5 years 125 mg 4 times daily; dose doubled in severe infection

Child 5–12 years 250 mg 4 times daily; dose doubled in severe infection

Child 12–18 years 500 mg 4 times daily; dose doubled in severe infection

• **By intramuscular injection**

Child 1 month–18 years 25 mg/kg (max. 500 mg) every 6 hours

• **By intravenous injection or infusion**

Neonate under 7 days 30 mg/kg every 12 hours; dose doubled in severe infection

Neonate 7–21 days 30 mg/kg every 8 hours; dose doubled in severe infection

Neonate 21–28 days 30 mg/kg every 6 hours; dose doubled in severe infection

Child 1 month–18 years 25 mg/kg (max. 1 g) every 6 hours; dose doubled in severe infection

Uncomplicated community-acquired pneumonia (Table 1, section 5.1), invasive salmonellosis
• **By mouth**

Child 1 month–1 year 125 mg 4 times daily

Child 1–5 years 250 mg 4 times daily

Child 5–18 years 500 mg 4 times daily

• **By slow intravenous injection or by intravenous infusion**

Neonate under 7 days 50 mg/kg every 12 hours

Neonate 7–21 days 50 mg/kg every 8 hours

Neonate 21–28 days 50 mg/kg every 6 hours

Child 1 month–18 years 50 mg/kg (max. 1 g) every 6 hours

◻ **AMPICILLIN** (*continued*)

> **Listerial meningitis, group B streptococcal infection, enterococcal endocarditis** (in combination with another antibacterial, see Table 1, section 5.1)
>
> • **By intravenous infusion**
>
>> **Neonate under 7 days** 50 mg/kg every 12 hours; dose doubled in meningitis
>>
>> **Neonate 7–21 days** 50 mg/kg every 8 hours; dose doubled in meningitis
>>
>> **Neonate 21–28 days** 50 mg/kg every 6 hours; dose doubled in meningitis
>>
>> **Child 1 month–18 years** 50 mg/kg every 4–6 hours (max. 2 g every 4 hours)

Administration *Oral*: administer at least 30 minutes before food

Injection: displacement value may be significant when reconstituting injection, consult local guidelines. Dilute intravenous injection to a concentration of 50–100 mg/mL. May be further diluted with glucose 5% or 10% or sodium chloride 0.9% or 0.45% for infusion. Give over 30 minutes when using doses of greater than 50 mg/kg to avoid CNS toxicity including convulsions.

Ampicillin (Non-proprietary) [PoM]
Capsules, ampicillin 250 mg, net price 28 = £3.88; 500 mg, 28 = £19.68. Label: 9, 23
Brands include *Rimacillin*®

Oral suspension, ampicillin 125 mg/5 mL when reconstituted with water, net price 100 mL = £3.38; 250 mg/5 mL, 100 mL = £6.61. Label: 9, 23
Brands include *Rimacillin*®

Injection, powder for reconstitution, ampicillin (as sodium salt), net price 500-mg vial = £7.83
Dental prescribing on NHS Ampicillin Capsules and Oral Suspension may be prescribed

Penbritin® (Chemidex) [PoM]
Capsules, both grey/red, ampicillin (as trihydrate) 250 mg, net price 28-cap pack = £2.10; 500 mg, 28-cap pack = £5.28. Label: 9, 23

Syrup, apricot- caramel- and peppermint-flavoured, ampicillin (as trihydrate) for reconstitution with water, 125 mg/5 mL, net price 100 mL = £3.78; 250 mg/5 mL, 100 mL = £7.39. Label: 9, 23
Excipients include sucrose 3.6 g/5 mL

◢**With flucloxacillin**
Co-fluampicil (Non-proprietary) [PoM]
Capsules, co-fluampicil 250/250 (flucloxacillin 250 mg as sodium salt, ampicillin 250 mg as trihydrate), net price 28-cap pack = £14.43. Label: 9, 22
Brands include *Flu-Amp*®

Magnapen® (CP) [PoM]
Capsules, black/turquoise, co-fluampicil 250/250 (flucloxacillin 250 mg as sodium salt, ampicillin 250 mg as trihydrate), net price 20-cap pack = £4.00. Label: 9, 22

Syrup, co-fluampicil 125/125 (flucloxacillin 125 mg as magnesium salt, ampicillin 125 mg as trihydrate)/5 mL when reconstituted with water, net price 100 mL = £4.99. Label: 9, 22
Excipients include sucrose 3.14 g/5 mL

Injection 500 mg, powder for reconstitution, co-fluampicil 250/250 (flucloxacillin 250 mg as sodium salt, ampicillin 250 mg as sodium salt), net price per vial = £1.33
Electrolytes Na⁺ 1.3 mmol/vial

▲ **CO-AMOXICLAV**

A mixture of amoxicillin (as the trihydrate or as the sodium salt) and clavulanic acid (as potassium clavulanate); the proportions are expressed in the form x/y where x and y are the strengths in milligrams of amoxicillin and clavulanic acid respectively

Cautions see under Ampicillin and notes above; also caution in hepatic impairment (monitor hepatic function); maintain adequate hydration with high doses (particularly during parenteral therapy)
Cholestatic jaundice CSM has advised that cholestatic jaundice can occur either during or shortly after the use of co-amoxiclav. An epidemiological study has shown that the risk of acute liver toxicity was about 6 times greater with co-amoxiclav than with amoxicillin; these reactions have only rarely been reported in children. Jaundice is usually self-limiting and very rarely fatal. The duration of treatment should be appropriate to the indication and should not usually exceed 14 days

Hepatic impairment monitor liver function in liver disease. See also Cholestatic Jaundice above

Renal impairment *Oral*: use normal dose every 12 hours if estimated glomerular filtration rate 10–30 mL/minute/1.73 m². Use half normal dose every 12 hours if estimated glomerular filtration rate less than 10 mL/minute/1.73 m². *Augmentin-Duo*® not recommended if estimated glomerular filtration rate less than 30 mL/minute/1.73 m².

Intravenous: use normal initial dose and then use half normal dose every 12 hours if estimated glomerular filtration rate 10–30 mL/minute/1.73 m²; use normal initial dose and then use half normal dose every 24 hours if estimated glomerular filtration rate less than 10 mL/minute/1.73 m²

Pregnancy not known to be harmful

Breast-feeding trace amounts present in breast milk—not known to be harmful but be alert for hypersensitivity in the infant

Contra-indications penicillin hypersensitivity, history of co-amoxiclav-associated or penicillin-associated jaundice or hepatic dysfunction

Side-effects see under Ampicillin; hepatitis, cholestatic jaundice (see above); Stevens-Johnson syndrome, toxic epidermal necrolysis, exfoliative dermatitis, vasculitis reported; rarely prolongation of bleeding time, dizziness, headache, convulsions (particularly with high doses or in renal impairment); superficial staining of teeth with suspension, phlebitis at injection site

◁ **CO-AMOXICLAV (continued)**

Indication and dose

Infections due to beta-lactamase-producing strains (where amoxicillin alone not appropriate) including respiratory-tract infections, genito-urinary and abdominal infections, cellulitis, animal bites
* **By mouth, expressed as co-amoxiclav (see also under *Augmentin-Duo*® preparation below)**

    Neonate 0.25 mL/kg of *125/31* suspension 3 times daily

    Child 1 month–1 year 0.25 mL/kg of *125/31* suspension 3 times daily; dose doubled in severe infection

    Child 1–6 years 5 mL of *125/31* suspension 3 times daily *or* 0.25 mL/kg of *125/31* suspension 3 times daily; dose doubled in severe infection

    Child 6–12 years 5 mL of *250/62* suspension 3 times daily *or* 0.15 mL/kg of *250/62* suspension 3 times daily; dose doubled in severe infection

    Child 12–18 years one *250/125* strength tablet 3 times daily; increased in severe infections to one *500/125* strength tablet, 3 times daily

* **By intravenous injection over 3–4 minutes or by intravenous infusion, expressed as co-amoxiclav**

    Preterm neonate and neonate under 7 days 30 mg/kg every 12 hours

    Neonate 7–28 days 30 mg/kg every 8 hours

    Child 1–3 months 30 mg/kg every 8 hours

    Child 3 months–12 years 30 mg/kg every 8 hours increased in more serious infections to 30 mg/kg every 6 hours

    Child 12–18 years 1.2 g every 8 hours increased in more serious infections to 1.2 g every 6 hours

Severe dental infections (but not generally first-line, see notes above), expressed as co-amoxiclav
* **By mouth**

    Child 12–18 years one *250/125* strength tablet every 8 hours for 5 days

Administration for *intermittent intravenous infusion* dilute reconstituted solution to a concentration of 10mg/mL with Sodium Chloride 0.9% or Water for Injections; give over 30–40 minutes and complete infusion within 4 hours of reconstitution.

Co-amoxiclav (Non-proprietary) [PoM]
Tablets, co-amoxiclav 250/125 (amoxicillin 250 mg as trihydrate, clavulanic acid 125 mg as potassium salt), net price 21-tab pack = £3.04. Label: 9

Dental prescribing on NHS Co-amoxiclav 250/125 Tablets may be prescribed

Tablets, co-amoxiclav 500/125 (amoxicillin 500 mg as trihydrate, clavulanic acid 125 mg as potassium salt), net price 21-tab pack = £6.32. Label: 9

Oral suspension, co-amoxiclav 125/31 (amoxicillin 125 mg as trihydrate, clavulanic acid 31.25 mg as potassium salt)/5 mL when reconstituted with water, net price 100 mL = £3.07. Label: 9

Oral suspension, co-amoxiclav 250/62 (amoxicillin 250 mg as trihydrate, clavulanic acid 62.5 mg as potassium salt)/5 mL when reconstituted with water, net price 100 mL = £3.87. Label: 9

Injection 500/100, powder for reconstitution, co-amoxiclav 500/100 (amoxicillin 500 mg as sodium salt, clavulanic acid 100 mg as potassium salt), net price per vial = £1.21

Injection 1000/200, powder for reconstitution, co-amoxiclav 1000/200 (amoxicillin 1 g as sodium salt, clavulanic acid 200 mg as potassium salt), net price per vial = £2.42

Augmentin® (GSK) [PoM]
Tablets 375 mg, f/c, co-amoxiclav 250/125 (amoxicillin 250 mg as trihydrate, clavulanic acid 125 mg as potassium salt), net price 21-tab pack = £4.45. Label: 9

Tablets 625 mg, f/c, co-amoxiclav 500/125 (amoxicillin 500 mg as trihydrate, clavulanic acid 125 mg as potassium salt). Net price 21-tab pack = £8.49. Label: 9

Dispersible tablets, sugar-free, co-amoxiclav 250/125 (amoxicillin 250 mg as trihydrate, clavulanic acid 125 mg as potassium salt). Net price 21-tab pack = £10.22. Label: 9, 13

Suspension '125/31 SF', sugar-free, co-amoxiclav 125/31 (amoxicillin 125 mg as trihydrate, clavulanic acid 31 mg as potassium salt)/5 mL when reconstituted with water. Net price 100 mL (raspberry- and orange-flavoured) = £4.25. Label: 9
Excipients include aspartame 12.5 mg/5 mL (section 9.4.1)

Suspension '250/62 SF', sugar-free, co-amoxiclav 250/62 (amoxicillin 250 mg as trihydrate, clavulanic acid 62 mg as potassium salt)/5 mL when reconstituted with water. Net price 100 mL (raspberry- and orange-flavoured) = £5.97. Label: 9
Excipients include aspartame 12.5 mg/5 mL (section 9.4.1)

Injection 600 mg, powder for reconstitution, co-amoxiclav 500/100 (amoxicillin 500 mg as sodium salt, clavulanic acid 100 mg as potassium salt). Net price per vial = £1.38
Electrolytes Na⁺ 1.35 mmol, K⁺ 0.5 mmol/600-mg vial

Injection 1.2 g, powder for reconstitution, co-amoxiclav 1000/200 (amoxicillin 1 g as sodium salt, clavulanic acid 200 mg as potassium salt). Net price per vial = £2.76
Electrolytes Na⁺ 2.7 mmol, K⁺ 1 mmol/1.2-g vial

Augmentin-Duo® (GSK) [PoM]
Suspension '400/57', sugar-free, strawberry-flavoured, co-amoxiclav 400/57 (amoxicillin 400 mg as trihydrate, clavulanic acid 57 mg as potassium salt)/5 mL when reconstituted with water. Net price 35 mL = £4.38, 70 mL = £6.15. Label: 9
Excipients include aspartame 12.5 mg/5 mL (section 9.4.1)

Dose

Child 2 months–2 years 0.15 mL/kg twice daily, doubled in severe infection

Child 2–6 years (13–21 kg) 2.5 mL twice daily, doubled in severe infection

Child 7–12 years (22–40 kg) 5 mL twice daily, doubled in severe infections

5.1.1.4 Antipseudomonal penicillins

The carboxypenicillin, **ticarcillin**, is principally indicated for serious infections caused by *Pseudomonas aeruginosa* although it also has activity against certain other Gram-negative bacilli including *Proteus* spp. and *Bacteroides fragilis*.

Ticarcillin is now available only in combination with clavulanic acid (section 5.1.1.3); the combination (*Timentin®*) is active against beta-lactamase-producing bacteria resistant to ticarcillin.

Tazocin® contains the ureidopenicillin **piperacillin** with the beta-lactamase inhibitor tazobactam. Piperacillin is more active than ticarcillin against *Ps. aeruginosa*. The spectrum of activity of *Tazocin®* and *Timentin®* is comparable to that of the carbapenems, imipenem and meropenem (section 5.1.2).

These antipseudomonal penicillins may be used for the empirical treatment of septicaemia in immunocompromised children but otherwise should generally be reserved for serious infections resistant to other antibacterials. For pseudomonas septicaemias (especially in neutropenia or endocarditis) these antipseudomonal penicillins should be given with an aminoglycoside (e.g. gentamicin or netilmicin, section 5.1.4) since they have a synergistic effect.

Tazocin® is used in cystic fibrosis for the treatment of *Ps. aeruginosa* colonisation when ciprofloxacin and nebulised colistin have been ineffective, or in infective exacerbations, when it is combined with an aminoglycoside.

Owing to the sodium content of many of these antibiotics, high doses may lead to hypernatraemia.

PIPERACILLIN

Cautions see under Benzylpenicillin (section 5.1.1.1)

Contra-indications see under Benzylpenicillin (section 5.1.1.1)

Renal impairment reduce dose if estimated glomerular filtration rate less than 40 mL/minute/1.73 m² (child under 12 years) or if estimated glomerular filtration rate less than 80 mL/minute/1.73 m² (child 12–18 years); consult product literature

Pregnancy manufacturer advises use only if potential benefit outweighs risk

Breast-feeding present in milk—manufacturer advises use only if potential benefit outweighs risk

Side-effects see under Benzylpenicillin (section 5.1.1.1); also nausea, vomiting, diarrhoea; *less commonly* stomatitis, dyspepsia, constipation, jaundice, hypotension, headache, insomnia, and injection-site reactions; *rarely* abdominal pain, hepatitis, oedema, fatigue and eosinophilia; *very rarely* hypoglycaemia, hypokalaemia, pancytopenia, Stevens-Johnson syndrome, and toxic epidermal necrolysis

Licensed use *Tazocin®* not licensed for use in children under 12 years (except for children with neutropenia and complicated appendicitis)

Indication and dose

See preparations

◀ **With tazobactam**

Tazocin® (Lederle) [PoM]

Injection 2.25 g, powder for reconstitution, piperacillin 2 g (as sodium salt), tazobactam 250 mg (as sodium salt). Net price per vial = £7.96
Electrolytes Na⁺ 5.58 mmol/2.25-g vial

Injection 4.5 g, powder for reconstitution, piperacillin 4 g (as sodium salt), tazobactam 500 mg (as sodium salt). Net price per vial = £15.79
Electrolytes Na⁺ 11.16 mmol/4.5-g vial

Dose

(Expressed as a combination of piperacillin and tazobactam combined)

Lower respiratory tract, urinary tract, intra-abdominal and skin infections, and bacterial septicaemia
• By intravenous injection over 3–5 minutes or by intravenous infusion

Neonate 90 mg/kg every 8 hours

Child 1 month–12 years 90 mg/kg every 6–8 hours; (max 4.5 g every 6 hours)

Child 12–18 years 2.25–4.5 g every 6–8 hours, usually 4.5 g every 8 hours

Infections in children with neutropenia in combination with an aminoglycoside
• By intravenous injection over 3–5 minutes or by intravenous infusion

Child 1 month–18 years 90 mg/kg every 6 hours; (max 4.5 g every 6 hours)

Complicated appendicitis
• By intravenous injection over 3–5 minutes or by intravenous infusion

Child 2–12 years 112.5 mg/kg every 8 hours (max 4.5 g every 8 hours) for 5–14 days

Administration for *intravenous infusion*, dilute reconstituted solution to a concentration of 15–90 mg/mL with Glucose 5%, Sodium Chloride 0.9% or Compund Sodium Lactate, or to a concentration of 90 mg/mL with Water for Injections; give over 20–30 minutes

Important Generic preparations of piperacillin with tazobactam may have different compatibilities to *Tazocin®*—consult product literature

TICARCILLIN

Cautions see under Benzylpenicillin (section 5.1.1.1)

Hepatic impairment cholestatic jaundice, see under Co-amoxiclav

Renal impairment reduce dose if estimated glomerular filtration rate less than 60 mL/minute/ 1.73 m²

Pregnancy not known to be harmful

Breast-feeding trace amounts present in breast milk—not known to be harmful but be alert for hypersensitivity in the infant

Contra-indications see under Benzylpenicillin (section 5.1.1.1)

Side-effects see under Benzylpenicillin (section 5.1.1.1); also nausea, vomiting, coagulation disorders, haemorrhagic cystitis (more frequent in children), injection-site reactions, Stevens-Johnson syndrome, toxic epidermal necrolysis, hypokalaemia, eosinophilia

Indication and dose

See under preparation

◢**With clavulanic acid**

Note For a CSM warning on cholestatic jaundice possibly associated with clavulanic acid, see under Co-amoxiclav

Timentin® (GSK) ℗ᴏᴹ

Injection 3.2 g, powder for reconstitution, ticarcillin 3 g (as sodium salt), clavulanic acid 200 mg (as potassium salt). Net price per vial = £5.66
Electrolytes Na⁺ 16 mmol, K⁺ 1 mmol /3.2-g vial

Dose

(Expressed as a combination of ticarcillin and clavulanic acid)

Infections due to *Pseudomonas* and *Proteus* spp. see notes above
• By intravenous infusion

Preterm neonate body-weight under 2 kg 80 mg/kg every 12 hours

Preterm neonate body-weight over 2 kg and neonate 80 mg/kg every 8 hours, increased to every 6 hours in more severe infections

Child 1 month–18 years and body-weight under 40 kg 80 mg/kg every 8 hours, increased to every 6 hours in more severe infections

Child under 18 years and body-weight over 40 kg 80 mg/kg (max 3.2 g) every 6–8 hours, increased to every 4 hours in more severe infections

Administration Displacement value may be important, consult local guidelines. For intermittent infusion, dilute reconstituted solution further to a concentration of 16–32 mg/mL with glucose 5% *or* to a concentration of 32 mg/mL with water for injections; infuse over 30–40 minutes.

5.1.1.5 Mecillinams

Pivmecillinam has significant activity against many Gram-negative bacteria including *Escherichia coli*, klebsiella, enterobacter, and salmonellae. It is not active against *Pseudomonas aeruginosa* or enterococci. Pivmecillinam is hydrolysed to mecillinam, which is the active drug.

PIVMECILLINAM HYDROCHLORIDE

Cautions see under Benzylpenicillin (section 5.1.1.1); also liver and renal function tests required in long-term use; avoid in acute porphyria (section 9.8.2); **interactions:** Appendix 1 (penicillins)

Renal impairment reduce dose

Pregnancy not known to be harmful

Breast-feeding trace amounts in milk

Contra-indications see under Benzylpenicillin (section 5.1.1.1); also carnitine deficiency, oesophageal strictures, gastro-intestinal obstruction, infants under 3 months

Side-effects see under Benzylpenicillin (section 5.1.1.1); nausea, vomiting, dyspepsia; also reduced serum and total body carnitine (especially with long-term or repeated use)

Licensed use not licensed for use in children under 3 months

Indication and dose

Acute uncomplicated cystitis
• By mouth

Child body-weight over 40 kg initially 400 mg then 200 mg every 8 hours for 3 days

Chronic or recurrent bacteriuria

Child body-weight over 40 kg 400 mg every 6–8 hours

Urinary-tract infections

Child body-weight under 40 kg 5–10 mg/kg every 6 hours; total daily dose may alternatively be given in 3 divided doses

Salmonellosis not recommended therefore no dose stated

Counselling Tablets should be swallowed whole with plenty of fluid during meals while sitting or standing

Selexid® (LEO) ℗ᴏᴹ

Tablets, f/c, pivmecillinam hydrochloride 200 mg, net price 10-tab pack = £4.50. Label: 9, 21, 27, counselling, posture (see Dose above)

5 Infections

5.1.2 Cephalosporins, carbapenems, and other beta-lactams

Antibiotics in this section include the **cephalosporins**, such as cefotaxime, ceftazidime, cefuroxime, cefalexin and cefradine, the **monobactam**, aztreonam, and the **carbapenems**, imipenem (a thienamycin derivative), meropenem, and ertapenem.

5.1.2.1 Cephalosporins

The cephalosporins are broad-spectrum antibacterials which are used for the treatment of septicaemia, pneumonia, meningitis, biliary-tract infections, peritonitis, and urinary-tract infections. The pharmacology of the cephalosporins is similar to that of the penicillins, excretion being principally renal. Cephalosporins penetrate the cerebrospinal fluid poorly unless the meninges are inflamed; cefotaxime and ceftriaxone are suitable cephalosporins for infections of the CNS (e.g meningitis).

The principal side-effect of the cephalosporins is hypersensitivity and about 0.5–6.5% of penicillin-sensitive patients will also be allergic to the cephalosporins. Patients with a history of immediate hypersensitivity to penicillin should not receive a cephalosporin. If a cephalosporin is essential in these patients because a suitable alternative antibacterial is not available, then cefixime, cefotaxime, ceftazidime, ceftriaxone, or cefuroxime can be used with caution; cefaclor, cefadroxil, cefalexin, and cefradine should be avoided.

Cefradine (cephradine) has generally been replaced by the newer cephalosporins.

Cefuroxime is a 'second generation' cephalosporin that is less susceptible than the earlier cephalosporins to inactivation by beta-lactamases. It is, therefore, active against certain bacteria that are resistant to the other drugs and has greater activity against *Haemophilus influenzae* and *Neisseria gonorrhoeae*.

Cefotaxime, **ceftazidime** and **ceftriaxone** are 'third generation' cephalosporins with greater activity than the 'second generation' cephalosporins against certain Gram-negative bacteria. However, they are less active than cefuroxime against Gram-positive bacteria, most notably *Staphylococcus aureus*. Their broad antibacterial spectrum may encourage superinfection with resistant bacteria or fungi.

Ceftazidime has good activity against pseudomonas. It is also active against other Gram-negative bacteria.

Ceftriaxone has a longer half-life and therefore needs to be given only once daily. Indications include serious infections such as septicaemia, pneumonia, and meningitis. The calcium salt of ceftriaxone forms a precipitate in the gall bladder which may rarely cause symptoms but these usually resolve when the antibacterial is stopped. In neonates, ceftriaxone may displace bilirubin from plasma-albumin and should be avoided in neonates with unconjugated hyperbilirubinaemia, hypoalbuminaemia, acidosis or impaired bilirubin binding.

Orally active cephalosporins   The orally active 'first generation' cephalosporins, **cefalexin** (cephalexin), **cefradine**, and **cefadroxil** and the 'second generation' cephalosporin, **cefaclor**, have a similar antimicrobial spectrum. They are useful for urinary-tract infections which do not respond to other drugs or which occur in pregnancy, respiratory-tract infections, otitis media, sinusitis, and skin and soft-tissue infections. Cefaclor has good activity against *H. influenzae*, but it is associated with protracted skin reactions especially in children. Cefadroxil has a long duration of action and can be given twice daily; it has poor activity against *H. influenzae*. **Cefuroxime axetil**, an ester of the 'second generation' cephalosporin cefuroxime, has the same antibacterial spectrum as the parent compound; it is poorly absorbed and needs to be given with food to maximise absorption.

Cefixime has a longer duration of action than the other cephalosporins that are active by mouth. It is presently only licensed for acute infections.

Cefpodoxime proxetil is more active than the other oral cephalosporins against respiratory bacterial pathogens and it is licensed for upper and lower respiratory-tract infections.

For treatment of Lyme disease, see section 5.1.1.3.

Oral infections   The cephalosporins offer little advantage over the penicillins in dental infections, often being less active against anaerobes. Infections due to oral streptococci (often termed viridans streptococci) which become resistant to penicillin are usually also resistant to cephalosporins. This is of importance in

5

Infections

the case of children who have had rheumatic fever and are on long-term penicillin therapy. Cefalexin and cefradine have been used in the treatment of oral infections.

CEFACLOR

Cautions sensitivity to beta-lactam antibacterials (avoid if history of immediate hypersensitivity reaction, see also notes above and p. 308); false positive urinary glucose (if tested for reducing substances) and false positive Coombs' test; **interactions:** Appendix 1 (cephalosporins)

Renal impairment no dosage adjustment required, manufacturer advises caution

Pregnancy not known to be harmful

Breast-feeding present in milk in low concentration, considered compatible with breast-feeding

Contra-indications cephalosporin hypersensitivity

Side-effects diarrhoea and rarely antibiotic-associated colitis (CSM has warned both more likely with higher doses), nausea and vomiting, abdominal discomfort, headache; allergic reactions including rashes, pruritus, urticaria, serum sickness-like reactions with rashes, fever and arthralgia, and anaphylaxis; Stevens-Johnson syndrome, toxic epidermal necrolysis reported; disturbances in liver enzymes, transient hepatitis and cholestatic jaundice; other side-effects reported include eosinophilia and blood disorders (including thrombocytopenia, leucopenia, agranulocytosis, aplastic anaemia and haemolytic anaemia); reversible interstitial nephritis, hyperactivity, nervousness, sleep disturbances, hallucinations, confusion, hypertonia, and dizziness

Indication and dose

Infections due to sensitive Gram-positive and Gram-negative bacteria but see notes above

• By mouth

Child 1 month–12 years 20 mg/kg daily in 3 divided doses, doubled for severe infection (usual max. 1 g daily)
or

Child 1 month–1 year 62.5 mg 3 times daily; dose doubled for severe infections

Child 1–5 years 125 mg 3 times daily; dose doubled for severe infections

Child 5–12 years 250 mg 3 times daily; dose doubled for severe infections

Child 12–18 years 250 mg 3 times daily; dose doubled for severe infections (max. 4 g daily)

Asymptomatic carriage of *Haemophilus influenzae* or mild exacerbations in cystic fibrosis

• By mouth

Child 1 month–1 year 125 mg every 8 hours

Child 1–7 years 250 mg 3 times daily

Child 7–18 years 500 mg 3 times daily

Cefaclor (Non-proprietary) PoM
Capsules, cefaclor (as monohydrate) 250 mg, net price 21-cap pack = £4.52; 500 mg, 50-cap pack = £23.88. Label: 9
Brands include *Keftid®*

Suspension, cefaclor (as monohydrate) for reconstitution with water, 125 mg/5 mL, net price 100 mL = £8.33; 250 mg/5 mL, 100 mL = £9.33. Label: 9

Note Sugar-free versions are available and can be ordered by specifying 'sugar-free' on the prescription
Brands include *Keftid®*

Distaclor® (Flynn) PoM
Capsules, cefaclor (as monohydrate) 500 mg (violet/grey), net price 20 = £17.33. Label: 9

Suspension, both pink, cefaclor (as monohydrate) for reconstitution with water, 125 mg/5 mL, net price 100 mL = £4.13; 250 mg/5 mL, 100 mL = £8.26. Label: 9

Distaclor MR® (Flynn) PoM
Tablets, m/r, both blue, cefaclor (as monohydrate) 375 mg. Net price 14-tab pack = £6.93. Label: 9, 21, 25

Dose

Susceptible infections
Child 12–18 years 375 mg every 12 hours with food, dose doubled for pneumonia

Lower urinary-tract infections
Child 12–18 years 375 mg every 12 hours with food

CEFADROXIL

Cautions see under Cefaclor

Renal impairment reduce dose if estimated glomerular filtration rate less than 26 mL/minute/1.73 m²

Pregnancy not known to be harmful

Breast-feeding present in milk in low concentrations

Contra-indications see under Cefaclor

Side-effects see under Cefaclor

Indication and dose

Infections due to sensitive Gram-positive and Gram-negative bacteria but see notes above

• By mouth

Child 1 month–1 year 12.5 mg/kg twice daily

Child 1–6 years 250 mg twice daily

Child 6–18 years
Body-weight under 40 kg 500 mg twice daily;
Body-weight over 40 kg 0.5–1 g twice daily (1 g once daily for skin, soft tissue and uncomplicated urinary-tract infections)

◻ **CEFADROXIL (continued)**

Cefadroxil (Non-proprietary) PoM
Capsules, cefadroxil (as monohydrate) 500 mg, net price 20-cap pack = £5.25. Label: 9

Baxan® (Bristol-Myers Squibb) PoM
Capsules, cefadroxil (as monohydrate) 500 mg, net price 20-cap pack = £5.64. Label: 9

Suspension, cefadroxil (as monohydrate) for reconstitution with water, 125 mg/5 mL, net price 60 mL = £1.63; 250 mg/5 mL, 60 mL = £3.24; 500 mg/5 mL, 60 mL = £4.85. Label: 9

CEFALEXIN

(Cephalexin)

Cautions   see under Cefaclor
Renal impairment   reduce dose in moderate impairment
Pregnancy   not known to be harmful
Breast-feeding   present in milk in low concentrations, considered compatible with breast feeding
Contra-indications   see under Cefaclor
Side-effects   see under Cefaclor

Indication and dose

Infections due to sensitive Gram-positive and Gram-negative bacteria but see notes above
• **By mouth**

Neonate under 7 days 25 mg/kg (max. 125 mg) twice daily

Neonate 7–21 days 25 mg/kg (max. 125 mg) 3 times daily

Neonate 21–28 days 25 mg/kg (max. 125 mg) 4 times daily

Child 1 month–12 years 12.5 mg/kg twice daily; dose doubled in severe infection; max. 25 mg/kg 4 times daily (max. 1 g 4 times daily) or

Child 1 month–1 year 125 mg twice daily

Child 1–5 years 125 mg 3 times daily

Child 5–12 years 250 mg 3 times daily

Child 12–18 years 500 mg 2–3 times daily, increased to 1–1.5 g 3–4 times daily for severe infection

Prophylaxis of recurrent urinary-tract infection
• **By mouth**
Child 1 month–18 years 12.5mg/kg at night (max. 125mg at night)

Cefalexin (Non-proprietary) PoM
Capsules, cefalexin 250 mg, net price 28-cap pack = £2.07; 500 mg, 21-cap pack = £2.61. Label: 9

Tablets, cefalexin 250 mg, net price 28-tab pack = £2.27; 500 mg, 21-tab pack = £2.84. Label: 9

Oral suspension, cefalexin for reconstitution with water, 125 mg/5 mL, net price 100 mL = £1.83; 250 mg/5 mL, 100 mL = £2.27. Label: 9

Dental prescribing on NHS Cefalexin Capsules, Tablets, and Oral Suspension may be prescribed

Ceporex® (Galen) PoM
Capsules, both caramel/grey, cefalexin 250 mg, net price 28-cap pack = £4.02; 500 mg, 28-cap pack = £7.85. Label: 9

Tablets, all pink, f/c, cefalexin 250 mg, net price 28-tab pack = £4.02; 500 mg, 28-tab pack = £7.85. Label: 9

Syrup, all orange, cefalexin for reconstitution with water, 125 mg/5 mL, net price 100 mL = £1.43; 250 mg/5 mL, 100 mL = £2.87; 500 mg/5 mL, 100 mL = £5.57. Label: 9

Keflex® (Flynn) PoM
Capsules, cefalexin 250 mg (green/white), net price 28-cap pack = £1.76; 500 mg (pale green/dark green), 21-cap pack = £2.66. Label: 9

Tablets, both peach, cefalexin 250 mg, net price 28-tab pack = £2.09; 500 mg (scored), 21-tab pack = £2.47. Label: 9

Suspension, cefalexin for reconstitution with water, 125 mg/5 mL, net price 100 mL = 88p; 250 mg/5 mL, 100 mL = £1.51. Label: 9

CEFIXIME

Cautions   see under Cefaclor
Renal impairment   reduce dose if estimated glomerular filtration rate less than 20 mL/minute/1.73 m²
Pregnancy   not known to be harmful
Breast-feeding   manufacturer advises avoid—no information available
Contra-indications   see under Cefaclor
Side-effects   see under Cefaclor

Indication and dose

Acute infections due to sensitive Gram-positive and Gram-negative bacteria, but see notes above
• **By mouth**
Child 6 months–1 year 75 mg daily

Child 1–5 years 100 mg daily

Child 5–10 years 200 mg daily

Child 10–18 years 200–400 mg daily or 100–200 mg twice daily

Gonorrhoea [unlicensed indication, see also Table 1, section 5.1]
• **By mouth**
Child 12–18 years 400 mg as a single dose

5
Infections

◁ **CEFIXIME (continued)**

Suprax® (Rhône-Poulenc Rorer) [PoM]
Tablets, f/c, scored, cefixime 200 mg. Net price 7-tab pack = £13.23. Label: 9

Paediatric oral suspension, cefixime 100 mg/5 mL when reconstituted with water, net price 50 mL

(with double-ended spoon for measuring 3.75 mL or 5 mL since dilution not recommended) = £10.53, 100 mL = £18.91. Label: 9

CEFOTAXIME

Cautions see under Cefaclor
Renal impairment usual initial dose, then use half normal dose if estimated glomerular filtration rate less than 5 mL/minute/1.73 m^2

Pregnancy not known to be harmful

Breast-feeding present in milk in low concentration, considered compatible with breast-feeding

Contra-indications see under Cefaclor

Side-effects see under Cefaclor; rarely arrhythmias following rapid injection reported

Indication and dose

Infections due to sensitive Gram-positive and Gram-negative bacteria, surgical prophylaxis, Haemophilus epiglottitis and meningitis (Table 1, section 5.1) see also notes above

• **By intramuscular or by intravenous injection or intravenous infusion**

Neonate under 7 days 25 mg/kg every 12 hours; dose doubled in severe infection and meningitis

Neonate 7–21 days 25 mg/kg every 8 hours; dose doubled in severe infection and meningitis

Neonate 21–28 days 25 mg/kg every 6–8 hours; dose doubled in severe infection and meningitis

Child 1 month–18 years 50 mg/kg every 8–12 hours; increase to every 6 hours in very severe infections and meningitis (max. 12 g daily)
Important. If bacterial meningitis and especially if meningococcal disease is suspected the patient

should be transferred urgently to hospital. If benzylpenicillin cannot be given (e.g. because of an allergy), a single dose of cefotaxime may be given (if available) before urgent transfer to hospital. Suitable doses of cefotaxime by intravenous injection (or by intramuscular injection) are Child under 12 years 50 mg/kg; Child over 12 years 1 g; chloramphenicol (section 5.1.7) may be used if there is a history of anaphylaxis to penicillins or cephalosporins

Gonorrhoea
• **By intramuscular or by intravenous injection or intravenous infusion**

Child 12–18 years 500 mg as a single dose

Severe exacerbations of *Haemophilus influenzae* infection in cystic fibrosis
• **By intravenous injection or intravenous infusion**

Child 1 month–18 years 50 mg/kg every 6–8 hours (max. 12 g daily)

Administration Displacement value may be significant, consult local guidelines. For intermittent intravenous infusion dilute in glucose 5% or sodium chloride 0.9% or compound sodium lactate or water for injections; administer over 20–60 minutes; incompatible with alkaline solutions

Cefotaxime (Non-proprietary) [PoM]
Injection, powder for reconstitution, cefotaxime (as sodium salt), net price 500-mg vial = £2.14; 1-g vial = £4.31; 2-g vial = £8.57

CEFPODOXIME

Cautions see under Cefaclor
Renal impairment increase dose interval to every 24 hours if estimated glomerular filtration rate 10–40 mL/minute/1.73 m^2. Increase dose interval to every 48 hours if estimated glomerular filtration rate less than 10 mL/minute/1.73 m^2

Pregnancy not known to be harmful

Breast-feeding present in milk in low concentration

Contra-indications see under Cefaclor

Side-effects see under Cefaclor

Indication and dose

Upper respiratory-tract infections (but in pharyngitis and tonsillitis reserved for infections which are recurrent, chronic, or resistant to other antibacterials), lower respiratory-tract infections (including bronchitis and pneumonia), skin and soft tissue infections, uncomplicated urinary-tract infections
• **By mouth**

Child 15 days–6 months 4 mg/kg twice daily

Child 6 months–2 years 40 mg twice daily

Child 3–8 years 80 mg twice daily

Child 9–12 years 100 mg twice daily

Child 12–18 years 100 mg twice daily (increased to 200 mg twice daily in sinusitis, skin and soft tissue infections, uncomplicated upper urinary tract infections and if necessary in lower respiratory tract infections)

5 **Infections**

◻ **CEFPODOXIME** (*continued*)

Uncomplicated gonorrhoea
- **By mouth**
  Child 12–18 years 200 mg as a single dose

Orelox® (Hoechst Marion Roussel) (PoM)
Tablets, f/c, cefpodoxime 100 mg (as proxetil), net price 10-tab pack = £10.18. Label: 5, 9, 21
Oral suspension, cefpodoxime (as proxetil) for reconstitution with water, 40 mg/5 mL, net price 100 mL = £11.97. Label: 5, 9, 21
Excipients include aspartame (section 9.4.1)

CEFRADINE
(Cephradine)

Cautions see under Cefaclor
  Renal impairment reduce dose if estimated glomerular filtration rate less than 20 mL/minute/1.73 m^2
  Pregnancy not known to be harmful
  Breast-feeding present in milk in low concentrations
Contra-indications see under Cefaclor
Side-effects see under Cefaclor
Licensed use not licensed for use in children for prophylaxis in urinary-tract infections or for prevention of *Staphylococcus aureus* lung infection in cystic fibrosis

Indication and dose

Infections due to sensitive Gram-positive and Gram-negative bacteria but see notes above
- **By mouth**
  Child 1 month–12 years 12.5–25 mg/kg twice daily (total daily dose may alternatively be given in 3–4 divided doses)

  Child 12–18 years 0.5–1 g twice daily *or* 250–500 mg 4 times daily; up to 1 g 4 times daily in severe infections

- **By deep intramuscular injection or by intravenous injection over 3–5 minutes or by intravenous infusion**
  Child 1 month–12 years 12.5–25 mg/kg every 6 hours

  Child 12–18 years 0.5–1 g every 6 hours, increased to 2 g every 6 hours in severe infection

Surgical prophylaxis
- **By deep intramuscular injection or by intravenous injection over 3-5 minutes**
  Child 12–18 years 1–2 g at induction

Prevention of *Staphylococcus aureus* lung infection in cystic fibrosis
- **By mouth**
  Child 1 month–1 year 500 mg twice daily
  Child 1–7 years 1 g twice daily
  Child 7–18 years 2 g twice daily

Prophylaxis in urinary-tract infection
- **By mouth**
  Child 1 month–12 years 3 mg/kg at night.

Administration Displacement value may be significant when reconstituting injections, consult local guidelines. For continuous *or* intermittent intravenous infusion dilute reconstituted solution further in Glucose 5% *or* Glucose 10% or Sodium chloride 0.9% or Ringer's solution or Compound sodium lactate

Cefradine (Non-proprietary) (PoM)
Capsules, cefradine 250 mg, net price 20-cap pack = £3.97; 500 mg, 20-cap pack = £6.49. Label: 9
Brands include *Nicef®*
Dental prescribing on NHS Cefradine Capsules may be prescribed

Velosef® (Squibb) (PoM)
Capsules, cefradine 250 mg (orange/blue), net price 20-cap pack = £5.42; 500 mg (blue), 20-cap pack = £11.22. Label: 9
Syrup, cefradine 250 mg/5 mL when reconstituted with water. Net price 100 mL = £4.22. Label: 9
Dental prescribing on NHS *Velosef®* syrup may be prescribed as Cefradine Oral Solution
Injection, powder for reconstitution, cefradine. Net price 500-mg vial = 99p; 1-g vial = £1.95

CEFTAZIDIME

Cautions see under Cefaclor
  Renal impairment reduce dose if estimated glomerular filtration rate less than 50 mL/minute/1.73 m^2
  Pregnancy not known to be harmful
  Breast-feeding present in milk in low concentration, considered compatible with breast-feeding
Contra-indications see under Cefaclor
Side-effects see under Cefaclor
Licensed use nebulised route unlicensed

Indication and dose

Infections due to sensitive Gram-positive and Gram-negative bacteria but see notes above
- **By intravenous injection or infusion**

  Neonate under 7 days 25 mg/kg every 24 hours; dose doubled in severe infection and meningitis

  Neonate 7–21 days 25 mg/kg every 12 hours; dose doubled in severe infection and meningitis

  Neonate 21–28 days 25 mg/kg every 8 hours; dose doubled in severe infection and meningitis

  Child 1 month–18 years 25 mg/kg every 8 hours; dose doubled in severe infection, febrile neutropenia and meningitis (max. 6 g daily)

5 Infections

◻ **CEFTAZIDIME** (*continued*)

Pseudomonal lung infection in cystic fibrosis
- **By intravenous injection or infusion or by deep intramuscular injection**
    Child 1 month–18 years 50 mg/kg every 8 hours (max. 9 g daily)

Chronic *Burkholderia cepacia* infection in cystic fibrosis
- **By inhalation of nebulised solution**
    Child 1 month–18 years 1 g twice daily

Administration For parenteral administration, intravenous route recommended in children. Displacement value may be significant, consult local guidelines. For intermittent intravenous infusion dilute reconstituted solution further to a concentration of not more than 40 mg/mL in Glucose 5% or Glucose 10% or Sodium chloride 0.9% or Compound sodium lactate.

For nebulisation, dissolve dose in 3 mL of water for injection

Ceftazidime (Non-proprietary) ℗ᴼᴹ
Injection, powder for reconstitution, ceftazidime (as pentahydrate), with sodium carbonate, net price 1-g vial = £8.50; 2-g vial = £17.90

Fortum® (GSK) ℗ᴼᴹ
Injection, powder for reconstitution, ceftazidime (as pentahydrate), with sodium carbonate, net price 500-mg vial = £4.40, 1-g vial = £8.79, 2-g vial = £17.59, 3-g vial = £25.76
Electrolytes Na⁺ 2.3 mmol/g

Kefadim® (Flynn) ℗ᴼᴹ
Injection, powder for reconstitution, ceftazidime (as pentahydrate), with sodium carbonate, net price 1-g vial = £7.92; 2-g vial = £15.84
Electrolytes Na⁺ 2.3 mmol/g

CEFTRIAXONE

Cautions see under Cefaclor; preterm neonates; may displace bilirubin from serum albumin, administer over 60 minutes in neonates (see also Contra-indications); treatment longer than 14 days, renal failure, dehydration—risk of ceftriaxone precipitation in gall bladder
Hepatic impairment if hepatic impairment is accompanied by severe renal impairment, reduce dose and monitor plasma concentration
Renal impairment max. 50 mg/kg daily (max. 2 g daily) in severe renal impairment; also monitor plasma concentration if hepatic impairment accompanied by severe renal impairment
Pregnancy not known to be harmful
Breast-feeding present in milk in low concentration, considered compatible with breast-feeding
Contra-indications see under Cefaclor; neonates with jaundice, hypoalbuminaemia, acidosis or impaired bilirubin binding; concomitant treatment with calcium—risk of precipitation in urine and lungs of neonates (and possibly infants and older children)
Side-effects see under Cefaclor; calcium ceftriaxone precipitates in urine (particularly in very young, dehydrated or those who are immobilised) or in gall bladder—consider discontinuation if symptomatic; rarely prolongation of prothrombin time, pancreatitis

Indication and dose

Infections due to sensitive Gram-positive and Gram-negative bacteria
- **By intravenous infusion over 60 minutes**
    Neonate 20–50 mg/kg once daily

- **By deep intramuscular injection, or by intravenous injection over 2–4 minutes, or by intravenous infusion**
    Child 1 month–12 years
    Body-weight under 50 kg 50 mg/kg once daily; up to 80 mg/kg daily in severe infections and meningitis; doses of 50 mg/kg and over by intravenous infusion only

Body-weight 50 kg and over dose as for child 12–18 years

Child 12–18 years 1 g daily; 2–4 g daily in severe infections and meningitis; intramuscular doses over 1 g divided between more than one site; single intravenous doses above 1 g by intravenous infusion only

Uncomplicated gonorrhoea
- **By deep intramuscular injection**
    Child 12–18 years 250 mg as a single dose

Early syphilis [unlicensed indication]
- **By deep intramuscular injection**
    Child 12–18 years 500 mg daily for 10 days

Surgical prophylaxis
- **By deep intramuscular injection or by intravenous injection over at least 2–4 minutes, or (for colorectal surgery) by intravenous infusion**
    Child 12–18 years 1 g at induction; colorectal surgery, 2 g at induction; intramuscular doses over 1 g divided between more than one site

Prophylaxis of meningococcal meningitis Table 2, section 5.1

Administration Displacement value may be significant, consult local guidelines. For *intravenous infusion*, dilute reconstituted solution with Glucose 5% or 10% *or* Sodium Chloride 0.9%; give over at least 30 minutes (60 minutes in neonates). Not to be given with parenteral nutrition or infusion fluids containing calcium, even by different infusion lines.

For *intramuscular injection* ceftriaxone may be mixed with 1% Lidocaine Hydrochloride Injection to reduce pain at intramuscular injection site; final concentration 250–350 mg/mL.

⌐ **CEFTRIAXONE** (*continued*)

Ceftriaxone (Non-proprietary) PoM
Injection, powder for reconstitution, ceftriaxone (as sodium salt), net price 1-g vial = £10.17; 2-g vial = £20.36

Rocephin® (Roche) PoM
Injection, powder for reconstitution, ceftriaxone (as sodium salt), net price 250-mg vial = £2.55; 1-g vial = £10.17; 2-g vial = £20.36
Electrolytes Na⁺ 3.6 mmol/g

CEFUROXIME

Cautions see under Cefaclor

Renal impairment reduce parenteral dose if estimated glomerular filtration rate less than 20 mL/minute/1.73 m²

Pregnancy not known to be harmful

Breast-feeding present in milk in low concentration

Contra-indications see under Cefaclor

Side-effects see under Cefaclor

Indication and dose

Infections due to sensitive Gram-positive and Gram-negative bacteria

• **By mouth (as cefuroxime axetil),**

Child 3 months–2 years 10 mg/kg (max. 125 mg) twice daily

Child 2–12 years 15 mg/kg (max. 250 mg) twice daily

Child 12–18 years 250 mg twice daily; dose doubled in severe lower respiratory-tract infections, or if pneumonia suspected; dose reduced to 125mg twice daily in lower urinary-tract infection

• **By intravenous injection or infusion or by intramuscular injection**

Neonate under 7 days 25 mg/kg every 12 hours; dose doubled in severe infection, intravenous route only

Neonate 7–21 days 25 mg/kg every 8 hours; dose doubled in severe infection, intravenous route only

Neonate 21-28 days 25 mg/kg every 6 hours; dose doubled in severe infection, intravenous route only

Child 1 month–18 years 20 mg/kg (max. 750 mg) every 8 hours; increase to 50–60 mg/kg (max. 1.5 g) every 6–8 hours in severe infection and cystic fibrosis

Lyme disease
• **By mouth**

Child 12–18 years 500 mg twice daily for 20 days

Surgical prophylaxis
• **By intravenous injection**

Child 1 month–18 years 50 mg/kg (max. 1.5 g) at induction, up to 3 further doses of 30 mg/kg (max. 750 mg) may be given by *intramuscular or intravenous injection* every 8 hours for high-risk procedures

Administration Single doses over 750mg should be administered by the intravenous route only. Displacement value may be significant when reconstituting injection, consult local guidelines. For intermittent intravenous infusion, dilute reconstituted solution further in glucose 5% *or* sodium chloride 0.9% *or* compound sodium lactate; give over 30 minutes.

Cefuroxime (Non-proprietary) PoM
Tablets, cefuroxime (as axetil) 250 mg, net price 14-tab pack = £9.01. Label: 9, 21, 25

Zinacef® (GSK) PoM
Injection, powder for reconstitution, cefuroxime (as sodium salt). Net price 250-mg vial = 94p; 750-mg vial = £2.34; 1.5-g vial = £4.70
Electrolytes Na⁺ 1.8 mmol/750-mg vial

Zinnat® (GSK) PoM
Tablets, both f/c, cefuroxime (as axetil) 125 mg, net price 14-tab pack = £4.84; 250 mg, 14-tab pack = £9.67. Label: 9, 21, 25

Suspension, cefuroxime (as axetil) 125 mg/5 mL when reconstituted with water, net price 70 mL (tutti-frutti-flavoured) = £5.52. Label: 9, 21
Excipients include aspartame (section 9.4.1), sucrose 3.1 g/5 mL

5
Infections

5.1.2.2 Carbapenems

The carbapenems are beta-lactam antibacterials with a broad-spectrum of activity which includes many Gram-positive and Gram-negative bacteria, and anaerobes; **imipenem** and **meropenem** have good activity against *Pseudomonas aeruginosa*. The carbapenems are not active against meticillin-resistant *Staphylococcus aureus* and *Enterococcus faecium*.

Imipenem and meropenem are used for the treatment of severe hospital-acquired infections and polymicrobial infections caused by multiple-antibacterial resistant organisms (including septicaemia, hospital-acquired pneumonia, intra-abdominal infections, skin and soft-tissue infections, and complicated urinary-tract infections).

Ertapenem is licensed for treating abdominal and gynaecological infections and for community-acquired pneumonia, but it is not active against atypical respiratory pathogens and it has limited activity against penicillin-resistant pneumococci. Unlike the other carbapenems, ertapenem is not active against *Pseudomonas* or against *Acinetobacter* spp.

Imipenem is partially inactivated in the kidney by enzymatic activity and is therefore administered in combination with **cilastatin**, a specific enzyme inhibitor, which blocks its renal metabolism. Meropenem and ertapenem are stable to the renal enzyme which inactivates imipenem and therefore can be given without cilastatin.

Side-effects of imipenem with cilastatin are similar to those of other beta-lactam antibiotics; neurotoxicity has been observed at very high dosage, in renal failure, or in patients with CNS disease. Meropenem has less seizure-inducing potential and can be used to treat central nervous system infection. Ertapenem has been associated with seizures uncommonly.

ERTAPENEM

Cautions hypersensitivity to beta-lactam antibacterials (avoid if history of immediate hypersensitivity reaction, see also p. 308); renal impairment, CNS disorders—risk of seizures; **interactions:** Appendix 1 (ertapenem)

Renal impairment avoid if estimated glomerular filtration rate less than 30 mL/minute/1.73 m²

Pregnancy manufacturer advises avoid unless potential benefit outweighs risk

Contra-indications

Breast-feeding present in milk—manufacturer advises avoid

Side-effects diarrhoea, nausea, vomiting, headache, injection-site reactions, rash, pruritus, raised platelet count; *less commonly* dry mouth, taste disturbances, dyspepsia, abdominal pain, anorexia, constipation, melaena, antibiotic-associated colitis, hypotension, chest pain, oedema, pharyngeal discomfort, dyspnoea, dizziness, sleep disturbances, confusion, asthenia, seizures, vaginitis, raised glucose, petechiae; *rarely* dysphagia, cholecystitis, liver disorder (including jaundice), arrhythmia, increase in blood pressure, syncope, nasal congestion, cough, wheezing, hypersensitivity reactions, anxiety, depression, agitation, tremor, pelvic peritonitis, renal impairment, muscle cramp, scleral disorder, blood disorders (including neutropenia, thrombocytopenia, haemorrhage), hypoglycaemia, electrolyte disturbances; *very rarely* hallucinations

Indication and dose

Abdominal infections, acute gynaecological infections, community-acquired pneumonia
- **By intravenous infusion**

  Child 3 months–13 years 15 mg/kg every 12 hours (max. 1 g daily)

  Child 13–18 years 1 g once daily

Administration reconstitute 1 g with 10 mL Water for Injections or Sodium Chloride 0.9%; for *intermittent intravenous infusion*, dilute requisite dose in Sodium Chloride 0.9% to a final concentration not exceeding 20 mg/mL; incompatible with glucose solutions

Invanz® (MSD) PoM
Intravenous infusion, powder for reconstitution, ertapenem (as sodium salt), net price 1-g vial = £31.65
Electrolytes Na⁺ 6 mmol/1-g vial

IMIPENEM WITH CILASTATIN

Cautions CNS disorders (e.g. epilepsy); hypersensitivity to beta-lactam antibacterials (avoid if history of immediate hypersensitivity reaction, see also p. 308); **interactions:** Appendix 1 (imipenem with cilastatin)

Renal impairment not licensed for use in children with renal impairment. Reduce dose if estimated glomerular filtration rate less than 70 mL/minute/1.73 m²

Pregnancy manufacturer advises avoid unless potential benefit outweighs risk (toxicity in *animal* studies)

Breast-feeding present in milk but unlikely to be absorbed (however, manufacturer advises avoid)

Side-effects nausea, vomiting, diarrhoea (antibiotic-associated colitis reported), taste disturbances, tooth or tongue discoloration, hearing loss; blood disorders, positive Coombs' test; allergic reactions (with rash, pruritus, urticaria, Stevens-Johnson syndrome, fever, anaphylactic reactions, rarely toxic epidermal necrolysis, exfoliative dermatitis); myoclonic activity, convulsions, confusion and mental disturbances reported; slight increases in liver enzymes and bilirubin reported, rarely hepatitis; increases in serum creatinine and blood urea; red coloration of urine in children reported; local reactions: erythema, pain and induration, and thrombophlebitis

Licensed use not licensed for use in children under 3 months

⌐ **IMIPENEM WITH CILASTATIN (*continued*)**

Indication and dose

Aerobic and anaerobic Gram-positive and Gram-negative infections, hospital-acquired septicaemia Table 1, section 5.1; not indicated for CNS infections

• **By intravenous infusion**
expressed in terms of imipenem

Neonate under 7 days 20 mg/kg every 12 hours

Neonate 7–21 days 20 mg/kg every 8 hours

Neonate 21–28 days 20 mg/kg every 6 hours

Child 1–3 months 20 mg/kg every 6 hours

Child 3 months–18 years
Body-weight under 40 kg 15 mg/kg (max. 500 mg) every 6 hours
Body-weight over 40 kg 250–500 mg every 6 hours; less sensitive organisms up to 12.5 mg/kg (max. 1 g) every 6 hours; total daily dose may alternatively be given in 3 divided doses

Cystic fibrosis

• **By intravenous infusion**
Child 1 month–18 years
Body-weight under 40 kg 22.5 mg/kg every 6 hours
Body-weight over 40 kg 1 g every 6–8 hours

Administration for intermittent intravenous infusion dilute to a concentration of 5 mg (as imipenem)/mL in sodium chloride 0.9% *or* sodium chloride and glucose; give up to 500 mg over 20–30 minutes; give 1 g over 40–60 minutes

Primaxin® (MSD) [PoM]
Intravenous infusion, powder for reconstitution, imipenem (as monohydrate) 500 mg with cilastatin (as sodium salt) 500 mg, net price per vial = £12.00
Electrolytes Na⁺ 1.72 mmol/vial

■ **MEROPENEM**

Cautions hypersensitivity to beta-lactam antibacterials (avoid if history of immediate hypersensitivity reaction, see also p. 308); **interactions:** Appendix 1 (meropenem)

Hepatic impairment monitor transaminase and bilirubin concentrations

Renal impairment use normal dose every 12 hours if estimated glomerular filtration rate 26–50 mL/minute/1.73 m²; use half normal dose every 12 hours if estimated glomerular filtration rate 10–25 mL/minute/1.73 m²; use half normal dose every 24 hours if estimated glomerular filtration rate less than 10 mL/minute/1.73 m²

Pregnancy manufacturer advises use only if potential benefit outweighs risk—no information available

Breast-feeding unlikely to be absorbed (but manufacturer advises avoid unless potential benefit outweighs risk)

Side-effects nausea, vomiting, diarrhoea (antibiotic-associated colitis reported), abdominal pain, disturbances in liver function tests; headache; thrombocythaemia, positive Coombs' test; rash, pruritus, injection-site reactions; *less commonly* eosinophilia and thrombocytopenia; *rarely* convulsions; also reported paraesthesia, leucopenia, haemolytic anaemia, reduction in partial thromboplastin time, Stevens-Johnson syndrome, and toxic epidermal necrolysis

Licensed use not licensed for use in children for infection in neutropenia; not licensed for use in children under 3 months

Indication and dose

Aerobic and anaerobic Gram-positive and Gram-negative infections, hospital-acquired septicaemia Table 1, section 5.1

• **By intravenous injection over 5 minutes or by intravenous infusion**
Neonate under 7 days 20 mg/kg every 12 hours, dose doubled in severe infection

Neonate 7–28 days 20 mg/kg every 8 hours; dose doubled in severe infection

Child 1 month–12 years
Body-weight under 50 kg 10 mg/kg every 8 hours; dose doubled in hospital-acquired pneumonia, peritonitis, septicaemia and infections in neutropenic patients
Body-weight over 50 kg dose as for child 12–18 years

Child 12–18 years 500 mg every 8 hours; dose doubled in hospital-acquired pneumonia, peritonitis, septicaemia and infections in neutropenic patients

Meningitis

• **By intravenous injection over 5 minutes or by intravenous infusion**
Neonate under 7 days 40 mg/kg every 12 hours

Neonate 7–28 days 40 mg/kg every 8 hours

Child 1 month–12 years
Body-weight under 50 kg 40 mg/kg every 8 hours
Body-weight over 50 kg dose as for child 12–18 years

Child 12–18 years 2 g every 8 hours

Exacerbations of chronic lower respiratory-tract infections in cystic fibrosis

• **By intravenous injection over 5 minutes or by intravenous infusion**
Child 1 month–18 years 40 mg/kg every 8 hours (max. 2 g every 8 hours)

Administration Displacement value may be significant, consult local guidelines. For intermittent intravenous infusion dilute reconstituted solution further in glucose 5% *or* glucose 10% *or* sodium chloride 0.9% and give over 15–30 minutes

◻ **MEROPENEM** *(continued)*

Meronem® (AstraZeneca) ⟨PoM⟩
Injection, powder for reconstitution, meropenem
(as trihydrate), net price 500-mg vial = £8.60; 1-g
vial = £17.19
Electrolytes Na⁺ 3.9 mmol/g

5.1.2.3 Other beta-lactam antibiotics

Aztreonam is a monocyclic beta-lactam ('monobactam') antibiotic with an antibacterial spectrum limited to Gram-negative aerobic bacteria including *Pseudomonas aeruginosa*, *Neisseria meningitidis*, and *Haemophilus influenzae*; it should not be used alone for 'blind' treatment since it is not active against Gram-positive organisms. Aztreonam is also effective against *Neisseria gonorrhoeae* (but not against concurrent chlamydial infection). Side-effects are similar to those of the other beta-lactams although aztreonam may be less likely to cause hypersensitivity in penicillin-sensitive patients.

▲ AZTREONAM

Cautions hypersensitivity to beta-lactam antibiotics; **interactions:** Appendix 1 (aztreonam)

Hepatic impairment experience limited, monitor liver function

Renal impairment usual initial dose, then half normal dose if estimated glomerular filtration rate 10–30 mL/minute/1.73 m², usual initial dose, then one-quarter normal dose if estimated glomerular filtration rate less than 10 mL/minute/1.73 m²

Breast-feeding present in milk in low concentration, considered compatible with breast-feeding

Contra-indications aztreonam hypersensitivity

Pregnancy manufacturer advises avoid—crosses placenta and no further information available

Side-effects nausea, vomiting, diarrhoea, abdominal cramps; mouth ulcers, altered taste; jaundice and hepatitis; flushing; hypersensitivity reactions; blood disorders (including thrombocytopenia and neutropenia); rashes, injection-site reactions; *rarely* hypotension, seizures, asthenia, confusion, dizziness, headache, halitosis, and breast tenderness; *very rarely* antibiotic-associated colitis, gastro-intestinal bleeding, and toxic epidermal necrolysis

Licensed use not licensed for use in children under 7 days

Indication and dose

Gram-negative infections including *Pseudomonas aeruginosa*, *Haemophilus influenzae*, and *Neisseria meningitidis*

- **By intravenous injection over 3–5 minutes or by intravenous infusion**

Neonate under 7 days 30 mg/kg every 12 hours

Neonate 7–28 days 30 mg/kg every 6–8 hours

Child 1 month–2 years 30 mg/kg every 6–8 hours

Child 2–12 years 30 mg/kg every 6–8 hours increased to 50 mg/kg every 6–8 hours in severe infection and cystic fibrosis (max 2 g every 6 hours)

Child 12–18 years 1 g every 8 hours or 2 g every 12 hours; 2 g every 6–8 hours for severe infections (including systemic *Ps. aeruginosa* and lung infections in cystic fibrosis)

Administration Displacement value may be significant, consult local guidelines. For intermittent intravenous infusion, dilute reconstituted solution further in Glucose 5% *or* Sodium chloride 0.9% *or* Ringer's solution *or* Compound sodium lactate to a concentration of less than 20 mg/mL; to be given over 20–60 minutes

Azactam® (Squibb) ⟨PoM⟩
Injection, powder for reconstitution, aztreonam.
Net price 500-mg vial = £5.00; 1-g vial = £9.98; 2-g vial = £19.98

5.1.3 Tetracyclines

The tetracyclines are broad-spectrum antibiotics whose value has decreased owing to increasing bacterial resistance. In children over 12 years of age they are useful for infections caused by chlamydia (trachoma, psittacosis, salpingitis, urethritis, and lymphogranuloma venereum), rickettsia (including Q-fever), brucella (doxycycline with either streptomycin or rifampicin), and the spirochaete, *Borrelia burgdorferi* (Lyme disease—see section 5.1.1.3). They are also used in respiratory and genital mycoplasma infections, in acne, in destructive (refractory) periodontal disease, in exacerbations of chronic respiratory diseases (because of their activity against *Haemophilus influenzae*), and for leptospirosis in penicillin hypersensitivity (as an alternative to erythromycin).

Microbiologically, there is little to choose between the various tetracyclines, the only exception being **minocycline** which has a broader spectrum; it is active

(left margin: 5 Infections)

against *Neisseria meningitidis* and has been used for meningococcal prophylaxis but is no longer recommended because of side-effects including dizziness and vertigo (see Table 2, section 5.1 for current recommendations). Compared to other tetracyclines, minocycline is associated with a greater risk of lupus-erythematosus-like syndrome. Minocycline sometimes causes irreversible pigmentation.

For the role of tetracyclines in the management of meticillin-resistant *Staphylococcus aureus* (MRSA) infections, see p. 310.

Oral infections   In children over 12 years of age, tetracyclines can be effective against oral anaerobes but the development of resistance (especially by oral streptococci) has reduced their usefulness for the treatment of acute oral infections; they may still have a role in the treatment of destructive (refractory) forms of periodontal disease. Doxycycline has a longer duration of action than tetracycline or oxytetracycline and need only be given once daily; it is reported to be more active against anaerobes than some other tetracyclines.

For the use of doxycycline in the treatment of recurrent aphthous ulceration, oral herpes, or as an adjunct to gingival scaling and root planing for periodontitis, see section 12.3.1 and section 12.3.2.

Cautions   Tetracyclines should be used with caution in patients receiving potentially hepatotoxic drugs. Tetracyclines may increase muscle weakness in patients with myasthenia gravis, and exacerbate systemic lupus erythematosus. Antacids, and aluminium, calcium, iron, magnesium and zinc salts decrease the absorption of tetracyclines; milk also reduces the absorption of demeclocycline, oxytetracycline, and tetracycline. Other **interactions**: Appendix 1 (tetracyclines).

Hepatic impairment: avoid (or use with caution); tetracycline and demeclocycline max. 1 g daily in divided doses.

Renal impairment: with the exception of doxycycline and minocycline, the tetracyclines may exacerbate renal failure and should not be given to patients with mild, moderate, or severe renal impairment. Doxycycline or minocycline may be used cautiously (avoid excessive doses).

Pregnancy: avoid in pregnancy. In the first trimester, effects on skeletal development in *animal* studies. In the second and third trimester, dental discolouration.

Breast-feeding: avoid (although absorption and therefore discolouration of teeth in infant probably usually prevented by chelation with calcium in milk)

Contra-indications   Deposition of tetracyclines in growing bone and teeth (by binding to calcium) causes staining and occasionally dental hypoplasia, and they should be **not** be given to children under 12 years, or to pregnant or breast-feeding women. However, doxycycline may be used in children for treatment and post-exposure prophylaxis of anthrax when an alternative antibacterial cannot be given [unlicensed indication]. Tetracyclines should not be given to children with acute porphyria (section 9.8.2).

Side-effects   Side-effects of the tetracyclines include nausea, vomiting, diarrhoea (antibiotic-associated colitis reported occasionally), dysphagia, and oesophageal irritation. Other rare side-effects include hepatotoxicity, pancreatitis, blood disorders, photosensitivity (particularly with demeclocycline), and hypersensitivity reactions (including rash, exfoliative dermatitis, Stevens-Johnson syndrome, urticaria, angioedema, anaphylaxis, pericarditis). Headache and visual disturbances may indicate benign intracranial hypertension (discontinue treatment); bulging fontanelles have been reported in infants.

5 Infections

◢ TETRACYCLINE

Cautions   see notes above

Contra-indications   see notes above

Side-effects   see notes above; also reported, pancreatitis, acute renal failure, skin discoloration

Indication and dose

Susceptible infections   see notes above

• By mouth

Child 12–18 years 250 mg 4 times daily, increased in severe infections to 500 mg 3–4 times daily

Acne section 13.6.2

◁ **TETRACYCLINE (continued)**

Non-gonococcal urethritis
• **By mouth**

Child 12–18 years 500 mg 4 times daily for 7–14 days (21 days if failure or relapse after first course)

Tetracycline (Non-proprietary) PoM

Tablets, coated, tetracycline hydrochloride 250 mg, net price 28-tab pack = £8.85. Label: 7, 9, 23, counselling, posture

Dental prescribing on NHS Tetracycline Tablets may be prescribed

DEMECLOCYCLINE HYDROCHLORIDE

Cautions see notes above, but photosensitivity more common (avoid exposure to sunlight or sun lamps)

Contra-indications see notes above

Side-effects see notes above; also reversible nephrogenic diabetes insipidus, acute renal failure

Indication and dose

Susceptible infections see notes above
• **By mouth**

Child 12–18 years 150 mg 4 times daily or 300 mg twice daily

Ledermycin® (Goldshield) PoM

Capsules, red, demeclocycline hydrochloride 150 mg, net price 28-cap pack = £13.73. Label: 7, 9, 11, 23

DOXYCYCLINE

Cautions see notes above, but may be used in renal impairment; alcohol dependence; photosensitivity reported (avoid exposure to sunlight or sun lamps)

Contra-indications see notes above

Side-effects see notes above; also anorexia, flushing, tinnitus

Licensed use not licensed for use in children under 12 years

Indication and dose

Susceptible infections see notes above
• **By mouth**

Child 12–18 years 200 mg on first day, then 100 mg daily; severe infections (including refractory urinary-tract infections) 200 mg daily

Early syphilis
• **By mouth**

Child 12–18 years 100 mg twice daily for 14 days

Late latent syphilis
• **By mouth**

Child 12–18 years 100 mg twice daily for 28 days

Uncomplicated genital chlamydia, non-gonococcal urethritis, pelvic inflammatory disease Table 1, section 5.1
• **By mouth**

Child 12–18 years 100 mg twice daily for 7 days (14 days in pelvic inflammatory disease)

Anthrax (treatment or post-exposure prophylaxis) see also section 5.1.12
• **By mouth**

Child under 12 years (only if alternative antibacterial cannot be given) 2.5 mg/kg twice daily (max. 100 mg twice daily)

Child 12–18 years 100 mg twice daily

Acne section 13.6.2

Adjunct to gingival scaling and root planing for periodontitis section 12.3.1

Counselling Capsules should be swallowed whole with plenty of fluid during meals while sitting or standing
Note Doxycycline doses in BNF for Children may differ from those in product literature

Doxycycline (Non-proprietary) PoM

Capsules, doxycycline (as hyclate) 50 mg, net price 28-cap pack = £1.78; 100 mg, 8-cap pack = £1.15. Label: 6, 9, 11, 27, counselling, posture
Brands include *Doxylar®*
Dental prescribing on NHS Doxycycline Capsules 100 mg may be prescribed

Vibramycin-D® (Pfizer) PoM

Dispersible tablets, yellow, scored, doxycycline 100 mg, net price 8-tab pack = £4.91. Label: 6, 9, 11, 13

LYMECYCLINE

Cautions see notes above

Contra-indications see notes above

Side-effects see notes above

Indication and dose

Susceptible infections see notes above
• **By mouth**

Child 12–18 years 408 mg twice daily, increased to 1.224–1.632 g daily in severe infections

◁ **LYMECYCLINE** (*continued*)

Acne
- By mouth

    Child 12–18 years 408 mg daily for at least 8 weeks

Tetralysal 300® (Galderma) (PoM)

Capsules, red/yellow, lymecycline 408 mg (= tetracycline 300 mg). Net price 28-cap pack = £7.16, 56-cap pack = £14.26. Label: 6, 9

■ MINOCYCLINE

Cautions see notes above, but may be used in renal impairment; if treatment continued for longer than 6 months, monitor every 3 months for hepatotoxicity, pigmentation and for systemic lupus erythematosus—discontinue if these develop or if pre-existing systemic lupus erythematosus worsens

Contra-indications see notes above

Side-effects see notes above; also dizziness and vertigo (more common in women); *rarely* anorexia, tinnitus, impaired hearing, hyperaesthesia, paraesthesia, acute renal failure, pigmentation (sometimes irreversible), and alopecia; *very rarely* systemic lupus erythematosus, discoloration of conjunctiva, tears, and sweat

Indication and dose

Susceptible infections see notes above
- By mouth

    Child 12–18 years 100 mg twice daily

Acne section 13.6.2

Counselling Tablets or capsules should be swallowed whole with plenty of fluid while sitting or standing

Minocycline (Non-proprietary) (PoM)

Capsules, minocycline (as hydrochloride) 50 mg, net price 56-cap pack = £15.27; 100 mg, 28-cap pack = £13.09. Label: 6, 9, counselling, posture
Brands include *Aknemin®*

Tablets, minocycline (as hydrochloride) 50 mg, net price 28-tab pack = £3.96; 100 mg, 28-tab pack = £8.43. Label: 6, 9, counselling, posture

◀Modified release

Acnamino® MR (Dexcel) (PoM)

Capsules, m/r, buff/brown (enclosing pink and peach tablets), minocycline (as hydrochloride) 100 mg, net price 56-cap pack = £21.14. Label: 6, 25

Dose

Acne
- By mouth

    Child 12–18 years 1 capsule daily

Minocin MR® (Meda) (PoM)

Capsules, m/r, orange/brown (enclosing yellow and white pellets), minocycline (as hydrochloride) 100 mg. Net price 56-cap pack = £21.14. Label: 6, 25

Dose

Acne
- By mouth

    Child 12–18 years 1 capsule daily

Sebomin MR® (Actavis) (PoM)

Capsules, m/r, orange, minocycline (as hydrochloride) 100 mg, net price 56-cap pack = £21.14. Label: 6, 25

Dose

Acne
- By mouth

    Child 12–18 years 1 capsule daily

■ OXYTETRACYCLINE

Cautions see notes above

Contra-indications see notes above

Side-effects see notes above

Indication and dose

Susceptible infections see notes above
- By mouth

    Child 12–18 years 250–500 mg 4 times daily

Acne section 13.6.2

Oxytetracycline (Non-proprietary) (PoM)

Tablets, coated, oxytetracycline dihydrate 250 mg, net price 28-tab pack = £1.00. Label: 7, 9, 23
Brands include *Oxymycin®*
Dental prescribing on NHS Oxtetracycline Tablets may be prescribed

5.1.4 Aminoglycosides

These include amikacin, gentamicin, neomycin, streptomycin, and tobramycin. All are bactericidal and active against some Gram-positive and many Gram-negative organisms. Amikacin, gentamicin, and tobramycin are also active against *Pseudomonas aeruginosa*; streptomycin is active against *Mycobacterium tuberculosis* and is now almost entirely reserved for tuberculosis (section 5.1.9).

The aminoglycosides are not absorbed from the gut (although there is a risk of absorption in inflammatory bowel disease and liver failure) and must therefore be given by injection for systemic infections.

5

Infections

Excretion is principally via the kidney and accumulation occurs in renal impairment.

Most side-effects of this group of antibiotics are dose-related therefore care must be taken with dosage and whenever possible treatment should not exceed 7 days. The important side-effects are ototoxicity, and nephrotoxicity; they occur most commonly in children with renal failure.

If there is impairment of renal function (or high pre-dose serum concentrations) the interval between doses must be increased; if the renal impairment is severe the dose itself should be reduced as well.

Aminoglycosides may impair neuromuscular transmission and should not be given to children with myasthenia gravis; large doses given during surgery have been responsible for a transient myasthenic syndrome in patients with normal neuromuscular function.

Aminoglycosides should preferably not be given with potentially ototoxic diuretics (e.g. furosemide (frusemide)); if concurrent use is unavoidable administration of the aminoglycoside and of the diuretic should be separated by as long a period as practicable.

Once daily dosage   *Once daily administration* of aminoglycosides is more convenient, provides adequate serum concentrations, and has largely superseded *multiple-daily dose regimens* (given in 2–3 divided doses during the 24 hours). Local guidelines on dosage and serum concentrations should be consulted. A once-daily, high-dose regimen of an aminoglycoside should be avoided in children with endocarditis or extensive burns of more than 20% of the total body surface area, or in children over 1 month of age with a creatinine clearance of less than 20 mL/minute/1.73m^2. The *extended interval dose regimen* is used in neonates to reflect the changes in renal function that occur with increasing gestational and postnatal age (see Neonates below).

Serum concentrations   Serum concentration monitoring avoids both excessive and subtherapeutic concentrations thus preventing toxicity and ensuring efficacy. In children with normal renal function, aminoglycoside concentration should be measured initially after 3 or 4 doses for multiple daily dose regimens; children with renal impairment may require earlier and more frequent measurement of aminoglycoside concentration.

Blood samples should be taken approximately 1 hour after intramuscular or intravenous administration ('peak' concentration, not necessary for once daily dosing in children over 1 month) and also just before the next dose ('trough' concentration).

Serum-aminoglycoside concentration should be measured in all children and **must** be determined in infants, in neonates, in obesity, and in cystic fibrosis, *or* if high doses are being given, *or* if there is renal impairment.

Cystic fibrosis   A higher dose of parenteral aminoglycoside is often required in children with cystic fibrosis because renal clearance of the aminoglycoside is increased. For the role of aminoglycosides in the treatment of pseudomonal lung infections in cystic fibrosis see Table 1, section 5.1. Nebulised tobramycin is used for chronic pseudomonal lung infection in cystic fibrosis; however, resistance may develop, and some children do not respond to treatment. Gentamicin can be used similarly [unlicensed use].

Endocarditis   **Gentamicin** is used in combination with other antibiotics for the treatment of bacterial endocarditis (Table 1, section 5.1). Serum-gentamicin concentration should be determined twice each week (more often in renal impairment). **Streptomycin** may be used as an alternative in gentamicin-resistant enterococcal endocarditis.

Gentamicin is the aminoglycoside of choice in the UK and is used widely for the treatment of serious infections. It has a broad spectrum but is inactive against anaerobes and has poor activity against haemolytic streptococci and pneumococci. When used for the 'blind' therapy of undiagnosed serious infections it is usually given in conjunction with a penicillin or metronidazole (or both). Gentamicin is used together with another antibiotic for the treatment of endocarditis (see above and Table 1, section 5.1).

Loading and maintenance doses may be calculated on the basis of the patient's weight and renal function (e.g. using a nomogram); adjustments are then made according to serum-gentamicin concentrations. High doses are occasionally indicated for serious infections, especially in the neonate, children with cystic fibrosis or the immunocompromised patient; whenever possible treatment should not exceed 7 days.

Amikacin is more stable than gentamicin to enzyme inactivation. Amikacin is used in the treatment of serious infections caused by gentamicin-resistant Gram-negative bacilli.

Tobramycin has similar activity to gentamicin. It is slightly more active against *Ps. aeruginosa* but shows less activity against certain other Gram-negative bacteria. Tobramycin may be administered by nebuliser for the treatment of *Ps. aeruginosa* infection in cystic fibrosis (see Cystic Fibrosis, above).

Neomycin is too toxic for parenteral administration and can only be used for infections of the skin or mucous membranes or to reduce the bacterial population of the colon prior to bowel surgery or in hepatic failure. Oral administration may lead to malabsorption. Small amounts of neomycin may be absorbed from the gut in children with hepatic failure and, as these children may also be uraemic, cumulation may occur with resultant ototoxicity.

Neonates   As aminoglycosides are eliminated principally via the kidney, neonatal treatment must reflect the changes in glomerular filtration that occur with increasing gestational and postnatal age. In patients on single daily dose regimens it may become necessary to prolong the dose interval to more than 24 hours if the trough concentration is high.

GENTAMICIN

Cautions   neonates, infants (adjust dose and monitor renal, auditory and vestibular function together with serum gentamicin concentrations); avoid prolonged use; conditions characterised by muscular weakness; obesity (use ideal weight for height to calculate dose and monitor serum-gentamicin concentration closely); see also notes above; **interactions:** Appendix 1 (aminoglycosides)

Renal impairment   reduce dose frequency; monitor renal, auditory, and vestibular function; monitor serum-gentamicin concentrations; see notes above

Pregnancy   *second, third trimesters*: auditory or vestibular nerve damage; risk greatest with streptomycin; probably very small with gentamicin and tobramycin, but avoid unless essential (if given, serum-aminoglycoside concentration monitoring essential)

Contra-indications   myasthenia gravis

Side-effects   vestibular and auditory damage, nephrotoxicity; rarely, hypomagnesaemia on prolonged therapy, antibiotic-associated colitis; also reported, nausea, vomiting, rash, blood disorders; see also notes above

Licensed use   not licensed for nebulisation

Pharmacokinetics   *Extended interval dose regimen in neonates*: pre-dose ('trough') concentration should be less than 2 mg/litre
Once daily dose regimen: pre-dose ('trough') concentration should be less than 1 mg/litre
Multiple daily dose regimen: one hour ('peak') serum concentration should be 5–10 mg/litre (3–5 mg/litre for endocarditis, 8–12 mg/litre in cystic fibrosis); pre-dose ('trough') concentration should be less than 2 mg/litre (less than 1 mg/litre for endocarditis)
Intrathecal/intraventricular injection: cerebrospinal fluid concentration should not exceed 10 mg/litre

Indication and dose

Neonatal sepsis
- **Extended interval dose regimen by slow intravenous injection or intravenous infusion**

  Neonate less than 32 weeks postmenstrual age 4–5 mg/kg every 36 hours

  Neonate 32 weeks and over postmenstrual age 4–5 mg/kg every 24 hours

- **Multiple daily dose regimen by slow intravenous injection**

  Neonate less than 29 weeks postmenstrual age 2.5 mg/kg every 24 hours

  Neonate 29-35 weeks postmenstrual age 2.5 mg/kg every 18 hours

  Neonate over 35 weeks postmenstrual age 2.5 mg/kg every 12 hours

Septicaemia, meningitis and other CNS infections, biliary-tract infection, acute pyelonephritis, endocarditis (see notes above), pneumonia in hospital patients, adjunct in listerial meningitis (Table 1, section 5.1)
- **Once daily dose regimen (not for endocarditis or meningitis) by intravenous infusion**

  Child 1 month–18 years initially 7 mg/kg, then adjusted according to serum-gentamicin concentration

- **Multiple daily dose regimen by intramuscular or by slow intravenous injection over at least 3 minutes**

  Child 1 month–12 years 2.5 mg/kg every 8 hours

  Child 12–18 years 2 mg/kg every 8 hours

5

Infections

◁ **GENTAMICIN (continued)**

Pseudomonal lung infection in cystic fibrosis
- **By slow intravenous injection over at least 3 minutes or by intravenous infusion**

  Child 1 month–18 years 3 mg/kg every 8 hours

- **By inhalation of nebulised solution**

  Child 1 month–2 years 40 mg twice daily

  Child 2–8 years 80 mg twice daily

  Child 8–18 years 160 mg twice daily

Bacterial ventriculitis and CNS infection (supplement to systemic therapy)
- **By intrathecal or intraventricular injection, seek specialist advice**

  Neonate seek specialist advice

  Child 1 month–18 years 1 mg daily (increased if necessary to 5 mg daily)
  Note only preservative-free, intrathecal preparation should be used

Eye section 11.3.1

Ear section 12.1.1

Note Local guidelines may vary. See Pharmacokinetics above for serum-concentration monitoring. In obese or severely oedematous children use ideal weight for height to calculate the dose

Administration for *intravenous infusion*, dilute in Glucose 5% or Sodium Chloride 0.9%; give over 30 minutes

For *nebulisation*, dilute preservative-free preparation in 3 mL sodium chloride 0.9%. Administer after physiotherapy and bronchodilators

For *intrathecal* or *intraventricular injection*, use preservative-free intrathecal preparations only

Gentamicin (Non-proprietary) PoM
Injection, gentamicin (as sulphate), net price 40 mg/mL, 1-mL amp = £1.40, 2-mL amp = £1.54, 2-mL vial = £1.48

Paediatric injection, gentamicin (as sulphate) 10 mg/mL, net price 2-mL vial = £1.80

Intrathecal injection, gentamicin (as sulphate) 5 mg/mL, net price 1-mL amp = 74p

Cidomycin® (Sanofi-Aventis) PoM
Injection, gentamicin (as sulphate) 40 mg/mL. Net price 2-mL amp or vial = £1.48

Genticin® (Amdipharm) PoM
Injection, gentamicin (as sulphate) 40 mg/mL. Net price 2-mL amp = £1.40

Isotonic Gentamicin Injection (Baxter) PoM
Intravenous infusion, gentamicin (as sulphate) 800 micrograms/mL in sodium chloride intravenous infusion 0.9%. Net price 100-mL (80-mg) *Viaflex®* bag = £1.61
Electrolytes Na⁺ 15.4 mmol/100-mL bag

AMIKACIN

Cautions see under Gentamicin

Contra-indications see under Gentamicin

Side-effects see under Gentamicin

Pharmacokinetics *Multiple dose regimen*: one-hour ('peak') serum concentration should not exceed 30 mg/litre; pre-dose ('trough') concentration should be less than 10 mg/litre
Once daily dose regimen: pre-dose ('trough') concentration should be less than 5 mg/litre

Licensed use dose for cystic fibrosis not licensed

Indication and dose

  Neonatal sepsis
- **Extended interval dose regimen by slow intravenous injection over 3–5 minutes or by intravenous infusion**

  Neonate 15 mg/kg every 24 hours

- **Multiple daily dose regimen by intramuscular or by slow intravenous injection or by infusion**

  Neonate loading dose of 10 mg/kg then 7.5 mg/kg every 12 hours

Serious Gram-negative infections resistant to gentamicin
- **By slow intravenous injection over 3–5 minutes**

  Child 1 month–12 years 7.5 mg/kg every 12 hours

  Child 12–18 years 7.5 mg/kg every 12 hours, increased to 7.5 mg/kg every 8 hours in severe infections, max. 500 mg every 8 hours for up to 10 days (max. cumulative dose 15 g)

Once daily dose regimen (not for endocarditis or meningitis)
- **By intravenous injection or infusion**

  Child 1 month–18 years initially 15 mg/kg, then adjusted according to serum-amikacin concentration

Pseudomonal lung infection in cystic fibrosis
- **Multiple daily dose regimen by slow intravenous injection or infusion**

  Child 1 month–18 years 10 mg/kg every 8 hours (max. 500 mg every 8 hours)

Note Local dosage guidelines may vary. For monitoring guidelines see Pharmacokinetics above. In obese or severely oedematous children use ideal weight for height to calculate the dose

Administration for *intravenous infusion*, dilute with Glucose 5% *or* Sodium Chloride 0.9% *or* Compound Sodium Lactate; give over 30 minutes

Amikacin (Non-proprietary) PoM
Injection, amikacin (as sulphate) 250 mg/mL. Net price 2-mL vial = £10.14
Electrolytes Na⁺ 0.56 mmol/500-mg vial

◁ **AMIKACIN** (*continued*)

Amikin® (Bristol-Myers Squibb) PoM
Injection, amikacin (as sulphate) 250 mg/mL. Net price 2-mL vial = £10.14
Electrolytes Na⁺< 0.5 mmol/vial

Paediatric injection, amikacin (as sulphate) 50 mg/mL. Net price 2-mL vial = £2.36
Electrolytes Na⁺< 0.5 mmol/vial

◢ TOBRAMYCIN

Cautions see under Gentamicin
Specific cautions for inhaled treatment Other inhaled drugs should be administered before tobramycin; monitor for bronchospasm with initial dose, measure peak flow before and after nebulisation—if bronchospasm occurs, repeat test using bronchodilator; monitor renal function before treatment and then annually; severe haemoptysis

Contra-indications see under Gentamicin

Side-effects see under Gentamicin; *on inhalation*, mouth ulcers, taste disturbances, voice alteration, cough, bronchospasm (see Cautions)

Pharmacokinetics *Intravenous extended interval dose regimen in neonates or multiple daily dose regimen*: one-hour ('peak') serum concentration should not exceed 10 mg/litre (8–12 mg/litre in cystic fibrosis); pre-dose ('trough') concentration should be less than 2 mg/litre
Once daily dose regimen: pre-dose ('trough') concentration should be less than 1 mg/litre

Indication and dose

Neonatal sepsis
- **Extended interval dose regimen by intravenous injection over 3–5 minutes or by intravenous infusion**

  Neonate less than 32 weeks postmenstrual age 4–5 mg/kg every 36 hours

  Neonate 32 weeks and over postmenstrual age 4–5 mg/kg every 24 hours

- **Multiple daily dose regimen by intramuscular injection or by slow intravenous injection or by intravenous infusion**

  Neonate under 7 days 2 mg/kg every 12 hours

  Neonate 7–28 days 2–2.5 mg/kg every 8 hours

Septicaemia, meningitis and other CNS infections, biliary-tract infection, acute pyelonephritis, pneumonia in hospital patients
- **Multiple daily dose regimen by slow intravenous injection over 3–5 minutes**

  Child 1 month–12 years 2–2.5 mg/kg every 8 hours

  Child 12–18 years 1 mg/kg every 8 hours; in severe infections up to 5 mg/kg daily in divided

doses every 6–8 hours (reduced to 3 mg/kg daily as soon as clinically indicated)

- **Once daily dose regimen by intravenous infusion**

  Child 1 month–18 years initially 7 mg/kg, then adjusted according to serum-tobramycin concentration

Pseudomonal lung infection in cystic fibrosis
- **Multiple daily dose regimen by slow intravenous injection over 3–5 minutes**

  Child 1 month–18 years 8–10 mg/kg/daily in 3 divided doses

- **Once daily dose regimen by intravenous infusion over 30 minutes**

  Child 1 month–18 years initially 10 mg/kg (max. 660 mg), then adjusted according to serum-tobramycin concentration

Chronic pulmonary *Pseudomonas aeruginosa* infection in patients with cystic fibrosis
- **By inhalation of nebulised solution**

  Child 6–18 years 300 mg every 12 hours for 28 days, subsequent courses repeated after 28-day interval without tobramycin nebuliser solution

Note Local dosage guidelines may vary. In obese or severely oedematous children use ideal weight for height to calculate the dose. For serum concentration monitoring guidelines see Pharmacokinetics above

Administration for *intravenous infusion*, dilute with Glucose 5% *or* Sodium Chloride 0.9%; give over 20–60 minutes

Tobramycin (Non-proprietary) PoM
Injection, tobramycin (as sulphate) 40 mg/mL, net price 1-mL (40-mg) vial = £4.00, 2-mL (80-mg) vial = £4.16, 6-mL (240-mg) vial = £19.20

Bramitob® (Chiesi) PoM
Nebuliser solution, tobramycin 75 mg/mL, net price 56 x 4-mL (300-mg) unit = £1187.00

Tobi® (Chiron) PoM
Nebuliser solution, tobramycin 60 mg/mL, net price 56 × 5-mL (300-mg) unit = £1484.00

5 Infections

5.1.5 Macrolides

Erythromycin has an antibacterial spectrum that is similar but not identical to that of penicillin; it is thus an alternative in penicillin-allergic patients.

Indications for erythromycin include respiratory infections, whooping cough, legionnaires' disease, and campylobacter enteritis. It is active against many penicillin-resistant staphylococci but some are now also resistant to erythromycin; it has poor activity against *Haemophilus influenzae*. Erythromycin is also active against chlamydia and mycoplasmas.

Erythromycin causes nausea, vomiting, and diarrhoea in some children; in mild to moderate infections this can be avoided by giving a lower dose or the total dose in 4 divided doses but if a more serious infection, such as Legionella pneumonia, is suspected higher doses are needed.

Clarithromycin is an erythromycin derivative with slightly greater activity than the parent compound. Tissue concentrations are higher than with erythromycin. It is given twice daily.

Azithromycin is a macrolide with slightly less activity than erythromycin against Gram-positive bacteria but enhanced activity against some Gram-negative organisms including *H. influenzae*. Plasma concentrations are very low but tissue concentrations are much higher. It has a long tissue half-life and once daily dosage is recommended. For treatment of Lyme disease, see section 5.1.1.3. Azithromycin is also used in the treatment of trachoma [unlicensed indication] (section 11.3.1).

Azithromycin and clarithromycin cause fewer gastro-intestinal side-effects than erythromycin.

Spiramycin is also a macrolide (section 5.4.7).

Oral infections   Erythromycin is an alternative for oral infections in penicillin-allergic patients or where a beta-lactamase producing organism is involved. However, many organisms are now resistant to erythromycin or rapidly develop resistance; its use should therefore be limited to short courses. Metronidazole (section 5.1.11) may be preferred as an alternative to a penicillin.

ERYTHROMYCIN

Cautions   neonate under 2 weeks (risk of hypertrophic pyloric stenosis); predisposition to QT interval prolongation (including electrolyte disturbances, concomitant use of drugs that prolong QT interval); acute porphyria (section 9.8.2); **interactions:** Appendix 1 (macrolides)

Hepatic impairment   may cause idiosyncratic hepatotoxicity

Renal impairment   reduce dose in severe renal impairment (ototoxicity)

Pregnancy   not known to be harmful

Breast-feeding   only small amounts in milk—not known to be harmful

Side-effects   nausea, vomiting, abdominal discomfort, diarrhoea (antibiotic-associated colitis reported); less frequently urticaria, rashes and other allergic reactions; reversible hearing loss reported after large doses; cholestatic jaundice, pancreatitis, cardiac effects (including chest pain and arrhythmias), myasthenia-like syndrome, Stevens-Johnson syndrome, and toxic epidermal necrolysis also reported

Indication and dose

Susceptible infections in patients with penicillin hypersensitivity, oral infections (see notes above), campylobacter enteritis, respiratory-tract infections (including legionnaires' disease), skin infections, chlamydial ophthalmia

• By mouth

Neonate 12.5 mg/kg every 6 hours

Child 1 month–2 years 125 mg 4 times daily; dose doubled in severe infections

Child 2–8 years 250 mg 4 times daily; dose doubled in severe infections

Child 8–18 years 250–500 mg 4 times daily; dose doubled in severe infections
Note Total daily dose may be given in two divided doses

• By intermittent intravenous infusion

Neonate 10–12.5 mg/kg every 6 hours

Child 1 month–18 years 12.5 mg/kg (max. 1 g) every 6 hours

• By continuous intravenous infusion

Child 1 month–18 years 50 mg/kg daily (max. 4 g daily); mild infections (oral treatment not possible) 25 mg/kg daily

Early syphilis
• By mouth

Child 12–18 years 500 mg 4 times daily for 14 days

Uncomplicated genital chlamydia, non-gonococcal urethritis
• By mouth

Child 12–18 years 500 mg twice daily for 14 days

Prophylaxis against pneumococcal infection
• By mouth

Child 1 month–2 years 125 mg twice daily

Child 2–8 years 250 mg twice daily

Child 8–18 years 500 mg twice daily

Gastric stasis section 1.2

◁ **ERYTHROMYCIN** *(continued)*

Acne vulgaris section 13.6

Diphtheria, whooping cough prophylaxis Table 2, section 5.1

Prevention of group A streptococcal infection Table 2, section 5.1

Administration Dilute reconstituted solution further in glucose 5% (neutralised with Sodium bicarbonate) or sodium chloride 0.9% to a concentration of 1 mg/mL for continuous infusion and 1–5 mg/mL for intermittent infusion; give intermittent infusion over 20–60 minutes

Concentration of up to 10 mg/mL may be used in fluid-restriction if administered via a central venous catheter

Erythromycin (Non-proprietary) [PoM]
Capsules, enclosing e/c microgranules, erythromycin 250 mg, net price 28-cap pack = £5.95. Label: 5, 9, 25
Brands include *Tiloryth*®

Tablets, e/c, erythromycin 250 mg, net price 28 = £1.93. Label: 5, 9, 25

Dental prescribing on NHS Erythromycin Tablets e/c may be prescribed

Erythromycin Ethyl Succinate (Non-proprietary) [PoM]
Oral suspension, erythromycin (as ethyl succinate) for reconstitution with water 125 mg/5 mL, net price 100 mL = £1.71; 250 mg/5 mL, 100 mL = £2.36; 500 mg/5 mL, 100 mL = £3.82. Label: 9

Note Sugar-free versions are available and can be ordered by specifying 'sugar-free' on the prescription
Brands include *Primacine*®
Dental prescribing on NHS Erythromycin Ethyl Succinate Oral Suspension may be prescribed

Erythromycin Lactobionate (Non-proprietary) [PoM]
Intravenous infusion, powder for reconstitution, erythromycin (as lactobionate), net price 1-g vial = £9.98

Erymax® (Zeneus) [PoM]
Capsules, opaque orange/clear orange, enclosing orange and white e/c pellets, erythromycin 250 mg, net price 28-cap pack = £5.95, 112-cap pack = £23.80. Label: 5, 9, 25

Erythrocin® (Abbott) [PoM]
Tablets, both f/c, erythromycin (as stearate), 250 mg, net price 20 = £3.64; 500 mg, 20 = £7.28. Label: 9
Dental prescribing on NHS May be prescribed as Erythromycin Stearate Tablets

Erythroped® (Abbott) [PoM]
Suspension SF, sugar-free, banana-flavoured, erythromycin (as ethyl succinate) for reconstitution with water, 125 mg/5 mL (*Suspension PI SF*), net price 140 mL = £3.18; 250 mg/5 mL, 140 mL = £6.20; 500 mg/5 mL (*Suspension SF Forte*), 140 mL = £10.99. Label: 9

Erythroped A® (Abbott) [PoM]
Tablets, yellow, f/c, erythromycin 500 mg (as ethyl succinate). Net price 28-tab pack = £10.78. Label: 9
Dental prescribing on NHS May be prescribed as Erythromycin Ethyl Succinate Tablets

---

■ **AZITHROMYCIN**

Cautions see under Erythromycin; interactions: Appendix 1 (macrolides)

Pregnancy manufacturer advises use only if adequate alternatives not available

Breast-feeding present in milk; use only if no suitable alternative

Contra-indications

Hepatic impairment avoid, jaundice reported

Side-effects see under Erythromycin; also anorexia, dyspepsia, flatulence, dizziness, headache, drowsiness, convulsions, arthralgia, and disturbances in taste and smell; *rarely* constipation, hepatitis, hepatic failure, syncope, insomnia, agitation, anxiety, asthenia, paraesthesia, hyperactivity, thrombocytopenia, haemolytic anaemia, insterstitial nephritis, acute renal failure, photosensitivity, tooth and tongue discoloration

Licensed use not licensed for typhoid fever or prophylaxis of group A streptococcal infection

Indication and dose

Respiratory-tract infections, otitis media, skin and soft-tissue infections
- **By mouth**
  Child over 6 months 10 mg/kg once daily (max. 500 mg once daily) for 3 days
  or
  Body-weight 15–25 kg 200 mg once daily for 3 days
  Body-weight 26–35 kg 300 mg once daily for 3 days
  Body-weight 36–45 kg 400 mg once daily for 3 days
  Body-weight over 45 kg 500 mg once daily for 3 days

Infection in cystic fibrosis
- **By mouth**
  Child 6 months–18 years 10 mg/kg once daily (max. 500 mg once daily) for 3 days; course repeated after 1 week, then repeat as necessary

5

Infections

◻ **AZITHROMYCIN (continued)**

Chronic *Pseudomonas aeruginosa* infection in cystic fibrosis
- **By mouth**
  Child 6–18 years
  Body-weight 25–40 kg 250 mg 3 times a week
  Body-weight over 40 kg 500 mg 3 times a week

Uncomplicated genital chlamydial infections and non-gonococcal urethritis
- **By mouth**
  Child 12–18 years 1 g as a single dose

Mild to moderate typhoid due to multiple-antibacterial resistant organisms
- **By mouth**
  Child 6 months–18 years 10 mg/kg once daily (max. 500 mg) for 7 days

Prevention of group A streptococcal infection
Table 2, section 5.1

Azithromycin (Non-proprietary) (PoM)
Capsules, azithromycin (as dihydrate) 250 mg, net price 4-cap pack = £8.77, 6-cap pack = £13.16. Label: 5, 9, 23
[1] Tablets, azithromycin (as monohydrate hemi-ethanolate) 250 mg, net price 4-tab pack = £9.05; 500 mg, 3-tab pack = £9.19. Label: 5, 9
1. Azithromycin tablets can be sold to the public for the treatment of confirmed, asymptomatic *Chlamydia trachomatis* genital infection in those over 16 years of age, and for the epidemiological treatment of their sexual partners, subject to max. single dose of 1 g, max. daily dose 1 g, and a pack size of 1 g

Zithromax® (Pfizer) (PoM)
Capsules, azithromycin (as dihydrate) 250 mg, net price 4-cap pack = £8.95, 6-cap pack = £13.43. Label: 5, 9, 23

Oral suspension, cherry/banana-flavoured, azithromycin (as dihydrate) 200 mg/5 mL when reconstituted with water. Net price 15-mL pack = £5.08, 22.5-mL pack = £7.62, 30-mL pack = £13.80. Label: 5, 9
Dental prescribing on NHS May be prescribed as Azithromycin Oral Suspension 200 mg/5 mL

▸ **CLARITHROMYCIN**

Cautions see under Erythromycin; **interactions:** Appendix 1 (macrolides)
Hepatic impairment hepatic dysfunction including jaundice reported
Renal impairment use half normal dose if estimated glomerular filtration rate less than 30 mL/minute/1.73 m²; avoid *Klaricid XL®* if estimated glomerular filtration rate less than 30 mL/minute/1.73 m²
Pregnancy manufacturer advises avoid unless potential benefit outweighs risk
Breast-feeding manufacturer advises avoid unless potential benefit outweighs risk—present in milk

Side-effects see under Erythromycin; also dyspepsia, tooth and tongue discoloration, smell and taste disturbances, stomatitis, glossitis, and headache; *less commonly* hepatitis, arthralgia, and myalgia; *rarely* tinnitus; *very rarely* dizziness, insomnia, nightmares, anxiety, confusion, psychosis, paraesthesia, convulsions, hypoglycaemia, renal failure, leucopenia, and thrombocytopenia; on intravenous infusion, local tenderness, phlebitis

Licensed use intravenous route not licensed for use in children

Indication and dose

Respiratory-tract infections, mild to moderate skin and soft tissue infections, otitis media
- **By mouth**
  Neonate 7.5 mg/kg twice daily

  Child 1 month–12 years
  Body-weight under 8 kg 7.5 mg/kg twice daily
  Body-weight 8–11 kg 62.5 mg twice daily
  Body-weight 12–19 kg 125 mg twice daily
  Body-weight 20–29 kg 187.5 mg twice daily
  Body-weight 30–40 kg 250 mg twice daily

  Child 12–18 years 250 mg twice daily for 7 days, increased if necessary in severe infections to 500 mg every 12 hours for up to 14 days

- **By intravenous infusion into large proximal vein**
  Child 1 month–12 years 7.5 mg/kg every 12 hours
  Child 12–18 years 500 mg every 12 hours

Helicobacter pylori eradication section 1.3

Administration for intermittent intravenous infusion dilute reconstituted solution further in Glucose 5% *or* Sodium chloride 0.9% *or* Ringer's solution *or* Compound sodium lactate to a concentration of 2 mg/mL; give into large proximal vein over 60 minutes

Clarithromycin (Non-proprietary) (PoM)
Tablets, clarithromycin 250 mg, net price 14-tab pack = £3.55; 500 mg, 14-tab pack = £7.02. Label: 9

Clarosip® (Grünenthal) (PoM)
Granules, clarithromycin 125 mg/straw, net price 14-straw pack = £6.70; 187.5 mg/straw, 14-straw pack = £9.70; 250 mg/straw, 14-straw pack = £12.70. Label: 9, counselling, administration
Counselling. Place straw in cold or warm drink such as water, carbonated drink, or tea (but **not** full fat milk, milkshake, or drink with solid particles) and sip drink through straw; several sips may be required to obtain full dose

Klaricid® (Abbott) (PoM)
Tablets, both yellow, f/c, clarithromycin 250 mg, net price 14-tab pack = £7.43; 500 mg, 14-tab pack = £12.00, 20-tab pack = £17.14. Label: 9

Paediatric suspension, clarithromycin for reconstitution with water 125 mg/5 mL, net price 70 mL

◻ **CLARITHROMYCIN** (*continued*)

= £5.58, 100 mL = £9.60; 250 mg/5 mL, 70 mL = £11.16. Label: 9

Granules, clarithromycin 250 mg/sachet, net price 14-sachet pack = £11.68. Label: 9, 13

Intravenous infusion, powder for reconstitution, clarithromycin. Net price 500-mg vial = £11.46
Electrolytes Na⁺< 0.5 mmol/500-mg vial

Klaricid XL® (Abbott) [PoM]
Tablets, m/r, yellow, clarithromycin 500 mg, net price 7-tab pack = £6.72, 14-tab pack = £13.23. Label: 9, 21, 25
Dose
• **By mouth**
  Child 12–18 years 500 mg once daily (doubled in severe infections) for 7–14 days

5.1.6 Clindamycin

Clindamycin is active against Gram-positive cocci, including streptococci and penicillin-resistant staphylococci, and also against many anaerobes, especially *Bacteroides fragilis*. It is well concentrated in bone and excreted in bile and urine.

Clindamycin is recommended for staphylococcal joint and bone infections such as osteomyelitis, and intra-abdominal sepsis; it is an alternative to macrolides for erysipelas or cellulitis in penicillin-allergic patients. It is also used in combination with other antibacterials for cellulitis in immunocompromised children. Clindamycin can also be used for infections associated with meticillin-resistant *Staphylococcus aureus* (MRSA) in bone and joint infections, and skin and soft-tissue infections.

Clindamycin has been associated with antibiotic-associated colitis (section 1.5), which may be fatal. Although it can occur with most antibacterials, antibiotic-associated colitis occurs more frequently with clindamycin. Children should therefore discontinue treatment immediately if diarrhoea develops.

Oral infections   Clindamycin should not be used routinely for the treatment of oral infections because it may be no more effective than penicillins against anaerobes and there may be cross-resistance with erythromycin-resistant bacteria. Clindamycin can be used for the treatment of dentoalveolar abscess that has not responded to penicillin or to metronidazole.

CLINDAMYCIN

Cautions discontinue immediately if diarrhoea or colitis develops; monitor liver and renal function on prolonged therapy and in neonates and infants; avoid rapid intravenous administration; avoid in acute porphyria (section 9.8.2); **interactions**: Appendix 1 (clindamycin)

Pregnancy not known to be harmful

Breast-feeding amount probably too small to be harmful; bloody diarrhoea reported in 1 infant

Contra-indications diarrhoeal states; avoid injections containing benzyl alcohol in neonates (see under preparations below)

Side-effects diarrhoea (discontinue treatment), abdominal discomfort, oesophagitis, oesophageal ulcers, taste disturbances, nausea, vomiting, antibiotic-associated colitis; jaundice; leucopenia, eosinophilia, and thrombocytopenia reported; rash, pruritus, urticaria, anaphylactoid reactions, Stevens-Johnson syndrome, toxic epidermal necrolysis, exfoliative and vesiculobullous dermatitis reported; pain, induration, and abscess after intramuscular injection; thrombophlebitis after intravenous injection

Indication and dose

Staphylococcal bone and joint infections, peritonitis see notes above
• **By mouth**
  Neonate under 14 days 3–6 mg/kg 3 times daily
  Neonate 14–28 days 3–6 mg/kg 4 times daily

  Child 1 month–12 years 3–6 mg/kg 4 times daily (body-weight under 10 kg, minimum dose 37.5 mg 3 times daily)
  Child 12–18 years 150–300 mg 4 times daily; in severe infections 450 mg 4 times daily

• **By deep intramuscular injection or by intravenous infusion**
  Child 1 month–12 years 3.75–6.25 mg/kg 4 times daily; increased up to 10 mg/kg 4 times daily in severe infections; total daily dose may alternatively be given in 3 divided doses
  Child 12–18 years 150–675 mg 4 times daily; total daily dose may alternatively be given in 2–3 divided doses; in life-threatening infection up to 1.2 g 4 times daily; single doses above 600 mg by intravenous infusion only; single doses by intravenous infusion not to exceed 1.2 g

Staphylococcal lung infection in cystic fibrosis
• **By mouth**
  Child 1 month–18 years 5–7 mg/kg (max. 600 mg) 4 times daily

Treatment of falciparum malaria, see p. 395

Administration for *intravenous infusion*, dilute to a concentration of not more than 18 mg/mL with Glucose 5% *or* Sodium Chloride 0.9%; give over 10–60 minutes at a max. rate of 20 mg/kg/hour

5 Infections

◻ CLINDAMYCIN (*continued*)

Clindamycin (Non-proprietary) PoM
  Capsules, clindamycin (as hydrochloride) 150 mg,
  net price 24-cap pack = £24.87. Label: 9, 27,
  counselling, see above (diarrhoea)
  Dental prescribing on NHS Clindamycin Capsules may be
  prescribed

  Liquid, 75 mg/5 mL available from 'special-order'
  manufacturers or specialist importing companies,
  see p. 943

Dalacin C® (Pharmacia) PoM
  Capsules, clindamycin (as hydrochloride) 75 mg
  (lavender), net price 24-cap pack = £7.45; 150 mg,
  (lavender/maroon), 24-cap pack = £13.72. Label: 9,
  27, counselling, see above (diarrhoea)
  Dental prescribing on NHS May be prescribed as Clindamycin Capsules

  Injection, clindamycin (as phosphate) 150 mg/mL,
  net price 2-mL amp = £6.20; 4-mL amp = £12.35
  Excipients include benzyl alcohol (avoid in neonates, see
  Excipients, p. 3)

5.1.7 Some other antibacterials

Antibacterials discussed in this section include chloramphenicol, fusidic acid, glycopeptide antibiotics (vancomycin and teicoplanin), linezolid, the streptogramins (quinupristin and dalfopristin) and the polymyxin, colistin.

Chloramphenicol

Chloramphenicol is a potent broad-spectrum antibiotic; however, it is associated with serious haematological side-effects when given systemically and should therefore be reserved for the treatment of life-threatening infections, particularly those caused by *Haemophilus influenzae*, and also for typhoid fever. Chloramphenicol is also used in cystic fibrosis for the treatment of respiratory *Burkholderia cepacia* infection resistant to other antibacterials.

Grey baby syndrome may follow excessive doses in neonates with immature hepatic metabolism; monitoring of plasma concentrations is recommended.

Chloramphenicol eye drops (section 11.3.1) and chloramphenicol ear drops (section 12.1.1) are also available.

CHLORAMPHENICOL

Cautions avoid repeated courses and prolonged treatment; blood counts required before and periodically during treatment; monitor plasma-chloramphenicol concentration in neonates (see below); **interactions:** Appendix 1 (chloramphenicol)

Hepatic impairment avoid if possible—increased risk of bone-marrow depression; reduce dose and monitor plasma-chloramphenicol concentration

Renal impairment avoid in severe impairment unless no alternative; dose-related depression of haematopoiesis

Contra-indications acute porphyria (section 9.8.2)

Pregnancy neonatal grey-baby syndrome if used in third trimester

Breast-feeding use another antibiotic; may cause bone-marrow toxicity in infant; concentration in milk usually insufficient to cause 'grey-baby syndrome'

Side-effects blood disorders including reversible and irreversible aplastic anaemia (with reports of resulting leukaemia), peripheral neuritis, optic neuritis, headache, depression, urticaria, erythema multiforme, nausea, vomiting, diarrhoea, stomatitis, glossitis, dry mouth; nocturnal haemoglobinuria reported; grey syndrome (abdominal distension, pallid cyanosis, circulatory collapse) may follow excessive doses in neonates with immature hepatic metabolism (see Pharmacokinetics below)

Pharmacokinetics plasma concentration monitoring required in neonates and preferred in those under 4 years of age, and in hepatic impairment; recommended peak plasma concentration (approx. 1 hour after end of intravenous injection or infusion or 2 hours after oral administration) 15–25 mg/litre; pre-dose ('trough') concentration should not exceed 15 mg/litre

Indication and dose
See notes above
• **By intravenous injection**
  Neonate up to 14 days 12.5 mg/kg twice daily
  Neonate 14–28 days 12.5 mg/kg 2–4 times daily
  Note Check dosage carefully; overdosage can be fatal (see also pharmacokinetics above)

• **By mouth or by intravenous injection or infusion**
  Child 1 month–18 years 12.5 mg/kg every 6 hours; dose may be doubled in severe infections such as septicaemia, meningitis and epiglottitis providing plasma-chloramphenicol concentrations are measured and high doses reduced as soon as indicated

Administration Displacement value may be significant for injection, consult local guidelines. For intermittent intravenous infusion, dilute reconstituted solution further in glucose 5% *or* sodium chloride 0.9%

◁ **CHLORAMPHENICOL (continued)**

Chloramphenicol (Non-proprietary) PoM
Capsules, chloramphenicol 250 mg. Net price 60 = £377.00

▲ Extemporaneous formulations available see Extemporaneous Preparations, p. 8

Kemicetine® (Pharmacia) PoM
Injection, powder for reconstitution, chloramphenicol (as sodium succinate). Net price 1-g vial = £1.39
Electrolytes Na⁺ 3.14 mmol/g

Fusidic acid

Fusidic acid and its salts are narrow-spectrum antibiotics. The only indication for their use is in infections caused by penicillin-resistant staphylococci, especially osteomyelitis, as they are well concentrated in bone; they are also used for staphylococcal endocarditis. A second antistaphylococcal antibiotic is usually required to prevent emergence of resistance during treatment.

■ SODIUM FUSIDATE

Cautions monitor liver function with high doses, on prolonged therapy or in hepatic impairment; elimination may be reduced in hepatic impairment or biliary disease or biliary obstruction; **interactions:** Appendix 1 (fusidic acid)

Hepatic impairment impaired biliary excretion, avoid or reduce dose; possibly increased risk of hepatotoxicity, monitor liver function

Pregnancy not known to be harmful; manufacturer advises use only if potential benefit outweighs risk

Breast-feeding present in milk; manufacturer advises caution

Side-effects nausea, vomiting, reversible jaundice, especially after high dosage or rapid infusion (withdraw therapy if persistent); rarely hypersensitivity reactions, acute renal failure (usually with jaundice), blood disorders

Indication and dose

Penicillin-resistant staphylococcal infection including osteomyelitis, staphylococcal endocarditis in combination with other antibacterials see under Preparations, below

Sodium fusidate (LEO) PoM
Intravenous infusion, powder for reconstitution, sodium fusidate 500 mg (= fusidic acid 480 mg), with buffer, net price per vial (with diluent) = £70.04
Electrolytes Na⁺ 3.1 mmol/vial when reconstituted with buffer

Dose
As sodium fusidate
• By intravenous infusion

Neonate 10 mg/kg every 12 hours

Child 1 month–18 years 6–7 mg/kg (max. 500 mg) every 8 hours

Administration reconstitute with buffer solution provided; further dilute to 1 mg/mL with Sodium chloride 0.9% *or* Glucose 5% intravenous infusion (but see below); infuse over at least 6 hours via a superficial vein or 2 hours via a central venous line; incompatible in solution of pH less than 7.4

Fucidin® (LEO) PoM
Tablets, f/c, sodium fusidate 250 mg, net price 10-tab pack = £6.02. Label: 9
Dose
as sodium fusidate

Child 12–18 years 500 mg every 8 hours, dose doubled for severe infections

Skin infection as sodium fusidate
Child 12–18 years 250 mg every 12 hours for 5–10 days

Suspension, off-white, banana- and orange-flavoured, fusidic acid 250 mg/5 mL, net price 50 mL = £6.73. Label: 9, 21
Dose
As fusidic acid

Neonate 15 mg/kg 3 times daily

Child 1 month–1 year 15 mg/kg 3 times daily
Child 1–5 years 250 mg 3 times daily
Child 5–12 years 500 mg 3 times daily
Child 12–18 years 750 mg 3 times daily
Note Fusidic acid is incompletely absorbed and doses recommended for suspension are proportionately higher than those for sodium fusidate tablets

---

Vancomycin and teicoplanin

The glycopeptide antibiotics vancomycin and teicoplanin have bactericidal activity against aerobic and anaerobic Gram-positive bacteria including multi-resistant *Staphylococci*. However, there are reports of *Staphylococcus aureus* with reduced susceptibility to glycopeptides. There are increasing reports of glycopeptide-resistant *Enterococci*.

Vancomycin is used *by the intravenous route* in the prophylaxis and treatment of serious infections caused by Gram-positive cocci. Vancomycin is principally excreted via the kidney and dose reduction is necessary in renal impairment.

Penetration in to cerebrospinal fluid is poor; vancomycin may be administered by the intrathecal or intraventricular route for treatment of meningitis [unlicensed]. Vancomycin (added to dialysis fluid) is also used in the treatment of peritonitis associated with peritoneal dialysis [unlicensed route] (Table 1 section 5.1).

Vancomycin given *by mouth* for 7–10 days is effective in the treatment of *Clostridium difficile* infection (see also section 1.5); low doses (see below) are considered adequate (higher dose may be considered if the infection fails to respond or if it is severe). Vancomycin is also used by mouth in prophylaxis of neonatal necrotising enterocolitis. Vancomycin should **not** be given by mouth for systemic infections since it is not significantly absorbed.

Teicoplanin is similar to vancomycin but has a significantly longer duration of action allowing once-daily administration. Plasma concentration monitoring is not usually necessary, but may help optimise therapy. Unlike vancomycin, teicoplanin can be given by intramuscular as well as by intravenous injection; it is not given by mouth.

VANCOMYCIN

Cautions avoid rapid infusion (risk of anaphylactoid reactions, see Side-effects); rotate infusion sites; avoid if history of deafness; all patients require plasma-vancomycin measurement (after 3 or 4 doses if renal function normal, earlier if renal impairment), blood counts, urinalysis, and renal function tests; monitor auditory function in renal impairment; systemic absorption may follow oral administration especially in inflammatory bowel disorders or following multiple doses; **interactions**: Appendix 1 (vancomycin)

Renal impairment reduce dose—monitor plasma-vancomycin concentration and renal function regularly

Pregnancy manufacturer advises use only if potential benefit outweighs risk—plasma-vancomycin concentration monitoring essential to reduce risk of fetal toxicity

Breast-feeding present in milk—significant absorption following oral administration unlikely

Side-effects after parenteral administration: nephrotoxicity including renal failure and interstitial nephritis; ototoxicity (discontinue if tinnitus occurs); blood disorders including neutropenia (usually after 1 week or high cumulative dose), rarely agranulocytosis and thrombocytopenia; nausea; chills, fever; eosinophilia, anaphylaxis, rashes (including exfoliative dermatitis, Stevens-Johnson syndrome, toxic epidermal necrolysis, and vasculitis); phlebitis (irritant to tissue); on rapid infusion, severe hypotension (including shock and cardiac arrest), wheezing, dyspnoea, urticaria, pruritus, flushing of the upper body ('red man' syndrome), pain and muscle spasm of back and chest

Pharmacokinetics plasma concentration monitoring required; pre-dose ('trough') concentration should be 10–15 mg/litre (15–20 mg/litre for less sensitive strains of meticillin-resistant *Staphylococcus aureus*)

Licensed use not licensed for intraventricular use

Indication and dose

Infections due to Gram-positive bacteria including osteomyelitis, septicaemia and soft-tissue infections see notes above
- **By intravenous infusion**

  Neonate less than 29 weeks postmenstrual age 15 mg/kg every 24 hours

  Neonate 29–35 weeks postmenstrual age 15 mg/kg every 12 hours

  Neonate over 35 weeks postmenstrual age 15 mg/kg every 8 hours

  Child 1 month–18 years 15 mg/kg every 8 hours (maximum daily dose 2 g), adjusted according to plasma concentration

Clostridium difficile infection (see also notes above)
- **By mouth**

  Child 1 month–5 years 5 mg/kg 4 times daily for 7–10 days

  Child 5–12 years 62.5 mg 4 times daily for 7–10 days

  Child 12–18 years 125 mg 4 times daily for 7–10 days

Prophylaxis of necrotising enterocolitis in neonates
- **By mouth**

  Neonate 15 mg/kg 3 times daily

CNS infection e.g. ventriculitis
- **By intraventricular administration, seek specialist advice**

  Neonate 10 mg once every 24 hours

  Child 1 month–18 years 10 mg once every 24 hours
  Note for all children reduce to 5 mg daily if ventricular size reduced or increase to 15–20 mg once daily if ventricular size increased. Adjust dose according to CSF concentration after 3-4 days; aim for pre-dose ('trough') concentration less than 10 mg/litre. If CSF not draining freely reduce dose frequency to once every 2–3 days

◁ **VANCOMYCIN** (*continued*)

> **Peritonitis associated with peritoneal dialysis**
> Add to each bag of dialysis fluid to achieve a
> concentration of 20–25 mg/litre

Note Vancomycin doses in BNF for Children may differ
from those in product literature

Administration Displacement value may be significant, consult product literature and local
guidelines. For intermittent intravenous infusion,
the reconstituted preparation should be further
diluted in sodium chloride 0.9% *or* glucose 5% to
a concentration of up to 5 mg/mL; give over at
least 60 minutes (rate not to exceed 10 mg/min-
ute for doses over 500 mg); use continuous infusion only if intermittent not available (limited
evidence); 10 mg/mL can be used if infused via a
central venous line over at least 1 hour

Injection may be given orally; flavouring syrups
may be added to the solution at the time of
administration.

> Safe Practice For intraventricular administration, seek
> specialist advice

Vancomycin (Non-proprietary) PoM
Capsules, vancomycin (as hydrochloride) 125 mg,
net price 28-cap pack = £132.47; 250 mg, 28-cap
pack = £132.47. Label: 9

Injection, powder for reconstitution, vancomycin
(as hydrochloride), for use as an infusion, net price
500-mg vial = £8.05; 1-g vial = £16.11

Note Can be used to prepare solution for oral administration

Vancocin® (Flynn) PoM
Matrigel capsules, vancomycin (as hydrochloride)
125 mg, net price 28-cap pack = £88.31. Label: 9

Injection, powder for reconstitution, vancomycin
(as hydrochloride), for use as an infusion, net price
500-mg vial = £8.05; 1-g vial = £16.11

Note Can be used to prepare solution for oral administration

TEICOPLANIN

Cautions vancomycin sensitivity; blood counts
and liver and kidney function tests required—
monitor renal and auditory function on prolonged administration during renal impairment or
if other nephrotoxic or neurotoxic drugs given;
monitor serum-teicoplanin concentration if
severe sepsis or burns, deep-seated staphylococcal infection (including bone and joint infection), renal impairment, and in intravenous drug
abusers; **interactions:** Appendix 1 (teicoplanin)

Renal impairment reduce dose on day 4: use half
normal dose if estimated glomerular filtration rate
is 40–60 mL/minute/1.73 m² and use one-third
normal dose if estimated glomerular filtration rate
is less than 40 mL/minute/1.73 m²

Pregnancy manufacturer advises use only if
potential benefit outweighs risk

Breast-feeding no information available

Side-effects nausea, vomiting, diarrhoea; rash;
pruritus, fever, bronchospasm, rigors, urticaria,
angioedema, anaphylaxis; dizziness, headache;
blood disorders including eosinophilia, leucopenia, neutropenia, and thrombocytopenia; disturbances in liver enzymes, transient increase of
serum creatinine, renal failure; tinnitus, mild
hearing loss, and vestibular disorders also
reported; rarely exfoliative dermatitis, Stevens-
Johnson syndrome, toxic epidermal necrolysis;
local reactions include erythema, pain, thrombophlebitis, injection site abscess and rarely
flushing with infusion

Pharmacokinetics plasma-teicoplanin concentration is not measured routinely because there is no
clear relationship between plasma-teicoplanin
concentration and toxicity. However, the plasma-
teicoplanin concentration can be used to opti-

mise treatment in some patients (see Cautions).
Pre-dose ('trough') concentration should be
greater than 10 mg/litre (greater than 15–20 mg/
litre in endocarditis) but less than 60 mg/litre

Indication and dose

> Potentially serious Gram-positive infections
> including endocarditis, and serious infections
> due to Staphylococcus aureus
> • **By intravenous injection or intravenous infu-**
> **sion over 30 minutes**
>
> **Neonate** initially 16 mg/kg for one dose fol-
> lowed 24 hours later by 8 mg/kg once daily
> (intravenous infusion only)
>
> **Child 1 month–18 years** in moderate infections
> initially 10 mg/kg (max. 400 mg) every 12 hours
> for 3 doses, then 6 mg/kg (max. 200 mg) once
> daily; in severe infections or in neutropenia
> initially 10 mg/kg (max. 400 mg) every 12 hours
> for 3 doses then 10 mg/kg (max. 400 mg) once
> daily; after first 3 doses, subsequent doses can
> be given by intramuscular injection if necessary
> although intravenous route preferable for chil-
> dren

Administration For intermittent intravenous infusion, dilute reconstituted solution further in sodium chloride 0.9% *or* glucose 5% *or* compound
sodium lactate intravenous infusion; give over 30
minutes. Intermittent intravenous infusion preferred in neonates

Targocid® (Aventis Pharma) PoM
Injection, powder for reconstitution, teicoplanin,
net price 200-mg vial (with diluent) = £17.58; 400-
mg vial (with diluent) = £35.62
Electrolytes Na⁺< 0.5 mmol/200- and 400-mg vial

5

Infections

Linezolid

Linezolid, an oxazolidinone antibacterial, is active against Gram-positive bacteria including meticillin-resistant *Staphylococcus aureus* (MRSA), and glycopeptide-resistant enterococci. Resistance to linezolid can develop with prolonged treatment or if the dose is less than that recommended. Linezolid should be reserved for infections caused by Gram-positive bacteria when the organisms are resistant to other antibacterials or when patients cannot tolerate other antibacterials. Linezolid is **not** active against common Gram-negative organisms; it must be given in combination with other antibacterials for mixed infections that also involve Gram-negative organisms. There is limited information on use in children and expert advice should be sought. A higher incidence of blood disorders and optic neuropathy have been reported in patients receiving linezolid for more than the maximum recommended duration of 28 days.

LINEZOLID

Cautions monitor full blood count (including platelet count) weekly (see also CSM Advice below); unless close observation and blood-pressure monitoring possible, avoid in uncontrolled hypertension, phaeochromocytoma, carcinoid tumour, thyrotoxicosis, bipolar depression, schizophrenia, or acute confusional states; **interactions:** Appendix 1 (MAOIs)

Hepatic impairment no dose adjustment necessary but in severe hepatic impairment use only if potential benefit outweighs risk

Renal impairment no dose adjustment necessary but metabolites may accumulate if estimated glomerular filtration rate less than 30 mL/minute/1.73 m^2

Pregnancy manufacturer advises use only if potential benefit outweighs risk—no information available

CSM advice Haematopoietic disorders (including thrombocytopenia, anaemia, leucopenia, and pancytopenia) have been reported in patients receiving linezolid. It is recommended that full blood counts are monitored weekly. Close monitoring is recommended in patients who:

- receive treatment for more than 10–14 days;
- have pre-existing myelosuppression;
- are receiving drugs that may have adverse effects on haemoglobin, blood counts, or platelet function;
- have severe renal impairment.

If significant myelosuppression occurs, treatment should be stopped unless it is considered essential, in which case intensive monitoring of blood counts and appropriate management should be implemented.

CHM advice (optic neuropathy) Severe optic neuropathy may occur rarely, particularly if linezolid is used for longer than 28 days. The CHM recommends that:

- patients should be warned to report symptoms of visual impairment (including blurred vision, visual field defect, changes in visual acuity and colour vision) immediately;
- patients experiencing new visual symptoms (regardless of treatment duration) should be evaluated promptly, and referred to an ophthalmologist if necessary;
- visual function should be monitored regularly if treatment is required for longer than 28 days.

Monoamine oxidase inhibition Linezolid is a reversible, non-selective monoamine oxidase inhibitor (MAOI). Patients should avoid consuming large amounts of tyramine-rich foods (such as mature cheese, yeast extracts, undistilled alcoholic beverages, and fermented soya bean products). In addition, linezolid should not be given with another MAOI or within 2 weeks of stopping another MAOI. Unless close observation and blood-pressure monitoring is possible, avoid in those receiving SSRIs, 5HT$_1$ agonists ('triptans'), tricyclic antidepressants, sympathomimetics, dopaminergics, buspirone, pethidine and possibly other opioid analgesics. For other interactions see Appendix 1 (MAOIs)

Contra-indications see also Monoamine oxidase inhibition above

Breast-feeding manufacturer advises avoid—present in milk in animal studies

Side-effects diarrhoea (antibiotic-associated colitis reported), nausea, vomiting, taste disturbances, headache; *less commonly* thirst, dry mouth, glossitis, stomatitis, tongue discoloration, abdominal pain, dyspepsia, gastritis, constipation, pancreatitis, hypertension, fever, fatigue, dizziness, insomnia, hypoaesthesia, paraesthesia, tinnitus, polyuria, anaemia, leucopenia, thrombocytopenia, eosinophilia, electrolyte disturbances, blurred vision, rash, pruritus, diaphoresis, and injection-site reactions; *very rarely* renal failure, pancytopenia and Stevens-Johnson syndrome; also reported, lactic acidosis; peripheral and optic neuropathy reported on prolonged therapy

Licensed use not licensed for use in children

Indication and dose

Pneumonia, complicated skin and soft-tissue infections caused by Gram-positive bacteria (initiated under expert supervision)

- **By mouth or by intravenous infusion over 30–120 minutes**

  Neonate under 7 days 10 mg/kg every 12 hours, increase to every 8 hours if poor response

  Neonate over 7 days 10 mg/kg every 8 hours

  Child 1 month–12 years 10 mg/kg (max. 600 mg) every 8 hours

  Child 12–18 years 600 mg every 12 hours

Zyvox® (Pharmacia) ▼ PoM
Tablets, f/c, linezolid 600 mg, net price 10-tab pack = £445.00. Label: 9, 10, patient information leaflet

Suspension, yellow, linezolid 100 mg/5 mL when reconstituted with water, net price 150 mL (orange-

◻ **LINEZOLID** (*continued*)

flavoured) = £222.50. Label: 9, 10 patient information leaflet
Excipients include aspartame 20 mg/5 mL (section 9.4.1)

Intravenous infusion, linezolid 2 mg/mL, net price 300-mL *Excel®* bag = £44.50
Excipients include Na⁺ 5 mmol/300-mL bag, glucose 13.71 g/ 300-mL bag

---

Quinupristin and dalfopristin

A combination of the streptogramin antibiotics, **quinupristin** and **dalfopristin** (as *Synercid®*) is licensed in adults for infections due to Gram-positive bacteria; there is limited information on use in children and expert advice should be sought. The combination should be reserved for treating infections which have failed to respond to other antibacterials (e.g. meticillin-resistant *Staphylococcus aureus*, MRSA) or for patients who cannot be treated with other antibacterials. Quinupristin and dalfopristin are not active against *Enterococcus faecalis* and they need to be given in combination with other antibacterials for mixed infections which also involve Gram-negative organisms.

QUINUPRISTIN WITH DALFOPRISTIN

A mixture of quinupristin and dalfopristin (both as mesilate salts) in the proportions 3 parts to 7 parts

Cautions predisposition to cardiac arrhythmias (including congenital QT syndrome, concomitant use of drugs that prolong QT interval, cardiac hypertrophy, dilated cardiomyopathy, hypokalaemia, hypomagnesaemia, bradycardia); **interactions**: Appendix 1 (quinupristin with dalfopristin)

Hepatic impairment consider reducing dose to 5 mg/kg every 8 hours in moderate impairment, adjusted according to clinical response; avoid in severe hepatic impairment or if plasma-bilirubin concentration greater than 3 times upper limit of reference range

Pregnancy manufacturer advises avoid unless potential benefit outweighs risk—no information available

Contra-indications plasma-bilirubin concentration greater than 3 times upper limit of reference range

Breast-feeding manufacturer advises avoid— present in milk in *animal* studies

Side-effects nausea, vomiting, diarrhoea, headache, arthralgia, myalgia, asthenia, rash, pruritus, anaemia, leucopenia, eosinophilia, raised urea and creatinine; injection-site reactions on peripheral venous administration; less frequently oral candidiasis, stomatitis, constipation, abdominal pain, antibiotic-associated colitis, anorexia, peripheral oedema, hypotension, chest pain, arrhythmias, dyspnoea, hypersensitivity reactions (including anaphylaxis and urticaria), insomnia, anxiety, confusion, dizziness, paraesthesia, hypertonia, hepatitis, jaundice, pancreat-itis, gout; also reported, thrombocytopenia, pancytopenia, electrolyte disturbances

Licensed use not licensed for use in children

Indication and dose

Serious Gram-positive infections where no alternative antibacterial is suitable including hospital-acquired pneumonia, skin and soft-tissue infections, infections due to vancomycin-resistant *Enterococcus faecium* Dose expressed as a combination of quinupristin and dalfopristin (in a ratio of 3:7)

- **By intravenous infusion into central vein**

  Child 1 month–18 years 7.5 mg/kg every 8 hours for 7 days in skin and soft-tissue infections; for 10 days in hospital-acquired pneumonia; duration of treatment in *E. faecium* infection depends on site of infection

Administration Reconstitute 500 mg with 5 mL water for injections or glucose 5%; gently swirl vial without shaking to dissolve; allow to stand for at least 2 minutes until foam disappears; *for intravenous infusion* dilute requisite dose with glucose 5% intravenous infusion to a concentration of 5 mg/mL and give over 60 minutes via central venous catheter. In an emergency, first dose may be diluted to 2 mg/mL and given over 60 minutes via peripheral line; flush line with glucose 5% before and after infusion; incompatible with sodium chloride solutions

Synercid® (Nordic) ▣PoM

Intravenous infusion, powder for reconstitution, quinupristin (as mesilate) 150 mg, dalfopristin (as mesilate) 350 mg, net price 500-mg vial = £37.00
Electrolytes Na⁺ approx. 16 mmol/500-mg vial

Polymyxins

The polymyxin antibiotic, **colistin**, is active against Gram-negative organisms including *Pseudomonas aeruginosa*, *Acinetobacter baumanii*, and *Klebsiella pneumoniae*. It is **not** absorbed by mouth and is given by injection for a systemic effect. Intravenous administration of colistin should be reserved for Gram-negative infections resistant to other antibacterials; its major adverse effects are dose-related neurotoxicity and nephrotoxicity.

Colistin is used by mouth in bowel sterilisation regimens in neutropenic patients (usually with nystatin); it is **not** recommended for gastro-intestinal infections. It is also given by inhalation of a nebulised solution as an adjunct to standard antibacterial therapy in patients with cystic fibrosis.

Both colistin and polymyxin B are included in some preparations for topical application.

◢ **COLISTIN**

Cautions acute porphyria (section 9.8.2); risk of bronchospasm on inhalation—may be prevented or treated with a selective beta₂ agonist; **interactions:** Appendix 1 (polymyxins)

Renal impairment monitor plasma-colistin concentration during parenteral treatment. Reduce parenteral dose in moderate to severe impairment

Contra-indications myasthenia gravis

Pregnancy avoid—possible risk of fetal toxicity especially in second and third trimesters

Breast-feeding present in milk but poorly absorbed from gut; manufacturers advise avoid (or use only if potential benefit outweighs risk)

Side-effects neurotoxicity reported especially with excessive doses (including apnoea, perioral and peripheral paraesthesia, vertigo; rarely vasomotor instability, slurred speech, confusion, psychosis, visual disturbances); nephrotoxicity; hypersensitivity reactions including rash; injection-site reactions; inhalation may cause sore throat, sore mouth, cough, bronchospasm

Pharmacokinetics see notes above; plasma concentration monitoring required for intravenous treatment in renal impairment and cystic fibrosis; recommended 'peak' plasma-colistin concentration (approx. 30 minutes after intravenous injection or infusion) 10–15 mg/litre (125–200 units/mL); colistin sulphate may be absorbed from the gastro-intestinal tract in infants under 6 months old

Indication and dose

Pseudomonas aeruginosa infection in cystic fibrosis
• By slow intravenous injection into a totally implantable venous access device, or by intravenous infusion (but see notes above)
  Child 1 month–18 years
  Body-weight under 60 kg 16 666–25 000 units/kg every 8 hours

Body-weight over 60 kg 1–2 million units every 8 hours

• By inhalation of nebulised solution
  Child 1 month–2 years 500 000–1 million units twice daily
  Child 2–18 years 1–2 million units twice daily

Administration For *intravenous infusion*, dilute to a concentration of 40 000 units/mL with Sodium Chloride 0.9%; give over 30 minutes

For *slow intravenous injection* into a totally implantable venous access device, dilute to a concentration of 90 000 units/mL for child under 12 years (200 000 units/mL for child over 12 years)

For *nebulisation* administer required dose in 2–4 mL of sodium chloride 0.9% (or water for injections). Colistin must not be mixed with tobramycin as they are chemically unstable together; it may be mixed with gentamicin if used immediately

Colomycin® (Forest) ℞
Injection, powder for reconstitution, colistimethate sodium (colistin sulphomethate sodium). Net price 1 million-unit vial = £1.68; 2 million-unit vial = £3.09
Electrolytes (before reconstitution) Na⁺< 0.5 mmol/500 000-unit, 1 million-unit, and 2 million-unit vial
Note *Colomycin®* Injection (dissolved in physiological saline) may be used for nebulisation

Promixin® (Profile) ℞
Powder for nebuliser solution, colistimethate sodium (colistin sulphomethate sodium), net price 1 million-unit vial = £4.60.

Injection, powder for reconstitution, colistimethate sodium (colistin sulphomethate sodium), net price 1 million unit-vial = £2.30
Electrolytes (before reconstitution) Na⁺< 0.5 mmol/1 million-unit vial

5.1.8 Sulphonamides and trimethoprim

The importance of the sulphonamides has decreased as a result of increasing bacterial resistance and their replacement by antibacterials which are generally more active and less toxic.

Sulfamethoxazole (sulphamethoxazole) and trimethoprim are used in combination (as **co-trimoxazole**) because of their synergistic activity. However, co-trimoxazole is associated with rare but serious side-effects e.g. Stevens-Johnson syndrome and blood dyscrasias, notably bone marrow depression and agranulocytosis (see CSM recommendations below). Co-trimoxazole should be avoided in children less than 6 weeks of age (except for treatment and prophylaxis of *pneumocystis pneumonia*) because of the risk of kernicterus. There is a risk of haemolytic anaemia if used in children with glucose-6-phosphate dehydrogenase (G6PD) deficiency (section 9.1.5).

> **CSM recommendations**
> Co-trimoxazole should be limited to the role of drug of choice in *Pneumocystis jiroveci* (*Pneumocystis carinii*) pneumonia; it is also indicated for *toxoplasmosis* and *nocardiasis*. It should now only be considered for use in *acute exacerbations of chronic bronchitis* and *infections of the urinary tract* when there is good bacteriological evidence of sensitivity to co-trimoxazole and good reason to prefer this combination to a single antibacterial; similarly it should only be used in *acute otitis media in children* when there is good reason to prefer it.

Trimethoprim can be used alone for urinary- and respiratory-tract infections and for shigellosis and invasive salmonella infections. Trimethoprim has side-effects similar to co-trimoxazole but they are less severe and occur less frequently.

For *topical preparations* of sulphonamides used in the treatment of burns see section 13.10.1.1.

◢ CO-TRIMOXAZOLE

A mixture of trimethoprim and sulfamethoxazole in the proportions of 1 part to 5 parts

Cautions maintain adequate fluid intake; avoid in blood disorders (unless under specialist supervision); monitor blood counts on prolonged treatment; discontinue immediately if blood disorders or rash develop; predisposition to folate deficiency; asthma; G6PD deficiency (section 9.1.5); avoid in infants under 6 weeks (except for treatment or prophylaxis of pneumocystis pneumonia); **interactions:** Appendix 1 (trimethoprim, sulfamethoxazole)

Hepatic impairment manufacturer advises avoid in severe liver disease

Renal impairment use half normal dose if estimated glomerular filtration rate 15–30 mL/minute/$1.73\,m^2$; avoid if estimated glomerular filtration rate less than $15\,mL/minute/1.73\,m^2$ and if plasma-sulfamethoxazole concentration cannot be monitored

Pregnancy teratogenic risk (trimethoprim a folate antagonist) in first trimester neonatal haemolysis and methaemoglobinaemia in 3rd trimester; fear of increased risk of kernicterus in neonates appears to be unfounded

Breast-feeding small risk of kernicterus in jaundiced infants and of haemolysis in G6PD-deficient infants (due to sulfamethoxazole)

Contra-indications acute porphyria (section 9.8.2)

Side-effects nausea, diarrhoea; headache, hyperkalaemia; rash (*very rarely* including Stevens-Johnson syndrome, toxic epidermal necrolysis, photosensitivity)—discontinue immediately; *less commonly* vomiting; *very rarely* glossitis, stomatitis, anorexia, liver damage (including jaundice and hepatic necrosis), pancreatitis, antibiotic-associated colitis, myocarditis, cough and shortness of breath, pulmonary infiltrates, aseptic meningitis, depression, convulsions, peripheral neuropathy, ataxia, tinnitus, vertigo, hallucinations, hypoglycaemia, blood disorders (including leucopenia, thrombocytopenia, megaloblastic anaemia, eosinophilia), hyponatraemia, renal disorders including interstitial nephritis, arthralgia, myalgia, vasculitis, systemic lupus erythematosus, and uveitis; rhabdomyolysis reported in HIV-infected patients

Pharmacokinetics plasma concentration monitoring may be required with high doses or during moderate to severe renal impairment; seek expert advice

Licensed use not licensed for use in children under 6 weeks

Indication and dose

> Treatment of susceptible infections (but see notes above) dose expressed as co-trimoxazole
> - **By mouth**
>   Child 6 weeks–12 years 24 mg/kg twice daily *or*
>   Child 6 weeks–6 months 120 mg twice daily
>   Child 6 months–6 years 240 mg twice daily
>   Child 6–12 years 480 mg twice daily
>   Child 12–18 years 960 mg twice daily
>
> - **By intravenous infusion**
>   Child 6 weeks–18 years 18 mg/kg every 12 hours; increased in severe infection to 27 mg/kg (max. 1.44 g) every 12 hours

> Treatment of *Pneumocystis jiroveci* (*P. carinii*) infections (undertaken where facilities for appropriate monitoring available—consult microbiologist and product literature)
> - **By mouth or by intravenous infusion**
>   Child 6 weeks–18 years 60 mg/kg every 12 hours for 14 days; total daily dose may alternatively be given in 3–4 divided doses
>   Note oral route preferred

> Prophylaxis of *Pneumocystis jiroveci* (*P. carinii*) infections
> - **By mouth**
>   Child 1 month–18 years $450\,mg/m^2$ (max 960 mg) twice daily for three days of the week (either consecutively or on alternate days)
>   Note dose regimens may vary, consult local guidelines

Note 480 mg of co-trimoxazole consists of sulfamethoxazole 400 mg and trimethoprim 80 mg

Administration for intermittent intravenous infusion may be further diluted in glucose 5% and 10% or sodium chloride 0.9% or Ringer's intravenous solution. Dilute contents of 1 ampoule (5 mL) to 125 mL, 2 ampoules (10 mL) to 250 mL or 3 ampoules (15 mL) to 500 mL; suggested

◁ **CO-TRIMOXAZOLE** (*continued*)

duration of infusion 60–90 minutes (but may be adjusted according to fluid requirements); if fluid restriction necessary, 1 ampoule (5 mL) may be diluted with 75 mL glucose 5% and the required dose infused over max. 60 minutes; check container for haze or precipitant during administration. In severe fluid restriction may be given undiluted via a central venous line

Co-trimoxazole (Non-proprietary) ▣PoM
Tablets, co-trimoxazole 480 mg, net price 28-tab pack = £13.83; 960 mg, 20 = £4.69. Label: 9
Brands include *Fectrim*®, *Fectrim*® *Forte*

Paediatric oral suspension, co-trimoxazole 240 mg/5 mL, net price 100 mL = £1.12. Label: 9

Oral suspension, co-trimoxazole 480 mg/5 mL. Net price 100 mL = £4.41. Label: 9

Strong sterile solution, co-trimoxazole 96 mg/mL. For dilution and use as an intravenous infusion. Net price 5-mL amp = £1.58, 10-mL amp = £3.06

Septrin® (GSK) ▣PoM
Tablets, co-trimoxazole 480 mg. Net price 20 = £3.10. Label: 9

Forte tablets, scored, co-trimoxazole 960 mg. Net price 20 = £4.69. Label: 9

Adult suspension, co-trimoxazole 480 mg/5 mL. Net price 100 mL (vanilla-flavoured) = £4.41. Label: 9

Paediatric suspension, sugar-free, co-trimoxazole 240 mg/5 mL. Net price 100 mL (banana- and vanilla-flavoured) = £2.45. Label: 9

Intravenous infusion, co-trimoxazole 96 mg/mL. To be diluted before use. Net price 5-mL amp = £1.48
Excipients include propylene glycol, sulphites

▮ TRIMETHOPRIM

Cautions predisposition to folate deficiency; manufacturer recommends blood counts on long-term therapy (but evidence of practical value unsatisfactory); neonates (specialist supervision required); acute porphyria (section 9.8.2); **interactions:** Appendix 1 (trimethoprim)

Renal impairment use half normal dose after 3 days if estimated glomerular filtration rate 15–30 mL/minute/1.73 m²; use half normal dose immediately if estimated glomerular filtration rate less than 15 mL/minute/1.73 m² (monitor plasma-trimethoprim concentration if estimated glomerular filtration rate less than 10 mL/minute/1.73 m²)

Breast-feeding present in milk—short-term use not known to be harmful

Blood disorders On long-term treatment, patients and their carers should be told how to recognise signs of blood disorders and advised to seek immediate medical attention if symptoms such as fever, sore throat, rash, mouth ulcers, purpura, bruising or bleeding develop

Contra-indications blood dyscrasias

Pregnancy teratogenic risk (folate antagonist) in first trimester; manufacturers advise avoid

Side-effects gastro-intestinal disturbances including nausea and vomiting, pruritus, rashes, hyperkalaemia, depression of haematopoiesis; rarely erythema multiforme, toxic epidermal necrolysis, photosensitivity and other allergic reactions including angioedema and anaphylaxis; aseptic meningitis reported

Licensed use not licensed for use in children under 6 weeks

Indication and dose

Urinary-tract infections; respiratory-tract infections
• By mouth

Neonate initially 3 mg/kg as a single dose then 1–2 mg/kg twice daily

Child 1 month–12 years 4 mg/kg (max. 200 mg) twice daily
or
Child 6 weeks–6 months 25 mg twice daily

Child 6 months–6 years 50 mg twice daily

Child 6–12 years 100 mg twice daily

Child 12–18 years 200 mg twice daily

Prophylaxis of urinary-tract infection
• By mouth

Neonate 2 mg/kg at night

Child 1 month–12 years 2 mg/kg (max. 100 mg) at night

Child 12–18 years 100 mg at night

Pneumocystis pneumonia see , p. 411

Trimethoprim (Non-proprietary) ▣PoM
Tablets, trimethoprim 100 mg, net price 28 = 98p; 200 mg, 14-tab pack = 90p. Label: 9
Brands include *Trimopan*®

Suspension, trimethoprim 50 mg/5 mL, net price 100 mL = £1.62. Label: 9

▮ 5.1.9 ▮ Antituberculosis drugs

Tuberculosis is treated in two phases—an *initial phase* using 4 drugs and a *continuation phase* using two drugs in fully sensitive cases. Treatment requires specialised knowledge, particularly where the disease involves resistant organisms or non-respiratory organs.

The regimens given below are recommended for the treatment of tuberculosis in the UK; variations occur in other countries. Either the unsupervised regimen or the supervised regimen described below should be used; the two regimens should **not** be used concurrently. Compliance with therapy is a major determinant of its success. Treatment needs to be carefully monitored in families in whom concordance may be problematic.

Initial phase   The concurrent use of 4 drugs during the initial phase is designed to reduce the bacterial population as rapidly as possible and to prevent the emergence of drug-resistant bacteria. The drugs are best given as combination preparations, provided the respective dose of each drug is appropriate, unless the child is unable to swallow the tablets or one of the components cannot be given because of resistance or intolerance. The treatment of choice for the initial phase is the daily use of isoniazid, rifampicin, pyrazinamide and ethambutol. However, care is needed in young children receiving ethambutol because of the difficulty in testing eyesight and in obtaining reports of visual symptoms (see below). Treatment should be started without waiting for culture results if clinical features or histology results are consistent with tuberculosis; treatment should be continued even if initial culture results are negative. The initial phase drugs should be continued for 2 months. Where a positive culture for *M. tuberculosis* has been obtained, but susceptibility results are not available after 2 months, treatment with rifampicin, isoniazid, pyrazinamide and ethambutol should be continued until full susceptibility is confirmed, even if this is for longer than 2 months.

Streptomycin is rarely used in the UK although it may be used in the initial phase of treatment if resistance to isoniazid has been established before therapy is commenced and ethambutol is contra-indicated.

Continuation phase   After the initial phase, treatment is continued for a further 4 months with isoniazid and rifampicin (preferably given as a combination preparation). Longer treatment is necessary for meningitis, direct spinal cord involvement, and for resistant organisms which may also require modification of the regimen.

Unsupervised treatment   The following regimen should be used for those who are likely to take antituberculous drugs reliably **without supervision**. Children and families who are unlikely to comply with daily administration of antituberculous drugs should be treated with the regimen described under Supervised Treatment.

Recommended dosage for standard unsupervised 6-month treatment

> **Isoniazid** (for 2-month initial and 4-month continuation phases)
> Child 1 month–18 years 5–10 mg/kg (max. 300 mg) once daily

> **Rifampicin** (for 2-month initial and 4–month continuation phase)
> Child 1 month–18 years 10 mg/kg once daily (max. 450 mg if body-weight under 50 kg; if body-weight 50 kg and over max. 600 mg)

> **Pyrazinamide** (for 2-month initial phase only)
> Child 1 month–18 years 35 mg/kg once daily (max. 1.5 g if body-weight under 50 kg; if body-weight 50 kg and over max. 2 g)

> **Ethambutol** (for 2-month initial phase only)
> Child 1 month–18 years 15 mg/kg once daily

Note In general, doses should be rounded up to facilitate administration of suitable volumes of liquid or an appropriate strength of tablet. The exception is ethambutol due to the risk of toxicity. Doses may also need to be recalculated to allow for weight gain in younger children.

The fixed-dose combination preparations (*Rifater*®, *Rifinah*®) are unlicensed for use in children. Consideration may be given to use of these preparations in older children, provided the respective dose of each drug is appropriate for the weight of the child.

Pregnancy and breast-feeding   The standard regimen (above) may be used during pregnancy and breast-feeding. Streptomycin should not be given in pregnancy.

Neonates   Congenital tuberculosis is acquired from maternal extrapulmonary sites at birth, particularly the genital tract; if infection is suspected, the baby will require treatment with isoniazid 10 mg/kg once daily, rifampicin 10 mg/kg once daily, pyrazinamide 35 mg/kg once daily, and ethambutol 15 mg/kg once daily. Isoniazid, rifampicin, pyrazinamide, and ethambutol are used for 2 months during the initial phase of treatment. After the initial phase, treatment is continued for a further 4 months with isoniazid and rifampicin.

5

Infections

Supervised treatment Drug administration needs to be **fully supervised** (directly observed therapy, DOT) in children or families who cannot comply reliably with the treatment regimen. These patients are given isoniazid, rifampicin, pyrazinamide and ethambutol (or streptomycin) 3 times a week under supervision for the first 2 months followed by isoniazid and rifampicin 3 times a week for a further 4 months.

Recommended dosage for intermittent supervised 6-month treatment

Isoniazid (for 2-month initial and 4-month continuation phases)
Child 1 month–18 years, 15 mg/kg (max. 900 mg) 3 times a week

Rifampicin (for 2-month initial and 4-month continuation phases)
Child 1 month–18 years, 15 mg/kg (max. 900 mg) 3 times a week

Pyrazinamide (for 2-month initial phase only)
Child 1 month–18 years, 50 mg/kg (max. 2 g 3 times a week if body-weight under 50 kg; max. 2.5 g 3 times a week if body-weight 50 kg and over)

Ethambutol (for 2-month initial phase only)
Child 1 month–18 years, 30 mg/kg 3 times a week

Note In general, doses should be rounded up to facilitate administration of suitable volumes of liquid or an appropriate strength of tablet. The exception is ethambutol due to the risk of toxicity. Doses may also need to be recalculated to allow for weight gain in younger children.

The fixed-dose combination preparations (*Rifater®*, *Rifinah®*) are unlicensed for use in children. Consideration may be given to use of these preparations in older children, provided the respective dose of each drug is appropriate for the weight of the child.

Immunocompromised patients Multi-resistant *Mycobacterium tuberculosis* may be present in immunocompromised children. The organism should always be cultured to confirm its type and drug sensitivity. Confirmed *M. tuberculosis* infection sensitive to first-line drugs should be treated with a standard 6-month regimen; after completing treatment, children should be closely monitored. The regimen may need to be modified if infection is caused by resistant organisms, and specialist advice is needed.

Specialist advice should be sought about tuberculosis treatment or chemoprophylaxis in a HIV-positive individual; care is required in choosing the regimen and in avoiding potentially hazardous interactions. Starting antiretroviral treatment in the first 2 months of antituberculosis treatment increases the risk of immune reconstitution syndrome.

Infection may also be caused by other mycobacteria e.g. *M. avium* complex in which case specialist advice on management is needed.

Corticosteroids A corticosteroid should be given (in addition to antituberculosis therapy) for meningeal or pericardial tuberculosis.

Prevention of tuberculosis Chemoprophylaxis may be required in children who are close contacts of a case of smear-positive pulmonary tuberculosis and who are severely immunosuppressed (including congenital immunodeficiencies, cytotoxic or immunosuppressive therapy) and in those who have evidence of latent tuberculosis and require treatment with immunosuppressants; expert advice should be sought.

Chemoprophylaxis involves use of either isoniazid alone for 6 months or of isoniazid and rifampicin for 3 months (see Table 2, section 5.1).

For prevention of tuberculosis in susceptible close contacts or those who have become tuberculin-positive, see Table 2, section 5.1. For advice on immunisation against tuberculosis and tuberculin testing, see section 14.4.

Monitoring Since isoniazid, rifampicin and pyrazinamide are associated with liver toxicity, *hepatic function* should be checked before treatment with these drugs. Those with pre-existing liver disease should have frequent checks particularly in the first 2 months. If there is no evidence of liver disease (and pretreatment liver function is normal), further checks are only necessary if the patient develops fever, malaise, vomiting, jaundice or unexplained deterioration during treatment. In view of the need to comply fully with antituberculous treatment on the one hand and to guard against serious liver damage on the other, children and their carers should be informed carefully how to recognise signs of liver disorders and advised to discontinue treatment and seek **immediate** medical attention should symptoms of liver disease occur.

Renal function should be checked before treatment with antituberculous drugs and appropriate dosage adjustments made. Streptomycin or ethambutol should preferably be avoided in patients with renal impairment, but if used, the dose should be reduced and the plasma-drug concentration monitored.

Visual acuity should be tested before ethambutol is used (see below).

> Major causes of treatment failure are incorrect prescribing by the physician and inadequate compliance by the child or their carer. Monthly tablet counts and urine examination (rifampicin imparts an orange-red coloration) may be useful indicators of compliance with treatment. Avoid both excessive and inadequate dosage. Treatment should be supervised by a specialist paediatrician.

Isoniazid is cheap and highly effective. Like rifampicin it should always be included in any antituberculous regimen unless there is a specific contra-indication. Its only common side-effect is peripheral neuropathy which is more likely to occur where there are pre-existing risk factors such as diabetes, chronic renal failure, malnutrition and HIV infection. In these circumstances, and in breast-fed infants treated with isoniazid, pyridoxine (section 9.6.2) should be given prophylactically from the start of treatment. Other side-effects such as hepatitis (important: see Monitoring above) and psychosis are rare.

Rifampicin, a rifamycin, is a key component of any antituberculous regimen. Like isoniazid it should always be included unless there is a specific contra-indication.

During the first two months ('initial phase') of rifampicin administration transient disturbance of liver function with elevated serum transaminases is common but generally does not require interruption of treatment. Occasionally more serious liver toxicity requires a change of treatment particularly in those with pre-existing liver disease (important: see Monitoring above).

On intermittent treatment six toxicity syndromes have been recognised—influenza-like, abdominal, and respiratory symptoms, shock, renal failure, and thrombocytopenic purpura—and can occur in 20 to 30% of patients.

Rifampicin induces hepatic enzymes which accelerate the metabolism of several drugs including oestrogens, corticosteroids, phenytoin, sulphonylureas, and anticoagulants; **interactions:** Appendix 1 (rifamycins). **Important:** the effectiveness of hormonal contraceptives is reduced and alternative family planning advice should be offered (section 7.3.1).

Rifabutin is indicated in adults for *prophylaxis* against *M. avium* complex infections in patients with a low CD4 count; it is also licensed in adults for the *treatment* of non-tuberculous mycobacterial disease and pulmonary tuberculosis. There is limited experience in children. As with rifampicin it induces hepatic enzymes and the effectiveness of hormonal contraceptives is reduced requiring alternative family planning methods.

Pyrazinamide is a bactericidal drug only active against intracellular dividing forms of *Mycobacterium tuberculosis*; it exerts its main effect only in the first two or three months. It is particularly useful in tuberculous meningitis because of good meningeal penetration. It is not active against *M. bovis*. Serious liver toxicity may occasionally occur (important: see Monitoring above).

Ethambutol is included in a treatment regimen if isoniazid resistance is suspected; it can be omitted if the risk of resistance is low.

Side-effects of ethambutol are largely confined to visual disturbances in the form of loss of acuity, colour blindness, and restriction of visual fields. These toxic effects are more common where excessive dosage is used or if the child's renal function is impaired. The earliest features of ocular toxicity are subjective and children and their carers should be advised to discontinue therapy immediately if deterioration in vision develops and promptly seek further advice. Early discontinuation of the drug is almost always followed by recovery of eyesight. Those who cannot understand warnings about visual side-effects should, if possible, be given an alternative drug. In particular, ethambutol should be used with caution in children until they are at least 5 years old and capable of reporting symptomatic visual changes accurately.

Where possible visual acuity should be tested by Snellen chart before treatment with ethambutol.

Streptomycin is now rarely used in the UK except for resistant organisms. Plasma-drug concentration should be measured in patients with impaired renal function in whom streptomycin must be used with great care. Side-effects increase after a cumulative dose of 100 g, which should only be exceeded in exceptional circumstances.

Drug-resistant tuberculosis should be treated by a specialist paediatrician with experience in such cases, and where appropriate facilities for infection-control exist. Second-line drugs available for infections caused by resistant organisms, or when first-line drugs cause unacceptable side-effects, include amikacin, capreomycin, cycloserine, newer macrolides (e.g. azithromycin and clarithromycin), quinolones (e.g. moxifloxacin) and protionamide (prothionamide; no longer on UK market). Availability of suitable formulations may limit choice in children.

CYCLOSERINE

Cautions monitor haematological, renal, and hepatic function; **interactions:** Appendix 1 (cycloserine)

Renal impairment reduce dose; avoid in severe impairment

Pregnancy manufacturer advises use only if potential benefit outweighs risk—crosses the placenta

Breast-feeding present in milk—amount too small to be harmful

Contra-indications epilepsy, depression, severe anxiety, psychotic states, alcohol dependence, acute porphyria (section 9.8.2)

Side-effects mainly neurological, including headache, dizziness, vertigo, drowsiness, tremor, convulsions, confusion, psychosis, depression (discontinue or reduce dose if symptoms of CNS toxicity); rashes, allergic dermatitis (discontinue or reduce dose); megaloblastic anaemia; changes in liver function tests; heart failure at high doses reported

Pharmacokinetics blood concentration should not exceed a peak concentration of 30 mg/litre (measured 3–4 hours after the dose); penetrates CNS

Licensed use licensed for use in children (age range not specified by manufacturer)

Indication and dose

Tuberculosis resistant to first-line drugs, used in combination with other drugs
- **By mouth**

Child 2–12 years initially 5 mg/kg twice daily, adjusted according to blood concentration and response

Child 12–18 years initially 250 mg twice daily for 2 weeks adjusted according to blood concentration and response to max. 500 mg twice daily

Cycloserine (King) ℗ℴ℧
Capsules, red/grey cycloserine 250 mg, net price 100-cap pack = £303.45. Label: 2, 8

ETHAMBUTOL HYDROCHLORIDE

Cautions test visual acuity before treatment and warn patients to report visual changes—see notes above; young children (see notes above)—routine ophthalmological monitoring recommended

Renal impairment reduce dose; if creatinine clearance less than 30 mL/minute/1.73 m² monitor plasma-ethambutol concentration; risk of optic nerve damage

Pregnancy not known to be harmful; see notes above

Breast-feeding amount too small to be harmful

Contra-indications optic neuritis, poor vision

Side-effects optic neuritis, red/green colour blindness, peripheral neuritis, rarely rash, pruritus, urticaria, thrombocytopenia

Pharmacokinetics 'peak' concentration (2–2.5 hours after dose) should be 2–6 mg/litre (7–

22 micromol/litre); 'trough' (pre-dose) concentration should be less than 1 mg/litre (4 micromol/litre); for advice on laboratory assay of ethambutol contact the Poisons Unit at New Cross Hospital (Tel (020) 7771 5360)

Indication and dose

Tuberculosis, used in combination with other drugs see notes above

Ethambutol (Non-proprietary) ℗ℴ℧
Tablets, ethambutol hydrochloride 100 mg (yellow), net price 56-tab pack = £11.51; 400 mg (grey), 56-tab pack = £42.74. Label: 8

◢Extemporaneous formulations available see Extemporaneous Preparations, p. 8

ISONIAZID

Cautions slow acetylator status (increased risk of side-effects); epilepsy; history of psychosis;

alcohol dependence, malnutrition, diabetes mellitus, HIV infection (risk of peripheral neuri-

◻ **ISONIAZID (*continued*)**

tis); acute porphyria (section 9.8.2); **interactions:** Appendix 1 (isoniazid)

Hepatic impairment use with caution; monitor liver function regularly and particularly frequently in the first 2 months

Renal impairment reduce dose if estimated glomerular filtration rate less than 10 mL/minute/ 1.73 m²; risk of peripheral neuropathy

Pregnancy not known to be harmful; see notes above

Breast-feeding monitor infant for possible toxicity; theoretical risk of convulsions and neuropathy; prophylactic pyridoxine advisable in mother and infant

Hepatic disorders Children and their carers should be told how to recognise signs of liver disorder, and advised to discontinue treatment and seek immediate medical attention if symptoms such as persistent nausea, vomiting, malaise or jaundice develop

Contra-indications drug-induced liver disease

Side-effects nausea, vomiting, constipation, dry mouth; peripheral neuritis with high doses (pyridoxine prophylaxis, see notes above), optic neuritis, convulsions, psychotic episodes, vertigo; hypersensitivity reactions including fever, erythema multiforme, purpura; blood disorders including agranulocytosis, haemolytic anaemia, aplastic anaemia; hepatitis; systemic lupus erythematosus-like syndrome, pellagra, hyperreflexia, difficulty with micturition, hyperglycaemia, and gynaecomastia reported; hearing loss and tinnitus (in children with end-stage renal impairment)

Indication and dose

> **Tuberculosis, used in combination with other drugs** see notes above

Isoniazid (Non-proprietary) PoM

Tablets, isoniazid 50 mg, net price 56-tab pack = £8.34; 100 mg, 28-tab pack = £8.29. Label: 8, 22

Injection, isoniazid 25 mg/mL, net price 2-mL amp = £11.04

◢ Extemporaneous formulations available see Extemporaneous Preparations, p. 8

▰ PYRAZINAMIDE

Cautions diabetes; **interactions:** Appendix 1 (pyrazinamide)

Hepatic disorders Children and their carers should be told how to recognise signs of liver disorder, and advised to discontinue treatment and seek immediate medical attention if symptoms such as persistent nausea, vomiting, malaise or jaundice develop

Hepatic impairment monitor hepatic function— idiosyncratic hepatotoxicity more common; avoid in severe hepatic impairment

Pregnancy manufacturer advises use only if potential benefit outweighs risk; see also notes above

Breast-feeding amount too small to be harmful

Contra-indications acute porphyria (section 9.8.2)

Side-effects hepatotoxicity including fever, anorexia, hepatomegaly, splenomegaly, jaundice, liver failure; nausea, vomiting, dysuria, arthralgia, sideroblastic anaemia, rash and occasionally photosensitivity

Licensed use not licensed

Indication and dose

> **Tuberculosis in combination with other drugs** see notes above

Pyrazinamide (Non-proprietary) PoM

Tablets, scored, pyrazinamide 500 mg. Label: 8
Available from 'special-order' manufacturers or specialist importing companies, see p. 943

◢ Extemporaneous formulations available see Extemporaneous Preparations, p. 8

▰ RIFABUTIN

Cautions see under Rifampicin; acute porphyria (section 9.8.2)

Hepatic impairment reduce dose in severe hepatic impairment

Renal impairment use half normal dose if estimated glomerular filtration rate less than 30 mL/ minute/1.73 m²

Pregnancy manufacturer advises avoid—no information available

Breast-feeding manufacturer advises avoid—no information available

Side-effects nausea, vomiting; leucopenia, thrombocytopenia, anaemia, rarely haemolysis; raised liver enzymes, jaundice, rarely hepatitis; uveitis following high doses or administration with drugs which raise plasma concentration— see also **interactions:** Appendix 1 (rifamycins); arthralgia, myalgia, influenza-like syndrome, dyspnoea; also hypersensitivity reactions including fever, rash, eosinophilia, bronchospasm, shock; skin, urine, saliva and other body secretions coloured orange-red; asymptomatic corneal opacities reported with long-term use

Licensed use not licensed for use in children

Indication and dose

> **Prophylaxis of *Mycobacterium avium* complex infections in immunosuppressed patients with low CD4 count** (see product literature) Also see notes above
>
> • By mouth
>
> **Child 1–12 years** 5 mg/kg (max. 300 mg) once daily
>
> **Child 12–18 years** 300 mg once daily

5

Infections

◻ RIFABUTIN (continued)

Treatment of non-tuberculous mycobacterial disease, in combination with other drugs
● By mouth

Child 1month–12 years 5 mg/kg once daily for up to 6 months after cultures negative

Child 12–18 years 450–600 mg once daily for up to 6 months after cultures negative

Treatment of pulmonary tuberculosis, in combination with other drugs
● By mouth

Child 12–18years 150–450 mg once daily for at least 6 months

Mycobutin® (Pharmacia) [PoM]
Capsules, red-brown, rifabutin 150 mg. Net price 30-cap pack = £90.38. Label: 8, 14, counselling, lenses, see under Rifampicin

◢ Extemporaneous formulations available see Extemporaneous Preparations, p. 8

RIFAMPICIN

Cautions liver function tests and blood counts in hepatic disorders, and on prolonged therapy, see also below; acute porphyria (section 9.8.2); **important:** advise those on hormonal contraceptives to use additional means (see also section 7.3.1); discolours soft contact lenses; see also notes above; **interactions:** Appendix 1 (rifamycins)

Note If treatment interrupted re-introduce with low dosage and increase gradually; discontinue permanently if serious side-effects develop

Hepatic disorders Children and their carers should be told how to recognise signs of liver disorder, and advised to discontinue treatment and seek immediate medical attention if symptoms such as persistent nausea, vomiting, malaise or jaundice develop

Hepatic impairment impaired elimination; monitor liver function; avoid or do not exceed 8 mg/kg daily

Pregnancy manufacturers advise very high doses teratogenic in *animal* studies in 3rd trimester; risk of neonatal bleeding may be increased; see also notes above

Breast-feeding amount too small to be harmful

Contra-indications jaundice

Side-effects gastro-intestinal symptoms including anorexia, nausea, vomiting, diarrhoea (antibiotic-associated colitis reported); headache, drowsiness; those occurring mainly on intermittent therapy include influenza-like symptoms (with chills, fever, dizziness, bone pain), respiratory symptoms (including shortness of breath), collapse and shock, haemolytic anaemia, disseminated intravascular coagulation and acute renal failure, thrombocytopenic purpura; alterations of liver function, jaundice; flushing, urticaria, and rashes; other side-effects reported include oedema, psychoses, adrenal insufficiency, muscular weakness and myopathy, exfoliative dermatitis, toxic epidermal necrolysis, Stevens-Johnson syndrome, pemphigoid reactions, leucopenia, eosinophilia, menstrual disturbances; urine, saliva, and other body secretions coloured orange-red; thrombophlebitis reported if infusion used for prolonged period

Licensed use not licensed for use in children for pruritus due to cholestasis

Indication and dose

Tuberculosis, in combination with other drugs see notes above

Prophylaxis of meningococcal meningitis and Haemophilus influenzae (type b) infection Table 2, section 5.1

Brucellosis, legionnaires disease, serious staphylococcal infections, in combination with other antibacterials
● By mouth or by intravenous infusion

Neonates 5–10 mg/kg twice daily

Child 1 month–1 year 5–10 mg/kg twice daily

Child 1–18 years 10 mg/kg (max. 600 mg) twice daily

Pruritus due to cholestasis
● By mouth

Child 1 month–18 years 5–10 mg/kg (max. 600 mg) once daily

Administration Owing to risk of contact sensitisation care must be taken to avoid contact during preparation and infusion. Displacement value may be significant, consult local reconstitution guidelines; reconstitute with solvent provided. May be further diluted with glucose 5% and 10% or sodium chloride 0.9% or Ringer's solution to a final concentration of 1.2 mg/mL; in fluid restricted patients up to 6 mg/mL may be used. Infuse over 2–3 hours.

Rifampicin (Non-proprietary) [PoM]
Capsules, rifampicin 150 mg, net price 20 = £4.17; 300 mg, 20 = £10.44. Label: 8, 14, 22, counselling, see contact lenses above

Rifadin® (Aventis Pharma) [PoM]
Capsules, rifampicin 150 mg (blue/red), net price 20 = £3.81; 300 mg (red), 20 = £7.62. Label: 8, 14, 22, counselling, see contact lenses above

Syrup, red, rifampicin 100 mg/5 mL (raspberry-flavoured). Net price 120 mL = £3.70. Label: 8, 14, 22, counselling, see contact lenses above
Excipients include sucrose

◁ **RIFAMPICIN** (*continued*)

Intravenous infusion, powder for reconstitution, rifampicin. Net price 600-mg vial (with solvent) = £7.98
Electrolytes Na⁺< 0.5 mmol/vial

Rimactane® (Sandoz) ꜰᴏᴍ
Capsules, rifampicin 150 mg (red), net price 60-cap pack = £11.35; 300 mg (red/brown), 60-cap pack = £22.69. Label: 8, 14, 22, counselling, see contact lenses above

◢Combined preparations
See notes above

Rifater® (Aventis Pharma) ꜰᴏᴍ
Tablets, pink, s/c, rifampicin 120 mg, isoniazid 50 mg, pyrazinamide 300 mg. Net price 20 = £4.39. Label: 8, 14, 22, counselling, see contact lenses above

Rifinah 150® (Aventis Pharma) ꜰᴏᴍ
Tablets, pink, s/c, rifampicin 150 mg, isoniazid 100 mg, net price 84-tab pack = £16.55. Label: 8, 14, 22, counselling, see contact lenses above

Rifinah 300® (Aventis Pharma) ꜰᴏᴍ
Tablets, orange, s/c, rifampicin 300 mg, isoniazid 150 mg, net price 56-tab pack = £21.87. Label: 8, 14, 22, counselling, see contact lenses above

◣ STREPTOMYCIN

Cautions see under Aminoglycosides, section 5.1.4; measure plasma-concentration in renal impairment; **interactions:** Appendix 1 (aminoglycosides)

Contra-indications see under Aminoglycosides, section 5.1.4

Side-effects see under Aminoglycosides, section 5.1.4; also hypersensitivity reactions, paraesthesia of mouth

Pharmacokinetics one-hour ('peak') concentration should be 15–40 mg/litre; pre-dose ('trough') concentration should be less than 5 mg/litre (less than 1 mg/litre in renal impairment)

Licensed use not licensed for use in children

Indication and dose

Tuberculosis, resistant to other treatment, in combination with other drugs
• By deep intramuscular injection
  Child 1 month–18 years 15 mg/kg (max. 1 g) once daily

Adjunct to doxycycline in brucellosis, expert advice essential
• By deep intramuscular injection
  Child 1 month–18 years 5–10 mg/kg every 6 hours; total daily dose may alternatively be given in 2–3 divided doses

Streptomycin Sulphate (Non-proprietary) ꜰᴏᴍ
Injection, powder for reconstitution, streptomycin (as sulphate), net price 1-g vial = £8.25
Available as an unlicensed preparation from UCB Pharma

5.1.10 Antileprotic drugs

Classification not used in *BNF for Children*.

5.1.11 Metronidazole

Metronidazole is an antimicrobial drug with high activity against anaerobic bacteria and protozoa. It is also used for surgical and gynaecological sepsis in which its activity against colonic anaerobes, especially *Bacteroides fragilis*, is important. Metronidazole by mouth is effective for the treatment of *Clostridium difficile* infection (see also section 1.5); it can be given by intravenous infusion if oral treatment is inappropriate. Metronidazole is well absorbed orally and the intravenous route is normally reserved for severe infections. Metronidazole by the rectal route is an effective alternative to the intravenous route when oral administration is not possible. Intravenous metronidazole is used for the treatment of established cases of tetanus; diazepam (section 10.2.2) and tetanus immunoglobulin (section 14.5) are also used.

Topical metronidazole (section 13.10.1.2) reduces the odour produced by anaerobic bacteria in fungating tumours; it is also used in the management of rosacea (section 13.6).

Oral infections Metronidazole is an alternative to a penicillin for the treatment of many oral infections where the patient is allergic to penicillin or the infection is due to beta-lactamase-producing anaerobes (Table 1, section 5.1). It is the drug of first choice for the treatment of acute necrotising ulcerative gingivitis (Vincent's infection) and pericoronitis; suitable alternatives are amoxicillin (section 5.1.1.3) and erythromycin (section 5.1.5). For these purposes treatment with metronidazole for 3 days is sufficient, but the duration of treatment may need to be longer

5

Infections

in pericoronitis. Tinidazole is licensed for the treatment of acute ulcerative gingivitis.

▲ METRONIDAZOLE

Cautions disulfiram-like reaction with alcohol, clinical and laboratory monitoring advised if treatment exceeds 10 days; **interactions:** Appendix 1 (metronidazole)

Hepatic impairment in severe liver disease reduce total daily dose to one-third, and give once daily; use with caution in hepatic encephalopathy

Pregnancy manufacturer advises avoidance of high-dose regimens; use only if potential benefit outweighs risk

Breast-feeding significant amount in milk; manufacturer advises avoid large single doses though otherwise compatible; may give milk a bitter taste

Side-effects gastro-intestinal disturbances (including nausea and vomiting), taste disturbances, furred tongue, oral mucositis, anorexia; *very rarely* hepatitis, jaundice, pancreatitis, drowsiness, dizziness, headache, ataxia, psychotic disorders, darkening of urine, thrombocytopenia, pancytopenia, myalgia, arthralgia, visual disturbances, rash, pruritus, and erythema multiforme; on prolonged or intensive therapy peripheral neuropathy, transient epileptiform seizures, and leucopenia

Licensed use not licensed for use in neonates or children under 1 year

Indication and dose

Protozoal infections section 5.4.2

Anaerobic infections (usually treated for 7 days and for 7–10 days in *Clostridium difficile* infection)
- By mouth

  Neonate initially 15 mg/kg then 7.5 mg/kg twice daily

  Child 1 month–12 years 7.5 mg/kg (max. 400 mg) every 8 hours

  Child 12–18 years 400 mg every 8 hours

- By rectum

  Child 1 month–1 year 125 mg 3 times daily for 3 days, then twice daily thereafter

  Child 1–5 years 250 mg 3 times daily for 3 days, then twice daily thereafter

  Child 5–12 years 500 mg 3 times daily, for 3 days, then twice daily thereafter

  Child 12–18 years 1 g 3 times daily for 3 days, then twice daily thereafter

- By intravenous infusion over 20–30 minutes

  Neonate 15 mg/kg as a single loading dose, followed after 24 hours by 7.5 mg/kg every 12 hours thereafter

  Child 1 month–18 years 7.5 mg/kg (max. 500 mg) every 8 hours

Pelvic inflammatory disease (see also Table 1, section 5.1)
- By mouth

  Child 12–18 years 400 mg twice daily for 14 days

Acute ulcerative gingivitis and other acute dental infections
- By mouth

  Child 1–3 years 50 mg every 8 hours

  Child 3–7 years 100 mg every 12 hours

  Child 7–10 years 100 mg every 8 hours

  Child 10–18 years 200 mg every 8 hours

Helicobacter pylori eradication section 1.3

Surgical prophylaxis
- By mouth or by intravenous infusion

  Child 1 month–12 years 7.5 mg/kg 2 hours before surgery; up to 3 further doses of 7.5 mg/kg may be given every 8 hours for high-risk procedures

  Child 12–18 years 400–500 mg 2 hours before surgery; up to 3 further doses of 400–500 mg may be given every 8 hours for high-risk procedures

- By rectum

  Child 5–10 years 500 mg 2 hours before surgery; up to 3 further doses of 500 mg may be given every 8 hours for high-risk procedures

  Child 10–18 years 1 g 2 hours before surgery; up to 3 further doses of 1 g may be given every 8 hours for high-risk procedures

Note Metronidazole doses in BNF for Children may differ from those in product literature

Metronidazole (Non-proprietary) PoM
Tablets, metronidazole 200 mg, net price 21-tab pack = £1.10; 400 mg, 21-tab pack = £1.29. Label: 4, 9, 21, 25, 27
Brands include *Vaginyl®*

Tablets, metronidazole 500 mg, net price 21-tab pack = £26.79. Label: 4, 9, 21, 25, 27

Suspension, metronidazole (as benzoate) 200 mg/ 5 mL. Net price 100 mL = £9.07. Label: 4, 9, 23
Brands include *Norzol®*

Intravenous infusion, metronidazole 5 mg/mL. Net price 20-mL amp = £1.56, 100-mL container = £3.41

Dental prescribing on NHS Metronidazole Tablets and Oral Suspension may be prescribed

Flagyl® (Winthrop) PoM
Tablets, both f/c, ivory, metronidazole 200 mg, net price 21-tab pack = £4.67; 400 mg, 14-tab pack = £6.60. Label: 4, 9, 21, 25, 27

Suppositories, metronidazole 500 mg, net price 10 = £15.80; 1 g, 10 = £24.00. Label: 4, 9

◯ **METRONIDAZOLE** (*continued*)

Flagyl S® (Winthrop) [PoM]
Suspension, orange- and lemon-flavoured, metro-nidazole (as benzoate) 200 mg/5 mL. Net price 100 mL = £11.63. Label: 4, 9, 23

Metrolyl® (Sandoz) [PoM]
Intravenous infusion, metronidazole 5 mg/mL, net price 100-mL Steriflex® bag = £1.22
Electrolytes Na⁺ 14.53 mmol/100-mL bag

Suppositories, metronidazole 500 mg, net price 10 = £12.34; 1 g, 10 = £18.34. Label: 4, 9

5.1.12 **Quinolones**

Nalidixic acid is effective in uncomplicated urinary-tract infections.

Ciprofloxacin is active against both Gram-positive and Gram-negative bacteria. It is particularly active against Gram-negative bacteria, including salmonella, shigella, campylobacter, neisseria, and pseudomonas. Ciprofloxacin has only moderate activity against Gram-positive bacteria such as *Streptococcus pneumoniae* and *Enterococcus faecalis*; it should not be used for pneumococcal pneumonia. It is active against chlamydia and some mycobacteria. Most anaerobic organisms are not susceptible. Ciprofloxacin is licensed in children over 1 year of age for pseudomonal infections in cystic fibrosis, for complicated urinary-tract infections, and for treatment and prophylaxis of inhalation anthrax. When the benefits of treatment outweigh the risks, ciprofloxacin is licensed in children over 1 year of age for severe infections of the respiratory tract and of the gastro-intestinal system (including typhoid fever). It is also used in the treatment of septicaemia caused by multi-resistant organisms (usually hospital acquired) and gonorrhoea (although resistance is increasing). Ciprofloxacin is also used in the prophylaxis of meningococcal disease.

Many staphylococci are resistant to quinolones and their use should be avoided in MRSA infections.

Ofloxacin eye drops are used in ophthalmic infections (section 11.3.1).

There is much less experience of the other quinolones in children; expert advice should be sought.

Anthrax   *Inhalation* or *gastro-intestinal anthrax* should be treated initially with either **ciprofloxacin** or, in children over 12 years, **doxycycline** [unlicensed indication] (section 5.1.3) combined with one or two other antibacterials (such as amoxicillin, benzylpenicillin, chloramphenicol, clarithromycin, clindamycin, imipenem with cilastatin, rifampicin [unlicensed indication], and vancomycin). When the condition improves and the sensitivity of the *Bacillus anthracis* strain is known, treatment may be switched to a single antibacterial. Treatment should continue for 60 days because germination may be delayed.

Cutaneous anthrax should be treated with either ciprofloxacin [unlicensed indication] or doxycycline [unlicensed indication] (section 5.1.3) for 7 days. Treatment may be switched to amoxicillin (section 5.1.1.3) if the infecting strain is susceptible. Treatment may need to be extended to 60 days if exposure is due to aerosol. A combination of antibacterials for 14 days is recommended for cutaneous anthrax with systemic features, extensive oedema, or lesions of the head or neck.

Ciprofloxacin or doxycycline may be given for *post-exposure prophylaxis*. If exposure is confirmed, antibacterial prophylaxis should continue for 60 days. Antibacterial prophylaxis may be switched to amoxicillin after 10–14 days if the strain of *B. anthracis* is susceptible. Vaccination against anthrax (section 14.4) may allow the duration of antibacterial prophylaxis to be shortened.

Cautions   Quinolones should be used with caution in children with a history of epilepsy or conditions that predispose to seizures, in G6PD deficiency (section 9.1.5), myasthenia gravis (risk of exacerbation). Exposure to excessive sunlight should be avoided (discontinue if photosensitivity occurs). The CSM has warned that quinolones may induce **convulsions** in patients with or without a history of convulsions; taking NSAIDs at the same time may also induce them. Other **interactions:** Appendix 1 (quinolones).

5

Infections

Quinolones cause arthropathy in the weight-bearing joints of immature *animals* and are therefore generally not recommended in children and growing adolescents. However, the significance of this effect in humans is uncertain and in some specific circumstances short-term use of a quinolone in children is justified. **Nalidixic acid** is used for resistant urinary-tract infections in children over 3 months of age.

Tendon damage

Tendon damage (including rupture) has been reported rarely in patients receiving quinolones. Tendon rupture may occur within 48 hours of starting treatment; cases have also been reported several months after stopping a quinolone. Healthcare professionals are reminded that:

- quinolones are contra-indicated in patients with a history of tendon disorders related to quinolone use;

- kidney, heart, or lung transplant recipients are more prone to tendon damage;

- the risk of tendon damage is increased by the concomitant use of corticosteroids;

- if tendinitis is suspected, the quinolone should be discontinued immediately.

Side-effects   Side-effects of the quinolones include nausea, vomiting, dyspepsia, abdominal pain, diarrhoea (rarely antibiotic-associated colitis), headache, dizziness, rash (very rarely Stevens-Johnson syndrome and toxic epidermal necrolysis). Less frequent side-effects include anorexia, sleep disturbances, asthenia, confusion, anxiety, depression, hallucinations, tremor, blood disorders (including eosinophilia, leucopenia, thrombocytopenia), arthralgia, myalgia, disturbances in vision and taste. Other side-effects reported rarely or very rarely include hepatic dysfunction (including jaundice and hepatitis), hypotension, vasculitis, dyspnoea, convulsions, psychoses, paraesthesia, renal failure, interstitial nephritis, tendon inflammation and damage (see also Tendon Damage above), photosensitivity, disturbances in hearing and smell. The drug should be **discontinued** if psychiatric, neurological or hypersensitivity reactions (including severe rash) occur.

◢ CIPROFLOXACIN

Cautions see notes above; avoid excessive alkalinity of urine and ensure adequate fluid intake (risk of crystalluria); **interactions:** Appendix 1 (quinolones)

Skilled tasks May impair performance of skilled tasks (e.g. driving)

Renal impairment reduce dose if estimated glomerular filtration rate less than 30 mL/minute/1.73 m^2—consult product literature

Breast-feeding amount probably too small to be harmful but manufacturer advises avoid

Contra-indications

Pregnancy avoid—arthropathy in *animal* studies; safer alternatives available

Side-effects see notes above; also flatulence, pain and phlebitis at injection site; *rarely* dysphagia, pancreatitis, chest pain, tachycardia, syncope, oedema, hot flushes, abnormal dreams, sweating, hyperglycaemia, and erythema nodosum; *very rarely* movement disorders, tinnitus, vasculitis, and tenosynovitis

Licensed use licensed for use in children over 1 year for complicated urinary-tract infections, for pseudomonal lower respiratory-tract infections in cystic fibrosis, for prophylaxis and treatment of inhalational anthrax; licensed for use in children over 1 year for other infections where the benefit is considered to outweigh the potential risks; not licensed for use in children for gastro-intestinal anthrax; not licensed for use in children for prophylaxis of meningococcal meningitis; not licensed for use in children under 1 year of age

Indication and dose

Complicated urinary-tract infections
- **By mouth**

  Neonate 7.5 mg/kg twice daily

  Child 1 month–1 year 5–7.5 mg/kg twice daily; dose doubled in severe infection

  Child 1–18 years 10 mg/kg twice daily; dose doubled in severe infection (max. 750 mg twice daily)

- **By intravenous infusion over 60 minutes**

  Neonate 5 mg/kg every 12 hours

  Child 1 month–1 year 4 mg/kg every 12 hours; dose doubled in severe infection

  Child 1–18 years 6 mg/kg every 8 hours; increased to 10 mg/kg every 8 hours in severe infection (max. 400 mg every 8 hours)

◻ **CIPROFLOXACIN** (*continued*)

Severe respiratory-tract infections, gastro-intestinal infections; see notes above
• **By mouth**
  Neonate 7.5 mg/kg twice daily

  Child 1 month–1 year 5–7.5 mg/kg twice daily; dose doubled in severe infection

  Child 1–18 years 20 mg/kg (max. 750 mg) twice daily

• **By intravenous infusion over 60 minutes**
  Neonate 5 mg/kg every 12 hours

  Child 1 month–1 year 4 mg/kg every 12 hours; dose doubled in severe infection

  Child 1–18 years 10 mg/kg (max. 400 mg) every 8 hours

Pseudomonal lower respiratory-tract infection in cystic fibrosis
• **By mouth**
  Child 1 month–1 year 15 mg/kg twice daily

  Child 1–18 years 20 mg/kg (max. 750 mg) twice daily

• **By intravenous infusion over 60 minutes**
  Child 1 month–1 year 4–8 mg/kg every 12 hours

  Child 1–18 years 10 mg/kg (max. 400 mg) every 8 hours

Gonorrhoea
• **By mouth**
  Child 12–18 years 500 mg as a single dose

Anthrax (treatment and post-exposure prophylaxis, see notes above)
• **By mouth**
  Child 1 month–18 years 15 mg/kg (max. 500 mg) twice daily

• **By intravenous infusion over 60 minutes**
  Child 1 month–18 years 10 mg/kg (max. 400 mg) every 12 hours

Eye infections section 11.3.1

Prophylaxis of meningococcal meningitis Table 2, section 5.1

Ciprofloxacin (Non-proprietary) ℗ℴℳ
Tablets, ciprofloxacin (as hydrochloride) 100 mg, net price 6-tab pack = £1.08; 250 mg, 10-tab pack = £1.12, 20-tab pack = £1.17; 500 mg, 10-tab pack = £1.19, 20-tab pack = £1.19; 750 mg, 10-tab pack = £1.99. Label: 7, 9, 25, counselling, driving

Intravenous infusion, ciprofloxacin (as lactate) 2 mg/mL, net price 50-mL bottle = £8.00, 100-mL bottle = £15.00, 200-mL bottle = £22.00

Ciproxin® (Bayer) ℗ℴℳ
Tablets, all f/c, ciprofloxacin (as hydrochloride) 250 mg (scored), net price 10-tab pack = £7.50, 20-tab pack = £15.00; 500 mg (scored), 10-tab pack = £14.20, 20-tab pack = £28.40; 750 mg, 10-tab pack = £20.00. Label: 7, 9, 25, counselling, driving

Suspension, strawberry-flavoured, ciprofloxacin for reconstitution with diluent provided, 250 mg/5 mL, net price 100 mL = £16.50. Label: 7, 9, 25, counselling, driving

Intravenous infusion, ciprofloxacin (as lactate) 2 mg/mL, in sodium chloride 0.9%, net price 50-mL bottle = £8.65, 100-mL bottle = £16.89, 200-mL bottle = £25.70
Electrolytes Na⁺ 15.4 mmol/100-mL bottle

▮ NALIDIXIC ACID

Cautions see notes above; avoid in acute porphyria (section 9.8.2); false positive urinary glucose (if tested for reducing substances); monitor blood counts, renal and liver function if treatment exceeds 2 weeks; **interactions:** Appendix 1 (quinolones)

Hepatic impairment manufacturer advises caution in liver disease

Renal impairment use with caution; avoid if estimated glomerular filtration rate less than 20 mL/minute/1.73 m²

Breast-feeding risk to infant very small but one case of haemolytic anaemia reported

Contra-indications

Pregnancy avoid—arthropathy in *animal* studies; safer alternatives available

Side-effects see notes above; also reported toxic psychosis, increased intracranial pressure, cranial nerve palsy, metabolic acidosis

Licensed use not licensed for use in children under 3 months of age

Indication and dose

Urinary tract infection resistant to other antibiotics
• **By mouth**
  Child 3 months–12 years 12.5 mg/kg 4 times daily for 7 days, reduced to 7.5 mg/kg 4 times daily in prolonged therapy or 15 mg/kg twice daily for prophylaxis

  Child 12–18 years 900 mg 4 times daily for 7 days, reduced in chronic infections to 600 mg 4 times daily

Uriben® (Rosemont) ℗ℴℳ
Suspension, pink, nalidixic acid 300 mg/5 mL, net price 150 mL (raspberry- and strawberry-flavoured) = £11.42. Label: 9, 11
Excipients include sucrose 450 mg/5mL

5.1.13 Urinary-tract infections

Urinary-tract infection is more common in adolescent girls than in boys; when it occurs in adolescent boys there is frequently an underlying abnormality of the renal tract. Recurrent episodes of infection are an indication for radiological investigation especially in children in whom untreated pyelonephritis may lead to permanent kidney damage.

Escherichia coli is the most common cause of urinary-tract infection; *Staphylococcus saprophyticus* is also common in sexually active young women. Less common causes include Proteus and Klebsiella spp. *Pseudomonas aeruginosa* infections usually occur in the hospital setting and may be associated with functional or anatomical abnormalities of the renal tract. *Staphylococcus epidermidis* and *Enterococcus faecalis* infection may complicate catheterisation or instrumentation.

> Whenever possible a specimen of urine should be collected for culture and sensitivity testing before starting antibacterial therapy. The antibacterial chosen should reflect current local bacterial sensitivity to antibacterials.

Urinary-tract infections in children require prompt antibacterial treatment to minimise the risk of renal scarring. Uncomplicated 'lower' urinary-tract infections in *children over 3 months* of age can be treated with trimethoprim, nitrofurantoin, a first generation cephalosporin, or amoxicillin for 3 days; children should be reassessed if they continue to be unwell 24–48 hours after the initial assessment.

Acute pyelonephritis in children over 3 months of age can be treated with a first generation cephalosporin or co-amoxiclav for 7–10 days. If the patient is severely ill, then the infection is best treated initially by intravenous injection of a broad-spectrum antibacterial such as cefotaxime or co-amoxiclav; gentamicin is an alternative.

Children under 3 months of age should be transferred to hospital and treated initially with intravenous antibacterials such as ampicillin with gentamicin, or cefotaxime alone, until the infection responds; full doses of oral antibacterials are then given for a further period.

Resistant infections Widespread bacterial resistance, especially to amoxicillin, ampicillin, and trimethoprim has increased the importance of urine culture before therapy. Alternatives for resistant organisms include co-amoxiclav (amoxicillin with clavulanic acid), an oral cephalosporin, pivmecillinam, or a quinolone.

Antibacterial prophylaxis Recurrent episodes of infection are an indication for imaging tests. *Antibacterial prophylaxis* with low doses of trimethoprim or nitrofurantoin may be considered for children with recurrent infection, significant urinary-tract anomalies, or significant kidney damage. Nitrofurantoin is contraindicated in children under 3 months of age because of the theoretical possibility of haemolytic anaemia.

Pregnancy Urinary-tract infection in *pregnancy* may be asymptomatic and requires prompt treatment to prevent progression to acute pyelonephritis. Penicillins and cephalosporins are suitable for treating urinary-tract infection during pregnancy. Nitrofurantoin may also be used but it should be avoided at term. Sulphonamides, quinolones, and tetracyclines should be avoided during pregnancy; trimethoprim should also preferably be avoided particularly in the first trimester.

Renal impairment In *renal failure* antibacterials normally excreted by the kidney accumulate with resultant toxicity unless the dose is reduced. This applies especially to the aminoglycosides which should be used with great caution; tetracyclines, methamine, and nitrofurantoin should be avoided altogether.

NITROFURANTOIN

Cautions anaemia; diabetes mellitus; electrolyte imbalance; vitamin B and folate deficiency; pulmonary disease; monitor lung and liver function on long-term therapy (discontinue if deterioration in lung function); susceptibility to peripheral neuropathy; false positive urinary glucose (if tested for reducing substances); urine may be coloured yellow or brown; **interactions:** Appendix 1 (nitrofurantoin)

Hepatic impairment cholestatic jaundice and chronic active hepatitis reported

Pregnancy may produce neonatal haemolysis if used at term

◻ **NITROFURANTOIN** (*continued*)

Contra-indications infants less than 3 months old, G6PD deficiency, acute porphyria (section 9.8.2)

Renal impairment avoid if estimated glomerular filtration rate less than 60 mL/minute/1.73 m²; risk of peripheral neuropathy; ineffective because of inadequate urine concentrations

Breast-feeding avoid; only small amounts in milk but enough to produce haemolysis in G6PD-deficient infants (section 9.1.5)

Side-effects anorexia, nausea, vomiting, and diarrhoea; acute and chronic pulmonary reactions (pulmonary fibrosis reported; possible association with lupus erythematosus-like syndrome); peripheral neuropathy; also reported, hypersensitivity reactions (including angioedema, anaphylaxis, sialadenitis, urticaria, rash and pruritus); rarely, cholestatic jaundice, hepatitis, exfoliative dermatitis, erythema multiforme, pancreatitis, arthralgia, blood disorders (including agranulocytosis, thrombocytopenia, and aplastic anaemia), benign intracranial hypertension, and transient alopecia

Indication and dose

Acute uncomplicated urinary tract infection
• **By mouth**

Child 3 months–12 years 750 micrograms/kg 4 times daily for 3–7 days

Child 12–18 years 50 mg 4 times daily for 3–7 days; increased to 100 mg 4 times daily in severe chronic recurrent infections

Prophylaxis of urinary tract infection (but see Cautions)
• **By mouth**

Child 3 months–12 years 1 mg/kg at night

Child 12–18 years 50–100 mg at night

Nitrofurantoin (Non-proprietary) ℞
Tablets, nitrofurantoin 50 mg, net price 28-tab pack = £1.84; 100 mg, 28-tab pack = £4.32 Label: 9, 14, 21

Oral suspension, nitrofurantoin 25 mg/5 mL, net price 300 mL = £65.00. Label: 9, 14, 21

Furadantin® (Goldshield) ℞
Tablets, all yellow, scored, nitrofurantoin 50 mg, net price 20 = £1.96; 100 mg, 20 = £3.62. Label: 9, 14, 21

Macrobid® (Goldshield) ℞
Capsules, m/r, blue/yellow, nitrofurantoin 100 mg (as nitrofurantoin macrocrystals and nitrofurantoin monohydrate). Net price 14-cap pack = £4.89. Label: 9, 14, 21, 25
Dose
Uncomplicated urinary-tract infection
Child 12–18 years 1 capsule twice daily with food

Genito-urinary surgical prophylaxis
Child 12–18 years 1 capsule twice daily on day of procedure and for 3 days after

Macrodantin® (Goldshield) ℞
Capsules, nitrofurantoin 50 mg (yellow/white), net price 30-cap pack = £3.05; 100 mg (yellow/white), 20 = £3.84. Label: 9, 14, 21

5 Infections

5.2 Antifungal drugs

Treatment of fungal infections

The systemic treatment of common fungal infections is outlined below; specialist treatment is required in most forms of systemic or disseminated fungal infections. For local treatment of fungal infections, see section 7.2.2 (genital), section 7.4.4 (bladder), section 11.3.2 (eye), section 12.1.1 (ear), section 12.3.2 (oropharynx), and section 13.10.2 (skin).

Aspergillosis Aspergillosis most commonly affects the respiratory tract but in severely immunocompromised patients, invasive forms can affect the sinuses, heart, brain, and skin. **Amphotericin** (liposomal formulation preferred if toxicity or renal impairment are concerns) or **voriconazole** can be used to treat aspergillosis. **Itraconazole** is an alternative for refractory infection or for patients who cannot tolerate amphotericin. Itraconazole is also used as an adjunct in the treatment of allergic bronchopulmonary aspergillosis. **Caspofungin** is licensed in children for invasive aspergillosis unresponsive to amphotericin or to itraconazole, or in children who cannot tolerate amphotericin or itraconazole; information on use in children is limited.

Candidiasis Many superficial candidal infections, including infections of the skin (section 13.10.2), are treated locally. Systemic antifungal treatment is required in widespread or intractable infection. Vaginal candidiasis can be treated with locally acting antifungals (section 7.2.2); alternatively, fluconazole can be given by mouth.

Oropharyngeal candidiasis generally responds to topical therapy (section 12.3.2). Fluconazole is given by mouth for unresponsive infections; it is reliably absorbed and is effective. Itraconazole can be used for fluconazole-resistant infections. Topical therapy may not be adequate in immunocompromised children and an oral triazole antifungal is preferred.

For *deep and disseminated candidiasis*, **amphotericin** can be given by intravenous infusion. **Fluconazole** is an alternative for *Candida albicans* infection in clinically stable children who have not received an azole antifungal recently. **Caspofungin** or **voriconazole** can be used for infections caused by fluconazole-resistant *Candida* spp. that have not responded to amphotericin, or in children intolerant of amphotericin. In refractory cases, **flucytosine** can be used with amphotericin.

Cryptococcosis   Cryptococcosis is uncommon but infection in the immunocompromised, especially HIV-infected children, can be life-threatening; cryptococcal meningitis is the most common form of fungal meningitis. The treatment of choice in cryptococcal meningitis is **amphotericin** by intravenous infusion with **flucytosine** by intravenous infusion for 2 weeks, followed by **fluconazole** by mouth for 8 weeks or until cultures are negative. In cryptococcosis, fluconazole is sometimes given alone as an alternative in AIDS patients with mild localised infection or in those who cannot tolerate amphotericin. Following successful treatment, fluconazole can be used for prophylaxis against relapse until immunity recovers.

Histoplasmosis   Histoplasmosis is rare in temperate climates; it can be life-threatening, particularly in HIV-infected children. **Itraconazole** can be used for the treatment of immunocompetent children with indolent non-meningeal infection including chronic pulmonary histoplasmosis. **Amphotericin** by intravenous infusion is preferred in children with fulminant or severe infections. Following successful treatment, itraconazole can be used for prophylaxis against relapse.

Skin and nail infections   Mild localised fungal infections of the skin (including tinea corporis, tinea cruris, and tinea pedis) respond to topical therapy (section 13.10.2). Systemic therapy is appropriate if topical therapy fails, if many areas are affected, or if the site of infection is difficult to treat such as in infections of the nails (onychomycosis) and of the scalp (tinea capitis).

Oral imidazole or triazole antifungals (particularly **itraconazole**) and **terbinafine** are used more frequently than griseofulvin because they have a broader spectrum of activity and require a shorter duration of treatment.

Tinea capitis is treated systemically; additional topical application of an antifungal (section 13.10.2) may reduce transmission. **Griseofulvin** is used for tinea capitis; it is effective against infections caused by *Trichophyton tonsurans* and *Microsporum spp.* Terbinafine is used for tinea capitis caused by *T. tonsurans* [unlicensed indication]. The role of terbinafine in the management of *Microsporum* infections is uncertain.

Pityriasis versicolor (section 13.10.2) may be treated with **itraconazole** by mouth if topical therapy is ineffective; **fluconazole** by mouth is an alternative. Oral **terbinafine** is **not** effective for pityriasis versicolor.

Antifungal treatment may not be necessary in asymptomatic children with tinea infection of the nails. If treatment is necessary, a systemic antifungal is more effective than topical therapy. **Terbinafine** and **itraconazole** have largely replaced griseofulvin for the systemic treatment of *onychomycosis*, particularly of the toenail; they should be used under specialist advice. Although terbinafine is not licensed for use in children, it is considered to be the drug of choice for onychomycosis. Itraconazole can be administered as intermittent 'pulse' therapy. For the role of topical antifungals in the treatment of onychomycosis, see section 13.10.2

Immunocompromised children   Immunocompromised children are at particular risk of fungal infections and may receive antifungal drugs prophylactically; oral imidazole or triazole antifungals are the drugs of choice for prophylaxis. **Fluconazole** is more reliably absorbed than itraconazole and ketoconazole and is considered less toxic than ketoconazole for long-term use.

Amphotericin by intravenous infusion is used for the empirical *treatment* of serious fungal infections. Fluconazole is used for treatment of *Candida albicans* infection.

Caspofungin is licensed for the empirical treatment of systemic fungal infections (such as those involving *Candida* spp. or *Aspergillus* spp.) in children with neutropenia.

Drugs used in fungal infections

Polyene antifungals   The polyene antifungals include amphotericin and nystatin; neither drug is absorbed when given by mouth. They are used for oral, oropharyngeal, and perioral infections by local application in the mouth (section 12.3.2).

Amphotericin by intravenous infusion is used for the treatment of systemic fungal infections and is active against most fungi and yeasts. It is highly protein bound and penetrates poorly into body fluids and tissues. When given parenterally amphotericin is toxic and side-effects are common. Lipid formulations of amphotericin (*Abelcet*®, *AmBisome*®, and *Amphocil*®) are significantly less toxic and are recommended when the conventional formulation of amphotericin is contra-indicated because of toxicity, especially nephrotoxicity, or when response to conventional amphotericin is inadequate; lipid formulations are more expensive.

Nystatin is used principally for *Candida albicans* infections of the skin (section 13.10.2) and mucous membranes, including oesophageal and intestinal candidiasis.

Imidazole antifungals   The imidazole antifungals include clotrimazole, econazole, sulconazole, and tioconazole. They are used for the local treatment of vaginal candidiasis (section 7.2.2) and for dermatophyte infections (section 13.10.2).

Ketoconazole is better absorbed by mouth than other imidazoles. It has been associated with fatal hepatotoxicity; the CSM has advised that prescribers should weigh the potential benefits of ketoconazole treatment against the risk of liver damage and should carefully monitor patients both clinically and biochemically. It should not be used by mouth for superficial fungal infections.

Miconazole (section 12.3.2) can be used locally for oral infections; it is also effective in intestinal infections. Systemic absorption may follow use of miconazole oral gel and may result in significant drug interactions.

Triazole antifungals   **Fluconazole** is very well absorbed after oral administration. It also achieves good penetration into the cerebrospinal fluid to treat fungal meningitis.

Itraconazole is active against a wide range of dermatophytes. There is limited information available on use in children. Itraconazole capsules require an acid environment in the stomach for optimal absorption.

Itraconazole has been associated with liver damage and should be avoided or used with caution in children with liver disease; fluconazole is less frequently associated with hepatotoxicity.

Voriconazole is a broad-spectrum antifungal drug which is licensed in adults for the treatment of life-threatening infections.

Echinocandin antifungals   **Caspofungin** is active against *Aspergillus* spp. and *Candida* spp. It is given by intravenous infusion for invasive infection resistant to other antifungals. **Micafungin** is licensed for the treatment of candidiasis.

Other antifungals   **Flucytosine** is used with amphotericin in a synergistic combination. Bone marrow depression can occur which limits its use, particularly in children with AIDS; weekly blood counts are necessary during prolonged therapy. Resistance to flucytosine can develop during therapy and sensitivity testing is essential before and during treatment.

Griseofulvin is effective for widespread or intractable dermatophyte infections but has been superseded by newer antifungals, particularly for nail infections. Griseofulvin is used in the treatment of tinea capitis. It is the drug of choice for

5 Infections

trichophyton infections in children. Duration of therapy is dependent on the site of the infection and may extend to a number of months.

Terbinafine is the drug of choice for fungal nail infections and is also used for ringworm infections where oral treatment is considered appropriate.

AMPHOTERICIN
(Amphotericin B)

Cautions when given parenterally, toxicity common (close supervision necessary and close observation required for at least 30 minutes after test dose; see Anaphylaxis below); hepatic and renal function tests, blood counts and plasma electrolyte (including plasma-potassium and magnesium concentration) monitoring required; corticosteroids (avoid except to control reactions); avoid rapid infusion (risk of arrhythmias); **interactions:** Appendix 1 (amphotericin)

Renal impairment use only if no alternative; nephrotoxicity may be reduced with use of lipid formulation

Pregnancy not known to be harmful, but manufacturers advise avoid unless potential benefit outweighs risk

Anaphylaxis The CSM has advised that anaphylaxis occurs rarely with any intravenous amphotericin product and a test dose is advisable before the first infusion; the patient should be carefully observed for at least 30 minutes after the test dose. Prophylactic antipyretics or hydrocortisone should only be used in patients who have previously experienced acute adverse reactions (in whom continued treatment with amphotericin is essential)

Side-effects when given parenterally, anorexia, nausea and vomiting, diarrhoea, epigastric pain; febrile reactions, headache, muscle and joint pain; anaemia; disturbances in renal function (including hypokalaemia and hypomagnesaemia) and renal toxicity; also cardiovascular toxicity (including arrhythmias, blood pressure changes), blood disorders, neurological disorders (including hearing loss, diplopia, convulsions, peripheral neuropathy, encephalopathy), abnormal liver function (discontinue treatment), rash, anaphylactoid reactions (see Anaphylaxis, above); pain and thrombophlebitis at injection site

Licensed use intravenous conventional formulation amphotericin (*Fungizone®*) is licensed for use in children (age range not specified by manufacturer); lipid formulations (*Abelcet®*, *Amphocil®*) are licensed for use in children (age range not specified by manufacturers); *Ambisome®* not licensed for use in children under 1 month

Indication and dose

Oral and perioral infections section 12.3.2

Systemic fungal infections
- By intravenous infusion
  see preparations
  Note Different preparations of intravenous amphotericin vary in their pharmacodynamics, pharmacokinetics, dosage, and administration; these preparations should **not** be considered interchangeable. To avoid confusion, prescribers should specify the brand to be dispensed.

Fungizone® (Squibb) [PoM]
Intravenous infusion, powder for reconstitution, amphotericin (as sodium deoxycholate complex), net price 50-mg vial = £4.12
Electrolytes Na⁺< 0.5 mmol/vial

Dose

Systemic fungal infection
- By intravenous infusion

  Neonate initial test dose of 100 micrograms/kg included as part of first dose of 1 mg/kg, then 1 mg/kg once daily (after 7 days, may be reduced to 1 mg/kg on alternate days)

  Child 1 month–18 years initial test dose of 100 micrograms/kg (max. 1 mg) included as part of first dose of 250 micrograms/kg daily; increased over 2–4 days, if tolerated, to 1 mg/kg daily; in severe infection max. 1.5 mg/kg daily or on alternate days
  Note prolonged treatment usually necessary; if interrupted for longer than 7 days, recommence at 250 micrograms/kg daily and increase gradually

  Administration For *intravenous infusion*, reconstitute each vial with 10 mL Water for Injections and shake immediately to produce a 5 mg/mL colloidal solution; dilute further in Glucose 5% to a concentration of 100 micrograms/mL (in fluid-restricted children, up to 400 micrograms/mL given via a central line); pH of glucose solution must not be below 4.2 (check each container—consult product literature for details of buffer); infuse over 4–6 hours, or if tolerated over a minimum of 2 hours (initial test dose given over 20–30 minutes); begin infusion immediately after dilution and protect from light; incompatible with Sodium Chloride solutions—flush existing intravenous line with Glucose 5% or use separate line; an in-line filter (pore size no less than 1 micron) may be used

---

◄ Lipid formulations

Abelcet® (Cephalon) [PoM]
Intravenous infusion, amphotericin 5 mg/mL as lipid complex with L-α-dimyristoylphosphatidyl-choline and L-α-dimyristoylphosphatidylglycerol, net price 20-mL vial = £82.13 (hosp. only)

Dose

Severe invasive candidiasis; severe systemic fungal infections in children not responding to conventional amphotericin or to other antifungal drugs or where toxicity or renal impairment precludes conventional amphotericin, including invasive aspergillosis, cryptococcal meningitis and disseminated cryptococcosis in children with HIV
- By intravenous infusion

  Child 1 month–18 years initial test dose of 100 micrograms/kg (max. 1 mg) then 5 mg/kg once daily

  Administration for *intravenous infusion*, allow suspension to reach room temperature, shake gently to ensure no yellow settlement, withdraw requisite dose (using 17–19 gauge needle) into one or more 20-mL syringes; replace needle on syringe with a 5-micron filter needle provided (fresh needle for each syringe) and dilute in Glucose 5% to a concentration of 2 mg/mL; preferably give *via* an infusion pump at a rate of 2.5 mg/kg/hour (initial test dose given over 15 minutes); an in-line filter (pore size no less than 15 micron) may be used; do not use sodium chloride or other electrolyte solutions—flush existing intravenous line with Glucose 5% or use separate line

◻ **AMPHOTERICIN (continued)**

AmBisome® (Gilead) PoM

Intravenous infusion, powder for reconstitution, amphotericin 50 mg encapsulated in liposomes, net price 50-mg vial = £96.69

Electrolytes Na$^+$< 0.5 mmol/vial

Excipients include sucrose 900 mg/vial

Dose

Severe systemic or deep mycoses where toxicity (particularly nephrotoxicity) precludes use of conventional amphotericin

• By intravenous infusion

Neonate initial test dose 100 micrograms/kg then 1 mg/kg once daily, increased if necessary to 3 mg/kg once daily; max. 5 mg/kg once daily

Child 1 month–18 years initial test dose 100 micrograms/kg (max. 1 mg) then 1 mg/kg once daily, increased if necessary in steps of 1 mg/kg daily to 3 mg/kg once daily; max. 5 mg/kg once daily

Suspected or proven infection in febrile neutropenic patients unresponsive to broad-spectrum antibacterials

• By intravenous infusion

Child 1 month–18 years initial test dose 100 micrograms/kg (max. 1 mg) then 3 mg/kg once daily until afebrile for 3 consecutive days; max. period of treatment 42 days; max. 5 mg/kg once daily

Visceral leishmaniasis see section 5.4.5 and product literature

Administration for *intravenous infusion*, reconstitute each vial with 12 mL Water for Injections and shake vigorously

to produce a preparation containing 4 mg/mL; withdraw requisite dose from vial and introduce into Glucose 5% through the 5-micron filter provided, to produce a final concentration of 0.2–2 mg/mL; infuse over 30–60 minutes (initial test dose given over 10 minutes); incompatible with sodium chloride solutions—flush existing intravenous line with Glucose 5% or use separate line

Amphocil® (Beacon) PoM

Intravenous infusion, powder for reconstitution, amphotericin as a complex with sodium cholesteryl sulphate, net price 50-mg vial = £104.10, 100-mg vial = £190.05

Electrolytes Na$^+$< 0.5 mmol/vial

Dose

Severe systemic or deep mycoses where toxicity or renal failure precludes use of conventional amphotericin

• By intravenous infusion

Child 1 month–18 years initial test dose 100 micrograms/kg (max. 2 mg) then 30 minutes later 1 mg/kg once daily, increased gradually if necessary to 3–4 mg/kg once daily; max. 6 mg/kg daily

Administration for *intravenous infusion*, initially reconstitute with Water for Injections (50 mg in 10 mL, 100 mg in 20 mL) shaking gently to dissolve (fluid may be opalescent) then dilute to a concentration of 625 micrograms/mL with Glucose 5% (1 volume of reconstituted solution with 7 volumes of infusion fluid); give at a rate of 1–2 mg/kg/hour or slower if not tolerated (for initial test dose use a 100 microgram/mL solution and give over 10 minutes); incompatible with sodium chloride or other electrolyte solutions, flush existing intravenous line with Glucose 5% or use separate line

---

▰ **CASPOFUNGIN**

Cautions interactions: Appendix 1 (caspofungin)

Hepatic impairment usual initial dose, then use 70% of normal maintenance dose in moderate hepatic impairment; no information available for severe hepatic impairment

Pregnancy manufacturer advises avoid unless essential—toxicity in *animal* studies

Contra-indications

Breast-feeding present in milk in *animal* studies—manufacturer advises avoid

Side-effects nausea, vomiting, abdominal pain, diarrhoea; tachycardia, flushing, hypotension; dyspnoea; fever, headache; anaemia, decrease in serum potassium, hypomagnesaemia; rash, pruritus, sweating; injection-site reactions; also reported, hepatic dysfunction, oedema, acute respiratory distress syndrome, hypersensitivity reactions (including anaphylaxis), and hypercalcaemia

Indication and dose

Invasive aspergillosis either unresponsive to amphotericin or itraconazole or in patients intolerant of amphotericin or itraconazole; invasive candidiasis (see notes above); empirical treatment of systemic fungal infections in patients with neutropenia

• By intravenous infusion

Child 1–18 years 70 mg/m^2 (max. 70 mg) on first day then 50 mg/m^2 (max. 70 mg) once daily; increased to 70 mg/m^2 (max. 70 mg) daily if lower dose tolerated but inadequate response

Administration for *intravenous infusion*, allow vial to reach room temperature; initially reconstitute 50 mg with 10.5 mL Water for Injections to produce a 5.2 mg/mL solution, or reconstitute 70 mg with 10.5 mL Water for Injections to produce a 7.2 mg/mL solution; mix gently to dissolve; dilute requisite dose to a final concentration not exceeding 500 micrograms/mL with Sodium Chloride 0.9% *or* Compound Sodium Lactate; give over 60 minutes; incompatible with glucose solutions

Cancidas® (MSD) ▼ PoM

Intravenous infusion, powder for reconstitution, caspofungin (as acetate), net price 50-mg vial = £327.67; 70-mg vial = £416.78

5

Infections

FLUCONAZOLE

Cautions concomitant use with hepatotoxic drugs, monitor liver function with high doses or extended courses—discontinue if signs or symptoms of hepatic disease (risk of hepatic necrosis); susceptibility to QT interval prolongation; **interactions**: Appendix 1 (antifungals, triazole)

Hepatic impairment toxicity with related drugs

Renal impairment usual initial dose then halve subsequent doses if estimated glomerular filtration rate less than 50 mL/minute/1.73m^2

Pregnancy manufacturer advises avoid—multiple congenital abnormalities reported with long-term high doses

Breast-feeding present in milk but amount probably too small to be harmful

Contra-indications acute porphyria (section 9.8.2)

Side-effects nausea, abdominal discomfort, diarrhoea, flatulence, headache, rash (discontinue treatment or monitor closely if infection invasive or systemic); less frequently dyspepsia, vomiting, taste disturbance, hepatic disorders, angioedema, anaphylaxis, dizziness, seizures, alopecia, pruritus, toxic epidermal necrolysis, Stevens-Johnson syndrome (severe cutaneous reactions more likely in AIDS patients); hyperlipidaemia, leucopenia, thrombocytopenia, and hypokalaemia reported

Licensed use not licensed for tinea infections in children, or for vaginal candidiasis in girls under 16 years, or for prevention of relapse of cryptococcal meningitis after completion of primary therapy in children with AIDS

Indication and dose

Mucosal candidiasis (except genital)
• By mouth or by intravenous infusion

Neonate under 2 weeks 3–6 mg/kg on first day then 3 mg/kg every 72 hours

Neonate 2–4 weeks 3–6 mg/kg on first day then 3 mg/kg every 48 hours

Child 1 month–12 years 3–6 mg/kg on first day then 3 mg/kg (max. 100 mg) daily for 7–14 days in oropharyngeal candidiasis (max. 14 days except in severely immunocompromised patients); for 14–30 days in other mucosal infections (e.g. oesophagitis, candiduria, non-invasive bronchopulmonary infections)

Child 12–18 years 50 mg daily (100 mg daily in unusually difficult infections) given for 7–14 days in oropharyngeal candidiasis (max. 14 days except in severely immunocompromised patients); for 14–30 days in other mucosal infections (e.g. oesophagitis, candiduria, non-invasive bronchopulmonary infections)

Vaginal candidiasis (see also Recurrent Vulvovaginal Candidiasis, section 7.2.2)
• By mouth
Child under 16 years (post-puberty) a single dose of 150 mg

Child 16–18 years a single dose of 150 mg

Candidal balanitis
• By mouth
Child 16–18 years a single dose of 150 mg

Tinea pedis, corporis, cruris, pityriasis versicolor, and dermal candidiasis
• By mouth
Child 1 month–18 years 3 mg/kg (max. 50 mg) daily for 2–4 weeks (for up to 6 weeks in tinea pedis); max. duration of treatment 6 weeks

Invasive candidal infections (including candidaemia and disseminated candidiasis) and cryptococcal infections (including meningitis)
• By mouth or by intravenous infusion

Neonate under 2 weeks 6–12 mg/kg every 72 hours, treatment continued according to response (at least 8 weeks for cryptococcal meningitis)

Neonate 2–4 weeks 6–12 mg/kg every 48 hours, treatment continued according to response (at least 8 weeks for cryptococcal meningitis)

Child 1 month–18 years 6–12 mg/kg (max. 800 mg) daily, treatment continued according to response (at least 8 weeks for cryptococcal meningitis)

Prevention of relapse of cryptococcal meningitis in AIDS patients after completion of primary therapy
• By mouth or by intravenous infusion
Child 1 month–18 years 6 mg/kg (max. 200 mg) daily

Prevention of fungal infections in immuno-compromised patients
• By mouth or by intravenous infusion

Neonate under 2 weeks according to extent and duration of neutropenia, 3–12 mg/kg every 72 hours

Neonate 2–4 weeks according to extent and duration of neutropenia, 3–12 mg/kg every 48 hours

Child 1 month–18 years according to extent and duration of neutropenia, 3–12 mg/kg (max. 400 mg) daily; 12 mg/kg (max. 400 mg) daily if high risk of systemic infections e.g. following bone-marrow transplantation; commence treatment before anticipated onset of neutropenia and continue for 7 days after neutrophil count in desirable range

Administration for *intravenous infusion*, give over 10–30 minutes; do not exceed an infusion rate of 5–10 mL/minute

◻ **FLUCONAZOLE** (*continued*)

Fluconazole (Non-proprietary) [PoM]
 [1]Capsules, fluconazole 50 mg, net price 7-cap pack = 98p; 150 mg, single-capsule pack = 91p; 200 mg, 7-cap pack = £2.02. Label: 9, (50 and 200 mg)
Dental prescribing on NHS Fluconazole Capsules 50 mg may be prescribed

Intravenous infusion, fluconazole 2 mg/mL, net price 25-mL bottle = £7.32; 100-mL bottle = £29.28

Diflucan® (Pfizer) [PoM]
 [1]Capsules, fluconazole 50 mg (blue/white), net price 7-cap pack = £16.61; 150 mg (blue), single-

capsule pack = £7.12; 200 mg (purple/white), 7-cap pack = £66.42. Label: 9, (50 and 200 mg)

Oral suspension, orange-flavoured, fluconazole for reconstitution with water, 50 mg/5 mL, net price 35 mL = £16.61; 200 mg/5 mL, 35 mL = £66.42. Label: 9
Dental prescribing on NHS May be prescribed as Fluconazole Oral Suspension 50 mg/5 mL

Intravenous infusion, fluconazole 2 mg/mL in sodium chloride intravenous infusion 0.9%, net price 25-mL bottle = £7.32; 100-mL bottle = £29.28
Electrolytes Na⁺ 15 mmol/100-mL bottle

◢ FLUCYTOSINE

Cautions blood disorders; liver- and kidney-function tests and blood counts required (weekly in renal impairment or blood disorders); **interactions:** Appendix 1 (flucytosine)

Renal impairment use normal dose every 12 hours if estimated glomerular filtration rate 20–40 mL/minute/1.73 m²; use normal dose every 24 hours if estimated glomerular filtration rate 10–20 mL/minute/1.73 m²; use initial normal dose if estimated glomerular filtration rate less than 10 mL/minute/1.73 m² and then adjust dose according to plasma-flucytosine concentration

Pregnancy teratogenic in *animal* studies; manufacturer advises use only if potential benefit outweighs risk

Breast-feeding manufacturer advises avoid—although risk to infant probably small

Side-effects nausea, vomiting, diarrhoea, rashes; less frequently cardiotoxicity, confusion, hallucinations, convulsions, headache, sedation, vertigo, alterations in liver function tests (hepatitis and hepatic necrosis reported), and toxic epidermal necrolysis; blood disorders including thrombocytopenia, leucopenia, and aplastic anaemia reported

Pharmacokinetics for plasma-concentration monitoring blood should be taken shortly before starting the next infusion. Plasma concentration for optimum response 25–50 mg/litre (200–400 micromol/litre)—should not be allowed to exceed 80 mg/litre (620 micromol/litre)

Licensed use tablets not licensed

Indication and dose

> Systemic yeast and fungal infections, adjunct to amphotericin in severe systemic candidiasis and in other severe or long-standing infections
> • **By intravenous infusion or by mouth**
>
> **Neonate** 50 mg/kg every 12 hours
>
> **Child 1 month–18 years** 50 mg/kg every 6 hours; extremely sensitive organisms, 25–37.5 mg/kg every 6 hours may be sufficient; treatment continued usually for not more than 7 days

> Cryptococcal meningitis (adjunct to amphotericin, see Cryptococcosis, p. 362)
> • **By intravenous infusion or by mouth**
>
> **Neonate** 50 mg/kg every 12 hours
>
> **Child 1 month–18 years** 25 mg/kg every 6 hours for 2 weeks

Administration for *intravenous infusion*, give over 20–40 minutes through a giving set with a 15-micron filter

Ancotil® (Valeant) [PoM]
 Intravenous infusion, flucytosine 10 mg/mL. Net price 250-mL infusion bottle = £30.33 (hosp. only)
Electrolytes Na⁺ 34.5 mmol/250-mL bottle

Note Flucytosine tablets may be available from 'special-order' manufacturers or specialist importing companies, see p. 943

◢ Extemporaneous formulations available see Extemporaneous Preparations, p. 8

◢ GRISEOFULVIN

Cautions interactions: Appendix 1 (griseofulvin)
Skilled tasks May impair performance of skilled tasks; effects of alcohol enhanced

Contra-indications systemic lupus erythematosus (risk of exacerbation); acute porphyria (section 9.8.2)

Hepatic impairment avoid in severe liver disease

Pregnancy avoid pregnancy *during* and for *1 month* after treatment (fetotoxicity and teratogenicity in *animals*); effective contraception required during and for at least 1 month after administration

(**important**: effectiveness of oral contraceptives reduced); also males should avoid fathering a child during and for at least 6 months after treatment

Breast-feeding avoid—no information available

Side-effects nausea, vomiting, diarrhoea; headache; less frequently hepatotoxicity, dizziness, confusion, fatigue, sleep disturbances, impaired co-ordination, peripheral neuropathy, leucopenia, systemic lupus erythematosus, rash (including rarely erythema multiforme, toxic epidermal necrolysis), and photosensitivity

---

1. Capsules can be sold to the public for vaginal candidiasis and associated candidal balanitis in those aged 16–18 years, in a container or packaging containing not more than 150 mg and labelled to show a max. dose of 150 mg

◻ **GRISEOFULVIN** (*continued*)

Licensed use tablets licensed for use in children (age range not specified by manufacturer); suspension not licensed

Indication and dose

Dermatophyte infections where topical therapy has failed or is inappropriate
* By mouth

    Child 1 month–12 years 10 mg/kg (max. 500 mg) once daily or in divided doses; in severe infection dose may be doubled, reducing when response occurs

    Child 12–18 years 500 mg once daily or in divided doses; in severe infection dose may be doubled, reducing when response occurs

Tinea capitis caused by *Trichophyton tonsurans*
* By mouth

    Child 1 month–12 years 15–20 mg/kg (max. 1 g) once daily or in divided doses

    Child 12–18 years 1 g once daily or in divided doses

Griseofulvin (Non-proprietary) PoM
Tablets, griseofulvin 125 mg, net price 20 = £6.76; 500 mg, 20 = £17.52. Label: 9, 21, counselling, skilled tasks

Suspension, griseofulvin 125 mg/5 mL. Label: 9, 21, counselling, skilled tasks
Available via specialist importing companies

◼ **ITRACONAZOLE**

Cautions absorption reduced in AIDS and neutropenia (monitor plasma-itraconazole concentration and increase dose if necessary); susceptibility to congestive heart failure (see also CSM advice, below); **interactions**: Appendix 1 (antifungals, triazole)

Hepatotoxicity Potentially life-threatening hepatotoxicity reported very rarely—discontinue if signs of hepatitis develop. Avoid or use with caution if history of hepatotoxicity with other drugs or in active liver disease. Monitor liver function if treatment continues for longer than one month, if receiving other hepatotoxic drugs, if history of hepatotoxicity with other drugs, or in hepatic impairment
Counselling Children or their carers should be told how to recognise signs of liver disorder and advised to seek prompt medical attention if symptoms such as anorexia, nausea, vomiting, fatigue, abdominal pain or dark urine develop

Hepatic impairment use only if potential benefit outweighs risk of hepatotoxicity (see hepatotoxicity above); dose reduction may be necessary

Renal impairment risk of congestive heart failure; bioavailability of oral formulations possibly reduced; use intravenous infusion with caution if estimated glomerular filtration rate 30–80 mL/minute/1.73 m^2 (monitor renal function); avoid intravenous infusion if estimated glomerular filtration rate less than 30 mL/minute/1.73 m^2

Pregnancy manufacturer advises use only in life-threatening situations (toxicity at high doses in *animal* studies); ensure effective contraception during treatment and until the next menstrual period following end of treatment

> CSM advice (heart failure) Following rare reports of heart failure, the CSM has advised caution when prescribing itraconazole to patients at high risk of heart failure. Those at risk include:
> * patients receiving high doses and longer treatment courses;
> * those with cardiac disease;
> * patients receiving treatment with negative inotropic drugs, e.g. calcium channel blockers.

Contra-indications acute porphyria (section 9.8.2)

Breast-feeding small amounts present in milk—may accumulate; manufacturer advises avoid

Side-effects *very rarely* nausea, vomiting, dyspepsia, abdominal pain, diarrhoea, constipation, jaundice, hepatitis (see also Hepatotoxicity

above), heart failure (see CSM advice above), pulmonary oedema, headache, dizziness, peripheral neuropathy (discontinue treatment), menstrual disorder, hypokalaemia, rash, pruritus, Stevens-Johnson syndrome, and alopecia; *with intravenous injection, very rarely* hypertension and hyperglycaemia

Licensed use *Sporanox*® capsules and *Sporanox*® *Pulse* are not licensed for use in children under 12 years; *Sporanox*® liquid and *Sporanox*® infusion are not licensed for use in children (age range not specified by manufacturer)

Indication and dose

Oropharyngeal candidiasis
* By mouth

    Child 1 month–12 years 3–5 mg/kg once daily; max. 100 mg daily (200 mg daily in AIDS or neutropenia) for 15 days

    Child 12–18 years 100 mg once daily (200 mg once daily in AIDS or neutropenia) for 15 days

Pityriasis versicolor
* By mouth

    Child 1 month–12 years 3–5 mg/kg (max. 200 mg) once daily for 7 days

    Child 12–18 years 200 mg once daily for 7 days

Tinea corporis and tinea cruris
* By mouth

    Child 1 month–12 years 3–5 mg/kg (max. 100 mg) once daily for 15 days

    Child 12–18 years *either* 100 mg once daily for 15 days *or* 200 mg once daily for 7 days

Tinea pedis and tinea manuum
* By mouth

    Child 1 month–12 years 3–5 mg/kg (max. 100 mg) once daily for 30 days

    Child 12–18 years *either* 100 mg once daily for 30 days *or* 200 mg twice daily for 7 days

5 Infections

▱ **ITRACONAZOLE** *(continued)*

Onychomycosis
● **By mouth**

Child 1–12 years course ('pulse') of 5 mg/kg (max. 200 mg) daily for 7 days; subsequent courses repeated after 21 day intervals; fingernails 2 courses, toenails 3 courses

Child 12–18 years *either* 200 mg once daily for 3 months *or* course ('pulse') of 200 mg twice daily for 7 days, subsequent courses repeated after 21-day intervals; fingernails 2 courses, toenails 3 courses

Systemic aspergillosis, candidiasis and cryptococcosis including cryptococcal meningitis where other antifungal drugs inappropriate or ineffective (limited information available)
● **By mouth**

Child 1 month–18 years 5 mg/kg (max. 200 mg) once daily; increased in invasive or disseminated disease and in cryptococcal meningitis to 5 mg/kg (max. 200 mg) twice daily

● **By intravenous infusion**

Child 1 month–18 years 2.5 mg/kg (max. 200 mg) every 12 hours for 2 days, then 2.5 mg/kg (max. 200 mg) once daily for max. 12 days

Histoplasmosis
● **By mouth**

Child 1 month–18 years 5 mg/kg (max. 200 mg) 1–2 times daily

Maintenance in AIDS patients to prevent relapse of underlying fungal infection and prophylaxis in neutropenia when standard therapy inappropriate
● **By mouth**

Child 1 month–18 years 5 mg/kg (max. 200 mg) once daily, increased to 5 mg/kg (max. 200 mg) twice daily if low plasma-itraconazole concentration (see Cautions)

Prophylaxis of deep fungal infections (when standard therapy inappropriate) in patients with haematological malignancy or undergoing bone-marrow transplantation who are expected to become neutropenic
● **By mouth (liquid preparation only)**

Child 1 month–18 years 2.5 mg/kg twice daily starting before transplantation or before chemotherapy (taking care to avoid interaction with cytotoxic drugs) and continued until neutrophil count recovers

Administration For *intravenous infusion*, dilute 250 mg with 50 mL Sodium Chloride 0.9% and give requisite dose through an in-line filter (0.2 micron) over 60 minutes

Sporanox® (Janssen-Cilag) ⒫ⓄⓂ
Capsules, blue/pink, enclosing coated beads, itraconazole 100 mg, net price 4-cap pack = £3.90; 15-cap pack = £20.96; 28-cap pack (*Sporanox®-Pulse*) = £27.30; 60-cap pack = £58.49. Label: 5, 9, 21, 25, counselling, hepatotoxicity

Oral liquid, sugar-free, cherry-flavoured, itraconazole 10 mg/mL, net price 150 mL (with 10-mL measuring cup) = £48.62. Label: 9, 23, counselling, administration, hepatotoxicity

Counselling Do not take with food; swish around mouth and swallow, do not rinse afterwards

Concentrate for intravenous infusion, itraconazole 10 mg/mL. For dilution before use. Net price 25-mL amp (with infusion bag and filter) = £66.43
Excipients include propylene glycol

▰ **KETOCONAZOLE**

Cautions predisposition to adrenocortical insufficiency; **interactions**: Appendix 1 (antifungals, imidazole)

Hepatotoxicity Potentially life-threatening hepatotoxicity reported very rarely; risk of hepatotoxicity greater if given for longer than 10 days. Monitor liver function before treatment, then on weeks 2 and 4 of treatment, then every month. Avoid or use with caution if abnormal liver function tests (avoid in active liver disease) or if history of hepatotoxicity with other drugs. For CSM advice see p. 363

Counselling Children and their carers should be told how to recognise signs of liver disorder and advised to seek prompt medical attention if symptoms such as anorexia, nausea, vomiting, fatigue, abdominal pain, jaundice, or dark urine develop

Pregnancy manufacturer advises avoid unless potential benefit outweighs risk (teratogenicity in *animal* studies)

Contra-indications acute porphyria (section 9.8.2)

Hepatic impairment avoid (see also Hepatotoxicity above)

Breast-feeding manufacturer advises avoid

Side-effects nausea, vomiting, abdominal pain; pruritus; *less commonly* diarrhoea, headache, dizziness, drowsiness, and rash; also reported fatal liver damage (see Hepatotoxicity above), dyspepsia, raised intracranial pressure, paraesthesia, adrenocortical insufficiency, erectile dysfunction, menstrual disorders, azoospermia (with high doses), gynaecomastia, thrombocytopenia, photophobia, photosensitivity, and alopecia

Indication and dose

Dermatophytoses and *Malassezia* folliculitis *either* resistant to fluconazole, terbinafine, or itraconazole *or* in patients intolerant of these antifungals; **chronic mucocutaneous, cutaneous, and oropharyngeal candidiasis** *either* resistant to fluconazole or itraconazole *or* in patients intolerant of these antifungals; see also CSM recommendations, p. 363
● **By mouth**

Child body-weight 15–30 kg 100 mg once daily

5

Infections

◁ **KETOCONAZOLE** (*continued*)

Child body-weight over 30 kg 200 mg once daily, increased if response inadequate to 400 mg once daily
Note Treatment continued until symptoms have cleared and cultures negative, but see Cautions (max. duration of treatment 4 weeks for *Malassezia* infection)

Nizoral® (Janssen-Cilag) [PoM]
Tablets, scored, ketoconazole 200 mg. Net price 30-tab pack = £14.59. Label: 5, 9, 21, Counselling, hepatotoxicity

◀Extemporaneous formulations available see Extemporaneous Preparations, p. 8

◢ MICAFUNGIN

Cautions monitor renal function; **interactions**: Appendix 1 (micafungin)
Hepatotoxicity Potentially life-threatening hepatotoxicity reported. Monitor liver function—discontinue if significant and persistent abnormalities in liver function tests develop. Use with caution in hepatic impairment (avoid if severe) or if receiving other hepatotoxic drugs. Risk of hepatic side-effects greater in children under 1 year of age

Renal impairment use with caution; deterioration in renal function

Pregnancy manufacturer advises avoid unless essential—toxicity in *animal* studies

Breast-feeding manufacturer advises use only if potential benefit outweighs risk—present in milk in *animal* studies

Side-effects nausea, vomiting, diarrhoea, abdominal pain, hepatomegaly; blood pressure changes, tachycardia; headache, fever; hypokalaemia, hypomagnesaemia, hypocalcaemia, leucopenia, anaemia, thrombocytopenia, renal failure; rash, phlebitis; *less commonly* dyspepsia, constipation, hepatitis and cholestasis (see also Hepatotoxicity above), taste disturbances, anorexia, palpitation, bradycardia, flushing, dyspnoea, sleep disturbances, anxiety, confusion, dizziness, tremor, pancytopenia, eosinophilia, hyponatraemia, hyperkalaemia, hypophosphataemia, hyperhidrosis, and pruritus; *rarely* haemolytic anaemia

Indication and dose

Invasive candidiasis
● By intravenous infusion

Neonate 2 mg/kg once daily (increased to 4 mg/kg daily if inadequate response) for at least 14 days

Child 1 month–18 years, body-weight under 40 kg 2mg/kg once daily (increased to 4 mg/kg daily if inadequate response) for at least 14 days

Child 1 month–18 years, body-weight over 40 kg 100 mg once daily (increased to 200 mg daily if inadequate response) for at least 14 days

Oesophageal candidiasis
● By intravenous infusion

Child 16–18 years, body-weight under 40 kg 3 mg/kg once daily

Child 16–18 years, body-weight over 40 kg 150 mg once daily

Prophylaxis of candidiasis in children undergoing bone-marrow transplantation or who are expected to become neutropenic for over 10 days
● By intravenous infusion

Neonate 1 mg/kg once daily; continue for at least 7 days after neutrophil count in desirable range

Child 1 month–18 years, body-weight under 40 kg 1 mg/kg once daily; continue for at least 7 days after neutrophil count in desirable range

Child 1 month–18 years, body-weight over 40 kg 50 mg once daily; continue for at least 7 days after neutrophil count in desirable range

Administration for *intravenous infusion* reconstitute each vial with 5 mL Glucose 5% *or* Sodium Chloride 0.9%; gently rotate vial, without shaking, to dissolve; dilute requisite dose to a concentration of 0.5–2mg/mL with Glucose 5% *or* Sodium Chloride 0.9%; protect from light; give over 60 minutes

Mycamine® (Astellas) ▼ [PoM]
Intravenous infusion, powder for reconstitution, micafungin (as sodium), net price 50-mg vial = £196.08; 100-mg vial = £341.00

◢ NYSTATIN

Side-effects nausea, vomiting, diarrhoea at high doses; oral irritation and sensitisation; rash (including urticaria) and rarely Stevens-Johnson syndrome reported

Licensed use suspension not licensed for treatment of intestinal candidiasis in neonates; suspension licensed for prophylaxis in neonates as once daily dose; tablets not licensed for use in children (age range not specified by manufacturer)

Indication and dose

Treatment of intestinal candidiasis
● By mouth

Neonate 100 000 units 4 times daily after feeds

Child 1 month–12 years 100 000 units 4 times daily; immunocompromised children may require higher doses (e.g. 500 000 units 4 times daily)

Child 12–18 years 500 000 units 4 times daily; doubled in severe infection

Oral infection section 12.3.2

◻ **NYSTATIN** (*continued*)

Skin infection section 13.10.2

Nystan® (Squibb) PoM
Tablets, brown, s/c, nystatin 500 000 units, net price 56-tab pack = £4.37. Label: 9

Suspension, yellow, nystatin 100 000 units/mL, net price 30 mL with pipette = £1.91. Label: 9, counselling, use of pipette
Excipients include alcohol

◤ TERBINAFINE

Cautions psoriasis (risk of exacerbation); autoimmune disease (risk of lupus-erythematosus-like effect) **interactions:** Appendix 1 (terbinafine)

Hepatic impairment manufacturer advises avoid—elimination reduced

Renal impairment use half normal dose if estimated glomerular filtration rate less than 50 mL/minute/1.73 m^2

Pregnancy manufacturer advises use only if benefit outweighs risk—no information available

Breast-feeding present in milk—manufacturer advises avoid

Side-effects abdominal discomfort, anorexia, nausea, diarrhoea; headache; rash and urticaria occasionally with arthralgia or myalgia; *less commonly* taste disturbance; *rarely* liver toxicity (including jaundice, cholestasis and hepatitis)—discontinue treatment, angioedema, dizziness, malaise, paraesthesia, hypoaesthesia, photosensitivity, serious skin reactions (including Stevens-Johnson syndrome and toxic epidermal necrolysis)—discontinue treatment if progressive skin rash; *very rarely* psychiatric disturbances, blood disorders (including incidence of leucopenia higher and thrombocytopenia), lupus erythematosus-like effect, and exacerbation of psoriasis

Licensed use not licensed for use in children

Indication and dose

Dermatophyte infections of the nails, ringworm infections (including tinea pedis, cruris, corporis, and capitis) where oral therapy appropriate (due to site, severity or extent)
• By mouth

Child over 1 year; body-weight 10–20 kg 62.5 mg once daily

Child body-weight 20–40 kg 125 mg once daily

Child body-weight over 40 kg 250 mg once daily

Note treatment usually for 4 weeks in tinea capitis, 2–6 weeks in tinea pedis, 2–4 weeks in tinea cruris, 4 weeks in tinea corporis, 6 weeks–3 months in nail infections (occasionally longer in toenail infections)

Fungal skin infections section 13.10.2

Terbinafine (Non-proprietary) PoM
Tablets, terbinafine (as hydrochloride) 250 mg, net price 14-tab pack = £2.70, 28-tab pack = £3.43. Label: 9

Lamisil® (Novartis) PoM
Tablets, off-white, scored, terbinafine (as hydrochloride) 250 mg, net price 14-tab pack = £23.16, 28-tab pack = £44.66. Label: 9

◤ VORICONAZOLE

Cautions electrolyte disturbances, cardiomyopathy, bradycardia, symptomatic arrhythmias, history of QT interval prolongation, concomitant use with other drugs that prolong QT interval; avoid exposure to sunlight; patients at risk of pancreatitis; monitor liver function before treatment and during treatment; haematological malignancy (increased risk of hepatic reactions); monitor renal function; **interactions:** Appendix 1 (antifungals, triazole)

Hepatic impairment in mild to moderate hepatic cirrhosis use usual initial dose then halve subsequent doses; no information available for severe hepatic cirrhosis—manufacturer advises use only if potential benefit outweighs risk

Renal impairment excipient in intravenous infusion solution may accumulate if estimated glomerular filtration rate less than 50 mL/minute/1.73 m^2—manufacturer advises use intravenous infusion only if potential benefit outweighs risk and monitor renal function; alternatively, use tablets or oral suspension (no dose adjustment required)

Pregnancy toxicity in *animal* studies—manufacturer advises avoid unless potential benefit out-

weighs risk; effective contraception required during treatment

Contra-indications acute porphyria (section 9.8.2)

Breast-feeding manufacturer advises avoid—no information available

Side-effects gastro-intestinal disturbances (including nausea, vomiting, abdominal pain, diarrhoea), jaundice; oedema, hypotension, chest pain; respiratory distress syndrome, sinusitis; headache, dizziness, asthenia, anxiety, depression, confusion, agitation, hallucinations, paraesthesia, tremor; influenza-like symptoms; hypoglycaemia; haematuria; blood disorders (including anaemia, thrombocytopenia, leucopenia, pancytopenia), acute renal failure, hypokalaemia; visual disturbances including altered perception, blurred vision, and photophobia; rash, pruritus, photosensitivity, alopecia, cheilitis; injection-site reactions; *less commonly* cholecystitis, pancreatitis, hepatitis, constipation, arrhythmias (including QT interval prolongation), syncope, raised serum cholesterol, hypersensitivity reactions (including flushing), ataxia, nystagmus, hypoaesthesia, adrenocortical insuffi-

◁ **VORICONAZOLE** (*continued*)

ciency, arthritis, blepharitis, optic neuritis, scleritis, glossitis, gingivitis, psoriasis, and Stevens-Johnson syndrome; *rarely* pseudomembranous colitis, convulsions, sleep disturbances, tinnitis, hearing disturbances, extrapyramidal effects, hypertonia, hypothyroidism, hyperthyroidism, discoid lupus erythematosus, toxic epidermal necrolysis, retinal haemorrhage, optic atrophy, and taste disturbances

Indication and dose

Invasive aspergillosis; serious infections caused by *Scedosporium* spp., *Fusarium* spp., or invasive fluconazole-resistant *Candida* spp. (including *C. krusei*)

• **By mouth**

Child 2–12 years (oral suspension recommended) 200 mg every 12 hours

Child 12–18 years, body-weight under 40 kg 200 mg every 12 hours for 2 doses then 100 mg every 12 hours, increased if necessary to 150 mg every 12 hours

Child 12–18 years, body-weight over 40 kg 400 mg every 12 hours for 2 doses then 200 mg every 12 hours, increased if necessary to 300 mg every 12 hours

• **By intravenous infusion**

Child 2–12 years 7 mg/kg every 12 hours (reduced to 4 mg/kg every 12 hours if not tolerated) for max. 6 months

Child 12–18 years 6 mg/kg every 12 hours for 2 doses, then 4 mg/kg every 12 hours (reduced to 3 mg/kg every 12 hours if not tolerated) for max. 6 months

Administration For *intravenous infusion*, reconstitute each 200 mg with 19 mL Water for Injections to produce a 10 mg/mL solution; dilute dose to concentration of 0.5–5 mg/mL with Glucose 5% *or* Sodium Chloride 0.9% *or* Compound Sodium Lactate and give at a rate not exceeding 3 mg/kg/hour

Vfend® (Pfizer) [PoM]

Tablets, f/c, voriconazole 50 mg, net price 28-tablet pack = £275.68; 200 mg, 28-tab pack = £1102.74. Label: 9, 11, 23

Oral suspension, voriconazole 200 mg/5 mL when reconstituted with water, net price 75 mL (orange-flavoured) = £551.37. Label: 9, 11, 23

Intravenous infusion, powder for reconstitution, voriconazole, net price 200-mg vial = £77.14
Excipients include sulphobutylether beta cyclodextrin sodium (risk of accumulation in renal impairment)
Electrolytes Na+ 9.47 mmol/vial

5.3 Antiviral drugs

5.3.1 HIV infection

5.3.2 Herpesvirus infections

5.3.3 Viral hepatitis

5.3.4 Influenza

5.3.5 Respiratory syncytial virus

The majority of virus infections resolve spontaneously in immunocompetent subjects. A number of specific treatments for viral infections are available, particularly for the immunocompromised. This section includes notes on herpes simplex and varicella-zoster, human immunodeficiency virus, cytomegalovirus, respiratory syncytial virus, viral hepatitis and influenza.

5.3.1 HIV infection

There is no cure for infection caused by the human immunodeficiency virus (HIV) but a number of drugs slow or halt disease progression. Drugs for HIV infection (antiretrovirals) increase life expectancy considerably but they may be associated with serious side-effects.

The natural progression of HIV disease is different in children compared to adults; drug treatment should only be undertaken by specialists within a formal paediatric HIV clinical network. Guidelines and dose regimens are under constant review and for this reason specific dose recommendations have not been included in *BNF for Children*.

Further information on the management of children with HIV can be obtained from the Children's HIV Association (CHIVA) www.chiva.org.uk; and further information on antiretroviral use and toxicity can be obtained from the Paediatric European Network for Treatment of AIDS (PENTA) website www.pentatrials.org.

Principles of treatment Treatment is aimed at suppressing viral replication for as long as possible; it should be started before the immune system is irreversibly damaged. The need for early drug treatment should, however, be balanced against the risk of toxicity. Commitment to treatment and strict adherence over many years are required; the regimen chosen should take into account convenience and the child's tolerance of treatment. The development of drug resistance is reduced by using a combination of drugs; such combinations should have synergistic or additive activity while ensuring that their toxicity is not additive. It is recommended that viral sensitivity to antiretroviral drugs is established before starting treatment or before switching drugs if the infection is not responding.

Initiation of treatment   Treatment is based on child's age, CD4 cell count, viral load, and symptoms. Treatment is started in all HIV infected children under 1 year of age regardless of clinical and immunological parameters. The choice of antiviral treatment for children should take into account the method and frequency of administration, risk of side-effects, compatibility of drugs with food, palatability, and the appropriateness of the formulation. Initiating treatment with a combination of drugs ('highly active antiretroviral therapy' which includes 2 nucleoside reverse transcriptase inhibitors with *either* a non-nucleoside reverse transcriptase inhibitor *or* a boosted protease inhibitor) is recommended. The metabolism of many antiretrovirals varies in young children; it may therefore be necessary to adjust the dose according to the plasma-drug concentration. Children who require treatment for both HIV and chronic hepatitis B should receive antivirals that are active against both diseases (section 5.3.3).

Switching therapy   Deterioration of the condition (including clinical, virological changes, and CD4 cell changes) may require a complete change of therapy. The choice of an alternative regimen depends on factors such as the response to previous treatment, tolerance, and the possibility of cross-resistance.

Pregnancy   Treatment of HIV infection in pregnancy aims to minimise the viral load and disease progression in the mother and reduce the risk of toxicity to the fetus (but the teratogenic potential of most antiretroviral drugs is unknown). Combination antiretroviral therapy represents optimal treatment but all options require **careful assessment** by a specialist. Combination antiretroviral therapy may be associated with a greater risk of preterm delivery. Consideration also needs to be given to preventing transmission of the infection to the neonate (see below).

Prevention of transmission to neonate   Zidovudine given in the perinatal period to the mother and the neonate reduces transmission to the baby. However, optimal treatment of the mother's HIV infection with combination treatment maximises the chance of preventing transmission. Local protocols and national guidelines (www.bhiva.org) should be consulted for recommendations on treatment during pregnancy and the perinatal period.

Breast-feeding   Breast-feeding by HIV-positive mothers may cause HIV infection in the infant and should be avoided.

Post-exposure prophylaxis   Children exposed to HIV infection through needle-stick injury or by another route should be sent to an accident and emergency department for post-exposure prophylaxis [unlicensed indication]. Antiretrovirals for prophylaxis are chosen on the basis of efficacy and potential for toxicity.

Drugs used for HIV infection   **Zidovudine**, a nucleoside reverse transcriptase inhibitor (or 'nucleoside analogue'), was the first anti-HIV drug to be introduced. Other nucleoside reverse transcriptase inhibitors include **abacavir, didanosine, emtricitabine, lamivudine, stavudine**, and **tenofovir**.

The protease inhibitors include **atazanavir, darunavir, fosamprenavir** (a prodrug of amprenavir), **indinavir, lopinavir, nelfinavir, ritonavir, saquinavir**, and **tipranavir**. Ritonavir in low doses boosts the activity of atazanavir, darunavir, fosamprenavir, indinavir, lopinavir, saquinavir, and tipranavir increasing the persistence of plasma concentrations of these drugs; at such a low dose, ritonavir has no intrinsic antiviral activity. A combination of lopinavir with low-dose ritonavir is available for use in children over 2 years. The protease inhibitors are metabolised by cytochrome P450 enzyme systems and therefore have a significant potential for drug interactions. Protease inhibitors are associated with lipodystrophy and metabolic effects (see below).

The non-nucleoside reverse transcriptase inhibitors **efavirenz, etravirine**, and **nevirapine** are active against the subtype HIV-1 but not HIV-2, a subtype that is rare in the UK. These drugs may interact with a number of drugs metabolised in the liver. Nevirapine is associated with a high incidence of rash (including Stevens-Johnson syndrome) and fatal hepatitis. Rash is also associated with efavirenz and etravirine but it is usually milder. Psychiatric or CNS disturbances are common with efavirenz. CNS disturbances are often self-limiting and can be reduced by taking the dose at bedtime (especially in the first 2–4 weeks of treatment). Efavirenz treatment has also been associated with an increased plasma cholesterol concentration. In adults, etravirine is licensed for use in regimens containing a boosted protease inhibitor for HIV infection resistant to other non-nucleoside reverse transcriptase inhibitors and protease inhibitors.

Enfuvirtide, which inhibits HIV from fusing to the host cell, is licensed for managing infection that has failed to respond to a regimen of other antiretroviral drugs. Enfuvirtide should be combined with other potentially active antiretroviral drugs; it is given by subcutaneous injection.

Maraviroc is an antagonist of the CCR5 chemokine receptor. It is used in patients exclusively infected with CCR5–tropic HIV.

Raltegravir is an inhibitor of HIV integrase. It is used for the treatment of HIV infection resistant to multiple antiretrovirals.

Immune reconstitution syndrome   Improvement in immune function as a result of antiretroviral treatment may provoke a marked inflammatory reaction against residual opportunistic organisms.

Lipodystrophy syndrome   Metabolic effects associated with antiretroviral treatment include *fat redistribution, insulin resistance* and *dyslipidaemia*; collectively these have been termed *lipodystrophy syndrome*. Children should be encouraged to lead a healthy lifestyle that reduces their long-term cardiovascular risk. Plasma lipids and blood glucose should be measured before starting antiretroviral therapy, after 3–6 months of treatment, and then at least annually. Insulin resistance and hyperglycaemia occur only rarely in children.

Fat redistribution (with loss of subcutaneous fat, increased abdominal fat, 'buffalo hump' and breast enlargement) is associated with regimens containing protease inhibitors and nucleoside reverse transcriptase inhibitors. Stavudine, and to a lesser extent zidovudine, are associated with a higher risk of lipoatrophy and should be used only if alternative regimens are not suitable.

Dyslipidaemia (with adverse effects on body lipids) is associated with antiretroviral treatment, particularly with protease inhibitors; in children, hypercholesterolaemia appears to be more common than hypertriglyceridaemia. Protease inhibitors are associated with insulin resistance and hyperglycaemia but they occur rarely in children. Of the protease inhibitors, atazanavir and darunavir are less likely to cause dyslipidaemia, while saquinavir and atazanavir are less likely to impair glucose tolerance.

Osteonecrosis   Osteonecrosis has been reported in children with advanced HIV disease or following long-term exposure to combination antiretroviral therapy.

Nucleoside reverse transcriptase inhibitors

Cautions   Nucleoside reverse transcriptase inhibitors should be used with caution in children with hepatic impairment (greater risk of hepatic side-effects, see also Lactic Acidosis below). However, some nucleoside reverse transcriptase inhibitors are used in children who also have chronic hepatitis B. They should also be used with caution in renal impairment and in pregnancy (see also p. 373).

Lactic acidosis   Life-threatening lactic acidosis associated with hepatomegaly and hepatic steatosis has been reported with nucleoside reverse transcriptase inhibitors. They should be used with caution in children with hepatomegaly, hepatitis (especially hepatitis C treated with interferon alfa and ribavirin), liver-enzyme abnormalities and with other risk factors for liver disease and hepatic steatosis. Treatment with the nucleoside reverse transcriptase inhibitor should be **discontinued** in case of symptomatic hyperlactataemia, lactic acidosis, progressive hepatomegaly or rapid deterioration of liver function. Stavudine, especially with didanosine, is associated with a higher risk of lactic acidosis and should be used only if alternative regimens are not suitable.

Side-effects Side-effects of the nucleoside reverse transcriptase inhibitors include gastro-intestinal disturbances (such as nausea, vomiting, abdominal pain, flatulence and diarrhoea), anorexia, pancreatitis, liver damage (see also Lactic Acidosis, above), dyspnoea, cough, headache, insomnia, dizziness, fatigue, blood disorders (including anaemia, neutropenia, and thrombocytopenia), myalgia, arthralgia, rash, urticaria, and fever. See notes above for Lipodystrophy Syndrome (p. 374) and Osteonecrosis (p. 374).

◢ ABACAVIR

Cautions see notes above; also test for HLA-B*5701 allele before treatment—risk of hypersensitivity reaction in presence of HLA-B*5701 allele; **interactions**: Appendix 1 (abacavir)

Hepatic impairment avoid in moderate hepatic impairment unless essential; avoid in severe hepatic impairment

Renal impairment manufacturer advises avoid in end-stage renal disease

Hypersensitivity reactions Life-threatening hypersensitivity reactions reported (more common in Caucasians)—characterised by fever or rash and possibly nausea, vomiting, diarrhoea, abdominal pain, dyspnoea, cough, lethargy, malaise, headache, and myalgia; less frequently mouth ulceration, oedema, hypotension, sore throat, acute respiratory distress syndrome, anaphylaxis, paraesthesia, arthralgia, conjunctivitis, lymphadenopathy, lymphocytopenia and renal failure (CSM has identified hypersensitivity reactions presenting as sore throat, influenza-like illness, cough, and breathlessness); rarely myolysis; laboratory abnormalities may include raised liver function tests (see Lactic Acidosis above) and creatine kinase; symptoms usually appear in the first 6 weeks, but may occur at any time; monitor for symptoms every 2 weeks for 2 months; discontinue immediately if any symptom of hypersensitivity develops and do not rechallenge (risk of more severe hypersensitivity reaction); discontinue if hypersensitivity cannot be ruled out, even when other diagnoses possible—if rechallenge necessary it must be carried out in hospital setting; if abacavir is stopped for any reason other than hypersensitivity, exclude hypersensitivity reaction as the cause and rechallenge only if medical assistance is readily available; care needed with concomitant use of drugs which cause skin toxicity

Counselling Children and carers should be told the importance of regular dosing (intermittent therapy may increase the risk of sensitisation), how to recognise signs of hypersensitivity, and advised to seek immediate medical attention if symptoms develop or before re-starting treatment; children or their carers should be advised to keep Alert Card with them at all times

Contra-indications

Pregnancy manufacturer advises avoid (toxicity in *animal* studies); see also Pregnancy, p. 373

Breast-feeding avoid (see notes above)

Side-effects see notes above; also hypersensitivity reactions (see above); *very rarely* Stevens-Johnson syndrome and toxic epidermal necrolysis; rash and gastro-intestinal disturbances more common in children

Licensed use *Ziagen®* not licensed for use in children under 3 months; *Kivexa®* not licensed for use in children under 12 years; *Trizivir®* not licensed for use in children

Indication and dose

HIV infection in combination with other antiretroviral drugs

 For dose, consult Guidelines (see notes above)

Ziagen® (GSK) ▢PoM

Tablets, yellow, f/c, scored, abacavir (as sulphate) 300 mg, net price 60-tab pack = £221.81. Counselling, hypersensitivity reactions

Oral solution, sugar-free, banana and strawberry flavoured, abacavir (as sulphate) 20 mg/mL, net price 240-mL = £59.15. Counselling, hypersensitivity reactions
Excipients include propylene glycol

◢**With lamivudine**

For cautions, contra-indications and side-effects see under individual drugs

Kivexa® (GSK) ▢PoM

Tablets, orange, f/c, abacavir (as sulphate) 600 mg, lamivudine 300 mg, net price 30-tab pack = £373.94. Counselling, hypersensitivity reactions

◢**With lamivudine and zidovudine**

Note use only if child is stabilised (for 6–8 weeks) on the individual components in the same proportions. For cautions, contra-indications and side-effects see under individual drugs

Trizivir® (GSK) ▢PoM

Tablets, blue-green, f/c, abacavir (as sulphate) 300 mg, lamivudine 150 mg, zidovudine 300 mg, net price 60-tab pack = £540.40. Counselling, hypersensitivity reactions

◢ DIDANOSINE
(ddI, DDI)

Cautions see notes above; also history of pancreatitis (preferably avoid, otherwise extreme caution, see also below); peripheral neuropathy or hyperuricaemia (see under Side-effects); ophthalmological examination (including visual acuity, colour vision, and dilated fundus examination) recommended annually or if visual changes occur; **interactions**: Appendix 1 (didanosine)

Renal impairment reduce dose if estimated glomerular filtration rate less than 60 mL/minute/1.73 m^2; consult product literature

Hepatic impairment insufficient information but monitor for toxicity

Pregnancy manufacturer advises use only if potential benefit outweighs risk—no information available

Pancreatitis If symptoms of pancreatitis develop or if serum lipase is raised and pancreatitis is confirmed, discontinue treatment. Whenever possible avoid concomitant treatment with other drugs known to cause pan-

◁ **DIDANOSINE** *(continued)*

creatic toxicity (e.g. intravenous pentamidine isetionate); monitor closely if concomitant therapy unavoidable. Since significant elevations of triglycerides cause pancreatitis monitor closely if triglycerides elevated

Contra-indications

Breast-feeding avoid (see notes above)

Side-effects see notes above; also pancreatitis (less common in children, see also under cautions), liver failure, anaphylactic reactions, peripheral neuropathy (switch to another antiretroviral if peripheral neuropathy develops), diabetes mellitus, hypoglycaemia, acute renal failure, rhabdomyolysis, dry eyes, retinal and optic nerve changes, dry mouth, parotid gland enlargement, sialadenitis, alopecia, hyperuricaemia (suspend if raised significantly)

Licensed use tablets not licensed for use in children under 3 months; EC capsules not licensed for use in children under 6 years

Indication and dose

HIV infection in combination with other antiretroviral drugs

For dose, consult Guidelines (see notes above)

Videx® (Bristol-Myers Squibb) ▣

Tablets, with calcium and magnesium antacids, didanosine 25 mg, net price 60-tab pack = £26.60. Label: 23, counselling, administration, see below
Excipients include aspartame equivalent to phenylalanine 36.5 mg per tablet (section 9.4.1)

Note Antacids in formulation may affect absorption of other drugs—see **interactions**: Appendix 1 (antacids)

Administration to ensure sufficient antacid, each dose to be taken as at least 2 tablets (child under 1 year 1 tablet) chewed thoroughly, crushed or dispersed in water; clear apple juice may be added for flavouring; tablets to be taken 2 hours after lopinavir with ritonavir capsules and oral solution or atazanavir with ritonavir

Videx® EC capsules, enclosing e/c granules, didanosine 125 mg, net price 30-cap pack = £51.15; 200 mg, 30-cap pack = £81.84; 250 mg, 30-cap pack = £102.30; 400 mg, 30-cap pack = £163.68.
Label: 25, counselling, administration, see below

Administration capsules should be swallowed whole and taken at least 2 hours before or 2 hours after food

---

▲ EMTRICITABINE

Cautions see notes above; also on discontinuation, monitor patients with hepatitis B (risk of exacerbation of hepatitis); **interactions**: Appendix 1 (emtricitabine)

Renal impairment reduce dose or increase dosage interval if estimated glomerular filtration rate less than 50 mL/minute/1.73 m²; consult product literature

Pregnancy manufacturer advises use only if essential—no information available

Contra-indications

Breast-feeding avoid (see notes above)

Side-effects see notes above; also abnormal dreams, pruritus, and hyperpigmentation

Licensed use not licensed for use in children under 4 months

Indication and dose

HIV infection in combination with other antiretroviral drugs

For dose, consult Guidelines (see notes above)

Emtriva® (Gilead) ▣

Capsules, white/blue, emtricitabine 200 mg, net price 30-cap pack = £163.50

Oral solution, orange, emtricitabine 10 mg/mL, net price 170-mL pack (candy-flavoured) = £46.50
Electrolytes Na⁺ 460 micromol/mL

Note 240 mg oral solution ≡ 200 mg capsule; where appropriate the capsule may be used instead of the oral solution

◀ **With tenofovir**
See under Tenofovir

◀ **With efavirenz and tenofovir**
See under Tenofovir

▲ LAMIVUDINE
(3TC)

Cautions see notes above; **interactions**: Appendix 1 (lamivudine)

Renal impairment reduce dose if estimated glomerular filtration rate less than 50 mL/minute/1.73 m²; consult product literature

Pregnancy manufacturer advises avoid during first trimester; see also p. 373
Chronic hepatitis B Recurrent hepatitis in patients with chronic hepatitis B may occur on discontinuation of lamivudine. When treating chronic hepatitis B with lamivudine, monitor liver function tests every 3 months, and viral and serological markers of hepatitis B every 3–6 months, more frequently in patients with advanced liver disease or following transplantation (monitoring to continue after discontinuation)—consult product literature

Contra-indications

Breast-feeding avoid (see notes above)

Side-effects see notes above; also peripheral neuropathy, muscle disorders including rhabdomyolysis, nasal symptoms, alopecia

Licensed use *Epivir®* not licensed for use in children under 3 months; *Zeffix®* not licensed for use in children

Indication and dose

See preparations, below

◁ **LAMIVUDINE** *(continued)*

Epivir® (GSK) [PoM]
Tablets, f/c, lamivudine 150 mg (scored, white), net price 60-tab pack = £152.14; 300 mg (grey), 30-tab pack = £167.21

Oral solution, banana- and strawberry-flavoured, lamivudine 50 mg/5 mL, net price 240-mL pack = £41.41
Excipients include sucrose 1 g/5 mL
Dose

> HIV infection in combination with other antiretroviral drugs
>> For dose, consult Guidelines (see notes above)

Zeffix® (GSK) [PoM]
Tablets, brown, f/c, lamivudine 100 mg, net price 28-tab pack = £78.09

Oral solution, banana and strawberry flavoured, lamivudine 25 mg/5 mL, net price 240-mL pack = £22.79
Excipients include propylene glycol, sucrose 1 g/5 mL
Dose

> Chronic hepatitis B infection with *either* compensated liver disease (with evidence of viral replication and histology of active liver inflammation or fibrosis), *or* decompensated liver disease
> • **By mouth**
>> **Child 2–12 years** 3 mg/kg (max. 100 mg) once daily
>> **Child 12–18 years** 100 mg once daily
>> Note Children receiving lamivudine for concomitant HIV infection should continue to receive lamivudine in a dose appropriate for HIV infection

◀**With abacavir**
See under Abacavir

◀**With zidovudine**
See under Zidovudine

◀**With abacavir and zidovudine**
See under Abacavir

◢ STAVUDINE
(d4T)

Cautions see notes above; also history of peripheral neuropathy (see under Side-effects); history of pancreatitis or concomitant use with other drugs associated with pancreatitis; **interactions:** Appendix 1 (stavudine)

> **Renal impairment** reduce dose to 50% if estimated glomerular filtration rate 25–50 mL/minute/1.73 m²; reduce dose to 25% if estimated glomerular filtration rate less than 25 mL/minute/1.73 m²

> **Pregnancy** manufacturer advises use only if potential benefit outweighs risk

Contra-indications

> **Breast-feeding** avoid (see notes above)

Side-effects see notes above; also peripheral neuropathy (switch to another antiretroviral if peripheral neuropathy develops), abnormal dreams, cognitive dysfunction, drowsiness,

depression, pruritus; *less commonly* anxiety, gynaecomastia

Licensed use capsules not licensed for use in children under 3 months

Indication and dose

> HIV infection in combination with other antiretroviral drugs
>> For dose, consult Guidelines (see notes above)

Zerit® (Bristol-Myers Squibb) [PoM]
Capsules, stavudine 20 mg (brown), net price 56-cap pack = £148.05; 30 mg (light orange/dark orange), 56-cap pack = £155.25; 40 mg (dark orange), 56-cap pack = £159.94 (all hosp. only)

Oral solution, cherry-flavoured, stavudine for reconstitution with water, 1 mg/mL, net price 200 mL = £24.35

◢ TENOFOVIR DISOPROXIL

Cautions see notes above; also test renal function and serum phosphate before treatment, then every 4 weeks (more frequently if at increased risk of renal impairment) for 1 year and then every 3 months, interrupt treatment if renal function deteriorates or serum phosphate decreases; concomitant or recent use of nephrotoxic drugs; on discontinuation, monitor patients with hepatitis B (risk of exacerbation of hepatitis); **interactions:** Appendix 1 (tenofovir)

> **Renal impairment** increase dose interval if estimated glomerular filtration rate less than 50 mL/minute/1.73 m²; avoid *Atripla®* if estimated glomerular filtration rate less than 50 mL/minute/1.73 m²; avoid *Truvada®* if estimated glomerular filtration rate less than 30 mL/minute/1.73 m²

> **Pregnancy** manufacturer advises use only if potential benefit outweighs risk—no information available

Contra-indications

> **Breast-feeding** avoid (see notes above)

Side-effects see notes above; also hypophosphataemia; *rarely* renal failure; also reported nephrogenic diabetes insipidus, reduced bone density, hypokalaemia, myopathy, and rhabdomyolysis

Licensed use not licensed for use in children

5

Infections

◁ TENOFOVIR DISOPROXIL (*continued*)

Indication and dose

> HIV infection in combination with other antiretroviral drugs
>
> For dose, consult Guidelines (see notes above)

Viread® (Gilead) ▼ PoM

Tablets, f/c, blue, tenofovir disoproxil (as fumarate) 245 mg, net price 30-tab pack = £255.00. Label: 21, counselling, administration

Counselling Children with swallowing difficulties may disperse tablet in half a glass of water, orange juice, or grape juice (but bitter taste)

◢With emtricitabine

For **cautions**, **contra-indications**, and **side-effects** see under individual drugs

Truvada® (Gilead) PoM

Tablets, blue, f/c, tenofovir disoproxil (as fumarate) 245 mg, emtricitabine 200 mg, net price 30-tab pack = £418.50. Label: 21, Counselling, administration

Children with swallowing difficulties may disperse tablet in half a glass of water, orange juice, or grape juice (but bitter taste)

◢With efavirenz and emtricitabine

For **cautions**, **contra-indications**, and **side-effects** see under individual drugs

Atripla® (Gilead) PoM

Tablets, pink, f/c, efavirenz 600 mg, emtricitabine 200 mg, tenofovir disoproxil (as fumarate) 245 mg, net price 30-tab pack = £626.90. Label: 23, 25

▮ ZIDOVUDINE
(Azidothymidine, AZT)

Note The abbreviation AZT which is sometimes used for zidovudine has also been used for another drug

Cautions see notes above; also haematological toxicity particularly with high dose and advanced disease—monitor full blood count after 4 weeks of treatment, then every 3 months; vitamin B_{12} deficiency (increased risk of neutropenia); if anaemia or myelosuppression occur, reduce dose or interrupt treatment according to product literature, or consider other treatment; **interactions**: Appendix 1 (zidovudine)

Hepatic impairment accumulation may occur

Renal impairment reduce dose if estimated glomerular filtration rate less than 10 mL/minute/ 1.73 m^2; consult product literature

Pregnancy limited information available; manufacturer advises use only if clearly indicated; see also p. 373

Contra-indications abnormally low neutrophil count or haemoglobin concentration (consult product literature); neonates with hyperbilirubinaemia requiring treatment other than phototherapy, or with raised transaminase (consult product literature); acute porphyria (section 9.8.2)

Breast-feeding avoid (see notes above)

Side-effects see notes above; also anaemia (may require transfusion), taste disturbance, chest pain, influenza-like symptoms, paraesthesia, neuropathy, convulsions, dizziness, drowsiness, anxiety, depression, loss of mental acuity, myopathy, gynaecomastia, urinary frequency, sweating, pruritus, pigmentation of nails, skin and oral mucosa

Licensed use *Combivir®* is not licensed for use in children with body-weight under 14 kg

Indication and dose

> HIV infection in combination with other antiretroviral drugs; prevention of maternal-fetal HIV transmission
>
> For dose, consult Guidelines (see notes above including Prevention of Transmission to Neonate)

Administration for *intermittent intravenous infusion*, dilute to a concentration of 2 mg/mL or 4 mg/mL with Glucose 5% and give over 1 hour.

For administration *by mouth*, *Combivir®* tablets may be crushed and mixed with semi-solid food or liquid just before administration

Retrovir® (GSK) PoM

Capsules, zidovudine 100 mg (white/blue band), net price 100-cap pack = £110.98; 250 mg (blue/white/dark blue band), 40-cap pack = £110.98

Oral solution, sugar-free, strawberry-flavoured, zidovudine 50 mg/5 mL, net price 200-mL pack with 10-mL oral syringe = £22.20

Injection, zidovudine 10 mg/mL. For dilution and use as an intravenous infusion. Net price 20-mL vial = £11.14

◢With lamivudine

For **cautions**, **contra-indications**, and **side-effects** see under individual drugs

Combivir® (GSK) PoM

Tablets, f/c, zidovudine 300 mg, lamivudine 150 mg, net price 60-tab pack = £318.60

◢With abacavir and lamivudine

See under Abacavir

▮ Protease inhibitors

Cautions Protease inhibitors should be used with caution in diabetes (see also Lipodystrophy Syndrome, p. 374). Caution is also needed in children with haemophilia who may be at increased risk of bleeding and in hepatic impairment; the risk of hepatic side-effects is increased in children with chronic hepatitis B or C. Atazanavir, darunavir, fosamprenavir, and tipranavir may be used at usual doses in children with renal impairment, but other protease inhibitors should be used with caution in renal impairment. Indinavir is rarely used in children because of the risk of nephrolithiasis. Protease inhibitors should also be used with caution during pregnancy.

Contra-indications Protease inhibitors should not be given to patients with acute porphyria (section 9.8.2) or to women who are breast-feeding (see also Breast-feeding, p. 373).

Side-effects Side-effects of the protease inhibitors include gastro-intestinal disturbances (including diarrhoea, nausea, vomiting, abdominal pain, flatulence), anorexia, hepatic dysfunction, pancreatitis; blood disorders including anaemia, neutropenia, and thrombocytopenia; sleep disturbances, fatigue, headache, dizziness, paraesthesia, myalgia, myositis, rhabdomyolysis; taste disturbances; rash, pruritus, Stevens-Johnson syndrome, hypersensitivity reactions including anaphylaxis; see also Lipodystrophy Syndrome (p. 374) and Osteonecrosis (p. 374).

ATAZANAVIR

Cautions see notes above; concomitant use with drugs that prolong PR interval; cardiac conduction disorders; predisposition to QT interval prolongation (including electrolyte disturbances, concomitant use of drugs that prolong QT interval); **interactions:** Appendix 1 (atazanavir)

Hepatic impairment use with caution in mild impairment; avoid in moderate to severe impairment

Pregnancy manufacturer advises use only if potential benefit outweighs risk; theoretical risk of hyperbilirubinaemia in neonate if used at term

Contra-indications see notes above

Side-effects see notes above; also peripheral neurological symptoms; *less commonly* mouth ulcers, hypertension, syncope, chest pain, dyspnoea, abnormal dreams, amnesia, disorientation, depression, anxiety, weight changes, increased appetite, gynaecomastia, nephrolithiasis, urinary frequency, haematuria, proteinuria, arthralgia, and alopecia; *rarely* hepatosplenomegaly, oedema, palpitation, and abnormal gait; also reported cholelithiasis, cholecystitis, and torsade de pointes

Licensed use not licensed for use in children

Indication and dose

HIV infection in combination with other antiretroviral drugs

For dose, consult Guidelines (see notes above)

Reyataz® (Bristol-Myers Squibb) PoM
Capsules, atazanavir (as sulphate) 150 mg (dark blue/light blue), net price 60-cap pack = £315.69; 200 mg (dark blue), 60-cap pack = £315.69; 300 mg (red/blue), 30-cap pack = £315.69. Label: 5, 21

DARUNAVIR

Cautions see notes above; also sulphonamide sensitivity; **interactions:** Appendix 1 (daruanvir)

Hepatic impairment use with caution in mild to moderate hepatic impairment; avoid in severe hepatic impairment—no information available

Pregnancy manufacturer advises use only if potential benefit outweighs risk—no information available

Contra-indications see notes above

Side-effects see notes above; also haematemesis, myocardial infarction, chest pain, QT interval prolongation, syncope, tachycardia, bradycardia, palpitation, hypertension, flushing, peripheral oedema, dyspnoea, cough, peripheral neuropathy, anxiety, confusion, memory impairment, convulsions, depression, abnormal dreams, weight changes, pyrexia, hypothyroidism, osteoporosis, gynaecomastia, erectile dysfunction, reduced libido, dysuria, polyuria, nephrolithiasis, renal failure, arthralgia, visual disturbances, conjunctival hyperaemia, epistaxis, rhinorrhoea, throat irritation, dry mouth, mouth ulcers, stomatitis, nail discoloration, acne, seborrhoeic dermatitis, xeroderma, increased sweating, and alopecia

Licensed use not licensed for use in children

Indication and dose

In combination with other antiretroviral drugs, for HIV infection resistant to other protease inhibitors

For dose, consult Guidelines (see notes above)

Prezista® (Janssen-Cilag) ▼ PoM
Tablets, f/c, darunavir (as ethanolate) 300 mg (orange), net price 120-tab pack = £446.70; 400 mg (light orange), 60-tab pack = £297.80; 600 mg (orange), 60-tab pack = £446.70. Label: 21

FOSAMPRENAVIR

Note Fosamprenavir is a pro-drug of amprenavir

Cautions see notes above; **interactions**: Appendix 1 (fosamprenavir)

Hepatic impairment Manufacturer advises caution in mild hepatic impairment; reduce dose in moderate to severe hepatic impairment

Pregnancy Toxicity in *animal* studies; manufacturer advises use only if potential benefit outweighs risk

Rash Rash may occur, usually in the second week of therapy; discontinue permanently if severe rash with systemic or allergic symptoms or, mucosal involvement; if rash mild or moderate, may continue without interruption—rash usually resolves within 2 weeks and may respond to antihistamines

Contra-indications see notes above

Side-effects see notes above; also reported, rash including rarely Stevens-Johnson syndrome (see also Rash above)

Licensed use not licensed for use in children under 6 years and body-weight under 25 kg

Indication and dose

HIV infection in combination with other antiretroviral drugs

For dose, consult Guidelines (see notes above)

Note 700 mg fosamprenavir is equivalent to approx. 600 mg amprenavir

Telzir® (GSK) PoM

Tablets, f/c, pink, fosamprenavir (as calcium) 700 mg, net price 60-tab pack = £274.92

Oral suspension, fosamprenavir (as calcium) 50 mg/mL, net price 225-mL pack (grape-bubblegum-and peppermint-flavoured) (with 10-mL oral syringe) = £73.31. Counselling, administration

Excipients include propylene glycol

Administration In children, oral suspension should be taken with food

INDINAVIR

Cautions see notes above; ensure adequate hydration (risk of nephrolithiasis); children at risk of nephrolithiasis (monitor for nephrolithiasis); **interactions:** Appendix 1 (indinavir)

Hepatic impairment increased risk of nephrolithiasis; reduce dose in mild to moderate impairment; not studied in severe impairment

Pregnancy toxicity in *animal* studies, manufacturer advises use only if potential benefit outweighs risk; theoretical risk of hyperbilirubinaemia and renal stones in neonate if used at term

Contra-indications see notes above; also contra-indicated in neonates (risk of hyperbilirubinaemia)

Side-effects see notes above; also reported, dry mouth, hypoaesthesia, dry skin, hyperpigmentation, alopecia, paronychia, interstitial nephritis (with medullary calcification and cortical atrophy in asymptomatic severe leucocyturia), nephrolithiasis (may require interruption or discontinuation), dysuria, haematuria, crystalluria, proteinuria, pyuria, pyelonephritis; haemolytic anaemia

Licensed use not licensed for use in children under 4 years

Indication and dose

HIV infection in combination with nucleoside reverse transcriptase inhibitors

For dose, consult Guidelines (see notes above)

Crixivan® (MSD) PoM

Capsules, indinavir (as sulphate), 200 mg, net price 360-cap pack = £226.28; 400 mg, 180-cap pack = £226.28. Label: 27, counselling, administration

Counselling Administer 1 hour before or 2 hours after a meal; may be administered with a low-fat light meal (may be mixed with apple sauce); in combination with didanosine tablets, allow 1 hour between each drug (antacids in didanosine tablets reduce absorption of indinavir); in combination with low-dose ritonavir, give with food

Note Dispense in original container (contains desiccant)

LOPINAVIR WITH RITONAVIR

Cautions see notes above; concomitant use with drugs that prolong QT or PR interval; cardiac conduction disorders, structural heart disease; pancreatitis (see below); **interactions**: Appendix 1 (lopinavir, ritonavir)

Hepatic impairment avoid oral solution—high propylene glycol content; manufacturer advises avoid capsules and tablets in severe impairment

Renal impairment avoid oral solution due to high propylene glycol content; use tablets with caution in severe renal impairment

Pregnancy avoid oral solution due to high propylene glycol content; manufacturer advises use capsules and tablets only if potential benefit outweighs risk (toxicity in *animal* studies)

Pancreatitis Signs and symptoms suggestive of pancreatitis (including raised serum lipase) should be evaluated—discontinue if pancreatitis diagnosed

Contra-indications see notes above

Side-effects see notes and Cautions above; also electrolyte disturbances; *less commonly* dysphagia, appetite changes, weight changes, cholecystitis, hypertension, myocardial infarction, palpitation, thrombophlebitis, vasculitis, chest pain, oedema, dyspnoea, cough, agitation, anxiety, amnesia, ataxia, hypertonia, confusion, depression, abnormal dreams, extrapyramidal effects, neuropathy, influenza-like syndrome, Cushing's syndrome, hypothyroidism, menorrhagia, amenorrhoea, sexual dysfunction, breast enlargement, dehydration, nephritis, hypercalciuria, lactic acidosis, arthralgia, hyperuricaemia, abnormal vision, otitis media, tinnitus, dry mouth, sialadenitis, mouth ulceration, peridontitis, acne, alopecia, dry skin, sweating, skin discoloration, nail disorders; *rarely* prolonged PR interval

5 Infections

◁ **LOPINAVIR WITH RITONAVIR (continued)**

Licensed use not licensed for use in children under 2 years

Indication and dose

HIV infection in combination with other antiretroviral drugs

For dose, consult Guidelines (see notes above)

Kaletra® (Abbott) PoM

Tablets, pale yellow, f/c, lopinavir 100 mg, ritonavir 25 mg, net price 60-tab pack = £76.85. Label: 25

Tablets, yellow, f/c, lopinavir 200 mg, ritonavir 50 mg, net price 120-tab pack = £307.39. Label: 25

Oral solution, lopinavir 400 mg, ritonavir 100 mg/ 5 mL, net price 5 × 60-mL packs = £307.39. Label: 21
Excipients include propylene glycol 153 mg/mL (see Excipients, p. 3), alcohol 42%

Counselling Oral solution tastes bitter

NELFINAVIR

Cautions see notes above; **interactions:** Appendix 1 (nelfinavir)

Hepatic impairment manufacturer advises caution—no information available

Renal impairment manufacturer advises caution—no information available

Pregnancy manufacturer advises use only if potential benefit outweighs risk—no information available

Contra-indications see notes above

Side-effects see notes above; also reported, fever

Licensed use not licensed for use in children under 3 years

Indication and dose

HIV infection in combination with other antiretroviral drugs

For dose, consult Guidelines (see notes above)

Viracept® (Roche) PoM

Tablets, blue, f/c, nelfinavir (as mesilate) 250 mg, net price 300-tab pack = £273.16. Label: 21

RITONAVIR

Cautions see notes above; concomitant use with drugs that prolong PR interval; cardiac conduction disorders, structural heart disease; pancreatitis (see below); **interactions:** Appendix 1 (ritonavir)

Hepatic impairment avoid in decompensated liver disease; in severe hepatic impairment without decompensation, use 'booster' doses with caution (avoid treatment doses)

Pregnancy manufacturer advises use only if potential benefit outweighs risk—toxicity in *animal* studies

Pancreatitis Signs and symptoms suggestive of pancreatitis (including raised serum lipase) should be evaluated—discontinue if pancreatitis diagnosed

Contra-indications see notes above

Side-effects see notes and Cautions above; also diarrhoea (may impair absorption—close monitoring required), vasodilatation, cough, throat irritation, anxiety, perioral and peripheral paraesthesia, hyperaesthesia, fever, decreased blood-thyroxine concentration, electrolyte disturbances, raised uric acid, dry mouth, mouth ulcers, and sweating; *less commonly* increased prothrombin time and dehydration; syncope, postural hypotension, seizures, menorrhagia, and renal failure also reported

Licensed use not licensed for use in children under 2 years

Indication and dose

HIV infection in combination with other antiretroviral drugs; low doses used to increase effect of some protease inhibitors

For dose, consult Guidelines (see notes above)

Norvir® (Abbott) PoM

Capsules, ritonavir 100 mg, net price 84-cap pack = £94.35. Label 21
Excipients include alcohol 12%

Oral solution, sugar-free, ritonavir 400 mg/5 mL, net price 5 × 90-mL packs (with measuring cup) = £403.20. Label: 21, counselling, administration
Excipients include alcohol, propylene glycol

Counselling Oral solution contains 43% alcohol; bitter taste can be masked by mixing with chocolate milk; do not mix with water, measuring cup must be dry
Administration of ritonavir and didanosine should be separated by at least 2 hours

◀With lopinavir
See under Lopinavir with ritonavir

SAQUINAVIR

Cautions see notes above; concomitant use of garlic (avoid garlic capsules—reduces plasma-saquinavir concentration); **interactions:** Appendix 1 (saquinavir)

Hepatic impairment manufacturer advises caution in moderate impairment; avoid in severe impairment

Renal impairment dose adjustment possibly required if estimated glomerular filtration rate less than 30 mL/minute/1.73 m^2

Pregnancy manufacturer advises use only if potential benefit outweighs risk

Contra-indications see notes above

◁ SAQUINAVIR *(continued)*

Side-effects see notes above; also dyspnoea, increased appetite, peripheral neuropathy, convulsions, changes in libido, renal impairment, dry mouth, and alopecia

Licensed use not licensed for use in children under 16 years

Indication and dose

> HIV infection in combination with other antiretroviral drugs
>
> > For dose, consult Guidelines (see notes above)

Invirase® (Roche) ℞

> Capsules, brown/green, saquinavir (as mesilate) 200 mg, net price 270-cap pack = £240.06. Label: 21

> Tablets, orange, f/c, saquinavir (as mesilate) 500 mg, net price 120-tab pack = £266.73. Label: 21

TIPRANAVIR

Cautions see notes above; also patients at risk of increased bleeding from trauma, surgery, or other pathological conditions; concomitant use of drugs that increase risk of bleeding; **interactions:** Appendix 1 (tipranavir)

Hepatotoxicity Potentially life-threatening hepatotoxicity reported; monitor liver function before treatment then every 2 weeks for 1 month, then every 3 months. Discontinue if signs or symptoms of hepatitis develop or if liver-function abnormality develops (consult product literature)

Hepatic impairment monitor liver function in mild hepatic impairment; avoid in moderate or severe hepatic impairment—no information available

Pregnancy manufacturer advises use only if potential benefit outweighs risk—toxicity in *animal* studies

Contra-indications see notes above

Side-effects see notes above; also dyspnoea, anorexia, peripheral neuropathy, influenza-like symptoms, renal impairment, and photosensitivity; *rarely* dehydration

Licensed use not licensed for use in children

Indication and dose

> HIV infection resistant to other protease inhibitors, in combination with other antiretroviral drugs in children previously treated with antiretrovirals
>
> > For dose, consult Guidelines (see notes above)

Aptivus® (Boehringer Ingelheim) ▼ ℞

> Capsules, pink, tipranavir 250 mg, net price 120-cap pack = £490.00. Label: 5, 21
> Excipients include ethanol 100 mg per capsule

Non-nucleoside reverse transcriptase inhibitors

EFAVIRENZ

Cautions chronic hepatitis B or C (greater risk of hepatic side-effects); history of mental illness or seizures; **interactions:** Appendix 1 (efavirenz)

Hepatic impairment in mild to moderate liver disease, monitor for dose-related side-effects (e.g. CNS effects) and liver function; avoid in severe hepatic impairment

Renal impairment manufacturer advises caution in severe renal failure—no information available

Pregnancy manufacturer advises avoid unless no alternative available

Rash Rash, usually in the first 2 weeks, is the most common side-effect; discontinue if severe rash with blistering, desquamation, mucosal involvement or fever; if rash mild or moderate, may continue without interruption—rash usually resolves within 1 month

Psychiatric disorders Children or their carers should be advised to seek immediate medical attention if symptoms such as severe depression, psychosis or suicidal ideation occur

Contra-indications acute porphyria (section 9.8.2)

Breast-feeding avoid (see p. 373)

Side-effects rash including Stevens-Johnson syndrome (see Rash above); abdominal pain, diarrhoea, nausea, vomiting; anxiety, depression, sleep disturbances, abnormal dreams, dizziness, headache, fatigue, impaired concentration

(administration at bedtime especially in first 2–4 weeks reduces CNS effects); pruritus; *less commonly* pancreatitis, hepatitis, psychosis, mania, suicidal ideation, amnesia, ataxia, convulsions, and blurred vision; also reported hepatic failure, raised serum cholesterol (see Lipodystrophy syndrome, p. 374), gynaecomastia, photosensitivity; see also Osteonecrosis, p. 374

Licensed use capsules and oral solution not licensed for use in children under 3 years and body-weight under 13 kg; tablets not licensed for use in children with body-weight under 40 kg

Indication and dose

> HIV infection in combination with other antiretroviral drugs
>
> > For dose, consult Guidelines (see notes above)

Sustiva® (Bristol-Myers Squibb) ℞

> Capsules, efavirenz 50 mg (yellow/white), net price 30-cap pack = £17.41; 200 mg (yellow), 90-cap pack = £208.40. Label: 23
> Administration Capsules may be opened and contents added to food (contents have a peppery taste) [unlicensed use]

> Tablets, f/c, yellow, efavirenz 600 mg, net price 30-tab pack = £208.40. Label: 23

5 Infections

⌐ **EFAVIRENZ** (*continued*)

Oral solution, sugar-free, strawberry and mint flavour, efavirenz 30 mg/mL, net price 180-mL pack = £56.02

Note The bioavailability of *Sustiva*® oral solution is lower than that of the capsules and tablets; the oral solution is **not** interchangeable with either capsules or tablets on a milligram-for-milligram basis

◢With emtricitabine and tenofovir
See under Tenofovir

ETRAVIRINE

Cautions chronic hepatitis B or C (greater risk of hepatic side-effects); **interactions:** Appendix 1 (etravirine)

Hepatic impairment use with caution in moderate hepatic impairment; avoid in severe hepatic impairment—no information available

Pregnancy manufacturer advises use only if potential benefit outweighs risk

Rash Rash, usually in the second week, is the most common side-effect and appears more frequently in females; discontinue if severe rash; if rash mild or moderate, may continue without interruption—rash usually resolves within 2 weeks

Contra-indications acute porphyria (section 9.8.2)

Breast-feeding avoid (see p. 373)

Side-effects rash (rarely including Stevens-Johnson syndrome; see also Rash above); gastro-oesophageal reflux, nausea, vomiting, abdominal pain, flatulence, gastritis; hypertension; peripheral neuropathy; diabetes, hyperlipidaemia (see also Lipodystrophy Syndrome, p. 374); renal failure; thrombocytopenia; *less commonly* pancreatitis, haematemesis, stomatitis, hepatitis, myo-

cardial infarction, angina, atrial fibrillation, syncope, bronchospasm, amnesia, sleep disturbances, abnormal dreams, anxiety, gynaecomastia, blurred vision, dry mouth, and sweating; also reported, haemorrhagic stroke; see also Osteonecrosis, p. 374

Licensed use not licensed for use in children

Indication and dose

In combination with other antiretroviral drugs (including a boosted protease inhibitor) for HIV infection resistant to other non-nucleoside reverse transcriptase inhibitors and protease inhibitors

For dose, consult Guidelines (see notes above)

Administration for children with swallowing difficulties, tablets may be dispersed in a glass of water just before administration

Intelence® (Janssen-Cilag) ▼ PoM
Tablets, etravirine 100 mg, net price 120-tab pack = £319.82. Label: 21
Note Dispense in original container (contains desiccant)

NEVIRAPINE

Cautions chronic hepatitis B or C, high CD4 cell count, and females (all at greater risk of hepatic side-effects); **interactions:** Appendix 1 (nevirapine)

Hepatic impairment manufacturer advises caution in moderate hepatic impairment; avoid in severe hepatic impairment; see also Hepatic Disease, below

Pregnancy although manufacturers advise avoid, may be appropriate to use if clearly indicated; see also p. 373

Hepatic disease Potentially life-threatening hepatotoxicity including fatal fulminant hepatitis reported usually in first 6 weeks; close monitoring required during first 18 weeks; monitor liver function before treatment then every 2 weeks for 2 months then after 1 month and then regularly; discontinue permanently if abnormalities in liver function tests accompanied by hypersensitivity reaction (rash, fever, arthralgia, myalgia, lymphadenopathy, hepatitis, renal impairment, eosinophilia, granulocytopenia); suspend if severe abnormalities in liver function tests but no hypersensitivity reaction—discontinue permanently if significant liver function abnormalities recur; monitor patient closely if mild to moderate abnormalities in liver function tests with no hypersensitivity reaction

Rash Rash, usually in first 6 weeks, is most common side-effect; incidence reduced if introduced at low dose and dose increased gradually; monitor closely for skin reactions during first 18 weeks; discontinue permanently if severe rash or if rash accompanied by blistering, oral lesions, conjunctivitis, facial oedema, general malaise or hypersensitivity reactions; if rash mild or moderate may

continue without interruption but dose should not be increased until rash resolves

Counselling Children and carers should be told how to recognise hypersensitivity reactions and advised to discontinue treatment and seek immediate medical attention if severe skin reaction, hypersensitivity reactions or symptoms of hepatitis develop

Contra-indications acute porphyria (section 9.8.2); severe hepatic impairment; post-exposure prophylaxis

Breast-feeding avoid (see p. 373)

Side-effects rash including Stevens-Johnson syndrome and rarely, toxic epidermal necrolysis (see also Cautions above); nausea, hepatitis (see also Hepatic Disease above), headache; *less commonly* vomiting, abdominal pain, fatigue, fever, and myalgia; *rarely* diarrhoea, angioedema, anaphylaxis, hypersensitivity reactions (may involve hepatic reactions and rash, see Hepatic Disease above), arthralgia, anaemia, and granulocytopenia; *very rarely* neuropsychiatric reactions; see also Osteonecrosis, p. 374

Licensed use tablets, not licensed for use in children weighing less than 50 kg or with body surface area less than 1.25 m^2

5
Infections

◁ **NEVIRAPINE** *(continued)*

Indication and dose

> HIV infection in combination with other antiretroviral drugs
>
> For dose, consult Guidelines (see notes above)
>
> Note If treatment interrupted for more than 7 days reintroduce using low dose and increase dose cautiously

Viramune® (Boehringer Ingelheim) PoM
Tablets, nevirapine 200 mg, net price 60-tab pack = £160.00. Counselling, hypersensitivity reactions

Suspension, nevirapine 50 mg/5 mL, net price 240-mL pack = £50.40. Counselling, hypersensitivity reactions

---

Other antiretrovirals

ENFUVIRTIDE

Cautions chronic hepatitis B or C (possibly greater risk of hepatic side-effects)

Hepatic impairment manufacturer advises caution—no information available

Pregnancy manufacturer advises avoid

Hypersensitivity reactions Hypersensitivity reactions including rash, fever, nausea, vomiting, chills, rigors, low blood pressure, respiratory distress, glomerulonephritis, and raised liver enzymes reported; discontinue immediately if any signs or symptoms of systemic hypersensitivity develop and do not rechallenge

Counselling Children and carers should be told how to recognise signs of hypersensitivity, and advised to discontinue treatment and seek prompt medical attention if symptoms develop

Contra-indications

Breast-feeding avoid (see p. 373)

Side-effects injection-site reactions; pancreatitis, gastro-oesophageal reflux disease, anorexia, weight loss; hypertriglyceridaemia; peripheral neuropathy, asthenia, tremor, anxiety, nightmares, irritability, impaired concentration, vertigo; pneumonia, sinusitis, influenza-like illness; diabetes mellitus; haematuria; renal calculi, lymphadenopathy; myalgia; conjunctivitis; dry skin, acne, erythema, skin papilloma; *less commonly* hypersensitivity reactions (see Cautions); see also Osteonecrosis, p. 374

Licensed use not licensed for use in children under 6 years

Indication and dose

> HIV infection in combination with other antiretroviral drugs for resistant infection or for children intolerant to other antiretroviral regimens
>
> For dose, consult Guidelines (see notes above)

Administration for *subcutaneous injection*, reconstitute with 1.1 mL Water for Injections and allow to stand (for up to 45 minutes) to dissolve; do **not** shake or invert vial

Fuzeon® (Roche) PoM
Injection, powder for reconstitution, enfuvirtide 108 mg (= enfuvirtide 90 mg/mL when reconstituted with 1.1 mL Water for Injections), net price 108-mg vial = £19.13 (with solvent, syringe, and alcohol swabs). Counselling, hypersensitivity reactions

MARAVIROC

Cautions cardiovascular disease; chronic hepatitis B or C; **interactions:** Appendix 1 (maraviroc)

Hepatic impairment use with caution

Renal impairment if estimated glomerular filtration rate less than 80 mL/minute/1.73 m², consult product literature

Pregnancy manufacturer advises use only if potential benefit outweighs risk—toxicity in *animal* studies

Contra-indications

Breast-feeding avoid (see notes above, p. 373)

Side-effects nausea, vomiting, abdominal pain, dyspepsia, constipation, diarrhoea; cough; dizziness, paraesthesia, asthenia, sleep disturbances, headache, weight loss; muscle spasms, back pain; taste disturbances; rash, pruritus; *less commonly* pancreatitis, hepatic cirrhosis, rectal bleeding, myocardial infarction, myocardial ischaemia, bronchospasm, seizures, hallucinations, loss of consciousness, polyneuropathy, pancytopenia, neutropenia, lymphadenopathy, renal failure, polyuria, and myositis; see also Osteonecrosis, p. 374

Licensed use not licensed for use in children

Indication and dose

> CCR5–tropic HIV infection in combination with other antiretroviral drugs in children previously treated with antiretrovirals
>
> For dose, consult Guidelines (see notes above)

Celsentri® (Pfizer) ▼ PoM
Tablets, blue, f/c, maraviroc 150 mg, net price 60-tab pack = £551.10; 300 mg, 60-tab pack = £551.10

RALTEGRAVIR

Cautions risk factors for myopathy or rhabdomyolysis; chronic hepatitis B or C (greater risk of hepatic side-effects); **interactions:** Appendix 1 (raltegravir)

Hepatic impairment use with caution in severe hepatic impairment—no information available

Pregnancy manufacturer advises avoid—toxicity in *animal* studies

◻ **RALTEGRAVIR** (*continued*)

Contra-indications

Breast-feeding avoid see p. 373

Side-effects abdominal pain, flatulence, constipation, lipodystrophy (see Lipodystrophy Syndrome, p. 374); dizziness, asthenia; arthralgia; pruritis, hyperhidrosis; *less commonly* vomiting, gastritis, hepatitis, myocardial infarction, hypertriglyceridaemia, allodynia, headache, renal failure, anaemia, neutropenia, and muscle spasm; *also reported* rash (including Stevens-Johnson syndrome): see also Osteonecrosis, p. 374

Licensed use not licensed for use in children under 16 years

Indication and dose

In combination with other antiretroviral drugs for HIV infection resistant to multiple antiretrovirals

For dose, consult Guidelines (see notes above)

Isentress® (MSD) ▼ PoM

Tablets, pink, f/c, raltegravir (as potassium salt) 400 mg, net price 60-tab pack = £647.29. Label: 25

5.3.2 Herpesvirus infections

5.3.2.1 Herpes simplex and varicella–zoster infection

5.3.2.2 Cytomegalovirus infection

5.3.2.1 Herpes simplex and varicella–zoster infection

The two most important herpesvirus pathogens are herpes simplex virus (herpesvirus hominis) and varicella–zoster virus.

Herpes simplex infections Herpes infection of the mouth and lips and in the eye is generally associated with herpes simplex virus serotype 1 (HSV-1); other areas of the skin may also be infected, especially in immunodeficiency. Genital infection is most often associated with HSV-2 and also HSV-1. Treatment of herpes simplex infection should start as early as possible and usually within 5 days of the appearance of the infection.

In individuals with good immune function, mild infection of the eye (ocular herpes, section 11.3.3) and of the lips (herpes labialis or cold sores, section 13.10.3) is treated with a topical antiviral drug. Primary herpetic gingivostomatitis is managed by changes to diet and with analgesics (section 12.3.2). Severe infection, neonatal herpes infection or infection in immunocompromised individuals requires treatment with a systemic antiviral drug. Primary or recurrent genital herpes simplex infection is treated with an antiviral drug given by mouth. Persistance of a lesion or recurrence in an immunocompromised child may signal the development of resistance.

Specialist advice should be sought for systemic treatment of herpes simplex infection in pregnancy.

Varicella–zoster infections Regardless of immune function and the use of any immunoglobulins, neonates with *chickenpox* should be treated with a parenteral antiviral to reduce the risk of severe disease. Oral therapy is not recommended as absorption is variable.

Chickenpox in otherwise healthy children between 1 month and 12 years is usually mild and antiviral treatment is not usually required. Chickenpox is more severe in adolescents than in children; antiviral treatment started within 24 hours of the onset of rash may reduce the duration and severity of symptoms in otherwise healthy adolescents. Antiviral treatment is generally recommended in immunocompromised patients and those at special risk (e.g. because of severe cardiovascular or respiratory disease or chronic skin disorder); in such cases, an antiviral is given for 10 days with at least 7 days of parenteral treatment.

In pregnancy severe chickenpox may cause complications, especially varicella pneumonia. Specialist advice should be sought for the treatment of chickenpox during pregnancy.

Neonates and children who have been exposed to chickenpox and are at special risk of complications may require prophylaxis with varicella-zoster immunoglobulin (see under Specific Immunoglobulins, section 14.5).

In *herpes zoster* (shingles) systemic antiviral treatment can reduce the severity and duration of pain, reduce complications, and reduce viral shedding. Treatment with the antiviral should be started within 72 hours of the onset of rash and is usually continued for 7–10 days. Immunocompromised patients at high risk of disseminated or severe infection should be treated with a parenteral antiviral drug. Chronic pain which persists after the rash has healed (postherpetic neuralgia) requires specific management (section 4.7.3).

Choice **Aciclovir** is active against herpesviruses but does not eradicate them. Uses of aciclovir include systemic treatment of varicella–zoster and the systemic and topical treatment of herpes simplex infections of the skin (section 13.10.3) and mucous membranes (section 7.2.2). It is used by mouth for severe herpetic stomatitis (see also p. 657). Aciclovir eye ointment (section 11.3.3) is used for herpes simplex infections of the eye; it is combined with systemic treatment for ophthalmic zoster.

Famciclovir, a prodrug of penciclovir, is similar to aciclovir and is licensed in adults for use in herpes zoster and genital herpes; there is limited information available on use in children. Penciclovir itself is used as a cream for herpes simplex labialis (section 13.10.3).

Valaciclovir is an ester of aciclovir, licensed in adults for herpes zoster and herpes simplex infections of the skin and mucous membranes (including genital herpes); it is also licensed in children over 12 years for preventing cytomegalovirus disease following renal transplantation. Valaciclovir may be used for the treatment of mild herpes zoster in immunocompromised children over 12 years; treatment should be initiated under specialist supervision. Valaciclovir once daily may reduce the risk of transmitting genital herpes to heterosexual partners—specialist advice should be sought.

5 Infections

ACICLOVIR
(Acyclovir)

Cautions maintain adequate hydration (especially with infusion or high doses, or during renal impairment); **interactions:** Appendix 1 (aciclovir)

Renal impairment risk of neurological reactions increased; use normal *intravenous* dose every 12 hours if estimated glomerular filtration rate 25–50 mL/minute/1.73 m² (every 24 hours if estimated glomerular filtration rate 10–25 mL/minute/1.73 m²); consult product literature for intravenous dose if estimated glomerular filtration rate less than 10 mL/minute/1.73 m². For *herpes zoster*, use normal oral dose every 8 hours if estimated glomerular filtration rate 10–25 mL/minute/1.73 m² (every 12 hours if estimated glomerular filtration rate less than 10 mL/minute/1.73 m²). For *herpes simplex*, use normal oral dose every 12 hours if estimated glomerular filtration rate less than 10 mL/minute/1.73 m²

Pregnancy not known to be harmful but manufacturers advise avoid unless potential benefit outweighs risk; limited absorption from topical preparations

Breast-feeding significant amount in milk after systemic administration; not known to be harmful but manufacturers advise caution

Side-effects nausea, vomiting, abdominal pain, diarrhoea, headache, fatigue, rash, urticaria, pruritus, photosensitivity; *very rarely* hepatitis, jaundice, dyspnoea, neurological reactions (including dizziness, confusion, hallucinations, convulsions, ataxia, dysarthria, and drowsiness), acute renal failure, anaemia, thrombocytopenia, and leucopenia; on *intravenous infusion*, severe local inflammation (sometimes leading to ulceration), and *very rarely* agitation, tremors, psychosis and fever

Licensed use tablets and suspension not licensed for treatment of herpes zoster in children (age range not specified by manufacturer); intravenous infusion not licensed for herpes zoster in children under 18 years; tablets and suspension not licensed for attenuation of chickenpox (if varicella-zoster immunoglobulin not indicated) in children under 18 years

Indication and dose

Herpes simplex treatment

- **By mouth**

   Child 1 month–2 years 100 mg 5 times daily, usually for 5 days (longer if new lesions appear during treatment or if healing incomplete); dose doubled if immunocompromised or if absorption impaired

   Child 2–18 years 200 mg 5 times daily, usually for 5 days (longer if new lesions appear during treatment or if healing incomplete); dose doubled if immunocompromised or if absorption impaired

- **By intravenous infusion**

   Neonate 20 mg/kg every 8 hours for 14 days (21 days if CNS involvement)

   Child 1–3 months with disseminated herpes simplex 20 mg/kg every 8 hours for 14 days (21 days if CNS involvement)

   Child 3 months–12 years 250 mg/m² every 8 hours usually for 5 days, dose doubled if CNS

◻ **ACICLOVIR** (*continued*)

involvement (given for up to 21 days) or if immunosuppressed

Child 12–18 years 5 mg/kg every 8 hours usually for 5 days, dose doubled if CNS involvement (given for up to 21 days) or if immunosuppressed
Note To avoid excessive dose in obese patients parenteral dose should be calculated on the basis of ideal weight for height

Herpes simplex prophylaxis in the immuno-compromised
• **By mouth**

Child 1 month–2 years 100–200 mg 4 times daily

Child 2–18 years 200–400 mg 4 times daily

Chickenpox and herpes zoster infection
• **By mouth**

Child 1 month–2 years 200 mg 4 times daily for 5 days

Child 2–6 years 400 mg 4 times daily for 5 days

Child 6–12 years 800 mg 4 times daily for 5 days

Child 12–18 years 800 mg 5 times daily for 7 days

• **By intravenous infusion**

Neonate 10–20 mg/kg every 8 hours for at least 7 days

Child 1–3 months 10–20 mg/kg every 8 hours for at least 7 days

Child 3 months–12 years 250 mg/m^2 every 8 hours usually for 5 days, dose doubled if immunocompromised

Child 12–18 years 5 mg/kg every 8 hours usually for 5 days, dose doubled if immunocompromised
Note To avoid excessive dose in obese patients parenteral dose should be calculated on the basis of ideal weight for height

Attenuation of chickenpox if varicella–zoster immunoglobulin not indicated
• **By mouth**

Child 1 month–18 years 10 mg/kg 4 times daily for 7 days starting 1 week after exposure

Herpesvirus skin infections section 13.10.3

Herpesvirus eye infections section 11.3.3

Administration for *intravenous infusion*, reconstitute to 25 mg/mL with Water for Injections or Sodium Chloride 0.9% then dilute to concentration of 5 mg/mL with Sodium Chloride 0.9% *or* Sodium Chloride and Glucose *or* Compound Sodium Lactate and give over 1 hour; alternatively, may be administered in a concentration of 25 mg/mL using a suitable infusion pump and central venous access and given over 1 hour

Aciclovir (Non-proprietary) ᴘᴏᴹ
Tablets, aciclovir 200 mg, net price 25-tab pack = £4.01; 400 mg, 56-tab pack = £9.28; 800 mg, 35-tab pack = £11.42. Label: 9
Brands include *Virovir*®
Dental prescribing on NHS Aciclovir Tablets 200 mg or 800 mg may be prescribed

Dispersible tablets, aciclovir 200 mg, net price 25-tab pack = £2.21; 400 mg, 56-tab pack = £7.15; 800 mg, 35-tab pack = £6.54. Label: 9

Suspension, aciclovir 200 mg/5 mL, net price 125 mL = £29.56; 400 mg/5 mL, 100 mL = £33.02. Label: 9
Dental prescribing on NHS Aciclovir Oral Suspension 200 mg/5 mL may be prescribed

Intravenous infusion, powder for reconstitution, aciclovir (as sodium salt). Net price 250-mg vial = £9.13; 500-mg vial = £20.22
Electrolytes Na⁺ 1.1 mmol/250-mg vial

Intravenous infusion, aciclovir (as sodium salt), 25 mg/mL, net price 10-mL (250-mg) vial = £10.37; 20-mL (500-mg) vial = £19.21; 40-mL (1-g) vial = £40.44
Electrolytes Na⁺ 1.16 mmol/250-mg vial

Zovirax® (GSK) ᴘᴏᴹ
Tablets, all dispersible, f/c, aciclovir 200 mg, net price 25-tab pack = £18.80; 800 mg (scored, *Shingles Treatment Pack*), 35-tab pack = £69.85. Label: 9

Suspension, both off-white, sugar-free, aciclovir 200 mg/5 mL (banana-flavoured), net price 125 mL = £29.53; 400 mg/5 mL (*Double Strength Suspension*, orange-flavoured), 100 mL = £33.01. Label: 9

Intravenous infusion, powder for reconstitution, aciclovir (as sodium salt). Net price 250-mg vial = £10.15; 500-mg vial = £18.81
Electrolytes Na⁺ 1.1 mmol/250-mg vial

5 Infections

◣ **VALACICLOVIR**

Note Valaciclovir is a pro-drug of aciclovir
Cautions see under Aciclovir

Hepatic impairment manufacturer advises caution with high doses used for preventing cytomegalovirus disease—no information available in children

Renal impairment for *herpes zoster*, 1 g every 12 hours if estimated glomerular filtration rate 15–30 mL/minute/1.73 m^2 (every 24 hours if estimated glomerular filtration rate less than 15 mL/

minute/1.73 m^2); for *treatment of herpes simplex*, 500 mg every 24 hours if estimated glomerular filtration rate less than 15 mL/minute/1.73 m^2; for *suppression of herpes simplex*, 250 mg (500 mg in immunocompromised) every 24 hours if estimated glomerular filtration rate less than 15 mL/minute/1.73 m^2; reduce dose according to estimated glomerular filtration rate for *cytomegalovirus prophylaxis* following renal transplantation (consult product literature)

◻ **VALACICLOVIR (continued)**

Side-effects see under Aciclovir but neurological reactions more frequent with high doses

Licensed use not licensed for use in children except for CMV prophylaxis in children over 12 years

Indication and dose

Herpes zoster in immunocompromised
• **By mouth**
Child 12–18 years 1 g 3 times daily for 7 days

Treatment of herpes simplex
• **By mouth**
Child 12–18 years first episode, 500 mg twice daily for 5 days (longer if new lesions appear during treatment or if healing incomplete); recurrent infection, 500 mg twice daily for 5 days

Suppression of herpes simplex
• **By mouth**
Child 12–18 years 500 mg daily in 1–2 divided doses (in immunocompromised or HIV-positive patients, 500 mg twice daily)

Prevention of cytomegalovirus disease following renal transplantation (preferably starting within 72 hours of transplantation)
• **By mouth**
Child 12–18 years 2 g 4 times daily usually for 90 days

Valtrex® (GSK) [PoM]
Tablets, f/c, valaciclovir (as hydrochloride) 250 mg, net price 60-tab pack = £130.87; 500 mg, 10-tab pack = £21.86, 42-tab pack = £91.61. Label: 9

5.3.2.2 Cytomegalovirus infection

Recommendations for the optimum maintenance therapy of cytomegalovirus (CMV) infections and the duration of treatment are subject to rapid change.

Ganciclovir is related to aciclovir but it is more active against cytomegalovirus; it is also much more toxic than aciclovir and should therefore be prescribed under specialist supervision and only when the potential benefit outweighs the risks. Ganciclovir is administered by intravenous infusion for the *initial treatment* of CMV infection. The use of ganciclovir may also be considered for symptomatic congenital CMV infection. Ganciclovir causes profound myelosuppression when given with zidovudine; the two should not normally be given together particularly during initial ganciclovir therapy. The likelihood of ganciclovir resistance increases in patients with a high viral load or in those who receive the drug over a long duration; cross-resistance to cidofovir is common.

Valaciclovir (section 5.3.2.1) is licensed for use in children over 12 years for prevention of cytomegalovirus disease following renal transplantation.

Foscarnet is also active against cytomegalovirus; it is toxic and can cause renal impairment.

Cidofovir is given in combination with probenecid for CMV retinitis in AIDS patients when ganciclovir and foscarnet are contra-indicated. Cidofovir is nephrotoxic. There is limited information on its use in children.

For local treatment of CMV retinitis, see section 11.3.3.

GANCICLOVIR

Cautions close monitoring of full blood count (severe deterioration may require correction and possibly treatment interruption); history of cytopenia; low platelet count; potential carcinogen and teratogen; radiotherapy; ensure adequate hydration during intravenous administration; vesicant—infuse into vein with adequate flow preferably using plastic cannula; possible risk of long-term carcinogenic or reproductive toxicity; **interactions:** Appendix 1 (ganciclovir)

Renal impairment reduce dose if estimated glomerular filtration rate less than 70 mL/minute/1.73 m²; consult product literature

Contra-indications hypersensitivity to ganciclovir or aciclovir; abnormally low haemoglobin, neutrophil, or platelet counts (consult product literature)

Pregnancy avoid—teratogenic risk (ensure effective contraception during treatment and barrier contraception for males during and for at least 90 days after treatment)

Breast-feeding avoid—no information available

Side-effects diarrhoea, nausea, vomiting, dyspepsia, abdominal pain, constipation, flatulence, dysphagia, hepatic dysfunction; dyspnoea, chest pain, cough; headache, insomnia, convulsions, dizziness, neuropathy, depression, anxiety, con-

◻ **GANCICLOVIR (continued)**

fusion, abnormal thinking, fatigue, weight loss, anorexia; infection, fever, night sweats; anaemia, leucopenia, thrombocytopenia, pancytopenia, renal impairment; myalgia, arthralgia; macular oedema, retinal detachment, vitreous floaters, eye pain; ear pain, taste disturbance; dermatitis, pruritus; injection-site reactions; *less commonly* mouth ulcers, pancreatitis, arrhythmias, hypotension, anaphylactic reactions, psychosis, tremor, male infertility, haematuria, disturbances in hearing and vision, and alopecia

Licensed use not licensed for use in children

Indication and dose

> Life-threatening or sight-threatening cytomegalovirus infections in immunocompromised patients only; prevention of cytomegalovirus disease during immunosuppressive therapy following organ transplantation
> • **By intravenous infusion**
> > **Child 1 month–18 years** initially (induction) 5 mg/kg every 12 hours for 14–21 days for treatment or for 7–14 days for prevention; maintenance (for patients at risk of relapse of retinitis), 6 mg/kg daily on 5 days per week *or* 5 mg/kg daily until adequate recovery of

immunity; if retinitis progresses initial induction treatment may be repeated

> **Congenital cytomegalovirus infection of the CNS**
> • **By intravenous infusion**
> > **Neonate** 6 mg/kg every 12 hours for 6 weeks

> **Local treatment of CMV retinitis** section 11.3.3

Administration for *intravenous infusion*, reconstitute with Water for Injections (500 mg/10 mL) then dilute to a concentration of not more than 10 mg/mL with Glucose 5% *or* Sodium Chloride 0.9% *or* Compound Sodium Lactate and give over 1 hour

Cymevene® (Roche) ⒫ₒₘ
Intravenous infusion, powder for reconstitution, ganciclovir (as sodium salt). Net price 500-mg vial = £31.60
Electrolytes Na⁺ 2 mmol/500-mg vial
Caution in handling Ganciclovir is toxic and personnel should be adequately protected during handling and administration; if solution comes into contact with skin or mucosa, wash off immediately with soap and water

---

◢ **FOSCARNET SODIUM**

Cautions monitor electrolytes, particularly calcium and magnesium; monitor serum creatinine every second day during induction and every week during maintenance; ensure adequate hydration; avoid rapid infusion; **interactions:** Appendix 1 (foscarnet)

Renal impairment reduce dose; consult product literature

Contra-indications

Pregnancy avoid

Breast-feeding avoid—present in milk in *animal* studies

Side-effects nausea, vomiting, diarrhoea (occasionally constipation and dyspepsia), abdominal pain, anorexia; changes in blood pressure and ECG; headache, fatigue, mood disturbances (including psychosis), asthenia, paraesthesia, convulsions, tremor, dizziness, and other neurological disorders; rash; impairment of renal function including acute renal failure; hypocalcaemia (sometimes symptomatic) and other electrolyte disturbances; abnormal liver function tests; decreased haemoglobin concentration, leucopenia, granulocytopenia, thrombocytopenia; thrombophlebitis if given undiluted by peripheral vein; genital irritation and ulceration (due

to high concentrations excreted in urine); isolated reports of pancreatitis

Licensed use not licensed for use in children

Indication and dose

> **CMV retinitis**
> • **By intravenous infusion**
> > **Child 1 month–18 years** induction 60 mg/kg every 8 hours for 2–3 weeks then maintenance 60 mg/kg daily, increased to 90–120 mg/kg if tolerated; if retinitis progresses on maintenance dose, repeat induction regimen

> **Mucocutaneous herpes simplex infection**
> • **By intravenous infusion**
> > **Child 1 month–18 years** 40 mg/kg every 8 hours for 2–3 weeks or until lesions heal

Administration for *intravenous infusion*, give undiluted solution via a central venous catheter; alternatively dilute to a concentration of 12 mg/mL with Glucose 5% *or* Sodium Chloride 0.9% for administration via a peripheral vein; give over at least 1 hour

Foscavir® (AstraZeneca) ⒫ₒₘ
Intravenous infusion, foscarnet sodium hexahydrate 24 mg/mL, net price 250-mL bottle = £34.49

5

Infections

5.3.3 Viral hepatitis

Treatment for viral hepatitis should be initiated by a specialist in hepatology or infectious diseases. The management of uncomplicated acute viral hepatitis is largely symptomatic. Hepatitis B and hepatitis C viruses are major causes of chronic hepatitis. For details on immunisation against hepatitis A and B infections, see section 14.4 (active immunisation) and section 14.5 (passive immunisation).

Chronic hepatitis B **Interferon alfa** (section 8.2.4), **peginterferon alfa-2a**, **lamivudine** (section 5.3.1), and **adefovir dipivoxil** have a role in the treatment of chronic hepatitis B in adults but their role in children has not been established. Specialist supervision is required for the management of chronic hepatitis B.

Tenofovir, or a combination of tenofovir with either emtricitabine or lamivudine, may be used with other antiretrovirals, as part of 'highly active antiretroviral therapy' (section 5.3.1) in children who require treatment for both HIV and chronic hepatitis B. If children infected with both HIV and chronic hepatitis B only require treatment for chronic hepatitis B, they should receive antivirals that are not active against HIV. Management of these children should be co-ordinated between HIV and hepatology specialists.

Chronic hepatitis C Treatment should be considered for children with moderate or severe liver disease. Specialist supervision is required and the regimen is chosen according to the genotype of the infecting virus and the viral load. A combination of **ribavirin** (section 5.3.5) and **interferon alfa** (section 8.2.4) is licensed for use in children over 3 years with chronic hepatitis C. A combination of **peginterferon alfa** (BNF Section 8.2.4) and ribavirin is preferred.

5.3.4 Influenza

For advice on immunisation against influenza, see section 14.4.

Oseltamivir and **zanamivir** reduce replication of influenza A and B viruses by inhibiting viral neuraminidase. They are most effective for the treatment of influenza if started within a few hours of the onset of symptoms; oseltamivir is licensed for use within 48 hours of the first symptoms while zanamivir is licensed for use within 36 hours of the first symptoms. In otherwise healthy individuals they reduce the duration of symptoms by about 1–1.5 days. For further information on the treatment of influenza, see NICE guidance, p. 391.

Oseltamivir and zanamivir are licensed for post-exposure prophylaxis of influenza when influenza is circulating in the community. Oseltamivir should be given within 48 hours of exposure to influenza while zanamivir should be given within 36 hours of exposure to influenza (see also NICE guidance, p. 391). Oseltamivir and zanamivir are also licensed for use in exceptional circumstances (e.g. when vaccination does not cover the infecting strain) to prevent influenza in an epidemic.

Oseltamivir in children under 1 year of age Safety data on the use of oseltamivir in children under 1 year of age is limited and it is not licensed for use in this age group. Furthermore, oseltamivir may be ineffective in neonates and very young infants because they may not be able to metabolise oseltamivir to its active form. In exceptional circumstances, oseltamivir can be used (under specialist supervision) for the treatment or post-exposure prophylaxis of influenza in children under 1 year of age. The Department of Health has advised (May 2009) that, during a pandemic, treatment with oseltamivir can be overseen by healthcare professionals experienced in assessing children.

Amantadine is licensed for prophylaxis and treatment of influenza A in children over 10 years of age, but it is no longer recommended (see NICE guidance, p. 391).

Information on pandemic influenza, avian influenza, and swine influenza can be found at www.dh.gov.uk/pandemicflu and at www.hpa.org.uk.

NICE guidance

Oseltamivir, zanamivir, and amantadine for prophylaxis and treatment of influenza (September 2008 and February 2009)

The drugs described here are not a substitute for vaccination, which remains the most effective way of preventing illness from influenza.

- Amantadine is **not** recommended for prophylaxis or treatment of influenza.

- Oseltamivir or zanamivir are **not** recommended for seasonal prophylaxis against influenza.

- When influenza is circulating in the community[1], either oseltamivir or zanamivir is recommended (in accordance with UK licensing) for post-exposure prophylaxis in at-risk children who are not effectively protected by influenza vaccine, and who have been in close contact with someone suffering from influenza-like illness in the same household or residential setting. Oseltamivir should be given within 48 hours of exposure to influenza while zanamivir should be given within 36 hours of exposure to influenza.

- When influenza is circulating in the community[1], oseltamivir or zanamivir is recommended (in accordance with UK licensing) for the treatment of influenza in at-risk children who can start treatment within 48 hours (within 36 hours for zanamivir) of the onset of symptoms.

- During local outbreaks of influenza-like illness, when there is a high level of certainty that influenza is present, either oseltamivir or zanamivir may be used for post-exposure prophylaxis or treatment in at-risk children (regardless of influenza vaccination) living in long-term residential or nursing homes.

At-risk children are those who have one or more of the following conditions:
- chronic respiratory disease (including asthma);
- chronic heart disease;
- chronic renal disease;
- chronic liver disease;
- chronic neurological disease;
- immunosuppression;
- diabetes mellitus.

This guidance does not cover the circumstances of a pandemic, an impending pandemic, or a widespread epidemic of a new strain of influenza to which there is little or no immunity in the community.

5 Infections

OSELTAMIVIR

Cautions

Renal impairment reduce dose by 50% if estimated glomerular filtration rate $10–30 \, mL/minute/1.73 \, m^2$; avoid if estimated glomerular filtration rate less than $10 \, mL/minute/1.73 \, m^2$

Pregnancy avoid unless potential benefit outweighs risk

Breast-feeding avoid unless potential benefit outweighs risk; present in milk in *animal* studies

Side-effects nausea, vomiting, abdominal pain, diarrhoea; headache; conjunctivitis; *less commonly* rash; also reported hepatitis, arrhythmias, neuropsychiatric disorders, visual disturbances, Stevens-Johnson syndrome, and toxic epidermal necrolysis

Licensed use not licensed for use in children under 1 year

Indication and dose

Prevention of influenza
- **By mouth**

    Child under 1 year (under specialist supervision, see notes above) 2 mg/kg once daily for 10 days for post-exposure prophylaxis

    Child 1–13 years

    Body-weight under 15 kg 30 mg once daily for 10 days for post-exposure prophylaxis; for up to 6 weeks during an epidemic

    Body-weight 15–23 kg 45 mg once daily for 10 days for post-exposure prophylaxis; for up to 6 weeks during an epidemic

    Body-weight 23–40 kg 60 mg once daily for 10 days for post-exposure prophylaxis; for up to 6 weeks during an epidemic

    Body-weight over 40 kg 75 mg once daily for 10 days for post-exposure prophylaxis; for up to 6 weeks during an epidemic

1. National surveillance schemes, including those run by the Health Protection Agency, should be used to indicate when influenza is circulating in the community.

◻ OSELTAMIVIR *(continued)*

Child 13–18 years 75 mg once daily for 10 days for post-exposure prophylaxis; for up to 6 weeks during an epidemic

Treatment of influenza
● By mouth
Child under 1 year (see notes above) 2 mg/kg twice daily for 5 days

Child 1–13 years
Body-weight under 15 kg 30 mg twice daily for 5 days
Body-weight 15–23 kg 45 mg twice daily for 5 days
Body-weight 23–40 kg 60 mg twice daily for 5 days
Body-weight over 40 kg 75 mg twice daily for 5 days
Child 13–18 years 75 mg twice daily for 5 days

Administration if suspension not available, capsules can be opened and the contents mixed with a small amount of sweetened food, such as yoghurt, just before administration

¹**Tamiflu®** (Roche) ▼ PoM
Capsules, oseltamivir (as phosphate) 30 mg (yellow), net price 10-cap pack = £8.18; 45 mg (grey), 10-cap pack = £16.36; 75 mg (grey-yellow), 10-cap pack = £16.36. Label: 9

Suspension, sugar-free, tutti-frutti-flavoured, oseltamivir (as phosphate) for reconstitution with water, 60 mg/5 mL, net price 75 mL = £16.36. Label: 9
Excipients include sorbitol 1.7 g/5 mL
1. NHS except for the treatment and prophylaxis of influenza as indicated in the notes above and NICE guidance; endorse prescription 'SLS'

◢ ZANAMIVIR

Cautions asthma and chronic pulmonary disease (risk of bronchospasm—short-acting bronchodilator should be available; avoid in severe asthma unless close monitoring possible and appropriate facilities available to treat bronchospasm); uncontrolled chronic illness; other inhaled drugs should be administered before zanamivir
Pregnancy only use if potential benefit outweighs risk—no information available

Contra-indications
Breast-feeding avoid—present in milk in *animal* studies
Side-effects *very rarely* bronchospasm, respiratory impairment, angioedema, urticaria, and rash; also reported neuropsychiatric disorders

Indication and dose
Post-exposure prophylaxis of influenza
● By inhalation of powder
Child 5–18 years 10 mg once daily for 10 days

Prevention of influenza during an epidemic
● By inhalation of powder
Child 5–18 years 10 mg once daily for up to 28 days

Treatment of influenza
● By inhalation of powder
Child 5–18 years 10 mg twice daily for 5 days

¹**Relenza®** (GSK) PoM
Dry powder for inhalation disks containing 4 blisters of zanamivir 5 mg/blister, net price 5 disks with *Diskhaler®* device = £16.36
1. NHS except for the treatment and prophylaxis of influenza as indicated in the notes above and NICE guidance; endorse prescription 'SLS'

5.3.5 Respiratory syncytial virus

Ribavirin (tribavirin) inhibits a wide range of DNA and RNA viruses. It is licensed for administration by inhalation for the treatment of severe bronchiolitis caused by the respiratory syncytial virus (RSV) in infants, especially when they have other serious diseases. However, there is no evidence that ribavirin produces clinically relevant benefit in RSV bronchiolitis. Ribavirin is given by mouth with peginterferon alfa or interferon alfa for the treatment of chronic hepatitis C infection (see Viral Hepatitis, section 5.3.3). Ribavirin is also effective in Lassa fever and has also been used parenterally in the treatment of life-threatening RSV, parainfluenza virus, and adenovirus infections in immunocompromised children [unlicensed indications].

Palivizumab is a monoclonal antibody licensed for preventing serious lower respiratory-tract disease caused by respiratory syncytial virus in children at high risk of the disease; it should be prescribed under specialist supervision and on the basis of the likelihood of hospitalisation. Palivizumab should be considered for children under 6 months with haemodynamically significant left-to-right shunt congenital heart disease or who have pulmonary hypertension. It should also be considered for children under 2 years *either* with chronic lung disease who are using oxygen at home (or have been on prolonged oxygen treatment) *or* with severe congenital immunodeficiency. Palivizumab may also be used for the first 6–12 months of life in a child born at under 35 weeks gestation, if the child is considered by the specialist to be at special risk of hospitalisation. It is licensed for monthly use during the RSV season; the first dose should be administered before the start of the RSV season.

◢ PALIVIZUMAB

Cautions moderate to severe acute infection or febrile illness; thrombocytopenia; serum-palivizumab concentration may be reduced after cardiac surgery

Contra-indications hypersensitivity to humanised monoclonal antibodies

Side-effects fever, injection-site reactions, nervousness; *less commonly* diarrhoea, vomiting, constipation, haemorrhage, rhinitis, cough, wheeze, pain, drowsiness, asthenia, hyperkinesia, leucopenia, and rash; *rarely* apnoea, hypersensitivity reactions (including anaphylaxis)

Licensed use not licensed in children with congenital immunodeficiency or in children born at 35 weeks gestation or less and older than 6 months (licensed in children under 6 months)

Indication and dose

Prevention of serious disease caused by respiratory syncytial virus infection (see notes above)

• **By intramuscular injection (preferably in anterolateral thigh)**

Neonate 15 mg/kg once a month during season of RSV risk

Child 1 month–2 years 15 mg/kg once a month during season of RSV risk (child undergoing cardiac bypass surgery, 15 mg/kg as soon as stable after surgery, then once a month during season of risk); injection volume over 1 mL should be divided between 2 or more sites

Synagis® (Abbott) ▼ PoM
Injection, powder for reconstitution, palivizumab, net price 50-mg vial = £360.40; 100-mg vial = £663.11

◢ RIBAVIRIN

(Tribavirin)

Cautions

Specific cautions for inhaled treatment Maintain standard supportive respiratory and fluid management therapy; monitor electrolytes closely; monitor equipment for precipitation; pregnant women (and those planning pregnancy) should avoid exposure to aerosol

Specific cautions for systemic treatment Exclude pregnancy before treatment in females of childbearing age; effective contraception essential during treatment and for 4 months after treatment in females and for 7 months after treatment in males of childbearing age; routine monthly pregnancy tests recommended; condoms must be used if partner of male patient is pregnant (ribavirin excreted in semen); cardiac disease (assessment including ECG recommended before and during treatment—discontinue if deterioration); determine full blood count, platelets, electrolytes, serum creatinine, liver function tests and uric acid before starting treatment and then on weeks 2 and 4 of treatment, then as indicated clinically—adjust dose if adverse reactions or laboratory abnormalities develop (consult product literature); eye examination recommended before oral treatment; eye examination also recommended during oral treatment if pre-existing ophthalmological disorder or if decrease in vision reported—discontinue treatment if ophthalmological disorder deteriorates or if new ophthalmological disorder develops; test thyroid function before treatment and then every 3 months

Interactions: Appendix 1 (ribavirin)

Hepatic impairment no dosage adjustment required; use oral ribavirin with caution in severe hepatic dysfunction or decompensated cirrhosis

Renal impairment plasma-ribavirin concentration increased; manufacturer advises avoid oral ribavirin if estimated glomerular filtration rate less than 50 mL/minute/1.73 m^2; manufacturer advises use intravenous preparation with caution if estimated glomerular filtration rate less than 30 mL/minute/1.73 m^2

Contra-indications

Pregnancy avoid (**important teratogenic risk**: see Cautions)

Breast-feeding avoid

Specific contra-indications for systemic treatment Severe cardiac disease, including unstable or uncontrolled cardiac disease in previous 6 months; haemoglobinopathies; severe debilitating medical conditions; severe hepatic dysfunction or decompensated cirrhosis; autoimmune disease (including autoimmune hepatitis); history of severe psychiatric condition

Side-effects

Specific side-effects for inhaled treatment Worsening respiration, bacterial pneumonia, and pneumothorax reported; rarely non-specific anaemia and haemolysis
Specific side-effects for systemic treatment Haemolytic anaemia (anaemia may be improved by epoetin); also (in combination with peginterferon alfa or interferon alfa) nausea, vomiting, dyspepsia, abdominal pain, peptic ulcer, flatulence, diarrhoea, constipation, colitis, pancreatitis, growth retardation (including decrease in height and weight), appetite changes, weight loss, pulmonary embolism, chest pain, tachycardia, palpitation, syncope, cerebrovascular disease, peripheral oedema, changes in blood pressure, flushing, Raynaud's disease, hypertriglyceridaemia, dyspnoea, cough, interstitial pneumonitis, sleep disturbances, abnormal dreams, asthenia, impaired concentration and memory, psychoses, anxiety, depression, suicidal ideation, dizziness, hyperkinesia, tremor, hypertonia, seizures, ataxia, dysphonia, peripheral neuropathy, influenza-like symptoms, headache, hyperglycaemia, thyroid disorders, menstrual disturbances, virilism, testicular pain, micturition disorders, leucopenia, thrombocytopenia, aplastic anaemia, lymphadenopathy, hypocalcaemia, renal failure, hyperuricaemia, myalgia, arthralgia, systemic lupus erythematosus, vasculitis, sarcoidosis, eye changes (including blurred vision and retinopathy), rhinitis, tinnitus, hearing impairment, dry mouth, stomatitis, glossitis, taste disturbance, pharyngitis, gingivitis, tooth disorders, rash (including very rarely Stevens-Johnson syndrome and toxic epidermal necrolysis), pruritus, urticaria, photosensitivity, psoriasis, alopecia, dry skin, skin discoloration, increased sweating

◻ **RIBAVIRIN** (*continued*)

Licensed use inhalation licensed for use in children (age range not specified by manufacturer); intravenous preparation not licensed

Indication and dose

Bronchiolitis
- **By aerosol inhalation or nebulisation (via small particle aerosol generator)**
  Child 1 month–2 years inhale solution containing 20 mg/mL for 12–18 hours for at least 3 days; max. 7 days

Life-threatening RSV, parainfluenza virus, and adenovirus infection in immunocompromised children (seek expert advice)
- **By intravenous infusion over 15 minutes**
  Child 1 month–18 years 33 mg/kg as a single dose, then 16 mg/kg every 6 hours for 4 days, then 8 mg/kg every 8 hours for 3 days

Chronic hepatitis C (in combination with interferon alfa or peginterferon alfa) in previously untreated children without liver decompensation
- **By mouth**
  Child over 3 years; body-weight under 47 kg 15 mg/kg daily in 2 divided doses

Child body-weight 47–50 kg 200 mg in the morning and 400 mg in the evening

Child body-weight 50–65 kg 400 mg twice daily

Child body-weight 65–86 kg 400 mg in the morning and 600 mg in the evening

Child body-weight 86–105 kg 600 mg twice daily

Child body-weight over 105 kg 600 mg in the morning and 800 mg in the evening

Rebetol® (Schering-Plough) ℗
Capsules, ribavirin 200 mg, net price 84-cap pack = £275.65, 140-cap pack = £459.42, 168-cap pack = £551.30. Label: 21

Oral solution, ribavirin 200 mg/5 mL, net price 100 mL (bubble-gum-flavoured) = £69.71. Label: 21

Virazole® (Valeant) ℗
Inhalation ribavirin 6 g for reconstitution with 300 mL water for injections. Net price 3 × 6-g vials = £349.00

Intravenous infusion, 100 mg/mL, 10-mL amp
Available on a named-patient basis from Valeant

5.4 Antiprotozoal drugs

5.4.1 Antimalarials
5.4.2 Amoebicides
5.4.3 Trichomonacides
5.4.4 Antigiardial drugs
5.4.5 Leishmaniacides
5.4.6 Trypanocides
5.4.7 Drugs for toxoplasmosis
5.4.8 Drugs for pneumocystis pneumonia

Advice on specific problems available from:

Advice for healthcare professionals

HPA (Health Protection Agency) Malaria Reference Laboratory   (020) 7636 3924 (prophylaxis only)
www.hpa.org.uk/infections/topics_az/malaria

National Travel Health Network and Centre   0845 602 6712

Travel Medicine Team, Health Protection, Scotland (registered users of Travax only)   (0141) 300 1100 (weekdays 2–4 p.m. only)
www.travax.nhs.uk
(for registered users of the NHS Travax website only)

Birmingham   (0121) 424 0357

Liverpool   (0151) 705 3100

London   0845 155 5000 (treatment)

Oxford   (01865) 225 430

Advice for travellers

Hospital for Tropical Diseases, Travel Healthline   020 7950 7799
www.fitfortravel.nhs.uk

WHO advice on international travel and health
www.who.int/ith

National Travel Health Network and Centre (NaTHNaC)
www.nathnac.org/travel/index.htm

5.4.1 Antimalarials

Recommendations on the prophylaxis and treatment of malaria reflect guidelines agreed by UK malaria specialists. Choice will depend on the age of the child (see below).

The centres listed above should be consulted for advice on special problems.

Treatment of malaria

If the infective species is **not known**, or if the infection is **mixed**, initial treatment should be as for *falciparum malaria* with quinine, *Malarone®* (proguanil with atovaquone), or *Riamet®* (artemether with lumefantrine). Falciparum malaria can progress rapidly in unprotected children and antimalarial treatment should be considered in those with features of severe malaria and possible exposure, even if the initial blood tests for the organism are negative.

Falciparum malaria (treatment)

Falciparum malaria (malignant malaria) is caused by *Plasmodium falciparum*. In most parts of the world *P. falciparum* is now resistant to chloroquine which should not therefore be given for treatment.

Quinine, *Malarone®* (proguanil with atovaquone), or *Riamet®* (artemether with lumefantrine) can be given *by mouth* if the child can swallow and retain tablets and there are no serious manifestations (e.g. impaired consciousness); quinine should be given *by intravenous infusion* (see below) if the child is seriously ill or unable to take tablets. **Mefloquine** is now rarely used for treatment because of concerns about resistance.

Oral. **Quinine** is well tolerated by children although the salts are bitter.

The dosage regimen for quinine *by mouth* is:
10 mg/kg (of quinine salt[1]; max. 600 mg) every 8 hours for 7 days
together with or followed by
either **clindamycin** 7–13 mg/kg (max. 450 mg) every 8 hours for 7 days [unlicensed indication]
or, in children over 12 years, **doxycycline** 200 mg once daily for 7 days

If the parasite is likely to be sensitive, **pyrimethamine** with **sulfadoxine** as a single dose [unlicensed] may be given instead of either clindamycin or doxycycline together with or after a course of quinine.

The dose regimen for pyrimethamine with sulfadoxine by mouth is:
Child up to 4 years and body-weight over 5 kg pyrimethamine 12.5 mg with sulfadoxine 250 mg as a single dose

Child 5–6 years pyrimethamine 25 mg with sulfadoxine 500 mg as a single dose

Child 7–9 years pyrimethamine 37.5 mg with sulfadoxine 750 mg as a single dose

Child 10–14 years pyrimethamine 50 mg with sulfadoxine 1 g as a single dose

Child 14–18 years pyrimethamine 75 mg with sulfadoxine 1.5 g as a single dose

Alternatively, *Malarone®*, or *Riamet®* may be given instead of quinine. It is not necessary to give clindamycin, doxycycline, or pyrimethamine with sulfadoxine after *Malarone®* or *Riamet®* treatment.

The dose regimen for *Malarone®* *by mouth* is:
Child body-weight 5–8 kg, 2 'paediatric' tablets once daily for 3 days

Child body-weight 9–10 kg, 3 'paediatric' tablets once daily for 3 days

Child body-weight 11–20 kg, 1 'standard' tablet once daily for 3 days

Child body-weight 21–30 kg, 2 'standard' tablets once daily for 3 days

Child body-weight 31–40 kg, 3 'standard' tablets once daily for 3 days

Child body-weight over 40 kg, 4 'standard' tablets once daily for 3 days

---

1. Valid for quinine hydrochloride, dihydrochloride, and sulphate; not valid for quinine bisulphate which contains a correspondingly smaller amount of quinine.

The dose regimen for *Riamet*® *by mouth* is:

Child body-weight 5–15 kg 1 tablet initially, followed by 5 further doses of 1 tablet each given at 8, 24, 36, 48, and 60 hours (total 6 tablets over 60 hours)

Child body-weight 15–25 kg 2 tablets initially, followed by 5 further doses of 2 tablets each given at 8, 24, 36, 48, and 60 hours (total 12 tablets over 60 hours)

Child body-weight 25–35 kg 3 tablets initially, followed by 5 further doses of 3 tablets each given at 8, 24, 36, 48, and 60 hours (total 18 tablets over 60 hours)

Child 12–18 years and body-weight over 35 kg, 4 tablets initially followed by 5 further doses of 4 tablets each given at 8, 24, 36, 48, and 60 hours (total 24 tablets over 60 hours)

Parenteral. If the child is seriously ill or unable to swallow tablets, **quinine** should be given *by intravenous infusion.* The dose regimen for quinine *by intravenous infusion* is calculated on a mg/kg basis:

Neonates and children, loading dose[1,2] of 20 mg/kg (up to maximum 1.4 g) of quinine salt[3] infused over 4 hours *then 8 hours after the start of the loading dose*, maintenance dose of 10 mg/kg[4] (up to maximum 700 mg) of quinine salt[3] infused over 4 hours every 8 hours (until child can swallow tablets to complete the 7-day course *together with or followed by either* clindamycin or doxycycline as above).

Specialist advice should be sought in difficult cases (e.g. very high parasite count, deterioration on optimal doses of quinine, infection acquired in quinine-resistant areas of south-east Asia) because intravenous **artesunate** may be available for 'named-patient' use.

Pregnancy   Falciparum malaria is particularly dangerous in pregnancy, especially in the last trimester. The treatment doses of oral and intravenous quinine given above (including the loading dose) can safely be given in pregnancy. Clindamycin [unlicensed indication] should be given for 7 days with or after quinine. Doxycycline should be avoided in pregnancy (affects teeth and skeletal development in fetus); pyrimethamine with sulfadoxine, *Malarone*®, and *Riamet*® are also best avoided until more information is available.

Benign malarias (treatment)

Benign malaria is usually caused by *Plasmodium vivax* and less commonly by *P. ovale* and *P. malariae*. **Chloroquine**[5] is the drug of choice for the treatment of benign malarias (but chloroquine-resistant *P. vivax* infection has been reported from Indonesia, New Guinea and some adjacent islands).

Chloroquine alone is adequate for *P. malariae* infections but in the case of *P. vivax* and *P. ovale*, a *radical cure* (to destroy parasites in the liver and thus prevent relapses) is required. This is achieved with **primaquine**[6] given after the chloroquine.

The dosage regimen of chloroquine *by mouth* for benign malaria in children is:

initial dose of 10 mg/kg of base (max. 620 mg) *then*

a single dose of 5 mg/kg of base (max. 310 mg) after 6–8 hours *then*

a single dose of 5 mg/kg of base (max. 310 mg) daily for 2 days

For a *radical cure*, **primaquine**[6] [unlicensed] is then given to children over 6 months of age; specialist advice should be sought for children under 6 months of age. Primaquine is given in a dose of 250 micrograms/kg (max. 15 mg) daily for 14

---

1. In intensive care units the loading dose can alternatively be given as quinine salt[3] 7 mg/kg infused over 30 minutes followed immediately by 10 mg/kg over 4 hours then (after 8 hours) maintenance dose as described.
2. **Important:** the loading dose of 20 mg/kg should **not** be used if the patient has received quinine or mefloquine during the previous 12 hours
3. Valid for quinine hydrochloride, dihydrochloride, and sulphate; not valid for quinine bisulphate which contains a correspondingly smaller amount of quinine.
4. Maintenance dose should be reduced to 5–7 mg/kg of quinine salt in children with severe renal impairment, severe hepatic impairment, or if parenteral treatment is required for more than 48 hours.
5. For the treatment of chloroquine-resistant benign malaria *Malarone*® [unlicensed indication], quinine, or *Riamet*® [unlicensed indication] can be used; as with chloroquine, primaquine should be given for radical cure.
6. Before starting primaquine, blood should be tested for glucose-6-phosphate dehydrogenase (G6PD) activity since the drug can cause haemolysis in G6PD-deficient patients. Specialist advice should be obtained in G6PD deficiency. In mild G6PD deficiency, primaquine in a dose of 750 micrograms/kg (max. 45 mg) once a week for 8 weeks, has been found useful and without undue harmful effects.

5 Infections

days in *P. ovale* infection or 500 micrograms/kg (max. 30 mg) daily for 14 days in *P. vivax* infection.

Pregnancy   Treatment doses of chloroquine can be given for benign malaria. In the case of *P. vivax* or *P. ovale*, however, the radical cure with primaquine should be **postponed** until the pregnancy is over; instead chloroquine should be continued at a dose of 10 mg/kg (max. 310 mg) each week during the pregnancy.

Prophylaxis against malaria

The recommendations on prophylaxis reflect guidelines agreed by UK malaria specialists; the advice is aimed at residents of the UK who travel to endemic areas. The choice of drug for a particular child should take into account:

- risk of exposure to malaria;
- extent of drug resistance;
- efficacy of the recommended drugs;
- side-effects of the drugs;
- patient-related factors (e.g. age, pregnancy, renal or hepatic impairment, compliance with prophylactic regimen).

Prophylactic doses are based on guidelines agreed by UK malaria experts and may differ from advice in product literature. **Weight is a better guide than age**. If in doubt obtain advice from specialist centre, see p. 394.

Protection against bites   **Prophylaxis is not absolute**, and breakthrough infection can occur with any of the drugs recommended. Personal protection against being bitten is very important. Mosquito nets impregnated with permethrin provide the most effective barrier protection against insects (infants should sleep with a mosquito net stretched over the cot or baby carrier); mats and vaporised insecticides are also useful. Diethyltoluamide (DEET) 20–50% in lotions, sprays, or roll-on formulations is safe and effective when applied to the skin of adults and children over 2 months of age. It can also be used during pregnancy and breast-feeding. The duration of protection varies according to the concentration of DEET and is longest for DEET 50%. Long sleeves and trousers worn after dusk also provide protection.

Length of prophylaxis   In order to determine tolerance and to establish habit, prophylaxis should generally be started one week (preferably 2–3 weeks in the case of mefloquine) before travel into an endemic area (or if not possible at earliest opportunity up to 1 or 2 days before travel); *Malarone®* or doxycycline prophylaxis should be started 1–2 days before travel. Prophylaxis should be continued for **4 weeks after leaving** (except for *Malarone®* prophylaxis which should be stopped 1 week after leaving).

In those requiring long-term prophylaxis, chloroquine and proguanil may be used for periods of over 5 years. Mefloquine is licensed for use up to 1 year (although it has been used for up to 3 years without undue problems). Doxycycline can be used for up to 2 years. *Malarone®* is licensed for use for up to 28 days but can be used for up to 1 year (and possibly longer) with caution. Specialist advice should be sought for long-term prophylaxis.

Return from malarial region   It is important to be aware that **any illness** that occurs within 1 year and **especially within 3 months of return might be malaria** even if all recommended precautions against malaria were taken. Travellers and carers of children should be **warned** of this and told that if they develop any illness **particularly within 3 months** of their return they should go **immediately** to a doctor and specifically mention their exposure to malaria.

Epilepsy   Both chloroquine and mefloquine are unsuitable for malaria prophylaxis in children with a history of epilepsy. In areas *without chloroquine resistance*, proguanil alone is recommended; in areas *with chloroquine resistance*, doxycycline or *Malarone®* may be considered. The metabolism of doxycycline may be influenced by antiepileptics (see **interactions**: Appendix 1 (tetracyclines)).

Asplenia   Asplenic children (or those with severe splenic dysfunction) are at particular risk of severe malaria. If travel to malarious areas is unavoidable, rigorous precautions are required against contracting the disease.

Renal impairment Avoidance (or dosage reduction) of proguanil is recommended since it is excreted by the kidneys. *Malarone*® should not be used for prophylaxis in children with estimated glomerular filtration rate less than 30 mL/minute/1.73 m². Chloroquine is only partially excreted by the kidneys and reduction of the dose for prophylaxis is not required except in severe impairment. Mefloquine is considered to be appropriate to use in renal impairment and does not require dosage reduction. Doxycycline is also considered to be appropriate.

Pregnancy Travel to malarious areas should be avoided during pregnancy; if travel is unavoidable, effective prophylaxis must be used. Chloroquine and proguanil can be given in the usual doses during pregnancy, but these drugs are not appropriate for most areas because their effectiveness has declined, particularly in sub-saharan Africa; in the case of proguanil, folic acid 5 mg daily should be given. The centres listed on p. 394 should be consulted for advice on prophylaxis in chloroquine-resistant areas. The manufacturer advises that prophylaxis with mefloquine should be avoided as a matter of principle but studies of mefloquine in pregnancy (including use in the first trimester) indicate that it can be considered for travel to chloroquine-resistant areas. Doxycycline is contra-indicated during pregnancy. *Malarone*® should be avoided during pregnancy unless there is no suitable alternative.

Breast-feeding Prophylaxis is required in **breast-fed infants**; although antimalarials are present in milk, the amounts are too variable to give reliable protection.

Specific recommendations

Where a journey requires two regimens, the regimen for the higher risk area should be used for the whole journey. Those travelling to remote or little-visited areas may require expert advice.

> Risk may vary in different parts of a country—check under all risk levels

> **Important** Settled immigrants and their carers (or long-term visitors) to the UK may be unaware that they will have **lost some of their immunity** and also that the areas where they previously lived **may now be malarious**

North Africa, the Middle East, and Central Asia

Very low risk Risk *very low* in Algeria, Egypt (but *low risk* in El Faiyum, see below), Georgia (south-east, July–October), Kyrgystan (but *low risk* in south-west, see below), Libya, rural Morocco, most tourist areas of Turkey (but *low risk* in Adana and border with Syria, see below), Uzbekistan (extreme south-east only):

> chemoprophylaxis not recommended but avoid mosquito bites and consider malaria if fever presents

Low risk Risk *low* in Armenia (June–October), Azerbaijan (southern border areas, June–September), Egypt (El Faiyum only, June–October), Iran (northern border with Azerbaijan, May–October; *variable risk* in rural south-east provinces; see below), rural north Iraq (May–November), Kyrgystan (south-west, May–October), north border of Syria (May–October), Turkey (plain around Adana and east of there, border with Syria, March–November), Turkmenistan (south-east only, June–October):

preferably

> chloroquine *or* (if chloroquine not appropriate) proguanil hydrochloride

Variable risk Risk *variable* and *chloroquine resistance present* in Afghanistan (below 2000 m, May–November), Iran (rural south-east provinces, March–November, see also *Low risk* above), Oman (remote rural areas only), Saudi

Arabia (south-west and rural areas of western region; no risk in Mecca, Medina, Jeddah, or high-altitude areas of Asir Province), Tajikistan (June–October), Yemen (no risk in Sana'a):

> chloroquine + proguanil hydrochloride *or* (if chloroquine + proguanil not appropriate and child over 12 years) doxycycline

Sub-Saharan Africa

No chemoprophylaxis recommended for Cape Verde (some risk on São Tiago) and Mauritius (but avoid mosquito bites and consider malaria if fever presents)

Very high risk   Risk *very high* (or *locally very high*) and *chloroquine resistance very widespread* in Angola, Benin, Botswana (northern half, November–June), Burkina Faso, Burundi, Cameroon, Central African Republic, Chad, Comoros, Congo, Democratic Republic of the Congo (formerly Zaïre), Djibouti, Equatorial Guinea, Eritrea, Ethiopia (below 2000 m; no risk in Addis Ababa), Gabon, Gambia, Ghana, Guinea, Guinea-Bissau, Ivory Coast, Kenya, Liberia, Madagascar, Malawi, Mali, Mauritania (all year in south; July–October in north), Mozambique, Namibia (all year along Kavango and Kunene rivers; November–June in northern third), Niger, Nigeria, Principe, Rwanda, São Tomé, Senegal, Sierra Leone, Somalia, South Africa (low-altitude areas of Mpumalanga and Limpopo Provinces, Kruger National Park, and north-east KwaZulu-Natal as far south as Jozini), Sudan, Swaziland, Tanzania, Togo, Uganda, Zambia, Zimbabwe (all year in Zambezi valley; November–June in other areas below 1200 m; risk negligible in Harare and Bulawayo):

> mefloquine *or* doxycycline (if child over 12) *or* *Malarone*®

Note In Zimbabwe and neighbouring countries, pyrimethamine with dapsone (also known as *Deltaprim*®) prophylaxis is used by local residents (sometimes with chloroquine—this regimen is not recommended).

South Asia

Low risk   Risk *low* in Bangladesh (but *high risk* in Chittagong Hill Tracts, see below), India (Kerala [southern states], Tamil Nadu, Karnataka, Southern Andhra Pradesh [including Hyderabad and Mumbai], Rajasthan [including Jaipur], Uttar Pradesh [including Agra], Haryana, Uttaranchal, Himachal Pradesh, Jammu, Kashmir, Punjab, Delhi; *variable risk* in other areas, see below; *high risk* in Assam), Sri Lanka (but *variable risk* north of Vavuniya, see below):

> chemoprophylaxis not recommended but avoid mosquito bites and consider malaria if fever present

Variable risk   Risk *variable* and *chloroquine resistance usually moderate* in southern districts of Bhutan, India (*low risk* in some areas, see above; *high risk* in Assam, see below), Nepal (below 1500 m, especially Terai districts; no risk in Kathmandu), Pakistan (below 2000 m), Sri Lanka (north of Vavuniya; *low risk* in other areas, see above):

> chloroquine + proguanil hydrochloride *or* (if chloroquine + proguanil not appropriate) mefloquine *or* doxycycline *or* *Malarone*®

High risk   Risk *high* and *chloroquine resistance high* in Bangladesh (only in Chittagong Hill Tracts; *low risk* in other areas, see above), India (Assam only; see also *low risk* and *variable risk* above):

> mefloquine *or* doxycycline (if child over 12) *or* *Malarone*® *or* (if mefloquine, doxycycline, or *Malarone*® not appropriate) chloroquine + proguanil hydrochloride

5

Infections

South-East Asia

Very low risk Risk *very low* in Bali, Brunei, main tourist areas of China (but *substantial risk* in Yunnan and Hainan, see below; *chloroquine prophylaxis* appropriate for other remote areas), Hong Kong, Korea (both North and South), Malaysia (both East and West including Cameron Highlands, but *substantial risk* in Sabah [except Kota Kinabalu], and *variable risk* in deep forests, see below), Singapore, Thailand (Bangkok, main tourist centres, Chang Ri, Kwai Bridge—**important**: regional risk exists, see under *Great risk*, below), Vietnam (cities, coast between Ho Chi Minh and Hanoi, and Mekong River until close to Cambodian border; *substantial risk* in other areas, see below):

> chemoprophylaxis not recommended but avoid mosquito bites and consider malaria if fever presents

Variable risk Risk *variable* and *some chloroquine resistance* in Indonesia (very low risk in Bali, and cities but *substantial risk* in Irian Jaya [West Papua] and Lombok, see below), rural Philippines below 600 m (no risk in cities, Cebu, Bohol, and Catanduanes), deep forests of peninsular Malaysia and Sarawak (but *substantial risk* in Sabah, see below):

> chloroquine + proguanil hydrochloride *or* (if chloroquine + proguanil not appropriate) mefloquine *or* doxycycline *or* Malarone®

Substantial risk Risk *substantial* and *drug resistance common* in Cambodia (no risk in Phnom Penh; for western provinces, see below), China (Yunnan and Hainan; *chloroquine prophylaxis* appropriate for other remote areas; see also *Very low risk* above), East Timor, Irian Jaya [West Papua], Laos (no risk in Vientiane), Lombok, Malaysia (Sabah; see also *Very low risk* and *Variable risk* above), Myanmar (formerly Burma; see also *Great risk* below), Vietnam (*very low risk* in some areas, see above):

> mefloquine *or* doxycycline (if child over 12) *or* Malarone®

Great risk and drug resistance present Risk *great* and *widespread chloroquine and mefloquine resistance present* in western provinces of Cambodia, borders of Thailand with Cambodia, Laos and Myanmar (*very low risk* in Chang Ri and Kwai Bridge, see above), Myanmar (eastern Shan State):

> doxycycline (if child over 12) *or* Malarone®

Oceania

Risk Risk *high* and *chloroquine resistance high* in Papua New Guinea (below 1800 m), Solomon Islands, Vanuatu:

> doxycycline (if child over 12) *or* mefloquine *or* Malarone®

Central and South America and the Caribbean

Variable to low risk Risk *variable to low* in Argentina (rural areas along northern borders only), rural Belize (except Belize district), Costa Rica (Limon Province except Puerto Limon and northern canton of Pococci), Dominican Republic, El Salvador (Santa Ana province in west), Guatemala (below 1500 m), Haiti, Honduras, Mexico (states of Oaxaca and Chiapas), Nicaragua, Panama (west of Panama Canal but *variable to high risk* east of Panama Canal, see below), rural Paraguay:

> chloroquine *or* (if chloroquine not appropriate) proguanil hydrochloride

Variable to high risk Risk *variable to high and chloroquine resistance present* in rural areas of Bolivia (below 2500 m; see below for Amazon basin area), Ecuador (below 1500 m; no malaria in Galapagos Islands and Guayaquil; see below for Esmeraldas Province), Panama (east of Panama Canal), Peru (rural areas east of the Andes and west of the Amazon basin area below 1500 m; see below for Amazon basin area), Venezuela (north of Orinoco river; *high risk* south of and including Orinoco river and Amazon basin area, see below; Caracas free of malaria):

> chloroquine + proguanil hydrochloride *or* (if chloroquine + proguanil not appropriate) mefloquine *or* doxycycline (if child over 12) *or Malarone®*

High risk   Risk *high* and *marked chloroquine resistance* in Bolivia (Amazon basin area; see also *variable to high risk* above), Brazil (throughout 'Legal Amazon' area which includes the Amazon basin area, Mato Grosso and Maranhao only; elsewhere *very low risk*—no chemoprophylaxis), Colombia (most areas below 800 m), Ecuador (Esmeraldas Province; *variable to high risk* in other areas, see above), French Guiana, all interior regions of Guyana, Peru (Amazon basin area; see also *variable to high risk* above), Suriname (except Paramaribo and coast), Venezuela (Amazon basin area, areas south of and including Orinoco river; see also *variable to high risk* above):

> mefloquine *or* doxycycline (if child over 12) *or Malarone®*

Standby treatment [unlicensed]

> Children and their carers visiting remote, malarious areas for prolonged periods should carry standby treatment if they are likely to be more than 24 hours away from medical care. Self-medication should be **avoided** if medical help is accessible.
>
> In order to avoid excessive self-medication, the traveller should be provided with **written instructions** that urgent medical attention should be sought if fever (38°C or more) develops 7 days (or more) after arriving in a malarious area and that self-treatment is indicated if medical help is not available within 24 hours of fever onset.
>
> In view of the continuing emergence of resistant strains and of the different regimens required for different areas expert advice should be sought on the best treatment course for an individual traveller. A drug used for chemoprophylaxis should not be considered for standby treatment for the same traveller.

Artemether with lumefantrine

Artemether with lumefantrine is licensed for the *treatment of acute uncomplicated falciparum malaria.*

ARTEMETHER WITH LUMEFANTRINE

Cautions electrolyte disturbances, concomitant use with other drugs known to cause QT-interval prolongation; monitor patients unable to take food (greater risk of recrudescence); **interactions**: Appendix 1 (artemether with lumefantrine)

Hepatic impairment manufacturer advises caution in severe impairment—monitor ECG and plasma potassium concentration

Renal impairment manufacturer advises caution in severe impairment—monitor ECG and plasma potassium concentration

Pregnancy toxicity in *animal* studies with artemether; manufacturer advises use only if potential benefit outweighs risk

Skilled tasks Dizziness may affect performance of skilled tasks

Contra-indications history of arrhythmias, of clinically relevant bradycardia, and of congestive heart failure accompanied by reduced left ventricular ejection fraction; family history of sudden death or of congenital QT interval prolongation

Breast-feeding Manufacturer advises avoid breast-feeding for at least 1 week after last dose; present in milk in *animal* studies

Side-effects abdominal pain, anorexia, diarrhoea, vomiting, nausea; palpitation, prolonged QT interval; cough; headache, dizziness, sleep disturbances, asthenia, paraesthesia; arthralgia, myalgia; pruritus, rash; *less commonly* ataxia, hypoaesthesia, clonus

◁ **ARTEMETHER WITH LUMEFANTRINE (continued)**

Indication and dose

Treatment of acute uncomplicated falciparum malaria see p. 395

Treatment of benign malaria see p. 396

Administration tablets may be crushed just before administration

Riamet® (Novartis) ▼ PoM
Tablets, yellow, artemether 20 mg, lumefantrine 120 mg, net price 24-tab pack = £22.50. Label: 21, counselling, skilled tasks

---

Chloroquine

Chloroquine is used for the *prophylaxis of malaria* in areas of the world where the *risk of chloroquine-resistant falciparum malaria is still low*. It is also used with proguanil when chloroquine-resistant falciparum malaria is present but this regimen may not give optimal protection (see specific recommendations by country, p. 398).

Chloroquine is **no longer recommended** for the *treatment of falciparum malaria* owing to widespread resistance, nor is it recommended if the infective species is *not known* or if the infection is *mixed*; in these cases treatment should be with quinine, *Malarone®*, or *Riamet®* (for details, see p. 395). It is still recommended for the *treatment of benign malarias* (for details, see p. 396).

CHLOROQUINE

Cautions moderate or severe hepatic impairment; may exacerbate psoriasis, neurological disorders (avoid for prophylaxis if history of epilepsy, see notes above), may aggravate myasthenia gravis, severe gastro-intestinal disorders, G6PD deficiency (see section 9.1.5); ophthalmic examination with long-term therapy; avoid concurrent therapy with hepatotoxic drugs—other **interactions:** Appendix 1 (chloroquine and hydroxychloroquine)

Renal impairment mild to moderate, reduce dose (but for malaria prophylaxis see, p. 398); severe, avoid (but for malaria prophylaxis see p. 398)

Pregnancy *first, third trimesters:* benefit of prophylaxis and treatment in malaria outweighs risk; **important:** *see also* Falciparum Malaria (Treatment), Benign Malarias (Treatment), and Prophylaxis Against Malaria

Breast-feeding amount probably too small to be harmful when used for malaria prophylaxis; inadequate for reliable protection against malaria in breast-fed infant, *see* p. 398; avoid breast-feeding when used for rheumatic diseases

Side-effects gastro-intestinal disturbances, headache; also hypotension, convulsions, visual disturbances, depigmentation or loss of hair, skin reactions (rashes, pruritus); rarely, bone-marrow suppression, hypersensitivity reactions such as urticaria and angioedema; other side-effects (not usually associated with malaria prophylaxis or treatment), see under Antimalarials, section 10.1.3; very toxic in **overdosage**—immediate advice from poisons centres essential (see also p. 41)

Indication and dose

Prophylaxis of malaria
• By mouth
Dose (expressed as chloroquine base) preferably started 1 week before entering endemic area and continued for 4 weeks after leaving (see notes above)

Child up to 12 weeks, body-weight under 6 kg 37.5 mg once weekly

Child 12 weeks–1 year, body-weight 6–10 kg 75 mg once weekly

Child 1–4 years, body-weight 10–16 kg 112.5 mg once weekly

Child 4–8 years, body-weight 16–25 kg 150 mg once weekly (or 155 mg once weekly if tablets used)

Child 8–13 years, body-weight 25–45 kg 225 mg once weekly (or 232.5 mg once weekly if tablets used)

Child over 13 years, body-weight over 45 kg 310 mg once weekly
Counselling Warn travellers about **importance** of avoiding mosquito bites, **importance** of taking prophylaxis regularly, and **importance** of immediate visit to doctor if ill within 1 year and **especially** within 3 months of return. For details, see notes above

Treatment of benign malaria see p. 396

Note Chloroquine doses in BNFC may differ from those in product literature

¹Avloclor® (AstraZeneca) PoM
Tablets, scored, chloroquine phosphate 250 mg (≡ chloroquine base 155 mg). Net price 20-tab pack = £1.22. Label: 5, counselling, prophylaxis, see above

---

1. Can be sold to the public provided it is licensed and labelled for the prophylaxis of malaria. Drugs for malaria prophylaxis not prescribable on the NHS; health authorities may investigate circumstances under which antimalarials are prescribed

◻ **CHLOROQUINE (continued)**

[1]**Malarivon®** (Wallace Mfg) PoM

Syrup, chloroquine phosphate 80 mg/5 mL (≡ chloroquine base 50 mg/5 mL), net price 75 mL = £3.35. Label: 5, counselling, prophylaxis, see above

[2]**Nivaquine®** (Sanofi-Aventis)

Syrup, golden, chloroquine sulphate 68 mg/5 mL (≡ chloroquine base 50 mg/5 mL), net price 100 mL = £5.15. Label: 5, counselling, prophylaxis, see above

◢**With proguanil**

For cautions and side-effects of proguanil see Proguanil; for dose see Chloroquine and Proguanil

Paludrine/Avloclor® (AstraZeneca)

Tablets, travel pack of 14 tablets of chloroquine phosphate 250 mg (≡ chloroquine base 155 mg) and 98 tablets of proguanil hydrochloride 100 mg, net price 112-tab pack = £8.79. Label: 5, 21, counselling, prophylaxis, see above

Mefloquine

Mefloquine is used for the *prophylaxis of malaria* in areas of the world where there is a *high risk of chloroquine-resistant falciparum malaria* (for details, see specific recommendations by country, p. 398).

Mefloquine is now rarely used for the *treatment of falciparum malaria* because of increased resistance. It is rarely used for the treatment of benign malarias because better tolerated alternatives are available. Mefloquine should not be used for treatment if it has been used for prophylaxis.

The CSM has advised that travellers should be informed about adverse reactions of mefloquine and, if they occur, medical advice should be sought on alternative antimalarials before the next dose is due; the patient information leaflet, which describes adverse reactions should always be provided when dispensing mefloquine.

MEFLOQUINE

Cautions cardiac conduction disorders; epilepsy (avoid for prophylaxis); not recommended in infants under 3 months (5 kg); **interactions:** Appendix 1 (mefloquine)

Hepatic impairment avoid for chemoprophylaxis in severe liver disease

Pregnancy (see Prophylaxis against Malaria, p. 398)—manufacturer advises **avoid** pregnancy during and for 3 months after (teratogenicity in *animal* studies)

Breast-feeding present in milk but risk to infant minimal

Skilled tasks Dizziness or a disturbed sense of balance may affect performance of skilled tasks; effects may persist for up to 3 weeks

Contra-indications hypersensitivity to quinine; avoid for prophylaxis if history of psychiatric disorders (including depression) or convulsions

Side-effects nausea, vomiting, diarrhoea, abdominal pain; dizziness, loss of balance, headache, sleep disorders (insomnia, drowsiness, abnormal dreams); *less commonly* circulatory disorders (hypotension and hypertension), chest pain, tachycardia, palpitation, bradycardia, cardiac conduction disorders, dyspnoea, fatigue, fever, loss of appetite, neuropsychiatric reactions (including sensory and motor neuropathies, tremor, ataxia, anxiety, depression, panic attacks, agitation, hallucinations, psychosis, convulsions), leucopenia or leucocytosis, thrombocytopenia, muscle weakness, myalgia, arthralgia, visual disturbances, tinnitus and vestibular disorders, rash (including Stevens-Johnson syndrome), urticaria, pruritus, alopecia; *rarely* suicidal ideation; *very rarely* AV block, pneumonitis, and encephalopathy

Licensed use not licensed for use in children under 5 kg body-weight and under 3 months

Indication and dose

Prophylaxis of malaria preferably started 2½ weeks before entering endemic area and continued for 4 weeks after leaving (see notes above)

• **By mouth**

Child body-weight 5–16 kg 62.5 mg once weekly

Child body-weight 16–25 kg 125 mg once weekly

Child body-weight 25–45 kg 187.5 mg once weekly

Child body-weight over 45 kg 250 mg once weekly

Long-term chemoprophylaxis Mefloquine prophylaxis can be taken for up to 1 year

Counselling See CSM advice in notes above. Also warn travellers and carers of children travelling about **importance** of avoiding mosquito bites, **importance** of taking prophylaxis regularly, and **importance** of immediate visit to doctor if ill within 1 year and **especially** within 3 months of return. For details, see notes above

Note Mefloquine doses in BNFC may differ from those in product literature

1. Can be sold to the public provided it is licensed and labelled for the prophylaxis of malaria. Drugs for malaria prophylaxis not prescribable on the NHS; health authorities may investigate circumstances under which antimalarials are prescribed

2. Drugs for malaria prophylaxis not prescribable on the NHS; health authorities may investigate circumstances under which antimalarials prescribed

◁ **MEFLOQUINE** *(continued)*

Administration Tablet may be crushed and mixed with food such as jam or honey just before administration

[1]**Lariam®** (Roche) PoM
Tablets, scored, mefloquine (as hydrochloride) 250 mg. Net price 8-tab pack = £14.53. Label: 21, 25, 27, counselling, skilled tasks, prophylaxis, see above

---

Primaquine

Primaquine is used to eliminate the liver stages of *P. vivax* or *P. ovale following chloroquine treatment* (for details, see p. 396).

PRIMAQUINE

Cautions G6PD deficiency (test blood, see under Benign Malarias (treatment), p. 396); systemic diseases associated with granulocytopenia (e.g. juvenile idiopathic arthritis, lupus erythematosus); **interactions:** Appendix 1 (primaquine)

Pregnancy risk of neonatal haemolysis and methaemoglobinaemia in third trimester; see also Benign Malarias (treatment)

Side-effects nausea, vomiting, anorexia, abdominal pain; *less commonly* methaemoglobinaemia, haemolytic anaemia especially in G6PD deficiency, leucopenia

Licensed use not licensed

Indication and dose

Adjunct in the treatment of *Plasmodium vivax* and *P. ovale* malaria (eradication of liver stages) for dose see Benign Malarias, p. 396

Primaquine (Non-proprietary)
Tablets, primaquine (as phosphate) 7.5 mg or 15 mg
Available from 'special-order' manufacturers or specialist importing companies, see p. 943

Proguanil

Proguanil is used (usually *with chloroquine*, but occasionally *alone*) for the *prophylaxis of malaria*, (for details, see specific recommendations by country, p. 398).

Proguanil used alone is not suitable for the *treatment of malaria*; however, *Malarone®* (a combination of atovaquone with proguanil) is licensed for the treatment of acute uncomplicated falciparum malaria.

Malarone® is also used for the *prophylaxis of falciparum malaria* in areas of widespread mefloquine or chloroquine resistance. *Malarone®* is also used as an alternative to mefloquine or doxycycline. *Malarone®* is particularly suitable for short trips to highly chloroquine-resistant areas because it needs to be taken only for 7 days after leaving an endemic area.

PROGUANIL HYDROCHLORIDE

Cautions interactions: Appendix 1 (proguanil)

Renal impairment (see notes under Prophylaxis against malaria). Use half normal dose if estimated glomerular filtration rate 20–60 mL/minute/1.73 m². Use one-quarter normal dose on alternate days if estimated glomerular filtration rate 10–20 mL/minute/1.73 m². Use one-quarter normal dose once weekly if estimated glomerular filtration rate less than 10 mL/minute/1.73 m²; increased risk of haematological toxicity.

Pregnancy benefit of prophylaxis in malaria outweighs risk. Adequate folate supplements should be given to mother; see also Prophylaxis Against Malaria

Breast-feeding amount probably too small to be harmful when used for malaria prophylaxis; inadequate for reliable protection against malaria in breast-fed infant

Side-effects mild gastric intolerance, diarrhoea, and constipation; occasionally mouth ulcers and stomatitis; *very rarely* cholestasis, vasculitis, skin reactions and hair loss

Indication and dose

Prophylaxis of malaria preferably started 1 week before entering endemic area and continued for 4 weeks after leaving (see notes above)

• By mouth

Child up to 12 weeks, body-weight under 6 kg 25 mg once daily

Child 12 weeks–1 year, body-weight 6–10 kg 50 mg once daily

Child 1–4 years, body-weight 10–16 kg 75 mg once daily

Child 4–8 years, body-weight 16–25 kg 100 mg once daily

Child 8–13 years, body-weight 25–45 kg 150 mg once daily

---

1. Drugs for malaria prophylaxis not prescribable on the NHS; health authorities may investigate circumstances under which antimalarials prescribed

◁ **PROGUANIL HYDROCHLORIDE** (*continued*)

> **Child over 13 years, body-weight over 45 kg**
> 200 mg once daily
> Counselling Warn travellers and carers of children
> travelling about **importance** of avoiding mosquito
> bites, **importance** of taking prophylaxis regularly, and
> **importance** of immediate visit to doctor if ill within 1
> year and **especially** within 3 months of return. For
> details, see notes above
> Note Proguanil doses in BNFC may differ from those in
> product literature

Administration Tablets may be crushed and mixed with food such as milk, jam or honey just before administration

[1]**Paludrine®** (AstraZeneca)
Tablets, scored, proguanil hydrochloride 100 mg. Net price 98-tab pack = £7.43. Label: 21, counselling, prophylaxis, see above

◢**With chloroquine**
See under Chloroquine

■ **PROGUANIL HYDROCHLORIDE WITH ATOVAQUONE**

Cautions diarrhoea or vomiting (reduced absorption of atovaquone); efficacy not evaluated in cerebral or complicated malaria (including hyperparasitaemia, pulmonary oedema or renal failure); **interactions**: see Appendix 1 (proguanil, atovaquone)

Renal impairment avoid for malaria prophylaxis and, if possible for treatment, if estimated glomerular filtration rate less than 30 mL/minute/1.73 m²

Pregnancy manufacturer advises avoid unless essential

Breast-feeding use only if no suitable alternative available; see also Breast-feeding, p. 398

Side-effects abdominal pain, nausea, vomiting, diarrhoea; cough; headache, dizziness, insomnia, abnormal dreams, depression, anorexia, fever; rash, pruritus; *less frequently* mouth ulcers, stomatitis, anxiety, blood disorders, hyponatraemia, palpitation, and hair loss; also reported hepatitis, cholestasis, tachycardia, hallucinations, panic attacks, vasculitis, and Stevens-Johnson syndrome

Indication and dose

See preparations

Counselling Warn travellers about **importance** of avoiding mosquito bites, **importance** of taking prophylaxis regularly, and **importance** of immediate visit to doctor if ill within 1 year and **especially** within 3 months of return. For details, see notes above

[1]**Malarone®** (GSK) [PoM]
Tablets ('standard'), pink, f/c, proguanil hydrochloride 100 mg, atovaquone 250 mg. Net price 12-tab pack = £25.21. Label: 21, counselling, prophylaxis, see above

Dose
Prophylaxis of malaria started 1–2 days before entering endemic area and continued for 1 week after leaving
• By mouth
  Child body-weight over 40 kg 1 tablet daily

Treatment of malaria
• By mouth
  Child body-weight 11–21 kg 1 tablet daily for 3 days
  Child body-weight 21–31 kg 2 tablets once daily for 3 days
  Child body-weight 31–40 kg 3 tablets once daily for 3 days
  Child body-weight over 40 kg 4 tablets once daily for 3 days

[1]**Malarone® Paediatric** (GSK) [PoM]
Paediatric tablets, pink, f/c proguanil hydrochloride 25 mg, atovaquone 62.5 mg, net price 12-tab pack = £6.26. Label: 21, counselling, prophylaxis, see above

Dose
Prophylaxis of malaria started 1–2 days before entering endemic area and continued for 1 week after leaving
• By mouth
  Child body-weight 11–21 kg 1 tablet once daily
  Child body-weight 21–31 kg 2 tablets once daily
  Child body-weight 31–40 kg 3 tablets once daily
  Child body-weight over 40 kg use *Malarone®* ('standard') tablets, see above

Treatment of malaria
• By mouth
  Child body-weight 5–9 kg 2 tablets once daily for 3 days
  Child body-weight 9–11 kg 3 tablets once daily for 3 days
  Child body-weight 11 kg and over use *Malarone®* ('standard') tablets, see above

Administration tablets may be crushed and mixed with food or milky drink just before administration

■ **Pyrimethamine**

Pyrimethamine should not be used alone, but is used with sulfadoxine.

Pyrimethamine with sulfadoxine is not recommended for the *prophylaxis of malaria*, but can be used in the treatment of *falciparum malaria* with (or following) *quinine*.

---

1. Drugs for malaria prophylaxis not prescribable on the NHS; health authorities may investigate circumstances under which antimalarials prescribed

PYRIMETHAMINE WITH SULFADOXINE

Cautions see under Pyrimethamine (section 5.4.7) and under Co-trimoxazole (section 5.1.8); not recommended for prophylaxis (severe side-effects on long-term use); **interactions:** Appendix 1 (pyrimethamine, sulphonamides)

Pregnancy possible teratogenic risk in *first trimester* as pyrimethamine is a folate antagonist; in *third trimester*—risk of neonatal haemolysis and methaemoglobinaemia; fears of increased risk of neonatal kernicterus appear unfounded

Breast-feeding small risk of neonatal kernicterus in jaundiced infants; risk of haemolysis in G6PD-deficient child due to sulfadoxine

Contra-indications see under Pyrimethamine (section 5.4.7) and under Co-trimoxazole (section 5.1.8); sulphonamide allergy

Side-effects see under Pyrimethamine (section 5.4.7) and under Co-trimoxazole (section 5.1.8); pulmonary infiltrates (e.g. eosinophilic or allergic alveolitis) reported—discontinue if cough or shortness of breath

Licensed use not licensed for use in children of body-weight under 5 kg

Indication and dose

Adjunct to quinine in treatment of *Plasmodium falciparum* malaria see p. 395

Prophylaxis not recommended by UK malaria experts

Pyrimethamine with sulfadoxine (Non-proprietary) ℗ｅ

Tablets, scored, pyrimethamine 25 mg, sulfadoxine 500 mg, net price 3-tab pack = 74p
Note Also known as *Fansidar®*
Available from 'special-order' manufacturers or specialist importing companies, see p. 943

Quinine

Quinine is not suitable for the *prophylaxis of malaria*.

Quinine is used for the *treatment of falciparum malaria* or if the infective species is *not known* or if the infection is *mixed* (for details see p. 395).

QUININE

Cautions cardiac disease (including atrial fibrillation, conduction defects, heart block)—monitor ECG during parenteral treatment; monitor blood glucose and electrolyte concentration during parenteral treatment; G6PD deficiency (see section 9.1.5); **interactions:** Appendix 1 (quinine)

Renal impairment reduce parenteral maintenance dose for malaria treatment, see p. 396

Pregnancy risk of teratogenesis with high doses in *first trimester*, but in malaria benefit of treatment outweighs risk

Contra-indications haemoglobinuria, myasthenia gravis, optic neuritis, tinnitus

Side-effects cinchonism, including tinnitus, headache, hot and flushed skin, nausea, abdominal pain, rashes, visual disturbances (including temporary blindness), confusion; cardiovascular effects (see Cautions); hypersensitivity reactions including angioedema; hypoglycaemia (especially after parenteral administration); blood disorders (including thrombocytopenia and intravascular coagulation); acute renal failure; photosensitivity; very toxic in **overdosage**—immediate advice from poisons centres essential (see also p. 41)

Licensed use injection not licensed

Indication and dose

Treatment of malaria see p. 395

Note Quinine (anhydrous base) 100 mg ≡ quinine bisulphate 169 mg ≡ quinine dihydrochloride 122 mg ≡ quinine hydrochloride 122 mg ≡ quinine sulphate 121 mg. Quinine bisulphate 300-mg tablets are available but provide less quinine than 300 mg of the dihydrochloride, hydrochloride, or sulphate

Administration for *intravenous infusion*, dilute to a concentration of 2 mg/mL (max. 30 mg/mL in fluid restriction) with Glucose 5% *or* Sodium Chloride 0.9% and give over 4 hours

Quinine Sulphate (Non-proprietary) ℗ｅ
Tablets, coated, quinine sulphate 200 mg, net price 28-tab pack = £1.95; 300 mg, 28-tab pack = £1.88

Quinine Dihydrochloride (Non-proprietary) ℗ｅ
Injection, quinine dihydrochloride 300 mg/mL. For dilution and use as an infusion. 1- and 2-mL amps
Available from 'special-order' manufacturers or specialist importing companies, see p. 943
Note Intravenous injection of quinine is so hazardous that it has been superseded by infusion

---

Tetracyclines

Doxycycline (section 5.1.3) is used in children over 12 years for the *prophylaxis of malaria* in areas of *widespread mefloquine or chloroquine resistance*. Doxycycline is also used as an alternative to mefloquine or *Malarone®* (for details, see specific recommendations by country, see p. 398).

Doxycycline is also used as an *adjunct to quinine in the treatment of falciparum malaria* (for details see p. 395).

◢ DOXYCYCLINE

Cautions section 5.1.3

Contra-indications section 5.1.3

Side-effects section 5.1.3

Licensed use not licensed for use in children under 12 years

Indication and dose

> Prophylaxis of malaria preferably started 1–2 days before entering endemic area and continued for 4 weeks after leaving (see notes above)
> * **By mouth**
>   **Child over 12 years** 100 mg once daily

Treatment of falciparum malaria see p. 395

◢Preparations
Section 5.1.3

5.4.2 Amoebicides

Metronidazole is the drug of choice for *acute invasive amoebic dysentery* since it is very effective against vegetative forms of *Entamoeba histolytica* which can cause ulceration of the large intestine. **Tinidazole** is also effective. Metronidazole and tinidazole are also active against amoebae which may have migrated to the liver. Treatment with metronidazole (or tinidazole) is followed by a 10-day course of diloxanide furoate.

Diloxanide furoate is the drug of choice for asymptomatic patients with *E. histolytica* cysts in the faeces; metronidazole and tinidazole are relatively ineffective. Diloxanide furoate is relatively free from toxic effects and the usual course is of 10 days, given alone for chronic infections or following metronidazole or tinidazole treatment.

For *amoebic abscesses* of the liver **metronidazole** is effective; tinidazole is an alternative. Aspiration of the abscess is indicated where it is suspected that it may rupture or where there is no improvement after 72 hours of metronidazole; the aspiration may need to be repeated. Aspiration aids penetration of metronidazole and, for abscesses with large volume of pus, if carried out in conjunction with drug therapy, may reduce the period of disability.

Diloxanide furoate is not effective against hepatic amoebiasis, but a 10-day course should be given at the completion of metronidazole or tinidazole treatment to destroy any amoebae in the gut.

◢ DILOXANIDE FUROATE

Contra-indications

Pregnancy manufacturer advises avoid—no information available

Breast-feeding manufacturer advises avoid—no information available

Side-effects flatulence, vomiting, urticaria, pruritus

Licensed use not licensed for use in children under 25 kg body-weight

Indication and dose

> Chronic amoebiasis and as adjunct to metronidazole or tinidazole in acute amoebiasis
> * **By mouth**
>   **Child 1 month–12 years** 6.6 mg/kg 3 times daily for 10 days
>   **Child 12–18 years** 500 mg 3 times daily for 10 days

Diloxanide (Sovereign) [PoM]
Tablets, diloxanide furoate 500 mg, net price 30-tab pack = £42.95. Label: 9

◢Extemporaneous formulations available see Extemporaneous Preparations, p. 8

5

Infections

◼ METRONIDAZOLE

Cautions section 5.1.11
Side-effects section 5.1.11
Indication and dose
  Anaerobic infections section 5.1.11

  Invasive intestinal amoebiasis
  • By mouth
    Child 1–3 years 200 mg 3 times daily for 5 days
    Child 3–7 years 200 mg 4 times daily for 5 days
    Child 7–10 years 400 mg 3 times daily for 5 days
    Child 10–18 years 800 mg 3 times daily for 5 days

  Extra-intestinal amoebiasis (including liver abscess)
  • By mouth
    Child 1–3 years 100–200 mg 3 times daily for 5–10 days
    Child 3–7 years 100–200 mg 4 times daily for 5–10 days
    Child 7–10 years 200–400 mg 3 times daily for 5–10 days
    Child 10–18 years 400–800 mg 3 times daily for 5–10 days

  Urogenital trichomoniasis
  • By mouth
    Child 1–3 years 50 mg 3 times daily for 7 days
    Child 3–7 years 100 mg twice daily for 7 days
    Child 7–10 years 100 mg 3 times daily for 7 days
    Child 10–18 years 200 mg 3 times daily for 7 days *or* 400–500 mg twice daily for 5–7 days, *or* 2 g as a single dose

  Giardiasis
  • By mouth
    Child 1–3 years 500 mg once daily for 3 days
    Child 3–7 years 600–800 mg once daily for 3 days
    Child 7–10 years 1 g once daily for 3 days
    Child 10–18 years 2 g once daily for 3 days *or* 400 mg 3 times daily for 5 days *or* 500 mg twice daily for 7–10 days

◀ Preparations
Section 5.1.11

◼ TINIDAZOLE

Cautions see under Metronidazole (section 5.1.11); avoid in acute porphyria (section 9.8.2); **interactions:** Appendix 1 (tinidazole)
Pregnancy manufacturer advises avoid in first trimester
Breast-feeding present in milk—manufacturer advises avoid breast-feeding during and for 3 days after stopping treatment
Side-effects see under Metronidazole (section 5.1.11)
Licensed use licensed for use in children (age range not specified by manufacturer)
Indication and dose
  Intestinal amoebiasis
  • By mouth
    Child 1 month–12 years 50–60 mg/kg (max. 2 g) once daily for 3 days
    Child 12–18 years 2 g once daily for 2–3 days

  Amoebic involvement of liver
  • By mouth
    Child 1 month–12 years 50–60 mg/kg (max. 2 g) once daily for 5 days
    Child 12–18 years 1.5–2 g once daily for 3–6 days

  Urogenital trichomoniasis and giardiasis
  • By mouth
    Child 1 month–12 years single dose of 50–75 mg/kg (max. 2 g) (repeated once if necessary)
    Child 12–18 years single dose of 2 g (repeated once if necessary)

Fasigyn® (Pfizer) ▢PoM
  Tablets, f/c, tinidazole 500 mg. Net price 20-tab pack = £13.80. Label: 4, 9, 21, 25

▮ 5.4.3 Trichomonacides

Metronidazole (section 5.4.2) is the treatment of choice for *Trichomonas vaginalis* infection. Contact tracing is recommended and sexual contacts should be treated simultaneously. If metronidazole is ineffective, **tinidazole** (section 5.4.2) may be tried.

▮ 5.4.4 Antigiardial drugs

Metronidazole (section 5.4.2) is the treatment of choice for *Giardia lamblia* infections. **Tinidazole** (section 5.4.2) may be used as an alternative to metronidazole.

5.4.5 Leishmaniacides

Cutaneous leishmaniasis frequently heals spontaneously but if skin lesions are extensive or unsightly, treatment is indicated, as it is in visceral leishmaniasis (kala-azar). Leishmaniasis should be treated under specialist supervision.

Sodium stibogluconate, an organic pentavalent antimony compound, is the treatment of choice for visceral leishmaniasis. The dose is 20 mg/kg daily (max. 850 mg) for at least 20 days by intramuscular or intravenous injection; the dosage varies with different geographical regions and expert advice should be obtained. Skin lesions can also be treated with sodium stibogluconate.

Amphotericin is used with or after an antimony compound for visceral leishmaniasis unresponsive to the antimonial alone; side-effects may be reduced by using liposomal amphotericin (*AmBisome®*—section 5.2) at a dose of 1–3 mg/kg daily for 10–21 days to a cumulative dose of 21–30 mg/kg *or* at a dose of 3 mg/kg for 5 consecutive days followed by a single dose of 3 mg/kg 6 days later. Other lipid formulations of amphotericin (*Abelcet®* and *Amphocil®*) are also likely to be effective but less information is available.

Pentamidine isetionate (pentamidine isethionate) (section 5.4.8) has been used in antimony-resistant visceral leishmaniasis, but although the initial response is often good, the relapse rate is high; it is associated with serious side-effects. Other treatments include paromomycin [unlicensed], available from 'special-order' manufacturers or specialist importing companies, see p. 943

SODIUM STIBOGLUCONATE

Cautions intravenous injections must be given slowly over 5 minutes (to reduce risk of local thrombosis) and stopped if coughing or substernal pain; mucocutaneous disease (see below); monitor ECG before and during treatment; heart disease (withdraw if conduction disturbances occur); treat intercurrent infection (e.g. pneumonia)

Hepatic impairment use with caution in hepatic disease

Pregnancy manufacturer advises use only if potential benefit outweighs risk

Breast-feeding amount probably too small to be harmful

Mucocutaneous disease Successful treatment of mucocutaneous leishmaniasis may induce severe inflammation around the lesions (may be life-threatening if pharyngeal or tracheal involvement)—may require corticosteroid

Contra-indications

Renal impairment manufacturer advises avoid in severe impairment

Side-effects anorexia, nausea, vomiting, abdominal pain; ECG changes; coughing (see Cautions); headache, lethargy, arthralgia, myalgia; *rarely* jaundice, flushing, bleeding from nose or gum, substernal pain (see Cautions), vertigo, fever, sweating, and rash; also reported pancreatitis and anaphylaxis; pain and thrombosis on intravenous administration, intramuscular injection also painful

Licensed use licensed for use in children (age range not specified by manufacturer)

Indication and dose

Leishmaniasis for dose, see notes above

Administration injection should be filtered immediately before administration using a filter of 5 microns or less; see also Cautions above

Pentostam® (GSK) [PoM]

Injection, sodium stibogluconate equivalent to pentavalent antimony 100 mg/mL. Net price 100-mL bottle = £66.43

5.4.6 Trypanocides

The prophylaxis and treatment of trypanosomiasis is difficult and differs according to the strain of organism. Expert advice should therefore be obtained.

5.4.7 Drugs for toxoplasmosis

Most infections caused by *Toxoplasma gondii* are self-limiting, and treatment is not necessary. Exceptions are children with eye involvement (toxoplasma choroidoretinitis), and those who are immunosuppressed. Toxoplasmic encephalitis is a common complication of AIDS. The treatment of choice is a combination of **pyrimethamine** and **sulfadiazine** (sulphadiazine), given for several weeks (expert advice **essential**). Pyrimethamine is a folate antagonist, and adverse reactions to this combination are relatively common (folinic acid supplements (see p. 501) and weekly blood counts needed). Alternative regimens use combinations of pyrimethamine with clindamycin or clarithromycin or azithromycin. Long-term secondary prophylaxis is required after treatment of toxoplasmosis in immunocompromised patients; prophylaxis should continue until immunity recovers.

If toxoplasmosis is acquired in pregnancy, transplacental infection may lead to severe disease in the fetus; specialist advice should be sought on management. Spiramycin may reduce the risk of transmission of maternal infection to the fetus. When there is evidence of placental or fetal infection, pyrimethamine may be given with sulfadiazine and folinic acid after the first trimester.

In neonates without signs of toxoplasmosis, but born to mothers known to have become infected, spiramycin is given while awaiting laboratory results. If toxoplasmosis is confirmed in the infant, pyrimethamine and sulfadiazine are given for 12 months, together with folinic acid.

PYRIMETHAMINE

Cautions blood counts required with prolonged treatment; history of seizures—avoid large loading doses; **interactions:** Appendix 1 (pyrimethamine)

Hepatic impairment manufacturer advises caution

Renal impairment manufacturer advises caution

Pregnancy theoretical teratogenic risk in first trimester (folate antagonist); adequate folate supplement should be given to mother

Breast-feeding present in milk—avoid breast-feeding during toxoplasmosis treatment; avoid other folate antagonists

Side-effects depression of haematopoiesis with high doses, rashes, insomnia

Licensed use not licensed for use in children under 5 years

Indication and dose

Toxoplasmosis in pregnancy (in combination with sulfadiazine and folinic acid (section 8.1)), see notes above

• By mouth

Child 12–18 years 50 mg once daily until delivery

Congenital toxoplasmosis (in combination with sulfadiazine and folinic acid (section 8.1)),
• By mouth

Neonate 1 mg/kg twice daily for 2 days, *then* 1 mg/kg once daily for 6 months, *then* 1 mg/kg 3 times a week for 6 months

Malaria no dose stated because not recommended alone

Daraprim® (GSK) PoM ◢

Tablets, scored, pyrimethamine 25 mg. Net price 30-tab pack = £2.17

◢Extemporaneous formulations available see Extemporaneous Preparations, p. 8

SPIRAMYCIN

Cautions cardiac disease, arrhythmias (including predisposition to QT interval prolongation)

Hepatic impairment use with caution

Breast-feeding present in breast milk

Contra-indications sensitivity to other macrolides

Side-effects gastro-intestinal disturbances including nausea, vomiting, diarrhoea; dizziness, headache; rash; hepatotoxicity; *rarely*, prolongation of QT interval, thrombocytopenia and vasculitis

Licensed use not licensed

Indication and dose

Toxoplasmosis in pregnancy see notes above
• By mouth

Child 12–18 years 1.5 g twice daily until delivery

Chemoprophylaxis of congenital toxoplasmosis
• By mouth

Neonate 50 mg/kg twice daily

Spiramycin (Non-proprietary)

Tablets, spiramycin 750 000 units (250 mg); 1.5 million units (500 mg); 3 million units (1 g)

Syrup, spiramycin 75 000 units/mL (25 mg/mL)

Note 3000 units ≡ 1 mg spiramycin

Available from 'special-order' manufacturers or specialist importing companies, see p. 943

■ SULFADIAZINE

Cautions see under Co-trimoxazole, section 5.1.8

Pregnancy risk of neonatal haemolysis and methaemoglobinaemia in third trimester; fear of increased risk of kernicterus in neonates appears to be unfounded

Breast-feeding small risk of kernicterus in jaundiced infants and of haemolysis in G6PD-deficient infants

Contra-indications see under Co-trimoxazole, section 5.1.8

Renal impairment use with caution; avoid in severe renal impairment; high risk of crystalluria

Side-effects see under Co-trimoxazole, section 5.1.8

Licensed use not licensed for use in toxoplasmosis

Indication and dose

Toxoplasmosis in pregnancy (in combination with pyrimethamine and folinic acid (section 8.1)), see notes above
- **By mouth**

  Child 12–18 years 1 g 3 times daily until delivery

Congenital toxoplasmosis (in combination with pyrimethamine and folinic acid (section 8.1))
- **By mouth**

  Neonate 50 mg/kg twice daily for 12 months

Sulfadiazine (Non-proprietary) PoM
    Tablets, sulfadiazine 500 mg, net price 56-tab pack = £57.15. Label: 9, 27

◢ Extemporaneous formulations available see Extemporaneous Preparations, p. 8

5.4.8 Drugs for pneumocystis pneumonia

Pneumonia caused by *Pneumocystis jiroveci* (*Pneumocystis carinii*) occurs in immunosuppressed children; it is a common cause of pneumonia in AIDS. Pneumocystis pneumonia should be generally be treated by those experienced in its management. Blood gas measurement is used to assess disease severity.

Treatment

Mild to moderate disease　**Co-trimoxazole** (section 5.1.8) in high dosage is the drug of choice for the treatment of mild to moderate pneumocystis pneumonia.

A combination of **dapsone** with **trimethoprim** 5 mg/kg every 6–8 hours (section 5.1.8) is given by mouth for the treatment of mild to moderate disease [unlicensed indication] in children who cannot tolerate co-trimoxazole.

A combination of **clindamycin** (section 5.1.6) and **primaquine** (section 5.4.1) may be used in the treatment of mild to moderate disease [unlicensed indication]; this combination is associated with considerable toxicity.

Inhaled **pentamidine isetionate** is sometimes used for mild disease. It is better tolerated than parenteral pentamidine but systemic absorption may still occur.

Severe disease　**Co-trimoxazole** (section 5.1.8) in high dosage, given by mouth or by intravenous infusion, is the drug of choice for the treatment of severe pneumocystis pneumonia. **Pentamidine isetionate** given by intravenous infusion is an alternative for children who cannot tolerate co-trimoxazole, or who have not responded to it. Pentamidine isetionate is a potentially toxic drug that can cause severe hypotension during or immediately after infusion.

Corticosteroid treatment can be lifesaving in those with severe pneumocystis pneumonia (see Adjunctive Therapy below).

Adjunctive therapy　In moderate to severe pneumocystis infections associated with HIV infection, prednisolone (section 6.3.2) is given by mouth in a dose of 2 mg/kg (max. 80 mg daily) for 5 days (alternatively, hydrocortisone may be given parenterally); the dose is then reduced over the next 16 days and then stopped. Corticosteroid treatment should ideally be started at the same time as the anti-pneumocystis therapy and certainly no later than 24–72 hours afterwards. The corticosteroid should be withdrawn before anti-pneumocystis treatment is complete.

Prophylaxis

Prophylaxis against pneumocystis pneumonia should be given to all children with a history of the infection. Prophylaxis against pneumocystis pneumonia should also be considered for severely immunocompromised children. Prophylaxis

5 Infections

should continue until immunity recovers sufficiently. It should not be discontinued if the child has oral candidiasis, continues to lose weight, or is receiving cytotoxic therapy or long-term immunosuppressant therapy.

Co-trimoxazole (section 5.1.8) by mouth is the drug of choice for prophylaxis against pneumocystis pneumonia. Co-trimoxazole may be used in infants born to mothers with a high risk of transmission of infection.

Intermittent inhalation of **pentamidine isetionate** is used for prophylaxis against pneumocystis pneumonia in children unable to tolerate co-trimoxazole. It is effective but children may be prone to extrapulmonary infection. Alternatively, **dapsone** can be used.

DAPSONE

Cautions cardiac or pulmonary disease; anaemia (treat severe anaemia before starting); susceptibility to haemolysis including G6PD deficiency (section 9.1.5); avoid in acute porphyria (section 9.8.2); **interactions:** Appendix 1 (dapsone)

Pregnancy neonatal haemolysis and methaemoglobinaemia reported in third trimester; folic acid 5 mg daily should be given to mother throughout pregnancy

Breast-feeding haemolytic anaemia; although significant amount in milk, risk to infant very small unless infant is G6PD deficient

Blood disorders On long-term treatment, children and their carers should be told how to recognise signs of blood disorders and advised to seek immediate medical attention if symptoms such as fever, sore throat, rash, mouth ulcers, purpura, bruising or bleeding develop

Side-effects haemolysis, methaemoglobinaemia, neuropathy, allergic dermatitis (rarely including toxic epidermal necrolysis and Stevens-Johnson syndrome), anorexia, nausea, vomiting, tachycardia, headache, insomnia, psychosis, hepatitis, agranulocytosis; dapsone syndrome (rash with fever and eosinophilia)—discontinue immediately (may progress to exfoliative dermatitis,

hepatitis, hypoalbuminaemia, psychosis and death)

Licensed use not licensed for treatment of *P. jiroveci* pneumonia; monotherapy not licensed for children for prophylaxis of *P. jiroveci* pneumonia

Indication and dose

Treatment of *Pneumocystis jiroveci (P. carinii)* pneumonia (in combination with trimethoprim)
- **By mouth**
  Child 1 month–12 years 2 mg/kg (max. 100 mg) once daily
  Child 13–18 years 100 mg once daily

Prophylaxis of *Pneumocystis jiroveci (P. carinii)* pneumonia
- **By mouth**
  Child 1 month–18 years 2 mg/kg (max. 100 mg) once daily

Dapsone (Non-proprietary) ▢PoM▢
Tablets, dapsone 50 mg, net price 28-tab pack = £23.01; 100 mg 28-tab pack = £33.74. Label: 8

PENTAMIDINE ISETIONATE

Cautions risk of severe hypotension following administration (establish baseline blood pressure and administer with child lying down; monitor blood pressure closely during administration, and at regular intervals, until treatment concluded); hypokalaemia, hypomagnesaemia, coronary heart disease, bradycardia, history of ventricular arrhythmias, concomitant use with other drugs known to prolong Q-T interval; hypertension or hypotension; hyperglycaemia or hypoglycaemia; leucopenia, thrombocytopenia, or anaemia; carry out laboratory monitoring according to product literature; care required to protect personnel during handling and administration; **interactions:** Appendix 1 (pentamidine isetionate)

Hepatic impairment use with caution

Renal impairment reduce dose for pneumocystis pneumonia if estimated glomerular filtration rate less than 10 mL/minute/1.73 m^2; consult product literature

Pregnancy manufacturer advises avoid unless essential

Breast-feeding manufacturer advises avoid unless essential

Side-effects severe reactions, sometimes fatal, due to hypotension, hypoglycaemia, pancreatitis,

and arrhythmias; also leucopenia, thrombocytopenia, acute renal failure, hypocalcaemia; also reported: azotaemia, abnormal liver-function tests, anaemia, hyperkalaemia, nausea and vomiting, dizziness, syncope, flushing, hyperglycaemia, rash, and taste disturbances; Stevens-Johnson syndrome reported; on inhalation, bronchoconstriction (may be prevented by prior use of bronchodilators), cough and shortness of breath; discomfort, pain, induration, abscess formation, and muscle necrosis at injection site

Licensed use *nebuliser solution* not licensed for use in children

Indication and dose

Pneumocystis jiroveci (Pneumocystis carinii) pneumonia
- **By intravenous infusion**
  Child 1 month–18 years 4 mg/kg once daily for at least 14 days

- **By inhalation of nebulised solution (using suitable equipment—consult product literature)**
  Child 1 month–18 years 600 mg once daily for 3 weeks; secondary prevention, 300 mg every 4 weeks *or* 150 mg every 2 weeks

◁ **PENTAMIDINE ISETIONATE** (*continued*)

Visceral leishmaniasis (kala-azar, section 5.4.5)
- **By deep intramuscular injection**

  Child 1–18 years 3–4 mg/kg on alternate days to max. total of 10 injections; course may be repeated if necessary

Cutaneous leishmaniasis
- **By deep intramuscular injection**

  Child 1–18 years 3–4 mg/kg once or twice weekly until condition resolves (but see also section 5.4.5)

Trypanosomiasis
- **By deep intramuscular injection or intravenous infusion**

  Child 1–18 years 4 mg/kg daily or on alternate days to total of 7–10 injections

Administration Direct intravenous injection should be avoided whenever possible and **never** given rapidly; intramuscular injections should be deep and preferably given into the buttock.

For *intravenous infusion*, reconstitute 300 mg with 3–5 mL Water for Injections (displacement value may be significant), then dilute required dose with 50–250 mL Glucose 5% *or* Sodium Chloride 0.9%; give over at least 60 minutes

Pentacarinat® (Sanofi-Aventis) PoM

Injection, powder for reconstitution, pentamidine isetionate, net price 300-mg vial = £30.45

Nebuliser solution, pentamidine isetionate, net price 300-mg bottle = £32.15

Caution in handling Pentamidine isetionate is toxic and personnel should be adequately protected during handling and administration—consult product literature

5.5 Anthelmintics

- 5.5.1 Drugs for threadworms
- 5.5.2 Ascaricides
- 5.5.3 Drugs for tapeworm infections
- 5.5.4 Drugs for hookworms
- 5.5.5 Schistosomicides
- 5.5.6 Filaricides
- 5.5.7 Drugs for cutaneous larva migrans
- 5.5.8 Drugs for strongyloidiasis

Advice on prophylaxis and treatment of helminth infections is available from the following specialist centres:

Birmingham	(0121) 424 0357
Scottish Centre for Infection and Environmental Health (registered users of Travax only)	(0141) 300 1100 (weekdays 2–4 p.m. only)
Liverpool	(0151) 708 9393
London	(020) 7387 9300 (treatment advice only)

5.5.1 Drugs for threadworms
(pinworms, *Enterobius vermicularis*)

Anthelmintics are effective in threadworm infections, but their use needs to be combined with hygienic measures to break the cycle of auto-infection. All members of the family require treatment.

Adult threadworms do not live for longer than 6 weeks and for development of fresh worms, ova must be swallowed and exposed to the action of digestive juices in the upper intestinal tract. Direct multiplication of worms does not take place in the large bowel. Adult female worms lay ova on the perianal skin which causes pruritus; scratching the area then leads to ova being transmitted on fingers to the mouth, often via food eaten with unwashed hands. Washing hands and scrubbing nails before each meal and after each visit to the toilet is essential. A bath taken immediately after rising will remove ova laid during the night.

Mebendazole is the drug of choice for treating threadworm infection in children over 6 months. It is given as a single dose; as reinfection is very common, a second dose may be given after 2 weeks.

Piperazine is available in combination with sennosides as a single-dose preparation.

◢ MEBENDAZOLE

Cautions interactions: Appendix 1 (mebendazole)

Pregnancy manufacturer advises avoid—toxicity in *animal* studies

Breast-feeding amount present in milk too small to be harmful but manufacturer advises avoid
Note The patient information leaflet in the *Vermox®* pack includes the statement that it is not suitable for women known to be pregnant or for children under 2 years

Side-effects *very rarely* abdominal pain, diarrhoea; convulsions (in infants) and rash (including Stevens-Johnson syndrome and toxic epidermal necrolysis) reported

Licensed use not licensed for use in children under 2 years

Indication and dose

Threadworms
● By mouth
  Child 6 months—18 years 100 mg as a single dose; if reinfection occurs second dose may be needed after 2 weeks

Whipworms, roundworms (section 5.5.2), hookworms (section 5.5.4)
● By mouth
  Child 1—18 years 100 mg twice daily for 3 days

¹**Mebendazole** (Non-proprietary) ⓅoM
Tablets, chewable, mebendazole 100 mg
1. Mebendazole tablets can be sold to the public if supplied for oral use in the treatment of enterobiasis in children over 2 years provided its container or package is labelled to show a max. single dose of 100 mg and it is supplied in a container or package containing not more than 800 mg

Vermox® (Janssen-Cilag) ⓅoM
Tablets, orange, scored, chewable, mebendazole 100 mg. Net price 6-tab pack = £1.42

Suspension, mebendazole 100 mg/5 mL. Net price 30 mL = £1.65

◢ PIPERAZINE

Cautions epilepsy

Hepatic impairment manufacturer advises avoid

Renal impairment use with caution; avoid in severe renal impairment; risk of neurotoxicity

Pregnancy not known to be harmful but manufacturer advises avoid in first trimester

Breast-feeding present in milk—manufacturer advises avoid breast-feeding for 8 hours after dose (express and discard milk during this time)
Note Packs on sale to the general public carry a warning to avoid in epilepsy, liver or kidney disease, and to seek medical advice in pregnancy

Side-effects nausea, vomiting, colic, diarrhoea, allergic reactions including urticaria, bronchospasm, and rare reports of arthralgia, fever, Stevens-Johnson syndrome and angioedema; rarely dizziness, muscular inco-ordination ('worm wobble'); drowsiness, nystagmus, vertigo, blurred vision, confusion and clonic contractions in children with neurological or renal abnormalities

Indication and dose
See under preparation, below

◢With sennosides
For cautions, contra-indications, side-effects of senna see section 1.6.2

Pripsen® (Thornton & Ross)
Oral powder, piperazine phosphate 4 g, total sennosides (calculated as sennoside B) 15.3 mg/sachet. Net price two-dose sachet pack = £1.53. Label: 13

Dose
(Stirred into milk or water)

Threadworms
● By mouth
  Child 3 months–1 year 1 level 2.5-mL spoonful as a single dose in the morning, repeated after 14 days
  Child 1–6 years 1 level 5-mL spoonful as a single dose in the morning, repeated after 14 days
  Child 6–18 years content of 1 sachet as a single dose (in the morning), repeated after 14 days

Roundworms first dose as for threadworms; repeat at monthly intervals for up to 3 months if reinfection risk

5.5.2 Ascaricides
(common roundworm infections)

Mebendazole (section 5.5.1) is effective against *Ascaris lumbricoides* and is generally considered to be the drug of choice.

Levamisole [unlicensed] (available from 'special-order' manufacturers or specialist importing companies, see p. 943) is an alternative. It is very well tolerated; mild nausea or vomiting has been reported in about 1% of treated patients.

Piperazine may be given in a single dose, see Piperazine, above.

◢ LEVAMISOLE

Cautions epilepsy; juvenile idiopathic arthritis; Sjögren's syndrome

Hepatic impairment use with caution—dose adjustment may be necessary

Pregnancy embryotoxic in *animal* studies, avoid if possible

Breast-feeding no information available

Contra-indications blood disorders

◁ **LEVAMISOLE** (*continued*)

Side-effects nausea, vomiting, diarrhoea; dizziness, headache; on *prolonged treatment* taste disturbances, insomnia, convulsions, influenza-like syndrome, blood disorders, vasculitis, arthralgia, myalgia, rash

Licensed use not licensed

Indication and dose

> Roundworm (*Ascaris lumbricoides*)
> • By mouth
>> **Child 1 month–18 years** 2.5–3 mg/kg (max. 150 mg) as a single dose

> Hookworm
> • By mouth
>> **Child 1 month–18 years** 2.5 mg/kg (max. 150 mg) as a single dose repeated after 7 days if severe

> Nephrotic syndrome (specialist supervision section 6.3.2)
> • By mouth
>> **Child 1 month–18 years** 2.5 mg/kg (max. 150 mg) on alternate days

Levamisole (Non-proprietary) [PoM]
Tablets, levamisole (as hydrochloride) 50 mg
Label: 4
Available from 'special-order' manufacturers or specialist importing companies, see p. 943

5.5.3 Drugs for tapeworm infections

Taenicides

Niclosamide [unlicensed] (available from 'special-order' manufacturers or specialist importing companies, see p. 943) is the most widely used drug for tapeworm infections and side-effects are limited to occasional gastro-intestinal upset, lightheadedness, and pruritus; it is not effective against larval worms. Fears of developing cysticercosis in *Taenia solium* infections have proved unfounded. All the same, an antiemetic can be given before treatment and a laxative can be given 2 hours after niclosamide.

Praziquantel [unlicensed] is available from Merck (*Cysticide®*); it is as effective as niclosamide and is given to children over 4 years of age as a single dose of 5–10 mg/kg after a light breakfast (*or* as a single dose of 25 mg/kg for *Hymenolepis nana*).

Hydatid disease

Cysts caused by *Echinococcus granulosus* grow slowly and asymptomatic children do not always require treatment. Surgical treatment remains the method of choice in many situations. **Albendazole** [unlicensed] (available from 'special-order' manufacturers or specialist importing companies, see p. 943 is used in conjunction with surgery to reduce the risk of recurrence or as primary treatment in inoperable cases. Albendazole is given to children over 2 years of age in a dose of 7.5 mg/kg twice daily (max. 400 mg twice daily) for 28 days followed by 14-day break and then repeated for up to 2–3 cycles. Alveolar echinococcosis due to *E. multilocularis* is usually fatal if untreated. Surgical removal with albendazole cover is the treatment of choice, but where effective surgery is impossible, repeated cycles of albendazole (for a year or more) may help. Careful monitoring of liver function is particularly important during drug treatment.

5.5.4 Drugs for hookworms
(ancylostomiasis, necatoriasis)

Hookworms live in the upper small intestine and draw blood from the point of their attachment to their host. An iron-deficiency anaemia may occur and, if present, effective treatment of the infection requires not only expulsion of the worms but treatment of the anaemia.

Mebendazole (section 5.5.1) has a useful broad-spectrum activity, and is effective against hookworms. **Albendazole** [unlicensed] (available from 'special-order' manufacturers or specialist importing companies, see p. 943) given as a single dose of 400 mg in children over 2 years, is an alternative. **Levamisole** is also effective (section 5.5.2).

5 Infections

5.5.5 Schistosomicides
(bilharziasis)

Adult *Schistosoma haematobium* worms live in the genito-urinary veins and adult *S. mansoni* in those of the colon and mesentery. *S. japonicum* is more widely distributed in veins of the alimentary tract and portal system.

Praziquantel [unlicensed] is available from Merck (*Cysticide*®) and is effective against all human schistosomes. In children over 4 years the dose is 20 mg/kg followed after 4–6 hours by a further dose of 20 mg/kg (20 mg/kg 3 times daily for one day for *S. japonicum* infections). No serious adverse effects have been reported. Of all the available schistosomicides, it has the most attractive combination of effectiveness, broad-spectrum activity, and low toxicity.

5.5.6 Filaricides

Diethylcarbamazine [unlicensed] (available from 'special-order' manufacturers or specialist importing companies, see p. 943) is effective against microfilariae and adult worms of *Loa loa*, *Wuchereria bancrofti*, and *Brugia malayi*. To minimise reactions, treatment in children over 1 month is commenced with a dose of diethylcarbamazine citrate 1 mg/kg in divided doses on the first day and increased gradually over 3 days to 6 mg/kg daily (3 mg/kg daily if child under 10 years) in divided doses; length of treatment varies according to infection type, and usually gives a radical cure for these infections. Close medical supervision is necessary particularly in the early phase of treatment. In heavy infections there may be a febrile reaction, and in heavy *Loa loa* infection there is a small risk of encephalopathy. In such cases treatment must be given under careful in-patient supervision and stopped at the first sign of cerebral involvement (and specialist advice sought).

Ivermectin [unlicensed] (available from 'special-order' manufacturers or specialist importing companies, see p. 943) is very effective in *onchocerciasis* and it is now the drug of choice. In children over 5 years, a single dose of 150 micrograms/kg by mouth produces a prolonged reduction in microfilarial levels. Retreatment at intervals of 6 to 12 months depending on symptoms must be given until the adult worms die out. Reactions are usually slight and most commonly take the form of temporary aggravation of itching and rash. Diethylcarbamazine or suramin should no longer be used for onchocerciasis because of their toxicity.

5.5.7 Drugs for cutaneous larva migrans
(creeping eruption)

Dog and cat hookworm larvae may enter human skin where they produce slowly extending itching tracks usually on the foot. Single tracks can be treated with topical tiabendazole (no commercial preparation available). Multiple infections respond to **ivermectin**, **albendazole** or **tiabendazole** (thiabendazole) by mouth (all unlicensed and available from 'special-order' manufacturers or specialist importing companies, see p. 943).

5.5.8 Drugs for strongyloidiasis

Adult forms of *Strongyloides stercoralis* live in the gut and produce larvae which penetrate the gut wall and invade the tissues, setting up a cycle of auto-infection. **Ivermectin** [unlicensed] in a dose of 200 micrograms/kg daily for 2 days is the treatment of choice for chronic *Strongyloides* infection in children over 5 years. **Albendazole** [unlicensed] is an alternative in children over 2 years given in a dose of 400 mg twice daily for 3 days, repeated after 3 weeks if necessary.

Both of these drugs are available from 'special-order' manufacturers or specialist importing companies, see p. 943.

6 Endocrine system

6.1 Drugs used in diabetes...**418**
6.1.1 Insulins 418
6.1.2 Oral antidiabetic drugs 429
6.1.3 Diabetic ketoacidosis... 432
6.1.4 Treatment of hypoglycaemia 433
6.1.5 Treatment of diabetic nephropathy and neuropathy..................................... 435
6.1.6 Diagnostic and monitoring agents for diabetes mellitus 435

6.2 Thyroid and antithyroid drugs...**438**
6.2.1 Thyroid hormones.. 438
6.2.2 Antithyroid drugs.. 439

6.3 Corticosteroids...**442**
6.3.1 Replacement therapy 442
6.3.2 Glucocorticoid therapy 443

6.4 Sex hormones...**453**
6.4.1 Female sex hormones 454
6.4.2 Male sex hormones and antagonists.. 455
6.4.3 Anabolic steroids 459

6.5 Hypothalamic and pituitary hormones **459**
6.5.1 Hypothalamic and anterior pituitary hormones including growth hormone .. 459
6.5.2 Posterior pituitary hormones and antagonists 464

6.6 Drugs affecting bone metabolism **467**
6.6.1 Calcitonin 467
6.6.2 Bisphosphonates 468

6.7 Other endocrine drugs..**470**
6.7.1 Bromocriptine and other dopaminergic drugs 470
6.7.2 Drugs affecting gonadotrophins 470
6.7.3 Metyrapone 470
6.7.4 Somatomedins 471

6 Endocrine system

This chapter includes advice on the drug management of the following:
> Adrenal suppression during illness, trauma or surgery, p. 445
> Serious infections in patients taking corticosteroids, p. 446
> Nephrotic syndrome, p. 445
> Delayed puberty, p. 453
> Precocious puberty, p. 457
> Diabetes insipidus, p. 464

For hormonal contraception, see section 7.3.

6.1 Drugs used in diabetes

6.1.1 Insulins
6.1.2 Oral antidiabetic drugs
6.1.3 Diabetic ketoacidosis
6.1.4 Treatment of hypoglycaemia
6.1.5 Treatment of diabetic nephropathy and neuropathy
6.1.6 Diagnostic and monitoring agents for diabetes mellitus

Diabetes mellitus occurs because of a lack of insulin or resistance to its action. It is diagnosed by measuring fasting or random blood-glucose concentration (and occasionally by oral glucose tolerance test). Although there are many subtypes, the two principle classes of diabetes are type 1 diabetes and type 2 diabetes.

Type 1 diabetes, (formerly referred to as insulin-dependent diabetes mellitus (IDDM)), is due to a deficiency of insulin following autoimmune destruction of pancreatic beta cells and is the most common form of diabetes in children. Children with type 1 diabetes require administration of insulin.

Type 2 diabetes, (formerly referred to as non-insulin-dependent diabetes mellitus (NIDDM)), is rare in children but the incidence is increasing, particularly in adolescents, as obesity increases. It results from reduced secretion of insulin or from peripheral resistance to the action of insulin. Although children may be controlled on diet alone, many require oral antidiabetic drugs or insulin to maintain satisfactory control. There is limited information available on the use of oral anti-diabetic drugs in children (see section 6.1.2). In overweight individuals, type 2 diabetes may be prevented by losing weight and increasing physical activity.

Maturity-onset diabetes of the young (MODY) describes a number of rare disease states, distinct from type 2 diabetes, that are also characterised by impaired glucose tolerance. A sulphonylurea such as gliclazide (p. 430) may be effective in certain forms of MODY.

Treatment of diabetes   Treatment should be aimed at alleviating symptoms and minimising the risk of long-term complications (see below).

Diabetes is a strong risk factor for cardiovascular disease later in life. Other risk factors for cardiovascular disease (smoking, hypertension, obesity and hyperlipidaemia) should be addressed. The use of an ACE inhibitor (section 2.5.5.1) and of a lipid-regulating drug (section 2.12) can be beneficial in children with diabetes and a high cardiovascular disease risk. For reference to the use of an ACE inhibitor in the management of diabetic nephropathy, see section 6.1.5.

Prevention of diabetic complications   Although rare, retinopathy, neuropathy and nephropathy can occur in children with diabetes. Screening for complications should begin 5 years after diagnosis of diabetes or from 12 years of age. Optimal glycaemic control in both type 1 diabetes and type 2 diabetes reduces, in the long term, the risk of microvascular complications including retinopathy, development of proteinuria and to some extent neuropathy.

A measure of the total glycated (or glycosylated) haemoglobin (HbA_1) or a specific fraction (HbA_{1c}) provides a good indication of long-term glycaemic control. The ideal HbA_{1c} concentration is between 6.5 and 7.5% but this cannot always be achieved, and for those using insulin there are significantly increased risks of severe hypoglycaemia.

Tight control of blood pressure in hypertensive children with type 2 diabetes may reduce mortality significantly and protects visual acuity (by reducing considerably the risks of maculopathy and retinal photocoagulation) (see also section 2.5).

Driving   Information on the requirements for driving vehicles by individuals receiving treatment for diabetes is available in the BNF (section 6.1) or from the DVLA at www.dvla.gov.uk/medical.aspx.

6.1.1 Insulins

Insulin is a polypeptide hormone that plays a key role in the regulation of carbohydrate, fat, and protein metabolism. There are differences in the amino-acid sequence of animal insulins, human insulins, and the human insulin analogues. Human sequence insulin may be produced semisynthetically by enzymatic modification of porcine insulin (emp) or biosynthetically by recombinant DNA technology using bacteria (crb, prb) or yeast (pyr).

Immunological resistance to insulin action is uncommon. Preparations of human sequence insulin should theoretically be less immunogenic than other insulin preparations, but no real advantage has been shown in trials.

Insulin is inactivated by gastro-intestinal enzymes, and must therefore be given by injection; the subcutaneous route is ideal in most circumstances. Insulin is usually injected into the thighs, buttocks, or abdomen; absorption from a limb site can be increased if the limb is used in strenuous exercise after the injection. Generally, subcutaneous insulin injections cause few problems; fat hypertrophy does however occur and is a factor in poor glycaemic control. Fat hypertrophy can be minimised by using different injection sites in rotation. Local allergic reactions are rare.

Insulin should be given to all children with type 1 diabetes; it may also be needed to treat type 2 diabetes either when other methods cannot control the condition or during periods of acute illness or peri-operatively. Insulin is required in all instances of ketoacidosis (section 6.1.3), which can develop rapidly in children.

Management of diabetes with insulin   The aim of treatment is to achieve the best possible control of blood-glucose concentration without making the child or carer obsessional and to avoid disabling hypoglycaemia; close co-operation is needed between the child or carer and the medical team to achieve good control and thereby reduce the risk of complications. Mixtures of insulin preparations may be required and appropriate combinations have to be determined for the individual child. Treatment should be started with several doses of short-acting insulin (soluble insulin or a rapid-acting insulin analogue) given throughout the day with a longer-acting insulin given once a day. Alternatively, for those who have difficulty with, or prefer not to use, multiple daily injection regimens or in whom such regimens fail to achieve adequate glycaemic control, a mixture of premixed short- and medium-acting insulins can be given twice daily. The dose of insulin is increased gradually taking care to avoid troublesome hypoglycaemia. The proportion of the short-acting soluble component can be increased in those with excessive postprandial hyperglycaemia.

Initiation of insulin may be followed by a partial remission phase or 'honeymoon period' when lower doses of insulin are required than are subsequently necessary to maintain glycaemic control.

Insulin preparations can be divided into 3 types:

*   those of **short** duration which have a relatively rapid onset of action, namely soluble insulin and the rapid-acting insulin analogues, insulin aspart, insulin glulisine, and insulin lispro (section 6.1.1.1);

*   those with an **intermediate** action, e.g. isophane insulin (section 6.1.1.2); and

*   those whose action is slower in onset and lasts for **long** periods, e.g. protamine zinc insulin, insulin detemir, and insulin glargine (section 6.1.1.2)

The duration of action of a particular type of insulin can vary from one child to another, and needs to be assessed individually.

Examples of insulin regimens

*   Multiple injection regimen: either soluble insulin or a rapid-acting insulin before meals and long–acting insulin at bedtime; suitable for those who wish to have flexibility. Long-acting insulin analogues (insulin detemir or insulin glargine) may be useful for this regimen;

*   Three-times-daily combination of soluble insulin and isophane insulin in the morning, soluble insulin or a rapid-acting insulin analogue only before evening meal, and isophane insulin or long-acting insulin analogue only at bedtime; suitable for children who have at least 2 hours between the last 2 injections of the day;

*   Twice-daily mixture of soluble insulin and isophane insulin: either mixed before administration or given as a pre-mixed combination e.g. 30:70 of soluble insulin: isophane insulin;

*   Twice-daily isophane insulin: soluble insulin is added when necessary;

*   Continuous subcutaneous insulin infusion (see below).

6 Endocrine system

Insulin requirements   Most prepubertal children require around 0.6–0.8 units/kg/day of insulin after the initial temporary remission phase. Unless the child has a very sedentary life-style, a requirement for higher doses may indicate poor compliance, poor absorption of insulin from the injection site (e.g. because of lipohypertrophic sites), or the beginning of puberty. During puberty up to 1.5–2 units/kg/day of insulin may be required, especially during growth spurts. Around 1 year after menarche or after the growth spurt in boys, the dose may need to be adjusted to avoid excessive weight gain. Insulin requirements can be *increased* by infection, stress, and accidental or surgical trauma. Insulin requirements can be *reduced* in very active individuals and in those with renal or hepatic impairment, some endocrine disorders (e.g. Addison's disease, hypopituitarism) or coeliac disease. Insulin requirements should be assessed frequently in all these circumstances.

Pregnancy and breast-feeding   During pregnancy and breast-feeding, insulin requirements may alter and doses should be assessed frequently by an experienced diabetes physician. The dose of insulin generally needs to be increased in the second and third trimesters of pregnancy. The short-acting insulin analogues, insulin aspart and insulin lispro, are not known to be harmful, and may be used during pregnancy and breast-feeding. The safety of long-acting insulin analogues in pregnancy has not been established, therefore isophane insulin is recommended where longer-acting insulins are needed.

Insulin administration   Insulin is generally given by *subcutaneous injection* half-an-hour before a meal, except for rapid-acting insulins, which should be given immediately before, with, or even immediately after a meal (section 6.1.1.1). Injection devices ('pens') (section 6.1.1.3), which hold the insulin in a cartridge and meter the required dose, are convenient to use. The conventional syringe and needle is less popular with children and carers, but may be required for insulins not available in cartridge form.

For intensive insulin regimens multiple subcutaneous injections (3 to 4 times daily) are usually recommended.

Short-acting insulins (soluble insulin, insulin aspart, insulin glulisine, and insulin lispro) can also be given by *continuous subcutaneous infusion* using a portable infusion pump. This device delivers a continuous basal insulin infusion and patient-activated bolus doses at meal times. This technique is appropriate only for children who suffer recurrent hypoglycaemia or marked morning rise in blood-glucose concentration despite optimised multiple-injection regimens. Children on subcutaneous insulin infusion must be highly motivated, able to monitor their blood-glucose concentration or have it monitored by a carer, and have expert training, advice, and supervision from an experienced healthcare team.

NICE guidance

Continuous subcutaneous insulin infusion for the treatment of diabetes mellitus (type 1) (July 2008)

Continuous subcutaneous insulin infusion is recommended as an option in children over 12 years with type 1 diabetes:

- who suffer repeated or unpredictable hypoglycaemia, whilst attempting to achieve optimal glycaemic control with multiple-injection regimens, **or**

- whose glycaemic control remains inadequate (HbA_{1c} over 8.5%) despite optimised multiple-injection regimens (including the use of long-acting insulin analogues where appropriate).

Continuous subcutaneous insulin infusion is also recommended as an option for children under 12 years with type 1 diabetes for whom multiple-injection regimens are considered impractical or inappropriate. Children on insulin pumps should undergo a trial of multiple-injection therapy between the ages of 12 and 18 years.

Soluble insulin by the *intravenous route* is reserved for urgent treatment e.g in diabetic ketoacidosis, and for fine control in serious illness and in the perioperative period (see under Diabetes and Surgery, below).

Monitoring   All carers and children need to be trained to monitor blood-glucose concentrations (section 6.1.6). Since blood-glucose concentrations vary substantially throughout the day, 'normoglycaemia' cannot always be achieved throughout a 24-hour period without causing damaging hypoglycaemia. It is therefore best to recommend that children should maintain a blood-glucose concentration of between 4 and 9 mmol/litre for most of the time (4–7 mmol/litre before meals and less than 9 mmol/litre after meals), while accepting that on occasions, for brief periods, it will be above these values; efforts should be made to prevent the blood-glucose concentration from falling below 4 mmol/litre. Carers and children should be advised to look for 'peaks' and 'troughs' of blood glucose, and to adjust the insulin dosage only once or twice weekly. Overall it is ideal to aim for an HbA_{1c} (glycosylated haemoglobin) concentration of 6.5–7.5% or less (reference range 4–6%) but this is not always possible without causing disabling hypoglycaemia. Measurement of serum-fructosamine concentration can also be used for assessment of control; this is simpler and cheaper but the measurement of HbA_{1c} is generally more reliable.

The intake of energy and of simple and complex carbohydrates should be adequate to allow normal growth and development but obesity must be avoided. The carbohydrate intake needs to be regulated and should be distributed throughout the day. Fine control of blood glucose can be achieved by moving portions of carbohydrate from one meal to another without altering the total intake.

Hypoglycaemia   Hypoglycaemia is a potential problem for all children using insulin, and they and their carers should be given careful instruction on how to avoid it.

Loss of warning of hypoglycaemia is common among insulin-treated children and can be a serious hazard, especially for cyclists and drivers. Very tight control of diabetes lowers the blood-glucose concentration needed to trigger hypoglycaemic symptoms; increase in the frequency of hypoglycaemic episodes reduces the warning symptoms experienced by the child.

To restore the warning signs, episodes of hypoglycaemia must be minimised; this involves appropriate adjustment of insulin type, dose, and frequency, together with suitable timing and quantity of meals and snacks.

Diabetes and surgery   Children with type 1 diabetes should undergo surgery in centres with facilities for the care of children with diabetes.

Children with type 1 diabetes who require surgery:

- should be admitted to hospital for general anaesthesia;
- should receive insulin, even if they are fasting, to avoid ketoacidosis;
- should receive glucose infusion when fasting before an anaesthetic to prevent hypoglycaemia.

Elective surgery   Surgery in children with diabetes is best scheduled early on the list, preferably in the morning. If glycaemic control is poor it is advisable to admit the child well in advance of surgery. On the *evening before surgery*, blood-glucose should be measured frequently, especially before meals and snacks and at bedtime; urine should be tested for ketones. The usual evening or bedtime insulin and bedtime snack should be given. Ketosis or severe hypoglycaemia require correction, preferably by overnight intravenous infusion (section 6.1.3 and section 6.1.4), and the surgery may need to be postponed.

For *surgery scheduled for the morning*, the usual morning dose of insulin should be omitted. Early on the day of the operation, intravenous infusion of fluids and insulin should be started (see Intravenous Fluids and Continuous Insulin Infusion below).

For *surgery scheduled for the afternoon*, one-third of the usual morning dose of insulin should be given in the morning as short-acting (or soluble) insulin. Intravenous fluids and insulin infusion should be started by midday.

For *emergency surgery*, intravenous fluids and an insulin infusion should be started immediately (see Intravenous Fluids and Continuous Insulin Infusion below). If ketoacidosis is present the recommendations for diabetic ketoacidosis should be followed (section 6.1.3).

For *minor procedures that require fasting*, a slight modification of the usual regimen may be all that is necessary e.g. for early morning procedures delay insulin and food until immediately after the procedure. In all cases the advice of a doctor or anaesthetist experienced in the management of children with diabetes should be sought.

6 Endocrine system

Intravenous fluids and continuous insulin infusion Blood-glucose and plasma-electrolyte concentrations must be measured frequently in a child receiving intravenous support. Intravenous infusion should be continued until after the child starts to eat and drink. The following infusions should be used and adjusted according to the child's fluid and electrolyte requirements:

- Constant infusion of sodium chloride 0.45% and glucose 5% intravenous infusion together with potassium chloride 20 mmol/litre (provided that plasma-potassium concentration is not raised) at a rate determined by factors such as volume depletion and age; the amount of potassium chloride infused is adjusted according to plasma electrolyte measurements;
- Constant infusion of soluble insulin 1 unit/mL in sodium chloride 0.9% intravenous infusion initially at a rate of 0.025 units/kg/hour (up to 0.05 units/kg/hour if the child is unwell), then adjusted to blood-glucose concentration;
- Blood-glucose concentration should be maintained between 5 and 12 mmol/litre. If the glucose concentration falls below 5 mmol/litre, glucose 10% intravenous infusion may be required; conversely, if the glucose concentration persistently exceeds 15 mmol/litre, sodium chloride 0.9% intravenous infusion should be substituted;
- If the child develops overt hypoglycaemia (blood-glucose less than 3 mmol/litre) then the insulin infusion should be suspended for up to 30 minutes.

The usual subcutaneous insulin regimen should be started before the first meal (but the dose may need to be 10–20% higher than usual if the child is still bedbound or unwell) and the intravenous insulin infusion stopped 1 hour later. If glycaemic control is not adequately achieved, additional insulin can be given in the following ways:

- additional doses of soluble insulin at any of the 4 injection times (before meals or bedtime) *or*
- temporary addition of intravenous insulin infusion to subcutaneous regimen *or*
- complete reversion to intravenous insulin infusion (particularly if the child is unwell).

Neonatal diabetes Neonatal diabetes is a rare condition that presents with acidosis, dehydration, hyperglycaemia and rarely ketosis; it responds to continuous insulin infusion (0.02 to 0.125 units/kg/hour); the dose should be adjusted according to blood glucose concentrations. When the neonate is stable, treatment can be switched to subcutaneous insulin given once or twice a day. Treatment is normally required for 4-6 weeks in transient forms but may be required permanently in some cases.

Neonatal hyperglycaemia Newborn babies are relatively intolerant of glucose, especially in the first week of life and if premature. If intravenous glucose is necessary e.g. for total parenteral nutrition, infuse at a lower rate for 6–12 hours and the glucose intolerance should resolve. Insulin is not needed for such transient glucose intolerance, but may be needed if blood-glucose concentration is persistently high.

6.1.1.1 Short-acting insulins

Soluble insulin is a short-acting form of insulin. For maintenance regimens it is usual to inject it 15 to 30 minutes before meals.

Soluble insulin is the most appropriate form of insulin for use in diabetic emergencies and at the time of surgery. It can be given intravenously and intramuscularly, as well as subcutaneously.

When injected subcutaneously, soluble insulin has a rapid onset of action (30 to 60 minutes), a peak action between 2 and 4 hours, and a duration of action of up to 8 hours.

When injected intravenously, soluble insulin has a very short half-life of only about 5 minutes and its effect disappears within 30 minutes.

The human insulin analogues, **insulin aspart**, **insulin glulisine**, and **insulin lispro**, have a faster onset (10–20 minutes) and shorter duration of action (2–5 hours) than soluble insulin; as a result, compared with soluble insulin, fasting and preprandial blood-glucose concentrations are a little higher, postprandial blood-glucose concentration is a little lower, and hypoglycaemia occurs slightly less frequently. There is no evidence to justify switching from conventional insulin to a human insulin analogue if glycaemic control is adequate; they should only be used in children in preference to soluble insulin when a fast onset of action is required, e.g. in very young children who refuse food and when timing of injections in relation to meals is difficult. They may also be useful in children susceptible to pre-lunch hypoglycaemia and those who eat late in the evening and are prone to nocturnal hypoglycaemia. Insulin aspart and insulin lispro can be administered by subcutaneous infusion (see Insulin Administration above). They can also be administered intravenously and can be used as alternatives to soluble insulin for diabetic emergencies and at the time of surgery.

◢ INSULIN

(Insulin Injection; Neutral Insulin; Soluble Insulin)

A sterile solution of insulin (i.e. bovine or porcine) or of human insulin; pH 6.6–8.0

Cautions see notes above; **interactions:** Appendix 1 (antidiabetics)

Renal impairment may need dose reduction; insulin requirements fall; compensatory response to hypoglycaemia is impaired

Pregnancy insulin requirements should be assessed frequently by an experienced diabetes physician; see also Pregnancy and Breast-feeding p. 420 above

Side-effects see notes above; transient oedema; local reactions and fat hypertrophy at injection site; rarely hypersensitivity reactions including urticaria, rash; overdose causes hypoglycaemia

Indication and dose

Hyperglycaemia, surgery in children with diabetes

• By intravenous infusion

Neonate 0.01–0.1 units/kg/hour, adjusted according to blood-glucose concentration, see also notes above

Child 1 month–18 years 0.025–0.1 units/kg/hour, adjusted according to blood-glucose concentration, see also notes above

Diabetes mellitus

• By subcutaneous injection

According to requirements (see notes above)
Note Rotate injection site to reduce local reactions and fat hypertrophy

Administration For *intravenous infusion*, dilute to a concentration of 1 unit/mL with Sodium Chloride 0.9% and mix thoroughly; insulin may be adsorbed by plastics, flush giving set with 5 mL of infusion fluid containing insulin.
Neonatal intensive care, dilute 5 units to a final volume of 50 mL with infusion fluid; an intra-venous infusion rate of 0.1 mL/kg/hour provides a dose of 0.01 units/kg/hour

◢Highly purified animal
Counselling Show container to child or carer and confirm the expected version is dispensed

Hypurin® Bovine Neutral (Wockhardt) ℗ₒₘ
Injection, soluble insulin (bovine, highly purified) 100 units/mL. Net price 10-mL vial = £18.48; cartridges (for *Autopen® Classic*) 5 × 3 mL = £27.72

Hypurin® Porcine Neutral (Wockhardt) ℗ₒₘ
Injection, soluble insulin (porcine, highly purified) 100 units/mL. Net price 10-mL vial = £16.80; cartridges (for *Autopen® Classic*) 5 × 3 mL = £25.20

◢Human sequence
Counselling Show container to child or carer and confirm the expected version is dispensed

Actrapid® (Novo Nordisk) ℗ₒₘ
Injection, soluble insulin (human, pyr) 100 units/mL. Net price 10-mL vial = £7.48

Note Not recommended for use in subcutaneous insulin infusion pumps—may precipitate in catheter or needle

Humulin S® (Lilly) ℗ₒₘ
Injection, soluble insulin (human, prb) 100 units/mL. Net price 10-mL vial = £16.50; 5 × 3-mL cartridge (for *Autopen® Classic* or *HumaPen®*) = £28.12

Insuman® Rapid (Aventis Pharma) ℗ₒₘ
Injection, soluble insulin (human, crb) 100 units/mL, net price 5 × 3-mL cartridge (for *OptiPen® Pro 1*) = £23.43; 5 × 3-mL *Insuman® Rapid OptiSet®* prefilled disposable injection devices (range 2–40 units, allowing 2-unit dosage adjustment) = £27.90

Note Not recommended for use in subcutaneous insulin infusion pumps

◢Mixed preparations
See Biphasic Isophane Insulin (section 6.1.1.2)

◢ INSULIN ASPART

(Recombinant human insulin analogue)

Cautions see under Insulin; use only if benefit likely compared to soluble insulin

Pregnancy see under Insulin;

Side-effects see under Insulin

Indication and dose

Diabetes mellitus

• By subcutaneous injection

Immediately before meals or when necessary shortly after meals, according to requirements

• By subcutaneous infusion, intravenous injection or intravenous infusion

According to requirements

◻ INSULIN ASPART (*continued*)

Administration for *intravenous infusion*, dilute to a concentration of 0.05–1 unit/mL with Glucose 5% *or* Sodium Chloride 0.9% and mix thoroughly; insulin may be adsorbed by plastics, flush giving set with 5 mL of infusion fluid containing insulin.

NovoRapid® (Novo Nordisk) [PoM]
Injection, insulin aspart (recombinant human insulin analogue) 100 units/mL, net price 10-mL vial =

£17.27; *Penfill®* cartridge (for *Innovo®* and *NovoPen®* devices) 5 × 3-mL = £29.43; 5 × 3-mL *FlexPen®* prefilled disposable injection devices (range 1–60 units, allowing 1-unit dosage adjustment) = £32.00
Counselling Show container to child or carer and confirm the expected version is dispensed

◼ INSULIN GLULISINE
(Recombinant human insulin analogue)
Cautions see under Insulin

Pregnancy see under Insulin

Side-effects see under Insulin

Licensed use not licensed for children under 6 years

Indication and dose
Diabetes mellitus
• **By subcutaneous injection**
Immediately before meals or when necessary shortly after meals, according to requirements

• **By subcutaneous infusion**
According to requirements

Apidra® (Sanofi-Aventis) ▼ [PoM]
Injection, insulin glulisine (recombinant human insulin analogue) 100 units/mL, net price 10-mL vial = £17.27; 5 × 3-mL cartridge (for *OptiPen® Pro 1* and *Autopen® 24*) = £29.45; 5 × 3-mL *OptiClik®* cartridge (for *OptiClik® Pen* [NHS]) = £31.50; 5 × 3-mL *Apidra® Optiset®* prefilled disposable injection devices (range 2–40 units, allowing 2-unit dosage adjustment) = £29.45; 5 × 3-mL *Apidra® SoloStar®* prefilled disposable injection devices (range 1–80 units, allowing 1-unit dosage adjustment) = £25.00
Counselling Show container to patient and confirm that patient is expecting the version dispensed
Note The *Scottish Medicines Consortium* (p. 4) has advised (October 2008) that *Apidra®* is accepted for restricted use within NHS Scotland for the treatment of children over 6 years with diabetes mellitus in whom the use of a short-acting insulin analogue is appropriate

◼ INSULIN LISPRO
(Recombinant human insulin analogue)
Cautions see under Insulin; children under 12 years (use only if benefit likely compared to soluble insulin)

Pregnancy see under Insulin;

Side-effects see under Insulin

Indication and dose
Diabetes mellitus
• **By subcutaneous injection**
Shortly before meals or when necessary shortly after meals, according to requirements

• **By subcutaneous infusion, or intravenous injection, or intravenous infusion**
According to requirements

Administration For *intravenous infusion*, dilute to a concentration of 0.1–1 unit/mL with Glucose 5%

or Sodium Chloride 0.9% and mix thoroughly; insulin may be adsorbed by plastics, flush giving set with 5 mL of infusion fluid containing insulin.

Humalog® (Lilly) [PoM]
Injection, insulin lispro (recombinant human insulin analogue) 100 units/mL. Net price 10-mL vial = £17.28; 5 × 3-mL cartridge (for *Autopen® Classic* or *HumaPen®*) = £29.46; 5 × 3-mL *Humalog®-Pen* prefilled disposable injection devices (range 1–60 units, allowing 1-unit dosage adjustment) = £29.46; 5 × 3-mL *Humalog® KwikPen* prefilled disposable injection devices (range 1–60 units, allowing 1-unit dosage adjustment) = £29.46
Counselling Show container to child or carer and confirm the expected version is dispensed

6.1.1.2 Intermediate- and long-acting insulins

When given by subcutaneous injection, intermediate- and long-acting insulins have an onset of action of approximately 1–2 hours, a maximal effect at 4–12 hours, and a duration of 16–35 hours. Some are given twice daily in conjunction with short-acting (soluble) insulin, and others are given once daily. Soluble insulin can be mixed with intermediate and long-acting insulins (except insulin detemir and insulin glargine), essentially retaining the properties of the two components, although there may be some blunting of the initial effect of the soluble insulin component (especially on mixing with protamine zinc insulin, see below).

Close monitoring of blood glucose is essential when introducing a change to the insulin regimen; the total daily dose as well as any concomitant treatment may need to be adjusted.

Endocrine system

6

Isophane insulin is a suspension of insulin with protamine; it is of particular value for initiation of twice-daily insulin regimens. Isophane can be mixed with soluble insulin before injection but ready-mixed preparations may be more appropriate (**biphasic isophane insulin**, **biphasic insulin aspart**, or **biphasic insulin lispro**).

Insulin zinc suspension (30% amorphous, 70% crystalline) has a more prolonged duration of action.

Protamine zinc insulin is usually given once daily with short-acting (soluble) insulin. It has the drawback of binding with the soluble insulin when mixed in the same syringe and is now rarely used.

Insulin detemir and **insulin glargine** are human insulin analogues with prolonged duration of action; insulin detemir is given once or twice daily and insulin glargine is given once daily. There is little evidence to justify switching from conventional intermediate- or long-acting insulin to a human insulin analogue if glycaemic control is adequate. NICE (December 2002) has recommended that insulin glargine should be available as an option for patients with type 1 diabetes.

NICE (May 2008) has recommended that, if insulin is required in patients with type 2 diabetes, insulin glargine may be considered for those:

- who require assistance with injecting insulin *or*

- whose lifestyle is significantly restricted by recurrent symptomatic hypoglycaemia *or*

- who would otherwise need twice-daily basal insulin injections in combination with oral antidiabetic drugs.

A trial of insulin glargine may be offered to those who have experienced significant nocturnal hypoglycaemia when treated with isophane insulin.

INSULIN DETEMIR

(Recombinant human insulin analogue—long-acting)

Cautions see under Insulin (section 6.1.1.1)

Pregnancy see under Insulin; limited evidence of safety

Side-effects see under Insulin (section 6.1.1.1)

Licensed use not licensed for use in children under 6 years

Indication and dose

Diabetes mellitus
- **By subcutaneous injection**

    Child over 6 years According to requirements

Levemir® (Novo Nordisk) PoM

Injection, insulin detemir (recombinant human insulin analogue) 100 units/mL, net price 5 × 3-mL cartridge (for *NovoPen®* devices) = £39.00; 5 × 3-mL *FlexPen®* prefilled disposable injection device (range 1–60 units, allowing 1-unit dosage adjustment) = £39.00; 5 × 3-mL *Levemir InnoLet®* prefilled disposable injection devices (range 1–50 units, allowing 1-unit dosage adjustment) = £44.85

Counselling Show container to child or carer and confirm the expected version is dispensed

---

INSULIN GLARGINE

(Recombinant human insulin analogue—long acting)

Cautions see under Insulin (section 6.1.1.1)

Pregnancy see under Insulin; limited evidence of safety

Side-effects see under Insulin (section 6.1.1.1)

Licensed use not licensed for use in children under 6 years

Indication and dose

Diabetes mellitus
- **By subcutaneous injection**

    According to requirements

Lantus® (Aventis Pharma) PoM

Injection, insulin glargine (recombinant human insulin analogue) 100 units/mL, net price 10-mL vial = £26.00; 5 × 3-mL cartridge (for *OptiPen® Pro 1* and *Autopen® 24*) = £39.00; 5 × 3-mL *OptiClik®* cartridge (for *OptiClik® Pen* NHS) = £42.00; 5 × 3-mL *Lantus® OptiSet®* prefilled disposable injection

devices (range 2–40 units, allowing 2-unit dosage adjustment) = £39.00; 5 × 3-mL *Lantus® SoloStar®* prefilled disposable injection devices (range 1–80 units, allowing 1-unit dosage adjustment) = £42.00

Note The *Scottish Medicines Consortium* (p. 4) has advised (October 2002) that insulin glargine is accepted for restricted use within NHS Scotland for the treatment of type 1 diabetes:

- in those who are at risk of or experience unacceptable frequency or severity of nocturnal hypoglycaemia on attempting to achieve better hypoglycaemic control during treatment with other insulins

- as a once daily insulin therapy for patients who require a carer to administer their insulin.

It is **not** recommended for routine use in patients with type 2 diabetes unless they suffer from recurrent episodes of hypoglycaemia or require assistance with their insulin injections.

Counselling Show container to child or carer and confirm the expected version is dispensed

6 Endocrine system

■ INSULIN ZINC SUSPENSION

(Insulin Zinc Suspension (Mixed)—long acting)
A sterile neutral suspension of bovine insulin or of human insulin in the form of a complex obtained by the addition of a suitable zinc salt; consists of rhombohedral crystals (10–40 microns) and of particles of no uniform shape (not exceeding 2 microns)

Cautions see under Insulin (section 6.1.1.1)

Side-effects see under Insulin (section 6.1.1.1)

Indication and dose

> Diabetes mellitus
> • **By subcutaneous injection**
> According to requirements

◢Highly purified animal

Hypurin® Bovine Lente (Wockhardt) (PoM)
Injection, insulin zinc suspension (bovine, highly purified) 100 units/mL. Net price 10-mL vial = £18.48

Counselling Show container to child or carer and confirm the expected version is dispensed

■ ISOPHANE INSULIN

(Isophane Insulin Injection; Isophane Prot-amine Insulin Injection; Isophane Insulin (NPH)—intermediate acting)
A sterile suspension of bovine or porcine insulin or of human insulin in the form of a complex obtained by the addition of protamine sulphate or another suitable protamine

Cautions see under Insulin (section 6.1.1.1)

Side-effects see under Insulin (section 6.1.1.1); protamine may cause allergic reactions

Indication and dose

> Diabetes mellitus
> • **By subcutaneous injection**
> According to requirements

◢Highly purified animal
Counselling Show container to child or carer and confirm the expected version is dispensed

Hypurin® Bovine Isophane (Wockhardt) (PoM)
Injection, isophane insulin (bovine, highly purified) 100 units/mL. Net price 10-mL vial = £18.48; cartridges (for *Autopen® Classic*) 5 × 3 mL = £27.72

Hypurin® Porcine Isophane (Wockhardt) (PoM)
Injection, isophane insulin (porcine, highly purified) 100 units/mL. Net price 10-mL vial = £16.80; cartridges (for *Autopen® Classic*) 5 × 3 mL = £25.20

◢Human sequence
Counselling Show container to child or carer and confirm the expected version is dispensed

Insulatard® (Novo Nordisk) (PoM)
Injection, isophane insulin (human, pyr) 100 units/mL. Net price 10-mL vial = £7.48; *Insulatard Penfill®* cartridge (for *Innovo®*, or *Novopen®* devices) 5 × 3 mL = £20.08; 5 × 3-mL *Insulatard InnoLet®* prefilled disposable injection devices (range 1–50 units, allowing 1-unit dosage adjustment) = £20.40

Humulin I® (Lilly) (PoM)
Injection, isophane insulin (human, prb) 100 units/mL. Net price 10-mL vial = £16.50; 5 × 3-mL cartridge (for *Autopen® Classic* or *HumaPen®*) = £29.94; 5 × 3-mL *Humulin I-Pen®* prefilled disposable injection devices (range 1–60 units, allowing 1-unit dosage adjustment) = £29.94

Insuman® Basal (Aventis Pharma) (PoM)
Injection, isophane insulin (human, crb) 100 units/mL, net price 5-mL vial = £5.84; 5 × 3-mL cartridge (for *OptiPen® Pro 1*) = £23.43; 5 × 3-mL *Insuman® Basal OptiSet®* prefilled disposable injection devices (range 2–40 units, allowing 2-unit dosage adjustment) = £27.90

◢Mixed preparations
See Biphasic Isophane Insulin (p. 427)

■ PROTAMINE ZINC INSULIN

(Protamine Zinc Insulin Injection—long acting)
A sterile suspension of insulin in the form of a complex obtained by the addition of a suitable protamine and zinc chloride; this preparation was included in BP 1980 but is not included in BP 1988

Cautions see under Insulin (section 6.1.1.1); see also notes above

Side-effects see under Insulin (section 6.1.1.1); protamine may cause allergic reactions

Indication and dose

> Diabetes mellitus
> • **By subcutaneous injection**
> According to requirements

Hypurin® Bovine Protamine Zinc (Wockhardt) (PoM)
Injection, protamine zinc insulin (bovine, highly purified) 100 units/mL. Net price 10-mL vial = £18.48

Counselling Show container to child or carer and confirm the expected version is dispensed

6 Endocrine system

Biphasic insulins

Biphasic insulins are pre-mixed insulin preparations containing various combinations of short-acting (soluble) or rapid-acting (analogue) insulin and an intermediate-acting insulin.

The percentage of short-acting insulin varies from 10% to 50%. These preparations should be administered by subcutaneous injection up to 15 minutes before or soon after a meal.

◢ BIPHASIC INSULIN ASPART
(Intermediate-acting insulin)

Cautions see under Insulin and Insulin Aspart (section 6.1.1.1)

Side-effects see under Insulin (section 6.1.1.1); protamine may cause allergic reactions

Indication and dose

Diabetes mellitus
- **By subcutaneous injection**
  Up to 10 minutes before or soon after a meal, according to requirements

NovoMix® 30 (Novo Nordisk) PoM
Injection, biphasic insulin aspart (recombinant human insulin analogue), 30% insulin aspart, 70% insulin aspart protamine, 100 units/mL, net price 5 × 3-mL *Penfill®* cartridges (for *Innovo®* and *NovoPen®* devices) = £29.43; 5 × 3-mL *FlexPen®* prefilled disposable injection devices (range 1–60 units, allowing 1-unit dosage adjustment) = £32.00

Counselling Show container to child or carer and confirm the expected version is dispensed; the proportions of the two components should be checked **carefully** (the order in which the proportions are stated may not be the same in other countries)

◢ BIPHASIC INSULIN LISPRO
(Intermediate-acting insulin)

Cautions see under Insulin and Insulin Lispro (section 6.1.1.1)

Side-effects see under Insulin (section 6.1.1.1); protamine may cause allergic reactions

Indication and dose

Diabetes mellitus
- **By subcutaneous injection**
  Up to 15 minutes before or soon after a meal, according to requirements

Humalog® Mix25 (Lilly) PoM
Injection, biphasic insulin lispro (recombinant human insulin analogue), 25% insulin lispro, 75% insulin lispro protamine, 100 units/mL, net price 5 × 3-mL cartridge (for *Autopen® Classic* or *HumaPen®*) = £29.46; 5 × 3-mL prefilled disposable injection devices (range 1–60 units, allowing 1-unit dosage adjustment) = £30.98; 5 × 3-mL *Humalog® Mix25 KwikPen* prefilled disposable injection

devices (range 1–60 units allowing 1-unit dosage adjustment) = £30.98

Counselling Show container to child or carer and confirm the expected version is dispensed; the proportions of the two components should be checked **carefully** (the order in which the proportions are stated may not be the same in other countries)

Humalog® Mix50 (Lilly) PoM
Injection, biphasic insulin lispro (recombinant human insulin analogue), 50% insulin lispro, 50% insulin lispro protamine, 100 units/mL, net price 5 × 3-mL cartridge (for *Autopen® Classic* or *HumaPen®*) = £29.46; 5 × 3-mL prefilled disposable injection devices (range 1–60 units, allowing 1-unit dosage adjustment) = £29.46; 5 × 3-mL *Humalog® Mix50 KwikPen* prefilled disposable injection devices (range 1–60 units, allowing 1-unit dosage adjustment) = £30.98

Counselling Show container to child or carer and confirm the expected version is dispensed; the proportions of the two components should be checked **carefully** (the order in which the proportions are stated may not be the same in other countries)

◢ BIPHASIC ISOPHANE INSULIN
(Biphasic Isophane Insulin Injection—intermediate acting)

A sterile buffered suspension of either porcine or human insulin complexed with protamine sulphate (or another suitable protamine) in a solution of insulin of the same species

Cautions see under Insulin (section 6.1.1.1)

Side-effects see under Insulin (section 6.1.1.1); protamine may cause allergic reactions

Indication and dose

Diabetes mellitus
- **By subcutaneous injection**
  According to requirements

◢Highly purified animal

Counselling Show container to child or carer and confirm the expected version is dispensed; the proportions of the two components should be checked **carefully** (the order in which the proportions are stated may not be the same in other countries)

Hypurin® Porcine 30/70 Mix (Wockhardt) PoM
Injection, biphasic isophane insulin (porcine, highly purified), 30% soluble, 70% isophane, 100 units/mL. Net price 10-mL vial = £16.80; cartridges (for *Autopen® Classic*) 5 × 3 mL = £25.20

◢Human sequence

Counselling Show container to child or carer and confirm the expected version is dispensed; the proportions of the

6

Endocrine system

◁ **BIPHASIC ISOPHANE INSULIN** (*continued*)

two components should be checked **carefully** (the order in which the proportions are stated may not be the same in other countries)

Mixtard® 30 (Novo Nordisk) PoM

Injection, biphasic isophane insulin (human, pyr), 30% soluble, 70% isophane, 100 units/mL. Net price 10-mL vial = £7.48; *Mixtard 30 Penfill*® cartridge (for *Innovo* or *Novopen*® devices) 5 × 3 mL = £20.08; 5 × 3-mL *Mixtard 30 InnoLet*® prefilled disposable injection devices (range 1–50 units allowing 1-unit dosage adjustment) = £19.87

Humulin M3® (Lilly) PoM

Injection, biphasic isophane insulin (human, prb), 30% soluble, 70% isophane, 100 units/mL. Net price 10-mL vial = £16.50; 5 × 3-mL cartridge (for *Autopen*® *Classic* or *HumaPen*®) = £28.12

Insuman® Comb 15 (Aventis Pharma) PoM

Injection, biphasic isophane insulin (human, crb), 15% soluble, 85% isophane, 100 units/mL, net price 5 × 3-mL *Insuman*® *Comb 15 OptiSet*® prefilled disposable injection devices (range 2–40 units, allowing 2-unit dosage adjustment) = £27.90

Insuman® Comb 25 (Aventis Pharma) PoM

Injection, biphasic isophane insulin (human, crb), 25% soluble, 75% isophane, 100 units/mL, net price 5-mL vial = £5.84; 5 × 3-mL cartridge (for *OptiPen*® *Pro 1*) = £23.43; 5 × 3-mL *Insuman*® *Comb 25 OptiSet*® prefilled disposable injection devices (range 2–40 units, allowing 2-unit dosage adjustment) = £27.90

Insuman® Comb 50 (Aventis Pharma) PoM

Injection, biphasic isophane insulin (human, crb), 50% soluble, 50% isophane, 100 units/mL, net price; 5 × 3-mL cartridge (for *OptiPen*® *Pro 1*) = £23.43; 5 × 3-mL *Insuman*® *Comb 50 OptiSet*® prefilled disposable injection devices (range 2–40 units, allowing 2-unit dosage adjustment) = £27.90

6.1.1.3 Hypodermic equipment

Carers and children should be advised on the safe disposal of lancets, single-use syringes, and needles. Suitable arrangements for the safe disposal of contaminated waste must be made before these products are prescribed for patients who are carriers of infectious diseases.

◀ **Injection devices**

Autopen® (Owen Mumford)

Injection device; *Autopen*® *24* (for use with Sanofi-Aventis 3-mL insulin cartridges), allowing 1-unit dosage adjustment, max. 21 units (single-unit version) *or* 2 unit dosage adjustment, max. 42 units (2-unit version), net price (both) = £15.55; *Autopen*® *Classic* (for use with Lilly and Wockhardt 3-mL insulin cartridges), allowing 1-unit dosage adjustment, max. 21 units (single-unit version) *or* 2 unit dosage adjustment, max. 42 units (2-unit version), net price (all) = £15.79

HumaPen® Luxura (Lilly)

Injection device, for use with *Humulin*® and *Humalog*® 3-mL cartridges; allowing 1-unit dosage adjustment, max. 60 units, net price = £26.36 (available in burgundy and champagne)

HumaPen® Luxura HD (Lilly)

Injection device, for use with *Humulin*® and *Humalog*® 3-mL cartridges; allowing 0.5-unit dosage adjustment, max. 30 units, net price = £26.36

NovoPen® (Novo Nordisk)

Injection device; for use with *Penfill*® insulin cartridges; *NovoPen*® *Junior* (for 3-mL cartridges), allowing 0.5-unit dosage adjustment, max. 35 units, net price = £24.60 (available in green and yellow); *NovoPen*® *3 Demi* (for 3-mL cartridges), allowing 0.5-unit dosage adjustment, max. 35 units, net price = £25.03; *NovoPen*® *4* (for 3-mL cartridges), allowing 1-unit dosage adjustment, max. 60 units, net price = £26.36 (available in silver and blue)

OptiClik® (Sanofi-Aventis)

Injection device, for use with *Lantus OptiClik*® insulin cartridges, allowing 1-unit dosage adjustment, max. 80 units, net price = £20.13 (available in blue and grey)

OptiPen® Pro 1 (Aventis Pharma)

Injection device, for use with *Insuman*® insulin cartridges; allowing 1-unit dosage adjustment, max. 60 units, net price = £22.00

SQ-PEN® (Medical House)

Needle-free insulin delivery device for use with any 10-mL vial *or* any 3-mL cartridge of insulin, allowing 1-unit dosage adjustment, max. 50 units, net price *starter pack* (*SQ-PEN*® device, 1 practice nozzle, 1 nozzle, 1 3-mL adaptor, 1 10-mL adaptor) = £147.83, *3-month consumables pack* for 10-mL adaptor (7 nozzles, 5 × 10-mL insulin vial adaptors) = £18.08, for 3-mL adaptor (7 nozzles, 15 × 3-mL insulin cartridge adaptors) = £30.82; *vial adaptor pack* (6 insulin vial adaptors) = £7.66, *cartridge adaptor pack* (6 insulin cartridge adaptors) = £7.66; nozzle pack (6 nozzles) = £10.03

◀ **Lancets**

Lancets—sterile, single use (Drug Tariff)

BD Micro-Fine®+ 100 = £3.16, 200 = £6.13; *Cleanlet Fine*® 100 = £3.19, 200 = £6.13; [1] *Finepoint*® 100 = £3.48; [1] *FreeStyle*® 200 = £6.89; [1] *GlucoMen*® Fine 100 = £3.48, 200 = £6.74; *Hypoguard Supreme*® 100 = £2.75; [1] *Microlet*® (formerly *Ascencia Microlet*®) 100 = £3.69, 200 = £7.03; [1] *Milward Steri-Let*®, 23 gauge, 100 = £3.00, 200 = £5.70, 28 gauge, 100 = £3.30, 200 = £5.70; [1] *Monolet*® 100 = £3.28, 200 = £6.24; *Monolet*® Extra 100 = £3.28; *MPD Ultra Thin*®, 100 = £3.30, 200 = £6.50; *Multiclix*® 204 = £9.02; [1] *One Touch UltraSoft*® 100 = £3.56; [2] *Softclix*® 200 = £7.20; [2] *Softclix XL*® 50 = £1.80; *Thin Lancets*, 200 = £7.02; [1] *Unilet ComforTouch*® 100 = £3.60, 200 = £6.83; [1] *Unilet General Purpose Superlite*® 100 = £3.67, 200 = £6.96; *Unistik 3 Comfort*®, 23-gauge, 100 = £6.24, 200 = £12.20; *Unistik 3 Extra*®, 21-gauge, 100 = £6.24, 200 = £12.20; *Unistik 3 Normal*®, 23-gauge, 100 = £6.24, 200 = £12.20; *Universal*®, 200 = £6.32; *Vitrex Soft*®, 23-gauge, 100 = £3.00, 200 = £5.70; *Vitrex Gentle*® 28-gauge, 100 = £3.19, 200 = £6.13; *WaveSense Ultra-Thin*® 28-gauge, 100 = £6.90, 33-gauge, 200 = £6.90

Compatible finger-pricking devices (unless indicated otherwise, see footnotes), all ᴺᴴˢ: *B-D Optimus*®, *Glucolet*®, *Monojector*®, *Penlet II*®, *Soft Touch*®

1. ᴺᴴˢ *Autolet*® and ᴺᴴˢ *Autolet Impression*® are also compatible finger-pricking devices
2. Use ᴺᴴˢ *Softclix*® finger-pricking device

◀ **Needles**

Hypodermic Needle, Sterile single use (Drug Tariff)

For use with reusable glass syringe, sizes 0.5 mm (25G), 0.45 mm (26G), 0.4 mm (27G). Net price 100-needle pack = £2.68

Brands include *Microlance*®, *Monoject*®

Needles for Prefilled and Reusable Pen Injectors (Drug Tariff)

Screw on, needle length 6.1 mm or less, net price 100-needle pack = £12.53; 6.2–9.9 mm, 100-needle pack = £8.89; 10 mm or more, 100-needle pack = £8.89

Brands include *BD Micro-Fine®+*, *Comfort Point®*, *NovoFine®*, *Novofine Autocover®*, *Unifine® Pentips*

Snap on, needle length 6.1 mm or less, net price 100-needle pack = £12.02; 6.2–9.9 mm, 100-needle pack = £8.52; 10 mm or more, 100-needle pack = £8.52

Brands include *Penfine®*

◄Syringes

Hypodermic Syringe (Drug Tariff)

Calibrated glass with Luer taper conical fitting, for use with U100 insulin. Net price 0.5 mL and 1 mL = £15.18

Brands include *Abcare®*

Pre-Set U100 Insulin Syringe (Drug Tariff)

Calibrated glass with Luer taper conical fitting, supplied with dosage chart and strong box, for blind patients. Net price 1 mL = £21.99

U100 Insulin Syringe with Needle (Drug Tariff)

Disposable with fixed or separate needle for single use or single patient-use, colour coded orange. Needle length 8 mm, diameters 0.33 mm (29G), 0.3 mm (30G), net price 10 (with needle), 0.3 mL = £1.35, 0.5 mL = £1.40; needle length 12 mm, diameters 0.45 mm (26G), 0.4 mm (27G), 0.36 mm (28G), 0.33 mm (29G), net price 10 (with needle), 0.3 mL = £1.45; 0.5 mL = £1.30; 1 mL = £1.29

Brands include *BD Micro-Fine®+*, *Clinipak®*, *Insupak®*, *Monoject® Ultra*, *Omnikan®*, *Plastipak®*

◄Accessories

Needle Clipping (Chopping) Device (Drug Tariff)

Consisting of a clipper to remove needle from its hub and container from which cut-off needles cannot be retrieved; designed to hold 1200 needles, not suitable for use with lancets. Net price = £1.32

Brands include *BD Safe-Clip®*

Sharpsguard (Drug Tariff)

Net price 1-litre sharpsbin = 85p

6.1.2 Oral antidiabetic drugs

6.1.2.1 Sulphonylureas
6.1.2.2 Biguanides
6.1.2.3 Other antidiabetic drugs

Oral antidiabetic drugs are used for the treatment of type 2 diabetes mellitus. They should be prescribed only if the child fails to respond adequately to restriction of energy and carbohydrate intake and an increase in physical activity. They should be used to augment the effect of diet and exercise, and not to replace them.

In children, type 2 diabetes does not usually occur until adolescence and information on the use of oral antidiabetic drugs in children is limited. Treatment with oral antidiabetic drugs should be initiated under specialist supervision **only**; the initial dose should be at the lower end of the adult dose range and then adjusted according to response.

Metformin (section 6.1.2.2) is the oral antidiabetic drug of choice because there is most experience with this drug in children. If dietary changes and metformin do not control the diabetes adequately, either a sulphonylurea (section 6.1.2.1) or insulin (section 6.1.1) can be added.

Alternatively, oral therapy may be substituted with insulin.

When insulin is added to oral therapy, it is generally given at bedtime as isophane insulin, and when insulin replaces an oral regimen it is generally given as twice-daily injections of a biphasic insulin (or isophane insulin mixed with soluble insulin). Weight gain and hypoglycaemia may be complications of insulin therapy but weight gain can be reduced if the insulin is given in combination with metformin.

Pregnancy and breast-feeding   During pregnancy, women with either pre-existing or gestational diabetes may be treated with metformin [unlicensed use], either alone or in combination with insulin (section 6.1.1). Women with gestational diabetes should discontinue hypoglycaemic treatment after giving birth. Metformin can be continued during breast-feeding for those with pre-existing diabetes.

Other oral hypoglycaemic drugs, including sulphonylureas, are contra-indicated in pregnancy and breast-feeding.

6.1.2.1 Sulphonylureas

The sulphonylureas are not the first choice oral antidiabetics in children. They act mainly by augmenting insulin secretion and consequently are effective only when some residual pancreatic beta-cell activity is present; during long-term administration they also have an extrapancreatic action. All can cause hypoglycaemia but this is uncommon and usually indicates excessive dosage. Sulphonylurea-induced hypoglycaemia can persist for many hours and must always be treated in hospital.

6 Endocrine system

Sulphonylureas are considered for children in whom metformin is contra-indicated or not tolerated. Several sulphonylureas are available but experience in children is limited; choice is determined by side-effects and the duration of action as well as the child's age and renal function. The long-acting sulphonylureas chlorpropamide and glibenclamide are associated with a greater risk of hypoglycaemia and for this reason are generally avoided in children. Shorter-acting alternatives, such as **tolbutamide**, may be preferred.

Insulin therapy should be instituted temporarily during intercurrent illness (such as coma, infection, and trauma). Sulphonylureas should be omitted on the morning of surgery; insulin is often required because of the ensuing hyperglycaemia in these circumstances.

Sulphonylureas can be useful in the management of certain forms of maturity-onset diabetes of the young (MODY); there is most experience with gliclazide.

Cautions   Sulphonylureas encourage weight gain and should be prescribed only if poor control and symptoms persist despite adequate attempts at dieting; metformin (section 6.1.2.2) is considered the drug of choice in children.

Contra-indications   Sulphonylureas should be avoided where possible in acute porphyria (section 9.8.2). They should not be used while breast-feeding and insulin therapy should be substituted during pregnancy. Sulphonylureas are contra-indicated in the presence of ketoacidosis.

Side-effects   Side-effects of sulphonylureas are generally mild and infrequent and include gastro-intestinal disturbances such as nausea, vomiting, diarrhoea and constipation.

Sulphonylureas can occasionally cause a disturbance in liver function, which rarely leads to cholestatic jaundice, hepatitis, and hepatic failure. Hypersensitivity reactions can occur, usually in the first 6–8 weeks of therapy. They consist mainly of allergic skin reactions which progress rarely to erythema multiforme or exfoliative dermatitis, fever, and jaundice; photosensitivity has rarely been reported with chlorpropamide and glipizide. Blood disorders are also rare but include leucopenia, thrombocytopenia, agranulocytosis, pancytopenia, haemolytic anaemia, and aplastic anaemia.

GLIBENCLAMIDE

Cautions see notes above; **interactions:** Appendix 1 (antidiabetics)

Hepatic impairment increased risk of hypoglycaemia in severe liver disease; avoid or use small dose; can produce jaundice

Renal impairment avoid in severe impairment

Contra-indications see notes above

Side-effects see notes above

Licensed use not licensed for use in children

Indication and dose

Type 2 diabetes mellitus, maturity-onset diabetes of the young (specialist management only, see notes above)
* By mouth

Child 12–18 years initially 2.5 mg daily with or immediately after breakfast, adjusted according to response, max. 15 mg daily

Glibenclamide (Non-proprietary) PoM
Tablets, glibenclamide 2.5 mg, net price 28-tab pack = 85p; 5 mg, 28-tab pack = 88p

GLICLAZIDE

Cautions see notes above; **interactions:** Appendix 1 (antidiabetics)

Hepatic impairment increased risk of hypoglycaemia in severe liver disease; avoid or use small dose; can produce jaundice

Renal impairment reduce initial dose and monitor closely; avoid in severe impairment

Contra-indications see notes above

Side-effects see notes above

Licensed use not licensed for use in children

Indication and dose

Type 2 diabetes mellitus, maturity-onset diabetes of the young (specialist management only, see notes above)
* By mouth

Child 12–18 years initially 20 mg once daily with breakfast, adjusted according to response; up to 160 mg as a single dose; max. 160 mg twice daily

◻ **GLICLAZIDE** (*continued*)

Gliclazide (Non-proprietary) ⒫ᴼᴹ
Tablets, scored, gliclazide 80 mg, net price 28-tab
pack = £1.07, 60-tab pack = £1.71
Brands include *DIAGLYK*®

Diamicron® (Servier) ⒫ᴼᴹ
Tablets, scored, gliclazide 80 mg, net price 60-tab
pack = £4.56

◼ TOLBUTAMIDE

Cautions see notes above; **interactions:** Appendix 1 (antidiabetics)

Hepatic impairment increased risk of hypoglycaemia in severe liver disease; avoid or use small dose; can produce jaundice

Renal impairment avoid if possible; if no alternative reduce dose and monitor closely

Contra-indications see notes above

Side-effects see notes above; also headache, tinnitus

Licensed use not licensed in children

Indication and dose

Type 2 diabetes mellitus (see notes above), **specialist management only**

• **By mouth**

Child 12–18 years 0.5–1.5 g (max. 2 g) daily in divided doses with or immediately after meals *or* as a single dose with or immediately after breakfast

Tolbutamide (Non-proprietary) ⒫ᴼᴹ
Tablets, tolbutamide 500 mg. Net price 28-tab pack = £1.51

◢Extemporaneous formulations available see Extemporaneous Preparations, p. 8

6.1.2.2   Biguanides

Metformin, the only available biguanide, has a different mode of action from the sulphonylureas, and is not interchangeable with them. It exerts its effect mainly by decreasing gluconeogenesis and by increasing peripheral utilisation of glucose; since it acts only in the presence of endogenous insulin it is effective only if there are some residual functioning pancreatic islet cells.

Metformin is the drug of first choice in children with type 2 diabetes, in whom strict dieting has failed to control diabetes. When the combination of strict diet and metformin treatment fails, other options to be considered under specialist management only, include:

• combining with insulin (section 6.1.1) but weight gain and hypoglycaemia can be problems (weight gain minimised if insulin given at night);

• combining with a sulphonylurea (section 6.1.2.1) (reports of increased hazard with this combination remain unconfirmed).

Insulin treatment is almost always required in medical and surgical emergencies; insulin should also be substituted before elective surgery (omit metformin on the morning of surgery and give insulin if required).

Hypoglycaemia does not usually occur with metformin; other advantages are the lower incidence of weight gain and lower plasma-insulin concentration. It does not exert a hypoglycaemic action in non-diabetic subjects unless given in overdose.

Gastro-intestinal side-effects are initially common with metformin, and may persist in some children, particularly when high doses are given. A slow increase in dose may improve tolerability.

Very rarely, metformin can provoke lactic acidosis which is most likely to occur in children with renal impairment, see Lactic Acidosis below.

◼ METFORMIN HYDROCHLORIDE

Cautions see notes above; determine renal function before treatment and once or twice annually during treatment; **interactions:** Appendix 1 (antidiabetics)

Lactic acidosis Metformin should be used cautiously in renal impairment because of the increased risk of lactic acidosis: it is contra-indicated in children with significant renal impairment. To reduce the risk of lactic acidosis, metformin should be stopped or temporarily withdrawn in

those at risk of tissue hypoxia or sudden deterioration in renal function, such as those with dehydration, severe infection, shock, sepsis, acute heart failure, respiratory failure, or hepatic impairment

Contra-indications ketoacidosis, use of iodine-containing X-ray contrast media (do not restart metformin until renal function returns to normal) and use of general anaesthesia (suspend met-

6   Endocrine system

⌁ **METFORMIN HYDROCHLORIDE (continued)**

formin on the morning of surgery and restart when renal function returns to normal)

Hepatic impairment see Lactic Acidosis above

Renal impairment see Lactic Acidosis above

Pregnancy used in pregnancy for both pre-existing and gestational diabetes—see also Pregnancy and Breast-feeding, p. 429; manufacturer advises avoid

Breast-feeding may be used during breast-feeding—see also Pregnancy and Breast-feeding, p. 429; manufacturer advises avoid

Side-effects anorexia, nausea, vomiting, diarrhoea (usually transient), abdominal pain, taste disturbance; *rarely* lactic acidosis (withdraw treatment), decreased vitamin-B_{12} absorption, erythema, pruritus and urticaria; hepatitis also reported

Licensed use not licensed in children under 10 years

Indication and dose

> Diabetes mellitus (see notes above) specialist supervision **only**
> * **By mouth**
>> **Child 8–10 years** initially 200 mg once daily adjusted according to response at intervals of at least 1 week; max. 2 g daily in 2–3 divided doses
>>
>> **Child 10–18 years** initially 500 mg once daily adjusted according to response at intervals of at least 1 week; max. 2 g daily in 2–3 divided doses

Metformin (Non-proprietary) [PoM]
Tablets, coated, metformin hydrochloride 500 mg, net price 28-tab pack = 88p, 84-tab pack= £1.37; 850 mg, 56-tab pack = £1.24. Label: 21

Oral solution, sugar-free, metformin hydrochloride 500 mg/5 mL, net price 100 mL = £62.41. Label: 21
Brands include *Metsol*®

Glucophage® (Merck) [PoM]
Tablets, f/c, metformin hydrochloride 500 mg, net price 84-tab pack = £2.88; 850 mg, 56-tab pack = £3.20. Label: 21

6.1.2.3 Other antidiabetic drugs

There is little experience of the use of **acarbose** in children. It has been used in older children; therapy should be initiated by an appropriate expert.

The use of nateglinide in combination with a sulphonylurea is generally reserved for the management of some subtypes of *maturity-onset diabetes of the young* or other syndromes of diabetes and requires specialist management.

6.1.3 Diabetic ketoacidosis

The management of diabetic ketoacidosis involves the replacement of fluid and electrolytes and the administration of insulin. Guidelines for the Management of Diabetic Ketoacidosis, published by the British Society of Paediatric Endocrinology and Diabetes[1], should be followed. Clinically well children who are dehydrated up to 5% usually respond to oral rehydration and subcutaneous insulin. For those who do not respond, or are clinically unwell, or are dehydrated by more than 5%, insulin and replacement fluids are best given by intravenous infusion.

To restore circulating volume, give 10 mL/kg **sodium chloride 0.9%** as a bolus, repeat as necessary up to a maximum of 30 mL/kg. Further fluid requirements should be given by intravenous infusion at a rate that corrects losses over 48 hours; initially use **sodium chloride 0.9%**, changing to **sodium chloride 0.45% and glucose 5%** after 6 hours if response is adequate and plasma sodium concentration is stable. **Potassium chloride** is included in the infusion unless anuria is suspected, adjust according to plasma-potassium concentration. Insulin infusion is necessary to switch off ketogenesis and reverse acidosis; it should not be started until at least 1 hour after the start of intravenous rehydration fluids. **Soluble insulin** should be diluted (and **mixed thoroughly**) with **sodium chloride 0.9%** intravenous infusion to a concentration of 1 unit/mL and infused at a rate of 0.1 units/kg/hour. Insulin is continued until the metabolic disturbance is brought under control. **Sodium bicarbonate** infusion (1.26% or 2.74%) is rarely necessary and is used only in cases of extreme acidosis (blood pH less than 6.9) and shock since the acid-base disturbance is normally corrected by the insulin.

Blood glucose is expected to decrease by about 5 mmol/litre/hour; if the response is inadequate the insulin infusion rate can be increased. If the rate of decrease exceeds 5 mmol/litre/hour or blood glucose falls to 14–17 mmol/litre, **glucose intravenous infusion 5% or 10%** should be added to the replacement fluids.

Endocrine system

6

The insulin infusion rate can be reduced to no less than 0.05 units/kg/hour when blood-glucose concentration is 14–17 mmol/litre *and* blood pH is greater than 7.3 *and* a glucose infusion has been started (see above); it is continued until the child is ready to take food by mouth. Subcutaneous insulin can then be started. The insulin infusion should not be stopped until 1 hour after starting subcutaneous soluble or long-acting insulin or 10 minutes after starting subcutaneous insulin aspart, or insulin glulisine, or insulin lispro.

Hyperosmolar hyperglycaemic state or hyperosmolar hyperglycaemic nonketotic coma occurs rarely in children. Treatment is similar to that of diabetic ketoacidosis, although lower rates of insulin infusion and slower rehydration may be required.

6.1.4 Treatment of hypoglycaemia

Prompt treatment of hypoglycaemia in children from any cause is essential as severe hypoglycaemia may cause subsequent neurological damage. Hyperinsulinism, fatty acid oxidation disorders and glycogen storage disease are less common causes of acute hypoglycaemia in children.

Initially glucose 10–20 g is given by mouth either in liquid form or as granulated sugar or sugar lumps. Approximately 10 g of glucose is available from 2 teaspoons of sugar, 3 sugar lumps, *Glucogel®* (formerly known as *Hypostop® Gel*, glucose 10 g/25 g tube, available from BBI Healthcare), and non-diet versions of *Lucozade® Energy Original* 55 mL, *Coca-Cola®* 100 mL, and *Ribena® Blackcurrant* 18 mL (to be diluted). If necessary this can be repeated in 10–15 minutes. After initial treatment, a snack providing sustained availability of carbohydrate (e.g. a sandwich, fruit, milk, or biscuits) or the next meal, if it is due, can prevent blood-glucose concentration from falling again.

Hypoglycaemia which causes unconsciousness or seizures is an emergency. **Glucagon**, a polypeptide hormone produced by the alpha cells of the islets of Langerhans, increases blood-glucose concentration by mobilising glycogen stored in the liver. In hypoglycaemia, if sugar cannot be given by mouth, glucagon can be given by injection. Carbohydrates should be given as soon as possible to restore liver glycogen; glucagon is not appropriate for chronic hypoglycaemia. Glucagon can be issued to parents or carers of insulin-treated children for emergency use in hypoglycaemic attacks. It is often advisable to prescribe it on an 'if necessary' basis for hospitalised insulin-treated children, so that it can be given rapidly by the nurses during a hypoglycaemic emergency. If not effective in 10 minutes intravenous glucose should be given.

Alternatively, 5 mL/kg of glucose intravenous infusion 10% (500 mg/kg of glucose) (section 9.2.2) can be given intravenously into a large vein through a large-gauge needle; care is required since this concentration is irritant especially if extravasation occurs. Glucose intravenous infusion 50% is **not** recommended, as it is very viscous and hypertonic. Close monitoring is necessary, particularly in the case of an overdose with a long-acting insulin because further administration of glucose may be required. Children whose hypoglycaemia is caused by an oral antidiabetic drug should be transferred to hospital because the hypoglycaemic effects of these drugs can persist for many hours.

Glucagon is not effective in the treatment of hypoglycaemia due to fatty acid oxidation or glycogen storage disorders.

Neonatal hypoglycaemia   Neonatal hypoglycaemia at birth is treated with **glucose intravenous infusion 10%** given at a rate of 5 mL/kg/hour. An initial dose of 2.5 mL/kg over 5 minutes may be required if hypoglycaemia is severe enough to cause loss of consciousness or seizures. Mild asymptomatic persistent hypoglycaemia may respond to a single dose of **glucagon**. Glucagon has also been used in the short-term management of endogenous hyperinsulinism.

6

Endocrine system

GLUCAGON

Cautions see notes above, insulinoma, glucagonoma; ineffective in chronic hypoglycaemia, starvation, and adrenal insufficiency; delayed hypoglycaemia when used as a diagnostic test—deaths reported (ensure a meal is eaten before discharge)

Contra-indications phaeochromocytoma

Side-effects nausea, vomiting, diarrhoea, hypokalaemia, rarely hypersensitivity reactions

Licensed use unlicensed for growth hormone test and hyperinsulinism

◁ **GLUCAGON** (*continued*)

Indication and dose

Hypoglycaemia associated with diabetes
• **By subcutaneous, intramuscular, or intra-venous injection**

Neonate 20 micrograms/kg

Child 1 month–2 years 500 micrograms

Child 2–18 years, body-weight less than 25 kg
500 micrograms; body-weight over 25 kg 1 mg

Endogenous hyperinsulinism
• **By intramuscular or intravenous injection**

Neonate 200 micrograms/kg (max. 1 mg) as a single dose

Child 1 month–2 years 1 mg as a single dose

• **By continuous intravenous infusion**

Neonate 1–18 micrograms/kg/hour, adjusted according to response (max. 50 micrograms/kg/hour)

Child 1 month–2 years 1–10 micrograms/kg/hour, increased if necessary
Administration Do not add to infusion fluids containing calcium—precipitation may occur

Diagnosis of growth hormone secretion specialist centre only (section 6.5.1)
• **By intramuscular injection**

Child 1month–18 years 100 micrograms/kg (max. 1 mg) as a single dose; dose may vary, consult local guidelines

Beta-blocker poisoning, see p. 41

Note 1 unit of glucagon = 1 mg of glucagon

[1]**GlucaGen® HypoKit** (Novo Nordisk) [PoM]
Injection, powder for reconstitution, glucagon (rys) as hydrochloride with lactose, net price 1-mg vial with prefilled syringe containing water for injection = £11.52
1. [PoM] restriction does not apply where administration is for saving life in emergency

---

Chronic hypoglycaemia

Diazoxide is useful in the management of chronic hypoglycaemia due to excessive insulin secretion, either from a tumour involving the islets of Langerhans or from persisting hyperinsulinaemic hypoglycaemia of infancy (nesidioblastosis, see also glucagon above). Diazoxide has no place in the management of acute hypoglycaemia. **Chlorothiazide** 3–5mg/kg twice daily (section 2.2.1) reduces diazoxide-induced sodium and water retention and has the added benefit of potentiating the glycaemic effect of diazoxide.

If diazoxide and chlorothiazide fail to suppress excessive glucose requirements in chronic hypoglycaemia then **octreotide** or **nifedipine** (section 2.6.2) can be added. Octreotide suppresses secretion of growth hormone, but growth is unlikely to be affected in the long term.

▌ DIAZOXIDE

Cautions ischaemic heart disease; monitor blood pressure, during prolonged use monitor white cell and platelet count, and regularly assess growth, bone, and psychological development; avoid the intravenous route if possible; extravasation can cause tissue necrosis and single doses of 300 mg have been associated with angina and cerebral and myocardial infarction; **interactions**: Appendix 1 (diazoxide)

Renal impairment increased sensitivity to hypotensive and hyperglycaemic effect; dose reduction may be required

Pregnancy prolonged use in second or third trimesters may produce alopecia and impaired glucose tolerance in neonate; inhibits uterine activity

Contra-indications see section 2.5.1

Side-effects anorexia, nausea, vomiting, hyperuricaemia, sodium and water retention, hyperglycaemia, hypotension, oedema, tachycardia, arrhythmias, extrapyramidal effects; hypertrichosis on prolonged treatment

Licensed use chronic intractable hypoglycaemia (for use in hypertensive crisis see section 2.5.1)

Indication and dose

Chronic intractable hypoglycaemia
• **By mouth or by intravenous injection**

Neonate initially 5 mg/kg twice daily to establish response, adjust dose according to response; usual maintenance dose 1.5–3 mg/kg 2–3 times daily; up to 7 mg/kg 3 times daily may be required in some cases, higher doses unlikely to be beneficial

Child 1 month–18 years initially 1.7 mg/kg 3 times daily then adjusted according to response; usual maintenance dose 1.5–3mg/kg 2–3 times daily; up to 5 mg/kg 3 times daily may be required in some cases, higher doses unlikely to be beneficial

Eudemine® (UCB Pharma) [PoM]
Tablets, diazoxide 50 mg. Net price 20 = £9.29

Injection, see section 2.5.1

◢Extemporaneous formulations available see Extemporaneous Preparations, p. 8

▲ OCTREOTIDE

Cautions avoid abrupt withdrawal of short-acting octreotide—see Side-effects below; in insulinoma (risk of increased depth and duration of hypo-glycaemia—monitor closely when initiating treatment and changing doses); diabetes mellitus (antidiabetic requirements may be reduced); monitor thyroid function on long-term therapy; **interactions:** Appendix 1 (octreotide)

Pregnancy possible effect on fetal growth, avoid unless benefit outweighs risk

Breast-feeding no information, avoid unless essential

Side-effects anorexia, nausea, vomiting, abdominal pain, bloating, flatulence, diarrhoea, and steatorrhoea; postprandial glucose tolerance may be impaired, rarely persistent hyperglycaemia with chronic administration; hypoglycaemia has also been reported; reduced gall bladder motility and bile flow; gallstones reported after long-term treatment; abrupt withdrawal of subcutaneous octreotide is associated with biliary colic and pancreatitis; pain and irritation at injection site—sites should be rotated; rarely, pancreatitis shortly after administration, altered liver function tests, hepatitis and transient alopecia

Licensed use not licensed in children

Indication and dose

Persistent hyperinsulinaemic hypoglycaemia unresponsive to diazoxide and glucose
• **By subcutaneous injection**

Neonate initially 2–5 micrograms/kg every 6–8 hours, adjusted according to response; up to 7 micrograms/kg every 4 hours may rarely be required

Child 1 month–18 years initially 1–2 micrograms/kg every 4–6 hours, dose adjusted according to response; up to 7 micrograms/kg every 4 hours may rarely be required

Bleeding from oesophageal or gastric varices
• **By continuous intravenous infusion**

Child 1 month–18 years 1 microgram/kg/hour, higher doses may be required initially; when no active bleeding reduce dose over 24 hours; usual max. 50 micrograms/hour

Administration *Intravenous infusion*, dilute with sodium chloride 0.9% to a concentration of 10-50%

Sandostatin® (Novartis) (PoM)
Injection, octreotide (as acetate) 50 micrograms/mL, net price 1-mL amp = £3.72; 100 micrograms/mL, 1-mL amp = £6.99; 200 micrograms/mL 5-mL vial = £69.66; 500 micrograms/mL, 1-mL amp = £33.87

6.1.5 Treatment of diabetic nephropathy and neuropathy

Diabetic nephropathy

Regular review of diabetic children over 12 years of age should include an annual test for microalbuminuria (the earliest sign of nephropathy). If reagent strip tests (*Micral-Test II®* (JHS) or *Microbumintest®* (JHS)) are used and prove positive, the result should be confirmed by laboratory analysis of a urine sample. Microalbuminuria can occur transiently during puberty; if it persists (at least 3 positive tests) treatment with an ACE inhibitor (section 2.5.5.1) or an angiotensin-II receptor antagonist (section 2.5.5.2) under specialist guidance should be considered; to minimise the risk of renal deterioration, blood pressure should be carefully controlled (section 2.5).

ACE inhibitors can potentiate the hypoglycaemic effect of insulin and oral anti-diabetic drugs; this effect is more likely during the first weeks of combined treatment and in children with renal impairment.

For the treatment of hypertension in diabetes, see section 2.5.

Diabetic neuropathy

Clinical neuropathy is rare in children whose diabetes is well controlled.

6.1.6 Diagnostic and monitoring agents for diabetes mellitus

Blood monitoring

Blood **glucose** monitoring using a meter gives a direct measure of the glucose concentration at the time of the test and can detect hypoglycaemia as well as hyperglycaemia. Carers and children should be properly trained in the use of blood glucose monitoring systems and the appropriate action to take on the

6

Endocrine system

results obtained. Inadequate understanding of the normal fluctuations in blood glucose can lead to confusion and inappropriate action.

Note In the UK blood-glucose concentration is expressed in mmol/litre and Diabetes UK advises that these units should be used for self-monitoring of blood glucose. In other European countries units of mg/100 mL (or mg/dL) are commonly used.

It is advisable to check that the meter is pre-set in the correct units.

If the blood glucose level is high or if the child is unwell, blood **ketones** should be measured according to local guidelines in order to detect diabetic ketoacidosis (section 6.1.3). Children and their carers should be trained in the use of blood ketone monitoring systems and to take appropriate action on the results obtained, including when to seek medical attention.

◀ Test strips

Active® (Roche Diagnostics)
Reagent strips, for blood glucose monitoring, range 0.6–33.3 mmol/litre, for use with *Glucotrend®* and *Accu-Chek® Active* NHS meters only. Net price 50-strip pack = £14.76

Advantage Plus® (Roche Diagnostics)
Reagent strips, for blood glucose monitoring, range 0.6–33.3 mmol/litre, for use with *Accu-Chek® Advantage* NHS meter only. Net price 50-strip pack = £14.76

Ascensia® Autodisc (Bayer Diabetes Care)
Sensor discs, for blood glucose monitoring, range 0.6–33.3 mmol/litre, for use with *Ascensia Breeze®* and *Ascensia Esprit® 2* NHS meters only. Net price 5 × 10-disc pack = £14.62

Aviva® (Roche Diagnostics)
Sensor strips, for blood glucose monitoring, range 0.6–33.3 mmol/litre, for use with *Accu-Chek® Aviva* NHS meter only. Net price 50-strip pack = £14.49

BM-Accutest® (Roche Diagnostics)
Reagent strips, for blood glucose monitoring, range 1.1–33.3 mmol/litre, for use with *Accutrend®* NHS meters only. Net price 50-strip pack = £14.31

Breeze 2® (Bayer Diabetes Care)
Sensor disks, for blood glucose monitoring, range 0.6–33.3 mmol/litre, for use with the *Breeze 2®* NHS meter only. Net price 5 × 10-disc pack = £14.34

Compact® (Roche Diagnostics)
Reagent strips, for blood glucose monitoring, range 0.6–33.3 mmol/litre, for use with *Accu-Chek® Compact* and *Accu-Chek® Compact Plus* NHS meters only. Net price 3 × 17-strip pack = £14.88

Contour® (Bayer Diabetes Care)
Sensor strips, for blood glucose monitoring, range 0.6–33.3 mmol/litre, for use with *Contour®* NHS meter only. Net price 50-strip pack = £14.45
Note Formerly *Ascensia® Microfill*

FreeStyle® (Abbott)
Sensor strips, for blood glucose monitoring, range 1.1–27.8 mmol/litre, for use with *FreeStyle®* NHS meter only. Net price 50-strip pack = £14.62

FreeStyle Lite® (Abbott)
Sensor strips, for blood glucose monitoring, range 1.1–27.8 micromol/litre, for use with *FreeStyle® Lite* NHS meter only. Net price 50-strip pack = £14.62

GlucoMen® (Menarini Diagnostics)
Sensor strips, for blood glucose monitoring, range 1.1–33.3 mmol/litre, for use with *GlucoMen® Glycó* and *GlucoMen® PC* NHS meters only. Net price 50-strip pack = £13.67

GlucoMen® LX (Menarini Diagnostics)
Sensor strips, for blood glucose monitoring, range 1.1–33.3 mmol/litre, for use with *GlucoMen® LX* NHS meter only. Net price 50-strip pack = £14.33

GlucoMen® Visio Sensor (Menarini Diagnostics)
Sensor strips, for blood glucose monitoring, range 1.1–33.3 mmol/litre, for use with *GlucoMen® Visio* NHS meter. Net price 50-strip pack = £14.53

Hypoguard® Supreme (Hypoguard)
Reagent strips, for blood glucose monitoring, range 2.2–27.7 mmol/litre, for use with *Hypoguard® Supreme* NHS meters. Net price 50-strip pack = £12.00

MediSense G2® (Abbott)
Sensor strips, for blood glucose monitoring, range 1.1–33.3 mmol/litre, for use with *MediSense Precision QID®* NHS meter only. Net price 50-strip pack = £13.67

MediSense® Soft-Sense Plus (Abbott)
Sensor strips, for blood glucose monitoring, range 1.7–25 mmol/litre, for use with *Optium Xceed* meter only. Net price 50-strip pack = £14.52

One Touch® (LifeScan)
Reagent strips, for blood glucose monitoring, range 1.1–33.3 mmol/litre, for use with *One Touch® II, Profile* and *Basic* NHS meters only. Net price 50-strip pack = £14.37

One Touch® Ultra (LifeScan)
Sensor strips, for blood glucose monitoring, range 1.1–33.3 mmol/litre, for use with *One Touch® Ultra, One Touch Ultra 2®* NHS, *One Touch UltraSmart®* NHS, and *One Touch UltraEasy®* NHS meters only. Net price 50-strip pack = £14.53

One Touch® Vita (LifeScan)
Sensor strips, for blood glucose monitoring, range 1.1–33.3 mmol/litre for use with *One Touch® Vita* NHS meter only. Net price 50-strip pack = £14.53

Optium® β-ketone test strips (Abbott)
Reagent Strips, for blood ketone monitoring, range 0–8.0 mmol/litre, for use with *Optium®* NHS or *Optium Xceed* NHS meters only. Net price 10-strip pack = £19.55

Optium® Plus (Abbott)
Sensor strips (formerly *Medisense® Optium Plus*), for blood glucose monitoring, range 1.1–33.3 mmol/litre, for use with *Optium Xceed* NHS meter only. Net price 50-strip pack = £14.53

PocketScan® (LifeScan)
Reagent strips, for blood glucose monitoring, range 1.1–33.3 mmol/litre, for use with *PocketScan®* NHS meter only. Net price 50-strip pack = £14.19

Prestige® (Home Diagnostics)
Reagent strips, for blood glucose monitoring, range 1.4–33.3 mmol/litre, for use with *Prestige®* NHS meter only. Net price 50-strip pack = £14.23

TRUEone® (Home Diagnostics)
Sensor strips with meter, for blood glucose monitoring, range 1.1–33.3 mmol/litre. Meter built into top of sensor strip pot. Net price 50-strip and meter pack = £14.25

TRUEtrack® (Home Diagnostics)
Sensor strips, for blood glucose monitoring, range 1.1–33.3 mmol/litre, for use with *TRUEtrack®* 〔NHS〕 meter only. Net price 50-strip pack = £13.97

WaveSense Jazz® (WaveSense)
Reagent strips, for blood glucose monitoring, range 1.1–33.3 mmol/litre, for use with *WaveSense Jazz®* 〔NHS〕 meter only. Net price 50-strip pack = £14.45

◀ Meters

Accu-Chek® Aviva (Roche Diagnostics) 〔NHS〕
Meter, for blood glucose monitoring (for use with *Aviva®* test strips). *Accu-Chek® Aviva* system = £12.99

Accu-Chek® Compact Plus (Roche Diagnostics) 〔NHS〕
Meter, for blood glucose monitoring (for use with *Compact Plus®* test strips). *Accu-Chek® Compact Plus* system = £12.99

Breeze 2® (Bayer Diabetes Care) 〔NHS〕
Meter, for blood glucose monitoring (for use with *Breeze 2®* sensor discs) = £10.29

Contour® (Bayer Diabetes Care) 〔NHS〕
Meter, for blood glucose monitoring (for use with *Ascensia® Microfill* sensor strips) = £10.29

FreeStyle® (Abbott) 〔NHS〕
Meters, for blood glucose monitoring (for use with *FreeStyle®* and *FreeStyle Lite®* test strips). *FreeStyle Lite®* meter = £7.79; *FreeStyle Freedom Lite®* meter = £5.99

GlucoMen® LX (Menarini Diagnostics)
Meter, for blood glucose monitoring (for use with *GlucoMen® LX* sensor strips) = £12.99

GlucoMen® Visio (Menarini Diagnostics) 〔NHS〕
Meter, for blood glucose monitoring (for use with *GlucoMen® Visio Sensor* strips) = £12.99

Hypoguard® Supreme (Hypoguard) 〔NHS〕
Meters, for blood glucose monitoring (for use with *Hypoguard® Supreme* test strips). *Hypoguard® Supreme Plus* meter = £35.00; *Hypoguard® Supreme Extra* meter = £45.00

One Touch Ultra® 2 (LifeScan)
Meter, for blood glucose monitoring (for use with *One Touch Ultra®* sensor strips) = £12.99

One Touch UltraEasy® (LifeScan)
Meter, for blood glucose monitoring (for use with *One Touch Ultra®* sensor strips) = £12.99

One Touch UltraSmart® (LifeScan)
Meter, for blood glucose monitoring (for use with *One Touch Ultra®* sensor strips) = £19.99

One Touch® Vita (LifeScan)
Meter, for blood glucose monitoring (for use with *One Touch® Vita* sensor strips) = £16.99

Optium® Xceed (Abbott) 〔NHS〕
Meter, for blood glucose monitoring (for use with *MediSense® Soft-Sense Plus*, and *Optium® Plus* test strips) and for blood ketone monitoring (for use with *Optium®* β-ketone test strips). Net price starter pack = £9.00

Prestige® (Home Diagnostics) 〔NHS〕
Meter, for blood glucose monitoring (for use with *Prestige®* test strips) = £5.63

TRUEtrack® (Home Diagnostics) 〔NHS〕
Meter, for blood glucose monitoring (for use with *TRUEtrack®* test strips) = £5.63

WaveSense Jazz® (WaveSense) 〔NHS〕
Meter, for blood glucose monitoring (for use with *WaveSense Jazz®* reagent strips) = £24.99

Urinalysis

Tests for glucose range from reagent strips specific to glucose to reagent tablets which detect all reducing sugars. *Clinitest®* is rarely used now; *Clinistix®* is suitable for screening purposes only. It is rarely necessary for children to test themselves for ketones unless they become unwell—see also Blood Monitoring, p. 435.

Microalbuminuria can be detected with *Micral-Test II®* 〔NHS〕 or *Microbumintest®* 〔NHS〕 but this should be followed by confirmation in the laboratory, since false positive results are common.

◀ Glucose

Clinistix® (Bayer Diabetes Care)
Reagent strips, for detection of glucose in urine. Net price 50-strip pack = £3.25

Clinitest® (Bayer Diabetes Care)
Reagent tablets, for detection of glucose and other reducing substances in urine. Net price 36-tab pack = £2.00

Diabur-Test 5000® (Roche Diagnostics)
Reagent strips, for detection of glucose in urine. Net price 50-strip pack = £2.79

Diastix® (Bayer Diabetes Care)
Reagent strips, for detection of glucose in urine. Net price 50-strip pack = £2.76

Medi-Test® Glucose (BHR)
Reagent strips, for detection of glucose in urine. Net price 50-strip pack = £2.30

◀ Ketones

Ketostix® (Bayer Diabetes Care)
Reagent strips, for detection of ketones in urine. Net price 50-strip pack = £2.92

Ketur Test® (Roche Diagnostics)
Reagent strips, for detection of ketones in urine. Net price 50-strip pack = £2.68

◀ Protein

Albustix® (Bayer Diabetes Care)
Reagent strips, for detection of protein in urine. Net price 50-strip pack = £4.10

Medi-Test® Protein 2 (BHR)
Reagent strips, for detection of protein in urine. Net price 50-strip pack = £3.22

◀ Other reagent strips available for urinalysis include:

Combur-3 Test® 〔NHS〕 (glucose and protein—Roche Diagnostics), *Clinitek Microalbumin®* 〔NHS〕 (albumin and

6ᵉ Endocrine system

creatinine—Bayer Diagnostics), *Ketodiastix®* [NHS] (glucose and ketones—Bayer Diagnostics), *Medi-Test Combi 2®* [NHS] (glucose and protein—BHR), *Micral-Test II®* [NHS] (albumin—Roche Diagnostics), *Micro-* *albustix®* [NHS] (albumin and creatinine—Bayer Diagnostics), *Microbumintest®* [NHS] (albumin—Bayer Diagnostics), *Uristix®* [NHS] (glucose and protein—Bayer Diagnostics)

Oral glucose tolerance test

The oral glucose tolerance test is now rarely needed for the diagnosis of diabetes when symptoms of hyperglycaemia are present. However, it is used for the investigation of insulin resistance, glycogen storage disease, and excessive growth hormone secretion. A dose of 1.75 g/kg (max. 75 g) of anhydrous glucose is used. It is also used to establish the presence of gestational diabetes; this generally involves giving anhydrous glucose 75 g (equivalent to Glucose BP 82.5 g) by mouth to the fasting patient, and measuring blood-glucose concentrations at intervals. The appropriate amount of glucose should be given with 200–300 mL fluid. Alternatively anhydrous glucose 75 g can be given as 113 mL *Polycal®* (Nutricia Clinical) with extra fluid to administer a total volume of 200–300 mL.

6.2 Thyroid and antithyroid drugs

6.2.1 Thyroid hormones
6.2.2 Antithyroid drugs

6.2.1 Thyroid hormones

Thyroid hormones are used in hypothyroidism (juvenile myxoedema), and also in diffuse non-toxic goitre, congenital or neonatal hypothyroidism, and Hashimoto's thyroiditis (lymphadenoid goitre). Neonatal hypothyroidism requires prompt treatment to facilitate normal development.

Levothyroxine sodium (thyroxine sodium) is the treatment of choice for *maintenance* therapy.

Doses for congenital hypothyroidism and juvenile myxoedema should be titrated according to clinical response, growth assessment, and measurement of plasma thyroxine and thyroid-stimulating hormone concentrations. In congenital hypothyroidism higher initial doses (up to 15 micrograms/kg daily; max. 50 micrograms daily) may benefit mental development.

Liothyronine sodium has a similar action to levothyroxine but is more rapidly metabolised and has a more rapid effect; 20–25 micrograms is equivalent to approximately 100 micrograms of levothyroxine. Its effects develop after a few hours and disappear within 24 to 48 hours of discontinuing treatment. It may be used in *severe hypothyroid states* when a rapid response is desired.

Liothyronine by intravenous injection is the treatment of choice in *hypothyroid coma*. Adjunctive therapy includes intravenous fluids, hydrocortisone, and treatment of infection; assisted ventilation is often required.

LEVOTHYROXINE SODIUM
(Thyroxine sodium)

Cautions panhypopituitarism or predisposition to adrenal insufficiency (initiate corticosteroid therapy before starting levothyroxine), cardiovascular disorders (pre-therapy ECG may be valuable), long-standing hypothyroidism, diabetes insipidus, diabetes mellitus (dose of antidiabetic drugs including insulin may need to be increased); **interactions:** Appendix 1 (thyroid hormones)

Pregnancy dose adjustment may be necessary, monitor maternal serum thyrotrophin

Breast-feeding minimal amount present in breast milk; unlikely to affect tests for neonatal hypothyroidism

Contra-indications thyrotoxicosis

Side-effects usually at excessive dosage include diarrhoea, vomiting; anginal pain, arrhythmias, palpitation, tachycardia; tremor, restlessness, excitability, insomnia, headache, flushing, sweating, fever, heat intolerance, weight-loss, muscle cramp, and muscular weakness; transient hair loss; hypersensitivity reactions including rash, pruritus and oedema also reported

◁ **LEVOTHYROXINE SODIUM** (*continued*)

Indication and dose

Hypothyroidism (in cardiac disease reduce dose by 50% and increase more slowly)

Note Levothyroxine equivalent to 100 micrograms/m²/day can be used as a guide to the requirements in children

- **By mouth**

  Neonate initially 10–15 micrograms/kg once daily (max. 50 micrograms daily), adjusted in steps of 5 micrograms/kg every 2 weeks or as necessary; usual maintenance dose 20–50 micrograms daily

  Child 1 month–2 years initially 5 micrograms/kg once daily (max. 50 micrograms daily) adjusted in steps of 10–25 micrograms daily every 2–4 weeks until metabolism normalised; usual maintenance dose 25–75 micrograms daily

Child 2–12 years initially 50 micrograms once daily adjusted in steps of 25 micrograms daily every 2–4 weeks until metabolism normalised; usual maintenance dose 75–100 micrograms daily

Child 12–18 years initially 50 micrograms once daily adjusted in steps of 25–50 micrograms daily every 3–4 weeks until metabolism normalised; usual maintenance dose 100–200 micrograms daily

Levothyroxine (Non-proprietary) ℗ⓞℳ
Tablets, levothyroxine sodium 25 micrograms, net price 28-tab pack = £1.80; 50 micrograms, 28-tab pack = £1.10; 100 micrograms, 28-tab pack = £1.22
Brands include *Eltroxin*®

Oral solution, levothyroxine sodium 25 micrograms/5 mL, net price 100 mL = £42.75; 50 micrograms/5 mL, 100 mL = £44.90; 100 micrograms/5 mL, 100 mL = £52.75
Brands include *Evotrox*® (sugar-free)

LIOTHYRONINE SODIUM
(ʟ-Tri-iodothyronine sodium)

Cautions see under Levothyroxine Sodium; also cardiovascular disease (dose reduction may be necessary); **interactions:** Appendix 1 (thyroid hormones)

Pregnancy does not cross the placenta in significant amounts; dose adjustments may be necessary, monitor maternal serum thyrotropin

Contra-indications see under Levothyroxine Sodium

Side-effects see under Levothyroxine Sodium

Licensed use unlicensed for use in children

Indication and dose

See Levothyroxine and notes above

Hypothyroidism
- **By mouth**

  Child 12–18 years initially 10–20 micrograms daily gradually increased to 60 micrograms daily in 2–3 divided doses

- **By slow intravenous injection**
  (replacement for oral levothyroxine)
  Convert **daily** levothyroxine dose to liothyronine (see below) and give in 2–3 divided doses, adjusted according to response
  Note 2 micrograms liothyronine equivalent to approx. 8 micrograms levothyroxine

Hypothyroid coma
- **By slow intravenous injection**

  Child 1 month–12 years 2–10 micrograms every 12 hours or up to every 4 hours if necessary

  Child 12–18 years 5–20 micrograms repeated every 12 hours or up to every 4 hours if necessary; *alternatively* initially 50 micrograms then 25 micrograms every 8 hours reducing to 25 micrograms twice daily

Liothyronine sodium (Goldshield) ℗ⓞℳ
Tablets, scored, liothyronine sodium 20 micrograms, net price 28-tab pack = £20.00

Triiodothyronine (Goldshield) ℗ⓞℳ
Injection, powder for reconstitution, liothyronine sodium (with dextran). Net price 20-microgram amp = £37.92

6 Endocrine system

6.2.2 Antithyroid drugs

Antithyroid drugs are used for hyperthyroidism either to prepare children for thyroidectomy or for long-term management. In the UK carbimazole is the most commonly used drug. Propylthiouracil can be used in those who suffer sensitivity reactions to carbimazole as sensitivity is not necessarily displayed to both drugs. Both drugs act primarily by interfering with the synthesis of thyroid hormones.

Treatment in children should be undertaken by a specialist.

> **CSM warning (neutropenia and agranulocytosis)**
> Doctors are reminded of the importance of recognising bone marrow suppression induced by carbimazole and the need to stop treatment promptly.
> 1. Children and their carers should be asked to report symptoms and signs suggestive of infection, especially sore throat.
> 2. A white blood cell count should be performed if there is any clinical evidence of infection.
> 3. Carbimazole should be stopped promptly if there is clinical or laboratory evidence of neutropenia.

Carbimazole or **propylthiouracil** are initially given in large doses to block thyroid function. This dose is continued until the child becomes euthyroid, usually after 4 to 8 weeks, and is then gradually reduced to a maintenance dose of 30–60% of the initial dose. Alternatively high-dose treatment is continued in combination with levothyroxine replacement (*blocking-replacement regimen*); this is particularly useful when dose adjustment proves difficult or relapse is a problem. Treatment is usually continued for 12 to 24 months. The blocking-replacement regimen is **not** suitable during pregnancy. Hypothyroidism should be avoided particularly during pregnancy as it can cause fetal goitre.

When substituting, carbimazole 1 mg is considered equivalent to propylthiouracil 10 mg but the dose may need adjusting according to response.

Rashes and pruritus are common with carbimazole but they can be treated with antihistamines without discontinuing therapy; alternatively propylthiouracil can be substituted. If a child on carbimazole develops a sore throat it should be reported immediately because of the rare complication of agranulocytosis (see CSM warning, above).

Iodine has been used as an adjunct to antithyroid drugs for 10 to 14 days before partial thyroidectomy; however, there is little evidence of a beneficial effect. Iodine should not be used for long-term treatment because its antithyroid action tends to diminish.

Radioactive sodium iodide (^{131}I) solution is used increasingly for the treatment of thyrotoxicosis at all ages, particularly where medical therapy or compliance is a problem, in patients with cardiac disease, and in patients who relapse after thyroidectomy.

Propranolol (section 2.4) is useful for rapid relief of thyrotoxic symptoms and can be used in conjunction with antithyroid drugs or as an adjunct to radioactive iodine. Beta-blockers are also useful in neonatal thyrotoxicosis and in supraventricular arrhythmias due to hyperthyroidism. Propranolol has been used in conjunction with iodine to prepare mildly thyrotoxic patients for surgery but it is preferable to make the patient euthyroid with carbimazole. Laboratory tests of thyroid function are not altered by beta-blockers. Most experience in treating thyrotoxicosis has been gained with propranolol but **atenolol** (section 2.4) is also used.

Thyrotoxic crisis ('thyroid storm') requires emergency treatment with intravenous administration of fluids, propranolol and hydrocortisone as sodium succinate, as well as oral iodine solution and carbimazole or propylthiouracil which may need to be administered by nasogastric tube.

Neonatal hyperthyroidism is treated with carbimazole or propylthiouracil, usually for 8 to 12 weeks. In severe symptomatic disease iodine may be needed to block the thyroid and propranolol required to treat peripheral symptoms.

Pregnancy and breast-feeding Radioactive iodine therapy is contra-indicated during pregnancy. Propylthiouracil and carbimazole can be given but the blocking-replacement regimen (see above) is **not** suitable. Both propylthiouracil and carbimazole cross the placenta and in high doses can cause fetal goitre and hypothyroidism—the lowest dose that will control the hyperthyroid state should be used (requirements in Graves' disease tend to fall during pregnancy). Rarely, carbimazole has been associated with congenital defects , including aplasia cutis of the neonate.

Carbimazole and propylthiouracil are present in breast milk but this does not preclude breast-feeding as long as neonatal development is closely monitored and the lowest effective dose is used.

CARBIMAZOLE

Cautions

Hepatic impairment manufacturers advise caution in mild to moderate hepatic impairment; avoid in severe hepatic impairment

Pregnancy see notes above

Breast-feeding see notes above

Side-effects nausea, mild gastro-intestinal disturbances, taste disturbance, hepatic disorders (including hepatitis and jaundice), headache; fever, malaise; rash, pruritus, arthralgia; *rarely* myopathy, alopecia, bone marrow suppression (including pancytopenia and agranulocytosis, see **CSM warning** above), hypersensitivity reactions

Indication and dose

Hyperthyroidism (including Graves' disease), thyrotoxic crisis, thyrotoxicosis
• **By mouth**

> **Neonate** initially 250 micrograms/kg 3 times daily until euthyroid then adjust as necessary (see notes above); higher initial doses (up to 1 mg/kg daily) are occasionally required, particularly in thyrotoxic crisis

> **Child 1 month–12 years** initially 250 micrograms/kg (max. 10 mg) 3 times daily until

> euthyroid then adjusted as necessary (see notes above); higher initial doses occasionally required, particularly in thyrotoxic crisis

> **Child 12–18 years** initially 10 mg 3 times daily until euthyroid then adjusted as necessary (see notes above); higher initial doses occasionally required, particularly in thyrotoxic crisis
> Counselling Warn child and carers to tell doctor **immediately** if sore throat, mouth ulcers, bruising, fever, malaise, or non-specific illness develops

Carbimazole (Non-proprietary) (PoM)
Tablets, carbimazole 5 mg, net price 100-tab pack = £5.51; 20 mg, 100-tab pack = £19.12. Counselling, blood disorder symptoms

Neo-Mercazole® (Amdipharm) (PoM)
Tablets, both pink, carbimazole 5 mg, net price 100-tab pack = £5.15; 20 mg, 100-tab pack = £19.12. Counselling, blood disorder symptoms
Administration tablets may be crushed in water and used immediately

◢ Extemporaneous formulations available see Extemporaneous Preparations, p. 8

IODINE AND IODIDE

Cautions not for long-term treatment

Pregnancy avoid if possible, neonatal goitre and hypothyroidism may occur

Contra-indications

Breast-feeding possibly concentrated in milk—avoid; risk of neonatal goitre and hypothyroidism

Side-effects hypersensitivity reactions including coryza-like symptoms, headache, lacrimation, conjunctivitis, pain in salivary glands, laryngitis, bronchitis, rashes; on prolonged treatment depression, insomnia, impotence; goitre in infants of mothers taking iodides

Indication and dose

See under preparation

Aqueous Iodine Oral Solution
(Lugol's Solution), iodine 5%, potassium iodide 10% in purified water, freshly boiled and cooled,

total iodine 130 mg/mL. Net price 100 mL = £1.19. Label: 27

Dose

Neonatal thyrotoxicosis
• **By mouth**
> **Neonate** 0.05–0.1 mL 3 times daily

Thyrotoxicosis (pre-operative)
• **By mouth**
> **Neonate** 0.1–0.3 mL 3 times daily

> **Child 1 month–18 years** 0.1–0.3 mL 3 times daily

Thyrotoxic crisis
• **By mouth**
> **Child 1 month–1 year** 0.2–0.3 mL 3 times daily

Administration Dilute well with milk or water

PROPYLTHIOURACIL

Cautions see under Carbimazole

Hepatic impairment consider dose reduction

Renal impairment estimated glomerular filtration rate 10–50 mL/minute/1.73 m^2, use 75% of normal dose; estimated glomerular filtration rate less than 10 mL/minute/1.73 m^2, use 50% of normal dose

Pregnancy see notes above

Breast-feeding see notes above

Side-effects see under Carbimazole; leucopenia; rarely cutaneous vasculitis, thrombocytopenia, aplastic anaemia, hypoprothrombinaemia,

hepatitis, encephalopathy, hepatic necrosis, nephritis, lupus erythematous-like syndromes

Licensed use not licensed for use in children under 6 years of age

Indication and dose

Hyperthyroidism (including Graves' disease), thyrotoxic crisis, thyrotoxicosis
• **By mouth**

> **Neonate** initially 2.5–5 mg/kg twice daily until euthyroid then adjusted as necessary (see notes above); higher doses occasionally required, particularly in thyrotoxic crisis

6

Endocrine system

◻ **PROPYLTHIOURACIL** (*continued*)

Child 1 month–1 year initially 2.5 mg/kg 3 times daily until euthyroid then adjusted as necessary (see notes above); higher doses occasionally required, particularly in thyrotoxic crisis

Child 1–5 years initially 25 mg 3 times daily until euthyroid then adjusted as necessary (see notes above); higher doses occasionally required, particularly in thyrotoxic crisis

Child 5–12 years initially 50 mg 3 times daily until euthyroid then adjusted as necessary (see notes above); higher doses occasionally required, particularly in thyrotoxic crisis

Child 12–18 years initially 100 mg 3 times daily administered until euthyroid then adjusted as necessary (see notes above); higher doses occasionally required, particularly in thyrotoxic crisis

Propylthiouracil (Non-proprietary) [PoM]
Tablets, propylthiouracil 50 mg. Net price 56-tab pack = £34.85

◢Extemporaneous formulations available see Extemporaneous Preparations, p. 8

◢ **PROPRANOLOL HYDROCHLORIDE**

Cautions see section 2.4
Contra-indications see section 2.4
Side-effects see section 2.4
Licensed use see section 2.4

Indication and dose

Hyperthyroidism with autonomic symptoms, thyrotoxicosis, thyrotoxic crisis
• By mouth

Neonate initially 250–500 micrograms/kg every 6–8 hours, adjusted according to response

Child 1 month–18 years initially 250–500 micrograms/kg every 8 hours, then adjusted according to response; doses up to 1 mg/kg every 8 hours occasionally required, max. 40 mg every 8 hours

• By intravenous injection over 10 minutes

Neonate initially 20–50 micrograms/kg every 6–8 hours, adjusted according to response

Child 1 month–18 years initially 25–50 micrograms/kg (max. 5 mg) every 6–8 hours, adjusted according to response

◢Preparations
See section 2.4

6.3 Corticosteroids

6.3.1 Replacement therapy
6.3.2 Glucocorticoid therapy

6.3.1 Replacement therapy

The adrenal cortex normally secretes hydrocortisone (cortisol) which has glucocorticoid activity and weak mineralocorticoid activity. It also secretes the mineralocorticoid aldosterone.

In deficiency states, physiological replacement is best achieved with a combination of **hydrocortisone** (section 6.3.2) and the mineralocorticoid **fludrocortisone**; hydrocortisone alone does not usually provide sufficient mineralocorticoid activity for complete replacement.

In *Addison's disease* or following adrenalectomy, **hydrocortisone** by mouth is usually required. This is given in 2–3 divided doses, the larger in the morning and the smaller in the evening, mimicking the normal diurnal rhythm of cortisol secretion. The optimum daily dose is determined on the basis of clinical response. Glucocorticoid therapy is supplemented by fludrocortisone.

In *acute adrenocortical insufficiency*, **hydrocortisone** is given intravenously (preferably as sodium succinate) every 6 to 8 hours in sodium chloride intravenous infusion 0.9%.

In *hypopituitarism*, glucocorticoids should be given as in adrenocortical insufficiency, but since production of aldosterone is also regulated by the renin-angiotensin system a mineralocorticoid is not usually required. Additional replacement therapy with levothyroxine (section 6.2.1) and sex hormones (section 6.4) should be given as indicated by the pattern of hormone deficiency.

In *congenital adrenal hyperplasia*, the pituitary gland increases production of corticotropin to compensate for reduced formation of cortisol; this results in excessive adrenal androgen production. Treatment is aimed at suppressing corticotropin using hydrocortisone (section 6.3.2). Careful and continual dose titration is required to avoid growth retardation and toxicity; for this reason potent, synthetic glucocorticoids such as dexamethasone are usually reserved for use in adolescents. The dose is adjusted according to clinical response and measurement of adrenal androgens and 17-hydroxyprogesterone. Salt-losing forms of congenital adrenal hyperplasia (where there is a lack of aldosterone production) require mineralocorticoid replacement. Mineralocorticoid replacement may also be beneficial even when salt-losing symptoms are not evident.

FLUDROCORTISONE ACETATE

Cautions section 6.3.2; **interactions:** Appendix 1 (corticosteroids)

Contra-indications section 6.3.2

Side-effects section 6.3.2

Indication and dose

Mineralocorticoid replacement in adrenocortical insufficiency
• **By mouth**

Neonate initially 100 micrograms once daily, adjusted according to response; usual range 50–300 micrograms daily

Child 1 month–18 years initially 50–100 micrograms once daily; maintenance 50–300 micrograms once daily, adjusted according to response

Florinef® (Squibb) [PoM]
Tablets, scored, fludrocortisone acetate 100 micrograms. Net price 100-tab pack = £5.36. Label: 10, steroid card

◢ Extemporaneous formulations available see Extemporaneous Preparations, p. 8
Note Bioavailability uncertain, tablets may result in more reliable absorption and may be dispersed in water

6.3.2 Glucocorticoid therapy

In comparing the relative potencies of corticosteroids in terms of their anti-inflammatory (glucocorticoid) effects it should be borne in mind that high glucocorticoid activity in itself is of no advantage unless it is accompanied by relatively low mineralocorticoid activity (see Disadvantages of Corticosteroids below). The mineralocorticoid activity of **fludrocortisone** (section 6.3.1) is so high that its anti-inflammatory activity is of no clinical relevance. The table below shows equivalent anti-inflammatory doses.

Equivalent anti-inflammatory doses of corticosteroids
This table takes no account of mineralocorticoid effects, nor does it take account of variations in duration of action
Prednisolone 1 mg ≡ Betamethasone 150 micrograms
≡ Cortisone acetate 5 mg
≡ Deflazacort 1.2 mg
≡ Dexamethasone 150 micrograms
≡ Hydrocortisone 4 mg
≡ Methylprednisolone 800 micrograms
≡ Triamcinolone 800 micrograms

The relatively high mineralocorticoid activity of **cortisone** and **hydrocortisone**, and the resulting fluid retention, make them unsuitable for disease suppression on a long-term basis. However, they can be used for adrenal replacement therapy (section 6.3.1); hydrocortisone is preferred because cortisone requires conversion in the liver to hydrocortisone. Hydrocortisone is used on a short-term basis by intravenous injection for the emergency management of some conditions. The relatively moderate anti-inflammatory potency of hydrocortisone also makes it a useful topical corticosteroid for the management of inflammatory skin conditions because side-effects (both topical and systemic) are less marked (section 13.4); cortisone is not active topically.

Prednisolone has predominantly glucocorticoid activity and is the corticosteroid most commonly used by mouth for long-term disease suppression.

6

Endocrine system

Betamethasone and **dexamethasone** have very high glucocorticoid activity in conjunction with insignificant mineralocorticoid activity. This makes them particularly suitable for high-dose therapy in conditions where fluid retention would be a disadvantage.

Betamethasone and dexamethasone also have a long duration of action and this, coupled with their lack of mineralocorticoid action makes them particularly suitable for conditions which require suppression of corticotropin (corticotrophin) secretion. Some esters of betamethasone and of **beclometasone** (beclomethasone) exert a considerably more marked topical effect (e.g. on the skin or the lungs) than when given by mouth; use is made of this to obtain topical effects whilst minimising systemic side-effects (e.g. for skin applications and asthma inhalations).

Deflazacort has a high glucocorticoid activity; it is derived from prednisolone.

Use of corticosteroids

Dosages of corticosteroids vary widely in different diseases and in different children. If the use of a corticosteroid can save or prolong life, as in exfoliative dermatitis, pemphigus, acute leukaemia or acute transplant rejection, high doses may need to be given, because the complications of therapy are likely to be less serious than the effects of the disease itself.

When long-term corticosteroid therapy is used in some chronic diseases, the adverse effects of treatment may become greater than the disabilities caused by the disease. To minimise side-effects the maintenance dose should be kept as low as possible.

When potentially less harmful measures are ineffective corticosteroids are used topically for the treatment of inflammatory conditions of the skin (section 13.4). Corticosteroids should be avoided or used only under specialist supervision in psoriasis (section 13.5).

Corticosteroids are used both topically (by rectum) and systemically (by mouth or intravenously) in the management of ulcerative colitis and Crohn's disease (section 1.5 and section 1.7.2).

Use can be made of the mineralocorticoid activity of fludrocortisone to treat postural hypotension in autonomic neuropathy.

High-dose corticosteroids should be avoided for the management of septic shock. However, low-dose hydrocortisone can be used in septic shock (section 2.7.1) that is resistant to volume expansion and catecholamines, and is accompanied by suspected or proven adrenal insufficiency.

The suppressive action of glucocorticoids on the hypothalamic-pituitary-adrenal axis is greatest and most prolonged when they are given at night. In most adults a single dose of 1 mg of dexamethasone at night is sufficient to inhibit corticotropin secretion for 24 hours. This is the basis of the 'overnight dexamethasone suppression test' for diagnosing Cushing's syndrome.

Betamethasone and dexamethasone are also appropriate for conditions where water retention would be a disadvantage.

A corticosteroid can be used in the management of raised intracranial pressure or cerebral oedema that occurs as a result of malignancy (see also p. 26); high doses of betamethasone or dexamethasone are generally used. However, a corticosteroid should **not** be used for the management of head injury or stroke because it is unlikely to be of benefit and may even be harmful

In acute hypersensitivity reactions such as angioedema of the upper respiratory tract and anaphylactic shock, corticosteroids are indicated as an adjunct to emergency treatment with adrenaline (epinephrine) (section 3.4.3). In such cases hydrocortisone (as sodium succinate) by intravenous injection may be required.

In the management of asthma, corticosteroids are preferably used by inhalation (section 3.2) but systemic therapy along with bronchodilators is required for the emergency treatment of severe acute asthma (section 3.1.1).

Dexamethasone should not be used routinely for the prophylaxis and treatment of chronic lung disease in neonates because of an association with adverse neurological effects.

Corticosteroids may be useful in conditions such as auto-immune hepatitis, rheumatoid arthritis, and sarcoidosis; they may also lead to remissions of acquired haemolytic anaemia (section 9.1.3) and thrombocytopenic purpura (section 9.1.4).

High doses of a corticosteroid (usually prednisolone) are used in the treatment of *glomerular kidney disease*, including *nephrotic syndrome*. The condition frequently recurs; a corticosteroid given in high doses and for prolonged periods may delay relapse but the higher incidence of adverse effects limits the overall benefit. Those who suffer frequent relapses may be treated with prednisolone given in a low dose (daily or on alternate days) for 3–6 months; the dose should be adjusted to minimise effects on growth and development. Other drugs used in the treatment of glomerular kidney disease include levamisole (section 5.5.2), cyclophosphamide and chlorambucil (section 8.1.1), and ciclosporin (section 8.2.2). *Congenital nephrotic syndrome* may be resistant to corticosteroids and immunosuppressants; indometacin (section 10.1.1) and an ACE inhibitor such as captopril (section 2.5.5.1) have been used.

Corticosteroids can improve the prognosis of serious conditions such as systemic lupus erythematosus and polyarteritis nodosa; the effects of the disease process may be suppressed and symptoms relieved, but the underlying condition is not cured, although it may ultimately remit. It is usual to begin therapy in these conditions at fairly high dose and then to reduce the dose to the lowest commensurate with disease control.

For other references to the use of corticosteroids see Prescribing in Palliative Care (p. 28), section 8.2.2 (immunosuppression), section 10.1.2 (rheumatic diseases), section 11.4 (eye), section 12.1.1 (otitis externa), section 12.2.1 (allergic rhinitis), and section 12.3.1 (aphthous ulcers).

Administration

Whenever possible *local treatment* with creams, intra-articular injections, inhalations, eye-drops, or enemas should be used in preference to *systemic treatment*. The suppressive action of a corticosteroid on cortisol secretion is least when it is given as a single dose in the morning. In an attempt to reduce pituitary-adrenal suppression further, the total dose for two days can sometimes be taken as a single dose on alternate days; alternate-day administration has not been very successful in the management of asthma (section 3.2). Pituitary-adrenal suppression can also be reduced by means of intermittent therapy with short courses. In some conditions it may be possible to reduce the dose of corticosteroid by adding a small dose of an immunosuppressive drug (section 8.2.1).

Cautions and contra-indications of corticosteroids

Adrenal suppression

During prolonged therapy with corticosteroids, adrenal atrophy develops and can persist for years after stopping. Abrupt withdrawal after a prolonged period can lead to acute adrenal insufficiency, hypotension, or death (see Withdrawal of Corticosteroids, below). Withdrawal can also be associated with fever, myalgia, arthralgia, rhinitis, conjunctivitis, painful itchy skin nodules, and weight loss.

To compensate for a diminished adrenocortical response caused by prolonged corticosteroid treatment, any significant intercurrent illness, trauma, or surgical procedure requires a temporary increase in corticosteroid dose, or if already stopped, a temporary re-introduction of corticosteroid treatment. To avoid a precipitous fall in blood pressure during anaesthesia or in the immediate post-operative period, anaesthetists **must** know whether a patient is taking or has been taking a corticosteroid. A regimen for corticosteroid replacement may be necessary before and after surgery.

Children on long-term corticosteroid treatment should carry a Steroid Treatment Card (see p. 449) which gives guidance on minimising risk and provides details of prescriber, drug, dosage and duration of treatment.

6 Endocrine system

Infections

Prolonged courses of corticosteroids increase susceptibility to infections and severity of infections; clinical presentation of infections may also be atypical. Serious infections, e.g. *septicaemia* and *tuberculosis*, may reach an advanced stage before being recognised, and *amoebiasis* or *strongyloidiasis* may be activated or exacerbated (exclude before initiating a corticosteroid in those at risk or with suggestive symptoms). Fungal or viral *ocular infections* may also be exacerbated (see also section 11.4.1).

Chickenpox Unless they have had chickenpox, children receiving oral or parenteral corticosteroids for purposes other than replacement should be regarded as being *at risk of severe chickenpox* (see Steroid Treatment Card). Manifestations of fulminant illness include pneumonia, hepatitis and disseminated intravascular coagulation; rash is not necessarily a prominent feature.

Passive immunisation with varicella–zoster immunoglobulin (section 14.5) is needed for exposed non-immune children receiving systemic corticosteroids or for those who have used them within the previous 3 months. Confirmed chickenpox warrants specialist care and urgent treatment (section 5.3.2.1). Corticosteroids should not be stopped and dosage may need to be increased.

Topical, inhaled or rectal corticosteroids are less likely to be associated with an increased risk of severe chickenpox.

Measles Children taking corticosteroids, and their carers, should be advised to take particular care to avoid exposure to measles and to seek urgent medical advice if exposure occurs. Prophylaxis with intramuscular normal immunoglobulin (section 14.5) may be needed.

Withdrawal of corticosteroids

The CSM has recommended that *gradual* withdrawal of systemic corticosteroids should be considered in those whose disease is unlikely to relapse and have:

- recently received repeated courses (particularly if taken for longer than 3 weeks);
- taken a short course within 1 year of stopping long-term therapy;
- other possible causes of adrenal suppression;
- received more than 40 mg daily prednisolone (or equivalent) [in adults];
- been given repeat doses in the evening;
- received more than 3 weeks' treatment.

Systemic corticosteroids may be stopped abruptly in those whose disease is unlikely to relapse *and* who have received treatment for 3 weeks or less *and* who are not included in the patient groups described above.

During corticosteroid withdrawal the dose may be reduced rapidly down to physiological doses (equivalent to prednisolone 5 mg/m^2 daily) and then reduced more slowly. Assessment of the disease may be needed during withdrawal to ensure that relapse does not occur.

Psychiatric reactions

Systemic corticosteroids, particularly in high doses, are linked to psychiatric reactions including euphoria, nightmares, insomnia, irritability, mood lability, suicidal thoughts, psychotic reactions, and behavioural disturbances. A serious paranoid state or depression with risk of suicide can be induced, particularly in children with a history of mental disorder. These reactions frequently subside on reducing the dose or discontinuing the corticosteroid but they may also require specific management. Children and their carers should be advised to seek medical advice if psychiatric symptoms (especially depression and suicidal thoughts) occur and they should also be alert to the rare possibility of such reactions during withdrawal of corticosteroid treatment.

Systemic corticosteroids should be prescribed with care in those predisposed to psychiatric reactions, including those who have previously suffered corticosteroid-induced psychosis, or who have a personal or family history of psychiatric disorders.

Advice to children and carers

A patient information leaflet should be supplied to every patient when a systemic corticosteroid is prescribed. Children and carers should especially be advised of the following (for details, see Infections, Adrenal Suppression, and Psychiatric Reactions above and Withdrawal of Corticosteroids below):

- **Immunosupression** Prolonged courses of corticosteroids can increase susceptibility to infection and serious infections can go unrecognised. Unless already immune, children are at risk of severe **chickenpox** and should avoid close contact with people who have chickenpox or shingles. Similarly, precautions should also be taken against contracting **measles**;

- **Adrenal suppression** If the corticosteroid is given for longer than 3 weeks, treatment must not be stopped abruptly. Adrenal suppression can last for a year or more after stopping treatment and the child or carer must mention the course of corticosteroid when receiving treatment for any illness or injury;

- **Mood and behaviour changes** Corticosteroid treatment, especially with high doses, can alter mood and behaviour early in treatment—the child can become confused, irritable and suffer from delusion and suicidal thoughts. These effects can also occur when corticosteroid treatment is being withdrawn. Medical advice should be sought if worrying psychological changes occur;

- **Other serious effects** Serious gastro-intestinal, musculoskeletal, and ophthalmic effects which require medical help can also occur; for details see Side-effects of Corticosteroids, p. 448.

Steroid treatment cards (see p. 449) should be issued where appropriate. Doctors and pharmacists can obtain supplies of the card from:

England and Wales

3M Security Printing and Systems Limited
Gorse Street, Chadderton

Oldham, OL9 9QH.

Tel: (0161) 683 2189
Fax: (0161) 683 2188

Email: nhsforms@spsl.uk.com

Scotland

Banner Business Supplies Ltd
Unit 2, Kingsthorne Park, Nettlehill Road, Houstoun Industrial Estate

Livingston, EH54 5DB.

Tel: (01506) 448 440
Fax: (01506) 448 400

Email: cust.serv.scotland@bbslimited.co.uk

Pregnancy and breast-feeding

The benefit of treatment with corticosteroids during preganancy and breast-feeding outweighs the risk; pregnant women with fluid retention should be monitored closely.

Following a review of the data on the safety of systemic corticosteroids used in pregnancy and breast-feeding the CSM concluded:

- corticosteroids vary in their ability to cross the placenta; betamethasone and dexamethasone cross the placenta readily while 88% of prednisolone is inactivated as it crosses the placenta;

- there is no convincing evidence that systemic corticosteroids increase the incidence of congenital abnormalities such as cleft palate or lip;

- when administration is prolonged or repeated during pregnancy, systemic corticosteroids increase the risk of intra-uterine growth restriction; there is no evidence of intra-uterine growth restriction following short-term treatment (e.g. prophylactic treatment for neonatal respiratory distress syndrome);

- any adrenal suppression in the neonate following prenatal exposure usually resolves spontaneously after birth and is rarely clinically important;

- prednisolone appears in small amounts in breast milk but maternal doses of up to 40 mg daily are unlikely to cause systemic effects in the infant; infants should be monitored for adrenal suppression if the mothers are taking a higher dose.

Other cautions and contra-indications

Other cautions include: growth restriction—possibly irreversible, frequent monitoring required if history of tuberculosis (or X-ray changes), hypertension, congestive heart failure, hepatic impairment (side-effects more common), renal impairment, diabetes mellitus including family history, osteoporosis (including family history), ocular herpes simplex—risk of corneal perforation, severe affective disorders (particularly if history of steroid-induced psychosis—see also Psychiatric Reactions above), epilepsy, peptic ulcer, hypothyroidism, history of steroid myopathy, ulcerative colitis, diverticulitis, recent intestinal anastomoses, thromboembolic disorders, myasthenia gravis; **interactions**: Appendix 1 (corticosteroids)

Other contra-indications include: systemic infection (unless specific therapy given); avoid live virus vaccines in those receiving immunosuppressive doses (serum antibody response diminished)

Side-effects of corticosteroids

Overdosage or prolonged use can exaggerate some of the normal physiological actions of corticosteroids leading to mineralocorticoid and glucocorticoid side-effects.

Corticosteroids suppress growth and can affect the development of puberty. It is important to use the lowest effective dose; alternate-day regimens may be appropriate and limit growth reduction. For the effect of corticosteroids given in pregnancy, see Pregnancy and Breast-feeding, p. 447.

Mineralocorticoid side-effects include hypertension, sodium and water retention, and potassium, and calcium loss. They are most marked with fludrocortisone, but are significant with cortisone, hydrocortisone, corticotropin, and tetracosactide (tetracosactrin). Mineralocorticoid actions are negligible with the high potency glucocorticoids, betamethasone and dexamethasone, and occur only slightly with methylprednisolone, prednisolone, and triamcinolone.

Glucocorticoid side-effects include diabetes and osteoporosis (section 6.6); in addition high doses are associated with avascular necrosis of the femoral head. Muscle wasting (proximal myopathy) can also occur. Corticosteroid therapy is also weakly linked with peptic ulceration (the potential advantage of soluble or enteric-coated preparations to reduce the risk is speculative only). See also Psychiatric Reactions, p. 446.

High doses of corticosteroids can cause Cushing's syndrome, with moon face, striae, and acne; it is usually reversible on withdrawal of treatment, but this must always be gradually tapered to avoid symptoms of acute adrenal insufficiency (**important**: see also Adrenal Suppression, p. 445).

Side-effects can be minimised by using the lowest effective dose for the minimum period possible.

Other side effects include: *gastro-intestinal effects*: dyspepsia, abdominal distension, acute pancreatitis, oesophageal ulceration and candidiasis; *musculoskeletal effects*: muscle weakness, vertebral and long bone fractures, tendon rupture; *endocrine effects*: menstrual irregularities and amenorrhoea, hirsutism, weight gain, negative nitrogen and calcium balance, increased appetite; increased susceptibility to and severity of infection, reactivation of dormant tuberculosis; *neuropsychiatric effects*: psychological dependence, insomnia, increased intracranial pressure with papilloedema (usually after withdrawal), aggravation of schizophrenia, aggravation of epilepsy; *ophthalmic effects*: glaucoma, papilloedema, posterior subcapsular cataracts, corneal or scleral thinning and exacerbation of ophthalmic viral or fungal disease, increased intra-ocular pressure, exophthalmos; *also* impaired healing, petechiae, ecchymoses, facial erythema, suppression of skin test reactions, urticaria, hyperhidrosis, skin atrophy, bruising, telangiectasia, myocardial rupture following recent myocardial infarction, congestive heart failure, leucocytosis, hyperglycaemia, hypersensitivity reactions (including anaphylaxis), thromboembolism, nausea, malaise, hiccups, headache, vertigo.

For other references to the side-effects of corticosteroids see section 1.5 (gastro-intestinal system), section 3.2 (asthma), section 11.4 (eye) and section 13.4 (skin).

STEROID TREATMENT CARD

I am a patient on STEROID treatment which must not be stopped suddenly

- If you have been taking this medicine for more than three weeks, the dose should be reduced gradually when you stop taking steroids unless your doctor says otherwise.

- Read the patient information leaflet given with the medicine.

- Always carry this card with you and show it to anyone who treats you (for example a doctor, nurse, pharmacist or dentist). For one year after you stop the treatment, you must mention that you have taken steroids.

- If you become ill, or if you come into contact with anyone who has an infectious disease, consult your doctor promptly. If you have never had chickenpox, you should avoid close contact with people who have chickenpox or shingles. If you do come into contact with chickenpox, see your doctor urgently.

- Make sure that the information on the card is kept up to date.

BETAMETHASONE

Cautions see notes above

Pregnancy transient effect on fetal movements and heart rate

Contra-indications see notes above

Side-effects see notes above

Licensed use *Betnesol*® tablets not licensed for use as mouthwash

Indication and dose

Ear (section 12.1.1); eye (section 11.4.1); nose (section 12.2.1); mouth (section 12.3.1)

Suppression of inflammatory and allergic disorders; congenital adrenal hyperplasia; see also notes above

- **By slow intravenous injection or by intravenous infusion**

  Child 1 month–1 year initially 1 mg repeated up to 4 times in 24 hours according to response

Child 1–6 years initially 2 mg repeated up to 4 times in 24 hours according to response

Child 6–12 years initially 4 mg repeated up to 4 times in 24 hours according to response

Child 12–18 years initially 4–20 mg repeated up to 4 times in 24 hours according to response

Administration For *intravenous infusion*, dilute with Glucose 5% or Sodium Chloride 0.9%

Betnesol® (UCB Pharma) [PoM]
Injection, betamethasone 4 mg (as sodium phosphate) /mL. Net price 1-mL amp = £1.22. Label: 10, steroid card

DEFLAZACORT

Cautions see notes above

Contra-indications see notes above

Side-effects see notes above

Indication and dose

Inflammatory and allergic disorders
- **By mouth**

  Child 1 month–12 years 0.25–1.5 mg/kg once daily or on alternate days; up to 2.4 mg/kg (max. 120 mg) daily has been used in emergency situations

  Child 12–18 years 3–18 mg once daily or on alternate days; up to 2.4 mg/kg (max. 120 mg) daily has been used in emergency situations

Nephrotic syndrome
- **By mouth**

  Child 1 month–18 years initially 1.5 mg/kg once daily (max. 120 mg) reduced to lowest effective dose for maintenance

Calcort® (Shire) [PoM]
Tablets, deflazacort 6 mg, net price 60-tab pack = £16.46. Label: 5, 10, steroid card

DEXAMETHASONE

Cautions see notes above

Contra-indications see notes above

Side-effects see notes above; also perineal irritation may follow intravenous administration of the phosphate ester

Licensed use not licensed for use in bacterial meningitis

Indication and dose

Croup (see p. 169); nausea and vomiting with chemotherapy (section 8.1); rheumatic disease (section 10.1.2); eye (see p. 625); see also notes above

Note Dexamethasone 1 mg ≡ dexamethasone phosphate 1.2 mg ≡ dexamethasone sodium phosphate 1.3 mg

Inflammatory and allergic disorders
- **By mouth (as dexamethasone)**

  Child 1 month–18 years 10–100 micrograms/ kg daily in 1–2 divided doses, adjusted according to response; up to 300 micrograms/kg daily may be required in emergency situations

- **By intramuscular injection or slow intravenous injection or infusion (as dexamethasone phosphate)**

  Child 1 month–12 years 100–400 micrograms/ kg daily in 1–2 divided doses; max. 24 mg daily

  Child 12–18 years initially 0.5–24 mg daily

Life-threatening cerebral oedema
- **By intravenous injection (as dexamethasone phosphate)**

  Child under 35 kg body-weight initially 20 mg, then 4 mg every 3 hours for 3 days, then 4 mg every 6 hours for 1 day, then 2 mg every 6 hours for 4 days, then decrease by 1 mg daily

  Child over 35 kg body-weight initially 25 mg, then 4 mg every 2 hours for 3 days, then 4 mg every 4 hours for 1 day, then 4 mg every 6 hours for 4 days, then decrease by 2 mg daily

6 Endocrine system

◻ **DEXAMETHASONE (continued)**

Bacterial meningitis (see section 5.1)

- **By slow intravenous injection (as dexamethasone phosphate)**

    Child 2 months–18 years 150 micrograms/kg every 6 hours for 4 days starting before or with first dose of antibacterial

Physiological replacement

- **By mouth or by slow intravenous injection (as dexamethasone)**

    Child 1 month–18 years 250–500 micrograms/m^2 every 12 hours, adjusted according to response

Administration for administration *by mouth* tablets may be dispersed in water or injection solution given by mouth

For *intravenous infusion* dilute with Glucose 5% or Sodium Chloride 0.9%; give over 15–20 minutes

Dexamethasone (Non-proprietary) PoM

Tablets, dexamethasone 500 micrograms, net price 20 = 70p; 2 mg, 20 = £1.75. Label: 10, steroid card, 21
Available from Chemidex and Organon

Oral solution, sugar-free, dexamethasone (as dexamethasone sodium phosphate) 2 mg/5 mL, net price 150-mL = £42.30. Label: 10, steroid card, 21
Brands include *Dexsol®*

Injection, dexamethasone phosphate (as dexamethasone phosphate) 4 mg/mL, net price 1-mL amp = £1.00, 2-mL vial = £1.98; 24 mg/mL, 5-mL vial = £16.66. Label: 10, steroid card
Available from Hospira

Injection, dexamethasone (as dexamethasone sodium phosphate) 4 mg/mL, net price 1-mL amp = 91p, 2-mL vial = £1.27. Label: 10, steroid card
Available from Organon

▲ HYDROCORTISONE

Cautions see notes above

Contra-indications see notes above

Side-effects see notes above; also phosphate ester associated with paraesthesia and pain (particularly in the perineal region)

Indication and dose

Adrenocortical insufficiency (section 6.3.1); shock (section 2.7.1), see also notes above; hypersensitivity reactions e.g. anaphylactic shock, angioedema (section 3.4.3); inflammatory bowel disease (section 1.5.2); haemorrhoids (section 1.7.2); rheumatic disease (section 10.1.2); eye (section 11.4.1); skin (section 13.4)

Congenital adrenal hyperplasia (see also section 6.3.1)

- **By mouth**

    Neonate 6–7 mg/m^2 every 8 hours, adjusted according to response

    Child 1 month–18 years 5–6.5 mg/m^2 every 8 hours, adjusted according to response; usual maintenance 4–5 mg/m^2 every 8 hours but higher doses may be needed

Acute adrenocortical insufficiency (*Addisonian crisis*) see also notes above and section 6.3.1

- **By slow intravenous administration**

    Neonate initially 10 mg as a slow intravenous injection then 100 mg/m^2 daily as a continuous infusion or in divided doses every 6–8 hours; adjusted according to response; when stable reduce over 4–5 days to oral maintenance dose

    Child 1 month–12 years initially 2–4 mg/kg as a slow intravenous injection or infusion then 2–4 mg/kg every 6 hours; adjusted according to response; when stable reduce over 4–5 days to oral maintenance dose

    Child 12–18 years 100 mg every 6 to 8 hours by slow intravenous injection or infusion

Adrenal hypoplasia, Addison's disease, chronic maintenance or replacement therapy

- **By mouth**

    Neonate usual dose 4–5 mg/m^2 every 8 hours; higher doses may be needed

    Child 1 month–18 years usual dose 4–5 mg/m^2 every 8 hours; higher doses may be needed
    Note larger doses given in the morning and smaller doses in the evening

Inflammatory bowel disease—induction of remission (see also section 1.5)

- **By intravenous injection**

    Child 2–18 years 2.5 mg/kg (max. 100 mg) every 6 hours

- **By continuous intravenous infusion**

    Child 2–18 years 10 mg/kg daily (max. 400 mg daily)

Severe acute asthma (see p. 168)

Acute hypersensitivity reactions, angioedema

- **By intramuscular or intravenous injection**

    Child under 6 months initially 25 mg 3 times daily, adjusted according to response

    Child 6 months–6 years initially 50 mg 3 times daily, adjusted according to response

    Child 6–12 years initially 100 mg 3 times daily, adjusted according to response

    Child 12–18 years initially 200 mg 3 times daily, adjusted according to response

6

Endocrine system

◁ **HYDROCORTISONE (continued)**

Hypotension resistant to inotropic treatment and volume replacement (limited evidence)
• **By intravenous injection**

Neonate initially 2.5 mg/kg repeated if necessary after 4 hours, then 2.5 mg/kg every 6 hours for 48 hours or until blood pressure recovers, then dose reduced gradually over at least 48 hours

Child 1 month–18 years 1 mg/kg (max. 100 mg) every 6 hours

Administration for *intravenous administration*, dilute with Glucose 5% or Sodium Chloride 0.9%; for *intermittent infusion* give over 20–30 minutes. For administration *by mouth*, injection solution may be swallowed [unlicensed use] but consider phosphate content; alternatively *Corlan®* pellets (section 12.3.1) may be swallowed [unlicensed use]—pellets should not be cut as may not provide appropriate dose

Hydrocortisone® (Non-proprietary) (PoM)
Tablets, scored, hydrocortisone 10 mg, net price 30-tab pack = £30.50; 20 mg, 30-tab pack = £32.00. Label: 10, steroid card, 21

¹**Efcortesol®** (Sovereign) (PoM) ◢
Injection, hydrocortisone 100 mg (as sodium phosphate)/mL, net price 1-mL amp = 75p, 5-mL amp = £4.48. Label: 10, steroid card

Note Paraesthesia and pain (particularly in the perineal region) may follow intravenous injection of the phosphate ester
1. (PoM) restriction does not apply where administration is for saving life in emergency

¹**Solu-Cortef®** (Pharmacia) (PoM)
Injection, powder for reconstitution, hydrocortisone (as sodium succinate). Net price 100-mg vial = 92p, 100-mg vial with 2-mL amp water for injections = £1.16. Label: 10, steroid card
1. (PoM) restriction does not apply where administration is for saving life in emergency

◢Extemporaneous formulations available see Extemporaneous Preparations, p. 8

METHYLPREDNISOLONE

Cautions see notes above; rapid intravenous administration of large doses associated with cardiovascular collapse

Contra-indications see notes above

Side-effects see notes above

Indication and dose

See also notes above; immunosuppression (section 8.2.2); rheumatic disease (section 10.1.2); skin (section 13.4)

Inflammatory and allergic disorders
• **By mouth, slow intravenous injection or by intravenous infusion**

Child 1 month–18 years 0.5–1.7 mg/kg daily in 2–4 divided doses depending on condition and response

Treatment of graft rejection reactions
• **By intravenous injection**

Child 1 month–18 years 10–20 mg/kg or 400–600 mg/m² (max. 1 g) once daily for 3 days

Severe erythema multiforme (Stevens-Johnson syndrome), lupus nephritis, systemic onset juvenile idiopathic arthritis (section 10.1.2.1)
• **By intravenous injection**

Child 1 month–18 years 10–30 mg/kg (max. 1 g) once daily or on alternate days for up to 3 doses

Administration intravenous injection given over 30 minutes; for intravenous infusion may be diluted with sodium chloride intravenous infusion 0.9% or 0.45%, or glucose intravenous infusion 5% or 10%

Medrone® (Pharmacia) (PoM)
Tablets, scored, methylprednisolone 2 mg (pink), net price 30-tab pack = £3.23; 4 mg, 30-tab pack = £6.19; 16 mg, 30-tab pack = £17.17; 100 mg (blue), 20-tab pack = £48.32. Label: 10, steroid card, 21

Solu-Medrone® (Pharmacia) (PoM)
Injection, powder for reconstitution, methylprednisolone (as sodium succinate) (all with solvent). Net price 40-mg vial = £1.58; 125-mg vial = £4.75; 500-mg vial = £9.60; 1-g vial = £17.30; 2-g vial = £32.86. Label: 10, steroid card

◢Intramuscular depot
Depo-Medrone® (Pharmacia) (PoM)
Injection (aqueous suspension), methylprednisolone acetate 40 mg/mL. Net price 1-mL vial = £2.87; 2-mL vial = £5.15; 3-mL vial = £7.47. Label: 10, steroid card
Dose
• **By deep intramuscular injection into gluteal muscle** seek specialist advice

PREDNISOLONE

Cautions see notes above

Contra-indications see notes above

Side-effects see notes above

Indication and dose

See also notes above

Asthma see p. 184

◁ **PREDNISOLONE** (*continued*)

Autoimmune inflammatory disorders (including juvenile idiopathic arthritis, connective tissue disorders and systemic lupus erythematosus)
• **By mouth**

Child 1 month–18 years initially 1–2 mg/kg once daily (usual max. 60 mg daily), then reduced after a few days if appropriate

Autoimmune hepatitis
• **By mouth**

Child 1 month–18 years initially 2 mg/kg once daily (max. 40 mg daily) then reduced to minimum effective dose

Corticosteroid replacement therapy
• **By mouth**

Child 12–18 years 5 mg/m² daily in 1–2 divided doses adjusted according to response

Ear section 12.1.1

Infantile spasms
• **By mouth**

Child 1 month–2 years initially 10 mg 4 times daily for 14 days (if seizures not controlled after 7 days increase to 20 mg 3 times daily for 7 days); reduce dose gradually over 15 days until stopped (patients taking 40 mg daily, reduce dose in steps of 10 mg every 5 days, then stop; patients taking 60 mg daily, reduce dose to 40 mg daily for 5 days, then 20 mg daily for 5 days, then 10 mg daily for 5 days, then stop)

Eye section 11.4.1

Idiopathic thrombocytopenic purpura
• **By mouth**

Child 1–10 years 1–2 mg/kg daily for max. 14 days *or* 4 mg/kg daily for max. 4 days

Immunosuppression see p. 520

Inflammatory bowel disease see p. 73

Nephrotic syndrome
• **By mouth**

Child 1 month–18 years initially 60 mg/m² once daily (max. 80 mg daily) for 4–6 weeks until proteinuria ceases then 40 mg/m² on alternate days for 4–6 weeks, then withdraw by reducing dose gradually; prevention of relapse 0.5–1 mg/kg once daily or on alternate days for 3–6 months

Pneumocystis pneumonia see p. 411

Rheumatic disease see p. 607

Prednisolone (Non-proprietary) ℗

Tablets, prednisolone 1 mg, net price 28-tab pack = 88p; 5 mg, 28-tab pack = 98p; 25 mg, 56-tab pack = £20.00. Label: 10, steroid card, 21

Tablets, both e/c, prednisolone 2.5 mg (brown), net price 30-tab pack = £4.81; 5 mg (red), 30-tab pack = £4.88. Label: 5, 10, steroid card, 25
Brands include *Deltacortril Enteric*®

Soluble tablets, prednisolone 5 mg (as sodium phosphate), net price 30-tab pack = £7.45. Label: 10, steroid card, 13, 21

6.4 **Sex hormones**

6.4.1 Female sex hormones
6.4.2 Male sex hormones and antagonists
6.4.3 Anabolic steroids

Sex hormone replacement therapy is indicated in children for the treatment of gonadotrophin deficiency, gonadal disorders, or delayed puberty that interferes with quality of life. Indications include constitutional delay in puberty, congenital or acquired hypogonadotrophic hypogonadism, hypergonadotrophic hypogonadism (Turner's syndrome, Klinefelter's syndrome), endocrine disorders (Cushing's syndrome or hyperprolactinaemia), and chronic illnesses, such as cystic fibrosis or sickle-cell disease, that may affect the onset of puberty.

Replacement therapy is generally started at the appropriate age for the development of puberty and should be managed by a paediatric endocrinologist. Patients with constitutional delay, chronic illness, or eating disorders may need only small doses of hormone supplements for 4 to 6 months to induce puberty and endogenous sex hormone production, which is then sustained. Patients with organic causes of hormone deficiency will require life-long replacement, adjusted to allow normal development.

Inadequate treatment may lead to poor bone mineralisation, resulting in fractures and osteoporosis.

6

Endocrine system

6.4.1 Female sex hormones

6.4.1.1 Oestrogens
6.4.1.2 Progestogens

6.4.1.1 Oestrogens

Oestrogens are necessary for the development of female secondary sexual characteristics. If onset of puberty is delayed because of organic pathology, puberty can be induced with ethinylestradiol in increasing doses, guided by breast staging and uterine scans. Cyclical progestogen replacement is added after 12–18 months of oestrogen treatment (see section 6.4.1.2). Once the adult dosage of oestrogen has been reached (20 micrograms ethinylestradiol daily), it may be more convenient to provide replacement either as a low-dose oestrogen containing oral contraceptive formulation [unlicensed indication] (see section 7.3.1) or as a combined oestrogen and progestogen hormone replacement therapy preparation [unlicensed indication] (see BNF section 6.4.1.2). There is limited experience in the use of transdermal patches or gels in children; compliance and skin irritation are sometimes a problem.

Ethinylestradiol is occasionally used, under **specialist supervision**, for the management of hereditary haemorrhagic telangiectasia (but evidence of benefit is limited), for the prevention of tall stature, and in tests of growth hormone secretion (see below). Side-effects include nausea and fluid retention.

Topical oestrogen creams are used in the treatment of labial adhesions (see section 7.2.1)

ETHINYLESTRADIOL
(Ethinyloestradiol)

Cautions see Combined Hormonal Contraceptives (section 7.3.1); **interactions**: Appendix 1 (Oestrogens)

Contra-indications cardiovascular disease (sodium retention with oedema), personal or family history of thromboembolism, acute porphyria; see also Combined Hormonal Contraceptives (section 7.3.1)

Hepatic impairment contra-indicated in liver disease including disorders of hepatic excretion (e.g. Dubin-Johnson or Rotor syndromes), infective hepatitis (until liver function returns to normal), and jaundice

Pregnancy contra-indicated

Breast-feeding contra-indicated

Side-effects nausea, vomiting, headache, breast tenderness, changes in body weight, fluid retention, depression, chorea, skin reactions, chloasma, hypertension, may irritate contact lenses, impairment of liver function, hepatic tumours, rarely photosensitivity; see also Combined Hormonal Contraceptives (section 7.3.1)

Licensed use unlicensed for use in children

Indication and dose
See notes above

Induction of sexual maturation in girls
• **By mouth**
Initially 2 micrograms daily, increasing every 6 months to 5 micrograms, then to 10 micrograms, and then to 20 micrograms daily
Note after 12–18 months of treatment give progestogen for 7 days of each 28-day cycle

Maintenance of sexual maturation in girls
• **By mouth**
20 micrograms daily with cyclical progestogen for 7 days of each 28-day cycle

Prevention of tall stature in girls
• **By mouth**
Girls 2–12 years 20–50 micrograms daily

Pituitary priming before growth hormone secretion test in girls
• **By mouth**
Girls with bone age above 10 years 100 micrograms daily for 3 days before test

Ethinylestradiol (Non-proprietary) ▣
Tablets, ethinylestradiol (unlicensed) 10 micrograms, net price 21-tab pack = £15.55; 50 micrograms, 21-tab pack = £18.55; 1 mg, 28-tab pack = £34.53

Note 2 microgram tablets available from 'special-order' manufacturers or specialist-importing companies, see p. 943

6.4.1.2 Progestogens

There are two main groups of progestogen, *progesterone and its analogues* (dydrogesterone and medroxyprogesterone) and *testosterone analogues* (norethisterone and norgestrel). The newer progestogens (desogestrel, norgestimate, and gestodene) are all derivatives of norgestrel; levonorgestrel is the active isomer of norgestrel and has twice its potency. Progesterone and its analogues are less androgenic than the testosterone derivatives and neither progesterone nor dydrogesterone causes virilisation.

In delayed puberty cyclical progestogen is added after 12–18 months of oestrogen therapy (section 6.4.1.1) to establish a menstrual cycle; usually levonorgestrel 30 micrograms or norethisterone 5 mg daily are used for the last 7 days of each 28 day cycle.

Norethisterone is also used to postpone menstruation during a cycle; treatment is started 3 days before the expected onset of menstruation.

▲ NORETHISTERONE

Cautions conditions that may worsen with fluid retention e.g. epilepsy, hypertension, migraine, asthma, cardiac or renal dysfunction; susceptibility to thromboembolism (particular caution with high dose); history of depression; diabetes (monitor closely); **interactions:** Appendix 1 (progestogens)

Hepatic impairment caution; avoid if severe

Breast-feeding higher doses may suppress lactation and alter milk composition; use lowest effective dose

Contra-indications history of liver tumours, severe liver impairment; severe arterial disease, undiagnosed vaginal bleeding; acute porphyria (section 9.8.2); history during pregnancy of idiopathic jaundice, severe pruritus, or pemphigoid gestationis

Pregnancy contra-indicated

Side-effects menstrual disturbances, premenstrual-like syndrome (including bloating, fluid retention, breast tenderness), weight gain, nausea, headache, dizziness, insomnia, drowsiness, depression; skin reactions (including urticaria, pruritus, rash, and acne), hirsutism and alopecia; jaundice and anaphylactoid reactions also reported

Licensed use not licensed for use in children

Indication and dose

See notes above

Induction and maintenance of sexual maturation in females (combined with an oestrogen after 12–24 months oestrogen therapy)
• **By mouth**
5 mg once daily for the last 7 days of a 28-day cycle

Postponement of menstruation
• **By mouth**
5 mg 3 times daily, starting 3 days before expected onset of menstruation

Norethisterone (Non-proprietary) PoM
Tablets, norethisterone 5 mg, net price 30-tab pack = £2.65

Primolut N® (Schering Health) PoM
Tablets, norethisterone 5 mg. Net price 30-tab pack = £2.01

Utovlan® (Pharmacia) PoM
Tablets, norethisterone 5 mg, net price 30-tab pack = £1.40, 90-tab pack = £4.21

6.4.2 Male sex hormones and antagonists

Androgens cause masculinisation; they are used as replacement therapy in androgen deficiency, in delayed puberty, and in those who are hypogonadal due to either pituitary or testicular disease.

When given to patients with hypopituitarism androgens can lead to normal sexual development and potency but not to fertility. If fertility is desired, the usual treatment is with gonadotrophins or pulsatile gonadotrophin-releasing hormone (section 6.5.1) which stimulates spermatogenesis as well as androgen production.

Intramuscular depot preparations of **testosterone esters** are preferred for replacement therapy. Testosterone enantate or propionate or alternatively *Sustanon®*, which consists of a mixture of testosterone esters and has a longer duration of action, can be used. For induction of puberty, depot testosterone injections are given monthly and the doses increased every 6 to 12 months according to response. Single ester testosterone injections may need to be given more frequently. Testosterone enantate is unlicensed in children. Implants of testosterone can be used for hypogonadism; the implants are replaced every 4 to 5 months.

Oral **testosterone undecanoate** is used for induction of puberty. An alternative approach that promotes growth rather than sexual maturation uses oral oxandrolone (section 6.4.3).

Chorionic gonadotrophin (section 6.5.1) has also been used in delayed puberty in the male to stimulate endogenous testosterone production, but has little advantage over testosterone.

6 Endocrine system

Caution should be used when androgens or chorionic gonadotrophin are used in treating boys with delayed puberty since the fusion of epiphyses is hastened and may result in short stature.

Testosterone patches and topical gel are also available but experience of their use in children under 15 years is limited. Topical testosterone is applied to the penis in the treatment of microphallus; an extemporaneously prepared cream should be used because the alcohol in proprietary gel formulations causes irritation.

TESTOSTERONE AND ESTERS

Cautions cardiac impairment, hypertension, epilepsy, migraine, diabetes mellitus, skeletal metastases (risk of hypercalcaemia); **interactions**: Appendix 1 (testosterone)

Hepatic impairment avoid if possible—fluid retention and dose-related toxicity

Renal impairment caution—potential for fluid retention

Contra-indications history of primary liver tumours, hypercalcaemia, nephrosis

Pregnancy avoid; causes masculinisation of female fetus

Breast-feeding avoid; may cause masculinisation in the female infant or precocious development in the male infant; high doses suppress lactation

Side-effects headache, depression, gastro-intestinal bleeding, nausea, cholestatic jaundice, changes in libido, gynaecomastia, polycythaemia, anxiety, asthenia, paraesthesia, hypertension, electrolyte disturbances including sodium retention with oedema and hypercalcaemia, weight gain; increased bone growth; androgenic effects such as hirsutism, male-pattern baldness, seborrhoea, acne, pruritus; excessive frequency and duration of penile erection, precocious sexual development and premature closure of epiphyses in pre-pubertal males, suppression of spermatogenesis in males and virilism in females; *rarely* liver tumours; sleep apnoea also reported; *with patches and gel*, local irritation and allergic reactions

Licensed use *Sustanon®* and *Virormone®* licensed for use in children; *Andropatch®* licensed for use in children over 15 years

Indication and dose

See also under preparations; specialist use only

Induction and maintenance of sexual maturation in males
* **By mouth (as testosterone undecanoate)**

  Child over 12 years 40 mg on alternate days increasing according to response up to 120 mg daily

* **By deep intramuscular injection of testosterone enantate or propionate**

  Child over 12 years 25–50 mg/m^2 every month increasing dose every 6–12 months according to response

* **Patch**

  Child over 15 years apply to clean, dry, unbroken skin on back, abdomen, upper arms or thighs, removing after 24 hours and siting replacement patch on a different area (with an interval of 7 days before using the same site);

initially apply patches equivalent to testosterone 5 mg/24 hours (2.5 mg/24 hours in non-virilised patients) at night (approx. 10 p.m.), then adjust to 2.5–7.5 mg every 24 hours according to plasma-testosterone concentration

Treatment of microphallus
* **Topically**

  Apply 3 times daily for 3 weeks
  Note Use only specially manufactured preparation (see notes above)

◢**Oral**

Restandol® Testocaps (Organon) [PoM]
Capsules, orange, testosterone undecanoate 40 mg in oily solution. Net price 30-cap pack = £8.89; 60-cap pack = £17.79. Label: 21, 25

◢**Intramuscular**

Testosterone Enantate (Cambridge) [PoM]
Injection (oily), testosterone enantate 250 mg/mL. Net price 1-mL amp = £11.01

Sustanon 100® (Organon) [PoM]
Injection (oily), testosterone propionate 20 mg, testosterone phenylpropionate 40 mg, and testosterone isocaproate 40 mg/mL. Net price 1-mL amp = £1.09
Excipients include arachis (peanut) oil, benzyl alcohol (see Excipients p. 3)

Dose
Delayed puberty in males
* **By intramuscular injection**

  1 mL every month for 3 doses

Pituitary priming prior to growth hormone secretion test
* **By deep intramuscular injection**

  1 mL 3–5 days before test

Sustanon 250® (Organon) [PoM]
Injection (oily), testosterone propionate 30 mg, testosterone phenylpropionate 60 mg, testosterone isocaproate 60 mg, and testosterone decanoate 100 mg/mL. Net price 1-mL amp = £2.55
Excipients include arachis (peanut) oil, benzyl alcohol (see Excipients p. 3)

Virormone® (Nordic) [PoM]
Injection, testosterone propionate 50 mg/mL. Net price 2-mL amp = 45p

◁ **TESTOSTERONE AND ESTERS** (*continued*)

◢ Implant

Testosterone (Organon) [PoM]
Implant, testosterone 100 mg, net price = £7.40;
200 mg = £13.79

Dose

Maintenance of sexual maturation in males
　Child over 16 years 100–600 mg; 600 mg usually
　maintains plasma-testosterone concentration within
　the normal range for 4–5 months

◢ Cream

Testosterone
Cream, testosterone 5% (other strengths available)
Available from 'special-order' manufacturers or specialist
importing companies, see p. 943

◢ Transdermal preparations

Andropatch® (GSK) [PoM]
Patches, self-adhesive, releasing testosterone
approx. 2.5 mg/24 hours, net price 60-patch pack =
£49.10; releasing testosterone approx. 5 mg/
24 hours, net price 30-patch pack = £49.10. Counselling, administration

Anti-androgens and precocious puberty

The gonadorelin stimulation test (section 6.5.1) is used to distinguish between *gonadotrophin-dependent (central) precocious puberty* and *gonadotrophin-independent precocious puberty*. Treatment requires specialist management.

Gonadorelin analogues, used in the management of gonadotrophin-dependent precocious puberty, delay development of secondary sexual characteristics and growth velocity.

Testolactone and **cyproterone** are used in the management of gonadotrophin-independent precocious puberty, resulting from McCune-Albright syndrome, familial male precocious puberty (testotoxicosis), hormone-secreting tumours, and ovarian and testicular disorders. Testolactone inhibits the aromatisation of testosterone, the rate limiting step in oestrogen synthesis. Cyproterone is a progestogen with anti-androgen properties.

Spironolactone (section 2.2.3) is sometimes used in combination with testolactone because it has some androgen receptor blocking properties.

High blood concentration of sex hormones may activate release of gonadotrophin releasing hormone, leading to development of secondary, central gonadotrophin-dependent precocious puberty. This may require the addition of gonadorelin analogues to prevent progression of pubertal development and skeletal maturation.

CYPROTERONE ACETATE

Cautions blood counts initially and throughout treatment; monitor adrenocortical function regularly; diabetes mellitus (see also Contra-indications)
Skilled tasks Fatigue and lassitude may impair performance of skilled tasks (e.g. driving)

Hepatic impairment monitor hepatic function regularly—dose-related toxicity, see side-effects below

Contra-indications hepatic disease, severe diabetes (with vascular changes); sickle-cell anaemia, malignant or wasting disease, severe depression, history of thrombo-embolic disorders

Side-effects fatigue and lassitude, breathlessness, weight changes, reduced sebum production (may clear acne), changes in hair pattern, gynaecomastia (rarely leading to galactorrhoea and benign breast nodules); rarely hypersensitivity reactions, rash and osteoporosis; inhibition of spermatogenesis (see notes above); hepatotoxicity reported (including jaundice, hepatitis and hepatic failure)
Hepatotoxicity Direct hepatic toxicity including jaundice, hepatitis and hepatic failure have been reported (usually after several months) with cyproterone acetate 200–300 mg daily. Liver function tests should be performed before treatment and whenever symptoms suggestive of hepatotoxicity occur—if confirmed cyproterone should normally be withdrawn unless the hepatotoxicity can be explained by another cause such as metastatic disease (in which case cyproterone should be continued only if the perceived benefit exceeds the risk)

Licensed use unlicensed for use in children

Indication and dose

Gonadotrophin-independent precocious puberty) (specialist use only; see also notes above)
　• **By mouth**
　Initially 25 mg twice daily, adjusted according to response

Cyproterone Acetate (Non-proprietary) [PoM]
Tablets, cyproterone acetate 50 mg, net price 56-tab pack = £31.54. Label: 21, counselling, driving
Note 10 mg tablets available from 'special-order' manufacturers or specialist-importing companies, see p. 943

Androcur® (Schering Health) [PoM]
Tablets, scored, cyproterone acetate 50 mg. Net price 56-tab pack = £25.89. Label: 21, counselling, driving

6 Endocrine system

TESTOLACTONE

Cautions interactions: Appendix 1 (testolactone)

Contra-indications

Pregnancy avoid

Breast-feeding no information available

Side-effects nausea, vomiting, anorexia, diarrhoea; hypertension; peripheral neuropathy; weight changes; changes in hair pattern; rarely hypersensitivity reactions, rash

Indication and dose

Gonadotrophin-independent precocious puberty (specialist use only; see also notes above)

- **By mouth**
  5 mg/kg 3–4 times daily; up to 10 mg/kg 4 times daily may be required

Testolactone [PoM]
Tablets, testolactone 50 mg
Available from 'special-order' manufacturers or specialist importing companies, see p. 943

GOSERELIN

Cautions monitor bone mineral density

Contra-indications undiagnosed vaginal bleeding

Pregnancy manufacturer advises avoid

Breast-feeding manufacturer advises avoid

Side-effects changes in blood pressure, headache, mood changes including depression, hypersensitivity reactions including urticaria, pruritus, rash, asthma and anaphylaxis; changes in scalp and body hair, weight changes, withdrawal bleeding, ovarian cysts (may require withdrawal), breast swelling and tenderness (males and females), visual disturbances, paraesthesia, local reactions at injection site

Licensed use not licensed for use in children

Indication and dose

Gonadotrophin-dependent precocious puberty
see notes above; for doses, see under preparations below
Note Injections may be required more frequently in some cases

Administration Rotate injection site to prevent atrophy and nodule formation

Zoladex® (AstraZeneca) [PoM]
Implant, goserelin 3.6 mg (as acetate) in *Safe-System®* syringe applicator. Net price each = £84.14
Dose

- **Implant, by subcutaneous injection into anterior abdominal wall**
  3.6 mg every 4 weeks

Zoladex® LA (AstraZeneca) [PoM]
Implant, goserelin 10.8 mg (as acetate) in *Safe-System®* syringe applicator. Net price each = £267.48
Dose

- **Implant, by subcutaneous injection into anterior abdominal wall**
  10.8 mg every 12 weeks

LEUPRORELIN ACETATE

Cautions see Goserelin

Contra-indications see Goserelin

Pregnancy avoid—teratogenic in *animal* studies

Breast-feeding manufacturer advises avoid

Side-effects see Goserelin

Licensed use not licensed for use in children

Indication and dose

Gonadotrophin-dependent precocious puberty
see notes above; for doses, see under preparations below
Note Injections may be required more frequently in some cases

Administration Rotate injection site to prevent atrophy and nodule formation

Prostap® SR (Wyeth) [PoM]
Injection (microsphere powder for reconstitution), leuprorelin acetate, net price 3.75-mg vial with 1-mL vehicle-filled syringe = £125.40
Dose

- **By subcutaneous or by intramuscular injection**
  3.75 mg every four weeks (half this dose is sometimes used in children with body-weight under 20 kg)

Prostap® 3 (Wyeth) [PoM]
Injection (microsphere powder for reconstitution), leuprorelin acetate, net price 11.25-mg vial with 2-mL vehicle-filled syringe = £376.20
Dose

- **By subcutaneous or by intramuscular injection**
  11.25 mg every 12 weeks

TRIPTORELIN

Cautions see Goserelin

Contra-indications see Goserelin

Pregnancy manufacturer advises avoid

Breast-feeding manufacturer advises avoid

Side-effects see Goserelin; also gastro-intestinal disturbances; asthenia; arthralgia

6 Endocrine system

◻ **TRIPTORELIN** (*continued*)

Indication and dose

> Gonadotrophin-dependent precocious puberty
>
> see notes above; for doses see under preparations below

Administration rotate injection site to prevent atrophy and nodule formation

Decapeptyl® SR (Ipsen) (PoM)

Injection, (powder for suspension), m/r, triptorelin (as acetate), net price 11.25-mg vial (with diluent) = £207.00

Dose

• **By intramuscular injection**

> 11.25 mg every 3 months
>
> Note Each vial includes an overage to allow accurate administration of 11.25 mg dose

Gonapeptyl® Depot (Ferring) (PoM)

Injection (powder for suspension), triptorelin (as acetate), net price 3.75-mg prefilled syringe (with prefilled syringe of vehicle) = £85.00

Dose

• **By subcutaneous or by intramuscular injection**

> **Body-weight under 20 kg** initially 1.875 mg on days 0, 14, and 28, then 1.875 mg every 4 weeks
>
> **Body-weight 20–30 kg** initially 2.5 mg on days 0, 14, and 28, then 2.5 mg every 4 weeks
>
> **Body-weight over 30 kg** initially 3.75 mg on days 0, 14, and 28, then 3.75 mg every 4 weeks; discontinue when bone maturation consistent with age over 12 years in girls and over 13 years in boys
>
> Note may be given every 3 weeks if necessary

6.4.3 Anabolic steroids

Anabolic steroids have some androgenic activity but in girls they cause less virilisation than androgens. They are used in the treatment of some *aplastic anaemias* (section 9.1.3). Oxandrolone is used to stimulate late pre-pubertal growth prior to induction of sexual maturation in boys with short stature and in girls with Turner's syndrome; specialist management is required.

OXANDROLONE

Cautions see Testosterone (section 6.4.2); **interactions:** Appendix 1 (oxandrolone)

Contra-indications see Testosterone (section 6.4.2)

Side-effects see Testosterone (section 6.4.2)

Indication and dose

> Stimulation of late pre-pubertal growth in boys with short stature
>
> • **By mouth**
>
> > **Boys 10–18 years (or appropriate age)** 1.25–2.5 mg daily for 3–6 months

> Stimulation of late pre-pubertal growth in girls with Turner's syndrome
>
> • **By mouth**
>
> > **Girls** in combination with growth hormone 0.625–2.5 mg daily

Oxandrolone

Tablets, oxandrolone 2.5 mg

Available from 'special-order' manufacturers or specialist importing companies, see p. 943

6.5 Hypothalamic and pituitary hormones

6.5.1 Hypothalamic and anterior pituitary hormones including growth hormone

6.5.2 Posterior pituitary hormones and antagonists

> Use of preparations in these sections requires detailed prior investigation of the patient and *should be reserved for specialist centres.*

6.5.1 Hypothalamic and anterior pituitary hormones including growth hormone

Anterior pituitary hormones

Corticotrophins

Tetracosactide (tetracosactrin), an analogue of corticotropin (adrenocorticotrophic hormone, ACTH), is used to test adrenocortical function; failure of plasma-cortisol concentration to rise after administration of tetracosactide indicates adrenocortical insufficiency. A low-dose test is considered by some clin-

6 Endocrine system

icians to be more sensitive when used to confirm established, partial adrenal suppression.

Tetracosactide should be used with caution in patients with allergic disorders e.g. asthma and should be given only if no other ACTH preparations have been given previously. Tetracosactide depot injection (*Synacthen Depot*®) is also used in the treatment of infantile spasms (see Infantile spasms, section 4.8.1) but it is contra-indicated in neonates because of the presence of benzyl alcohol in the injection. Corticotropin-releasing factor, corticorelin, (also known as corticotropin-releasing hormone, CRH) is used to test anterior pituitary function and secretion of corticotropin.

▲ TETRACOSACTIDE
(Tetracosactrin)

Cautions as for corticosteroids, section 6.3.2; **important:** risk of anaphylaxis (medical supervision; consult product literature); **interactions:** Appendix 1 (corticosteroids)

Contra-indications as for corticosteroids, section 6.3.2; avoid injections containing benzyl alcohol in neonates (see under preparations)

Pregnancy avoid

Breast-feeding avoid

Side-effects as for corticosteroids, section 6.3.2

Licensed use not licensed for low-dose test for adrenocortical insufficiency or treatment of infantile spasms

Indication and dose

See notes above and under preparations below

Synacthen® (Alliance) [PoM]
Injection, tetracosactide 250 micrograms (as acetate)/mL. Net price 1-mL amp = £2.93

Dose

Diagnosis of adrenocortical insuffiency (30-minute test)
• By intramuscular or intravenous injection
  Standard-dose test 145 micrograms/m^2 (max. 250 micrograms) as a single dose

  Low-dose test 300 nanograms/m^2 as a single dose
  Administration may be diluted in sodium chloride 0.9% to 250 nanograms/mL

Synacthen Depot® (Alliance) [PoM]
Injection (aqueous suspension), tetracosactide acetate 1 mg/mL, with zinc phosphate complex. Net price 1-mL amp = £4.18
Excipients include benzyl alcohol (avoid in neonates, see Excipients p. 3)

Dose

Infantile spasms
• By intramuscular injection
  Child 1 month–2 years initially 500 micrograms on alternate days, adjusted according to response

▲ CORTICORELIN
(Corticotrophin-releasing hormone, CRH)

Contra-indications

Pregnancy contra-indicated

Breast-feeding contra-indicated

Side-effects flushing of face, neck and upper body, hypotension, mild sensation of taste or smell

Licensed use not licensed

Indication and dose

Test of anterior pituitary function
• By intravenous injection over 30 seconds
  Child 1 month–18 years 1 microgram/kg (max. 100 micrograms) as a single dose

CRH Ferring® (Shire) [PoM]
Injection, corticorelin 100 micrograms

Gonadotrophins

Gonadotrophins are occasionally used in the treatment of hypogonadotrophic hypogonadism and associated oligospermia. There is no justification for their use in primary gonadal failure.

Chorionic gonadotrophin is used in the investigation of testicular function in suspected primary hypogonadism and incomplete masculinisation. It has also been used in delayed puberty in boys to stimulate endogenous testosterone production, but it has little advantage over testosterone (section 6.4.2).

▲ CHORIONIC GONADOTROPHIN
(Human Chorionic Gonadotrophin; HCG)

A preparation of a glycoprotein fraction secreted by the placenta and obtained from the urine of pregnant women having the action of the pituitary luteinising hormone

Cautions cardiac or renal impairment, asthma, epilepsy, migraine; prepubertal boys (risk of pre-

◁ **CHORIONIC GONADOTROPHIN (continued)**

mature epiphyseal closure or precocious puberty)

Contra-indications androgen-dependent tumours

Side-effects oedema (reduce dose), headache, tiredness, mood changes, gynaecomastia, local reactions

Licensed use unlicensed in children for test of testicular function

Indication and dose

Test of testicular function

• **By intramuscular injection**

Short stimulation test:

Child 1 month–18 years 1500–2000 units once daily for 3 days

Prolonged stimulation test:

Child 1 month–18 years 1500–2000 units twice weekly for 3 weeks

Hypogonadotrophic hypogonadism

• **By intramuscular injection**

Child 1 month–18 years 1000–2000 units twice weekly, adjusted to response

Undescended testes

• **By intramuscular injection**

Child 7–18 years initially 500 units 3 times weekly (1000 units twice weekly if over 17 years); adjusted to response; up to 4000 units 3 times weekly may be required; continue for 1–2 months after testicular descent

Choragon® (Ferring) [PoM]
Injection, powder for reconstitution, chorionic gonadotrophin. Net price 5000-unit amp (with solvent) = £3.26. For intramuscular injection

Pregnyl® (Organon) [PoM]
Injection, powder for reconstitution, chorionic gonadotrophin. Net price 1500-unit amp = £2.20; 5000-unit amp = £3.27 (both with solvent). For subcutaneous or intramuscular injection

Growth hormone

Growth hormone is used to treat proven deficiency of the hormone, Prader-Willi syndrome, Turner's syndrome, growth disturbance in children born small for gestational age, and chronic renal insufficiency (see NICE guidance below). Growth hormone is also used in Noonan syndrome and idiopathic short stature [unlicensed indications] under specialist management. Treatment should be initiated and monitored by a paediatrician with expertise in managing growth-hormone disorders; treatment can be continued under a shared-care protocol by a general practitioner.

Growth hormone of human origin (HGH; somatotrophin) has been replaced by a growth hormone of human sequence, **somatropin**, produced using recombinant DNA technology.

> **NICE guidance**
>
> Somatropin in children with growth failure (May 2002)
> Treatment with somatropin is recommended for children with:
>
> • proven growth-hormone deficiency;
>
> • Turner's syndrome;
>
> • Prader-Willi syndrome;
>
> • chronic renal insufficiency before puberty.
>
> Treatment should be discontinued if the response is poor (i.e. an increase in growth velocity of less than 50% from baseline) in the first year of therapy.
>
> In children with chronic renal insufficiency, treatment should be stopped after renal transplantation and not restarted for at least a year

Mecasermin, a human insulin-like growth factor-I (rhIGF-I), is licensed to treat growth failure in children with severe primary insulin-like growth factor-I deficiency (section 6.7.4).

SOMATROPIN

(Synthetic Human Growth Hormone)

Cautions diabetes mellitus (adjustment of anti-diabetic therapy may be necessary), papilloedema (see under Side-effects), relative deficiencies of other pituitary hormones (notably hypo-thyroidism—manufacturers recommend periodic thyroid function tests but limited evidence of clinical value), history of malignant disease, disorders of the epiphysis of the hip (monitor for limping), resolved intracranial hypertension

6

Endocrine system

◁ **SOMATROPIN** (continued)

(monitor closely), initiation of treatment close to puberty not recommended in child born small for gestational age; Silver-Russell syndrome; rotate subcutaneous injection sites to prevent lipoatrophy; **interactions:** Appendix 1 (somatropin)

Breast-feeding no information available but absorption from milk unlikely

Contra-indications evidence of tumour activity (complete antitumour therapy and ensure intracranial lesions inactive before starting); not to be used after renal transplantation or for growth promotion in children with closed epiphyses (or near closure in Prader-Willi syndrome); severe obesity or severe respiratory syndrome in Prader-Willi syndrome

Pregnancy interrupt treatment if pregnancy occurs

Side-effects headache, funduscopy for papilloedema recommended if severe or recurrent headache, visual problems, nausea and vomiting occur—if papilloedema confirmed consider benign intracranial hypertension (rare cases reported); fluid retention (peripheral oedema), arthralgia, myalgia, carpal tunnel syndrome, paraesthesia, antibody formation, hypothyroidism, insulin resistance, hyperglycaemia, hypoglycaemia, reactions at injection site; leukaemia in children with growth hormone deficiency also reported

Licensed use Genotropin® and Omnitrope® not licensed for use in Noonan syndrome; Humatrope®, Nutropin Aq®, and Saizen® not licensed for use in Prader–Willi syndrome, Noonan syndrome, or growth disturbance in children born small for gestational age; Norditropin® not licensed for use in Prader–Willi syndrome or Noonan syndrome; Zomacton® not licensed for use in chronic renal insufficiency, Prader–Willi syndrome, Noonan syndrome or growth disturbance in children born small for gestational age

Indication and dose

Gonadal dysgenesis (Turner's syndrome)
• **By subcutaneous injection**
    45–50 micrograms/kg daily or 1.4 mg/m² daily

Deficiency of growth hormone
• **By subcutaneous or intramuscular injection**
    23–39 micrograms/kg daily or 0.7–1 mg/m² daily

Prader-Willi syndrome
• **By subcutaneous injection**
    Children with growth velocity greater than 1 cm/year in combination with energy-restricted diet, 35 micrograms/kg daily or 1 mg/m² daily; max. 2.7 mg daily

Chronic renal insufficiency (renal function decreased to less than 50%)
• **By subcutaneous injection**
    45–50 micrograms/kg daily or 1.4 mg/m² daily (higher doses may be needed) adjusted if necessary after 6 months

Growth disturbance in children born small for gestational age whose growth has not caught up by 4 years of age or later; Noonan syndrome
• **By subcutaneous injection**
    35 micrograms/kg daily or 1 mg/m² daily

Genotropin® (Pharmacia) PoM
Injection, two-compartment cartridge containing powder for reconstitution, somatropin (rbe) and diluent, net price 5.3-mg (16-unit) cartridge = £122.87, 12-mg (36-unit) cartridge = £278.20. For use with Genotropin® Pen JHS device (available free of charge from clinics). For subcutaneous injection

MiniQuick injection, two-compartment single-dose syringe containing powder for reconstitution, somatropin (rbe) and diluent, net price 0.2-mg (0.6-unit) syringe = £4.64; 0.4-mg (1.2-unit) syringe = £9.27; 0.6-mg (1.8-unit) syringe = £13.91; 0.8-mg (2.4-unit) syringe = £18.55; 1-mg (3-unit) syringe = £23.18; 1.2-mg (3.6-unit) syringe = £27.82; 1.4-mg (4.2-unit) syringe = £32.46; 1.6-mg (4.8-unit) syringe = £37.09; 1.8-mg (5.4-unit) syringe = £41.73; 2-mg (6-unit) syringe = £46.37. For subcutaneous injection

Humatrope® (Lilly) PoM
Injection, powder for reconstitution, somatropin (rbe), net price 6-mg (18-unit) cartridge = £137.25; 12-mg (36-unit) cartridge = £274.50; 24-mg (72-unit) cartridge = £549.00; all supplied with diluent. For subcutaneous or intramuscular injection; cartridges for subcutaneous injection

Norditropin® (Novo Nordisk) PoM
SimpleXx injection, somatropin (epr) 3.3 mg (10 units)/mL, net price 1.5-mL (5-mg, 15-unit) cartridge = £115.90; 6.7 mg (20 units)/mL, 1.5-mL (10-mg, 30-unit) cartridge = £231.80; 10 mg (30 units)/mL, 1.5-mL (15-mg, 45-unit) cartridge = £347.70. For use with appropriate NordiPen® JHS device (available free of charge from clinics). For subcutaneous injection

NutropinAq (Ipsen) PoM
Injection, Somatropin (rbe), net price 10 mg (30 units) 2-mL cartridge = £230.00. For use with NutropinAq® Pen JHS device (available free of charge from clinics). For subcutaneous injection

Omnitrope® (Sandoz) ▼ PoM
Injection, somatropin (rbe) 3.3 mg (10 units)/mL, net price 1.5 mL (5-mg, 15-unit) cartridge = £91.33; 6.7 mg (20 units)/mL, 1.5 mL (10-mg, 30-unit) cartridge = £182.66. For use with Omnitrope Pen 5® JHS and Omnitrope Pen 10® JHS devices respectively (available free of charge from clinics). For subcutaneous injection

Note Biosimilar medicine, see p. 2

Saizen® (Serono) PoM
Injection, powder for reconstitution, somatropin (rmc), net price 1.33-mg (4-unit) vial (with diluent) = £29.28; 3.33-mg (10-unit) vial (with diluent) = £73.20. For subcutaneous or intramuscular injection
Excipients include benzyl alcohol (avoid in neonates, see Excipients, p. 3)

◁ **SOMATROPIN** (*continued*)

Click.easy®, powder for reconstitution, somatropin (rmc), net price 8-mg (24-unit) vial (in *Click.easy®* device with diluent) = £185.44. For use with *One.click®* ⟨NHS⟩ autoinjector device *or Cool.Click®* ⟨NHS⟩ needle-free device (both available free of charge from clinics). For subcutaneous injection

Zomacton® (Ferring) ⟨PoM⟩
Injection, powder for reconstitution, somatropin (rbe), net price 4-mg (12-unit) vial (with diluent) = £81.32. For use with *ZomaJet 2* ⟨NHS⟩ needle-free device or with *Auto-Jector®* ⟨NHS⟩ (both available free of charge from clinics) or with needles and syringes. For subcutaneous injection
Excipients include benzyl alcohol (avoid in neonates, see Excipients, p. 3)

Hypothalamic hormones

Gonadorelin when injected intravenously in post-pubertal girls leads to a rapid rise in plasma concentrations of both luteinising hormone (LH) and follicle-stimulating hormone (FSH). It has not proved to be very helpful, however, in distinguishing hypothalamic from pituitary lesions. It is used in the assessment of delayed or precocious puberty.

Protirelin is a hypothalamic releasing hormone which stimulates the release of thyrotrophin from the pituitary. It is indicated for the diagnosis of mild hyper-thyroidism or hypothyroidism, but its use has been superseded by immunoassays for thyroid-stimulating hormone. Together with other tests protirelin may also be used to confirm hypopituitarism and hypothalamic disease in children with marginally lowered thyrotrophin.

Other growth hormone stimulation tests involve the use of insulin, glucagon, arginine, and clonidine [all unlicensed uses]. The tests should be carried out in specialist centres.

GONADORELIN
(Gonadotrophin-releasing hormone; GnRH; LH–RH)

Cautions   pituitary adenoma

Contra-indications

Pregnancy   avoid

Breast-feeding   avoid

Side-effects   rarely nausea, headache, abdominal pain, increased menstrual bleeding; rarely, hypersensitivity reaction on repeated administration of large doses; irritation at injection site

Licensed use   not licensed for use in children under 1 year

Indication and dose

Assessment of anterior pituitary function; assessment of delayed puberty
• By subcutaneous or intravenous injection
   Child 1–18 years 2.5 micrograms/kg (max. 100 micrograms) as a single dose

HRF® (Intrapharm) ⟨PoM⟩
Injection, powder for reconstitution, gonadorelin. Net price 100-microgram vial (with diluent) = £13.72 (hosp. only)
Excipients include benzyl alcohol (avoid in neonates, see Excipients p. 3)

PROTIRELIN
(Thyrotrophin-releasing hormone; TRH)

Cautions   severe hypopituitarism, myocardial ischaemia, bronchial asthma and obstructive air-ways disease

Pregnancy   use with caution as limited information available

Breast-feeding   breast enlargement and leakage of milk reported

Side-effects   after rapid intravenous administration desire to micturate, flushing, dizziness, nausea, abnormal taste; transient increase in pulse rate and blood pressure; rarely broncho-spasm

Indication and dose

Assessment of thyroid function and thyroid stimulating hormone reserve
• By intravenous injection
   Neonate 1 microgram/kg as a single dose; dose may vary—consult local protocol

   Child 1 month–18 years 1 microgram/kg (max. 200 micrograms) as a single dose; dose may vary—consult local protocol

Diagnosis of hypopituitarism and hypothalamic disease
• By intravenous injection
   Neonate 7 micrograms/kg as a single dose (unlicensed dose); dose may vary—consult local protocol

   Child 1 month–18 years 7 micrograms/kg (max. 200 micrograms) as a single dose (unlicensed dose); dose may vary—consult local protocol

Protirelin (Cambridge) ⟨PoM⟩
Injection, protirelin 100 micrograms/mL. Net price 2-mL amp = £14.43

6   Endocrine system

6.5.2 Posterior pituitary hormones and antagonists

Posterior pituitary hormones

Diabetes insipidus   Diabetes insipidus is caused by either a deficiency of anti-diuretic hormone (ADH, vasopressin) secretion (cranial, neurogenic, or pituitary diabetes insipidus) or by failure of the renal tubules to react to secreted antidiuretic hormone (nephrogenic diabetes insipidus).

Vasopressin (antidiuretic hormone, ADH) is used in the treatment of *pituitary diabetes insipidus* as is its analogue **desmopressin**. Dosage is tailored to produce a regular diuresis every 24 hours to avoid water intoxication. Treatment may be required permanently or for a limited period only in diabetes insipidus following trauma or pituitary surgery.

Desmopressin is more potent and has a longer duration of action than vasopressin; unlike vasopressin it has no vasoconstrictor effect. It is given by mouth or intranasally for maintenance therapy, and by injection in the postoperative period or in unconscious patients. Desmopressin is also used in the differential diagnosis of diabetes insipidus; following an intramuscular or intranasal dose, restoration of the ability to concentrate urine after water deprivation confirms a diagnosis of pituitary diabetes insipidus. Failure to respond suggests nephrogenic diabetes insipidus. Fluid input must be managed carefully to avoid hyponatraemia; this test is not usually recommended in young children.

In *nephrogenic* and *partial pituitary diabetes insipidus* benefit may be gained from the paradoxical antidiuretic effect of thiazides (section 2.2.1) e.g. chlorothiazide 10–20 mg/kg (max. 500 mg) twice daily.

Other uses   Desmopressin is also used to boost factor VIII concentration in mild to moderate haemophilia and in von Willebrand's disease; it is also used to test fibrinolytic response. For a comment on use of desmopressin in nocturnal enuresis see section 7.4.2.

Vasopressin infusion is used to control variceal bleeding in portal hypertension, before introducing more definitive treatment. Terlipressin, a derivative of vasopressin, and octreotide are used similarly but experience in children is limited.

VASOPRESSIN

Cautions heart failure, hypertension, asthma, epilepsy, migraine or other conditions which might be aggravated by water retention; renal impairment (see also Contra-indications); avoid fluid overload

Pregnancy oxytocic effect in third trimester

Breast-feeding not known to be harmful

Contra-indications vascular disease (especially disease of coronary arteries) unless extreme caution, chronic nephritis (until reasonable blood nitrogen concentrations attained)

Side-effects fluid retention, pallor, tremor, sweating, vertigo, headache, nausea, vomiting, belching, abdominal cramps, desire to defaecate, hypersensitivity reactions (including anaphylaxis), constriction of coronary arteries (may cause anginal attacks and myocardial ischaemia), peripheral ischaemia and rarely gangrene

Licensed use not licensed for use in children

Indication and dose

Adjunct in acute massive haemorrhage of gastro-intestinal tract or oesophageal varices (specialist use only)

- **By continuous intravenous infusion (may also be infused directly into the superior mesenteric artery)**

  Child 1 month–18 years initially 0.3 units/kg (max. 20 units) over 20–30 minutes *then* 0.3 units/kg/hour, adjusted according to response (max. 1 unit/kg/hour); if bleeding stops, continue at same dose for 12 hours, then withdraw gradually over 24–48 hours; max. duration of treatment 72 hours

Administration for *intravenous infusion* dilute with Glucose 5% or Sodium Chloride 0.9% to a concentration of 0.2–1 unit/mL

◢Synthetic vasopressin

Pitressin® (Goldshield) PoM
Injection, argipressin (synthetic vasopressin) 20 units/mL. Net price 1-mL amp = £17.14 (hosp. only)

DESMOPRESSIN

Cautions see under Vasopressin; less pressor activity, but still considerable caution in cardio-

vascular disease and in hypertension (not indicated for nocturnal enuresis or nocturia in these

◻ **DESMOPRESSIN** (*continued*)

circumstances); also considerable caution in cystic fibrosis; in nocturia and nocturnal enuresis limit fluid intake from 1 hour before dose until 8 hours afterwards; in nocturia periodic blood pressure and weight checks needed to monitor for fluid overload; **interactions:** Appendix 1 (desmopressin)

Renal impairment use with caution, antidiuretic effect reduced

Pregnancy small oxytocic effect in third trimester; increased risk of pre-eclampsia

Breast-feeding concentration too low to be harmful

For cautions specifically relating to the use of desmopressin in nocturnal enuresis see section 7.4.2

Hyponatraemic convulsions The CSM has advised that patients being treated for primary nocturnal enuresis should be warned to avoid fluid overload (including during swimming) and to stop taking desmopressin during an episode of vomiting or diarrhoea (until fluid balance normal). The risk of hyponatraemic convulsions can also be minimised by keeping to the recommended starting doses and by avoiding concomitant use of drugs which increase secretion of vasopressin (e.g. tricyclic antidepressants)

Contra-indications cardiac insufficiency and other conditions treated with diuretics; psychogenic polydipsia and polydipsia in alcohol dependence

Side-effects fluid retention, and hyponatraemia (in more serious cases with convulsions) on administration without restricting fluid intake; stomach pain, headache, nausea, vomiting, allergic reactions, and emotional disturbance in children also reported; epistaxis, nasal congestion, rhinitis with nasal spray

Licensed use *intranasal* preparations not licensed for use in children for assessment of antidiuretic hormone secretion, for fibrinolytic response testing, or for haemophilia and von Willebrand's disease; *Desmomelt*® and *Desmotab*® not licensed for use in children for treatment of diabetes insipidus; *Octim*® preparations not licensed for use in children for renal function testing or for treatment or diagnosis of diabetes insipidus

Indication and dose

Assessment of antidiuretic hormone secretion (congenital deficiency suspected) (specialist use only)
- **Intranasally**
  Child 1 month–2 years initially 100–500 nanograms as a single dose

Assessment of antidiuretic hormone secretion (congenital deficiency not suspected) (specialist use only)
- **Intranasally**
  Child 1 month–2 years 1–5 micrograms as a single dose

Test for suspected diabetes insipidus (water deprivation test) (specialist use only)
- **Intranasally**
  Neonate not recommended, use trial of treatment

  Child 1 month–2 years 5–10 micrograms as a single dose; not usually recommended, see notes above

  Child 2–12 years 10–20 micrograms as a single dose, see notes above

  Child 12–18 years 20 micrograms as a single dose, see notes above

- **By subcutaneous or intramuscular injection**
  Neonate not recommended, use trial of treatment

  Child 1 month–2 years 400 nanograms as a single dose; not usually recommended, see notes above

  Child 2–12 years 0.5–1 microgram as a single dose, see notes above

  Child 12–18 years 1–2 micrograms as a single dose, see notes above

Diabetes insipidus, treatment (specialist use only)
- **By mouth**
  (as desmopressin acetate)
  Neonate initially 1–4 micrograms 2–3 times daily, adjusted according to response

  Child 1 month–2 years initially 10 micrograms 2–3 times daily, adjusted according to response (range 30-150 micrograms daily)

  Child 2–12 years initially 50 micrograms 2–3 times daily, adjusted according to response (range 100-800 micrograms daily)

  Child 12–18 years initially 100 micrograms 2–3 times daily, adjusted according to response (range 0.2–1.2 mg daily)

- **Sublingually**
  (as desmopressin base)
  Child 2–18 years initially 60 micrograms 3 times daily, adjusted according to response (range 40–240 micrograms 3 times daily)

- **Intranasally**
  (as desmopressin acetate)
  Neonate initially 100–500 nanograms, adjusted according to response (range 1.25–10 micrograms daily in 1–2 divided doses)

  Child 1 month–2 years initially 2.5–5 micrograms 1–2 times daily, adjusted according to response

  Child 2–12 years initially 5–20 micrograms 1–2 times daily, adjusted according to response

  Child 12–18 years initially 10–20 micrograms 1–2 times daily, adjusted according to response

6

Endocrine system

◻ **DESMOPRESSIN** *(continued)*

• **By subcutaneous or intramuscular injection**

Neonate initially 100 nanograms once daily, adjusted according to response (intramuscular route only)

Child 1 month–12 years initially 400 nanograms once daily, adjusted according to response

Child 12–18 years initially 1–4 micrograms once daily, adjusted according to response

Primary nocturnal enuresis (if urine concentrating ability normal) (specialist use only)
• **By mouth**
(as desmopressin acetate)

Child 5–18 years (preferably over 7 years) 200 micrograms at bedtime, increased to 400 micrograms at bedtime only if lower dose not effective (**important:** see also Cautions), reassess after 3 months by withdrawing treatment for at least 1 week

• **Sublingually**
(as desmopressin base)

Child 5–18 years (preferably over 7 years) 120 micrograms at bedtime, increased to 240 micrograms at bedtime only if lower dose not effective (**important:** see also Cautions); reassess after 3 months by withdrawing treatment for at least 1 week

Fibrinolytic response testing (specialist use only)
• **By intravenous injection over 20 minutes or by subcutaneous injection**

Child 2–18 years 300 nanograms/kg as a single dose; blood sampled after 20 minutes for fibrinolytic activity

Mild to moderate haemophilia and von Willebrand's disease (specialist use only)
• **By intravenous infusion over 20 minutes or by subcutaneous injection**

Child 1 month–18 years 300 nanograms/kg as a single dose immediately before surgery or after trauma; may be repeated at intervals of 12 hours if no tachycardia

• **Intranasally**

Child 1–18 years 4 micrograms/kg as a single dose, for pre-operative use give 2 hours before procedure

Renal function testing (specialist use only)
• **Intranasally**

Child 1 month–1 year 10 micrograms (empty bladder at time of administration and restrict fluid intake to 50% at next 2 feeds to avoid fluid overload)

Child 1–15 years 20 micrograms (empty bladder at time of administration and restrict fluid intake to 500 mL from 1 hour before until 8 hours after administration to avoid fluid overload)

Child 15–18 years 40 micrograms (empty bladder at time of administration and restrict

fluid intake to 500 mL from 1 hour before until 8 hours after administration to avoid fluid overload)

• **By subcutaneous or intramuscular injection**

Child 1 month–1 year 400 micrograms (empty bladder at time of administration and restrict fluid intake to 50% at next 2 feeds to avoid fluid overload)

Child 1–18 years 2 micrograms (empty bladder at time of administration and restrict fluid intake to 500 mL from 1 hour before until 8 hours after administration to avoid fluid overload)

Desmopressin acetate (Non-proprietary) ⟮PoM⟯
Nasal spray, desmopressin acetate 10 micrograms/ metered spray, net price 6-mL unit (60 metered sprays) = £27.04. Counselling, fluid intake, see above
Brands include *Presinex®*
Note Children requiring dose of less than 10 micrograms should be given *DDAVP®* intranasal solution

DDAVP® (Ferring) ▼ ⟮PoM⟯
Tablets, both scored, desmopressin acetate 100 micrograms, net price 90-tab pack = £45.48; 200 micrograms, 90-tab pack = £90.96. Counselling, fluid intake, see above
Note Tablets may be crushed

Sublingual tablets, (*DDAVP® Melt*), desmopressin (as acetate) 60 micrograms, net price 100-tab pack = £50.53; 120 micrograms, 100-tab pack = £101.07; 240 micrograms, 100-tab pack = £202.14. Label: 26, counselling, fluid intake, see notes above

Intranasal solution, desmopressin acetate 100 micrograms/mL. Net price 2.5-mL dropper bottle and catheter = £9.72. Counselling, fluid intake, see above
Administration May be diluted with sodium chloride 0.9% to a concentration of 10 micrograms/mL

Injection, desmopressin acetate 4 micrograms/mL. Net price 1-mL amp = £1.10
Administration May be administered orally [unlicensed]; for intravenous infusion, to be diluted to a concentration not less than 1 microgram/mL as adheres to surfaces if very dilute; for higher doses used in mild to moderate haemophilia and von Willebrand's disease may be diluted with 30–50 mL sodium chloride 0.9% intravenous infusion

Desmotabs® (Ferring) ⟮PoM⟯
Tablets, scored, desmopressin acetate 200 micrograms, net price 30-tab pack = £30.34. Counselling, fluid intake, see above
Note tablets may be crushed

Desmomelt® (Ferring) ▼ ⟮PoM⟯
Sublingual tablets desmopressin (as acetate) 120 micrograms, net price 30-tab pack = £30.34; 240 micrograms, 30-tab pack = £60.68. Label: 26, counselling, fluid intake, see above

Desmospray® (Ferring) ⟮PoM⟯
Nasal spray, desmopressin acetate 10 micrograms/ metered spray. Net price 6-mL unit (60 metered

◁ **DESMOPRESSIN** (*continued*)

sprays) = £26.04. Counselling, fluid intake, see above

Note Children requiring dose of less than 10 micrograms should be given *DDAVP® intranasal solution*

Low dose Desmospray® [PoM]
Nasal spray, desmopressin acetate 2.5 micrograms/metered spray
Available from Ferring on a named-patient basis

Octim® (Ferring) [PoM]
Nasal spray, desmopressin acetate 150 micrograms/metered spray, net price 2.5-mL unit (25 metered sprays) = £600.00. Counselling, fluid intake, see above

Injection, desmopressin acetate 15 micrograms/mL, net price 1-mL amp = £20.00
Administration for *intravenous infusion* dilute with 50 mL of Sodium Chloride 0.9% and give over 20 minutes

---

◢ TERLIPRESSIN

Cautions see under Vasopressin

Contra-indications see under Vasopressin

Side-effects see under Vasopressin, but effects milder

Licensed use unlicensed for use in children

Indication and dose

> Adjunct in acute massive haemorrhage of gastro-intestinal tract or oesophageal varices (specialist use only)
> • **By intravenous injection**
> **Child 12–18 years** initially 2 mg then 1–2 mg every 4–6 hours until bleeding is controlled; max. duration of treatment 72 hours

Glypressin® (Ferring) [PoM]
Injection, terlipressin, powder for reconstitution. Net price 1-mg vial with 5 mL diluent = £19.44 (hosp. only)

6.6 Drugs affecting bone metabolism

6.6.1 Calcitonin
6.6.2 Bisphosphonates

The two main disorders of bone metabolism that occur in children are rickets and osteoporosis. The two most common forms of rickets are Vitamin D deficiency rickets (section 9.6.4) and hypophosphataemic rickets (section 9.5.2). See also calcium (section 9.5.1.1).

◢ Osteoporosis

Osteoporosis in children may be primary (e.g. *osteogenesis imperfecta* and *idiopathic juvenile osteoporosis*), or secondary (e.g. due to inflammatory disorders, immobilisation, or corticosteroids); specialist management is required.

Corticosteroid-induced osteoporosis To reduce the risk of osteoporosis doses of oral corticosteroids should be as low as possible and courses of treatment as short as possible.

6.6.1 Calcitonin

Calcitonin is involved with parathyroid hormone in the regulation of bone turnover and hence in the maintenance of calcium balance and homeostasis. **Calcitonin (salmon)** (**salcatonin**, synthetic or recombinant salmon calcitonin) is used to lower the plasma-calcium concentration in some patients with hypercalcaemia (notably when associated with malignant disease).

◢ CALCITONIN (SALMON)/SALCATONIN

Cautions history of allergy (skin test advised); renal impairment; heart failure; children—use for short periods only and monitor bone growth

Pregnancy avoid unless essential, toxicity in *animal* studies

Breast-feeding avoid unless essential, may inhibit lactation

Contra-indications hypocalaemia

◻ **CALCITONIN (SALMON)/SALCATONIN** *(continued)*

Side-effects nausea, vomiting, diarrhoea, abdominal pain, flushing, dizziness, headache, taste disturbances; musculoskeletal pain; with nasal spray nose and throat irritation, rhinitis, sinusitis and epistaxis; *less commonly* diuresis, oedema, cough, visual disturbances, injection-site reactions, rash, hypersensitivity reactions including pruritus

Licensed use not licensed in children

Indication and dose

> Hypercalcaemia (experience limited in children) (specialist use only)
>
> • **By subcutaneous or intramuscular injection**
>
> **Child 1 month–18 years** 2.5–5 units/kg every 12 hours, max. 400 units every 6–8 hours, adjusted according to response (no additional benefit with over 8 units/kg every 6 hours)
>
> • **By slow intravenous infusion**
>
> **Child 1 month–18 years** 5–10 units/kg over at least 6 hours

> Osteoporosis (specialist use only)
>
> Refer for specialist advice, experience very limited

Administration for *intravenous infusion*, dilute injection solution (e.g. 400 units in 500 mL) with Sodium Chloride 0.9% and give over at least 6 hours; glass or hard plastic containers should not be used; some loss of potency on dilution and administration—use diluted solution without delay

Miacalcic® (Novartis) [PoM]
Nasal spray ▼, calcitonin (salmon) 200 units/metered spray, net price 2-mL unit (approx. 14 metered sprays) = £20.99

Injection, calcitonin (salmon) 50 units/mL, net price 1-mL amp = £4.27; 100 units/mL, 1-mL amp = £8.55; 200 units/mL, 2-mL vial = £30.75

---

6 Endocrine system

6.6.2 Bisphosphonates

Bisphosphonates are adsorbed on to hydroxyapatite crystals in bone, slowing both their rate of growth and dissolution, and therefore reducing the rate of bone turnover.

A bisphosphonate such as **disodium pamidronate** is used in the management of severe forms of *osteogenesis imperfecta* and other causes of osteoporosis in children to reduce the number of fractures; the long-term effects of bisphosphonates in children have not been established. Single doses of biphosphonates are also used to manage hypercalaemia (section 9.5.1.2). Treatment should be initiated under specialist advice **only**.

Osteonecrosis of the jaw Osteonecrosis of the jaw has been reported in adult patients receiving intravenous bisphosphonates and, rarely, in those taking oral bisphosphonates. Adequate oral hygiene should be maintained during and after treatment with bisphosphonates. Ideally in children with concomitant risk factors (such as cancer, chemotherapy treatment, corticosteroid treatment, or poor oral hygiene), remedial dental work should be carried out before starting bisphosphonate treatment.

ALENDRONIC ACID

Cautions upper gastro-intestinal disorders (dysphagia, symptomatic oesophageal disease, gastritis, duodenitis, or ulcers—see also under Contra-indications and Side-effects); history (within 1 year) of ulcers, active gastro-intestinal bleeding, or surgery of the upper gastro-intestinal tract; correct disturbances of calcium and mineral metabolism (e.g. vitamin-D deficiency, hypocalcaemia) before starting and monitor serum-calcium concentration during treatment; consider preventive dental treatment before initiating bisphosphonate (risk of osteonecrosis of the jaw, see notes above); exclude other causes of osteoporosis; atypical stress fractures reported (discontinue unless benefits of continued treatment clearly outweigh risks); **interactions:** Appendix 1 (bisphosphonates)

Renal impairment avoid if estimated glomerular filtration rate is less than 35 mL/minute/1.73 m^2

Contra-indications abnormalities of oesophagus and other factors which delay emptying (e.g. stricture or achalasia), hypocalcaemia,

Pregnancy manufacturer advises avoid

Breast-feeding no information available

Side-effects oesophageal reactions (see below), abdominal pain and distension, dyspepsia, regurgitation, melaena, diarrhoea or constipation, flatulence, musculoskeletal pain, headache; *rarely* rash, pruritus, erythema, photosensitivity, uveitis, scleritis, transient decrease in serum phosphate; nausea, vomiting, gastritis, peptic ulceration, hypersensitivity reactions (including urticaria and angioedema), and atypical stress fractures with long term use also reported; myalgia, malaise, and fever at initiation of treatment; *very rarely* severe skin reactions (including Stevens-Johnson syndrome), osteonecrosis (see notes above)

Oesophageal reactions Severe oesophageal reactions (oesophagitis, oesophageal ulcers, oesophageal stricture

◻ **ALENDRONIC ACID** (*continued*)

and oesophageal erosions) have been reported; patients should be advised to stop taking the tablets and to seek medical attention if they develop symptoms of oesophageal irritation such as dysphagia, new or worsening heartburn, pain on swallowing or retrosternal pain

Licensed use not licensed for use in children

Indication and dose

See notes above, specialist use only

Counselling Swallow the tablets whole with a full glass of water on an empty stomach at least 30 minutes before breakfast (and any other oral medication); stand or sit

upright for at least 30 minutes and do not lie down until after eating breakfast. Do not take the tablets at bedtime or before rising.

Fosamax® (MSD) [PoM]
Tablets, alendronic acid (as sodium alendronate) 10 mg, 28-tab pack = £23.12. Counselling, administration

Fosamax® Once Weekly (MSD) [PoM]
Tablets, alendronic acid (as sodium alendronate) 70 mg, net price 4-tab pack = £22.80. Counselling, administration

▰ DISODIUM PAMIDRONATE

Disodium pamidronate was formerly called aminohydroxy-propylidenediphosphonate disodium (APD)

Cautions cardiac disease; previous thyroid surgery (risk of hypocalcaemia); monitor serum electrolytes, calcium, and phosphate—possibility of convulsions due to electrolyte changes; ensure adequate hydration; avoid concurrent use with other bisphosphonates; consider preventive dental treatment before initiating bisphosphonate (risk of osteonecrosis of the jaw, see notes above); **interactions**: Appendix 1 (bisphosphonates)

Hepatic impairment manufacturer advises caution in severe impairment—no information available

Renal impairment monitor renal function in renal disease or predisposition to renal impairment (e.g. in tumour-induced hypercalcaemia)

Skilled tasks Patients should be warned against driving, cycling, or performing skilled tasks immediately after treatment (somnolence or dizziness can occur)

Contra-indications

Pregnancy manufacturer advises avoid—toxicity in *animal* studies

Breast-feeding manufacturer advises avoid

Side-effects hypophosphataemia, transient rise in body temperature, fever and influenza-like symptoms (sometimes accompanied by malaise, rigors, fatigue, and flushes); arthralgia, myalgia, bone pain, nausea, vomiting, headache, lymphocytopenia, hypomagnesaemia; *rarely* muscle

cramps, anorexia, abdominal pain, diarrhoea, constipation, dyspepsia, agitation, confusion, dizziness, insomnia, somnolence, lethargy, anaemia, leucopenia, hypotension or hypertension, rash, pruritus, symptomatic hypocalcaemia (paraesthesia, tetany), hyperkalaemia or hypokalaemia, hypernatraemia; osteonecrosis (see notes above); isolated cases of seizures, hallucinations, thrombocytopenia, haematuria, acute renal failure, deterioration of renal disease, conjunctivitis and other ocular symptoms; atrial fibrillation, and reactivation of herpes simplex and zoster also reported; also local reactions at injection site

Licensed use not licensed for use in children

Indication and dose

See notes above, specialist use only

Disodium pamidronate (Non-proprietary) [PoM]
Concentrate for intravenous infusion, disodium pamidronate 3 mg/mL, net price 5-mL vial = £27.50, 10-mL vial = £55.00; 6 mg/mL, 10-mL vial = £95.00; 9 mg/mL, 10-mL vial = £165.00

Aredia Dry Powder® (Novartis) [PoM]
Injection, powder for reconstitution, disodium pamidronate, for use as an infusion. Net price 15-mg vial = £29.83; 30-mg vial = £59.66; 90-mg vial = £170.45 (all with diluent)

▰ RISEDRONATE SODIUM

Cautions oesophageal abnormalities and other factors which delay transit or emptying (e.g. stricture or achalasia—see also under Side-effects); correct hypocalcaemia before starting, correct other disturbances of bone and mineral metabolism (e.g. Vitamin-D deficiency) at onset of treatment; consider preventive dental treatment before initiating bisphosphonate (risk of osteonecrosis of the jaw, see notes above); **interactions**: Appendix 1 (bisphosphonates)

Renal impairment avoid if estimated glomerular filtration rate is less than 30 mL/minute/1.73 m²

Contra-indications hypocalcaemia (see Cautions above)

Pregnancy manufacturer advises avoid

Breast-feeding manufacturer advises avoid

Side-effects gastro-intestinal effects (including abdominal pain, dyspepsia, nausea, diarrhoea, constipation); dizziness, headache; influenza-like symptoms, musculoskeletal pain; *rarely* oesophageal stricture, oesophagitis, oesophageal ulcer, dysphagia, gastritis, duodenitis, glossitis, peripheral oedema, weight loss, myasthenia, arthralgia, apnoea, bronchitis, sinusitis, rash, nocturia, amblyopia, corneal lesion, dry eye, tinnitus, iritis; *very rarely* hypersensitivity reactions including angioedema, osteonecrosis (see notes above)

Licensed use not licensed for use in children

Indication and dose

See notes above, specialist use only

Counselling Swallow tablets whole with full glass of water; on rising, take on an empty stomach at least 30 minutes

6

Endocrine system

◻ **RISEDRONATE SODIUM** (*continued*)

before first food or drink of the day or, if taking at any other time of the day, avoid food and drink for at least 2 hours before or after risedronate (particularly avoid calcium containing products e.g. milk, also avoid iron and mineral supplements and antacids); stand or sit upright for at least 30 minutes; do not take tablets at bedtime or before rising

Actonel® (Procter & Gamble Pharm.) ⟨PoM⟩
Tablets, f/c, risedronate sodium 5 mg (yellow), net price 28-tab pack = £19.10; 30 mg (white), 28-tab

pack = £152.81. Counselling, administration, food, and calcium (see above)

Actonel Once a Week® (Procter & Gamble Pharm.) ⟨PoM⟩
Tablets, f/c, risedronate sodium 35 mg (orange), net price 4-tab pack = £20.30. Counselling, administration, food and calcium (see above)

▰ SODIUM CLODRONATE

Cautions monitor renal and hepatic function and white cell count; also monitor serum calcium and phosphate periodically; renal dysfunction reported in patients receiving concomitant NSAIDs; maintain adequate fluid intake during treatment; consider preventive dental treatment before initiating bisphosphonate (risk of osteo-necrosis of the jaw, see notes above); **interactions:** Appendix 1 (bisphosphonates)

Renal impairment use half normal dose if estimated glomerular filtration rate 10–30 mL/minute/1.73 m²; avoid if estimated glomerular filtration rate less than 10 mL/minute/1.73 m²

Contra-indications acute gastro-intestinal inflammatory conditions

Pregnancy manufacturer advises avoid

Breast-feeding no information available

Side-effects nausea, diarrhoea; skin reactions; bronchospasm; *very rarely* osteonecrosis (see notes above)

Licensed use not licensed for use in children

Indication and dose

See notes above, specialist use only

Counselling Avoid food for 1 hour before and after oral treatment, particularly calcium-containing products e.g. milk; also avoid iron and mineral supplements and antacids; maintain adequate fluid intake

Bonefos® (Bayer) ⟨PoM⟩
Capsules, yellow, sodium clodronate 400 mg. Net price 120-cap pack = £161.97. Counselling, food and calcium

Tablets, f/c, scored, sodium clodronate 800 mg. Net price 60-tab pack = £169.62. Counselling, food and calcium

Clasteon® (Beacon) ⟨PoM⟩
Capsules, blue/white, sodium clodronate 400 mg, net price 30-cap pack = £40.49, 120-cap pack = £161.97. Counselling, food and calcium

Loron® (Roche) ⟨PoM⟩
Loron 520® tablets, f/c, scored, sodium clodronate 520 mg. Net price 60-tab pack = £161.99. Label: 10, patient information leaflet., Counselling, food and calcium

---

6.7 Other endocrine drugs

6.7.1 Bromocriptine and other dopaminergic drugs
6.7.2 Drugs affecting gonadotrophins
6.7.3 Metyrapone
6.7.4 Somatomedins

6.7.1 Bromocriptine and other dopaminergic drugs

Classification not used in BNF for Children

6.7.2 Drugs affecting gonadotrophins

Classification not used in BNF for Children. See section 6.4.3 for use in precocious puberty.

6.7.3 Metyrapone

Metyrapone is a competitive inhibitor of 11β-hydroxylation in the adrenal cortex; the resulting inhibition of cortisol (and to a lesser extent aldosterone) production leads to an increase in ACTH production which, in turn, leads to increased synthesis and release of cortisol precursors. It is used as a test of anterior pituitary function.

Most types of *Cushing's syndrome* are treated surgically. Metyrapone may be useful to control the symptoms of the disease or to prepare the child for surgery. The dosages used are either low, and tailored to cortisol production, or high, in which case corticosteroid replacement therapy is also needed.

Ketoconazole (section 5.2) is also used by specialists for the management of *Cushing's syndrome* [unlicensed indication].

◢ METYRAPONE

Cautions gross hypopituitarism (risk of precipitating acute adrenal failure); hypertension on long-term administration; hypothyroidism or hepatic impairment (delayed response); many drugs interfere with diagnostic estimation of steroids; avoid in acute porphyria (section 9.8.2)
Skilled tasks Drowsiness may affect the performance of skilled tasks (e.g. driving)

Contra-indications adrenocortical insufficiency (see Cautions)

Pregnancy contra-indicated

Breast-feeding contra-indicated

Side-effects occasional nausea, vomiting, dizziness, headache, hypotension, sedation; rarely abdominal pain, allergic skin reactions, hypoadrenalism, hirsutism

Licensed use licensed for use in children

Indication and dose

Differential diagnosis of ACTH-dependent Cushing's syndrome
● **By mouth**
  Child 1 month–18 years 15 mg/kg (or 300 mg/m²) every 4 hours for 6 doses; minimum dose 250 mg every 4 hours, max. 750 mg every 4 hours

Management of Cushing's syndrome
● **By mouth**
  Range 250 mg–6 g daily, adjusted according to cortisol production; see notes above

Metopirone® (Alliance) PoM
Capsules, ivory, metyrapone 250 mg. Net price 100-tab pack = £41.44. Label: 21, counselling, driving

6.7.4 Somatomedins

Somatomedins are a group of polypeptide hormones structurally related to insulin and commonly known as insulin-like growth factors (IGFs). **Mecasermin**, a human insulin-like growth factor-I (rhIGF-I), is the principal mediator of the somatotropic effects of human growth hormone and is used to treat growth failure in children with severe primary insulin-like growth factor-I deficiency.

◢ MECASERMIN

(Recombinant human insulin-like growth factor-I; rhIGF-I)

Cautions correct hypothyroidism before initiating treatment; diabetes mellitus (adjustment of anti-diabetic therapy may be necessary), monitor ECG before and on termination of treatment (and during treatment if ECG abnormal), papilloedema (see under Side-effects), monitor for disorders of the epiphysis of the hip (monitor for limping), monitor for signs of tonsillar hypertrophy (snoring, sleep apnoea, and chronic middle ear effusions)

Pregnancy manufacturer advises avoid unless essential; contraception advised in women of child-bearing potential

Contra-indications evidence of tumour activity (discontinue treatment)

Breast-feeding manufacturer advises avoid

Side-effects headache, funduscopy for papilloedema recommended if severe or recurrent headache, visual problems, nausea and vomiting occur—if papilloedema confirmed consider benign intracranial hypertension (rare cases reported); cardiomegaly, ventricular hypertrophy, tachycardia; convulsions, sleep apnoea, night terrors, dizziness, nervousness; tonsillar hypertrophy (see Cautions above); hypoglycaemia (especially in first month, and in younger children), hyperglycaemia, gynaecomastia; arthralgia, myalgia; visual disturbance, impaired hearing; antibody formation; injection-site reactions (rotate site)

Indication and dose

Growth failure in children with severe primary insulin-like growth factor-I deficiency
● **By subcutaneous injection**
  Child 2–18 years initially 40 micrograms/kg twice daily for 1 week, if tolerated increase dose in steps of 40 micrograms/kg to max. 120 micrograms/kg twice daily; discontinue if no response within 1 year

Counselling Dose should be administered just before or after food; do not increase dose if a dose is missed
Note Reduce dose if hypoglycaemia occurs despite adequate food intake; withhold injection if patient unable to eat

Increlex® (Ipsen) ▼ PoM
Injection, mecasermin 10 mg/mL, net price 4-mL vial = £384.00. Counselling, administration
Excipients include benzyl alcohol (avoid in neonates, see Excipients, p. 3)

6 Endocrine system

7 Obstetrics, gynaecology, and urinary-tract disorders

7.1 Drugs used in obstetrics **472**

7.2 Treatment of vaginal and vulval conditions **472**
7.2.1 Preparations for vaginal and vulval changes 472
7.2.2 Vaginal and vulval infections 473

7.3 Contraceptives **475**
7.3.1 Combined hormonal contraceptives... 475
7.3.2 Progestogen-only contraceptives 484
7.3.3 Spermicidal contraceptives.. 488
7.3.4 Contraceptive devices 488
7.3.5 Emergency contraception 490

7.4 Drugs for genito-urinary disorders **491**
7.4.1 Drugs for urinary retention 491
7.4.2 Drugs for urinary frequency, enuresis, and incontinence 492
7.4.3 Drugs used in urological pain.. 494
7.4.4 Bladder instillations and urological surgery................................. 494
7.4.5 Drugs for erectile dysfunction... 495

7.1 Drugs used in obstetrics

This section is not included in *BNF for Children*. See BNF for management of obstetrics.

For the management of ductus arteriosus, see section 2.14

7.2 Treatment of vaginal and vulval conditions

7.2.1 Preparations for vaginal and vulval changes
7.2.2 Vaginal and vulval infections

Pre-pubertal girls may be particularly susceptible to vulvovaginitis. Barrier preparations (section 13.2.2) applied after cleansing can be useful when the symptoms are due to non-specific irritation, but systemic drugs are required in the treatment of bacterial infection (section 5.1) or threadworm infestation (section 5.5.1). Intravaginal preparations, particularly those that require the use of an applicator, are not generally suitable for young girls; topical preparations may be useful in some adolescent girls.

In older girls symptoms are often restricted to the vulva, but infections almost invariably involve the vagina, which should also be treated; treatment should be as for adults (see BNF section 7.2).

7.2.1 Preparations for vaginal and vulval changes

Topical oestrogen creams containing **estriol** 0.01% (*Ortho-Gynest®*) are used in the treatment of labial adhesions (for details of preparation, see BNF section 7.2.1); treatment is usually restricted to symptomatic cases. Estriol cream should be applied to the adhesions once or twice daily for 2–6 weeks; adhesions may recur following treatment.

7.2.2 Vaginal and vulval infections

Effective specific treatments are available for the common vaginal infections.

Fungal infections

Vaginal fungal infections are not normally a problem in younger girls but can occur in adolescents. *Candidal vulvitis* can be treated locally with cream but is almost invariably associated with vaginal infection which should also be treated. *Vaginal candidiasis*, rare in girls before puberty, can be treated with antifungal pessaries or cream inserted high into the vagina (including during menstruation), however, these are not recommended for pre-pubertal girls and treatment with an external cream may be more appropriate. Single-dose intravaginal preparations offer an advantage when compliance is a problem. Local irritation can occur on application of vaginal antifungal products.

Imidazole drugs (clotrimazole, econazole, and miconazole) are effective against candida in short courses of 1 to 3 days according to the preparation used; treatment can be repeated if initial course fails to control symptoms or if symptoms recur. Vaginal applications may be supplemented with antifungal cream for vulvitis and to treat other superficial sites of infection.

Oral treatment of vaginal infection with fluconazole (section 5.2) may be considered for girls post-puberty.

Vulvovaginal candidiasis in pregnancy Vulvovaginal candidiasis is common during pregnancy and can be treated with vaginal application of an imidazole (such as clotrimazole), and a topical imidazole cream for vulvitis. Pregnant women need a longer duration of treatment, usually about 7 days, to clear the infection. There is limited absorption of imidazoles from the skin and vagina. Oral antifungal treatment should be avoided during pregnancy.

Recurrent vulvovaginal candidiasis Recurrent vulvovaginal candidiasis is very rare in children, but can occur if there are predisposing factors such as antibacterial therapy, pregnancy, diabetes mellitus, and possibly oral contraceptive use. Reservoirs of infection can also lead to recontamination and should be treated; these include other skin sites such as the digits, nail beds, and umbilicus, as well as the gastro-intestinal tract and the bladder. The sexual partner may also be the source of re-infection and, if symptomatic, should be treated with cream at the same time.

Treatment against candida may need to be extended for 6 months in recurrent vulvovaginal candidiasis. Some recommended regimens suitable for older children [all unlicensed] include:

- fluconazole (section 5.2) by mouth 100 mg (as a single dose) every week for 6 months
- clotrimazole vaginally 500-mg pessary (as a single dose) every week for 6 months.

PREPARATIONS FOR VAGINAL AND VULVAL CANDIDIASIS

Note Intravaginal preparations, particularly those that require use of an applicator, should be avoided in young girls unless there is no other alternative

Side-effects occasional local irritation

Licensed use consult product literature for the licensing status of individual preparations

Indication and dose
See notes above.

Clotrimazole (Non-proprietary)
Cream (topical), clotrimazole 1%, net price 20 g = £1.92, 50 g = £3.84
Condoms: effect on latex condoms and diaphragms not yet known

Dose
> Apply to anogenital area 2–3 times daily

Pessary, clotrimazole 500 mg, net price 1 pessary with applicator = £3.16

Dose
> Insert 1 pessary at night as a single dose; can be repeated once if necessary

Canesten® (Bayer Consumer Care)
Cream (topical), clotrimazole 1%. Net price 20 g = £2.14; 50 g = £3.80
Excipients include benzyl alcohol, cetostearyl alcohol, polysorbates
Condoms: damages latex condoms and diaphragms

Dose
> Apply to anogenital area 2–3 times daily

7 Obstetrics, gynaecology, and urinary-tract disorders

⌒ **PREPARATIONS FOR VAGINAL AND VULVAL CANDIDIASIS** (*continued*)

Thrush Cream (topical), clotrimazole 2%, net price
20 g = £3.99
Excipients include benzyl alcohol, cetostearyl alcohol, poly-
sorbates
Condoms: damages latex condoms and diaphragms
Dose

Apply to anogenital area 2–3 times daily

Vaginal cream (*10% VC®*) PoM, clotrimazole 10%.
Net price 5-g applicator pack = £5.62
Excipients include benzyl alcohol, cetostearyl alcohol, poly-
sorbates
Condoms: damages latex condoms and diaphragms
Dose

Insert 5 g at night as a single dose; may be repeated
once if necessary

Note Brands for sale to the public include *Canesten®
Internal Cream*

Cream Combi, clotrimazole 10% vaginal cream and
2% topical cream, net price 5-g vaginal cream (with
applicator) and 10-g topical cream = £5.76
Excipients include benzyl alcohol, cetostearyl alcohol, polysorbates
Condoms: damages latex condoms and diaphragms
Dose

See under individual components

Pessaries, clotrimazole 200 mg, 3 pessaries with
applicator = £3.63
Condoms: damages latex condoms and diaphragms
Dose

Insert 200 mg for 3 nights; course may be repeated
once if necessary

Pessary, clotrimazole 500 mg. Net price 1 with
applicator = £3.25
Excipients none as listed in section 13.1.3
Condoms: damages latex condoms and diaphragms
Dose

Insert 1 pessary at night as a single dose; may be
repeated once if necessary

Combi, clotrimazole 500-mg pessary and cream
(topical) 2%. Net price 1 pessary and 10-g cream
= £5.21
Condoms: damages latex condoms and diaphragms
Dose

See under individual components

Ecostatin® (Squibb)
Cream (topical), econazole nitrate 1%. Net price
15 g = £1.49; 30 g = £2.75
Excipients include butylated hydroxyanisole, fragrance
Condoms: damages latex condoms and diaphragms
Dose

Apply to anogenital area twice daily

Pessaries PoM, econazole nitrate 150 mg. Net price
3 with applicator = £3.35
Excipients none as listed in section 13.1.3
Condoms: damages latex condoms and diaphragms
Dose

Insert 1 pessary for 3 nights; course may be repeated
once if necessary

Pessary (*Ecostatin 1®*) PoM, econazole nitrate
150 mg, formulated for single-dose therapy. Net
price 1 pessary with applicator = £3.35
Excipients none as listed in section 13.1.3
Condoms: damages latex condoms and diaphragms
Dose

Insert 1 pessary at night as a single dose; may be
repeated once if necessary

Twinpack PoM, econazole nitrate 150-mg pessaries
and cream 1%. Net price 3 pessaries and 15 g
cream = £4.35
Condoms: damages latex condoms and diaphragms
Dose

See under individual components

Gyno-Daktarin® (Janssen-Cilag) PoM
Ovule (= vaginal capsule) (*Gyno-Daktarin 1®*),
miconazole nitrate 1.2 g in a fatty basis. Net price 1
ovule = £3.12
Excipients include hydroxybenzoates (parabens)
Condoms: damages latex condoms and diaphragms
Dose

Insert 1 ovule at night as a single dose; can be repeated
once if necessary

Gyno-Pevaryl® (Janssen-Cilag) PoM
Pessaries, econazole nitrate 150 mg. Net price 3
pessaries = £2.95
Excipients none as listed in section 13.1.3
Condoms: damages latex condoms and diaphragms
Dose

Insert 1 pessary for 3 nights; course can be repeated
once if necessary

Pessary (*Gyno-Pevaryl 1®*), econazole nitrate
150 mg, formulated for single-dose therapy. Net
price 1 pessary with applicator = £3.13
Excipients none as listed in section 13.1.3
Condoms: damages latex condoms and diaphragms
Dose

Insert 1 pessary at night as a single dose; can be
repeated once if necessary

Nizoral® (Janssen-Cilag) PoM
Cream (topical), ketoconazole 2%. Net price 30 g =
£3.54
Excipients include polysorbates, propylene glycol, stearyl
alcohol
Condoms: effect on latex condoms and diaphragms not yet
known
Dose

Apply to anogenital area once or twice daily

Other infections

Trichomonal infections commonly involve the lower urinary tract as well as the
genital system and need systemic treatment with metronidazole (section 5.1.11)
or tinidazole (section 5.4.2).

Bacterial infections with Gram-negative organisms are particularly common in
association with gynaecological operations and trauma. Metronidazole is effec-

tive against certain Gram-negative organisms, especially *Bacteroides* spp. and can be used prophylactically in gynaecological surgery.

Clindamycin cream and metronidazole gel are indicated for bacterial vaginosis.

The antiviral drugs aciclovir, famciclovir, and valaciclovir can be used in the treatment of genital infection due to *herpes simplex virus*, the HSV type 2 being a major cause of genital ulceration. They have a beneficial effect on virus shedding and healing, generally giving relief from pain and other symptoms. See section 5.3 for systemic preparations, and section 13.10.3 for topical preparations.

◢ PREPARATIONS FOR OTHER VAGINAL INFECTIONS

Dalacin® (Pharmacia) PoM
    Cream, clindamycin 2% (as phosphate). Net price 40-g pack with 7 applicators = £10.86
    Excipients include benzyl alcohol, cetostearyl alcohol, polysorbates, propylene glycol
    Condoms: damages latex condoms and diaphragms
    Side-effects irritation, cervicitis and vaginitis; poorly absorbed into the blood—very low likelihood of systemic effects (section 5.1.6)
    Licensed use Not licensed for use in pre-pubertal children

Dose

    Bacterial vaginosis
        Insert 5-g applicatorful at night for 3–7 nights

Zidoval® (3M) PoM
    Vaginal gel, metronidazole 0.75%. Net price 40-g pack with 5 applicators = £4.31
    Excipients include disodium edetate, hydroxybenzoates (parabens), propylene glycol
    Cautions not recommended during menstruation; some absorption may occur, see section 5.1.11 for systemic effects
    Side-effects local effects including irritation, candidiasis, abnormal discharge, pelvic discomfort
    Licensed use Not licensed for use in pre-pubertal children

Dose

    Bacterial vaginosis
        Insert 5-g applicatorful at night for 5 nights

7.3 Contraceptives

7.3.1 Combined hormonal contraceptives

7.3.2 Progestogen-only contraceptives

7.3.3 Spermicidal contraceptives

7.3.4 Contraceptive devices

7.3.5 Emergency contraception

The Fraser Guidelines[1] should be followed when prescribing contraception for women under 16 years. The UK Medical Eligibility Criteria for Contraceptive Use (available at www.ffprhc.org.uk) is published by The Faculty of Sexual and Reproductive Healthcare; it categories the risks of using contraceptive methods with pre-existing medical conditions.

Hormonal contraception is the most effective method of fertility control, but has major and minor side-effects, especially for certain groups of women. Hormonal contraception should only be used by adolescents after menarche.

Intra-uterine devices are a highly effective method of contraception but may produce undesirable local side-effects. They may be used in women of all ages irrespective of parity but are less appropriate for those with an increased risk of pelvic inflammatory disease.

Barrier methods alone (condoms, diaphragms, and caps) are less effective but can be very reliable for well-motivated couples if used in conjunction with a **spermicide**. Occasionally sensitivity reactions occur. A female condom (*Femidom®*) is also available; it is prelubricated but does not contain a spermicide.

7.3.1 Combined hormonal contraceptives

Oral contraceptives containing an oestrogen and a progestogen ('combined oral contraceptives') are the most effective preparations for general use. Advantages of combined oral contraceptives include:

- reliable and reversible;
- reduced dysmenorrhoea and menorrhagia;
- reduced incidence of premenstrual tension;
- less symptomatic fibroids and functional ovarian cysts;
- less benign breast disease;
- reduced risk of ovarian and endometrial cancer;
- reduced risk of pelvic inflammatory disease.

1. See Department of Health Guidance (July 2004): Best practice guidance for doctors and other health professionals on the provision of advice and treatment to young people under 16 on contraception, sexual and reproductive health. Available at www.dh.gov.uk

7 Obstetrics, gynaecology, and urinary-tract disorders

Combined oral contraceptives containing a fixed amount of an oestrogen and a progestogen in each active tablet are termed 'monophasic'; those with varying amounts of the two hormones according to the stage of the cycle are termed 'biphasic' and 'triphasic'. A transdermal patch and a vaginal ring, both containing an oestrogen with a progestogen are also available.

Choice The oestrogen content of combined oral contraceptives ranges from 20 to 40 micrograms. Generally a preparation with the lowest oestrogen and progestogen content which gives good cycle control and minimal side-effects in the individual woman is chosen.

- *Low strength preparations* (containing ethinylestradiol 20 micrograms) are particularly appropriate for women with risk factors for circulatory disease, provided a combined oral contraceptive is otherwise suitable.

- *Standard strength preparations* (containing ethinylestradiol 30 or 35 micrograms or in 30–40 microgram *phased* preparations) are appropriate for standard use—but see Risk of Venous Thromboembolism below. Phased preparations are generally reserved for women who *either* do not have withdrawal bleeding *or* who have breakthrough bleeding with monophasic products.

The progestogens desogestrel, drospirenone, and gestodene (in combination with ethinylestradiol) may be considered for women who have side-effects (such as acne, headache, depression, weight gain, breast symptoms, and breakthrough bleeding) with other progestogens. However, women should be advised that desogestrel and gestodene have also been associated with an increased risk of *venous thromboembolism*. Drospirenone, a derivative of spironolactone, has anti-androgenic and anti-mineralocorticoid activity; it should be used with care if an increased plasma-potassium concentration might be hazardous.

The progestogen norelgestromin is combined with ethinylestradiol in a transdermal patch.

The vaginal contraceptive ring contains the progestogen etonogestrel combined with ethinylestradiol.

Risk of venous thromboembolism There is an increased risk of venous thromboembolic disease (particularly during the first year) in users of oral contraceptives but this risk is considerably smaller than that associated with pregnancy (about 60 cases of venous thromboembolic disease per 100 000 pregnancies). In all cases the risk of venous thromboembolism increases with age and in the presence of other risk factors for venous thromboembolism (e.g. obesity).

The incidence of venous thromboembolism in healthy, non-pregnant women who are not taking an oral contraceptive is about 5–10 cases per 100 000 women per year. For those using combined oral contraceptives containing second-generation progestogens e.g. levonorgestrel, this incidence is about 15 per 100 000 women per year of use. The risk of venous thromboembolism with transdermal patches may be slightly increased compared with combined oral contraceptives that contain levonorgestrel. Some studies have reported a greater risk of venous thromboembolism in women using combined oral contraceptives containing the third-generation progestogens desogestrel and gestodene; the incidence in these women is about 25 per 100 000 women per year of use. The absolute risk of venous thromboembolism in women using combined oral contraceptives containing these third-generation progestogens is very small and well below the risk associated with pregnancy. The incidence of venous thromboembolism in women using a combined oral contraceptive containing drospirenone is the same range as that for users of combined oral contraceptives containing other progestogens, including levonorgestrel. The risk of venous thromboembolism with vaginal ring use compared to the risk with other combined hormonal contraceptives is unknown.

Provided that women are informed of the relative risks of venous thromboembolism and accept them, the choice of oral contraceptive is for the woman together with the prescriber jointly to make in light of her individual medical history and any contra-indications.

Travel Women taking oral contraceptives, or using the patch, or vaginal ring are at an increased risk of deep-vein thrombosis during travel involving long periods of immobility (over 5 hours). The risk may be reduced by appropriate exercise during the journey and possibly by wearing graduated compression hosiery.

Missed pill   The critical time for loss of contraceptive protection is when a pill is omitted at the *beginning* or *end* of a cycle (which lengthens the pill-free interval).

If a woman forgets to take a pill, it should be taken as soon as she remembers, and the next one taken at the normal time (even if this means taking 2 pills together). A missed pill is one that is 24 or more hours late. If a woman misses only one pill, she should take an active pill as soon as she remembers and then resume normal pill-taking. No additional precautions are necessary.

If a woman misses 2 or more pills (especially from the first 7 in a packet), she may not be protected. She should take an active pill as soon as she remembers and then resume normal pill-taking. In addition, she must either abstain from sex or use an additional method of contraception such as a condom for the next 7 days. If these 7 days run beyond the end of the packet, the next packet should be started at once, omitting the pill-free interval (or, in the case of *everyday* (ED) pills, omitting the 7 inactive tablets).

Emergency contraception (section 7.3.5) is recommended if 2 or more combined oral contraceptive tablets are missed from the first 7 tablets in a packet and unprotected intercourse has occurred since finishing the last packet.

Note The Faculty of Sexual and Reproductive Healthcare offers 2 different types of missed pill advice depending on the ethinylestradiol content of the contraceptive pill. The missed pill information above offers the same advice regardless of the ethinylestradiol content of the contraceptive pill; it is a simplified, more cautious version of advice issued by The Faculty of Sexual and Reproductive Healthcare.

Delayed application or detached patch   If a patch is partly detached for less than 24 hours, reapply to the same site or replace with a new patch immediately; no additional contraception is needed and the next patch should be applied on the usual change day. If a patch remains detached for more than 24 hours or if the user is not aware when the patch became detached then stop the current contraceptive cycle and start a new cycle by applying a new patch, giving a new 'Day 1'; an additional non-hormonal contraceptive must be used concurrently for the first 7 days of the new cycle.

If application of a new patch at the start of a new cycle is delayed, contraceptive protection is lost. A new patch should be applied as soon as remembered giving a new 'Day 1'; additional non-hormonal methods of contraception should be used for the first 7 days of the new cycle. If intercourse has occurred during this extended patch-free interval, a possibility of fertilisation should be considered. If application of a patch in the middle of the cycle is delayed (i.e. the patch is not changed on day 8 or day 15):

- for up to 48 hours, apply a new patch immediately; next patch change day remains the same and no additional contraception is required.
- for more than 48 hours, contraceptive protection may have been lost. Stop the current cycle and start a new 4-week cycle immediately by applying a new patch giving a new 'Day 1'; additional non-hormonal contraception should be used for the first 7 days of the new cycle.

If the patch is not removed at the end of the cycle (day 22), remove it as soon as possible and start the next cycle on the usual 'change day', the day after day 28; no additional contraception is required.

Expulsion, delayed insertion or removal, or broken vaginal ring   If the vaginal ring is expelled for *less than 3 hours*, rinse the ring with cool water and reinsert immediately; no additional contraception is needed.

If the ring remains outside the vagina for *more than 3 hours* or if the user is not aware when the ring was expelled, contraceptive protection may be reduced:

- if ring expelled during week 1 or 2 of cycle, rinse ring with cool water and reinsert; use additional precautions (barrier methods) for next 7 days
- if ring expelled during week 3 of cycle, either insert a new ring to start a new cycle *or* allow a withdrawal bleed and insert a new ring no later than 7 days after ring was expelled; latter option only available if ring was used continuously for at least 7 days prior to expulsion

If insertion of a new ring at the start of a new cycle is delayed, contraceptive

7

Obstetrics, gynaecology, and urinary-tract disorders

protection is lost. A new ring should be inserted as soon as possible; additional precautions (barrier methods) should be used for the first 7 days of the new cycle. If intercourse occurred during the extended ring-free interval, pregnancy should be considered.

No additional contraception is required if the removal of the ring is delayed by up to 1 week (4 weeks of continuous use). The 7-day ring-free interval should be observed and subsequently a new ring should be inserted. Contraceptive protection may be reduced with continuous use of the ring for more than 4 weeks—pregnancy should be ruled out before inserting a new ring.

If the ring breaks during use, remove it and insert a new ring immediately; additional precautions (barrier methods) should be used for the first 7 days of the new cycle.

Diarrhoea and vomiting   Vomiting and persistent, severe diarrhoea can interfere with the absorption of combined oral contraceptives. If vomiting occurs within 2 hours of taking a combined oral contraceptive another pill should be taken as soon as possible. In cases of persistent vomiting or severe diarrhoea lasting more than 24 hours, additional precautions should be used during and for 7 days after recovery (see also under Missed pill, above). If the vomiting and diarrhoea occurs during the last 7 tablets, the next pill-free interval should be omitted (in the case of ED tablets the inactive ones should be omitted).

Interactions   The effectiveness of both *combined* and *progestogen-only* oral contraceptives can be considerably reduced by interaction with drugs that induce hepatic enzyme activity (e.g. **carbamazepine, griseofulvin, modafinil, nelfinavir, nevirapine, oxcarbazepine, phenytoin, phenobarbital, primidone, ritonavir, St John's Wort, topiramate**, and, above all, **rifabutin** and **rifampicin**). A condom together with a long-acting method, such as an injectable contraceptive, may be more suitable for patients with HIV infection or at risk of HIV infection; advice on the possibility of interaction with antiretroviral drugs should be sought from HIV specialists.

For a *short course of an enzyme-inducing drug*, the dose of combined oral contraceptives should be adjusted to provide ethinylestradiol 50 micrograms or more daily [unlicensed use]; furthermore, additional contraceptive precautions should be taken whilst taking the enzyme-inducing drug and for 4 weeks after stopping it.

Women requiring a *long-term course of an enzyme-inducing drug* should be encouraged to consider a contraceptive method that is unaffected by the interacting drug. In women unable to use an alternative method of contraception (for rifampicin and rifabutin see also below), a regimen of combined oral contraceptives should be taken which provides a daily intake of ethinylestradiol 50 micrograms or more [unlicensed use]; 'tricycling' (i.e. taking 3 or 4 packets of monophasic tablets without a break followed by a short tablet-free interval of 4 days) is recommended (but women should be warned of uncertainty about the effectiveness of this regimen). **Rifampicin** and **rifabutin** are such potent enzyme-inducing drugs that an alternative method of contraception (such as an IUD) is **always** recommended. Since enzyme activity does not return to normal for several weeks after stopping an enzyme-inducing drug, appropriate contraceptive measures are required for 4 to 8 weeks after stopping.

The effectiveness of contraceptive patches and vaginal rings can also be reduced by drugs that induce hepatic enzyme activity. Additional contraceptive precautions are required whilst taking the enzyme-inducing drug and for 4 weeks after stopping. If concomitant administration runs beyond the 3 weeks of patch or vaginal ring use, a new treatment cycle should be started immediately without a patch-free or ring-free break. For women taking enzyme-inducing drugs over a long period, another method of contraception should be considered.

Some antibacterials that do not induce liver enzymes (e.g. ampicillin, doxycycline) may reduce the efficacy of *combined* oral contraceptives by impairing the bacterial flora responsible for recycling ethinylestradiol from the large bowel. Additional contraceptive precautions should be taken whilst taking a short course of an antibacterial drug that is not enzyme-inducing and for 7 days after stopping. If these 7 days run beyond the end of a packet the next packet should be started immediately without a break (in the case of ED tablets the inactive ones should be omitted). If the antibacterial course *exceeds 3 weeks*, the bacterial flora develop antibacterial resistance and additional precautions become unnecessary unless a new antibacterial is prescribed; additional precautions are also unnecessary if a woman starting a *combined* oral contraceptive has been on a course of antibacterial therapy for 3 weeks or more.

It is possible that some antibacterials affect the efficacy of contraceptive patches and vaginal rings. Additional contraceptive precautions are recommended during concomitant use and for 7 days after discontinuation of an antibacterial that is not enzyme-inducing (except tetracycline with contraceptive patch use, and amoxicillin or doxycycline with vaginal ring use). If concomitant administration runs beyond the 3 weeks of patch or vaginal ring use, a new treatment cycle should be started immediately without a patch-free or ring-free break. If the antibacterial course exceeds 3 weeks, additional precautions become unnecessary unless a new antibacterial is prescribed; additional precautions are also unnecessary if a woman starting a contraceptive patch or vaginal ring has been on a course of antibacterial therapy for 3 weeks or more.

Surgery   Oestrogen-containing contraceptives should preferably be discontinued (and adequate alternative contraceptive arrangements made) 4 weeks before major elective surgery and all surgery to the legs or surgery which involves prolonged immobilisation of a lower limb; they should normally be recommenced at the first menses occurring at least 2 weeks after full mobilisation. A depot injection of a progestogen-only contraceptive may be offered and the oestrogen-containing contraceptive restarted later—if preferred before the next injection would be due. When discontinuation of an oestrogen-containing contraceptive is not possible, e.g. after trauma or if a patient admitted for an elective procedure is still on an oestrogen-containing contraceptive, thromboprophylaxis (with heparin and graduated compression hosiery) is advised. These recommendations do not apply to minor surgery with short duration of anaesthesia, e.g. laparoscopic sterilisation or tooth extraction, or to women using oestrogen-free hormonal contraceptives (whether by mouth or by injection).

Reason to stop immediately   Combined hormonal contraceptives should be stopped (pending investigation and treatment), if any of the following occur:

- sudden severe chest pain (even if not radiating to left arm);
- sudden breathlessness (or cough with blood-stained sputum);
- unexplained swelling or severe pain in calf of one leg;
- severe stomach pain;
- serious neurological effects including unusual severe, prolonged headache especially if first time or getting progressively worse *or* sudden partial or complete loss of vision *or* sudden disturbance of hearing or other perceptual disorders *or* dysphasia *or* bad fainting attack or collapse *or* first unexplained epileptic seizure *or* weakness, motor disturbances, very marked numbness suddenly affecting one side or one part of body;
- hepatitis, jaundice, liver enlargement;
- very high blood pressure;
- prolonged immobility after surgery or leg injury;
- detection of a risk factor which contra-indicates treatment (see Cautions and Contra-indications under Combined Hormonal Contraceptives below).

◣ COMBINED HORMONAL CONTRACEPTIVES

Cautions   see notes above; also risk factors for venous thromboembolism (see below and also notes above), arterial disease and migraine, see below; personal or family history of hypertriglyceridaemia (increased risk of pancreatitis); hyperprolactinaemia (seek specialist advice); history of severe depression especially if induced by hormonal contraceptive; undiagnosed breast mass; gene mutations associated with breast cancer (e.g. BRCA 1); sickle-cell disease; inflammatory bowel disease including Crohn's disease; reduced efficacy of contraceptive patch in women with body-weight ≥ 90 kg; **interactions**: see above and Appendix 1 (oestrogens, progestogens)

Risk factors for venous thromboembolism See also notes above. Use with **caution** if any of following factors present but **avoid** if two or more factors present:

- *family history of venous thromboembolism* in first-degree relative aged under 45 years (avoid contraceptive containing desogestrel or gestodene, *or* avoid if known prothrombotic coagulation abnormality e.g. factor V Leiden or antiphospholipid antibodies (including lupus anticoagulant));
- *obesity*—caution if overweight according to BMI (adjusted for age and gender), avoid if obese;
- *long-term immobilisation* e.g. in a wheelchair (avoid if confined to bed or leg in plaster cast);
- *history of superficial thrombophlebitis;*
- *smoking.*

Risk factors for arterial disease Use with **caution** if any one of following factors present but **avoid** if two or more factors present:

- *family history of arterial disease* in first degree relative aged under 45 years (avoid if atherogenic lipid profile);

◻ **COMBINED HORMONAL CONTRACEPTIVES (continued)**

7 Obstetrics, gynaecology, and urinary-tract disorders

- *diabetes mellitus* (avoid if diabetes complications present);

- *hypertension* (avoid if blood pressure very high);

- *smoking* (avoid if smoking 40 or more cigarettes daily);

- *obesity*—caution if overweight according to BMI (adjusted for age and gender), avoid if obese;

- *migraine without aura* (avoid if *migraine with aura* (focal symptoms), *or* severe migraine frequently lasting over 72 hours despite treatment, *or* migraine treated with ergot derivatives).

Migraine Women should report any increase in headache frequency or onset of focal symptoms (discontinue immediately and refer urgently to neurology expert if focal neurological symptoms not typical of aura persist for more than 1 hour—see also Reason to stop immediately in notes above)

Contra-indications see notes above; also personal history of venous or arterial thrombosis, severe or multiple risk factors for arterial disease or for venous thromboembolism (see above), heart disease associated with pulmonary hypertension or risk of embolus; sclerosing treatment for varicose veins; migraine (but see above); transient cerebral ischaemic attacks without headaches; systemic lupus erythematosus; acute porphyria (section 9.8.2); gallstones; active trophoblastic disease (until return to normal of urine- and plasma-gonadotrophin concentration); history of haemolytic uraemic syndrome or history during pregnancy of chorea, pemphigoid gestationis; history of breast cancer but can be used after 5 years if no evidence of disease and non-hormonal methods unacceptable; undiagnosed vaginal bleeding

Hepatic impairment avoid in active liver disease including disorders of hepatic excretion (e.g. Dubin-Johnson or Rotor syndromes), infective hepatitis (until liver function returns to normal), liver tumours, and if history of pruritus or cholestatic jaundice during pregnancy

Pregnancy avoid but epidemiological evidence for combined oral contraceptives suggests no harmful effects on fetus

Breast-feeding avoid until weaning or for 6 months after birth (adverse effects on lactation)

Side-effects see notes above; also nausea, vomiting, abdominal cramps, changes in body-weight, liver impairment, hepatic tumours; fluid retention, thrombosis (more common when factor V Leiden present or in blood groups A, B, and AB; see also notes above), hypertension, changes in lipid metabolism; headache, depression, chorea, nervousness, irritability; changes in libido, breast tenderness, enlargement, and secretion; reduced menstrual loss, 'spotting' in early cycles, absence of withdrawal bleeding, amenorrhoea after discontinuation, changes in vaginal discharge, cervical erosion; contact lenses may irritate, visual disturbances; leg cramps; skin reactions, chloasma, photosensitivity; rarely gallstones and systemic lupus erythematosus

Breast cancer There is a small increase in the risk of having breast cancer diagnosed in women taking the combined oral contraceptive pill; this relative risk may be due to an earlier diagnosis. In users of combined oral contraceptive pills the cancers are more likely to be localised to the breast. The most important factor for diagnosing breast cancer appears to be the age at which the contraceptive is stopped rather than the duration of use; any increase in the rate of diagnosis diminishes gradually during the 10 years after stopping and disappears by 10 years.

Cervical cancer Use of combined oral contraceptives for 5 years or longer is associated with a small increased risk of cervical cancer; the risk diminishes after stopping and disappears by about 10 years. The risk of cervical cancer with transdermal patches and vaginal rings is not yet known

Note The possible small increase in the risk of breast cancer and cervical cancer should be weighed against the protective effect against cancers of the ovary and endometrium

Licensed use consult product literature for the licensing status of individual preparations

Indication and dose

Contraception, menstrual symptoms (section 6.4.1.2)

- **By mouth**

  Each tablet should be taken at approximately same time each day; if delayed by longer than 24 hours contraceptive protection may be lost

  21-day combined (monophasic) preparations, 1 tablet daily for 21 days; subsequent courses repeated after a 7-day interval (during which withdrawal bleeding occurs); first course usually started on day 1 of cycle—if starting on day 4 of cycle or later, additional precautions (barrier methods) necessary during first 7 days

  Every day (ED) combined (monophasic) preparations, 1 *active* tablet starting on day 1 of cycle (see also under preparations below)—if starting on day 4 of cycle or later, additional precautions (barrier methods) necessary during first 7 days; withdrawal bleeding occurs when *inactive* tablets being taken; subsequent courses repeated without interval

  Biphasic and triphasic preparations, see under individual preparations below

  Changing to combined preparation containing different progestogen *21-day combined preparations*: continue current pack until last tablet and start first tablet of new brand the next day. If a 7-day break is taken before starting new brand, additional precautions (barrier methods) should be used during first 7 days of taking the new brand.

  Every Day (ED) combined preparations: start the new brand (first tablet of a *21-day preparation* or the first *active* tablet of an *ED preparation*) the day after taking the last *active* tablet of previous brand (omitting the *inactive* tablets).

  Changing from progestogen-only tablet Start on day 1 of menstruation or any day if amenorrhoea present and pregnancy has been excluded.

  Secondary amenorrhoea (exclude pregnancy) Start any day, additional precautions (barrier methods) necessary during first 7 days.

  After childbirth (not breast-feeding) Start 3 weeks after birth (increased risk of thrombosis if started earlier); later than 3 weeks postpartum additional precautions (barrier methods) necessary for first 7 days.

  Not recommended if woman breast-feeding—oral progestogen-only contraceptive preferred.

  After abortion or miscarriage Start same day.

◻ **COMBINED HORMONAL CONTRACEPTIVES (continued)**

- **By transdermal application**

  Apply first patch on day 1 of cycle, change patch on days 8 and 15; remove third patch on day 22 and apply new patch after 7-day patch-free interval to start subsequent contraceptive cycle

  Note If first patch applied later than day 1, additional precaution (abstinence or barrier methods) should be used for the next 7 days

  Changing from combined oral contraception Apply patch on the first day of withdrawal bleeding; if no withdrawal bleeding within 5 days of taking last *active* tablet, rule out pregnancy before applying first patch. Unless patch is applied on first day of withdrawal bleeding, additional precautions (barrier methods) should be used concurrently for first 7 days

  Changing from progestogen-only method From an implant, apply first patch on the day implant removed; from an injection, apply first patch when next injection due; from oral progestogen, first patch may be started on any day after stopping pill. For all methods additional precautions (barrier methods) should be used concurrently for first 7 days

  After childbirth (not breast-feeding) Start 4 weeks after birth; if started later than 4 weeks after birth additional precautions (barrier methods) should be used for first 7 days

  After abortion or miscarriage Before 20 weeks' gestation start immediately; no additional contraception required if started immediately. After 20 weeks' gestation start on day 21 after abortion or on the first day of first spontaneous menstruation; additional precautions (barrier methods) should be used for first 7 days after applying the patch

- **By vagina**

  Insert ring into vagina on day 1 of cycle and leave in for 3 weeks; remove ring on day 22; subsequent courses repeated after 7-day ring-free interval (during which withdrawal bleeding occurs)

  Note If first ring inserted later than day 1, additional precaution (abstinence or barrier methods) should be used for the next 7 days

  Changing from combined hormonal contraception Insert the ring at the latest on the day after the usual tablet-free, patch-free, or placebo-tablet interval. If previous contraceptive used correctly and pregnancy unlikely, can switch to ring on any day of cycle

  Changing from progestogen-only method From an implant or intra-uterine progestogen-only device, insert ring on the day implant or intra-uterine progestogen-only device removed; from an injection, insert ring when injection next due; from oral preparation, first ring may be inserted on any day after stopping pill. For all methods additional precautions (barrier methods) should be used concurrently for first 7 days

  After first trimester abortion Start immediately

  After childbirth (not breast-feeding) or second trimester abortion Start 4 weeks after birth or abortion; if started later than 4 weeks after birth or abortion additional precautions (barrier methods) should be used for first 7 days

Low strength (oral)

◢ **Ethinylestradiol with Norethisterone**

Loestrin 20® (Galen) [PoM]

Tablets, blue, norethisterone acetate 1 mg, ethinylestradiol 20 micrograms. Net price 3 × 21-tab pack = £2.70

Dose

> 1 tablet daily for 21 days; subsequent courses repeated after 7-day tablet-free interval (during which withdrawal bleeding occurs); for starting routines see under Dose above

◢ **Ethinylestradiol with Desogestrel**

See Risk of Venous Thromboembolism in notes above before prescribing

Mercilon® (Organon) [PoM]

Tablets, desogestrel 150 micrograms, ethinylestradiol 20 micrograms. Net price 3 × 21-tab pack = £7.97

Dose

> 1 tablet daily for 21 days; subsequent courses repeated after 7-day tablet-free interval (during which withdrawal bleeding occurs); for starting routines see under Dose above

◢ **Ethinylestradiol with Gestodene**

See Risk of Venous Thromboembolism in notes above before prescribing

Femodette® (Schering Health) [PoM]

Tablets, s/c, gestodene 75 micrograms, ethinylestradiol 20 micrograms, net price 3 × 21-tab pack = £9.45

Dose

> 1 tablet daily for 21 days; subsequent courses repeated after 7-day tablet-free interval (during which withdrawal bleeding occurs); for starting routines see under Dose above

Sunya 20/75® (Stragen) [PoM]

Tablets, s/c, gestodene 75 micrograms, ethinylestradiol 20 micrograms, net price 3 × 21-tab pack = £6.62

Dose

> 1 tablet daily for 21 days; subsequent courses repeated after 7-day tablet-free interval (during which withdrawal bleeding occurs); for starting routines see under Dose above

Low strength (vaginal)

◢ **Ethinylestradiol with Etonogestrel**

NuvaRing® (Organon) ▼ [PoM]

Vaginal ring, releasing ethinylestradiol approx. 15 micrograms/24 hours and etonogestrel approx. 120 micrograms/24 hours, net price 3-ring pack = £27.00. Counselling, administration

Dose

> 1 ring to be inserted into the vagina for 3 weeks, removed on day 22; subsequent courses repeated after 7-day ring-free interval (during which withdrawal bleeding occurs); for starting routines see under Dose above

Counselling The presence of the ring should be checked regularly. In case of expulsion see Expulsion, Delayed Insertion or Removal, or Broken Vaginal Ring, p. 477

Standard strength (oral)

◢ **Ethinylestradiol with Levonorgestrel**

Logynon® (Schering Health) [PoM]

6 light brown tablets, ethinylestradiol 30 micrograms, levonorgestrel 50 micrograms;

5 white tablets, ethinylestradiol 40 micrograms, levonorgestrel 75 micrograms;

7 Obstetrics, gynaecology, and urinary-tract disorders

◁ **COMBINED HORMONAL CONTRACEPTIVES (continued)**

10 ochre tablets, ethinylestradiol 30 micrograms, levonorgestrel 125 micrograms.
Net price 3 × 21-tab pack = £4.12

Dose

> 1 tablet daily for 21 days, starting with light brown tablet marked 1 on day 1 of cycle; repeat after 7-day tablet-free interval

Logynon ED® (Schering Health) [PoM]
6 light brown tablets, ethinylestradiol 30 micrograms, levonorgestrel 50 micrograms;

5 white tablets, ethinylestradiol 40 micrograms, levonorgestrel 75 micrograms;

10 ochre tablets, ethinylestradiol 30 micrograms, levonorgestrel 125 micrograms;

7 white, inactive tablets.
Net price 3 × 28-tab pack = £4.12

Dose

> 1 tablet daily for 28 days, starting on day 1 of cycle with active tablet (withdrawal occurs when inactive tablets being taken); subsequent courses repeated without interval; for starting routines see under Dose above

Microgynon 30® (Schering Health) [PoM]
Tablets, s/c, levonorgestrel 150 micrograms, ethinylestradiol 30 micrograms. Net price 3 × 21-tab pack = £2.99

Dose

> 1 tablet daily for 21 days; subsequent courses repeated after 7-day tablet-free interval (during which withdrawal bleeding occurs); for starting routines see under Dose above

Microgynon 30 ED® (Schering Health) [PoM]
Tablets, beige, levonorgestrel 150 micrograms, ethinylestradiol 30 micrograms, white inactive tablets. Net price 3 × 28-tab (7 are inactive) pack = £2.69

Dose

> 1 tablet daily for 28 days starting on day 1 of cycle with active tablet (withdrawal bleeding occurs when inactive tablets being taken); subsequent courses repeated without interval; for starting routines see also under Dose above

Ovranette® (Wyeth) [PoM]
Tablets, levonorgestrel 150 micrograms, ethinylestradiol 30 micrograms. Net price 3 × 21-tab pack = £2.29

Dose

> 1 tablet daily for 21 days; subsequent courses repeated after 7-day tablet-free interval (during which withdrawal bleeding occurs); for starting routines see under Dose above

◀ **Ethinylestradiol with Norethisterone**
BiNovum® (Janssen-Cilag) [PoM]
7 white tablets, ethinylestradiol 35 micrograms, norethisterone 500 micrograms;

14 peach tablets, ethinylestradiol 35 micrograms, norethisterone 1mg.
Net price 3 × 21-tab pack = £2.08

Dose

> 1 tablet daily for 21 days, starting with white tablet on day 1 of cycle; repeat after 7-day tablet-free interval

Brevinor® (Pharmacia) [PoM]
Tablets, blue, norethisterone 500 micrograms, ethinylestradiol 35 micrograms. Net price 3 × 21-tab pack = £1.99

Dose

> 1 tablet daily for 21 days; subsequent courses repeated after 7-day tablet-free interval (during which withdrawal bleeding occurs); for starting routines see under Dose above

Loestrin 30® (Galen) [PoM]
Tablets, pale green, norethisterone acetate 1.5 mg, ethinylestradiol 30 micrograms. Net price 3 × 21-tab pack = £3.90

Dose

> 1 tablet daily for 21 days; subsequent courses repeated after 7-day tablet-free interval (during which withdrawal bleeding occurs); for starting routines see under Dose above

Norimin® (Pharmacia) [PoM]
Tablets, norethisterone 1 mg, ethinylestradiol 35 micrograms. Net price 3 × 21-tab pack = £2.28

Dose

> 1 tablet daily for 21 days; subsequent courses repeated after 7-day tablet-free interval (during which withdrawal bleeding occurs); for starting routines see under Dose above

Ovysmen® (Janssen-Cilag) [PoM]
Tablets, norethisterone 500 micrograms, ethinylestradiol 35 micrograms. Net price 3 × 21-tab pack = £1.58

Dose

> 1 tablet daily for 21 days; subsequent courses repeated after 7-day tablet-free interval (during which withdrawal bleeding occurs); for starting routines see under Dose above

Synphase® (Pharmacia) [PoM]
7 blue tablets, ethinylestradiol 35 micrograms, norethisterone 500 micrograms;

9 white tablets, ethinylestradiol 35 micrograms, norethisterone 1 mg;

5 blue tablets, ethinylestradiol 35 micrograms, norethisterone 500 micrograms.
Net price 21-tab pack = £1.20

Dose

> 1 tablet daily for 21 days, starting with blue tablet marked 1 on day 1 of cycle; repeat after 7-day tablet-free interval

TriNovum® (Janssen-Cilag) [PoM]
7 white tablets, ethinylestradiol 35 micrograms, norethisterone 500 micrograms;

7 light peach tablets, ethinylestradiol 35 micrograms, norethisterone 750 micrograms;

7 peach tablets, ethinylestradiol 35 micrograms, norethisterone 1 mg.
Net price 3 × 21-tab pack = £2.89

Dose

> 1 tablet daily for 21 days, starting with white tablet on day 1 of cycle; repeat after 7-day tablet-free interval

◁ **COMBINED HORMONAL CONTRACEPTIVES** (*continued*)

◢**Ethinylestradiol with Norgestimate**

Cilest® (Janssen-Cilag) (PoM)

Tablets, blue, norgestimate 250 micrograms, ethinylestradiol 35 micrograms. Net price 3 × 21-tab pack = £5.97, 6 × 21-tab pack = £11.94

Dose

1 tablet daily for 21 days; subsequent courses repeated after 7-day tablet-free interval (during which withdrawal bleeding occurs); for starting routines see under Dose above

◢**Ethinylestradiol with Desogestrel**

See Risk of Venous Thromboembolism in notes above before prescribing

Marvelon® (Organon) (PoM)

Tablets, desogestrel 150 micrograms, ethinylestradiol 30 micrograms. Net price 3 × 21-tab pack = £6.70

Dose

1 tablet daily for 21 days; subsequent courses repeated after 7-day tablet-free interval (during which withdrawal bleeding occurs); for starting routines see under Dose above

◢**Ethinylestradiol with Drospirenone**

Yasmin® (Bayer) (PoM)

Tablets, f/c, yellow, drospirenone 3 mg, ethinylestradiol 30 micrograms. Net price 3 × 21-tab pack = £14.70

Cautions use with care if increased concentration of plasma-potassium might be hazardous; renal impairment—avoid if estimated glomerular filtration rate less than 30 mL/minute/1.73 m²

Dose

1 tablet daily for 21 days; subsequent courses repeated after 7-day tablet-free interval (during which withdrawal bleeding occurs); for starting routines see under Dose above

Note The *Scottish Medicines Consortium* has advised (March 2003) that *Yasmin®* is not recommended

◢**Ethinylestradiol with Gestodene**

See Risk of Venous Thromboembolism in notes above before prescribing

Femodene® (Schering Health) (PoM)

Tablets, s/c, gestodene 75 micrograms, ethinylestradiol 30 micrograms. Net price 3 × 21-tab pack = £7.18

Dose

1 tablet daily for 21 days; subsequent courses repeated after 7-day tablet-free interval (during which withdrawal bleeding occurs); for starting routines see under Dose above

Femodene® ED (Schering Health) (PoM)

Tablets, s/c, gestodene 75 micrograms, ethinylestradiol 30 micrograms. Net price 3 × 28-tab (7 are inactive) pack = £7.18

Dose

1 tablet daily for 28 days, starting on day 1 of cycle with active tablet (withdrawal bleeding occurs when inactive tablets being taken); subsequent courses repeated without interval; for starting routines see under Dose above

Katya 30/75® (Stragen) (PoM)

Tablets, s/c, gestodene 75 micrograms, ethinylestradiol 30 micrograms. Net price 3 × 21-tab pack = £5.03

Dose

1 tablet daily for 21 days; subsequent courses repeated after 7-day tablet-free interval (during which withdrawal bleeding occurs); for starting routines see under Dose above

Triadene® (Schering Health) (PoM)

6 beige tablets, ethinylestradiol 30 micrograms, gestodene 50 micrograms;

5 dark brown tablets, ethinylestradiol 40 micrograms, gestodene 70 micrograms;

10 white tablets, ethinylestradiol 30 micrograms, gestodene 100 micrograms.

Net price 3 × 21-tab pack = £9.54

Dose

1 tablet daily for 21 days, starting with beige tablet marked 'start' on day 1 of cycle; repeat after 7-day tablet-free interval

◢**Mestranol with Norethisterone**

Norinyl-1® (Pharmacia) (PoM)

Tablets, norethisterone 1 mg, mestranol 50 micrograms. Net price 3 × 21-tab pack = £2.19

Dose

1 tablet daily for 21 days; subsequent courses repeated after 7-day tablet-free interval (during which withdrawal bleeding occurs); for starting routines see under Dose above

◢**Ethinylestradiol with cyproterone acetate**

See Co-cyprindiol (section 13.6.2)

Standard strength (transdermal)

◢**Ethinylestradiol with Norelgestromin**

Evra® (Janssen-Cilag) (PoM)

Patches, self-adhesive (releasing ethinylestradiol approx. 33.9 micrograms/24 hours and norelgestromin approx. 203 micrograms/24 hours); net price 9-patch pack = £16.26. Counselling, administration

Dose

1 patch to be applied once weekly for three weeks, followed by a 7-day patch-free interval; subsequent courses repeated after 7-day patch-free interval (during which withdrawal bleeding occurs); for starting routines see under Dose above

Note Adhesives or bandages should not be used to hold patch in place. If patch no longer sticky do not reapply but use a new patch.

The *Scottish Medicines Consortium* has advised (September 2003) that *Evra®* patches should be restricted for use in women who are likely to comply poorly with combined oral contraceptives

7

Obstetrics, gynaecology, and urinary-tract disorders

7.3.2 Progestogen-only contraceptives

    7.3.2.1 Oral progestogen-only contraceptives
    7.3.2.2 Parenteral progestogen-only contraceptives
    7.3.2.3 Intra-uterine progestogen-only device

7.3.2.1 Oral progestogen-only contraceptives

Oral progestogen-only preparations may offer a suitable alternative when oestrogens are contra-indicated (including those patients with venous thrombosis or a past history or predisposition to venous thrombosis), but have a higher failure rate than combined preparations. They are suitable for heavy smokers, and for those with hypertension, valvular heart disease, diabetes mellitus, and migraine. Menstrual irregularities (oligomenorrhoea, menorrhagia) are more common but tend to resolve on long-term treatment.

Interactions Effectiveness of oral progestogen-only preparations is not affected by antibacterials that do not induce liver enzymes. The efficacy of oral progestogen-only preparations is, however, reduced by enzyme-inducing drugs and an additional or alternative contraceptive method is recommended during treatment with an enzyme-inducing drug and for at least 4 weeks afterwards—see p. 478 and Appendix 1 (progestogens).

Surgery All progestogen-only contraceptives (including those given by injection) are suitable for use as an alternative to combined oral contraceptives before major elective surgery, before all surgery to the legs, or before surgery which involves prolonged immobilisation of a lower limb.

Starting routine One tablet daily, on a continuous basis, starting on day 1 of cycle and taken at the same time each day (if delayed by longer than 3 hours (12 hours for *Cerazette®*) contraceptive protection may be lost). Additional contraceptive precautions are not necessary when initiating treatment.

Changing from a combined oral contraceptive Start on the day following completion of the combined oral contraceptive course without a break (or in the case of ED tablets omitting the inactive ones).

After childbirth Start any time after 3 weeks postpartum (increased risk of breakthrough bleeding if started earlier)—lactation is not affected.

Missed pill The following advice is now recommended by family planning organisations:

'If you forget a pill, take it as soon as you remember and carry on with the next pill at the right time. If the pill was more than 3 hours (12 hours for *Cerazette®*) overdue you are not protected. Continue normal pill-taking but you must also use another method, such as the condom, for the next 2 days.'

The Faculty of Sexual and Reproductive Healthcare recommends emergency contraception (see p. 490) if one or more progestogen-only contraceptive tablets are missed or taken more than 3 hours (12 hours for *Cerazette®*) late and unprotected intercourse has occurred before 2 further tablets have been correctly taken.

Diarrhoea and vomiting Vomiting and persistent, severe diarrhoea can interfere with the absorption of oral progestogen-only contraceptives. If vomiting occurs within 2 hours of taking an oral progestogen-only contraceptive, another pill should be taken as soon as possible. If a replacement pill is not taken within 3 hours (12 hours for *Cerazette®*) of the normal time for taking the progestogen-only pill, or in cases of persistent vomiting or very severe diarrhoea, additional precautions should be used during illness and for 2 days after recovery (see also under Missed pill above).

ORAL PROGESTOGEN-ONLY CONTRACEPTIVES

(Progestogen-only pill, 'POP')

Cautions arterial disease; sex-steroid dependent cancer; past ectopic pregnancy; malabsorption syndromes; active trophoblastic disease (until return to normal of urine- and plasma-gonadotrophin concentration); functional ovarian cysts; **interactions:** see notes above and Appendix 1 (progestogens)

Hepatic impairment caution in active liver disease, recurrent cholestatic jaundice, and history of jaundice in pregnancy; avoid in liver tumour

Breast-feeding progestogen-only contraceptives do not affect lactation—start 3 weeks after birth or later

Other conditions The product literature advises caution in patients with history of thromboembolism, hypertension,

◻ **ORAL PROGESTOGEN-ONLY CONTRACEPTIVES** (*continued*)

diabetes mellitus and migraine; evidence for caution in these conditions is unsatisfactory

Contra-indications   undiagnosed vaginal bleeding; severe arterial disease; acute porphyria (section 9.8.2); history of breast cancer but can be used after 5 years if no evidence of disease and non-hormonal contraceptive methods unacceptable

Pregnancy   avoid but epidemiological evidence suggests no harmful effects of oral contraceptives on fetus

Side-effects   menstrual irregularities (see also notes above); nausea, vomiting, headache, dizziness, breast discomfort, depression, skin disorders, disturbance of appetite, weight changes, changes in libido

Breast cancer There is a small increase in the risk of having breast cancer diagnosed in women using, or who have recently used, a progestogen-only contraceptive pill; this relative risk may be due to an earlier diagnosis. The most important risk factor appears to be the age at which the contraceptive is stopped rather than the duration of use; the risk disappears gradually during the 10 years after stopping and there is no excess risk by 10 years. The CSM has advised that a possible small increase in the risk of breast cancer should be weighed against the benefits

Licensed use   consult product literature for the licensing status of individual preparations

Indication and dose

Contraception

● **By mouth**

1 tablet daily at same time each day, starting on day 1 of cycle then continuously; if administration delayed for 3 hours (12 hours for *Cerazette*®) or more it should be regarded as a 'missed pill', see notes above

Cerazette® (Organon) [PoM]
Tablets, f/c, desogestrel 75 micrograms. Net price 3 × 28-tab pack = £8.85
The *Scottish Medicines Consortium* has advised (September 2003) that *Cerazette*® should be restricted for use in women who cannot tolerate oestrogen-containing contraceptives or in whom these preparations are contra-indicated

Femulen® (Pharmacia) [PoM]
Tablets, etynodiol diacetate 500 micrograms. Net price 3 × 28-tab pack = £3.31

Micronor® (Janssen-Cilag) [PoM]
Tablets, norethisterone 350 micrograms. Net price 3 × 28-tab pack = £1.76

Norgeston® (Bayer) [PoM]
Tablets, s/c, levonorgestrel 30 micrograms. Net price 35-tab pack = 98p

Noriday® (Pharmacia) [PoM]
Tablets, norethisterone 350 micrograms. Net price 3 × 28-tab pack = £2.10

7.3.2.2   Parenteral progestogen-only contraceptives

Medroxyprogesterone acetate (*Depo-Provera*®) is a long-acting progestogen given by intramuscular injection; it is as effective as the combined oral preparations but because of its prolonged action it should never be given without *full counselling backed by the patient information leaflet.* It may be used as a short-term or long-term contraceptive for women who have been counselled about the likelihood of menstrual disturbance and the potential for a delay in return to full fertility. Delayed return of fertility and irregular cycles may occur after discontinuation of treatment but there is no evidence of permanent infertility. Heavy bleeding has been reported in patients given medroxyprogesterone acetate in the immediate puerperium; delaying the first injection until 6 weeks after the birth may minimise bleeding problems. If the woman is not breast-feeding, the first injection may be given within 5 days postpartum (she should be warned that the risk of heavy or prolonged bleeding may be increased). The manufacturer advises that in women who are breast-feeding, the first dose should be delayed until 6 weeks after the birth — however, evidence suggests no harmful effect to infant if given earlier; the benefits of using medroxyprogesterone acetate in breast-feeding women outweigh any risks

Reduction in bone mineral density and, rarely, osteoporosis and osteoporotic fractures have also been reported with medroxyprogesterone acetate. The reduction in bone mineral density occurs in the first 2–3 years of use and then stabilises. See also CSM advice below.

CSM advice
The CSM has advised that:
● in adolescents, medroxyprogesterone acetate (*Depo-Provera*®) be used only when other methods of contraception are inappropriate;
● in all women, benefits of using medroxyprogesterone acetate beyond 2 years should be evaluated against risks;
● in women with risk factors for osteoporosis a method of contraception other than medroxyprogesterone acetate should be considered.

7 Obstetrics, gynaecology, and urinary-tract disorders

Norethisterone enantate (*Noristerat*®) is a long-acting progestogen given as an oily injection which provides contraception for 8 weeks; it is used as short-term interim contraception e.g. before vasectomy becomes effective.

An **etonogestrel-releasing implant** (*Implanon*®), consisting of a single flexible rod, is also available; the rod is inserted subdermally into the lower surface of the upper arm and it provides effective contraception for up to 3 years. The manufacturer advises that in heavier women, blood etonogestrel concentrations are lower and therefore the implant may not provide effective contraception during the third year; they advise that earlier replacement should be considered in such patients—however evidence to support this recommendation is lacking. Local reactions such as bruising and itching can occur at the insertion site. The contraceptive effect of *Implanon*® is rapidly reversed on removal of the implant. *The doctor or nurse administering (or removing) the system should be fully trained in the technique and should provide full counselling reinforced by the patient information leaflet.*

The cautions, contra-indications, and side-effects of oral progestogen-only contraceptives apply to parenteral progestogen-only contraceptives, except that parenteral preparations reliably inhibit ovulation and therefore protect against ectopic pregnancy and functional ovarian cysts.

Interactions Effectiveness of parenteral progestogen-only contraceptives is not affected by antibacterials that do not induce liver enzymes. However, effectiveness of norethisterone and etonogestrel (but not medroxyprogesterone acetate) may be reduced by enzyme-inducing drugs; additional contraceptive precautions should be taken whilst taking the enzyme-inducing drug and for 4 weeks after stopping it *or* an alternative contraceptive method should be considered if *long-term* use of the enzyme-inducing drug is contemplated.

PARENTERAL PROGESTOGEN-ONLY CONTRACEPTIVES

Cautions see notes above and under preparations; possible risk of breast cancer, see oral progestogen-only contraceptives (section 7.3.2.1); history during pregnancy of pruritus or of deterioration of otosclerosis, disturbances of lipid metabolism; **interactions:** see notes above and Appendix 1 (progestogens)
Counselling Full counselling backed by *patient information leaflet* required before administration

Contra-indications see notes above; history of breast cancer but can be used after 5 years if no evidence of disease and non-hormonal contraceptive methods unacceptable

Side-effects see notes above; injection-site reactions
Cervical cancer Use of injectable progestogen-only contraceptives is associated with a small increased risk of cervical cancer; this increased risk may be similar to that seen with combined oral contraceptives, see p. 479. The risk of cervical cancer with other progestogen-only contraceptives is not known.

Licensed use consult product literature for the licensing status of individual preparations

Indication and dose

Contraception see also notes above and under preparations (roles vary according to preparation)
For dose see under preparations

◢ **Injectable preparations**

Depo-Provera® (Pfizer) [PoM]
Injection (aqueous suspension), medroxyprogesterone acetate 150 mg/mL, net price 1-mL prefilled syringe = £6.01, 1-mL vial = £6.01. Counselling, see patient information leaflet
Dose
• By deep intramuscular injection
150 Mg within first 5 days of cycle or within first 5 days after parturition (delay until 6 weeks after parturition if

breast-feeding); for long-term contraception, repeated every 12 weeks (if interval greater than 12 weeks and 5 days, rule out pregnancy before next injection and advise patient to use additional contraceptive measures (e.g. barrier) for 14 days after the injection)

Noristerat® (Schering Health) [PoM]
Injection (oily), norethisterone enantate 200 mg/mL, net price 1-mL amp = £3.59. Counselling, see patient information leaflet
Dose
• By deep intramuscular injection
Given very slowly *into gluteal muscle*, short-term contraception, 200 mg within first 5 days of cycle or immediately after parturition (duration 8 weeks); may be repeated once after 8 weeks (withhold breast-feeding for neonates with severe or persistent jaundice requiring medical treatment)

◢ Implants

Implanon® (Organon) [PoM]
Implant, containing etonogestrel 68 mg in each flexible rod, net price = £81.00. Counselling, see patient information leaflet
Dose
• By subdermal implantation
No previous hormonal contraceptive, 1 implant inserted during first 5 days of cycle; parturition or abortion in second trimester, 1 implant inserted between days 21–28 after delivery or abortion (if inserted after 28 days additional precautions necessary for next 7 days); abortion in first trimester, 1 implant inserted immediately; changing from another method of contraception, consult product literature; remove within 3 years of insertion

7.3.2.3 Intra-uterine progestogen-only device

The progestogen-only intra-uterine system, *Mirena*®, releases **levonorgestrel** directly into the uterine cavity. It is used as a contraceptive, for the treatment of primary menorrhagia and for the prevention of endometrial hyperplasia during oestrogen replacement therapy. This may therefore be a contraceptive method of choice for women who have excessively heavy menses.

The effects of the progestogen-only intra-uterine system are mainly local and hormonal including prevention of endometrial proliferation, thickening of cervical mucus, and suppression of ovulation in some women (in some cycles). In addition to the progestogenic activity, the intra-uterine system itself may contribute slightly to the contraceptive effect. Return of fertility after removal is rapid and appears to be complete.

Advantages of the progestogen-only intra-uterine system over copper intra-uterine devices are that there may be an improvement in any dysmenorrhoea and a reduction in blood loss; there is also evidence that the frequency of pelvic inflammatory disease may be reduced (particularly in the youngest age groups who are most at risk).

In primary menorrhagia, menstrual bleeding is reduced significantly within 3–6 months of inserting the progestogen-only intra-uterine system, probably because it prevents endometrial proliferation. Another treatment should be considered if menorrhagia does not improve within this time (section 6.4.1.2).

Cautions and contra-indications   Generally the cautions and contra-indications for the progestogen-only intra-uterine system are as for standard intra-uterine devices (section 7.3.4), but the risk of ectopic pregnancy is considerably smaller. Although the progestogen-only intra-uterine system produces little systemic progestogenic activity, it is usually avoided for 5 years after any evidence of breast cancer. However, the system can be considered for a woman in long-term remission from breast cancer who has menorrhagia and requires effective contraception. Since levonorgestrel is released close to the site of the main contraceptive action (on cervical mucus and endometrium) progestogenic side-effects and interactions are less likely; in particular, enzyme-inducing drugs are unlikely to significantly reduce the contraceptive effect of the progestogen-only intra-uterine system and additional contraceptive precautions are not required.

Side-effects   Initially, changes in the pattern and duration of menstrual bleeding (spotting or prolonged bleeding) are common; endometrial disorders should be ruled out before insertion and the patient should be fully counselled (and provided with a patient information leaflet). Improvement in progestogenic side-effects, such as mastalgia and mood changes, and in the bleeding pattern usually occurs a few months after insertion and bleeding may often become very light or absent. Functional ovarian cysts (usually asymptomatic) can occur and usually resolve spontaneously (ultrasound monitoring recommended).

INTRA-UTERINE PROGESTOGEN-ONLY SYSTEM

Cautions   see notes above; advanced uterine atrophy; not suitable for emergency contraception; **interactions:** see notes above and Appendix 1 (progestogens)

Hepatic impairment   caution in active liver disease and liver tumour

Pregnancy   remove system—teratogenicity cannot be excluded

Breast-feeding   progestogen-only contraceptives do not affect lactation

Contra-indications   see notes above

Side-effects   see notes above; also abdominal pain; peripheral oedema; nervousness; salpingitis and pelvic inflammatory disease; pelvic pain, back pain; *rarely* hirsutism, hair loss, pruritus, migraine, rash

Licensed use   not licensed for use in women under 18 years

Indication and dose
> See under preparation

Mirena® (Bayer) [PoM]
Intra-uterine system, T-shaped plastic frame (impregnated with barium sulphate and with threads attached to base) with polydimethylsiloxane reservoir releasing levonorgestrel 20 micrograms/24 hours. Net price = £83.16. Counselling, see patient information leaflet

Dose
> Contraception and menorrhagia
> Insert into uterine cavity within 7 days of onset of menstruation (anytime if replacement) or immediately after first-trimester termination by curettage; post-partum insertions should be delayed until 6 weeks after delivery; effective for 5 years

7 Obstetrics, gynaecology, and urinary-tract disorders

◁ **INTRA-UTERINE PROGESTOGEN-ONLY SYSTEM (continued)**

Prevention of endometrial hyperplasia during oestrogen replacement therapy
  Insert during last days of menstruation or withdrawal
  bleeding or anytime if amenorrhoeic; effective for 4
  years

7.3.3 Spermicidal contraceptives

Spermicidal contraceptives are useful additional safeguards but do **not** give
adequate protection if used alone unless fertility is already significantly diminished. They have two components: a spermicide and a vehicle which itself may
have some inhibiting effect on sperm activity. They are suitable for use with
barrier methods, such as diaphragms or caps; however spermicidal contraceptives are not generally recommended for use with condoms, as there is no
evidence of any additional protection compared with non-spermicidal lubricants.

Spermicidal contraceptives are not suitable for use in those with or at high risk of
sexually transmitted diseases (including HIV); high frequency use of the spermicide nonoxinol '9' has been associated with genital lesions, which may increase
the risk of acquiring these infections.

> **CSM advice**
> Products such as petroleum jelly (*Vaseline*®), baby oil and oil-based vaginal
> and rectal preparations are likely to damage condoms and contraceptive
> diaphragms made from latex rubber, and may render them less effective as a
> barrier method of contraception and as a protection from sexually transmitted
> diseases (including HIV).

Gygel® (Marlborough)
  Gel, nonoxinol '9' 2%, net price 30 g = £4.25
  Excipients include hydroxybenzoates (parabens), propylene
  glycol, sorbic acid
  Condoms: No evidence of harm to latex condoms and
  diaphragms

7.3.4 Contraceptive devices

Intra-uterine devices

The intra-uterine device (IUD) is a suitable contraceptive for women of all ages;
however it is less appropriate for those with an increased risk of pelvic inflammatory disease e.g. women under 25 years (see below).

Smaller devices have been introduced to minimise side-effects; these consist of a
plastic carrier wound with copper wire or fitted with copper bands; some also
have a central core of silver to prevent fragmentation of the copper. The intra-
uterine device *Gyne-T 380*® (Janssen-Cilag) is no longer available, but some
women may have the device in place until 2009. The intra-uterine devices
Multiload® *Cu250* and *Multiload*® *Cu250 Short* (Organon) have been discontinued,
but some women may have the devices in place until 2011.

A frameless, copper-bearing intra-uterine device (*GyneFix*®) is also available. It
consists of a knotted, polypropylene thread with 6 copper sleeves; the device is
anchored in the uterus by inserting the knot into the uterine fundus. *The healthcare
professional inserting (or removing) the device should be fully trained in the technique
and should provide full counselling backed by the patient information leaflet.*

The timing and technique of fitting an intra-uterine device are critical for its
subsequent performance and call for proper training and experience. Devices
should not be fitted during the heavy days of the period; they are best fitted after
the end of menstruation and before the calculated time of implantation. The main
excess risk of infection occurs in the first 20 days after insertion and is believed to
be related to existing carriage of a sexually transmitted disease. Women under 25
years are at a higher risk of sexually transmitted diseases, and pre-insertion
screening (for chlamydia, and depending on sexual history and local prevalence
of disease, *Neisseria gonorrhoeae*) should be performed. If results are unavailable at
the time of fitting an intra-uterine device for emergency contraception, appro-

priate prophylactic antibacterial cover should be given. The woman should be advised to attend *as an emergency* if she experiences sustained pain during the next 20 days.

An intra-uterine device should not be removed in mid-cycle unless an additional contraceptive was used for the previous 7 days. If removal is essential post-coital contraception should be considered.

If an intra-uterine device fails and the woman wishes to continue to full-term the device should be removed in the first trimester if possible.

◢ INTRA-UTERINE CONTRACEPTIVE DEVICES

Cautions see notes above; also anaemia, menorrhagia (progestogen intra-uterine system might be preferable, section 7.3.2.3), endometriosis, severe primary dysmenorrhoea, history of pelvic inflammatory disease, diabetes, fertility problems, nulliparity and young age, severely scarred uterus (including after endometrial resection) or severe cervical stenosis; valvular heart disease or history of endocarditis (Table 2, section 5.1); drug- or disease-induced immunosuppression (risk of infection—avoid if marked immunosuppression); epilepsy (risk of seizure at time of insertion); increased risk of expulsion if inserted before uterine involution; gynaecological examination before insertion, 6–8 weeks after then annually but counsel women to see doctor promptly in case of significant symptoms, especially pain; anticoagulant therapy (avoid if possible)

Contra-indications severe anaemia, recent sexually transmitted infection (if not fully investigated and treated), unexplained uterine bleeding, distorted or small uterine cavity, genital malignancy, active trophoblastic disease (until return to normal of urine- and plasma-gonadotrophin concentration), pelvic inflammatory disease, established or marked immunosuppression; *copper devices:* copper allergy, Wilson's disease, medical diathermy

Pregnancy remove device; if pregnancy occurs, increased likelihood that it may be ectopic

Side-effects uterine or cervical perforation, displacement, expulsion; pelvic infection may be exacerbated, menorrhagia, dysmenorrhoea, allergy; *on insertion*: pain (alleviated by NSAID such as ibuprofen 30 minutes before insertion) and bleeding, occasionally epileptic seizure and vasovagal attack

Indication and dose
See notes above

Flexi-T 300® (FP)
Intra-uterine device, copper wire, surface area approx. 300 mm² wound on vertical stem of T-shaped plastic carrier, impregnated with barium sulphate for radio-opacity, monofilament thread attached to base of vertical stem; preloaded in inserter, net price = £9.47
For uterine length over 5 cm; replacement every 5 years (see also notes above)

Flexi-T® + 380 (FP)
Intra-uterine device, copper wire, surface area approx. 380 mm² wound on vertical stem of T-shaped plastic carrier with copper sleeve on each arm, impregnated with barium sulphate for radio-opacity, monofilament thread attached to base of vertical stem; preloaded in inserter, net price = £10.06
For uterine length over 6 cm; replacement every 5 years (see also notes above)

GyneFix® (FP)
Intra-uterine device, 6 copper sleeves with surface area of 330 mm² on polypropylene thread, net price = £26.64
Suitable for all uterine sizes; replacement every 5 years

Load® 375 (Durbin)
Intra-uterine device, copper wire, surface area approx. 375 mm², wound on vertical stem of U-shaped plastic carrier, impregnated with barium sulphate for radio-opacity, monofilament thread attached to base of vertical stem; preloaded in inserter, net price = £8.00
For uterine length over 7 cm; replacement every 5 years (see also notes above)

Mini TT 380® Slimline (Durbin)
Intra-uterine device, copper wire, wound on vertical stem of T-shaped plastic carrier with copper sleeves fitted flush on to distal portion of each horizontal arm, total surface area approx. 380 mm², impregnated with barium sulphate for radio-opacity, thread attached to base of vertical stem; easy-loading system, no capsule, net price = £11.70
For minimum uterine length 5 cm; replacement every 5 years (see also notes above)

Multiload® Cu375 (Organon)
Intra-uterine device, as *Load® 375*, with copper surface area approx. 375 mm² and vertical stem length 3.5 cm, net price = £9.24
For uterine length 6–9 cm; replacement every 5 years (see notes above)

Nova-T® 380 (Schering Health)
Intra-uterine device, copper wire with silver core, surface area approx. 380 mm² wound on vertical stem of T-shaped plastic carrier, impregnated with barium sulphate for radio-opacity, threads attached to base of vertical stem, net price = £13.50
For uterine length 6.5–9 cm; replacement every 5 years (see also notes above)

T-Safe® CU 380 A (FP)
Intra-uterine device, copper wire, wound on vertical stem of T-shaped plastic carrier with copper collar on the distal portion of each arm, total surface area approx. 380 mm², impregnated with barium sulphate for radio-opacity, threads attached to base of vertical stem, net price = £10.29
For uterine length 6.5–9 cm; replacement every 10 years (see also notes above)

TT 380® Slimline (Durbin)
Intra-uterine device, copper wire wound on vertical stem of T-shaped plastic carrier, with copper sleeves fitted flush on to distal portion of each horizontal arm, total surface area approx. 380 mm², impregnated with barium sulphate for radio-opacity, thread attached to base of vertical stem; easy-loading system, no capsule, net price = £11.70
For uterine length 6.5–9 cm; replacement every 10 years (see also notes above)

7 Obstetrics, gynaecology, and urinary-tract disorders

⌒ INTRA-UTERINE CONTRACEPTIVE DEVICES (*continued*)

UT 380 Short® (Durbin)
Intra-uterine device, copper wire wound on vertical stem of T-shaped plastic carrier, total surface area approx. 380 mm², impregnated with barium sulphate for radio-opacity, thread attached to base of vertical stem; net price = £10.53
For uterine length 5–7 cm; replacement every 5 years (see also notes above)

UT 380 Standard® (Durbin)
Intra-uterine device, copper wire, surface area approx. 380 mm², wound on vertical stem of T-shaped plastic carrier, impregnated with barium sulphate for radio-opacity, thread attached to base of vertical stem; net price = £10.53
For uterine length 6.5–9 cm; replacement every 5 years (see also notes above)

Other contraceptive devices

◢**Rubber contraceptive caps**
Type A Contraceptive Pessary
Opaque rubber, sizes 1 (50 mm), 2 (55 mm), 3 (60 mm), 4 (65 mm), 5 (75 mm), net price = £6.85

Type B Contraceptive Pessary
Opaque rubber, sizes 22 to 31 mm (rising in steps of 3 mm), net price = £8.46

Type C Contraceptive Pessary
Opaque rubber, sizes 1 to 3 (42, 48, and 54 mm), net price = £7.26

◢**Silicone contraceptive caps**
Silicone Contraceptive Pessary
Silicone, sizes 22, 26, and 30 mm, net price = £15.00
Brands include *FemCap®*

◢**Rubber contraceptive diaphragms**
Type A Diaphragm with Flat Metal Spring
Transparent rubber with flat metal spring, sizes 55–95 mm (rising in steps of 5 mm), net price = £5.78
Brands include *Reflexions®*

Type B Diaphragm with Coiled Metal Spring
Opaque rubber with coiled metal spring, sizes 60–100 mm (rising in steps of 5 mm), net price = £6.59

Type C Arcing Spring Diaphragm
Opaque rubber with arcing spring, sizes 60–95 mm (rising in steps of 5 mm), net price = £7.49

◢**Silicone contraceptive diaphragms**
Type B Diaphragm with Coiled Metal Spring
Silicone with coiled metal spring, sizes 60–90 mm (rising in steps of 5 mm), net price = £8.35
Brands include *Milex Omniflex®*

Type C Arcing Spring diaphragm
Silicone with arcing spring, sizes 60–90 mm (rising in steps of 5 mm), net price = £8.35
Brands include *Milex Arcing Style®*

7.3.5 Emergency contraception

Hormonal methods

Hormonal emergency contraception involves the use of **levonorgestrel**. It is effective if taken within 72 hours (3 days) of unprotected intercourse; taking the dose as soon as possible increases efficacy. Levonorgestrel may also be used between 72 and 120 hours after unprotected intercourse [unlicensed use] but efficacy decreases with time. Hormonal emergency contraception is less effective than insertion of an intra-uterine device (see below).

If vomiting occurs within 2 hours of taking levonorgestrel, a replacement dose should be given. If an anti-emetic is required domperidone is preferred.

When prescribing hormonal emergency contraception the doctor should explain:

- that the next period may be early or late;
- that a barrier method of contraception needs to be used until the next period;
- the need to return promptly if any lower abdominal pain occurs because this could signify an ectopic pregnancy (and also in 3 to 4 weeks if the subsequent menstrual bleed is abnormally light, heavy or brief, or is absent, or if she is otherwise concerned).

Interactions The effectiveness of hormonal emergency contraception is reduced by enzyme-inducing drugs; a copper intra-uterine device can be offered instead or the dose of levonorgestrel should be increased to a total of 3 mg taken as a single dose [unlicensed dose—advise women accordingly]. There is no need to increase the dose for emergency contraception if the patient is taking antibacterials that are not enzyme inducers.

◢ LEVONORGESTREL

Cautions see notes above; past ectopic pregnancy; severe malabsorption syndromes; active trophoblastic disease (until return to normal of urine- and plasma-gonadotrophin concentration); **interactions**: see notes above and Appendix 1 (progestogens)

Pregnancy avoid but no evidence of harm to fetus; see also notes above

Breast-feeding progestogen-only contraceptives do not affect lactation

Contra-indications acute porphyria (section 9.8.2)

◻ **LEVONORGESTREL** (*continued*)

Side-effects   menstrual irregularities (see also notes above), nausea, low abdominal pain, fatigue, headache, dizziness, breast tenderness, vomiting

Licensed use   consult product literature

Indication and dose

Emergency contraception

● **By mouth**

1.5 mg as a single dose as soon as possible after coitus (preferably within 12 hours but no later than after 72 hours)

[1]**Levonelle® One Step** (Schering Health)

Tablets, levonorgestrel 1.5 mg, net price 1-tab pack = £13.83

1. Can be sold to women over 16 years; when supplying emergency contraception to the public, pharmacists should refer to guidance issued by the Royal Pharmaceutical Society of Great Britain

Levonelle® 1500 (Schering Health) PoM

Tablets, levonorgestrel 1.5 mg, net price 1-tab pack = £5.11

Intra-uterine device

Insertion of an intra-uterine device is more effective than the hormonal methods of emergency contraception. A copper intra-uterine contraceptive device (section 7.3.4) can be inserted up to 120 hours (5 days) after unprotected intercourse; sexually transmitted diseases should be tested for and insertion of the device should usually be covered by antibacterial prophylaxis (e.g. azithromycin 1 g as a single dose). If intercourse has occurred more than 5 days previously, the device can still be inserted up to 5 days after the earliest likely calculated ovulation (i.e. within the minimum period before implantation).

7.4 Drugs for genito-urinary disorders

7.4.1 Drugs for urinary retention
7.4.2 Drugs for urinary frequency, enuresis, and incontinence
7.4.3 Drugs used in urological pain
7.4.4 Bladder instillations and urological surgery
7.4.5 Drugs for erectile dysfunction

For drugs used in the treatment of urinary-tract infections see section 5.1.13.

7.4.1 Drugs for urinary retention

Acute retention is painful and is treated by catheterisation.

Chronic retention is painless and often long-standing. Clean intermittent catheterisation may be considered. After the cause has been established and treated, drugs may be required to increase detrusor muscle tone.

Alpha-blockers such as doxazosin and tamsulosin can be used in some cases of dysfunctional voiding.

Alpha-blockers

The selective alpha-blockers **doxazosin** and **tamsulosin** can be used to improve bladder emptying in children with dysfunctional voiding where the post-void residual urine volume is significant; treatment should be under specialist advice only. Alpha-blockers can reduce blood pressure rapidly after the first dose and should be introduced with caution.

◢ DOXAZOSIN

Cautions   see under doxazosin (section 2.5.4)

Contra-indications   see under doxazosin (section 2.5.4)

Side-effects   see under doxazosin (section 2.5.4)

Licensed use   not licensed for use in children

Indication and dose

Dysfunctional voiding (see notes above)

● **By mouth**

Child 4–12 years initially 0.5 mg daily increased at monthly intervals according to response; maximum 2 mg daily

Child 12–18 years initially 1 mg daily, dose may be doubled at intervals of 1 month according to response; usual maintenance 2–4 mg daily; max. 8 mg daily

Hypertension section 2.5.4

◢**Preparations**
Section 2.5.4

◾ TAMSULOSIN HYDROCHLORIDE

Cautions care with initial dose (postural hypotension); cataract surgery (risk of intra-operative floppy iris syndrome); **interactions:** Appendix 1 (alpha-blockers)

    Renal impairment use with caution if estimated glomerular filtration rate less than 10 mL/minute/ $1.73 \, m^2$

Contra-indications history of postural hypotension

    Hepatic impairment avoid in severe impairment

Side-effects dizziness, headache, asthenia; abnormal ejaculation; *less commonly* nausea, vomiting, constipation, diarrhoea, palpitation, postural hypotension, syncope, rhinitis, rash, pruritus, and urticaria; *very rarely* angioedema and priapism; also drowsiness, blurred vision, dry mouth, and oedema

Licensed use not licensed for use in children

Indication and dose

> Dysfunctional voiding (see notes above)
> * By mouth
>> Child 12–18 years 400 micrograms once daily

Tamsulosin hydrochloride (Non-proprietary) ℗ₒₘ
    Capsules, m/r, tamsulosin hydrochloride 400 micrograms, net price 30-cap pack = £6.11. Label: 25
    Brands include *Bazetham® MR, Contiflo® XL, Diffundox® XL, Omnic® MR, Stronazon® MR, Tabphyn® MR*

Flomaxtra® XL (Astellas) ℗ₒₘ
    Tablets, m/r, tamsulosin hydrochloride 400 micrograms, net price 30-tab pack = £17.55. Label: 25

7.4.2   Drugs for urinary frequency, enuresis, and incontinence

Urinary incontinence

Involuntary detrusor contractions cause urgency and urge incontinence, usually with frequency and nocturia. Antimuscarinic drugs reduce these contractions and increase bladder capacity; **oxybutynin** also has a direct relaxant effect on urinary smooth muscle. Oxybutynin can be considered first for children under 12 years. Side-effects limit the use of oxybutynin but they may be reduced by starting at a lower dose and then slowly titrating upwards; alternatively oxybutynin can be given by intravesicular instillation. **Tolterodine** is also effective for urinary incontinence; it can be considered for children over 12 years, or for younger children who have failed to respond to oxybutynin. Modified-release preparations of oxybutynin and tolterodine are available; they may have fewer side-effects. Antimuscarinic treatment should be reviewed soon after it is commenced, and then at regular intervals; a response generally occurs within 6 months but occasionally may take longer. Children with nocturnal enuresis may require specific additional measures if night-time symptoms also need to be controlled (see p. 493).

Cautions Antimuscarinic drugs should be used with caution in autonomic neuropathy and in hepatic or renal impairment. Antimuscarinics can worsen hyperthyroidism, congestive heart failure, arrhythmias, and tachycardia. For **interactions** see Appendix 1 (antimuscarinics).

Contra-indications Antimuscarinic drugs should be avoided in myasthenia gravis, significant bladder outflow obstruction or urinary retention, severe ulcerative colitis, toxic megacolon, and in gastro-intestinal obstruction or intestinal atony.

Side-effects Side-effects of antimuscarinic drugs include dry mouth, gastro-intestinal disturbances including constipation, blurred vision, dry eyes, drowsiness, difficulty in micturition (less commonly urinary retention), palpitation, and skin reactions (including dry skin, rash, and photosensitivity); also headache, diarrhoea, angioedema, arrhythmias, and tachycardia. Central nervous system stimulation, such as restlessness, disorientation, hallucination, and convulsions may occur. Antimuscarinic drugs may reduce sweating leading to heat sensations and fainting in hot environments or in patients with fever.

◾ OXYBUTYNIN HYDROCHLORIDE

Cautions see also notes above; also acute porphyria (section 9.8.2); **interactions:** Appendix 1 (antimuscarinics)

    Hepatic impairment manufacturer advises caution

    Renal impairment manufacturer advises caution

Pregnancy manufacturer advises avoid unless potential benefit outweighs risk

Breast-feeding present in milk—manufacturer advises avoid

Contra-indications see notes above

◻ OXYBUTYNIN HYDROCHLORIDE (*continued*)

Side-effects see notes above; also dizziness; *less commonly* anorexia, facial flushing; *rarely* night terrors

Licensed use not licensed for use in children under 5 years; intravesical instillation not licensed

Indication and dose

Urinary frequency, urgency and incontinence, neurogenic bladder instability
- **By mouth**

  Child 2–5 years 1.25–2.5 mg 2–3 times daily;

  Child 5–12 years 2.5–3 mg twice daily, increased to 5 mg 2–3 times daily

  Child 12–18 years 5 mg 2–3 times daily, increased if necessary to max. 5 mg 4 times daily

- **By intravesical instillation**

  Child 2–18 years 5 mg 2–3 times daily

Nocturnal enuresis associated with overactive bladder
- **By mouth**

  Child 7–18 years 2.5–3 mg twice daily increased to 5 mg 2–3 times daily (last dose before bedtime)

Oxybutynin Hydrochloride (Non-proprietary) ℗oM
Tablets, oxybutynin hydrochloride 2.5 mg, net price 56-tab pack = £7.24; 3 mg, 56-tab pack = £9.15;

5 mg, 56-tab pack = £10.21, 84-tab pack = £2.96. Label: 3

Intravesical instillation, oxybutynin (as hydrochloride) 5 mg/30 mL.
Available from 'special-order' manufacturers or specialist importing companies, see p. 943

Cystrin® (Sanofi-Synthelabo) ℗oM
Tablets, oxybutynin hydrochloride 3 mg, net price 56-tab pack = £9.15; 5 mg (scored), 84-tab pack = £22.88. Label: 3

Ditropan® (Sanofi-Synthelabo) ℗oM
Tablets, both blue, scored, oxybutynin hydrochloride 2.5 mg, net price 84-tab pack = £6.86; 5 mg, 84-tab pack = £13.34. Label: 3

Elixir, oxybutynin hydrochloride 2.5 mg/5 mL. Net price 150-mL pack= £5.74. Label: 3

◢ Modified release
Lyrinel® XL (Janssen-Cilag) ℗oM
Tablets, m/r, oxybutynin hydrochloride 5 mg (yellow), net price 30-tab pack = £11.48; 10 mg (pink), 30-tab pack = £22.95. Label: 3, 25

Dose

Neurogenic bladder instability
- **By mouth**

  Child 6–18 years initially 5 mg once daily adjusted according to response in steps of 5 mg at weekly intervals; max. 15 mg once daily

Note Children taking immediate-release oxybutynin may be transferred to the nearest equivalent daily dose of *Lyrinel® XL*

◢ TOLTERODINE TARTRATE

Cautions see notes above; also history of QT-interval prolongation; concomitant use with other drugs known to prolong QT interval; **interactions:** see Appendix 1 (antimuscarinics)

Contra-indications see notes above

Hepatic impairment reduce dose; avoid *Detrusitol ®XL* in hepatic impairment

Renal impairment reduce dose if estimated glomerular filtration rate less than 30 mL/minute/1.73 m²; avoid *Detrusitol® XL* if estimated glomerular filtration rate less than 30 mL/minute/1.73 m²

Pregnancy manufacturer advises avoid—toxicity in *animal* studies

Breast-feeding manufacturer advises avoid—no information available

Side-effects see notes above; also chest pain, peripheral oedema; sinusitis, bronchitis; paraesthesia, fatigue, vertigo, weight gain; flushing also reported

Licensed use not licensed for use in children under 18 years

Indication and dose

Urinary frequency, urgency, incontinence
- **By mouth**

  Child 2–18 years 1 mg once daily, increase according to response; max. 2 mg twice daily

Detrusitol® (Pharmacia) ℗oM
Tablets, f/c, tolterodine tartrate 1 mg, net price 56-tab pack = £29.03; 2 mg, 56-tab pack = £30.56

◢ Modified release
Detrusitol® XL (Pharmacia) ℗oM
Capsules, blue, m/r, tolterodine tartrate 4 mg, net price 28-cap pack = £29.03. Label: 25
Note Children stabilised on immediate-release tolteridone 2 mg twice daily may be transferred to *Detrusitol® XL* 4 mg once daily

Nocturnal enuresis

Nocturnal enuresis is common in young children but persists in as many as 5% by 10 years of age. Treatment is not appropriate in children under 5 years and it is usually not needed in those aged under 7 years and in cases where the child and parents are not anxious about the bedwetting; however, children over 10 years usually require prompt treatment. An **enuresis alarm** should be first-line treatment for well-motivated, well supported children aged over 7 years because alarms have a lower relapse rate than drug treatment when discontinued. Use of

7

Obstetrics, gynaecology, and urinary-tract disorders

an alarm can be combined with drug therapy if either method alone is unsuccessful.

Drug therapy is not usually appropriate for children under 7 years of age; it can be used when alternative measures have failed, preferably on a short-term basis, for example to cover periods away from home, or if the child and family are anxious about the condition. The possible side-effects of the various drugs should be borne in mind when they are prescribed.

Desmopressin (section 6.5.2), an analogue of vasopressin, is used for nocturnal enuresis; it is given by oral or by sublingual administration. Particular care is needed to avoid fluid overload and treatment should not be continued for longer than 3 months without interrupting treatment for one week for full reassessment. When stopping treatment with desmopressin gradual withdrawal may be considered. Desmopressin should not be given intranasally for nocturnal enuresis due to an increased incidence of side-effects.

Tricyclics (section 4.3.1) such as **amitriptyline**, **imipramine**, and less often **nortriptyline** can be used, but behavioural disturbances can occur and relapse is common after withdrawal. Treatment should not normally exceed 3 months unless a full physical examination is made and the child is fully reassessed; toxicity following overdosage with tricyclics is of particular concern.

Nocturnal enuresis associated with daytime symptoms (overactive bladder) can be managed by antimuscarinic drugs (see Urinary incontinence, p. 492), with the addition of desmopressin if necessary.

7.4.3 Drugs used in urological pain

Lidocaine (lignocaine) gel is a useful topical application in *urethral pain* or to relieve the discomfort of catheterisation (section 15.2).

Alkalinisation of urine

Alkalinisation of urine can be undertaken with **potassium citrate**. The alkalinising action may relieve the discomfort of *cystitis* caused by lower urinary tract infections.

POTASSIUM CITRATE

Cautions cardiac disease; **interactions**: Appendix 1 (potassium salts)

Renal impairment close monitoring required—high risk of hyperkalaemia; avoid in severe impairment

Side-effects hyperkalaemia on prolonged high dosage, mild diuresis

Indication and dose

Relief of discomfort in mild urinary-tract infections, alkalinisation of urine for dose see preparations below

Potassium Citrate Mixture BP
(Potassium Citrate Oral Solution)
Oral solution, potassium citrate 30%, citric acid monohydrate 5% in a suitable vehicle with a lemon flavour. Extemporaneous preparations should be recently prepared according to the following formula: potassium citrate 3 g, citric acid monohydrate 500 mg, syrup 2.5 mL, quillaia tincture 0.1 mL, lemon spirit 0.05 mL, double-strength chloroform water 3 mL, water to 10 mL. Contains about 28 mmol K^+/10 mL. Label: 27

Dose
• By mouth
  Child 1–6 years 5 mL 3 times daily well diluted with water
  Child 6–18 years 10 mL 3 times daily well diluted with water

Note Proprietary brands of potassium citrate are on sale to the public for the relief of discomfort in mild urinary-tract infections

7.4.4 Bladder instillations and urological surgery

Bladder infection   Various solutions are available as irrigations or washouts.

Aqueous **chlorhexidine** (section 13.11.2) can be used in the management of common infections of the bladder but it is ineffective against most *Pseudomonas* spp. Solutions containing chlorhexidine 1 in 5000 (0.02%) are used, but they may irritate the mucosa and cause burning and haematuria (in which case they should be discontinued); sterile **sodium chloride solution 0.9%** (physiological saline) is usually adequate and is preferred as a mechanical irrigant.

Dissolution of blood clots   Clot retention is usually treated by irrigation with sterile **sodium chloride solution 0.9%** but sterile **sodium citrate solution for bladder irrigation 3%** may also be helpful.

Maintenance of indwelling urinary catheters

The deposition which occurs in catheterised patients is usually chiefly composed of phosphate and to minimise this the catheter (if latex) should be changed at least as often as every 6 weeks. If the catheter is to be left for longer periods a silicone catheter should be used together with the appropriate use of catheter maintenance solutions. Repeated blockage usually indicates that the catheter needs to be changed.

CATHETER PATENCY SOLUTIONS

Chlorhexidine 0.02%

Brands include *Uriflex C*®, 100-mL sachet = £2.40; *Uro-Tainer Chlorhexidine*®, 100-mL sachet = £2.60

Sodium chloride 0.9%

Brands include *OptiFlo S*®, 50- and 100-mL sachets = £3.20; *Uriflex S*®, 100-mL sachet = £2.40; *Uriflex SP*®, with integral drug additive port, 100-mL sachet = £2.40; *Uro-Tainer Sodium Chloride*®, 50- and 100-mL sachets = £3.23; *Uro-Tainer M*®, with integral drug additive port, 50- and 100-mL sachets = £2.90

Solution G

Citric acid 3.23%, magnesium oxide 0.38%, sodium bicarbonate 0.7%, disodium edetate 0.01%. Brands include *OptiFlo G*®, 50- and 100-mL sachets = £3.40; *Uriflex G*®, 100-mL sachet = £2.40; *Uro-Tainer*® *Twin Suby G*, 2 × 30-mL = £4.42

Solution R

Citric acid 6%, gluconolactone 0.6%, magnesium carbonate 2.8%, disodium edetate 0.01%. Brands include *OptiFlo R*®, 50- and 100-mL sachets = £3.40; *Uriflex R*®, 100-mL sachet = £2.40; *Uro-Tainer*® *Twin Solutio R*, 2 × 30-mL = £4.42

7.4.5 Drugs for erectile dysfunction

This section is not included in *BNF for Children*. Adolescents presenting with erectile dysfunction should be referred to a specialist.

7

Obstetrics, gynaecology, and urinary-tract disorders

8 Malignant disease and immunosuppression

8.1 Cytotoxic drugs **496**
8.1.1 Alkylating drugs 502
8.1.2 Cytotoxic antibiotics 505
8.1.3 Antimetabolites 507
8.1.4 Vinca alkaloids and etoposide 511
8.1.5 Other antineoplastic drugs 513

8.2 Drugs affecting the immune response **517**
8.2.1 Antiproliferative immunosuppressants 518
8.2.2 Corticosteroids and other immunosuppressants 520
8.2.3 Rituximab and alemtuzumab 525
8.2.4 Other immunomodulating drugs 526

8.3 Sex hormones and hormone antagonists in malignant disease **527**

8.1 Cytotoxic drugs

8.1.1 Alkylating drugs
8.1.2 Cytotoxic antibiotics
8.1.3 Antimetabolites
8.1.4 Vinca alkaloids and etoposide
8.1.5 Other antineoplastic drugs

The management of childhood cancer is complex and is generally confined to specialist regional centres, and some associated shared-care units, affiliated to the Children's Cancer and Leukaemia Group (CCLG). The Group, together with other national and international organisations, develops and co-ordinates treatment protocols. In children, cytotoxic drugs are almost always administered in the context of a formal protocol.

Cytotoxic drugs have both anti-cancer activity and the potential for damage to normal tissue. In children, chemotherapy is almost always started with curative intent, but may be continued as palliation if the disease is refractory.

Chemotherapy with a combination of two or more cytotoxic drugs aims to reduce the development of resistance and to improve cytotoxic effect. Treatment protocols generally incorporate a series of treatment courses at defined intervals with clear criteria for starting each course, such as adequate bone-marrow recovery and renal or cardiac function. The principal component of treatment for leukaemias in children is cytotoxic therapy, whereas solid tumours may be managed with surgery or radiotherapy in addition to chemotherapy.

Guidelines on handling cytotoxic drugs:
1. Trained personnel should reconstitute cytotoxics;
2. Reconstitution should be carried out in designated areas;
3. Protective clothing (including gloves, gowns, and masks) should be worn;
4. The eyes should be protected and means of first aid should be specified;
5. Pregnant staff should avoid exposure to cytotoxic drugs (all females of child-bearing age should be informed of the reproductive hazard);
6. Use local procedures for dealing with spillages and safe disposal of waste material, including syringes, containers, and absorbent material;
7. Staff exposure to cytotoxic drugs should be monitored.

Only medical or nursing staff who have received appropriate training should administer parenteral cytotoxics. In most instances central venous access will be required for the intravenous administration of cytotoxics to children; care is required to avoid the risk of extravasation (see Side-effects of Cytotoxic Drugs and their Management).

> **Intrathecal chemotherapy**
> A Health Service Circular (HSC 2003/010) provides guidance on the introduction of safe practice in NHS Trusts where intrathecal chemotherapy is administered; written local guidance covering all aspects of national guidance must be available.
>
> Copies, and further information may be obtained from:
>
> Department of Health
>
> PO Box 777
>
> London SE1 6XH
>
> Fax: 01623 724524
>
> www.dh.gov.uk

> Because of the complexity of dosage regimens in the treatment of malignant disease, dose statements have been omitted from many of the drug entries in this chapter.

Side-effects of cytotoxic drugs and their management

Side-effects common to most cytotoxic drugs are discussed below whilst side-effects characteristic of a particular drug or class of drugs (e.g. neurotoxicity with vinca alkaloids) are mentioned in the appropriate sections. Manufacturers' product literature should be consulted for full details of side-effects of individual drugs.

Extravasation of intravenous drugs   A number of cytotoxic drugs will cause severe local tissue irritation and necrosis if leakage into the extravascular compartment occurs. For information on the prevention and management of extravasation injury, see section 10.3.

Gastro-intestinal effects   Management of gastro-intestinal effects of cytotoxic drugs includes the use of antacids, H_2-receptor antagonists, and proton pump inhibitors to protect the gastric mucosa, laxatives to treat constipation, and enteral and parenteral nutritional support.

Oral mucositis   Good oral hygiene keeps the mouth clean and moist and helps to prevent mucositis; prevention is more effective than treatment of the complication. Good oral hygiene measures for children over 6 months include brushing teeth with a soft small brush with fluoride toothpaste 2–3 times daily, and rinsing the mouth frequently. Daily fluoride supplements (section 9.5.3) can be used on the advice of the child's dental team. For children under 6 months or when it is not possible to brush teeth, carers should be instructed how to clean the mouth using an oral sponge moistened with water or with an antimicrobial solution such as diluted chlorhexidine. Mucositis related to chemotherapy can be extremely painful and may, in some circumstances, require opioid analgesia (section 4.7.2). Secondary infection with candida is frequent; treatment with a systemically absorbed antifungal, such as fluconazole (section 5.2), is effective.

Nausea and vomiting   Nausea and vomiting cause considerable distress to many children who receive chemotherapy, and to a lesser extent abdominal radiotherapy, and may lead to refusal of further treatment; prophylaxis of nausea and vomiting is therefore extremely important. Symptoms may be acute (occurring within 24 hours of treatment), delayed (first occurring more than 24 hours after treatment), or anticipatory (occurring prior to subsequent doses). Delayed and anticipatory symptoms are more difficult to control than acute symptoms and require different management.

Susceptibility to nausea and vomiting may increase with repeated exposure to the cytotoxic drug.

Drugs may be divided according to their emetogenic potential and some examples are given below, but the symptoms vary according to the dose, to other drugs administered, and to the individual's susceptibility to emetogenic stimuli.

Mildly emetogenic treatment—fluorouracil, etoposide, low doses of methotrexate, the vinca alkaloids, and abdominal radiotherapy.

Moderately emetogenic treatment—carboplatin, doxorubicin, intermediate and low doses of cyclophosphamide, mitoxantrone (mitozantrone), and high doses of methotrexate.

Highly emetogenic treatment—cisplatin, dacarbazine, and high doses of alkylating drugs.

Anti-emetic drugs, when given regularly, help prevent or ameliorate emesis associated with chemotherapy in children.

Prevention of acute symptoms For patients at *low risk of emesis*, pretreatment with metoclopramide (or less commonly domperidone) continued for up to 24 hours after chemotherapy, is often effective (section 4.6); a $5HT_3$ antagonist (section 4.6) may also be of benefit.

For patients at *high risk of emesis* or when other treatment is inadequate, a $5HT_3$ antagonist (section 4.6) is often highly effective. The addition of dexamethasone and other anti-emetics may also be required.

Prevention of delayed symptoms Dexamethasone, given by mouth, is the drug of choice for preventing delayed symptoms; it is used alone or with metoclopramide. The $5HT_3$ antagonists may have a role in preventing uncontrolled symptoms.

Prevention of anticipatory symptoms Good symptom control is the best way to prevent anticipatory symptoms. Lorazepam can be helpful for its amnesiac, sedative, and anxiolytic effects.

Bone-marrow suppression All cytotoxic drugs except vincristine and bleomycin cause bone-marrow depression. This commonly occurs 7 to 10 days after administration, but is delayed for certain drugs, such as melphalan. Peripheral blood counts must be checked before each treatment. The duration and severity of neutropenia can be reduced by the use of granulocyte-colony stimulating factors (section 9.1.6); their use should be reserved for children who have previously experienced severe neutropenia.

Infection in a child with neutropenia requires immediate broad-spectrum antibacterial treatment that covers all likely pathogens (Table 1, section 5.1). Antifungal treatment (section 5.2) may be required in a child with prolonged neutropenia or fever lasting longer than 4–5 days. Chickenpox and measles can be particularly hazardous in immunocompromised children. Varicella–zoster immunoglobulin (section 14.5) is indicated if the child does not have immunity against varicella and has had close contact with infectious chickenpox or herpes zoster. Antiviral prophylaxis (section 5.3.2.1) can be considered in addition to varicella–zoster immunoglobulin or as an alternative if varicella–zoster immunoglobulin is inappropriate. If an immunocompromised child has come into close contact with an infectious individual with measles, normal immunoglobulin (section 14.5) should be given.

Alopecia Reversible hair loss is a common complication, although it varies in degree between drugs and individual patients.

Pregnancy and reproductive function Before using cytotoxic drugs during pregnancy consideration should be given to both the prognosis of the patient and the fetal risk. The rapidly dividing cells of the fetus are potentially susceptible to the effects of cytotoxic drugs. Although antimetabolites are thought to be the strongest teratogens, specific risk assessment of individual cytotoxics is not possible with the available data. All of the long-term effects of cytotoxic exposure are not fully known.

The use of cytotoxic drugs during the first trimester is associated with the greatest risk of harm to the fetus; spontaneous abortion and teratogenicity are possible. If at all possible cytotoxic drugs should be avoided before week 10 of pregnancy.

In the second and third trimesters the risk of teratogenicity is negligible, but growth and developmental effects are possible. In the third trimester early induction of delivery may be considered. If cytotoxic drugs are unavoidable in older girls with reproductive potential, contraceptive advice should be offered where appropriate. Regimens containing an alkylating drug carry the risk of causing permanent male sterility (but may not affect sexual potency).

Long-term and delayed toxicity   Cytotoxic drugs may produce specific organ-related toxicity in children (e.g. cardiotoxicity with doxorubicin or nephrotoxicity with cisplatin and ifosfamide). Manifestations of such toxicity may not appear for several months or even years after cancer treatment. Careful follow-up of survivors of childhood cancer is therefore vital; national and local guidelines have been developed to facilitate this.

Thromboembolism   Venous thromboembolism can be a complication of cancer itself, but chemotherapy can also increase the risk.

Tumour lysis syndrome   Tumour lysis syndrome occurs secondary to spontaneous or treatment related rapid destruction of malignant cells. Features include hyperkalaemia, hyperuricaemia, and hyperphosphataemia with hypocalcaemia; renal damage and arrhythmias can follow. Early recognition of patients at risk and initiation of prophylaxis or therapy for tumour lysis syndrome is essential.

Drugs for cytotoxic-induced side-effects

Anthracycline-induced cardiotoxicity

The anthracycline cytotoxic drugs are associated with dose-related, cumulative, and potentially life-threatening cardiotoxic side-effects.

Dexrazoxane, an iron chelator, is licensed in adults for the prevention of chronic cumulative cardiotoxicity caused by doxorubicin or epirubicin treatment in advanced or metastatic cancer patients who have previously received anthracycline therapy. In practice, dexrazoxane is used for any patient receiving anthracycline therapy with evidence of subclinical cardiotoxicity thought to be secondary to anthracycline therapy, or for those children at risk of anthracycline-induced cardiotoxicity. Children receiving dexrazoxane should continue to be monitored for cardiac toxicity. The myelosuppressive effects of dexrazoxane may be additive to those of chemotherapy.

DEXRAZOXANE

Cautions   monitor full blood count; heart failure, uncontrolled angina, symptomatic cardiac valvulopathy

Renal impairment   reduce dose by 50% if creatinine clearance less than 40 mL/minute/1.73 m²

Contra-indications

Pregnancy   manufacturer advises avoid unless essential; ensure effective contraception during and for 3 months after treatment in men and women

Breast-feeding   discontinue breast-feeding

Side-effects   gastro-intestinal disturbances; blood disorders (including anaemia, leucopenia, and neutropenia); injection site reactions including phlebitis

Licensed use   not licensed for use in children

Indication and dose

> Prevention of antracycline-induced cardiotoxicity (see notes above)
> - **By intravenous infusion, 30 minutes prior to anthracycline administration**
>   10–20 times the doxorubicin-equivalent dose (depending on treatment protocol) *or* 10 times the epirubicin-equivalent dose

Administration   for *intravenous infusion* reconstitute each vial with 25 mL Water for injections then dilute contents of each vial with 25–100 mL Compound sodium lactate. Give over 15 minutes

Cardioxane® (Novartis) ▼ PoM
Intravenous infusion, powder for reconstitution, dexrazoxane (as hydrochloride), net price 500-mg vial = £156.57

Hyperuricaemia

Hyperuricaemia, which may be present in high-grade lymphoma and leukaemia, can be markedly worsened by chemotherapy and is associated with acute renal failure.

Allopurinol is used routinely in children at low to moderate risk of hyperuricaemia. It should be started 24 hours before treatment; patients should be adequately hydrated (consideration should be given to omitting phosphate and potassium from hydration fluids). The dose of mercaptopurine or azathioprine should be reduced if allopurinol is given concomitantly (see Appendix 1).

Rasburicase is a recombinant urate oxidase used in children who are at high-risk of developing hyperuricaemia. It rapidly reduces plasma uric acid and may be of particular value in reducing complications following treatment of leukaemias or bulky lymphomas.

ALLOPURINOL

Cautions ensure adequate fluid intake; for hyperuricaemia associated with cancer therapy, allopurinol treatment should be started before cancer therapy; **interactions:** Appendix 1 (allopurinol)

Hepatic impairment reduce dose, monitor liver function

Renal impairment manufacturer advises reduce dose or increase dose interval in severe impairment; if monitoring possible, adjust dose to maintain plasma-oxipurinol concentration below 100 micromol/litre

Pregnancy toxicity not reported; manufacturer advises use only if no safer alternative and disease carries risk for mother or child

Breast-feeding present in milk—not known to be harmful

Side-effects rashes (**withdraw** therapy; if rash mild re-introduce cautiously but **discontinue** immediately if recurrence—hypersensitivity reactions occur rarely and include exfoliation, fever, lymphadenopathy, arthralgia, and eosinophilia resembling Stevens-Johnson or Lyell's syndrome, vasculitis, hepatitis, renal impairment, and very rarely seizures); gastro-intestinal disorders; rarely malaise, headache, vertigo, drowsiness, visual and taste disturbances, hypertension, alopecia, hepatotoxicity, paraesthesia and neuropathy, blood disorders (including leuco-penia, thrombocytopenia, haemolytic anaemia and aplastic anaemia)

Indication and dose

Prophylaxis of hyperuricaemia associated with cancer chemotherapy, prophylaxis of hyperuricaemic nephropathy, enzyme disorders causing increased serum urate e.g. Lesch-Nyhan syndrome
• By mouth
   Child 1 month–15 years 10–20 mg/kg daily (max. 400 mg daily), preferably after food
   Child 15–18 years initially 100 mg daily, increased according to response; max. 900 mg daily (doses over 300 mg daily given in divided doses); preferably after food

Allopurinol (Non-proprietary) [PoM]
Tablets, allopurinol 100 mg, net price 28-tab pack = 97p; 300 mg, 28-tab pack = £1.10. Label: 8, 21, 27
Brands include *Caplenal®, Cosuric®, Rimapurinol®*

Zyloric® (GSK) [PoM]
Tablets, allopurinol 100 mg, net price 100-tab pack = £10.19; 300 mg, 28-tab pack = £7.31. Label: 8, 21, 27

◀Extemporaneous formulations available see Extemporaneous Preparations, p. 8

RASBURICASE

Cautions monitor closely for hypersensitivity; atopic allergies; may interfere with test for uric acid—consult product literature

Contra-indications G6PD deficiency (section 9.1.5)

Pregnancy manufacturer advises avoid—no information available

Breast-feeding manufacturer advises avoid—no information available

Side-effects fever; nausea, vomiting; less frequently diarrhoea, headache, hypersensitivity reactions (including rash, bronchospasm and anaphylaxis); haemolytic anaemia, methaemoglobinaemia

Licensed use not licensed for use in children

Indication and dose

Prophylaxis and treatment of acute hyperuricaemia with initial chemotherapy for haematological malignancy
• By intravenous infusion
   Consult local treatment protocol for details

Administration Consult local treatment protocol for details
For *intravenous infusion*, reconstitute with solvent provided then dilute requisite dose with Sodium Chloride 0.9% to 50 mL; give over 30 minutes; use immediately

Fasturtec (Sanofi-Synthelabo) ▼ [PoM]
Intravenous infusion, powder for reconstitution, rasburicase, net price 1.5-mg vial (with solvent) = £57.89; 7.5-mg vial (with solvent) = £241.20

Methotrexate-induced mucositis and myelosuppression

Folinic acid (given as calcium folinate) is used to counteract the folate-antagonist action of methotrexate and thus speed recovery from methotrexate-induced mucositis or myelosuppression.

The calcium salt of **levofolinic acid**, a single isomer of folinic acid, is also used following methotrexate administration. The dose of calcium levofolinate is generally half that of calcium folinate.

The efficacy of high dose methotrexate is enhanced by delaying initiation of folinic acid for at least 24 hours, local protocols define the correct time. Folinic acid is normally continued until the plasma-methotrexate concentration falls to 100–200 nanomol/litre (45–90 micrograms/mL).

In the treatment of methotrexate overdose, folinate should be administered immediately; other measures to enhance the elimination of methotrexate are also necessary.

CALCIUM FOLINATE
(Calcium leucovorin)

Cautions avoid simultaneous administration of methotrexate; **not** indicated for pernicious anaemia or other megaloblastic anaemias due to vitamin B$_{12}$ deficiency; **interactions:** Appendix 1 (folates)

Pregnancy manufacturer advises use only if potential benefit outweighs risk

Breast-feeding manufacturer advises caution—no information available

> Safe Practice Intrathecal injection **contra-indicated**

Side-effects hypersensitivity reactions; *rarely* pyrexia after parenteral use

Licensed use not licensed for use in children for treatment of methotrexate overdose, megaloblastic anaemia due to folate deficiency or metabolic disorders leading to folate deficiency

Indication and dose

Reduction of methotrexate-induced toxicity
• **By mouth, by intravenous injection over 2 minutes, or by intravenous infusion**
 See notes above. Consult local treatment protocol for details

Methotrexate overdose
• **By intravenous infusion**
 See notes above. Consult local treatment protocol for details

Megaloblastic anaemia due to folate deficiency
• **By mouth**
 Child up to 12 years 250 microgram/kg once daily
 Child 12–18 years 15 mg once daily

Metabolic disorders leading to folate deficiency
• **By mouth or by intravenous infusion**
 Child up to 18 years 15 mg once daily; larger doses may be required in older children

Prevention of megaloblastic anaemia associated with pyrimethamine and sulfadiazine treatment of congenital toxoplasmosis
• **By mouth**
 Neonate 5 mg 3 times a week (increased up to 20 mg 3 times a week if neutropenic)
 Child 1 month–1 year 10 mg 3 times a week

Administration Consult local treatment protocol for details

For *intravenous infusion*, dilute with Glucose 5% *or* Sodium Chloride 0.9%, give over at least 30 minutes

For administration *by mouth*, the injection solution may be given orally

Calcium Folinate (Non-proprietary) ℗⚬ℳ
Tablets, scored, folinic acid (as calcium salt) 15 mg, net price 10-tab pack = £39.20, 30-tab pack = £85.74
Brands include *Refolinon*®
Note Not all strengths and pack sizes are available from all manufacturers

Injection, folinic acid (as calcium salt) 3 mg/mL, net price 1-mL amp = £4.00, 10-mL amp = £4.62; 7.5 mg/mL, net price 2-mL amp = £7.80; 10 mg/mL, net price 5-mL vial = £19.41, 10-mL vial = £35.09, 30-mL vial = £94.69, 35-mL vial = £90.98
Note Not all strengths and pack sizes are available from all manufacturers

Injection, powder for reconstitution, folinic acid (as calcium salt), net price 15-mg vial = £4.46; 30-mg vial = £8.36

CALCIUM LEVOFOLINATE
(Calcium levoleucovorin)

Cautions see Calcium Folinate

Side-effects see Calcium Folinate

Indication and dose

Reduction of methotrexate-induced toxicity
• **By intramuscular injection, by intravenous injection over at least 3 minutes, or by intravenous infusion**
 See notes above. Consult local treatment protocol for details

Methotrexate overdose
• **By intramuscular injection, by intravenous injection over at least 3 minutes, or by intravenous infusion**
 See notes above. Consult local treatment protocol for details

Administration Consult local treatment protocol for details.
For *intravenous infusion*, dilute with Glucose 5% *or* Sodium Chloride 0.9%

Isovorin® (Wyeth) ▼ ℗⚬ℳ
Injection, levofolinic acid (as calcium salt) 10 mg/mL, net price 2.5-mL vial = £12.09, 5-mL vial = £26.00, 17.5-mL vial = £84.63

Urothelial toxicity

Haemorrhagic cystitis is a common manifestation of urothelial toxicity which occurs with the oxazaphosphorines, cyclophosphamide and ifosfamide; it is caused by the metabolite acrolein. Adequate hydration is essential to reduce the risk of urothelial toxicity. **Mesna** reacts specifically with acrolein in the urinary tract, preventing toxicity. Mesna is given for the same duration as cyclophosphamide or ifosfamide. It is generally given intravenously; the dose of mesna is equal to or greater than that of the oxazaphosphorine. For the role of nebulised mesna as a mucolytic in cystic fibrosis, see section 3.7.

MESNA

Cautions

Pregnancy not known to be harmful

Contra-indications hypersensitivity to thiol-containing compounds

Side-effects nausea, vomiting, colic, diarrhoea, fatigue, headache, limb and joint pains, depression, irritability, rash, hypotension and tachycardia; rarely hypersensitivity reactions (more common in patients with auto-immune disorders)

Licensed use not licensed for use in children

Indication and dose

Urothelial toxicity following oxazaphosphorine therapy

• **By intravenous injection or by continuous intravenous infusion**

See notes above. Consult local treatment protocol for details

---

Mucolytic in cystic fibrosis section 3.7

Administration Consult local treatment protocol for details

For *intravenous infusion*, dilute with Glucose 5% *or* Sodium Chloride 0.9%

Mesna (Baxter) [PoM]

Tablets, f/c, mesna 400 mg, net price 10-tab pack = £23.20; 600 mg, 10-tab pack = £30.10

Injection, mesna 100 mg/mL. Net price 4-mL amp = £1.95; 10-mL amp = £4.38

Note For oral administration contents of ampoule are taken in a flavoured drink such as orange juice or cola which may be stored in a refrigerator for up to 24 hours in a sealed container

8.1.1 Alkylating drugs

Extensive experience is available with these drugs, which are among the most widely used in cancer chemotherapy. They act by damaging DNA, thus interfering with cell replication. In addition to the side-effects common to many cytotoxic drugs (section 8.1), problems associated specifically with alkylating drugs include:

• an adverse effect on gametogenesis which may be reversible, particularly in females; amenorrhoea may also occur, which also may be reversible;

• a marked increase in the incidence of secondary tumours and leukaemia, particularly when alkylating drugs are combined with extensive irradiation;

• fluid retention with oedema and dilutional hyponatraemia in younger children; the risk of this complication is higher in the first 2 days and also when given with concomitant vinca alkaloids;

• urothelial toxicity with intravenous use; adequate hydration may reduce this risk; mesna (section 8.1) provides further protection against urotoxic effects of cyclophosphamide and ifosfamide.

BUSULFAN

(Busulphan)

Cautions see section 8.1 and notes above; monitor full blood count regularly throughout treatment; monitor liver function; previous mediastinal or pulmonary radiation therapy; avoid in acute porphyria (section 9.8.2); **interactions:** Appendix 1 (busulfan)

Hepatic impairment manufacturer advises monitor liver function—no information available

Contra-indications

Pregnancy avoid (teratogenic in *animals*); manufacturers advise effective contraception during and for 6 months after treatment in men or women; *see also* section 8.1

Breast-feeding discontinue breast-feeding

Side-effects see section 8.1 and notes above; also hepatotoxicity (including hepatic veno-occlusive disease, hyperbilirubinaemia, jaundice, and fibrosis); cardiac tamponade in thalassaemia; pneumonia, skin hyperpigmentation; *rarely* progressive pulmonary fibrosis, seizures, aplastic anaemia, visual disturbances, hypersensitivity reactions (including urticaria, erythema); *very rarely* myasthenia gravis, gynaecomastia

Licensed use *Busilvex®* not licensed for chronic granulocytic leukaemia

◁ **BUSULFAN** (*continued*)

Indication and dose

Chronic granulocytic leukaemia
* **By mouth**
  Consult local treatment protocol for details

Conditioning treatment before haematopoietic stem-cell transplantation
* **By mouth or by intravenous infusion**
  Consult local treatment protocol for details

Administration Consult local treatment protocol for details

For *intravenous infusion*, dilute to a concentration of 500 micrograms/mL with Glucose 5% *or* Sodium Chloride 0.9%; give through a central venous catheter over 2 hours

Busilvex® (Fabre) ▼ ℗oM
Concentrate for intravenous infusion, busulfan 6 mg/mL, net price 10-mL vial = £201.25

Myleran® (GSK) ℗oM
Tablets, f/c, busulfan 2 mg, net price 25-tab pack = £5.20

Busulfan
Capsules, busulfan 25 mg
Available from 'special-order' manufacturers or specialist importing companies, p. 943

◢Extemporaneous formulations available see Extemporaneous Preparations, p. 8

◤ CHLORAMBUCIL

Cautions see section 8.1 and notes above; monitor full blood count regularly throughout treatment; increased seizure risk in children with nephrotic syndrome or history of epilepsy; avoid in acute porphyria (section 9.8.2)

Hepatic impairment manufacturer advises consider dose reduction in severe hepatic impairment—limited information available

Contra-indications

Pregnancy avoid; manufacturer advises effective contraception during treatment in men or women; *see also* section 8.1

Breast-feeding discontinue breast-feeding

Side-effects see section 8.1 and notes above; also *less commonly* skin rash (possible progression to Stevens-Johnson syndrome and toxic epidermal necrolysis); *rarely* seizures, hepatotoxicity and jaundice; *very rarely* irreversible bone-marrow suppression, pulmonary fibrosis, tremor, peripheral neuropathy, sterile cystitis, sterility in prepubertal and pubertal males

Licensed use not licensed for use in nephrotic syndrome

Indication and dose

Hodgkin's disease
* **By mouth**
  Consult local treatment protocol for details

Non-Hodgkin's lymphoma
* **By mouth**
  Consult local treatment protocol for details

Relapsing steroid-sensitive nephrotic syndrome; initiated in specialist centres (see also section 6.3.2, p. 445)
* **By mouth**
  Child 3 months–18 years 200 micrograms/kg once daily for 8 weeks

Leukeran® (GSK) ℗oM
Tablets, f/c, brown, chlorambucil 2 mg, net price 25-tab pack = £8.36

◢Extemporaneous formulations available see Extemporaneous Preparations, p. 8

◤ CYCLOPHOSPHAMIDE

Cautions see section 8.1 and notes above; avoid in acute porphyria (section 9.8.2); **interactions:** Appendix 1 (cyclophosphamide)

Hepatic impairment reduce dose—consult local treatment protocol for details

Renal impairment reduce dose—consult local treatment protocol for details

Contra-indications haemorrhagic cystitis

Pregnancy avoid; manufacturer advises effective contraception during and for at least 3 months after treatment in men or women; see also section 8.1

Breast-feeding discontinue breast-feeding during and for 36 hours after stopping treatment

Side-effects see section 8.1 and notes above; *also* anorexia; cardiotoxicity at high doses; interstitial pulmonary fibrosis; inappropriate secretion of anti-diuretic hormone, disturbances of carbohydrate metabolism; urothelial toxicity; pigmenta-

tion of palms, nails and soles; *rarely* hepatotoxicity

Licensed use not licensed for use in children

Indication and dose

Acute lymphoblastic leukaemia, non-Hodgkin's lymphoma, retinoblastoma, neuroblastoma, rhabdomyosarcoma, soft-tissue sarcomas, Ewing tumour, neuroectodermal tumours (including medulloblastoma), infant brain tumours, ependymona, high-dose conditioning for bone marrow transplantation
* **By mouth or by intravenous infusion**
  Consult local treatment protocol for details

Steroid-sensitive nephrotic syndrome see also section 6.3.2, p. 445
* **By mouth**
  Child 3 months–18 years 2–3 mg/kg once daily for eight weeks

◻ **CYCLOPHOSPHAMIDE** (*continued*)

• **By intravenous infusion**

Child 3 months–18 years 500 mg/m² once a month for six months

Administration Consult local treatment protocol for details

For *intravenous infusion*, dilute with Glucose 5% *or* Sodium Chloride 0.9% *or* 0.18% with Glucose 4%; give over at least one hour

Cyclophosphamide (Non-proprietary) ⒫ᵒᴹ
Tablets, s/c, cyclophosphamide (anhydrous) 50 mg, net price 20 = £2.49. Label: 27

Injection, powder for reconstitution, cyclophosphamide, net price 500-mg vial = £2.88; 1-g vial = £5.04

Cyclophosphamide (Baxter) ⒫ᵒᴹ
Tablets, s/c, cyclophosphamide 50 mg, net price 100-tab pack = £12.00. Label: 23, 25, 27

Injection, powder for reconstitution, cyclophosphamide. Net price 200-mg vial = £1.86; 500-mg vial = £3.54; 1-g vial = £6.18

◀ Extemporaneous formulations available see Extemporaneous Preparations, p. 8

▟ IFOSFAMIDE

Cautions see section 8.1 and notes above; ensure satisfactory electrolyte balance, and renal function before each course (risk of tubular dysfunction, Fanconi's syndrome, or diabetes insipidus if renal toxicity not treated promptly); risk of urothelial toxicity (see notes above); **interactions:** Appendix 1 (ifosfamide)

Renal impairment avoid

Contra-indications bone marrow aplasia, myelosuppression; urinary tract obstruction; acute infection (including urinary-tract infection); urothelial damage

Hepatic impairment avoid

Pregnancy avoid (teratogenic and carcinogenic in *animals*), manufacturer advises adequate contraception during and for at least 6 months after treatment in men or women; see also section 8.1

Breast-feeding discontinue breast-feeding

Side-effects see section 8.1 and notes above; *also* drowsiness, confusion, disorientation, restlessness, psychosis; urothelial toxicity causing haemorrhagic cystitis and dysuria, renal toxicity (see Cautions above); *less commonly* severe

encephalopathy; *rarely* diarrhoea, constipation, convulsions, anorexia; *very rarely* jaundice, thrombophlebitis, syndrome of inappropriate antidiuretic hormone secretion

Indication and dose

Rhabdomyosarcoma, soft-tissue sarcomas, Ewing tumour, germ cell tumour, osteogenic sarcoma
• **By intravenous infusion**
Consult local treatment protocol for details

Administration Consult local treatment protocol for details

For *intravenous infusion*, dilute reconstituted solution to a max. concentration of 40 mg/mL with Glucose 5% *or* Sodium Chloride 0.9%; give over 30–120 minutes. Ensure adequate hydration and concurrent administration of mesna (see notes above and section 8.1).

Ifosfamide (Baxter) ⒫ᵒᴹ
Injection, powder for reconstitution, ifosfamide. Net price 1-g vial = £27.03; 2-g vial = £45.49 (hosp. only)

▟ MELPHALAN

Cautions see section 8.1 and notes above; monitor full blood count before and throughout treatment; for high-dose intravenous administration establish adequate hydration (see notes above), consider use of prophylactic anti-infective agents; haematopoietic stem cell transplantation essential for high dose treatment (consult local treatment protocol for details); **interactions:** Appendix 1 (melphalan)

Renal impairment reduce dose initially—consult product literature

Contra-indications

Pregnancy avoid; manufacturer advises adequate contraception during treatment in men or women; see also section 8.1

Breast-feeding discontinue breast-feeding

Side-effects see section 8.1 and notes above

Licensed use childhood neuroblastoma; oral use not licensed in children

Indication and dose

High intravenous dose with haematopoietic stem cell transplantation in the treatment of childhood neuroblastoma and some other advanced embryonal tumours
• **Intravenous infusion**
Consult local treatment protocol for details

Administration For *intravenous infusion* in Sodium Chloride 0.9%. Reconstitute with the solvent provided and inject slowly into the tubing of a fast running infusion; alternatively, reconstituted solution can be diluted in infusion fluid to a concentration not greater than 0.45 mg/mL. Max. 90 minutes between reconstitution and completion of administration. Incompatible with glucose infusion

Alkeran® (GSK) ⒫ᵒᴹ
Injection, powder for reconstitution, melphalan 50 mg (as hydrochloride). Net price 50-mg vial (with solvent-diluent) = £27.61

8.1.2 **Cytotoxic antibiotics**

Cytotoxic antibiotics are widely used. Many act as radiomimetics and simultaneous use of radiotherapy should be **avoided** as it may enhance toxicity markedly.

Daunorubicin, **doxorubicin**, and **epirubicin** are anthracycline antibiotics. **Mitoxantrone** (mitozantrone) is an anthracycline derivative.

All anthracycline antibiotics have been associated with varying degrees of cardiac toxicity—this may be idiosyncratic and reversible, but is commonly related to total cumulative dose and is irreversible. Cardiac function should be monitored before and at regular intervals throughout treatment and afterwards. Anthracycline antibiotics should not normally be used in children with left ventricular dysfunction. Epirubicin and mitoxantrone are considered less toxic, and may be suitable for children who have received high cumulative doses of other anthracyclines.

BLEOMYCIN

Cautions   see section 8.1; ensure monitoring of pulmonary function—investigate any shortness of breath before initiation; caution in handling—irritant to tissues

Renal impairment   reduce dose in renal impairment—consult local treatment protocol for details

Contra-indications   acute pulmonary infection or significantly reduced lung function

Pregnancy   avoid (teratogenic and carcinogenic in *animal* studies); see also section 8.1

Breast-feeding   discontinue breast-feeding

Side-effects   see section 8.1, less bone marrow suppression; anorexia; pulmonary toxicity e.g. pulmonary fibrosis (usually dose-related and delayed); fever (directly following administration), fatigue; dermatological and mucous membrane toxicity, localised skin hyperpigmentation; rarely cardiorespiratory collapse and hyperpyrexia

Licensed use   not licensed for use in children

Indication and dose

> Some germ cell tumours, Hodgkin's lymphoma
> • By intravenous infusion
>   Consult local treatment protocol for details

Administration   Consult local treatment protocol for details

For *intravenous infusion* dilute with a suitable volume of Sodium Chloride 0.9% (e.g. up to 100 mL) into established intravenous line

Bleomycin (Non-proprietary) (PoM)
Injection, powder for reconstitution, bleomycin (as sulphate). Net price 15 000-unit vial = £15.56
Note To conform to the European Pharmacopoeia vials previously labelled as containing '15 units' of bleomycin are now labelled as containing 15 000 units. The amount of bleomycin in the vial has not changed.
Brands include *Bleo-Kyowa*®

DACTINOMYCIN
(Actinomycin D)

Cautions   see section 8.1 and notes above; caution in handling—irritant to tissues

Hepatic impairment   consider dose reduction if raised serum bilirubin or biliary obstruction (consult local treatment protocol for details)

Contra-indications

Pregnancy   avoid (teratogenic in *animal* studies); see also section 8.1

Breast-feeding   discontinue breast-feeding

Side-effects   see section 8.1 and notes above; *less commonly* cheilitis, dysphagia; fever, malaise, lethargy; anaemia, hypoglycaemia; myalgia; acne; *rarely* hepatotoxicity (possibly dose-related)

Licensed use   not licensed for use in children under 12 years

Indication and dose

> Wilms' tumour, childhood rhabdomyosarcoma and other soft tissue sarcomas, Ewing's sarcoma
> • By intravenous injection
>   Consult local treatment protocol for details

Administration   Consult local treatment protocol for details

For *slow intravenous injection*, give 500 micrograms/mL solution over 2–3 minutes

Cosmegen Lyovac® (Ovation) (PoM)
Injection, powder for reconstitution, dactinomycin, net price 500-microgram vial = £6.75

DAUNORUBICIN

Cautions   see section 8.1 and notes above; caution in handling—irritant to tissues

Hepatic impairment   reduce dose according to serum bilirubin concentration (consult local treatment protocol for details)

Renal impairment   reduce dose in renal impairment—consult local treatment protocol for details

Contra-indications

Pregnancy   avoid (teratogenic and carcinogenic in *animal* studies), see also section 8.1

Breast-feeding   discontinue breast-feeding

Side-effects   see section 8.1 and notes above, leucopenia, less commonly mucositis; cardiac

8

Malignant disease and immunosuppression

◁ **DAUNORUBICIN (continued)**

toxicity (usually 1–6 months after initiation of therapy); fever; red urine discolouration

Licensed use liposomal preparation not licensed for use in children

Indication and dose

Acute myelogenous leukaemia, acute lympho-cytic leukaemia
• **By intravenous infusion**
Consult local treatment protocol for details

Daunorubicin (Non-proprietary) PoM

Injection, powder for reconstitution, daunorubicin (as hydrochloride), net price 20-mg vial = £44.76

Administration Dilute with Sodium Chloride 0.9% and give into the tubing or side-arm of a fast flowing infusion—consult local treatment protocol for details

◀Lipid formulation

DaunoXome® (Diatos) PoM

Concentrate for intravenous infusion, daunorubicin encapsulated in liposomes. For dilution before use. Net price 50-mg vial = £137.67

Administration Consult local treatment protocol for details

DOXORUBICIN HYDROCHLORIDE

Cautions see section 8.1 and notes above; caution in handling—irritant to tissues; **interactions:** Appendix 1 (doxorubicin)

Hepatic impairment reduce dose according to bilirubin concentration, consult local treatment protocol for details

Contra-indications

Pregnancy avoid (teratogenic and toxic in *animal* studies); manufacturer of liposomal product advises effective contraception during and for at least 6 months after treatment in men or women; see also section 8.1

Breast-feeding discontinue breast-feeding

Side-effects see section 8.1 and notes above; red urine discoloration; thrombophlebitis over injection site; less commonly bronchospasm, fever, amenorrhoea, and skin rash

Licensed use not licensed for use in children

Indication and dose

Paediatric malignancies including Ewing's sar-coma, osteogenic sarcoma, Wilms' tumour, neuroblastoma, retinoblastoma, some liver tumours, acute lymphoblastic leukaemia, Hodgkin's lymphoma, non-Hodgkin's lymph-oma
• **By intravenous infusion**
Consult local treatment protocol for details

Administration Consult local treatment protocol for details

For *intravenous infusion*, dilute with Sodium Chloride 0.9%; give preferably through a central venous catheter

Doxorubicin (Non-proprietary) PoM

Injection, powder for reconstitution, doxorubicin hydrochloride, net price 10-mg vial = £18.72; 50-mg vial = £96.86

Note The brand name *Adriamycin®* was formerly used

Injection, doxorubicin hydrochloride 2 mg/mL, net price 5-mL vial = £20.60, 25-mL vial = £103.00, 100-mL vial = £412.00

EPIRUBICIN HYDROCHLORIDE

Cautions see section 8.1 and notes above; caution in handling—irritant to tissues

Hepatic impairment reduce dose according to bilirubin concentration (consult local treatment protocol for details)

Contra-indications

Pregnancy avoid (carcinogenic in *animal* studies); see also section 8.1

Breast-feeding discontinue breast-feeding

Side-effects see section 8.1 and notes above; red urine discolouration; anaphylaxis

Licensed use not licensed for use in children

Indication and dose

Recurrent acute lymphoblastic leukaemia, rhabdomyosarcoma, other soft tissue tumours of childhood
• **Intravenous infusion**
Consult local treatment protocol for details

Administration Consult local treatment protocol for details

For *intravenous infusion*, dilute with Sodium Chloride 0.9%; give preferably through a central venous catheter

Pharmorubicin® Rapid Dissolution (Pharmacia) PoM
Injection, powder for reconstitution, epirubicin hydrochloride. Net price 50-mg vial = £96.54

Pharmorubicin® Solution for Injection (Pharmacia) PoM

Injection, epirubicin hydrochloride 2 mg/mL, net price 5-mL vial = £19.31, 25-mL vial = £96.54, 100-mL vial = £386.16

■ MITOXANTRONE
(Mitozantrone)

Cautions see section 8.1 and notes above

Hepatic impairment manufacturer advises caution in severe hepatic impairment

Contra-indications

Pregnancy avoid; manufacturer advises effective contraception during and for at least 6 months after treatment in men or women; see also section 8.1

Breast-feeding discontinue breast feeding

Side-effects see section 8.1 and notes above; transient blue-green discoloration of urine; less commonly gastro-intestinal bleeding, anorexia, allergic reactions, dyspnoea, fatigue, fever, amenorrhoea, and transient blue discoloration of skin and nails

Licensed use not licensed for use in children

Indication and dose

Acute myeloid leukaemia, recurrent acute lymphoblastic leukaemia
• **By intravenous infusion**
Consult local treatment protocol for details

Administration Consult local treatment protocol for details

For *intravenous infusion*, dilute with at least 50 mL Glucose 5% *or* Sodium Chloride 0.9% *or* Sodium Chloride 0.18% and Glucose 4%; give over 6 hours through a central venous catheter

Mitoxantrone (Non-proprietary) PoM
Concentrate for intravenous infusion, mitoxantrone (as hydrochloride) 2 mg/mL, net price 10-mL vial = £100.00

Onkotrone® (Baxter) PoM
Concentrate for intravenous infusion, mitoxantrone (as hydrochloride) 2 mg/mL, net price 10-mL vial = £121.85, 12.5-mL vial = £152.33, 15-mL vial = £203.04

8.1.3 Antimetabolites

Antimetabolites are incorporated into new nuclear material or they combine irreversibly with vital cellular enzymes and prevent normal cellular division. **Cytarabine, fludarabine, mercaptopurine, methotrexate,** and **tioguanine** are commonly used in paediatric chemotherapy.

Methotrexate inhibits the enzyme dihydrofolate reductase, essential for the synthesis of purines and pyrimidines. It is given by mouth, intravenously, intramuscularly, or intrathecally. Methotrexate causes myelosuppression, mucositis, and rarely pneumonitis. It is **contra-indicated** in significant renal impairment because it is excreted primarily by the kidney. It is also contra-indicated in patients with severe hepatic impairment. It should also be **avoided** in the presence of significant pleural effusion or ascites because it can accumulate in these fluids, and its subsequent return to the circulation may cause myelosuppression. Systemic toxicity may follow intrathecal administration and blood counts should be carefully monitored. Folinic acid (section 8.1) following methotrexate administration helps to prevent methotrexate-induced mucositis and myelosuppression.

Cytarabine acts by interfering with pyrimidine synthesis. It is given subcutaneously, intravenously, or intrathecally. It is a potent myelosuppressant and requires careful haematological monitoring. A liposomal formulation of cytarabine for intrathecal use is available for lymphomatous meningitis.

Fludarabine is generally well tolerated but does cause myelosuppression, which may be cumulative.

> **Fludarabine** has a potent and prolonged immunosuppressive effect. Children treated with fludarabine are more prone to serious bacterial, opportunistic fungal, and viral infections, and prophylactic therapy is recommended in children at risk. To prevent potentially fatal transfusion-related graft-versus-host reaction, only irradiated blood products should be administered. Prescribers should consult specialist literature when using highly immunosuppressive drugs.

Clofarabine is licensed for the treatment of acute lymphoblastic leukaemia in children who have relapsed or are refractory after receiving at least two previous regimens. It is given by intravenous infusion.

Nelarabine is licensed for the treatment of T-cell acute lymphoblastic leukaemia and T-cell lymphoblastic lymphoma in children who have relapsed or who are refractory after receiving at least two previous regimens. It is given by intravenous infusion. Neurotoxicity is common with nelarabine, and close monitoring for

8

Malignant disease and immunosuppression

neurological events is strongly recommended—discontinue treatment if neurotoxicity occurs.

Mercaptopurine is used as maintenance therapy for acute lymphoblastic leukaemia and in the management of ulcerative colitis and Crohn's disease (section 1.5). Azathioprine, which is metabolised to mercaptopurine, is generally used as an immunosuppressant (section 8.2.1 and section 10.1.3). The dose of both drugs should be reduced if the child is receiving allopurinol since it interferes with their metabolism. For the role of thiopurine methyltransferase (TPMT) in the metabolism of azathioprine see section 8.2.1.

Tioguanine (thioguanine) is given by mouth for the treatment of acute lymphoblastic leukaemia; it is given at various stages of treatment in short-term cycles. Tioguanine has a lower incidence of gastro-intestinal side-effects than mercaptopurine. Long-term therapy with tioguanine is no longer recommended because of the high risk of liver toxicity.

▲ CLOFARABINE

Cautions see section 8.1

Hepatic impairment manufacturer advises caution in mild to moderate impairment; avoid in severe impairment

Renal impairment manufacturer advises caution in mild to moderate impairment; avoid in severe impairment

Contra-indications

Pregnancy manufacturer advises avoid (teratogenic in *animal* studies); see also section 8.1

Breast-feeding discontinue breast-feeding

Side-effects see section 8.1; also jaundice, tachycardia, flushing, hypotension, pericardial effusion, haematoma, dyspnoea, cough, anxiety, agitation, dizziness, drowsiness, headache, paraesthesia, peripheral neuropathy, restlessness, rash, pruritus, increased sweating

Licensed use not licensed for use in children under 1 year

Indication and dose

> Relapsed or refractory acute lymphoblastic leukaemia
> * **By intravenous infusion**
> Consult local treatment protocol for details

Administration Consult local treatment protocol for details

For *intravenous infusion*, filter requisite dose through a 0.2-micron filter and dilute with Sodium Chloride 0.9%; give over 2 hours

Evoltra® (Bioenvision) ▼ PoM
Concentrate for intravenous infusion, clofarabine 1 mg/mL, net price 20-mL vial = £1200.00
Electrolytes Na⁺ 3.08 mmol/vial

▲ CYTARABINE

Cautions see section 8.1 and notes above; **interactions:** Appendix 1 (cytarabine)

Hepatic impairment reduce dose

Renal impairment reduce dose for high dose regimens or avoid, consult local treatment protocol for details

Contra-indications

Pregnancy avoid (teratogenic in *animal* studies); see also section 8.1

Breast-feeding discontinue breast-feeding

Side-effects see section 8.1 and notes above; 'cytarabine syndrome'—6–12 hours after intravenous administration—characterised by fever and malaise, myalgia, bone pain, maculopapular rash, and occasionally chest pain; *less commonly* conjunctivitis (consider prophylactic corticosteroid eye drops), neurotoxicity, renal and hepatic dysfunction, jaundice; *rarely* severe spinal cord toxicity following intrathecal administration

Licensed use *Depocyte®* intrathecal injection not licensed for use in children

Indication and dose

> Acute lymphoblastic leukaemia, acute myeloid leukaemia, non-Hodgkin's lymphoma
> * **By intravenous injection, by intravenous infusion, or by subcutaneous injection**
> Consult local treatment protocol for details

> Meningeal leukaemia, meningeal neoplasms
> * **By intrathecal injection**
> Consult local treatment protocol for details

> Note Based on weight or body-surface area, children may tolerate higher doses of cytarabine than adults

Administration Consult local treatment protocol for details

For *intravenous injection* or *intravenous infusion* dilute with Water for Injections *or* Sodium Chloride 0.9% *or* Glucose 5%; do not give high strength (100 mg/mL) intrathecally

Cytarabine (Non-proprietary) PoM
Injection (for intravenous, subcutaneous or intrathecal use), cytarabine 20 mg/mL, net price 5-mL vial = £4.00

Injection (for intravenous or subcutaneous use), cytarabine 20 mg/mL, net price 5-mL vial = £3.90, 25-mL vial = £19.50

Injection (for intravenous or subcutaneous use), cytarabine 100 mg/mL, net price 1-mL vial = £4.00; 5-mL vial = £20.00; 10-mL vial = £39.00; 20-mL vial = £77.50

◢ **Lipid formulation for intrathecal use**
DepoCyte® (Napp) ▼ PoM
Intrathecal injection, cytarabine encapsulated in liposomes, net price 50-mg vial = £1223.75

■ FLUDARABINE PHOSPHATE

Cautions see section 8.1 and notes above; monitor for signs of haemolysis; monitor for neurological toxicity; worsening of existing and increased susceptibility to skin cancer; **interactions:** Appendix 1 (fludarabine)

Renal impairment reduce dose by up to 50% if creatinine clearance 30–70 mL/minute/1.73 m²; avoid if creatinine clearance less than 30 mL/minute/1.73 m²

Contra-indications haemolytic anaemia

Pregnancy avoid (teratogenic in *animal* studies); manufacturer advises effective contraception during and for at least 6 months after treatment in men or women; see also section 8.1

Breast-feeding discontinue breast-feeding

Side-effects see section 8.1 and notes above; also diarrhoea, anorexia; oedema; pneumonia, cough; peripheral neuropathy, visual disturbances; chills, fever, malaise, weakness; rash; *less commonly* gastro-intestinal haemorrhage, pulmonary toxicity (including pulmonary infiltrates, pneumonitis, and fibrosis), and confusion; *rarely* heart failure, arrhythmia, coma, seizures, agitation, myelodysplastic syndrome, acute myeloid leukaemia, optic neuropathy, blindness, Stevens-Johnson syndrome, toxic epidermal necrolysis, skin cancer, and haemorrhagic cystitis

Licensed use not licensed for use in children

Indication and dose

> Poor prognosis or relapsed acute myeloid leukaemia, relapsed acute lymphoblastic leukaemia, conditioning before bone marrow transplantation
> * **By mouth, by intravenous injection, or by intravenous infusion**
>   Consult local treatment protocol for details

Administration Consult local treatment protocol for details

Reconstitute each 50 mg powder with 2 mL Water for Injections

For *intravenous injection*, dilute requisite dose with 10 mL Sodium Chloride 0.9%

For *intravenous infusion*, dilute requisite dose with 100–125 mL Sodium Chloride 0.9%; give over 30 minutes

Fludara® (Bayer) (PoM)
Tablets, f/c, pink, fludarabine phosphate 10 mg, net price 15-tab pack = £279.00, 20-tab pack = £372.00

Injection, powder for reconstitution, fludarabine phosphate. Net price 50-mg vial = £156.00

■ MERCAPTOPURINE

Cautions see section 8.1 and notes above; monitor liver function; **interactions:** Appendix 1 (mercaptopurine)

Hepatic impairment may need dose reduction; avoid if jaundice or hepatomegaly; consult local treatment protocol for details

Renal impairment manufacturer advises consider reducing dose

Contra-indications

Pregnancy avoid (teratogenic); see also section 8.1

Breast-feeding discontinue breast-feeding

Side-effects see section 8.1 and notes above; gastro-intestinal effects less common; hepatotoxicity (more frequent at higher doses); rarely intestinal ulceration, pancreatitis, fever, crystalluria with haematuria, rash, and hyperpigmentation

Licensed use not licensed for use in children for acute lymphoblastic lymphoma or T-cell non-Hodgkins lymphoma

Indication and dose

> Acute lymphoblastic leukaemia, lymphoblastic lymphomas
> * **By mouth**
>   Consult local treatment protocol for details

> Severe ulcerative colitis and Crohn's disease section 1.5.3

Puri-Nethol® (GSK) (PoM)
Tablets, yellow, scored, mercaptopurine 50 mg. Net price 25-tab pack = £18.78

Mercaptopurine
Capsules, mercaptopurine 10 mg
Available from 'special-order' manufacturers or specialist importing companies, p. 943

◢ Extemporaneous formulations available see Extemporaneous Preparations, p. 8

■ METHOTREXATE

Cautions see section 8.1 and section 10.1.3; monitor renal and hepatic function; peptic ulceration, ulcerative colitis, diarrhoea, and ulcerative stomatitis; porphyria (section 9.8.2); **interactions:** Appendix 1 (methotrexate)

Hepatic impairment consult local treatment protocol for details; avoid for all indications in severe hepatic impairment

Renal impairment reduce dose; risk of nephrotoxicity at high doses (reduced if adequate hydra-

tion and urinary pH of 6.5–7); manufacturers advise avoid in severe renal impairment

Contra-indications

Pregnancy avoid (teratogenic; fertility may be reduced during therapy but this may be reversible); manufacturer advises effective contraception during and for at least 3 months after treatment in men or women; see also section 8.1

Breast-feeding discontinue breast-feeding

8

Malignant disease and immunosuppression

◁ **METHOTREXATE** (*continued*)

Side-effects see section 8.1; also anorexia, abdominal discomfort, dyspepsia, gastro-intestinal ulceration and bleeding, diarrhoea, toxic megacolon, hepatotoxicity (see Cautions above); hypotension, pericarditis, pericardial tamponade, thrombosis; pulmonary oedema, pleuritic pain, pulmonary fibrosis, interstitial pneumonitis (see also Pulmonary Toxicity, p. 611); anaphylactic reactions, urticaria; dizziness, fatigue, chills, fever, drowsiness, malaise, headache, mood changes, abnormal cranial sensations, neurotoxicity, confusion, psychosis, paraesthesia, cerebral oedema; precipitation of diabetes; menstrual disturbances, vaginitis, cystitis, reduced libido, impotence; haematuria, dysuria, renal failure; osteoporosis, arthralgia, myalgia, vasculitis; conjunctivitis, blepharitis, visual disturbances; rash, pruritus, Stevens-Johnson syndrome, toxic epidermal necrolysis, photosensitivity, changes in nail and skin pigmentation, telangiectasia, acne, furunculosis, ecchymosis; injection-site reactions

Indication and dose

Maintenance and remission of acute lymphoblastic leukaemia, lymphoblastic lymphoma
• **By mouth**
Consult local treatment protocol for details

Safe Practice To avoid error with low-dose methotrexate, it is recommended that:
• the child or their carer is carefully advised of the **dose** and **frequency** and the reason for taking methotrexate and any other prescribed medicine (e.g. folic acid);
• only one strength of methotrexate tablet (usually 2.5 mg) is prescribed and dispensed;
• the prescription and the dispensing label clearly show the dose and frequency of methotrexate administration;
• the child or their carer is warned to report immediately the onset of any feature of blood disorders (e.g. sore throat, bruising, and mouth ulcers), liver toxicity (e.g. nausea, vomiting, abdominal discomfort, and dark urine), and respiratory effects (e.g. shortness of breath).

Treatment of early stage Burkitt's lymphoma, non-Hodgkin's lymphoma, osteogenic sarcoma, some CNS tumours including infant brain tumours, acute lymphoblastic leukaemia
• **By intravenous injection or infusion**
Consult local treatment protocol for details

Meningeal leukaemia, treatment and prevention of CNS involvement of leukaemia
• **By intrathecal injection**
Consult local treatment protocol for details

Severe Crohn's disease section 1.5.3

Rheumatic disease section 10.1.3

Psoriasis section 13.5.3

Administration Consult local treatment protocol for details
For *intravenous infusion*, dilute with Glucose 5% *or* Sodium Chloride 0.9%
For *intrathecal injection*, use low-volume preservative-free preparation

Methotrexate (Non-proprietary) (PoM)
Injection, methotrexate (as sodium salt) 2.5 mg/mL, net price 2-mL vial = £1.68
Injection, methotrexate (as sodium salt) 25 mg/mL, net price 2-mL vial = £2.62, 20-mL vial = £25.07
Injection, methotrexate 100 mg/mL (not for intrathecal use), net price 10-mL vial = £78.33, 50-mL vial = £380.07

◀Oral preparations
Section 10.1.3

NELARABINE

Cautions see section 8.1 and notes above; previous or concurrent intrathecal chemotherapy or craniospinal irradiation (increased risk of neurotoxicity)
Skilled tasks Drowsiness may affect performance of skilled tasks (e.g. cycling or driving)

Contra-indications

Pregnancy avoid (teratogenic in *animal* studies); manufacturer advises effective contraception during and for at least 3 months after treatment in men and women; see also section 8.1

Breast-feeding discontinue breast-feeding

Side-effects see section 8.1 and notes above; also constipation, diarrhoea; confusion, seizures, drowsiness, peripheral neurological disorders, demyelination, hypoesthesia, paraesthesia, ataxia, tremor, headache, asthenia, fatigue, pyrexia;

hypoglycaemia, electrolyte disturbances; arthralgia; benign and malignant tumours also reported

Indication and dose

T-cell acute lymphoblastic leukaemia, T-cell lymphoblastic lymphoma
• **By intravenous infusion**
Consult local treatment protocol for details

Administration Consult local treatment protocol for details
For *intravenous infusion*, give over 1–2 hours

Atriance® (GSK) ▼ (PoM)
Intravenous infusion, nelarabine 5 mg/mL, net price 50-mL vial = £222.00
Electrolytes Na⁺ 3.75 mmol/vial

◢ TIOGUANINE
(Thioguanine)

Cautions see section 8.1 and notes above; monitor liver function weekly—discontinue if liver toxicity develops; **interactions**: Appendix 1 (tioguanine)

Hepatic impairment reduce dose; consult local treatment protocol for details

Renal impairment reduce dose; consult local treatment protocol for details

Contra-indications

Pregnancy avoid (teratogenicity reported when men receiving tioguanine have fathered children); ensure effective contraception during treatment in men or women; see also section 8.1

Breast-feeding discontinue breast-feeding

Side-effects see section 8.1; also stomatitis and hepatotoxicity; *rarely* intestinal necrosis and perforation

Indication and dose

Infant acute lymphoblastic leukaemia
- **By mouth**
  Consult local treatment protocol for details

Lanvis® (GSK) ▣PoM▢
Tablets, yellow, scored, tioguanine 40 mg. Net price 25-tab pack = £45.41

◢Extemporaneous formulations available see Extemporaneous Preparations, p. 8

▌8.1.4▐ Vinca alkaloids and etoposide

The vinca alkaloids, **vinblastine** and **vincristine** are used to treat a variety of cancers including leukaemias, lymphomas, and some solid tumours.

Neurotoxicity, usually as peripheral or autonomic neuropathy, occurs with all vinca alkaloids and is a limiting side-effect of vincristine; it occurs less often with vinblastine. Children with neurotoxicity commonly have peripheral paraesthesia, loss of deep tendon reflexes, abdominal pain, and constipation; ototoxicity has been reported. If symptoms of neurotoxicity are severe, doses should be reduced, but children generally tolerate vincristine better than adults. Motor weakness can also occur and dose reduction or discontinuation of therapy may be appropriate if motor weakness increases. Recovery from neurotoxic effects is usually slow but complete.

Myelosuppression is the dose-limiting side-effect of vinblastine; vincristine causes negligible myelosuppression. The vinca alkaloids may cause reversible alopecia. They cause severe local irritation and care must be taken to avoid extravasation. Constipation is common with vinblastine and vincristine; prophylactic use of laxatives may be considered.

> **Safe Practice**
> Vinblastine and vincristine are for **intravenous administration only**. Inadvertent intrathecal administration can cause severe neurotoxicity, which is usually fatal.
>
> The National Patient Safety Agency has advised (August 2008) that teenage patients treated in an adolescent unit should receive their vinca alkaloid dose in a 50 mL minibag. Teenagers and children treated in a child unit may receive their vinca alkaloid dose in a syringe.

Etoposide, usually given by slow intravenous infusion, is used to treat acute leukaemias, lymphomas, and some solid tumours. Etoposide may also be given by mouth but it is unpredictably absorbed.

◢ ETOPOSIDE

Cautions see section 8.1 and notes above; **interactions**: Appendix 1 (etoposide)

Renal impairment consult specialist literature and local treatment protocol for details

Contra-indications see section 8.1

Hepatic impairment avoid in severe impairment

Pregnancy avoid (teratogenic in *animal* studies); see also section 8.1

Breast-feeding discontinue breast-feeding

Side-effects see section 8.1, dose limiting myelosuppression, mucositis more common if given with doxorubicin; anaphylaxis associated with concentrated infusions; hypotension associated with rapid infusion; irritant to tissues if extravasated

Licensed use not licensed for use in children

Indication and dose

Stage 4 neuroblastoma, germ-cell tumours, intracranial germ-cell tumours, rhabdomyosarcoma, soft-tissue sarcomas, neuroectodermal tumours (including medulloblastoma), relapsed Hodgkin's disease, non-Hodgkin's lymphoma, Ewing tumour, acute lymphoblastic leukaemia, acute myeloid leukaemia
- **By mouth or by intravenous infusion**
  Consult local treatment protocol for details

8

Malignant disease and immunosuppression

◻ **ETOPOSIDE** (*continued*)

Administration Consult local treatment protocol for details

For *intravenous infusion*, dilute with Sodium Chloride 0.9%. Use nylon filters and PVC bags or glass bottles. Inspect solution regularly for precipitate

Etoposide (Non-proprietary) (PoM)
Concentrate for intravenous infusion, etoposide 20 mg/mL, net price 5-mL vial = £12.15, 10-mL vial = £29.00, 25-mL vial = £60.75
Brands include *Eposin®*

Etopophos® (Bristol-Myers Squibb) (PoM)
Injection, powder for reconstitution, etoposide (as phosphate), net price 100-mg vial = £27.78 (hosp. only)

Vepesid® (Bristol-Myers Squibb) (PoM)
Capsules, both pink, etoposide 50 mg, net price 20 = £105.97; 100 mg, 10-cap pack = £92.60 (hosp. only). Label: 23

▰ **VINBLASTINE SULPHATE**

Cautions see section 8.1 and notes above; caution in handling; **interactions**: Appendix 1 (vinblastine)

Hepatic impairment dose reduction may be necessary, consult local treatment protocol for details

Contra-indications see section 8.1 and notes above

Pregnancy avoid (limited experience suggests fetal harm; teratogenic in *animal* studies); see also section 8.1

Breast-feeding discontinue breast-feeding

⌐ Safe Practice Intrathecal injection **contra-indicated** ⌐

Side-effects see section 8.1 and notes above; abdominal pain, constipation, leucopenia, muscle pain; less commonly peripheral neuropathy; rarely paralytic ileus; irritant to tissues if extravasated

Licensed use licensed for use in children (age range not specified by manufacturer)

Indication and dose

Hodgkin's disease and other lymphomas
• **By intravenous injection**
Consult local treatment protocol for details

Administration Consult local treatment protocol for details

For *intravenous injection*, dilute solution containing 1 mg/mL with Sodium Chloride 0.9%; give into the tubing of a fast-running Sodium Chloride 0.9% infusion

For child over 10 years, dilute to at least 20 mL to avoid inadvertent intrathecal use.

Vinblastine (Non-proprietary) (PoM)
Injection, vinblastine sulphate 1 mg/mL. Net price 10-mL vial = £13.09

Velbe® (Genus) (PoM)
Injection, powder for reconstitution, vinblastine sulphate. Net price 10-mg amp = £14.15

▰ **VINCRISTINE SULPHATE**

Cautions see section 8.1 and notes above; neuromuscular disease; ileus; caution in handling; **interactions**: Appendix 1 (vincristine)

Hepatic impairment dose reduction may be necessary, consult local treatment protocol for details

Contra-indications see section 8.1 and notes above

Pregnancy avoid (teratogenicity and fetal loss in *animal* studies); see also section 8.1

Breast-feeding discontinue breast-feeding

⌐ Safe Practice Intrathecal injection **contra-indicated** ⌐

Side-effects see section 8.1 and notes above; constipation (see notes above), paralytic ileus may occur in young children; dose-limiting neuromuscular effects (see notes above); rarely convulsions followed by coma; irritant to tissues if extravasated

Licensed use licensed for use in children (age range not specified by manufacturer)

Indication and dose

Acute leukaemias, lymphomas, paediatric solid tumours
• **By intravenous injection**
Consult local treatment protocol for details

Administration Consult local treatment protocol for details

For *intravenous injection*, dilute solution containing 1 mg/mL with Sodium Chloride 0.9%; give into the tubing of a fast-running Sodium Chloride 0.9% infusion

For child over 10 years dilute to at least 20 mL to avoid inadvertent intrathecal use

Vincristine (Non-proprietary) (PoM)
Injection, vincristine sulphate 1 mg/mL. Net price 1-mL vial = £10.92; 2-mL vial = £21.17; 5-mL vial = £44.16

Oncovin® (Genus) (PoM)
Injection, vincristine sulphate 1 mg/mL, net price 1-mL vial = £14.18; 2-mL vial = £28.05

8.1.5 Other antineoplastic drugs

Amsacrine

Amsacrine has an action and toxic effects similar to those of doxorubicin (section 8.1.2) and is given *intravenously*. It is occasionally used in acute myeloid leukaemia.

AMSACRINE

Cautions see section 8.1 and notes above; consider monitoring cardiac function; monitor electrolytes (fatal arrhythmias possible if hypokalaemia); previous treatment with anthracyclines; also caution in handling—irritant to skin and tissues

Hepatic impairment reduce dose—25% initially, up to 50% in severe impairment

Renal impairment manufacturer advises reduce initial dose by 20–30%

Pregnancy avoid (teratogenic and toxic in *animal* studies); may reduce fertility; see also section 8.1

Breast-feeding discontinue breast-feeding

Side-effects see section 8.1 mucositis, phlebitis; less commonly diarrhoea, cardiotoxicity, haematuria, renal impairment, hepatotoxicity, skin rash; rarely acute renal failure, grand mal seizures

Licensed use not licensed for use in children

Indication and dose

Acute myeloid leukaemia
- **By intravenous infusion**
  Consult local treatment protocol for details

Administration Consult local treatment protocol for details

For *intravenous infusion*, dilute with Glucose 5%; give over 60–90 minutes through central venous catheter

Amsidine® (Goldshield) (PoM)
Concentrate for intravenous infusion, amsacrine 5 mg (as lactate)/mL, when reconstituted by mixing two solutions. Net price 1.5-mL (75-mg) amp with 13.5-mL diluent vial = £54.08 (hosp. only)

Note Use glass apparatus for reconstitution

Asparaginase

Asparaginase is used almost exclusively in the treatment of acute lymphoblastic leukaemia. Hypersensitivity reactions may occur and facilities for the management of anaphylaxis should be available. A number of different preparations of asparaginase exist and only the product specified in the treatment protocol should be used. **Crisantaspase** is the enzyme asparaginase produced by *Erwinia chrysanthemi*. Preparations of asparaginase derived from *Escherichia coli* are also available. Children who are hypersensitive to asparaginase derived from one organism may tolerate asparaginase derived from another organism but cross-sensitivity occurs in about 20–30% of individuals.

CRISANTASPASE

Cautions see section 8.1 and notes above
Pregnancy avoid; see also section 8.1
Breast-feeding discontinue breast-feeding

Side-effects see section 8.1 and notes above; fever, CNS depression, neurotoxicity; hyperglycaemia, liver dysfunction, coagulation disorders, altered plasma lipid concentration, pancreatitis

Indication and dose

Acute lymphoblastic leukaemia, acute myeloid leukaemia, non-Hodgkin's lymphoma
- **By intravenous, intramuscular or subcutaneous injection**
  Consult local treatment protocol for details

Erwinase® (EUSA Pharma) (PoM)
Injection, powder for reconstitution, crisantaspase. Net price 10 000-unit vial = £194.77

◀ Preparations
Preparations of asparaginase derived from *Escherichia coli* are available but they are not licensed, they include: *Medac®* asparaginase, *Elspar®* asparaginase, and *Oncaspar®* pegaspargase.

Dacarbazine and temozolomide

Dacarbazine is a component of a commonly used combination for Hodgkin's disease (ABVD—doxorubicin [previously *Adriamycin®*], bleomycin, vinblastine, and dacarbazine). It is given *intravenously*.

Temozolomide is structurally related to dacarbazine and is used in children for second-line treatment of malignant glioma.

8 Malignant disease and immunosuppression

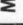
Malignant disease and immunosuppression

8

DACARBAZINE

Cautions see section 8.1; caution in handling

Hepatic impairment dose reduction may be required in combined hepatic and renal impairment; avoid in severe impairment

Renal impairment dose reduction may be required in combined renal and hepatic impairment; manufacturer advises avoid in severe renal impairment

Contra-indications

Pregnancy avoid (carcinogenic and teratogenic in *animal* studies); ensure effective contraception during and for at least 6 months after treatment in men or women; see also section 8.1

Breast-feeding discontinue breast-feeding

Side-effects see section 8.1; *also* anorexia; *less commonly* facial flushing, confusion, headache, seizures, facial paraesthesia, influenza-like symptoms, blurred vision, renal impairment, rash; *rarely* diarrhoea, hepatotoxicity including liver necrosis and hepatic vein thrombosis, photosensitivity, irritant to skin and tissues, injection-site reactions

Indication and dose

Hodgkin's disease, paediatric solid tumours
● **By intravenous injection or by intravenous infusion**
Consult local treatment protocol for details

Administration Consult local treatment protocol for details

For *slow intravenous injection*, reconstitute vial with Water for Injections to produce solution containing 10 mg/mL; give over 2–3 minutes.

For *intravenous infusion*, further dilute reconstituted solution in 125–250 mL Glucose 5% *or* Sodium Chloride 0.9%; give over 15–30 minutes. Protect infusion set from light throughout administration to reduce pain

Dacarbazine (Non-proprietary) ℗oM
Injection, powder for reconstitution, dacarbazine (as citrate), net price 100-mg vial = £5.05; 200-mg vial = £7.16; 500-mg vial = £16.50; 600-mg vial = £22.50; 1-g vial = £31.80

TEMOZOLOMIDE

Cautions see section 8.1; **interactions:** Appendix 1 (temozolomide)

Hepatic impairment use with caution in severe impairment

Renal impairment use with caution in severe impairment

Contra-indications

Pregnancy avoid (teratogenic and embryotoxic in *animal* studies); manufacturer advises adequate contraception during treatment; see also section 8.1; also men should avoid fathering a child during and for at least 6 months after treatment

Breast-feeding discontinue breast-feeding

Side-effects see section 8.1

Licensed use not licensed for treatment of malignant gliomas in children under 3 years

Indication and dose

Treatment of malignant gliomas
● **By mouth**
Consult local treatment protocol for details

Temodal® (Schering-Plough) ℗oM
Capsules, temozolomide 5 mg (green/white), net price 5-cap pack = £17.30; 20 mg (yellow/white), 5-cap pack = £69.20; 100 mg (pink/white), 5-cap pack = £346.00; 140 mg (blue/white), 5-cap pack = £484.40; 180 mg (orange/white), 5-cap pack = £622.80; 250 mg (white), 5-cap pack = £865.00. Label: 23, 25

Imatinib

Imatinib, a tyrosine kinase inhibitor, has recently been licensed in children for the treatment of newly diagnosed Philadelphia-chromosome-positive chronic myeloid leukaemia when bone marrow transplantation is not considered first line treatment, and for Philadelphia-chromosome-positive chronic myeloid leukaemia in chronic phase after failure of interferon alfa, or in accelerated phase, or in blast crisis.

IMATINIB

Cautions see section 8.1; cardiac disease; monitor for fluid retention; monitor liver function (see also Hepatic Impairment, below); **interactions:** Appendix 1 (imatinib)

Hepatic impairment start with minimum recommended dose; reduce dose further if not tolerated; consult local treatment protocol

Renal impairment start with minimum recommended dose; reduce dose further if not tolerated; consult local treatment protocol

Contra-indications

Pregnancy manufacturer advises avoid unless potential benefit outweighs risk; see also section 8.1

Breast-feeding discontinue breast-feeding

Side-effects see section 8.1; *also* abdominal pain, appetite changes, constipation, diarrhoea, flatulence, gastro-oesophageal reflux, taste disturbance, weight changes, dry mouth; oedema (including pulmonary oedema, pleural effusion, and ascites), flushing, haemorrhage; cough, dys-

◁ **IMATINIB** (*continued*)

pnoea; dizziness, headache, insomnia, hypoaesthesia, paraesthesia, fatigue; influenza-like symptoms; cramps, arthralgia; visual disturbances, lacrimation, conjunctivitis, dry eyes; epistaxis; dry skin, sweating, rash, pruritus, photosensitivity; *less commonly* gastric ulceration, pancreatitis, hepatic dysfunction (rarely hepatic failure, hepatic necrosis), dysphagia, heart failure, tachycardia, palpitation, syncope, hypertension, hypotension, cold extremities, cough, acute respiratory failure, depression, drowsiness, anxiety, peripheral neuropathy, tremor, migraine, impaired memory, vertigo, gynaecomastia, menorrhagia, irregular menstruation, sexual dysfunction, electrolyte disturbances, renal failure, urinary frequency, gout, tinnitus, hearing loss; skin hyperpigmentation; *rarely* intestinal obstruction, gastro-intestinal perforation, inflammatory bowel disease, arrhythmia, atrial fibrillation, myocardial infarction, angina, pulm-

onary fibrosis, pulmonary hypertension, increased intracranial pressure, convulsions, confusion, haemolytic anaemia, aseptic necrosis of bone, cataract, glaucoma, angioedema, exfoliative dermatitis, and Stevens-Johnson syndrome

Indication and dose

Chronic phase and advanced phase chronic myeloid leukaemia
• By mouth
Consult local treatment protocol for details

Glivec® (Novartis) ▼ PoM
Tablets, f/c, imatinib (as mesilate) 100 mg (yellow-brown, scored), net price 60-tab pack = £802.04; 400 mg (yellow), 30-tab pack = £1604.08. Label: 21, 27

Counselling Tablets may be dispersed in water or apple juice

Mitotane

Mitotane is used in children for the symptomatic treatment of advanced or inoperable adrenocortical carcinoma. It selectively inhibits the activity of the adrenal cortex, necessitating corticosteroid replacement therapy (section 6.3.1); the dose of glucocorticoid should be increased in case of shock, trauma, or infection. Neuro-psychological impairment can occur, possibly secondary to hypothyroidism, and growth retardation has also been reported in children treated with mitotane.

▲ MITOTANE

Cautions see notes above; risk of accumulation in overweight patients; monitor plasma-mitotane concentration—consult product literature; **interactions:** Appendix 1 (mitotane)
Skilled tasks Central nervous system toxicity may affect performance of skilled tasks
Counselling Children and their carers should be warned to contact doctor immediately if injury, infection, or illness occurs (because of the risk of acute adrenal insufficiency)

Hepatic impairment manufacturer advises caution in mild to moderate impairment—monitoring of plasma-mitotane concentration recommended; avoid in severe impairment

Renal impairment manufacturer advises caution in mild to moderate renal impairment—monitoring of plasma-mitotane concentration recommended; avoid in severe renal impairment

Contra-indications

Pregnancy manufacturer advises avoid—effective contraception should be used during and after treatment; see also section 8.1

Breast-feeding discontinue breast-feeding

Side-effects see section 8.1 and notes above; also gastro-intestinal disturbances (including nausea, vomiting, diarrhoea, epigastric discomfort), ano-

rexia, liver disorders; hypercholesterolaemia, hypertriglyceridaemia; ataxia, confusion, asthenia, myasthenia, paraesthesia, drowsiness, neuropathy, cognitive impairment, movement disorder, dizziness, headache, gynaecomastia; prolonged bleeding time, leucopenia, thrombocytopenia, anaemia; rash; *rarely* hypersalivation, hypertension, postural hypotension, flushing, pyrexia, haematuria, proteinuria, haemorrhagic cystitis, hypouricaemia, visual disturbances and ocular disorders

Licensed use not licensed for use in children

Indication and dose

Symptomatic treatment of advanced or inoperable adrenocortical carcinoma
• By mouth
Consult local treatment protocol for details

Lysodren® (HRA Pharma) PoM
Tablets, scored, mitotane 500 mg, net price 100-tab pack = £460.40. Label: 2, 10, 21, counselling, skilled tasks, adrenal suppression

---

Platinum compounds

Carboplatin is used in the treatment of a variety of paediatric malignancies; it is given by intravenous infusion. Carboplatin can be given in an outpatient setting and is better tolerated than cisplatin; nausea and vomiting are less severe and nephrotoxicity, neurotoxicity, and ototoxicity are much less of a problem. Carboplatin is, however, more myelosuppressive than cisplatin.

8 Malignant disease and immunosuppression

Cisplatin is of value in children with a variety of malignancies; it is given by intravenous infusion. Cisplatin requires intensive intravenous hydration; routine use of intravenous fluids containing potassium or magnesium may also be required to help control hypokalaemia and hypomagnesaemia. Treatment may be complicated by severe nausea and vomiting; delayed vomiting may occur and is difficult to control. Cisplatin has dose-related and potentially cumulative side-effects including nephrotoxicity, neurotoxicity, and ototoxicity. Baseline testing of renal function and hearing is required; for children with pre-existing renal or hearing impairment or marked bone-marrow suppression, consideration should be given to withholding treatment or using another drug.

CARBOPLATIN

Cautions see section 8.1 and notes above; consider therapeutic drug monitoring; **interactions**: Appendix 1 (platinum compounds)

Renal impairment reduce dose and monitor haematological parameters and renal function; avoid if creatinine clearance less than 20 mL/minute/1.73 m²

Contra-indications

Pregnancy avoid (teratogenic and embryotoxic in *animal* studies); see also section 8.1

Breast-feeding discontinue breast-feeding

Side-effects see section 8.1 and notes above; less commonly nephrotoxicity and ototoxicity

Licensed use not licensed for use in children

Indication and dose

Stage 4 neuroblastoma, germ cell tumours, low-grade gliomas (including astrocytomas), neuroectodermal tumours (including medulloblastoma), rhabdomyosarcoma (metastatic and non-metastatic disease), soft-tissue sarcomas, retinoblastoma, high risk Wilms' tumour, some liver tumours
• By intravenous infusion
  Consult local treatment protocol for details

Administration Consult local treatment protocol for details

For *intravenous infusion*, dilute with Glucose 5% *or* Sodium Chloride 0.9% to a concentration no lower than 500 microgram/mL; give over at least 1 hour as dictated by fluid volume.

Carboplatin (Non-proprietary) PoM
Injection, carboplatin 10 mg/mL, net price 5-mL vial = £22.04, 15-mL vial = £56.29, 45-mL vial = £168.85, 60-mL vial = £260.00

Paraplatin® (Bristol-Myers Squibb) PoM
Concentrate for intravenous infusion, carboplatin 10 mg/mL, net price 5-mL vial = £21.26, 60-mL vial = £244.88

CISPLATIN

Cautions see section 8.1 and notes above; monitor full blood count, renal function, audiology, and plasma electrolytes; **interactions**: Appendix 1 (platinum compounds)

Renal impairment avoid if possible—nephrotoxic and neurotoxic

Contra-indications

Pregnancy avoid (teratogenic and toxic in *animal* studies); see also section 8.1

Breast-feeding discontinue breast-feeding

Side-effects see section 8.1 and notes above; ototoxicity (may be particularly severe in children); nephrotoxicity; hypomagnesaemia, hypokalaemia, hypophosphataemia, hypocalcaemia, hyperuricaemia; less commonly peripheral neuropathy

Licensed use not licensed for use in children

Indication and dose

Osteogenic sarcoma, stage 4 neuroblastoma, some liver tumours, infant brain tumours, intracranial germ-cell tumours
• By intravenous infusion
  Consult local treatment protocol for details

Administration Consult local treatment protocol for details

For *intravenous infusion*, dilute in Sodium Chloride 0.9% *or* Sodium Chloride 0.45% and Glucose 2.5%; give over at least 24 hours (48 hours for infant brain tumours). Do not refrigerate (risk of precipitation).

Ensure adequate intravenous hydration and urinary output, at least 3 hours before, during, and for at least 24 hours after administration. Mannitol routinely used to aid diuresis.

Cisplatin (Non-proprietary) PoM
Injection, cisplatin 1 mg/mL, net price 10-mL vial = £5.85, 50-mL vial = £24.50, 100-mL vial = £50.22
Brands include *Platinex®*

Injection, powder for reconstitution, cisplatin, net price 50-mg vial = £17.00

Malignant disease and immunosuppression

8

Procarbazine

Procarbazine is most often used in Hodgkin's disease. It is given *by mouth*. It is a weak monoamine-oxidase inhibitor and dietary restriction is rarely considered necessary. Alcohol ingestion may cause a disulfiram-like reaction.

PROCARBAZINE

Cautions see section 8.1 and notes above; **interactions:** Appendix 1 (procarbazine)

Hepatic impairment consider dose reduction; avoid in severe impairment

Renal impairment manufacturer advises use with caution; avoid in severe renal impairment

Contra-indications

Pregnancy avoid (teratogenic in *animal* studies and isolated reports in humans); see also section 8.1

Breast-feeding discontinue breast-feeding

Side-effects see section 8.1 and notes above; hypersensitivity rash (discontinue treatment)

Indication and dose

Hodgkin's lymphoma, gliomas
- **By mouth**
  Consult local treatment protocol for details

Procarbazine (Cambridge) ⊡PoM⊡
Capsules, ivory, procarbazine (as hydrochloride) 50 mg, net price 50-cap pack = £181.04. Label: 4

◢Extemporaneous formulations available see Extemporaneous Preparations, p. 8

Tretinoin

Tretinoin is licensed for the induction of remission in acute promyelocytic leukaemia. It is used in previously untreated children as well as in those who have relapsed after standard chemotherapy or who are refractory to it.

TRETINOIN

Note Tretinoin is the acid form of vitamin A

Cautions monitor full blood count and coagulation profile, liver function, serum calcium and plasma lipids before and during treatment; increased risk of thrombo-embolism during first month of treatment; **interactions:** Appendix 1 (retinoids)

Hepatic impairment reduce dose; consult local treatment protocol for details

Renal impairment mild impairment—reduce dose; consult local treatment protocol for details

Contra-indications

Pregnancy teratogenic; exclude pregnancy before starting treatment; effective contraception must be used for at least 1 month before oral treatment, during treatment and for at least 1 month after stopping (oral progestogen-only contraceptives **not** considered sufficiently effective); see also section 8.1

Breast-feeding discontinue breast-feeding

Side-effects retinoic acid syndrome (fever, dyspnoea, acute respiratory distress, pulmonary infiltrates, pleural effusion, hyperleukocytosis, hypotension, oedema, weight gain, hepatic, renal and multi-organ failure) requires immediate treatment—consult product literature; gastrointestinal disturbances, pancreatitis; arrhythmias, flushing, oedema; headache, benign intracranial hypertension (children particularly susceptible—consider dose reduction if intractable headache), shivering, dizziness, confusion, anxiety, depression, insomnia, paraesthesia, visual and hearing disturbances (children particularly susceptible to nervous system effects); raised liver enzymes, serum creatinine and lipids; bone and chest pain, alopecia, erythema, rash, pruritus, sweating, dry skin and mucous membranes, cheilitis; thromboembolism, hypercalcaemia, and genital ulceration reported

Indication and dose

Acute promyelocytic leukaemia
- **By mouth**
  Consult treatment protocol for details

Vesanoid® (Roche) ⊡PoM⊡
Capsules, yellow/brown, tretinoin 10 mg. Net price 100-cap pack = £170.52. Label: 21, 25

8.2 Drugs affecting the immune response

8.2.1   Antiproliferative immunosuppressants

8.2.2   Corticosteroids and other immunosuppressants

8.2.3   Rituximab and alemtuzumab

8.2.4   Other immunomodulating drugs

Immunosuppressant therapy

Immunosuppressants are used to suppress rejection in organ transplant recipients and to treat a variety of chronic inflammatory and autoimmune diseases. Solid organ transplant patients are usually maintained on a calcineurin inhibitor

8   Malignant disease and immunosuppression

(ciclosporin or tacrolimus), combined with an antiproliferative drug (azathioprine or mycophenolate mofetil) and a corticosteroid. Specialist management is required and other immunomodulators may be used to initiate treatment or to treat rejection.

> **Bioavailability**
> Different formulations of the same immunosuppressant may vary in bioavailability and to avoid reduced effect or excessive side-effects, it is important not to change formulation except on the advice of a transplant specialist.

Impaired immune responsiveness   Infections in the immunocompromised child can be severe and show atypical features. Specific local protocols should be followed for the management of infection. Corticosteroids may suppress clinical signs of infection and allow diseases such as septicaemia or tuberculosis to reach an advanced stage before being recognised. Children should be up-to-date with their childhood vaccinations before initiation of immunosuppressant therapy (e.g. before transplantation); vaccination with varicella-zoster vaccine (section 14.4) is also necessary during this period—**important:** for advice on measles and chickenpox (varicella) exposure, see Immunoglobulins (section 14.5). For advice on the use of live vaccines in individuals with impaired immune response, see section 14.1. For general comments and warnings relating to corticosteroids and immunosuppressants, see section 6.3.2 (under Prednisolone).

Pregnancy   Transplant patients immunosuppressed with azathioprine should not discontinue it on becoming pregnant; there is no evidence that azathioprine is teratogenic. However, there have been reports of premature birth and low birthweight following exposure to azathioprine, particularly in combination with corticosteroids. Spontaneous abortion has been reported following maternal or paternal exposure.

There is less experience of ciclosporin in pregnancy but it does not appear to be any more harmful than azathioprine. The use of these drugs during pregnancy needs to be supervised in specialist units.

Manufacturers contra-indicate the use of tacrolimus and mycophenolate in pregnancy.

8.2.1 Antiproliferative immunosuppressants

Azathioprine is widely used for transplant recipients and it is also used to treat a number of auto-immune conditions (see section 10.1.3), usually when corticosteroid therapy alone provides inadequate control. It is metabolised to mercaptopurine, and doses should be reduced to one quarter of the original dose when allopurinol is given concurrently.

Blood tests and monitoring for signs of myelosuppression are essential in long-term treatment with azathioprine. The enzyme thiopurine methyltransferase (TPMT) metabolises azathioprine; the risk of myelosuppression is increased in those with a low activity of the enzyme, particularly in the very few individuals who are homozygous for low TPMT activity.

Mycophenolate mofetil is metabolised to mycophenolic acid which has a more selective mode of action than azathioprine. It is used in combination with a corticosteroid and either ciclosporin or tacrolimus for the prophylaxis of acute rejection in transplant recipients. Compared with similar regimens incorporating azathioprine, mycophenolate mofetil may reduce the risk of acute rejection episodes; the risk of opportunistic infections (particularly due to tissue-invasive cytomegalovirus) and the occurrence of blood disorders such as leucopenia may be higher. Children may suffer a high incidence of side-effects, particularly gastrointestinal effects, calling for temporary reduction in dose or interruption of treatment.

> **NICE guidance (immunosuppressive therapy for renal transplantation in children and adolescents)**
> See p. 521

Cyclophosphamide (section 8.1.1) is less commonly prescribed as an immunosuppressant.

AZATHIOPRINE

Cautions monitor for toxicity throughout treatment; monitor full blood count weekly (more frequently with higher doses or if hepatic or renal impairment) for first 4 weeks (manufacturer advises weekly monitoring for 8 weeks but evidence of practical value unsatisfactory), thereafter reduce frequency of monitoring to at least every 3 months; **interactions:** Appendix 1 (azathioprine)

Bone marrow suppression Children and their carers should be warned to report immediately any signs or symptoms of bone marrow suppression e.g. inexplicable bruising or bleeding, infection

Hepatic impairment may need dose reduction

Renal impairment reduce dose and monitor full blood count

Pregnancy see section 8.2; treatment should not normally be initiated during pregnancy

Breast-feeding teratogenic metabolite present in milk in low concentration but no evidence of harm in small studies—consider if potential benefit outweighs risk

Contra-indications hypersensitivity to azathioprine or mercaptopurine

Side-effects hypersensitivity reactions (including malaise, dizziness, vomiting, diarrhoea, fever, rigors, myalgia, arthralgia, rash, hypotension and interstitial nephritis—calling for immediate withdrawal); dose-related bone marrow suppression (see also Cautions); liver impairment, cholestatic jaundice, hair loss and increased susceptibility to infections and colitis in patients also receiving corticosteroids; nausea; rarely pancreatitis, pneumonitis, hepatic veno-occlusive disease

Indication and dose

Suppression of transplant rejection
- **By mouth, or (if oral route not possible) by intravenous infusion (see also note below)** Consult local treatment protocol for details

  Child 1 month–18 years maintenance, 1–3 mg/kg once daily, adjusted according to response;

total daily dose may alternatively be given in 2 divided doses

Severe ulcerative colitis and Crohn's disease section 1.5.3

Inflammatory arthritis, vasculitis, auto-immune conditions when corticosteroid therapy alone has proved inadequate section 10.1.3

Administration Consult local treatment protocol for details

For *intravenous injection*, give over at least 1 minute

For *intravenous infusion*, dilute to a concentration of 0.25–2.5 mg/mL in Glucose 5% *or* Sodium Chloride 0.9% *or* Sodium Chloride and Glucose; give over 30–60 minutes

Note Intravenous injection is alkaline and very irritant. Intravenous route should therefore be used **only** if oral route not feasible and discontinued as soon as oral route can be tolerated. To reduce irritation flush line with sodium chloride 0.9% *or* glucose 4%/sodium chloride 0.18%.

Azathioprine (Non-proprietary) PoM
Tablets, azathioprine 25 mg, net price 28-tab pack = £6.27; 50 mg, 56-tab pack = £6.41. Label: 21
Brands include *Azamune*®

Imuran® (GSK) PoM
Tablets, both f/c, azathioprine 25 mg (orange), net price 100-tab pack = £10.99; 50 mg (yellow), 100-tab pack = £7.99. Label: 21

Injection, powder for reconstitution, azathioprine (as sodium salt). Net price 50-mg vial = £15.38

◢Extemporaneous formulations available see Extemporaneous Preparations, p. 8

MYCOPHENOLATE MOFETIL

Cautions full blood counts every week for 4 weeks then twice a month for 2 months then every month in the first year (consider interrupting treatment if neutropenia develops); active gastro-intestinal disease (risk of haemorrhage, ulceration and perforation); delayed graft function; increased susceptibility to skin cancer (avoid exposure to strong sunlight); possible decreased effectiveness of vaccination—avoid live vaccines; **interactions:** Appendix 1 (mycophenolate mofetil)

Bone marrow suppression Children and their carers should be warned to report immediately any signs or symptoms of bone marrow suppression e.g. infection or inexplicable bruising or bleeding

Renal impairment manufacturer advises consider dose reduction if estimated glomerular filtration rate less than 25 mL/minute/1.73 m²

Contra-indications

Pregnancy manufacturer advises avoid—congenital malformations reported; effective contra-

ception required before treatment, during treatment, and for 6 weeks after discontinuation of treatment

Breast-feeding manufacturer advises avoid—present in milk in *animal* studies

Side-effects gastro-intestinal disturbances (including diarrhoea, vomiting, and abdominal pain), gastro-intestinal ulceration and bleeding, oesophagitis, abnormal liver function tests, hepatitis, jaundice, pancreatitis; oedema, tachycardia, hypertension, hypotension, vasodilation; cough, dyspnoea; insomnia, agitation, tremor, dizziness, headache; influenza-like syndrome, infections (viral, bacterial and fungal); hyperglycaemia; renal impairment; increased risk of malignancies particularly of the skin; blood disorders (including leucopenia, anaemia, thrombocytopenia, pancytopenia), disturbances of electrolytes and blood lipids; arthralgia; alopecia, acne, and rash; progressive multifocal leucoencephalopathy reported

◻ **MYCOPHENOLATE MOFETIL (continued)**

Licensed use by mouth, in combination with a corticosteroid and ciclosporin, for children 2 years and older for the prophylaxis of acute transplant rejection in renal transplantation

Indication and dose

Prophylaxis of acute rejection in renal transplantation in combination with a corticosteroid and ciclosporin

- **By mouth or by intravenous infusion**
  Consult local treatment protocol for details

  Child 1 month–18 years 600 mg/m^2 twice daily (max. 2 g daily)

Prophylaxis of acute rejection in renal transplantation in combination with a corticosteroid and tacrolimus

- **By mouth or by intravenous infusion**
  Consult local treatment protocol for details

  Child 1 month–18 years 300 mg/m^2 twice daily (max. 2 g daily)

Prophylaxis of acute rejection in hepatic transplantation in combination with a corticosteroid and ciclosporin or tacrolimus

- **By mouth or by intravenous infusion**
  Consult local treatment protocol for details

  Child 1 month–18 years 10 mg/kg twice daily, increased to 20 mg/kg twice daily (max. 2 g daily)

  Note Tablets and capsules not appropriate for dose titration in children with body surface area less than 1.25 m^2

Administration For *intravenous infusion*, dilute reconstituted solution to a concentration of 6 mg/mL in Glucose 5%; infuse over 2 hours

CellCept® (Roche) ⒫ⓄⓂ
Capsules, blue/brown, mycophenolate mofetil 250 mg, net price 100-cap pack = £87.33

Tablets, lavender, mycophenolate mofetil 500 mg, net price 50-tab pack = £87.33

Oral suspension, mycophenolate mofetil 1 g/5 mL when reconstituted with water, net price 175 mL = £122.25

Intravenous infusion, powder for reconstitution, mycophenolate mofetil (as hydrochloride), net price 500-mg vial = £9.69

8.2.2 Corticosteroids and other immunosuppressants

The corticosteroids prednisolone and dexamethasone are widely used in paediatric oncology; they have a marked antitumour effect. Dexamethasone is preferred for acute lymphoblastic leukaemia whilst prednisolone may be used for Hodgkin's disease, non-Hodgkin's lymphoma, and B-cell lymphoma and leukaemia.

Dexamethasone is the corticosteroid of choice in paediatric supportive and palliative care. For children who are not receiving a corticosteroid as a component of their chemotherapy, dexamethasone may be used to reduce raised intracranial pressure (see p. 28), or to help control emesis when combined with an appropriate anti-emetic (see p. 27). For more information on glucocorticoid therapy, including the disadvantages of treatment, see section 6.3.2.

The corticosteroids are also powerful immunosuppressants. They are used to prevent organ transplant rejection, and in high dose to treat rejection episodes.

Ciclosporin (ciclosporin), a calcineurin inhibitor, is a potent immunosuppressant which is virtually non-myelotoxic but markedly nephrotoxic. It may be used in organ and tissue transplantation, for prevention of graft rejection following bone marrow, kidney, liver, pancreas, heart, lung, and heart-lung transplantation, and for prophylaxis and treatment of graft-versus-host disease. Ciclosporin also has a role in steroid-sensitive and steroid-resistant nephrotic syndrome; in corticosteroid-sensitive nephrotic syndrome it may be given with prednisolone (section 6.3).

Tacrolimus is also a calcineurin inhibitor. Although not chemically related to ciclosporin it has a similar mode of action and side-effects.

Both ciclosporin and tacrolimus may affect glucose metabolism in children. Hypertrichosis may be a concern with ciclosporin.

Sirolimus is a potent non-calcineurin inhibiting immunosuppressant.

Basiliximab is a monoclonal antibody that prevents T-lymphocyte proliferation; it is used for prophylaxis of acute rejection in allogeneic renal transplantation. It is given with ciclosporin and corticosteroid immunosuppression regimens; its use should be confined to specialist centres.

Antithymocyte immunoglobulin (rabbit) is used for the prophylaxis of organ rejection in renal and heart allograft recipients and for the treatment of cortico-steroid-resistant allograft rejection in renal transplantation. Tolerability may be increased by pretreatment with an intravenous corticosteroid and antihistamine; an antipyretic drug such as paracetamol may also be beneficial.

NICE guidance

Immunosuppressive therapy for renal transplantation in children and adolescents (April 2006)
NICE has recommended that for induction therapy in the prophylaxis of organ rejection, either basiliximab or daclizumab [discontinued] are options for combining with a calcineurin inhibitor. For each individual, ciclosporin or tacrolimus is chosen as the calcineurin inhibitor on the basis of side-effects. Mycophenolate mofetil is recommended as part of an immunosuppressive regimen **only if**:

- the calcineurin inhibitor is not tolerated, particularly if nephrotoxicity endangers the transplanted kidney; *or*
- there is very high risk of nephrotoxicity from the calcineurin inhibitor, requiring a reduction in the dose of the calcineurin inhibitor or its avoidance.

Mycophenolic acid is not recommended as part of an immunosuppressive regimen for renal transplantation in children or adolescents.

Sirolimus [not licensed for use in children] is recommended as a component of immunosuppressive regimen **only if** intolerance necessitates the withdrawal of a calcineurin inhibitor.

These recommendations may not be consistent with the marketing author-isation of some of the products.

ANTITHYMOCYTE IMMUNOGLOBULIN (RABBIT)

Cautions see notes above; monitor blood count

Pregnancy manufacturer advises use only if potential benefit outweighs risk—no information available

Contra-indications infection

Breast-feeding manufacturer advises avoid—no information available

Side-effects nausea, vomiting, dysphagia, diarr-hoea; hypotension; infusion-related reactions (including cytokine release syndrome and anaphylaxis, see notes above); serum sickness; fever, shivering, increased susceptibility to infec-tion; increased susceptibility to malignancy; lymphopenia, neutropenia, thrombocytopenia; myalgia; pruritus; rash

Indication and dose

Heart transplantation
- **By intravenous infusion over at least 6 hours**

  Child 1 month–18 years 1–2.5 mg/kg daily for 3–5 days starting the day of transplantation
  Note To avoid excessive dosage in obese patients, calculate dose on the basis of ideal body weight

Renal transplantation
- **By intravenous infusion over at least 6 hours**

  Child 1–18 years 1–1.5 mg/kg daily for 3–9 days starting the day of transplantation
  Note To avoid excessive dosage in obese patients, calculate dose on the basis of ideal body weight

Corticosteroid-resistant renal graft rejection
- **By intravenous infusion over at least 6 hours**

  Child 1–18 years 1.5 mg/kg daily for 7–14 days
  Note To avoid excessive dosage in obese patients, calculate dose on the basis of ideal body weight

Administration For *continuous intravenous infusion* reconstitute each vial with 5 mL water for injec-tion to produce a solution of 5 mg/mL; gently rotate to dissolve. Dilute requisite dose with Glucose 5% *or* Sodium Chloride 0.9% to an approx. concentration of 0.5 mg/mL; begin infu-sion immediately after dilution; give through an in-line filter (pore size 0.22 micron); incompatible with heparin and hydrocortisone glucose infu-sion—precipitation reported

Thymoglobuline® (Genzyme) ▼ PoM
Intravenous infusion, powder for reconstitution, rabbit anti-human thymocyte immunoglobulin, net price 25-mg vial = £168.18

◢ BASILIXIMAB

Contra-indications

Pregnancy avoid; adequate contraception must be used during treatment and for 16 weeks after last dose

Breast-feeding avoid

Side-effects severe hypersensitivity reactions and cytokine release syndrome reported

Indication and dose

> Prophylaxis of acute rejection in allogeneic renal transplantation used in combination with ciclosporin and corticosteroid-containing immunosuppression regimens
> * **By intravenous injection or by intravenous infusion**
>   Consult local treatment protocol for details
>   **Child over 1 year, body-weight under 35 kg** 10 mg within 2 hours before transplant surgery and 10 mg 4 days after surgery

> **Child body-weight over 35 kg** 20 mg within 2 hours before transplant surgery and 20 mg 4 days after surgery

Note withhold second dose if severe hypersensitivity or graft loss occurs

Administration For *intravenous infusion*, dilute reconstituted solution to a concentration not exceeding 400 micrograms/mL, with Glucose 5% or Sodium Chloride 0.9%; give over 20–30 minutes

Simulect® (Novartis) [PoM]
Injection, powder for reconstitution, basiliximab, net price 10-mg vial = £758.69, 20-mg vial = £842.38 (both with water for injections). For intravenous infusion

◢ CICLOSPORIN

(Cyclosporin)

Cautions monitor kidney function (see also below); monitor liver function (see also below); monitor blood pressure—discontinue if hypertension develops that cannot be controlled by antihypertensives; hyperuricaemia; monitor serum potassium especially in renal dysfunction (risk of hyperkalaemia); monitor serum magnesium; measure blood lipids before treatment and thereafter as appropriate; acute porphyria (section 9.8.2); monitor whole blood ciclosporin concentration (trough level dependent on indication—consult local treatment protocol for details); use with tacrolimus specifically contra-indicated; for patients other than transplant recipients, preferably avoid other immunosuppressants (increased risk of infection and malignancies, including lymphoma and skin cancer); avoid excessive exposure to UV light, including sunlight; **interactions:** Appendix 1 (ciclosporin)
Additional cautions in nephrotic syndrome *Contra-indicated* in uncontrolled hypertension, uncontrolled infections, and malignancy; in long-term management, perform renal biopsies every 1–2 years
Additional cautions Atopic Dermatitis and Psoriasis, section 13.5.3; Rheumatoid Arthritis, section 10.1.3

Hepatic impairment dosage adjustment based on bilirubin and liver enzymes may be needed

Renal impairment dose as in normal renal function but dose dependent increase in serum creatinine and urea during first few weeks may necessitate discontinuation (exclude rejection if kidney transplant); in nephrotic syndrome reduce dose by 25–50% if serum creatinine more than 30% above baseline on more than one measurement

Pregnancy see section 8.2; crosses placenta

Breast-feeding present in milk—manufacturer advises avoid

Side-effects gastro-intestinal disturbances, gingival hyperplasia, hepatic dysfunction, anorexia; hypertension; tremor, headache, paraesthesia, fatigue; renal dysfunction (renal structural changes on long-term administration; see also under Cautions), hyperuricaemia, hyperkalaemia, hypomagnesaemia, hyperlipidaemia, hypercholesterolaemia; muscle cramps, myalgia; hypertrichosis; *less commonly* oedema, weight gain, encephalopathy, anaemia, thrombocytopenia, rash; *rarely* pancreatitis, motor polyneuropathy, menstrual disturbances, gynaecomastia, micro-angiopathic haemolytic anaemia, haemolytic uraemic syndrome, hyperglycaemia, muscle weakness, myopathy; visual disturbances secondary to benign intracranial hypertension (discontinue), also anaphylaxis reported with infusion

Indication and dose

> Prevention of graft rejection following bone-marrow, kidney, liver, pancreas, heart, lung, and heart-lung transplantation, prophylaxis and treatment of graft-versus-host disease
> * **By mouth or by intravenous infusion**
>   Consult local treatment protocols for details

> Nephrotic syndrome see also section 6.3.2, p. 445
> * **By mouth**
>   **Child 1 month–18 years** 3 mg/kg twice daily, increase if necessary in corticosteroid-resistant disease; for maintenance reduce to lowest effective dose according to whole blood-ciclosporin concentrations, proteinuria, and renal function

> Refractory ulcerative colitis section 1.5.3

> Severe psoriasis, severe eczema section 13.5.3

Conversion Any conversion between brands should be undertaken very carefully and the manufacturer contacted for further information. Currently only *Neoral®* remains available for oral use; *Sandimmun®* capsules and oral solution and *SangCya®* oral solution are available on named-patient basis only for children who cannot be transferred to another brand of oral ciclosporin

> Because of differences in bioavailability, the brand of ciclosporin to be dispensed should be specified by the prescriber

◁ **CICLOSPORIN** (*continued*)

Neoral® (Novartis) [PoM]

Capsules, ciclosporin 10 mg (yellow/white), net price 60-cap pack = £18.98; 25 mg (blue/grey), 30-cap pack = £19.10; 50 mg (yellow/white), 30-cap pack = £37.40; 100 mg (blue/grey), 30-cap pack = £70.99. Counselling, administration

Oral solution, yellow, sugar-free, ciclosporin 100 mg/mL, net price 50 mL = £106.37. Counselling, administration

Counselling Total daily dose should be taken in 2 divided doses. Avoid grapefruit or grapefruit juice for 1 hour before dose

Mix solution with orange juice (or squash) or apple juice (to improve taste) or with water immediately before taking (and rinse with more to ensure total dose). Do not mix with grapefruit juice. Keep medicine measure away from other liquids (including water)

Sandimmun® (Novartis) [PoM]

Concentrate for intravenous infusion (oily), ciclosporin 50 mg/mL. To be diluted before use. Net price 1-mL amp = £1.94; 5-mL amp = £9.17

Excipients include polyoxyl castor oil (risk of anaphylaxis, see Excipients, p. 3)

Administration For *intravenous infusion*, dilute to a concentration of 0.5–2.5 mg/mL with Glucose 5% *or* Sodium Chloride 0.9%; give over 2–6 hours; not to be used with PVC equipment; observe patient for signs of anaphylaxis for at least 30 minutes after starting infusion and at frequent intervals thereafter

◤ SIROLIMUS

Cautions monitor kidney function when given with ciclosporin; Afro-Caribbean patients may require higher doses; **interactions**: Appendix 1 (sirolimus)

Hepatic impairment monitor blood-sirolimus trough concentration

Contra-indications

Pregnancy manufacturer advises avoid (toxicity in *animal* studies); effective contraception must be used during treatment and for 12 weeks after stopping

Breast-feeding discontinue breast-feeding

Side-effects abdominal pain, diarrhoea, stomatitis, abnormal liver-function tests (elevated transaminases)—oedema, tachycardia, hypercholesterolaemia, hypertriglyceridaemia, venous thromboembolism; pneumonitis; pyrexia, increased susceptibility to infection (especially urinary-tract infection); proteinuria, haemolytic uraemic syndrome; anaemia, thrombocytopenia, thrombotic thrombocytopenic purpura, leucopenia, neutropenia, hypokalaemia, hypophosphataemia, hyperglycaemia, lymphocele; arthralgia, osteonecrosis; epistaxis; acne, rash, impaired healing; *less commonly* pancreatitis, pulmonary embolism, pulmonary haemorrhage, pericardial effusion, nephrotic syndrome, increased susceptibility to lymphoma and other malignancies particularly of the skin, and pancytopenia; *rarely* interstitial lung disease, hepatic necrosis, lymphoedema, and hypersensitivity reactions including anaphylactic reactions, angiodema, exfoliative dermatitis, and hypersensitivity vasculitis

Licensed use not licensed for use in children

Indication and dose

See NICE guidance, p. 521

● By mouth

  Consult local treatment protocols for details

Rapamune® (Wyeth) ▼ [PoM]

Tablets, coated, sirolimus 1 mg (white), net price 30-tab pack = £90.00; 2 mg (yellow), 30-tab pack = £180.00

Oral solution, sirolimus 1mg/mL, net price 60 mL = £169.00. Counselling, administration

Administration food may affect absorption (give at the same time with respect to food). Mix solution with at least 60 mL water or orange juice in a glass or plastic container immediately before taking; refill container with at least 120 mL of water or orange juice and drink immediately (to ensure total dose). Do not mix with any other liquids

◤ TACROLIMUS

Cautions see under Ciclosporin; also monitor ECG (**important**: also echocardiography, see CSM warning below), visual status, blood glucose, haematological and neurological parameters; monitor whole blood 'trough' concentration of tacrolimus (especially during episodes of diarrhoea)—consult local treatment protocol for details; **interactions**: Appendix 1 (tacrolimus)

Skilled tasks May affect performance of skilled tasks (e.g. driving)

Hepatic impairment reduce dose in severe impairment

Contra-indications hypersensitivity to macrolides; avoid concurrent administration with ciclosporin (care if patient has previously received ciclosporin)

Pregnancy crosses placenta; association with pre-term delivery and intra-uterine growth retardation; contra-indicated by manufacturer; exclude pregnancy before starting—if contraception needed non-hormonal methods should be used

Breast-feeding avoid—present in milk following systemic administration

Side-effects include gastro-intestinal disturbances including dyspepsia, and inflammatory and ulcerative disorders; hepatic dysfunction, jaundice, bile-duct and gall-bladder abnormalities; hypertension (less frequently hypotension), tachycardia, angina, arrhythmias, thromboembolic and ischaemic events, rarely myocardial hypertrophy, cardiomyopathy (**important**: see CSM warning below); dyspnoea, pleural effusion, tremor, headache, insomnia, paraesthesia, confusion, depression, dizziness, anxiety, convulsions, incoordination, encephalopathy, psychosis; visual and hearing abnormalities; haematological effects including anaemia, leucocytosis, leucopenia, thrombocytopenia, coagulation disorders; altered acid-base balance and glucose metabolism, electrolyte disturbances including hyperkalaemia (less frequently hypokalaemia); altered renal function including

◁ **TACROLIMUS** *(continued)*

increased serum creatinine; hypophosphataemia; hypercalcaemia, hyperuricaemia; muscle cramps, arthralgia; pruritus, alopecia, rash, sweating, acne, photosensitivity; susceptibility to lymphoma and other malignancies particularly of the skin; *less commonly* ascites, pancreatitis, atelectasis, kidney damage and renal failure, myasthenia, hirsutism, *rarely* Stevens-Johnson syndrome
CSM warning Cardiomyopathy has been reported in children given tacrolimus after transplantation. Children should be monitored carefully by echocardiography for hypertrophic changes; dose reduction or discontinuation should be considered if these occur

Licensed use *Advagraf®* not licensed for use in children

Indication and dose

See under preparation

Atopic eczema (topical use) section 13.5.3

Administration For *continuous intravenous infusion* over 24 hours, dilute to a concentration of 4–100 micrograms/mL with Glucose 5% *or* Sodium Chloride 0.9%, to a total volume between 20–500 mL; incompatible with PVC

MHRA/CHM advice (December 2008) *Prograf®* and *Advagraf®* (tacrolimus): serious medication errors
It is important to note the correct use of these medicines:
- *Prograf®* is an immediate-release formulation that is taken twice daily, once in the morning and once in the evening;
- *Advagraf®* is a prolonged-release formulation that is taken once daily in the morning
Prograf® and *Advagraf®* are not interchangeable; switching between *Prograf®* and *Advagraf®* requires careful therapeutic monitoring.
Substitution should be made only under the close supervision of a transplant specialist.

Prograf® (Astellas) [PoM]
Capsules, tacrolimus 500 micrograms (yellow), net price 50-cap pack = £65.69; 1 mg (white), 50-cap pack = £85.22, 100-cap pack = £170.43; 5 mg (greyish-red), 50-cap pack = £314.84. Label: 23, counselling, driving

Concentrate for intravenous infusion, tacrolimus 5 mg/mL. To be diluted before use. Net price 1-mL amp = £62.05
Excipients include polyoxyl castor oil (risk of anaphylaxis, see Excipients, p. 3)

Dose
Prophylaxis of graft rejection following liver transplantation, commencing 12 hours after completion of surgery
- By mouth
  Consult local treatment protocol for details
  Child 1 month–18 years initially 150 micrograms/kg twice daily, adjusted according to whole blood concentration
- By continuous intravenous infusion (only if oral route inappropriate)
  Consult local treatment protocol for details
  Child 1 month–18 years 50 micrograms/kg over 24 hours for up to 7 days (then transfer to oral therapy), adjusted according to whole blood concentration

Allograft rejection resistant to conventional immunosuppressive regimen following liver transplantation
Consult local treatment protocol for details

Prophylaxis of graft rejection following kidney transplantation, commencing within 24 hours of completion of surgery
- By mouth
  Consult local treatment protocol for details
  Child 1 month–18 years initially 150 micrograms/kg twice daily adjusted according to whole blood concentration
  Note A lower dose of 100 micrograms/kg twice daily has been used in adolescents to prevent very high 'trough' concentrations
- By continuous intravenous infusion (only if oral route inappropriate)
  Consult local treatment protocol for details
  Child 1 month–18 years 75–100 micrograms/kg over 24 hours for up to 7 days (then transfer to oral therapy), adjusted according to whole blood concentration

Allograft rejection resistant to conventional immunosuppressive regimen following kidney transplantation
Consult local treatment protocol for details

Prophylaxis of graft rejection following heart transplantation *without antibody induction*
- By continuous intravenous infusion
  Consult local treatment protocol for details
  Child 1 month–18 years initially 30–50 micrograms/kg daily over 24 hours for up to 7 days (then transfer to oral therapy), adjusted according to whole blood concentration
- By mouth
  Consult local treatment protocols for details
  Child 1 month–18 years 150 micrograms/kg twice daily as soon as clinically possible (give 8–12 hours after discontinuation of intravenous infusion), adjusted according to whole blood concentration

Prophylaxis of graft rejection following heart transplantation *following antibody induction*
- By mouth
  Consult local treatment protocol for details
  Child 1 month–18 years 50–150 micrograms/kg twice daily, adjusted according to whole blood concentration

Allograft rejection resistant to conventional immunosuppressive regimen following heart transplantation
Consult local treatment protocol for details

Important *Prograf®* and *Advagraf®* are not interchangeable (see MHRA/CHM advice, above); tacrolimus trough levels should be measured before conversion and within 2 weeks of conversion to *Advagraf®*, and if necessary dose adjustment made to maintain similar systemic exposure

◢ Modified release
Advagraf® is not licensed for use in children

Advagraf® (Astellas) [PoM]
Capsules, m/r, tacrolimus 500 micrograms (yellow/orange), net price 50-cap pack = £42.22; 1 mg (white/orange), 50-cap pack = £84.43, 100-cap pack = £168.87; 5 mg (red/orange), 50-cap pack = £422.17. Label: 23, 25, counselling, driving

Dose *Prograf®* and *Advagraf®* are not interchangeable (see MHRA/CHM advice, above); tacrolimus trough levels should be measured before conversion and within 2 weeks of conversion to *Advagraf®*, and if necessary dose adjustment made to maintain similar systemic exposure

◢ Extemporaneous formulations available see Extemporaneous Preparations, p. 8

8 Malignant disease and immunosuppression

8.2.3 Rituximab and alemtuzumab

Rituximab, a monoclonal antibody which causes lysis of B lymphocytes, has been used as a component of the treatment of post-transplantation lymphoproliferative disease, non-Hodgkin's lymphoma, Hodgkin's lymphoma, and severe cases of resistant immune modulated disease including idiopathic thrombocytopenia purpura, haemolytic anaemia, and systemic lupus erythematosus. Full resuscitation facilities should be at hand and as with other cytotoxics, treatment should be undertaken under the close supervision of a specialist.

Rituximab should be used with caution in children receiving cardiotoxic chemotherapy or with a history of cardiovascular disease; in adults exacerbation of angina, arrhythmia, and heart failure have been reported. Transient hypotension occurs frequently during infusion and antihypertensives may need to be withheld for 12 hours before infusion.

Infusion-related side-effects (including cytokine release syndrome) are reported commonly with rituximab and occur predominantly during the first infusion; they include fever and chills, nausea and vomiting, allergic reactions (such as rash, pruritus, angioedema, bronchospasm and dyspnoea), flushing and tumour pain. Children should be given an analgesic and an antihistamine before each dose of rituximab to reduce these effects. Premedication with a corticosteroid should also be considered. The infusion may have to be stopped temporarily and the infusion-related effects treated—consult product literature or local treatment protocol for appropriate management. Evidence of pulmonary infiltration and features of tumour lysis syndrome should be sought if infusion-related effects occur.

Fatalities following **severe** cytokine release syndrome (characterised by severe dyspnoea) and associated with features of tumour lysis syndrome have occurred 1–2 hours after infusion of rituximab. Children with a high tumour burden as well as those with pulmonary insufficiency or infiltration are at increased risk and should be monitored **very closely** (and a slower rate of infusion considered).

Alemtuzumab, another monoclonal antibody that causes lysis of B lymphocytes, has been used in children for conditioning therapy before allogeneic bone marrow transplantation. In common with rituximab, it causes infusion-related side-effects including cytokine release syndrome (see above) and premedication with an analgesic, an antihistamine, and a corticosteroid is recommended.

8 Malignant disease and immunosuppression

◢ ALEMTUZUMAB

Cautions see notes above—for full details (including monitoring) consult product literature or local treatment protocol

Contra-indications for full details consult product literature or local treatment protocol

　Pregnancy avoid; manufacturer advises effective contraception for 6 months after treatment in men or women

　Breast-feeding avoid; manufacturer advises avoid breast-feeding during treatment and for at least 4 weeks after treatment

Side-effects see notes above—for full details (including monitoring and management of side-effects) consult product literature

Licensed use not licensed for use in children under 17 years

Indication and dose

　See notes above
　● **By intravenous infusion**
　　Consult local treatment protocol for details

Administration For *intravenous infusion*, dilute with Glucose 5% *or* Sodium Chloride 0.9%. Add requisite dose through a low protein binding 5-micron filter to 100-mL infusion fluid; infuse over 2 hours

MabCampath® (Bayer) ▼ [PoM]
Concentrate for intravenous infusion, alemtuzumab 30 mg/mL, net price 1-mL amp = £274.83

◢ RITUXIMAB

Cautions see notes above—but for full details (including monitoring) consult product literature or local treatment protocol

Contra-indications

　Pregnancy avoid unless potential benefit to mother outweighs risk of B-lymphocyte depletion

in fetus—effective contraception (in both sexes) required during and for 12 months after treatment

　Breast-feeding avoid breast-feeding during and for 12 months after treatment

Side-effects see notes above—but for full details (including monitoring and management of side-effects) consult product literature

◁ **RITUXIMAB** (*continued*)

Licensed use not licensed for use in children

Indication and dose

See notes above

● **By intravenous infusion**
Consult local treatment protocol for details

Administration For *intravenous infusion*, dilute to a concentration of 1–4 mg/mL with Glucose 5% *or*

Sodium Chloride 0.9%; gently invert bag to avoid foaming

MabThera® (Roche) ⟨PoM⟩
Concentrate for intravenous infusion, rituximab 10 mg/mL, net price 10-mL vial = £174.63, 50-mL vial = £873.15

8.2.4 Other immunomodulating drugs

Interferon alfa

Interferon alfa has shown some antitumour effect and may have a role in inducing early regression of life-threatening corticosteroid-resistant haemangiomas of infancy. Interferon alfa preparations are also used in the treatment of chronic hepatitis B, and chronic hepatitis C ideally in combination with ribavirin (section 5.3.3). Interferon alfa should always be used under the close supervision of a specialist. Side-effects are dose-related, but commonly include anorexia, nausea, influenza-like symptoms, and lethargy. Ocular side-effects and depression (including suicidal behaviour) have also been reported. Myelosuppression may occur, particularly affecting granulocyte counts. Cardiovascular problems (hypotension, hypertension, and arrhythmias), nephrotoxicity and hepatotoxicity have been reported and monitoring of hepatic function is recommended. Hypertriglyceridaemia, sometimes severe, has been observed; monitoring of lipid concentration is recommended. Other side-effects include hypersensitivity reactions, thyroid abnormalities, hyperglycaemia, alopecia, psoriasiform rash, confusion, coma and seizures, and reversible motor problems in young children. Rarely pulmonary infiltrates, pneumonitis, and pneumonia have occurred; respiratory symptoms should be investigated and if pulmonary infiltrates are suspected or lung function is impaired the discontinuation of interferon alfa should be considered.

INTERFERON ALFA

Cautions consult product literature and local treatment protocol for details; **interactions:** Appendix 1 (interferons)

Hepatic impairment close monitoring in mild to moderate impairment; avoid if severe

Renal impairment close monitoring required; manufacturers advise avoid in severe impairment

Contra-indications consult product literature and local treatment protocol for details; avoid injections containing benzyl alcohol in neonates (see under preparations below)

Pregnancy manufacturers recommend avoid unless compelling reasons; effective contraception required in both sexes if receiving treatment

Breast-feeding manufacturers advise avoid

Side-effects see notes above, consult product literature and local treatment protocols for details

Licensed use not licensed for use in children for chronic active hepatitis B; *Roferon-A®* not licensed for use in children

Indication and dose

Induction of early regression of life-threatening corticosteroid resistant haemangiomata of infancy

● **By subcutaneous injection**
Consult local treatment protocol for details

Chronic active hepatitis B infection see under preparations below

Chronic active hepatitis C infection see under preparations below

IntronA® (Schering-Plough) ⟨PoM⟩
Injection, interferon alfa-2b (rbe) 10 million units/mL, net price 1-mL vial = £43.17, 2.5-mL vial = £108.00. For subcutaneous injection or intravenous infusion

Injection pen, interferon alfa-2b (rbe), net price 15 million units/mL, 1.5-mL cartridge = £77.76; 25 million units/mL, 1.5-mL cartridge = £129.60; 50 million units/mL, 1.5-mL cartridge = £259.20. For subcutaneous injection

Note Each 1.5-mL multidose cartridge delivers 6 doses of 0.2 mL i.e. a total of 1.2 mL

Dose

Chronic active hepatitis B
● **By subcutaneous injection**
Child 2–18 years 5–10 million units/m^2 3 times weekly

Chronic active hepatitis C (in combination with oral ribavirin, see p. 393)
● **By subcutaneous injection**
Child 3–18 years 3 million units/m^2 3 times weekly

Roferon-A® (Roche) ⟨PoM⟩
Injection, interferon alfa-2a (rbe). Net price 6 million units/mL, 0.5-mL (3 million-unit) prefilled syringe = £15.07; 9 million units/mL, 0.5-mL (4.5 million-unit) prefilled syringe = £22.60; 12 mil-

◁ **INTERFERON ALFA** (*continued*)

lion units/mL, 0.5-mL (6 million-unit) prefilled syringe = £30.12; 18 million units/mL, 0.5-mL (9 million-unit) prefilled syringe = £45.19; 36 million units/mL, 0.5-mL (18 million-unit) prefilled syringe = £90.39; 30 million units/mL, 0.6-mL (18 million-unit) cartridge = £90.39, for use with *Roferon* pen device. For subcutaneous injection

(cartridges, vials, and prefilled syringes) and intramuscular injection (cartridges and vials)

Excipients include benzyl alcohol (avoid in neonates, see Excipients, p. 3)

Dose

Chronic active hepatitis B

• **By subcutaneous injection**

Child 2–18 years 2.5–5 million units/m² 3 times weekly; up to 10 million units/m² has been used 3 times weekly

---

Interferon gamma

Interferon gamma-1b is used to reduce the frequency of serious infection in chronic granulomatous disease and in severe malignant osteopetrosis.

INTERFERON GAMMA-1b
(Immune interferon)

Cautions seizure disorders (including seizures associated with fever); cardiac disease (including ischaemia, congestive heart failure, and arrhythmias); monitor before and during treatment: haematological tests (including full blood count, differential white cell count, and platelet count), blood chemistry tests (including renal and liver function tests) and urinalysis; avoid simultaneous administration of foreign proteins including immunological products (risk of exaggerated immune response); **interactions:** Appendix 1 (interferons)

Driving May impair ability to perform skilled tasks; effects may be enhanced by alcohol

Hepatic impairment manufacturer advises caution in severe liver disease

Renal impairment manufacturer advises caution in severe impairment—risk of accumulation

Pregnancy manufacturer recommends avoid unless compelling reasons; effective contraception should be used by men and women

Breast-feeding manufacturer advises avoid—no information available

Side-effects nausea, vomiting; headache, fatigue, fever; myalgia, arthralgia; rash, injection-site reactions; *rarely* confusion and systemic lupus erythematosus; also reported, neutropenia, thrombocytopenia, and raised liver enzymes

Indication and dose

See notes above and under Preparations below

Immukin® (Boehringer Ingelheim) PoM
Injection, recombinant human interferon gamma-1b 200 micrograms/mL, net price 0.5-mL vial = £88.00

Dose

• **By subcutaneous injection**

Body surface area 0.5 m² or less 1.5 micrograms/kg 3 times a week

Body surface area greater than 0.5 m² 50 micrograms/m² 3 times a week

Not recommended for infant under 6 months with chronic granulomatous disease

---

8.3 Sex hormones and hormone antagonists in malignant disease

Classification not used in *BNF for Children*.

9 Nutrition and blood

9.1 Anaemias and some other blood disorders **528**
9.1.1 Iron-deficiency anaemias 529
9.1.2 Drugs used in megaloblastic anaemias 533
9.1.3 Drugs used in hypoplastic, haemolytic, and renal anaemias 535
9.1.4 Drugs used in platelet disorders 541
9.1.5 G6PD deficiency 542
9.1.6 Drugs used in neutropenia 543

9.2 Fluids and electrolytes **546**
9.2.1 Oral preparations for fluid and electrolyte imbalance 546
9.2.2 Parenteral preparations for fluid and electrolyte imbalance 551

9.3 Intravenous nutrition **558**

9.4 Oral nutrition **561**
9.4.1 Foods for special diets 561
9.4.2 Enteral nutrition 562

9.5 Minerals **565**
9.5.1 Calcium and magnesium 565
9.5.2 Phosphorus 569
9.5.3 Fluoride 571
9.5.4 Zinc 573

9.6 Vitamins **574**
9.6.1 Vitamin A 574
9.6.2 Vitamin B group 575
9.6.3 Vitamin C 578
9.6.4 Vitamin D 578
9.6.5 Vitamin E 582
9.6.6 Vitamin K 583
9.6.7 Multivitamin preparations 584

9.7 Bitters and tonics **585**

9.8 Metabolic disorders **586**
9.8.1 Drugs used in metabolic disorders 586
9.8.2 Acute porphyrias 597

9.1 Anaemias and some other blood disorders

9.1.1 Iron-deficiency anaemias
9.1.2 Drugs used in megaloblastic anaemias
9.1.3 Drugs used in hypoplastic, haemolytic, and renal anaemias
9.1.4 Drugs used in platelet disorders
9.1.5 G6PD deficiency
9.1.6 Drugs used in neutropenia

Before initiating treatment for anaemia it is essential to determine which type is present. Iron salts may be harmful and result in iron overload if given alone to patients with anaemias other than those due to iron deficiency.

9.1.1 Iron-deficiency anaemias

9.1.1.1 Oral iron
9.1.1.2 Parenteral iron

Treatment with an iron preparation is justified only in the presence of a demonstrable iron-deficiency state. Before starting treatment, it is important to exclude any serious underlying cause of the anaemia (e.g. gastro-intestinal bleeding). The possibility of thalassaemia should be considered in children of Mediterranean or Indian subcontinent descent.

Prophylaxis with an iron preparation may be appropriate in those with a poor diet, malabsorption, menorrhagia, pregnancy, in haemodialysis patients, and in the management of low birth-weight infants such as preterm neonates.

9.1.1.1 Oral iron

Iron salts should be given by mouth unless there are good reasons for using another route.

Ferrous salts show only marginal differences between one another in efficiency of absorption of iron. Haemoglobin regeneration rate is little affected by the type of salt used provided sufficient iron is given, and in most patients the speed of response is not critical. Choice of preparation is thus usually decided by formulation, palatability, incidence of side-effects and cost.

Treatment of iron-deficiency anaemia   The oral dose of **elemental iron** to treat deficiency is 3–6 mg/kg (max. 200 mg) daily given in 2–3 divided doses. Iron supplementation may also be required to produce an optimum response to erythropoietins in iron-deficient children with chronic renal failure or in preterm neonates. (See also Prophylaxis of iron deficiency, below.)

Prescribing Express the dose in terms of elemental iron and iron salt and select the most appropriate preparation; specify both the iron salt and formulation on the prescription. The iron content of artificial formula feeds should also be considered.

Iron content of different iron salts		
Iron salt	Amount	Content of ferrous iron
Ferrous fumarate	200 mg	65 mg
Ferrous gluconate	300 mg	35 mg
Ferrous sulphate	300 mg	60 mg
Ferrous sulphate, dried	200 mg	65 mg
Sodium feredetate	190 mg	27.5 mg

Therapeutic response The haemoglobin concentration should rise by about 100–200 mg/100 mL (1–2 g/litre) per day *or* 2 g/100 mL (20 g/litre) over 3–4 weeks. When the haemoglobin is in the normal range, treatment should be continued for a further 3 months to replenish the iron stores. Epithelial tissue changes such as atrophic glossitis and koilonychia are usually improved, but the response is often slow. The most common reason for lack of response in children is poor compliance; poor absorption is rare in children.

Prophylaxis of iron deficiency   In neonates, haemoglobin and haematocrit concentrations change rapidly. These changes are not due to iron deficiency and cannot be corrected by iron supplementation. Similarly, neonatal anaemia resulting from repeated blood sampling does not respond to iron therapy.

All babies, including preterm neonates, are born with substantial iron stores but these stores can become depleted unless dietary intake is adequate. All babies require an iron intake of 400–700 nanograms daily to maintain body stores. Iron in breast milk is well absorbed but that in artificial feeds or in cow's milk is less so. Most artificial formula feeds are sufficiently fortified with iron to prevent deficiency and their iron content should be taken into account when considering further iron supplementation.

Dose Prophylactic iron supplementation (elemental iron 5 mg daily) may be required in babies of low birth-weight who are solely breast-fed; supplementation

9

Nutrition and blood

is started 4–6 weeks after birth and continued until mixed feeding is established.

Infants with a poor diet may become anaemic in the second year of life, particularly if cow's milk, rather than fortified formula feed, is a major part of the diet.

Compound preparations Some oral preparations contain **ascorbic acid** to aid absorption of the iron but the therapeutic advantage of such preparations is minimal and cost may be increased.

There is no justification for the inclusion of other ingredients, such as the **B group of vitamins**, except **folic acid** for pregnant women, see p. 534.

Side-effects Gastro-intestinal irritation can occur with iron salts. Nausea and epigastric pain are dose-related but the relationship between dose and altered bowel habit (constipation or diarrhoea) is less clear. Oral iron can exacerbate diarrhoea in patients with inflammatory bowel disease.

Iron preparations taken orally can be constipating and occasionally lead to faecal impaction.

If side-effects occur, the dose may be reduced; alternatively, another iron salt may be used but an improvement in tolerance may simply be a result of a lower content of elemental iron. The incidence of side-effects due to ferrous sulphate is no greater than with other iron salts when compared on the basis of equivalent amounts of elemental iron.

Iron preparations are an important cause of accidental overdose in children and as little as 20 mg/kg of elemental iron can lead to symptoms of toxicity. For the treatment of **iron overdose**, see Emergency Treatment of Poisoning, p. 42.

Counselling Although iron preparations are best absorbed on an empty stomach, they may be taken after food to reduce gastro-intestinal side-effects; they may discolour stools.

FERROUS SULPHATE

Cautions interactions: Appendix 1 (iron)
Side-effects see notes above

Indication and dose

Iron-deficiency anaemia, prophylaxis of iron deficiency See notes above and preparations

Ferrous Sulphate (Non-proprietary)
Tablets, coated, dried ferrous sulphate 200 mg (65 mg iron), net price 28-tab pack = £1.44
Dose
Child 6–18 years prophylactic, 1 tablet daily; therapeutic, 1 tablet 2–3 times daily, see notes above

Ironorm® Drops (Wallace Mfg)
Oral drops, ferrous sulphate 625 mg (125 mg iron)/5 mL. Net price 15 mL = £3.35
Dose
Child 1 month–6 years prophylactic 0.3 mL daily, but see notes above
Child 6–18 years prophylactic 0.6 mL daily

FERROUS FUMARATE

Cautions interactions: Appendix 1 (iron)
Side-effects see notes above

Indication and dose

Iron-deficiency anaemia, prophylaxis of iron deficiency See notes above and preparations

Fersaday® (Goldshield)
Tablets, brown, f/c, ferrous fumarate 322 mg (100 mg iron). Net price 28-tab pack = 79p
Dose
Child 12–18 years prophylactic, 1 tablet daily; therapeutic, 1 tablet twice daily

Fersamal® (Goldshield)
Tablets, brown, ferrous fumarate 210 mg (68 mg iron). Net price 20 = 29p
Dose
Child 12–18 years 1–2 tablets 3 times daily, but see notes above

Syrup, brown, ferrous fumarate approx. 140 mg (45 mg iron)/5 mL. Net price 200 mL = £3.11
Dose
Preterm neonate see notes above
Neonate see notes above
Child 1 month–6 years 2.5–5 mL twice daily, but see notes above
Child 6–18 years 10 mL twice daily, but see notes above

◁ **FERROUS FUMARATE** (*continued*)

Galfer® (Thornton & Ross)
Capsules, red/green, ferrous fumarate 305 mg
(100 mg iron). Net price 20 = 36p

Dose
> **Child 12–18 years** prophylactic, 1 capsule daily;
> therapeutic, 1 capsule twice daily

Syrup, brown, sugar-free ferrous fumarate 140 mg
(45 mg iron)/5 mL. Net price 300 mL = £4.86

Dose
> **Preterm neonate and body-weight up to 3 kg** prophy-
> lactic, 0.5 mL daily, see notes above

> **Neonate** prophylactic and therapeutic, 0.25 mL/kg
> twice daily (total daily dose may alternatively be
> given in 3 divided doses), see notes above

> **Child 1 month–12 years** prophylactic and therapeutic,
> 0.25 mL/kg twice daily (total daily dose may alterna-
> tively be given in 3 divided doses); max 20 mL daily,
> see notes above

> **Child 12–18 years** prophylactic, 10 mL once daily;
> therapeutic, 10 mL 1–2 times daily

■ FERROUS GLUCONATE

Cautions interactions: Appendix 1 (iron)
Side-effects see notes above

Indication and dose
> Iron-deficiency anaemia See notes above and
> preparation

Ferrous Gluconate (Non-proprietary)
Tablets, red, coated, ferrous gluconate 300 mg
(35 mg iron). Net price 20 = 73p

Dose
> **Child 6–12 years** prophylactic and therapeutic, 1–3
> tablets daily
> **Child 12–18 years** prophylactic, 2 tablets daily; ther-
> apeutic, 4–6 tablets daily in divided doses

■ POLYSACCHARIDE-IRON COMPLEX

Cautions interactions: Appendix 1 (iron)
Side-effects see notes above

Indication and dose
> Iron-deficiency anaemia, prophylaxis of iron
> deficiency See notes above and preparation

Niferex® (Tillomed)
Elixir, brown, sugar-free, polysaccharide-iron complex equivalent to 100 mg of iron/5 mL. Net price
240-mL pack = £6.06; ⟨NHS⟩¹ 30-mL dropper bottle
for paediatric use = £2.16. Counselling, use of
dropper

Dose
> **Neonate** (from dropper bottle) 1 drop (approx.
> 500 micrograms iron) per 450 g body-weight 3 times
> daily, see notes above

> **Child 1 month–2 years** (from dropper bottle) 1 drop
> (approx. 500 micrograms iron) per 450 g body-weight
> 3 times daily, see notes above

> **Child 2–6 years** therapeutic, 2.5 mL daily

> **Child 6–12 years** therapeutic, 5 mL daily

> **Child 12–18 years** prophylactic, 2.5 mL daily; thera-
> peutic, 5 mL 1–2 times daily (5 mL once daily if
> required during second and third trimester of
> pregnancy)

1. except 30 mL paediatric dropper bottle for prophylaxis
and treatment of iron deficiency in infants born prematurely; endorse prescription 'SLS'

■ SODIUM FEREDETATE
(Sodium ironedetate)

Cautions interactions: Appendix 1 (iron)
Side-effects see notes above
Licensed use not licensed for prophylaxis of iron
deficiency

Indication and dose
> Iron-deficiency anaemia, prophylaxis of iron
> deficiency See notes above and preparation

Sytron® (Link)
Elixir, sugar-free, sodium feredetate 190 mg
equivalent to 27.5 mg of iron/5 mL. Net price
100 mL = 89p

Dose
> **Neonate** prophylactic, 1 mL daily, see notes above;
> therapeutic, up to 2.5 mL twice daily (smaller doses
> should be used initially), see notes above

> **Child 1 month–1 year** prophylactic, 1 mL daily, see
> notes above; therapeutic, up to 2.5 mL twice daily
> (smaller doses should be used initially), see notes
> above

> **Child 1–5 years** therapeutic, 2.5 mL 3 times daily

> **Child 5–12 years** therapeutic, 5 mL 3 times daily

> **Child 12–18 years** therapeutic, 5 mL increasing gra-
> dually to 10 mL 3 times daily

9.1.1.2 Parenteral iron

Iron can be administered parenterally as iron dextran, iron sucrose, or as ferric carboxymaltose. Parenteral iron is generally reserved for use when oral therapy is unsuccessful because the child cannot tolerate oral iron, or does not take it reliably, or if there is continuing blood loss, or in malabsorption.

Many children with chronic renal failure who are receiving haemodialysis (and some who are receiving peritoneal dialysis) also require iron by the intravenous route on a regular basis (see also Erythropoietins, section 9.1.3).

With the exception of children with severe renal failure receiving haemodialysis, parenteral iron does not produce a faster haemoglobin response than oral iron provided that the oral iron preparation is taken reliably and is absorbed adequately.

Anaphylactoid reactions can occur with parenteral iron complexes; depending on the preparation, a small test dose may be required, see preparations for details; facilities for cardiopulmonary resuscitation must be available. If children complain of acute symptoms particularly nausea, back pain, breathlessness, or develop hypotension, the infusion should be stopped.

FERRIC CARBOXYMALTOSE

A ferric carboxymaltose complex containing 5% (50 mg/mL) of iron

Cautions hypersensitivity can occur with parenteral iron and facilities for cardiopulmonary resuscitation must be available; oral iron should not be given concomitantly; allergic disorders including asthma and eczema; infection (discontinue if ongoing bacteraemia)

Hepatic impairment use with caution; avoid in conditions where iron overload increases risk of impairment

Pregnancy avoid in first trimester; crosses the placenta in *animal* studies; may influence skeletal development

Side-effects gastro-intestinal disturbances; headache, dizziness; rash; injection-site reactions; *less commonly* hypotension, flushing, chest pain, peripheral oedema, fatigue, paraesthesia, malaise, pyrexia, rigors, myalgia, arthralgia, back pain, pruritus, and urticaria

Licensed use not licensed for use in children under 14 years

Indication and dose

Iron-deficiency anaemia see notes above
- **By slow intravenous injection or by intravenous infusion**
  Calculated according to body-weight and iron deficit, consult product literature

Ferinject® (Syner-Med) ▼ [PoM]
Injection, iron (as ferric carboxymaltose) 50 mg/mL, net price 2-mL vial = £21.75, 10-mL vial = £108.75
Electrolytes Na$^+$ 0.24 mmol/mL

IRON DEXTRAN

A complex of ferric hydroxide with sucrose containing 5% (50 mg/mL) of iron

Cautions oral iron not to be given until 5 days after last injection

Pregnancy avoid in first trimester

Anaphylaxis Anaphylactic reactions can occur with parenteral iron and a test dose is recommended before *each* dose; the patient should be carefully observed for 60 minutes after the first test dose and for 15 minutes after subsequent test doses. Facilities for cardiopulmonary resuscitation must be available; risk of allergic reactions increased in immune or inflammatory conditions

Contra-indications history of allergic disorders including asthma and eczema; infection; active rheumatoid arthritis

Hepatic impairment avoid in severe impairment

Renal impairment avoid in acute renal failure

Side-effects *less commonly* nausea, vomiting, abdominal pain, flushing, dyspnoea, anaphylactic reactions (see Anaphylaxis above), numbness, cramps, blurred vision, pruritus, and rash; *rarely* diarrhoea, chest pain, hypotension, angioedema, arrhythmias, tachycardia, dizziness, restlessness, fatigue, seizures, tremor, impaired consciousness, myalgia, arthralgia, sweating, and injection-site reactions; *very rarely* hypertension, palpitation, headache, paraesthesia, haemolysis, and transient deafness

Licensed use not licensed for use in children under 14 years

Indication and dose

Iron-deficiency anaemia see notes above
- **By slow intravenous injection or by intravenous infusion**
  Calculated according to body-weight and iron deficit, consult product literature

CosmoFer® (Vitaline) [PoM]
Injection, iron (as iron dextran) 50 mg/mL, net price 2-mL amp = £7.97; 10-mL amp = £39.85

9 Nutrition and blood

■ IRON SUCROSE

A complex of ferric hydroxide with sucrose containing 2% (20 mg/mL) of iron

Cautions oral iron therapy should not be given until 5 days after last injection; infection (discontinue if ongoing bacteraemia)

Pregnancy avoid in first trimester

Hepatic impairment use with caution; avoid in conditions where iron overload increases risk of impairment

Anaphylaxis Anaphylactic reactions can occur with parenteral iron and a test dose is recommended before the first dose; the patient should be carefully observed for 15 minutes. Facilities for cardiopulmonary resuscitation must be available

Contra-indications history of allergic disorders including asthma, eczema and anaphylaxis

Side-effects taste disturbances; *less commonly* nausea, vomiting, abdominal pain, diarrhoea, hypotension, tachycardia, flushing, palpitation, chest pain, bronchospasm, dyspnoea, headache, dizziness, fever, myalgia, pruritus, rash, and injection-site reactions; *rarely* peripheral oedema, anaphylactic reactions (see Anaphylaxis above), fatigue, asthenia, and paraesthesia; confusion, arthralgia, and increased sweating also reported

Licensed use not licensed for use in children

Indication and dose

Iron-deficiency anaemia see notes above

• **By slow intravenous injection or by intravenous infusion**

Calculated according to body-weight and iron deficit, consult product literature

Venofer® (Syner-Med) ⟦PoM⟧
Injection, iron (as iron sucrose) 20 mg/mL, net price 5-mL amp = £7.08

9.1.2 Drugs used in megaloblastic anaemias

Megaloblastic anaemias are rare in children; they may result from a lack of either vitamin B_{12} or folate, and it is essential to establish in every case which deficiency is present and the underlying cause. In emergencies, when delay might be dangerous, it is sometimes necessary to administer both substances after the bone marrow test while plasma assay results are awaited. Normally, however, appropriate treatment should be instituted only when the results of tests are available.

Vitamin B_{12} is used in the treatment of megaloblastosis caused by *prolonged nitrous oxide anaesthesia*, which inactivates the vitamin, and in the rare disorders of *congenital transcobalamin II deficiency*, *methylmalonic acidaemia* and *homocystinuria* (see section 9.8.1).

Vitamin B_{12} should be given prophylactically after *total ileal resection*.

Apart from dietary deficiency, all other causes of vitamin B_{12} deficiency are attributable to malabsorption. There is little place for the use of low-dose vitamin B_{12} orally and none for vitamin B_{12} intrinsic factor complexes given by mouth. Vitamin B_{12} in large oral doses [unlicensed] may be effective.

Hydroxocobalamin has completely replaced cyanocobalamin as the form of vitamin B_{12} of choice for therapy; it is retained in the body longer than cyanocobalamin and thus for maintenance therapy can be given at intervals of up to 3 months. Treatment is generally initiated with frequent administration of intramuscular injections to replenish the depleted body stores. Thereafter, maintenance treatment, which is usually for life, can be instituted. There is no evidence that doses larger than those recommended provide any additional benefit in vitamin B_{12} neuropathy.

Folic acid has few indications for long-term therapy since most causes of folate deficiency are self-limiting or will yield to a short course of treatment. It should not be used in undiagnosed megaloblastic anaemia unless vitamin B_{12} is administered concurrently otherwise neuropathy may be precipitated (see above).

In *folate-deficient megaloblastic anaemia* (e.g. because of poor nutrition, pregnancy, or treatment with antiepileptics), daily folic acid supplementation for 4 months brings about haematological remission and replenishes body stores; higher doses may be necessary in malabsorption states. In pregnancy, folic acid 5 mg daily is continued to term.

For prophylaxis in *chronic haemolytic states, malabsorption* or *in renal dialysis,* folic acid is given daily or sometimes weekly, depending on the diet and the rate of haemolysis.

For *prophylaxis in pregnancy,* see Prevention of Neural Tube Defects below.

Folic acid is actively excreted in breast milk and is well absorbed by the infant. It is also present in cow's milk and artificial formula feeds but is heat labile. Serum and

9

Nutrition and blood

red cell folate concentrations fall after delivery and urinary losses are high, particularly in low birth-weight neonates. Although symptomatic deficiency is rare in the absence of malabsorption or prolonged diarrhoea, it is common for neonatal units to give supplements of folic acid to all preterm neonates from 2 weeks of age until full-term corrected age is reached, particularly if heated breast milk is used without an artificial formula fortifier.

Folinic acid is also effective in the treatment of folate-deficient megaloblastic anaemia but it is normally only used in association with cytotoxic drugs (see section 8.1); it is given as calcium folinate.

Prevention of neural tube defects Folic acid supplements taken before and during pregnancy can reduce the occurrence of neural tube defects. The risk of a neural tube defect occurring in a child should be assessed and folic acid given as follows:

Women at a low risk of conceiving a child with a neural tube defect should be advised to take folic acid as a medicinal or food supplement at a dose of 400 micrograms daily before conception and until week 12 of pregnancy. Women who have not been taking folic acid and who suspect they are pregnant should start at once and continue until week 12 of pregnancy.

Couples are at a high risk of conceiving a child with a neural tube defect if either partner has a neural tube defect (or either partner has a family history of neural tube defects), if they have had a previous pregnancy affected by a neural tube defect, or if the woman has coeliac disease (or other malabsorption state), diabetes mellitus, sickle-cell anaemia, or is taking antiepileptic medicines (see also section 4.8.1).

Women in the high risk group who wish to become pregnant (or who are at risk of becoming pregnant) should be advised to take folic acid 5 mg daily and continue until week 12 of pregnancy (women with sickle-cell disease should continue taking their normal dose of folic acid 5 mg daily throughout pregnancy).

There is **no** justification for prescribing multiple-ingredient vitamin preparations containing vitamin B_{12} or folic acid.

HYDROXOCOBALAMIN

Cautions should not be given before diagnosis fully established but see also notes above; **interactions** Appendix 1 (hydroxocobalamin)

Side-effects itching, exanthema; fever, chills, hot flushes; nausea, dizziness; initial hypokalaemia; rarely acneform and bullous eruptions; anaphylaxis

Licensed use licensed for use in children (age not specified by manufacturers); not licensed for use in inborn errors of metabolism

Indication and dose

Macrocytic anaemia without neurological involvement
• By intramuscular injection
  Child 1 month–18 years initially 250 micrograms–1 mg 3 times a week for 2 weeks then 250 micrograms once weekly until blood count normal, then 1 mg every 3 months

Macrocytic anaemia with neurological involvement
• By intramuscular injection
  Child 1 month–18 years initially 1 mg on alternate days until no further improvement, then 1 mg every 2 months

Prophylaxis of macrocytic anaemias associated with vitamin B_{12} deficiency
• By intramuscular injection
  Child 1 month–18 years 1 mg every 2–3 months

Leber's optic atrophy
• By intramuscular injection
  initially 1 mg daily for 2 weeks, then 1 mg twice weekly until no further improvement, thereafter 1 mg every 1–3 months

Congenital transcobalamin II deficiency
• By intramuscular injection
  Neonate 1 mg 3 times a week, reduce after 1 year to 1 mg once weekly or as appropriate

  Child 1 month–18 years 1 mg 3 times a week, reduce after 1 year to 1 mg once weekly or as appropriate

Methylmalonic acidaemia and homocystinuria
• By intramuscular injection
  Child 1 month–18 years initially 1 mg daily for 5–7 days, reduce according to response to maintenance dose of up to 1 mg once or twice weekly

◁ **HYDROXOCOBALAMIN** *(continued)*

Methylmalonic acidaemia, maintenance once intramuscular response established
• **By mouth**

Child 1 month–18 years 5–10 mg once or twice weekly

Note Some children do not respond to the oral route

Hydroxocobalamin (Non-proprietary) ℗ℴℳ
Injection, hydroxocobalamin 1 mg/mL. Net price 1-mL amp = £2.46
Brands include *Cobalin-H®* ᴺᴴˢ, *Neo-Cytamen®* ᴺᴴˢ

Injection, hydroxocobalamin 2.5 mg/mL, 2 mL
Available from 'special-order' manufacturers or specialist importing companies, see p. 943

Administration For administration *by mouth*, injection solution may be given orally; it will not have prolonged effect via this route

Note The BP directs that when Vitamin B₁₂ injection is prescribed or demanded hydroxocobalamin injection shall be dispensed or supplied
Powder available from specialist importing companies

FOLIC ACID

Cautions should never be given alone for vitamin B₁₂ deficiency states (may precipitate subacute combined degeneration of the spinal cord); **interactions**: Appendix 1 (folates)

Side-effects rarely gastro-intestinal disturbances

Licensed use unlicensed for limiting methotrexate toxicity

Indication and dose

Folate supplementation in neonates (see notes above)
• **By mouth**

Neonate 50 micrograms once daily *or* 500 micrograms once weekly

Megaloblastic anaemia due to folate deficiency (see notes above)
• **By mouth**

Neonate initially 500 micrograms/kg once daily for up to 4 months

Child 1 month–1 year initially 500 micrograms/kg once daily (max. 5 mg) for up to 4 months; up to 10 mg daily may be required in malabsorption states

Child 1–18 years 5 mg daily for 4 months; (until term in pregnant women); up to 15 mg daily may be required in malabsorption states

Haemolytic anaemia; metabolic disorders
• **By mouth**

Child 1 month–12 years 2.5–5 mg once daily

Child 12–18 years 5–10 mg once daily

Prophylaxis of folate deficiency in dialysis
• **By mouth**

Child 1 month–12 years 250 microgram/kg (max. 10 mg) once daily

Child 12–18 years 5–10 mg once daily

Prevention of methotrexate side-effects in juvenile idiopathic arthritis
• **By mouth**

Child 2–18 years 1 mg daily *or* 5 mg once weekly, adjusted according to local guidelines

Prevention of methotrexate side-effects in severe Crohn's disease or severe psoriasis
• **By mouth**

See section 1.5.3 and section 13.5.3

Prevention of neural tube defects
• **By mouth**

See notes above

¹**Folic Acid** (Non-proprietary) ℗ℴℳ
Tablets, folic acid 400 micrograms, net price 90-tab pack = £2.32; 5 mg, 28-tab pack = 88p
Syrup, folic acid 2.5 mg/5 mL, net price 150 mL = £9.16; 400 micrograms/5 mL, 150 mL = £1.40
Brands include *Folicare®*, *Lexpec®* (sugar-free)
1. Can be sold to the public provided daily doses do not exceed 500 micrograms

9.1.3 Drugs used in hypoplastic, haemolytic, and renal anaemias

Anabolic steroids (see BNF, section 6.4.3), pyridoxine, antilymphocyte immunoglobulin, and various corticosteroids are used in hypoplastic and haemolytic anaemias.

Antilymphocyte globulin given intravenously through a central line over 12–18 hours each day for 5 days produces a response in about 50% of cases of acquired *aplastic anaemia*; the response rate may be increased when ciclosporin is given as well. Severe reactions are common in the first 2 days and profound immunosuppression can occur; antilymphocyte globulin should be given under specialist supervision with appropriate resuscitation facilities. Alternatively, oxymetholone tablets (available from 'special-order' manufacturers or specialist importing companies, see p. 943) may be used in aplastic anaemia at a dose of 1–5 mg/kg daily for 3 to 6 months.

It is unlikely that dietary deficit of **pyridoxine** (section 9.6.2) produces clinically relevant haematological effects. However, certain forms of *sideroblastic anaemia* respond to pharmacological doses, possibly reflecting its role as a co-enzyme during haemoglobin synthesis. Pyridoxine is indicated in both *idiopathic acquired* and *hereditary sideroblastic anaemias*. Although complete cures have not been reported, some increase in haemoglobin can occur with high doses. *Reversible sideroblastic anaemias* respond to treatment of the underlying cause but pyridoxine is indicated in pregnancy, haemolytic anaemias, or during isoniazid treatment.

Corticosteroids (section 6.3) have an important place in the management of haematological disorders including *autoimmune haemolytic anaemia*, *idiopathic thrombocytopenias* (section 9.1.4) and *neutropenias*, and *major transfusion reactions*. They are also used in chemotherapy schedules for many types of *lymphoma*, *lymphoid leukaemias*, and *paraproteinaemias*, including *multiple myeloma*.

Erythropoietins

Epoetins (recombinant human erythropoietins) are used to treat the anaemia associated with erythropoietin deficiency in chronic renal failure, see below.

Epoetin beta is also used for the prevention of anaemia in preterm neonates of low birth-weight; a therapeutic response may take several weeks. Only unpreserved formulations should be used as other preparations may contain benzyl alcohol (see Excipients, p. 3).

There is insufficient information to support the use of erythropoietins in children with leukaemia or in those receiving cancer chemotherapy.

Darbepoetin is a glycosylated derivative of epoetin; it persists longer in the body and can be administered less frequently than epoetin.

Other factors, such as iron or folate deficiency, that contribute to the anaemia of chronic renal failure should be corrected before treatment and monitored during therapy. Supplemental iron may improve the response in resistant patients and in preterm neonates (see section 9.1.1.1). Aluminium toxicity, concurrent infection, or other inflammatory disease can impair the response to erythropoietin.

> **Erythropoietins—haemoglobin concentration**
> In chronic kidney disease, the use of erythropoietins can be considered in a child with anaemia. The aim of treatment is to relieve symptoms of anaemia and to avoid the need for blood transfusion. The optimum haemoglobin concentration is dependent on the child's age and factors such as symptoms, co-morbidities, and patient preferences. The haemoglobin concentration should not be increased beyond that which provides adequate control of symptoms of anaemia. In *adults*, overcorrection of haemoglobin concentration with erythropoietins in those with chronic kidney disease may increase the risk of serious cardiovascular events and death; haemoglobin concentrations higher than 12 g/100 mL should be avoided in children.
> For MHRA/CHM advice relating to adults, see *BNF* section 9.1.3.

> **CSM advice (pure red cell aplasia)**
> There have been very rare reports of pure red cell aplasia in patients treated with epoetin alfa. The CSM has advised that in patients developing lack of efficacy with epoetin alfa, with a diagnosis of pure red cell aplasia, treatment with epoetin alfa must be discontinued and testing for erythropoietin antibodies considered. Patients who develop pure red cell aplasia should **not** be switched to another form of erythropoietin.

DARBEPOETIN ALFA

Cautions see Epoetin

Hepatic impairment manufacturer advises caution

Pregnancy no evidence of harm in *animal* studies—manufacturer advises caution

Contra-indications see Epoetin

Breast-feeding manufacturer advises avoid—no information available

Side-effects see Epoetin; also, oedema, injection-site pain; isolated reports of pure red cell aplasia particularly following subcutaneous administration in patients with chronic renal faliure (discontinue therapy)—see also CSM advice above

◌ **DARBEPOETIN ALFA** (*continued*)

Indication and dose

> Symptomatic anaemia associated with chronic renal failure in children on dialysis (see also notes above)
>
> • **By intravenous or subcutaneous injection**
>
>   **Child 11–18 years** initially 450 nanograms/kg once weekly adjusted according to response by approx. 25% at intervals of at least 4 weeks; maintenance dose, given once weekly *or* once every 2 weeks

> Symptomatic anaemia associated with chronic renal failure in children not on dialysis (see also notes above)
>
> • **By intravenous or subcutaneous injection**
>
>   **Child 11–18 years** *by subcutaneous or intravenous injection*, initially 450 nanograms/kg once weekly *or by subcutaneous injection*, initially 750 nanograms/kg once every 2 weeks; adjusted according to response by approx. 25% at intervals of at least 4 weeks; maintenance dose, given subcutaneously or intravenously once weekly *or* subcutaneously once every 2 weeks *or* subcutaneously once every month

Note Reduce dose by approximately 25% if rise in haemoglobin concentration exceeds 2 g/100 mL over 4 weeks or if haemoglobin concentration exceeds 12 g/100 mL; if haemoglobin concentration continues to rise, despite dose reduction, suspend treatment until haemoglobin concentration decreases and then restart at a dose approximately 25% lower than the previous dose. When changing route give same dose then adjust according to weekly or fortnightly haemoglobin measurements. Adjust doses not more frequently than every 2 weeks during maintenance treatment. Subcutaneous route preferred in patients not on haemodialysis

Aranesp® (Amgen) [PoM]
Injection, prefilled syringe, darbepoetin alfa, 25 micrograms/mL, net price 0.4 mL (10 micrograms) = £15.59; 40 micrograms/mL, 0.375 mL (15 micrograms) = £23.38, 0.5 mL (20 micrograms) = £31.17; 100 micrograms/mL, 0.3 mL (30 micrograms) = £46.76, 0.4 mL (40 micrograms) = £62.34, 0.5 mL (50 micrograms) = £77.93; 200 micrograms/mL, 0.3 mL (60 micrograms) = £93.51, 0.4 mL (80 micrograms) = £124.68, 0.5 mL (100 micrograms) = £155.85, 0.65 mL (130 micrograms) = £202.61; 500 micrograms/mL, 0.3 mL (150 micrograms) = £233.78, 0.6 mL (300 micrograms) = £467.55, 1 mL (500 micrograms) = £779.25

Injection (*Aranesp®* SureClick), prefilled disposable injection device, darbepoetin alfa, 40 micrograms/mL, net price 0.5 mL (20 micrograms) = £31.17; 100 micrograms/mL, net price 0.4 mL (40 micrograms) = £62.34; 200 micrograms/mL, net price 0.3 mL (60 micrograms) = £93.51, 0.4mL (80 micrograms) = £124.68, 0.5 mL (100 micrograms) = £155.85, 0.65 mL (130 micrograms) = £202.61; 500 micrograms/mL, net price 0.3 mL (150 micrograms) = £233.78, 0.6 mL (300 micrograms) = £467.55, 1 mL (500 micrograms) = £779.25

▲ **EPOETIN ALFA, BETA, and ZETA**
(Recombinant human erythropoietins)

Note The prescriber must specify which epoetin is required, see also Biosimilar medicines, p. 2

Cautions see notes above; also inadequately treated or poorly controlled blood pressure (monitor closely blood pressure, reticulocyte counts, haemoglobin, and electrolytes), interrupt treatment if blood pressure uncontrolled; sudden stabbing migraine-like pain is warning of hypertensive crisis; sickle-cell disease (lower target haemoglobin concentration may be appropriate); ischaemic vascular disease; thrombocytosis (monitor platelet count for first 8 weeks); epilepsy; malignant disease; increase in heparin dose may be needed

Hepatic impairment manufacturers advise caution in chronic impairment

Pregnancy no evidence of harm; benefits probably outweigh risks of anaemia and blood transfusion

Breast-feeding unlikely to be present in milk; effect on infant minimal

Contra-indications pure red cell aplasia following erythropoietin therapy (see also CSM advice above); uncontrolled hypertension; avoid injections containing benzyl alcohol in neonates (see under preparations, below)

Side-effects diarrhoea, nausea, vomiting; dose-dependent increase in blood pressure or aggravation of hypertension; in isolated patients with normal or low blood pressure, hypertensive crisis with encephalopathy-like symptoms and generalised tonic-clonic seizures requiring immediate medical attention; dose-dependent increase in platelet count (but thrombocytosis rare) regressing during treatment; influenza-like symptoms (may be reduced if intravenous injection given over 5 minutes); cardiovascular events; shunt thrombosis especially if tendency to hypotension or arteriovenous shunt complications; *very rarely* sudden loss of efficacy because of pure red cell aplasia, particularly following subcutaneous administration in patients with chronic renal failure (discontinue erythropoietin therapy)—see also CSM advice above, hyperkalaemia, hypersensitivity reactions (including anaphylaxis and angioedema), skin reactions, and peripheral oedema also reported

Licensed use *Eprex®* 20 000–unit, 30 000–unit, and 40 000–unit prefilled syringes not licensed for use in children; *NeoRecormon®* Multidose Injection and *Reco-Pen* not licensed for use in children under 3 years

Indication and dose

> See under preparations, below

◀ Epoetin alfa

Binocrit® (Sandoz) ▼ [PoM]
Injection, prefilled syringe, epoetin alfa, net price 1000 units = £5.09; 2000 units = £10.18; 3000 units = £15.27; 4000 units = £20.36; 5000 units = £25.46;

⌓ EPOETIN ALFA, BETA, and ZETA (*continued*)

6000 units = £30.55; 8000 units = £40.73;
10 000 units = £50.91

Note Biosimilar Medicine, p. 2

Dose

Symptomatic anaemia associated with chronic renal failure in children on haemodialysis (see also notes above)

• By intravenous injection over 1–5 minutes

Child 1 month–18 years initially 50 units/kg 3 times weekly adjusted according to response in steps of 25 units/kg 3 times weekly at intervals of at least 4 weeks; maintenance dose, body-weight under 10 kg usually 75–150 units/kg 3 times weekly, body-weight 10–30 kg usually 60–150 units/kg 3 times weekly, body-weight over 30 kg usually 30–100 units/kg 3 times weekly

Note Reduce dose by approximately 25% if rise in haemoglobin concentration exceeds 2 g/100 mL over 4 weeks or if haemoglobin concentration exceeds 12 g/100 mL; if haemoglobin concentration continues to rise, despite dose reduction, suspend treatment until haemoglobin concentration decreases and then restart at a dose approximately 25% lower than the previous dose

Eprex® (Janssen-Cilag) [PoM]

Injection, prefilled syringe, epoetin alfa, net price 1000 units = £6.29; 2000 units = £12.57; 3000 units = £18.86; 4000 units = £25.14; 5000 units = £31.43; 6000 units = £37.71; 8000 units = £50.28; 10 000 units = £62.85; 20 000 units = £125.70; 30 000 units = £226.26; 40 000 units = £301.68. An auto-injector device is available for use with pre-filled syringes

Dose

Symptomatic anaemia associated with chronic renal failure in children on haemodialysis (see also notes above)

• By intravenous injection over 1–5 minutes

Child 1 month–18 years initially 50 units/kg 3 times weekly adjusted according to response in steps of 25 units/kg 3 times weekly at intervals of at least 4 weeks; maintenance dose, body-weight under 10 kg usually 75–150 units/kg 3 times weekly, body-weight 10–30 kg usually 60–150 units/kg 3 times weekly, body-weight 30–60 kg usually 30–100 units/kg 3 times weekly, body-weight over 60 kg usually 75–300 units/kg 3 times weekly (as a single dose or in divided doses)

Note Reduce dose by approximately 25% if rise in haemoglobin concentration exceeds 2 g/100 mL over 4 weeks or if haemoglobin concentration exceeds 12 g/100 mL; if haemoglobin concentration continues to rise, despite dose reduction, suspend treatment until haemoglobin concentration decreases and then restart at a dose approximately 25% lower than the previous dose

◀Epoetin beta

NeoRecormon® (Roche) [PoM]

Injection, prefilled syringe, epoetin beta, net price 500 units = £3.90; 1000 units = £7.79; 2000 units = £15.59; 3000 units = £23.38; 4000 units = £31.17; 5000 units = £38.97; 6000 units = £46.76; 10 000 units = £77.93; 20 000 units = £155.87; 30 000 units = £233.81

Excipients include phenylalanine up to 300 micrograms/syringe (section 9.4.1)

Multidose injection, powder for reconstitution, epoetin beta, net price 50 000-unit vial = £419.01; 100 000-unit vial = £838.01 (both with solvent)

Excipients include phenylalanine up to 5 mg/vial (section 9.4.1), benzyl alcohol (avoid in neonates, see Excipients p. 3)

Note Avoid contact of reconstituted injection with glass; use only plastic materials

Reco-Pen, (for subcutaneous use), double-chamber cartridges (containing epoetin beta and solvent), net price 10 000-unit cartridge = £77.93; 20 000-unit cartridge = £155.87; for use with *Reco-Pen* injection device and needles (both available free from Roche)

Excipients include phenylalanine up to 500 micrograms/cartridge (section 9.4.1), benzyl alcohol (avoid in neonates, see Excipients, p. 3)

Dose

Symptomatic anaemia associated with chronic renal failure (see also notes above)

• By subcutaneous injection

Child 1 month–18 years initially 20 units/kg 3 times weekly for 4 weeks, increased according to response at intervals of 4 weeks in steps of 20 units/kg 3 times weekly; total weekly dose may be divided into daily doses; maintenance dose, initially reduce dose by half then adjust according to response at intervals of 1–2 weeks; total weekly maintenance dose may be given as a single dose or in 3 or 7 divided doses; max. 720 units/kg weekly

• By intravenous injection over 2 minutes

Child 1 month–18 years initially 40 units/kg 3 times weekly for 4 weeks, increased according to response to 80 units/kg 3 times weekly after 4 weeks, with further increases if needed at intervals of 4 weeks in steps of 20 units/kg 3 times weekly; maintenance dose, initially reduce dose by half then adjust according to response at intervals of 1–2 weeks; max. 720 units/kg weekly

Note Reduce dose by approximately 25% if rise in haemoglobin concentration exceeds 2 g/100 mL over 4 weeks or if haemoglobin concentration approaches or exceeds 12 g/100 mL; if haemoglobin concentration continues to rise, despite dose reduction, suspend treatment until haemoglobin concentration decreases and then restart at a dose approximately 25% lower than the previous dose. Subcutaneous route preferred in patients not on haemodialysis

Prevention of anaemias of prematurity in neonates with birth-weight of 0.75–1.5 kg and gestational age under 34 weeks

• By subcutaneous injection (of single-dose, unpreserved injection)

Neonate 250 units/kg 3 times weekly preferably starting within 3 days of birth and continued for 6 weeks

◀Epoetin zeta

Retacrit® (Hospira) ▼ [PoM]

Injection, prefilled syringe, epoetin zeta, net price 1000 units = £5.66; 2000 units = £11.31; 3000 units = £16.97; 4000 units = £22.63; 5000 units = £28.28; 6000 units = £33.94; 8000 units = £45.25; 10 000 units = £56.57; 20 000 units = £113.13; 30 000 units = £169.70; 40 000 units = £226.26

Excipients include phenylalanine up to 500 micrograms/syringe (section 9.4.1)

Note Biosimilar Medicine, p. 2

Dose

Symptomatic anaemia associated with chronic renal failure in children on haemodialysis (see also notes above)

• By intravenous injection over 1–5 minutes

Child 1 month–18 years initially 50 units/kg 3 times weekly adjusted according to response in steps of 25 units/kg 3 times weekly at intervals of at least 4 weeks; maintenance dose, body-weight under 10 kg usually 75–150 units/kg 3 times weekly, body-weight 10–30 kg usually 60–150 units/kg 3 times weekly, body-weight over 30 kg usually 30–100 units/kg 3 times weekly

Note Avoid increasing haemoglobin concentration at a rate exceeding 2 g/100 mL over 4 weeks

Sickle-cell disease

Sickle-cell disease is caused by a structural abnormality of haemoglobin resulting in deformed, less flexible red blood cells. Acute complications in the more severe forms include *sickle-cell crisis*, where infarction of the microvasculature and blood supply to organs results in severe pain. Sickle-cell crisis requires hospitalisation, intravenous fluids, analgesia (section 4.7) and treatment of any concurrent infection. Chronic complications include skin ulceration, renal failure and increased susceptibility to infection. Pneumococcal vaccine (section 14.4), haemophilus influenzae type b vaccine (section 14.4), an annual influenza vaccine (section 14.4) and prophylactic penicillin (Table 2, section 5.1) reduce the risk of infection. Hepatitis B vaccine (section 14.4) should be considered if the child is not immune.

In most forms of sickle-cell disease, varying degrees of haemolytic anaemia are present accompanied by increased erythropoiesis; this may increase folate requirements and folate supplementation may be necessary (section 9.1.2).

Hydroxycarbamide (hydroxyurea) may reduce the rate of crises and the need for blood transfusions. Hydroxycarbamide should be considered, in consultation with a specialist centre, for children who have recurrent episodes of acute pain (more than 3 admissions in the previous 12 months, or who are very symptomatic in the community) or who have had 2 or more episodes of acute sickle chest syndrome in the last 2 years (or 1 episode requiring ventilatory support). Beneficial effects of hydroxycarbamide may not become evident for several months. Myelosuppression, nausea, and skin reactions are the most common adverse effects.

HYDROXYCARBAMIDE
(Hydroxyurea)

Cautions see section 8.1 and notes above; also monitor renal and hepatic function before and during treatment; monitor full blood count before treatment, then every 2 weeks for the first 2 months and then every 2 months thereafter (or every 2 weeks if on max. dose); leg ulcers (review treatment if cutaneous vasculitic ulcerations develop); **interactions:** Appendix 1 (hydroxycarbamide)

Renal impairment reduce initial dose by 50% if estimated glomerular filtration rate less than 60 mL/minute/1.73 m²; avoid if estimated glomerular filtration rate less than 30 mL/minute/ 1.73 m²

Hepatic impairment avoid if severe

Contra-indications

Pregnancy avoid (teratogenic in *animal* studies); manufacturer advises effective contraception before and during treatment; see also section 8.1

Breast-feeding discontinue breast-feeding

Side-effects see section 8.1 and notes above; also dizziness, headache; *rarely* reduced sperm count and activity; fever, amenorrhoea, bleeding, and hypomagnesaemia also reported

Indication and dose

Sickle-cell disease (see notes above)
- **By mouth**

  Child 2–18 years initially 10–15 mg/kg once daily, increased every 12 weeks in steps of 5 mg/kg daily according to response; usual dose 15–30 mg/kg daily (max. 35 mg/kg daily)

Siklos (Nordic) ▼ [PoM]
Tablets, scored, f/c, hydroxycarbamide 1 g, net price 30-tab pack = £500.00

◢Extemporaneous formulations available see Extemporaneous Preparations, p. 8

Iron overload

Severe tissue iron overload can occur in aplastic and other refractory anaemias, mainly as the result of repeated blood transfusions. It is a particular problem in refractory anaemias with hyperplastic bone marrow, especially *thalassaemia major*, where excessive iron absorption from the gut and inappropriate iron therapy can add to the tissue siderosis.

Iron overload associated with haemochromatosis can be treated with repeated venesection. Venesection may also be used for patients who have received multiple transfusions and whose bone marrow has recovered. Where venesection is contra-indicated, and in thalassaemia, the long-term administration of the iron chelating compound **desferrioxamine mesilate** is useful. Subcutaneous infusions of desferrioxamine are given over 8–12 hours, 3–7 times a week; the dose should reflect the degree of iron overload. The initial dose should not exceed 30 mg/kg. For established overload the dose is usually between 20 and 50 mg/kg daily.

Desferrioxamine (up to 2 g per unit of blood) may also be given at the time of blood transfusion, provided that the desferrioxamine is **not** added to the blood and is **not** given through the same line as the blood (but the two may be given through the same cannula).

Iron excretion induced by desferrioxamine is enhanced by ascorbic acid (vitamin C, section 9.6.3) 100–200 mg daily by mouth; it should be given separately from food since it also enhances iron absorption. Ascorbic acid should not be given to children with cardiac dysfunction; in children with normal cardiac function ascorbic acid should be introduced 1 month after starting desferrioxamine.

Desferrioxamine infusion can be used to treat *aluminium overload* in dialysis patients; theoretically 100 mg of desferrioxamine binds with 4.1 mg of aluminium.

Deferasirox, an oral iron chelator, is licensed for the treatment of chronic iron overload in children over 6 years with thalassaemia major who receive frequent blood transfusions (more than 7 mL/kg/month of packed blood cells). It is also licensed for chronic iron overload when desferrioxamine is contra-indicated or inadequate in children with thalassaemia major who receive infrequent blood transfusions (less than 7 mL/kg/month of packed red blood cells), in children with other anaemias, and in children aged 2 to 5 years.

Deferiprone, an oral iron chelator, is licensed for the treatment of iron overload in children over 6 years of age with thalassaemia major in whom desferrioxamine is contra-indicated or is inadequate. Blood dyscrasias, particularly agranulocytosis, have been reported with deferiprone.

DEFERASIROX

Cautions eye and ear examinations required before treatment and annually during treatment; monitor body-weight, height and sexual development annually; monitor serum-ferritin concentration monthly; risk of gastro-intestinal ulceration and haemorrhage; history of liver cirrhosis; test liver function before treatment, then every 2 weeks during the first month, and then monthly; measure baseline serum creatinine and monitor renal function weekly during the first month of treatment and monthly thereafter; test for proteinuria monthly; **interactions:** Appendix 1 (deferasirox)

Hepatic impairment manufacturer advises caution—no information available; avoid in severe impairment

Renal impairment reduce dose by 10 mg/kg if serum creatinine increased above age-appropriate limits *or* estimated glomerular filtration rate less than 90 mL/minute/1.73 m² on 2 consecutive occasions—interrupt treatment if deterioration in renal function persists after dose reduction; avoid if estimated glomerular filtration rate less than 60 mL/minute/1.73 m²

Pregnancy manufacturer advises avoid unless potential benefit outweighs risk—toxicity in *animal* studies

Breast-feeding manufacturer advises avoid—present in milk in *animal* studies

Side-effects gastro-intestinal disturbances (including ulceration and haemorrhage); headache; proteinuria; pruritus; rash; *less commonly* oedema, hepatitis, cholelithiasis, fatigue, anxiety, sleep disorder, dizziness, pyrexia, pharyngitis, glucosuria, renal tubulopathy, disturbances of hearing and vision (including lens opacity and maculopathy), and skin pigmentation; hepatic failure, acute renal failure, blood disorders (including agranulocytosis, neutropenia, and thrombocytopenia), hypersensitivity reactions (including anaphylaxis and angioedema) also reported

Indication and dose

Chronic iron overload
• By mouth

Child 2–18 years initially 10–30 mg/kg once daily according to serum-ferritin concentration and amount of transfused blood (consult product literature); maintenance, adjust dose every 3–6 months in steps of 5–10 mg/kg according to serum-ferritin concentration; max. 30 mg/kg daily
Note dose should be rounded to nearest whole tablet size

Exjade® (Novartis) ▼ [PoM]
Dispersible tablets, deferasirox 125 mg, net price 28-tab pack = £117.60; 250 mg, 28-tab pack = £235.20; 500 mg, 28-tab pack = £470.40. Label: 13, 22, counselling, administration

Counselling Tablets may be dispersed in water, orange juice, or apple juice; if necessary, resuspend residue and swallow

DEFERIPRONE

Cautions monitor neutrophil count weekly and discontinue treatment if neutropenia develops
Blood disorders Patients or their carers should be told how to recognise signs of neutropenia and advised to seek immediate medical attention if symptoms such as fever or sore throat develop

Hepatic impairment manufacturer advises monitor liver function—interrupt treatment if persistent elevation in serum alanine aminotransferase

Renal impairment manufacturer advises caution—no information available

◁ **DEFERIPRONE** (*continued*)

Contra-indications history of agranulocytosis or recurrent neutropenia

Pregnancy manufacturer advises avoid before intended conception and during pregnancy—teratogenic and embryotoxic in *animal* studies; contraception advised in girls of child-bearing potential

Breast-feeding manufacturer advises avoid—no information available

Side-effects gastro-intestinal disturbances (reducing dose and increasing gradually may improve tolerance), increased appetite; headache; red-brown urine discoloration; neutropenia, agranulocytosis; zinc deficiency; arthropathy

Licensed use see notes above

Indication and dose

Iron overload in thalassaemia major
• By mouth
    Child 6-18 years 25 mg/kg 3 times daily (max. 100 mg/kg daily)

Ferriprox® (Swedish Orphan) (PoM)
    Tablets, f/c, scored, deferiprone 500 mg, net price 100-tab pack = £152.39. Label: 14, counselling, blood disorders

    Oral solution, red, deferiprone 100 mg/mL, net price 500 mL = £152.39. Label: 14, counselling, blood disorders

▲ **DESFERRIOXAMINE MESILATE**
(Deferoxamine Mesilate)

Cautions eye and ear examinations before treatment and at 3-month intervals during treatment; monitor body-weight and height in children at 3-month intervals—risk of growth restriction with excessive doses; aluminium-related encephalopathy (may exacerbate neurological dysfunction); **interactions**: Appendix 1 (desferrioxamine)

Pregnancy teratogenic in *animal* studies, manufacturer advises use only if potential benefit outweighs risk

Breast-feeding manufacturer advises use only if potential benefit outweighs risk—no information available

Side-effects hypotension (especially when given too rapidly by intravenous injection), disturbances of hearing and vision (including lens opacity and retinopathy); injection site reactions, gastro-intestinal disturbances, asthma, fever, headache, arthralgia and myalgia; very rarely anaphylaxis, acute respiratory distress syndrome, neurological disturbances (including dizziness, neuropathy and paraesthesia), Yersinia and mucormycosis infections, rash, renal impairment, and blood dyscrasias

Indication and dose

Chronic iron overload see notes above

Aluminium overload in dialysis patients
• By intravenous infusion
    Child 1 month-18 years 5 mg/kg once weekly

Iron poisoning
    see Emergency Treatment of Poisoning, p. 42

Administration For *intravenous* or *subcutaneous infusion*, reconstitute powder with Water for Injection to a concentration of 100 mg/mL; dilute with Glucose 5% or Sodium Chloride 0.9%. In *haemodialysis* or *haemofiltration* administer over the last hour of dialysis (may be given via the dialysis fistula). *Intraperitoneal*: may be added to dialysis fluid. In CAPD give prior to the last exchange of the day.
Note For full details and warnings relating to administration, consult product literature

Desferrioxamine mesilate (Non-proprietary) (PoM)
    Injection, powder for reconstitution, desferrioxamine mesilate, net price 500-mg vial = £4.26; 2-g vial = £17.05

Desferal® (Novartis) (PoM)
    Injection, powder for reconstitution, desferrioxamine mesilate, net price 500-mg vial = £4.44, 2-g vial = £17.77

9.1.4 **Drugs used in platelet disorders**

Idiopathic thrombocytopenic purpura Acute idiopathic thrombocytopenic purpura is usually self-limiting in children. A corticosteroid such as prednisolone (p. 452) is sometimes used if idiopathic thrombocytopenic purpura does not resolve spontaneously or if it is associated with severe cutaneous symptoms or mucous membrane bleeding; corticosteroid treatment should not be continued longer than 14 days regardless of the response.

Immunoglobulin preparations (section 14.5) may be used in idiopathic thrombocytopenic purpura or where a temporary rapid rise in platelets is needed, as in pregnancy or pre-operatively; they are often used in preference to a corticosteroid. Anti-D immunoglobulin is licensed for the management of idiopathic thrombocytopenic purpura.

Other therapy that has been tried under specialist supervision in refractory idiopathic thrombocytopenic purpura includes azathioprine (section 8.2.1), cyclophosphamide (section 8.1.1), vincristine (section 8.1.4), and ciclosporin (section 8.2.2). Rituximab is also used in specialist centres but experience of its use in children is limited. For patients with chronic severe thrombocytopenia refractory to other therapy, tranexamic acid (section 2.11) may be given to reduce the severity of haemorrhage.

Splenectomy is considered in chronic thrombocytopenic purpura if a satisfactory platelet count is not achieved with regular immunoglobulin infusions, if there is a relapse on withdrawing or reducing the dose of corticosteroid, and if other therapies are considered inappropriate.

Thrombocythaemia Anagrelide reduces platelets in essential thrombocythaemia in patients at risk of thrombo-haemorrhagic events who have not responded adequately to other drugs or who cannot tolerate other drugs.

ANAGRELIDE

Cautions cardiovascular disease—assess cardiac function before and during treatment; concomitant aspirin in patients at risk of haemorrhage; monitor full blood count (monitor platelet count every 2 days for 1 week, then weekly until maintenance dose established), liver function, serum creatinine, and urea; **interactions:** Appendix 1 (anagrelide)

Skilled tasks Dizziness may affect performance of skilled tasks (e.g. driving)

Hepatic impairment manufacturer advises caution in mild hepatic impairment; avoid in moderate to severe impairment

Renal impairment manufacturer advises avoid if estimated glomerular filtration rate less than 50 mL/minute/1.73 m^2

Contra-indications

Pregnancy manufacturer advises avoid (toxicity in *animal* studies)

Breast-feeding manufacturer advises avoid—no information available

Side-effects gastro-intestinal disturbances; palpitation, tachycardia, fluid retention; headache, dizziness, fatigue; anaemia; rash; *less commonly* pancreatitis, gastro-intestinal haemorrhage, congestive heart failure, hypertension, arrhythmias, syncope, chest pain, dyspnoea, sleep disturbances, paraesthesia, hypoaesthesia, depression, nervousness, confusion, amnesia, fever, weight changes, impotence, blood disorders, myalgia, arthralgia, epistaxis, dry mouth, alopecia, skin discoloration, and pruritus; *rarely* gastritis, colitis, postural hypotension, angina, myocardial infarction, vasodilatation, pulmonary infiltrates, migraine, drowsiness, impaired co-ordination, dysarthria, asthenia, tinnitus, renal failure, nocturia, visual disturbances, and gingival bleeding; allergic alveolitis also reported

Licensed use not licensed for use in children

Indication and dose

Essential thrombocythaemia in at-risk children who have not responded adequately to other therapy or who are intolerant of it (initiated under specialist supervision)

• **By mouth**

Child 7–18 years initially 500 micrograms daily adjusted according to response in steps of 500 micrograms daily at weekly intervals to max. 10 mg daily (max. single dose 2.5 mg); usual dose range 1–3 mg daily in divided doses

Xagrid® (Shire) ▼ PoM

Capsules, anagrelide (as hydrochloride), 500 micrograms, net price 100-cap pack= £337.14. Counselling, skilled tasks, see above

9.1.5 G6PD deficiency

Glucose 6-phosphate dehydrogenase (G6PD) deficiency is highly prevalent in individuals originating from most parts of Africa, from most parts of Asia, from Oceania, and from Southern Europe; it can also occur, rarely, in any other individuals. G6PD deficiency is more common in males than it is in females.

Individuals with G6PD deficiency are susceptible to developing acute haemolytic anaemia on taking a number of common drugs. They are also susceptible to developing acute haemolytic anaemia upon ingestion of fava beans (broad beans, *Vicia faba*); this is termed *favism* and can be more severe in children or when the fresh fava beans are eaten raw.

9 Nutrition and blood

When prescribing drugs for children with G6PD deficiency, the following three points should be kept in mind:

- G6PD deficiency is genetically heterogeneous; susceptibility to the haemolytic risk from drugs varies; thus, a drug found to be safe in some G6PD-deficient individuals may not be equally safe in others;

- manufacturers do not routinely test drugs for their effects in G6PD-deficient individuals;

- the risk and severity of haemolysis is almost always dose-related.

The lists below should be read with these points in mind. Ideally, information about G6PD deficiency should be available before prescribing a drug listed below. However, in the absence of this information, the possibility of haemolysis should be considered, especially if the child belongs to a group in which G6PD deficiency is common.

A very few G6PD-deficient individuals with chronic non-spherocytic haemolytic anaemia have haemolysis even in the absence of an exogenous trigger. These children must be regarded as being at high risk of severe exacerbation of haemolysis following administration of any of the drugs listed below.

Drugs with *definite* risk of haemolysis in most G6PD-deficient individuals

Dapsone and other sulphones (higher doses for dermatitis herpetiformis more likely to cause problems)

Methylthioninium chloride (methylene blue)

Niridazole [not on UK market]

Nitrofurantoin

Pamaquin [not on UK market]

Primaquine (30 mg weekly for 8 weeks has been found to be without undue harmful effects in African and Asian people, see section 5.4.1)

Quinolones (including ciprofloxacin, moxifloxacin, nalidixic acid, norfloxacin, and ofloxacin)

Sulphonamides (including co-trimoxazole; some sulphonamides, e.g. sulfadiazine, have been tested and found not to be haemolytic in many G6PD-deficient individuals)

Drugs with *possible* risk of haemolysis in some G6PD-deficient individuals

Aspirin (acceptable up to a dose of at least 1 g daily in most G6PD-deficient individuals)

Chloroquine (acceptable in acute malaria and malaria chemoprophylaxis)

Menadione, water-soluble derivatives (e.g. menadiol sodium phosphate)

Probenecid [not on UK market]

Quinidine (acceptable in acute malaria) [not on UK market]

Quinine (acceptable in acute malaria)

Rasburicase

Note Naphthalene in mothballs also causes haemolysis in individuals with G6PD-deficiency.

9.1.6 Drugs used in neutropenia

Recombinant human granulocyte-colony stimulating factor (rhG-CSF) stimulates the production of neutrophils and may reduce the duration of chemotherapy-induced neutropenia and thereby reduce the incidence of associated sepsis; there is as yet no evidence that it improves overall survival. **Filgrastim** (unglycosylated rhG-CSF) and **lenograstim** (glycosylated rhG-CSF) have similar effects; both have been used in a variety of clinical settings, including cytotoxic-induced neutropenia, and neutropenia following bone marrow transplantation, but they do not have

9

Nutrition and blood

any clear-cut routine indications. In congenital neutropenia filgrastim usually elevates the neutrophil count with appropriate clinical response. Prolonged use may be associated with an increased risk of myeloid malignancy.

Treatment with recombinant human growth factors should only be prescribed by those experienced in their use.

Neonatal neutropenia Filgrastim and lenograstim have been used to abolish sepsis-induced neutropenia in preterm neonates. The majority of studies have used filgrastim. The effects on survival and long-term outcome are unclear.

Cautions Recombinant human granulocyte-colony stimulating factors should be used with caution in patients with pre-malignant or malignant myeloid conditions. Full blood counts (including differential white cell count and platelet count) should be monitored. Treatment should be withdrawn in patients who develop signs of pulmonary infiltration. There have been reports of pulmonary infiltrates leading to acute respiratory distress syndrome—patients with a history of pulmonary infiltrates or pneumonia may be at higher risk.

Side-effects Side-effects of granulocyte-colony stimulating factors include gastro-intestinal disturbances (including nausea, vomiting, and diarrhoea), mucositis, anorexia, headache, asthenia, fever, musculoskeletal pain, bone pain, rash, alopecia, injection-site reactions, thrombocytopenia, and leucocytosis. Less frequent side-effects include chest pain, hypersensitivity reactions (including anaphylaxis and bronchospasm) and arthralgia. There have been reports of pulmonary side-effects, particularly interstitial pneumonia (see Cautions above), cutaneous vasculitis, and acute febrile neutrophilic dermatosis.

FILGRASTIM
(Recombinant human granulocyte-colony stimulating factor, G-CSF)

Cautions see notes above; also regular morphological and cytogenetic bone-marrow examinations recommended in severe congenital neutropenia (possible risk of myelodysplastic syndromes or leukaemia); secondary acute myeloid leukaemia, sickle-cell disease; monitor spleen size (risk of rupture); osteoporotic bone disease (monitor bone density if given for more than 6 months); **interactions:** Appendix 1 (filgrastim)

Pregnancy toxicity in *animal* studies; manufacturer advises use only if potential benefit outweighs risk

Breast-feeding manufacturer advises avoid—no information available

Contra-indications severe congenital neutropenia (Kostman's syndrome) with abnormal cytogenetics

Side-effects see notes above; also splenic enlargement, hepatomegaly, transient hypotension, epistaxis, urinary abnormalities (including dysuria, proteinuria, and haematuria), osteoporosis, exacerbation of rheumatoid arthritis, anaemia, transient decrease in blood glucose, and raised uric acid

Licensed use not licensed for treatment of glycogen storage disease or neonatal neutropenia

Indication and dose

Cytotoxic-induced neutropenia
- Preferably by subcutaneous injection or by intravenous infusion (over 30 minutes)

  Child 1 month–18 years 5 micrograms/kg daily started not less than 24 hours after cytotoxic chemotherapy, continued until neutrophil count in normal range, usually for up to 14 days (up to 38 days in acute myeloid leukaemia)

Myeloablative therapy followed by bone-marrow transplantation
- By intravenous infusion over 30 minutes or over 24 hours or by subcutaneous infusion over 24 hours

  Child 1 month–18 years 10 micrograms/kg daily, started not less than 24 hours following cytotoxic chemotherapy (and within 24 hours of bone-marrow infusion), then adjusted according to absolute neutrophil count (consult product literature and local protocol)

Mobilisation of peripheral blood progenitor cells for autologous infusion, used alone
- By subcutaneous injection or by subcutaneous infusion over 24 hours

  Child 1 month–18 years 10 micrograms/kg daily for 5–7 days

Mobilisation of peripheral blood progenitor cells for autologous infusion following adjunctive myelosuppressive chemotherapy (to improve yield)
- By subcutaneous injection

  Child 1 month–18 years 5 micrograms/kg daily, started the day after completion of chemotherapy and continued until neutrophil count in normal range; for timing of leucopheresis consult product literature

Mobilisation of peripheral blood progenitor cells in normal donors for allogeneic infusion
- By subcutaneous injection

  Child over 16 years 10 micrograms/kg daily for 4–5 days; for timing of leucopheresis consult product literature

◻ **FILGRASTIM** (*continued*)

Severe chronic neutropenia
- **By subcutaneous injection**

 Child 1 month–18 years in severe congenital neutropenia, initially 12 micrograms/kg daily in single or divided doses (initially 5 micrograms/kg daily in idiopathic or cyclic neutropenia), adjusted according to response (consult product literature and local protocol)

Persistent neutropenia in HIV infection
- **By subcutaneous injection**

 Child 1 month–18 years initially 1 microgram/kg daily, increased as necessary until absolute neutrophil count in normal range (usual max. 4 micrograms/kg daily), then adjusted to maintain absolute neutrophil count in normal range (consult product literature)

Neonatal neutropenia
- **By subcutaneous injection**

 Neonate 10 micrograms/kg daily, discontinue if white cell count exceeds 50×10^9/litre

Glycogen storage disease type 1b
- **By subcutaneous injection**
 5 micrograms/kg daily, adjusted as necessary

Administration For *subcutaneous* or *intravenous injection* or *infusion*, dilute with Glucose 5% to a concentration of not less than 15 micrograms/mL (concentration of 100 micrograms/mL adequate for subcutaneous use in neonates); to dilute to a concentration of 2–15 micrograms/mL, add albumin solution (human serum albumin) to produce a final albumin solution of 2 mg/mL; not compatible with Sodium Chloride solutions

Neupogen® (Amgen) (PoM)
Injection, filgrastim 30 million units (300 micrograms)/mL; net price 1-mL vial = £68.41

Injection (Singleject®), filgrastim 60 million units (600 micrograms)/mL, net price 0.5-mL prefilled syringe = £68.41; 96 million units (960 micrograms)/mL, 0.5-mL prefilled syringe = £109.11

Ratiograstim® (Ratiopharm UK) ▼ (PoM)
Injection, prefilled syringe, filgrastim, net price 30 million units (300 micrograms)/0.5 ml = £62.25; 48 million units (480 micrograms)/0.8 ml = £99.29
Note Biosimilar medicine p. 2

█ **LENOGRASTIM**
(Recombinant human granulocyte-colony stimulating factor, rHuG-CSF)

Cautions see notes above; also sickle-cell disease; monitor spleen size (risk of rupture)

Pregnancy toxicity in *animal* studies; manufacturer advises use only if potential benefit outweighs risk

Breast-feeding manufacturer advises avoid—no information available

Side-effects see notes above; also splenic rupture and toxic epidermal necrolysis

Licensed use not licensed for use in children for cytotoxic-induced neutropenia, mobilisation of peripheral blood progenitor cells (monotherapy or adjunctive therapy), or following peripheral stem cells transplantation

Indication and dose

Following peripheral stem cells or bone-marrow transplantation
- **By intravenous infusion over 30 minutes or by subcutaneous injection**

 Child 2–18 years 150 micrograms/m² daily started the day after transplantation, continued until neutrophil count stable in acceptable range (max. 28 days)

Cytotoxic-induced neutropenia
- **By subcutaneous injection**

 Child 2–18 years 150 micrograms/m² daily started the day after completion of chemotherapy, continued until neutrophil count stable in acceptable range (max. 28 days)

Mobilisation of peripheral blood progenitor cells, used alone
- **By subcutaneous injection**

 Child 2–18 years 10 micrograms/kg daily for 4–6 days (5–6 days in healthy donors)

Mobilisation of peripheral blood progenitor cells following adjunctive myelosuppressive chemotherapy (to improve yield)
- **By subcutaneous injection**

 Child 2–18 years 150 micrograms/m² daily, started 1–5 days after completion of chemotherapy and continued until neutrophil count in acceptable range; for timing of leucopheresis consult product literature

Administration For *intravenous infusion*, dilute reconstituted solution to a concentration of not less than 2 micrograms/mL (*Granocyte-13*) or 2.5 micrograms/mL (*Granocyte-34*) with Sodium Chloride 0.9%

Granocyte® (Chugai) (PoM)
Injection, powder for reconstitution, lenograstim, net price 13.4 million-unit (105-microgram) vial = £42.00; 33.6 million-unit (263-microgram) vial = £67.09 (both with 1-mL prefilled syringe water for injections)
Excipients include phenylalanine (section 9.4.1)

9

Nutrition and blood

9.2 Fluids and electrolytes

9.2.1 Oral preparations for fluid and electrolyte imbalance
9.2.2 Parenteral preparations for fluid and electrolyte imbalance

The following tables give a selection of useful electrolyte values:

Electrolyte concentrations—intravenous fluids

Intravenous infusion	Millimoles per litre				
	Na⁺	K⁺	HCO₃⁻	Cl⁻	Ca²⁺
Normal plasma values	142	4.5	26	103	2.5
Sodium Chloride 0.9%	150	—	—	150	—
Compound Sodium Lactate (Hartmann's)	131	5	29	111	2
Sodium Chloride 0.45% and Glucose 5%	75	—	—	75	—
Potassium Chloride 0.15% and Glucose 5%	—	20	—	20	—
Potassium Chloride 0.15% and Sodium Chloride 0.9%	150	20	—	170	—
Potassium Chloride 0.3% and Glucose 5%	—	40	—	40	—
Potassium Chloride 0.3% and Sodium Chloride 0.9%	150	40	—	190	—
To correct metabolic acidosis					
Sodium Bicarbonate 1.26%	150	—	150	—	—
Sodium Bicarbonate 8.4% for cardiac arrest	1000	—	1000	—	—
Sodium Lactate (m/6)	167	—	167	—	—

Electrolyte content—gastro-intestinal secretions

Type of fluid	Millimoles per litre				
	H⁺	Na⁺	K⁺	HCO₃⁻	Cl⁻
Gastric	40–60	20–80	5–20	—	100–150
Biliary	—	120–140	5–15	30–50	80–120
Pancreatic	—	120–140	5–15	70–110	40–80
Small bowel	—	120–140	5–15	20–40	90–130

Faeces, vomit, or aspiration should be saved and analysed where possible if abnormal losses are suspected; where this is impracticable the approximations above may be helpful in planning replacement therapy

9.2.1 Oral preparations for fluid and electrolyte imbalance

9.2.1.1 Oral potassium
9.2.1.2 Oral sodium and water
9.2.1.3 Oral bicarbonate

Sodium and potassium salts, which may be given by mouth to prevent deficiencies or to treat established deficiencies of mild or moderate degree, are discussed in this section. Oral preparations for removing excess potassium and preparations for oral rehydration therapy are also included here. Oral bicarbonate, for metabolic acidosis, is also described in this section.

For reference to calcium, magnesium, and phosphate, see section 9.5.

9.2.1.1 Oral potassium

Compensation for potassium loss is especially necessary:

- in children in whom secondary hyperaldosteronism occurs, e.g. renal artery stenosis, renal tubule disorder, the nephrotic syndrome, and severe heart failure;

- in children with excessive losses of potassium in the faeces, e.g. chronic diarrhoea associated with intestinal malabsorption or laxative abuse;

- in those taking digoxin or anti-arrhythmic drugs, where potassium depletion may induce arrhythmias.

Measures to compensate for potassium loss may be required during long-term administration of drugs known to induce potassium loss (e.g. corticosteroids).

9 Nutrition and blood

Potassium supplements are **seldom required** with the small doses of diuretics given to treat hypertension; **potassium-sparing diuretics** (rather than potassium supplements) are recommended for prevention of hypokalaemia due to diuretics such as furosemide (frusemide) or the thiazides when these are given to eliminate oedema.

Dosage If potassium salts are used for the *prevention of hypokalaemia*, then doses of potassium chloride 1–2 mmol/kg (usual max. 50 mmol potassium) daily by mouth are suitable in patients taking a normal diet. *Smaller doses* must be used if there is *renal insufficiency* otherwise there is **danger of hyperkalaemia**. Potassium salts cause nausea and vomiting therefore poor compliance is a major limitation to their effectiveness (small divided doses may minimise gastric irritation); where appropriate, potassium-sparing diuretics are preferable (see also above). Regular monitoring of plasma-potassium concentration is essential in those receiving potassium supplements. When there is *established potassium depletion* larger doses may be necessary, the quantity depending on the severity of any continuing potassium loss (monitoring of plasma-potassium concentration and specialist advice would be required). Potassium depletion is frequently associated with chloride depletion and with metabolic alkalosis, and these disorders require correction.

Administration Potassium salts are preferably given as a liquid (or effervescent) preparation, rather than modified-release tablets; they should be given as the chloride (the use of effervescent potassium tablets BPC 1968 should be restricted to *hyperchloraemic states*, section 9.2.1.3). Potassium chloride solutions suitable for use by mouth in neonates are available from 'special-order' manufacturers or specialist importing companies, see p. 943; they should be used with care because they are hypertonic and can damage the gastric mucosa.

Salt substitutes A number of salt substitutes which contain significant amounts of potassium chloride are readily available as health food products (e.g. *LoSalt*® and *Ruthmol*®). These should not be used by patients with renal failure as potassium intoxication may result.

◢ POTASSIUM CHLORIDE

Cautions intestinal stricture, history of peptic ulcer, hiatus hernia (for modified-release preparations); **important:** special hazard if given with drugs liable to raise plasma-potassium concentration such as potassium-sparing diuretics, ACE inhibitors, or ciclosporin, for other **interactions:** Appendix 1 (potassium salts)

Renal impairment close monitoring required—high risk of hyperkalaemia; avoid in severe impairment

Contra-indications plasma-potassium concentration above 5 mmol/litre

Side-effects nausea and vomiting (severe symptoms may indicate obstruction), oesophageal or small bowel ulceration

Indication and dose

Potassium depletion
• By mouth

> **Neonate** 0.5–1 mmol/kg K^+ twice daily (total daily dose may alternatively be given in 3 divided doses), adjusted according to plasma-potassium concentration

> **Child 1 month–18 years** 0.5–1 mmol/kg K^+ twice daily (total daily dose may alternatively be given in 3 divided doses), adjusted according to plasma-potassium concentration

Note Do not confuse Effervescent Potassium Tablets BPC 1968 (section 9.2.1.3) with effervescent potassium chloride tablets. Effervescent Potassium Tablets BPC 1968 do not contain chloride ions and their use should be restricted to hyperchloraemic states (section 9.2.1.3).

Kay-Cee-L® (Geistlich)
Syrup, sugar-free, red, potassium chloride 7.5% (1 mmol/mL each of K^+ and Cl^-), net price 500 mL = £3.74. Label: 21

Sando-K® (HK Pharma)
Tablets, effervescent, potassium bicarbonate and chloride equivalent to potassium 470 mg (12 mmol of K^+) and chloride 285 mg (8 mmol of Cl^-). Net price 20 = £1.53. Label: 13, 21

◢Modified-release preparations
Avoid unless effervescent tablets or liquid preparations inappropriate

Slow-K® (Alliance) ◢
Tablets, m/r, orange, s/c, potassium chloride 600 mg (8 mmol each of K^+ and Cl^-). Net price 20 = 54p. Label: 25, 27, counselling, swallow whole with fluid during meals while sitting or standing

---

◢ Management of hyperkalaemia

Acute severe hyperkalaemia calls for urgent treatment with intravenous infusion of **soluble insulin** (0.3–0.6 units/kg/hour in neonates and 0.05–0.2 units/kg/hour in children over 1 month) with **glucose** 0.5–1 g/kg/hour (5–10 mL/kg of glucose 10%; 2.5–5 mL/kg of glucose 20% via a central venous catheter may also be considered). If insulin cannot be used, **salbutamol** (section 3.1.1.1) can be given

9

Nutrition and blood

by intravenous infusion but it has a slower onset of action and may be less effective for reducing plasma-potassium concentration.

Calcium gluconate (section 9.5.1.1) is given by slow intravenous injection to manage cardiac excitability caused by hyperkalaemia.

The correction of causal or compounding acidosis with sodium bicarbonate infusion (section 9.2.2.1) should be considered (**important**: preparations of sodium bicarbonate and calcium salts should not be administered in the same line—risk of precipitation). Intravenous furosemide can also be given but is less effective in children with renal impairment. Drugs exacerbating hyperkalaemia should be reviewed and stopped as appropriate; dialysis may occasionally be required.

Ion-exchange resins may be used to remove excess potassium in *mild hyperkalaemia* or in *moderate hyperkalaemia* when there are no ECG changes. Calcium polystyrene sulphonate is preferred unless plasma-calcium concentrations are high.

POLYSTYRENE SULPHONATE RESINS

Cautions impaction of resin with excessive dosage or inadequate dilution; monitor for electrolyte disturbances (stop if plasma-potassium concentration below 5 mmol/litre); pregnancy and breast-feeding; sodium-containing resin in congestive heart failure, hypertension, renal impairment, and oedema; **interactions:** Appendix 1 (polystyrene sulphonate resins)

Contra-indications obstructive bowel disease; oral administration or reduced gut motility in neonates; avoid calcium-containing resin in hyperparathyroidism, multiple myeloma, sarcoidosis, or metastatic carcinoma

Side-effects rectal ulceration following rectal administration; colonic necrosis reported following enemas containing sorbitol; sodium retention, hypercalcaemia, gastric irritation, anorexia, nausea and vomiting, constipation (discontinue treatment—avoid magnesium-containing laxatives), diarrhoea; calcium-containing resin can cause hypercalcaemia (in dialysed patients and occasionally in those with renal impairment), hypomagnesaemia

Licensed use licensed for use in children

Indication and dose

Hyperkalaemia associated with anuria or severe oliguria, and in dialysis patients
• By mouth

Neonate not recommended

Child 1 month–18 years 125–250 mg/kg (max. 15 g) 3–4 times daily

• By rectum

Neonate 125–250 mg/kg repeated as necessary every 6–8 hours. Irrigate colon to remove resin after 6–12 hours

Child 1 month–18 years 125–250 mg/kg repeated as necessary every 6–8 hours. Irrigate colon to remove resin after 6–12 hours

Administration By mouth: administer in water or as a paste—do not give with fruit squash, which has a high potassium content.

By rectum: mix 1 g of resin with 5–10 mL of a methylcellulose solution. Water may be used but retention is more difficult.

Calcium Resonium® (Sanofi-Synthelabo)
Powder, buff, calcium polystyrene sulphonate. Net price 300 g = £47.55. Label: 13

Resonium A® (Sanofi-Synthelabo)
Powder, buff, sodium polystyrene sulphonate. Net price 454 g = £70.24. Label: 13

9.2.1.2 Oral sodium and water

Sodium chloride is indicated in states of sodium depletion. In preterm neonates in the first few weeks of life and in chronic conditions associated with mild or moderate degrees of sodium depletion, e.g. in salt-losing bowel or renal disease, oral supplements of sodium chloride (section 9.2.1.3) may be sufficient. Sodium chloride solutions suitable for use by mouth in neonates are available from 'special-order' manufacturers or specialist importing companies, see p. 943; they should be used with care because they are hypertonic. Supplementation with sodium chloride may be required to replace losses in children with cystic fibrosis particularly in warm weather.

Nutrition and blood

9

■ SODIUM CHLORIDE

Indication and dose

See also section 9.2.2

Sodium supplementation in neonates
● **By mouth**

Preterm neonate 2 mmol/100 mL of formula feed or 3–4 mmol/100 mL of breast milk, consult dietician

Sodium replacement
● **By mouth**

Child 1 month–18 years According to requirements, generally 1–2 mmol/kg daily in divided doses, higher doses may be needed in severe depletion

Chronic renal loss
● **By mouth**

Child 1 month–18 years 1–2 mmol/kg daily in divided doses, adjusted according to requirements

Slow Sodium® (HK Pharma)
Tablets, m/r, sodium chloride 600 mg (approx. 10 mmol each of Na^+ and Cl^-). Net price 100-tab pack = £6.05. Label: 25

Capsules available from 'special-order' manufacturers or specialist importing companies, see p. 943

◢Extemporaneous formulations available see Extemporaneous Preparations, p. 8

Oral rehydration therapy (ORT)

Diarrhoea in children is usually self-limiting, however, in children under 6 months of age, and more particularly in those under 3 months, symptoms of dehydration may be less obvious and there is a risk of rapid and severe deterioration. Intestinal absorption of sodium and water is enhanced by glucose (and other carbohydrates). Replacement of fluid and electrolytes lost through diarrhoea can therefore be achieved by giving solutions containing sodium, potassium, and glucose or another carbohydrate such as rice starch.

Oral rehydration solutions should:

● enhance the absorption of water and electrolytes;

● replace the electrolyte deficit adequately and safely;

● contain an alkalinising agent to counter acidosis;

● be slightly hypo-osmolar (about 250 mmol/litre) to prevent the possible induction of osmotic diarrhoea;

● be simple to use in hospital and at home;

● be palatable and acceptable, especially to children;

● be readily available.

It is the policy of the World Health Organization (WHO) to promote a single oral rehydration solution but to use it flexibly (e.g. by giving extra water between drinks of oral rehydration solution to moderately dehydrated infants).

Oral rehydration solutions used in the UK are lower in sodium (50–60 mmol/litre) than the WHO formulation since, in general, patients suffer less severe sodium loss.

Rehydration should be rapid over 3 to 4 hours (except in hypernatraemic dehydration in which case rehydration should occur more slowly over 12 hours). The patient should be reassessed after initial rehydration and if still dehydrated rapid fluid replacement should continue.

Once rehydration is complete further dehydration is prevented by encouraging the patient to drink normal volumes of an appropriate fluid and by replacing continuing losses with an oral rehydration solution; in infants, breast-feeding or formula feeds should be offered between oral rehydration drinks.

For intravenous rehydration see section 9.2.2.

■ ORAL REHYDRATION SALTS (ORS)

Licensed use *Dioralyte® Relief* not licensed for use in children under 3 months

Indication and dose

Fluid and electrolyte loss in diarrhoea see notes above
● **By mouth**

Child 1 month–1 year 1–1½ times usual feed volume

◻ **ORAL REHYDRATION SALTS (ORS)** (*continued*)

Child 1–12 years 200 mL after every loose motion

Child 12–18 years 200–400 mL after every loose motion

◢**UK formulations**

Note After reconstitution any unused solution should be discarded no later than 1 hour after preparation unless stored in a refrigerator when it may be kept for up to 24 hours.

Dioralyte® (Sanofi-Aventis)

Oral powder, sodium chloride 470 mg, potassium chloride 300 mg, disodium hydrogen citrate 530 mg, glucose 3.56 g/sachet, net price 6-sachet pack = £2.11, 20-sachet pack (black currant- or citrus-flavoured or natural) = £6.99

Note Reconstitute 1 sachet with 200 mL of water (freshly boiled and cooled for infants); 5 sachets reconstituted with 1 litre of water provide Na$^+$ 60 mmol, K$^+$ 20 mmol, Cl$^-$ 60 mmol, citrate 10 mmol, and glucose 90 mmol

Dioralyte® Relief (Sanofi-Aventis)

Oral powder, sodium chloride 350 mg, potassium chloride 300 mg, sodium citrate 580 mg, cooked rice powder 6 g/sachet, net price 6-sachet pack (apricot-, black currant- or raspberry-flavoured) = £2.35, 20-sachet pack (apricot-flavoured) = £7.42

Note Reconstitute 1 sachet with 200 mL of water (freshly boiled and cooled for infants); 5 sachets when reconsti-

tuted with 1 litre of water provide Na$^+$ 60 mmol, K$^+$ 20 mmol, Cl$^-$ 50 mmol and citrate 10 mmol; contains aspartame (section 9.4.1)

Electrolade® (Actavis)

Oral powder, sodium chloride 236 mg, potassium chloride 300 mg, sodium bicarbonate 500 mg, anhydrous glucose 4 g/sachet (banana-, black currant-, lemon and lime-, or orange-flavoured). Net price 6-sachet (plain or multiflavoured) pack = £1.33, 20-sachet (single- or multiflavoured) pack = £4.99

Note Reconstitute 1 sachet with 200 mL of water (freshly boiled and cooled for infants); 5 sachets when reconstituted with 1 litre of water provide Na$^+$ 50 mmol, K$^+$ 20 mmol, Cl$^-$ 40 mmol, HCO$_3$$^-$ 30 mmol, and glucose 111 mmol

◢**WHO formulation**

Oral Rehydration Salts (Non-proprietary)

Oral powder, sodium chloride 2.6 g, potassium chloride 1.5 g, sodium citrate 2.9 g, anhydrous glucose 13.5 g. To be dissolved in sufficient water to produce 1 litre (providing Na$^+$ 75 mmol, K$^+$ 20 mmol, Cl$^-$ 65 mmol, citrate 10 mmol, glucose 75 mmol/litre)

Note Recommended by the WHO and the United Nations Children's Fund but not commonly used in the UK

9.2.1.3 Oral bicarbonate

Sodium bicarbonate is given by mouth for *chronic acidotic states* such as uraemic acidosis or renal tubular acidosis. The dose for correction of metabolic acidosis is not predictable and the response must be assessed. For *severe metabolic acidosis*, sodium bicarbonate can be given intravenously (section 9.2.2).

Sodium supplements may increase blood pressure or cause fluid retention and pulmonary oedema in those at risk; hypokalaemia may be exacerbated.

Sodium bicarbonate may affect the stability or absorption of other drugs if administered at the same time. If possible, allow 1–2 hours before administering other drugs orally.

Where *hyperchloraemic acidosis* is associated with potassium deficiency, as in some renal tubular and gastro-intestinal disorders it may be appropriate to give oral **potassium bicarbonate**, although acute or severe deficiency should be managed by intravenous therapy.

◢ **SODIUM BICARBONATE**

Cautions see notes above; avoid in respiratory acidosis; **interactions:** Appendix 1 (antacids)

Indication and dose

Renal acidosis (see also notes above)
• By mouth

Neonate initially 1–2 mmol/kg daily in divided doses

Child 1 month–18 years initially 1–2 mmol/kg daily in divided doses, adjusted according to response

Metabolic acidosis section 9.2.2.1

Renal hyperkalaemia section 9.2.2.1

Sodium Bicarbonate (Non-proprietary)

Capsules, sodium bicarbonate 500 mg (approx. 6 mmol each of Na$^+$ and HCO$_3$$^-$), net price 56-cap pack = £13.07

Tablets, sodium bicarbonate 600 mg, net price 100 tabs = £2.48

Important Oral solutions of sodium bicarbonate are required occasionally; these need to be obtained from 'special-order' manufacturers or specialist importing companies, see p. 943, and the strength of sodium bicarbonate should be stated on the prescription

9 Nutrition and blood

■ POTASSIUM BICARBONATE

Cautions cardiac disease, **interactions:** Appendix 1 (potassium salts)

Renal impairment close monitoring required— high risk of hyperkalaemia; avoid in severe impairment

Contra-indications hypochloraemia; plasma-potassium concentration above 5 mmol/litre

Side-effects nausea and vomiting

Potassium Tablets, Effervescent (Non-proprietary)
Effervescent tablets, potassium bicarbonate 500 mg, potassium acid tartrate 300 mg, each tablet providing 6.5 mmol of K^+. To be dissolved in water before administration. Net price 56 = £28.20.
Label: 13, 21

Note These tablets do not contain chloride; for effervescent tablets containing potassium and chloride, see under Potassium Chloride, section 9.2.1.1

9.2.2 Parenteral preparations for fluid and electrolyte imbalance

9.2.2.1 Electrolytes and water
9.2.2.2 Plasma and plasma substitutes

9.2.2.1 Electrolytes and water

Solutions of electrolytes are given intravenously, to meet normal fluid and electrolyte requirements or to replenish substantial deficits or continuing losses when it is not possible or desirable to use the oral route. When intravenous administration is not possible, fluid (as sodium chloride 0.9% or glucose 5%) can also be given subcutaneously by hypodermoclysis.

In an individual patient the nature and severity of the electrolyte imbalance must be assessed from the history and clinical and biochemical examination. Sodium, potassium, chloride, magnesium, phosphate, and water depletion can occur singly and in combination with or without disturbances of acid-base balance; for reference to the use of magnesium and phosphates, see section 9.5.

Isotonic solutions may be infused safely into a peripheral vein. Solutions more concentrated than plasma, for example 15% glucose, are best given through an indwelling catheter positioned in a large vein.

Maintenance fluid requirements in children are usually derived from the relationship that exists between body-weight and metabolic rate; the figures in the table below may be used as a guide outside the neonatal period. The glucose requirement is that needed to minimise gluconeogenesis from amino acids obtained as substrate from muscle breakdown. Maintenance fluids are intended only to provide hydration for a short period until enteral or parenteral nutrition can be established.

It is usual to meet these requirements by using a standard solution of sodium chloride and glucose. Solutions containing 20 mmol/litre of potassium chloride meet usual potassium requirements when given in the suggested volumes; adjustments may be needed if there is an inability to excrete fluids or electrolytes, excessive renal loss or continuing extra-renal losses. The exact requirements depend upon the nature of the clinical situation and types of losses incurred; see Caution on dilutional hyponatraemia below.

Fluid requirements for children over 1 month:	
Body-weight	**24-hour fluid requirement**
Under 10 kg	100 mL/kg
10–20 kg	100 mL/kg for the first 10 kg
	+ 50 mL/kg for each 1 kg body-weight over 10 kg
Over 20 kg	100 mL/kg for the first 10 kg
	+ 50 mL/kg for each 1 kg body-weight between 10–20 kg
	+ 20 mL/kg for each 1 kg body-weight over 20 kg
	(max. 2 litres in females, 2.5 litres in males)

Important The baseline fluid requirements shown in the table above should be adjusted to take account of factors that reduce water loss (e.g. increased antidiuretic hormone, renal failure, hypothermia, and high ambient humidity) or increase water loss (e.g. pyrexia or burns).

9

Nutrition and blood

Caution During parenteral hydration, fluids and electrolytes should be monitored closely and any disturbance corrected by slow infusion of an appropriate solution. The volume of fluid infused should take into account the possibility of reduced fluid loss owing to increased antidiuretic hormone and factors such as renal failure, hypothermia, and high humidity.

Dilutional hyponatraemia is a rare but potentially fatal risk of parenteral hydration. It may be caused by inappropriate use of hypotonic fluids such as sodium chloride 0.18% and glucose 4% intravenous infusion, especially in the postoperative period when antidiuretic hormone secretion is increased. Dilutional hyponatraemia is characterized by a rapid fall in plasma-sodium concentration leading to cerebral oedema and seizures; any child with severe hyponatraemia or rapidly changing plasma-sodium concentration should be referred urgently to a paediatric high dependency facility.

> **Safe practice**
> Sodium chloride 0.18% and glucose 4% intravenous infusion fluid should not generally be used for fluid replacement in children because of the risk of hyponatraemia; availability of this infusion should be restricted to critical care and specialist wards, such as renal, liver, and cardiac units. Local guidelines on intravenous fluids should be consulted.

Replacement therapy: initial intravenous replacement fluid is generally required if the child is over 10% dehydrated, or if 5–10% dehydrated and oral or enteral rehydration is not tolerated or possible. Oral rehydration is adequate, if tolerated, in the majority of those less than 10% dehydrated. Subsequent fluid and electrolyte requirements are determined by clinical assessment of fluid balance.

Neonates Neonates lose water through the skin and nose, particularly if preterm or if the skin is damaged. The basic fluid requirement for a term baby in average ambient humidity is 40–60 mL/kg/day plus urinary losses. Preterm babies have very high transepidermal losses particularly in the first few days of life; they may need more fluid replacement than full term babies and up to 180 mL/kg/day may be required. Local guidelines for fluid management in the neonatal period should be consulted.

Intravenous sodium

Intravenous sodium chloride in isotonic (0.9%) solution provides the most important extracellular ions in near physiological concentration and is indicated in *sodium depletion*. It may be given for initial treatment of acute fluid loss and to replace ongoing gastro-intestinal losses from the upper gastro-intestinal tract. Intravenous sodium chloride is commonly given as a component of maintenance and replacement therapy, usually in combination with other electrolytes and glucose, see notes above. Sodium chloride solutions should be used cautiously in renal insufficiency, cardiac failure, cardio-respiratory diseases, hepatic cirrhosis and in children receiving glucocorticoids. Hyponatraemia with serious consequences may occur if maintenance and replacement fluids do not meet sodium requirements (see Caution, dilutional hyponatraemia, above).

Chronic hyponatraemia should ideally be corrected by fluid restriction. However, if sodium chloride is required, the deficit should be corrected slowly to avoid the risk of osmotic demyelination syndrome; the rise in plasma-sodium concentration should be no more than 10 mmol/litre in 24 hours.

Sodium chloride and glucose solutions are indicated when there is combined *water and sodium depletion*. A 1:1 mixture of isotonic sodium chloride and 5% glucose allows some of the water (free of sodium) to enter body cells which suffer most from dehydration while the sodium salt with a volume of water determined by the normal plasma Na^+ remains extracellular. Maintenance fluid should accurately reflect daily requirements and close monitoring is required to avoid fluid and electrolyte imbalance. Illness or injury increase the secretion of antidiuretic hormone and therefore the ability to excrete excess water may be impaired. Injudicious use of hypotonic solutions such as sodium chloride 0.18% and glucose 4% may also cause dilutional hyponatraemia especially in children (see Caution on dilutional hyponatraemia, above); if necessary, guidance should be sought from a clinician experienced in the management of fluid and electrolytes.

Combined sodium, potassium, chloride, and water depletion may occur, for example, with severe diarrhoea or persistent vomiting; replacement is carried out with sodium chloride intravenous infusion 0.9% and glucose intravenous infusion 5% with potassium as appropriate.

Compound sodium lactate (Hartmann's solution) can be used instead of isotonic sodium chloride solution during surgery or in the initial management of the injured or wounded.

Neonates   The sodium requirement for most healthy neonates is 3 mmol/kg daily. Preterm neonates, particularly below 30 weeks gestation, may require up to 6 mmol/kg daily. *Hyponatraemia* may be caused by excessive renal loss of sodium; it may also be dilutional and restriction of fluid intake may be appropriate. Sodium supplementation is likely to be required if the serum sodium concentration is significantly reduced.

Hypernatraemia may also occur, most often due to dehydration (e.g. breast milk insufficiency). Severe hypernatraemia and hyponatraemia can cause fits and rarely brain damage. Sodium in drug preparations, delivered via continuous infusions, or in infusions to maintain the patency of intravascular or umbilical lines, can result in significant amounts of sodium being delivered, (e.g. 1 mL/hour of 0.9% sodium chloride infused over 24 hours is equivalent to 3.6 mmol/day of sodium).

■ SODIUM CHLORIDE

Cautions   restrict intake in impaired renal function, cardiac failure, hypertension, peripheral and pulmonary oedema, toxaemia of pregnancy; see also notes above

Side-effects   administration of large doses may give rise to sodium accumulation and oedema

Indication and dose

Electrolyte imbalance see notes above, also section 9.2.1.2

Sodium Chloride (Non-proprietary) PoM
Intravenous infusion, usual strength sodium chloride 0.9% (9 g, 150 mmol each of Na^+ and Cl^-/litre), this strength being supplied when normal saline for injection is requested. Net price 2-mL amp = 29p; 5-mL amp = 35p; 10-mL amp = 46p; 20-mL amp = £1.04; 50-mL amp = £2.01
In hospitals, 500- and 1000-mL packs, and sometimes other sizes, are available
Note The term 'normal saline' should **not** be used to describe sodium chloride intravenous infusion 0.9%; the term 'physiological saline' is acceptable but it is preferable to give the composition (i.e. sodium chloride intravenous infusion 0.9%).

◢With other ingredients
Note See above for warning on hyponatraemia

Sodium Chloride and Glucose (Non-proprietary) PoM
Intravenous infusion, sodium chloride 0.18% (Na^+ and Cl^- each 30 mmol/litre), glucose 4%
In hospitals, usually 500-mL packs and sometimes other sizes are available

Intravenous infusion, sodium chloride 0.45% (Na^+ and Cl^- each 75 mmol/litre), glucose 5%
In hospitals, usually 500-mL packs and sometimes other sizes are available

Intravenous infusion, sodium chloride 0.9% (Na^+ and Cl^- each 150 mmol/litre), glucose 5%
In hospitals, usually 500-mL packs and sometimes other sizes are available

Ringer's Solution (Non-proprietary) PoM
Calcium chloride (dihydrate) 322 micrograms, potassium chloride 300 micrograms, sodium chloride 8.6 mg/mL, providing the following ions (in mmol/litre), Ca^{2+} 2.2, K^+ 4, Na^+ 147, Cl^- 156
In hospitals, 500- and 1000-mL packs, and sometimes other sizes, are available

Sodium Lactate, Compound (Non-proprietary) PoM
(Hartmann's Solution; Ringer-Lactate Solution)
Intravenous infusion, sodium chloride 0.6%, sodium lactate 0.32%, potassium chloride 0.04%, calcium chloride 0.027% (containing Na^+ 131 mmol, K^+ 5 mmol, Ca^{2+} 2 mmol, HCO_3^- (as lactate) 29 mmol, Cl^- 111 mmol/litre)
In hospitals, 500- and 1000-mL packs, and sometimes other sizes, are available

---

▬ Intravenous glucose

Glucose solutions are used mainly to replace water deficit and should be given alone only when there is no significant loss of electrolytes; prolonged administration of glucose solutions without electrolytes can lead to hyponatraemia and other electrolyte disturbances. Water depletion (dehydration) tends to occur when losses are not matched by a comparable intake, as may occur in coma or dysphagia.

Water loss rarely exceeds electrolyte losses but this can occur in fevers, hyperthyroidism, and in uncommon water-losing renal states such as diabetes insipidus or hypercalcaemia. The volume of glucose solution needed to replace deficits varies with the severity of the disorder; the rate of infusion should be adjusted to return the plasma-sodium concentration to normal over 48 hours.

Glucose solutions are also used to correct and prevent hypoglycaemia and to provide a source of energy in those too ill to be fed adequately by mouth; glucose solutions are a key component of parenteral nutrition (section 9.3).

Glucose solutions are given with insulin for the emergency management of *hyperkalaemia* (see p. 547). They are also given, after correction of hyperglycaemia, during treatment of diabetic ketoacidosis, when they must be accompanied by continuous insulin infusion (section 6.1.3).

Injections containing more than 10% glucose can be irritant and should be given into a central venous line; however, solutions containing up to 12.5% can be administered for a short period into a peripheral line.

GLUCOSE
(Dextrose Monohydrate)
Note Glucose BP is the monohydrate but Glucose Intravenous Infusion BP is a sterile solution of anhydrous glucose or glucose monohydrate, potency being expressed in terms of anhydrous glucose

Side-effects glucose injections especially if hypertonic may have a low pH and may cause venous irritation and thrombophlebitis

Indication and dose

Fluid replacement see notes above

Provision of energy section 9.3

Hypoglycaemia section 6.1.4

Glucose (Non-proprietary) ⒫ⓄⓂ
Intravenous infusion, glucose or anhydrous glucose (potency expressed in terms of anhydrous glucose), usual strengths 5% (50 mg/mL) and 10% (100 mg/mL); 25% solution, net price 25-mL amp = £2.21; 50% solution[1], 20-mL amp = 95 p, 50-mL amp = £1.63
In hospitals, 500- and 1000-mL packs, and sometimes other sizes and strengths, are available; also available *Min-I-Jet® Glucose*, 50% in 50-mL disposable syringe[1]
1. ⒫ⓄⓂ restriction does not apply where administration is for saving life in emergency

Intravenous potassium

Potassium chloride and sodium chloride intravenous infusion is the initial treatment for the correction of *severe hypokalaemia* and when sufficient potassium cannot be taken by mouth. Ready-mixed infusion solutions should be used when possible (see under Safe Practice below); for peripheral intravenous infusion, the concentration of potassium should not usually exceed 40 mmol/litre. Potassium infusions should be given slowly over at least 2–3 hours and at a rate not exceeding 0.2 mmol/kg/hour with specialist advice and ECG monitoring in difficult cases. Higher concentrations of potassium chloride or faster infusion rates may be given in very severe depletion, but require specialist advice.

Repeated measurements of plasma-potassium concentration are necessary to determine whether further infusions are required and to avoid the development of hyperkalaemia, which is especially likely in renal impairment.

Initial potassium replacement therapy should **not** involve glucose infusions, because glucose may cause a further decrease in the plasma-potassium concentration.

> Safe Practice
> Potassium overdose can be fatal. Ready-mixed infusion solutions containing potassium should be used. Exceptionally, if potassium chloride concentrate is used for preparing an infusion, the infusion solution should be **thoroughly mixed**. Local policies on avoiding inadvertent use of potassium chloride concentrate should be followed.

POTASSIUM CHLORIDE

Cautions for peripheral intravenous infusion the concentration of solution should not usually exceed 3 g (40 mmol)/litre; specialist advice and ECG monitoring (see notes above); **interactions:** Appendix 1 (potassium salts)

Renal impairment close monitoring required— high risk of hyperkalaemia; avoid in severe impairment

Contra-indications plasma-potassium concentration above 5 mmol/litre

◻ **POTASSIUM CHLORIDE** (*continued*)

Side-effects rapid infusion toxic to heart

Indication and dose

Electrolyte imbalance see also oral potassium supplements, section 9.2.1.1

• **By slow intravenous infusion**
depending on the deficit or the daily maintenance requirements, see also notes above

Neonate 1–2 mmol/kg daily

Child 1 month–18 years 1–2 mmol/kg daily

Administration see notes above

Potassium Chloride and Glucose (Non-proprietary) [PoM]

Intravenous infusion, usual strengths potassium chloride 0.3% (3 g, 40 mmol each of K^+ and Cl^-/litre) or 0.15% (1.5 g, 20 mmol each of K^+ and Cl^-/litre) with 5% of anhydrous glucose
In hospitals, 500- and 1000-mL packs, and sometimes other sizes, are available

Potassium Chloride and Sodium Chloride (Non-proprietary) [PoM]

Intravenous infusion, usual strength potassium chloride 0.15% (1.5 g/litre) with sodium chloride 0.9% (9 g/litre), containing K^+ 20 mmol, Na^+ 150 mmol, and Cl^- 170 mmol/litre
In hospitals, 500- and 1000-mL packs, and sometimes other sizes, are available

Potassium Chloride, Sodium Chloride, and Glucose (Non-proprietary) [PoM]

Intravenous infusion, sodium chloride 0.45% (4.5 g, Na^+ 75 mmol/litre) with 5% of anhydrous glucose and usually sufficient potassium chloride to provide K^+ 10–40 mmol/litre (to be specified by the prescriber)
In hospitals, 500- and 1000-mL packs, and sometimes other sizes, are available

Potassium Chloride (Non-proprietary) [PoM]

Sterile concentrate, potassium chloride 15% (150 mg, approximately 2 mmol each of K^+ and Cl^-/mL). Net price 10-mL amp = 48p
Solutions containing 10 and 20% of potassium chloride are also available in both 5- and 10-mL ampoules
Important Must be diluted with **not less** than 50 times its volume of Sodium Chloride 0.9% or other suitable diluent and **mixed well**; see Safe Practice, above

---

Bicarbonate and trometamol

Sodium bicarbonate is used to control severe *metabolic acidosis* (pH < 7.1) particularly that caused by loss of bicarbonate (as in renal tubular acidosis or from excessive gastro-intestinal losses). Mild metabolic acidosis associated with volume depletion should first be managed by appropriate fluid replacement because acidosis usually resolves as tissue and renal perfusion are restored. In more severe metabolic acidosis or when the acidosis remains unresponsive to correction of anoxia or hypovolaemia, sodium bicarbonate (1.26%) can be infused over 3–4 hours with plasma-pH and electrolyte monitoring. In severe shock (section 2.7.1), for example in cardiac arrest, metabolic acidosis can develop without sodium depletion; in these circumstances sodium bicarbonate is best given intravenously as a small volume of hypertonic solution, such as 8.4%; plasma pH and electrolytes should be monitored. For *chronic acidotic states*, sodium bicarbonate can be given by mouth (section 9.2.1.3).

Trometamol (tris(hydroxymethyl)aminomethane, THAM), an organic buffer, corrects metabolic acidosis by causing an increase in urinary pH and an osmotic diuresis. It is indicated when sodium bicarbonate is unsuitable as in carbon dioxide retention, hypernatraemia, or renal impairment. Respiratory support may be required because trometamol induces respiratory depression. It is also used during cardiac bypass surgery and, very rarely, in cardiac arrest.

SODIUM BICARBONATE

Indication and dose

Metabolic acidosis see also notes above

• **By slow intravenous injection of a strong solution (up to 8.4%), or by continuous intravenous infusion of a weaker solution (usually 1.26%)**
an amount appropriate to the body base deficit

Renal hyperkalaemia
• **By slow intravenous injection**

Neonate 1 mmol/kg daily

Child 1 month–18 years 1 mmol/kg daily

Renal acidosis section 9.2.1.3

Sodium Bicarbonate [PoM]

Intravenous infusion, usual strength sodium bicarbonate 1.26% (12.6 g, 150 mmol each of Na^+ and HCO_3^-/litre); various other strengths available
In hospitals, 500- and 1000-mL packs, and sometimes other sizes, are available

Administration For *peripheral infusion* dilute 8.4% solution at least 1 in 10; for *central line infusion* dilute 1 in 5 with Glucose 5% or 10% *or* Sodium Chloride 0.9%. Extravasation can cause severe tissue damage

◁ **SODIUM BICARBONATE** (*continued*)

Min-I-Jet® Sodium Bicarbonate (UCB Pharma) PoM
Intravenous injection, sodium bicarbonate in disposable syringe, net price 4.2%, 10 mL = £5.82; 8.4%, 10 mL = £6.00, 50 mL = £8.14

◤ TROMETAMOL

(Tris(hydroxymethyl)aminomethane, THAM)

Cautions extravasation can cause severe tissue damage

Renal impairment use with caution, may cause hyperkalaemia

Pregnancy little information available, hypoglycaemia may harm fetus

Breast-feeding no information available

Contra-indications anuria; chronic respiratory acidosis

Side-effects respiratory depression; hypoglycaemia; hyperkalaemia in renal impairment; liver necrosis reported following administration via umbilical vein in neonates

Licensed use unlicensed preparation

Indication and dose

Metabolic acidosis
• By intravenous infusion
  an amount appropriate to the body base deficit

◢Preparations
Available from 'special-order' manufacturers or specialist importing companies, see p. 943

◤ Water

Water for Injections PoM
Net price 1-mL amp = 18p; 2-mL amp = 18p; 5-mL amp = 33p; 10-mL amp = 33p; 20-mL amp = 92p; 50-mL amp = £1.91; 100-mL vial = 23p

9.2.2.2 Plasma and plasma substitutes

Albumin solutions, prepared from whole blood, contain soluble proteins and electrolytes but no clotting factors, blood group antibodies, or plasma cholinesterases; they may be given without regard to the recipient's blood group.

Albumin is usually used after the acute phase of illness to correct a plasma-volume deficit; hypoalbuminaemia itself is not an appropriate indication. The use of albumin solutions in acute plasma or blood loss may be wasteful; plasma substitutes are more appropriate. Concentrated albumin solutions may also be used to obtain a diuresis in hypoalbuminaemic patients (e.g. in nephrotic syndrome).

Recent evidence does not support the previous view that the use of albumin increases mortality.

> Plasma and plasma substitutes are often used in very ill children whose condition is unstable. Therefore, close monitoring is required and fluid and electrolyte therapy should be adjusted according to the child's condition at all times.

◤ ALBUMIN SOLUTION

(Human Albumin Solution)

A solution containing protein derived from plasma, serum, or normal placentas; at least 95% of the protein is albumin. The solution may be isotonic (containing 3.5–5% protein) or concentrated (containing 15–25% protein).

Cautions history of cardiac or circulatory disease (administer slowly to avoid rapid rise in blood pressure and cardiac failure, and monitor cardiovascular and respiratory function); increased capillary permeability; correct dehydration when administering concentrated solution

Contra-indications cardiac failure; severe anaemia

Side-effects hypersensitivity reactions (including anaphylaxis) with nausea, vomiting, increased salivation, fever, tachycardia, hypotension and chills reported

Indication and dose
See under preparations, below

◢Isotonic solutions
Indications: acute or sub-acute loss of plasma volume e.g. in burns, pancreatitis, trauma, and complications of surgery; plasma exchange
Available as: *Human Albumin Solution 4.5%* (50-, 100-, 250- and 400-mL bottles—Baxter); Human Albumin Solution 5% (250- and 500-mL bottles—Baxter); *Octalbin®* 5% (100- and 250-mL bottles—Octapharm); *Zenalb®* 4.5% (50-, 100-, 250-, and 500-mL bottles—BPL)

9 Nutrition and blood

◁ **ALBUMIN SOLUTION** (*continued*)

◢Concentrated solutions (20%)

Indications: severe hypoalbuminaemia associated with low plasma volume and generalised oedema where salt and water restriction with plasma volume expansion are required; adjunct in the treatment of hyperbilirubinaemia by exchange

transfusion in the newborn; paracentesis of large volume ascites associated with portal hypertension

Available as: *Human Albumin Solution 20%* (50- and 100-mL vials—Baxter); *Flexbumin®* 20% (50- and 100-mL bags—Baxter); *Octalbin®* 20% (50- and 100-mL bottles—Octapharm); *Zenalb®* 20% (50- and 100-mL bottles—BPL)

Plasma substitutes

Gelatin and the **etherified starches** (**pentastarch** and **tetrastarch**) are macromolecular substances which are metabolised slowly; they may be used at the outset to expand and maintain blood volume in shock arising from conditions such as burns or septicaemia. Plasma substitutes may be used as an immediate short-term measure to treat haemorrhage until blood is available. They are rarely needed when shock is due to sodium and water depletion because, in these circumstances, the shock responds to water and electrolyte repletion; see also section 2.7.1 for the management of shock.

Plasma substitutes should **not** be used to maintain plasma volume in conditions such as burns or peritonitis where there is loss of plasma protein, water, and electrolytes over periods of several days or weeks. In these situations, plasma or plasma protein fractions containing large amounts of albumin should be given.

Large volumes of *some* plasma substitutes can increase the risk of bleeding through depletion of coagulation factors.

> Plasma and plasma substitutes are often used in very ill children whose condition is unstable. Therefore, close monitoring is required and fluid and electrolyte therapy should be adjusted according to the child's condition at all times.
>
> The use of plasma substitutes in children requires specialist supervision due to the risk of fluid overload; use is best restricted to an intensive care setting.

Cautions   Plasma substitutes should be used with caution in cardiac disease, liver disease, or renal impairment; urine output should be monitored. Care should be taken to avoid haematocrit concentration from falling below 25–30% and the child should be monitored for hypersensitivity reactions.

Side-effects   Hypersensitivity reactions may occur including, rarely, severe anaphylactoid reactions. Transient increase in bleeding time may occur.

◢ GELATIN

Note The gelatin is partially degraded

Cautions see notes above

  Pregnancy manufacturer of *Geloplasma®* advises avoid at the end of pregnancy

Side-effects see notes above

Indication and dose

  Low blood volume in hypovolaemic shock, burns and cardiopulmonary bypass

  • By intravenous infusion

    initially 10–20 mL/kg of a 3.5–4% solution (see notes above)

Gelofusine® (Braun) ᴾᵒᴹ

Intravenous infusion, succinylated gelatin (modified fluid gelatin, average molecular weight 30 000) 40 g (4%), Na⁺ 154 mmol, Cl⁻ 124 mmol/litre, net price 500-mL *Ecobag®* = £4.70; 1-litre *Ecobag®* = £9.45

Contains traces of calcium

Geloplasma® (Fresenius Kabi) ᴾᵒᴹ

Intravenous infusion, partially hydrolysed and succinylated gelatin (modified liquid gelatin) (as

anhydrous gelatin) 30 g (3%) , Na⁺ 150 mmol, K⁺ 5 mmol, Mg²⁺ 1.5 mmol, Cl⁻ 100 mmol, lactate 30 mmol/litre, net price 500-mL bag = £5.05

Haemaccel® (KoRa) ᴾᵒᴹ

Intravenous infusion, polygeline (gelatin derivative, average molecular weight 30 000) 35 g (3.5%), Na⁺ 145 mmol, K⁺ 5.1 mmol, Ca²⁺ 6.25 mmol, Cl⁻ 145 mmol/litre, net price 500-mL bottle = £5.00

Isoplex® (IS Pharmaceuticals) ᴾᵒᴹ

Intravenous infusion, succinylated gelatin (modified fluid gelatin, average molecular weight 30 000) 40 g (4%), Na⁺ 145 mmol, K⁺ 4 mmol, Mg²⁺ 0.9 mmol, Cl⁻ 105 mmol, lactate 25 mmol/litre, net price 500-mL bag = £7.53; 1-litre bag = £14.54

Volplex® (IS Pharmaceuticals) ᴾᵒᴹ

Intravenous infusion, succinylated gelatin (modified fluid gelatin, average molecular weight 30 000) 40 g (4%), Na⁺ 154 mmol, Cl⁻ 125 mmol/litre, net price 500-mL bag = £4.70; 1-litre bag = £9.09

■ ETHERIFIED STARCH

A starch composed of more than 90% of amylopectin that has been etherified with hydroxyethyl groups; the terms tetrastarch and pentastarch reflect the degree of etherification

Cautions see notes above

Side-effects see notes above; also pruritus, raised serum amylase

Indication and dose

Low blood volume
• **By intravenous infusion**
according to the child's condition (see notes above)

◀Pentastarch

HAES-steril® (Fresenius Kabi) (PoM)
Intravenous infusion, pentastarch (weight average molecular weight 200 000) 10% in sodium chloride intravenous infusion 0.9%, net price, 500 mL = £16.50

Hemohes® (Braun) (PoM)
Intravenous infusion, pentastarch (weight average molecular weight 200 000), net price (both in sodium chloride intravenous infusion 0.9%) 6%, 500 mL = £12.50; 10%, 500 mL = £16.50

◀Tetrastarch

Tetraspan® (Braun) (PoM)
Intravenous infusion, hydroxyethyl starch (weight average molecular weight 130 000) 6% in sodium chloride 0.625%, containing Na^+ 140 mmol, K^+ 4 mmol, Mg^{2+} 1 mmol, Cl^- 118 mmol, Ca^{2+} 2.5 mmol, acetate 24 mmol, malate 5 mmol/litre, net price 500-mL bag = £13.50

Volulyte® (Fresenius Kabi) (PoM)
Intravenous infusion, hydroxyethyl starch (weight average molecular weight 130 000) 6% in sodium chloride intravenous infusion 0.6%, containing Na^+ 137 mmol, K^+ 4 mmol, Mg^{2+} 1.5 mmol, Cl^- 110 mmol, acetate 34 mmol/litre, net price 500-mL bag = £13.50

Voluven® (Fresenius Kabi) (PoM)
Intravenous infusion, hydroxyethyl starch (weight average molecular weight 130 000) 6% in sodium chloride intravenous infusion 0.9%, net price 500-mL bag = £12.50

◀Hypertonic solution

HyperHAES® (Fresenius Kabi) (PoM)
Intravenous infusion, hydroxyethyl starch (weight average molecular weight 200 000) 6% in sodium chloride intravenous infusion 7.2%, net price 250-mL bag = £28.00

Cautions see notes above; also diabetes

9.3 Intravenous nutrition

When adequate feeding through the alimentary tract is not possible, nutrients may be given by intravenous infusion. This may be in addition to oral or enteral tube feeding—**supplemental parenteral nutrition**, or may be the sole source of nutrition—**total parenteral nutrition** (TPN). Complete enteral starvation is undesirable and total parenteral nutrition is a last resort.

Indications for parenteral nutrition include prematurity; severe or prolonged disorders of the gastro-intestinal tract; preparation of undernourished patients for surgery, chemotherapy, or radiation therapy; major surgery, trauma, or burns; prolonged coma or inability to eat; and some patients with renal or hepatic failure. The composition of proprietary preparations used in children is given in the table Proprietary Infusion Fluids for Parenteral Feeding, p. 559.

Parenteral nutrition requires the use of a solution containing amino acids, glucose, lipids, electrolytes, trace elements, and vitamins. This is now commonly provided by the pharmacy in the form of an amino-acid, glucose, electrolyte bag, and a separate lipid infusion or, in older children a single 'all-in-one' bag. If the patient is able to take small amounts by mouth, vitamins may be given orally.

The nutrition solution is infused through a central venous catheter inserted under full surgical precautions. Alternatively, infusion through a peripheral vein may be used for supplementary as well as total parenteral nutrition, depending on the availability of peripheral veins; factors prolonging cannula life and preventing thrombophlebitis include the use of soft polyurethane paediatric cannulas and use of nutritional solutions of low osmolality and neutral pH. Nutritional fluids should be given by a dedicated intravenous line; if not possible, compatibility with any drugs or fluids should be checked as precipitation of components may occur. Extravasation of parenteral nutrition solution can cause severe tissue damage and injury; the infusion site should be regularly monitored.

Nutrition and blood

9

Proprietary Infusion Fluids for Parenteral Feeding

Preparation	Nitrogen g/litre	[1,2]Energy kJ/litre	Electrolytes mmol/litre					Other components/litre
			K+	Mg2+	Na+	Acet-	Cl-	
ClinOleic 20% (Baxter) Net price 100 mL = £6.28; 250 mL = £10.08; 500 mL = £13.88		8360						purified olive and soya oil 200 g, glycerol 22.5 g, egg phosphatides 12 g
Glamin (Fresenius Kabi) Net price 250 mL = £14.16; 500 mL = £26.38	22.4				62			
Intralipid 10% (Fresenius Kabi) Net price 100 mL = £4.70; 500 mL = £10.30		4600						soya oil 100 g, glycerol 22 g, purified egg phospholipids 12 g, phosphate 15 mmol
Intralipid 20% (Fresenius Kabi) Net price 100 mL = £7.05; 250 mL = £11.60; 500 mL = £15.45		8400						soya oil 200 g, glycerol 22 g, purified egg phospholipids 12 g, phosphate 15 mmol
Intralipid 30% (Fresenius Kabi) Net price 333 mL = £17.30		12600						soya oil 300 g, glycerol 16.7 g, purified egg phospholipids 12 g, phosphate 15 mmol
Lipofundin MCT/LCT 10% (Braun) Net price 100 mL = £7.70; 500 mL = £12.90		4430						soya oil 50 g, medium chain triglycerides 50 g
Lipofundin MCT/LCT 20% (Braun) Net price 100 mL = £12.51; 250 mL = £11.30; 500 mL = £19.18		8000						soya oil 100 g, medium chain triglycerides 100 g
[3]Primene 10% (Baxter) Net price 100 mL = £5.78, 250 mL = £7.92	15						19	
Synthamin 9 (Baxter) Net price 500 mL = £6.66; 1000 mL = £12.34	9.1		60	5	70	100	70	acid phosphate 30 mmol
Synthamin 9 EF (electrolyte-free) (Baxter) Net price 500 mL = £6.66; 1000 mL = £12.34	9.1					44	22	
Vamin 9 Glucose (Fresenius Kabi) Net price 100 mL = £3.80; 500 mL = £7.70; 1000 mL = £13.40	9.4	1700	20	1.5	50		50	Ca2+ 2.5 mmol, anhydrous glucose 100 g
Vaminolact (Fresenius Kabi) Net price 100 mL = £4.20; 500 mL = £9.70	9.3							

Before starting intravenous nutrition the patient should be clinically stable and renal function and acid-base status should be assessed. Appropriate biochemical tests should have been carried out beforehand and serious deficits corrected. Nutritional and electrolyte status must be monitored throughout treatment. The nutritional components of parenteral nutrition regimens are usually increased gradually over a number of days to prevent metabolic complications and to allow metabolic adaptation to the infused nutrients. The solutions are usually infused over 24 hours but this may be gradually reduced if long-term nutrition is required. Home parenteral nutrition is usually infused over 12 hours overnight.

Complications of long-term parenteral nutrition include gall bladder sludging, gall stones, cholestasis and abnormal liver function tests. For details of the prevention and management of parenteral nutrition complications, specialist literature should be consulted.

1. *Note*. 1000 kcal = 4200 kJ; 1000 kJ= 238.8 kcal. All entries are PoM
2. Excludes protein- or amino acid-derived energy
3. For use in neonates and children only

Protein (nitrogen) is given as mixtures of essential and non-essential synthetic L-amino acids. Ideally, all essential amino acids should be included with a wide variety of non-essential ones to provide sufficient nitrogen together with electrolytes (see also section 9.2.2). Solutions vary in their composition of amino acids; they often contain an energy source (usually glucose) and electrolytes. Solutions for use in neonates and children under 1 year of age are based on the amino acid profile of umbilical cord blood (*Primene®*) or breast milk (*Vaminolact®*) and contain amino acids that are essential in this age group; these amino acids may not be present in sufficient quantities in preparations designed for older children and adults.

Energy requirements must be met if amino acids are to be utilised for tissue maintenance. An appropriate energy to protein ratio is essential and requirements will vary depending on the child's age and condition. A mixture of carbohydrate and fat energy sources (usually 30–50% as fat) gives better utilisation of amino acids than glucose alone.

Glucose is the preferred source of carbohydrate, but frequent monitoring of blood glucose is required particularly during initiation and build-up of the regimen; insulin may be necessary. Glucose above a concentration of 12.5% must be infused through a central venous catheter to avoid thrombosis; the maximum concentration of glucose that should normally be infused in fluid restricted children is 20–25%.

In parenteral nutrition regimens, it is necessary to provide adequate **phosphate** in order to allow phosphorylation of glucose and to prevent hypophosphataemia. Neonates, particularly preterm neonates, and young children also require phosphorus and calcium to ensure adequate bone mineralisation. The compatibility and solubility of calcium and phosphorus salts is complex and unpredictable; precipitation is a risk and specialist pharmacy advice should be sought.

Fat (lipid) emulsions have the advantages of a high energy to fluid volume ratio, neutral pH, and iso-osmolarity with plasma, and provide essential fatty acids. Several days of adaptation may be required to attain maximal utilisation. Reactions include occasional febrile episodes (usually only with 20% emulsions) and rare anaphylactic responses. Interference with biochemical measurements such as those for blood gases and calcium may occur if samples are taken before fat has been cleared. Regular monitoring of plasma cholesterol and triglyceride is necessary to ensure clearance from the plasma, particularly in conditions where fat metabolism may be disturbed e.g. infection. Emulsions containing 20% or 30% fat should be used in neonates as they are cleared more efficiently. **Additives may only be mixed with fat emulsions where compatibility is known**.

Electrolytes are usually provided as the chloride salts of potassium and sodium. Acetate salts can be used to reduce the amount of chloride infused; hyperchloraemic acidosis or hypochloraemic alkalosis can occur in preterm neonates or children with renal impairment.

> **Administration**. Because of the complex requirements relating to parenteral nutrition full details relating to administration have been omitted. In all cases *specialist pharmacy advice, product literature and other specialist literature should be consulted.*

Supplementary preparations

> Compatibility with the infusion solution must be ascertained before adding supplementary preparations.

Addiphos® (Fresenius Kabi) [PoM]
Solution, sterile, phosphate 40 mmol, K^+ 30 mmol, Na^+ 30 mmol/20 mL. For addition to *Vamin®* solutions and glucose intravenous infusions. Net price 20-mL vial = £1.53

Additrace® (Fresenius Kabi) [PoM]
Solution, trace elements for addition to *Vamin®* solutions and glucose intravenous infusions, traces of Fe^{3+}, Zn^{2+}, Mn^{2+}, Cu^{2+}, Cr^{3+}, Se^{4+}, Mo^{6+}, F^-, I^-. For children over 40 kg. Net price 10-mL amp = £2.31

Cernevit® (Baxter) [PoM]
Solution, dl-alpha tocopherol 11.2 units, ascorbic acid 125 mg, biotin 69 micrograms, colecalciferol 220 units, cyanocobalamin 6 micrograms, folic acid 414 micrograms, glycine 250 mg, nicotinamide 46 mg, pantothenic acid (as dexpanthenol) 17.25 mg, pyridoxine hydrochloride 5.5 mg, retinol (as palmitate) 3500 units, riboflavin (as dihydrated sodium phosphate) 4.14 mg, thiamine (as cocarboxylase tetrahydrate) 3.51 mg. Dissolve in 5 mL water for injections. Net price per vial = £3.32

Decan® (Baxter) [PoM]
Solution, trace elements for addition to infusion solutions, Fe^{2+}, Zn^{2+}, Cu^{2+}, Mn^{2+}, F^-, Co^{2+} I^-, Se^{4+}, Mo^{6+}, Cr^{3+}. For children over 40 kg. Net price 40-mL vial = £2.00

Dipeptiven® (Fresenius Kabi) [PoM]
Solution, N(2)-L-alanyl-L-glutamine 200 mg/mL (providing L-alanine 82 mg, L-glutamine 134.6 mg). For addition to infusion solutions containing amino acids. Net price 50 mL = £16.40, 100 mL = £30.50
Dose
Amino acid supplement for hypercatabolic or hypermetabolic states
300–400 mg/kg daily; max. 400 mg/kg daily, dose not to exceed 20% of total amino acid intake

Glycophos® Sterile Concentrate (Fresenius Kabi) [PoM]
Solution, sterile, phosphate 20 mmol, Na^+ 40 mmol/20 mL. For addition to Vamin® and Vaminolact® solutions, and glucose intravenous infusions. Net price 20-mL vial = £4.60

Peditrace® (Fresenius Kabi) [PoM]
Solution, trace elements for addition to Vaminolact®, Vamin® 14 Electrolyte-Free solutions

and glucose intravenous infusions, traces of Zn^{2+}, Cu^{2+}, Mn^{2+}, Se^{4+}, F^-, I^-. For use in neonates (when kidney function established, usually second day of life), infants, and children. Net price 10-mL vial = £4.18
Cautions reduced biliary excretion especially in cholestatic liver disease or in markedly reduced urinary excretion (careful biochemical monitoring required); total parenteral nutrition exceeding 1 month (measure serum manganese concentration and check liver function before commencing treatment and regularly during treatment)—discontinue if manganese concentration raised or if cholestasis develops

Solivito N® (Fresenius Kabi) [PoM]
Solution, powder for reconstitution, biotin 60 micrograms, cyanocobalamin 5 micrograms, folic acid 400 micrograms, glycine 300 mg, nicotinamide 40 mg, pyridoxine hydrochloride 4.9 mg, riboflavin sodium phosphate 4.9 mg, sodium ascorbate 113 mg, sodium pantothenate 16.5 mg, thiamine mononitrate 3.1 mg. Dissolve in water for injections or glucose intravenous infusion for adding to glucose intravenous infusion or Intralipid®; dissolve in Vitlipid N® or Intralipid® for adding to Intralipid® only. Net price per vial = £2.32

Vitlipid N® (Fresenius Kabi) [PoM]
Emulsion, adult, vitamin A 330 units, ergocalciferol 20 units, dl-alpha tocopherol 1 unit, phytomenadione 15 micrograms/mL. For addition to Intralipid®. For adults and children over 11 years. Net price 10-mL amp = £2.32

Emulsion, infant, vitamin A 230 units, ergocalciferol 40 units, dl-alpha tocopherol 0.7 unit, phytomenadione 20 micrograms/mL. For addition to Intralipid®. Net price 10-mL amp = £2.32

9.4 Oral nutrition

9.4.1 Foods for special diets
9.4.2 Enteral nutrition

9.4.1 Foods for special diets

Preparations that have been modified to eliminate a particular constituent from a food or are nutrient mixtures formulated as food substitutes for children who either cannot tolerate or cannot metabolise certain common constituents of food.

Coeliac disease Intolerance to gluten in coeliac disease is managed by completely eliminating gluten from the diet. A range of gluten-free products is available for prescription—see Appendix 2 (p. 910).

Phenylketonuria Phenylketonuria (hyperphenylalaninaemia, PKU), which results from the inability to metabolise phenylalanine, is managed by restricting dietary intake of phenylalanine to a small amount sufficient for tissue building and repair. Some rare forms of phenylketonuria are caused by a deficiency of tetrahydrobiopterin. Treatment involves oral supplementation of **tetrahydrobiopterin**; in some severe cases, the addition of the neurotransmitter precursors, levodopa (L-dopa, section 4.9.1) and 5-hydroxytryptophan, is also necessary.

Sapropterin, a synthetic form of tetrahydrobiopterin, is licensed as an adjunct to dietary restriction of phenylalanine in the management of patients with phenylketonuria and tetrahydrobiopterin deficiency.

Aspartame (used as a sweetener in some foods and medicines) contributes to the phenylalanine intake and may affect control of phenylketonuria. If alternatives are

9

Nutrition and blood

unavailable, children with phenylketonuria should not be denied access to appropriate medication; the amount of aspartame consumed can be taken in to account in the management of the condition. Where the presence of aspartame in a preparation is specified in the product literature, aspartame is listed as an excipient in the relevant product entry in *BNF for Children*; the child or carer should be informed of this.

For further information on special dietary products used in the management of metabolic diseases, see Appendix 2

▲ TETRAHYDROBIOPTERIN

Cautions

Renal impairment use with caution—accumulation of metabolites

Pregnancy crosses the placenta; use only if benefit outweighs risk

Breast-feeding present in milk, effects unknown

Side-effects diarrhoea, urinary frequency, disturbed sleep

Licensed use not licensed in the UK

Indication and dose

Monotherapy in tetrahydrobiopterin-sensitive phenylketonuria (specialist use only)
• **By mouth**
Child 1 month–18 years 10 mg/kg twice daily (total daily dose may alternatively be given in 3 divided doses), adjusted according to response

In combination with neurotransmitter precursors for tetrahydrobiopterin-sensitive phenylketonuria (specialist use only)
• **By mouth**
Child 1 month–2 years initially 250–750 micrograms/kg 4 times daily (total daily dose may alternatively be given in 3 divided doses), adjusted according to response; max. 7 mg/kg daily

Child 2–18 years initially 250–750 micrograms/kg 4 times daily (total daily dose may alternatively be given in 3 divided doses), adjusted according to response; usual max. 10 mg/kg daily

Tetrahydrobiopterin (Non-proprietary)
Tablets, tetrahydrobiopterin 10 mg and 50 mg
Available from 'special-order' manufacturers or specialist importing companies, see p. 943

▲ SAPROPTERIN DIHYDROCHLORIDE

Note Sapropterin is a synthetic form of tetrahydrobiopterin

Cautions monitor blood-phenylalanine concentration before and after first week of treatment—if unsatisfactory response increase dose at weekly intervals to max. dose and monitor blood-phenylalanine concentration weekly; discontinue treatment if unsatisfactory response after 1 month; monitor blood-phenylalanine and tyrosine concentrations 1–2 weeks after dose adjustment and during treatment; history of convulsions

Hepatic impairment manufacturer advises caution—no information available

Renal impairment manufacturer advises caution—no information available

Pregnancy manufacturer advises caution—consider only if dietary management inadequate

Contra-indications

Breast-feeding manufacturer advises avoid—on information available

Side-effects diarrhoea, vomiting, abdominal pain; nasal congestion, cough, pharyngolaryngeal pain; headache

Indication and dose

Phenylketonuria (specialist use only)
• **By mouth**
Child 4–18 years initially 10 mg/kg once daily, preferably in the morning, adjusted according to response; usual dose 5–20 mg/kg daily

Tetrahydrobiopterin deficiency (specialist use only)
• **By mouth**
Child 4–18 years initially 2–5 mg/kg once daily, preferably in the morning, adjusted according to response; max. 20 mg/kg daily; total daily dose may alternatively be given in 2–3 divided doses

Kuvan® (Merck Serono) ▼ PoM
Dispersible tablets, sapropterin dihydrochloride 100 mg, net price 30-tab pack = £597.22, 120-tab pack = £2388.88. Label: 13, 21, counselling, tablets should be dissolved in water and taken within 20 minutes

9.4.2 Enteral nutrition

Children have higher nutrient requirements per kg body-weight, different metabolic rates, and physiological responses compared to adults. They have low nutritional stores and are particularly vulnerable to growth and nutritional problems during critical periods of development. Major illness, operations, or trauma impose increased metabolic demands and can rapidly exhaust nutritional reserves.

Every effort should be made to optimise oral food intake before beginning enteral tube feeding; this may include change of posture, special seating, feeding equipment, oral desensitisation, food texture changes, thickening of liquids, increasing energy density of food, treatment of reflux or oesophagitis, as well as using age-specific nutritional supplements.

Enteral tube feeding has a role in both short-term rehabilitation and long-term nutritional management in paediatrics. It can be used as supportive therapy, in which the enteral feed supplies a proportion of the required nutrients, or as primary therapy, in which the enteral feed delivers all the necessary nutrients. Most children receiving tube feeds should also be encouraged to take oral food and drink. Tube feeding should be considered in the following situations:

- unsafe swallowing and risk of aspiration;

- inability to consume at least 60% of energy needs by mouth;

- total feeding time of more than 4 hours per day;

- weight loss or no weight gain for a period of 3 months (less for younger children and infants);

- weight for height (or length) less than 2nd percentile for age and sex.

Most feeds for enteral use (Appendix 2) contain protein derived from cows' milk or soya. Elemental feeds containing protein hydrolysates or free amino acids can be used for children who have diminished ability to break down protein, for example in inflammatory bowel disease or pancreatic insufficiency.

Even when nutritionally complete feeds are given, water and electrolyte balance should be monitored. Haematological and biochemical parameters should also be monitored, particularly in the clinically unstable child. Extra minerals (e.g. magnesium and zinc) may be needed in patients where gastro-intestinal secretions are being lost. Additional vitamins may also be needed. Feeds containing vitamin K may affect the INR in children receiving warfarin—see **interactions**: Appendix 1 (vitamins).

Choosing the best formula for children depends on several factors including: nutritional requirements, gastro-intestinal function, underlying disease, nutrient restrictions, age, and feed characteristics (nutritional composition, viscosity, osmolality, availability and cost). Children have specific dietary requirements and in many situations liquid feeds prepared for adults are totally unsuitable and should not be given. Expert advice from a dietician should be sought before prescribing enteral feeds for a child.

Infant formula feeds   Child 0–12 months. Term infants with normal gastro-intestinal function are given either breast milk or normal infant formula during the first year of life. The average intake is between 150 mL and 200 mL/kg/day. Infant milk formulas are based on whey- or casein-dominant protein, lactose with or without maltodextrin, amylose, vegetable oil and milk fat. The composition of all normal and soya infant formulas have to meet The Infant Formula and Follow-on Formula Regulations (England and Wales) 2007, which enact the European Community Regulations 2006/141/EC; the composition of other enteral and specialist feeds has to meet the Commission Directive (1999/21/EC) on Dietary Foods for Special Medical Purposes.

A high-energy feed (Appendix 2, p. 885), which contains 9–11% of energy derived from protein can be used for infants who fail to grow adequately. Alternatively, energy supplements (Appendix 2, p. 904) may be added to normal infant formula to achieve a higher energy content (but this will reduce the protein to energy ratio) or the normal infant formula concentration may be increased slightly. Care should be taken not to present an osmotic load of more than 500 milliosmols/kg water to the normal functioning gut, otherwise osmotic diarrhoea will result. Concentrating or supplementing feeds should not be attempted without the advice of a paediatric dietician.

Enteral feeds   Child 1–6 years (body–weight 8–20 kg). Ready-to-use feeds (Appendix 2, p. 885) based on caseinates, maltodextrin and vegetable oils (with or without added medium chain triglyceride (MCT) oil or fibre) are well tolerated and effective in improving nutritional status in this age group. Although originally designed for children 1–6 years (body–weight 8–20 kg), some products have ACBS approval for use in children weighing up to 30 kg (approx. 10 years of age). Enteral feeds formulated for children 1–6 years are low in sodium and potassium; electrolyte intake and biochemical status should be monitored. Older children in this age range taking small feed volumes may need to be given additional micronutrients. Fibre-enriched feeds may be helpful for children with chronic constipation or diarrhoea.

Child 7–12 years (body-weight 21–45 kg). Depending on age, weight, clinical condition and nutritional requirements, ready-to-use feeds (Appendix 2, p. 885) formulated for 7–12 year olds may be given at appropriate rates.

Child over 12 years (body-weight over 45 kg). As there are no standard enteral feeds formulated for this age group, adult formulations are used. The intake of protein, electrolytes, vitamins, and trace minerals should be carefully assessed and monitored.

Note Adult feeds containing more than 6 g/100 mL protein or 2 g/100 mL fibre should be used with caution and expert advice.

Specialised formula   It is essential that any infant who is intolerant of breast milk or normal infant formula, or whose condition requires nutrient-specific adaptation, is prescribed an adequate volume of a nutritionally complete replacement formula (see Appendix 2, p. 896). In the first 4 months of life, a volume of 150–200 mL/kg/day is recommended. After 6 months, should the formula still be required, a volume of 600 mL/day should be maintained, in addition to solid food.

Products for cow's milk protein intolerance or lactose intolerance. There are a number of infant formulas formulated for cow's milk protein intolerance or lactose intolerance; these feeds may contain a residual amount of lactose (less than 1 g/100 mL formula)—sometimes described as clinically lactose-free or 'lactose-free' by manufacturers. If the total daily intake of these formulas is low, it may be necessary to supplement with calcium, and a vitamin and mineral supplement.

Soya-based infant formulas have a high phytoestrogen content and this may be a long-term reproductive health risk. The Chief Medical Officer has advised that soya-based infant formulas should not be used as the first choice for the management of infants with proven cow's milk sensitivity, lactose intolerance, galacto-kinase deficiency and galactosaemia. Most UK paediatricians with expertise in inherited metabolic disease still advocate soya-based formulations for infants with galactosaemia as there are concerns about the residual lactose content of low lactose formulas and protein hydrolysates based on cow's milk protein.

Low lactose infant formulations, based on whole cow's milk protein, are unsuitable for children with cow's milk protein intolerance. Liquid soya milks purchased from supermarkets and health food stores are not nutritionally complete and should never be used for infants under 1 year of age.

Protein hydrolysate formulas. Non-milk, peptide-based feeds containing hydrolysates of casein, whey, meat and soya protein, are suitable for infants with disaccharide or whole protein intolerance. The total daily intake of electrolytes, vitamins and minerals should be carefully assessed and modified to meet the child's nutritional requirements; these feeds have a high osmolality when given at recommended dilution and need gradual and careful introduction.

Elemental (amino acid based formula). Specially formulated elemental feeds containing essential and non-essential amino acids are available for use in infants and children under 6 years with proven whole protein intolerance. Adult elemental formula may be used for children over 6 years; the intake of electrolytes, vitamins and minerals should be carefully assessed and modified to meet nutritional requirements. These feeds have a high osmolality when given at the recommended concentration and therefore need gradual and careful introduction.

Modular feeds. Modular feeds (Appendix 2, p. 901) are based on individual protein, fat, carbohydrate, vitamin and mineral components or modules which can be combined to meet the specific needs of a child. Modular feeds are used when nutritionally complete specialised formula are not tolerated, or if the fluid and nutrient requirements change e.g. in gastro-intestinal, renal or liver disease. The main advantage of modular feeds is their flexibility; disadvantages include their complexity and preparation difficulties. Modular feeds should not be used without the supervision of a paediatric dietician.

Specialised formula. Highly specialised formulas are designed to meet the specific requirements in various clinical conditions such as renal and liver diseases. When using these formulas, both the biochemical status of the child and their growth parameters need to be monitored.

Feed thickeners   **Carob based thickeners** (Appendix 2, p. 909) may be used to thicken feeds for infants under 1 year with significant gastro-oesophageal reflux. Breast-fed infants can be given the thickener mixed to a paste with water or breast-milk prior to feeds.

Pre-thickened formula Milk-protein- or casein-dominant infant formula, which contains small quantities of pre-gelatinized starch, is recommended primarily for infants with mild gastro-oesophageal reflux. Pre-thickened formula is prepared in the same way as normal infant formula and flows through a standard teat. The feeds do not thicken on standing but thicken in the stomach when exposed to acid pH.

Starched based thickeners can be used to thicken liquids and feeds for children over 1 year of age with dysphagia.

Dietary supplements for oral use   (Appendix 2, p. 890) Three types of prescribable fortified dietary supplements are available: fortified milk and non-milk tasting (juice-style) drinks, and fortified milk-based semi-solid preparations. The recommended daily quantity is age-dependent. The following is a useful guide: 1–2 years, 200 kcal (840 kJ); 3–5 years, 400 kcal (1680 kJ); 6–11 years, 600 kcal (2520 kJ); and over 12 years, 800 kcal (3360 kJ). Supplements containing 1.5 kcal/mL are high in protein and should not be used for children under 3 years of age. Many supplements are high in sugar or maltodextrin; care should be taken to prevent prolonged contact with teeth. Ideally supplements should be administered after meals or at bedtime so as not to affect appetite.

Products for metabolic diseases   There is a large range of disease-specific infant formulas and amino acid-based supplements available for use in children with metabolic diseases (see under specific metabolic diseases, Appendix 2, p. 912). Some of these formulas are nutritionally incomplete and supplementation with vitamins and other nutrients may be necessary. Many of the product names are similar; to prevent metabolic complications in children who cannot tolerate specific amino acids it is important to ensure the correct supplement is supplied.

Preparations (Borderline substances)   See Appendix 2.

9.5   Minerals

9.5.1 Calcium and magnesium
9.5.2 Phosphorus
9.5.3 Fluoride
9.5.4 Zinc

See section 9.1.1 for iron salts.

9.5.1   Calcium and magnesium

9.5.1.1 Calcium supplements
9.5.1.2 Hypercalcaemia and hypercalciuria
9.5.1.3 Magnesium

9.5.1.1   Calcium supplements

Calcium supplements are usually only required where dietary calcium intake is deficient. This dietary requirement varies with age and is relatively greater in childhood, pregnancy, and lactation, due to an increased demand. Hypocalcaemia may be caused by vitamin D deficiency (section 9.6.4), impaired metabolism, a failure of secretion (hypoparathyroidism), or resistance to parathyroid hormone (pseudohypoparathyroidism).

Mild asymptomatic hypocalcaemia may be managed with oral calcium supplements. *Severe symptomatic hypocalcaemia* requires an intravenous infusion of calcium gluconate 10% over 5 to 10 minutes, repeating the dose if symptoms

9
Nutrition and blood

persist; in exceptional cases it may be necessary to maintain a continuous calcium infusion over a day or more. Calcium chloride injection is also available, but is more irritant; care should be taken to prevent extravasation.

For the role of calcium gluconate in temporarily reducing the toxic effects of *hyperkalaemia*, see p. 547.

Persistent hypocalcaemia requires oral calcium supplements and either a vitamin D analogue (alfacalcidol or calcitriol) for hypoparathyroidism and pseudohypoparathyroidism or natural vitamin D (calciferol) if due to vitamin D deficiency (section 9.6.4). It is important to monitor plasma and urinary calcium during long-term maintenance therapy.

Neonates Hypocalcaemia is common in the first few days of life, particularly following birth asphyxia or respiratory distress. Late onset at 4–10 days after birth may be secondary to vitamin D deficiency, hypoparathyroidism or hypomagnesaemia and may be associated with seizures.

◢ CALCIUM SALTS

Cautions sarcoidosis; history of nephrolithiasis; avoid calcium chloride in respiratory acidosis or respiratory failure; **interactions**: Appendix 1 (antacids, calcium salts)

Renal impairment use with caution, risk of hypercalcaemia and renal calculi

Contra-indications conditions associated with hypercalcaemia and hypercalciuria (e.g. some forms of malignant disease)

Side-effects gastro-intestinal disturbances, constipation; bradycardia, arrhythmias; with injection, peripheral vasodilatation, fall in blood pressure, injection-site reactions, severe tissue damage with extravasation

Indication and dose

See notes above; calcium deficiency
* **By mouth**

  Neonate 0.25 mmol/kg 4 times a day, adjusted to response

  Child 1 month–4 years 0.25 mmol/kg 4 times a day, adjusted to response

  Child 5–12 years 0.2 mmol/kg 4 times a day, adjusted to response

  Child 12–18 years 10 mmol 4 times a day, adjusted to response

Acute hypocalcaemia, urgent correction; hyperkalaemia (prevention of arrhythmias)
* **By slow intravenous injection over 5–10 minutes**

  Neonate 0.11 mmol/kg (0.5 mL/kg of calcium gluconate 10%) as a single dose. [Some units use a dose of 0.46 mmol/kg (2 mL/kg calcium gluconate 10%) for hypocalcaemia in line with US practice]

  Child 1 month–18 years 0.11 mmol/kg (0.5 mL/kg calcium gluconate 10%), max 4.5 mmol (20 mL calcium gluconate 10%)

Acute hypocalcaemia, maintenance
* **By continuous intravenous infusion**

  Neonate 0.5 mmol/kg daily over 24 hours, adjusted to response, use oral route as soon as possible due to risk of extravasation

  Child 1 month–2 years 1 mmol/kg daily (usual max 8.8 mmol) over 24 hours, use oral route as soon as possible due to risk of extravasation

  Child 2–18 years 8.8 mmol over 24 hours, use oral route as soon as possible due to risk of extravasation

◢ Oral preparations

Calcium Gluconate (Non-proprietary)
Tablets, calcium gluconate 600 mg (calcium 53.4 mg or Ca^{2+} 1.35 mmol), net price 20 = £1.43. Label: 24

Effervescent tablets, calcium gluconate 1 g (calcium 89 mg or Ca^{2+} 2.23 mmol), net price 28-tab pack = £8.83. Label: 13

Note Each tablet usually contains 4.46 mmol Na^+

Calcium Lactate (Non-proprietary)
Tablets, calcium lactate 300 mg (calcium 39 mg or Ca^{2+} 1 mmol), net price 84 = £3.01

Adcal® (Strakan)
Chewable tablets, fruit flavour, calcium carbonate 1.5 g (calcium 600 mg or Ca^{2+} 15 mmol), net price 100-tab pack = £7.25. Label: 24

Cacit® (Procter & Gamble Pharm.)
Tablets, effervescent, pink, calcium carbonate 1.25 g, providing calcium citrate when dispersed in water (calcium 500 mg or Ca^{2+} 12.5 mmol), net price 76-tab pack = £12.54. Label: 13

Calcichew® (Shire)
Tablets (chewable), orange flavour, calcium carbonate 1.25 g (calcium 500 mg or Ca^{2+} 12.5 mmol), net price 100-tab pack = £9.33. Label: 24

Forte tablets (chewable), orange flavour, scored, calcium carbonate 2.5 g (calcium 1 g or Ca^{2+} 25 mmol), net price 60-tab pack = £13.16. Label: 24
Excipients include aspartame (section 9.4.1)

Nutrition and blood

9

◻ **CALCIUM SALTS** (*continued*)

Calcium-500 (Martindale)
Tablets, pink, f/c, calcium carbonate 1.25 g (calcium 500 mg or Ca²⁺ 12.5 mmol), net price 100-tab pack = £9.46. Label: 25

Calcium-Sandoz® (Alliance)
Syrup, orange flavour, calcium glubionate 1.09 g, calcium lactobionate 727 mg (calcium 108.3 mg or Ca²⁺ 2.7 mmol)/5 mL, net price 300 mL = £3.39

Sandocal® (Novartis Consumer Health)
Sandocal-400 tablets, effervescent, orange flavour, calcium lactate gluconate 930 mg, calcium carbonate 700 mg, anhydrous citric acid 1.189 g, providing calcium 400 mg (Ca²⁺ 10 mmol), net price 5 × 20-tab pack = £6.87. Label: 13
Excipients include aspartame (section 9.4.1)

Sandocal-1000 tablets, effervescent, orange flavour, calcium lactate gluconate 2.263 g, calcium carbonate 1.75 g, anhydrous citric acid 2.973 g providing 1 g calcium (Ca²⁺ 25 mmol), net price 3 × 10-tab pack = £6.17. Label: 13
Excipients include aspartame (section 9.4.1)

◢**Parenteral preparations**
Calcium Gluconate (Non-proprietary) [PoM]
Injection, calcium gluconate 10% (calcium 8.4 mg or Ca²⁺ 226 micromol)/mL. Net price 10-mL amp = 60p

Administration For *intravenous infusion* dilute to at least 45 micromol/mL with Glucose 5% *or* Sodium Chloride 0.9%. Maximum administration rate 45 micromol/kg/hour (or in neonates max. 22 micromol/kg/hour). May be given more concentrated via a central venous catheter. May be used undiluted (10% calcium gluconate) in emergencies. Avoid extravasation; should not be given by intramuscular injection. Incompatible with sodium bicarbonate and phosphate solutions.

Calcium Chloride (Non-proprietary) [PoM]
Injection, calcium chloride dihydrate 10% (calcium 27.3 mg or Ca²⁺ 680 micromol/mL), net price 10-mL disposable syringe = £4.64
Brands include *Minijet® Calcium Chloride 10%*

Injection, calcium chloride dihydrate 13.4% (calcium 36 mg or Ca²⁺ 910 micromol/mL), net price 10–mL amp = £14.94

◢**With vitamin D**
Section 9.6.4

9.5.1.2 Hypercalcaemia and hypercalciuria

Severe hypercalcaemia Severe hypercalcaemia calls for urgent treatment before detailed investigation of the cause. Dehydration should be corrected first with intravenous infusion of **sodium chloride 0.9%**. Drugs (such as thiazides and vitamin D compounds) which promote hypercalcaemia, should be discontinued and dietary calcium should be restricted.

If *severe hypercalcaemia persists* drugs which inhibit mobilisation of calcium from the skeleton may be required. The **bisphosphonates** are useful and disodium pamidronate (section 6.6.2) is probably the most effective.

Corticosteroids (section 6.3) are widely given, but may only be useful where hypercalcaemia is due to sarcoidosis or vitamin D intoxication; they often take several days to achieve the desired effect.

Calcitonin (section 6.6.1) is relatively non-toxic, but its effect can wear off after a few days despite continued use; it is rarely effective where bisphosphonates have failed to reduce serum calcium adequately.

After treatment of severe hypercalcaemia the underlying cause must be established. *Further treatment* is governed by the same principles as for initial therapy. Salt and water depletion and drugs promoting hypercalcaemia should be avoided; oral administration of a bisphosphonate may be useful. Parathyroidectomy may be indicated for hyperparathyroidism.

Hypercalciuria Hypercalciuria should be investigated for an underlying cause, which should be treated. Reducing dietary calcium intake may be beneficial but severe restriction of calcium intake has not proved beneficial and may even be harmful.

9.5.1.3 Magnesium

Magnesium is an essential constituent of many enzyme systems, particularly those involved in energy generation; the largest stores are in the skeleton.

Magnesium salts are not well absorbed from the gastro-intestinal tract, which explains the use of magnesium sulphate (section 1.6.4) as an osmotic laxative.

Magnesium is excreted mainly by the kidneys and is therefore retained in renal failure, but significant *hypermagnesaemia* (causing muscle weakness and arrhythmias) is rare.

9

Nutrition and blood

Hypomagnesaemia Since magnesium is secreted in large amounts in the gastro-intestinal fluid, excessive losses in diarrhoea, stoma or fistula are the most common causes of *hypomagnesaemia*; deficiency may also occur as a result of treatment with certain drugs. Hypomagnesaemia often causes secondary hypocalcaemia (with which it may be confused), particularly in neonates, and also hypokalaemia and hyponatraemia.

Symptomatic *hypomagnesaemia* is associated with a deficit of 0.5–1 mmol/kg. Magnesium is given initially by intravenous infusion or by intramuscular injection of **magnesium sulphate**; the intramuscular injection is painful. Plasma magnesium concentration should be measured to determine the rate and duration of infusion and the dose should be reduced in renal impairment. To prevent *recurrence of the deficit*, magnesium may be given by mouth in divided doses. For maintenance (e.g. in intravenous nutrition), parenteral doses of magnesium are of the order of 0.2–0.4 mmol/kg (usual max. 20 mmol) Mg^{2+} daily.

Arrhythmias Magnesium sulphate has also been recommended for the emergency treatment of *serious arrhythmias*, especially in the presence of hypokalaemia (when hypomagnesaemia may also be present) and when salvos of rapid ventricular tachycardia show the characteristic twisting wave front known as *torsade de pointes* (see also section 2.3.1).

MAGNESIUM SULPHATE

Cautions see notes above; in severe hypomagnesaemia administer initially via controlled infusion device (preferably syringe pump); monitor blood pressure, respiratory rate, urinary output and for signs of overdosage (loss of patellar reflexes, weakness, nausea, sensation of warmth, flushing, drowsiness, double vision, and slurred speech); **interactions**: Appendix 1 (magnesium, parenteral)

Renal impairment avoid or reduce dose; increased risk of toxicity

Pregnancy sufficient may cross the placenta in mothers treated with high doses e.g. in pre-eclampsia, causing hypotonia and respiratory depression in newborns

Breast-feeding present in breast milk; may cause diarrhoea in breast-fed babies

Side-effects generally associated with hypermagnesaemia, nausea, vomiting, thirst, flushing of skin, hypotension, arrhythmias, coma, respiratory depression, drowsiness, confusion, loss of tendon reflexes, muscle weakness

Licensed use 20% injection licensed for use in children. Other strengths unlicensed

Indication and dose

(See also notes above)

Neonatal hypocalcaemia
- By deep intramuscular injection or intravenous infusion

  Neonate 0.4 mmol/kg Mg^{2+} (100 mg/kg magnesium sulphate) 12 hourly for 2–3 doses

Hypomagnesaemia
- By intravenous injection over at least 10 minutes

  Neonate 0.4 mmol/kg Mg^{2+} (100 mg/kg magnesium sulphate) 6–12 hourly as necessary

Child 1 month–12 years 0.2 mmol/kg Mg^{2+} (50 mg/kg magnesium sulphate) 12 hourly as necessary

Child 12–18 years 4 mmol Mg^{2+} (1 g magnesium sulphate) 12 hourly as necessary

Acute severe asthma section 3.1

Persistent pulmonary hypertension section 2.5.1

Torsade de pointes (consult local guidelines)
- By intravenous injection over 10–15 minutes
  Child 1 month–18 years 0.1–0.2 mmol/kg (25–50 mg/kg magnesium sulphate); max. 8 mmol (2 g magnesium sulphate); dose repeated once if necessary

Administration Dilute to 10% (100 mg in 1 mL) with Glucose 5 *or* 10%, Sodium Chloride 0.45 *or* 0.9% *or* Glucose and Sodium Chloride combinations. Up to 20% solution may be given in fluid restriction. Rate of administration should not exceed 10 mg/kg/minute of magnesium sulphate

Note Magnesium sulphate 1 g equivalent to Mg^{2+} approx. 4 mmol

Magnesium Sulphate (Non-proprietary) ▣PoM▣
Injection, magnesium sulphate 20% (Mg^{2+} approx. 0.8 mmol/mL), net price 20-mL (4-g) amp = £2.75; 50% (Mg^{2+} approx. 2 mmol/mL), 2-mL (1-g) amp = £3.80, 4-mL (2-g) prefilled syringe = £6.40; 5-mL (2.5-g) amp = £3.00, 10-mL (5-g) amp = £3.35; 10-mL (5-g) prefilled syringe = £4.95
Brands include *Min-I-Jet® Magnesium Sulphate 50%*

◢ MAGNESIUM-ʟ-ASPARTATE

Cautions see under Magnesium Sulphate

Renal impairment avoid or reduce dose; increased risk of toxicity

Side-effects diarrhoea; see also under Magnesium Sulphate

Licensed use classified as a Food for Special Medical Purposes for use in children over 2 years

Indication and dose

Hypomagnesaemia
- **By mouth**

  Child 1 month–2 years initially 0.2 mmol/kg of Mg^{2+} 3 times daily dissolved in water, dose adjusted as required

Child 2–10 years half a sachet (5 mmol Mg^{2+}) daily dissolved in 100 mL of water, dose adjusted as required

Child 10–18 years one sachet (10 mmol Mg^{2+}) daily dissolved in 200 mL of water, dose adjusted as required

Magnaspartate® (KoRa)
Oral powder, magnesium-ʟ-aspartate 6.5 g (10 mmol Mg^{2+})/sachet, net price 10-sachet pack = £7.50
Excipients include sucrose

◢ MAGNESIUM GLYCEROPHOSPHATE

Cautions see under Magnesium Sulphate

Renal impairment avoid or reduce dose; increased risk of toxicity

Side-effects diarrhoea; see also under Magnesium Sulphate

Licensed use not licensed for use

Indication and dose

Hypomagnesaemia
- **By mouth**

  Child 1 month–12 years initially 0.2 mmol/kg Mg^{2+} 3 times daily, dose adjusted as required

  Child 12–18 years initially 4–8 mmol Mg^{2+} 3 times daily, dose adjusted as required

Administration tablets may be dispersed in water

Magnesium Glycerophosphate (Non-proprietary)
Tablets, magnesium glycerophosphate 1 g (approximately magnesium 97 mg or Mg^{2+} 4 mmol)
Available from 'special-order' manufacturers or specialist importing companies, see p. 943

Liquid, magnesium glycerophosphate 250 mg/mL (approximately magnesium 24.25 mg or Mg^{2+} 1 mmol/mL)
Available from 'special-order' manufacturers or specialist importing companies, see p. 943

◢ Extemporaneous formulations available see Extemporaneous Preparations, p. 8

9.5.2 Phosphorus

9.5.2.1 Phosphate supplements

9.5.2.2 Phosphate-binding agents

9.5.2.1 Phosphate supplements

Oral phosphate supplements may be required in addition to vitamin D in children with hypophosphataemic vitamin D-resistant rickets (section 9.6.4). Diarrhoea is a common side-effect and should prompt a reduction in dosage.

Phosphate infusion is occasionally needed in phosphate deficiency arising from use of parenteral nutrition deficient in phosphate supplements; phosphate depletion also occurs in severe diabetic ketoacidosis. It is difficult to provide detailed guidelines for the treatment of *severe hypophosphatemia* because the extent of total body deficits and response to therapy are difficult to predict. High doses of phosphate may result in a transient serum elevation followed by redistribution into intracellular compartments or bone tissue; excessive doses may cause hypocalcaemia and metastatic calcification. It is essential to monitor plasma concentrations of calcium, phosphate, potassium and other electrolytes. It is recommended that severe hypophosphataemia be treated intravenously as large doses of oral phosphate may cause diarrhoea; intestinal absorption may be unreliable and dose adjustment may be necessary.

Phosphate is not the first choice for the treatment of hypercalcaemia because of the risk of precipitation of calcium phosphate in the kidney and other tissues. If used, the child should be well hydrated and electrolytes monitored.

Neonates Phosphate deficiency may occur in very low-birthweight infants and may compromise bone growth if not corrected. Parenterally fed infants may be at risk of phosphate deficiency due to the limited solubility of phosphate. Some units routinely supplement expressed breast milk with phosphate, although the effect on the osmolality of the milk should be considered.

9

Nutrition and blood

PHOSPHATE

Cautions see notes above, also cardiac disease, diabetes mellitus, dehydration; avoid extravasation with parenteral forms, severe tissue necrosis; sodium and potassium concentrations of preparations

Renal impairment reduce dose in renal impairment, monitor closely

Contra-indications hyperphosphataemia

Side-effects nausea, diarrhoea; hypotension, oedema; hypocalcaemia; acute renal failure; phlebitis; tissue necrosis on extravasation

Indication and dose

Hypophosphataemia, including hypophosphataemic rickets and osteomalacia (see notes above)
• **By mouth**

Neonate 1 mmol/kg daily in 1–2 divided doses, or as a supplement in breast milk

Child 1 month–5 years 2–3 mmol/kg (max. 48 mmol) phosphate daily in 2–4 divided doses, adjusted as necessary

Child 5–18 years 2–3 mmol/kg (max. 97 mmol) phosphate daily in 2–4 divided doses, adjusted as necessary
Administration Caution, solubility in breast milk is limited to 1.2 mmol in 100 mL if calcium also added, contact pharmacy department for details

• **By intravenous infusion (see administration below)**

Neonate 1 mmol/kg phosphate daily, adjusted as necessary

Child 1 month–2 years 0.7 mmol/kg phosphate daily, adjusted as necessary

Child 2–18 years 0.4 mmol/kg phosphate daily, adjusted as necessary
Administration (see also Important, below) Dilute injection with Sodium Chloride 0.9% or 0.45% or Glucose 5% or 10%. Administration rate of phosphate should not exceed 0.05 mmol/kg/hour. In emergencies in intensive care faster rates may be used—seek specialist advice

> Important Some phosphate injection preparations also contain potassium. For peripheral intravenous administration the *concentration* of potassium should not usually exceed 40 mmol/litre. The infusion solution should be **thoroughly mixed**. Local policies on avoiding inadvertent use of potassium concentrate should be followed. The potassium content of some phosphate preparations may also limit the *rate* at which they may be administered, see section 9.2.2.1.

◢Oral
Phosphate-Sandoz® (HK Pharma)
Tablets, effervescent, anhydrous sodium acid phosphate 1.936 g, sodium bicarbonate 350 mg, potassium bicarbonate 315 mg, equivalent to phosphorus 500 mg (phosphate 16.1 mmol), sodium 468.8 mg (Na^+ 20.4 mmol), potassium 123 mg (K^+ 3.1 mmol). Net price 20 = £3.29. Label: 13

◢Extemporaneous formulations available see Extemporaneous Preparations, p. 8
Various strengths and salts available, caution electrolyte load

◢Injection
Phosphates (Fresenius Kabi) ⒫ⓄⓂ
Intravenous infusion, phosphates (providing phosphate 100 mmol/litre, potassium 19 mmol/litre, sodium 162 mmol/litre), net price 500 mL (*Polyfusor®*) = £3.75.

Potassium acid phosphate (Non-proprietary) ⒫ⓄⓂ
Injection, 13.6% (1 mmol/mL phosphate, 1 mmol/mL potassium) 10 mL ampoule
Note See also Important, above

Dipotassium hydrogen phosphate (Non-proprietary)
⒫ⓄⓂ
Injection, 17.42% (1 mmol/mL phosphate and 2 mmol/mL potassium) 10 mL ampoule
Note See also Important, above

Disodium hydrogen phosphate (Non-proprietary) ⒫ⓄⓂ
Injection, 17.42% (0.6 mmol/mL phosphate and 1.2 mmol/mL sodium) 10 mL ampoule

9.5.2.2 Phosphate-binding agents

Calcium-containing preparations are used as phosphate-binding agents in the management of hyperphosphataemia complicating renal failure. Aluminium-containing preparations are rarely used and have a high risk of aluminium accumulation.

Sevelamer is licensed for the treatment of hyperphosphataemia in adults on haemodialysis or peritoneal dialysis. Although experience is limited in children sevelamer may be useful when hypercalcaemia prevents the use of calcium carbonate.

ALUMINIUM HYDROXIDE

Cautions hyperaluminaemia; see also notes above; **interactions**: Appendix 1 (antacids)

Side-effects see section 1.1.1

Alu-Cap® (3M)
Capsules, green/red, dried aluminium hydroxide 475 mg (low Na^+). Net price 120-cap pack = £3.75

Dose
Hyperphosphataemia
• **By mouth**
Child 5–12 years 1–2 capsules 3–4 times daily, adjusted as necessary
Child 12–18 years 1–5 capsules 3–4 times daily, adjusted as necessary

9 Nutrition and blood

▲ CALCIUM SALTS

Cautions see notes above; **interactions:** Appendix 1 (antacids, calcium salts)

Contra-indications hypercalcaemia, hypercalciuria

Side-effects hypercalcaemia

Indication and dose

Phosphate binding in renal failure and hyperphosphataemia
* **By mouth**

Child 1 month–1 year 120 mg calcium carbonate 3–4 times daily with feeds, adjusted as necessary

Child 1–6 years 300 mg calcium carbonate 3–4 times daily prior to or with meals, adjusted as necessary

Child 6–12 years 600 mg calcium carbonate 3–4 times daily prior to or with meals, adjusted as necessary

Child 12–18 years 1.25 g calcium carbonate 3–4 times daily prior to or with meals, adjusted as necessary

Adcal®
Section 9.5.1.1

Calcichew®
Section 9.5.1.1

Calcium-500
Section 9.5.1.1

Phosex® (Vitaline)
Tablets, yellow, calcium acetate 1 g (calcium 250 mg or Ca^{2+} 6.2 mmol), net price 180-tab pack = £19.79. Label: 25, counselling, with meals

Dose
Phosphate-binding agent (with meals) in renal failure, according to the requirements of the patient

◄ Extemporaneous formulations available see Extemporaneous Preparations, p. 8

▲ SEVELAMER

Cautions gastro-intestinal disorders; **interactions:** Appendix 1 (sevelamer)

Pregnancy manufacturer advises use only if potential benefit outweighs risk

Breast-feeding manufacturer advises use only if potential benefit outweighs risk

Contra-indications bowel obstruction

Side-effects gastro-intestinal disturbances; *very rarely* intestinal obstruction

Licensed use not licensed for use in children under 18 years

Indication and dose

Hyperphosphataemia in patients on haemodialysis or peritoneal dialysis
* **By mouth**

Child 12–18 years initially 0.8–1.6 g 3 times daily with meals, then adjusted according to plasma-phosphate concentration

Renagel® (Genzyme) PoM
Tablets, f/c, sevelamer 800 mg, net price 180-tab pack = £122.76. Label: 25, counselling, with meals

9.5.3 Fluoride

Availability of adequate fluoride confers significant resistance to dental caries. It is now considered that the topical action of fluoride on enamel and plaque is more important than the systemic effect.

Where the fluoride content of the drinking water is less than 700 micrograms per litre (0.7 parts per million), daily administration of fluoride tablets or drops is a suitable means of supplementation. Systemic fluoride supplements should not be prescribed without reference to the fluoride content of the local water supply. Infants need not receive fluoride supplements until the age of 6 months.

Dentifrices which incorporate sodium fluoride or monofluorophosphate are also a convenient source of fluoride.

Individuals who are either particularly caries prone or medically compromised may be given additional protection by use of fluoride rinses or by application of fluoride gels. Rinses may be used daily or weekly; daily use of a less concentrated rinse is more effective than weekly use of a more concentrated one. High-strength gels must be applied on a regular basis under professional supervision; extreme caution is necessary to prevent the child from swallowing any excess. Less concentrated gels are available for home use. Varnishes are also available and are particularly valuable for young or disabled children since they adhere to the teeth and set in the presence of moisture.

9

Nutrition and blood

Fluoride mouthwash, oral drops, tablets, and toothpaste are prescribable on form FP10D (GP14 in Scotland, WP10D in Wales; for details see preparations below).

There are also arrangements for health authorities to supply fluoride tablets in the course of pre-school dental schemes, and they may also be supplied in school dental schemes.

Fluoride gels are not prescribable on form FP10D (GP14 in Scotland, WP10D in Wales).

FLUORIDES

Note Sodium fluoride 2.2 mg provides approx. 1 mg fluoride ion

Contra-indications not for areas where drinking water is fluoridated

Side-effects occasional white flecks on teeth with recommended doses; rarely yellowish-brown discoloration if recommended doses are exceeded

Indication and dose

Prophylaxis of dental caries—see notes above

Note Dose expressed as fluoride ion (F−):
Water content less than F− 300 micrograms/litre (0.3 parts per million)

• **By mouth**

Child 6 months–3 years F− 250 micrograms daily

Child 3–6 years F− 500 micrograms daily

Child 6 years and over F− 1 mg daily

Water content between F− 300 and 700 micrograms/litre (0.3–0.7 parts per million)

Child 3–6 years F− 250 micrograms daily

Child 6 years and over F− 500 micrograms daily

Water content above F− 700 micrograms/litre (0.7 parts per million), supplements not advised

Note These doses reflect the recommendations of the British Dental Association, the British Society of Paediatric Dentistry and the British Association for the Study of Community Dentistry (*Br Dent J* 1997; **182**: 6–7)

◢Tablets

Counselling Tablets should be sucked or dissolved in the mouth and taken preferably in the evening
There are arrangements for health authorities to supply fluoride tablets in the course of pre-school dental schemes, and they may also be supplied in school dental schemes.

En-De-Kay® (Manx)
Fluotabs 3–6 years, orange-flavoured, scored, sodium fluoride 1.1 mg (F− 500 micrograms). Net price 200-tab pack = £2.38

Fluotabs 6+ years, orange-flavoured, scored, sodium fluoride 2.2 mg (F− 1 mg). Net price 200-tab pack = £2.38

Dental prescribing on NHS May be prescribed as Sodium Fluoride Tablets

Fluor-a-day® (Dental Health)
Tablets, buff, sodium fluoride 1.1 mg (F− 500 micrograms), net price 200-tab pack = £2.41; 2.2 mg (F− 1 mg), 200-tab pack = £2.41

Dental prescribing on NHS May be prescribed as Sodium Fluoride Tablets

FluoriGard® (Colgate-Palmolive)
Tablets 0.5, purple, grape-flavoured, scored, sodium fluoride 1.1 mg (F− 500 micrograms). Net price 200-tab pack = £1.91

Tablets 1.0, orange, orange-flavoured, scored, sodium fluoride 2.2 mg (F− 1 mg). Net price 200-tab pack = £1.91

Dental prescribing on NHS May be prescribed as Sodium Fluoride Tablets

◢Oral drops

Note Fluoride supplements not considered necessary below 6 months of age (see notes above)

En-De-Kay® (Manx)
Fluodrops® (= paediatric drops), sugar-free, sodium fluoride 550 micrograms (F− 250 micrograms)/0.15 mL. Net price 60 mL = £2.38

Dental prescribing on NHS Corresponds to Sodium Fluoride Oral Drops DPF 0.37% equivalent to sodium fluoride 80 micrograms (F− 36 micrograms)/drop

◢Mouthwashes

Rinse mouth for 1 minute and spit out
Counselling Avoid eating, drinking, or rinsing mouth for 15 minutes after use

Duraphat® (Colgate-Palmolive)
Weekly dental rinse (= mouthwash), blue, sodium fluoride 0.2%. Net price 150 mL = £2.37. Counselling, see above

Dose

Child 6 years and over for *weekly* use, rinse with 10 mL

Dental prescribing on NHS May be prescribed as Sodium Fluoride Mouthwash 0.2%

En-De-Kay® (Manx)
Daily fluoride mouthrinse (= mouthwash), blue, sodium fluoride 0.05%. Net price 250 mL = £1.51

Dose

Child 6 years and over for *daily* use, rinse with 10 mL

Dental prescribing on NHS May be prescribed as Sodium Fluoride Mouthwash 0.05%

Fluorinse [PoM] (= mouthwash), red, sodium fluoride 2%. Net price 100 mL = £4.97. Counselling, see above

Dose

Child 8 years and over for *daily* use, dilute 5 drops to 10 mL of water; for *weekly* use, dilute 20 drops to 10 mL

Dental prescribing on NHS May be prescribed as Sodium Fluoride Mouthwash 2%

9 Nutrition and blood

◻ **FLUORIDES** (*continued*)

FluoriGard® (Colgate-Palmolive)
Daily dental rinse (= mouthwash), blue, sodium fluoride 0.05%. Net price 500 mL = £3.14. Counselling, see above

Dose

> **Child 6 years and over** for *daily* use, rinse with 10 mL

> Dental prescribing on NHS May be prescribed as Sodium Fluoride Mouthwash 0.05%

◀ **Gels**

FluoriGard® (Colgate-Palmolive)
Gel-Kam (= gel), stannous fluoride 0.4% in glycerol basis. Net price 100 mL = £2.97. Counselling, see below

Dose

> **Child over 3 years** for *daily* use, using a toothbrush, apply on to all tooth surfaces

> Counselling Swish between teeth for 1 minute before spitting out. Avoid eating, drinking, or rinsing mouth for at least 30 minutes after use

◀ **Toothpastes**

Duraphat® (Colgate-Palmolive) PoM
Duraphat® '2800 ppm' toothpaste, sodium fluoride 0.619%. Net price 75 mL = £3.26. Counselling, see below

Dose

> **Child over 10 years** apply 1 cm twice daily using a toothbrush
> Counselling Brush teeth for 1 minute before spitting out. Avoid drinking or rinsing mouth for 30 minutes after use

> Dental prescribing on NHS May be prescribed as Sodium Fluoride Toothpaste 0.619%

Duraphat® '5000 ppm' toothpaste, sodium fluoride 1.1%. Net price 51 g = £4.45. Counselling, see below

Dose

> **Child over 16 years** apply 2 cm 3 times daily after meals using a toothbrush
> Counselling Brush teeth for 3 minutes before spitting out

> Dental prescribing on NHS May be prescribed as Sodium Fluoride Toothpaste 1.1%

9.5.4 Zinc

Zinc supplements should be given only when there is good evidence of deficiency (hypoproteinaemia spuriously lowers plasma-zinc concentration) or in zinc-losing conditions. Zinc deficiency can occur as a result of inadequate diet or malabsorption; excessive loss of zinc can occur in trauma, burns, and protein-losing conditions. A zinc supplement is given until clinical improvement occurs, but it may need to be continued in severe malabsorption, metabolic disease, or in zinc-losing states. Zinc is used in the treatment of Wilson's disease (section 9.8.1) and acrodermatitis enteropathica, a rare inherited abnormality of zinc absorption.

Parenteral nutrition regimens usually include trace amounts of zinc (section 9.3). If necessary, further zinc can be added to some intravenous feeding regimens.

▌ ZINC SULPHATE

Cautions interactions: Appendix 1 (zinc)

Renal impairment accumulation may occur in acute renal failure

Pregnancy crosses placenta, risk theoretically minimal but no information available

Breast-feeding present in breast milk, risk theoretically minimal but no information available

Side-effects abdominal pain, dyspepsia, nausea, vomiting, diarrhoea, gastric irritation, gastritis; irritability, headache, lethargy

Licensed use *Solvazinc®* not licensed in Wilson's disease or acrodermatitis enteropathica

Solvazinc® (KoGEN)
Effervescent tablets, yellow-white, zinc sulphate monohydrate 125 mg (45 mg zinc), net price 30 = £4.32. Label: 13, 21

Dose

Zinc deficiency (see notes above)
● By mouth

> **Neonate** 1 mg/kg elemental zinc daily

> **Child under 10 kg** half a tablet daily in water after food, adjusted as necessary

> **Child 10–30 kg** half a tablet 1–3 times daily in water after food, adjusted as necessary

> **Child over 30 kg** 1 tablet 1–3 times daily in water after food, adjusted as necessary

Acrodermatitis enteropathica
● By mouth

> **Neonate** 0.5–1 mg/kg elemental zinc twice daily (total daily dose may alternatively be given in 3 divided doses), adjusted as necessary

> **Child 1 month–18 years** 0.5–1 mg/kg elemental zinc twice daily (total daily dose may alternatively be given in 3 divided doses), adjusted as necessary

9

Nutrition and blood

9.6 Vitamins

9.6.1 Vitamin A
9.6.2 Vitamin B group
9.6.3 Vitamin C
9.6.4 Vitamin D
9.6.5 Vitamin E
9.6.6 Vitamin K
9.6.7 Multivitamin preparations

Vitamins are used for the prevention and treatment of specific deficiency states or where the diet is known to be inadequate; they may be prescribed in the NHS to prevent or treat deficiency but not as dietary supplements. Except for iron-deficiency anaemia, a primary vitamin or mineral deficiency due to simple dietary inadequacy is rare in the developed world. Some children may be at risk of developing deficiencies because of an inadequate intake, impaired vitamin synthesis or malabsorption in disease states such as cystic fibrosis and Crohn's disease.

The use of vitamins as general 'pick-me-ups' is of unproven value and the 'fad' for mega-vitamin therapy with water-soluble vitamins, such as ascorbic acid and pyridoxine, is unscientific and can be harmful. Many vitamin supplements are described as 'multivitamin' but few contain the whole range of essential vitamins and many contain relatively high amounts of vitamins A and D. Care should be taken to ensure the correct dose is not exceeded.

Dietary reference values for vitamins are available in the Department of Health publication:

Dietary Reference Values for Food Energy and Nutrients for the United Kingdom: Report of the Panel on Dietary Reference Values of the Committee on Medical Aspects of Food Policy. *Report on Health and Social Subjects 41*. London: HMSO, 1991

Dental patients It is unjustifiable to treat stomatitis or glossitis with mixtures of vitamin preparations; this delays diagnosis and correct treatment.

Most patients who develop a nutritional deficiency despite an adequate intake of vitamins have malabsorption and if this is suspected the patient should be referred to a medical practitioner.

9.6.1 Vitamin A

Deficiency of vitamin A (retinol) is associated with ocular defects (particularly xerophthalmia) and an increased susceptibility to infections, but deficiency is rare in the UK (even in disorders of fat absorption).

Vitamin A supplementation may be required in children with liver disease, particularly cholestatic liver disease, due to the malabsorption of fat soluble vitamins. In those with complete biliary obstruction an intramuscular dose once a month may be appropriate.

Treatment is sometimes initiated with very high doses of vitamin A and the child should be monitored closely; very high doses are associated with acute toxicity.

Preterm neonates have low plasma concentrations of vitamin A and are usually given vitamin A supplements, often as part of an oral multivitamin preparation (section 9.6.7) once enteral feeding has been established.

Massive overdose can cause rough skin, dry hair, an enlarged liver, and a raised erythrocyte sedimentation rate and raised serum calcium and serum alkaline phosphatase concentrations.

Pregnancy In view of evidence suggesting that high levels of vitamin A may cause birth defects, women who are (or may become) pregnant are advised not to take vitamin A supplements (including tablets and fish-liver oil drops), except on the advice of a doctor or an antenatal clinic; nor should they eat liver or products such as liver paté or liver sausage.

◢ VITAMIN A
(Retinol)

Cautions see notes above; **interactions**: Appendix 1 (vitamins)

Pregnancy teratogenic; see notes above

Breast-feeding toxicity likely if mother taking high doses

Side-effects see notes above

◻ **VITAMIN A** (*continued*)

Licensed use preparations containing only vitamin A are not licensed

Indication and dose

See also notes above

Vitamin A deficiency
• **By mouth**

Neonate 5000 units daily

Child 1 month–1 year 5000 units daily with or
after food

Child 1–18 years 10 000 units daily with or after
food

Note Higher doses may be used initially for treatment of
severe deficiency

**Prevention of deficiency in complete biliary
obstruction**
• **By intramuscular injection**

Neonate 50 000 units once a month

Child 1 month–1 year 50 000 units once a
month

Arovit® (Non-proprietary)
Oral solution, vitamin A 150 000 units/mL
Available from 'special-order' manufacturers or specialist
importing companies, see p. 943

Aquasol-A® (Non-proprietary)
Injection, vitamin A (as palmitate) 50 000 units/
mL, 2-mL amp
Available from 'special-order' manufacturers or specialist
importing companies, see p. 943

◢ VITAMINS A and D

Cautions see notes above and section 9.6.4; prolonged excessive ingestion of vitamins A and D
can lead to hypervitaminosis; **interactions:**
Appendix 1 (vitamins)

Pregnancy see notes above

Side-effects see notes above and section 9.6.4

Licensed use not licensed in children under 6
months of age

Indication and dose

See notes above and section 9.6.4

Prevention of vitamin A and D deficiency see
individual preparations for dose information

◢Vitamins A and D
Vitamins A and D (Non-proprietary)
Capsules, vitamin A 4000 units, vitamin D
400 units. Net price 84 = £3.14
Note May be difficult to obtain
Dose

Child 1–18 years 1 capsule daily

◢Vitamins A, C and D
Healthy Start Children's Vitamin Drops (Non-proprietary)
Oral drops, vitamin A 5000 units, vitamin D
2000 units, ascorbic acid 150 mg/mL
Available free of charge to children under 4 years through
the Healthy Start Scheme; otherwise available direct to
the public from maternity and child health clinics; community pharmacists may have difficulty obtaining supplies
Dose
Prevention of vitamin deficiency
• **By mouth**
Child 1 month–5 years 5 drops daily (5 drops contain
vitamin A approx. 700 units, vitamin D approx.
300 units, ascorbic acid approx. 20 mg)

Note *Healthy Start Vitamins for women* (containing ascorbic
acid, vitamin D, and folic acid) are also available to women
during pregnancy and until their baby is one year old,
through the Healthy Start Scheme

9.6.2 Vitamin B group

Deficiency of the B vitamins, other than deficiency of vitamin B_{12} (section 9.1.2), is
rare in the UK and is usually treated by preparations containing thiamine (B_1),
riboflavin (B_2), and nicotinamide, which is used in preference to nicotinic acid, as
it does not cause vasodilatation. Other members (or substances traditionally
classified as members) of the vitamin B complex such as aminobenzoic acid,
biotin, choline, inositol, and pantothenic acid or panthenol may be included in
vitamin B preparations but there is no evidence of their value as supplements;
however they can be used in the management of certain metabolic disorders

(section 9.8.1). Anaphylaxis has been reported with parenteral B vitamins (see MHRA/CHM advice, below).

As with other vitamins of the B group, pyridoxine (B_6) deficiency is rare, but it may occur during isoniazid therapy (section 5.1.9) or penicillamine treatment in Wilson's disease (section 9.8.1) and is characterised by peripheral neuritis. High doses of **pyridoxine** are given in some metabolic disorders, such as hyperoxaluria, cystathioninuria and homocystinuria; folic acid supplementation may also be beneficial in these disorders (section 9.1.2). Pyridoxine is also used in sideroblastic anaemia (section 9.1.3). Rarely, seizures in the neonatal period or during infancy respond to pyridoxine treatment; pyridoxine should be tried in all cases of early-onset intractable seizures and status epilepticus. Pyridoxine has been tried for a wide variety of other disorders, but there is little sound evidence to support the claims of efficacy, and overdosage induces toxic effects.

A number of mitochondrial disorders may respond to treatment with certain B vitamins but these disorders require specialist management. **Thiamine** is used in the treatment of maple syrup urine disease, mitochondrial respiratory chain defects and, together with riboflavin, in the treatment of congenital lactic acidosis; riboflavin is also used in glutaric acidaemias and cytochrome oxidase deficiencies; biotin (section 9.8.1) is used in carboxylase defects.

Nicotinic acid inhibits the synthesis of cholesterol and triglyceride (section 2.12). Folic acid and vitamin B_{12} are used in the treatment of megaloblastic anaemia (section 9.1.2). Folinic acid (available as calcium folinate) is used in association with cytotoxic therapy (section 8.1).

◢ RIBOFLAVIN
(Riboflavine, vitamin B_2)

Cautions see notes above

Pregnancy crosses the placenta but no adverse effects reported, information at high doses limited

Breast-feeding present in breast milk but no adverse effects reported, information at high doses limited

Side-effects bright yellow urine

Licensed use not licensed in children

Indication and dose

See also notes above

Metabolic diseases
• By mouth

Neonate 50 mg 1–2 times daily, adjusted according to response

Child 1 month–18 years 50–100 mg 1–2 times daily, adjusted according to response, up to 400 mg daily has been used

Riboflavin (Non-proprietary)
Tablets, 10 mg, 50 mg and 100 mg
Available from 'special-order' manufacturers or specialist importing companies, see p. 943

◢ Oral vitamin B complex preparations
See below

◢ Extemporaneous formulations available see Extemporaneous Preparations, p. 8

◢ THIAMINE
(Vitamin B_1)

MHRA/CHM advice (September 2007) Although potentially serious allergic adverse reactions may rarely occur during, or shortly after, parenteral administration, the CHM has recommended that:

1. This should not preclude the use of parenteral thiamine in patients where this route of administration is required, particularly in patients at risk of Wernicke-Korsakoff syndrome where treatment with thiamine is essential;

2. Intravenous administration should be by infusion over 30 minutes;

3. Facilities for treating anaphylaxis (including resuscitation facilities) should be available when parenteral thiamine is administered.

Cautions anaphylactic shock may occasionally follow injection (see MHRA/CHM advice above)

Contra-indications

Breast-feeding severely thiamine-deficient mothers should avoid breast-feeding as toxic methyl-glyoxal present in milk

Side-effects hypersensitivity reactions to injection

Licensed use not licensed in children

Indication and dose

See also notes above

Maple syrup urine disease
• By mouth

Neonate 5 mg/kg daily, adjusted as necessary

Child 1 month–18 years 5 mg/kg daily, adjusted as necessary

◻ **THIAMINE** (*continued*)

Metabolic disorders including congenital lactic acidosis
• **By mouth or by intravenous infusion over 30 minutes**

Neonate 50–200 mg once daily (total dose may alternatively be given in 2–3 divided doses), adjusted as necessary

Child 1 month–18 years 100–300 mg once daily (total dose may alternatively be given in 2–3 divided doses), adjusted as necessary; up to 2 g daily may be necessary

Thiamine (Non-proprietary)
Tablets, thiamine hydrochloride 50 mg, net price 20 = £1.31; 100 mg, 20 = £1.50
Brands include *Benerva*® ⃞Hs

Injection, 50 mg/mL, 2-mL vial; 100 mg/mL, 2-mL vial

Injection (intramuscular), 100 mg/mL, 5-mL vial
Available from 'special-order' manufacturers or specialist importing companies, see p. 943
Note Some preparations may contain phenol as a preservative

◢Oral vitamin B complex preparations
See below

▰ PYRIDOXINE HYDROCHLORIDE
(Vitamin B₆)

Cautions see notes above; risk of cardiovascular collapse with intravenous injection; **interactions:** Appendix 1 (vitamins)

Side-effects sensory neuropathy reported with high doses given for extended periods

Licensed use not licensed for use in children

Indication and dose
See also notes above

Metabolic diseases including cystathioninuria and homocystinuria
• **By mouth**

Neonate 50–100 mg 1–2 times daily

Child 1 month–18 years 50–250 mg 1–2 times daily

Treatment of isoniazid-induced neuropathy
• **By mouth**

Neonate 5–10 mg daily

Child 1 month–12 years 10–20 mg 2–3 times daily

Child 12–18 years 30–50 mg 2–3 times daily

Prevention of isoniazid-induced neuropathy
• **By mouth**

Neonate 5 mg daily

Child 1 month–12 years 5–10 mg daily

Child 12–18 years 10 mg daily

Prevention of penicillamine-induced neuropathy in Wilson's disease (see notes above)
• **By mouth**

Child 1–12 years 5–10 mg daily

Child 12–18 years 10 mg daily

Pyridoxine-dependent seizures
• **By intravenous injection or by mouth**

Neonate initial test dose 50–100 mg by intravenous injection, may be repeated; if responsive followed by an oral maintenance dose of 50–100 mg once daily, adjusted as necessary

Child 1 month–12 years initial test dose 50–100 mg daily; if responsive followed by an oral dose of 20–50 mg 1–2 times daily, adjusted as necessary; doses up to 30 mg/kg or 1 g daily have been used

Pyridoxine (Non-proprietary)
Tablets, pyridoxine hydrochloride 10 mg, net price 20 = 34p; 20 mg, 20 = 34p; 50 mg, 28 = 76p

Injection, 25 mg/mL, 2 mL vial
Available from 'special-order' manufacturers or specialist importing companies, see p. 943

◢ Extemporaneous formulations available see Extemporaneous Preparations, p. 8

▰ NICOTINAMIDE

Indication and dose
See notes above, Acne vulgaris see section 13.6.1

Nicotinamide (Non-proprietary)
Tablets, nicotinamide 50 mg. Net price 20 = £1.37

▰ Oral vitamin B complex preparations
Note Other multivitamin preparations are in section 9.6.7.

Vitamin B Tablets, Compound ◢
Tablets, nicotinamide 15 mg, riboflavin 1 mg, thiamine hydrochloride 1 mg. Net price 20 = 7p

Vitamin B Tablets, Compound, Strong ◢
Tablets, brown, f/c or s/c, nicotinamide 20 mg, pyridoxine hydrochloride 2 mg, riboflavin 2 mg, thiamine hydrochloride 5 mg. Net price 28-tab pack = £2.00

9

Nutrition and blood

Vigranon B® (Wallace Mfg) [NHS] [◄]
Syrup, thiamine hydrochloride 5 mg, riboflavin
2 mg, nicotinamide 20 mg, pyridoxine hydrochloride 2 mg, panthenol 3 mg/5 mL. Net price
150 mL = £2.41

Dose

Treatment of deficiency
• By mouth
    Child 1 month–1 year 5 mL 3 times daily

    Child 1–12 years 10 mL 3 times daily
    Child 12–18 years 10–15 mL 3 times daily

Prophylaxis of deficiency
• By mouth
    Child 1 month–1 year 5 mL once daily
    Child 1–12 years 5 mL twice daily
    Child 12–18 years 5 mL 3 times daily

9.6.3 Vitamin C
(Ascorbic acid)

Vitamin C therapy is essential in scurvy, but less florid manifestations of vitamin C
deficiency have been reported. Vitamin C is used to enhance the excretion of iron
one month after starting desferrioxamine therapy (section 9.1.3); it is given
separately from food as it also enhances iron absorption. Vitamin C is also used
in the treatment of some inherited metabolic disorders, particularly mitochondrial
disorders; specialist management of these conditions is required.

Severe scurvy causes gingival swelling and bleeding margins as well as petechiae
on the skin. This is, however, exceedingly rare and a child with these signs is more
likely to have leukaemia. Investigation should not be delayed by a trial period of
vitamin treatment.

Claims that vitamin C ameliorates colds or promotes wound healing have not
been proved.

ASCORBIC ACID
(Vitamin C)

Cautions interactions: Appendix 1 (vitamins)

Contra-indications hyperoxaluria

Side-effects nausea, diarrhoea; headache, fatigue; hyperoxaluria

Licensed use not licensed for metabolic disorders

Indication and dose

Treatment of scurvy
• By mouth
    Child 1 month–4 years 125–250 mg daily in 1–2
    divided doses

    Child 4–12 years 250–500 mg daily in 1–2
    divided doses

    Child 12–18 years 500 mg–1 g daily in 1–2
    divided doses

Adjunct to desferrioxamine (see notes above)
• By mouth
    Child 1 month–18 years 100–200 mg daily 1
    hour before food

Metabolic disorders (tyrosinaemia type III; transient tyrosinaemia of the newborn; glutathione
synthase deficiency; Hawkinsinuria)
• By mouth
    Neonate 50–200 mg daily, adjusted as necessary

    Child 1 month–18 years 200–400 mg daily in 1–
    2 divided doses, adjusted as necessary; up to 1 g
    daily may be required

Ascorbic Acid (Non-proprietary)
Tablets, ascorbic acid 50 mg, net price 28 = £1.21;
100 mg, 28 = £1.26; 200 mg, 28 = £1.27; 500 mg
(label: 24), 28 = £3.12
Excipients may include aspartame
Brands include *Redoxon®* [NHS]

Injection, ascorbic acid 100 mg/mL. Net price 5-
mL amp = £2.51
Excipients include metabisulphite
Available from UCB Pharma

9.6.4 Vitamin D

Note The term Vitamin D is used for a range of compounds including ergocalciferol (calciferol, vitamin
D₂), colecalciferol (vitamin D₃), dihydrotachysterol, alfacalcidol (1α-hydroxycholecalciferol), and
calcitriol (1,25-dihydroxycholecalciferol).

Symptomatic deficiency of vitamin D is uncommon in the United Kingdom, but
may occur in certain ethnic groups, and rarely in association with malabsorption.
The amount of vitamin D required in infancy is related to the stores built up *in
utero* and subsequent exposure to sunlight. The amount of vitamin D in breast
milk varies and some breast-fed babies, particularly if preterm or born to vitamin
D deficient mothers, may become deficient. Most formula milk and supplement
feeds contain adequate vitamin D to prevent deficiency.

9 Nutrition and blood

Simple, nutritional vitamin D deficiency can be prevented by oral supplementation of 400 units of **ergocalciferol** (calciferol, vitamin D$_2$) or **colecalciferol** (vitamin D$_3$) daily, using multi-vitamin drops (section 9.6.7), manufactured 'special' solutions, or as calcium and ergocalciferol tablets (although the calcium is unnecessary); excessive supplementation may cause hypercalcaemia.

Inadequate bone mineralisation can be caused by a deficiency, or a lack of action of vitamin D or its active metabolite. In childhood this causes bowing and distortion of bones (rickets); initial high doses of vitamin D should be reduced after a few weeks, as there is a significant risk of hypercalcaemia (see caution below).

Poor bone mineralisation in neonates and young children may also be due to inadequate intake of phosphate or calcium particularly during long-term parenteral nutrition—supplementation with phosphate (section 9.5.2.1) or calcium (section 9.5.1.1) may be required.

Hypophosphataemic rickets occurs due to abnormal phosphate excretion; treatment with high doses of oral phosphate (section 9.5.2.1), and hydroxylated (activated) forms of vitamin D allow bone mineralisation and optimise growth.

Nutritional deficiency of vitamin D is best treated with colecalciferol or ergocalciferol. Preparations containing calcium and colecalciferol are also occasionally used in children where there is evidence of combined calcium and vitamin D deficiency. Vitamin D deficiency caused by *intestinal malabsorption* or *chronic liver disease* usually requires vitamin D in pharmacological doses, such as **ergocalciferol** in doses of up to 40 000 units daily; the hypocalcaemia of *hypoparathyroidism* often requires higher doses in order to achieve normocalcaemia and alfacalcidol is generally preferred.

Vitamin D supplementation is often given in combination with calcium supplements for persistent hypocalcaemia in neonates, and in chronic renal disease.

Vitamin D requires hydroxylation, by the kidney and liver, to its active form therefore the hydroxylated derivatives **alfacalcidol** or **calcitriol** should be prescribed if patients with *severe liver or renal impairment* require vitamin D therapy. Alfacalcidol is generally preferred in children as there is more experience of its use and appropriate formulations are available. Calcitriol is unlicensed for use in children and is generally reserved for those with severe liver disease.

Important. All patients receiving pharmacological doses of vitamin D or its analogues should have their plasma-calcium concentration checked at intervals (initially once or twice weekly) and whenever nausea or vomiting occur. Breast milk from women taking pharmacological doses of vitamin D can cause hypercalcaemia if given to an infant.

ERGOCALCIFEROL
(Calciferol, Vitamin D$_2$)

Cautions monitor plasma calcium in patients receiving high doses and in renal impairment; **interactions**: Appendix 1 (vitamins)

Pregnancy avoid excessive supplementation; high doses teratogenic in *animals* but therapeutic doses unlikely to be harmful

Breast-feeding avoid excessive supplementation; may cause hypercalcaemia in infant—monitor serum-calcium concentration

Contra-indications hypercalcaemia; metastatic calcification

Side-effects symptoms of overdosage include anorexia, lassitude, nausea and vomiting, diarrhoea, constipation, weight loss, polyuria, sweating, headache, thirst, vertigo, and raised concentrations of calcium and phosphate in plasma and urine

Licensed use Calcium and Ergocalciferol tablets not licensed for use in children under 6 years

Indication and dose

See also notes above

Nutritional vitamin-D deficiency rickets
• By mouth

Child 1–6 months 3000 units daily, adjusted as necessary

Child 6 months–12 years 6000 units daily, adjusted as necessary

Child 12–18 years 10 000 units daily, adjusted as necessary

9

Nutrition and blood

◁ **ERGOCALCIFEROL** (*continued*)

Nutritional or physiological supplement; prevention of rickets

• **By mouth**

Neonate 400 units daily

Child 1 month–18 years 400–600 units daily

Vitamin D deficiency in intestinal malabsorption or in chronic liver disease

• **By mouth or by intramuscular injection**

Child 1–12 years 10 000–25 000 units daily, adjusted as necessary

Child 12–18 years 10 000–40 000 units daily, adjusted as necessary

◢**Pharmacological strengths**

(see notes above)
The BP directs that when calciferol is prescribed or demanded, colecalciferol or ergocalciferol should be dispensed or supplied

Ergocalciferol (Non-proprietary)

Tablets, ergocalciferol 250 micrograms (10 000 units), net price 100 = £21.99; 1.25 mg (50 000 units), 100 = £30.34

Note May be difficult to obtain
Important When the strength of the tablets ordered or prescribed is not clear, the intention of the prescriber or purchaser with respect to the strength (expressed in micrograms or milligrams per tablet) should be ascertained.

Solution ergocalciferol 3000 units/mL
Excipients may include peanut oil
Available from 'special-order' manufacturers or specialist importing companies, see p. 943

Injection, colecalciferol or ergocalciferol, 7.5 mg (300 000 units)/mL in oil. Net price 1-mL amp = £7.44, 2-mL amp = £8.93

◢**Daily supplements**

Note There is no plain vitamin D tablet available for treating simple deficiency (see notes above). Alternatives include vitamins capsules (section 9.6.7), preparations of vitamins A and D (section 9.6.1), and calcium and ergocalciferol tablets (see below).
For cautions, contra-indications, and side-effects of calcium, see section 9.5.1

Calcium and Ergocalciferol (Non-proprietary) (**Calcium and Vitamin D**)

Tablets, calcium lactate 300 mg, calcium phosphate 150 mg (calcium 97 mg or Ca^{2+} 2.4 mmol), ergocalciferol 10 micrograms (400 units). Net price 28-tab pack = £2.38. Counselling, crush before administration or may be chewed

---

■ **ALFACALCIDOL**

(1α-Hydroxycholecalciferol)

Cautions see under Ergocalciferol; also nephrolithiasis

Contra-indications see under Ergocalciferol

Side-effects see under Ergocalciferol; also *rarely* nephrocalcinosis, pruritus, rash, urticaria

Indication and dose

See also notes above

Hypophosphataemic rickets; persistent hypocalcaemia due to hypoparathyroidism or pseudohypoparathyroidism

• **By mouth or by intravenous injection**

Child 1 month–12 years 25–50 nanograms/kg (max. 1 microgram) once daily, adjusted as necessary

Child 12–18 years 1 microgram once daily, adjusted as necessary

Persistent neonatal hypocalcaemia

• **By mouth or by intravenous injection**

Neonate 50–100 nanograms/kg once daily, adjusted as necessary (up to 2 micrograms/kg daily may be needed in resistant cases)

Prevention of vitamin D deficiency in renal or cholestatic liver disease

• **By mouth or by intravenous injection**

Neonate 20 nanograms/kg once daily, adjusted as necessary

Child 1 month–12 years, body-weight under 20 kg 15–30 nanograms/kg (max. 500 nanograms) once daily; **body-weight over 20 kg** 250–500 nanograms once daily, adjusted as necessary

Child 12–18 years 250–500 nanograms once daily, adjusted as necessary

Alfacalcidol (Non-proprietary) ▢PoM

Capsules, alfacalcidol 250 nanograms, net price 30-cap pack = £5.08; 500 nanograms 30-cap pack = £9.99; 1 microgram 30-cap pack = £13.89

One-Alpha® (LEO) ▢PoM

Capsules, alfacalcidol 250 nanograms (white), net price 30-cap pack = £3.37; 500 nanograms (red), 30-cap pack = £6.27; 1 microgram (brown), 30-cap pack = £8.75
Excipients include sesame oil

Oral drops, sugar-free, alfacalcidol 2 micrograms/mL (1 drop contains approx. 100 nanograms), net price 10 mL = £22.49
Excipients include alcohol

Note The concentration of alfacalcidol in *One-Alpha®* drops is **10 times greater** than that of the former presentation *One-Alpha®* solution.

Injection, alfacalcidol 2 micrograms/mL, net price 0.5-mL amp = £2.16, 1-mL amp = £4.11

Note Contains propylene glycol and should be used with caution in small preterm neonates

◢ CALCITRIOL

(1,25-Dihydroxycholecalciferol)

Cautions see under Ergocalciferol; monitor plasma calcium, phosphate, and creatinine during dosage titration

Contra-indications see under Ergocalciferol

Side-effects see under Ergocalciferol

Licensed use not licensed for use in children

Indication and dose

See also notes above

Vitamin D dependent rickets; hypophosphataemic rickets; persistent hypocalcaemia due to hypoparathyroidism or pseudo-hypoparathyroidism (limited experience)

* **By mouth**

    Child 1 month–12 years initially 15 nanograms/kg (max. 250 nanograms) once daily, increased if necessary in steps of 5 nanograms/kg daily (max. 250 nanograms) every 2–4 weeks

    Child 12–18 years initially 250 nanograms once daily increased if necessary in steps of 5 nanograms/kg daily (max. 250 nanograms step) every 2–4 weeks; usual dose 0.5–1 microgram daily

Hypocalcaemia in dialysis patients (limited experience)

* **By intravenous injection**

    Child 12–18 years initially 250–500 nanograms (approx. 10 nanograms/kg) 3 times a week, increased if necessary in steps of 2–5 nanograms/kg every 2–4 weeks; usual dose 0.5–3 micrograms 3 times a week

Administration For administration *by mouth*, injection solution may be given orally or contents of capsule administered by oral syringe; capsules contain approx. 0.168 mL of fluid

For administration *by intravenous injection*, injection may be given via catheter after dialysis

Calcitriol (Non-proprietary) [PoM]

Capsules, calcitriol 250 nanograms, net price 30-cap pack = £5.87, 100-cap pack = £19.15; 500 nanograms, 30-cap pack =£10.50, 100-cap pack = £34.24

Rocaltrol® (Roche) [PoM]

Capsules, calcitriol 250 nanograms (red/white), net price 20 = £3.83; 500 nanograms (red), 20 = £6.85

Calcijex® (Abbott) [PoM]

Injection, calcitriol 1 microgram/mL, net price 1-mL amp = £5.14; 2 micrograms/mL, 1-mL amp = £10.28

◢ COLECALCIFEROL

(Cholecalciferol, vitamin D₃)

Cautions see under Ergocalciferol

Contra-indications see under Ergocalciferol

Side-effects see under Ergocalciferol

Licensed use *Adcal-D3®*, *Calceos®*, and *Calcichew®D3* not licensed for use in children under 12 years; *Cacit®D3* not licensed for use in children (age range not specified by manufacturers); *Calcichew®D3 Forte*, *Calfovit D3®*, and *Natecal D3®* not licensed for use in children under 18 years

Indication and dose

See under Ergocalciferol and notes above—alternative to Ergocalciferol, see also Pharmacological Strengths

◢ Extemporaneous formulations available see Extemporaneous Preparations, p. 8

◢ **With calcium**

For cautions, contra-indications, and side-effects of calcium, see section 9.5.1

Adcal-D₃® (Strakan)

Tablets (chewable), lemon or tutti-frutti flavour, calcium carbonate 1.5 g (calcium 600 mg or Ca²⁺ 15 mmol), colecalciferol 10 micrograms (400 units), net price 56-tab pack = £4.06, 112-tab pack = £7.99. Label: 24

Dissolve (effervescent tablets), lemon flavour, calcium carbonate 1.5 g (calcium 600 mg or Ca²⁺ 15 mmol), colecalciferol 10 micrograms (400 units), net price 56-tab pack = £4.99. Label: 13

Cacit® D3 (Procter & Gamble Pharm.)

Granules, effervescent, lemon flavour, calcium carbonate 1.25 g (calcium 500 mg or Ca²⁺ 12.5 mmol), colecalciferol 11 micrograms (440 units)/sachet, net price 30-sachet pack = £4.31. Label: 13

Calceos® (Galen)

Tablets (chewable), lemon flavour, calcium carbonate 1.25 g (calcium 500 mg or Ca²⁺ 12.5 mmol), colecalciferol 10 micrograms (400 units), net price 60-tab pack = £3.90. Label: 24

Calcichew® D3 (Shire)

Tablets (chewable), orange flavour, calcium carbonate 1.25 g (calcium 500 mg or Ca²⁺ 12.5 mmol), colecalciferol 5 micrograms (200 units), net price 100-tab pack = £15.02. Label: 24
Excipients include aspartame (section 9.4.1)

Calcichew® D3 Forte (Shire)

Tablets (chewable), lemon flavour, calcium carbonate 1.25 g (calcium 500 mg or Ca²⁺ 12.5 mmol), colecalciferol 10 micrograms (400 units), net price 100-tab pack = £7.50. Label: 24
Excipients include aspartame (section 9.4.1)

Calfovit D3® (Menarini)

Powder, lemon flavour, calcium phosphate 3.1 g (calcium 1.2 g or Ca²⁺ 30 mmol), colecalciferol 20 micrograms (800 units), net price 30-sachet pack = £4.32. Label: 13, 21

Natecal D3® (Chiesi)

Tablets, (aniseed, peppermint, and molasses flavour), calcium carbonate 1.5 g (calcium 600 mg or

9

Nutrition and blood

◁ **COLECALCIFEROL (continued)**

Ca²⁺ 15 mmol), colecalciferol 10 micrograms (400 units), net price 60-tab pack = £3.85. Label: 24
Excipients include aspartame (section 9.4.1)

Sandocal®+D 600 (Novartis Consumer Health)
Tablets, effervescent, orange flavour, calcium lactate gluconate 1.36 g, calcium carbonate 1.05 g,

providing calcium 600 mg (Ca²⁺ 15 mmol), colecalciferol concentrate 4 mg, providing colecalciferol 10 micrograms (400 units), net price 60-tab pack = £5.35, 100-tab pack = £8.75. Label: 13
Excipients include aspartame (section 9.4.1)

9.6.5 Vitamin E
(Tocopherols)

The daily requirement of vitamin E has not been well defined. Vitamin E supplements are given to children with fat malabsorption such as in cystic fibrosis and cholestatic liver disease. In children with abetalipoproteinaemia abnormally low vitamin E concentrations may occur in association with neuromuscular problems; this usually responds to high doses of vitamin E. Some neonatal units still administer a single intramuscular dose of vitamin E at birth to preterm neonates to reduce the risk of complications; no trials of long-term outcome have been carried out. The intramuscular route should also be considered in children with severe liver disease when response to oral therapy is inadequate.

Vitamin E has been tried for various other conditions but there is little scientific evidence of its value.

ALPHA TOCOPHERYL ACETATE
(Vitamin E)

Cautions predisposition to thrombosis; increased risk of necrotising enterocolitis in preterm neonates (see administration); **interactions:** Appendix 1 (vitamins)

Pregnancy avoid high doses in first trimester

Breast-feeding excreted in breast milk, minimal risk although caution with large doses

Side-effects diarrhoea and abdominal pain, particularly with high doses

Indication and dose

Vitamin E deficiency
• By mouth

> Neonate 10 mg/kg once daily

> Child 1 month–18 years 2–10 mg/kg daily, up to 20 mg/kg has been used

Malabsorption in cystic fibrosis
• By mouth (with food and pancreatic enzymes)

> Child 1 month–1 year 50 mg once daily, adjusted as necessary

> Child 1–12 years 100 mg once daily, adjusted as necessary

> Child 12–18 years 100–200 mg once daily, adjusted as necessary

Vitamin E deficiency in cholestasis and severe liver disease
• By mouth

> Neonate 10 mg/kg daily

> Child 1 month–12 years initially 100 mg daily, adjusted according to response; up to 200 mg/kg daily may be required

> Child 12–18 years initially 200 mg daily, adjusted according to response; up to 200 mg/kg daily may be required

• By intramuscular injection

> Neonate 10 mg/kg once a month

> Child 1 month–18 years 10 mg/kg (max. 100 mg) once a month

Malabsorption in abetalipoproteinaemia
• By mouth

> Neonate 100 mg/kg once daily

> Child 1 month–18 years 50–100 mg/kg once daily

Vitamin E Suspension (Cambridge)
Suspension, alpha tocopheryl acetate 100 mg/mL. Net price 100 mL = £25.08
Excipients include sucrose
Administration consider dilution in neonates due to high osmolality (see Cautions)
Note Tablets containing tocopheryl acetate are available from 'special-order' manufacturers or specialist importing companies, see p. 943

Vitamin E Injection (Roche)
Injection tocopheryl acetate 50 mg/mL, 2-mL ampoule
Available from 'special-order' manufacturers or specialist importing companies, see p. 943

9.6.6 Vitamin K

Vitamin K is necessary for the production of blood clotting factors and proteins necessary for the normal calcification of bone.

Because vitamin K is fat soluble, children with fat malabsorption, especially in biliary obstruction or hepatic disease, may become deficient. For oral administration to prevent vitamin K deficiency in malabsorption syndromes, a water-soluble preparation, **menadiol sodium phosphate** (see Contra-indications below) must be used.

Oral coumarin anticoagulants act by interfering with vitamin K metabolism in the hepatic cells and their effects can be antagonised by giving vitamin K (see also section 2.8.2).

Vitamin K deficiency bleeding Neonates are relatively deficient in vitamin K and those who do not receive supplements are at risk of serious bleeds (haemorrhagic disease), including intracranial bleeding. The Chief Medical Officer and the Chief Nursing Officer have recommended that all newborn babies should receive vitamin K to prevent vitamin K deficiency bleeding (haemorrhagic disease of the newborn). Local protocols may vary and an appropriate regimen should be selected after discussion with parents in the antenatal period.

Vitamin K (as phytomenadione) 1 mg may be given by a single intramuscular injection at birth; this prevents vitamin K deficiency bleeding in virtually all babies; preterm neonates may be given 400 micrograms/kg (max. 1 mg). The intravenous route is preferred by some in preterm neonates of very low birth-weight but it does not provide the prolonged protection of the intramuscular injection, and any babies receiving intravenous vitamin K should be given subsequent oral doses, as described below.

Babies considered at particular risk of vitamin K deficiency bleeding should receive intramuscular vitamin K at birth; this includes those experiencing birth asphyxia or bleeding problems, those born to mothers with liver disease or taking enzyme inducing anticonvulsant drugs (carbamazepine, phenobarbital, phenytoin), rifampicin or warfarin. In infants with cholestatic disease, vitamin K must be given either intramuscularly or intravenously because oral absorption is likely to be impaired.

Alternatively, in healthy babies who are not at particular risk of bleeding disorders, vitamin K may be given by mouth, and arrangements must be in place to ensure the appropriate regimen is followed. Two doses of a colloidal (mixed micelle) preparation of phytomenadione 2 mg should be given in the first week, the first dose being given at birth. For exclusively breast-fed babies, a third dose of phytomenadione 2 mg is given at 1 month of age; the third dose is omitted in formula-fed babies because formula feeds contain vitamin K.

MENADIOL SODIUM PHOSPHATE

Cautions G6PD deficiency (section 9.1.5) and vitamin E deficiency (risk of haemolysis); **interactions**: Appendix 1 (vitamins)

Contra-indications neonates and infants, late pregnancy

Indication and dose

See notes above

Supplementation in vitamin K malabsorption
• **By mouth**
    Child 1–12 years 5–10 mg daily, adjusted as necessary

    Child 12–18 years 10–20 mg daily, adjusted as necessary

Menadiol Phosphate (Cambridge)
    Tablets, menadiol sodium phosphate equivalent to 10 mg of menadiol phosphate. Net price 100-tab pack = £48.25

◢Extemporaneous formulations available see Extemporaneous Preparations, p. 8

PHYTOMENADIONE
(Vitamin K₁)

Cautions intravenous injections should be given very slowly—risk of vascular collapse (see also below); **interactions**: Appendix 1 (vitamins)

Indication and dose

Neonatal prophylaxis of vitamin-K deficiency bleeding see notes above

9

Nutrition and blood

◻ **PHYTOMENADIONE** (*continued*)

Neonatal hypoprothrombinaemia or vitamin-K deficiency bleeding
• **By intravenous injection**

  Neonate 1 mg repeated 8 hourly if necessary

Neonatal biliary atresia and liver disease
• **By mouth**

  Neonate 1 mg daily

Reversal of coumarin anticoagulation when continued anticoagulation required or if no significant bleeding (see also section 2.8.2)—seek specialist advice
• **By intravenous injection**

  Child 1 month–18 years 15–30 micrograms/kg (max. 1 mg) as a single dose, repeated as necessary

Reversal of coumarin anticoagulation when anticoagulation not required or if significant bleeding; treatment of haemorrhage associated with vitamin-K deficiency (see also section 2.8.2)—seek specialist advice
• **By intravenous injection**

  Child 1 month–18 years 250–300 micrograms/kg (max. 10 mg) as a single dose

Konakion® (Roche) [PoM]
Tablets, s/c, phytomenadione 10 mg, net price 10-tab pack = £1.65. To be chewed or allowed to dissolve slowly in the mouth. Label: 24

◀**Colloidal formulation**
Konakion® MM (Roche) [PoM]
Injection, phytomenadione 10 mg/mL in a mixed micelles vehicle. Net price 1-mL amp = 40p
Excipients include glycocholic acid 54.6 mg/amp, lecithin
Cautions reduce dose in liver impairment (glycocholic acid may displace bilirubin); reports of anaphylactoid reactions
Administration *Konakion® MM* may be administered by slow intravenous injection or by intravenous infusion in glucose 5%; **not** for intramuscular injection

Konakion® MM Paediatric (Roche) ▼ [PoM]
Injection, phytomenadione 10 mg/mL in a mixed micelles vehicle, net price 0.2-mL amp = £1.00
Excipients include glycocholic acid 10.9 mg/amp, lecithin
Cautions parenteral administration in premature infants body-weight less than 2.5 kg (increased risk of kernicterus)
Administration *Konakion® MM Paediatric* may be administered *by mouth* or *by intramuscular injection* or *by intravenous injection*. For *intravenous injection*, may be diluted with Glucose 5% if necessary

---

9.6.7 Multivitamin preparations

Multivitamin supplements are used in children with vitamin deficiencies and also in malabsorption conditions such as cystic fibrosis or liver disease. To avoid potential toxicity, the content of all vitamin preparations, particularly vitamin A, should be considered when used together with other supplements. Supplementation is not required if nutrient enriched feeds are used; consult a dietician for further advice.

◢ MULTIVITAMIN PREPARATIONS

Cautions see individual vitamins; vitamin A concentration of preparations varies

Contra-indications see individual vitamins

Side-effects see individual vitamins

Licensed use *Dalivit®* not licensed for use in children under 6 weeks

Indication and dose

  See under preparations below

Vitamins
Capsules, ascorbic acid 15 mg, nicotinamide 7.5 mg, riboflavin 500 micrograms, thiamine hydrochloride 1 mg, vitamin A 2500 units, vitamin D 300 units. Net price 20 = 22p
Dose
  Prevention of deficiency
  • By mouth
    Child 1–12 years 1 capsule daily
    Child 12–18 years 2 capsules daily

  Cystic fibrosis: prevention of deficiency
  • By mouth
    Child 1–18 years 2–3 capsules daily

Abidec® (Chefaro UK)
Drops, vitamins A, B group, C, and D. Net price 25 mL (with dropper) = £2.08
Note Contains 1333 units of vitamin A (as palmitate) per 0.6 mL dose
  Excipients include arachis (peanut) oil and sucrose
Dose
  Prevention of deficiency
  • By mouth
    Preterm neonate 0.6 mL daily
    Neonate 0.3 mL daily

    Child 1 month–1 year 0.3 mL daily
    Child 1–18 years 0.6 mL daily

◁ **MULTIVITAMIN PREPARATIONS (*continued*)**

Cystic fibrosis: prevention of deficiency
• By mouth
Child 1 month–1 year 0.6 mL daily
Child 1–18 years 1.2 mL daily

Dalivit® (LPC)
Oral drops, vitamins A, B group, C, and D, net price
25 mL = £2.98, 50 mL = £4.85
Note Contains 5000 units of vitamin A (as palmitate) per
0.6 mL dose
Excipients include sucrose

Dose

Prevention of deficiency
• By mouth
Neonate (including preterm) 0.3 mL daily

Child 1 month–1 year 0.3 mL daily
Child 1–18 years 0.6 mL daily

Cystic fibrosis: prevention of deficiency
• By mouth
Child 1 month–1 year 0.6 mL daily
Child 1–18 years 1 mL daily

Vitamin and mineral supplements and adjuncts to synthetic diets

Forceval® (Alliance)
Capsules, brown/red, vitamins (ascorbic acid
60 mg, biotin 100 micrograms, cyanocobalamin
3 micrograms, folic acid 400 micrograms, nicotinamide 18 mg, pantothenic acid 4 mg, pyridoxine
2 mg, riboflavin 1.6 mg, thiamine 1.2 mg, vitamin A
2500 units, vitamin D_2 400 units, vitamin E 10 mg,
minerals and trace elements (calcium 100 mg,
chromium 200 micrograms, copper 2 mg, iodine
140 micrograms, iron 12 mg, magnesium 30 mg,
manganese 3 mg, molybdenum 250 micrograms,
phosphorus 77 mg, potassium 4 mg, selenium
50 micrograms, zinc 15 mg), net price 15-cap pack
= £2.83, 30-cap pack = £4.94, 90-cap pack =
£11.93. Label: 25

Dose

Vitamin and mineral deficiency and as adjunct in
synthetic diets
Child 12–18 years 1 capsule daily one hour after a
meal

Junior capsules, brown, vitamins (ascorbic acid
25 mg, biotin 50 micrograms, cyanocobalamin
2 micrograms, folic acid 100 micrograms, nicotinamide 7.5 mg, pantothenic acid 2 mg, pyridoxine
1 mg, riboflavin 1 mg, thiamine 1.5 mg, vitamin A
1250 units, vitamin D_2 200 units, vitamin E 5 mg,
vitamin K_1 25 micrograms), minerals and trace
elements (chromium 50 micrograms, copper 1 mg,
iodine 75 micrograms, iron 5 mg, magnesium 1 mg,
manganese 1.25 mg, molybdenum 50 micrograms,
selenium 25 micrograms, zinc 5 mg), net price 30-
cap pack = £3.52, 60-cap pack = £6.69

Dose

Vitamin and mineral deficiency and as adjunct in
synthetic diets
Child 5–12 years 2 junior capsules daily

Ketovite® (Paines & Byrne)
Tablets [PoM], yellow, ascorbic acid 16.6 mg, riboflavin 1 mg, thiamine hydrochloride 1 mg, pyridoxine
hydrochloride 330 micrograms, nicotinamide
3.3 mg, calcium pantothenate 1.16 mg, alpha tocopheryl acetate 5 mg, inositol 50 mg, biotin
170 micrograms, folic acid 250 micrograms, aceto-
menaphthone 500 micrograms, net price 100-tab
pack = £4.17

Dose

Prevention of vitamin deficiency in disorders of
carbohydrate or amino-acid metabolism and adjunct
in restricted, specialised, or synthetic diets
Child 1 month–18 years 1 tablet 3 times daily; dose
adjusted according to condition, diet, or age; use with
Ketovite® Liquid for complete vitamin supplementation

Administration may be crushed immediately before use

Liquid, pink, sugar-free, vitamin A 2500 units,
ergocalciferol 400 units, choline chloride 150 mg,
cyanocobalamin 12.5 micrograms/5 mL, net price
150-mL pack = £2.70

Dose

Prevention of vitamin deficiency in disorders of
carbohydrate or amino-acid metabolism and adjunct
in restricted, specialised, or synthetic diets
Child 1 month–18 years 5 mL daily; dose adjusted
according to condition, diet, or age; use with *Ketovite®
Tablets* for complete vitamin supplementation

Administration may be mixed with milk, cereal, or fruit
juice

9.7 Bitters and tonics

Classification not included in *BNF for Children*.

9.8 Metabolic disorders

9.8.1 Drugs used in metabolic disorders
9.8.2 Acute porphyrias

This section covers drugs used in metabolic disorders and not readily classified elsewhere.

9.8.1 Drugs used in metabolic disorders

Metabolic disorders should be managed under the guidance of a specialist. As many preparations are unlicensed and may be difficult to obtain, arrangements for continued prescribing and supply should be made in primary care.

General advice on the use of medicines in metabolic disorders can be obtained from
Alder Hey Children's Hospital
Medicines Information Centre
Tel: (0151) 252 5381

and
Great Ormond Street Hospital for Children
Pharmacy
Tel: (020) 7405 9200

Wilson's disease

Penicillamine is used in Wilson's disease (hepatolenticular degeneration) to aid the elimination of copper ions; it is also used for cystinuria. Children who are hypersensitive to penicillin may react rarely to penicillamine.

Trientine is used for the treatment of Wilson's disease only, in patients intolerant of penicillamine; it is **not** an alternative to penicillamine in other diseases such as cystinuria. Penicillamine-induced systemic lupus erythematosus may not resolve on transfer to trientine.

Zinc prevents the absorption of copper in Wilson's disease. Symptomatic patients should be treated initially with a chelating agent because zinc has a slow onset of action. When transferring from chelating treatment to zinc maintenance therapy, chelating treatment should be co-administered for 2–3 weeks until zinc produces its maximal effect.

PENICILLAMINE

Cautions concomitant nephrotoxic drugs (increased risk of toxicity); monitor urine for proteinuria; monitor blood and platelet count regularly (see below); neurological involvement; **interactions:** Appendix 1 (penicillamine)

Renal impairment reduce dose and monitor renal function or avoid—consult product literature

Pregnancy fetal abnormalities reported rarely; avoid if possible

Breast-feeding manufacturer advises avoid unless potential benefit outweighs risk—no information available

Blood counts and urine tests Consider withdrawal if platelet count falls below 120 000/mm³ or white blood cells below 2500/mm³ or if 3 successive falls within reference range (can restart at reduced dose when counts return to within reference range but permanent withdrawal necessary if recurrence of leucopenia or thrombocytopenia)

Counselling Warn child and carer to tell doctor immediately if sore throat, fever, infection, non-specific illness, unexplained bleeding and bruising, purpura, mouth ulcers, or rashes develop

Contra-indications lupus erythematosus

Side-effects initially nausea, anorexia, fever, and skin reactions; taste loss (mineral supplements not recommended); blood disorders including thrombocytopenia, leucopenia, agranulocytosis and aplastic anaemia; proteinuria, rarely haematuria (withdraw immediately); haemolytic anaemia, pancreatitis, cholestatic jaundice, nephrotic syndrome, lupus erythematosus-like syndrome, myasthenia gravis-like syndrome, neuropathy (especially if neurological involvement in Wilson's disease—prophylactic pyridoxine recommended, see section 9.6.2, p. 577), polymyositis (rarely with cardiac involvement), dermatomyositis, mouth ulcers, stomatitis, alopecia, bronchiolitis and pneumonitis, pemphigus, Goodpasture's syndrome, and Stevens-Johnson syndrome also reported; male and female breast enlargement reported; in non-rheumatoid conditions rheumatoid arthritis-like syndrome also reported; late rashes (consider withdrawing treatment)

Indication and dose

Wilson's disease
- **By mouth**

  Child 1 month–12 years 2.5 mg/kg twice daily before food, increased at 1–2 week intervals to 10 mg/kg twice daily

  Child 12–18 years 0.75–1 g twice daily before food, max. 2 g daily for 1 year; usual maintenance dose 0.75–1 g daily

◁ **PENICILLAMINE** (*continued*)

Cystinuria
• **By mouth**

Child 1 month–12 years 5–10 mg/kg twice daily before food, adjusted to maintain urinary cystine below 200 mg/litre; maintain adequate fluid intake

Child 12–18 years 0.5–1.5 g twice daily before food, adjusted to maintain urinary cystine below 200 mg/litre; maintain adequate fluid intake

Penicillamine (Non-proprietary) ℗ᴏᴹ

Tablets, penicillamine 125 mg, net price 56-tab pack = £13.19; 250 mg, 56-tab pack = £16.96. Label: 6, 22, counselling, blood disorder symptoms (see above)

Distamine® (Alliance) ℗ᴏᴹ

Tablets, all f/c, penicillamine 125 mg, net price 100 = £8.62; 250 mg, 100 = £14.82. Label: 6, 22, counselling, blood disorder symptoms (see above)

◤ TRIENTINE DIHYDROCHLORIDE

Cautions see notes above; **interactions:** Appendix 1 (trientine)

Pregnancy teratogenic in *animal* studies—use only if benefit outweighs risk; monitor maternal and neonatal serum-copper concentrations

Side-effects nausea, rash; rarely anaemia

Indication and dose

Wilson's disease in patients intolerant of penicillamine
• **By mouth**

Child 2–12 years 0.6–1.5 g daily in 2–4 divided doses before food, adjusted according to

response; reduce dose and increase frequency if nausea is a problem

Child 12–18 years 1.2–2.4 g daily in 2–4 divided doses before food, adjusted according to response; reduce dose and increase frequency if nausea is a problem

Trientine Dihydrochloride (Univar) ℗ᴏᴹ

Capsules, trientine dihydrochloride 300 mg. Label: 6, 22

◤ ZINC ACETATE

Cautions portal hypertension (risk of hepatic decompensation when switching from chelating agent); monitor full blood count and serum cholesterol; **interactions:** Appendix 1 (zinc)

Pregnancy usual dose 25 mg 3 times daily adjusted according to plasma-copper concentration and urinary copper excretion

Contra-indications breast-feeding

Side-effects gastric irritation (usually transient; may be reduced if first dose taken mid-morning or with a little protein); *less commonly* sideroblastic anaemia and leucopenia

Indication and dose

Wilson's disease
Note dose expressed as elemental zinc
• **By mouth**

Child 1–6 years 25 mg twice daily

Child 6–16 years body-weight under 57 kg, 25 mg 3 times daily; body-weight 57 kg or over, 50 mg 3 times daily

Child 16–18 years 50 mg 3 times daily

Wilzin® (Orphan Europe) ▼ ℗ᴏᴹ

Capsules, zinc (as acetate) 25 mg (blue), net price 250-cap pack = £132.00; 50 mg (orange), 250-cap pack = £242.00. Label: 23

Administration capsules may be opened and the contents mixed with water

Carnitine deficiency

Carnitine is available for the management of primary carnitine deficiency due to inborn errors of metabolism, or of secondary deficiency in haemodialysis patients.

Carnitine is also used in the treatment of some organic acidaemias; however, use in fatty acid oxidation is controversial.

◤ CARNITINE

Cautions diabetes mellitus; monitoring of free and acyl carnitine in blood and urine recommended

Renal impairment accumulation of metabolites may occur with chronic oral administration in severe renal impairment

Pregnancy appropriate to use; no evidence of teratogenicity in *animal* studies

Side-effects nausea, vomiting, abdominal pain, diarrhoea, fishy body odour; side-effects may be dose-related—monitor tolerance during first week and after any dose increase

Licensed use not licensed for use by intravenous infusion; oral liquid (10%) not licensed in children under 12 years; Paediatric solution (30%) not licensed in children over 12 years; not licensed for use in organic acidaemias

9

Nutrition and blood

◁ **CARNITINE** (*continued*)

Indication and dose

Primary deficiency and organic acidaemias
- **By mouth**

  Neonate 50 mg/kg twice daily, higher doses up to 200 mg/kg daily occasionally required

  Child 1 month–18 years 50 mg/kg twice daily, higher doses up to 200 mg/kg daily or 3 g daily occasionally required

- **By intravenous infusion**

  Neonate initially 100 mg/kg over 30 minutes followed by a continuous infusion of 4 mg/kg/hour

  Child 1 month–18 years initially 100 mg/kg over 30 minutes followed by a continuous infusion of 4mg/kg/hour

- **By slow intravenous injection over 2–3 minutes**

  Neonate 100 mg/kg/daily in 2–4 divided doses

  Child 1 month–18 years 100 mg/kg/daily in 2–4 divided doses

Secondary deficiency in dialysis patients
- **By slow intravenous injection over 2–3 minutes**

  Child 1 month –18 years 20 mg/kg after each dialysis session, adjusted according to plasma-carnitine concentration

- **By mouth**
  (maintenance therapy if benefit gained from first intravenous course)

  Child 1 month–18 years 1 g daily

Administration For *intravenous infusion*, dilute injection with Sodium Chloride 0.9% or Glucose 5% or 10%.

Carnitor® (Sigma-Tau) PoM
Oral liquid, L-carnitine 100 mg/mL (10%), net price 10 × 10-mL (1-g) single-dose bottle = £35.00

Paediatric solution, L-carnitine 300 mg/mL (30%), net price 20 mL = £21.00

Injection, L-carnitine 200 mg/mL, net price 5-mL amp = £11.90

Fabry's disease

Agalsidase alfa and **agalsidase beta**, enzymes produced by recombinant DNA technology, are licensed for long-term enzyme replacement therapy in Fabry's disease (a lysosomal storage disorder caused by deficiency of alpha-galactosidase A).

AGALSIDASE ALFA and BETA

Cautions interactions: Appendix 1 (agalsidase alfa and beta)

Pregnancy use with caution

Breast-feeding use with caution—no information available

Infusion-related reactions Infusion-related reactions very common; manage by slowing the infusion rate or interrupting the infusion, or minimise by pre-treatment with an antihistamine, antipyretic, or corticosteroid—consult product literature

Side-effects gastro-intestinal disturbances, taste disturbances; tachycardia, bradycardia, palpitation, hypertension, hypotension, chest pain, oedema, flushing; dyspnoea, cough, wheezing, hoarseness, rhinorrhoea; headache, fatigue, dizziness, asthenia, paraesthesia, syncope, neuropathic pain, tremor, sleep disturbances; influenza-like symptoms, nasopharyngitis; pain in extremities; eye irritation; tinnitus, vertigo; hypersensitivity reactions, pruritus, urticaria, rash, acne; *less commonly* bronchospasm, angioedema, cold extremities, parosmia, ear pain and swelling, skin discoloration, and injection-site reactions

Indication and dose

Fabry's disease (specialist use only)
see under preparations

Fabrazyme® (Genzyme) PoM
Intravenous infusion, powder for reconstitution, agalsidase beta, net price 5-mg vial = £325.50; 35-mg vial = £2269.20

Dose

Fabry's disease (specialist use only)
- **By intravenous infusion**
  Child 8–18 years 1 mg/kg every 2 weeks

Administration for *intravenous infusion*, reconstitute initially with Water for Injections (5 mg in 1.1 mL, 35 mg in 7.2 mL) to produce a solution containing 5 mg/mL; dilute with Sodium Chloride 0.9% (for doses less than 35 mg dilute with at least 50 mL; doses 35–70 mg dilute with at least 100 mL; doses 70–100 mg dilute with at least 250 mL; doses greater than 100 mg dilute with 500 mL) and give through an in-line low protein-binding 0.2 micron filter at an initial rate of no more than 15 mg/hour; for subsequent infusions, infusion rate may be increased gradually once tolerance has been established

Replagal® (Shire) PoM
Concentrate for intravenous infusion, agalsidase alfa 1 mg/mL, net price 1-mL vial = £356.85; 3.5-mL vial = £1161.57

Dose

Fabry's disease (specialist use only)
- **By intravenous infusion**
  Child 7–18 years 200 micrograms/kg every 2 weeks

Administration for *intravenous infusion*, dilute requisite dose with 100 mL Sodium Chloride 0.9% and give over 40 minutes using an in-line filter; use within 3 hours of dilution

Gaucher's disease

Imiglucerase, an enzyme produced by recombinant DNA technology, is administered as enzyme replacement therapy in Gaucher's disease, a familial disorder affecting principally the liver, spleen, bone marrow, and lymph nodes.

Miglustat, an inhibitor of glucosylceramide synthase, is licensed in adults for the treatment of mild to moderate type I Gaucher's disease in patients for whom imiglucerase is unsuitable; it is given by mouth.

IMIGLUCERASE

Cautions monitor for imiglucerase antibodies; when stabilised, monitor all parameters and response to treatment at intervals of 6–12 months

Pregnancy manufacturer advises use only if potential benefit outweighs risk—no information available

Breast-feeding no information available

Side-effects hypersensitivity reactions (including urticaria, angioedema, hypotension, flushing, tachycardia); *less commonly* nausea, vomiting, diarrhoea, abdominal cramps, fatigue, headache, dizziness, paraesthesia, fever, arthralgia, injection-site reactions

Indication and dose

Gaucher's disease type I (specialist use only)
- **By intravenous infusion**

  Neonate 60 units/kg once every 2 weeks, adjusted according to response

  Child 1 month–18 years 60 units/kg once every 2 weeks, adjusted according to response

Gaucher's disease type III (specialist use only)
- **By intravenous infusion**

  Neonate 120 units/kg once every 2 weeks, adjusted according to response

  Child 1 month–18 years 120 units/kg once every 2 weeks, adjusted according to response

Administration For *intravenous infusion*, initially reconstitute with Water for Injections (200 units in 5.1 mL, 400 units in 10.2 mL) to a concentration of 40 units/mL; dilute requisite dose with Sodium Chloride 0.9% to a final volume of 100–200 mL; give over 1–2 hours *or* at a rate not exceeding 1 unit/kg/minute; administer within 3 hours of reconstitution

Cerezyme® (Genzyme) ℗
Intravenous infusion, powder for reconstitution, imiglucerase, net price 200-unit vial = £553.35; 400-unit vial = £1106.70
Electrolytes Na⁺ 0.62 mmol/200-unit vial, 1.24 mmol/400-unit vial

Mucopolysaccharidosis

Laronidase, an enzyme produced by recombinant DNA technology, is licensed for long-term replacement therapy in the treatment of non-neurological manifestations of mucopolysaccharidosis I, a lysosomal storage disorder caused by deficiency of alpha-L-iduronidase.

Idursulfase, an enzyme produced by recombinant DNA technology, is licensed for long-term replacement therapy in mucopolysaccharidosis II (Hunter syndrome), a lysosomal storage disorder caused by deficiency of iduronate-2-sulfatase.

Galsulfase, a recombinant form of human N-acetylgalactosamine-4-sulfatase, is licensed for long-term replacement therapy in mucopolysaccharidosis VI (Maroteaux-Lamy syndrome).

Infusion-related reactions often occur with administration of laronidase, idursulfase, and galsulfase; they can be managed by slowing the infusion rate or interrupting the infusion, and can be minimised by pre-treatment with an antihistamine and an antipyretic. Recurrent infusion-related reactions may require pre-treatment with a corticosteroid—consult product literature for details.

GALSULFASE

Cautions respiratory disease; acute febrile or respiratory illness (consider delaying treatment)

Pregnancy manufacturer advises avoid unless essential

Infusion-related reactions See notes above

Contra-indications

Breast-feeding manufacturer advises avoid—no information available

Side-effects abdominal pain, umbilical hernia, gastroenteritis; chest pain, hypertension; dyspnoea, apnoea, nasal congestion; rigors, malaise, areflexia; pharyngitis; conjunctivitis, corneal opacity; ear pain; facial oedema

9

Nutrition and blood

◁ **GALSULFASE (***continued***)**

Indication and dose

> Mucopolysaccharidosis VI (specialist use only)
> • **By intravenous infusion**
> **Child 5–18 years** 1 mg/kg once weekly

Administration for *intravenous infusion*, dilute requisite dose with Sodium Chloride 0.9% to a final volume of 250 mL and mix gently; infuse through a 0.2 micron in-line filter; give approx. 2.5% of the total volume over 1 hour, then infuse remaining volume over next 3 hours; if body-weight under 20 kg and at risk of fluid overload, dilute requisite dose in 100 mL Sodium Chloride 0.9% and give over at least 4 hours

Naglazyme® (BioMarin) ▼ [PoM]
Concentrate for intravenous infusion, galsulfase 1 mg/mL, net price 5-mL vial = £982.00

IDURSULFASE

Cautions severe respiratory disease; acute febrile respiratory illness (consider delaying treatment)

Breast-feeding no information available
Infusion-related reactions See notes above

Contra-indications women of child-bearing potential

Pregnancy manufacturer advises avoid—no information available

Side-effects gastro-intestinal disturbances, swollen tongue; arrhythmia, chest pain, cyanosis, peripheral oedema, hypertension, hypotension, flushing, pulmonary embolism; bronchospasm, cough, wheezing, tachypnoea, dyspnoea; headache, dizziness, tremor; pyrexia; arthralgia; increased lacrimation; facial oedema, urticaria, pruritus, rash, infusion-site swelling, erythema, and eczema; anaphylaxis also reported

Indication and dose

> Mucopolysaccharidosis II (specialist use only)
> • **By intravenous infusion**
> **Child 5–18 years** 500 micrograms/kg once weekly

Administration for *intravenous infusion*, dilute requisite dose in 100 mL Sodium Chloride 0.9% and mix gently (do not shake); give over 3 hours (gradually reduced to 1 hour if no infusion-related reactions)

Elaprase® (Shire) ▼ [PoM]
Concentrate for intravenous infusion, idursulfase 2 mg/mL, net price 3-mL vial = £1985.00

LARONIDASE

Cautions monitor immunoglobulin G (IgG) antibody concentration; **interactions:** Appendix 1 (laronidase)

Pregnancy manufacturer advises avoid unless essential—no information available

Breast-feeding manufacturer advises avoid—no information available
Infusion-related reactions See notes above

Side-effects nausea, vomiting, diarrhoea, abdominal pain; cold extremities, pallor, flushing, tachycardia, blood pressure changes; dyspnoea, cough, angioedema, anaphylaxis; headache, paraesthesia, dizziness, fatigue, restlessness; influenza-like symptoms; musculoskeletal pain, pain in extremities; rash, pruritus, urticaria, alopecia, infusion-site reactions; bronchospasm and respiratory arrest also reported

Indication and dose

> Non-neurological manifestations of mucopoly-saccharidosis I (specialist use only)
> • **By intravenous infusion**
> **Child 1 month–18 years** 100 units/kg once weekly

Administration for *intravenous infusion*, dilute with Sodium Chloride 0.9%; body-weight under 20 kg, dilute to 100 mL, body-weight over 20 kg dilute to 250 mL; give through in-line filter (0.22 micron) initially at a rate of 2 units/kg/hour then increase gradually every 15 minutes to max. 43 units/kg/hour

Aldurazyme (Genzyme) [PoM]
Concentrate for intravenous infusion, laronidase 100 units/mL, net price 5-mL vial = £460.35
Electrolytes Na$^+$ 1.29 mmol /5-mL vial

Pompe disease

Alglucosidase alfa, an enzyme produced by recombinant DNA technology, is licensed for long-term replacement therapy in Pompe disease, a lysosomal storage disorder caused by deficiency of acid alpha-glucosidase.

The *Scottish Medicines Consortium* (p. 4) has advised (February 2007) that alglucosidase alfa (*Myozyme®*) is **not** recommended for use within NHS Scotland for the treatment of Pompe disease.

9 **Nutrition and blood**

ALGLUCOSIDASE ALFA

Cautions cardiac and respiratory dysfunction—monitor closely; monitor immunoglobulin G (IgG) antibody concentration

Pregnancy manufacturer advises avoid unless essential—no information available

Infusion-related reactions Infusion-related reactions very common, calling for use of antihistamine, antipyretic or corticosteroid; consult product literature for details

Contra-indications

Breast-feeding manufacturer advises avoid—no information available

Side-effects nausea, vomiting; flushing, tachycardia, blood pressure changes, cold extremities, cyanosis, facial oedema; cough, tachypnoea, bronchospasm; headache, agitation, tremor, irritability, restlessness, paraesthesia, dizziness; pyrexia; antibody formation; sweating, rash, pruritus, and urticaria; anaphylaxis

Indication and dose

Pompe disease (specialist use only)
• By intravenous infusion

   Child 1 month –18 years 20 mg/kg every 2 weeks

Administration for *intravenous infusion*, reconstitute 50 mg with 10.3 mL water for injections to produce 5 mg/mL solution; gently rotate vial without shaking; dilute requisite dose with sodium chloride 0.9% to give a final concentration of 0.5–4 mg/mL; give through a low protein-binding in-line filter (0.2 micron) at an initial rate of 1 mg/kg/hour increased by 2 mg/kg/hour every 30 minutes to max. 7 mg/kg/hour

Myozyme® (Genzyme) ▼ PoM
Intravenous infusion, powder for reconstitution, alglucosidase alfa, net price 50-mg vial = £368.59

Urea cycle disorders

Sodium benzoate and **sodium phenylbutyrate** are used in the management of urea cycle disorders. Both, either singly or in combination, are indicated as adjunctive therapy in all patients with neonatal-onset disease and in those with late-onset disease who have a history of hyperammonaemic encephalopathy. Sodium benzoate is also used in non-ketotic hyperglycinaemia. In anuric states dialysis is necessary to treat hyperammonaemia.

Gastro-intestinal side-effects of sodium benzoate or sodium phenylbutyrate may be reduced by giving smaller doses more frequently. The preparations contain significant amounts of sodium; therefore, they should be used with caution in children with congestive heart failure, renal insufficiency and clinical conditions involving sodium retention with oedema.

The long-term management of urea cycle disorders includes oral maintenance treatment with sodium benzoate and sodium phenylbutyrate combined with a low protein diet and other drugs such as **arginine** or **citrulline**, depending on the specific disorder.

Carglumic acid is licensed for the treatment of hyperammonaemia due to *N*-acetylglutamate synthase deficiency.

ARGININE

Cautions monitor plasma pH and chloride

Contra-indications not to be used in the treatment of arginase deficiency

Pregnancy no information available

Breast-feeding no information available

Side-effects intravenous injection only: nausea, vomiting; flushing, hypotension; headache, numbness; hyperchloraemic metabolic acidosis; irritation at injection-site

Licensed use injection and tablets not licensed in children; powder licensed for urea cycle disorders in children

Indication and dose

Acute hyperammonaemia in carbamylphosphate synthetase deficiency, ornithine carbamyl transferase deficiency (specialist use only)
• By intravenous infusion

   Neonate initially 200 mg/kg over 90 minutes followed by 8 mg/kg/hour

   Child 1 month–18 years initially 200 mg/kg over 90 minutes followed by 8 mg/kg/hour

Maintenance treatment of hyperammonaemia in carbamylphosphate synthetase deficiency, ornithine carbamyl transferase deficiency (specialist use only)
• By mouth

   Neonate 100 mg/kg daily in 3–4 divided doses

   Child 1 month–18 years 100 mg/kg daily in 3–4 divided doses

Acute hyperammonaemia in citrullinaemia, arginosuccinic aciduria (specialist use only)
• By intravenous infusion

   Neonate initially 600 mg/kg over 90 minutes followed by 25 mg/kg/hour

   Child 1 month–18 years initially 600 mg/kg over 90 minutes followed by 25 mg/kg/hour

9

Nutrition and blood

◁ **ARGININE (continued)**

Maintenance treatment of hyperammonaemia in citrullinaemia, arginosuccinic aciduria (specialist use only)
• By mouth

Neonate 100–175 mg/kg 3–4 times daily, with food, adjusted according to response

Child 1 month–18 years 100–175 mg/kg 3–4 times daily, with food, adjusted according to response

L-Arginine (Non-proprietary)
Tablets, L-arginine (as hydrochloride) 500 mg,

Oral solution, L-arginine 100 mg/mL
Available from 'special-order' manufacturers or specialist importing companies, see p. 943

Powder, L-arginine (as hydrochloride), net price 100 g = £10.64
Available from SHS
Prescribe as a borderline substance (ACBS). For use as a supplement in urea cycle disorders other than arginase deficiency, such as hyperammonaemia types I and II, citrullinaemia, arginosuccinic aciduria, and deficiency of N-acetyl glutamate synthetase

Injection, L-arginine (as hydrochloride) 500 mg/mL, 10-mL ampoules; 100 mg/mL, 200-mL amp
Available from 'special-order' manufacturers or specialist importing companies, see p. 943
Note Other strengths may be available from 'special-order' manufacturers or specialist importing companies, see p. 943

Administration dilute to a concentration of 20 mg/mL with Sodium Chloride 0.9% or 0.45%, or Glucose 5% or 10%; max. concentration 100 mg/mL; may be given orally

CARGLUMIC ACID

Cautions

Pregnancy manufacturer advises avoid unless essential—no information available

Contra-indications

Breast-feeding manufacturer advises avoid—present in milk in *animal* studies

Side-effects sweating

Indication and dose

Hyperammonaemia due to *N*-acetyl glutamate synthase deficiency (initiated under specialist supervision)
• By mouth

Neonate initially 50–125 mg/kg twice daily immediately before feeds, adjusted according to

plasma-ammonia concentration; maintenance 5–50 mg/kg twice daily; total daily dose may alternatively be given in 3–4 divided doses

Child 1 month–18 years initially 50–125 mg/kg twice daily immediately before food, adjusted according to plasma-ammonia concentration; maintenance 5–50 mg/kg twice daily; total daily dose may alternatively be given in 3–4 divided doses

Carbaglu® (Orphan Europe) ℞
Dispersible tablets, carglumic acid 200 mg, net price 5-tab pack = £243.00, 60-tab pack = £2914.00. Label: 13

CITRULLINE

Cautions

Pregnancy no information available

Breast-feeding no information available

Indication and dose

Carbamyl phosphate synthase deficiency, ornithine carbamyl transferase deficiency
• By mouth

Neonate 150 mg/kg daily in 3–4 divided doses, adjusted according to response

Child 1 month–18 years 150 mg/kg daily in 3–4 divided doses, adjusted according to response

Citrulline Powder (Non-proprietary)
Powder, L-citrulline 100 g
Available from 'special-order' manufacturers or specialist importing companies, see p. 943
Administration May be mixed with drinks or taken as a paste

SODIUM BENZOATE

Cautions see notes above; neonates (risk of kernicterus and increased side-effects); **interactions:** Appendix 1 (sodium benzoate)

Pregnancy no information available

Breast-feeding no information available

Side-effects nausea, vomiting, anorexia; irritability, lethargy, coma

Licensed use not licensed for use in children

Indication and dose

Acute hyperammonaemia due to urea cycle disorders (specialist use only)
• By intravenous infusion

Neonate initially 250 mg/kg over 90 minutes followed by 20 mg/kg/hour, adjusted according to response

Child 1 month–18 years initially 250 mg/kg over 90 minutes followed by 20 mg/kg/hour, adjusted according to response

9 Nutrition and blood

◻ **SODIUM BENZOATE** (*continued*)

Maintenance treatment of hyperammonaemia due to urea cycle disorders; non-ketotic hyperglycinaemia (specialist use only)
• **By mouth**

Neonate 50–150 mg/kg 3–4 times daily, with food, adjusted according to response

Child 1 month–18 years 50–150 mg/kg 3–4 times daily, with food, adjusted according to response

Administration for administration *by mouth*, oral solution or powder may be administered in fruit drinks; less soluble in acidic drinks

Sodium Benzoate (Non-proprietary) ⒫ₒₘ
Tablets, sodium benzoate 500 mg
Available from 'special-order' manufacturers or specialist importing companies, see p. 943

Capsules, sodium benzoate 50 mg; 250 mg; 400 mg; 500 mg
Available from 'special-order' manufacturers or specialist importing companies, see p. 943

Oral solution, sodium benzoate 100 mg/mL; 200 mg/mL; 300 mg/mL
Available from 'special-order' manufacturers or specialist importing companies, see p. 943

Powder
Available from 'special-order' manufacturers or specialist importing companies, see p. 943

Injection, sodium benzoate 200 mg/mL, 5-mL amp
Note Contains Na^+ 1.4 mmol /mL
Available from 'special-order' manufacturers or specialist importing companies, see p. 943

Administration for *intravenous infusion*, dilute to a concentration of 20 mg/mL with Sodium Chloride 0.9% or 0.45%, *or* Glucose 5% or 10%; max. concentration 50 mg/mL

▰ **SODIUM PHENYLBUTYRATE**

Cautions congestive heart failure, hepatic and renal impairment; **interactions:** Appendix 1 (sodium phenylbutyrate)

Contra-indications

Pregnancy avoid

Breast-feeding avoid

Side-effects amenorrhoea and irregular menstrual cycles, decreased appetite, body odour, taste disturbances; less commonly nausea, vomiting, abdominal pain, peptic ulcer, pancreatitis, rectal bleeding, arrhythmia, oedema, syncope, depression, headache, rash, weight gain, renal tubular acidosis, aplastic anaemia, ecchymoses

Licensed use injection not licensed for use in children

Indication and dose

Acute hyperammonaemia due to urea cycle disorders (specialist use only)
• **By continuous intravenous infusion**

Neonate initially 250 mg/kg over 90 minutes followed by 20 mg/kg/hour adjusted according to response

Child 1 month–18 years initially 250 mg/kg over 90 minutes followed by 20 mg/kg/hour adjusted according to response

Maintenance treatment of hyperammonaemia due to urea cycle disorders (specialist use only)
• **By mouth**

Neonate 75–150 mg/kg 3–4 times daily, with food

Child 1 month–18 years 75–150 mg/kg 3–4 times daily, with food (max. 20 g daily)
Administration Oral dose may be mixed with fruit drinks, milk, or feeds

Sodium Phenylbutyrate (Non-proprietary) ⒫ₒₘ
Injection, sodium phenylbutyrate 200 mg/mL, 5-mL amp

Note Contains Na^+ 1.1 mmol /mL
Available from 'special-order' manufacturers or specialist importing companies, see p. 943

Administration for *intravenous infusion*, dilute to a concentration of 20 mg/mL (max. 50 mg/mL) with Glucose 5% or 10%

Ammonaps® (Swedish Orphan) ⒫ₒₘ
Tablets, sodium phenylbutyrate 500 mg. Contains Na^+ 2.7 mmol/tablet. Net price 250-tab pack = £493.00

Granules, sodium phenylbutyrate 940 mg/g. Contains Na^+ 5.4 mmol/g. Net price 266-g pack = £860.00

Note Granules should be mixed with food before taking

▰ **Nephropathic cystinosis**

Mercaptamine (cysteamine) is available for the treatment of nephropathic cystinosis. The oral dose is increased over several weeks to avoid intolerance.

Mercaptamine eye drops are used in the management of ocular symptoms arising from the deposition of cystine crystals in the eye.

Phosphocysteamine is a pro-drug of mercaptamine; it is available from specialist centres only, as a powder or specially manufactured capsule. Mercaptamine does not contain phosphate, therefore, if transferring from phosphocysteamine to mercaptamine phosphate supplements may need to be initiated or adjusted. Mercaptamine 1 mg is approximately equivalent to 3 mg of phosphocysteamine.

Both mercaptamine and phosphocysteamine have a very unpleasant taste and smell, which can affect compliance.

9

Nutrition and blood

All patients receiving mercaptamine and phosphocysteamine should be registered (contact local specialist centre for details).

> **Safe Practice**
> Mercaptamine has been confused with mercaptopurine; care must be taken to ensure the correct drug is prescribed and dispensed.

◢ MERCAPTAMINE
(Cysteamine)

Cautions leucocyte-cystine concentration and haematological monitoring required—consult product literature; dose of phosphate supplement may need to be adjusted

Contra-indications hypersensitivity to mercaptamine or penicillamine

Pregnancy avoid

Breast-feeding avoid

Side-effects breath and body odour, nausea, vomiting, diarrhoea, anorexia, lethargy, fever, rash; also reported dehydration, hypertension, abdominal discomfort, gastroenteritis, drowsiness, encephalopathy, headache, nervousness, depression; anaemia, leucopenia, *rarely* gastrointestinal ulceration and bleeding, seizures, hallucinations, urticaria, interstitial nephritis

Licensed use eye drops not licensed

Indication and dose

Nephropathic cystinosis (specialist use only)
* By mouth

Neonate initially 2–3 mg/kg 4 times daily, increased over 4–6 weeks to 12.5 mg/kg 4 times daily

Child 1 month–12 years or under 50 kg initially 2–3 mg/kg 4 times daily, increased over 4–6 weeks to 12.5 mg/kg 4 times daily

Child 12–18 years or over 50 kg initially 100 mg 4 times daily, increased over 4–6 weeks to 500 mg 4 times daily

Cystagon® (Orphan Europe) [PoM]
Capsules, mercaptamine (as bitartrate) 50 mg, net price 100-cap pack = £59.00; 150 mg, 100-cap pack = £162.00

Note For child under 6 years at risk of aspiration, capsules can be opened and contents sprinkled on food (at a temperature suitable for eating); avoid adding to acidic drinks (e.g. orange juice)

◢ **Eye drops**
Mercaptamine (Non-proprietary)
Eye drops, mercaptamine 0.11%, 10 mL
Available from 'special-order' manufacturers or specialist importing companies, see p. 943

◢ Other metabolic disorders

Other metabolic disorders and the drugs used in their management include:

Amino acid disorders: maple syrup urine disease (thiamine section 9.6.2); tyrosinaemia type III, hawkinsinuria (Vitamin C, section 9.6.3); tyrosinaemia type I (nitisinone).

Mitochondrial disorders: isolated carboxylase defects, defects of biotin metabolism (biotin, see below); mitochondrial myopathies (ubidecarenone); congenital lactic acidosis (riboflavine and thiamine, section 9.6.2); respiratory chain defects (thiamine, section 9.6.2); pyruvate dehydrogenase defects (sodium dichloroacetate)

Neimann-Pick type C disease: miglustat is available for the treatment of progressive neurological manifestations of Neimann-Pick type C disease, a neurodegenerative disorder characterised by impaired intracellular lipid trafficking.

Homocystinuria and defects in cobalamin metabolism: betaine, pyridoxine (section 9.6.2), hydroxocobalamin (section 9.1.2)

Tetrahydrofolate reductase deficiency: betaine, folic acid (section 9.1.2)

The *Scottish Medicines Consortium* (p. 4) has advised (February 2009) that betaine anhydrous powder (*Cystadane®*) is **not** recommended for use as adjunctive treatment of homocystinuria.

◢ BETAINE

Cautions monitor plasma-methionine concentration before and during treatment—interrupt treatment if symptoms of cerebral oedema occur

Pregnancy manufacturer advises avoid unless essential—limited information available

Breast-feeding manufacturer advises caution—no information available

Side-effects *less commonly* gastro-intestinal disorders, anorexia, reversible cerebral oedema (see Cautions), agitation, depression, personality disorder, sleep disturbances, urinary incontinence, alopecia, and urticaria

◻ **BETAINE** *(continued)*

Indication and dose

Adjunctive treatment of homocystinuria (specialist use only)

• **By mouth**

Neonate 50 mg/kg twice daily, dose and frequency adjusted according to response; max. 75 mg/kg twice daily

Child 1 month–10 years 50 mg/kg twice daily, dose and frequency adjusted according to response; max. 75 mg/kg twice daily

Child 10–18 years 3 g twice daily, adjusted according to response; max. 10 g twice daily

Administration Powder should be mixed with water, juice, milk, formula, or food until completely dissolved and taken immediately; measuring spoons are provided to measure 1 g, 150 mg, and 100 mg of *Cystadane*® powder

Betaine (Non-proprietary) ⒫ᴼᴹ
Powder (for oral solution), betaine anhydrous 500 mg/mL when reconstituted.
Available from 'special-order' manufacturers or specialist importing companies, see p. 943

Tablets, betaine anhydrous 500 mg
Available from 'special-order' manufacturers or specialist importing companies, see p. 943

Cystadane® (Orphan Europe) ⒫ᴼᴹ
Powder, betaine (anhydrous), net price 180 g = £314.00

◼ BIOTIN

(Vitamin H)

Cautions

Pregnancy no information available

Breast-feeding no information available

Indication and dose

Isolated carboxylase defects

• **By mouth or by slow intravenous injection**

Neonate 5 mg once daily, adjusted according to response; usual maintenance 10–50 mg daily, higher doses may be required

Child 1 month–18 years 10 mg once daily, adjusted according to response; usual maintenance 10–50 mg daily but up to 100 mg daily may be required

Defects of biotin metabolism

• **By mouth or by slow intravenous injection**

Neonate 10 mg once daily adjusted according to response; usual maintenance 5–20 mg daily but higher doses may be required

Child 1 month–18 years 10 mg once daily adjusted according to response; usual maintenance 5–20 mg daily but higher doses may be required

Biotin (Non-proprietary) ⒫ᴼᴹ
Tablets, biotin 5 mg, 20-tab pack

Injection, biotin 5 mg/mL
Available from 'special order' manufacturers or specialist importing companies, see p. 943

Administration For administration *by mouth*, tablets may be crushed and mixed with food or drink

◼ MIGLUSTAT

Cautions monitor cognitive and neurological function, growth, and platelet count

Hepatic impairment manufacturer advises caution—no information available

Renal impairment child 12–18 years, initially 200 mg twice daily if estimated glomerular filtration rate 50–70 mL/minute/1.73 m²; child 12–18 years, initially 100 mg twice daily if estimated glomerular filtration rate 30–50 mL/minute/1.73 m²; avoid if estimated glomerular filtration rate less than 30 mL/minute/1.73 m²; child under 12 years—consult product literature

Contra-indications

Pregnancy manufacturer advises avoid (toxicity in *animal* studies)—effective contraception must be used during treatment; also men should avoid fathering a child during and for 3 months after treatment

Breast-feeding manufacturer advises avoid—no information available

Side-effects diarrhoea, flatulence, abdominal pain, dyspepsia, constipation, nausea, vomiting, anorexia, weight changes; tremor, dizziness, headache, peripheral neuropathy, ataxia, hypoaesthesia, paraesthesia, insomnia, fatigue, asthenia; decreased libido; thrombocytopenia; muscle spasm

Indication and dose

Neimann-Pick type C disease (specialist supervision only)

• **By mouth**

Child 4–12 years

Body surface area less than 0.47 m² 100 mg once daily

Body surface area 0.47–0.73 m² 100 mg twice daily

Body surface area 0.73–0.88 m² 100 mg three times daily

Body surface area 0.88–1.25 m² 200 mg twice daily

Body surface area greater than 1.25 m² 200 mg three times daily

Child 12–18 years 200 mg three times daily

Zavesca® (Actelion) ⒫ᴼᴹ
Capsules, miglustat 100 mg, net price 84-cap pack = £4015.00 (hospital only)

NITISINONE
(NTBC)

Cautions slit-lamp examination of eyes recommended before treatment; monitor liver function regularly; monitor platelet and white blood cell count every 6 months

Pregnancy manufacturer advises avoid unless potential benefit outweighs risk (toxicity in *animal* studies)

Contra-indications

Breast-feeding manufacturer advises avoid—adverse effect in *animal* studies

Side-effects thrombocytopenia, leucopenia, granulocytopenia; conjunctivitis, photophobia, corneal opacity, keratitis, eye pain; *less commonly* leucocytosis, blepharitis, pruritus, exfoliative dermatitis, and erythematous rash

Indication and dose

Hereditary tyrosinaemia type I (in combination with dietary restriction of tyrosine and phenylalanine)
• By mouth

Neonate initially 500 micrograms/kg twice daily, adjusted according to response; max. 2 mg/kg daily

Child 1 month–18 years initially 500 micrograms/kg twice daily, adjusted according to response; max. 2 mg/kg daily

Administration capsules can be opened and the contents suspended in a small amount of water or formula diet and taken immediately

Orfadin® (Swedish Orphan) [PoM]
Capsules, nitisinone 2 mg, net price 60-cap pack = £564.00; 5mg, 60-cap pack = £1127.00; 10mg, 60-cap pack = £2062.00

SODIUM DICHLOROACETATE

Cautions

Pregnancy no information available

Breast-feeding no information available

Side-effects polyneuropathy on prolonged use; abnormal oxalate metabolism; metabolic acidosis

Indication and dose

Pyruvate dehydrogenase defects
• By mouth

Neonate initially 12.5 mg/kg 4 times daily, adjusted according to response; up to 200 mg/kg daily may be required

Child 1 month–18 years initially 12.5 mg/kg 4 times daily, adjusted according to response; up to 200 mg/kg daily may be required

Sodium dichloroacetate (Non-proprietary) [PoM]
Powder (for oral solution), sodium dichloroacetate 50 mg/mL when reconstituted with water
Available from 'special-order' manufacturers or specialist importing companies, see p. 943

UBIDECARENONE
(Ubiquinone, Co-enzyme Q10)

Cautions may reduce insulin requirement in diabetes mellitus; **interactions**: Appendix 1 (ubidecarenone)

Hepatic impairment reduce dose in moderate and severe liver disease

Side-effects nausea, diarrhoea, heartburn; rarely headache, irritability, agitation, dizziness

Licensed use not licensed for the treatment of mitochondrial disorders

Indication and dose

Mitochondrial disorders
• By mouth

Neonate initially 5 mg once or twice daily with food, adjusted according to response, up to 200 mg daily may be required

Child 1 month–18 years initially 5 mg once or twice daily with food, adjusted according to response, up to 300 mg daily may be required

Ubidecarenone (Non-proprietary) [PoM]
Oral solution ubidecarenone 50 mg/10mL

Tablets, ubidecarenone 10 mg

Capsules, ubidecarenone 10 mg, 30 mg
Available from 'special-order' manufacturers or specialist importing companies, see p. 943

9.8.2 Acute porphyrias

The acute porphyrias (acute intermittent porphyria, variegate porphyria, hereditary coproporphyria, and 5-aminolaevulinic acid dehydratase deficiency porphyria) are hereditary disorders of haem biosynthesis; they have a prevalence of about 1 in 10 000 of the population.

Great care must be taken when prescribing for patients with acute porphyria, since certain drugs can induce acute porphyric crises. Since acute porphyrias are hereditary, relatives of affected individuals should be screened and advised about the potential danger of certain drugs. Acute attacks of porphyria are exceptionally rare before puberty. When acute porphyria is suspected in a child, support from an expert porphyria service should be sought.

Treatment of serious or life-threatening conditions should not be withheld from patients with acute porphyria. When there is no safe alternative, urinary porphobilinogen excretion should be measured regularly; if it increases or symptoms occur, the drug can be withdrawn and the acute attack treated. If an acute porphyric attack occurs during pregnancy, contact an expert porphyria service for further advice.

Haem arginate is administered by short intravenous infusion as haem replacement in moderate, severe, or unremitting acute porphyria crises.

Supplies of haem arginate may be obtained outside office hours from the on-call pharmacist at:

St Thomas' Hospital, London
Tel: (020) 7188 7188

HAEM ARGINATE
(Human hemin)

Cautions

Pregnancy manufacturer advises avoid unless essential

Breast-feeding manufacturer advises avoid unless essential—no information available

Side-effects rarely hypersensitivity reactions and fever; pain and thrombophlebitis at injection site

Indication and dose

Acute porphyrias (acute intermittent porphyria, porphyria variegata, hereditary coproporphyria)

• **By intravenous infusion**

Child 1 month–18 years 3 mg/kg once daily (max. 250 mg daily) for 4 days; if response inadequate, repeat 4-day course with close biochemical monitoring

Normosang® (Orphan Europe) ▼ PoM
Concentrate for intravenous infusion, haem arginate 25 mg/mL, net price 10-mL amp = £338.50
Administration administer over at least 30 minutes; dilute requisite dose in 100 mL Sodium Chloride 0.9% in glass bottle; administer within 1 hour after dilution; max. concentration 2.5 mg/mL

Drugs unsafe for use in acute porphyrias

The following list contains drugs on the UK market that have been classified as 'unsafe' in porphyria because they have been shown to be porphyrinogenic in animals or *in vitro*, or have been associated with acute attacks in patients. Absence of a drug from the following lists does not necessarily imply that the drug is safe. For many drugs no information about porphyria is available.

An up-to-date list of drugs considered **safe** in acute porphyrias is available at www.wmic.wales.nhs.uk/porphyria_info.php.

Further information may be obtained from www.porphyria-europe.com and also from:

Welsh Medicines Information Centre
University Hospital of Wales
Cardiff, CF14 4XW.
Tel: (029) 2074 2979/3877

Note Quite modest changes in chemical structure can lead to changes in porphyrinogenicity but where possible general statements have been made about groups of drugs; these should be checked first.

Unsafe drug groups (check first)

Amphetamines	Ergot derivatives[6]	Protease inhibitors[8]
Anabolic steroids	Gold salts	Statins[9]
Antidepressants[1]	Hormone replacement therapy[5]	Sulphonamides[10]
Antihistamines[2]	Imidazole antifungals[7]	Sulphonylureas[11]
Barbiturates[3]	Non-nucleoside reverse transcri-	Tetracyclines
Calcium channel blockers[4]	ptase inhibitors[8]	Triazole antifungals[7]
Contraceptives, hormonal[5]	Progestogens[5]	

Unsafe drugs (check groups above first)

Aceclofenac	Ethosuximide	Oxycodone[17]
Alcohol	Etomidate	Pentazocine[17]
Amiodarone	Fenfluramine	Pentoxifylline (oxpentifylline)
Azapropazone	Flupentixol	Phenoxybenzamine
Bosentan	Griseofulvin	Phenytoin
Bromocriptine	Halothane	Pivmecillinam
Buspirone	Hydralazine	Porfimer
Busulfan	Indapamide	Potassium canrenoate[18]
Cabergoline	Isometheptene mucate	Probenecid
Carbamazepine	Isoniazid	Pyrazinamide
Carisoprodol	Ketamine	Rifabutin [19]
Chloral hydrate [12]	Ketorolac	Rifampicin [19]
Chlorambucil[13]	Lidocaine (lignocaine)[16]	Spironolactone
Chloramphenicol	Mebeverine	Sulfinpyrazone
Chloroform[14]	Mefenamic acid[13]	Sulpiride
Clindamycin	Meprobamate	Tamoxifen
Clonidine	Methyldopa	Temoporfin
Cocaine	Metoclopramide[13]	Theophylline[20]
Colistin	Metolazone	Tiagabine
Cyclophosphamide[13]	Metronidazole[13]	Tinidazole
Cycloserine	Metyrapone	Topiramate
Danazol	Mifepristone	Tramadol[17]
Dapsone	Minoxidil [13]	Triclofos[12]
Dexfenfluramine	Nalidixic acid	Trimethoprim
Diazepam[15]	Nitrofurantoin	Valproate[15]
Diclofenac	Orphenadrine	Xipamide
Erythromycin	Oxcarbazepine	Zidovudine[8]
Etamsylate	Oxybutynin	Zuclopenthixol

1. Includes tricyclic (and related) and MAOIs; fluoxetine and mianserin thought to be safe.
2. Alimemazine (trimeprazine), chlorphenamine, desloratadine, fexofenadine, ketotifen, loratadine, and promethazine thought to be safe.
3. Includes primidone and thiopental.
4. Diltiazem may be used with caution if safer alternative not available.
5. Progestogens are more porphyrinogenic than oestrogens; oestrogens may be safe at least in replacement doses. Progestogens should be avoided whenever possible by all young women susceptible to acute porphyria; however, when non-hormonal contraception is inappropriate, progestogens may be used with extreme caution if the potential benefit outweighs risk. The risk of an acute attack is greatest in young women who have had a previous attack. Long-acting progestogen preparations should never be used in those at risk of acute porphyria.
6. Includes ergometrine (oxytocin probably safe) and pergolide.
7. Applies to oral and intravenous use; topical antifungals are thought to be safe due to low systemic exposure.
8. Contact Welsh Medicines Information Centre for further advice.
9. Rosuvastatin thought to be safe.
10. Includes co-trimoxazole and sulfasalazine.
11. Glipizide is thought to be safe.
12. Although evidence of hazard is uncertain, manufacturer advises avoid.
13. May be used with caution if safer alternative not available.
14. Small amounts in medicines probably safe.
15. Status epilepticus has been treated successfully with intravenous diazepam.
16. When used for local anaesthesia, bupivacaine, lidocaine (lignocaine), procaine, prilocaine, and tetracaine are thought to be safe.
17. Buprenorphine, codeine, diamorphine, dihydrocodeine, fentanyl, methadone, morphine, and pethidine are thought to be safe.
18. Evidence of hazard uncertain—contact Welsh Medicines Information Centre for further advice
19. Rifamycins have been used in a few patients without evidence of harm—use with caution if safer alternative not available.
20. Includes aminophylline.

9 Nutrition and blood

10 Musculoskeletal and joint diseases

10.1 Drugs used in rheumatic diseases **599**
10.1.1 Non-steroidal anti-inflammatory drugs 600
10.1.2 Corticosteroids 607
10.1.3 Drugs that suppress the rheumatic disease process 608
10.1.4 Cytotoxic-induced hyperuricaemia 613
10.1.5 Other drugs for rheumatic diseases 614

10.2 Drugs used in neuromuscular disorders **614**
10.2.1 Drugs that enhance neuromuscular transmission 614
10.2.2 Skeletal muscle relaxants 616

10.3 Drugs for the relief of soft-tissue inflammation **618**
10.3.1 Enzymes 619
10.3.2 Rubefacients and other topical antirheumatics 619

This chapter also includes advice on the drug management of the following:
  dental and orofacial pain, p. 600
  extravasation, p. 618
  myasthenia gravis, p. 614
  soft-tissue and other musculoskeletal disorders, below
  juvenile idiopathic arthritis and other inflammatory disorders, below

For treatment of septic arthritis see Table 1, section 5.1.

10.1 Drugs used in rheumatic diseases

10.1.1 Non-steroidal anti-inflammatory drugs
10.1.2 Corticosteroids
10.1.3 Drugs that suppress the rheumatic disease process
10.1.4 Cytotoxic-induced hyperuricaemia
10.1.5 Other drugs for rheumatic diseases

Juvenile idiopathic arthritis and other inflammatory disorders

Rheumatic diseases require symptomatic treatment to relieve pain, swelling, and stiffness, together with treatment to control and suppress disease activity. Treatment of juvenile idiopathic arthritis may involve non-steroidal anti-inflammatory drugs (NSAIDs) (section 10.1.1), a disease modifying antirheumatic drug (DMARD) (section 10.1.3) usually methotrexate or etanercept, and intra-articular, intravenous, or oral corticosteroids (section 10.1.2).

Soft-tissue and musculoskeletal disorders

The management of children with soft-tissue injuries and strains, and musculo-skeletal disorders, may include temporary rest together with the local application of heat or cold, local massage and physiotherapy. For pain relief, **paracetamol** (section 4.7.1) is often adequate and should be used first. Alternatively, the lowest effective dose of a **NSAID** (e.g. ibuprofen) can be used. If pain relief with either drug is inadequate, both paracetamol (in a full dose appropriate for the child) and a low dose of a NSAID may be required.

10.1.1 Non-steroidal anti-inflammatory drugs

In *single doses* non-steroidal anti-inflammatory drugs (NSAIDs) have analgesic activity comparable to that of paracetamol (section 4.7.1), but paracetamol is preferred.

In regular *full dosage* NSAIDs have both a lasting analgesic and an anti-inflammatory effect which makes them particularly useful for the treatment of continuous or regular pain associated with inflammation.

Choice Differences in anti-inflammatory activity between NSAIDs are small, but there is considerable variation in individuals' tolerance to these drugs and their response to them. A large proportion of children will respond to any NSAID; of the others, those who do not respond to one may well respond to another. Pain relief starts soon after taking the first dose and a full analgesic effect should normally be obtained within a week, whereas an anti-inflammatory effect may not be achieved (or may not be clinically assessable) for up to 3 weeks. However, in juvenile idiopathic arthritis NSAIDs may take 4–12 weeks to be effective. If appropriate responses are not obtained within these times, another NSAID should be tried. The availability of appropriate formulations needs to be considered when prescribing NSAIDs for children.

NSAIDs reduce the production of prostaglandins by inhibiting the enzyme cyclo-oxygenase. They vary in their selectivity for inhibiting different types of cyclo-oxygenase; selective inhibition of cyclo-oxygenase-2 reduces gastro-intestinal intolerance. However, in children gastro-intestinal symptoms are rare in those taking NSAIDs for short periods. The role of selective inhibitors of cyclo-oxygenase-2 is undetermined in children.

Ibuprofen and **naproxen** are propionic acid derivatives used in children:

Ibuprofen combines anti-inflammatory, analgesic, and antipyretic properties. It has fewer side-effects than other NSAIDs but its anti-inflammatory properties are weaker.

Naproxen combines good efficacy with a low incidence of side-effects.

Diclofenac, indometacin, mefenamic acid, and **piroxicam** have properties similar to those of propionic acid derivatives:

Diclofenac has actions and side-effects similar to those of naproxen.

Indometacin (indomethacin) has an action equal to or superior to that of naproxen, but with a high incidence of side-effects including headache, dizziness, and gastro-intestinal disturbances. It is rarely used in children and should be reserved for when other NSAIDs have been unsuccessful.

Mefenamic acid has minor anti-inflammatory properties. It has occasionally been associated with diarrhoea and haemolytic anaemia which require discontinuation of treatment.

Piroxicam is as effective as naproxen and has a long duration of action which permits once-daily administration. However, it has more gastro-intestinal side-effects than most other NSAIDs, and is associated with more frequent serious skin reactions (**important:** see CHMP advice, p. 606).

Meloxicam is a selective inhibitor of cyclo-oxygenase-2. Its use may be considered in adolescents intolerant to other NSAIDs.

Ketorolac can be used for the short-term management of postoperative pain (section 15.1.4.2).

Etoricoxib, a selective inhibitor of cyclo-oxygenase-2, is licensed for the relief of pain in osteoarthritis, rheumatoid arthritis, ankylosing spondylitis, and acute gout in children aged 16 years and over. For concerns about the cardiovascular safety of cyclo-oxygenase-2 selective inhibitors (see below).

For the role of **aspirin** in children, see section 2.9.

Dental and orofacial pain Most mild to moderate dental pain and inflammation is effectively relieved by **ibuprofen** or **diclofenac**. In an appraisal of the relative safety in adults of 7 non-selective NSAIDs, the CSM assessed ibuprofen to have the lowest risk of serious gastro-intestinal side-effects (see below).

For further information on the management of dental and orofacial pain, see p. 246.

10 Musculoskeletal and joint diseases

Cautions and contra-indications   NSAIDs should be used with caution in children with a history of hypersensitivity to any NSAID—which includes those in whom attacks of asthma, angioedema, urticaria or rhinitis have been precipitated by any NSAID. NSAIDs should also be used with caution during pregnancy (see below) and breast-feeding (see individual drug monographs), and in coagulation defects. Caution may also be required in children with allergic disorders.

In patients with renal, cardiac, or hepatic impairment, caution is required since the use of NSAIDs may result in deterioration of renal function (see also under Side-effects below); the dose should be kept as **low as possible** and renal function should be **monitored**. In *mild renal impairment* the **lowest effective dose** should be used for the **shortest possible duration** and renal function **monitored**; sodium and water retention may occur, as may deterioration in renal function possibly leading to renal failure. In *moderate to severe renal impairment* NSAIDs should be avoided if possible.

All NSAIDs are contra-indicated in severe heart failure. The selective inhibitor of cyclo-oxygenase-2, etoricoxib, is contra-indicated in ischaemic heart disease, cerebrovascular disease, peripheral arterial disease, and moderate or severe heart failure. Etoricoxib should be used with caution in children with a history of cardiac failure, left ventricular dysfunction, hypertension, in children with oedema for any other reason, and in children with risk factors for heart disease.

NSAIDs and cardiovascular events

The role of cyclo-oxygenase-2 selective inhibitors is undetermined in children. Cyclo-oxygenase-2 selective inhibitors are associated with an increased risk of thrombotic events (e.g. myocardial infarction and stroke) and should not be used in preference to non-selective NSAIDs except when specifically indicated (i.e. for children at a particularly high risk of developing gastro-duodenal ulcers or bleeding) *and* after assessing their cardiovascular risk.

Non-selective NSAIDs may also be associated with a small increased risk of thrombotic events, particularly when used at high doses and for long-term treatment. In adults, **diclofenac** (150 mg daily) and **ibuprofen** (2.4 g daily) are associated with an increased risk of thrombotic events. The increased risk for diclofenac is similar to that of **etoricoxib**. **Naproxen** (in adults, 1 g daily) is associated with a lower thrombotic risk, and lower doses of ibuprofen (in adults, 1.2 g daily or less) have not been associated with an increased risk of myocardial infarction. A small increased thrombotic risk cannot be excluded for other NSAIDs, or in children.

The CHM has advised (October 2006) that the lowest effective dose of NSAID or cyclo-oxygenase-2 selective inhibitor should be prescribed for the shortest period of time to control symptoms, and that the need for long-term treatment should be reviewed periodically.

Most manufacturers advise avoiding NSAIDs during pregnancy or avoiding them unless the potential benefit outweighs risk. Ibuprofen and diclofenac are generally considered safe during the first and second trimesters. In the third trimester, NSAIDs are associated with a risk of closure of fetal ductus arteriosus and possibly persistent pulmonary hypertension of the newborn; also, labour may be delayed and its duration may be increased.

NSAIDs are generally contra-indicated if there is active or previous gastro-intestinal ulceration or bleeding; however, some children may require NSAIDs for effective relief of pain and stiffness, and prophylaxis or treatment of NSAID-associated peptic ulcers may be necessary (see section 1.3).

For **interactions** of NSAIDs, see Appendix 1 (NSAIDs).

Side-effects   The side-effects of NSAIDs vary in severity and frequency. Gastro-intestinal discomfort, nausea, diarrhoea, and occasionally bleeding and ulceration may occur. Other side-effects include hypersensitivity reactions (particularly rashes, angioedema, and bronchospasm), headache, dizziness, nervousness, depression, drowsiness, insomnia, vertigo, hearing disturbances such as tinnitus, photosensitivity, and haematuria. Blood disorders have also occurred. Fluid retention may occur (rarely precipitating congestive heart failure); blood pressure may be raised. Renal failure may be provoked by NSAIDs especially in patients with pre-existing renal impairment (**important**, see also under Cautions above). Rarely, papillary necrosis or interstitial fibrosis associated with NSAIDs can lead to renal failure. Hepatic damage, alveolitis, pulmonary eosinophilia, pancreatitis, eye changes, Stevens-Johnson syndrome and toxic epidermal necrolysis are other rare side-effects. Induction of or exacerbation of colitis has been reported. Aseptic meningitis has been reported rarely with NSAIDs; children with connective tissue disorders such as systemic lupus erythematosus may be especially susceptible.

Overdosage: see Emergency Treatment of Poisoning, p. 36.

Gastro-intestinal side-effects

All NSAIDs are associated with gastro-intestinal toxicity. In adults, evidence on the relative safety of NSAIDs indicates differences in the risks of serious upper gastro-intestinal side-effects. **Ibuprofen** is associated with the *lowest risk*; **piroxicam**, **indometacin**, **naproxen**, and **diclofenac** are associated with *intermediate risks* (possibly higher in the case of piroxicam, see also CHMP advice, p. 606). **Selective inhibitors of cyclo-oxygenase-2** are associated with a *lower risk* of serious upper gastro-intestinal side-effects than non-selective NSAIDs.

Children appear to tolerate NSAIDs better than adults and gastro-intestinal side-effects are less common; use of drugs such as **ranitidine** or **omeprazole** may not be necessary.

Asthma

All NSAIDs have the potential to worsen asthma, either acutely or as a gradual worsening of symptoms; consider both prescribed NSAIDs and those that are purchased over the counter.

■ DICLOFENAC SODIUM

Cautions see notes above; **interactions:** Appendix 1 (NSAIDs)

Hepatic impairment increased risk of gastro-intestinal bleeding and fluid retention; avoid in severe liver disease

Breast-feeding amount too small to be harmful

Contra-indications see notes above; acute porphyria (section 9.8.2); avoid injections containing benzyl alcohol in neonates (see preparations below)

Intravenous use Additional contra-indications include concomitant NSAID or anticoagulant use (including low-dose heparin), history of haemorrhagic diathesis, history of confirmed or suspected cerebrovascular bleeding, operations with high risk of haemorrhage, history of asthma, moderate or severe renal impairment, hypovolaemia, dehydration

Rectal route Additional contra-indications include ulcerative or acute inflammatory conditions of the anus, rectum, or sigmoid colon

Side-effects see notes above; suppositories may cause rectal irritation; injection site reactions

Licensed use not licensed for use in children under 1 year; *suppositories* not licensed for use in children under 6 years except for use in children over 1 year for juvenile idiopathic arthritis; solid dose forms containing more than 25 mg not licensed for use in children; *diclofenac potassium tablets* not licensed for use in children under 14 years; *injection* not licensed for use in children

Indication and dose

Inflammation and mild to moderate pain
• **By mouth or by rectum**

  Child 6 months–18 years 0.3–1 mg/kg (max. 50 mg) 3 times daily

Postoperative pain
• **By rectum**

  Child 6–18 years 0.5–1 mg/kg (max. 75 mg) twice daily for max. 4 days; total daily dose may alternatively be given in 3 divided doses

• **By intravenous infusion or deep intramuscular injection into gluteal muscle**

  Child 2–18 years 0.3–1 mg/kg once or twice daily for max. 2 days (max. 150 mg daily)

Pain and inflammation in rheumatic disease including juvenile idiopathic arthritis
• **By mouth**

  Child 6 months–18 years 1.5–2.5 mg/kg (max. 75 mg) twice daily; total daily dose may alternatively be given in 3 divided doses

Administration for *intravenous infusion*, dilute 75 mg with 100–500 mL Glucose 5% *or* Sodium Chloride 0.9% (previously buffered with 0.5 mL Sodium Bicarbonate 8.4% solution *or* with 1 mL Sodium Bicarbonate 4.2% solution); give over 30–120 minutes

Diclofenac Sodium (Non-proprietary) ▣ℙ₀ℳ
Tablets, both e/c, diclofenac sodium 25 mg, net price 84-tab pack = £1.19; 50 mg, 84-tab pack = £1.36. Label: 5, 25
Brands include *Defenac®*, *Dicloflex®*, *Diclozip®*, *Fenactol®*, *Flamrase®*

Dispersible tablets, sugar-free, diclofenac sodium 10 mg
Available from 'special-order' manufacturers or specialist importing companies, see p. 943

Suppositories, diclofenac sodium 100 mg, net price 10 = £3.06
Brands include *Econac®*

◻ **DICLOFENAC SODIUM** (*continued*)

Voltarol® (Novartis) ℗ₒₘ

Tablets, e/c, diclofenac sodium 25 mg (yellow), net price 84-tab pack = £3.67; 50 mg (brown), 84-tab pack = £5.71. Label: 5, 25

Dispersible tablets, sugar-free, pink, diclofenac, equivalent to diclofenac sodium 50 mg, net price 21-tab pack = £6.19. Label: 13, 21

Injection, diclofenac sodium 25 mg/mL, net price 3-mL amp = 83p

Excipients include benzyl alcohol (avoid in neonates unless there is no safer alternative, see Excipients, p. 3), propylene glycol

Suppositories, diclofenac sodium 12.5 mg, net price 10 = 71p; 25 mg, 10 = £1.26; 50 mg, 10 = £2.07; 100 mg, 10 = £3.70

◢**Diclofenac potassium**

¹**Voltarol® Rapid** (Novartis) ℗ₒₘ

Tablets, s/c, diclofenac potassium 25 mg (red), net price 30-tab pack = £4.33; 50 mg (brown), 30-tab pack = £8.28

Dose

Rheumatic disease, musculoskeletal disorders, postoperative pain

Child 14–18 years 75–100 mg daily in 2–3 divided doses

1. 12.5 mg tablets can be sold to the public for the treatment of headache, dental pain, period pain, rheumatic and muscular pain, backache and the symptoms of cold and flu (including fever), in patients aged over 14 years subject to max. single dose of 25 mg, max. daily dose of 75 mg for max. 3 days, and max. pack size of 18 × 12.5 mg

◢**Modified release**

Diclomax SR® (Provalis) ℗ₒₘ

Capsules, m/r, yellow, diclofenac sodium 75 mg, net price 56-cap pack = £12.10. Label: 21, 25

Diclomax Retard® (Provalis) ℗ₒₘ

Capsules, m/r, diclofenac sodium 100 mg, net price 28-tab pack = £8.70. Label: 21, 25

Motifene® 75 mg (Daiichi Sankyo) ℗ₒₘ

Capsules, e/c, m/r, diclofenac sodium 75 mg (enclosing e/c pellets containing diclofenac sodium 25 mg and m/r pellets containing diclofenac sodium 50 mg), net price 56-cap pack = £8.00. Label: 25

Voltarol® 75 mg SR (Novartis) ℗ₒₘ

Tablets, m/r, pink, diclofenac sodium 75 mg, net price 28-tab pack = £8.08; 56-tab pack = £16.15. Label: 21, 25

Note Other brands of modified-release tablets containing diclofenac sodium 75 mg include *Defenac® SR, Dexomon® 75 SR, Dicloflex® 75 SR, Fenactol® 75 mg SR, Flamatak® 75 MR, Flamrase® SR, Flexotard® MR 75, Rheumatac® Retard 75, Rhumalgan® CR, Slofenac® SR, Volsaid® Retard 75*

Voltarol® Retard (Novartis) ℗ₒₘ

Tablets, m/r, red, diclofenac sodium 100 mg, net price 28-tab pack = £11.84. Label: 21, 25

Note Other brands of modified-release tablets containing diclofenac sodium 100 mg include *Defenac® Retard, Dexomon® Retard 100, Dicloflex® Retard, Fenactol® Retard 100 mg, Flamatak® 100 MR, Flamrase® SR, Rhumalgan® CR, Slofenac® SR, Volsaid® Retard 100*

■ **ETORICOXIB**

Cautions see notes above; also dehydration; monitor blood pressure before treatment, 2 weeks after initiation and periodically during treatment; **interactions:** Appendix 1 (NSAIDs)

Hepatic impairment increased risk of gastrointestinal bleeding and fluid retention; max. 60 mg daily in mild impairment; max. 60 mg on alternate days or 30 mg once daily in moderate impairment; avoid in severe impairment

Renal impairment see notes above; avoid if estimated glomerular filtration rate less than 30 mL/minute/1.73 m²

Contra-indications see notes above; inflammatory bowel disease; uncontrolled hypertension (persistently above 140/90 mmHg)

Breast-feeding manufacturer advises avoid—present in milk in *animal* studies

Side-effects see notes above; also flatulence, palpitation, fatigue, influenza-like symptoms, ecchymosis; *less commonly* dry mouth, taste disturbance, mouth ulcer, constipation, appetite and weight change, atrial fibrillation, transient ischaemic attack, chest pain, flushing, cough, dyspnoea, epistaxis, anxiety, mental acuity impaired, paraesthesia, electrolyte disturbance,

myalgia and arthralgia; *very rarely* confusion and hallucinations

Indication and dose

Osteoarthritis

• **By mouth**

Child 16–18 years 30 mg once daily, increased if necessary to 60 mg once daily

Rheumatoid arthritis and ankylosing spondylitis

• **By mouth**

Child 16–18 years 90 mg once daily

Acute gout

• **By mouth**

Child 16–18 years 120 mg once daily for max. 8 days

Arcoxia® (MSD) ▼ ℗ₒₘ

Tablets, f/c, etoricoxib 30 mg (blue-green), net price 28-tab pack = £13.99; 60 mg (dark green), 28-tab pack = £20.11; 90 mg (white), 28-tab pack = £22.96; 120 mg (pale green), 7-tab pack = £5.74

10

Musculoskeletal and joint diseases

■ IBUPROFEN

Cautions see notes above; **interactions:** Appendix 1 (NSAIDs)

Hepatic impairment increased risk of gastro-intestinal bleeding and can cause fluid retention; avoid in severe liver disease

Breast-feeding amount too small to be harmful, but some manufacturers advise avoid

Contra-indications see notes above

Side-effects see notes above; **overdosage:** see Emergency Treatment of Poisoning, p. 36

Licensed use not licensed for use in children under 3 months or body-weight under 5 kg

Indication and dose

> Mild to moderate pain, pain and inflammation of soft-tissue injuries, pyrexia with discomfort
> • By mouth
>
> **Child 1–3 months** 5 mg/kg 3–4 times daily
>
> **Child 3–6 months** 50 mg 3 times daily; max. 30 mg/kg daily in 3–4 divided doses
>
> **Child 6 months–1 year** 50 mg 3–4 times daily; max. 30 mg/kg daily in 3–4 divided doses
>
> **Child 1–4 years** 100 mg 3 times daily; max. 30 mg/kg daily in 3–4 divided doses
>
> **Child 4–7 years** 150 mg 3 times daily; max. 30 mg/kg daily in 3–4 divided doses
>
> **Child 7–10 years** 200 mg 3 times daily; max. 30 mg/kg (max. 2.4 g) daily in 3–4 divided doses
>
> **Child 10–12 years** 300 mg 3 times daily; max. 30 mg/kg (max. 2.4 g) daily in 3–4 divided doses
>
> **Child 12–18 years** initially 300–400 mg 3–4 times daily; increased if necessary to max. 600 mg 4 times daily; maintenance dose of 200–400 mg 3 times daily may be adequate

> Pain and inflammation in rheumatic disease including juvenile idiopathic arthritis
> • By mouth
>
> **Child 3 months–18 years** 30–40 mg/kg (max. 2.4 g) daily in 3–4 divided doses; in systemic juvenile idiopathic arthritis up to 60 mg/kg (max. 2.4 g) daily [unlicensed] in 4–6 divided doses

> Post-immunisation pyrexia in infants (see also p. 727)
> • By mouth
>
> **Child 2–3 months** 50 mg as a single dose repeated once after 6 hours if necessary

Closure of patent ductus arteriosus in neonates see section 2.14

¹ Ibuprofen (Non-proprietary) [PoM]
Tablets, coated, ibuprofen 200 mg, net price 84-tab pack = £2.07; 400 mg, 84-tab pack = £2.31; 600 mg, 84-tab pack = £3.96. Label: 21
Brands include *Arthrofen®*, *Ebufac®*, *Rimafen®*

Oral suspension, ibuprofen 100 mg/5 mL, net price 100 mL = £1.44, 150 mL = £2.71, 500 mL = £8.88. Label: 21

Note Sugar-free versions are available and can be ordered by specifying 'sugar-free' on the prescription
Brands include *Calprofen®*, *Fenpaed®*, *Feverfen®*, *Nurofen® for Children*, *Orbifen® for Children*
Dental prescribing on NHS Ibuprofen Tablets and Ibuprofen Oral Suspension Sugar-free may be prescribed

Brufen® (Abbott) [PoM]
Tablets, f/c, ibuprofen 200 mg, net price 100-tab pack = £4.08; 400 mg, 100-tab pack = £8.16; 600 mg, 100-tab pack = £12.24. Label: 21

Syrup, orange, ibuprofen 100 mg/5 mL, net price 500 mL (orange-flavoured) = £8.88. Label: 21

Granules, effervescent, ibuprofen 600 mg/sachet, net price 20–sachet pack = £6.80. Label: 13, 21
Contains sodium approx. 9 mmol/sachet

◢ Modified release
Brufen Retard® (Abbott) [PoM]
Tablets, m/r, ibuprofen 800 mg, net price 56-tab pack = £6.74. Label: 25, 27
Dose
> Pain and inflammation
> • By mouth
>
> **Child 12–18 years** 2 tablets daily as a single dose, preferably in the early evening, increased in severe cases to 3 tablets daily in 2 divided doses

Fenbid® (Goldshield) [PoM]
Spansule® (= capsule m/r), maroon/pink, enclosing off-white pellets, ibuprofen 300 mg, net price 120-cap pack = £9.64. Label: 25
Dose
> Pain and inflammation
> • By mouth
>
> **Child 12–18 years** initially 2 capsules twice daily, increased in severe cases to 3 capsules twice daily; then 1–2 capsules twice daily

■ INDOMETACIN
(Indomethacin)

Cautions see notes above; also epilepsy, psychiatric disturbances; during prolonged therapy ophthalmic and blood examinations particularly advisable; avoid rectal administration in proctitis and haemorrhoids; **interactions:** Appendix 1 (NSAIDs)
Skilled tasks Dizziness may affect performance of skilled tasks (e.g. driving)

Hepatic impairment increased risk of gastro-intestinal bleeding and can cause fluid retention; avoid in severe liver disease

Breast-feeding amount probably too small to be harmful—manufacturer advises avoid

Contra-indications see notes above

---

1. Can be sold to the public under certain circumstances; for exemptions see *Medicines, Ethics and Practice*, No. 32, London, Pharmaceutical Press, 2008 (and subsequent editions as available)

◻ **INDOMETACIN (continued)**

Side-effects see notes above; frequently gastro-intestinal disturbances (including diarrhoea), headache, dizziness, and light-headedness; also gastro-intestinal ulceration and bleeding; rarely, drowsiness, confusion, insomnia, convulsions, psychiatric disturbances, depression, syncope, blood disorders (particularly thrombocytopenia), hypertension, hyperglycaemia, blurred vision, corneal deposits, peripheral neuropathy, and intestinal strictures; suppositories may cause rectal irritation and occasional bleeding

Licensed use not licensed for use in children

Indication and dose

> Relief of pain and inflammation in rheumatic diseases including juvenile idiopathic arthritis
> * By mouth
>   **Child 1 month –18 years** 0.5–1 mg/kg twice daily; higher doses may be used under specialist supervision

Closure of patent ductus arteriosus in prema-ture babies section 2.14

Indometacin (Non-proprietary) PoM

Capsules, indometacin 25 mg, net price 28-cap pack = £1.59; 50 mg, 28-cap pack = £1.93. Label: 21, counselling, driving, see above
Brands include *Rimacid*®

Suppositories, indometacin 100 mg, net price 10 = £14.46. Counselling, driving, see above

Suspension, indometacin 5 mg/mL
Available from 'special-order' manufacturers or specialist importing companies, see p. 943

◢ Modified release
Indometacin m/r preparations PoM

Capsules, m/r, indometacin 75 mg. Label: 21, 25, counselling, driving, see above
Brands include *Indolar SR*®, *Pardelprin*®, *Slo-Indo*®

◢ MEFENAMIC ACID

Cautions see notes above; epilepsy; acute por-phyria (section 9.8.2); **interactions**: Appendix 1 (NSAIDs)

Hepatic impairment increased risk of gastro-intestinal bleeding and can cause fluid retention; avoid in severe liver disease

Breast-feeding amount too small to be harmful but manufacturer advises avoid

Contra-indications see notes above; inflamm-atory bowel disease

Side-effects see notes above; also diarrhoea or rashes (withdraw treatment), vomiting, flatu-lence, constipation, ulcerative stomatitis; fatigue; *less commonly* paraesthesia; *rarely* hypotension, palpitation, and glucose intolerance, thrombocy-topenia, haemolytic anaemia (positive Coombs' test), and aplastic anaemia reported

Indication and dose

> Acute pain including dysmenorrhoea, menorr-hagia
> * By mouth
>   **Child 6 months–12 years** not recommended
>   **Child 12–18 years** 500 mg 3 times daily

Mefenamic Acid (Non-proprietary) PoM

Capsules, mefenamic acid 250 mg, net price 20 = 79p. Label: 21

Tablets, mefenamic acid 500 mg, net price 28-tab pack = £1.97. Label: 21

Suspension, mefenamic acid 50 mg/5 mL, net price 125 mL = £79.99. Label: 21
Excipients include ethanol

Ponstan® (Chemidex) PoM

Capsules, blue/ivory, mefenamic acid 250 mg, net price 100-cap pack = £8.17. Label: 21

Forte tablets, yellow, mefenamic acid 500 mg, net price 100-tab pack = £15.72. Label: 21

◢ MELOXICAM

Cautions see notes above; **interactions**: Appen-dix 1 (NSAIDs)

Hepatic impairment increased risk of gastro-intestinal bleeding and can cause fluid retention; avoid in severe liver disease

Breast-feeding no information available—manu-facturer advises avoid

Contra-indications see notes above; renal failure (unless receiving dialysis); severe heart failure

Side-effects see notes above

Licensed use not licensed for use in children under 15 years

Indication and dose

> Relief of pain and inflammation in juvenile idiopathic arthritis and other musculoskeletal disorders in children intolerant to other NSAIDs
> * By mouth
>   **Child 12–18 years and body-weight under 50 kg** 7.5 mg once daily
>   **Child 12–18 years and body-weight over 50 kg** 15 mg once daily

Administration *Mobic*® tablets may be dispersed in water

10
Musculoskeletal and joint diseases

◁ **MELOXICAM** (*continued*)

Meloxicam (Non-proprietary) PoM
   Tablets, meloxicam 7.5 mg, net price 30-tab pack = £2.85; 15 mg, 30-tab pack = £3.52

Mobic® (Boehringer Ingelheim) PoM
   Tablets, yellow, scored, meloxicam 7.5 mg, net price 30-tab pack = £9.30; 15 mg, 30-tab pack = £12.93. Label: 21

■ NAPROXEN

Cautions see notes above; **interactions:** Appendix 1 (NSAIDs)

   Hepatic impairment increased risk of gastro-intestinal bleeding and can cause fluid retention; avoid in severe liver disease

   Breast-feeding amount too small to be harmful but manufacturer advises avoid

Contra-indications see notes above

Side-effects see notes above

Licensed use not licensed for use in children under 5 years for juvenile idiopathic arthritis; not licensed for use in children under 16 years for musculoskeletal disorders or dysmenorrhoea

Indication and dose

> Pain and inflammation in musculoskeletal disorders, dysmenorrhoea
> * By mouth
>> **Child 1 month–18 years** 5 mg/kg twice daily (max. 1 g daily)
>
> Juvenile idiopathic arthritis
> * By mouth
>> **Child 2–18 years** 5–7.5 mg/kg twice daily (max. 1 g daily)

[1]**Naproxen** (Non-proprietary) PoM
   Tablets, naproxen 250 mg, net price 28-tab pack = £1.29; 500 mg, 28-tab pack = £1.71. Label: 21
   Brands include *Arthroxen®*

   Tablets, e/c, naproxen 250 mg, net price 56-tab pack = £4.99; 375 mg, 56-tab pack = £6.96; 500 mg, 56-tab pack = £6.88. Label: 5, 25

   Suspension, naproxen 25 mg/mL
   Available from 'special-order' manufacturers or specialist importing companies, see p. 943

1. Can be sold to the public for the treatment of primary dysmenorrhoea in women aged 15–50 years subject to max. single dose of 500 mg, max. daily dose of 750 mg for max. 3 days, and a max. pack size of 9 × 250 mg tablets; for exemptions see *Medicines, Ethics and Practice*, No. 32, London, Pharmaceutical Press, 2008 (and subsequent editions as available)

Naprosyn® (Roche) PoM
   Tablets, yellow, scored, naproxen 250 mg, net price 56-tab pack = £4.55; 500 mg, 56-tab pack = £9.09. Label: 21

   Tablets, e/c, (*Naprosyn EC®*), naproxen 250 mg, net price 56-tab pack = £4.55; 375 mg, 56-tab pack = £6.82; 500 mg, 56-tab pack = £9.09. Label: 5, 25

Synflex® (Roche) PoM
   Tablets, blue, naproxen sodium 275 mg, net price 60-tab pack = £7.54. Label: 21

   Note 275 mg naproxen sodium ≡ 250 mg naproxen

■ PIROXICAM

Cautions see notes above and CHMP advice below; **interactions:** Appendix 1 (NSAIDs)

   Hepatic impairment increased risk of gastro-intestinal bleeding and can cause fluid retention; avoid in severe liver disease

   Breast-feeding amount too small to be harmful

Contra-indications see notes above

Side-effects see notes above; pain at injection site (occasionally tissue damage)

Licensed use capsules and non-dispersible tablets not licensed for use in children

Indication and dose

> Relief of pain and inflammation in juvenile idiopathic arthritis
> * By mouth
>> **Child 6–18 years and body-weight under 15 kg** 5 mg daily
>>
>> **Child 6–18 years and body-weight 16–25 kg** 10 mg daily
>>
>> **Child 6–18 years and body-weight 26–45 kg** 15 mg daily
>>
>> **Child 6–18 years and body-weight over 46 kg** 20 mg daily

> **CHMP advice**
>
> Piroxicam (June 2007) The CHMP has recommended restrictions on the use of piroxicam because of the increased risk of gastro-intestinal side effects and serious skin reactions. The CHMP has advised that:
> * piroxicam should be initiated only by physicians experienced in treating inflammatory or degenerative rheumatic diseases
> * piroxicam should not be used as first-line treatment
> * in adults, use of piroxicam should be limited to the symptomatic relief of osteoarthritis, rheumatoid arthritis, and ankylosing spondylitis
> * piroxicam dose should not exceed 20 mg daily
> * piroxicam should no longer be used for the treatment of acute painful and inflammatory conditions
> * treatment should be reviewed 2 weeks after initiating piroxicam, and periodically thereafter
> * concomitant administration of a gastro-protective agent (section 1.3) should be considered
>
> **Note** Topical preparations containing piroxicam are not affected by these restrictions

Piroxicam (Non-proprietary) PoM
   Capsules, piroxicam 10 mg, net price 56-cap pack = £2.07; 20 mg, 28-cap pack = £1.99. Label: 21

◻ **PIROXICAM (continued)**

Dispersible tablets, piroxicam 10 mg, net price 56-tab pack = £9.96; 20 mg, 28-tab pack = £35.07. Label: 13, 21

Feldene® (Pfizer) [PoM]

Capsules, piroxicam 10 mg (maroon/blue), net price 56-cap pack = £7.20; 20 mg (maroon), 28-cap pack = £7.20. Label: 21

Tablets, (*Feldene Melt®*), piroxicam 20 mg, net price 28-tab pack = £9.83. Label: 10, patient information leaflet, 21

Excipients include aspartame equivalent to phenylalanine 140 micrograms/tablet (section 9.4.1)

Note Tablets may be halved [unlicensed] to give 10-mg dose; tablet placed on tongue and allowed to dissolve or may be swallowed

Brexidol® (Chiesi) [PoM]

Tablets, yellow, scored, piroxicam (as betadex) 20 mg, net price 30-tab pack = £14.66. Label: 21

10.1.2 Corticosteroids

10.1.2.1 Systemic corticosteroids

The general actions, uses, and cautions of corticosteroids are described in section 6.3. In children with rheumatic diseases corticosteroids should be reserved for specific indications (e.g. when other anti-inflammatory drugs are unsuccessful) and should be used only under the supervision of a specialist.

Systemic corticosteroids may be considered for the management of juvenile idiopathic arthritis in systemic disease or when several joints are affected. Systemic corticosteroids may also be considered in severe, possibly life-threatening conditions such as systemic lupus erythematosus, systemic vasculitis, juvenile dermatomyositis, Behçet's disease, and polyarticular joint disease.

In severe conditions, short courses ('pulses') of high-dose intravenous methylprednisolone or a pulsed oral corticosteroid may be particularly effective for providing rapid relief, and has fewer long-term adverse effects than continuous treatment.

Corticosteroid doses should be reduced with care because of the possibility of relapse if the reduction is too rapid. If complete discontinuation of corticosteroids is not possible, consideration should be given to alternate-day (or alternate high-dose, low-dose) administration; on days when no corticosteroid is given, or a lower dose is given, an additional dose of a NSAID may be helpful. In some conditions, alternative treatment using an antimalarial or concomitant use of an immunosuppressant drug, such as azathioprine, methotrexate or cyclophosphamide may prove useful; in less severe conditions treatment with a NSAID alone may be adequate.

Administration of corticosteroids may result in suppression of growth and may affect the development of puberty. The risk of corticosteroid-induced osteoporosis should be considered for those on long-term corticosteroid treatment (section 6.6); corticosteroids may also increase the risk of osteopenia in those unable to exercise. For the disadvantages of corticosteroid treatment see section 6.3.2.

10.1.2.2 Local corticosteroid injections

Corticosteroids are injected locally for an anti-inflammatory effect. In inflammatory conditions of the joints, including juvenile idiopathic arthritis, they are given by *intra-articular injection* as an adjunct to long-term therapy to reduce swelling and deformity in one or a few joints. Aseptic precautions (e.g. a no-touch technique) are essential, as is a clinician skilled in the technique; infected areas should be avoided and general anaesthesia, or local anaesthesia, or conscious sedation should be used. Occasionally an acute inflammatory reaction develops after an intra-articular or soft-tissue injection of a corticosteroid. This may be a reaction to the microcrystalline suspension of the corticosteroid used, but must be distinguished from sepsis introduced into the injection site.

Triamcinolone hexacetonide is preferred for intra-articular injection because it is almost insoluble and has a long-acting (depot) effect. Triamcinolone acetonide and methylprednisolone may also be considered for intra-articular injection into larger joints, whilst hydrocortisone acetate should be reserved for smaller joints or for soft-tissue injections. Intra-articular corticosteroid injections can cause

10 Musculoskeletal and joint diseases

flushing and may affect the hyaline cartilage. Each joint should usually be treated no more than 3–4 times in one year.

A smaller amount of corticosteroid may also be injected directly into soft tissues for the relief of inflammation in conditions such as *tennis* or *golfer's elbow* or *compression neuropathies*. In *tendinitis*, injections should be made into the tendon sheath and not directly into the tendon (due to the absence of a true tendon sheath and a high risk of rupture, the Achilles tendon should not be injected).

Corticosteroid injections are also injected into soft tissues for the treatment of skin lesions (see section 13.4).

■ LOCAL CORTICOSTEROID INJECTIONS

Cautions see notes above and consult product literature; see also section 6.3.2

Contra-indications see notes above and consult product literature; avoid injections containing benzyl alcohol in neonates (see preparation below)

Side-effects see notes above and consult product literature

Licensed use triamcinolone acetonide not licensed for use in children under 6 years

Indication and dose

See under preparations

◢ Hydrocortisone acetate

Hydrocortistab® (Sovereign) PoM

Injection (aqueous suspension), hydrocortisone acetate 25 mg/mL, net price 1-mL amp = £5.72

Dose

- **By intra-articular or intrasynovial injection** (for details consult product literature)

  Child 1 month–12 years 5–30 mg according to size of child and joint

  Child 12–18 years 5–50 mg according to size of child and joint

  Note Where appropriate may be repeated at intervals of 21 days; not more than 3 joints should be treated on any one day

◢ Methylprednisolone acetate

Depo-Medrone® (Pharmacia) PoM

Injection (aqueous suspension), methylprednisolone acetate 40 mg/mL, net price 1-mL vial = £2.87; 2-mL vial = £5.15; 3-mL vial = £7.47

Depo-Medrone® with Lidocaine (Pharmacia) PoM

Injection (aqueous suspension), methylprednisolone acetate 40 mg, lidocaine hydrochloride 10 mg/mL, net price 1-mL vial = £3.28; 2-mL vial = £5.88

◢ Triamcinolone hexacetonide

Available from 'special-order' manufacturers or specialist importing companies, see p. 943

◢ Triamcinolone acetonide

Adcortyl® Intra-articular/Intradermal (Squibb) PoM

Injection (aqueous suspension), triamcinolone acetonide 10 mg/mL, net price 1-mL amp = £1.02; 5-mL vial = £4.14

Excipients include benzyl alcohol (avoid in neonates, see Excipients, p. 3)

Dose

- **By intra-articular injection or intrasynovial injection** (for details consult product literature)

  Child 1–18 years 500 micrograms/kg for smaller joints, max. 20 mg for small joints and max. 10 mg for finger and toe joints; 1 mg/kg for larger joints (max. 40 mg), may be repeated for relapse

Kenalog® Intra-articular/Intramuscular (Squibb) PoM

Injection (aqueous suspension), triamcinolone acetonide 40 mg/mL, net price 1-mL vial = £1.70; 1-mL prefilled syringe = £2.11; 2-mL prefilled syringe = £3.66

Note Intramuscular needle with prefilled syringe should be replaced for intra-articular injection

Dose

- **By intra-articular or intrasynovial injection** (for details consult product literature)

  Child 1–18 years 1 mg/kg for larger joints (max. 40 mg), 500 micrograms/kg for smaller joints, max. 20 mg for small joints and max. 10 mg for finger and toe joints; may be repeated for relapse

10.1.3 Drugs that suppress the rheumatic disease process

Certain drugs such as methotrexate, etanercept, and sulfasalazine may suppress the disease process in *juvenile idiopathic arthritis* (juvenile chronic arthritis); these drugs are known as disease-modifying antirheumatic drugs (DMARDs). In children, disease-modifying antirheumatic drugs should generally be used under specialist supervision.

Some children with juvenile idiopathic arthritis do not require disease-modifying antirheumatic drugs. Methotrexate is effective in juvenile idiopathic arthritis; sulfasalazine is an alternative but should be avoided in *systemic-onset juvenile idiopathic arthritis*. Gold and penicillamine are no longer used. For the role of adalimumab and etanercept in *polyarticular juvenile idiopathic arthritis*, see p. 611.

Unlike NSAIDs, disease-modifying antirheumatic drugs can affect the progression of disease but they may require 3–6 months of treatment for a full therapeutic response. Response to a disease-modifying antirheumatic drug may allow the dose of the NSAID to be reduced.

Disease-modifying antirheumatic drugs can improve not only the symptoms of inflammatory joint disease but also extra-articular manifestations such as vasculitis. They reduce the erythrocyte sedimentation rate and C-reactive protein.

Antimalarials

The antimalarial **hydroxychloroquine** is rarely used to treat juvenile idiopathic arthritis. Hydroxychloroquine can also be useful for systemic or discoid lupus erythematosus, particularly involving the skin and joints, and in sarcoidosis.

Retinopathy (see below) rarely occurs provided that the recommended doses are not exceeded.

Mepacrine is used on rare occasions to treat discoid lupus erythematosus [unlicensed].

Cautions Hydroxychloroquine should be used with caution in hepatic impairment and in renal impairment (see hydroxychloroquine sulphate, below). Hydroxychloroquine should be used with caution in neurological disorders (especially in those with a history of epilepsy), in severe gastro-intestinal disorders, in G6PD deficiency (section 9.1.5), and in acute porphyria. Hydroxychloroquine may exacerbate psoriasis and aggravate myasthenia gravis. Concurrent use of hepatotoxic drugs should be avoided; other **interactions**: Appendix 1 (chloroquine and hydroxychloroquine).

Pregnancy and breast-feeding It is not necessary to withdraw an antimalarial drug during pregnancy if the rheumatic disease is well controlled. Hydroxychloroquine is present in breast milk and breast-feeding should be avoided when it is used to treat rheumatic disease.

> Screening for ocular toxicity
> Hydroxychloroquine is rarely associated with ocular toxicity. The British Society for Paediatric and Adolescent Rheumatology recommends that children should have their vision tested before long-term treatment with hydroxychloroquine and have an annual review of visual acuity. Children should be referred to an ophthalmologist if there is visual impairment, changes in visual acuity, or blurred vision. The Royal College of Ophthalmologists has recommended that a locally agreed protocol between the prescribing doctor and ophthalmologist be established to monitor the vision of these children.

Note To avoid excessive dosage in obese children, the dose of hydroxychloroquine should be calculated on the basis of lean body weight; ocular toxicity is unlikely with doses under 5–6.5 mg/kg or max. 400 mg daily.

Side-effects The side-effects of hydroxychloroquine include gastro-intestinal disturbances, headache, and skin reactions (rashes, pruritus); those occurring less frequently include ECG changes, convulsions, visual changes, retinal damage (see above), keratopathy, ototoxicity, hair depigmentation, hair loss, and discoloration of skin, nails, and mucous membranes. Side-effects that occur rarely include blood disorders (including thrombocytopenia, agranulocytosis, and aplastic anaemia), mental changes (including emotional disturbances and psychosis), myopathy (including cardiomyopathy and neuromyopathy), acute generalised exanthematous pustulosis, exfoliative dermatitis, Stevens-Johnson syndrome, photosensitivity, and hepatic damage; angioedema and bronchospasm have also been reported. **Important**: very toxic in overdosage—immediate advice from poisons centres essential (see also p. 41).

HYDROXYCHLOROQUINE SULPHATE

Cautions see notes above

Renal impairment Manufacturer advises caution and monitoring of plasma-hydroxychloroquine concentration in severe reanl impairment

Pregnancy manufacturer advises avoid but see also notes above

Breast-feeding avoid—risk of toxicity in infant

Side-effects see notes above

◻ **HYDROXYCHLOROQUINE SULPHATE** (*continued*)

Licensed use Juvenile idiopathic arthritis, systemic and discoid lupus erythematosus, dermatological conditions caused or aggravated by sunlight

Indication and dose

Juvenile idiopathic arthritis, systemic and discoid lupus erythematosus, dermatological conditions caused or aggravated by sunlight
• **By mouth**
  Child 1 month–18 years 5–6.5 mg/kg (max. 400 mg) once daily

Plaquenil® (Sanofi-Synthelabo) [PoM]
Tablets, f/c, hydroxychloroquine sulphate 200 mg, net price 60-tab pack = £5.46. Label: 5, 21

◢Extemporaneous formulations available see Extemporaneous Preparations, p. 8

Drugs affecting the immune response

Methotrexate, given as a once weekly dose, is the disease-modifying antirheumatic drug of choice in the treatment of juvenile idiopathic arthritis and also has a role in juvenile dermatomyositis, vasculitis, uveitis, systemic lupus erythromatosus, localised scleroderma, and sarcoidosis. For these indications it is given by the intramuscular, subcutaneous, or oral routes. Absorption from intramuscular or subcutaneous routes may be more predictable than from the oral route; if the oral route is ineffective subcutaneous administration is generally preferred. Regular full blood counts (including differential white cell count and platelet count), renal and liver function tests are required. Folic acid may reduce mucosal or gastro-intestinal side-effects of methotrexate. The dosage regimen for folic acid has not been established—in children over 2 years a dose of 5 mg weekly may be given, usually at least 24 hours after the dose of methotrexate.

Azathioprine may be used in children for vasculitis which has failed to respond to other treatments, for the management of severe cases of *systemic lupus erythematosus* and other connective tissue disorders, in conjunction with corticosteroids for patients with severe or progressive renal disease, and in cases of *polymyositis* which are resistant to corticosteroids. Azathioprine has a corticosteroid-sparing effect in patients whose corticosteroid requirements are excessive.

Ciclosporin (cyclosporin) is rarely used in juvenile idiopathic arthritis, connective tissue diseases, vasculitis, and uveitis; it may be considered if the condition has failed to respond to other treatments.

▲ AZATHIOPRINE

Cautions see section 8.2.1
Contra-indications see section 8.2.1
Side-effects see section 8.2.1

Indication and dose

Juvenile idiopathic arthritis, vasculitis, auto-immune conditions usually when corticosteroid therapy alone has proved inadequate
• **By mouth**
  Child 1 month–18 years initially 1 mg/kg daily, adjusted according to response to max. 3 mg/kg daily (consider withdrawal if no improvement within 3 months)

Inflammatory bowel disease section 1.5.3

Transplantation rejection section 8.2.1

◢Preparations
Section 8.2.1

▲ METHOTREXATE

Cautions section 8.1.3; see advice below (blood count, gastro-intestinal, liver, and pulmonary toxicity); extreme caution in blood disorders (avoid if severe); risk of accumulation in pleural effusion or ascites—drain before treatment; full blood count and liver function tests before starting treatment repeated fortnightly for at least the first 4 weeks and at this frequency after any change in dose until therapy stabilised, thereafter monthly; regular renal function tests are also necessary; children or their carers should report all symptoms and signs suggestive of infection, especially sore throat; treatment with folinic acid (as calcium folinate, section 8.1) may be required in acute toxicity; check immunity to varicella-zoster and consider vaccination (section 14.4) before initiating therapy; acute porphyria (section 9.8.2); **interactions**: see below and Appendix 1 (methotrexate)
Blood count Bone marrow suppression can occur abruptly; factors likely to increase toxicity include renal impairment and concomitant use with another anti-folate drug. A clinically significant drop in white cell count or

◻ **METHOTREXATE** (*continued*)

platelet count calls for immediate withdrawal of methotrexate and introduction of supportive therapy

Gastro-intestinal toxicity Withdraw treatment if stomatitis develops—may be first sign of gastro-intestinal toxicity

Liver toxicity Persistent 2–fold rise in liver transaminases
may necessitate dose reduction or rarely discontinuation;
abrupt withdrawal should be avoided as this can lead to
disease flare

Pulmonary toxicity Acute pulmonary toxicity is rare in
children treated for juvenile idiopathic arthritis, but children and carers should seek medical attention if dyspnoea, cough or fever develops; discontinue if pneumonitis suspected.

NSAIDs Children and carers should be advised to avoid
self-medication with over-the-counter ibuprofen

Hepatic impairment dose-related toxicity—
avoid in non-malignant conditions

Contra-indications see section 8.1.3 and cautions
above

Side-effects section 8.1.3; chronic pulmonary
fibrosis; blood dyscrasias (including fatalities);
liver cirrhosis

Licensed use not licensed for use in children for
non-malignant conditions

Indication and dose

> Juvenile idiopathic arthritis, juvenile dermato-
> myositis, vasculitis, uveitis, systemic lupus
> erythematosus, localised scleroderma, sarcoi-
> dosis
>
> • By mouth, subcutaneous injection, or intra-
>   muscular injection
>
>   **Child 1 month–18 years** 10–15 mg/m² once
>   weekly initially, increased if necessary to max.
>   25 mg/m² once weekly

Safe Practice Note that the above dose is a **weekly** dose.
To avoid error with low-dose methotrexate, it is recommended that:

• the child or their carer is carefully advised of the
  dose and **frequency** and the reason for taking
  methotrexate and any other prescribed medicine
  (e.g. folic acid);

• only one strength of methotrexate tablet (usually
  2.5 mg) is prescribed and dispensed;

• the prescription and the dispensing label clearly
  show the dose and frequency of methotrexate
  administration;

• the child or their carer is warned to report immediately the onset of any feature of blood disorders
  (e.g. sore throat, bruising, and mouth ulcers), liver
  toxicity (e.g. nausea, vomiting, abdominal discomfort, and dark urine), and respiratory effects (e.g.
  shortness of breath).

Severe Crohn's disease section 1.5.3

Malignant disease section 8.1.3

Psoriasis section 13.5.3

Methotrexate (Non-proprietary) ▣ᴾᵒᴹ

Tablets, yellow, methotrexate 2.5 mg, net price 28-
tab pack = £3.27. Counselling, dose, NSAIDs
Brands include *Maxtrex®*

Tablets, yellow, methotrexate 10 mg, net price 20-
tab pack (Hospira) = £11.44; (Pharmacia, *Maxtrex®*)
= £9.03. Counselling, dose, NSAIDs

Suspension
Available from 'special-order' manufacturers or specialist
importing companies, see p. 943

◢Parenteral preparations
See also section 8.1.3

Metoject® (Medac) ▣ᴾᵒᴹ

Injection, prefilled syringe, methotrexate (as
disodium salt) 10 mg/mL, net price 0.75 mL
(7.5 mg) = £14.85, 1 mL (10 mg) = £15.29, 1.5 mL
(15 mg) = £16.57, 2 mL (20 mg) = £17.84, 2.5 mL
(25 mg) = £18.48

▰ **Cytokine modulators**

Cytokine modulators should be used under specialist supervision.

Adalimumab, **etanercept**, and **infliximab** inhibit the activity of tumour necrosis
factor alpha (TNF-α).

NICE guidance

Etanercept for the treatment of juvenile idiopathic arthritis (March 2002)
Etanercept is recommended in children aged 4–17 years with active polyarticular-course juvenile idiopathic arthritis who have not responded adequately to methotrexate or who are intolerant of it. Etanercept should be used
under specialist supervision according to the guidelines of the British Society
for Paediatric and Adolescent Rheumatology [previously the British Paediatric
Rheumatology Group].

Etanercept should be withdrawn if severe side-effects develop or if there is no
response after 6 months or if the initial response is not maintained. A decision
to continue therapy beyond 2 years should be based on disease activity and
clinical effectiveness in individual cases.

Prescribers of etanercept should register consenting patients with the Biolo-
gics Registry of the British Society for Paediatric and Adolescent Rheumatology.

10

Musculoskeletal and joint diseases

Side-effects Adalimumab, etanercept, and infliximab have been associated with infections, sometimes severe, including tuberculosis, septicaemia, and hepatitis B reactivation. Other side-effects include nausea, abdominal pain, worsening heart failure, hypersensitivity reactions (including angioedema, bronchospasm, urticaria, and anaphylaxis), fever, headache, depression, antibody formation (including lupus erythematosus-like syndrome), pruritus, injection-site reactions, and blood disorders (including anaemia, leucopenia, thrombocytopenia, pancytopenia, aplastic anaemia).

ADALIMUMAB

Cautions predisposition to infection; monitor for infections before, during, and for 5 months after treatment (see also Tuberculosis below); do not initiate until active infections are controlled; discontinue if new serious infection develops; hepatitis B virus—monitor for active infection; children should be brought up to date with current immunisation schedule (section 14.1) before initiating therapy; mild heart failure (discontinue if symptoms develop or worsen—avoid in moderate or severe heart failure); demyelinating CNS disorders (risk of exacerbation); history of malignancy; monitor for non-melanoma skin cancer before and during treatment, especially in children with history of PUVA treatment for psoriasis or extensive immunosuppressant therapy; **interactions**: Appendix 1 (adalimumab)

Tuberculosis Children should be evaluated for tuberculosis before treatment. Active tuberculosis should be treated with standard treatment (section 5.1.9) for at least 2 months before starting adalimumab. Children who have previously received adequate treatment for tuberculosis can start adalimumab but should be monitored every 3 months for possible recurrence. In those without active tuberculosis but who were previously not treated adequately, chemoprophylaxis should ideally be completed before starting adalimumab. In children at high risk of tuberculosis who cannot be assessed by tuberculin skin test, chemoprophylaxis can be given concurrently with adalimumab. Children and their carers should be advised to seek medical attention if symptoms suggestive of tuberculosis (e.g. persistent cough, weight loss, and fever) develop

Contra-indications severe infection (see also Cautions)

Pregnancy avoid; manufacturer advises adequate contraception during and for at least 5 months after last dose

Breast-feeding manufacturer advises avoid for at least 5 months after last dose

Side-effects see under Cytokine Modulators, above and Cautions above; also mouth ulceration, stomatitis, diarrhoea, cough, dizziness, fatigue, paraesthesia, musculoskeletal pain, rash, and pruritus; *less commonly* vomiting, dyspepsia, constipation, rectal bleeding, arrhythmias, syncope, chest pain, hyperlipidaemia, hypertension, flushing, dyspnoea, dysphonia, appetite disorders, anxiety, tremor, sleep disturbances, influenza-like symptoms, menstrual disorders, electrolyte disturbances, haematuria, renal impairment, hyperuricaemia, eye disorders, and skin papilloma, alopecia; *rarely* pancreatitis, colitis, oesophagitis, gastritis, hepatitis, cholelithiasis, palpitation, myocardial infarction, vascular occlusion, pleural effusion, demyelinating disorders, facial palsy, thyroid disorders, malignancy, rhabdomyolysis, hearing loss, tinnitus, and erythema multiforme; also reported intestinal perforation, vasculitis, and interstitial lung disease

Indication and dose

Active polyarticular juvenile idiopathic arthritis (in combination with methotrexate or alone if methotrexate inappropriate) in children who have not responded adequately to one or more disease-modifying antirheumatic drug

• By subcutaneous injection

Child 13–17 years 40 mg on alternate weeks; review treatment if no response within 12 weeks

Humira® (Abbott) ▼ PoM

Injection, adalimumab, net price 40-mg prefilled pen or prefilled syringe = £357.50. Counselling, tuberculosis

ETANERCEPT

Cautions predisposition to infection (avoid if predisposition to septicaemia); significant exposure to herpes zoster virus—interrupt treatment and consider varicella–zoster immunoglobulin; hepatitis B virus—monitor for active infection; monitor for worsening hepatitis C infection; heart failure (risk of exacerbation); demyelinating CNS disorders (risk of exacerbation); history of blood disorders; **interactions**: Appendix 1 (etanercept)

Tuberculosis Children should be evaluated for tuberculosis before treatment. Active tuberculosis should be treated with standard treatment (section 5.1.9) for at least 2 months before starting etanercept. Children who have previously received adequate treatment for tuberculosis can start etanercept but should be monitored every 3 months for possible recurrence. In those without active tuberculosis but who were previously not treated adequately, chemoprophylaxis should ideally be completed

before starting etanercept. In children at high risk of tuberculosis who cannot be assessed by tuberculin skin test, chemoprophylaxis can be given concurrently with etanercept. Children and their carers should be advised to seek medical attention if symptoms suggestive of tuberculosis (e.g. persistent cough, weight loss, and fever) develop

Blood disorders Children and their carers should be advised to seek medical attention if symptoms suggestive of blood disorders (such as fever, sore throat, bruising, or bleeding) develop

Contra-indications active infection; avoid injections containing benzyl alcohol in neonates (see preparations below)

Pregnancy manufacturer advises avoid—no information available

Breast-feeding manufacturer advises avoid—present in milk in *animal* studies

◁ **ETANERCEPT** *(continued)*

Side-effects see under Cytokine Modulators, p. 612; also *less commonly* interstitial lung disease, rash; *rarely* demyelinating disorders, seizures, Stevens-Johnson syndrome, and cutaneous vasculitis; *very rarely* toxic epidermal necrolysis; *also reported* appendicitis, cholecystitis, gastritis, gastro-intestinal haemorrhage, intestinal obstruction, liver damage, oesophagitis, pancreatitis, ulcerative colitis, vomiting, cerebral ischaemia, hypertension, hypotension, myocardial infarction, thrombophlebitis, thromboembolism, asthma, dyspnoea, aseptic meningitis, confusion, paresis, paraesthesia, vertigo, lymphadenopathy, diabetes mellitus, haematuria, malignancy, renal calculi, renal impairment, bone fracture, bursitis, polymyositis, scleritis, and cutaneous ulcer

Indication and dose

Polyarticular-course juvenile idiopathic arthritis in children who have had an inadequate response to methotrexate or who cannot tolerate it

• **By subcutaneous injection**

Child 4–18 years 400 micrograms/kg (max. 25 mg) twice weekly, with an interval of 3–4 days between doses

Severe plaque psoriasis section 13.5.3

Enbrel® (Wyeth) ▼ PoM
Injection, powder for reconstitution, etanercept, net price 25-mg vial (with solvent) = £89.38. Label: 10, alert card, counselling, tuberculosis and blood disorders

Paediatric injection, powder for reconstitution, etanercept, net price 25-mg vial (with solvent) = £89.38. Label: 10, alert card, counselling, tuberculosis and blood disorders
Excipients include benzyl alcohol (avoid in neonates, see Excipients, p. 3)

Injection, etanercept, net price 25-mg prefilled syringe = £89.38. Label: 10, alert card, counselling, tuberculosis and blood disorders

Sulfasalazine

Sulfasalazine (sulphasalazine) has a beneficial effect in suppressing the inflammatory activity associated with some forms of juvenile idiopathic arthritis; it is generally not used in systemic-onset disease. Sulfasalazine may cause haematological abnormalities including leucopenia, neutropenia, and thrombocytopenia and close monitoring of full blood counts (including differential white cell count and platelet count) is necessary initially, and at monthly intervals during the first 3 months (liver-function tests also being performed at monthly intervals for the first 3 months). Although the manufacturer recommends renal function tests, evidence of practical value is unsatisfactory. For use of sulfasalazine also see section 1.5.1, aminosalicylates.

SULFASALAZINE
(Sulphasalazine)

Cautions see section 1.5.1 and notes above

Contra-indications see section 1.5.1

Side-effects see section 1.5.1 and notes above

Licensed use not licensed for use in children for juvenile idiopathic arthritis

Indication and dose

Juvenile idiopathic arthritis (see also notes above)

• **By mouth**

Child 2–18 years initially 5 mg/kg twice daily for 1 week, then 10 mg/kg twice daily for 1 week, then 20 mg/kg twice daily for 1 week, maintenance dose 20–25 mg/kg twice daily; Child 2–12 years max. 2 g daily, Child 12–18 years max. 3 g daily

◀Preparations
Section 1.5.1

10.1.4 Cytotoxic-induced hyperuricaemia

This section is not included in *BNF for Children*. For the role of allopurinol and rasburicase in the prophylaxis of hyperuricaemia associated with cancer chemotherapy and in enzyme disorders causing increased serum urate, see section 8.1. The management of gout in adolescents requires specialist supervision.

10

Musculoskeletal and joint diseases

Classification not used in *BNF for Children*.

10.2 Drugs used in neuromuscular disorders

10.2.1 Drugs that enhance neuromuscular transmission
10.2.2 Skeletal muscle relaxants

10.2.1 Drugs that enhance neuromuscular transmission

Anticholinesterases are used as first-line treatment in *ocular myasthenia gravis* and as an adjunct to immunosuppressant therapy for *generalised myasthenia gravis*.

Corticosteroids are used when anticholinesterases do not control symptoms completely. A second-line immunosuppressant such as azathioprine is frequently used to reduce the dose of corticosteroid.

Plasmapheresis or infusion of intravenous immunoglobulin [unlicensed indication] may induce temporary remission in severe relapses, particularly where bulbar or respiratory function is compromised or before thymectomy.

Anticholinesterases

Anticholinesterase drugs enhance neuromuscular transmission in voluntary and involuntary muscle in myasthenia gravis. They prolong the action of acetylcholine by inhibiting the action of the enzyme acetylcholinesterase. Excessive dosage of these drugs can impair neuromuscular transmission and precipitate cholinergic crises by causing a depolarising block. This may be difficult to distinguish from a worsening myasthenic state.

Muscarinic side-effects of anticholinesterases include increased sweating, increased salivary and gastric secretions, increased gastro-intestinal and uterine motility, and bradycardia. These parasympathomimetic effects are antagonised by atropine.

Edrophonium has a very brief action and it is therefore used mainly for the diagnosis of myasthenia gravis. However, such testing should be performed only by those experienced in its use; other means of establishing the diagnosis are available. A single test-dose usually causes substantial improvement in muscle power (lasting about 5 minutes) in patients with the disease (if respiration already impaired, *only* in conjunction with someone skilled at intubation).

Edrophonium can also be used to determine whether a patient with myasthenia is receiving inadequate or excessive treatment with cholinergic drugs. If treatment is excessive an injection of edrophonium will either have no effect or will intensify symptoms (if respiration already impaired, give *only* in conjunction with someone skilled at intubation). Conversely, transient improvement may be seen if the patient is being inadequately treated. The test is best performed just before the next dose of anticholinesterase.

Neostigmine produces a therapeutic effect for up to 4 hours. Its pronounced muscarinic action is a disadvantage, and simultaneous administration of an antimuscarinic drug such as atropine or propantheline may be required to prevent colic, excessive salivation, or diarrhoea. In severe disease neostigmine can be given every 2 hours. In infants, neostigmine by either subcutaneous or intramuscular injection is preferred for the short-term management of myasthenia.

Pyridostigmine is less powerful and slower in action than neostigmine but it has a longer duration of action. It is preferable to neostigmine because of its smoother action and the need for less frequent dosage. It is particularly preferred in patients whose muscles are weak on waking. It has a comparatively mild gastro-intestinal effect but an antimuscarinic drug may still be required. It is inadvisable to use excessive doses because acetylcholine receptor down regulation may occur. Immunosuppressant therapy may be considered if high doses of pyridostigmine are needed. Neostigmine and pyridostigmine should be given to neonates 30 minutes before feeds to improve suckling.

Neostigmine and edrophonium are also used to reverse the actions of the non-depolarising neuromuscular blocking drugs (section 15.1.6).

▲ NEOSTIGMINE

Cautions asthma (*extreme* caution), bradycardia, arrhythmias, recent myocardial infarction, epilepsy, hypotension, parkinsonism, vagotonia, peptic ulceration, hyperthyroidism; atropine or other antidote to muscarinic effects may be necessary (particularly when neostigmine is given by injection), but not given routinely because it may mask signs of overdosage; **interactions**: Appendix 1 (parasympathomimetics)

Renal impairment may need dose reduction

Pregnancy manufacturer advises use only if potential benefit outweighs risk

Breast-feeding amount probably too small to be harmful; monitor infant

Contra-indications intestinal or urinary obstruction

Side-effects nausea, vomiting, increased salivation, diarrhoea, abdominal cramps (more marked with higher doses); signs of overdosage include bronchoconstriction, increased bronchial secretions, lacrimation, excessive sweating, involuntary defaecation and micturition, miosis, nystagmus, bradycardia, heart block, arrhythmias, hypotension, agitation, excessive dreaming, and weakness eventually leading to fasciculation and paralysis

Indication and dose

Treatment of myasthenia gravis
* **By mouth (as neostigmine bromide)**

  Neonate initially 1–2 mg, then 1–5 mg every 4 hours, give 30 minutes before feeds

Child up to 6 years initially 7.5 mg repeated at suitable intervals throughout the day, total daily dose 15–90 mg

Child 6–12 years initially 15 mg repeated at suitable intervals throughout the day, total daily dose 15–90 mg

Child 12–18 years initially 15–30 mg repeated at suitable intervals throughout the day, total daily dose 75–300 mg (but max. most can tolerate is 180 mg daily)

* **By subcutaneous or intramuscular injection (as neostigmine metilsulfate)**

  Neonate 150 micrograms/kg every 6–8 hours, 30 minutes before feeds, increased to max. 300 micrograms/kg every 4 hours, if necessary [unlicensed]

  Child 1 month–12 years 200–500 micrograms repeated at suitable intervals throughout the day

  Child 12–18 years 1–2.5 mg repeated at suitable intervals throughout the day

Neostigmine (Non-proprietary) ⒫ⓞⓜ
Tablets, scored, neostigmine bromide 15 mg, net price 20 = £7.29

Injection, neostigmine metilsulfate 2.5 mg/mL, net price 1-mL amp = 57p

▲ EDROPHONIUM CHLORIDE

Cautions see under Neostigmine; have resuscitation facilities; *extreme* caution in respiratory distress (see notes above) and in asthma
Note Severe cholinergic reactions can be counteracted by injection of atropine sulphate (which should always be available)

Contra-indications see under Neostigmine

Side-effects see under Neostigmine

Licensed use not licensed for use in children under 1 year as a diagnostic test for myasthenia gravis

Indication and dose

Diagnostic test for myasthenia gravis
* **By intravenous injection**

  Child 1 month–12 years 20 micrograms/kg followed after 30 seconds (if no adverse reaction has occurred) by 80 micrograms/kg

Child 12–18 years 2 mg followed after 30 seconds (if no adverse reaction has occurred) by 8 mg

Detection of overdosage or underdosage of cholinergic drugs
* **By intravenous injection**

  Child 1 month–12 years 20 micrograms/kg (preferably just before next dose of anticholinesterase, see notes above)

  Child 12–18 years 2 mg (preferably just before next dose of anticholinesterase, see notes above)

Edrophonium (Cambridge) ⒫ⓞⓜ
Injection, edrophonium chloride 10 mg/mL, net price 1-mL amp = £7.89

▲ PYRIDOSTIGMINE BROMIDE

Cautions see under Neostigmine; weaker muscarinic action

Contra-indications see under Neostigmine

Side-effects see under Neostigmine

Indication and dose

Treatment of myasthenia gravis
* **By mouth**

  Neonate initially 1–1.5 mg/kg, increased gradually to max. 10 mg, repeated throughout the day, give 30–60 minutes before feeds

10

Musculoskeletal and joint diseases

◁ **PYRIDOSTIGMINE BROMIDE** (*continued*)

Child 1 month –12 years initially 1–1.5 mg/kg/day, increased gradually to 7 mg/kg/day in 6 divided doses; usual total daily dose 30–360 mg

Child 12–18 years 30–120 mg, repeated throughout the day; usual total daily dose 0.3–1.2 g (but consider immunosuppressant therapy if total daily dose exceeds 360 mg, down-regulation of acetylcholine receptors possible if total daily dose exceeds 450 mg; see notes above)

Mestinon® (Valeant) ⟨PoM⟩
Tablets, scored, pyridostigmine bromide 60 mg, net price 20 = £4.81

◀ Extemporaneous formulations available see Extemporaneous Preparations, p. 8

Immunosuppressant therapy

A course of **corticosteroids** (section 6.3) is an established treatment in severe cases of myasthenia gravis and may be particularly useful when antibodies to the acetylcholine receptor are present in high titre. Short courses of high-dose ('pulsed') methylprednisolone followed by maintenance therapy with oral corticosteroids may also be useful.

Corticosteroid treatment is usually initiated under specialist supervision. For disadvantages of corticosteroid treatment, see section 6.3.2. Transient but very serious worsening of symptoms can occur in the first 2–3 weeks, especially if the corticosteroid is started at a high dose. Once remission has occurred (usually after 2–6 months), the dose of prednisolone should be reduced slowly to the minimum effective dose.

10.2.2 Skeletal muscle relaxants

The drugs described below are used for the relief of chronic muscle spasm or spasticity associated with neurological damage; they are not indicated for spasm associated with minor injuries. They act principally on the central nervous system with the exception of dantrolene, which has a peripheral site of action. They differ in action from the muscle relaxants used in anaesthesia (section 15.1.5), which block transmission at the neuromuscular junction.

The underlying cause of spasticity should be treated and any aggravating factors (e.g. pressure sores, infection) remedied. Skeletal muscle relaxants are effective in most forms of spasticity except the rare alpha variety. The major disadvantage of treatment with these drugs is that reduction in muscle tone can cause a loss of splinting action of the spastic leg and trunk muscles and sometimes lead to an increase in disability.

Dantrolene acts directly on skeletal muscle and produces fewer central adverse effects. It is generally used in resistant cases. The dose should be increased slowly.

Baclofen inhibits transmission at spinal level and also depresses the central nervous system. The dose should be increased slowly to avoid the major side-effects of sedation and muscular hypotonia (other adverse events are uncommon).

Diazepam has undoubted efficacy in some children. Sedation and occasionally extensor hypotonus are disadvantages. Other benzodiazepines also have muscle-relaxant properties.

◣ BACLOFEN

Cautions psychiatric illness, respiratory impairment, epilepsy; history of peptic ulcer (avoid oral route in active peptic ulceration); diabetes; hypertonic bladder sphincter; avoid abrupt withdrawal (risk of hyperactive state, may exacerbate spasticity, and precipitate autonomic dysfunction including hyperthermia, psychiatric reactions and convulsions, see also under Withdrawal below); **interactions:** Appendix 1 (muscle relaxants)
Withdrawal CSM has advised that serious side-effects can occur on abrupt withdrawal; to minimise risk, discontinue by gradual dose reduction over at least 1–2 weeks (longer if symptoms occur)
Skilled tasks Drowsiness may affect performance of skilled tasks (e.g. driving); effects of alcohol enhanced

Renal impairment use smaller doses; excreted by kidney

Pregnancy manufacturer advises use only if potential benefit outweighs risk (toxicity in *animal* studies)

Breast-feeding amount too small to be harmful

Musculoskeletal and joint diseases — **10**

◻ **BACLOFEN** (*continued*)

Side-effects gastro-intestinal disturbances, dry mouth; hypotension, respiratory or cardiovascular depression; sedation, drowsiness, confusion, dizziness, ataxia, hallucinations, nightmares, headache, euphoria, insomnia, depression, anxiety, agitation, tremor; seizure; urinary disturbances; myalgia; nystagmus; visual disorders; rash, hyperhidrosis; *rarely* taste disturbances, abdominal pain, paraesthesia, erectile dysfunction, dysarthria; *very rarely* hypothermia

Indication and dose

Chronic severe spasticity of voluntary muscle
* **By mouth**

Child 1–10 years 0.75–2 mg/kg daily *or* 2.5 mg 4 times daily increased gradually according to age to maintenance: Child 1–2 years 10–20 mg daily in divided doses, Child 2–6 years 20–30 mg daily in divided doses, Child 6–10 years 30–60 mg daily in divided doses

Child 10–18 years 5 mg 3 times daily increased gradually; max. 2.5 mg/kg *or* 100 mg daily

Severe chronic spasticity of cerebral origin unresponsive to oral antispastic drugs (or oral therapy not tolerated), as alternative to ablative neurosurgical procedures—specialist use only
* **By intrathecal injection**

Child 4–18 years initial *test dose* 25 micrograms over at least 1 minute via catheter or lumbar puncture, increased in 25-microgram steps (not more often than every 24 hours) to max. 100 micrograms to determine appropriate dose *then dose-titration phase*, most often using infu-sion pump (implanted into chest wall or abdominal wall tissues) to establish *maintenance dose* (ranging from 24 micrograms to 1.2 mg daily in children under 12 years or 1.4 mg daily for those over 12 years) retaining some spasticity to avoid sensation of paralysis

---

Safe Practice Consult product literature for details on dose testing and titration—important to monitor patients closely in appropriately equipped and staffed environment during screening and immediately after pump implantation. Resuscitation equipment must be available for immediate use

---

Baclofen (Non-proprietary) ⒫ₒₘ
Tablets, baclofen 10 mg, net price 84-tab pack = £1.65. Label: 2, 8

Oral solution, baclofen 5 mg/5 mL, net price 300 mL = £8.95. Label: 2, 8
Brands include *Lyflex*® (sugar-free)

Lioresal® (Novartis) ⒫ₒₘ
Tablets, scored, baclofen 10 mg, net price 84-tab pack = £10.84. Label: 2, 8
Excipients include gluten

Liquid, sugar-free, raspberry-flavoured, baclofen 5 mg/5 mL, net price 300 mL = £8.95. Label: 2, 8

◢**By intrathecal injection**
Lioresal® (Novartis) ⒫ₒₘ
Intrathecal injection, baclofen, 50 micrograms/mL, net price 1-mL amp (for test dose) = £2.74; 500 micrograms/mL, 20-mL amp (for use with implantable pump) = £60.77; 2 mg/mL, 5-mL amp (for use with implantable pump) = £60.77

▊ DANTROLENE SODIUM

Cautions impaired cardiac and pulmonary function; therapeutic effect may take a few weeks to develop—discontinue if no response within 45 days; **interactions**: Appendix 1 (muscle relaxants)

Hepatotoxicity Potentially life-threatening hepatotoxicity reported, usually if doses greater than 400 mg daily used, in females, if history of liver disorders, or concomitant use of hepatotoxic drugs; test liver function before and at intervals during therapy—discontinue if abnormal liver function tests or symptoms of liver disorder (counselling, see below); re-introduce only if complete reversal of hepatotoxicity

Counselling Children and their carers should be told how to recognise signs of liver disorder and advised to seek prompt medical attention if symptoms such as anorexia, nausea, vomiting, fatigue, abdominal pain, dark urine, or pruritus develop

Skilled tasks Drowsiness may affect performance of skilled tasks (eg. driving); effects of alcohol enhanced

Breast-feeding present in milk—manufacturer advises avoid

Contra-indications hepatic impairment (may cause severe liver damage); acute muscle spasm; avoid when spasticity is useful, for example, locomotion

Pregnancy avoid use in chronic spasticity—embryotoxic in *animal* studies

Side-effects diarrhoea (withdraw if severe, discontinue treatment if recurs on re-introduction), nausea, vomiting, anorexia, hepatotoxicity (see above), abdominal pain; pericarditis; pleural effusion, respiratory depression; headache, drowsiness, dizziness, asthenia, fatigue, seizures, fever, chills; speech and visual disturbances; rash; *less commonly* dysphagia, constipation, exacerbation of cardiac insufficiency, tachycardia, erratic blood pressure, dyspnoea, depression, confusion, nervousness, insomnia, increased urinary frequency, urinary incontinence or retention, haematuria, crystalluria, and increased sweating

Licensed use not licensed for use in children

Indication and dose

Chronic severe spasticity of voluntary muscle
* **By mouth**

Child 5–12 years initially 500 micrograms/kg once daily; after 7 days increase to 500 micrograms/kg/dose 3 times daily; every 7 days increase by further 500 micrograms/kg/dose until satisfactory response; max. 2 mg/kg 3–4 times daily (max. total daily dose 400 mg)

Child 12–18 years initially 25 mg once daily; increase to 3 times daily after 7 days; every 7 days increase by further 500 micrograms/kg/dose until satisfactory response; max. 2 mg/kg 3–4 times daily (max. total daily dose 400 mg)

10

Musculoskeletal and joint diseases

◁ **DANTROLENE SODIUM** (*continued*)

Malignant hyperthermia section 15.1.8

Dantrium® (Procter & Gamble Pharm.) [PoM]
Capsules, orange/brown, dantrolene sodium
25 mg, net price 20 = £2.46; 100 mg, 20 = £8.61.
Label: 2, counselling, driving, hepatotoxicity

◢ DIAZEPAM

Cautions see section 4.8.2

Contra-indications see section 4.8.2

Side-effects see section 4.8.2; also hypotonia

Indication and dose

Muscle spasm in cerebral spasticity or in
postoperative skeletal muscle spasm
• By mouth

Child 1–12 months initially 250 microgram/kg
twice daily

Child 1–5 years initially 2.5 mg twice daily

Child 5–12 years initially 5 mg twice daily

Child 12–18 years initially 10 mg twice daily;
max. total daily dose 40 mg

Tetanus
• By intravenous injection

Child 1 month–18 years 100–300 micrograms/
kg repeated every 1–4 hours

• By intravenous infusion (or by nasoduodenal
tube)

Child 1 month–18 years 3–10 mg/kg over 24
hours, adjusted according to response

Status epilepticus section 4.8.2

Febrile convulsions section 4.8.3

Peri-operative use section 15.1.4.1

Administration for *continuous intravenous infusion*
of diazepam emulsion, dilute to a concentration
of max. 400 micrograms/mL with Glucose 5% or
10%; max. 6 hours between addition and completion of infusion; diazepam adsorbed by plastics of infusion bags and giving sets
For *continuous intravenous infusion* of diazepam
solution, dilute to a concentration of max.
50 micrograms/mL with Glucose 5% or Sodium
Chloride 0.9%; diazepam adsorbed by plastics of
infusion bags and giving sets

◢Oral preparations
Section 15.1.4.1

◢Parenteral preparations
Section 4.8.2

10.3 Drugs for the relief of soft-tissue inflammation

10.3.1 Enzymes
10.3.2 Rubefacients and other topical antirheumatics

Extravasation

Local guidelines for the management of extravasation should be followed
where they exist or specialist advice sought.

Extravasation injury follows leakage of drugs or intravenous fluids from the veins
or inadvertent administration into the subcutaneous or subdermal tissue. It must
be dealt with **promptly** to prevent tissue necrosis.

Acidic or alkaline preparations and those with an osmolarity greater than that of
plasma can cause extravasation injury; excipients including alcohol and polyethylene glycol have also been implicated. Cytotoxic drugs commonly cause
extravasation injury. Very young children are at increased risk. Those receiving
anticoagulants are more likely to lose blood into surrounding tissues if extravasation occurs, while those receiving sedatives or analgesics may not notice the early
signs or symptoms of extravasation.

Prevention of extravasation Precautions should be taken to avoid extravasation; ideally, drugs likely to cause extravasation injury should be given through a
central line and children receiving repeated doses of hazardous drugs peripherally
should have the cannula resited at regular intervals. Attention should be paid to
the manufacturers' recommendations for administration. Placing a glyceryl trinitrate patch or using glyceryl trinitrate ointment distal to the cannula may
improve the patency of the vessel in children with small veins or in those
whose veins are prone to collapse.

Children or their carers should be asked to report any pain or burning at the site of injection immediately.

Management of extravasation   If extravasation is suspected the infusion should be stopped immediately but the cannula should not be removed until after an attempt has been made to aspirate the area (through the cannula) in order to remove as much of the drug as possible. Aspiration is sometimes possible if the extravasation presents with a raised bleb or blister at the injection site and is surrounded by hardened tissue, but it is often unsuccessful if the tissue is soft or soggy. **Corticosteroids** are usually given to treat inflammation, although there is little evidence to support their use in extravasation. Hydrocortisone or dexamethasone (section 6.3.2) can be given either locally by subcutaneous injection or intravenously at a site distant from the injury. **Antihistamines** (section 3.4.1) and **analgesics** (section 4.7) may be required for symptom relief.

The management of extravasation beyond these measures is not well standardised and calls for specialist advice. Treatment depends on the nature of the offending substance; one approach is to localise and neutralise the substance whereas another is to spread and dilute it. The first method may be appropriate following extravasation of vesicant drugs and involves administration of an antidote (if available) and the application of cold compresses 3–4 times a day (consult specialist literature for details of specific antidotes). Spreading and diluting the offending substance involves infiltrating the area with physiological saline, applying warm compresses, elevating the affected limb, and administering hyaluronidase (section 10.3.1). A saline flush-out technique (involving flushing the subcutaneous tissue with physiological saline) may be effective but requires specialist advice. Hyaluronidase should **not** be administered following extravasation of vesicant drugs (unless it is either specifically indicated or used in the saline flush-out technique).

10.3.1 Enzymes

Hyaluronidase is used for the management of extravasation For preparations, see *BNF section 10.3.1.*

10.3.2 Rubefacients and other topical antirheumatics

Classification not used in *BNF for Children.*

10

Musculoskeletal and joint diseases

11 Eye

11.1 Administration of drugs to the eye **620**

11.2 Control of microbial contamination **621**

11.3 Anti-infective eye preparations **621**
11.3.1 Antibacterials 622
11.3.2 Antifungals 624
11.3.3 Antivirals 625

11.4 Corticosteroids and other anti-inflammatory preparations **625**
11.4.1 Corticosteroids 625
11.4.2 Other anti-inflammatory preparations 627

11.5 Mydriatics and cycloplegics **629**

11.6 Treatment of glaucoma **630**

11.7 Local anaesthetics **635**

11.8 Miscellaneous ophthalmic preparations **636**
11.8.1 Tear deficiency, ocular lubricants, and astringents 636
11.8.2 Ocular diagnostic and peri-operative preparations 639

11.9 Contact lenses **640**

11.1   Administration of drugs to the eye

Drugs are most commonly administered to the eye by topical application as eye drops or eye ointments. Where a higher drug concentration is required within the eye, a local injection may be necessary.

Eye-drop dispenser devices are available to aid the instillation of eye drops from plastic bottles especially by the visually impaired or otherwise physically limited patients; they may be useful in children in whom normal application is difficult.

Eye drops and eye ointments   Eye drops are generally instilled into the pocket formed by gently pulling down the lower eyelid and keeping the eye closed for as long as possible after application; in neonates and infants it may be more appropriate to administer the drop in the inner angle of the open eye. One drop is all that is needed. A small amount of eye ointment is applied similarly; the ointment melts rapidly and blinking helps to spread it.

When two different eye-drop preparations are used at the same time of day, dilution and overflow may occur when one immediately follows the other. The carer or child should therefore leave an interval of at least 5 minutes between the two. Eye ointment should be applied after drops. Both drops and ointment may cause transient blurred vision.

Systemic effects may arise from absorption of drugs into the general circulation from conjunctival vessels or from the nasal mucosa after the excess preparation has drained down through the tear ducts. The extent of systemic absorption following ocular administration is highly variable; nasal drainage of drugs is associated with eye drops much more often than with eye ointments. Pressure on the lacrimal punctum for at least a minute after applying eye drops reduces nasolacrimal drainage and therefore decreases systemic absorption from the nasal mucosa.

For warnings relating to eye drops and contact lenses, see section 11.9.

Eye lotions   These are solutions for the irrigation of the conjunctival sac. They act mechanically to flush out irritants or foreign bodies as a first-aid treatment. Sterile sodium chloride 0.9% solution (section 11.8.1) is usually used. Clean water will suffice in an emergency.

Other preparations   Subconjunctival injection may be used to administer anti-infective drugs, mydriatics, or corticosteroids for conditions not responding to topical therapy. The drug diffuses through the cornea and sclera to the anterior and posterior chambers and vitreous humour. However, because the dose-volume is limited, this route is suitable only for drugs which are readily soluble.

Drugs such as antimicrobials and corticosteroids may be administered systemically to treat an eye condition.

Preservatives and sensitisers   Information on preservatives and on substances identified as skin sensitisers (section 13.1.3) is provided under preparation entries.

11.2 Control of microbial contamination

Preparations for the eye should be sterile when issued. Eye drops in multiple-application containers include a preservative but care should nevertheless be taken to avoid contamination of the contents during use.

Eye drops in multiple-application containers for *home use* should not be used for more than 4 weeks after first opening (unless otherwise stated).

Eye drops for use in *hospital wards* are normally discarded 1 week after first opening (24 hours if preservative-free). Individual containers should be provided for each child, and for each eye if there are special concerns about contamination. Containers used before an operation should be discarded at the time of the operation and fresh containers supplied. A fresh supply should also be provided upon discharge from hospital; in specialist ophthalmology units it may be acceptable to issue eye-drop bottles that have been dispensed to the patient on the day of discharge.

In *out-patient departments* single-application packs should preferably be used; if multiple-application packs are used, they should be discarded at the end of each day. In clinics for eye diseases and in accident and emergency departments, where the dangers of infection are high, single-application packs should be used; if a multiple-application pack is used, it should be discarded after single use.

Diagnostic dyes (section 11.8.2) should be used only from single-application packs.

In *eye surgery* single-application containers should be used if possible; if a multiple-application pack is used, it should be discarded after single use. Preparations used during intra-ocular procedures and others that may penetrate into the anterior chamber must be isotonic and without preservatives and buffered if necessary to a neutral pH. Specially formulated fluids should be used for intra-ocular surgery; large volume intravenous infusion preparations are not suitable for this purpose. For all surgical procedures, a previously unopened container is used for each patient.

11.3 Anti-infective eye preparations

11.3.1 Antibacterials
11.3.2 Antifungals
11.3.3 Antivirals

Eye infections   Most acute superficial eye infections can be treated topically. Blepharitis and conjunctivitis are often caused by staphylococci; keratitis and endophthalmitis may be bacterial, viral, or fungal.

Bacterial *blepharitis* is treated by lid hygiene and application of antibacterial eye drops to the conjunctival sac or to the lid margins. Systemic treatment may be required and may be necessary for 3 months or longer.

Most cases of acute bacterial conjunctivitis are self-limiting; where treatment is appropriate, antibacterial eye drops or an eye ointment are used. A poor response might indicate viral or allergic conjunctivitis or antibiotic resistance.

Corneal ulcer and *keratitis* require specialist treatment, usually under inpatient care, and may call for intensive topical, subconjunctival, or systemic administration of antimicrobials.

Endophthalmitis is a medical emergency which also calls for specialist management and often requires parenteral, subconjunctival, or intra-ocular administration of antimicrobials.

For reference to the treatment of *crab lice of the eyelashes*, see section 13.10.4

11.3.1 Antibacterials

Bacterial infections are generally treated topically with eye drops and eye ointments; systemic treatment is sometimes appropriate in blepharitis.

Chloramphenicol has a broad spectrum of activity and is the drug of choice for *superficial eye infections*. Chloramphenicol eye drops are well tolerated and the recommendation that chloramphenicol eye drops should be avoided because of an increased risk of aplastic anaemia is not well founded.

Other antibacterials with a broad spectrum of activity include the quinolones, **ciprofloxacin**, **levofloxacin**, and **ofloxacin**; the aminoglycosides, **gentamicin** and **neomycin** are also active against a wide variety of bacteria. Gentamicin, quinolones, and **polymyxin B** are effective for infections caused by *Pseudomonas aeruginosa*.

Ciprofloxacin eye drops are licensed for *corneal ulcers*; intensive application (especially in the first 2 days) is required throughout the day and night.

Trachoma, which results from chronic infection with *Chlamydia trachomatis*, can be treated with **azithromycin** by mouth [unlicensed indication].

Fusidic acid is useful for staphylococcal infections.

Propamidine isetionate is of little value in bacterial infections but is specific for the rare but potentially devastating condition of *acanthamoeba keratitis* (see also section 11.9).

Other antibacterial eye drops may be prepared aseptically in a specialist manufacturing unit from material supplied for injection, see section 11.8.

Neonates   Antibacterial eye drops are used to treat acute bacterial conjunctivitis in neonates (ophthalmia neonatorum); where possible the causative micro-organism should be identified. **Chloramphenicol** or **neomycin** eye drops are used to treat mild conjunctivitis; more serious infections also require a systemic antibacterial. Failure to respond to initial treatment requires further investigation; chlamydial infection is one of the most frequent causes of neonatal conjunctivitis and should be considered.

Gonococcal eye infections are treated with a single-dose of **ceftriaxone**. *Chlamydial eye infections* should be managed with oral **erythromycin**. **Gentamicin** eye drops together with appropriate systemic antibacterials are used in the treatment of *pseudomonal eye infections*; high-strength gentamicin eye drops (1.5%) [unlicensed] are available for severe infections.

With corticosteroids   Many antibacterial preparations also incorporate a corticosteroid but such mixtures should **not** be used unless a patient is under close specialist supervision. In particular they should not be prescribed for undiagnosed 'red eye' which is sometimes caused by the herpes simplex virus and may be difficult to diagnose (section 11.4).

Administration   Frequency of application depends on the severity of the infection and the potential for irreversible ocular damage; antibacterial eye preparations are usually administered as follows.

Eye drops. Apply 1 drop at least every 2 hours in severe infection then reduce frequency as infection is controlled and continue for 48 hours after healing. For less severe infection 3–4 times daily is generally sufficient.

Eye ointment. Apply *either* at night (if eye drops used during the day) *or* 3–4 times daily (if eye ointment used alone).

CHLORAMPHENICOL

Side-effects transient stinging; see also notes above

Indication and dose

See notes above

[1]**Chloramphenicol** (Non-proprietary) [PoM]

Eye drops, chloramphenicol 0.5%. Net price 10 mL = £1.39

Eye ointment, chloramphenicol 1%. Net price 4 g = £1.63

1. Chloramphenicol 0.5% eye drops can be sold to the public (in max. pack size 10 mL) for treatment of acute bacterial conjunctivitis in adults and children over 2 years; max. duration of treatment 5 days

Chloromycetin® (Goldshield) [PoM]

Redidrops (= eye drops), chloramphenicol 0.5%. Net price 5 mL = £1.65; 10 mL = £1.85
Excipients include phenylmercuric acetate

Ophthalmic ointment (= eye ointment), chloramphenicol 1%. Net price 4 g = £1.85

◀Single use

Minims® Chloramphenicol (Chauvin) [PoM]

Eye drops, chloramphenicol 0.5%. Net price 20 × 0.5 mL = £4.92

CIPROFLOXACIN

Cautions not recommended for children under 1 year

Pregnancy Manufacturer advises caution

Breast-feeding Manufacturer advises caution but unlikely to appear in milk

Side-effects local burning and itching; lid margin crusting; hyperaemia; taste disturbances; corneal staining, keratitis, lid oedema, lacrimation, photophobia, corneal infiltrates; nausea and visual disturbances reported

Licensed use not licensed for use in children under 1 year

Indication and dose

Superficial bacterial infections

See notes above

Corneal ulcer

Apply eye drops throughout day and night, day 1 apply every 15 minutes for 6 hours then every 30 minutes, day 2 apply every hour, days 3–14 apply every 4 hours (max. duration of treatment 21 days)

Apply eye ointment throughout day and night; apply 1.25 cm ointment every 1–2 hours for 2 days then every 4 hours for next 12 days

Ciloxan® (Alcon) [PoM]

Ophthalmic solution (= eye drops), ciprofloxacin (as hydrochloride) 0.3%. Net price 5 mL = £4.94
Excipients include benzalkonium chloride

Eye ointment, ciprofloxacin (as hydrochloride) 0.3%. Net price 3.5 g = £5.49

FUSIDIC ACID

Indication and dose

See under preparation below

Fucithalmic® (LEO) [PoM]

Eye drops, m/r, fusidic acid 1% in gel basis (liquifies on contact with eye). Net price 5 g = £2.09
Excipients include benzalkonium chloride, disodium edetate

Dose

Apply twice daily

GENTAMICIN

Indication and dose

See notes above

Genticin® (Roche) [PoM]

Drops (for ear or eye), gentamicin 0.3% (as sulphate). Net price 10 mL = £1.78
Excipients include benzalkonium chloride

Gentamicin (Non-proprietary) [PoM]

Eye drops, gentamicin 1.5%, 10 mL, available as a manufactured special from Moorfields Eye Hospital, see also 'special-order' manufacturers or specialist importing companies, p. 943

LEVOFLOXACIN

Contra-indications

Pregnancy manufacturer advises avoid—systemic quinolones have caused arthropathy in *animal* studies

Breast-feeding manufacturer advises avoid

Side-effects transient ocular irritation, visual disturbances, lid margin crusting, lid or conjunctival oedema, hyperaemia, conjunctival follicles, photophobia, headache, rhinitis

Licensed use not licensed for use in children under 1 year

Indication and dose

See notes above

Oftaquix® (Kestrel Ophthalmics) ▼ [PoM]

Eye drops, levofloxacin 0.5%, net price 5 mL = £6.95

11

Eye

◾ NEOMYCIN SULPHATE

Licensed use *Neosporin*® not licensed for use in children under 2 years

Indication and dose

See notes above and under preparations below

Neomycin (Non-proprietary) [PoM]
Eye drops, neomycin sulphate 0.5% (3500 units/mL). Net price 10 mL = £3.11
Available from 'special-order' manufacturers or specialist importing companies, see p. 943

Eye ointment, neomycin sulphate 0.5% (3500 units/g). Net price 3 g = £2.44
Available from 'special-order' manufacturers or specialist importing companies, see p. 943

◢With other antibacterials

Neosporin® (PLIVA) [PoM]
Eye drops, gramicidin 25 units, neomycin sulphate 1700 units, polymyxin B sulphate 5000 units/mL. Net price 5 mL = £4.86
Excipients include thiomersal

Dose

Apply 2–4 times daily or more frequently if required

◢With hydrocortisone
Section 12.1.1

◾ OFLOXACIN

Cautions not to be used for more than 10 days

Pregnancy manufacturer advises use only if benefit outweighs risk; systemic quinolones have caused arthropathy in animal studies

Breast-feeding manufacturer advises avoid

Side-effects local irritation including photophobia; dizziness, numbness, nausea and headache reported

Licensed use not licensed for use in neonates

Indication and dose

Local treatment of infections (but see notes above)

Apply every two to four hours for the first two days then reduce frequency to four times daily (max. 10 days treatment)

Exocin® (Allergan) [PoM]
Ophthalmic solution (= eye drops), ofloxacin 0.3%. Net price 5 mL = £2.17
Excipients include benzalkonium chloride

◾ POLYMYXIN B SULPHATE

Indication and dose

See notes above

◢With other antibacterials

Polyfax® (PLIVA) [PoM]
Eye ointment, polymyxin B sulphate 10 000 units, bacitracin zinc 500 units/g. Net price 4 g = £3.26

Polytrim® (PLIVA) [PoM]
Eye drops, trimethoprim 0.1%, polymyxin B sulphate 10 000 units/mL. Net price 5 mL = £3.05
Excipients include benzalkonium chloride

Eye ointment, trimethoprim 0.5%, polymyxin B sulphate 10 000 units/g. Net price 4 g = £2.90

◾ PROPAMIDINE ISETIONATE

Indication and dose

See under preparations below

Brolene® (Aventis Pharma)
Eye drops, propamidine isetionate 0.1%. Net price 10 mL = £2.80
Excipients include benzalkonium chloride

Dose

Local treatment of infections (but see notes above)
apply 4 times daily

Note Eye drops containing propamidine isetionate 0.1% also available from Typharm (*Golden Eye Drops*)

Eye ointment, dibromopropamidine isetionate 0.15%. Net price 5 g = £2.92

Dose

Local treatment of infections (but see notes above)
Apply 1–2 times daily

Note Eye ointment containing dibromopropamidine isetionate 0.15% also available from Typharm (*Golden Eye Ointment*)

▰ 11.3.2 Antifungals

Fungal infections of the cornea are rare. Orbital mycosis is rarer, and when it occurs it is usually because of a direct spread of infection from the paranasal sinuses. Debility or immunosuppression may encourage fungal proliferation. The spread of infection through blood occasionally produces a metastatic endophthalmitis.

Many different fungi are capable of producing ocular infection; they may be identified by appropriate laboratory procedures.

Antifungal preparations for the eye are not generally available. Treatment is normally carried out at specialist centres, but requests for information about supplies of preparations not available commercially should be addressed to the Strategic Health Authority (or equivalent in Scotland or Northern Ireland), or to the nearest hospital ophthalmology unit, see also 'special-order' manufacturers or specialist importing companies, p. 943.

11.3.3 Antivirals

Herpes simplex infections producing, for example, dendritic corneal ulcer can be treated with **aciclovir**.

For systemic treatment of CMV retinitis, see section 5.3.

ACICLOVIR
(Acyclovir)

Side-effects local irritation and inflammation, superficial punctate keratopathy; *rarely* blepharitis; *very rarely* hypersensitivity reactions including angioedema

Indication and dose

Local treatment of herpes simplex infections
Apply 5 times daily (continue for at least 3 days after complete healing)

Zovirax® (GSK) ℗ₒₘ [PoM]
Eye ointment, aciclovir 3%. Net price 4.5 g = £9.92
Tablets, see section 5.3.2.1
Injection, see section 5.3.2.1
Cream, see section 13.10.3

11.4 Corticosteroids and other anti-inflammatory preparations

11.4.1 Corticosteroids
11.4.2 Other anti-inflammatory preparations

11.4.1 Corticosteroids

Corticosteroids administered locally to the eye or given by mouth are effective for treating anterior segment inflammation in uveitis (section 11.5) and following surgery.

Topical corticosteroids should normally only be used under expert supervision; three main dangers are associated with their use:

- a 'red eye', where the diagnosis is unconfirmed, may be due to herpes simplex virus, and a corticosteroid may aggravate the condition, leading to corneal ulceration, with possible damage to vision and even loss of the eye. Bacterial, fungal and amoebic infections pose a similar hazard;

- 'steroid glaucoma' may follow the use of corticosteroid eye preparations in susceptible individuals;

- a 'steroid cataract' may follow prolonged use.

Other side-effects of ocular corticosteroids include thinning of the cornea and sclera. Prolonged use in neonates and infants can cause adrenal suppression.

Products combining a corticosteroid with an antimicrobial are used after ocular surgery to reduce inflammation and prevent infection: use of combination products is otherwise rarely justified.

Systemic corticosteroids (section 6.3.2) may be useful for ocular conditions. The risk of producing a 'steroid cataract' increases with the dose and duration of corticosteroid use.

▌ BETAMETHASONE

Cautions see notes above

Side-effects see notes above

Indication and dose

Local treatment of inflammation (short-term)

Apply eye drops every 1–2 hours until controlled then reduce frequency; eye ointment 2–4 times daily or at night when used with eye drops

Betnesol® (UCB Pharma) ℗ℴ𝕄
Drops (for ear, eye, or nose), betamethasone sodium phosphate 0.1%. Net price 10 mL = £2.32
Excipients include benzalkonium chloride, disodium edetate

Eye ointment, betamethasone sodium phosphate 0.1%. Net price 3 g = £1.41

Vistamethasone® (Martindale) ℗ℴ𝕄
Drops (for ear, eye, or nose), betamethasone sodium phosphate 0.1%. Net price 5 mL = £1.02; 10 mL = £1.16
Excipients include benzalkonium chloride

◢With neomycin
Betnesol-N® (UCB Pharma) ℗ℴ𝕄 ◢
Drops (for ear, eye, or nose), see section 12.1.1

Eye ointment, betamethasone sodium phosphate 0.1%, neomycin sulphate 0.5%. Net price 3 g = £1.28
Note May be difficult to obtain

Vistamethasone N® (Martindale) ℗ℴ𝕄 ◢
Drops (for ear, eye, or nose), see section 12.1.1

▌ DEXAMETHASONE

Cautions see notes above

Side-effects see notes above

Indication and dose

Local treatment of inflammation (short-term)

Apply eye drops 4–6 times daily; severe conditions every 30–60 minutes until controlled then reduce frequency

Maxidex® (Alcon) ℗ℴ𝕄
Eye drops, dexamethasone 0.1%, hypromellose 0.5%. Net price 5 mL = £1.49; 10 mL = £2.95
Excipients include benzalkonium chloride, disodium edetate, polysorbate 80

◢Single use
Minims® Dexamethasone (Chauvin) ℗ℴ𝕄
Eye drops, dexamethasone sodium phosphate 0.1%. Net price 20 × 0.5 mL = £6.95
Excipients include disodium edetate

◢With antibacterials
Maxitrol® (Alcon) ℗ℴ𝕄 ◢
Eye drops, dexamethasone 0.1%, hypromellose 0.5%, neomycin 0.35% (as sulphate), polymyxin B sulphate 6000 units/mL. Net price 5 mL = £1.77
Excipients include benzalkonium chloride, polysorbate 20

Eye ointment, dexamethasone 0.1%, neomycin 0.35% (as sulphate), polymyxin B sulphate 6000 units/g. Net price 3.5 g = £1.52
Excipients include hydroxybenzoates (parabens), wool fat

Sofradex® (Sanofi-Aventis) ℗ℴ𝕄 ◢
Drops (for ear or eye), see section 12.1.1

▌ FLUOROMETHOLONE

Cautions see notes above

Side-effects see notes above

Licensed use not licensed for use in children under 2 years

Indication and dose

Local treatment of inflammation (short-term)

Apply 2–4 times daily (initially every hour for 24–48 hours then reduce frequency)

FML® (Allergan) ℗ℴ𝕄
Ophthalmic suspension (= eye drops), fluorometholone 0.1%, polyvinyl alcohol (*Liquifilm®*) 1.4%. Net price 5 mL = £1.71; 10 mL = £2.95
Excipients include benzalkonium chloride, disodium edetate, polysorbate 80

▌ HYDROCORTISONE ACETATE

Cautions see notes above

Side-effects see notes above

Indication and dose

Local treatment of inflammation (short-term)

Apply eye drops 4 times daily; apply eye ointment twice daily or at night

Hydrocortisone (Non-proprietary) ℗ℴ𝕄
Eye drops, hydrocortisone acetate 1%. Net price 10 mL = £3.21

Eye ointment, hydrocortisone acetate 0.5%, net price 3 g = £2.40; 1%, 3 g = £2.42; 2.5%, 3 g = £6.55

▌ PREDNISOLONE

Cautions see notes above

Side-effects see notes above

Indication and dose

Local treatment of inflammation (short-term)

Apply every 1–2 hours until controlled then reduce frequency

11 Eye

⌐ **PREDNISOLONE** *(continued)*

Pred Forte® (Allergan) PoM
Eye drops, prednisolone acetate 1%. Net price 5 mL
= £1.52; 10 mL = £3.05
Excipients include benzalkonium chloride, disodium edetate,
polysorbate 80

Predsol® (UCB Pharma) PoM
Drops (for ear or eye), prednisolone sodium phos-
phate 0.5%. Net price 10 mL = £2.00
Excipients include benzalkonium chloride, disodium edetate

◀Single use
Minims® Prednisolone Sodium Phosphate (Chau-
vin) PoM
Eye drops, prednisolone sodium phosphate 0.5%.
Net price 20 × 0.5 mL = £5.75
Excipients include disodium edetate

◀With neomycin
Predsol-N® (UCB Pharma) PoM ◣
Drops (for ear or eye), see section 12.1.1

11.4.2 Other anti-inflammatory preparations

Topical preparations of **antihistamines** such as eye drops containing **antazoline**
(with xylometazoline as *Otrivine-Antistin®*), **azelastine**, **epinastine**, **ketotifen**, and
olopatadine may be used for allergic conjunctivitis.

Sodium cromoglicate and **nedocromil sodium** eye drops may be useful for
vernal keratoconjunctivitis and other allergic forms of conjunctivitis.

Lodoxamide eye drops are used for allergic conjunctival conditions including
seasonal allergic conjunctivitis.

Emedastine eye drops are licensed for seasonal allergic conjunctivitis.

▲ ANTAZOLINE SULPHATE

Indication and dose
Allergic conjunctivitis
See preparation below

Otrivine-Antistin® (Novartis Consumer Health)
Eye drops, antazoline sulphate 0.5%, xylomet-
azoline hydrochloride 0.05%. Net price 10 mL =
£2.35
Excipients include benzalkonium chloride, disodium edetate
Dose
> Child 5–18 years apply 2–3 times daily

Note Xylometazoline is a sympathomimetic; it should be
avoided in angle-closure glaucoma; absorption of antazoline and xylometazoline may result in systemic side-
effects and the possibility of interaction with other drugs,
see Appendix 1 (antihistamines and sympathomimetics)

▲ AZELASTINE HYDROCHLORIDE

Side-effects mild transient irritation; bitter taste
reported

Indication and dose
Allergic conjunctivitis, seasonal allergic conjunctivitis
> Child 4–18 years apply twice daily, increased if
> necessary to 4 times daily

Perennial conjunctivitis
> Child 12–18 years apply twice daily, increased if
> necessary to 4 times daily; max. duration of
> treatment 6 weeks

Optilast® (Viatris) PoM
Eye drops, azelastine hydrochloride 0.05%. Net
price 8 mL = £6.40
Excipients include benzalkonium chloride, disodium edetate
Note Azelastine 0.05% eye drops can be sold to the public
(in max. pack size of 6 mL) for treatment of seasonal and
perennial allergic conjunctivitis in children over 12 years

▲ EMEDASTINE

Side-effects transient burning or stinging; blurred
vision, local oedema, keratitis, irritation, dry eye,
lacrimation, corneal infiltrates (discontinue) and
staining; photophobia; headache, and rhinitis
occasionally reported

Indication and dose
Seasonal allergic conjunctivitis
> Child 3–18 years apply twice daily

Emadine® (Alcon) PoM
Eye drops, emedastine 0.05% (as difumarate), net
price 5 mL = £7.69
Excipients include benzalkonium chloride

11
Eye

EPINASTINE HYDROCHLORIDE

Side-effects burning; *less commonly* dry mouth, taste disturbance; nasal irritation, rhinitis; headache, blepharoptosis, conjunctival oedema and hyperaemia, dry eye, local irritation, photophobia, visual disturbance; pruritus

Indication and dose

Seasonal allergic conjunctivitis

Child 12–18 years apply twice daily; max. duration of treatment 8 weeks

Relestat® (Allergan) PoM
Eye drops, epinastine hydrochloride 500 micrograms/mL, net price 5 mL = £9.90
Excipients include benzalkonium chloride, disodium edetate

KETOTIFEN

Side-effects transient burning or stinging, punctate corneal epithelial erosion; *less commonly* dry eye, subconjunctival haemorrhage, photophobia; headache, drowsiness, skin reactions, and dry mouth also reported

Indication and dose

Seasonal allergic conjunctivitis

Child 3–18 years apply twice daily

Zaditen® (Novartis) PoM
Eye drops, ketotifen (as fumarate) 250 micrograms/mL, net price 5 mL = £9.75
Excipients include benzalkonium chloride

LODOXAMIDE

Side-effects mild transient burning, stinging, itching, and lacrimation; flushing and dizziness reported

Indication and dose

Allergic conjunctivitis

Child 4–18 years apply 4 times daily

Alomide® (Alcon) PoM
Ophthalmic solution (= eye drops), lodoxamide 0.1% (as trometamol). Net price 10 mL = £5.48
Excipients include benzalkonium chloride, disodium edetate
Note Lodoxamide 0.1% eye drops can be sold to the public for treatment of allergic conjunctivitis in children over 4 years

NEDOCROMIL SODIUM

Side-effects transient burning and stinging; distinctive taste reported

Indication and dose

Seasonal and perennial allergic conjunctivitis

Child 6–18 years apply twice daily increased if necessary to 4 times daily; max. 12 weeks treatment for seasonal allergic conjunctivitis

Vernal keratoconjunctivitis

Child 6–18 years apply 4 times daily

Rapitil® (Aventis Pharma) PoM
Eye drops, nedocromil sodium 2%. Net price 5 mL = £5.12
Excipients include benzalkonium chloride, disodium edetate

OLOPATADINE

Side-effects local irritation; less commonly keratitis, dry eye, local oedema, photophobia; headache, asthenia, dizziness; dry nose also reported

Indication and dose

Seasonal allergic conjunctivitis

Child 3–18 years apply twice daily; max. duration of treatment 4 months

Opatanol® (Alcon) PoM
Eye drops, olopatadine (as hydrochloride) 1 mg/mL, net price 5 mL = £4.11
Excipients include benzalkonium chloride

SODIUM CROMOGLICATE
(Sodium cromoglycate)

Side-effects transient burning and stinging

Indication and dose

Allergic conjunctivitis, vernal keratoconjunctivitis

apply eye drops 4 times daily

¹**Sodium Cromoglicate** (Non-proprietary) PoM
Eye drops, sodium cromoglicate 2%. Net price 13.5 mL = £2.01
Brands include *Hay-Crom® Aqueous, Opticrom® Aqueous, Vividrin®*
1. Sodium cromoglicate 2% eye drops can be sold to the public (in max. pack size of 10 mL) for treatment of acute seasonal and perennial allergic conjunctivitis

11.5 Mydriatics and cycloplegics

Antimuscarinics dilate the pupil and paralyse the ciliary muscle; they vary in potency and duration of action.

Short-acting, relatively weak mydriatics, such as **tropicamide** 0.5% (action lasts for 4–6 hours), facilitate the examination of the fundus of the eye. **Cyclopentolate** 1% (action up to 24 hours) or **atropine** (action up to 7 days) are preferable for producing cycloplegia for refraction in young children; tropicamide may be preferred in neonates. Atropine ointment 1% is sometimes preferred for children under 5 years because systemic absorption from the ointment is reduced. **Phenyl-ephrine** 2.5% is used for mydriasis in diagnostic or therapeutic procedures; mydriasis occurs within 60–90 minutes and lasts up to 5–7 hours. Phenylephrine 10% drops are contra-indicated in children owing to the risk of systemic effects.

Mydriatics and cycloplegics are used in the treatment of anterior uveitis, usually as an adjunct to corticosteriods (section 11.4.1). Atropine is used in anterior uveitis mainly to prevent posterior synechiae and to relieve ciliary spasm, often in combination with phenylephrine eye drops; cyclopentolate or **homatropine** (action up to 3 days) can also be used and may be preferred because they have a shorter duration of action.

Cautions and contra-indications   Darkly pigmented irides are more resistant to pupillary dilatation and caution should be exercised to avoid overdosage. Mydriasis can precipitate acute angle-closure glaucoma in the very few children who are predisposed to the condition because of a shallow anterior chamber. Atropine, cyclopentolate, and homatropine should be used with caution in children under 3 months owing to the possible association between cycloplegia and the development of amblyopia; also, neonates are at increased risk of systemic toxicity.
Skilled tasks Children may not be able to undertake skilled tasks for 1–2 hours after mydriasis.

Side-effects   Ocular side-effects of mydriatics and cycloplegics include transient stinging and raised intra-ocular pressure; on prolonged administration, local irritation, hyperaemia, oedema, and conjunctivitis can occur. Contact dermatitis can occur with the antimuscarinic mydriatic drugs, especially atropine.

Toxic systemic reactions to atropine and cyclopentolate can occur in neonates and children; see section 1.2 for systemic side-effects of antimuscarinic drugs.

Antimuscarinics

◢ ATROPINE SULPHATE

Cautions risk of systemic effects with eye drops in infants under 3 months—eye ointment preferred; see also notes above

Side-effects see notes above

Licensed use not licensed for use in children for uveitis

Indication and dose

Cyclopegia

   Child 3 months–18 years apply drops or ointment twice daily for 3 days before procedure

Anterior uveitis

   Child 2–18 years 1 drop up to 4 times daily

Atropine (Non-proprietary) PoM
Eye drops, atropine sulphate 0.5%, net price 10 mL = £2.32; 1%, 10 mL = 98p

Eye ointment, atropine sulphate 1%. Net price 3 g = £2.97

Isopto Atropine® (Alcon) PoM
Eye drops, atropine sulphate 1%, hypromellose 0.5%. Net price 5 mL = 99p
Excipients include benzalkonium chloride

◢Single use
Minims® Atropine Sulphate (Chauvin) PoM
Eye drops, atropine sulphate 1%. Net price 20 × 0.5 mL = £4.92

◢ CYCLOPENTOLATE HYDROCHLORIDE

Cautions see notes above

Side-effects see notes above

Indication and dose

   See notes above

Cyclopegia

   Child 3 months–12 years 1 drop of 1% eye drops 30–60 minutes before examination

   Child 12–18 years 1 drop of 0.5% eye drops 30–60 minutes before examination

11
Eye

◁ **CYCLOPENTOLATE HYDROCHLORIDE** (*continued*)

Uveitis

> **Child 3 months–18 years** 1 drop of 0.5% eye
> drops (1% for deeply pigmented eyes) 2–4 times
> daily

Mydrilate® (Intrapharm) [PoM]
> Eye drops, cyclopentolate hydrochloride 0.5%, net
> price 5 mL = 97p; 1%, 5 mL = £1.19
> **Excipients** include benzalkonium chloride

◀**Single use**
Minims® Cyclopentolate Hydrochloride (Chauvin)
[PoM]
> Eye drops, cyclopentolate hydrochloride 0.5% and
> 1%. Net price 20 × 0.5 mL (both) = £4.92

HOMATROPINE HYDROBROMIDE

Cautions see notes above

Side-effects see notes above

Licensed use not licensed for use in children
under 3 months

Indication and dose
> See notes above
>
> > **Child 3 months–2 years** (0.5% only) 1 drop daily
> > or on alternate days adjusted according to
> > response
> >
> > **Child 2–18 years** 1 drop twice daily adjusted
> > according to response

Homatropine (Non-proprietary) [PoM]
> Eye drops, homatropine hydrobromide 1%, net
> price 10 mL = £2.14; 2%, 10 mL = £2.26
> Available without preservatives as manufactured
> specials from Moorfields Eye Hospital
>
> Eye drops, homatropine 0.125% and 0.5%, 10 mL,
> available as a manufactured special from Moor-
> fields Eye Hospital, see also 'special-order' manu-
> facturers or specialist importing companies, p. 943
> **Excipients** include chlorhexidine

TROPICAMIDE

Cautions see notes above

Side-effects see notes above

Indication and dose
> See notes above
>
> > **Funduscopy**
> >
> > **Neonate and child** apply 0.5% eye drops 20
> > minutes before examination

Mydriacyl® (Alcon) [PoM]
> Eye drops, tropicamide 0.5%, net price 5 mL =
> £1.36; 1%, 5 mL = £1.68
> **Excipients** include benzalkonium chloride, disodium edetate

◀**Single use**
Minims® Tropicamide (Chauvin) [PoM]
> Eye drops, tropicamide 0.5% and 1%. Net price 20
> × 0.5 mL (both) = £5.75

Sympathomimetics

PHENYLEPHRINE HYDROCHLORIDE

Cautions cardiovascular disease (avoid or use
2.5% strength only); tachycardia; hyperthyroidism; diabetes; susceptibility to angle-closure
glaucoma; see also notes above

Contra-indications 10% drops in neonates and
children

Side-effects eye pain and stinging; blurred vision,
photophobia; systemic effects include palpitations, arrhythmias, hypertension, coronary artery
spasm

Indication and dose
> **Mydriasis**
> See notes above

◀**Single use**
Minims® Phenylephrine Hydrochloride (Chauvin)
> Eye drops, phenylephrine hydrochloride 2.5%, net
> price 20 × 0.5 mL = £5.75
> **Excipients** include disodium edetate, sodium metabisulphite

11.6 Treatment of glaucoma

Glaucoma describes a group of disorders characterised by a loss of visual field
associated with cupping of the optic disc and optic nerve damage and is generally
associated with raised intra-ocular pressure.

Glaucoma is rare in children and should always be managed by a specialist.
Primary congenital glaucoma is the most common form of glaucoma in children,
followed by *secondary glaucomas*, such as following hereditary anterior segment

malformations; *juvenile open-angle glaucoma* is less common and usually occurs in older children. *Primary angle closure glaucoma* (acute closed-angle glaucoma, narrow angle glaucoma) is very rare in children; it results from blockage of aqueous humour flow into the anterior chamber and is a medical emergency that requires urgent reduction of intra-ocular pressure, see below.

Treatment of glaucoma is determined by the pathophysiology and usually involves controlling raised intra-ocular pressure with surgery and drug therapy. Drugs that reduce intra-ocular pressure by different mechanisms are available for managing glaucoma. A topical beta-blocker or a prostaglandin analogue can be used. It may be necessary to combine these drugs or add others, such as miotics, sympathomimetics, or carbonic anhydrase inhibitors, to control intra-ocular pressure.

For urgent reduction of intra-ocular pressure and before surgery, **mannitol** 20% (up to 500 mL) is given by slow intravenous infusion until the intra-ocular pressure has been satisfactorily reduced (see section 2.2.5). **Acetazolamide** by intravenous injection can also be used for the emergency management of raised intra-ocular pressure.

Standard antiglaucoma therapy is used if supplementary treatment is required after iridotomy, iridectomy, or a drainage operation in either primary open-angle or acute closed-angle glaucoma.

Beta-blockers

Topical application of a beta-blocker to the eye reduces intra-ocular pressure effectively in *primary open-angle glaucoma*, probably by reducing the rate of production of aqueous humour. Administration by mouth also reduces intra-ocular pressure but this route is not used since side-effects may be troublesome.

Cautions, contra-indications and side-effects   Systemic absorption may follow topical application to the eye; therefore, eye drops containing a beta-blocker are contra-indicated in bradycardia, heart block, or uncontrolled heart failure. **Important:** avoid in asthma, see CSM advice below. Consider also other cautions, contra-indications and side-effects of beta-blockers (p. 113). Local side-effects of eye drops include ocular stinging, burning, pain, itching, erythema, dry eyes and allergic reactions including anaphylaxis and blepharoconjunctivitis; occasionally corneal disorders have been reported.

CSM advice The CSM has advised that beta-blockers, even those with apparent cardioselectivity, should not be used in patients with asthma or a history of obstructive airways disease, unless no alternative treatment is available. In such cases the risk of inducing bronchospasm should be appreciated and appropriate precautions taken.

Interactions   Since systemic absorption may follow topical application the possibility of interactions, in particular with drugs such as verapamil, should be borne in mind. See also Appendix 1 (beta-blockers).

◢ BETAXOLOL HYDROCHLORIDE

Cautions see notes above

Contra-indications see notes above

Side-effects see notes above

Licensed use not licensed for use in children

Indication and dose

> See notes above
>   Apply twice daily

Betoptic® (Alcon) [PoM]

Ophthalmic solution (= eye drops), betaxolol (as hydrochloride) 0.5%, net price 5 mL = £2.00
Excipients include benzalkonium chloride, disodium edetate

Ophthalmic suspension (= eye drops), m/r, betaxolol (as hydrochloride) 0.25%, net price 5 mL = £2.80
Excipients include benzalkonium chloride, disodium edetate

Unit dose eye drop suspension, m/r, betaxolol (as hydrochloride) 0.25%, net price 50 × 0.25 mL = £14.49

◢ CARTEOLOL HYDROCHLORIDE

Cautions see notes above

Contra-indications see notes above

Side-effects see notes above

Licensed use not licensed for use in children

Indication and dose

> See notes above
>   Apply twice daily

Teoptic® (Novartis) [PoM]

Eye drops, carteolol hydrochloride 1%, net price 5 mL = £4.60; 2%, 5 mL = £5.40
Excipients include benzalkonium chloride

◢ LEVOBUNOLOL HYDROCHLORIDE

Cautions see notes above

Contra-indications see notes above

Side-effects see notes above; anterior uveitis occasionally reported

Licensed use not licensed for use in children

Indication and dose

See notes above
> Apply once or twice daily

Levobunolol (Non-proprietary) ᴘᴏᴹ
Eye drops, levobunolol hydrochloride 0.5%. Net price 5 mL = £2.68

Betagan® (Allergan) ᴘᴏᴹ
Eye drops, levobunolol hydrochloride 0.5%, polyvinyl alcohol (*Liquifilm®*) 1.4%. Net price 5-mL = £1.85
Excipients include benzalkonium chloride, disodium edetate, sodium metabisulphite

Unit dose eye drops, levobunolol hydrochloride 0.5%, polyvinyl alcohol (*Liquifilm®*) 1.4%. Net price 30 × 0.4 mL = £9.98
Excipients include disodium edetate

◢ TIMOLOL MALEATE

Cautions see notes above

Contra-indications see notes above

Side-effects see notes above

Licensed use not licensed for use in children

Indication and dose

See notes above
> Apply twice daily; long-acting preparations, see under preparations below

Timolol (Non-proprietary) ᴘᴏᴹ
Eye drops, timolol (as maleate) 0.25%, net price 5 mL = £2.30; 0.5%, 5 mL = £1.95

Timoptol® (MSD) ᴘᴏᴹ
Eye drops, in *Ocumeter®* metered-dose unit, timolol (as maleate) 0.25%, net price 5 mL = £3.12; 0.5%, 5 mL = £3.12
Excipients include benzalkonium chloride

Unit dose eye drops, timolol (as maleate) 0.25%, net price 30 × 0.2 mL = £8.45; 0.5%, 30 × 0.2 mL = £9.65

◢ **Once-daily preparations**

Nyogel® (Novartis) ᴘᴏᴹ
Eye gel (= eye drops), timolol (as maleate) 0.1%, net price 5 g = £2.85
Excipients include benzalkonium chloride

Dose

> **Child 12–18 years** apply once daily

Timoptol®-LA (MSD) ᴘᴏᴹ
Ophthalmic gel-forming solution (= eye drops), timolol (as maleate) 0.25%, net price 2.5 mL = £3.12; 0.5%, 2.5 mL = £3.12
Excipients include benzododecinium bromide

Dose

> Apply eye drops once daily

◢ **With dorzolamide**
See under Dorzolamide

Prostaglandin analogues

Latanoprost and **travoprost** are prostaglandin analogues which increase uveoscleral outflow; **bimatoprost** is a related drug. They are used to reduce intra-ocular pressure. They are not licensed for use in children. Children receiving prostaglandin analogues should be managed by a specialist and monitored for any changes to eye coloration since an increase in the brown pigment in the iris can occur; particular care is required in those with mixed coloured irides and those receiving treatment to one eye only.

Sympathomimetics

Dipivefrine is a pro-drug of adrenaline. It is claimed to pass more rapidly than adrenaline through the cornea and is then converted to the active form. Adrenaline (epinephrine) probably acts both by reducing the rate of production of aqueous humour and by increasing the outflow through the trabecular meshwork. It is contra-indicated in angle-closure glaucoma because it is a mydriatic, unless an iridectomy has been carried out. Side-effects include severe smarting and redness of the eye; adrenaline should be used with caution in children with hypertension and heart disease.

Apraclonidine (section 11.8.2) is an alpha$_2$-adrenoceptor agonist. Eye drops containing apraclonidine 0.5% are used for a short period to delay laser treatment or surgery for glaucoma in patients not adequately controlled by another drug; eye drops containing 1% are used for control of intra-ocular pressure after anterior segment laser surgery.

Brimonidine is an alpha$_2$-adrenoceptor agonist that reduces intra-ocular pressure; it should be used with caution in children because it has been associated with severe systemic side-effects.

◢ DIPIVEFRINE HYDROCHLORIDE

Contra-indications see notes above

Side-effects see notes above

Licensed use not licensed for use in children

Indication and dose

> See notes above
>   Apply twice daily

Propine® (Allergan) PoM

Eye drops, dipivefrine hydrochloride 0.1%, net price 5 mL = £3.81, 10 mL = £4.77

Excipients include benzalkonium chloride, disodium edetate

Carbonic anhydrase inhibitors and systemic drugs

The **carbonic anhydrase inhibitors**, acetazolamide, brinzolamide, and dorzolamide, reduce intra-ocular pressure by reducing aqueous humour production. Systemic use of acetazolamide also produces weak diuresis.

Acetazolamide is given by mouth or, rarely in children, by intravenous injection (intramuscular injections are painful because of the alkaline pH of the solution). It is used as an adjunct to other treatment for reducing intra-ocular pressure. Acetazolamide is a sulphonamide; blood disorders, rashes, and other sulphonamide-related side-effects occur occasionally. It is not generally recommended for long-term use; electrolyte disturbances and metabolic acidosis that occur may be corrected by administering potassium bicarbonate (as effervescent potassium tablets, section 9.2.1.3).

Dorzolamide and **brinzolamide** are topical carbonic anhydrase inhibitors. They are unlicensed in children but are used in those resistant to beta-blockers or those in whom beta-blockers are contra-indicated. They are used alone or as an adjunct to a topical beta-blocker. Systemic absorption may rarely give rise to sulphonamide-like side-effects and may require discontinuation if severe.

The **osmotic diuretics**, intravenous hypertonic **mannitol** (section 2.2.5), or **glycerol** by mouth, are useful short-term ocular hypotensive drugs.

◢ ACETAZOLAMIDE

Cautions not generally recommended for prolonged use but if given monitor blood count and plasma electrolyte concentration; pulmonary obstruction (risk of acidosis); avoid extravasation at injection site (risk of necrosis); **interactions:** Appendix 1 (diuretics)

Pregnancy manufacturer advises avoid, especially in first trimester (toxicity in *animal* studies)

Breast-feeding amount too small to be harmful

Contra-indications hypokalaemia, hyponatraemia, hyperchloraemic acidosis; sulphonamide hypersensitivity

Hepatic impairment avoid in severe impairment

Renal impairment avoid; metabolic acidosis

Side-effects nausea, vomiting, diarrhoea, taste disturbance; loss of appetite, paraesthesia, flushing, headache, dizziness, fatigue, irritability, depression; thirst, polyuria; metabolic acidosis and electrolyte disturbances on long-term therapy; occasionally, drowsiness, confusion, hearing disturbances, urticaria, melaena, glycosuria, haematuria, abnormal liver function, renal calculi, blood disorders including agranulocytosis and thrombocytopenia, rashes including Stevens-Johnson syndrome and toxic epidermal necrolysis; rarely, photosensitivity, liver damage, flaccid paralysis, convulsions; transient myopia reported

Licensed use not licensed for use in children for treatment of glaucoma

Indication and dose

Reduction of intra-ocular pressure in open-angle glaucoma, secondary glaucoma, perioperatively in angle-closure glaucoma
- **By mouth or by intravenous injection**

  Child 1 month–12 years 5 mg/kg 2–4 times daily, adjusted according to response, max. 750 mg daily

  Child 12–18 years 250 mg 2–4 times daily

Epilepsy
- **By mouth or slow intravenous injection**

  Neonate initially 2.5 mg/kg 2–3 times daily, followed by 5–7 mg/kg 2–3 times daily (maintenance dose)

  Child 1 month–12 years initially 2.5 mg/kg 2–3 times daily, followed by 5–7 mg/kg 2–3 times daily, max. 750 mg daily (maintenance dose)

  Child 12–18 years 250 mg 2–4 times daily

Raised intracranial pressure
- **By mouth or slow intravenous injection**

  Child 1 month–12 years initially 8 mg/kg 3 times daily, increased as necessary to max. 100 mg/kg daily

11

Eye

◻ **ACETAZOLAMIDE** (*continued*)

Diamox® (Goldshield) [PoM]
Tablets, acetazolamide 250 mg. Net price 112-tab pack = £12.68. Label: 3

Sodium Parenteral (= injection), powder for reconstitution, acetazolamide (as sodium salt). Net price 500-mg vial = £14.76

◢Modified release
Diamox® SR (Goldshield) [PoM]
Capsules, m/r, orange, enclosing orange f/c pellets, acetazolamide 250 mg. Net price 30-cap pack = £13.88. Label: 3, 25

Dose

> Child 12–18 years glaucoma, 1–2 capsules daily

◢Extemporaneous formulations available see Extemporaneous Preparations, p. 8

◢ BRINZOLAMIDE

Cautions systemic absorption follows topical application; neonates and infants with immature renal tubules—risk of metabolic acidosis; **interactions**: Appendix 1 (brinzolamide)

Hepatic impairment manufacturer advises caution—no information available

Pregnancy manufacturer advises avoid unless essential—embryotoxic in *animal* studies

Contra-indications hyperchloraemic acidosis

Renal impairment avoid if estimated glomerular filtration rate less than 30 mL/minute/1.73 m²

Breast-feeding manufacturer advises avoid—no information available

Side-effects local irritation, taste disturbance; less commonly nausea, dyspepsia, dry mouth, chest pain, epistaxis, haemoptysis, dyspnoea, rhinitis, pharyngitis, bronchitis, paraesthesia, depression, dizziness, headache, dermatitis, alopecia, corneal erosion

Licensed use not licensed for use in children

Indication and dose

> Adjunct to beta-blockers or used alone in raised intra-ocular pressure in ocular hypertension and in open-angle glaucoma if beta-blocker alone inadequate or inappropriate
>
> > Apply twice daily increased to 3 times daily if necessary

Azopt® (Alcon) [PoM]
Eye drops, brinzolamide 10 mg/mL, net price 5 mL = £6.90
Excipients include benzalkonium chloride, disodium edetate

◢ DORZOLAMIDE

Cautions systemic absorption follows topical application; history of renal calculi; neonates and infants with immature renal tubules—risk of metabolic acidosis; chronic corneal defects, history of intra-ocular surgery; **interactions**: Appendix 1 (dorzolamide)

Hepatic impairment manufacturer advises caution—no information available

Contra-indications hyperchloraemic acidosis

Renal impairment avoid if estimated glomerular filtration rate less than 30 mL/minute/1.73 m²

Pregnancy manufacturer advises avoid—embryotoxic in *animal* studies

Breast-feeding manufacturer advises avoid—no information available

Side-effects nausea, bitter taste; headache, asthenia; ocular irritation, blurred vision, lacrimation, conjunctivitis, superficial punctuate keratitis, eyelid inflammation; *less commonly* iridocyclitis; *rarely* hypersensitivity reactions (including urticaria, angioedema, bronchospasm), dizziness, paraesthesia, urolithiasis, eyelid crusting, transient myopia, corneal oedema, epistaxis, dry mouth, throat irritation; also reported metabolic acidosis

Licensed use not licensed for use in children

Indication and dose

> Raised intra-ocular pressure in ocular hypertension, open-angle glaucoma, pseudo-exfoliative glaucoma *either* as adjunct to beta-blocker *or* used alone in patients unresponsive to beta-blockers or if beta-blockers contra-indicated
>
> > Used alone, apply 3 times daily; with topical beta-blocker, apply twice daily

Trusopt® (MSD) [PoM]
Ophthalmic solution (= eye drops), in *Ocumeter® Plus* metered-dose unit, dorzolamide (as hydrochloride) 2%, net price 5 mL = £6.33
Excipients include benzalkonium chloride

Unit dose eye drops, dorzolamide (as hydrochloride) 2%, net price 60 × 0.2 mL = £24.18

◢With timolol
For cautions, contra-indications, and side-effects of timolol, see section 11.6, Beta-blockers

Cosopt® (MSD) [PoM]
Ophthalmic solution (= eye drops), dorzolamide (as hydrochloride) 2%, timolol (as maleate) 0.5%, net price 5 mL = £10.05
Excipients include benzalkonium chloride

Unit dose eye drops, dorzolamide (as hydrochloride) 2%, timolol (as maleate) 0.5%, net price 60 × 0.2 mL = £28.59

Dose

> Raised intra-ocular pressure in open-angle glaucoma, or pseudoexfoliative glaucoma when beta-blockers alone not adequate
>
> > Apply twice daily

Miotics

Pilocarpine is a miotic used in the management of raised intra-ocular pressure. The small pupil is an unfortunate side-effect of these drugs (except when pilocarpine is used temporarily before an operation for angle-closure glaucoma). Miotics act by opening up the inefficient drainage channels in the trabecular meshwork which may be occluded by contraction or spasm of the ciliary muscle.

Cautions A darkly pigmented iris may require higher concentration of the miotic or more frequent administration and care should be taken to avoid over-dosage. Retinal detachment has occurred in susceptible individuals and those with retinal disease; therefore fundus examination is advised before starting treatment with a miotic. Care is also required in conjunctival or corneal damage. Intra-ocular pressure and visual fields should be monitored in those with chronic simple glaucoma and those receiving long-term treatment with a miotic. Miotics should be used with caution in cardiac disease, hypertension, asthma, peptic ulceration and urinary-tract obstruction.

Counselling Blurred vision may affect performance of skilled tasks (e.g. driving) particularly at night or in reduced lighting

Contra-indications Miotics are contra-indicated in conditions where pupillary constriction is undesirable such as acute iritis, anterior uveitis and some forms of secondary glaucoma. They should be avoided in acute inflammatory disease of the anterior segment.

Side-effects Ciliary spasm leads to headache and browache which may be more severe in the initial 2–4 weeks of treatment. Ocular side-effects include burning, itching, smarting, blurred vision, conjunctival vascular congestion, myopia, lens changes with chronic use, vitreous haemorrhage, and pupillary block. Systemic side-effects are rare following application to the eye.

PILOCARPINE

Cautions see notes above
Contra-indications see notes above
Side-effects see notes above
Licensed use not licensed for use in children
Indication and dose
See also notes above

Raised intra-ocular pressure in ocular hypertension and open-angle glaucoma
   Child 1 month–2 years 1 drop of 0.5% or 1% solution 3 times daily
   Child 2–18 years 1 drop 4 times daily

Pre-operatively in goniotomy and trabeculotomy
   Child 1 month–18 years apply 1% or 2% solution once daily

Dry mouth (section 12.3.5)

Pilocarpine Hydrochloride (Non-proprietary) ⒫ℴ𝓂
Eye drops, pilocarpine hydrochloride 0.5%, net price 10 mL = £1.39; 1%, 10 mL = £2.71; 2%, 10 mL = £2.59; 3%, 10 mL = £1.77; 4%, 10 mL = £3.46

◢Single use
Minims® Pilocarpine Nitrate (Chauvin) ⒫ℴ𝓂
Eye drops, pilocarpine nitrate 2%, net price 20 × 0.5 mL = £4.92

11
Eye

11.7 Local anaesthetics

Oxybuprocaine and **tetracaine** (amethocaine) are widely used topical local anaesthetics. **Proxymetacaine** causes less initial stinging and is particularly useful for children. Oxybuprocaine or a combined preparation of lidocaine (lignocaine) and fluorescein is used for tonometry. Tetracaine produces more profound anaesthesia and is suitable for use before minor surgical procedures, such as the removal of corneal sutures. It has a temporary disruptive effect on the corneal epithelium. **Lidocaine**, with or without adrenaline (epinephrine), is injected into the eyelids for minor surgery, while retrobulbar or peribulbar injections are used for surgery of the globe itself. Local anaesthetics should never be used for the management of ocular symptoms.

Caution Local anaesthetic eye drops should be avoided in preterm neonates because of the immaturity of the metabolising enzyme system.

LIDOCAINE HYDROCHLORIDE
(Lignocaine hydrochloride)

Contra-indications avoid in preterm neonates

Indication and dose

Local anaesthetic
Use as required

Minims® Lignocaine and Fluorescein (Chauvin) (PoM)
Eye drops, lidocaine hydrochloride 4%, fluorescein sodium 0.25%. Net price 20 × 0.5 mL = £6.93

OXYBUPROCAINE HYDROCHLORIDE

Contra-indications avoid in preterm neonates

Indication and dose

Local anaesthetic
Use as required

Minims® Benoxinate (Oxybuprocaine) Hydro-chloride (Chauvin) (PoM)
Eye drops, oxybuprocaine hydrochloride 0.4%. Net price 20 × 0.5 mL = £4.92

PROXYMETACAINE HYDROCHLORIDE

Contra-indications avoid in preterm neonates

Indication and dose

Local anaesthetic
Use as required

Minims® Proxymetacaine (Chauvin) (PoM)
Eye drops, proxymetacaine hydrochloride 0.5%.
Net price 20 × 0.5 mL = £6.95

◀With fluorescein
Minims® Proxymetacaine and Fluorescein (Chauvin)
(PoM)
Eye drops, proxymetacaine hydrochloride 0.5%,
fluorescein sodium 0.25%. Net price 20 × 0.5 mL =
£7.95

TETRACAINE HYDROCHLORIDE
(Amethocaine hydrochloride)

Contra-indications avoid in preterm neonates

Indication and dose

Local anaesthetic
Use as required

Minims® Amethocaine Hydrochloride (Chauvin) (PoM)
Eye drops, tetracaine hydrochloride 0.5% and 1%.
Net price 20 × 0.5 mL (both) = £5.75

11 Eye

11.8 Miscellaneous ophthalmic preparations

Certain eye drops, e.g. amphotericin, ceftazidime, cefuroxime, colistin, desferri-oxamine, dexamethasone, gentamicin and vancomycin, may be prepared asepti-cally in a specialist manufacturing unit from material supplied for injection.

Preparations may also be available from Moorfields Eye Hospital as manufactured specials, see also 'special-order' manufacturers or specialist importing companies, p. 943.

11.8.1 Tear deficiency, ocular lubricants, and astringents

Chronic soreness of the eyes associated with reduced or abnormal tear secretion often responds to tear replacement therapy. The severity of the condition and the child's preference will often guide the choice of preparation.

Hypromellose is the traditional choice of treatment for tear deficiency. It may need to be instilled frequently (e.g. hourly) for adequate relief. Ocular surface mucin is often abnormal in tear deficiency and the combination of hypromellose with a mucolytic such as **acetylcysteine** can be helpful.

The ability of **carbomers** to cling to the eye surface may help reduce frequency of application to 4 times daily.

Polyvinyl alcohol increases the persistence of the tear film and is useful when the ocular surface mucin is reduced.

Sodium Hyaluronate eye drops are also used in the management of tear deficiency.

Sodium chloride 0.9% drops are sometimes useful in tear deficiency, and can be used as 'comfort drops' by contact lens wearers, and to facilitate lens removal. Special presentations of sodium chloride 0.9% and other irrigation solutions are used routinely for intra-ocular surgery and in first-aid for removal of harmful substances.

Eye ointments containing a **paraffin** may be used to lubricate the eye surface, especially in cases of recurrent corneal epithelial erosion. They may cause temporary visual disturbance and are best suited for application before sleep. Ointments should not be used during contact lens wear.

◢ ACETYLCYSTEINE

Indication and dose

Tear deficiency, impaired or abnormal mucus production
  Apply 3–4 times daily

Ilube® (Alcon) PoM
Eye drops, acetylcysteine 5%, hypromellose 0.35%. Net price 10 mL = £4.63
Excipients include benzalkonium chloride, disodium edetate

◢ CARBOMERS
(Polyacrylic acid)
Synthetic high molecular weight polymers of acrylic acid cross-linked with either allyl ethers of sucrose or allyl ethers of pentaerithrityl

Licensed use some preparations not licensed for use in children

Indication and dose

Dry eyes including keratoconjunctivitis sicca, unstable tear film
  Apply 3–4 times daily or as required

GelTears® (Chauvin)
Gel (= eye drops), carbomer 980 (polyacrylic acid) 0.2%, net price 10 g = £2.80
Excipients include benzalkonium chloride

Liposic® (Bausch & Lomb)
Gel (= eye drops), carbomer 980 (polyacrylic acid) 0.2%, net price 10 g = £2.96
Excipients include cetrimide

Viscotears® (Novartis)
Liquid gel (= eye drops), carbomer 980 (polyacrylic acid) 0.2%, net price 10 g = £3.12
Excipients include cetrimide

Liquid gel (= eye drops), carbomer 980 (polyacrylic acid) 0.2%, net price 30 × 0.6-mL single-dose units = £5.75

◢ CARMELLOSE SODIUM

Indication and dose

Dry eye conditions
  Apply as required

Optive® (Allergan)
Eye drops, carmellose sodium 0.5%, glycerol, net price 10 mL = £7.49

◢Single use
Celluvisc® (Allergan)
Eye drops, carmellose sodium 0.5%, net price 30 × 0.4 mL = £5.75, 90 × 0.4 mL = £15.53; 1%, 30 × 0.4 mL = £5.75, 60 × 0.4 mL = £10.99

◢ HYDROXYETHYLCELLULOSE

Indication and dose

Tear deficiency
  Apply as required

Minims® Artificial Tears (Chauvin)
Eye drops, hydroxyethylcellulose 0.44%, sodium chloride 0.35%. Net price 20 × 0.5 mL = £5.75

11

Eye

HYPROMELLOSE

Indication and dose

Tear deficiency

Apply as required

Note The Royal Pharmaceutical Society of Great Britain has stated that where it is not possible to ascertain the strength of hypromellose prescribed, the prescriber should be contacted to clarify the strength intended.

Hypromellose (Non-proprietary)

Eye drops, hypromellose 0.3%, net price 10 mL = £1.63

Brands include *Artelac*®

Isopto Alkaline® (Alcon)

Eye drops, hypromellose 1%, net price 10 mL = 99p

Excipients include benzalkonium chloride

Isopto Plain® (Alcon)

Eye drops, hypromellose 0.5%, net price 10 mL = 85p

Excipients include benzalkonium chloride

Tears Naturale® (Alcon)

Eye drops, dextran '70' 0.1%, hypromellose 0.3%, net price 15 mL = £1.68

Excipients include benzalkonium chloride, disodium edetate

◢Single use

Artelac® **SDU** (Pharma-Global)

Eye drops, hypromellose 0.32%, net price 30 × 0.5 mL = £13.95

LIQUID PARAFFIN

Indication and dose

Dry eye conditions

Apply as required

Lacri-Lube® (Allergan)

Eye ointment, white soft paraffin 57.3%, liquid paraffin 42.5%, wool alcohols 0.2%. Net price 3.5 g = £2.28, 5 g = £2.96

Lubri-Tears® (Alcon)

Eye ointment, white soft paraffin 60%, liquid paraffin 30%, wool fat 10%. Net price 5 g = £2.29

PARAFFIN, YELLOW, SOFT

Indication and dose

See notes above

Apply 2 hourly as required

Simple Eye Ointment

Ointment, liquid paraffin 10%, wool fat 10%, in yellow soft paraffin. Net price 4 g = £3.03

POLYVINYL ALCOHOL

Indication and dose

Tear deficiency

Apply as required

Liquifilm Tears® (Allergan)

Ophthalmic solution (= eye drops), polyvinyl alcohol 1.4%. Net price 15 mL = £1.93

Excipients include benzalkonium chloride, disodium edetate

Ophthalmic solution (= eye drops), polyvinyl alcohol 1.4%, povidone 0.6%. Net price 30 × 0.4 mL = £5.35

Sno Tears® (Chauvin)

Eye drops, polyvinyl alcohol 1.4%. Net price 10 mL = £1.06

Excipients include benzalkonium chloride, disodium edetate

SODIUM CHLORIDE

Indication and dose

Irrigation, including first-aid removal of harmful substances

Use as required

Sodium Chloride 0.9% Solutions

See section 13.11.1

Balanced Salt Solution

Solution (sterile), sodium chloride 0.64%, sodium acetate 0.39%, sodium citrate 0.17%, calcium chloride 0.048%, magnesium chloride 0.03%, potassium chloride 0.075%

For intra-ocular or topical irrigation during surgical procedures

Brands include *Iocare*®

◢Single use

Minims® **Saline** (Chauvin)

Eye drops, sodium chloride 0.9%. Net price 20 × 0.5 mL = £4.92

11

Eye

▲ SODIUM HYALURONATE

Indication and dose

Dry eye conditions
Apply as required

Oxyal® (Kestrel Ophthalmics)
Eye drops, sodium hyaluronate 0.15%, net price
10 ml = £4.15

Vismed® Multi (TRB Chemedica)
Eye drops, sodium hyaluronate 0.18%, net price
10 mL = £6.81

◀Single use
Clinitas® (Altacor)
Eye drops, sodium hyaluronate 0.4%, net price 30 ×
0.5 mL = £5.70

Ocusan® (Agepha)
Eye drops, sodium hyaluronate 0.2%, net price 20 ×
0.5 mL = £5.25

Vismed® (TRB Chemedica)
Eye drops, sodium hyaluronate 0.18%, net price 20
× 0.3 mL = £5.10

11.8.2 Ocular diagnostic and peri-operative preparations

Ocular diagnostic preparations

Fluorescein sodium is used in diagnostic procedures and for locating damaged areas of the cornea due to injury or disease.

▲ FLUORESCEIN SODIUM

Indication and dose

Detection of lesions and foreign bodies
sufficient to stain damaged areas

Minims® Fluorescein Sodium (Chauvin)
Eye drops, fluorescein sodium 1% or 2%. Net price
20 × 0.5 mL (both) = £4.92

◀With local anaesthetic
Section 11.7

Ocular peri-operative drugs

Drugs used to prepare the eye for surgery and drugs that are injected into the anterior chamber at the time of surgery are included here.

Sodium hyaluronate is used during surgical procedures on the eye.

Apraclonidine, an alpha$_2$-adrenoceptor agonist, reduces intra-ocular pressure possibly by reducing the production of aqueous humour. It is used for short-term treatment only.

Balanced Salt Solution is used routinely in intra-ocular surgery (section 11.8.1).

▲ ACETYLCHOLINE CHLORIDE

Licensed use not licensed for use in children

Indication and dose

Cataract surgery, penetrating keratoplasty, iridectomy, other anterior segment surgery requiring rapid complete miosis
consult product literature

Miochol-E® (Novartis) [PoM]
Solution for intra-ocular irrigation, acetylcholine chloride 1%, mannitol 3% when reconstituted. Net price 2 mL-vial = £9.10

▲ APRACLONIDINE

Note Apraclonidine is a derivative of clonidine

Cautions history of angina, severe coronary insufficiency, recent myocardial infarction, heart failure, cerebrovascular disease, vasovagal attack, chronic renal failure; depression; pregnancy and breast-feeding; monitor intra-ocular pressure and visual fields; loss of effect may occur over time; suspend treatment if reduction in vision occurs in end-stage glaucoma; monitor for excessive

reduction in intra-ocular pressure following peri-operative use; **interactions:** Appendix 1 (alpha$_2$-adrenoceptor stimulants)
Skilled tasks Drowsiness may affect performance of skilled tasks (e.g. driving)

Contra-indications history of severe or unstable and uncontrolled cardiovascular disease

11

Eye

◻ **APRACLONIDINE** (*continued*)

Side-effects dry mouth, taste disturbance; hyperaemia, ocular pruritus, discomfort and lacrimation (withdraw if ocular intolerance including oedema of lids and conjunctiva); headache, asthenia, dry nose; lid retraction, conjunctival blanching and mydriasis reported after peri-operative use; since absorption may follow topical application systemic effects (see Clonidine Hydrochloride, section 2.5.2) may occur

Licensed use 0.5% drops not licensed for use in children under 12 years; 1% drops not licensed for use in children

Indication and dose

See preparations below

Iopidine® (Alcon) [PoM]

Ophthalmic solution (= eye drops), apraclonidine 1% (as hydrochloride). Net price 12 × 2 single use 0.25-mL units = £81.90

Dose

Control or prevention of postoperative elevation of intra-ocular pressure after anterior segment laser surgery

apply 1 drop 1 hour before laser procedure then 1 drop immediately after completion of procedure

Ophthalmic solution (= eye drops), apraclonidine 0.5% (as hydrochloride). Net price 5 mL = £11.45
Excipients include benzalkonium chloride

Dose

Short-term adjunctive treatment of chronic glaucoma in patients not adequately controlled by another drug (see note below)

Child 12–18 years apply 1 drop 3 times daily usually for max. 1 month

Note May not provide additional benefit if patient already using two drugs that suppress the production of aqueous humour

---

▌ DICLOFENAC SODIUM

Licensed use not licensed for use in children

Indication and dose

Inhibition of intra-operative miosis during cataract surgery (but does not possess intrinsic mydriatic properties), postoperative inflammation in cataract surgery, strabismus surgery, argon laser trabeculoplasty

consult product literature

Voltarol® Ophtha Multidose (Novartis) [PoM]

Eye drops, diclofenac sodium 0.1%, net price 5 mL = £6.68
Excipients include benzalkonium chloride, disodium edetate, propylene glycol

◄Single use
Voltarol® Ophtha (Novartis) [PoM]

Eye drops, diclofenac sodium 0.1%. Net price pack of 5 single-dose units = £4.00, 40 single-dose units = £32.00

▌ FLURBIPROFEN SODIUM

Licensed use not licensed for use in children

Indication and dose

Inhibition of intra-operative miosis (but does not possess intrinsic mydriatic properties), control of postoperative and post-laser trabeculoplasty inflammation (if corticosteroids contra-indicated)

consult product literature

Ocufen® (Allergan) [PoM]

Ophthalmic solution (= eye drops), flurbiprofen sodium 0.03%, polyvinyl alcohol (*Liquifilm®*) 1.4%. Net price 40 × 0.4 mL = £37.15

▌ KETOROLAC TROMETAMOL

Licensed use not licensed for use in children

Indication and dose

Prophylaxis and reduction of inflammation and associated symptoms following ocular surgery

consult product literature

Acular® (Allergan) [PoM]

Eye drops, ketorolac trometamol 0.5%. Net price 5 mL = £5.00
Excipients include benzalkonium chloride, disodium edetate

11.9 Contact lenses

Note Some recommendations in this section involve non-licensed indications.

Some children and adolescents prefer to wear contact lenses rather than spectacles for both cosmetic and medical reasons. Visual defects are corrected by either rigid ('hard' or gas permeable) lenses or soft (hydrogel) lenses; soft lenses are the most popular type, because they are the most comfortable, but they may not give the best vision. Lenses should usually be worn for a specified number of hours each day. Continuous (extended) wear involves much greater risks to eye health and is not recommended except where medically indicated.

Contact lenses require meticulous care. Poor compliance with directions for use, and with daily cleaning and disinfection, can result in complications including ulcerative keratitis and conjunctival problems (such as purulent or papillary conjunctivitis). One-day disposable lenses, which are worn only once and therefore require no maintenance or storage, are becoming increasingly popular.

Acanthamoeba keratitis, a sight-threatening condition, is associated with ineffective lens cleaning and disinfection or the use of contaminated lens cases. The condition is especially associated with the use of soft lenses (including frequently replaced lenses). Acanthamoeba keratitis is treated, by specialists, with intensive use of polihexanide (polyhexamethylene biguanide), propamidine isetionate (section 11.3.1), chlorhexidine, and neomycin (section 11.3.1) drops, sometimes used in combination.

Contact lenses and drug treatment   Special care is required in prescribing eye preparations for contact lens users. Some drugs and preservatives in eye preparations can accumulate in hydrogel lenses and can cause adverse reactions. Therefore, unless medically indicated, the lenses should be removed before instillation and not worn during the period of treatment. Alternatively, unpreserved drops can be used. Eye drops may, however, be instilled over rigid corneal contact lenses. Ointment preparations should never be used in conjunction with contact lens wear; oily eye drops should also be avoided.

Many drugs given systemically can also have adverse effects on contact lens wear. These include oral contraceptives (particularly those with a higher oestrogen content), drugs which reduce blink rate (e.g. anxiolytics, hypnotics, antihistamines, and muscle relaxants), drugs which reduce lacrimation (e.g. antihistamines, antimuscarinics, phenothiazines and related drugs, some beta-blockers, diuretics, and tricyclic antidepressants), and drugs which increase lacrimation (including ephedrine and hydralazine). Other drugs that can affect contact lens wear are isotretinoin (can cause conjunctival inflammation), aspirin (salicylic acid appears in tears and can be absorbed by contact lenses—leading to irritation), and rifampicin and sulfasalazine (can discolour lenses).

11

Eye

12 Ear, nose, and oropharynx

12.1 Drugs acting on the ear...642
12.1.1 Otitis externa 642
12.1.2 Otitis media 646
12.1.3 Removal of ear wax.. 647
12.2 Drugs acting on the nose 647
12.2.1 Drugs used in nasal allergy 648
12.2.2 Topical nasal decongestants.. 651
12.2.3 Nasal preparations for infection 653
12.3 Drugs acting on the oropharynx...................................654
12.3.1 Drugs for oral ulceration and inflammation.................... 654
12.3.2 Oropharyngeal anti-infective drugs 657
12.3.3 Lozenges and sprays 659
12.3.4 Mouthwashes and gargles.. 659
12.3.5 Treatment of dry mouth 661

> This chapter also includes advice on the drug management of the following:
> allergic rhinitis, p. 648
> nasal polyps, p. 648
> oropharyngeal infections, p. 657
> periodontitis, p. 655

12.1 Drugs acting on the ear

12.1.1 Otitis externa
12.1.2 Otitis media
12.1.3 Removal of ear wax

12.1.1 Otitis externa

Otitis externa is an inflammatory reaction of the lining of the ear canal usually associated with an underlying seborrhoeic dermatitis or eczema; it is important to exclude an underlying chronic otitis media before treatment is commenced. Many cases recover after thorough cleansing of the external ear canal by suction or dry mopping.

A frequent problem in resistant cases is the difficulty in applying lotions and ointments satisfactorily to the relatively inaccessible affected skin. The most effective method is to introduce a ribbon gauze dressing or sponge wick soaked with **corticosteroid** ear drops or with an astringent such as **aluminium acetate** solution. When this is not practical, the ear should be gently cleansed with a probe covered in cotton wool and the patient encouraged to lie with the affected ear uppermost for ten minutes after the canal has been filled with a liberal quantity of the appropriate solution.

Secondary infection in otitis externa may be of bacterial, fungal, or viral origin. If infection is present, a topical anti-infective which is not used systemically (such as **neomycin** or **clioquinol**) may be used, but for only about a week because excessive use may result in fungal infections that are difficult to treat. Sensitivity to the anti-infective or solvent may occur and resistance to antibacterials is a possibility with prolonged use. **Aluminium acetate** ear drops are also effective against bacterial infection and inflammation of the ear. **Chloramphenicol** may be used, but the ear drops contain propylene glycol and cause hypersensitivity reactions in about 10% of patients. Solutions containing an anti-infective and a corticosteroid (such as *Locorten-Vioform®*) are used for treating children when infection is present with inflammation and eczema. **Clotrimazole** 1% solution is used topically to treat fungal infection in otitis externa.

In view of reports of ototoxicity in patients with a perforated tympanic membrane (eardrum), the CSM has stated that treatment with a topical aminoglycoside antibiotic is contra-indicated in those with a tympanic perforation. However, many specialists do use these drops cautiously in the presence of a perforation in children with otitis media (section 12.1.2) and where other measures have failed for otitis externa.

A solution of **acetic acid** 2% acts as an antifungal and antibacterial in the external ear canal and may be used to treat mild otitis externa. More severe cases require treatment with an anti-inflammatory preparation with or without an anti-infective drug. A proprietary preparation containing acetic acid 2% (*EarCalm®* spray) is on sale to the public for children over 12 years.

For severe pain associated with otitis externa, a simple analgesic, such as **paracetamol** (section 4.7.1) or **ibuprofen** (section 10.1.1), can be used. A systemic antibacterial (Table 1, section 5.1) can be used if there is spreading cellulitis or if the child is systemically unwell. When a resistant staphylococcal infection (a boil) is present in the external auditory canal, oral **flucloxacillin** (section 5.1.1.2) is the drug of choice; oral **ciprofloxacin** (section 5.1.12) or a systemic aminoglycoside may be needed for pseudomonal infections, particularly in children with diabetes or compromised immunity.

The skin of the pinna adjacent to the ear canal is often affected by eczema. A topical corticosteroid (section 13.4) cream or ointment is then required, but prolonged use should be avoided.

Administration   To administer ear drops, lay the child down with the head turned to one side; for an infant pull the earlobe back and down, for an older child pull the earlobe back and up.

Astringent preparations

▲ ALUMINIUM ACETATE

Licensed use not licensed

Indication and dose

Inflammation in otitis externa (see notes above)
  Insert into meatus or apply on a ribbon gauze dressing or sponge wick which should be kept saturated with the ear drops

Aluminium Acetate (Non-proprietary)
  Ear drops 13%, aluminium sulphate 2.25 g, calcium carbonate 1 g, tartaric acid 450 mg, acetic acid (33%) 2.5 mL, purified water 7.5 mL
  Available as manufactured special

  Ear drops 8%, dilute 8 parts aluminium acetate ear drops (13%) with 5 parts purified water. Must be freshly prepared

---

Anti-inflammatory preparations

Corticosteroids

Topical corticosteroids are used to treat inflammation and eczema in otitis externa.

Cautions   Prolonged use of topical corticosteroid ear preparations should be avoided.

Contra-indications   Corticosteroid ear preparations should be avoided in the presence of an untreated ear infection. If infection is present, the corticosteroid should be used in combination with a suitable anti-infective (see notes above).

Side-effects   Local sensitivity reactions may occur.

� BETAMETHASONE SODIUM PHOSPHATE

Cautions see notes above
Contra-indications see notes above
Side-effects see notes above
Licensed use licensed for use in children (age range not specified by manufacturers)

Indication and dose

Eczematous inflammation in otitis externa (see notes above); for dose, see under preparations

Eye section 11.4.1

Nose section 12.2.1 and section 12.2.3

Betnesol® (UCB Pharma) PoM
Drops (for ear, eye, or nose), betamethasone sodium phosphate 0.1%. Net price 10 mL = £2.32
Excipients include benzalkonium chloride, disodium edetate

Dose
Ear, instil 2–3 drops every 2–3 hours; reduce frequency when relief obtained

Vistamethasone® (Martindale) PoM
Drops (for ear, eye, or nose), betamethasone sodium phosphate 0.1%. Net price 5 mL = £1.02; 10 mL = £1.16
Excipients include benzalkonium chloride, disodium edetate

Dose
Ear, instil 2–3 drops every 3–4 hours; reduce frequency when relief obtained

◢With antibacterial
Betnesol-N® (UCB Pharma) PoM
Drops (for ear, eye, or nose), betamethasone sodium phosphate 0.1%, neomycin sulphate 0.5%. Net price 10 mL = £2.39
Excipients include benzalkonium chloride, disodium edetate

Dose
Ear, instil 2–3 drops 3–4 times daily

Vistamethasone N® (Martindale) PoM
Drops (for ear, eye, or nose), betamethasone sodium phosphate 0.1%, neomycin sulphate 0.5%. Net price 5 mL = £1.09; 10 mL = £1.20
Excipients include thiomersal

Dose
Ear, instil 2–3 drops every 3–4 hours; reduce frequency when relief obtained

▢ DEXAMETHASONE

Cautions see notes above
Contra-indications see notes above
Side-effects see notes above
Licensed use licensed for use in children (age range not specified by manufacturers)

Indication and dose

Eczematous inflammation in otitis externa (see notes above); for dose, see under preparations

◢With antibacterial
Otomize® (GSK Consumer Healthcare) PoM
Ear spray, dexamethasone 0.1%, neomycin sulphate 3250 units/mL, glacial acetic acid 2%. Net price 5-mL pump-action aerosol unit = £4.24
Excipients include hydroxybenzoates (parabens)

Dose
Ear, apply 1 metered spray 3 times daily

Sofradex® (Sanofi-Aventis) PoM ◢
Drops (for ear or eye), dexamethasone (as sodium metasulphobenzoate) 0.05%, framycetin sulphate 0.5%, gramicidin 0.005%. Net price 10 mL = £5.21
Excipients include polysorbate 80

Dose
Ear, instil 2–3 drops 3–4 times daily; *eye*, section 11.4.1

▢ FLUMETASONE PIVALATE

(Flumethasone Pivalate)
Cautions see notes above
Contra-indications see notes above
Side-effects see notes above

Indication and dose

Eczematous inflammation in otitis externa (see notes above); for dose, see under preparation

◢With antibacterial
Locorten-Vioform® (Amdipharm) PoM
Ear drops, flumetasone pivalate 0.02%, clioquinol 1%. Net price 7.5 mL = £1.47
Contra-indications iodine sensitivity

Dose
Child 2–18 years instil 2–3 drops into the ear twice daily for 7–10 days

Note Clioquinol stains skin and clothing

▢ HYDROCORTISONE

Cautions see notes above

Contra-indications see notes above

Side-effects see notes above

Licensed use *Otosporin®* not licensed for use in children under 3 years; *other preparations* licensed for use in children (age range not specified by manufacturers)

◁ **HYDROCORTISONE (***continued***)**

Indication and dose

Eczematous inflammation in otitis externa (see notes above); for dose, see under preparations

◢**With antibacterial**

Gentisone® HC (Amdipharm) PoM

Ear drops, hydrocortisone acetate 1%, gentamicin 0.3% (as sulphate). Net price 10 mL = £3.69
Excipients include benzalkonium chloride, disodium edetate

Dose

Ear, instil 2–4 drops 3–4 times daily and at night

Otosporin® (GSK) PoM ◢

Ear drops, hydrocortisone 1%, neomycin sulphate 3400 units, polymyxin B sulphate 10 000 units/mL. Net price 5 mL = £2.00; 10 mL = £4.00
Excipients include cetostearyl alcohol, hydroxybenzoates (parabens), polysorbate 20

Dose

Child 3–18 years instil 3 drops into the ear 3–4 times daily

◢ **PREDNISOLONE SODIUM PHOSPHATE**

Cautions see notes above

Contra-indications see notes above

Side-effects see notes above

Licensed use licensed for use in children (age range not specified by manufacturers)

Indication and dose

Eczematous inflammation in otitis externa (see notes above); for dose, see under preparations

Eye section 11.4.1

Predsol® (UCB Pharma) PoM

Drops (for ear or eye), prednisolone sodium phosphate 0.5%. Net price 10 mL = £2.00
Excipients include benzalkonium chloride, disodium edetate

Dose

Ear, instil 2–3 drops every 2–3 hours; reduce frequency when relief obtained

◢**With antibacterial**

Predsol-N® (UCB Pharma) PoM

Drops (for ear or eye), prednisolone sodium phosphate 0.5%, neomycin sulphate 0.5%. Net price 10 mL = £2.36
Excipients include benzalkonium chloride, disodium edetate

Dose

Ear, instil 2–3 drops 3–4 times daily

◢ **Anti-infective preparations**

◢ **CHLORAMPHENICOL** ◢

Cautions avoid prolonged use (see notes above)

Side-effects high incidence of sensitivity reactions to vehicle

Licensed use licensed for use in children (age range not specified by manufacturers)

Indication and dose

Bacterial infection in otitis externa (but see notes above); for dose, see under preparation

Chloramphenicol (Non-proprietary) PoM ◢

Ear drops, chloramphenicol in propylene glycol, net price 5%, 10 mL = £1.83; 10%, 10 mL = £5.62
Excipients include propylene glycol

Dose

Ear, instil 2–3 drops 2–3 times daily

◢ **CLOTRIMAZOLE**

Side-effects occasional local irritation or sensitivity

Licensed use licensed for use in children (age range not specified by manufacturer)

Indication and dose

Fungal infection in otitis externa (see notes above); for dose, see under preparation

Canesten® (Bayer Consumer Care)

Solution, clotrimazole 1% in polyethylene glycol 400 (macrogol 400). Net price 20 mL = £2.43

Dose

Ear, apply 2–3 times daily continuing for at least 14 days after disappearance of infection

◢ **FRAMYCETIN SULPHATE**

Cautions avoid prolonged use (see notes above)

Contra-indications perforated tympanic membrane (see p. 643)

Side-effects local sensitivity

12

Ear, nose, and oropharynx

◁ **FRAMYCETIN SULPHATE** (*continued*)

Indication and dose

Bacterial infection in otitis externa (see notes above)

Eye section 11.3.1

◀**With corticosteroid**
Sofradex®
see Dexamethasone, p. 644

▰ GENTAMICIN

Cautions avoid prolonged use (see notes above)
Contra-indications perforated tympanic membrane (but see p. 643 and section 12.1.2)
Side-effects local sensitivity
Licensed use licensed for use in children (age range not specified by manufacturer)

Indication and dose

Bacterial infection in otitis externa (see notes above); for dose, see under preparations

Genticin® (Amdipharm) [PoM]
Drops (for ear or eye), gentamicin 0.3% (as sulphate). Net price 10 mL = £1.78
Excipients include benzalkonium chloride

Dose
Ear, instil 2–3 drops 3–4 times daily and at night; eye, section 11.3.1

◀**With corticosteroid**
Gentisone® HC
see Hydrocortisone, p. 645

▰ NEOMYCIN SULPHATE

Cautions avoid prolonged use (see notes above)
Contra-indications perforated tympanic membrane (see p. 643)
Side-effects local sensitivity

Indication and dose

Bacterial infection in otitis externa (see notes above)

◀**With corticosteroid**
Betnesol-N® [PoM]
see Betamethasone, p. 644

Otomize®
see Dexamethasone, p. 644

Otosporin®
see Hydrocortisone, p. 645

Predsol-N®
see Prednisolone, p. 645

Vistamethasone N® [PoM]
see Betamethasone, p. 644

---

12 Ear, nose, and oropharynx

12.1.2 Otitis media

Acute otitis media Acute otitis media is the commonest cause of severe aural pain in young children and may occur with even minor upper respiratory tract infections. Children diagnosed with acute otitis media should not be prescribed antibacterials routinely as many infections, especially those accompanying coryza, are caused by viruses. Most uncomplicated cases resolve without antibacterial treatment and a **simple analgesic**, such as paracetamol, may be sufficient. In children without systemic features, a **systemic antibacterial** (Table 1, section 5.1) may be started after 72 hours if there is no improvement, or earlier if there is deterioration, if the child is systemically unwell, if the child is at high risk of serious complications (e.g. in immunosuppression, cystic fibrosis), if mastoiditis is present, or in children under 2 years of age with bilateral otitis media. Perforation of the tympanic membrane in children with *acute otitis media* usually heals spontaneously without treatment; if there is no improvement, e.g. pain or discharge persists, a systemic antibacterial (Table 1, section 5.1) can be given. Topical antibacterial treatment of acute otitis media is ineffective and there is no place for ear drops containing a local anaesthetic.

Otitis media with effusion Otitis media with effusion ('glue ear') occurs in about 10% of children and in 90% of children with cleft palates. Antimicrobials, corticosteroids, decongestants, and antihistamines have little place in the routine management of otitis media with effusion. If 'glue ear' persists for more than a month or two, the child should be referred for assessment and follow up because of the risk of long-term hearing impairment which can delay language development. Untreated or resistant glue ear may be responsible for some types of *chronic otitis media*.

Chronic otitis media   Opportunistic organisms are often present in the debris, keratin, and necrotic bone of the middle ear and mastoid in children with chronic otitis media. The mainstay of treatment is thorough cleansing with aural micro-suction, which may completely resolve long-standing infection. Cleansing may be followed by topical treatment as for otitis externa (section 12.1.1); this is particularly beneficial for discharging ears or infections of the mastoid cavity. Acute exacerbations of chronic infection may require treatment with an oral antibacterial (Table 1, section 5.1); a swab should be taken to identify infecting organisms and antibacterial sensitivity. Parenteral antibacterial treatment is required if *Pseudomonas aeruginosa* or *Proteus spp.* are present.

The CSM has stated that topical treatment with ototoxic antibacterials is contraindicated in the presence of a perforation (section 12.1.1). However, many specialists use ear drops containing **aminoglycosides** (e.g. neomycin) or **polymyxins** if the otitis media has failed to settle with systemic antibacterials; it is considered that the pus in the middle ear associated with otitis media carries a higher risk of ototoxicity than the drops themselves. **Ciprofloxacin** or **ofloxacin** ear drops (available from specialist importing companies) or eye drops used in the ear [unlicensed indication] are an effective alternative to aminoglycoside ear drops for chronic otitis media in patients with perforation of the tympanic membrane.

12.1.3 Removal of ear wax

Ear wax (cerumen) is a normal bodily secretion which provides a protective film on the meatal skin and need only be removed if it causes hearing loss or interferes with a proper view of the ear drum. Irrigation of the ear canal is generally best avoided in young children and in children with a history of recurrent otitis externa, a history of ear-drum perforation, previous ear surgery, or unilateral deafness.

Ear wax causing discomfort or impaired hearing may be softened with simple remedies such as **olive oil** ear drops or **almond oil** ear drops; **sodium bicarbonate** ear drops are also effective but may cause dryness of the ear canal. If the wax is hard and impacted the drops may be used twice daily for a few days before syringing or cleansing with aural microsuction. The child should lie with the affected ear uppermost for 5 to 10 minutes after a generous amount of the softening remedy has been introduced into the ear. Proprietary preparations containing organic solvents can irritate the meatal skin, and in most cases the simple remedies indicated above are just as effective and less likely to cause irritation. Docusate sodium or urea hydrogen peroxide are ingredients in a number of proprietary preparations for softening ear wax.

For administration of ear drops, see p. 643.

Almond Oil (Non-proprietary)
Ear drops, almond oil in a suitable container
Allow to warm to room temperature before use

Olive Oil (Non-proprietary)
Ear drops, olive oil in a suitable container
Allow to warm to room temperature before use

Sodium Bicarbonate (Non-proprietary)
Ear drops, sodium bicarbonate 5%, net price 10 mL = £1.25

Cerumol® (Thornton & Ross) ▰
Ear drops, chlorobutanol 5%, arachis (peanut) oil 57.3%. Net price 11 mL = £1.76

Exterol® (Dermal) ▰
Ear drops, urea–hydrogen peroxide complex 5% in glycerol. Net price 8 mL = £1.83

Molcer® (Wallace Mfg) ▰
Ear drops, docusate sodium 5%. Net price 15 mL = £1.90
Excipients include propylene glycol

Otex® (DDD) ▰
Ear drops, urea–hydrogen peroxide 5%. Net price 8 mL = £2.64

Waxsol® (Norgine) ▰
Ear drops, docusate sodium 0.5%. Net price 10 mL = £1.26

12.2 Drugs acting on the nose

12.2.1 Drugs used in nasal allergy
12.2.2 Topical nasal decongestants
12.2.3 Nasal preparations for infection

Rhinitis is often self-limiting but bacterial sinusitis may require treatment with antibacterials (Table 1, section 5.1). Many nasal preparations contain sympatho-

12

Ear, nose, and oropharynx

mimetic drugs (section 12.2.2) which can give rise to rebound congestion (*rhinitis medicamentosa*) and may damage the nasal cilia. **Sodium chloride 0.9% solution** may be used as a douche or 'sniff' following endonasal surgery.

Administration   To administer nasal drops, lay the child face-upward with the neck extended, instil the drops, then sit the child up and tilt the head forward.

Nasal polyps   Short-term use of corticosteroid nasal drops helps to shrink nasal polyps; to be effective, the drops must be administered with the child in the 'head down' position. A short course of a systemic corticosteroid (section 6.3.2) may be required initially to shrink large polyps. A corticosteroid nasal spray can be used to maintain the reduction in swelling and also for the initial treatment of small polyps.

12.2.1   Drugs used in nasal allergy

Mild allergic rhinitis is controlled by **antihistamines** (see also section 3.4.1) or topical **nasal corticosteroids**; systemic nasal decongestants (section 3.10) are not recommended for use in children. Topical nasal decongestants can be used for a short period to relieve congestion and allow penetration of a topical nasal corticosteroid.

More persistent symptoms can be relieved by topical nasal **corticosteroids** or **cromoglicate**; the topical antihistamine, **azelastine**, is useful for controlling breakthrough symptoms in allergic rhinitis. Azelastine is less effective than nasal corticosteroids, but probably more effective than sodium cromoglicate. In seasonal allergic rhinitis (e.g. hay fever), treatment should begin 2 to 3 weeks before the season commences and may have to be continued for several months; continuous long-term treatment may be required in perennial rhinitis.

Monteleukast (section 3.3.2) can be used in children with seasonal allergic rhinitis (unresponsive to other treatments) and concomitant asthma; montelukast is less effective than topical nasal corticosteroids.

Children with disabling symptoms of seasonal rhinitis (e.g. students taking important examinations), may be treated with oral **corticosteroids** (section 6.3.2) for short periods. Oral corticosteroids may also be used at the beginning of a course of treatment with a corticosteroid spray to relieve severe mucosal oedema and allow the spray to penetrate the nasal mucosa.

Sometimes allergic rhinitis is accompanied by vasomotor rhinitis. In this situation, the addition of topical nasal **ipratropium bromide** (section 12.2.2) can reduce watery rhinorrhoea.

Pregnancy   If a pregnant woman cannot tolerate the symptoms of allergic rhinitis, treatment with nasal beclometasone, budesonide, fluticasone propionate, or sodium cromoglicate may be considered.

Antihistamines

▲ AZELASTINE HYDROCHLORIDE

Side-effects   irritation of nasal mucosa; bitter taste (if applied incorrectly)

Indication and dose

Treatment of allergic rhinitis for dose, see under preparation

Rhinolast® (Viatris) [PoM]
Nasal spray, azelastine hydrochloride 140 micrograms (0.14 mL)/metered spray. Net price 22 mL (with metered pump) = £11.09
Excipients include sodium edetate

Dose

> **Child 5–18 years** apply 140 micrograms (1 spray) into each nostril twice daily

Note Preparations of azelastine hydrochloride can be sold to the public for nasal administration in aqueous form (other than by aerosol) for the treatment of seasonal allergic rhinitis or perennial allergic rhinitis in children over 5 years, subject to max. single dose of 140 micrograms per nostril, max. daily dose of 280 micrograms per nostril, and a pack size limit of 36 doses

Corticosteroids

Nasal preparations containing corticosteroids have a useful role in the prophylaxis and treatment of allergic rhinitis (see notes above). Preparations containing budesonide, fluticasone propionate, mometasone, or triamcinolone are preferred in children.

Cautions   Corticosteroid nasal preparations should be avoided in the presence of untreated nasal infections, and also after nasal surgery (until healing has occurred); they should also be avoided in pulmonary tuberculosis. Systemic absorption may follow nasal administration particularly if high doses are used or if treatment is prolonged; for cautions and side-effects of systemic corticosteroids, see section 6.3.2. The risk of systemic effects may be greater with nasal drops than with nasal sprays; drops are administered incorrectly more often than sprays. The CSM recommends that the height of children receiving prolonged treatment with nasal corticosteroids is monitored; if growth is slowed, referral to a paediatrician should be considered.

Side-effects   Local side-effects include dryness, irritation of nose and throat, and epistaxis. Nasal ulceration has been reported, and occurs commonly with nasal preparations containing fluticasone furoate or mometasone furoate. Nasal septal perforation (usually following nasal surgery) occurs very rarely. Raised intra-ocular pressure or glaucoma may occur rarely. Headache, smell and taste disturbances may also occur. Hypersensitivity reactions, including bronchospasm, have been reported.

BECLOMETASONE DIPROPIONATE
(Beclomethasone Dipropionate)

Cautions   see notes above

Side-effects   see notes above

Indication and dose

Prophylaxis and treatment of allergic and vasomotor rhinitis

Child 6–18 years apply 100 micrograms (2 sprays) into each nostril twice daily; max. total 400 micrograms (8 sprays) daily; when symptoms controlled, dose reduced to 50 micrograms (1 spray) into each nostril twice daily

Beclometasone (Non-proprietary) ᴘᴏᴹ

Nasal spray, beclometasone dipropionate 50 micrograms/metered spray. Net price 200-spray unit = £2.89

Brands include *Nasobec Aqueous®*

Beconase® (A&H) ᴘᴏᴹ

Nasal spray (aqueous suspension), beclometasone dipropionate 50 micrograms/metered spray. Net price 200-spray unit with applicator = £2.19

Excipients include benzalkonium chloride, polysorbate 80

BETAMETHASONE SODIUM PHOSPHATE

Cautions   see notes above

Side-effects   see notes above

Licensed use   licensed for use in children (age range not specified by manufacturer)

Indication and dose

Non-infected inflammatory conditions of nose for dose, see under preparations

Eye section 11.4.1

Ear section 12.1.1

Betnesol® (UCB Pharma) ᴘᴏᴹ

Drops (for ear, eye, or nose), betamethasone sodium phosphate 0.1%, net price 10 mL = £2.32

Excipients include benzalkonium chloride, disodium edetate

Dose

Nose, instil 2–3 drops into each nostril 2–3 times daily

Vistamethasone® (Martindale) ᴘᴏᴹ

Drops (for ear, eye, or nose), betamethasone sodium phosphate 0.1%. Net price 5 mL = £1.02, 10 mL = £1.16

Excipients include benzalkonium chloride, disodium edetate

Dose

Nose, instil 2–3 drops into each nostril twice daily

BUDESONIDE

Cautions   see notes above; interactions: Appendix 1 (corticosteroids)

Side-effects   see notes above

Indication and dose

See under preparations

12 Ear, nose, and oropharynx

◁ **BUDESONIDE** (*continued*)

Budesonide (Non-proprietary) PoM

Nasal spray, budesonide 100 micrograms/metered spray, net price 100-spray unit = £5.66

Dose

Prophylaxis and treatment of allergic and vasomotor rhinitis

Child 12–18 years apply 200 micrograms (2 sprays) into each nostril once daily in the morning *or* 100 micrograms (1 spray) into each nostril twice daily; when control achieved reduce to 100 micrograms (1 spray) into each nostril once daily

Nasal polyps

Child 12–18 years apply 100 micrograms (1 spray) into each nostril twice daily for up to 3 months

Rhinocort Aqua® (AstraZeneca) PoM

Nasal spray, budesonide 64 micrograms/metered spray. Net price 120-spray unit = £4.49
Excipients include disodium edetate, polysorbate 80, potassium sorbate

Dose

Rhinitis

Child 12–18 years 128 micrograms (2 sprays) into each nostril once daily in the morning *or* 64 micrograms (1 spray) into each nostril twice daily; when control achieved reduce to 64 micrograms (1 spray) into each nostril once daily; max. duration of treatment 3 months

Nasal polyps

Child 12–18 years 64 micrograms (1 spray) into each nostril twice daily for up to 3 months

---

▗ FLUNISOLIDE

Cautions see notes above

Side-effects see notes above

Indication and dose

Prophylaxis and treatment of allergic rhinitis

Child 5–14 years initially 25 micrograms (1 spray) into each nostril up to 3 times daily then reduced for maintenance

Child 14–18 years 50 micrograms (2 sprays) into each nostril twice daily, increased if necessary to max. 3 times daily then reduced for maintenance

Syntaris® (IVAX) PoM

Aqueous nasal spray, flunisolide 25 micrograms/metered spray. Net price 240-spray unit with pump and applicator = £5.05
Excipients include benzalkonium chloride, butylated hydroxytoluene, disodium edetate, polysorbate 20, propylene glycol

---

▗ FLUTICASONE PROPIONATE

Cautions see notes above; **interactions:** Appendix 1 (corticosteroids)

Side-effects see notes above

Indication and dose

Prophylaxis and treatment of allergic rhinitis

Child 4–12 years 50 micrograms (1 spray) into each nostril once daily, preferably in the morning, increased to max. twice daily if required

Child 12–18 years 100 micrograms (2 sprays) into each nostril once daily, preferably in the morning, increased to max. twice daily if required; when control achieved reduce to 50 micrograms (1 spray) into each nostril once daily

Nasal polyps see *Flixonase Nasule®* below

Flixonase® (A&H) PoM

Aqueous nasal spray, fluticasone propionate 50 micrograms/metered spray. Net price 150-spray unit with applicator = £11.69
Excipients include benzalkonium chloride, polysorbate 80

Flixonase Nasule® (A&H) PoM

Nasal drops, fluticasone propionate 400 micrograms/unit dose, net price 28 × 0.4-mL units = £13.76
Excipients include polysorbate 20

Dose

Nasal polyps

Child 16–18 years instil 200 micrograms (approx. 6 drops) into each nostril once or twice daily; consider alternative treatment if no improvement after 4–6 weeks

Nasofan® (IVAX) PoM

Aqueous nasal spray, fluticasone propionate 50 micrograms/metered spray. Net price 150-spray unit = £10.52
Excipients include benzalkonium chloride, polysorbate 80

◀ **Fluticasone furoate**

Avamys® (GSK) ▼ PoM

Nasal spray, fluticasone furoate 27.5 micrograms/metered spray, net price 120-spray unit = £6.44
Excipients include benzalkonium chloride, disodium edetate, polysorbate 80

Dose

Prophylaxis and treatment of allergic rhinitis

Child 6–12 years 27.5 micrograms (1 spray) into each nostril once daily, increased if necessary to 55 micrograms (2 sprays) into each nostril once daily; when control achieved reduce to 27.5 micrograms (1 spray) into each nostril once daily

Child 12–18 years 55 micrograms (2 sprays) into each nostril once daily; when control achieved reduce to 27.5 micrograms (1 spray) into each nostril once daily

▲ MOMETASONE FUROATE

Cautions see notes above
Side-effects see notes above

Indication and dose
　See under preparation

Nasonex® (Schering-Plough) ⒫ⓄⓂ
　Nasal spray, mometasone furoate 50 micrograms/
　metered spray. Net price 140-spray unit = £7.83
　Excipients include benzalkonium chloride, polysorbate 80

Dose
　Prophylaxis and treatment of allergic rhinitis
　　Child 6–12 years 50 micrograms (1 spray) into each
　　nostril once daily
　　Child 12–18 years 100 micrograms (2 sprays) into
　　each nostril once daily, increased if necessary to max.
　　200 micrograms (4 sprays) into each nostril once daily;
　　when control achieved reduce to 50 micrograms (1
　　spray) into each nostril once daily

▲ TRIAMCINOLONE ACETONIDE

Cautions see notes above
Side-effects see notes above

Indication and dose
　Treatment of allergic rhinitis

Child 6–12 years 55 micrograms (1 spray) into each
　nostril once daily, increased if necessary to
　110 micrograms (2 sprays) into each nostril once
　daily; when control achieved reduce to
　55 micrograms (1 spray) into each nostril once
　daily; max. duration of treatment 3 months

Child 12–18 years 110 micrograms (2 sprays)
into each nostril once daily; when control
achieved, reduce to 55 micrograms (1 spray)
into each nostril once daily

Nasacort® (Aventis Pharma) ⒫ⓄⓂ
　Aqueous nasal spray, triamcinolone acetonide
　55 micrograms/metered spray. Net price 120-spray
　unit = £7.39
　Excipients include benzalkonium chloride, disodium edetate,
　polysorbate 80

＝＝＝ Cromoglicate

▲ SODIUM CROMOGLICATE

　(Sodium Cromoglycate)
Side-effects local irritation; rarely transient
bronchospasm
Licensed use licensed for use in children (age
range not specified by manufacturers)

Indication and dose
　Prophylaxis of allergic rhinitis for dose, see
　under preparations

Rynacrom® (Sanofi-Aventis)
　4% aqueous nasal spray, sodium cromoglicate 4%
　(5.2 mg/spray). Net price 22 mL with pump =
　£17.76
　Excipients include benzalkonium chloride, disodium edetate
Dose
　Nose, 1 spray into each nostril 2–4 times daily

Vividrin® (Pharma-Global)
　Nasal spray, sodium cromoglicate 2%. Net price
　15 mL = £10.35
　Excipients include benzalkonium chloride, edetic acid, poly-
　sorbate 80
Dose
　Nose, 1 spray into each nostril 4–6 times daily

12.2.2 Topical nasal decongestants

Sodium chloride 0.9% given as nasal drops may relieve nasal congestion by
helping to liquefy mucous secretions in children with rhinitis. In infants, 1–2 drops
of sodium chloride 0.9% solution in each nostril before feeds will help relieve
congestion and allow more effective suckling.

Inhalation of **warm moist air** is useful in the treatment of symptoms of acute
nasal congestion in infants and children, but the use of boiling water for steam
inhalation is dangerous for children and should **not** be recommended. Volatile
substances (section 3.8) such as menthol and eucalyptus may encourage inhalation of warm moist air.

Topical nasal decongestants containing sympathomimetics can cause rebound
congestion (*rhinitis medicamentosa*) following prolonged use (more than 7 days),
and are therefore of limited value in the treatment of nasal congestion.

Ephedrine nasal drops is the least likely of the sympathomimetic nasal
decongestants to cause rebound congestion and can provide relief for several
hours. The more potent sympathomimetic drugs **oxymetazoline** and **xylometazoline** are more likely to cause a rebound effect.

The CHM/MHRA has stated that non-prescription cough and cold medicines containing ephedrine, oxymetazoline, or xylometazoline can be considered in children aged 6–12 years after basic principals of best care have been tried; these medicines should not be used in children under 6 years of age (section 3.9.1). However, in special circumstances, some specialists prescribe nasal drops containing ephedrine or xylometazoline to children under 6 years of age for the short-term treatment of severe nasal obstruction that has not responded to sodium chloride 0.9% nose drops and inhalation of warm moist air.

Non-allergic watery rhinorrhoea often responds well to treatment with the antimuscarinic **ipratropium bromide**.

Recurrent, persistent bleeding may respond to the use of a sympathomimetic nasal spray; if infection is present, chlorhexidine and neomycin (*Naseptin®*) cream (section 12.2.3) may be effective.

Systemic nasal decongestants—see section 3.10.

Sinusitis and oral pain   Sinusitis affecting the maxillary antrum can cause pain in the upper jaw. Where this is associated with blockage of the opening from the sinus into the nasal cavity, it may be helpful to relieve the congestion with inhalation of warm moist air (section 3.8) or with **ephedrine nasal drops** (see above). For antibacterial treatment of sinusitis, see Table 1, section 5.1.

Sympathomimetics

EPHEDRINE HYDROCHLORIDE

Cautions   see notes above; also avoid excessive or prolonged use; caution in infants under 3 months (no good evidence of value—if irritation occurs might narrow nasal passage); **interactions:** Appendix 1 (sympathomimetics)

Side-effects   local irritation, nausea, headache; after excessive use tolerance with diminished effect, rebound congestion; cardiovascular effects also reported

Licensed use   not licensed for use in children under 3 months

Indication and dose

Nasal congestion (see notes above)

Child 1–3 months (on a specialist's advice only) instil 1–2 drops (0.25% strength) into each nostril 3–4 times daily, 15 minutes before feeds; max. duration 5 days

Child 3 months–18 years (on a specialist's advice only for children under 6 years) instil 1–2 drops (0.5% strength) into each nostril 3–4 times daily; max. duration 5 days (7 days in child over 12 years of age)

¹**Ephedrine** (Non-proprietary)
Nasal drops, ephedrine hydrochloride 0.5%, net price 10 mL = £1.25; 1%, 10 mL = £1.31

Note Ephedrine 0.25% nasal solution is prepared by diluting ephedrine 0.5% solution with sodium chloride 0.9% solution. Discard diluted solution after 1 week. The BP directs that if no strength is specified 0.5% drops should be supplied

Dental prescribing on NHS Ephedrine nasal drops may be prescribed

1. Can be sold to the public provided no more than 180 mg of ephedrine base (or salts) are supplied at one time, and pseudoephedrine salts are not supplied at the same time; for details see *Medicines, Ethics and Practice*, No. 32, London, Pharmaceutical Press, 2008 (and subsequent editions as available)

XYLOMETAZOLINE HYDROCHLORIDE

Cautions   see under Ephedrine Hydrochloride and notes above

Side-effects   see under Ephedrine Hydrochloride and notes above

Indication and dose

Nasal congestion for dose, see under preparations

Xylometazoline (Non-proprietary)
Nasal drops, xylometazoline hydrochloride 0.1%, net price 10 mL = £1.91

Dose

Child 12–18 years instil 2–3 drops into each nostril 2–3 times daily when required; max. duration 7 days

Brands include *Otradrops®, Otrivine®* ᴺᴴˢ

Paediatric nasal drops, xylometazoline hydrochloride 0.05%, net price 10 mL = £1.59

Dose

Child 3 months–12 years (on a specialist's advice only for children under 6 years) instil 1–2 drops into each nostril 1–2 times daily when required; max. duration 5 days

Brands include *Otradrops®, Otrivine®* ᴺᴴˢ, *Tixycolds®*

Nasal spray, xylometazoline hydrochloride 0.1%, net price 10 mL = £1.91

Dose

Child 12–18 years apply 1 spray into each nostril 2–3 times daily when required; max. duration 7 days

Brands include *Otraspray®, Otrivine®* ᴺᴴˢ

Ear, nose, and oropharynx

12

Antimuscarinic

▲ IPRATROPIUM BROMIDE

Cautions see section 3.1.2; avoid spraying near eyes

Side-effects epistaxis, nasal dryness, and irritation; less frequently nausea, headache, and pharyngitis; *very rarely* antimuscarinic effects such as gastro-intestinal motility disturbances, palpitations, and urinary retention

Indication and dose

> Rhinorrhoea associated with allergic and non-allergic rhinitis

> **Child 12–18 years** apply 42 micrograms (2 sprays) into each nostril 2–3 times daily

> **Asthma and reversible airways obstruction** section 3.1.2

Rinatec® (Boehringer Ingelheim) [PoM]
Nasal spray 0.03%, ipratropium bromide 21 micrograms/metered spray. Net price 180-dose unit = £4.55
Excipients include benzalkonium chloride, disodium edetate

12.2.3 Nasal preparations for infection

There is **no** evidence that topical anti-infective nasal preparations have any therapeutic value in rhinitis or sinusitis; for elimination of nasal staphylococci, see below. Acute complications such as periorbital cellulitis require hospital treatment. For systemic treatment of sinusitis, see Table 1, section 5.1.

Betnesol-N® (UCB Pharma) [PoM] ◢
Drops (for ear, eye, or nose), betamethasone sodium phosphate 0.1%, neomycin sulphate 0.5%. Net price 10 mL = £2.39
Excipients include benzalkonium chloride, disodium edetate

Dose

> *Nose*, instil 2–3 drops into each nostril 2–3 times daily

Note *Betnesol-N®* licensed for use in children (age range not specified by manufacturer)

Vistamethasone N® (Martindale) [PoM] ◢
Drops (for ear, eye, or nose), betamethasone sodium phosphate 0.1%, neomycin sulphate 0.5%. Net price 5 mL = £1.09, 10 mL = £1.20
Excipients include thiomersal

Dose

> *Nose*, instil 2–3 drops into each nostril twice daily

Note *Vistamethasone N®* licensed for use in children (age range not specified by manufacturer)

Nasal staphylococci

Elimination of organisms such as staphylococci from the nasal vestibule can be achieved by the use of a cream containing **chlorhexidine** and **neomycin** (*Naseptin®*), but re-colonisation frequently occurs. Coagulase-positive staphylococci are present in the noses of 40% of the population. A nasal ointment containing **mupirocin** is also available; it should probably be held in reserve for resistant infections. In hospitals or in care establishments, mupirocin nasal ointment should be reserved for the *eradication* (in both patients and staff) of nasal carriage of meticillin-resistant *Staphylococcus aureus* (MRSA). The ointment should be applied 3 times daily for 5 days and a sample taken 2 days after treatment to confirm eradication. The course may be repeated if the sample is positive (and the throat is not colonised). To avoid the development of resistance, the treatment course should not exceed 7 days and the course should not be repeated on more than one occasion. If the MRSA strain is mupirocin-resistant or does not respond after 2 courses, consider alternative products such as chlorhexidine and neomycin cream. For eradication of MRSA also consult local infection control policy. See section 13.10.1 for treatment of MRSA-infected open wounds. See section 5.1.1.2 for *treatment* of children with MRSA-positive throat swabs or systemic MRSA infection.

Bactroban Nasal® (GSK) [PoM]
Nasal ointment, mupirocin 2% (as calcium salt) in white soft paraffin basis. Net price 3 g = £5.80

Dose

> For eradication of nasal carriage of staphylococci, including meticillin-resistant *Staphylococcus aureus* (MRSA)
>
> > Apply 2–3 times daily to the inner surface of each nostril (see notes above)

Naseptin® (Alliance) [PoM]
Cream, chlorhexidine hydrochloride 0.1%, neomycin sulphate 0.5%, net price 15 g = £1.58
Excipients include arachis (peanut) oil, cetostearyl alcohol

Dose

> For eradication of nasal carriage of staphylococci
>
> > Apply to nostrils 4 times daily for 10 days

> For preventing nasal carriage of staphylococci
>
> > Apply to nostrils twice daily

12 Ear, nose, and oropharynx

12.3 Drugs acting on the oropharynx

12.3.1 Drugs for oral ulceration and inflammation
12.3.2 Oropharyngeal anti-infective drugs
12.3.3 Lozenges and sprays
12.3.4 Mouthwashes and gargles
12.3.5 Treatment of dry mouth

12.3.1 Drugs for oral ulceration and inflammation

Ulceration of the oral mucosa may be caused by trauma (physical or chemical), recurrent aphthous ulcers, infections, carcinoma, dermatological disorders, nutritional deficiencies, gastro-intestinal disease, haematopoietic disorders, and drug therapy. It is important to establish the diagnosis in each case as the majority of these lesions require specific management in addition to local treatment. Local treatment aims to protect the ulcerated area, to relieve pain, to reduce inflammation, or to control secondary infection. Children with an unexplained mouth ulcer of more than 3 weeks' duration require urgent referral to hospital to exclude secondary causes such as leukaemia.

Simple mouthwashes A **saline** mouthwash (section 12.3.4) may relieve the pain of traumatic ulceration. The mouthwash is made up with warm water and used at frequent intervals until the discomfort and swelling subsides.

Antiseptic mouthwashes Secondary bacterial infection may be a feature of any mucosal ulceration; it can increase discomfort and delay healing. Use of **chlorhexidine** mouthwash (section 12.3.4) is often beneficial and may accelerate healing of recurrent aphthous ulcers.

Mechanical protection **Carmellose gelatin paste** may relieve some discomfort arising from ulceration by protecting the ulcer site. As the paste adheres to dry mucosa, it is difficult to apply effectively to the tongue and oropharynx.

Corticosteroids Topical corticosteroid therapy may be used for some forms of oral ulceration; for aphthous ulcers it is most effective if applied in the 'prodromal' phase. Thrush or other types of candidiasis are recognised complications of corticosteroid treatment.

Hydrocortisone oromucosal tablets are useful in recurrent aphthous ulcers and erosive lichenoid lesions.

Triamcinolone dental paste is formulated to keep the corticosteroid in contact with the mucosa for long enough to permit penetration of the lesion. As the paste adheres to dry mucosa, it is difficult to apply effectively to the tongue and oropharynx.

Beclometasone dipropionate inhaler (p. 185) 50–100 micrograms sprayed twice daily on the oral mucosa is used to manage oral ulceration [unlicensed indication]. Alternatively, **betamethasone** soluble tablets dissolved in water, can be used as a mouthwash to treat oral ulceration.

Systemic corticosteroid therapy (section 6.3.2) is reserved for severe conditions such as pemphigus vulgaris.

Local analgesics Local analgesics have a limited role in the management of oral ulceration. When applied topically their action is of a relatively short duration and analgesia cannot be maintained continuously throughout the day. When local anaesthetics are used in the mouth, care must be taken not to produce anaesthesia of the pharynx before meals as this might lead to choking.

Benzydamine mouthwash or spray may be useful in reducing the discomfort associated with a variety of ulcerative conditions. It has also been found to be effective in reducing the discomfort of tonsillectomy and post-irradiation mucositis. Some children find the full-strength mouthwash causes some stinging and, for them, it should be diluted with an equal volume of water.

Flurbiprofen lozenges are licensed for the relief of sore throat in adolescents.

Choline salicylate dental gel has some analgesic action and may provide relief for recurrent aphthous ulcers in children over 16 years of age.

Periodontitis Low-dose **doxycycline** (*Periostat®*) is licensed as an adjunct to scaling and root planing for the treatment of periodontitis in children over 12 years; a low dose of doxycycline reduces collagenase activity without inhibiting bacteria associated with periodontitis. For anti-infectives used in the treatment of destructive (refractory) forms of periodontal disease, see section 12.3.2 and Table 1, section 5.1. For mouthwashes used for oral hygiene and plaque inhibition, see section 12.3.4.

BENZYDAMINE HYDROCHLORIDE

Side-effects occasional numbness or stinging; rarely hypersensitivity reactions

Licensed use *Difflam® Spray* licensed for use in children (age range not specified by manufacturer)

Indication and dose

Painful inflammatory conditions of oropharynx
for dose, see under preparations

Difflam® (3M)

Oral rinse, green, benzydamine hydrochloride 0.15%, net price 200 mL (*Difflam® Sore Throat Rinse*) = £2.63; 300 mL = £4.01

Dose

Child 12–18 years rinse or gargle, using 15 mL (dilute with an equal volume of water if stinging occurs) every 1½–3 hours as required, usually for not more than 7 days

Dental prescribing on NHS May be prescribed as Benzydamine Mouthwash 0.15%

Spray, benzydamine hydrochloride 0.15%. Net price 30-mL unit = £3.17

Dose

Child under 6 years 1 puff per 4 kg body-weight to max. 4 puffs onto affected area every 1½–3 hours

Child 6–12 years 4 puffs onto affected area every 1½–3 hours

Child 12–18 years 4–8 puffs onto affected area every 1½–3 hours

Dental prescribing on NHS May be prescribed as Benzydamine Oromucosal Spray 0.15%

CARMELLOSE SODIUM

Licensed use licensed for use in children (age range not specified by manufacturer)

Indication and dose

Mechanical protection of oral and perioral lesions for dose, see under preparation

Orabase® (ConvaTec)

Protective paste (= oral paste), carmellose sodium 16.7%, pectin 16.7%, gelatin 16.7%, in *Plastibase®*. Net price 30 g = £2.02; 100 g = £4.48

Dose

Apply a thin layer when necessary after meals

Dental prescribing on NHS May be prescribed as Carmellose Gelatin Paste

CORTICOSTEROIDS

Contra-indications untreated oral infection; manufacturer of triamcinolone contra-indicates use on tuberculous and viral lesions

Side-effects occasional exacerbation of local infection; thrush or other candidal infections

Licensed use *Adcortyl in Orabase®* licensed for use in children (age range not specified by manufacturer); *Corlan® Pellets* licensed for use in children (under 12 years—on medical advice only)

Indication and dose

Oral and perioral lesions for dose, see under preparations

Adcortyl in Orabase® (Squibb) PoM

Oral paste, triamcinolone acetonide 0.1% in adhesive basis. Net price 10 g = £1.18

Dose

Apply a thin layer 2–4 times daily for max. 5 days; do not rub in

Dental prescribing on NHS May be prescribed as Triamcinolone Dental Paste

Note A 5-g tube is on sale to the public for the treatment of common mouth ulcers for max. 5 days

Betnesol® (UCB Pharma) PoM

Soluble tablets, pink, scored, betamethasone 500 micrograms (as sodium phosphate), net price 100-tab pack = £5.17. Label: 10, steroid card, 13, 21

Dose

Oral ulceration

Child 12–18 years 500 micrograms dissolved in 20 ml water and rinsed around the mouth 4 times daily; not to be swallowed

Dental prescribing on NHS May be prescribed as Betamethasone Soluble Tablets 500 micrograms

12

Ear, nose, and oropharynx

◻ **CORTICOSTEROIDS (continued)**

Corlan® (UCB Pharma)
Pellets (= oromucosal tablets), hydrocortisone 2.5 mg (as sodium succinate). Net price 20 = £2.54

Dose
> 1 lozenge 4 times daily, allowed to dissolve slowly in the mouth in contact with the ulcer

Dental prescribing on NHS May be prescribed as Hydrocortisone Oromucosal Tablets

---

◢ DOXYCYCLINE

Cautions section 5.1.3; monitor for superficial fungal infection, particularly if predisposition to oral candidiasis

Contra-indications section 5.1.3

Side-effects section 5.1.3; fungal superinfection

Indication and dose
> See under preparations

> **Oral herpes** section 12.3.2

> **Other indications** section 5.1.3

Periostat® (Alliance) [PoM]
Tablets, f/c, doxycycline (as hyclate) 20 mg, net price 56-tab pack = £16.50. Label: 6, 11, 27, counselling, posture

Dose
> **Periodontitis (as an adjunct to gingival scaling and root planing)**
> **Child 12–18 years** 20 mg twice daily for 3 months

> **Counselling** Tablets should be swallowed whole with plenty of fluid, while sitting or standing
> **Dental prescribing on NHS** May be prescribed as Doxycycline Tablets 20 mg

◢ **Local application**
For severe recurrent aphthous ulceration, the contents of a 100 mg doxycycline capsule can be stirred into a small amount of water then rinsed around the mouth for 2–3 minutes 4 times daily usually for 3 days; it should preferably not be swallowed [unlicensed indication].
Note Doxycycline stains teeth; avoid in children under 12 years of age

---

◢ FLURBIPROFEN

Cautions see section 10.1.1

Contra-indications see section 10.1.1

Side-effects taste disturbance, mouth ulcers (move lozenge around mouth); see also section 10.1.1

Indication and dose
> **Relief of sore throat** for dose, see under preparation

Strefen® (Crookes)
Lozenges, flurbiprofen 8.75 mg, net price 16 = £2.24

Dose
> **Child 12–18 years** allow 1 lozenge to dissolve slowly in the mouth every 3–6 hours, max. 5 lozenges in 24 hours, for max. 3 days

---

◢ SALICYLATES

Cautions frequent application, especially in children, may give rise to salicylate poisoning

Contra-indications children under 16 years
Reyes syndrome The CHM has advised (April 2009) that topical oral pain relief products containing salicylate salts should not be used in children under 16 years, as a cautionary measure due to the theoretical risk of Reyes syndrome

Indication and dose
> **Mild oral and perioral lesions** for dose, see under preparations

◢ **Choline salicylate**
Choline Salicylate Dental Gel, BP
Oral gel, choline salicylate 8.7% in a flavoured gel basis, net price 15 g = £1.89
Brands include *Bonjela®* (sugar-free)

Dose
> **Child 16–18 years** apply ½-inch of gel with gentle massage not more often than every 3 hours

> **Dental prescribing on NHS** Choline Salicylate Dental Gel may be prescribed

◢ **Salicylic acid**
Pyralvex® (Norgine)
Oral paint, brown, rhubarb extract (anthraquinone glycosides 0.5%), salicylic acid 1%. Net price 10 mL with brush = £3.38

Dose
> **Child 16–18 years** apply 3–4 times daily

12.3.2 Oropharyngeal anti-infective drugs

Sore throat is usually a self-limiting condition often caused by viral infection which does not benefit from anti-infective treatment. Adequate analgesia may be all that is required. Systemic **antibacterials** (Table 1, section 5.1) should only be used in severe cases where there is concern for the child's overall clinical condition. Acute ulcerative gingivitis (Vincent's infection) requires treatment with oral **metronidazole** (section 5.1.11).

Benzydamine (section 12.3.1) may be beneficial in relieving pain and dysphagia in children, especially after tonsillectomy or the use of a nasogastric tube.

Oropharyngeal viral infections

Children with varicella–zoster infection often develop painful lesions in the mouth and throat. **Benzydamine** (section 12.3.1) may be used to provide local analgesia. **Chlorhexidine** mouthwash or gel (section 12.3.4) will control plaque accumulation if toothbrushing is painful and will also help to control secondary infection in general.

In severe herpetic stomatitis systemic **aciclovir** or **valaciclovir** (section 5.3.2.1) may be used for oral lesions associated with herpes zoster. Aciclovir and valaciclovir are also used to prevent frequently recurring herpes simplex lesions of the mouth particularly when associated with the initiation of erythema multiforme. For the treatment of labial herpes simplex infections, see section 13.10.3.

Herpes infections of the mouth in children aged over 12 years may also respond to rinsing the mouth with **doxycycline** (section 12.3.1).

Oropharyngeal fungal infections

Fungal infections of the mouth are usually caused by *Candida* spp. (candidiasis or candidosis). Different types of oropharyngeal candidiasis are managed as follows:

Thrush   Acute pseudomembranous candidiasis (thrush), is usually an acute infection but it may persist for months in patients receiving inhaled corticosteroids, cytotoxics, or broad-spectrum antibacterials. Thrush also occurs in patients with serious systemic disease associated with reduced immunity such as leukaemia, other malignancies, and HIV infection. Any predisposing condition should be managed appropriately. When thrush is associated with corticosteroid inhalers, rinsing the mouth with water (or cleaning a child's teeth) immediately after using the inhaler may avoid the problem. Treatment with **nystatin**, **amphotericin**, or **miconazole** may be needed. **Fluconazole** (section 5.2) is effective for unresponsive infections or if a topical antifungal drug cannot be used. Topical therapy may not be adequate in immunocompromised children and an oral triazole antifungal is preferred (section 5.2).

Acute erythematous candidiasis   Acute erythematous (atrophic) candidiasis is a relatively uncommon condition associated with corticosteroid and broad-spectrum antibacterial use and with HIV disease. It is usually treated with **fluconazole** (section 5.2).

Angular cheilitis   Angular cheilitis (angular stomatitis) is characterised by soreness, erythema and fissuring at the angles of the mouth. It may represent a nutritional deficiency or it may be related to orofacial granulomatosis or HIV infection. Both yeasts (*Candida* spp.) and bacteria (*Staphylococcus aureus* and beta-haemolytic streptococci) are commonly involved as interacting, infective factors. While the underlying cause is being identified and treated, it is often helpful to apply **miconazole** and **hydrocortisone** cream or ointment (see p. 674), **miconazole** cream (see p. 711), or **sodium fusidate** ointment (p. 709).

Immunocompromised patients   For advice on prevention of fungal infections in immunocompromised children see p. 362.

For the role of antiseptic mouthwashes in the prevention of oral candidiasis in immunocompromised children, see section 12.3.4.

Drugs used in oropharyngeal candidiasis   **Amphotericin** and **nystatin** are not absorbed from the gastro-intestinal tract and are applied locally (as lozenges or suspension) to the mouth for treating local fungal infections. **Miconazole** is used by local application (as an oral gel) in the mouth but it is also absorbed to the extent that potential interactions need to be considered. Miconazole also has

12 Ear, nose, and oropharynx

some activity against Gram-positive bacteria including streptococci and staphylococci. In neonates, nystatin oral suspension or miconazole oral gel is used for the treatment of oropharyngeal candidiasis; to prevent re-infection it is important to ensure that the mother's breast nipples and the teats of feeding bottles are cleaned adequately.

Fluconazole (section 5.2) given by mouth is reliably absorbed; it is used for infections that do not respond to topical therapy or when topical therapy cannot be used. **Itraconazole** (section 5.2) can be used for fluconazole-resistant infections.

If candidal infection fails to respond after 1 to 2 weeks of treatment with antifungal drugs the child should be sent for investigation to eliminate the possibility of underlying disease. Persistent infection may also be caused by re-infection from the genito-urinary or gastro-intestinal tract.

AMPHOTERICIN

Side-effects mild gastro-intestinal disturbances reported

Licensed use *lozenges* not licensed for use in children

Indication and dose

Oral and perioral fungal infections for doses, see under preparations

Fungilin® (Squibb) [PoM]
Lozenges, yellow, amphotericin 10 mg. Net price 60-lozenge pack = £3.67. Label: 9, 24, counselling, after food

Dose

Allow 1 lozenge to dissolve slowly in the mouth 4 times daily for 10–15 days (continued for 48 hours after lesions have resolved); increase to 8 daily if infection severe

Dental prescribing on NHS May be prescribed as Amphotericin Lozenges

MICONAZOLE

Cautions avoid in acute porphyria (section 9.8.2); interactions: Appendix 1 (antifungals, imidazole)

Pregnancy manufacturer advises avoid if possible—toxicity at high doses in *animal* studies

Breast-feeding manufacturer advises caution—no information available

Contra-indications impaired swallowing reflex

Hepatic impairment avoid

Side-effects nausea and vomiting, *very rarely* diarrhoea (usually on long-term treatment), hepatitis, rash, toxic epidermal necrolysis, and Stevens-Johnson syndrome

Licensed use not licensed for use in children under 4 months of age or during first 5–6 months of life of an infant born pre-term

Indication and dose

Prevention and treatment of oral and intestinal fungal infections
• By mouth

Neonate (oral fungal infections only) 1 mL 2–4 times daily smeared around the mouth after feeds

Child 1 month–2 years 2.5 mL twice daily smeared around the mouth after food

Child 2–6 years 5 mL twice daily after food; retain near lesions before swallowing

Child 6–12 years 5 mL 4 times daily after food; retain near lesions before swallowing

Child 12–18 years 5–10 mL 4 times daily after food; retain near lesions before swallowing
Note Treatment should be continued for 48 hours after lesions have healed

Localised lesions

Child 6–18 years smear small amount on affected area with clean finger 4 times daily for 5–7 days (orthodontic appliances should be removed at night and brushed with gel); continue treatment for 48 hours after lesions have healed

¹**Daktarin®** (Janssen-Cilag) [PoM]
Oral gel, sugar-free, orange-flavoured, miconazole 24 mg/mL (20 mg/g). Net price 15-g tube = £2.45, 80-g tube = £4.65. Label: 9, counselling, hold in mouth, after food
Dental prescribing on NHS May be prescribed as Miconazole Oromucosal Gel
1. 15-g tube can be sold to the public

NYSTATIN

Side-effects oral irritation and sensitisation, nausea reported; see also section 5.2

Licensed use *suspension* not licensed for use in neonates for the treatment of candidiasis

◁ **NYSTATIN** (*continued*)

Indication and dose

Oral and perioral fungal infections

Neonate 100 000 units 4 times daily after feeds

Child 1 month–18 years 100 000 units 4 times daily after food

Note Treatment is usually given for 7 days, and continued for 48 hours after lesions have healed.

Intestinal fungal infections section 5.2

Skin infections section 13.10.2

Nystan® (Squibb) PoM
Oral suspension, yellow, nystatin 100 000 units/mL. Net price 30 mL with pipette = £1.91. Label: 9, counselling, use of pipette, hold in mouth, after food

Dental prescribing on NHS May be prescribed as Nystatin Oral Suspension

12.3.3 Lozenges and sprays

There is no convincing evidence that antiseptic lozenges and sprays have a beneficial action and they sometimes irritate and cause sore tongue and sore lips. Some preparations also contain local anaesthetics which relieve pain but may cause sensitisation.

12.3.4 Mouthwashes and gargles

Superficial infections of the mouth are often helped by warm mouthwashes which have a mechanical cleansing effect and cause some local hyperaemia. However, to be effective, they must be used frequently and vigorously. Mouthwashes may not be suitable for children under 7 years (risk of the solution being swallowed); the mouthwash or dental gel may be applied using a cotton bud.

A warm saline mouthwash is ideal for its cleansing effect and can be prepared either by dissolving half a teaspoonful of salt in a glassful of warm water or by diluting **compound sodium chloride mouthwash** with an equal volume of warm water. **Mouthwash solution-tablets** containing thymol are used to remove unpleasant tastes.

Mouthwashes containing an oxidising agent, such as **hydrogen peroxide**, may be useful in the treatment of acute ulcerative gingivitis (Vincent's infection). Hydrogen peroxide solution has also a mechanical cleansing effect arising from frothing when in contact with oral debris, but in concentrations greater than 1.5% may cause ulceration and tissue damage.

Chlorhexidine is an effective antiseptic which has the advantage of inhibiting plaque formation on the teeth. It does not, however, completely control plaque deposition and is not a substitute for effective toothbrushing. Moreover, chlorhexidine preparations do not penetrate significantly into stagnation areas and are therefore of little value in the control of dental caries or of periodontal disease once pocketing has developed. Chlorhexidine preparations are of little value in the control of acute necrotising ulcerative gingivitis. With prolonged use, chlorhexidine causes reversible brown staining of teeth and tongue. Chlorhexidine may be incompatible with some ingredients in toothpaste, causing an unpleasant taste in the mouth; allow at least 30 minutes between using the mouthwash and toothpaste.

Chlorhexidine can be used as a mouthwash, spray or gel for secondary infection in mucosal ulceration and for controlling gingivitis, as an adjunct to other oral hygiene measures. These preparations may also be used instead of toothbrushing where there is a painful periodontal condition (e.g. primary herpetic stomatitis) or if the child has a haemorrhagic disorder, or is disabled. Chlorhexidine mouthwash is used in the prevention of oral candidiasis in immunocompromised patients. Chlorhexidine mouthwash reduces the incidence of alveolar osteitis following tooth extraction. Chlorhexidine mouthwash should not be used for the prevention of endocarditis in children undergoing dental procedures.

CHLORHEXIDINE GLUCONATE

Side-effects mucosal irritation (if desquamation occurs, discontinue treatment or dilute mouthwash with an equal volume of water); taste disturbance; reversible brown staining of teeth, and of silicate or composite restorations; tongue discoloration; parotid gland swelling reported

Note Chlorhexidine gluconate may be incompatible with some ingredients in toothpaste; leave an interval of at least 30 minutes between using mouthwash and toothpaste

◁ **CHLORHEXIDINE GLUCONATE (continued)**

Licensed use licensed for use in children (age range not specified by manufacturer)

Indication and dose
> See under preparations below

Chlorhexidine (Non-proprietary)
Mouthwash, chlorhexidine gluconate 0.2%, net price 300 mL = £1.97
Dose
> Oral hygiene and plaque inhibition, oral candidiasis, gingivitis, and management of aphthous ulcers
> > Rinse mouth with 10 mL for about 1 minute twice daily

> Dental prescribing on NHS Chlorhexidine Mouthwash may be prescribed

Chlorohex® (Colgate-Palmolive)
Chlorohex 1200® mouthwash, chlorhexidine gluconate 0.12% (mint-flavoured). Net price 300 mL = £2.00
Dose
> Oral hygiene and plaque inhibition
> > Rinse mouth with 15 mL for about 30 seconds twice daily

Corsodyl® (GSK Consumer Healthcare)
Dental gel, chlorhexidine gluconate 1%. Net price 50 g = £1.21
Dose
> Oral hygiene and plaque inhibition and gingivitis
> > Brush on the teeth once or twice daily

> Oral candidiasis and management of aphthous ulcers
> > Apply to affected areas once or twice daily

> Dental prescribing on NHS May be prescribed as Chlorhexidine Gluconate Gel 1%

Mouthwash, chlorhexidine gluconate 0.2%. Net price 300 mL (original or mint) = £1.93, 600 mL (mint) = £3.85
Dose
> Oral hygiene and plaque inhibition, oral candidiasis, gingivitis, and management of aphthous ulcers
> > Rinse mouth with 10 mL for about 1 minute twice daily

Oral spray, chlorhexidine gluconate 0.2% (mint-flavoured). Net price 60 mL = £4.10
Dose
> Oral hygiene and plaque inhibition, oral candidiasis, gingivitis, and management of aphthous ulcers
> > Apply as required to tooth, gingival, or ulcer surfaces using up to 12 actuations (approx. 0.14 mL/actuation) twice daily

> Dental prescribing on NHS May be prescribed as Chlorhexidine Oral Spray

◢ **With chlorobutanol**
Eludril® (Fabre)
Mouthwash or gargle, chlorhexidine gluconate 0.1%, chlorobutanol 0.5% (mint-flavoured), net price 90 mL = £1.36, 250 mL = £2.83, 500 mL = £5.06
Dose
> Oral hygiene and plaque inhibition
> > Use 10–15 mL (diluted with warm water in measuring cup provided) 2–3 times daily

---

HEXETIDINE

Side-effects local irritation; *very rarely* taste disturbance and transient anaesthesia

Indication and dose
> Oral hygiene for dose, see preparation below

Oraldene® (McNeil)
Mouthwash or gargle, red or blue-green (mint-flavoured), hexetidine 0.1%. Net price 100 mL = £1.31; 200 mL = £2.02
Dose
> Child 6–18 years use 15 mL (undiluted) 2–3 times daily

HYDROGEN PEROXIDE

Side-effects hypertrophy of papillae of tongue on prolonged use

Indication and dose
> Oral hygiene (see notes above); for dose, see under preparations

Hydrogen Peroxide Mouthwash, BP
Mouthwash, consists of Hydrogen Peroxide Solution 6% (= approx. 20 volume) BP
Dose
> Rinse the mouth for 2–3 minutes with 15 mL diluted in half a tumblerful of warm water 2–3 times daily (see notes above)

> Dental prescribing on NHS Hydrogen Peroxide Mouthwash may be prescribed

Peroxyl® (Colgate-Palmolive)
Mouthwash, hydrogen peroxide 1.5%, net price 300 mL = £2.95
Dose
> Child 6–18 years, rinse the mouth with 10 mL for about 1 minute 3 times daily (after meals and at bedtime) for max. 7 days

▌ SODIUM CHLORIDE

Indication and dose

Oral hygiene (see notes above); for dose, see under preparation

mint emulsion 2.5 mL, double-strength chloroform water 50 mL, water to 100 mL

To be diluted with an equal volume of warm water

Dental prescribing on NHS Compound Sodium Chloride Mouthwash may be prescribed

Sodium Chloride Mouthwash, Compound, BP

Mouthwash, sodium bicarbonate 1%, sodium chloride 1.5% in a suitable vehicle with a peppermint flavour

Dose

Extemporaneous preparations should be prepared according to the following formula: sodium chloride 1.5 g, sodium bicarbonate 1 g, concentrated pepper-

---

▌ THYMOL

Indication and dose

Oral hygiene (see notes above); for dose, see under preparation

Mouthwash Solution-tablets

Consist of tablets which may contain antimicrobial, colouring, and flavouring agents in a suitable soluble effervescent basis to make a mouthwash

suitable for dental purposes. Net price 100-tab pack = £14.12

Dose

Dissolve 1 tablet in a tumblerful of warm water

Note Mouthwash Solution-tablets may contain ingredients such as thymol

Dental prescribing on NHS Mouthwash Solution-tablets may be prescribed

---

12.3.5 Treatment of dry mouth

Dry mouth (xerostomia) may be caused by drugs with antimuscarinic (anticholinergic) side-effects (e.g. antispasmodics and sedating antihistamines), by irradiation of the head and neck region or by damage to or disease of the salivary glands. Children with a persistently dry mouth may develop a burning or scalded sensation and have poor oral hygiene; they may develop dental caries, periodontal disease, and oral infections (particularly candidiasis). Dry mouth may be relieved in many patients by simple measures such as frequent sips of cool drinks or sucking pieces of ice or sugar-free fruit pastilles. Sugar-free chewing gum stimulates salivation in patients with residual salivary function.

Artificial saliva can provide useful relief of dry mouth. A properly balanced artificial saliva should be of a neutral pH and contain electrolytes (including fluoride) to correspond approximately to the composition of saliva. The acidic pH of some artificial saliva products may be inappropriate.

Local treatment

Artificial saliva products with **ACBS approval** may be prescribed for children with dry mouth as a result of having (or having undergone) radiotherapy, or sicca syndrome. SST tablets and *Salinum*® liquid may also be prescribed on the NHS.

AS Saliva Orthana® (AS Pharma)

Oral spray, gastric mucin (porcine) 3.5%, xylitol 2%, sodium fluoride 4.2 mg/litre, with preservatives and flavouring agents, pH neutral, net price 50-mL bottle = £4.92; 450-mL refill = £29.69

Dose

(ACBS) spray 2–3 times onto oral and pharyngeal mucosa, when required

Lozenges, mucin 65 mg, xylitol 59 mg, in a sorbitol basis, pH neutral, net price 45-lozenge pack = £3.50

Note *AS Saliva Orthana*® lozenges do not contain fluoride
Dental prescribing on NHS *AS Saliva Orthana*® Oral Spray and Lozenges may be prescribed

Biotène Oralbalance® (Anglian)

Saliva replacement gel, lactoperoxidase, lactoferrin, lysozyme, glucose oxidase, xylitol in a gel basis, net price 50-g tube = £4.10; 24 × 12.4 mL tube = £30.40 (for hospital use)

Dose

(ACBS) apply to gums and tongue as required

Note Avoid use with toothpastes containing detergents (including foaming agents)
Dental prescribing on NHS *Biotène Oralbalance*® Saliva Replacement Gel may be prescribed

12 Ear, nose, and oropharynx

BioXtra® (RIS Products)

Gel, lactoperoxidase, lactoferrin, lysozyme, whey colostrum, xylitol and other ingredients, net price 40-mL tube = £3.94, 50-mL spray = £3.94

Dose

(ACBS) apply to oral mucosa as required

Dental prescribing on NHS *BioXtra®* Gel may be prescribed

Glandosane® (Fresenius Kabi)

Aerosol spray, carmellose sodium 500 mg, sorbitol 1.5 g, potassium chloride 60 mg, sodium chloride 42.2 mg, magnesium chloride 2.6 mg, calcium chloride 7.3 mg, and dipotassium hydrogen phosphate 17.1 mg/50 g, pH 5.75, net price 50-mL unit (neutral, lemon or peppermint flavoured) = £4.48

Dose

(ACBS) spray onto oral and pharyngeal mucosa as required

Dental prescribing on NHS *Glandosane®* Aerosol Spray may be prescribed

Luborant® (Goldshield)

Oral spray, pink, sorbitol 1.8 g, carmellose sodium (sodium carboxymethylcellulose) 390 mg, dibasic potassium phosphate 48.23 mg, potassium chloride 37.5 mg, monobasic potassium phosphate 21.97 mg, calcium chloride 9.972 mg, magnesium chloride 3.528 mg, sodium fluoride 258 micrograms/60 mL, with preservatives and colouring agents. Net price 60-mL unit = £3.96

Dose

Saliva deficiency

2–3 sprays onto oral mucosa up to 4 times daily, or as directed

Note May be difficult to obtain

Dental prescribing on NHS *Luborant®* Oral Spray may be prescribed as Artificial Saliva

Salinum® (Crawford)

Liquid sugar free, linseed extract (containing polysaccharides), with dipotassium phosphate buffer and preservatives, pH 6–7, net price 300-mL bottle = £13.50

Dose

Symptomatic treatment of dry mouth

Approx. 2 mL rinsed around the mouth and then swallowed, when required

Saliveze® (Wyvern)

Oral spray, carmellose sodium (sodium carboxymethylcellulose), calcium chloride, magnesium chloride, potassium chloride, sodium chloride, and dibasic sodium phosphate, pH neutral, net price 50-mL bottle (mint-flavoured) = £3.50

Dose

(ACBS) 1 spray onto oral mucosa as required

Dental prescribing on NHS *Saliveze®* Oral Spray may be prescribed

Salivix® (KoGEN)

Pastilles, sugar-free, reddish-amber, acacia, malic acid and other ingredients. Net price 50-pastille pack = £3.50

Dose

(ACBS) suck 1 pastille when required

Dental prescribing on NHS *Salivix®* Pastilles may be prescribed

SST (Medac)

Tablets, sugar-free, citric acid, malic acid and other ingredients in a sorbitol base, net price 100-tab pack = £4.86

Dose

Symptomatic treatment of dry mouth in patients with impaired salivary gland function and patent salivary ducts

Allow 1 tablet to dissolve slowly in the mouth when required

Dental prescribing on NHS May be prescribed as Saliva Stimulating Tablets

13 Skin

13.1 Management of skin conditions **664**
13.1.1 Vehicles 664
13.1.2 Suitable quantities for prescribing 665
13.1.3 Excipients and sensitisation 665

13.2 Emollient and barrier preparations **665**
13.2.1 Emollients 666
13.2.2 Barrier preparations 670

13.3 Topical antipruritics **671**

13.4 Topical corticosteroids **672**

13.5 Preparations for eczema and psoriasis **681**
13.5.1 Preparations for eczema 681
13.5.2 Preparations for psoriasis 683
13.5.3 Drugs affecting the immune response 690

13.6 Acne and rosacea **692**
13.6.1 Topical preparations for acne 693
13.6.2 Oral preparations for acne 697

13.7 Preparations for warts and calluses **700**

13.8 Sunscreens and camouflagers **703**
13.8.1 Sunscreen preparations 703
13.8.2 Camouflagers 704

13.9 Shampoos and other preparations for scalp conditions **705**

13.10 Anti-infective skin preparations **707**
13.10.1 Antibacterial preparations 707
13.10.2 Antifungal preparations 710
13.10.3 Antiviral preparations 715
13.10.4 Parasiticidal preparations 715
13.10.5 Preparations for minor cuts and abrasions 719

13.11 Skin cleansers and antiseptics **719**
13.11.1 Alcohols and saline 720
13.11.2 Chlorhexidine salts 720
13.11.3 Cationic surfactants and soaps 721
13.11.4 Iodine 722
13.11.5 Phenolics 722
13.11.6 Oxidisers and dyes 722
13.11.7 Preparations for promotion of wound healing 723

13.12 Antiperspirants **723**

13.13 Topical circulatory preparations **724**

13

Skin

> This chapter also includes advice on the management of the following:
>   candidiasis, p. 711
>   dermatophytoses, p. 710
>   head lice, p. 716
>   nappy rash, p. 670
>   pityriasis versicolor, p. 711
>   scabies, p. 715

The British Association of Dermatologists' list of preferred unlicensed dermatological preparations (specials) is available at http://88.208.244.6/BAD/site/495/default.aspx

13.1 Management of skin conditions

When prescribing topical preparations for the treatment of skin conditions in children, the site of application, the condition being treated, and the child's (and carer's) preference for a particular vehicle all need to be taken into consideration.

Neonates Caution is required when prescribing topical preparations for neonates—their large body surface area in relation to body mass increases susceptibility to toxicity from systemic absorption of substances applied to the skin. Topical preparations containing potentially sensitising substances such as corticosteroids, aminoglycosides, iodine, and parasiticidal drugs should be avoided. Preparations containing alcohol should be avoided because they can dehydrate the skin, cause pain if applied to raw areas, and the alcohol can cause necrosis.

In *preterm neonates*, the skin is more fragile and offers a poor barrier, especially in the first fortnight after birth. Preterm infants, especially if below 32 weeks postmenstrual age, may also require special measures to maintain skin hydration.

13.1.1 Vehicles

The vehicle in topical preparations for the skin affects the degree of hydration, has a mild anti-inflammatory effect, and aids the penetration of the active drug. Therefore, the vehicle, as well as the active drug, should be chosen on the basis of their suitability for the child's skin condition.

Applications are usually viscous solutions, emulsions, or suspensions for application to the skin (including the scalp) or nails.

Collodions are painted on the skin and allowed to dry to leave a flexible film over the site of application.

Creams are emulsions of oil and water and are generally well absorbed into the skin. They may contain an antimicrobial preservative unless the active ingredient or basis is intrinsically bactericidal and fungicidal. Generally, creams are cosmetically more acceptable than ointments because they are less greasy and easier to apply.

Gels consist of active ingredients in suitable hydrophilic or hydrophobic bases; they generally have a high water content. Gels are particularly suitable for application to the face and scalp.

Lotions have a cooling effect and may be preferred to ointments or creams for application over a hairy area. Lotions in alcoholic basis can sting if used on broken skin. *Shake lotions* (such as calamine lotion) contain insoluble powders which leave a deposit on the skin surface.

Ointments are greasy preparations which are normally anhydrous and insoluble in water, and are more occlusive than creams. They are particularly suitable for chronic, dry lesions. The most commonly used ointment bases consist of soft paraffin or a combination of soft, liquid and hard paraffin. Some ointment bases have both *hydrophilic* and *lipophilic* properties; they may have occlusive properties on the skin surface, encourage hydration, and also be miscible with water; they often have a mild anti-inflammatory effect. *Water-soluble ointments* contain macrogols which are freely soluble in water and are therefore readily washed off; they have a limited but useful role where ready removal is desirable.

Pastes are stiff preparations containing a high proportion of finely powdered solids such as zinc oxide and starch suspended in an ointment. They are used for

13 Skin

circumscribed lesions such as those which occur in lichen simplex, chronic eczema, or psoriasis. They are less occlusive than ointments and can be used to protect inflamed, lichenified, or excoriated skin.

Dusting powders are used only rarely. They reduce friction between opposing skin surfaces. Dusting powders should not be applied to moist areas because they can cake and abrade the skin. Talc is a lubricant but it does not absorb moisture; it can cause respiratory irritation. Starch is less lubricant but absorbs water.

Dilution   The BP directs that creams and ointments should **not** normally be diluted but that should dilution be necessary care should be taken, in particular, to prevent microbial contamination. The appropriate diluent should be used and heating should be avoided during mixing; excessive dilution may affect the stability of some creams. Diluted creams should normally be used within 2 weeks of their preparation.

13.1.2 Suitable quantities for prescribing

Suitable quantities of dermatological preparations to be prescribed for specific areas of the body

Area of the body	Creams and Ointments	Lotions
Face	15–30 g	100 mL
Both hands	25–50 g	200 mL
Scalp	50–100 g	200 mL
Both arms or both legs	100–200 g	200 mL
Trunk	400 g	500 mL
Groins and genitalia	15–25 g	100 mL

The amounts shown above are usually suitable for children 12–18 years for twice daily application for 1 week; smaller quantities will be required for children under 12 years. These recommendations **do not apply** to corticosteroid preparations.

13.1.3 Excipients and sensitisation

Excipients in topical products rarely cause problems. If a patch test indicates allergy to an excipient, then products containing the substance should be avoided (see also Anaphylaxis, p. 198). The following excipients in topical preparations may rarely be associated with sensitisation; the presence of these excipients is indicated in the entries for topical products. See also Excipients, under General Guidance, p. 3.

Beeswax	Imidurea
Benzyl alcohol	Isopropyl palmitate
Butylated hydroxyanisole	*N*-(3-Chloroallyl)hexaminium chloride (quaternium
Butylated hydroxytoluene	15)
Cetostearyl alcohol (including cetyl and stearyl alcohol)	Polysorbates
	Propylene glycol
Chlorocresol	Sodium metabisulphite
Edetic acid (EDTA)	Sorbic acid
Ethylenediamine	Wool fat and related substances including lanolin[1]
Fragrances	
Hydroxybenzoates (parabens)	

1. Purified versions of wool fat have reduced the problem

13.2 Emollient and barrier preparations

13.2.1 Emollients
13.2.2 Barrier preparations

Borderline substances   The preparations marked 'ACBS' are regarded as drugs when prescribed in accordance with the advice of the Advisory Committee on Borderline Substances for the clinical conditions listed. Prescriptions issued in accordance with this advice and endorsed 'ACBS' will normally not be investigated. See Appendix 2 for listing by clinical condition.

13

Skin

13.2.1 Emollients

Emollients hydrate the skin, soften the skin, act as barrier to water and external irritants, and are indicated for all dry or scaling disorders. Their effects are short-lived and they should be applied frequently even after improvement occurs. They are useful in dry and eczematous disorders, and to a lesser extent in psoriasis (section 13.5.2); they should be applied immediately after washing or bathing to maximise the effect of skin hydration. Light emollients such as **aqueous cream** are suitable for many dry skin conditions but more greasy preparations, such as **white soft paraffin**, **emulsifying ointment**, and **liquid and white soft paraffin ointment**, are often more effective. The severity of the condition, the child's (or carer's) preference, and the site of application will often guide the choice of emollient. Some ingredients rarely cause sensitisation (section 13.1.3) and this should be suspected if an eczematous reaction occurs. Ointments may exacerbate acne and folliculitis.

> **Fire hazard with paraffin-based emollients**
> Emulsifying ointment *or* 50% Liquid Paraffin and 50% White Soft Paraffin Ointment in contact with dressings and clothing is easily ignited by a naked flame. The risk is greater when these preparations are applied to large areas of the body, and clothing or dressings become soaked with the ointment. Patients should be told to keep away from fire or flames, and not to smoke when using these preparations. The risk of fire should be considered when using large quantities of any paraffin-based emollient.

Preparations such as **aqueous cream** and **emulsifying ointment** can be used as soap substitutes; the preparation is rubbed on the skin before rinsing off completely. The addition of a bath oil (section 13.2.1.1) may also be helpful.

In the *neonate*, a preservative-free paraffin-based emollient hydrates the skin without affecting the normal skin flora; substances such as olive oil are also used. The development of blisters (epidermolysis bullosa) or ichthyosis may be alleviated by applying liquid and white soft paraffin ointment while awaiting dermatological investigation.

Preparations containing an antibacterial (section 13.10.1) should be avoided unless infection is present or is a frequent complication of the dry skin condition.

Urea is a keratin softener used in the treatment of dry, scaling conditions (including ichthyosis). It is occasionally used with other topical agents such as corticosteroids to enhance penetration of the skin.

◀ **Non-proprietary emollient preparations**

Aqueous Cream, BP
Cream, emulsifying ointment 30%, [1]phenoxyethanol 1% in freshly boiled and cooled purified water, net price 100 g = 47p
Excipients include cetostearyl alcohol
1. The BP permits use of alternative antimicrobials provided their identity and concentration are stated on the label

Emulsifying Ointment, BP
Ointment, emulsifying wax 30%, white soft paraffin 50%, liquid paraffin 20%, net price 100 g = 57p
Excipients include cetostearyl alcohol

Hydrous Ointment, BP
Ointment, (oily cream), dried magnesium sulphate 0.5%, phenoxyethanol 1%, wool alcohols ointment 50%, in freshly boiled and cooled purified water, net price 100 g = 40p

Liquid and White Soft Paraffin Ointment, NPF
Ointment, liquid paraffin 50%, white soft paraffin 50%, net price 250 g = £3.94

Paraffin, White Soft, BP
White petroleum jelly, net price 100 g = 48p

Paraffin, Yellow Soft, BP
Yellow petroleum jelly, net price 100 g = 34p

◀ **Proprietary emollient preparations**

Aveeno® (J&J)
Cream, colloidal oatmeal in emollient basis, net price 100 mL = £3.78, 300-mL pump pack = £6.80
Excipients include benzyl alcohol, cetyl alcohol, isopropyl palmitate
ACBS: For endogenous and exogenous eczema, xeroderma, and ichthyosis

Lotion, colloidal oatmeal in emollient basis, net price 400 mL = £6.42
Excipients include benzyl alcohol, cetyl alcohol, isopropyl palmitate
ACBS: as for *Aveeno®* Cream

Cetraben® (Genus)
Emollient cream, white soft paraffin 13.2%, light liquid paraffin 10.5%, net price 50-g pump pack = £1.17, 150-g pump pack = £2.88, 500-g pump pack = £5.61, 1.05-kg pump pack = £11.11
Excipients include cetostearyl alcohol, hydroxybenzoates (parabens)

Dermamist® (Alliance)
Spray application, white soft paraffin 10% in a basis containing liquid paraffin, fractionated coconut oil, net price 250-mL pressurised aerosol unit = £9.22
Excipients none as listed in section 13.1.3
Note Flammable

Diprobase® (Schering-Plough)
Cream, cetomacrogol 2.25%, cetostearyl alcohol 7.2%, liquid paraffin 6%, white soft paraffin 15%, water-miscible basis used for *Diprosone®* cream, net price 50 g = £1.34; 500-g pump pack= £6.76
Excipients include cetostearyl alcohol, chlorocresol

Ointment, liquid paraffin 5%, white soft paraffin 95%, basis used for *Diprosone®* ointment, net price 50 g = £1.34
Excipients none as listed in section 13.1.3

Doublebase® (Dermal)
Emollient shower gel, isopropyl myristate 15%, liquid paraffin 15%, net price 200 g = £5.45
Excipients none as listed in section 13.1.3

Gel, isopropyl myristate 15%, liquid paraffin 15%, net price 100 g = £2.77, 500 g = £6.09
Excipients none as listed in section 13.1.3

E45® (Crookes)
Cream, light liquid paraffin 12.6%, white soft paraffin 14.5%, hypoallergenic anhydrous wool fat (hypoallergenic lanolin) 1% in self-emulsifying monostearin, net price 50 g = £1.40, 125 g = £2.55, 350 g = £4.46, 500-g pump pack = £6.20
Excipients include cetyl alcohol, hydroxybenzoates (parabens)

Emollient Wash Cream, soap substitute, zinc oxide 5% in an emollient basis, net price 250-mL pump pack = £3.19
Excipients none as listed in section 13.1.3
ACBS: for endogenous and exogenous eczema, xeroderma, and ichthyosis

Lotion, light liquid paraffin 4%, cetomacrogol, white soft paraffin 10%, hypoallergenic anhydrous wool fat (hypoallergenic lanolin) 1% in glyceryl monostearate, net price 200 mL = £2.40, 500-mL pump pack = £4.50
Excipients include isopropyl palmitate, hydroxybenzoates (parabens), benzyl alcohol
ACBS: for symptomatic relief of dry skin conditions, such as those associated with atopic eczema and contact dermatitis

Emollin® (C D Medical)
Spray, liquid paraffin 50%, white soft paraffin 50% in aerosol basis, net price 240 mL = £5.98
Excipients none as listed in section 13.1.3

Epaderm® (Medlock)
Ointment, emulsifying wax 30%, yellow soft paraffin 30%, liquid paraffin 40%, net price 125 g = £3.62, 500 g = £6.14, 1 kg = £11.44
Excipients include cetostearyl alcohol

Hewletts® (Kestrel)
Cream, hydrous wool fat 4%, zinc oxide 8%, arachis (peanut) oil, oleic acid, white soft paraffin, net price 35 g = £1.43, 400 g = £6.69
Excipients include fragrance

Hydromol® (Alliance)
Cream, sodium pidolate 2.5%, liquid paraffin 13.8%, net price 50 g = £2.04, 100 g = £3.80, 500 g = £12.60
Excipients include cetostearyl alcohol, hydroxybenzoates (parabens)

Ointment, yellow soft paraffin 30%, emulsifying wax 30%, liquid paraffin 40%, net price 125 g = £2.79, 500 g = £4.74
Excipients include cetostearyl alcohol

Linola® Gamma (Linderma)
Cream, evening primrose oil 20%, net price 50 g = £2.83, 250 g = £8.20
Excipients include beeswax, hydroxybenzoates (parabens), propylene glycol
Cautions epilepsy (but hazard unlikely with topical preparations)

Lipobase® (Astellas)
Cream, fatty cream basis used for *Locoid Lipocream®*, net price 50 g = £2.08
Excipients include cetostearyl alcohol, hydroxybenzoates (parabens)
For dry skin conditions, also for use during treatment with topical corticosteroid and as diluent for *Locoid Lipocream®*

Oilatum® (Stiefel)
Cream, light liquid paraffin 6%, white soft paraffin 15%, net price 40 g = £1.79, 150 g = £3.38, 500-mL pump pack = £6.35, 1.05-litre pump pack = £14.67; *Oilatum® Junior* 150 g = £3.38, 350-mL pump pack = £4.65, 500-mL pump pack = £6.35, 1.05-litre pump pack = £14.67
Excipients include benzyl alcohol, cetostearyl alcohol

Shower emollient (gel), light liquid paraffin 70%, net price 150 g = £5.15
Excipients include fragrance

QV® (Crawford)
Cream, glycerol 10%, light liquid paraffin 10%, white soft paraffin 5%, net price 100 g = £1.95, 500 g = £5.60
Excipients include cetostearyl alcohol, hydroxybenzoates (parabens)

Lotion, white soft paraffin 5%, net price 250 mL = £3.00
Excipients include cetostearyl alcohol, hydroxybenzoates (parabens)

Wash, glycerol 10%, net price 200 mL = £2.50
Excipients include hydroxybenzoates (parabens)

Ultrabase® (Valeant)
Cream, water-miscible, containing liquid paraffin and white soft paraffin, net price 50 g = 89p, 500-g pump pack = £6.44
Excipients include fragrance, hydroxybenzoates (parabens), disodium edetate, stearyl alcohol

Unguentum M® (Almirall)
Cream, containing saturated neutral oil, liquid paraffin, white soft paraffin, net price 50 g = £1.41, 100 g = £2.78, 200-mL pump pack = £5.50, 500 g = £8.48
Excipients include cetostearyl alcohol, polysorbate 40, propylene glycol, sorbic acid

Zerobase® (Zeroderma)
Cream, liquid paraffin 11%, net price 500 g pump pack = £5.99
Excipients include cetostearyl alcohol, chlorocresol

13

Skin

◢Preparations containing urea

Aquadrate® (Alliance)
Cream, urea 10%, net price 30 g = £1.37, 100 g = £3.64
Excipients none as listed in section 13.1.3

Dose
> Apply thinly and rub into area when required

Balneum® Plus (Crookes)
Cream, urea 5%, lauromacrogols 3%, net price 100 g = £3.29, 175-g pump pack = £8.33, 500-g pump pack = £17.09
Excipients include benzyl alcohol, polysorbates

Dose
> Apply twice daily

Calmurid® (Galderma)
Cream, urea 10%, lactic acid 5%, net price 100 g = £7.36, 500-g pump pack = £28.37
Excipients none as listed in section 13.1.3

Dose
> Apply a thick layer for 3–5 minutes, massage into area, and remove excess, usually twice daily. Use half-strength cream for 1 week if stinging occurs

> Note Can be diluted with aqueous cream (life of diluted cream 14 days)

E45® Itch Relief Cream (Crookes)
Cream, urea 5%, macrogol lauryl ether 3%, net price 50 g = £2.55, 100 g = £3.47, 500 g = £17.09
Excipients include benzyl alcohol, polysorbates

Dose
> Apply twice daily

Eucerin® Intensive (Beiersdorf)
Cream, urea 10%, net price 100 mL = £7.59
Excipients include benzyl alcohol, isopropyl palmitate, wool fat

Dose
> Apply thinly and rub into area twice daily

Lotion, urea 10%, net price 250 mL = £7.93
Excipients include benzyl alcohol, isopropyl palmitate

Dose
> Apply sparingly and rub into area twice daily

Nutraplus® (Galderma)
Cream, urea 10%, net price 100 g = £4.37
Excipients include hydroxybenzoates (parabens), propylene glycol

Dose
> Apply 2–3 times daily

◢With antimicrobials

Dermol® (Dermal)
Cream, benzalkonium chloride 0.1%, chlorhexidine hydrochloride 0.1%, isopropyl myristate 10%, liquid paraffin 10%, net price 100-g tube = £3.22, 500-g pump pack = £7.45
Excipients include cetostearyl alcohol

Dose
> Apply to skin or use as soap substitute

Dermol® 500 Lotion, benzalkonium chloride 0.1%, chlorhexidine hydrochloride 0.1%, liquid paraffin 2.5%, isopropyl myristate 2.5%, net price 500-mL pump pack = £6.31
Excipients include cetostearyl alcohol

Dose
> Apply to skin or use as soap substitute

Dermol® 200 Shower Emollient, benzalkonium chloride 0.1%, chlorhexidine hydrochloride 0.1%, liquid paraffin 2.5%, isopropyl myristate 2.5%, net price 200 mL = £3.71
Excipients include cetostearyl alcohol

Dose
> Apply to skin or use as soap substitute

13.2.1.1 Emollient bath additives

Emollient bath additives should be added to bath water; some can be applied to wet skin undiluted and rinsed off. Hydration can be improved by soaking in the bath for 10–20 minutes. In dry skin conditions soap should be avoided (see section 13.2.1 for soap substitutes).

The quantities of bath additives recommended for older children are suitable for an adult-size bath. Proportionately less should be used for a child-size bath or a washbasin; recommended bath additive quantities for younger children reflect this.

> These preparations make skin and surfaces slippery—particular care is needed when bathing a child.

Alpha Keri Bath® (Novartis Consumer Health)
Bath oil, liquid paraffin 91.7%, oil-soluble fraction of wool fat 3%, net price 240 mL = £3.45, 480 mL = £6.43
Excipients include fragrance

Dose
> **Neonate** add 5 mL to bath water or apply to wet skin and rinse

> **Child 1 month–2 years** add 5 mL to bath water or apply to wet skin and rinse

> **Child 2–18 years** add 10–20 mL to bath water or apply to wet skin and rinse

13 Skin

Aveeno® (J&J)

Bath oil, colloidal oatmeal, white oat fraction in emollient basis, net price 250 mL = £4.28
Excipients include beeswax, fragrance
ACBS: for endogenous and exogenous eczema, xeroderma, and ichthyosis

Dose

> **Child 2–18 years** add 20–30 mL to bath water or apply to wet skin and rinse

Colloidal® bath additive, oatmeal, white oat fraction in emollient basis, net price 10 × 50-g sachets = £7.33; *Baby Bath Additive*®, 10 × 15-g sachets = £4.39
Excipients none as listed in section 13.1.3
ACBS: as for *Aveeno*® Bath oil

Dose

> **Child 1 month–12 years** add 15 g to bath water
> **Child 12–18 years** add 50 g to bath water

Balneum® (Crookes)

Balneum® bath oil, soya oil 84.75%, net price 200 mL = £2.48, 500 mL = £5.38, 1 litre = £10.39
Excipients include butylated hydroxytoluene, propylene glycol, fragrance

Dose

> **Neonate** add 5–15 mL to bath water; do not use undiluted
>
> **Child 1 month–2 years** add 5–15 mL to bath water; do not use undiluted
> **Child 2–18 years** add 20–60 mL to bath water; do not use undiluted

Balneum Plus® bath oil, soya oil 82.95%, mixed lauromacrogols 15%, net price 500 mL = £6.66
Excipients include butylated hydroxytoluene, propylene glycol, fragrance

Dose

> **Neonate** add 5 mL to bath water or apply to wet skin and rinse
>
> **Child 1 month–2 years** add 5 mL to bath water or apply to wet skin and rinse
> **Child 2–18 years** add 10–20 mL to bath water or apply to wet skin and rinse

Cetraben® (Genus)

Emollient bath additive, light liquid paraffin 82.8%, net price 500 mL = £5.25

Dose

> **Neonate** add ½ capful to bath water or apply to wet skin and rinse
>
> **Child 1 month–12 years** add ½–1 capful to bath water or apply to wet skin and rinse
> **Child 12–18 years** add 1–2 capfuls to bath water or apply to wet skin and rinse

Dermalo® (Dermal)

Bath emollient, acetylated wool alcohols 5%, liquid paraffin 65%, net price 500 mL = £3.60
Excipients none as listed in section 13.1.3

Dose

> **Neonate** add 5 mL to bath water or apply to wet skin and rinse
>
> **Child 1 month–12 years** add 5–10 mL to bath water or apply to wet skin and rinse
> **Child 12–18 years** add 15–20 mL to bath water or apply to wet skin and rinse

Diprobath® (Schering-Plough)

Bath additive, isopropyl myristate 39%, light liquid paraffin 46%, net price 500 mL = £6.97
Excipients none as listed in section 13.1.3

Dose

> **Neonate** add 5 mL to bath water; do not use undiluted
>
> **Child 1 month–12 years** add 10 mL to bath water; do not use undiluted
> **Child 12–18 years** add 25–50 mL to bath water; do not use undiluted

Doublebase® (Dermal)

Emollient bath additive, liquid paraffin 65%, net price 500 mL = £5.70
Excipients include cetostearyl alcohol

Dose

> **Neonate** add 5–10 mL to bath water
>
> **Child 1 month–12 years** add 5–10 mL to bath water
> **Child 12–18 years** add 15–20 mL to bath water

E45® (Crookes)

Emollient bath oil, cetyl dimeticone 5%, liquid paraffin 91%, net price 250 mL = £3.19, 500 mL = £5.11
Excipients none as listed in section 13.1.3
ACBS: for endogenous and exogenous eczema, xeroderma, and ichthyosis

Dose

> **Neonate** add 5 mL to bath water or apply to wet skin and rinse
>
> **Child 1 month–12 years** add 5–10 mL to bath water or apply to wet skin and rinse
> **Child 12–18 years** add 15 mL to bath water or apply to wet skin and rinse

Hydromol® (Alliance)

Bath and Shower Emollient, isopropyl myristate 13%, light liquid paraffin 37.8%, net price 350 mL = £3.80, 500 mL = £5.14, 1 litre = £9.00
Excipients none as listed in section 13.1.3

Dose

> **Neonate** add ½ capful to bath water or apply to wet skin and rinse
>
> **Child 1 month–12 years** add ½–2 capfuls to bath water or apply to wet skin and rinse
> **Child 12–18 years** add 1–3 capfuls to bath water or apply to wet skin and rinse

Imuderm® (Goldshield)

Bath oil, almond oil 30%, light liquid paraffin 69.6%, net price 250 mL = £3.75
Excipients include butylated hydroxyanisole

Dose

> **Neonate** add 7.5 mL to bath water or rub into dry skin until absorbed
>
> **Child 1 month–12 years** add 7.5–15 mL to bath water or rub into dry skin until absorbed
> **Child 12–18 years** add 15–30 mL to bath water or rub into dry skin until absorbed

13

Skin

Oilatum® (Stiefel)

Emollient bath additive (emulsion), acetylated wool alcohols 5%, liquid paraffin 63.4%, net price 250 mL = £2.75, 500 mL = £4.57
Excipients include isopropyl palmitate, fragrance

Dose

> Neonate add ½ capful to bath water or apply to wet skin and rinse

> Child 1 month–12 years add ½–2 capfuls to bath water or apply to wet skin and rinse

> Child 12–18 years add 1–3 capfuls to bath water or apply to wet skin and rinse

Junior emollient bath additive, light liquid paraffin 63.4%, net price 150 mL = £2.82, 250 mL = £3.25, 300 mL = £5.10, 500 mL = £5.75
Excipients include wool fat, isopropyl palmitate

Dose

> Neonate add ½ capful to bath water or apply to wet skin and rinse

> Child 1 month–12 years add ½–2 capfuls to bath water or apply to wet skin and rinse

> Child 12–18 years add 1–3 capfuls to bath water or apply to wet skin and rinse

QV® (Crawford)

Bath oil, light liquid paraffin 85.09%, net price 200 mL = £2.20, 500 mL = £4.50
Excipients include hydroxybenzoates (parabens)

Dose

> Child 1 month–1 year add 4 mL to bath water or apply to wet skin and rinse

> Child 1–12 years add 7 mL to bath water or apply to wet skin and rinse

> Child 12–18 years add 10 mL to bath water or apply to wet skin and rinse

◢**With antimicrobials**

Dermol® 600 (Dermal)

Bath emollient, benzalkonium chloride 0.5%, liquid paraffin 25%, isopropyl myristate 25%, net price 600 mL = £7.90
Excipients include polysorbate 60

Dose

> Child 1 month–2 years add 5–15 mL to bath water; do not use undiluted

> Child 2–18 years add 15–30 mL to bath water; do not use undiluted

Emulsiderm® (Dermal)

Liquid emulsion, liquid paraffin 25%, isopropyl myristate 25%, benzalkonium chloride 0.5%, net price 300 mL (with 15-mL measure) = £4.03, 1 litre (with 30-mL measure) = £12.55
Excipients include polysorbate 60

Dose

> Child 1 month–2 years add 5–10 mL to bath water or rub into dry skin until absorbed

> Child 2–18 years add 10–30 mL to bath water or rub into dry skin until absorbed

Oilatum® Plus (Stiefel)

Bath additive, benzalkonium chloride 6%, triclosan 2%, light liquid paraffin 52.5%, net price 500 mL = £6.98
Excipients include wool fat, isopropyl palmitate

Dose

> Child 6 months–1 year add 1 mL to bath water; do not use undiluted

> Child 1–18 years add 1–2 capfuls to bath water; do not use undiluted

◢**With tar**
Section 13.5.2

13.2.2 Barrier preparations

Barrier preparations often contain water-repellent substances such as **dimeticone** (dimethicone), natural oils, and paraffins, to help protect the skin from abrasion and irritation; they are used to protect intact skin around stomas and pressure sores, and as a barrier against nappy rash. In neonates, barrier preparations which do not contain potentially sensitising excipients (section 13.1.3) are preferred. Where the skin has broken down, barrier preparations have a limited role in protecting adjacent skin. **Zinc ointments** or barrier creams with zinc oxide or titanium salts, are used to aid healing of uninfected, excoriated skin.

Nappy rash (dermatitis)   The first line of treatment is to ensure that nappies are changed frequently and that tightly fitting water-proof pants are avoided. The rash may clear when left exposed to the air and a barrier preparation can be helpful. If the rash is associated with a yeast or fungal infection, an antifungal cream such as clotrimazole cream (section 13.10.2) is useful. A mild corticosteroid such as hydrocortisone 1% is useful in moderate to severe inflammation, but it should be avoided in neonates. The barrier preparation is applied after the corticosteroid preparation to prevent further damage. Hydrocortisone may be used in combination with antifungal and antibacterial drugs (section 13.4) if there is considerable inflammation, erosion, and infection. Preparations containing hydrocortisone should be applied for no more than a week; the hydrocortisone should be discontinued as soon as the inflammation subsides. The occlusive effect of nappies and water-proof pants may increase absorption of corticosteroid (for cautions, see section 13.4).

13 Skin

◢Non-proprietary barrier preparations

Zinc Cream, BP

Cream, zinc oxide 32%, arachis (peanut) oil 32%, calcium hydroxide 0.045%, oleic acid 0.5%, wool fat 8%, in freshly boiled and cooled purified water, net price 50 g = 50p

Zinc Ointment, BP

Ointment, zinc oxide 15%, in Simple Ointment BP 1988 (which contains wool fat 5%, hard paraffin 5%, cetostearyl alcohol 5%, white soft paraffin 85%), net price 25 g = 22p

Zinc and Castor Oil Ointment, BP

Ointment, zinc oxide 7.5%, castor oil 50%, arachis (peanut) oil 30.5%, white beeswax 10%, cetostearyl alcohol 2%, net price 25 g = 14p

◢Proprietary barrier preparations

Conotrane® (Astellas)

Cream, benzalkonium chloride 0.1%, dimeticone 22%, net price 100 g = 74p, 500 g = £3.51
Excipients include cetostearyl alcohol, fragrance

Drapolene® (Chefaro UK)

Cream, benzalkonium chloride 0.01%, cetrimide 0.2% in a basis containing white soft paraffin, cetyl alcohol and wool fat, net price 100 g = £1.54, 200 g = £2.50, 350 g = £3.75
Excipients include cetyl alcohol, chlorocresol, wool fat

Medicaid® (LPC)

Cream, cetrimide 0.5% in a basis containing light liquid paraffin, white soft paraffin, cetostearyl alcohol, glyceryl monostearate, net price 50 g = £1.69
Excipients include cetostearyl alcohol, fragrance, hydroxy-benzoates (parabens), wool fat

Metanium® (Ransom)

Ointment, titanium dioxide 20%, titanium peroxide 5%, titanium salicylate 3% in a basis containing dimeticone, light liquid paraffin, white soft paraffin, and benzoin tincture, net price 30 g = £2.01
Excipients none as listed in section 13.1.3

Morhulin® (Actavis)

Ointment, cod-liver oil 11.4%, zinc oxide 38%, in a basis containing liquid paraffin and yellow soft paraffin, net price 50 g = £1.72
Excipients include wool fat derivative

Siopel® (Centrapharm)

Barrier cream, dimeticone '1000' 10%, cetrimide 0.3%, arachis (peanut) oil, net price 50 g = £2.15
Excipients include butylated hydroxytoluene, cetostearyl alcohol, hydroxybenzoates (parabens)

Sprilon® (Ayrton Saunders)

Spray application, dimeticone 1.04%, zinc oxide 12.5%, in a basis containing wool alcohols, cetostearyl alcohol, dextran, white soft paraffin, liquid paraffin, propellants, net price 115-g pressurised aerosol unit = £3.54
Excipients include cetostearyl alcohol, hydroxybenzoates (parabens), wool fat

Note Flammable

Sudocrem® (Forest)

Cream, benzyl alcohol 0.39%, benzyl benzoate 1.01%, benzyl cinnamate 0.15%, hydrous wool fat (hypoallergenic lanolin) 4%, zinc oxide 15.25%, net price 30 g = £1.13, 60 g = £1.25, 125 g = £1.84, 250 g = £3.09, 400 g = £4.34
Excipients include beeswax (synthetic), propylene glycol, fragrance

Vasogen® (Forest)

Barrier cream, dimeticone 20%, calamine 1.5%, zinc oxide 7.5%, net price 50 g = 80p, 100 g = £1.36
Excipients include hydroxybenzoates (parabens), wool fat

13.3 Topical antipruritics

Pruritus may be caused by systemic disease (such as drug hypersensitivity, obstructive jaundice, endocrine disease, and certain malignant diseases), skin disease (e.g. eczema, psoriasis, urticaria, and scabies) or as a side-effect of opioid analgesics. Where possible the underlying cause should be treated. For the treatment of pruritus in palliative care, see Prescribing in Palliative Care, p. 27. Pruritus caused by cholestasis generally requires a bile acid sequestrant (section 1.9.2).

An **emollient** (section 13.2.1) may be of value where the pruritus is associated with dry skin. Preparations containing **calamine** or **crotamiton** are sometimes used but are of uncertain value.

A topical preparation containing **doxepin 5%** is licensed for the relief of pruritus in eczema in children over 12 years; it can cause drowsiness and there may be a risk of sensitisation.

Topical antihistamines and local anaesthetics (section 15.2) are only marginally effective and occasionally cause sensitisation. For *insect stings* and *insect bites*, a short course of a topical corticosteroid is appropriate. Short-term treatment with a **sedating antihistamine** (section 3.4.1) may help in insect stings and in intractable pruritus where sedation is desirable. Calamine preparations are of little value for the treatment of insect stings or bites.

In *pruritus ani*, the underlying cause such as faecal soiling, eczema, psoriasis, or helminth infection should be treated; for preparations used to relieve pruritus ani, see section 1.7.

13

Skin

CALAMINE

Indication and dose
Pruritus but see notes above

Calamine (Non-proprietary)
Aqueous cream, calamine 4%, zinc oxide 3%, liquid paraffin 20%, self-emulsifying glyceryl monostearate 5%, cetomacrogol emulsifying wax 5%, phenoxyethanol 0.5%, freshly boiled and cooled purified water 62.5%, net price 100 mL = 59p

Lotion (= cutaneous suspension), calamine 15%, zinc oxide 5%, glycerol 5%, bentonite 3%, sodium citrate 0.5%, liquefied phenol 0.5%, in freshly boiled and cooled purified water, net price 200 mL = 63p

Oily lotion (BP 1980), calamine 5%, arachis (peanut) oil 50%, oleic acid 0.5%, wool fat 1%, in calcium hydroxide solution, net price 200 mL = £1.57

CROTAMITON

Cautions avoid use near eyes and broken skin; use on doctor's advice for children under 3 years
Contra-indications acute exudative dermatoses
Indication and dose
Pruritus (including pruritus after scabies—section 13.10.4) see notes above
Apply 2–3 times daily (for pruritus after scabies in children under 3 years apply once daily only)

Eurax® (Novartis Consumer Health)
Cream, crotamiton 10%, net price 30 g = £2.27, 100 g = £3.95
Excipients include beeswax, fragrance, hydroxybenzoates (parabens), stearyl alcohol

Lotion, crotamiton 10%, net price 100 mL = £2.99
Excipients include cetyl alcohol, fragrance, propylene glycol, sorbic acid, stearyl alcohol

DOXEPIN HYDROCHLORIDE

Cautions glaucoma, urinary retention, severe liver impairment, mania; avoid application to large areas; **interactions**: Appendix 1 (antidepressants, tricyclic)
Driving Drowsiness may affect performance of skilled tasks (e.g. driving); effects of alcohol enhanced
Pregnancy manufacturer advises use only if potential benefit outweighs risk
Breast-feeding manufacturer advises use only if potential benefit outweighs risk
Side-effects drowsiness; local burning, stinging, irritation, tingling and rash; systemic side-effects such as antimuscarinic affects, headache, fever, dizziness, gastro-intestinal disturbances also reported

Indication and dose
Pruritus in eczema
Child 12–18 years apply thinly 3–4 times daily; usual max. 3 g per application; usual total max. 12 g daily; coverage should be less than 10% of body surface area

Depressive illness section 4.3.1

Xepin® (CHS) [PoM]
Cream, doxepin hydrochloride 5%, net price 30 g = £11.70. Label: 2, 10, patient information leaflet
Excipients include benzyl alcohol

13.4 Topical corticosteroids

Topical corticosteroids are used for the treatment of inflammatory conditions of the skin (other than those arising from an infection), particularly eczema (section 13.5.1), contact dermatitis, insect stings (p. 48), and eczema of scabies (section 13.10.4). Corticosteroids suppress the inflammatory reaction during use; they are not curative and on discontinuation a rebound exacerbation of the condition may occur. They are generally used to relieve symptoms and suppress signs of the disorder when other measures such as emollients are ineffective.

Children, especially infants, are particularly susceptible to side-effects. However, concern about the safety of topical corticosteroids in children should not result in the child being undertreated. The aim is to control the condition as well as possible; inadequate treatment will perpetuate the condition. Carers of young children should be advised that treatment should **not** necessarily be reserved to 'treat only the worst areas' and they may need to be advised that patient information leaflets may contain inappropriate advice for the child's condition.

In an acute flare-up of atopic eczema, it may be appropriate to use more potent formulations of topical corticosteroids for a short period to regain control of the condition. Continuous daily application of a mild corticosteroid such as hydrocortisone 1% is equivalent to a potent corticosteroid such as betamethasone 0.1% applied intermittently.

Topical corticosteroids are of no value in the treatment of *urticaria*. They may worsen ulcerated or secondarily infected lesions. They should not be used indiscriminately in *pruritus* (where they will only benefit if inflammation is causing the itch) and are **not** recommended for *acne vulgaris*.

Systemic or potent topical corticosteroids should be avoided or given only under specialist supervision in *psoriasis* because, although they may suppress the psoriasis in the short term, relapse or vigorous rebound occurs on withdrawal (sometimes precipitating severe pustular psoriasis). Topical use of potent corticosteroids on widespread psoriasis can lead to systemic as well as to local side-effects. It is reasonable, however, to prescribe a mild to moderate topical corticosteroid for a short period (2–4 weeks) for *flexural* and *facial psoriasis*, and to use a more potent corticosteroid such as betamethasone or fluocinonide for *psoriasis* of the *scalp*, *palms*, or *soles* (see below for cautions in psoriasis).

In general, the most potent topical corticosteroids should be reserved for recalcitrant dermatoses such as *chronic discoid lupus erythematosus, lichen simplex chronicus, hypertrophic lichen planus*, and *palmoplantar pustulosis*. Potent corticosteroids should generally be avoided on the face and skin flexures, but specialists occasionally prescribe them for use on these areas in certain circumstances.

When topical treatment has failed, intralesional corticosteroid injections (section 10.1.2.2) may be used. These are more effective than the very potent topical corticosteroid preparations and should be reserved for severe cases where there are localised lesions such as *keloid scars, hypertrophic lichen planus*, or *localised alopecia areata*.

Choice   Water-miscible corticosteroid *creams* are suitable for moist or weeping lesions whereas *ointments* are generally chosen for dry, lichenified or scaly lesions or where a more occlusive effect is required. *Lotions* may be useful when minimal application to a large or hair-bearing area is required or for the treatment of exudative lesions. *Occlusive polythene or hydrocolloid dressings* increase absorption, but also increase the risk of side-effects; they are therefore used only under supervision on a short-term basis for areas of very thick skin (such as the palms and soles). Disposable nappies and tight fitting pants increase the risk of side-effects by increasing absorption of the corticosteroid. The inclusion of urea or salicylic acid also increases the penetration of the corticosteroid.

'Wet-wrap bandaging' (section 13.5.1) increases absorption into the skin, but should be initiated only by a dermatologist and application supervised by a healthcare professional trained in the technique.

In the *BNF for Children*, topical corticosteroids for the skin are categorised as 'mild', 'moderately potent', 'potent' or 'very potent' (see p. 675); the **least potent** preparation which is effective should be chosen but dilution should be avoided whenever possible.

Topical hydrocortisone is usually used in children under 1 year of age. Moderately potent and potent topical corticosteroids should be used with great care in children and for short periods (1–2 weeks) only. A very potent corticosteroid should be initiated under the supervision of a specialist.

Appropriate topical corticosteroids for specific conditions are:

- *insect bites and stings*—mild corticosteroid such as hydrocortisone 1% cream;
- *severely inflamed nappy rash* in infant over 1 month (section 13.2.2)—mild corticosteroid such as hydrocortisone 0.5 or 1% for 5–7 days (combined with antimicrobial if infected);
- *mild to moderate eczema, flexural and facial eczema or psoriasis*—mild corticosteroid such as hydrocortisone 1%;
- *severe eczema of the face and neck*—moderately potent corticosteroid for 3–5 days only;
- *severe eczema on the trunk and limbs* in children over 1 year—moderately potent or potent corticosteroid for 1–2 weeks only, switching to a less potent preparation as the condition improves;
- *eczema affecting area with thickened skin* (e.g. soles of feet)—potent topical corticosteroid in combination with urea or salicylic acid (to increase penetration of corticosteroid).

13

Skin

Perioral lesions   **Hydrocortisone** cream 1% can be used for up to 7 days to treat uninfected inflammatory lesions on the lips and on the skin surrounding the mouth. **Hydrocortisone and miconazole** cream or ointment is useful where infection by susceptible organisms and inflammation co-exist, particularly for initial treatment (up to 7 days) e.g. in angular cheilitis (see also p. 657). Organisms susceptible to miconazole include *Candida* spp. and many Gram-positive bacteria including streptococci and staphylococci.

Cautions   Avoid prolonged use of a topical corticosteroid particularly on the face (and keep away from eyes). Use potent or very potent corticosteroids under specialist supervision; extreme caution is required in dermatoses of infancy including nappy rash—treatment should be limited to 5–7 days.

Psoriasis The use of potent or very potent corticosteroids in psoriasis can result in rebound relapse, development of generalised pustular psoriasis, and local and systemic toxicity, see notes above.

Contra-indications   Topical corticosteroids are contra-indicated in untreated bacterial, fungal, or viral skin lesions, in acne, and in perioral dermatitis; potent corticosteroids are contra-indicated in widespread plaque psoriasis (see notes above).

Side-effects   *Mild* and *moderately potent* topical corticosteroids are associated with few side-effects but particular care is required when treating neonates and infants, and in the use of *potent* and *very potent* corticosteroids. Absorption through the skin can rarely cause adrenal suppression and even Cushing's syndrome (section 6.3.2), depending on the area of the body being treated and the duration of treatment. Absorption of corticosteroid is greatest from severely inflamed skin, thin skin (especially on the face or genital area), from flexural sites (e.g. axillae groins), and in infants where skin surface area is higher in relation to body-weight; absorption is increased by occlusion.

Local side-effects include: spread and worsening of untreated infection; thinning of the skin which may be restored over a period after stopping treatment but the original structure may never return; irreversible striae atrophicae and telangiectasia; contact dermatitis; perioral dermatitis; acne, or worsening of acne or rosacea; mild depigmentation which may be reversible; hypertrichosis also reported.

Children and their carers should be reassured that side effects such as skin thinning and systemic effects rarely occur when topical corticosteroids are used appropriately.

> **Safe Practice**
> In order to minimise the side-effects of a topical corticosteroid, it is important to apply it **thinly** to affected areas **only**, no more frequently than **twice daily**, and to use the least potent formulation which is fully effective.

Application   Topical corticosteroid preparations should be applied no more frequently than twice daily; once daily is often sufficient.

Topical corticosteroids are spread thinly on the skin; the length of cream or ointment expelled from a tube may be used to specify the quantity to be applied to a given area of skin. This length can be measured in terms of a *fingertip unit* (the distance from the tip of the adult index finger to the first crease). One fingertip unit (approximately 500 mg) is sufficient to cover an area that is twice that of the flat adult palm.

If a child is using topical corticosteroids of different potencies, the child and their carers should be told when to use each corticosteroid. The potency of each topical corticosteroid (see Topical Corticosteroid Preparation Potencies, p. 675) should be included on the label with the directions for use. The label should be attached to the container (for example, the tube) rather than the outer packaging.

Mixing topical preparations on the skin should be avoided where possible; several minutes should elapse between application of different preparations.

Compound preparations   The advantages of including other substances (such as antibacterials or antifungals) with corticosteroids in topical preparations are uncertain, but such combinations may have a place where inflammatory skin conditions are associated with bacterial or fungal infection, such as infected eczema. In these cases the antimicrobial drug should be chosen according to the sensitivity of the infecting organism and used regularly for a short period (typically twice daily for 1 week). Longer use increases the likelihood of resistance and of sensitisation.

Topical corticosteroid potencies

Potency of a topical corticosteroid preparation depends upon the formulation as well as the corticosteroid. Therefore, proprietary names are shown below.

Mild

Hydrocortisone 0.1–2.5%, *Dioderm, Mildison, Synalar 1 in 10 Dilution*

Mild with antimicrobials *Canesten HC, Daktacort, Econacort, Fucidin H, Nystaform-HC, Timodine*

Mild with crotamiton *Eurax-Hydrocortisone*

Moderate

Betnovate-RD, Eumovate, Haelan, Modrasone, Synalar 1 in 4 Dilution, Ultralanum Plain

Moderate with antimicrobials *Trimovate*

Moderate with urea *Alphaderm, Calmurid HC*

Potent

Betamethasone valerate 0.1%, *Betcap, Bettamousse, Betnovate, Cutivate, Diprosone, Elocon*, Hydrocortisone butyrate, *Locoid, Locoid Crelo, Metosyn, Nerisone, Synalar*

Potent with antimicrobials *Aureocort, Betnovate-C, Betnovate-N, Fucibet, Lotriderm, Synalar C, Synalar N*

Potent with salicylic acid *Diprosalic*

Very potent

Dermovate, Nerisone Forte

HYDROCORTISONE

Cautions see notes above

Contra-indications see notes above

Side-effects see notes above

Indication and dose

Mild inflammatory skin disorders such as eczemas (but for over-the-counter preparations, see below)
Apply thinly 1–2 times daily

Nappy rash see notes above and section 13.2.2

◄Over-the-counter hydrocortisone preparations

Skin creams and ointments containing hydrocortisone (alone or with other ingredients) can be sold to the public for the treatment of allergic contact dermatitis, irritant dermatitis, insect bite reactions and mild to moderate eczema in children over 10 years, to be applied sparingly over the affected area 1–2 times daily for max. 1 week. Over-the-counter hydrocortisone preparations should not be sold without medical advice for children under 10 years or for pregnant women; they should **not** be sold for application to the face, anogenital region, broken or infected skin (including cold sores, acne, and athlete's foot).

Hydrocortisone (Non-proprietary) PoM

Cream, hydrocortisone 0.5%, net price, 15 g = £3.04, 30 g = £5.19; 1%, 15 g = £2.70, 30 g = £3.65, 50 g = £16.96; 2.5%, 15 g = £24.03. Label: 28, counselling, application, see p. 674. Potency: mild

Dental prescribing on NHS Hydrocortisone Cream 1% 15 g may be prescribed

Ointment, hydrocortisone 0.5%, net price 15 g = £3.57, 30 g = £5.23; 1%, 15 g = £2.55, 30 g = £3.55, 50 g = £25.22; 2.5%, 15 g = £32.53. Label: 28, counselling, application, see p. 674. Potency: mild
When hydrocortisone cream or ointment is prescribed and no strength is stated, the 1% strength should be supplied

◄Proprietary hydrocortisone preparations

Dioderm® (Dermal) PoM

Cream, hydrocortisone 0.1%, net price 30 g = £2.50. Label: 28, counselling, application, see p. 674. Potency: mild
Excipients include cetostearyl alcohol, propylene glycol

Note Although this contains only 0.1% hydrocortisone, the formulation is designed to provide a clinical activity comparable to that of Hydrocortisone Cream 1% BP

Mildison® (Astellas) PoM

Lipocream, hydrocortisone 1%, net price 30 g = £2.45. Label: 28, counselling, application, see p. 674. Potency: mild
Excipients include cetostearyl alcohol, hydroxybenzoates (parabens)

13

Skin

◻ **HYDROCORTISONE** (*continued*)

◀ Compound preparations
Compound preparations with coal tar see section 13.5.2

Alphaderm® (Alliance) [PoM]
Cream, hydrocortisone 1%, urea 10%, net price 30 g = £1.98; 100 g = £5.86. Label: 28, counselling, application, see p. 674. Potency: moderate
Excipients none as listed in section 13.1.3

Calmurid HC® (Galderma) [PoM]
Cream, hydrocortisone 1%, urea 10%, lactic acid 5%, net price 30 g = £2.80, 50 g = £4.67. Label: 28, counselling, application, see p. 674. Potency: moderate
Excipients none as listed in section 13.1.3

Note Manufacturer advises dilute to half-strength with aqueous cream for 1 week if stinging occurs then transfer to undiluted preparation (but see section 13.1.1 for advice to avoid dilution where possible)

¹**Eurax-Hydrocortisone®** (Novartis Consumer Health) [PoM]
Cream, hydrocortisone 0.25%, crotamiton 10%, net price 30 g = 87p. Label: 28, counselling, application, see p. 674. Potency: mild
Excipients include fragrance, hydroxybenzoates (parabens), propylene glycol, stearyl alcohol
1. A 15-g tube is on sale to the public for treatment of contact dermatitis and insect bites in children 10–18 years.

◀ With antimicrobials
See notes above for comment on compound preparations

¹**Canesten HC®** (Bayer Consumer Care) [PoM]
Cream, hydrocortisone 1%, clotrimazole 1%, net price 30 g = £2.42. Label: 28, counselling, application, see p. 674. Potency: mild
Excipients include benzyl alcohol, cetostearyl alcohol
1. A 15-g tube is on sale to the public for the treatment of athlete's foot and fungal infection of skin folds with associated inflammation in children 10–18 years.

Daktacort® (Janssen-Cilag) [PoM]
Cream¹, hydrocortisone 1%, miconazole nitrate 2%, net price 30 g = £2.08. Label: 28, counselling, application, see p. 674. Potency: mild
Excipients include butylated hydroxyanisole, disodium edetate

Ointment, hydrocortisone 1%, miconazole nitrate 2%, net price 30 g = £2.09. Label: 28, counselling, application, see p. 674.
Excipients none as listed in section 13.1.3

Dental prescribing on NHS May be prescribed as Miconazole and Hydrocortisone Cream or Ointment for max. 7 days
1. A 15-g tube is on sale to the public for the treatment of athlete's foot and candidal intertrigo in children 10–18 years

Econacort® (Squibb) [PoM]
Cream, hydrocortisone 1%, econazole nitrate 1%, net price 30 g = £2.25. Label: 28, counselling, application, see p. 674. Potency: mild
Excipients include butylated hydroxyanisole

Fucidin H® (LEO) [PoM]
Cream, hydrocortisone acetate 1%, fusidic acid 2%, net price 30 g = £5.30, 60 g = £10.60. Label: 28, counselling, application, see p. 674. Potency: mild
Excipients include butylated hydroxyanisole, cetyl alcohol, polysorbate 60, potassium sorbate

Ointment, hydrocortisone acetate 1%, sodium fusidate 2%, net price 30 g = £3.26, 60 g = £6.53. Label: 28, counselling, application, see p. 674. Potency: mild
Excipients include cetyl alcohol, wool fat

Nystaform-HC® (Typharm) [PoM]
Cream, hydrocortisone 0.5%, nystatin 100 000 units/g, chlorhexidine hydrochloride 1%, net price 30 g = £2.66. Label: 28, counselling, application, see p. 674. Potency: mild
Excipients include benzyl alcohol, cetostearyl alcohol, polysorbate '60'

Ointment, hydrocortisone 1%, nystatin 100 000 units/g, chlorhexidine acetate 1%, net price 30 g = £2.66. Label: 28, counselling, application, see p. 674. Potency: mild
Excipients none as listed in section 13.1.3

Timodine® (R&C) [PoM]
Cream, hydrocortisone 0.5%, nystatin 100 000 units/g, benzalkonium chloride solution 0.2%, dimeticone '350' 10%, net price 30 g = £2.38. Label: 28, counselling, application, see p. 674. Potency: mild
Excipients include butylated hydroxyanisole, cetostearyl alcohol, hydroxybenzoates (parabens), sodium metabisulphite, sorbic acid

---

▮ **HYDROCORTISONE BUTYRATE**

Cautions see notes above

Contra-indications see notes above

Side-effects see notes above

Indication and dose

Severe inflammatory skin disorders such as eczemas unresponsive to less potent corticosteroids, psoriasis see notes above

Child 1–18 years apply thinly 1–2 times daily

Locoid® (Astellas) [PoM]
Cream, hydrocortisone butyrate 0.1%, net price 30 g = £2.29, 100 g = £7.05. Label: 28, counselling, application, see p. 674. Potency: potent
Excipients include cetostearyl alcohol, hydroxybenzoates (parabens)

Lipocream, hydrocortisone butyrate 0.1%, net price 30 g = £2.41, 100 g = £7.38. Label: 28, counselling, application, see p. 674. Potency: potent
Excipients include benzyl alcohol, cetostearyl alcohol, hydroxybenzoates (parabens)

Note For bland cream basis see *Lipobase®*, section 13.2.1

Ointment, hydrocortisone butyrate 0.1%, net price 30 g = £2.29, 100 g = £7.05. Label: 28, counselling, application, see p. 674. Potency: potent
Excipients none as listed in section 13.1.3

13 **Skin**

◁ HYDROCORTISONE BUTYRATE (*continued*)

Scalp lotion, hydrocortisone butyrate 0.1%, in an aqueous isopropyl alcohol basis, net price 100 mL = £9.76. Label: 15, 28, counselling, application, see p. 674. Potency: potent
Excipients none as listed in section 13.1.3

Locoid Crelo® (Astellas) PoM
Lotion (topical emulsion), hydrocortisone butyrate 0.1% in a water-miscible basis, net price 100 g (with applicator nozzle) = £8.44. Label: 28, counselling, application, see p. 674. Potency: potent
Excipients include butylated hydroxytoluene, cetostearyl alcohol, hydroxybenzoates (parabens), propylene glycol

■ ALCLOMETASONE DIPROPIONATE

Cautions see notes above

Contra-indications see notes above

Side-effects see notes above

Licensed use licensed for use in children (age range not specified by manufacturer)

Indication and dose

Inflammatory skin disorders such as eczemas
Apply thinly 1–2 times daily

Modrasone® (PLIVA) PoM
Cream, alclometasone dipropionate 0.05%, net price 50 g = £2.68. Label: 28, counselling, application, see p. 674. Potency: moderate
Excipients include cetostearyl alcohol, chlorocresol, propylene glycol

Ointment, alclometasone dipropionate 0.05%, net price 50 g = £2.68. Label: 28, counselling, application, see p. 674. Potency: moderate
Excipients include beeswax, propylene glycol

■ BETAMETHASONE ESTERS

Cautions see notes above; use of more than 100 g per week of 0.1% preparation likely to cause adrenal suppression

Contra-indications see notes above

Side-effects see notes above

Licensed use *Betacap®*, *Betnovate®*, *Betnovate-C®*, and *Betnovate-RD®* not licensed for use in children under 1 year; *Bettamousse®* and *Fucibet® Lipid Cream* not licensed for use in children under 6 years; *Betnovate-N®* not licensed for use in children under 2 years; *Lotriderm®* not licensed for use in children under 12 years; *all other preparations* licensed for use in children (age range not specified by manufacturer)

Indication and dose

Severe inflammatory skin disorders such as eczemas unresponsive to less potent corticosteroids, psoriasis see notes above
Apply thinly 1–2 times daily

Betamethasone Valerate (Non-proprietary) PoM
Cream, betamethasone (as valerate) 0.1%, net price 30 g = £1.63, 100 g = £4.36. Label: 28, counselling, application, see p. 674. Potency: potent

Ointment, betamethasone (as valerate) 0.1%, net price 30 g = £1.70, 100 g = £4.15. Label: 28, counselling, application, see p. 674. Potency: potent

Betacap® (Dermal) PoM
Scalp application, betamethasone (as valerate) 0.1% in a water-miscible basis containing coconut oil derivative, net price 100 mL = £3.92. Label: 15, 28, counselling, application, see p. 674. Potency: potent
Excipients none as listed in section 13.1.3

Betnovate® (GSK) PoM
Cream, betamethasone (as valerate) 0.1% in a water-miscible basis, net price 30 g = £1.43, 100 g = £4.05. Label: 28, counselling, application, see p. 674. Potency: potent
Excipients include cetostearyl alcohol, chlorocresol

Ointment, betamethasone (as valerate) 0.1% in an anhydrous paraffin basis, net price 30 g = £1.43, 100 g = £4.05. Label: 28, counselling, application, see p. 674. Potency: potent
Excipients none as listed in section 13.1.3

Lotion, betamethasone (as valerate) 0.1%, net price 100 mL = £4.86. Label: 28, counselling, application, see p. 674. Potency: potent
Excipients include cetostearyl alcohol, hydroxybenzoates (parabens)

Scalp application, betamethasone (as valerate) 0.1% in a water-miscible basis, net price 100 mL = £5.30. Label: 15, 28, counselling, application, see p. 674. Potency: potent
Excipients none as listed in section 13.1.3

Betnovate-RD® (GSK) PoM
Cream, betamethasone (as valerate) 0.025% in a water-miscible basis (1 in 4 dilution of *Betnovate®* cream), net price 100 g = £3.34. Label: 28, counselling, application, see p. 674. Potency: moderate
Excipients include cetostearyl alcohol, chlorocresol

Ointment, betamethasone (as valerate) 0.025% in an anhydrous paraffin basis (1 in 4 dilution of *Betnovate®* ointment), net price 100 g = £3.34. Label: 28, counselling, application, see p. 674. Potency: moderate
Excipients none as listed in section 13.1.3

Bettamousse® (UCB Pharma) PoM
Foam (= scalp application), betamethasone valerate 0.12% (≡ betamethasone 0.1%), net price 100 g = £9.75. Label: 28, counselling, application, see p. 674. Potency: potent
Excipients include cetyl alcohol, polysorbate 60, propylene glycol, stearyl alcohol
Note Flammable

Diprosone® (Schering-Plough) PoM
Cream, betamethasone (as dipropionate) 0.05%, net price 30 g = £2.24, 100 g = £6.36. Label: 28, counselling, application, see p. 674. Potency: potent
Excipients include cetostearyl alcohol, chlorocresol

◁ **BETAMETHASONE ESTERS** (*continued*)

Ointment, betamethasone (as dipropionate) 0.05%, net price 30 g = £2.24, 100 g = £6.36. Label: 28, counselling, application, see p. 674. Potency: potent
Excipients none as listed in section 13.1.3

Lotion, betamethasone (as dipropionate) 0.05%, net price 30 mL = £2.83, 100 mL = £8.10. Label: 28, counselling, application, see p. 674. Potency: potent
Excipients none as listed in section 13.1.3

◢**With salicylic acid**
See notes above for comment on compound preparations

Diprosalic® (Schering-Plough) [PoM]
Ointment, betamethasone (as dipropionate) 0.05%, salicylic acid 3%, net price 30 g = £3.30, 100 g = £9.50. Label: 28, counselling, application, see p. 674. Potency: potent
Excipients none as listed in section 13.1.3
Dose
> Apply thinly 1–2 times daily; max. 60 g per week

Scalp application, betamethasone (as dipropionate) 0.05%, salicylic acid 2%, in an alcoholic basis, net price 100 mL = £10.50. Label: 28, counselling, application, see p. 674. Potency: potent
Excipients include disodium edetate
Dose
> Apply a few drops 1–2 times daily

◢**With antimicrobials**
See notes above for comment on compound preparations

Betnovate-C® (Chemidex) [PoM]
Cream, betamethasone (as valerate) 0.1%, clioquinol 3%, net price 30 g = £1.76. Label: 28, counselling, application, see p. 674. Potency: potent
Excipients include cetostearyl alcohol, chlorocresol

Note Stains clothing

Ointment, betamethasone (as valerate) 0.1%, clioquinol 3%, net price 30 g = £1.76. Label: 28, counselling, application, see p. 674. Potency: potent
Excipients none as listed in section 13.1.3

Note Stains clothing

Betnovate-N® (Chemidex) [PoM]
Cream, betamethasone (as valerate) 0.1%, neomycin sulphate 0.5%, net price 30 g = £1.76, 100 g = £4.88. Label: 28, counselling, application, see p. 674. Potency: potent
Excipients include cetostearyl alcohol, chlorocresol

Ointment, betamethasone (as valerate) 0.1%, neomycin sulphate 0.5%, net price 30 g = £1.76, 100 g = £4.88. Label: 28, counselling, application, see p. 674. Potency: potent
Excipients none as listed in section 13.1.3

Fucibet® (LEO) [PoM]
Cream, betamethasone (as valerate) 0.1%, fusidic acid 2%, net price 30 g = £5.62, 60 g = £11.23. Label: 28, counselling, application, see p. 674. Potency: potent
Excipients include cetostearyl alcohol, chlorocresol

Lipid cream, betamethasone (as valerate) 0.1%, fusidic acid 2%, net price 30 g = £5.62. Label: 28, counselling, application, see p. 674. Potency: potent
Excipients include cetostearyl alcohol, hydroxybenzoates (parabens)

Lotriderm® (PLIVA) [PoM]
Cream, betamethasone dipropionate 0.064% (≡ betamethasone 0.05%), clotrimazole 1%, net price 30 g = £6.34. Label: 28, counselling, application, see p. 674. Potency: potent
Excipients include benzyl alcohol, cetostearyl alcohol, propylene glycol

CLOBETASOL PROPIONATE

Cautions see notes above

Contra-indications see notes above

Side-effects see notes above

Licensed use not licensed for use in children under 1 year

Indication and dose
> Short-term treatment only of severe resistant inflammatory skin disorders such as recalcitrant eczemas unresponsive to less potent corticosteroids, psoriasis see notes above
> Apply thinly 1–2 times daily for up to 4 weeks; max. 50 g of 0.05% preparation per week

Dermovate® (GSK) [PoM]
Cream, clobetasol propionate 0.05%, net price 30 g = £2.86, 100 g = £8.39. Label: 28, counselling, application, see p. 674. Potency: very potent
Excipients include beeswax (or beeswax substitute), cetostearyl alcohol, chlorocresol, propylene glycol

Ointment, clobetasol propionate 0.05%, net price 30 g = £2.86, 100 g = £8.39. Label: 28, counselling, application, see p. 674. Potency: very potent
Excipients include propylene glycol

Scalp application, clobetasol propionate 0.05%, in a thickened alcoholic basis, net price 30 mL = £3.26, 100 mL = £11.06. Label: 15, 28, counselling, application, see p. 674. Potency: very potent
Excipients none as listed in section 13.1.3

CLOBETASONE BUTYRATE

Cautions see notes above

Contra-indications see notes above

Side-effects see notes above

Licensed use licensed for use in children (age range not specified by manufacturer)

Indication and dose
> Eczemas and dermatitis of all types; maintenance between courses of more potent corticosteroids
> Apply thinly 1–2 times daily

13 Skin

◁ **CLOBETASONE BUTYRATE** (*continued*)

[1]**Eumovate®** (GSK) ℞

Cream, clobetasone butyrate 0.05%, net price 30 g = £1.97, 100 g = £5.77. Label: 28, counselling, application, see p. 674. Potency: moderate
Excipients include beeswax substitute, cetostearyl alcohol, chlorocresol

Ointment, clobetasone butyrate 0.05%, net price 30 g = £1.97, 100 g = £5.77. Label: 28, counselling, application, see p. 674. Potency: moderate
Excipients none as listed in section 13.1.3

1. Cream can be sold to the public for short-term symptomatic treatment and control of patches of eczema and dermatitis (but not seborrhoeic dermatitis) in children over 12 years provided pack does not contain more than 15 g

◢**With antimicrobials**
See notes above for comment on compound preparations

Trimovate® (GSK) ℞

Cream, clobetasone butyrate 0.05%, oxytetracycline 3% (as calcium salt), nystatin 100 000 units/g, net price 30 g = £3.49. Label: 28, counselling, application, see p. 674. Potency: moderate
Excipients include cetostearyl alcohol, chlorocresol, sodium metabisulphite

Note Stains clothing

◢ **DIFLUCORTOLONE VALERATE**

Cautions see notes above

Contra-indications see notes above

Side-effects see notes above

Licensed use *Nerisone®* licensed for use in children (age range not specified by manufacturer); *Nerisone Forte®* not licensed for use in children under 4 years

Indication and dose

Severe inflammatory skin disorders such as eczemas unresponsive to less potent corticosteroids; high strength (0.3%), short-term treatment of severe exacerbations, psoriasis see notes above

Apply thinly 1–2 times daily for up to 4 weeks (0.1% preparations) or 2 weeks (0.3% preparations), reducing strength as condition responds; max. 60 g of 0.3% per week

Nerisone® (Meadow) ℞

Cream, diflucortolone valerate 0.1%, net price 30 g = £1.59. Label: 28, counselling, application, see p. 674. Potency: potent
Excipients include disodium edetate, hydroxybenzoates (parabens), stearyl alcohol

Oily cream, diflucortolone valerate 0.1%, net price 30 g = £2.56. Label: 28, counselling, application, see p. 674. Potency: potent
Excipients include beeswax

Ointment, diflucortolone valerate 0.1%, net price 30 g = £1.59. Label: 28, counselling, application, see p. 674. Potency: potent
Excipients none as listed in section 13.1.3

Nerisone Forte® (Meadow) ℞

Oily cream, diflucortolone valerate 0.3%, net price 15 g = £2.09. Label: 28, counselling, application, see p. 674. Potency: very potent
Excipients include beeswax

Ointment, diflucortolone valerate 0.3%, net price 15 g = £2.09. Label: 28, counselling, application, see p. 674. Potency: very potent
Excipients none as listed in section 13.1.3

◢ **FLUDROXYCORTIDE**

(Flurandrenolone)

Cautions see notes above

Contra-indications see notes above

Side-effects see notes above

Licensed use licensed for use in children (age range not specified by manufacturer)

Indication and dose

Inflammatory skin disorders such as eczemas
Apply thinly 1–2 times daily

Haelan® (Typharm) ℞

Cream, fludroxycortide 0.0125%, net price 60 g = £3.26. Label: 28, counselling, application, see p. 674. Potency: moderate
Excipients include cetyl alcohol, propylene glycol

Ointment, fludroxycortide 0.0125%, net price 60 g = £3.26. Label: 28, counselling, application, see p. 674. Potency: moderate
Excipients include beeswax, cetyl alcohol, polysorbate

Tape, polythene adhesive film impregnated with fludroxycortide 4 micrograms /cm^2, net price 7.5 cm × 50 cm = £9.27, 7.5 cm × 200 cm = £24.95

Dose

Chronic localised recalcitrant dermatoses (but not acute or weeping)

Cut tape to fit lesion, apply to clean, dry skin shorn of hair, usually for 12 hours daily

---

◢ **FLUOCINOLONE ACETONIDE**

Cautions see notes above

Contra-indications see notes above

Side-effects see notes above

Licensed use not licensed for use in children under 1 year

13

Skin

◁ **FLUOCINOLONE ACETONIDE** (*continued*)

Indication and dose

Severe inflammatory skin disorders such as
eczemas, psoriasis see notes above

Apply thinly 1–2 times daily, reducing strength
as condition responds

Synalar® (GP Pharma) (PoM)

Cream, fluocinolone acetonide 0.025%, net price
30 g = £3.76, 100 g = £10.68. Label: 28, counselling,
application, see p. 674. Potency: potent
Excipients include benzyl alcohol, cetostearyl alcohol, polysorbates, propylene glycol

Gel, fluocinolone acetonide 0.025%, net price 30 g
= £5.56. For use on scalp and other hairy areas.
Label: 28, counselling, application, see p. 674.
Potency: potent
Excipients include hydroxybenzoates (parabens), propylene
glycol

Ointment, fluocinolone acetonide 0.025%, net price
30 g = £3.76, 100 g = £10.68. Label: 28, counselling,
application, see p. 674. Potency: potent
Excipients include propylene glycol, wool fat

Synalar 1 in 4 Dilution® (GP Pharma) (PoM)

Cream, fluocinolone acetonide 0.00625%, net price
50 g = £4.40. Label: 28, counselling, application, see
p. 674. Potency: moderate
Excipients include benzyl alcohol, cetostearyl alcohol, polysorbates, propylene glycol

Ointment, fluocinolone acetonide 0.00625%, net
price 50 g = £4.40. Label: 28, counselling, application, see p. 674. Potency: moderate
Excipients include propylene glycol, wool fat

Synalar 1 in 10 Dilution® (GP Pharma) (PoM)

Cream, fluocinolone acetonide 0.0025%, net price
50 g = £4.16. Label: 28, counselling, application, see
p. 674. Potency: mild
Excipients include benzyl alcohol, cetostearyl alcohol, polysorbates, propylene glycol

◢**With antibacterials**
See notes above for comment on compound preparations

Synalar C® (GP Pharma) (PoM)

Cream, fluocinolone acetonide 0.025%, clioquinol
3%, net price 15 g = £2.42. Label: 28, counselling,
application, see p. 674. Potency: potent
Excipients include cetostearyl alcohol, disodium edetate,
hydroxybenzoates (parabens), polysorbates, propylene glycol

Ointment, fluocinolone acetonide 0.025%, clioquinol 3%, net price 15 g = £2.42. Label: 28, counselling, application, see p. 674. Potency: potent.
Note stains clothing
Excipients include propylene glycol, wool fat

Synalar N® (GP Pharma) (PoM)

Cream, fluocinolone acetonide 0.025%, neomycin
sulphate 0.5%, net price 30 g = £3.96. Label: 28,
counselling, application, see p. 674. Potency: potent
Excipients include cetostearyl alcohol, hydroxybenzoates
(parabens), polysorbates, propylene glycol

Ointment, fluocinolone acetonide 0.025%, neomycin sulphate 0.5%, in a greasy basis, net price
30 g = £3.96. Label: 28, counselling, application, see
p. 674. Potency: potent
Excipients include propylene glycol, wool fat

▋ FLUOCINONIDE

Cautions see notes above

Contra-indications see notes above

Side-effects see notes above

Licensed use not licensed for use in children
under 1 year

Indication and dose

Severe inflammatory skin disorders such as
eczemas unresponsive to less potent corticosteroids, psoriasis see notes above

Apply thinly 1–2 times daily

Metosyn® (GP Pharma) (PoM)

FAPG cream, fluocinonide 0.05%, net price 25 g =
£3.30, 100 g = £11.12. Label: 28, counselling,
application, see p. 674. Potency: potent
Excipients include propylene glycol

Ointment, fluocinonide 0.05%, net price 25 g =
£2.92, 100 g = £10.96. Label: 28, counselling,
application, see p. 674. Potency: potent
Excipients include propylene glycol, wool fat

▋ FLUOCORTOLONE

Cautions see notes above

Contra-indications see notes above

Side-effects see notes above

Licensed use licensed for use in children (age
range not specified by manufacturer)

Indication and dose

Severe inflammatory skin disorders such as
eczemas unresponsive to less potent corticosteroids, psoriasis see notes above

Apply thinly 1–2 times daily

Ultralanum Plain® (Meadow) (PoM)

Cream, fluocortolone caproate 0.25%, fluocorto-
lone pivalate 0.25%, net price 50 g = £2.95.
Label: 28, counselling, application, see p. 674.
Potency: moderate
Excipients include disodium edetate, fragrance, hydroxy-
benzoates (parabens), stearyl alcohol

Ointment, fluocortolone 0.25%, fluocortolone
caproate 0.25%, net price 50 g = £2.95. Label: 28,
counselling, application, see p. 674. Potency: moderate
Excipients include wool fat, fragrance

▋ FLUTICASONE PROPIONATE

Cautions see notes above

Contra-indications see notes above

Side-effects see notes above

Licensed use not licensed for use in children
under 3 months

◁ **FLUTICASONE PROPIONATE** (*continued*)

Indication and dose

Inflammatory skin disorders such as dermatitis and eczemas unresponsive to less potent corticosteroids, psoriasis see notes above
   Apply thinly 1–2 times daily

Cutivate® (GSK) PoM
Cream, fluticasone propionate 0.05%, net price 15 g = £2.41, 50 g = £7.11. Label: 28, counselling, application, see p. 674. Potency: potent
Excipients include cetostearyl alcohol, imidurea, propylene glycol

Ointment, fluticasone propionate 0.005%, net price 15 g = £2.41, 50 g = £7.11. Label: 28, counselling, application, see p. 674. Potency: potent
Excipients include propylene glycol

▌MOMETASONE FUROATE

Cautions see notes above

Contra-indications see notes above

Side-effects see notes above

Licensed use licensed for use in children (age range not specified by manufacturer)

Indication and dose

Severe inflammatory skin disorders such as eczemas unresponsive to less potent corticosteroids, psoriasis see notes above
   Apply thinly once daily (to scalp in case of lotion)

Elocon® (Schering-Plough) PoM
Cream, mometasone furoate 0.1%, net price 30 g = £4.54, 100 g = £13.07. Label: 28, counselling, application, see p. 674. Potency: potent
Excipients include propylene glycol, stearyl alcohol

Ointment, mometasone furoate 0.1%, net price 30 g = £4.54, 100 g = £13.07. Label: 28, counselling, application, see p. 674. Potency: potent
Excipients include propylene glycol

Scalp lotion, mometasone furoate 0.1% in an aqueous isopropyl alcohol basis, net price 30 mL = £4.54. Label: 28, counselling, application, see p. 674. Potency: potent
Excipients include propylene glycol

▌TRIAMCINOLONE ACETONIDE

Cautions see notes above

Contra-indications see notes above

Side-effects see notes above

Licensed use *Aureocort®* not licensed for use in children under 8 years

Indication and dose

Severe inflammatory skin disorders such as eczemas unresponsive to less potent corticosteroids, psoriasis see notes above
   Apply thinly 1–2 times daily

◢With antimicrobials
See notes above for comment on compound preparations

Aureocort® (Goldshield) PoM
Ointment, triamcinolone acetonide 0.1%, chlortetracycline hydrochloride 3%, in an anhydrous greasy basis containing wool fat and white soft paraffin, net price 15 g = £2.70. Label: 28, counselling, application, see p. 674. Potency: potent
Excipients include wool fat
Note Stains clothing

13 Skin

13.5 Preparations for eczema and psoriasis

   13.5.1 Preparations for eczema
   13.5.2 Preparations for psoriasis
   13.5.3 Drugs affecting the immune response

13.5.1 Preparations for eczema

The main types of eczema (dermatitis) in children are atopic, irritant and allergic contact; different types may co-exist. *Atopic eczema* is the most common type and it usually involves dry skin as well as infection and lichenification caused by scratching and rubbing. *Seborrhoeic dermatitis* (see below) is also common in infants.

Management of eczema involves the removal or treatment of contributory factors; known or suspected irritants and contact allergens should be avoided. Rarely, ingredients in topical medicinal products may sensitise the skin (section 13.1.3); *BNF for Children* lists active ingredients together with excipients that have been associated with skin sensitisation.

Skin dryness and the consequent irritant eczema requires **emollients** (section 13.2.1) applied regularly and liberally to the affected area; this can be supplemented with bath or shower emollients. The use of emollients should continue even if the eczema improves or if other treatment is being used.

Topical corticosteroids (section 13.4) are also required in the management of eczema; the potency of the corticosteroid should be appropriate to the severity and site of the condition, and the age of the child. Mild corticosteroids are generally used on the face and on flexures; the more potent corticosteroids are generally required for use on lichenified areas of eczema or for severe eczema on the scalp, limbs, and trunk. Treatment should be reviewed regularly, especially if a potent corticosteroid is required.

Bandages (including those containing **zinc** and **ichthammol**) are sometimes applied over topical corticosteroids or emollients to treat eczema of the limbs. Wet elasticated viscose stockinette is used for 'wet-wrap' bandaging over topical corticosteroids or emollients to cool the skin and relieve itching, but there is an increased risk of infection and excessive absorption of the corticosteroid; 'wet-wrap' bandaging should be used under specialist supervision.

For the role of topical **pimecrolimus** and **tacrolimus** in atopic eczema, see section 13.5.3.

Infection Bacterial infection (commonly with *Staphylococcus aureus* and occasionally with *Streptococcus pyogenes*) can exacerbate eczema. A topical antibacterial such as fusidic acid (section 13.10.1) may be used for small areas of mild infection; treatment should be limited to a short course (typically 1 week) to reduce the risk of drug resistance or skin sensitisation. Associated eczema is treated simultaneously with a moderately potent or potent topical corticosteroid which can be combined with an antimicrobial such as clioquinol.

Eczema involving moderate to severe, widespread, or recurrent infection requires the use of a systemic antibacterial (section 5.1, table 1) that is active against the infecting organism. Preparations that combine an antiseptic with an emollient application (section 13.2.1) and with a bath emollient (section 13.2.1.1) can also be used; antiseptic shampoos (section 13.9) can be used on the scalp.

Intertriginous eczema commonly involves candida and bacteria; it is best treated with a mild or moderately potent topical corticosteroid combined with a suitable antimicrobial drug. For the treatment of nappy rash, see section 13.2.2.

Widespread *herpes simplex infection* may complicate atopic eczema (eczema herpeticum) and treatment under specialist supervision with a systemic antiviral drug (section 5.3.2.1) is indicated. Secondary bacterial infection often exacerbates eczema herpeticum.

The management of *seborrhoeic dermatitis* is described below.

Management of other features of eczema *Lichenification*, which results from repeated scratching, is treated initially with a potent corticosteroid. Bandages containing **ichthammol** (to reduce pruritus) and other substances such as **zinc oxide** can be applied over the corticosteroid or emollient. **Coal tar** (section 13.5.2) and ichthammol can be useful in some cases of *chronic eczema*. *Discoid eczema*, with thickened plaques in chronic atopic eczema, is usually treated with a topical antiseptic preparation, a potent topical corticosteroid, and paste bandages containing zinc oxide and ichthammol.

A *non-sedating* antihistamine (section 3.4.1) may be of some value in relieving severe itching or urticaria associated with eczema. A *sedating* antihistamine (section 3.4.1) may be used at night if itching causes sleep disturbance, but a large dose may be needed and drowsiness may persist on the following day.

Exudative ('weeping') *eczema* requires a potent corticosteroid initially; infection may also be present and require specific treatment (see above). **Potassium permanganate** solution (1 in 10 000) can be used as a soak in exudating eczema for its antiseptic and astringent effects; treatment should be stopped when exudation stops.

Severe refractory eczema is best managed under specialist supervision; it may require phototherapy or drugs that act on the immune system (section 13.5.3).

Seborrhoeic dermatitis   *Seborrhoeic dermatitis* (*seborrhoeic eczema*) is associated with species of the yeast *Malassezia*. *Infantile seborrhoeic dermatitis* affects particularly the body folds, nappy area and scalp; it is treated with emollients and mild topical corticosteroids with suitable antimicrobials. Infantile seborrhoeic dermatitis affecting the scalp (*cradle cap*) is treated by hydrating the scalp using natural oils and the use of mild shampoo (section 13.9).

In older children, seborrhoeic dermatitis affects the scalp, paranasal areas, and eyebrows. Shampoos active against the yeast (including those containing ketoconazole and coal tar, section 13.9) and combinations of mild topical corticosteroids with suitable antimicrobials (section 13.4) are used to treat older children.

ICHTHAMMOL

Side-effects skin irritation

Licensed use no information available

Indication and dose

Chronic lichenified eczema

Child 1–18 years apply 1–3 times daily

Ichthammol Ointment, BP 1980
Ointment, ichthammol 10%, yellow soft paraffin 45%, wool fat 45%

Zinc and Ichthammol Cream, BP
Cream, ichthammol 5%, cetostearyl alcohol 3%, wool fat 10%, in zinc cream

Medicated bandages

Zinc paste bandages are also used with **coal tar** or **ichthammol** in chronic lichenified skin conditions such as chronic eczema (ichthammol often being preferred since its action is considered to be milder). They are also used with **calamine** in milder eczematous skin conditions (but the inclusion of **clioquinol** may lead to irritation in susceptible children).

Zinc Paste Bandage, BP 1993
Cotton fabric, plain weave, impregnated with suitable paste containing zinc oxide; requires additional bandaging. Net price 6 m × 7.5 cm = £3.24 (Mölnlycke—*Steripaste®* (15%), *excipients: include* polysorbate 80); £3.23 (Mölnlycke—*Zincaband®* (15%), *excipients: include* hydroxybenzoates); £3.35 (S&N Hlth—*Viscopaste PB7®* (10%), *excipients: include* cetostearyl alcohol, hydroxybenzoates)

Zinc Paste and Calamine Bandage
(Drug Tariff specification 5). Cotton fabric, plain weave, impregnated with suitable paste containing calamine and zinc oxide; requires additional bandaging. Net price 6 m × 7.5 cm = £3.33 (Mölnlycke—*Calaband®*)

Zinc Paste, Calamine, and Clioquinol Bandage, BP 1993
Cotton fabric, plain weave, impregnated with suitable paste containing calamine, clioquinol, and zinc oxide; requires additional bandaging. Net price 6 m × 7.5 cm = £3.33 (Mölnlycke—*Quinaband®* excipients: include hydroxybenzoates)

Zinc Paste and Ichthammol Bandage, BP 1993
Cotton fabric, plain weave, impregnated with suitable paste containing zinc oxide and ichthammol; requires additional bandaging. Net price 6 m × 7.5 cm = £3.38 (S&N Hlth—*Ichthopaste®* (6/2%), *excipients: include* cetostearyl alcohol)

Medicated stocking
Zipzoc® (S&N Hlth.)
Sterile rayon stocking impregnated with ointment containing zinc oxide 20%. 4-pouch carton = £12.52; 10-pouch carton = £31.30

13.5.2 Preparations for psoriasis

Psoriasis is characterised by epidermal thickening and scaling. It commonly affects extensor surfaces and the scalp. For mild psoriasis, reassurance and treatment with an emollient may be all that is necessary. *Guttate psoriasis* is a distinctive form of psoriasis that characteristically occurs in children and young adults, often following a streptococcal throat infection or tonsillitis.

Occasionally psoriasis is provoked or exacerbated by drugs such as lithium, chloroquine and hydroxychloroquine, beta-blockers, non-steroidal anti-inflammatory drugs, and ACE inhibitors. Psoriasis may not occur until the drug has been taken for weeks or months.

Emollients (section 13.2.1), in addition to their effects on dryness, scaling and cracking, may have an antiproliferative effect in psoriasis. They are particularly useful in *inflammatory psoriasis* and in *chronic stable plaque psoriasis*.

For *chronic stable plaque psoriasis* on extensor surfaces of trunk and limbs preparations containing **coal tar** are moderately effective, but the smell is unacceptable to some children. **Vitamin D** and its analogues are effective and cosmetically acceptable alternatives to preparations containing coal tar or dithranol.

13

Skin

Dithranol is the most effective topical antipsoriatic agent but it irritates and stains the skin and it should be used only under specialist supervision. Adverse effects of dithranol are minimised by using a 'short-contact technique' (see below) and by starting with low concentration preparations. **Tazarotene**, a topical retinoid for the treatment of mild to moderate plaque psoriasis, is not recommended for use in children under 18 years. These medications can irritate the skin particularly in the flexures and they are not suitable for the more inflammatory forms of psoriasis; their use should be suspended during an inflammatory phase of psoriasis. The efficacy and the irritancy of each substance varies between patients. If a substance irritates significantly, it should be stopped or the concentration reduced; if it is tolerated, its effects should be assessed after 4 to 6 weeks and treatment continued if it is effective.

Widespread *unstable psoriasis* of erythrodermic or generalised pustular type requires urgent specialist assessment. Initial topical treatment should be limited to using emollients frequently and generously. More localised acute or subacute *inflammatory psoriasis* with hot, spreading or itchy lesions, should be treated topically with emollients or with a corticosteroid of moderate potency.

Scalp psoriasis is usually scaly, and the scale may be thick and adherent. This requires softening with an emollient ointment, cream, or oil and usually combined with **salicylic acid** as a keratolytic.

Some preparations for psoriasis affecting the scalp combine salicylic acid with coal tar or **sulphur**. The preparation should be applied generously and left on for at least an hour, often more conveniently overnight, before washing it off. If a corticosteroid lotion or gel is required (e.g. for itch), it can be used in the morning.

Calcipotriol and **tacalcitol** are analogues of vitamin D that affect cell division and differentiation. **Calcitriol** is an active form of vitamin D. Vitamin D and its analogues are used as first-line treatment for plaque psoriasis; they do not smell or stain and they may be more acceptable than tar or dithranol products. Of the vitamin D analogues, tacalcitol and calcitriol are less likely to irritate.

Coal tar has anti-inflammatory properties that are useful in chronic plaque psoriasis; it also has antiscaling properties. Contact of coal tar products with normal skin is not normally harmful and preparations containing coal tar can be used for widespread small lesions; however, irritation, contact allergy, and sterile folliculitis can occur. Preparations containing up to 6% coal tar may be used on children 1 month to 2 years; preparations containing coal tar 10% may be used on children over 2 years with more severe psoriasis. For shampoo preparations containing coal tar, see section 13.9.

Dithranol is effective for chronic plaque psoriasis. Its major disadvantages are irritation (for which individual susceptibility varies) and staining of skin and of clothing. It should be applied to chronic extensor plaques only, carefully avoiding normal skin. Dithranol is not generally suitable for widespread small lesions nor should it be used in the flexures or on the face. Treatment should be started with a low concentration such as dithranol 0.1%, and the strength increased gradually every few days up to 3%, according to tolerance. Proprietary preparations are more suitable for home use; they are usually washed off after 20–30 minutes ('short contact' technique). Specialist nurses may apply intensive treatment with dithranol paste which is covered by stockinette dressings and usually retained overnight. Dithranol should be discontinued if even a low concentration causes acute inflammation; continued use can result in the psoriasis becoming unstable. When applying dithranol, hands should be protected by gloves or they should be washed thoroughly afterwards.

A topical **corticosteroid** (section 13.4) is not generally suitable as the sole treatment of extensive chronic plaque psoriasis; any early improvement is not usually maintained and there is a risk of the condition deteriorating or of precipitating an unstable form of psoriasis (e.g. erythrodermic psoriasis or generalised pustular psoriasis). However, it may be appropriate to treat psoriasis in specific sites such as the face and flexures usually with a mild corticosteroid, and psoriasis of the scalp, palms and soles with a potent corticosteroid.

Combining the use of a corticosteroid with another specific topical treatment may be beneficial in chronic plaque psoriasis; the drugs may be used separately at different times of the day or used together in a single formulation. *Eczema* co-existing with psoriasis may be treated with a corticosteroid, or coal tar, or both.

13 Skin

Systemic or potent topical corticosteroids should be avoided or used only under specialist supervision; although corticosteroids may suppress psoriasis in the short term, relapse or vigorous rebound occurs on withdrawal.

Phototherapy   Phototherapy is available in specialist centres under the supervision of a dermatologist. Narrow band ultraviolet B (UVB) radiation is usually effective for *chronic stable psoriasis* and for *guttate psoriasis*. It can be considered for children with moderately severe psoriasis in whom topical treatment has failed, but it may irritate inflammatory psoriasis. The use of phototherapy and photochemotherapy in children is limited by concerns over carcinogenicity and premature ageing.

Photochemotherapy combining long-wave ultraviolet A radiation with a psoralen (PUVA) is available in specialist centres under the supervision of a dermatologist. The psoralen, which enhances the effect of irradiation, is administered either by mouth or topically. PUVA is effective in most forms of psoriasis, including the *localised palmoplantar pustular psoriasis*. Early adverse effects include phototoxicity and pruritus. Higher cumulative doses exaggerate skin ageing, increase the risk of dysplastic and neoplastic skin lesions especially squamous cancer, and pose a theoretical risk of cataracts.

Phototherapy combined with coal tar, dithranol, topical vitamin D or vitamin D analogues, or oral acitretin, allows reduction of the cumulative dose of phototherapy required to treat psoriasis.

Systemic treatment   Systemic treatment is required for severe, resistant, unstable or complicated forms of psoriasis, and it should be initiated only under specialist supervision. Systemic drugs for psoriasis include acitretin and drugs that affect the immune response (section 13.5.3).

Acitretin, a metabolite of etretinate, is a retinoid (vitamin A derivative); it is prescribed by specialists. The main indication of acitretin is severe psoriasis resistant to other forms of therapy. It is also used in disorders of keratinisation such as severe *Darier's disease* (keratosis follicularis), and some forms of *ichthyosis*. Although a minority of cases of psoriasis respond well to acitretin alone, it is only moderately effective in many cases; adverse effects are a limiting factor. A therapeutic effect occurs after 2 to 4 weeks and the maximum benefit after 4 to 6 weeks or longer. Continuous treatment for longer than 6 months is not usually necessary in psoriasis. However, some patients, particularly those with severe ichthyosis, may benefit from longer treatment, provided that the lowest effective dose is used, patients are monitored carefully for adverse effects, and the need for treatment is reviewed regularly. Topical preparations containing keratolytics should normally be stopped before administration of acitretin. Liberal use of emollients should be encouraged and topical corticosteroids can be continued if necessary.

Acitretin is teratogenic; in females of child-bearing age, the possibility of pregnancy must be excluded before treatment and effective contraception must be used during treatment and for at least 3 years afterwards (oral progestogen-only contraceptives not considered effective). Common side-effects derive from its widespread but reversible effects on epithelia, such as dry and cracking lips, dry skin and mucosal surfaces, hair thinning, paronychia, and soft and sticky palms and soles. Liver function and blood-lipid concentration should be monitored before starting treatment, after 1 month, and then 3-monthly during treatment. Musculoskeletal development should also be monitored closely.

13 Skin

Topical preparations for psoriasis

Vitamin D and analogues

Calcipotriol, **calcitriol**, and **tacalcitol** are used for the management of *plaque psoriasis*. They should be avoided by those with calcium metabolism disorders, and used with caution in *generalised pustular* or *erythrodermic exfoliative psoriasis* (enhanced risk of hypercalcaemia). Local skin reactions (itching, erythema, burning, paraesthesia, dermatitis) are common. Hands should be washed thoroughly after application to avoid inadvertent transfer to other body areas. Aggravation of psoriasis has also been reported.

CALCIPOTRIOL

Cautions see notes above; avoid use on face; avoid excessive exposure to sunlight and sun-lamps

Pregnancy manufacturer advises avoid if possible

Breast-feeding no information available

Contra-indications see notes above

Side-effects see notes above; also photosensitivity; rarely facial or perioral dermatitis, skin atrophy

Licensed use Calcipotriol ointment, *Dovonex® Scalp Solution* and *Dovobet®* not licensed for use in children

Indication and dose

> Plaque psoriasis
>
> **Child 6–18 years** apply cream *or* ointment twice daily; 6–12 years max. 50 g weekly, over 12 years max. 75 g weekly (less with scalp solution, see below)
> Note Patient information leaflet for *Dovonex®* cream advises liberal application (but note max. recommended weekly dose, above)

Calcipotriol (Non-proprietary) (PoM)

Ointment, calcipotriol 50 micrograms/g, net price 120 g = £25.88

Dovonex® (LEO) (PoM)

Cream, calcipotriol 50 micrograms/g, net price 60 g = £12.02, 120 g = £24.04
Excipients include cetostearyl alcohol, disodium edetate

Scalp solution, calcipotriol 50 micrograms/mL, net price 60 mL = £13.04, 120 mL = £26.07
Excipients include propylene glycol

Dose

> Scalp psoriasis (specialist use only)
>
> **Child 6–12 years** apply to scalp twice daily; max. 30 mL weekly (less when used with cream or ointment, see below)
>
> **Child 12–18 years** apply to scalp twice daily; max. 45 mL weekly (less when used with cream or ointment, see below)

Note When preparations used together max. total calcipotriol 2.5 mg in any one week for child 6–12 years (e.g. scalp solution 20 mL with cream or ointment 30 g); max. 3.75 mg in any one week for child 12–18 years (e.g. scalp solution 30 mL with cream or ointment 45 g)

With betamethasone

For cautions, contra-indications, side-effects, and for comment on the limited role of corticosteroids in psoriasis, see section 13.4.

Dovobet® (LEO) (PoM)

Ointment, betamethasone 0.05% (as dipropionate), calcipotriol 50 micrograms/g, net price 60 g = £35.00, 120 g = £65.00. Label: 28
Excipients none as listed in section 13.1.3

Dose

> Stable plaque psoriasis (specialist use only)
>
> **Child 12–18 years** apply once daily to max. 30% of body surface for up to 4 weeks; max. 75 g weekly; subsequent courses repeated after an interval of at least 4 weeks

Note When different preparations containing calcipotriol used together, max. total calcipotriol 3.75 mg in any one week for child 12–18 years

CALCITRIOL

Cautions see notes above

Pregnancy avoid; use in restricted amounts if clearly necessary (significant systemic absorption); monitor urine and plasma-calcium concentration

Contra-indications see notes above; do not apply under occlusion

Hepatic impairment manufacturer advises avoid

Renal impairment manufacturer advises avoid—no information available

Breast-feeding manufacturer advises avoid

Side-effects see notes above

Indication and dose

> Mild to moderate plaque psoriasis
>
> **Child 12–18 years** apply twice daily; not more than 35% of body surface to be treated daily, max. 30 g daily

Silkis® (Galderma) (PoM)

Ointment, calcitriol 3 micrograms/g, net price 100 g = £16.34
Excipients none as listed in section 13.1.3

TACALCITOL

Cautions see notes above; avoid eyes; monitor plasma-calcium concentration if risk of hypercalcaemia or in renal impairment; if used in conjunction with UV treatment, UV radiation should be given in the morning and tacalcitol applied at bedtime

Pregnancy avoid if possible

Breast-feeding no information on presence in milk; avoid application to breast area

Contra-indications see notes above

Side-effects see notes above

Indication and dose

> Plaque psoriasis
>
> **Child 12–18 years** apply once daily preferably at bedtime; max. 10 g *ointment* or 10 mL *lotion* daily
> Note When lotion and ointment used together, max. total tacalcitol 280 micrograms in any one week (e.g. lotion 30 mL with ointment 40 g)

Curatoderm® (Almirall) (PoM)

Lotion, tacalcitol (as monohydrate) 4 micrograms/g, net price 30 mL = £12.73
Excipients include disodium edetate, propylene glycol

Ointment, tacalcitol (as monohydrate) 4 micrograms/g, net price 30 g = £13.40, 60 g = £23.14, 100 g = £30.86
Excipients none as listed in section 13.1.3

13 Skin

Tars

TARS

Cautions avoid eyes, mucosa, genital or rectal areas, and broken or inflamed skin; use suitable chemical protection gloves for extemporaneous preparation

Pregnancy no adverse effects reported

Breast-feeding no adverse effects reported

Contra-indications not for use in sore, acute, or pustular psoriasis or in presence of infection

Side-effects skin irritation and acne-like eruptions, photosensitivity; stains skin, hair, and fabric

Indication and dose

> Psoriasis and occasionally chronic atopic eczema
>
> Apply 1–3 times daily starting with low-strength preparations; proprietary preparations, see individual entries below
>
> Note For shampoo preparations see section 13.9

◢ Non-proprietary preparations
May be difficult to obtain. Patients may find newer proprietary preparations more acceptable

Coal Tar Paste, BP
Paste, strong coal tar solution 7.5%, in compound zinc paste

Zinc and Coal Tar Paste, BP
Paste, zinc oxide 6%, coal tar 6%, emulsifying wax 5%, starch 38%, yellow soft paraffin 45%
Excipients include cetostearyl alcohol

◢ Proprietary preparations
Carbo-Dome® (Sandoz)
Cream, coal tar solution 10%, in a water-miscible basis, net price 30 g = £4.77, 100 g = £16.38
Excipients include beeswax, hydroxybenzoates (parabens)

Dose
> Psoriasis
>
> Apply to skin 2–3 times daily

Clinitar® (CHS)
Cream, coal tar extract 1%, net price 100 g = £10.99
Excipients include cetostearyl alcohol, isopropyl palmitate, propylene glycol

Dose
> Psoriasis and eczema
>
> Apply to skin 1–2 times daily

Cocois® (UCB Pharma)
Scalp ointment, coal tar solution 12%, salicylic acid 2%, precipitated sulphur 4%, in a coconut oil emollient basis, net price 40 g (with applicator nozzle) = £6.22, 100 g = £11.69
Excipients include cetostearyl alcohol

Dose
> Scaly scalp disorders including psoriasis, eczema, seborrhoeic dermatitis and dandruff
>
> **Child 6–12 years** medical supervision required
>
> **Child 12–18 years** apply to scalp once weekly as necessary (if severe use daily for first 3–7 days), shampoo off after 1 hour

Exorex® (Forest)
Lotion, prepared coal tar 1% in an emollient basis, net price 100 mL = £8.11, 250 mL = £16.24
Excipients include hydroxybenzoates (parabens), polysorbate 80

Dose
> Psoriasis
>
> Apply to skin or scalp 2–3 times daily; product can be diluted with a few drops of water before applying

Psoriderm® (Dermal)
Cream, coal tar 6%, lecithin 0.4%, net price 225 mL = £9.85
Excipients include isopropyl palmitate, propylene glycol

Dose
> Psoriasis
>
> Apply to skin or scalp 1–2 times daily

Scalp lotion—section 13.9

Sebco® (Centrapharm)
Scalp ointment, coal tar solution 12%, salicylic acid 2%, precipitated sulphur 4%, in a coconut oil emollient basis, net price 40 g = £4.54, 100 g = £8.52
Excipients include cetostearyl alcohol

Dose
> Scaly scalp disorders including psoriasis, eczema, seborrhoeic dermatitis and dandruff
>
> **Child 6–12 years** medical supervision required
>
> **Child 12–18 years** apply to scalp as necessary (if severe use daily for first 3–7 days), shampoo off after 1 hour

◢ Bath preparations
Coal Tar Solution, BP
Solution, coal tar 20%, polysorbate '80' 5%, in alcohol (96%), net price 500 mL = £7.22
Excipients include polysorbates

Dose
> Use 100 mL in an adult-size bath, and proportionally less for a child's bath
>
> Note Strong Coal Tar Solution BP contains coal tar 40%

Pinetarsol® (Crawford)
Bath oil, tar 2.3% in a light liquid paraffin basis, net price 200 mL = £4.75, 500 mL = £7.95
Excipients include fragrance

Dose
> Eczema and psoriasis
>
> Use 15–30 mL in adult-size bath or apply directly to wet skin and rinse after a few minutes; can be used as a soap substitute

Gel, tar 1.6%, net price 100 g = £4.95

Dose
> Eczema and psoriasis
>
> Apply directly to wet skin and rinse after a few minutes; can be used as a soap substitute

13
Skin

◻ **TARS (continued)**

Solution, tar 2.3%, net price 200 mL = £4.45,
500 mL = £7.45

Dose

> **Eczema and psoriasis**
>
> Use 15–30 mL in adult-size bath *or* dilute 15 mL with 3
> litres of water and apply to affected areas *or* apply
> solution directly to wet skin and rinse after a few
> minutes; can be used as a soap substitute

Polytar Emollient® (Stiefel)

Bath additive, coal tar solution 2.5%, arachis
(peanut) oil extract of coal tar 7.5%, tar 7.5%, cade
oil 7.5%, liquid paraffin 35%, net price 500 mL =
£5.78

Excipients include isopropyl palmitate

Dose

> **Psoriasis, eczema, atopic and pruritic dermatoses**
>
> Use 2–4 capfuls (15–30 mL) in adult-size bath and
> proportionally less for a child's bath; soak for 20
> minutes

Psoriderm® (Dermal)

Bath emulsion, coal tar 40%, net price 200 mL =
£2.87

Excipients include polysorbate 20

Dose

> **Psoriasis**
>
> Use 30 mL in adult-size bath, and proportionally less
> for a child's bath; soak for 5 minutes

◢**With corticosteroids**

Alphosyl HC® (GSK Consumer Healthcare) [PoM]

Cream, coal tar extract 5%, hydrocortisone 0.5%,
allantoin 2%, net price 100 g = £3.54. Label: 28.
Potency: mild

Excipients include beeswax, cetyl alcohol, hydroxybenzoates
(parabens), isopropyl palmitate, wool fat

Dose

> **Psoriasis**
>
> **Child 5–18 years** apply thinly twice daily

Dithranol

◢ **DITHRANOL**

(Anthralin)

Cautions avoid use near eyes and sensitive areas
of skin; see also notes above

> **Pregnancy** no adverse effects reported
>
> **Breast-feeding** no adverse effects reported

Contra-indications hypersensitivity; acute and
pustular psoriasis

Side-effects local burning sensation and irritation; stains skin, hair, and fabrics

Licensed use *Dithrocream®* and *Psorin®* licensed
for use in children (age range not specified by
manufacturer); *Micanol®* licensed for use in
children, but not recommended for infants or
young children (age range not specified by
manufacturer)

Indication and dose

> **Subacute and chronic psoriasis**
>
> See notes above and under preparations
> Note Some of these dithranol preparations also con-
> tain coal tar or salicylic acid—for cautions, contra-
> indications, and side-effects see under Tars or under
> Salicylic Acid

◢**Non-proprietary preparations**

¹**Dithranol Ointment, BP** [PoM]

Ointment, dithranol, in yellow soft paraffin; usual
strengths 0.1–2%. Part of basis may be replaced by
hard paraffin if a stiffer preparation is required.
Label: 28

1. [PoM] if dithranol content more than 1%, otherwise may
be sold to the public

Dithranol Paste, BP

Paste, dithranol in zinc and salicylic acid (Lassar's)
paste. Usual strengths 0.1–1% of dithranol.
Label: 28

◢**Proprietary preparations**

Dithrocream® (Dermal)

Cream, dithranol 0.1%, net price 50 g = £3.94;
0.25%, 50 g = £4.23; 0.5%, 50 g = £4.87; 1%, 50 g =
£5.67; [PoM] 2%, 50 g = £7.10. Label: 28

Excipients include cetostearyl alcohol, chlorocresol

Dose

> For application to skin or scalp; 0.1–0.5% cream sui-
> table for overnight treatment, 1–2% cream for max.
> 1 hour

Micanol® (GP Pharma)

Cream, dithranol 1% in a lipid-stabilised basis, net
price 50 g = £13.48; [PoM] 3%, 50 g = £16.79.
Label: 28

Excipients none as listed in section 13.1.3

Dose

> For application to skin or scalp, apply 1% cream for up
> to 30 minutes once daily, if necessary 3% cream can be
> used under medical supervision

Note At the end of contact time, use plenty of lukewarm
(not hot) water to rinse off cream; soap may be used *after*
the cream has been rinsed off; use shampoo before
applying cream to scalp and if necessary after cream has
been rinsed off

Psorin® (LPC)

Ointment, dithranol 0.11%, coal tar 1%, salicylic
acid 1.6%, net price 50 g = £9.22, 100 g = £18.44.
Label: 28

Excipients include beeswax, wool fat

Dose

> For application to skin up to twice daily

Scalp gel, dithranol 0.25%, salicylic acid 1.6% in gel
basis containing methyl salicylate, net price 50 g
= £7.03. Label: 28

Excipients none as listed in section 13.1.3

Dose

> For application to scalp, initially apply on alternate
> days for 10–20 minutes; may be increased to daily
> application for max. 1 hour and then wash off

13 Skin

| Salicylic acid |

SALICYLIC ACID

For coal tar preparations containing salicylic acid, see under Tars p. 687; for dithranol preparations containing salicylic acid see under Dithranol, above

Cautions see notes above; avoid broken or inflamed skin

Salicylate toxicity Salicylate toxicity may occur particularly if applied on large areas of skin or on neonatal skin

Side-effects sensitivity, excessive drying, irritation, systemic effects after widespread use (see under Cautions)

Indication and dose

Hyperkeratotic skin disorders see under preparation

Acne section 13.6.1

Warts and calluses section 13.7

Scalp conditions section 13.9

Fungal nail infections section 13.10.2

Zinc and Salicylic Acid Paste, BP
Paste, (Lassar's Paste), zinc oxide 24%, salicylic acid 2%, starch 24%, white soft paraffin 50%, net price 25 g = 17p
Dose

Child 1 month–18 years apply twice daily

| Oral retinoids for psoriasis |

ACITRETIN

Note Acitretin is a metabolite of etretinate

Cautions in children use only in exceptional circumstances (premature epiphyseal closure reported); in females of childbearing age exclude pregnancy before starting (test for pregnancy within 2 weeks before treatment and monthly thereafter; start treatment on day 2 or 3 of menstrual cycle)—females of childbearing age (including those with history of infertility) should avoid pregnancy for at least 1 month before, during, and for at least 3 years after treatment; patients should avoid concomitant tetracycline or methotrexate, high doses of vitamin A (more than 4000–5000 units daily) and use of keratolytics, and should not donate blood during or for at least 1 year after stopping therapy (teratogenic risk); check liver function at start, after 1 month, then every 3 months; monitor plasma lipids; diabetes (can alter glucose tolerance—initial frequent blood glucose checks); radiographic assessment on long-term treatment; investigate atypical musculoskeletal symptoms; avoid excessive exposure to sunlight and unsupervised use of sunlamps; **interactions:** Appendix 1 (retinoids)

Contra-indications hyperlipidaemia

Hepatic impairment avoid—further impairment may occur

Renal impairment avoid; increased risk of toxicity

Pregnancy teratogenic; effective contraception must be used (see Cautions above)

Breast-feeding avoid

Side-effects dryness of mucous membranes (sometimes erosion), of skin (sometimes scaling, thinning, erythema especially of face, and pruritus), and of conjunctiva (sometimes conjunctivitis and decreased tolerance of contact lenses); sticky skin, dermatitis; other side-effects reported include palmoplantar exfoliation, epistaxis, epidermal and nail fragility, oedema, paronychia, granulomatous lesions, bullous eruptions, reversible hair thinning and alopecia, myalgia and arthralgia, occasional nausea, headache, malaise, drowsiness, rhinitis, sweating, taste disturbance, and gingivitis; benign intracranial hypertension (discontinue if severe headache, vomiting, diarrhoea, abdominal pain, and visual disturbance occur; **avoid** concomitant tetracyclines); photosensitivity, corneal ulceration, raised liver enzymes, rarely jaundice and hepatitis (**avoid** concomitant methotrexate); raised serum triglycerides or cholesterol; decreased night vision reported; skeletal hyperostosis and extraosseous calcification reported following long-term administration of etretinate (and premature epiphyseal closure in children, see Cautions)

Indication and dose

Harlequin ichthyosis (under expert supervision only)

• By mouth

Neonate 500 micrograms/kg once daily with food or milk (occasionally up to 1 mg/kg daily) with careful monitoring of musculoskeletal development

Severe extensive psoriasis resistant to other forms of therapy, palmoplantar pustular psoriasis, severe congenital ichthyosis, severe Darier's disease (keratosis follicularis) (all under expert supervision only)

• By mouth

Child 1 month–12 years 500 micrograms/kg once daily with food or milk (occasionally up to 1 mg/kg daily) to max. 35 mg daily with careful monitoring of musculoskeletal development (see also p. 685)

Child 12–18 years initially 25–30 mg daily (Darier's disease 10 mg daily) for 2–4 weeks, then adjusted according to response, usual range 25–50 mg daily; up to 75 mg daily for short periods in psoriasis and ichthyosis (see also p. 685)

13

Skin

◺ **ACITRETIN (continued)**

Neotigason® (Actavis) PoM
   Capsules, acitretin 10 mg (brown/white), net price
   60-cap pack = £25.25; 25 mg (brown/yellow), 60-
   cap pack = £58.59. Label: 10, patient information
   leaflet, 21

◄Extemporaneous formulations available see
Extemporaneous Preparations, p. 8

13.5.3 Drugs affecting the immune response

Drugs affecting the immune response are used for eczema or psoriasis.

Pimecrolimus by topical application is licensed for *mild to moderate atopic eczema*. **Tacrolimus** is licensed for topical use in *moderate to severe atopic eczema*. Both are drugs whose long-term safety and place in therapy is still being evaluated and they should not usually be considered first-line treatment unless there is a specific reason to avoid or reduce the use of topical corticosteroids. Short-term treatment with topical pimecrolimus or topical tacrolimus should be initiated only by prescribers experienced in treating atopic eczema; continuous long-term treatment should be avoided.

> **NICE guidance**
>
> Tacrolimus and pimecrolimus for atopic eczema (August 2004)
> Topical pimecrolimus and tacrolimus are options for atopic eczema not controlled by maximal topical corticosteroid treatment or if there is a risk of important corticosteroid side-effects (particularly skin atrophy).
>
> Topical pimecrolimus is recommended for moderate atopic eczema on the face and neck of children aged 2–16 years and topical tacrolimus is recommended for moderate to severe atopic eczema in children over 2 years. Pimecrolimus and tacrolimus should be used within their licensed indications.

For the role of topical corticosteroids in eczema, see section 13.5.1, and for comment on their limited role in psoriasis, see section 13.4. A systemic corticosteroid (section 6.3.2) such as prednisolone may be used in *severe* refractory eczema.

Systemic drugs acting on the immune system are generally used by **specialists** in a hospital setting.

Ciclosporin (cyclosporin) by mouth can be used for *severe psoriasis* and for *severe eczema*. **Azathioprine** (section 8.2.1) or **mycophenolate mofetil** (section 8.2.1) are also used for severe refractory eczema in children.

Methotrexate can be used for *severe resistant psoriasis*; the dose is given **once weekly** and adjusted according to severity of the condition and haematological and biochemical measurements. Folic acid (section 9.1.2) should be given to reduce the possibility of methotrexate toxicity. Folic acid can be given at a dose of 5 mg once weekly; alternative regimens may be used in some settings.

Etanercept (a cytokine modulator) is licensed in children over 8 years of age for the treatment of severe plaque psoriasis that is inadequately controlled by other systemic treatments and photochemotherapy, or when these other treatments cannot be used because of intolerance or contra-indications.

◣ **CICLOSPORIN**
(Cyclosporin)

Cautions see section 8.2.2
   Additional cautions in atopic dermatitis and psoriasis
   Contra-indicated in abnormal renal function, uncontrolled hypertension (see also below), infections not under control, and malignancy (see also below). Dermatological and physical examination, including blood pressure and renal function measurements required at least twice before starting. During treatment, monitor serum creatinine every 2 weeks for first 3 months then every month; reduce dose by 25–50% if serum creatinine increases more than 30% above baseline (even if within normal range) and discontinue if reduction not successful within one month. Discontinue if hypertension develops that cannot be controlled by dose reduction or antihyper-

tensive therapy. Avoid excessive exposure to sunlight and avoid use of UVB or PUVA. *In atopic dermatitis*, also allow herpes simplex infections to clear before starting (if they occur during treatment withdraw if severe); *Staphylococcus aureus* skin infections not absolute contra-indication providing controlled (but avoid erythromycin unless no other alternative—see also **interactions**: Appendix 1 (ciclosporin)); investigate lymphadenopathy that persists despite improvement in atopic dermatitis. *In psoriasis*, also exclude malignancies (including those of skin and cervix) before starting (biopsy any lesions not typical of psoriasis) and treat patients with malignant or pre-malignant conditions of skin only after appropriate treatment (and if no other option); discontinue if lymphoproliferative disorder develops

13 Skin

◻ **CICLOSPORIN** (*continued*)

Side-effects see section 8.2.2

Licensed use not licensed for use in children under 16 years for atopic eczema (dermatitis)

Indication and dose

> Short-term treatment (usually max. 8 weeks but may be used for longer by specialists) of severe atopic dermatitis where conventional therapy ineffective or inappropriate
> * **By mouth, administered in accordance with expert advice**
>
>   **Child 1 month–18 years** initially 1.25 mg/kg twice daily, if good initial response not achieved within 2 weeks, increase rapidly to max. 2.5 mg/kg twice daily; initial dose of 2.5 mg/kg twice daily if very severe

> Severe psoriasis where conventional therapy ineffective or inappropriate
> * **By mouth, administered in accordance with expert advice**
>
>   **Child 1 month–18 years** initially 1.25 mg/kg twice daily, increased gradually to

max. 2.5 mg/kg twice daily if no improvement within 1 month (discontinue if response still insufficient after 6 weeks); initial dose of 2.5 mg/kg twice daily justified if condition requires rapid improvement

Important For preparations and counselling and for advice on conversion between the preparations, see section 8.2.2

> Refractory ulcerative colitis section 1.5.3

> Transplantation and graft-versus-host disease section 8.2.2

◄ **Preparations**
Section 8.2.2

🔳 **METHOTREXATE**

Cautions see section 8.1.3, also photosensitivity—psoriasis lesions aggravated by UV radiation (skin ulceration reported)

Contra-indications see section 8.1.3

Side-effects see section 8.1.3

Licensed use not licensed for use in children with psoriasis

Indication and dose

> Severe uncontrolled psoriasis unresponsive to conventional therapy (specialist use only)
> * **By mouth**
>
>   **Child 2–18 years** initially 200 micrograms/kg (max. 10 mg) once **weekly** increased according to response to 400 micrograms/kg (max. 25 mg) once **weekly**

Safe Practice Note that the above dose is a **weekly** dose. To avoid error with low-dose methotrexate, it is recommended that:

* the child or their carer is carefully advised of the **dose** and **frequency** and the reason for taking methotrexate and any other prescribed medicine (e.g. folic acid);
* only one strength of methotrexate tablet (usually 2.5 mg) is prescribed and dispensed;
* the prescription and the dispensing label clearly show the dose and frequency of methotrexate administration;
* the child or their carer is warned to report immediately the onset of any feature of blood disorders (e.g. sore throat, bruising, and mouth ulcers), liver toxicity (e.g. nausea, vomiting, abdominal discomfort, and dark urine), and respiratory effects (e.g. shortness of breath).

> Malignant disease section 8.1.3

> Rheumatoid arthritis section 10.1.3

> Severe Crohn's disease section 1.5.3

◄ **Preparations**
Section 10.1.3

🔳 **PIMECROLIMUS**

Cautions UV light (avoid excessive exposure to sunlight and sunlamps), avoid other topical treatments except emollients at treatment site; alcohol consumption (risk of facial flushing and skin irritation)

Contra-indications contact with eyes and mucous membranes, application under occlusion, infection at treatment site; congenital epidermal barrier defects; generalised erythroderma; immuno-

deficiency; concomitant use with drugs that cause immunosuppression (may be prescribed in exceptional circumstances by specialists); application to malignant or potentially malignant skin lesions

Side-effects burning sensation, pruritus, erythema, skin infections (including folliculitis and *less commonly* impetigo, herpes simplex and zoster, molluscum contagiosum); *rarely* papilloma, skin

PIMECROLIMUS (*continued*)

discoloration, local reactions including pain, paraesthesia, peeling, dryness, oedema, and worsening of eczema; skin malignancy reported

Indication and dose

Short-term treatment of mild to moderate atopic eczema (including flares) when topical corticosteroids cannot be used; see also notes above

Child 2–18 years apply twice daily until symptoms resolve (stop treatment if eczema worsens or no response after 6 weeks)

Elidel® (Novartis) PoM

Cream, pimecrolimus 1%, net price 30 g = £19.69, 60 g = £37.41, 100 g = £59.07. Label: 4, 28

Excipients include benzyl alcohol, cetyl alcohol, propylene glycol, stearyl alcohol

TACROLIMUS

Cautions infection at treatment site, UV light (avoid excessive exposure to sunlight and sunlamps); alcohol consumption (risk of facial flushing and skin irritation)

Pregnancy manufacturer advises avoid unless essential; toxicity in *animal* studies following systemic administration

Contra-indications hypersensitivity to macrolides; congenital epidermal barrier defects; generalised erythroderma; immunodeficiency; concomitant use with drugs that cause immunosuppression (may be prescribed in exceptional circumstances by specialists); application to malignant or potentially malignant skin lesions; application under occlusion; avoid contact with eyes and mucous membranes

Breast-feeding avoid—present in milk following systemic administration

Side-effects application-site reactions including rash, irritation, pain, and paraesthesia; herpes simplex infection, Kaposi's varicelliform eruption; *less commonly* acne; rosacea, and skin malignancy also reported

Indication and dose

Short-term treatment of moderate to severe atopic eczema (including flares) either unresponsive to, or in children intolerant of conventional therapy; see also notes above

Child 2–16 years initially apply 0.03% ointment thinly twice daily for up to 3 weeks (consider other treatment if eczema worsens or if no improvement after 2 weeks) then reduce to once daily until lesion clears

Child 16–18 years initially apply 0.1% ointment thinly twice daily until lesion clears (consider other treatment if eczema worsens or if no improvement after 2 weeks); reduce to once daily or switch to 0.03% ointment if clinical condition allows

Other indications section 8.2.2

Protopic® (Astellas) PoM

Ointment, tacrolimus (as monohydrate) 0.03%, net price 30 g = £19.44, 60 g = £36.94; 0.1%, 30 g = £21.60, 60 g = £41.04. Label: 4, 11, 28

Excipients include beeswax

Cytokine modulators

ETANERCEPT

Cautions section 10.1.3

Contra-indications section 10.1.3

Side-effects section 10.1.3

Indication and dose

Severe plaque psoriasis

- **By subcutaneous injection**

Child 8–18 years 800 micrograms/kg (max. 50 mg) once weekly; max. treatment duration 24 weeks; discontinue if no response after 12 weeks

Polyarticular-course juvenile idiopathic arthritis

section 10.1.3

Preparations

Section 10.1.3

13.6 Acne and rosacea

13.6.1 Topical preparations for acne
13.6.2 Oral preparations for acne

Acne vulgaris Acne vulgaris commonly affects children around puberty and occasionally affects infants. Treatment of acne should be commenced early to prevent scarring; lesions may worsen before improving. The choice of treatment depends on age, severity, and whether the acne is predominantly inflammatory or comedonal.

Mild to moderate acne is generally treated with topical preparations, such as benzoyl peroxide, azelaic acid, and retinoids, (section 13.6.1).

For *moderate to severe inflammatory acne* or where topical preparations are not tolerated or are ineffective or where application to the site is difficult, systemic treatment (section 13.6.2) with oral antibacterials may be effective. **Co-cyprindiol** (cyproterone acetate with ethinylestradiol) has anti-androgenic properties and may be useful in young women with acne refractory to other treatments.

Severe acne, acne unresponsive to prolonged courses of oral antibacterials, acne with scarring, or acne associated with psychological problems calls for early referral to a consultant dermatologist who may prescribe oral **isotretinoin** (section 13.6.2).

Neonatal and infantile acne Inflammatory papules, pustules, and occasionally comedones may develop at birth or within the first month; most neonates with acne do not require treatment. Acne developing at 3–6 months of age may be more severe and persistent; lesions are usually confined to the face. Topical preparations containing benzoyl peroxide (at the lowest strength possible to avoid irritation), azelaic acid, adapalene, or tretinoin may be used if treatment for infantile acne is necessary. In infants with inflammatory acne, oral **erythromycin** (section 5.1.5) is used because topical preparations for acne are not well tolerated. In cases of erythromycin-resistant acne, oral isotretinoin (section 13.6.2) can be given on the advice of a consultant dermatologist.

Rosacea The adult form of rosacea rarely occurs in children. Persistent or repeated use of potent topical corticosteroids may cause periorificial rosacea (steroid acne). The pustules and papules of rosacea may be treated for at least 6 weeks with a topical **metronidazole** preparation (section 13.10.1.2), or a systemic antibacterial such as **erythromycin** (section 5.1.5), or for a child over 12 years, **oxytetracycline** (section 5.1.3). Tetracyclines are **contra-indicated** in children under 12 years of age.

13.6.1 Topical preparations for acne

In mild to moderate acne, comedones and inflamed lesions respond well to benzoyl peroxide (see below) or topical retinoids (see p. 695). Alternatively, topical application of an antibacterial such as erythromycin or clindamycin may be effective for inflammatory acne. However, topical antibacterials are probably no more effective than benzoyl peroxide and may promote the emergence of resistant organisms. If topical preparations prove inadequate oral preparations may be needed (section 13.6.2). The choice of product and formulation (gel, solution, lotion, or cream) is largely determined by skin type, patient preference, and previous usage of acne products.

13

Skin

Benzoyl peroxide and azelaic acid

Benzoyl peroxide is effective in mild to moderate acne. Both comedones and inflamed lesions respond well to benzoyl peroxide. The lower concentrations seem to be as effective as higher concentrations in reducing inflammation. It is usual to start with a lower strength and to increase the concentration of benzoyl peroxide gradually. Adverse effects include local skin irritation, particularly when therapy is initiated, but the scaling and redness often subside with a reduction in benzoyl peroxide concentration, frequency, and area of application. If the acne does not respond after 2 months then use of a topical antibacterial should be considered.

Azelaic acid has antimicrobial and anticomedonal properties. It may be used as an alternative to benzoyl peroxide or to a topical retinoid for treating mild to moderate comedonal acne, particularly of the face; azelaic acid is less likely to cause local irritation than benzoyl peroxide.

BENZOYL PEROXIDE

Cautions avoid contact with eyes, mouth, and mucous membranes; may bleach fabrics and hair; avoid excessive exposure to sunlight

Side-effects skin irritation (reduce frequency or suspend use until irritation subsides and re-introduce at reduced frequency)

Licensed use *Quinoderm®* is licensed for use in children; *all other preparations*, not licensed for use in treatment of infantile acne

Indication and dose

Acne vulgaris

Child 12–18 years apply 1–2 times daily preferably after washing with soap and water, start treatment with lower-strength preparations
Note May bleach clothing

Infantile acne

Neonate apply 1–2 times daily; start treatment with lower-strength preparations

Child 1 month–2 years apply 1–2 times daily; start treatment with lower-strength preparations

Acnecide® (Galderma)
Gel, benzoyl peroxide 5% in an aqueous gel basis, net price 60 g = £5.69
Excipients include propylene glycol

Brevoxyl® (Stiefel)
Cream, benzoyl peroxide 4% in an aqueous basis, net price 40 g = £3.30
Excipients include cetyl alcohol, fragrance, stearyl alcohol

PanOxyl® (Stiefel)
Aquagel (= aqueous gel), benzoyl peroxide 2.5%, net price 40 g = £1.76; 5%, 40 g = £1.92; 10%, 40 g = £2.13
Excipients include propylene glycol

Cream, benzoyl peroxide 5% in a non-greasy basis, net price 40 g = £1.89
Excipients include isopropyl palmitate, propylene glycol

Gel, benzoyl peroxide 5% in an aqueous alcoholic basis, net price 40 g = £1.51; 10%, 40 g = £1.69
Excipients include fragrance

Wash, benzoyl peroxide 10% in a detergent basis, net price 150 mL = £4.00
Excipients include imidurea

◢With antimicrobials

Duac® Once Daily (Stiefel) [PoM]
Gel, benzoyl peroxide 5%, clindamycin 1% (as phosphate) in an aqueous basis, net price 25 g = £9.95, 50 g = £19.90
Excipients include disodium edetate

Dose

Acne vulgaris

Child 12–18 years apply once daily in the evening

Quinoderm® (Ferndale)
Cream, benzoyl peroxide 5%, potassium hydroxyquinoline sulphate 0.5%, in an astringent vanishing-cream basis, net price 50 g = £2.21
Excipients include cetostearyl alcohol, edetic acid (EDTA)

Cream, benzoyl peroxide 10%, potassium hydroxyquinoline sulphate 0.5%, in an astringent vanishing-cream basis, net price 25 g = £1.30, 50 g = £2.49
Excipients include cetostearyl alcohol, edetic acid (EDTA)

Dose

Infantile acne, acne vulgaris, acneform eruptions, impetigo, folliculitis

apply 2–3 times daily

AZELAIC ACID

Cautions avoid contact with eyes, mouth, and mucous membranes

Side-effects local irritation (reduce frequency or discontinue temporarily); *less commonly* skin discoloration; *very rarely* photosensitisation

Licensed use not licensed for use in infantile acne

Indication and dose

See under preparations

Finacea® (Valeant) [PoM]
Gel, azelaic acid 15%, net price 30 g = £7.48
Excipients include disodium edetate, polysorbate 80, propylene glycol

Dose

Facial acne vulgaris

Child 14–18 years apply twice daily; discontinue if no improvement after 1 month

Skinoren® (Valeant) [PoM]
Cream, azelaic acid 20%, net price 30 g = £3.74
Excipients include propylene glycol

Dose

Acne vulgaris, infantile acne

Apply twice daily (sensitive skin, once daily for first week). Extended treatment may be required but manufacturer advises period of treatment should not exceed 6 months

13 Skin

Topical antibacterials for acne

In the treatment of mild to moderate inflammatory acne, topical antibacterials may be no more effective than topical benzoyl peroxide or tretinoin. Topical antibacterials are probably best reserved for children who wish to avoid oral antibacterials or who cannot tolerate them.

Topical preparations of **erythromycin** and **clindamycin** may be used to treat *inflamed lesions* in mild to moderate acne when topical benzoyl peroxide or tretinoin is ineffective or poorly tolerated. Topical benzoyl peroxide, azelaic acid, or retinoids used in combination with an antibacterial (topical or systemic) may be more effective than an antibacterial used alone. Topical antibacterials can produce mild irritation of the skin, and on rare occasions cause sensitisation.

Antibacterial resistance of *Propionibacterium acnes* is increasing; there is cross-resistance between erythromycin and clindamycin. To avoid development of resistance:

- when possible use non-antibiotic antimicrobials (such as benzoyl peroxide or azelaic acid);
- avoid concomitant treatment with different oral and topical antibacterials;
- if a particular antibacterial is effective, use it for repeat courses if needed (short intervening courses of benzoyl peroxide or azelaic acid may eliminate any resistant propionibacteria);
- do not continue treatment for longer than necessary (but treatment with a topical preparation should be continued for at least 6 months).

ANTIBACTERIALS

Cautions   some manufacturers advise preparations containing alcohol are not suitable for use with benzoyl peroxide

Indication and dose

Acne vulgaris for dose, see under preparations

Dalacin T® (Pharmacia) [PoM]
Topical solution, clindamycin 1% (as phosphate), in an aqueous alcoholic basis, net price (both with applicator) 30 mL = £4.34, 50 mL = £7.23
Excipients include propylene glycol

Dose
Apply twice daily

Lotion, clindamycin 1% (as phosphate) in an aqueous basis, net price 30 mL = £5.08, 50 mL = £8.47
Excipients include cetostearyl alcohol, hydroxybenzoates (parabens)

Dose
Apply twice daily

Stiemycin® (Stiefel) [PoM]
Solution, erythromycin 2% in an alcoholic basis, net price 50 mL = £8.00
Excipients include propylene glycol

Dose
Apply twice daily

Zindaclin® (Crawford) [PoM]
Gel, clindamycin 1% (as phosphate), net price 30 g = £8.66
Excipients include propylene glycol

Dose
Child 12–18 years apply once daily

Zineryt® (Astellas) [PoM]
Topical solution, powder for reconstitution, erythromycin 40 mg, zinc acetate 12 mg/mL when reconstituted with solvent containing ethanol, net price per pack of powder and solvent to provide 30 mL = £7.71, 90 mL = £22.24
Excipients none as listed in section 13.1.3

Dose
Apply twice daily

Topical retinoids and related preparations for acne

Topical **tretinoin** and its isomer **isotretinoin** are useful for treating comedones and inflammatory lesions in mild to moderate acne. Patients should be warned that some redness and skin peeling may occur initially but settles with time. Several months of treatment may be needed to achieve an optimal response and the treatment should be continued until no new lesions develop.

Tretinoin is used under specialist supervision to treat infantile acne, see Neonatal and Infantile Acne, p. 693.

Adapalene, a retinoid-like drug, is used for mild to moderate acne vulgaris and may also be used to treat infantile acne. It is less irritant than topical retinoids.

Cautions Topical retinoids should be avoided in severe acne involving large areas. Contact with eyes, nostrils, mouth and mucous membranes, eczematous, broken or sunburned skin should be avoided. Topical retinoids should be used with caution on sensitive areas such as the neck, and accumulation in angles of the nose should be avoided. Exposure to UV light (including sunlight, solariums) should be avoided; if sun exposure is unavoidable, an appropriate sunscreen (section 13.8.1) or protective clothing should be used. Use of retinoids with abrasive cleaners, comedogenic or astringent cosmetics should be avoided. Allow peeling (e.g. resulting from use of benzoyl peroxide) to subside before using a topical retinoid; alternating a preparation that causes peeling with a topical retinoid may give rise to contact dermatitis (reduce frequency of retinoid application).

Contra-indications Tretinoin is contra-indicated in children with personal or familial history of cutaneous epithelioma. Topical retinoids are contra-indicated in **pregnancy**; females of child-bearing age must use effective contraception (oral progestogen-only contraceptives not considered effective).

Side-effects Local reactions include burning, erythema, stinging, pruritus, dry or peeling skin (discontinue if severe). Increased sensitivity to UVB light or sunlight occurs. Temporary changes of skin pigmentation have been reported. Eye irritation and oedema, and blistering or crusting of skin have been reported rarely.

ADAPALENE

Cautions see notes above

Contra-indications see notes above

Side-effects see notes above

Licensed use not licensed for use in infantile acne

Indication and dose

Infantile acne

Neonate apply thinly once daily at night

Child 1 month–2 years apply thinly once daily at night

Mild to moderate acne vulgaris
Apply thinly once daily before retiring

Differin® (Galderma) [PoM]
Cream, adapalene 0.1%, net price 45 g = £11.40
Excipients include disodium edetate, hydroxybenzoates (parabens)

Gel, adapalene 0.1%, net price 45 g = £11.40
Excipients include disodium edetate, hydroxybenzoates (parabens), propylene glycol

TRETINOIN

Note Tretinoin is the acid form of vitamin A

Cautions see notes above

Contra-indications see notes above

Side-effects see notes above

Licensed use *Retin-A®* not licensed for use in infantile acne

Indication and dose

See under preparations

Malignant disease (section 8.1.5)

Retin-A® (Janssen-Cilag) [PoM]
Gel, tretinoin 0.01%, net price 60 g = £5.61; 0.025%, 60 g = £5.61
Excipients include butylated hydroxytoluene
Dose

Acne vulgaris, particularly that associated with oily skin
Apply thinly 1–2 times daily

◀With antibacterial
Aknemycin Plus® (Almirall) [PoM]
Solution, tretinoin 0.025%, erythromycin 4% in an alcoholic basis, net price 25 mL = £7.05
Excipients none as listed in section 13.1.3
Dose

Acne (all forms), particularly that associated with oily skin
Apply thinly 1–2 times daily

ISOTRETINOIN

Note Isotretinoin is an isomer of tretinoin
Important For **indications, cautions, contra-indications** and **side-effects** of isotretinoin **when given by mouth**, see p. 699

Cautions (*topical application* **only**) see notes above

Contra-indications (*topical application* **only**) see notes above

◁ **ISOTRETINOIN** (*continued*)

Indication and dose

> Acne vulgaris
>
>   Apply thinly 1–2 times daily

Isotrex® (Stiefel) [PoM]

> Gel, isotretinoin 0.05%, net price 30 g = £6.18
> **Excipients** include butylated hydroxytoluene

◀With antibacterial

Isotrexin® (Stiefel) [PoM]

> Gel, isotretinoin 0.05%, erythromycin 2% in etha-
> nolic basis, net price 30 g = £7.78
> **Excipients** include butylated hydroxytoluene

Other topical preparations for acne

Salicylic acid is available in various preparations for sale direct to the public for the treatment of mild acne. Other products are more suitable for acne; salicylic acid is used mainly for its keratolytic effect.

Preparations containing **sulphur** and **abrasive agents** are not considered beneficial in acne.

Topical **corticosteroids** should **not** be used in acne.

A topical preparation of **nicotinamide** is available for inflammatory acne.

NICOTINAMIDE

Cautions avoid contact with eyes and mucous membranes (including nose and mouth); reduce frequency of application if excessive dryness, irritation or peeling

Side-effects dryness of skin; also pruritus, erythema, burning and irritation

Licensed use licensed for use in children (age range not specified by manufacturer)

Indication and dose

> Inflammatory acne vulgaris see under preparations below

Nicam® (Dermal)

> Gel, nicotinamide 4%, net price 60 g = £7.42
> **Excipients** none as listed in section 13.1.3

Dose

> Apply twice daily; reduce to once daily or on alternate days if irritation occurs

SALICYLIC ACID

Cautions risk of significant systemic absorption in neonates; avoid contact with mouth, eyes, mucous membranes; systemic effects after excessive use

Side-effects local irritation

Licensed use licensed for use in children (age range not specified by manufacturer)

Indication and dose

> Acne vulgaris see under preparation

> Psoriasis section 13.5.2

> Warts and calluses section 13.7

> Fungal nail infections section 13.10.2

Acnisal® (Alliance)

> Topical solution, salicylic acid 2% in a detergent and emollient basis, net price 177 mL = £4.03.
> **Excipients** include benzyl alcohol

Dose

> Apply up to 3 times daily

13.6.2 Oral preparations for acne

Oral antibacterials for acne

Oral antibacterials may be used in *moderate to severe inflammatory acne* when topical treatment is not adequately effective or is inappropriate. Concomitant anticomedonal treatment with topical benzoyl peroxide or azelaic acid may also be required (section 13.6.1).

Tetracyclines should not be given to children under 12 years. In children over 12 years, either **oxytetracycline** or **tetracycline** (section 5.1.3) is usually given for acne in a dose of 500 mg twice daily. If there is no improvement after the first 3 months another oral antibacterial should be used. Maximum improvement usually occurs after 4 to 6 months but in more severe cases treatment may need to be continued for 2 years or longer.

13

Skin

Doxycycline and **lymecycline** (section 5.1.3) are alternatives to tetracycline in children over 12 years. Doxycycline can be used in a dose of 100 mg daily. Lymecycline is given in a dose of 408 mg daily.

Although **minocycline** is as effective as other tetracyclines for acne, it is associated with a greater risk of lupus erythematosus-like syndrome. Minocycline sometimes causes irreversible pigmentation; it is given in a dose of 100 mg once daily or 50 mg twice daily.

Erythromycin (section 5.1.5) in a dose of 500 mg twice daily for children over 12 years is an alternative for the management of moderate to severe acne with inflamed lesions, but propionibacteria strains resistant to erythromycin are becoming widespread and this may explain poor response. Infants with acne requiring oral treatment with erythromycin should be given 250 mg once daily *or* 125 mg twice daily; in cases of erythromycin-resistant *P. acnes* in infants, oral isotretinoin may be used on the advice of a consultant dermatologist.

Concomitant use of different topical and systemic antibacterials is undesirable owing to the increased likelihood of the development of bacterial resistance.

Hormone treatment for acne

Co-cyprindiol (cyproterone acetate with ethinylestradiol) contains an anti-androgen. It is no more effective than an oral broad-spectrum antibacterial but is useful in females of childbearing age who also wish to receive oral contraception.

Improvement of acne with co-cyprindiol probably occurs because of decreased sebum secretion which is under androgen control. Some females with moderately severe hirsutism may also benefit because hair growth is also androgen-dependent. Contra-indications of co-cyprindiol include pregnancy and a predisposition to thrombosis.

> CSM advice
> Venous thromboembolism occurs more frequently in women taking co-cyprindiol than those taking a low-dose combined oral contraceptive. The CSM has reminded prescribers that co-cyprindiol is licensed for use in women with severe acne which has not responded to oral antibacterials and for moderately severe hirsutism; it should not be used solely for contraception. It is contra-indicated in those with a personal or close family history of venous thromboembolism. Women with severe acne or hirsutism may have an inherently increased risk of cardiovascular disease.

CO-CYPRINDIOL

A mixture of cyproterone acetate and ethinylestradiol in the mass proportions 2000 parts to 35 parts, respectively

Cautions see under Combined Hormonal Contraceptives, section 7.3.1

Contra-indications see under Combined Hormonal Contraceptives, section 7.3.1

Side-effects see under Combined Hormonal Contraceptives, section 7.3.1

Licensed use licensed for use in females of childbearing age

Indication and dose

Severe acne in females of childbearing age refractory to prolonged oral antibacterial therapy (but see notes above), moderately severe hirsutism
• By mouth
  1 tablet daily for 21 days starting on day 1 of menstrual cycle and repeated after a 7-day interval, usually for several months; withdraw 3–4 months after acne or hirsutism completely resolved (repeat courses may be given if recurrence); long-term treatment may be necessary for severe symptoms

Co-cyprindiol (Non-proprietary) [PoM]
Tablets, co-cyprindiol 2000/35 (cyproterone acetate 2 mg, ethinylestradiol 35 micrograms), net price 21-tab pack = £3.74
Brands include *Acnocin*®, *Cicafem*®, *Clairette*®, *Diva*®

Dianette® (Schering Health) [PoM]
Tablets, beige, s/c, co-cyprindiol 2000/35 (cyproterone acetate 2 mg, ethinylestradiol 35 micrograms), net price 21-tab pack = £3.70

13 Skin

Oral retinoid for acne

The retinoid **isotretinoin** reduces sebum secretion. It is used for the systemic treatment of nodulo-cystic and conglobate acne, severe acne, acne with scarring, or for acne which has not responded to an adequate course of a systemic antibacterial. Isotretinoin is used for the treatment of severe infantile acne resistant to erythromycin.

Isotretinoin is a toxic drug that should be prescribed **only** by, or under the supervision of, a consultant dermatologist. It is given for at least 16 weeks; repeat courses are not normally required.

Side-effects of isotretinoin include severe dryness of the skin and mucous membranes, nose bleeds, and joint pains. The drug is **teratogenic** and must **not** be given to females of child-bearing age unless they practise effective contraception (oral progestogen-only contraceptives not considered effective) and then only after detailed assessment and explanation by the physician. They must also be registered with a pregnancy prevention programme (see under Contra-indications below).

Although a causal link between isotretinoin use and psychiatric changes (including suicidal ideation) has not been established, the possibility should be considered before initiating treatment; if psychiatric changes occur during treatment, isotretinoin should be stopped, the prescriber informed, and specialist psychiatric advice should be sought.

ISOTRETINOIN

Note Isotretinoin is an isomer of tretinoin

Cautions avoid blood donation during treatment and for at least 1 month after treatment; history of depression—monitor all patients for depression; measure hepatic function and serum lipids before treatment, 1 month after starting and then every 3 months (reduce dose or discontinue if transaminase or serum lipids persistently raised); discontinue if uncontrolled hypertriglyceridaemia or pancreatitis; diabetes; dry eye syndrome (associated with risk of keratitis); avoid keratolytics; **interactions:** Appendix 1 (retinoids)

Counselling Warn patient to avoid wax epilation (risk of epidermal stripping), dermabrasion, and laser skin treatments (risk of scarring) during treatment and for at least 6 months after stopping; patient should avoid exposure to UV light (including sunlight) and use sunscreen and emolient (including lip balm) preparations from the start of treatment

Renal impairment reduce initial dose and increase gradually, if necessary, up to max. 1 mg/kg daily as tolerated

Contra-indications hypervitaminosis A, hyperlipidaemia

Hepatic impairment avoid—further impairment may occur

Pregnancy (**important teratogenic risk**) exclude pregnancy before starting (perform pregnancy test 2–3 days before expected menstruation, start treatment on day 2 or 3 of menstrual cycle)—effective contraception must be practised at least 1 month before, during, and for at least 1 month after treatment (see also notes above)

Breast-feeding avoid

Side-effects dryness of skin (with dermatitis, scaling, thinning, erythema, pruritus), epidermal fragility (trauma may cause blistering), dryness of lips (sometimes cheilitis), dryness of eyes (with blepharitis and conjunctivitis), dryness of pharyngeal mucosa (with hoarseness), dryness of nasal mucosa (with epistaxis), headache, myalgia and arthralgia, raised plasma concentration of triglycerides, of glucose, of serum transaminases, and of cholesterol (risk of pancreatitis if triglycerides above 9 mmol/litre), haematuria and proteinuria, thrombocytopenia, thrombocytosis, neutropenia and anaemia; *rarely* mood changes (depression, suicidal ideation, aggressive behaviour, anxiety)—expert referral required, exacerbation of acne, acne fulminans, allergic skin reactions, and hypersensitivity, alopecia; *very rarely* nausea, inflammatory bowel disease, diarrhoea (discontinue if severe) benign intracranial hypertension (avoid concomitant tetracyclines) convulsions, malaise, drowsiness, dizziness, lymphadenopathy, increased sweating, hyperuricaemia, raised serum creatinine concentration and glomerulonephritis, hepatitis, tendinitis, bone changes (including reduced bone density, early epiphyseal closure, and skeletal hyperstosis following long-term administration), visual disturbances (papilloedema, corneal opacities, cataracts, decreased night vision, photophobia, blurred vision, colour blindness)—expert referral required and consider withdrawal, decreased tolerance to contact lenses and keratitis, impaired hearing, Gram-positive infections of skin and mucous membranes, allergic vasculitis and granulomatous lesions, paronychia, hirsutism, nail dystrophy, skin hyperpigmentation, photosensitivity

13

Skin

◻ **ISOTRETINOIN** (*continued*)

Indication and dose

Acne vulgaris under supervision of consultant dermatologist, see notes above
- **By mouth**

  Child 12–18 years 500 micrograms/kg once daily increased if necessary to 1 mg/kg (in 1–2 divided doses) for 16–24 weeks (repeat treatment course after a period of at least 8 weeks if failure or relapse after first course); max. cumulative dose 150 mg/kg per course

Severe infantile acne under supervision of a consultant dermatologist, see p. 693
- **By mouth**

  Child 1 month–2 years 200 micrograms/kg once daily increased if necessary to 1 mg/kg daily (in 1–2 divided doses) for 16–24 weeks; max. cumulative dose 150 mg/kg per course

Isotretinoin (Non-proprietary) ⒫ⓄⓂ
Capsules, isotretinoin 5 mg, net price 56-cap pack = £14.99; 20 mg, 56-cap pack = £39.99. Label: 10, patient information leaflet, 11, 21

Roaccutane® (Roche) ⒫ⓄⓂ
Capsules, isotretinoin 10 mg (brown-red), net price 30-cap pack = £17.46; 20 mg (brown-red/white), 30-cap pack = £25.02. Label: 10, patient information card, 11, 21
Excipients may include arachis (peanut) oil in *Roaccutane®* 20 mg capsules; *Roaccutane®* 5 mg capsules are discontinued, but those in circulation contain arachis (peanut) oil

◢Extemporaneous formulations available see Extemporaneous Preparations, p. 8

13.7 Preparations for warts and calluses

Warts (verruca vulgaris) are common, benign, self-limiting, and usually asymptomatic. They are caused by a human papillomavirus, which most frequently affects the hands, feet (plantar warts), and the anogenital region (see below); treatment usually relies on local tissue destruction and is required only if the warts are painful, unsightly, persistent, or cause distress. In immunocompromised children, warts may be more difficult to eradicate.

Preparations of **salicylic acid, formaldehyde, gluteraldehyde** or **silver nitrate** are used for the removal of warts on hands and feet. **Salicylic acid** is a useful keratolytic which may be considered first-line in the treatment of warts; it is also suitable for the removal of *corns and calluses*. Preparations of salicylic acid in a collodion basis are available but some children may develop an allergy to colophony in the formulation; collodion should be avoided in children allergic to elastic adhesive plaster. An ointment combining **salicylic acid** with **podophyllum resin** (*Posalfilin®*) is available for treating plantar warts. Cryotherapy causes pain, swelling, and blistering and may be no more effective than topical salicylic acid in the treatment of warts.

◢ **SALICYLIC ACID**

Cautions significant peripheral neuropathy, patients with diabetes at risk of neuropathic ulcers; protect surrounding skin and avoid broken skin; not suitable for application to face, anogenital region, or large areas

Side-effects skin irritation, see notes above

Licensed use not licensed for use in children under 2 years

Indication and dose

Warts on hands and feet (plantar)
For dose see preparations; apply carefully to wart and protect surrounding skin (e.g. with soft paraffin or specially designed plaster); rub wart surface gently with file or pumice stone once weekly; treatment may need to be continued for up to 3 months

Psoriasis section 13.5.2

Acne section 13.6.1

Fungal nail infections section 13.10.2

Cuplex® (Crawford)
Gel, salicylic acid 11%, lactic acid 4%, in a collodion basis, net price 5 g = £2.23. Label: 15
Dose
Apply twice daily
Note Contains colophony (see notes above)

Duofilm® (Stiefel)
Paint, salicylic acid 16.7%, lactic acid 16.7%, in flexible collodion, net price 15 mL (with applicator) = £2.25. Label: 15
Dose
Apply daily

Occlusal® (Alliance)
Cutaneous solution, salicylic acid 26% in polyacrylic solution, net price 10 mL (with applicator) = £3.39. Label: 15
Dose
Apply daily

13 Skin

◁ **SALICYLIC ACID** *(continued)*

Salactol® (Dermal)
Paint, salicylic acid 16.7%, lactic acid 16.7%, in flexible collodion, net price 10 mL (with applicator) = £1.79. Label: 15

Dose
Apply daily

Note Contains colophony (see notes above)

Salatac® (Dermal)
Gel, salicylic acid 12%, lactic acid 4% in a collodion basis, net price 8 g (with applicator) = £3.12. Label: 15

Dose
Apply daily

Verrugon® (Ransom)
Ointment, salicylic acid 50% in a paraffin basis, net price 6 g = £2.83

Dose
Apply daily

◀ **With podophyllum**

Posalfilin® (Norgine)
Ointment, podophyllum resin 20%, salicylic acid 25%, net price 10 g = £3.51

Dose
Plantar warts
Apply daily

Note Owing to the salicylic acid content, not suitable for anogenital warts; owing to the podophyllum content also contra-indicated in pregnancy and breast-feeding

▌ FORMALDEHYDE

Cautions see under Salicylic Acid

Side-effects see under Salicylic Acid

Licensed use licensed for use in children (age range not specified by manufacturer)

Indication and dose

Warts, particularly plantar warts for dose see preparation below

Veracur® (Typharm)
Gel, formaldehyde 0.75% in a water-miscible gel basis, net price 15 g = £2.41.

Dose
Apply twice daily

▌ GLUTARALDEHYDE

Cautions protect surrounding skin; not for application to face, mucosa, or anogenital areas

Side-effects rashes, skin irritation (discontinue if severe); stains skin brown

Licensed use licensed for use in children (age range not specified by manufacturer)

Indication and dose

Warts, particularly plantar warts
Apply twice daily

Glutarol® (Dermal)
Solution (= application), glutaraldehyde 10%, net price 10 mL (with applicator) = £2.17

▌ SILVER NITRATE

Cautions protect surrounding skin and avoid broken skin; not suitable for application to face, anogenital region, or large areas

Side-effects chemical burns on surrounding skin; stains skin and fabric

Licensed use no age range specified by manufacturer

Indication and dose

Common warts and verrucas
Apply moistened caustic pencil tip for 1–2 minutes; repeat after 24 hours up to max. 3 applications for warts *or* max. 6 applications for verrucas
Instructions in proprietary packs generally incorporate advice to remove dead skin before use by gentle filing and to cover with adhesive dressing after application

Umbilical granulomas
Apply moistened caustic pencil tip (usually containing silver nitrate 40%) for 1–2 minutes while protecting surrounding skin with soft paraffin

Silver nitrate (Non-proprietary)
Caustic pencil, tip containing silver nitrate 40%, potassium nitrate 60%, net price = 93p
Available from Bray

AVOCA® (Bray)
Caustic pencil, tip containing silver nitrate 95%, potassium nitrate 5%, net price, treatment pack (including emery file, 6 adhesive dressings and protector pads) = £1.94.

13
Skin

▌ **Anogenital warts**

Anogenital warts (condylomata acuminata) in children are often asymptomatic and require only a simple barrier preparation. If treatment is required it should be supervised by a hospital specialist. Persistent warts on genital skin may require treatment with cryotherapy or other forms of physical ablation under general anaesthesia.

Podophyllotoxin (the major active ingredient of podophyllum), or **imiquimod** are used to treat external anogenital warts; these preparations can cause considerable irritation of the treated area and are therefore suitable only for children who are able to cooperate with the treatment.

Severe systemic toxicity including gastro-intestinal, renal, haematological, and CNS effects may occur with excessive application of podophyllotoxin.

IMIQUIMOD

Cautions avoid normal or broken skin and open wounds; not suitable for internal genital warts; uncircumcised males (risk of phimosis or stricture of foreskin); autoimmune disease; immunosuppressed patients

Pregnancy no evidence of teratogenicity or toxicity in *animal* studies; manufacturer advises caution

Breast-feeding manufacturer advises no information available

Side-effects local reactions (including itching, burning sensation, erythema, erosion, oedema, excoriation, and scabbing); headache; influenza-like symptoms; myalgia; *less commonly* local ulceration and alopecia; *rarely* Stevens-Johnson syndrome and cutaneous lupus erythematosus-like effect; permanent hypopigmentation or hyperpigmentation reported

Licensed use not licensed for use in children

Indication and dose

> **External genital and perianal warts (for use under specialist supervision only)**
>
> Apply thinly 3 times a week at night until lesions resolve (max. 16 weeks)
> **Important** Should be rubbed in and allowed to stay on the treated area for 6–10 hours then washed off with mild soap and water (uncircumcised males treating warts under foreskin should wash the area daily). The cream should be washed off before sexual contact

Aldara® (3M) (PoM)
Cream, imiquimod 5%, net price 12-sachet pack = £51.32. Label: 10, patient information leaflet
Excipients include benzyl alcohol, cetyl alcohol, hydroxybenzoates (parabens), polysorbate 60, stearyl alcohol
Condoms: may damage latex condoms and diaphragms

PODOPHYLLOTOXIN

Cautions see notes above; avoid normal skin and open wounds; keep away from face; very irritant to eyes

Contra-indications

Pregnancy avoid

Breast-feeding avoid

Side-effects see notes above

Licensed use not licensed for use in children

Indication and dose

> See under preparations (for use under specialist supervision only)

Condyline® (Ardern) (PoM)
Solution, podophyllotoxin 0.5% in alcoholic basis, net price 3.5 mL (with applicators) = £14.49. Label: 15

Dose

> **Condylomata acuminata affecting the penis or the female external genitalia**
>
> **Child 2–18 years** (see notes above) apply twice daily for 3 consecutive days; treatment may be repeated at weekly intervals if necessary for a total of five 3-day treatment courses; direct medical supervision for lesions in the female and for lesions greater than 4 cm² in the male; max. 50 single applications ('loops') per session (consult product literature)

Warticon® (Stiefel) (PoM)
Cream, podophyllotoxin 0.15%, net price 5 g (with mirror) = £15.46
Excipients include butylated hydroxyanisole, cetyl alcohol, hydroxybenzoates (parabens), sorbic acid, stearyl alcohol

Dose

> **Condylomata acuminata affecting the penis or the female external genitalia**
>
> **Child 2–18 years** (see notes above) apply twice daily for 3 consecutive days; treatment may be repeated at weekly intervals if necessary for a total of four 3-day treatment courses; direct medical supervision for lesions greater than 4 cm²

Solution, blue, podophyllotoxin 0.5% in alcoholic basis, net price 3 mL (with applicators— *Warticon®* [for men]; with applicators and mirror—*Warticon Fem®* [for women]) = £12.88. Label: 15

Dose

> **Condylomata acuminata affecting the penis or the female external genitalia**
>
> **Child 2–18 years** (see notes above) apply twice daily for 3 consecutive days; treatment may be repeated at weekly intervals if necessary for a total of four 3-day treatment courses; direct medical supervision for lesions greater than 4 cm²; max. 50 single applications ('loops') per session (consult product literature)

13 Skin

13.8 Sunscreens and camouflagers

13.8.1 Sunscreen preparations
13.8.2 Camouflagers

13.8.1 Sunscreen preparations

Solar ultraviolet irradiation can be harmful to the skin. It is responsible for disorders such as *polymorphic light eruption, solar urticaria,* and it provokes the various *cutaneous porphyrias.* It also provokes (or at least aggravates) skin lesions of *lupus erythematosus* and may aggravate some other *dermatoses.* Certain drugs, such as demeclocycline, phenothiazines, or amiodarone, can cause photosensitivity. All these conditions (as well as *sunburn*) may occur after relatively short periods of exposure to the sun. Solar ultraviolet irradiation may provoke attacks of recurrent herpes labialis (but it is not known whether the effect of sunlight exposure is local or systemic).

The effects of exposure over longer periods include *ageing changes* and more importantly the initiation of *skin cancer.*

Solar ultraviolet radiation is approximately 200–400 nm in wavelength. The medium wavelengths (290–320 nm, known as UVB) cause *sunburn.* The long wavelengths (320–400 nm, known as UVA) are responsible for many *photosensitivity reactions* and *photodermatoses.* Both UVA and UVB contribute to long-term *photodamage* and to the changes responsible for *skin cancer* and ageing.

Sunscreen preparations contain substances that protect the skin against UVA and UVB radiation, but they are no substitute for covering the skin and avoiding sunlight. Protective clothing and sun avoidance (rather than the use of sunscreen preparations) are recommended for children under 6 months of age.

The sun protection factor (SPF, usually indicated in the preparation title) provides guidance on the degree of protection offered against UVB; it indicates the multiples of protection provided against burning, compared with unprotected skin; for example, an SPF of 8 should enable a child to remain 8 times longer in the sun without burning. However, in practice users do not apply sufficient sunscreen product and the protection is lower than that found in experimental studies. Some manufacturers use a star rating system to indicate the protection against UVA relative to protection against UVB for sunscreen products. However, the usefulness of the star rating system remains controversial. The EU Commission (September 2006) has recommended that the UVA protection factor for a sunscreen should be at least one-third of the sun protection factor (SPF); products that achieve this requirement will be labelled with a UVA logo alongside the SPF classification. Preparations that also contain reflective substances, such as titanium dioxide, provide the most effective protection against UVA.

Sunscreen preparations may rarely cause allergic reactions.

> For optimum photoprotection, sunscreen preparations should be applied **thickly** and **frequently** (approximately 2 hourly). In photodermatoses, they should be used from spring to autumn. As maximum protection from sunlight is desirable, preparations with the highest SPF should be prescribed.

Borderline substances   The preparations marked 'ACBS' cannot be prescribed on the NHS except for skin protection against ultraviolet radiation in abnormal cutaneous photosensitivity resulting from genetic disorders or photodermatoses, including vitiligo and those resulting from radiotherapy; chronic or recurrent herpes simplex labialis. Preparations with SPF less than 30 should not normally be prescribed. See also Appendix 2.

Delph® (Fenton)
  Lotion, (UVA and UVB protection; UVB-SPF 30), avobenzone 4%, octinoxate 4.8%, oxybenzone 1.5%, titanium dioxide 2.5%, net price 200 mL = £3.53. ACBS
  Excipients include cetostearyl alcohol, fragrance, hydroxybenzoates (parabens), imidurea

E45 Sun® (Crookes)
  Reflective Sunscreen (UVA and UVB protection; UVB-SPF 50), waterproof, titanium dioxide 6.4%, zinc oxide 16%, net price 150 mL = £7.09. ACBS
  Excipients include hydroxybenzoates (parabens), isopropyl palmitate

13

Skin

SpectraBan® (Stiefel)
Ultra lotion (UVA and UVB protection; UVB-SPF 28), water resistant, avobenzone 2%, oxybenzone 3%, padimate-O 8%, titanium dioxide 2%, net price 150 mL = £6.54. ACBS
Excipients include benzyl alcohol, disodium edetate, sorbic acid, fragrance

Sunsense® Ultra (Crawford)
Lotion (UVA and UVB protection; UVB-SPF 60), octinoxate 7.5%, oxybenzone 3%, titanium dioxide 3.5%, net price 50-mL bottle with roll-on applicator = £3.11, 125 mL = £5.10. ACBS
Excipients include butylated hydroxytoluene, cetyl alcohol, fragrance, hydroxybenzoates (parabens), propylene glycol

Uvistat® (LPC)
Cream (UVA and UVB protection; UVB-SPF 30), avobenzone 5%, bisoctrizole 1.5%, octinoxate 7.5%, octocri-

lene 4%, titanium dioxide 5.2%, net price 125 mL = £7.45. ACBS
Excipients include disodium edetate, hydroxybenzoates (parabens), propylene glycol

Cream (UVA and UVB protection; UVB-SPF 50), amiloxate 2%, avobenzone 5%, bisoctrizole 6%, octinoxate 10%, octocrilene 4%, titanium dioxide 4.8%, net price 125 mL = £8.45. ACBS
Excipients include disodium edetate, polysorbate 60, propylene glycol

Lipscreen (UVA and UVB protection; UVB-SPF 50), avobenzone 5%, bemotrizinol 3%, octinoxate 10%, octocrilene 4%, titanium dioxide 3%, net price 5 g = £2.99. ACBS
Excipients include butylated hydroxytoluene, hydroxybenzoates (parabens)

Photodamage

Actinic keratoses occur very rarely in healthy children; *actinic cheilitis* may occur on the lips of adolescents following excessive sun exposure.

Diclofenac gel (*Solaraze®*) and **fluorouracil** cream are licensed for the treatment of actinic keratoses but they are not licensed for use in children.

In children with photosensitivity disorders, such as erythropoietic protoporphyria, specialists may use **betacarotene**, **mepacrine**, **chloroquine** or **hydroxychloroquine** (section 10.1.3) to reduce skin reactions.

BETACAROTENE

Note Betacarotene is a precursor to vitamin A

Cautions monitor vitamin A intake; **interactions:** Appendix 1 (vitamins)

Renal impairment use with caution

Pregnancy partially converted to vitamin A, but does not give rise to abnormally high serum concentration; manufacturer advises use only if potential benefit outweighs risk

Breast-feeding use with caution, present in milk

Contra-indications

Hepatic impairment avoid

Side-effects loose stools; yellow discoloration of skin; *rarely,* bruising, arthralgia

Licensed use not licensed for use in UK

Indication and dose

Management of photosensitivity reactions in erythropoietic protoporphyria (specialist use only)
- By mouth
  Child 1–5 years 60–90 mg daily in single or divided doses

Child 5–9 years 90–120 mg daily in single or divided doses

Child 9–12 years 120–150 mg daily in single or divided doses

Child 12–16 years 150–180 mg daily in single or divided doses

Child 16–18 years 180–300 mg daily in single or divided doses

Note Protection not total—avoid strong sunlight and use sunscreen preparations; generally 2–6 weeks of treatment (resulting in yellow coloration of palms and soles) necessary before increasing exposure to sunlight; dose should be adjusted according to level of exposure to sunlight

Betacarotene (Non-proprietary)
Capsules, 15 mg, 25 mg are available from 'special-order' manufacturers or specialist importing companies, see p. 943. Label: 21

13.8.2 Camouflagers

Disfigurement of the skin can be very distressing and may have a marked psychological effect, especially in children. Cosmetic preparations may be used to camouflage unsightly scars, skin deformities, and pigment abnormalities, such as vitiligo and birthmarks.

Opaque cover foundation or cream is used to mask skin pigment abnormalities; careful application using a combination of dark- and light-coloured cover creams set with powder helps to minimise the appearance of skin deformities.

Borderline substances The preparations marked 'ACBS' cannot be prescribed on the NHS for postoperative scars and other deformities except as adjunctive therapy in the relief of emotional disturbances due to disfiguring skin disease, such as vitiligo.

13 Skin

Covermark® (Skin Camouflage Co.)
Classic foundation (masking cream), net price 15 mL (10 shades) = £10.75. ACBS
Excipients include beeswax, hydroxybenzoates (parabens), fragrance

Finishing powder, net price 60 g = £11.32. ACBS
Excipients include beeswax, hydroxybenzoates (parabens), fragrance

Dermacolor® (Fox)
Camouflage creme, (100 shades), net price 25 g = £9.05. ACBS
Excipients include beeswax, butylated hydroxytoluene, fragrance, propylene glycol, stearyl alcohol, wool fat

Fixing powder, (7 shades), net price 60 g = £7.68. ACBS
Excipients include fragrance

Keromask® (Lornamead)
Masking cream, (2 shades), net price 15 mL = £5.67. ACBS
Excipients include butylated hydroxyanisole, hydroxybenzoates (parabens), wool fat, propylene glycol

Finishing powder, net price 20 g = £5.67. ACBS
Excipients include butylated hydroxytoluene, hydroxybenzoates (parabens)

Veil® (Blake)
Cover cream (40 shades), net price 19 g = £19.65, 44 g = £29.22, 70 g = £36.90. ACBS
Excipients include hydroxybenzoates (parabens), wool fat derivative

Finishing powder, translucent, net price 35 g = £21.55. ACBS
Excipients include butylated hydroxyanisole, hydroxybenzoates (parabens)

13.9 Shampoos and other preparations for scalp conditions

The detergent action of shampoo removes grease (sebum) from hair. Prepubertal children produce very little grease and require shampoo less frequently than adults. Shampoos can be used as vehicles for medicinal products, but their usefulness is limited by the short time the product is in contact with the scalp and by their irritant nature.

Oils and ointments are very useful for scaly, dry scalp conditions; if a greasy appearance is cosmetically unacceptable, the preparation may be applied at night and washed out in the morning. Alcohol-based lotions are rarely used in children; alcohol causes painful stinging on broken skin and the fumes may exacerbate asthma.

Itchy, inflammatory, eczematous scalp conditions may be relieved by a simple emollient oil such as **olive oil** or **coconut oil** (arachis oil (ground nut oil, peanut oil) is best avoided in children under 5 years). In more severe cases a topical **corticosteroid** (section 13.4) may be required. Preparations containing **coal tar** are used for the common scaly scalp conditions of childhood including seborrhoeic dermatitis, dandruff (a mild form of seborrhoeic dermatitis), and psoriasis (section 13.5.2); **salicylic acid** is used as a keratolytic in some scalp preparations.

Shampoos containing antimicrobials such as **selenium sulphide** or **ketoconazole** are used for seborrhoeic dermatitis and dandruff in which yeast infection has been implicated, and for tinea capitis (ringworm of the scalp, section 13.10.2). Bacterial infection affecting the scalp (usually secondary to eczema, head lice, or ringworm) may be treated with shampoos containing antimicrobials such as **pyrithione zinc**, **cetrimide**, or **povidone–iodine**.

In neonates and infants, *cradle cap* (which is also a form of seborrhoeic eczema) can be treated by massaging **coconut oil** or **olive oil** into the scalp; a bland emollient such as **emulsifying ointment** can be rubbed onto the affected area once or twice daily before bathing and a mild shampoo used.

◀Shampoos

[1]Ketoconazole (Non-proprietary) ᴾᵒᴹ
Cream—section 13.10.2

Shampoo, ketoconazole 2%, net price 120 mL = £3.26
Excipients include imidurea
Brands include Dandrazol® 2% Shampoo, Nizoral®

Dose

Seborrhoeic dermatitis and dandruff
treatment, apply twice weekly for 2–4 weeks; prophylaxis, apply once every 1–2 weeks

Pityriasis versicolor
treatment, apply once daily for max. 5 days; prophylaxis, apply once daily for up to 3 days before sun exposure; leave preparation on for 3–5 minutes before rinsing

1. Can be sold to the public for the prevention and treatment of dandruff and seborrhoeic dermatitis of the scalp as a shampoo formulation containing ketoconazole max. 2%, in a pack containing max. 120 mL and labelled to show a max. frequency of application of once every 3 days

Alphosyl 2 in 1® (GSK Consumer Healthcare)
Shampoo, alcoholic coal tar extract 5%, net price
125 mL = £1.81, 250 mL = £3.43
Excipients include hydroxybenzoates (parabens), fragrance

Dose

> Dandruff
>> use once or twice weekly as necessary

> Psoriasis, seborrhoeic dermatitis, scaling and itching
>> use every 2–3 days

Capasal® (Dermal)
Shampoo, coal tar 1%, coconut oil 1%, salicylic
acid 0.5%, net price 250 mL = £4.91
Excipients none as listed in section 13.1.3

Dose

> Scaly scalp disorders including psoriasis, seborr-
> hoeic dermatitis, dandruff, and cradle cap
>> apply daily as necessary

Ceanel Concentrate® (Ferndale)
Shampoo, cetrimide 10%, undecenoic acid 1%,
phenylethyl alcohol 7.5%, net price 150 mL =
£3.40, 500 mL = £9.80
Excipients none as listed in section 13.1.3

Dose

> Scalp psoriasis, seborrhoeic dermatitis, dandruff
>> apply 3 times in first week then twice weekly

Clinitar® (CHS)
Shampoo, coal tar extract 2%, net price 100 g =
£2.50
Excipients include polysorbates, fragrance

Dose

> Scalp psoriasis, seborrhoeic dermatitis, and dandruff
>> apply up to 3 times weekly

Dermax® (Dermal)
Shampoo, benzalkonium chloride 0.5%, net price
250 mL = £5.95
Excipients none as listed in section 13.1.3

Dose

> Seborrhoeic scalp conditions associated with dan-
> druff and scaling
>> apply as necessary

Meted® (Alliance)
Shampoo, salicylic acid 3%, sulphur 5%, net price
120 mL = £3.80
Excipients include fragrance

Dose

> Scaly scalp disorders including psoriasis, seborr-
> hoeic dermatitis, and dandruff
>> apply at least twice weekly

Pentrax® (Alliance)
Shampoo, coal tar 4.3%, net price 120 mL = £3.80
Excipients none as listed in section 13.1.3

Dose

> Scaly scalp disorders including psoriasis, seborr-
> hoeic dermatitis, and dandruff
>> apply at least twice weekly

Polytar AF® (Stiefel)
Shampoo, arachis (peanut) oil extract of coal tar
0.3%, cade oil 0.3%, coal tar solution 0.1%, pine tar
0.3%, pyrithione zinc 1%, net price 250 mL = £6.52
Excipients include fragrance, imidurea

Dose

> Scaly scalp disorders including psoriasis, seborr-
> hoeic dermatitis, and dandruff
>> apply 2–3 times weekly for at least 3 weeks

Psoriderm® (Dermal)
Scalp lotion (= shampoo), coal tar 2.5%, lecithin
0.3%, net price 250 mL = £4.96
Excipients include disodium edetate

Dose

> Scalp psoriasis
>> use as necessary

Selsun® (Chattem UK)
Shampoo, selenium sulphide 2.5%, net price 50 mL
= £1.44, 100 mL = £1.96, 150 mL = £2.75
Excipients include fragrance

Cautions avoid using 48 hours before or after applying
hair colouring, straightening or waving preparations

Dose

> Seborrhoeic dermatitis and dandruff
>> **Child 5–18 years** apply twice weekly for 2 weeks then
>> once weekly for 2 weeks and then as necessary

> Pityriasis versicolor [unlicensed indication]
>> **Child 5–18 years** dilute shampoo with water and
>> apply to affected area, leave on for at least 30 minutes;
>> apply 2–7 times over a two-week period; repeat course
>> as necessary

T/Gel® (J&J)
Shampoo, coal tar extract 2%, net price 125 mL =
£3.18, 250 mL = £4.78
Excipients include fragrance, hydroxybenzoates (parabens),
imidurea, tetrasodium edetate

Dose

> Scalp psoriasis, seborrhoeic dermatitis, dandruff
>> apply as necessary

◀ **Other scalp preparations**
Cocois®
Section 13.5.2

Polytar® (Stiefel)
Liquid, arachis (peanut) oil extract of coal tar 0.3%,
cade oil 0.3%, coal tar solution 0.1%, oleyl alcohol
1%, tar 0.3%, net price 250 mL = £2.23
Excipients include fragrance, imidurea, polysorbate 80

Dose

> Scalp disorders including psoriasis, seborrhoea,
> eczema, pruritus, and dandruff
>> apply 1–2 times weekly

Polytar Plus® (Stiefel)
Liquid, ingredients as *Polytar®* liquid with hydro-
lysed animal protein 3%, net price 500 mL = £3.91
Excipients include fragrance, imidurea, polysorbate 80

Dose

> Scalp disorders including psoriasis, seborrhoea,
> eczema, pruritus, and dandruff
>> apply 1–2 times weekly

13.10 Anti-infective skin preparations

13.10.1 Antibacterial preparations
13.10.2 Antifungal preparations
13.10.3 Antiviral preparations
13.10.4 Parasiticidal preparations
13.10.5 Preparations for minor cuts and abrasions

13.10.1 Antibacterial preparations

Topical antibacterial preparations are used to treat localised bacterial skin infections caused by Gram-positive organisms (particularly by staphylococci or streptococci). Systemic antibacterial treatment (Table 1, section 5.1) is more appropriate for deep-seated skin infections.

Problems associated with the use of topical antibacterials include bacterial resistance, contact sensitisation, and superinfection. In order to minimise the development of resistance, antibacterials used systemically (e.g. fusidic acid) should not generally be chosen for topical use. **Neomycin** applied topically may cause sensitisation and cross-sensitivity with other aminoglycoside antibacterials such as gentamicin may occur. Topical antibacterials applied over large areas can cause systemic toxicity; ototoxicity with neomycin and with polymyxins is a particular risk for neonates and children with renal impairment.

Superficial bacterial infection of the skin may be treated with a topical antiseptic such as **povidine–iodine** (section 13.11.4) which also softens crusts.

Bacterial infections such as *impetigo* and *folliculitis* can be treated with a short course of topical **fusidic acid**; **mupirocin** should be used only to treat meticillin-resistant *Staphylococcus aureus*.

For extensive or long-standing impetigo, an oral antibacterial such as **flucloxacillin** (or **erythromycin** in children with penicillin-allergy), Table 1, section 5.1, should be used. A mild antiseptic such as **povidine–iodine** may help to soften crusts and clear exudate. Mild antiseptics may be useful in reducing the spread of infection, but there is little evidence to support the use of topical antiseptics alone in the treatment of impetigo.

Cellulitis, a rapidly spreading deeply seated inflammation of the skin and subcutaneous tissue, requires systemic antibacterial treatment (see Table 1, section 5.1); it often involves staphylococcal infection. Lower leg infections or infections spreading around wounds are almost always cellulitis. *Erysipelas*, a superficial infection with clearly defined edges (and often affecting the face), is also treated with a systemic antibacterial (see Table 1, section 5.1); it usually involves streptococcal infection.

Staphylococcal scalded-skin syndrome requires urgent treatment with a systemic antibacterial, such as flucloxacillin.

Mupirocin is not related to any other antibacterial in use; it is effective for skin infections, particularly those due to Gram-positive organisms but it is not indicated for pseudomonal infection. Although *Staphylococcus aureus* strains with low-level resistance to mupirocin are emerging, it is generally useful in infections resistant to other antibacterials. To avoid the development of resistance, mupirocin or fusidic acid should not be used for longer than 10 days and local microbiology advice should be sought before using it in hospital. In the presence of mupirocin-resistant MRSA infection, a topical antiseptic, such as povidone–iodine, chlorhexidine, or alcohol, can be used (section 13.11); their use should be discussed with the local microbiologist.

Mupirocin ointment contains macrogol; extensive absorption of macrogol through the mucous membranes or through application to thin or damaged skin may result in renal toxicity, especially in neonates. Mupirocin nasal ointment is formulated in a paraffin base and may be more suitable for the treatment of MRSA-infected open wound in neonates.

Metronidazole gel is used topically in children to reduce the odour associated with anaerobic infections and for the treatment of periorificial rosacea (section 13.6); oral metronidazole (section 5.1.11) is used to treat wounds infected with anaerobic bacteria.

13

Skin

Retapamulin can be used for impetigo and other superficial bacterial skin infections caused by *Staphylococcus aureus* and *Streptococcus pyogenes* that are resistant to first-line topical antibacterials. However, it is not effective against MRSA. The *Scottish Medicines Consortium* (p. 4) has advised (March 2008) that retapamulin (*Altargo®*) is **not** recommended for use within NHS Scotland for the treatment of superficial skin infections.

Silver sulfadiazine (silver sulphadiazine) is licensed for the prevention and treatment of infection in burns but the use of appropriate dressings may be more effective. Systemic effects may occur following extensive application of silver sulfadiazine; its use is not recommended in neonates.

13.10.1.1 Antibacterial preparations only used topically

MUPIROCIN

Side-effects local reactions including urticaria, pruritus, burning sensation, rash

Licensed use *Bactroban®* ointment licensed for use in children (age range not specified by manufacturer); *Bactroban®* cream not recommended for use in children under 1 year

Indication and dose

Bacterial skin infections (see also notes above)

Child 1 month–18 years apply up to 3 times daily for up to 10 days

Bactroban® (GSK) [PoM]

Cream, mupirocin (as mupirocin calcium) 2%, net price 15 g = £4.38
Excipients include benzyl alcohol, cetyl alcohol, stearyl alcohol

Ointment, mupirocin 2%, net price 15 g = £4.38
Excipients none as listed in section 13.1.3

Note Contains macrogol and manufacturer advises caution in renal impairment; may sting

Nasal ointment—section 12.2.3

NEOMYCIN SULPHATE

Cautions large areas—if large areas of skin are being treated ototoxicity may be a hazard in children, particularly in those with renal impairment

Contra-indications neonates

Side-effects sensitisation (see also notes above)

Licensed use *Neomycin Cream BPC*—no information available

Indication and dose

Bacterial skin infections see under preparations

Neomycin Cream BPC [PoM]

Cream, neomycin sulphate 0.5%, cetomacrogol emulsifying ointment 30%, chlorocresol 0.1%, disodium edetate 0.01%, in freshly boiled and cooled purified water, net price 15 g = £2.17
Excipients include cetostearyl alcohol, edetic acid (EDTA)

Dose

Apply up to 3 times daily (short-term use)

POLYMYXINS

Cautions large areas—if large areas of skin are being treated nephrotoxicity and neurotoxicity may be a hazard, particularly in children with renal impairment

Side-effects sensitisation (see also notes above)

Licensed use licensed for use in children (age range not specified by manufacturer)

Indication and dose

Bacterial skin infections see under preparation

Polyfax® (PLIVA) [PoM]

Ointment, polymyxin B sulphate 10 000 units, bacitracin zinc 500 units/g, net price 4 g = £3.26, 20 g = £4.62
Excipients none as listed in section 13.1.3

Dose

Apply twice daily or more frequently if required

RETAPAMULIN

Contra-indications contact with eyes and mucous membranes

Side-effects local reactions including irritation, erythema, pain, and pruritus

Indication and dose

Superficial bacterial skin infections (but see also notes above)

Child 9 months–18 years apply thinly twice daily for 5 days; review treatment if no response within 2–3 days

Altargo® (GSK) ▼ [PoM]

Ointment, retapamulin 1%, net price 5 g = £7.89.
Label: 28
Excipients include butylated hydroxytoluene

SILVER SULFADIAZINE
(Silver sulphadiazine)

Cautions G6PD deficiency; may inactivate enzymatic debriding agents—concomitant use may be inappropriate; **interactions:** Appendix 1 (sulphonamides)

Hepatic impairment severe, use with caution (see Large Areas, below)

Renal impairment severe, use with caution (see Large Areas, below)

Pregnancy avoid in third trimester, risk of neonatal haemolysis and methaemoglobinaemia

Breast-feeding small risk of kernicterus in jaundiced neonates and of haemolysis in G6PD deficient infant

Large areas Plasma-sulfadiazine concentrations may approach therapeutic levels with *side-effects* and *interactions* as for sulphonamides (see section 5.1.8) if large areas of skin are treated. Owing to the association of sulphonamides with severe blood and skin disorders treatment should be stopped immediately if blood disorders or rashes develop—but leucopenia developing 2–3 days after starting treatment of burns patients is reported usually to be self-limiting and silver sulfadiazine need not usually be discontinued provided blood counts are monitored carefully to ensure return to baseline within a few days. Argyria may also occur if large areas of skin are treated (or if application is prolonged).

Contra-indications sensitivity to sulphonamides; neonates

Side-effects allergic reactions including burning, itching and rashes; argyria reported following

prolonged use; leucopenia reported (monitor blood count)

Licensed use no age range specified by manufacturer but see contra-indications, above

Indication and dose

> Prophylaxis and treatment of infection in burn wounds, for conservative management of finger-tip injuries see under preparation

> Adjunct to short-term treatment of infection in pressure sores, adjunct to prophylaxis of infection in skin graft donor sites and extensive abrasions consult product literature for details

Flamazine® (S&N Hlth.) ℗ℴ𝕄
Cream, silver sulfadiazine 1%, net price 20 g = £2.91, 50 g = £3.85, 250 g = £10.32, 500 g = £18.27
Excipients include cetyl alcohol, polysorbates, propylene glycol

Dose
> Burns
> **Child 1 month–18 years** apply daily or more frequently if very exudative

> Finger-tip injuries
> **Child 1 month–18 years** apply every 2–3 days
Note apply with sterile applicator

13.10.1.2 Antibacterial preparations also used systemically

Sodium fusidate is a narrow-spectrum antibacterial used for staphylococcal infections. For the role of sodium fusidate in the treatment of impetigo see p. 707.

Metronidazole is used topically to treat rosacea and to reduce the odour associated with anaerobic infections; oral metronidazole (section 5.1.11) is used to treat wounds infected with anaerobic bacteria.

Angular cheilitis An ointment containing sodium fusidate is used in the fissures of angular cheilitis when associated with staphylococcal infection. For further information on angular cheilitis, see p. 657.

FUSIDIC ACID

Cautions see notes above; avoid contact with eyes

Side-effects rarely hypersensitivity reactions

Licensed use licensed for use in children (age range not specified by manufacturer)

Indication and dose

> Staphylococcal skin infections
> apply 3–4 times daily, usually for 7 days

> Penicillin-resistant staphylococcal infections
> section 5.1.7

> Staphylococcal eye infections
> section 11.3.1

Fucidin® (LEO) ℗ℴ𝕄
Cream, fusidic acid 2%, net price 15 g = £2.00, 30 g = £3.79
Excipients include butylated hydroxyanisole, cetyl alcohol

Ointment, sodium fusidate 2%, net price 15 g = £2.23, 30 g = £3.79
Excipients include cetyl alcohol, wool fat

Dental prescribing on NHS May be prescribed as Sodium Fusidate ointment

---

METRONIDAZOLE

Cautions avoid exposure to strong sunlight or UV light

Side-effects skin irritation

Licensed use *Metrotop®* licensed for use in children (age range not specified by manufacturer); *Acea®* and *Anabact®* not licensed for use in

children under 12 years; *Noritate®* not licensed for use in children under 16 years; *Metrogel®*, *Metrosa®*, *Rosiced®*, *Rozex®*, and *Zyomet®* not licensed for use in children

13
Skin

◁ **METRONIDAZOLE** (*continued*)

Indication and dose

Malodorous tumours and wounds
For dose see preparations

Rosacea (see also section 13.6)
For dose see preparations

Helicobacter pylori eradication
section 1.3

Anaerobic infections
section 5.1.11 and section 7.2.2

Protozoal infections
section 5.4.2

Acea® (Ferndale) PoM
Gel, metronidazole 0.75%, net price 40 g = £9.95
Excipients include disodium edetate, hydroxybenzoates
(parabens)
Dose
Acute inflammatory exacerbations of rosacea
Child 1–18 years apply thinly twice daily

Anabact® (CHS) PoM
Gel, metronidazole 0.75%, net price 15 g = £4.47,
30 g = £7.89
Excipients include hydroxybenzoates (parabens), propylene
glycol
Dose
Malodorous fungating tumours and skin ulcers
apply to clean wound 1–2 times daily and cover with
non-adherent dressing

Metrogel® (Galderma) PoM
Gel, metronidazole 0.75%, net price 40 g = £19.90
Excipients include hydroxybenzoates (parabens), propylene
glycol
Dose
Acute inflammatory exacerbations of rosacea
Child 1–18 years apply thinly twice daily

Malodorous fungating tumours
Apply to clean wound 1–2 times daily and cover with
non-adherant dressing

Metrosa® (Linderma) PoM
Gel, metronidazole 0.75%, net price 40 g = £19.90
Excipients include propylene glycol
Dose
Acute exacerbation of rosacea
Child 1–18 years apply thinly twice daily

Metrotop® (Medlock) PoM
Gel, metronidazole 0.8%, net price 15 g = £4.59
Excipients none as listed in section 13.1.3
Dose
Malodorous fungating tumours and skin ulcers
apply to clean wound 1–2 times daily and cover (flat
wounds, apply liberally; cavities, smear gel on paraffin
gauze and pack loosely)

Rosiced® (Fabre) PoM
Cream, metronidazole 0.75%, net price 30 g = £7.50
Excipients include propylene glycol
Dose
Inflammatory papules and pustules of rosacea
Child 1–18 years apply twice daily for 6 weeks (longer
if necessary)

Rozex® (Galderma) PoM
Cream, metronidazole 0.75%, net price 40 g =
£15.28
Excipients include benzyl alcohol, isopropyl palmitate
Gel, metronidazole 0.75%, net price 40 g = £15.28
Excipients include disodium edetate, hydroxybenzoates
(parabens), propylene glycol
Dose
Inflammatory papules, pustules and erythema of
rosacea
Child 1–18 years apply twice daily

Zyomet® (Goldshield) PoM
Gel, metronidazole 0.75%, net price 30 g = £12.00
Excipients include benzyl alcohol, disodium edetate, propy-
lene glycol
Dose
Acute inflammatory exacerbations of rosacea
Child 1–18 years apply thinly twice daily

13.10.2 Antifungal preparations

Most localised fungal infections are treated with topical preparations. To prevent relapse, local antifungal treatment should be continued for 1–2 weeks after the disappearance of all signs of infection. Systemic therapy (section 5.2) is necessary for nail or scalp infection or if the skin infection is widespread, disseminated or intractable. Specimens of scale, nail or hair should be sent for mycological examination before starting treatment, unless the diagnosis is certain.

Dermatophytoses Ringworm infection can affect the scalp (tinea capitis), body (tinea corporis), groin (tinea cruris), hand (tinea manuum), foot (tinea pedis, athlete's foot), or nail (tinea unguium, onychomycosis). Tinea capitis is a common childhood infection that requires systemic treatment with an oral antifungal (section 5.2); additional application of a topical antifungal, during the early stages of treatment, may reduce the risk of transmission. A topical antifungal can also be used to treat asymptomatic carriers of scalp ringworm.

13 Skin

Tinea corporis and tinea pedis infections in children respond to treatment with a topical **imidazole** (clotrimazole, econazole, ketoconazole, miconazole, or sulconazole) or **terbinafine** cream. Nystatin is less effective against tinea.

Compound benzoic acid ointment (Whitfield's ointment) has been used for ringworm infections but it is cosmetically less acceptable than proprietary preparations. Antifungal dusting powders are of little therapeutic value in the treatment of fungal skin infections and may cause skin irritation; they may have some role in preventing re-infection.

Antifungal treatment may not be necessary in asymptomatic children with tinea infection of the nails. If treatment is necessary, a systemic antifungal (section 5.2) is more effective than topical therapy. However, topical application of **amorolfine** or **tioconazole** may be useful for treating early onychomycosis when involvement is limited to mild distal disease in up to 2 nails, or for superficial white onychomycosis, or where there are contra-indications to systemic therapy. Chronic paronychia on the fingers (usually due to a candidal infection) should be treated with topical clotrimazole or nystatin, but these preparations should be used with caution in children who suck their fingers. Chronic paronychia of the toes (usually due to dermatophyte infection) can be treated with topical terbinafine.

Pityriasis versicolor   Pityriasis (tinea) versicolor can be treated with **ketoconazole** shampoo or **selenium sulphide** shampoo (section 13.9). Topical imidazole antifungals, **clotrimazole, econazole, ketoconazole, miconazole,** and **sulconazole,** and topical **terbinafine** are alternatives, but large quantities may be required.

If topical therapy fails, or if the infection is widespread, pityriasis versicolor is treated systemically with an azole antifungal (section 5.2). Relapse is common, especially in the immunocompromised.

Candidiasis   Candidal skin infections can be treated with topical imidazole antifungals **clotrimazole, econazole, ketoconazole, miconazole,** or **sulconazole**; topical terbinafine is an alternative. Topical application of **nystatin** is also effective for candidiasis but it is ineffective against dermatophytosis. Refractory candidiasis requires systemic treatment (section 5.2) generally with a triazole such as fluconazole; systemic treatment with griseofulvin or terbinafine is **not appropriate** for refractory candidiasis. For the treatment of oral candiasis see section 12.3.2 and for the management of nappy rash see section 13.2.2.

Angular cheilitis   Miconazole cream is used in the fissures of angular cheilitis when associated with *Candida*. For further information on angular cheilitis, see p. 657.

Cautions   Contact with eyes and mucous membranes should be avoided.

Side-effects   Occasional local irritation and hypersensitivity reactions include mild burning sensation, erythema, and itching. Treatment should be discontinued if symptoms are severe.

Compound topical preparations   Combination of an imidazole and a mild corticosteroid (such as hydrocortisone 1%) (section 13.4) may be of value in the treatment of eczematous intertrigo and, in the first few days only, of a severely inflamed patch of ringworm. Combination of a mild corticosteroid with either an imidazole or nystatin may be of use in the treatment of *intertriginous eczema* associated with candida.

◢ AMOROLFINE

Cautions see notes above; also avoid contact with ears; pregnancy and breast-feeding

Side-effects see notes above

Licensed use not licensed for use in children under 12 years

Indication and dose
See under preparations

Loceryl® (Galderma) PoM
Cream, amorolfine (as hydrochloride) 0.25%, net price 20 g = £4.83. Label: 10, patient information leaflet
Excipients include cetostearyl alcohol, disodium edetate
Dose
Fungal skin infections
apply once daily after cleansing in the evening for at least 2–3 weeks (up to 6 weeks for foot infection) continuing for 3–5 days after lesions have healed

13
Skin

◁ **AMOROLFINE (***continued***)**

Nail lacquer, amorolfine (as hydrochloride) 5%, net price 5-mL pack (with nail files, spatulas and cleansing swabs) = £18.71. Label: 10, patient information leaflet
Excipients none as listed in section 13.1.3

Dose

Fungal nail infections

apply to infected nails 1–2 times weekly after filing and cleansing; allow to dry (approx. 3 minutes); treat finger nails for 6 months, toe nails for 9–12 months (review at intervals of 3 months); avoid nail varnish or artificial nails during treatment

Note Use with caution in child likely to suck affected digits

BENZOIC ACID

Licensed use licensed for use in children (age range not specified by manufacturer)

Indication and dose

Ringworm (tinea) but see notes above; dose under preparation

Benzoic Acid Ointment, Compound, BP (Whitfield's ointment)
Ointment, benzoic acid 6%, salicylic acid 3%, in emulsifying ointment
Excipients include cetostearyl alcohol

Dose

Child 1 month–18 years apply twice daily

CLOTRIMAZOLE

Cautions see notes above

Side-effects see notes above

Licensed use licensed for use in children (age range not specified by manufacturer)

Indication and dose

Fungal skin infections
apply 2–3 times daily

Vaginal candidiasis section 7.2.2

Otitis externa section 12.1.1

Clotrimazole (Non-proprietary)
Cream, clotrimazole 1%, net price 20 g = £1.92

Canesten® (Bayer Consumer Care)
Cream, clotrimazole 1%, net price 20 g = £2.14, 50 g = £3.80
Excipients include benzyl alcohol, cetostearyl alcohol, polysorbate 60

Powder, clotrimazole 1%, net price 30 g = £1.52
Excipients none as listed in section 13.1.3

Solution, clotrimazole 1% in macrogol 400 (polyethylene glycol 400), net price 20 mL = £2.43. For hairy areas
Excipients none as listed in section 13.1.3

Spray, clotrimazole 1%, in 30% isopropyl alcohol, net price 40-mL atomiser = £4.99. Label: 15. For large or hairy areas
Excipients include propylene glycol

ECONAZOLE NITRATE

Cautions see notes above

Side-effects see notes above

Licensed use *Ecostatin®* not licensed for use in children under 1 year; *Pevaryl®*, no age range specified by manufacturer

Indication and dose

Fungal skin infections
apply twice daily

Fungal nail infections
apply once daily under occlusive dressing

Vaginal candidiasis section 7.2.2

Ecostatin® (Squibb)
Cream, econazole nitrate 1%, net price 15 g = £1.49; 30 g = £2.75
Excipients include butylated hydroxyanisole, fragrance

Pevaryl® (Janssen-Cilag)
Cream, econazole nitrate 1%, net price 30 g = £2.65
Excipients include butylated hydroxyanisole, fragrance

KETOCONAZOLE

Cautions see notes above; do **not** use within 2 weeks of a potent topical corticosteroid for seborrhoeic dermatitis—risk of skin sensitisation

Side-effects see notes above

Indication and dose

Tinea pedis
apply twice daily

Other fungal infections
apply 1–2 times daily

Systemic or resistant fungal infections section 5.2

Vulval candidiasis section 7.2.2

13 Skin

◻ **KETOCONAZOLE (continued)**

Nizoral® (Janssen-Cilag) [PoM]
[1]Cream, ketoconazole 2%, net price 30 g = £3.54
Excipients include cetyl alcohol, polysorbates, propylene glycol, stearyl alcohol

Note A 15-g tube is available for sale to the public for the treatment of tinea pedis, tinea cruris, and candidal intertrigo

Shampoo—section 13.9
1. [NHS] except for seborrhoeic dermatitis and pityriasis versicolor and endorsed 'SLS'

◼ MICONAZOLE NITRATE

Cautions see notes above

Side-effects see notes above

Licensed use Licensed for use in children (age range not specified by manufacturer)

Indication and dose

> Fungal skin infections
>
> > **Neonate** apply twice daily continuing for 10 days after lesions have healed
>
> > **Child 1 month–18 years** apply twice daily continuing for 10 days after lesions have healed
>
> Fungal nail infections
> apply 1–2 times daily

Oral and intestinal fungal infections section 12.3.2

Vaginal candidiasis section 7.2.2

Miconazole (Non-proprietary)
Cream, miconazole nitrate 2%, net price 20 g = £2.05, 45 g = £1.97
Dental prescribing on NHS Miconazole cream may be prescribed

Daktarin® (Janssen-Cilag)
Cream, miconazole nitrate 2%, net price 30 g = £1.93
Excipients include butylated hydroxyanisole

◼ NYSTATIN

Cautions see notes above

Side-effects see notes above

Licensed use licensed for use in children (age range not specified by manufacturer)

Indication and dose

> Skin infections due to *Candida* spp. for dose, see preparations

Intestinal candidiasis section 5.2

Oral fungal infections section 12.3.2

Nystaform® (Typharm) [PoM]
Cream, nystatin 100 000 units/g, chlorhexidine hydrochloride 1%, net price 30 g = £2.62
Excipients include benzyl alcohol, cetostearyl alcohol, polysorbate 60

Dose
> Apply 2–3 times daily continuing for 7 days after lesions have healed.

Tinaderm-M® (Schering-Plough) [PoM]
Cream, nystatin 100 000 units/g, tolnaftate 1%, net price 20 g = £1.83
Excipients include butylated hydroxytoluene, cetostearyl alcohol, hydroxybenzoates (parabens), fragrance

Dose
> Apply 2–3 times daily

◼ SALICYLIC ACID

Cautions avoid broken or inflamed skin
Salicylate toxicity Salicylate toxicity can occur particularly if applied on large areas of skin

Contra-indications children under 5 years

Side-effects see notes above

Licensed use not licensed for use in children under 5 years

Indication and dose

> Fungal nail infections, particularly tinea
> Apply twice daily and after washing
> **Note** Use with caution in child likely to suck affected digits

Hyperkeratotic skin disorders section 13.5.2

Acne vulgaris section 13.6.1

Warts and calluses section 13.7

Phytex® (Wynlit)
Paint, salicylic acid 1.46% (total combined), tannic acid 4.89% and boric acid 3.12% (as borotannic complex), in a vehicle containing alcohol and ethyl acetate, net price 25 mL (with brush) = £1.56
Excipients none as listed in section 13.1.3

Note Flammable

SULCONAZOLE NITRATE

Cautions see notes above

Side-effects see notes above; also blistering

Indication and dose

Fungal skin infections

apply 1–2 times daily continuing for 2–3 weeks after lesions have healed

Exelderm® (Centrapharm)

Cream, sulconazole nitrate 1%, net price 30 g = £3.90

Excipients include cetyl alcohol, polysorbates, propylene glycol, stearyl alcohol

TERBINAFINE

Cautions avoid contact with eyes

Pregnancy manufacturer advises avoid—studies in *animals* suggest no adverse effects

Breast-feeding manufacturer advises avoid—present in milk, but less than 5% of the dose is absorbed after topical application of terbinafine

Side-effects see notes above

Licensed use not licensed for use in children

Indication and dose

Fungal skin infections

Apply thinly 1–2 times daily for up to 1 week in tinea pedis, 1–2 weeks in tinea corporis and tinea cruris, 2 weeks in cutaneous candidiasis and pityriasis versicolor; review after 2 weeks

Systemic therapy section 5.2

¹**Terbinafine** (Non-proprietary) [PoM]

Cream, terbinafine hydrochloride 1%, net price 15 g = £4.86, 30 g = £8.76

1. Can be sold to the public for external use in children over 16 years for the treatment of tinea pedis and tinea cruris as a cream containing terbinafine hydrochloride max. 1% in a pack containing max. 15 g; also for the treatment of tinea pedis, tinea cruris, and tinea corporis as a spray containing terbinafine hydrochloride max. 1% in a pack containing max. 30 mL or as a gel containing terbinafine hydrochloride max. 1% in a pack containing max. 30 g

Lamisil® (Novartis Consumer Health) [PoM]

Cream, terbinafine hydrochloride 1%, net price 15 g = £4.86, 30 g = £8.76

Excipients include benzyl alcohol, cetyl alcohol, polysorbate 60, stearyl alcohol

TIOCONAZOLE

Cautions see notes above

Contra-indications

Pregnancy manufacturer advises avoid

Side-effects see notes above; also local oedema, dry skin, nail discoloration, periungual inflammation, nail pain, rash, exfoliation

Licensed use licensed for use in children (age range not specified by manufacturer)

Indication and dose

Fungal nail infections

apply to nails and surrounding skin twice daily for up to 6 months (may be extended to 12 months)

Trosyl® (Pfizer) [PoM]

Cutaneous solution, tioconazole 28%, net price 12 mL (with applicator brush) = £27.38

Excipients none as listed in section 13.1.3

Note Use with caution in child likely to suck affected digits

UNDECENOATES

Side-effects see notes above

Licensed use *Monphytol®* not licensed for use in children under 12 years; *Mycota®* licensed for use in children (age range not specified by manufacturer)

Indication and dose

See under preparations

Mycota® (Thornton & Ross)

Cream, zinc undecenoate 20%, undecenoic acid 5%, net price 25 g = £1.37

Excipients include fragrance

Dose

Treatment of athlete's foot

apply twice daily continuing for 7 days after lesions have healed

Prevention of athlete's foot

apply once daily

Powder, zinc undecenoate 20%, undecenoic acid 2%, net price 70 g = £1.93

Excipients include fragrance

Dose

Treatment of athlete's foot

apply twice daily continuing for 7 days after lesions have healed

Prevention of athlete's foot

apply once daily

Spray application, undecenoic acid 2.5%, dichlorophen 0.25% (pressurised aerosol pack), net price 100 mL = £2.19

Excipients include fragrance

Dose

Treatment of athlete's foot

apply twice daily continuing for 7 days after lesions have healed

Prevention of athlete's foot

apply once daily

13.10.3 Antiviral preparations

See section 12.3.2 for drugs used in *herpetic stomatitis*, section 13.5.1 for *eczema herpeticum*, and section 11.3.3 for viral infections of the *eye*.

Aciclovir cream is used for the treatment of initial and recurrent labial, cutaneous, and genital *herpes simplex infections* in children; treatment should begin as early as possible. Systemic treatment is necessary for buccal or vaginal infections or if cold sores recur frequently (for details of systemic use see section 5.3.2.1).

Herpes labialis　　**Aciclovir** cream can be used for the treatment of initial and recurrent labial herpes simplex infections (cold sores). It is best applied at the earliest possible stage, usually when prodromal changes of sensation are felt in the lip and before vesicles appear.

Penciclovir cream is also licensed for the treatment of herpes labialis; it needs to be applied more frequently than aciclovir cream. These creams should not be used in the mouth.

◢ ACICLOVIR

(Acyclovir)

Cautions　avoid contact with eyes and mucous membranes

Side-effects　transient stinging or burning; occasionally erythema, itching or drying of the skin

Licensed use　licensed for use in children (age range not specified by manufacturer)

Indication and dose

> **Herpes simplex infections**
>
> Apply to lesions every 4 hours (5 times daily) for 5–10 days, starting at first sign of attack

> **Herpes simplex and varicella–zoster infections** section 5.3.2.1

Eye infections section 11.3.3

Aciclovir (Non-proprietary) (PoM)
Cream, aciclovir 5%, net price 2 g = £1.10, 10 g = £2.16
Excipients include propylene glycol
Brands include *Zuvogen®* (*excipients* include cetyl alcohol, propylene glycol)
Dental prescribing on NHS Aciclovir Cream may be prescribed

Zovirax® (GSK) (PoM)
Cream, aciclovir 5%, net price 2 g = £3.98, 10 g = £14.82
Excipients include cetostearyl alcohol, propylene glycol

◢ PENCICLOVIR

Cautions　avoid contact with eyes and mucous membranes

Side-effects　transient stinging, burning, numbness; hypersensitivity reactions also reported

Licensed use　not licensed for use in children under 12 years

Vectavir® (Novartis Consumer Health) (PoM)
Cream, penciclovir 1%, net price 2 g = £4.20
Excipients include cetostearyl alcohol, propylene glycol

Dose

> **Herpes labialis**
>
> Apply to lesions every 2 hours during waking hours for 4 days, starting at first sign of attack

Dental prescribing on NHS May be prescribed as Penciclovir Cream

13.10.4 Parasiticidal preparations

Suitable quantities of parasiticidal preparations			
	Skin creams	Lotions	Cream rinses
Scalp (head lice)	—	50–100 mL	50–100 mL
Body (scabies)	30–60 g	100 mL	—
Body (crab lice)	30–60 g	100 mL	—
These amounts are usually suitable for a child 12–18 years for single application			

Scabies

Permethrin is used for the treatment of *scabies* (*Sarcoptes scabiei*); **malathion** can be used if permethrin is inappropriate.

Aqueous preparations are preferable; alcoholic lotions cause irritation of excoriated skin and the genitalia.

Benzyl benzoate is an irritant and should be avoided in children; it is less effective than malathion and permethrin.

Ivermectin (available from 'special-order' manufacturers or specialist importing

13

Skin

companies, see p. 943), is used in combination with topical drugs, for the treatment of hyperkeratotic (crusted or 'Norwegian') scabies that does not respond to topical treatment alone.

Application Although acaricides have traditionally been applied after a hot bath, this is **not** necessary and there is even evidence that a hot bath may increase absorption into the blood, removing them from their site of action on the skin.

All members of the affected household should be treated simultaneously. Treatment should be applied to the whole body including the scalp, neck, face, and ears. Particular attention should be paid to the webs of the fingers and toes and lotion brushed under the ends of nails. Malathion and permethrin should be applied twice, one week apart. It is important to warn users to reapply treatment to the hands if they are washed. Children with hyperkeratotic scabies may require 2 or 3 applications of acaricide on consecutive days to ensure that enough penetrates the skin crusts to kill all the mites.

Itching The *itch* and *eczema* of scabies persists for some weeks after the infestation has been eliminated and treatment for pruritus and eczema (section 13.5.1) may be required. Application of **crotamiton** can be used to control itching after treatment with more effective acaricides. A topical **corticosteroid** (section 13.4) may help to reduce itch and inflammation after scabies has been treated successfully; however, persistent symptoms suggest failure of scabies eradication. Oral administration of a **sedating antihistamine** (section 3.4.1) at night may also be useful.

Head lice

Malathion and **phenothrin** can be used against head lice (*Pediculus humanus capitis*) but lice in some districts have developed resistance; resistance to two or more parasiticidal preparations has also been reported. **Permethrin** is effective against head lice but no suitable preparation for a contact time of 12 hours exists. Careful application of **dimeticone**, which acts on the surface of head lice, is also effective. Benzyl benzoate is licensed for the treatment of head lice but it is not recommended for use in children.

Head lice infestation (pediculosis) should be treated using lotion or liquid formulations. Shampoos are diluted too much in use to be effective. Alcoholic formulations are effective but aqueous formulations are preferred in children, especially those with severe eczema or asthma. A contact time of 12 hours or overnight treatment is recommended for lotions and liquids; a 2-hour treatment is not sufficient to kill eggs.

In general, a course of treatment for head lice should be 2 applications of product 7 days apart to prevent lice emerging from any eggs that survive the first application.

The policy of rotating insecticides on a district-wide basis is now considered outmoded. To overcome the development of resistance, a mosaic strategy is required whereby, if a course of treatment fails to cure, a different insecticide is used for the next course. If a course of treatment with either permethrin or phenothrin fails, then a non-pyrethroid parasiticidal product should be used for the next course.

Wet combing methods Head lice can be mechanically removed by combing wet hair meticulously with a plastic detection comb (probably for at least 30 minutes each time) over the whole scalp at 4-day intervals for a minimum of 2 weeks; hair conditioner or vegetable oil can be used to facilitate the process. Several products are available and some are prescribable on the NHS.

Crab lice

Permethrin, **phenothrin**, and **malathion** are used to eliminate *crab lice* (*Pthirus pubis*); permethrin is not licensed for treatment of crab lice in children under 18 years. An aqueous preparation should be applied, allowed to dry naturally and washed off after 12 hours; a second treatment is needed after 7 days to kill lice emerging from surviving eggs. All surfaces of the body should be treated, including the scalp, neck, and face (paying particular attention to the eyebrows and other facial hair). A different insecticide should be used if a course of treatment fails. Alcoholic lotions are not recommended (owing to irritation of excoriated skin and the genitalia).

Aqueous **malathion** lotion is effective for *crab lice of the eye lashes* [unlicensed use].

Parasiticidal preparations

Dimeticone coats head lice and interferes with water balance in lice by preventing excretion of water; it is less active against eggs and treatment should be repeated after 7 days.

Malathion is recommended for *scabies, head lice* and *crab lice* (see notes above). The risk of systemic effects associated with 1–2 applications of malathion is considered to be very low; however, except in the treatment of hyperkeratotic scabies (see notes above), applications of lotion repeated at intervals of less than 1 week *or* application for more than 3 consecutive weeks should be **avoided** since the likelihood of eradication of lice is not increased.

Permethrin is effective for *scabies*. It is active against *head lice* but the formulation and licensed methods of application of the current products make them unsuitable for the treatment of head lice. Permethrin is also effective against *crab lice* but it is not licensed for this purpose in children under 18 years.

Phenothrin is recommended for *head lice* and *crab lice*.

DIMETICONE

Cautions avoid contact with eyes
Side-effects skin irritation
Licensed use not licensed for use in children under 6 months except under medical supervision

Indication and dose

Head lice
Rub into dry hair and scalp, allow to dry naturally, shampoo after 8 hours (or overnight); repeat application after 7 days

Hedrin® (Thornton & Ross)
Lotion, dimeticone 4%, net price 50 mL = £2.98, 120-mL spray pack = £7.14, 150 mL = £6.83
Note Patients should be told to keep their hair away from fire and flames during treatment

MALATHION

Cautions avoid contact with eyes; do not use on broken or secondarily infected skin; do not use lotion more than once a week for 3 consecutive weeks; alcoholic lotions **not** recommended for head lice in children with severe eczema or asthma, or for scabies or crab lice (see notes above)
Side-effects skin irritation and hypersensitivity reactions; chemical burns also reported
Licensed use not licensed for use in children under 6 months except under medical supervision

Indication and dose

See notes above and under preparations

Head lice
Rub 0.5% preparation into dry hair and scalp, allow to dry naturally, remove by washing after 12 hours; repeat application after 7 days (see also notes above)

Crab lice
Apply 0.5% aqueous preparation over whole body, allow to dry naturally, wash off after 12 hours or overnight; repeat application after 7 days

Scabies
Apply 0.5% preparation over whole body, and wash off after 24 hours; if hands are washed with soap within 24 hours, they should be retreated; see also notes above; repeat application after 7 days

Note For scabies, manufacturer recommends application to the body but not necessarily to the head and neck. However, application should be extended to the scalp, neck, face, and ears

Derbac-M® (SSL)
Liquid, malathion 0.5% in an aqueous basis, net price 50 mL = £2.27, 200 mL = £5.70
Excipients include cetostearyl alcohol, fragrance, hydroxybenzoates (parabens)
For crab lice, head lice, and scabies

◁ **MALATHION (continued)**

Prioderm® (SSL)
Lotion, malathion 0.5%, in an alcoholic basis, net price 50 mL = £2.22, 200 mL = £5.70. Label: 15
Excipients include fragrance
For head lice (alcoholic formulation, see notes above)

Cream shampoo NHS⬛ malathion 1%, net price 40 g = £2.77
Excipients include cetostearyl alcohol, fragrance, hydroxy-benzoates (parabens), sodium edetate, wool fat

Note Head and crab lice, not recommended, therefore no dose stated (product too diluted in use and insufficient contact time)

Quellada M® (GSK Consumer Healthcare)
Liquid, malathion 0.5% in an aqueous basis, net price 50 mL = £1.85, 200 mL = £4.62
Excipients include cetostearyl alcohol, fragrance, hydroxy-benzoates (parabens)
For crab lice, head lice, and scabies

Cream shampoo⬛ malathion 1%, net price 40 g = £2.18
Excipients include cetostearyl alcohol, fragrance, hydroxy-benzoates (parabens), sodium edetate, wool fat

Note Head and crab lice, not recommended, therefore no dose stated (product too diluted in use and insufficient contact time)

◢ PERMETHRIN

Cautions avoid contact with eyes; do not use on broken or secondarily infected skin

Side-effects pruritus, erythema, and stinging; rarely rashes and oedema

Licensed use *Dermal Cream* (scabies), not licensed for use in children under 2 months; children aged 2 months–2 years, medical supervison required; not licensed for treatment of crab lice in children under 18 years; *Creme Rinse* (head lice) not licensed for use in children under 6 months except under medical supervision

Indication and dose

See notes above

> **Scabies**
> Apply 5% preparation over whole body including face, neck, scalp and ears; wash off after 8-12 hours; if hands washed with soap within 8 hours of application, they should be treated again with cream (see notes above); repeat application after 7 days
> Note Manufacturer recommends application to the body but to exclude head and neck. However, application should be extended to the scalp, neck, face, and ears

Permethrin (Non-proprietary)
Cream, permethrin 5%, net price 30 g = £5.55

Lyclear® Creme Rinse (Chefaro UK) ⬛
Cream rinse, permethrin 1% in basis containing isopropyl alcohol 20%, net price 59 mL = £2.38, 2 × 59-mL pack = £4.32
Excipients include cetyl alcohol

Note Head lice, not recommended, therefore no dose stated (product too diluted in use and insufficient contact time)

Lyclear® Dermal Cream (Chefaro UK)
Dermal cream, permethrin 5%, net price 30 g = £5.71. Label: 10, patient information leaflet
Excipients include butylated hydroxytoluene, wool fat derivative

---

◢ PHENOTHRIN

Cautions avoid contact with eyes; do not use on broken or secondarily infected skin; do not use more than once a week for 3 weeks at a time; alcoholic preparations **not** recommended for head lice in severe eczema, in asthma, in small children, or for crab lice (see notes above)

Side-effects skin irritation

Licensed use not licensed for use in children under 6 months except under medical supervision

Indication and dose

See notes above and under preparations

Full Marks® (SSL)
Liquid, phenothrin 0.5% in an aqueous basis, net price 50 mL = £2.22, 200 mL = £5.70
Excipients include cetostearyl alcohol, fragrance, hydroxy-benzoates (parabens)

Dose

> **Head lice**
> apply to dry hair, allow to dry naturally; shampoo after 12 hours or next day, comb wet hair; repeat application after 7 days

Lotion, phenothrin 0.2% in basis containing isopropyl alcohol 69.3%, net price 50 mL = £2.22, 200 mL = £5.70. Label: 15
Excipients include fragrance

Dose

> **Crab lice and head lice**
> (alcoholic formulation, see notes above) apply to dry hair, allow to dry naturally; shampoo after 12 hours [unlicensed contact duration], comb wet hair; repeat application after 7 days

Mousse (= foam application) ⬛ phenothrin 0.5% in an alcoholic basis, net price 50 g = £2.53, 150 g = £6.11. Label: 15
Excipients include cetostearyl alcohol

Dose

> **Head lice**
> (alcoholic formulation, see notes above) apply to dry hair, shampoo after 30 minutes, comb wet hair—but product not recommended because contact time insufficient (longer contact time not recommended because of risk of irritation)

13 Skin

13.10.5 Preparations for minor cuts and abrasions

Cetrimide cream is used to treat minor cuts and abrasions. **Proflavine** cream may be used to treat infected wounds or burns, but has now been largely superseded by other antiseptics or suitable antibacterials.

Cetrimide Cream, BP
Cream, cetrimide 0.5% in a suitable water-miscible basis such as cetostearyl alcohol 5%, liquid paraffin 50% in freshly boiled and cooled purified water, net price 50 g = £1.11

Proflavine Cream, BPC
Cream, proflavine hemisulphate 0.1%, yellow beeswax 2.5%, chlorocresol 0.1%, liquid paraffin 67.3%, freshly boiled and cooled purified water 25%, wool fat 5%, net price 100 mL = 68p
Excipients include beeswax, wool fat

Note Stains clothing

Collodion

Flexible collodion may be used to seal minor cuts and wounds that have partially healed.

Collodion, Flexible, BP
Collodion, castor oil 2.5%, colophony 2.5% in a collodion basis, prepared by dissolving pyroxylin (10%) in a mixture of 3 volumes of ether and 1 volume of alcohol (90%), net price 10 mL = 25p.
Label: 15
Contra-indications allergy to colophony in elastic adhesive plasters and tape

Skin tissue adhesive

Tissue adhesives are used for closure of minor skin wounds and for additional suture support. They should be applied by an appropriately trained healthcare professional. Skin tissue adhesives may cause skin sensitisation.

Dermabond ProPen® (Ethicon)
Topical skin adhesive, sterile, octyl 2-cyanoacrylate, net price 0.5 mL = £18.38

Epiglu® (Schuco)
Tissue adhesive, sterile, ethyl-2-cyanoacrylate 954.5 mg/g, polymethylmethacrylate, net price 4 × 3-g vials = £149.50 (with dispensing pipettes and pallete)

Histoacryl® (Braun)
Tissue adhesive, sterile, enbucrilate, net price 5 × 200-mg unit (blue) = £32.00, 10 × 200-mg unit (blue) = £67.20, 5 × 500-mg unit (clear or blue) = £34.65, 10 × 500-mg unit (blue) = £69.30

LiquiBand® (MedLogic)
Tissue adhesive, sterile, enbucrilate, net price 0.5-g amp = £5.50

13.11 Skin cleansers and antiseptics

13.11.1 Alcohols and saline
13.11.2 Chlorhexidine salts
13.11.3 Cationic surfactants and soaps
13.11.4 Iodine
13.11.5 Phenolics
13.11.6 Oxidisers and dyes
13.11.7 Preparations for promotion of wound healing

Soap or detergent is used with water to cleanse intact skin but they can irritate infantile skin; emollient preparations such as aqueous cream or emulsifying ointment (section 13.2.1) that do not irritate the skin are best used in place of soap or detergent for cleansing dry or irritated skin.

An antiseptic is used for skin that is infected or that is susceptible to recurrent infection. Detergent preparations containing **chlorhexidine** or **povidone–iodine**, which should be thoroughly rinsed off, are used. Emollients may also contain antiseptics (section 13.2.1).

Antiseptics such as **chlorhexidine** or **povidone–iodine** are used on intact skin before surgical procedures; their antiseptic effect is enhanced by an alcoholic solvent. Antiseptic solutions containing **cetrimide** can be used if a detergent effect is also required. On neonatal skin, regular use of povidone–iodine and of preparations containing alcohol should be avoided.

13

Skin

For irrigating ulcers or wounds, lukewarm sterile **sodium chloride 0.9% solution** is used but tap water is often appropriate.

Potassium permanganate solution 1 in 10 000, a mild antiseptic with astringent properties, can be used as a soak for exudative eczematous areas (section 13.5.1); treatment should be stopped when the skin becomes dry. Potassium permanganate can stain skin and nails especially with prolonged use.

13.11.1 Alcohols and saline

ALCOHOL

Cautions flammable; avoid broken skin; patients have suffered severe burns when diathermy has been preceded by application of alcoholic skin disinfectants

Contra-indications neonates, see section 13.1

Indication and dose

Skin preparation before injection
apply to skin as necessary

Industrial Methylated Spirit, BP
Solution, 19 volumes of ethanol and 1 volume approved wood naphtha, net price '66 OP' (containing 95% by volume alcohol) 100 mL = 39p; '74 OP' (containing 99% by volume alcohol) 100 mL = 39p. Label: 15

Surgical Spirit, BP
Spirit, methyl salicylate 0.5 mL, diethyl phthalate 2%, castor oil 2.5%, in industrial methylated spirit, net price 100 mL = 20p. Label: 15

SODIUM CHLORIDE

Indication and dose

See notes above

Nebuliser diluent section 3.1.5

Sodium depletion section 9.2.1.2

Electrolyte imbalance section 9.2.2.1

Eye section 11.8.1

Oral hygiene section 12.3.4

Sodium Chloride (Non-proprietary)
Solution (sterile), sodium chloride 0.9%, net price 25 × 20-mL unit = £5.50, 200–mL can = £2.65, 1 litre = 97p

Flowfusor® (Fresenius Kabi)
Solution (sterile), sodium chloride 0.9%, net price 120-mL Bellows Pack = £1.53

Irriclens® (ConvaTec)
Solution in aerosol can (sterile), sodium chloride 0.9%, net price 240-mL can = £3.24

Irripod® (C D Medical)
Solution (sterile), sodium chloride 0.9%, net price 25 × 20-mL sachet = £5.50

Miniversol® (Aguettant)
Solution (sterile), sodium chloride 0.9%, net price 30 × 45-mL unit = £13.20; 30 × 100-mL unit = £19.50

Normasol® (Medlock)
Solution (sterile), sodium chloride 0.9%, net price 25 × 25-mL sachet = £5.98; 10 × 100-mL sachet = £7.27

Stericlens® (C D Medical)
Solution in aerosol can (sterile), sodium chloride 0.9%, net price 100-mL can = £1.94, 240-mL can = £2.95

Steripod® Sodium Chloride (Medlock)
Solution (sterile), sodium chloride 0.9%, net price 25 × 20-mL sachet = £7.36

13.11.2 Chlorhexidine salts

CHLORHEXIDINE

Cautions avoid contact with eyes, brain, meninges and middle ear; not for use in body cavities; alcoholic solutions not suitable before diathermy or for use on neonatal skin

Side-effects occasional sensitivity

Indication and dose

See under preparations

Bladder irrigation and catheter patency solutions section 7.4.4

Chlorhexidine 0.05% (Baxter)
2000 Solution (sterile), pink, chlorhexidine acetate 0.05%, net price 500 mL = 72p, 1000 mL = 77p
For cleansing and disinfecting wounds and burns

13 Skin

◻ **CHLORHEXIDINE** (*continued*)

Cepton® (LPC)

Skin wash (= solution), red, chlorhexidine gluconate 1%, net price 150 mL = £2.48
For use as skin wash in acne

Lotion, blue, chlorhexidine gluconate 0.1%, net price 150 mL = £2.48
For skin disinfection in acne

ChloraPrep® (Enturia)

Cutaneous solution, sterile, chlorhexidine gluconate 2% in isopropyl alcohol 70%, net price (single applicator) 0.67 mL = 30p, 1.5 mL = 55p, 3 mL = 85p, 10.5 mL = £2.92, 26 mL = £6.50
For skin disinfection before invasive procedures; Child under 2 months not recommended
Note Flammable

CX Antiseptic Dusting Powder® (Ecolab)

Dusting powder, sterile, chlorhexidine acetate 1%, net price 15 g = £2.68
For skin disinfection

Hibiscrub® (Regent Medical)

Cleansing solution, red, chlorhexidine gluconate 4%, perfumed, in a surfactant solution, net price 250 mL = £4.25, 500 mL = £5.25, 5 litres = £16.20
Excipients include fragrance
Use instead of soap for pre-operative hand and skin preparation and for general hand and skin disinfection

Hibisol® (Regent Medical)

Solution, chlorhexidine gluconate 0.5%, in isopropyl alcohol 70% with emollients, net price 500 mL = £5.25
To be used undiluted for hand and skin disinfection

Hibitane Obstetric® (Centrapharm)

Cream, chlorhexidine gluconate solution 5% (≡ 1% chlorhexidine gluconate), in a pourable water-miscible basis, net price 250 mL = £4.44
For use in obstetrics and gynaecology as an antiseptic and lubricant (for application to skin around vulva and perineum and to hands of midwife or doctor)

Hydrex® (Ecolab)

Solution, chlorhexidine gluconate solution 2.5% (≡ chlorhexidine gluconate 0.5%), in an alcoholic solution, net price 600 mL (clear) = £2.06; 600 mL (pink) = £2.06, 200-mL spray = £1.77, 500-mL spray = £3.01; 600 mL (blue) = £2.26
Note Flammable
For pre-operative skin disinfection

Surgical scrub, chlorhexidine gluconate 4% in a surfactant solution, net price 250 mL = £1.93, 500 mL = £2.05
For pre-operative hand and skin preparation and for general hand disinfection

Unisept® (Medlock)

Solution (sterile), pink, chlorhexidine gluconate 0.05%, net price 25 × 25-mL sachet = £5.40; 10 × 100-mL sachet = £6.67
For cleansing and disinfecting wounds and burns and swabbing in obstetrics

◀ **With cetrimide**

Tisept® (Medlock)

Solution (sterile), yellow, chlorhexidine gluconate 0.015%, cetrimide 0.15%, net price 25 × 25-mL sachet = £5.20; 10 × 100-mL sachet = £6.68
To be used undiluted for general skin disinfection and wound cleansing

Travasept 100® (Baxter)

Solution (sterile), yellow, chlorhexidine acetate 0.015%, cetrimide 0.15%, net price 500 mL = 72p, 1 litre = 77p
To be used undiluted in skin disinfection such as wound cleansing and obstetrics

---

Concentrates

Hibitane 5% Concentrate® (Regent Medical)

Solution, red, chlorhexidine gluconate 5%, in a perfumed aqueous solution, net price 5 litres = £14.50

Dose

Pre-operative skin preparation
Dilute 1 in 10 (0.5%) with alcohol 70%

General skin disinfection
Dilute 1 in 100 (0.05%) with water

Note Alcoholic solutions not suitable for use before diathermy (see Alcohol, p. 720) or on neonatal skin

---

13.11.3 Cationic surfactants and soaps

◀ **CETRIMIDE**

Cautions avoid contact with eyes; avoid use in body cavities

Side-effects skin irritation and occasionally sensitisation

Indication and dose

Skin disinfection

◀ **Preparations**
Ingredient of *Tisept®* and *Travasept® 100*, see above

13

Skin

13.11.4 Iodine

POVIDONE–IODINE

Cautions broken skin (see below)

Renal impairment avoid regular application to inflamed or broken skin or mucosa

Large open wounds The application of povidone–iodine to large wounds or severe burns may produce systemic adverse effects such as metabolic acidosis, hypernatraemia, and impairment of renal function

Contra-indications preterm neonate gestational age under 32 weeks; infants body-weight under 1.5 kg; regular use in neonates; thyroid disorders; concomitant lithium treatment

Pregnancy avoid regular use

Breast-feeding avoid

Side-effects rarely sensitivity; may interfere with thyroid function tests

Indication and dose

Skin disinfection see preparations

Betadine® (Mölnlycke)
Dry powder spray, povidone–iodine 2.5% in a pressurised aerosol unit, net price 150-g unit = £2.63
For skin disinfection, particularly minor wounds and infections; child under 2 years not recommended
Note Not for use in serous cavities

Ointment, povidone–iodine 10%, in a water-miscible basis, net price 20 g = £1.33, 80 g = £2.66
Excipients none as listed in section 13.1.3
For skin disinfection, particularly minor wounds and infections; child under 2 years not recommended

Savlon® Dry (Novartis Consumer Health)
Powder spray, povidone–iodine 1.14% in a pressurised aerosol unit, net price 50-mL unit = £2.39
For minor wounds

Videne® (Ecolab)
Alcoholic tincture, povidone–iodine 10%, net price 500 mL = £2.50
Dose

Apply undiluted in pre-operative skin disinfection

Note Flammable—caution in procedures involving hot wire cautery and diathermy; avoid use in neonates

Antiseptic solution, povidone–iodine 10% in aqueous solution, net price 500 mL = £2.50
Dose

Apply undiluted in pre-operative skin disinfection and general antisepsis

Surgical scrub, povidone–iodine 7.5% in aqueous solution, net price 500 mL = £2.50
Dose

Use as a pre-operative scrub for hand and skin disinfection

13.11.5 Phenolics

Triclosan has been used for disinfection of the hands and wounds, and for disinfection of the skin before surgery.

13.11.6 Oxidisers and dyes

HYDROGEN PEROXIDE

Cautions large or deep wounds; avoid on healthy skin and eyes; bleaches fabric; incompatible with products containing iodine or potassium permanganate

Licensed use licensed for use in children (age range not specified by manufacturer)

Indication and dose

Superficial bacterial skin infection see under preparation below

Crystacide® (GP Pharma)
Cream, hydrogen peroxide 1%, net price 10 g = £4.82, 25 g = £8.07, 40 g = £11.62
Dose
Superficial bacterial skin infection
apply 2–3 times daily for up to 3 weeks
Excipients include edetic acid (EDTA), propylene glycol

POTASSIUM PERMANGANATE

Cautions irritant to mucous membranes

Indication and dose

Cleansing and deodorising suppurating eczematous reactions (section 13.5.1) and wounds
for wet dressings or baths, use approx. 0.01% (1 in 10 000) solution
Note Stains skin and clothing

Potassium Permanganate Solution
Solution, potassium permanganate 0.1% (1 in 1000) in water
Note to be diluted 1 in 10 to provide a 0.01% (1 in 10 000) solution

13 **Skin**

◁ **POTASSIUM PERMANGANATE (continued)**

Permitabs® (Alliance)
Solution tablets, for preparation of topical solution, potassium permanganate 400 mg, net price 30-tab pack = £6.22

Note 1 tablet dissolved in 4 litres of water provides a 0.01% (1 in 10 000) solution

13.11.7 Preparations for promotion of wound healing

Desloughing agents Alginate, hydrogel, and hydrocolloid dressings (BNF Appendix 8) are effective in wound debridement. Sterile larvae (maggots) (LarvE®, Zoobiotic) are also used for managing sloughing wounds and are prescribable on the NHS.

Desloughing solutions and creams are of little clinical value. Substances applied to an open area are easily absorbed and perilesional skin is easily sensitised.

Growth factor A topical preparation of **becaplermin** (recombinant human platelet-derived growth factor) is used as an adjunct treatment of full-thickness, neuropathic, diabetic ulcers. It enhances the formulation of granulation tissue, thereby promoting wound healing.

For further information on wound management products and elastic hosiery, see BNF Appendix 8.

BECAPLERMIN
(Recombinant human platelet-derived growth factor)

Cautions malignant disease; avoid on sites with infection, malignancy, or peripheral arteriopathy

Side-effects pain; infections including cellulitis and osteomyelitis, local reactions including erythema; *rarely* bullous eruption, oedema, and hypertrophic granulation

Licensed use not licensed for use in children

Indication and dose

Full-thickness, neuropathic, diabetic ulcers (no larger than 5 cm²)

Apply thin layer daily and cover with gauze dressing moistened with physiological saline; max. duration of treatment 20 weeks (reassess if no healing after first 10 weeks)

Regranex® (Janssen-Cilag) [PoM]
Gel, becaplermin (recombinant human platelet-derived growth factor) 0.01%, net price 15 g = £255.75
Excipients include hydroxybenzoates (parabens)

13.12 Antiperspirants

Aluminium chloride is a potent antiperspirant used in the treatment of axillary, palmar, and plantar hyperhidrosis. Aluminium salts are also incorporated in preparations used for minor fungal skin infections associated with hyperhidrosis.

In more severe cases specialists use tap water or **glycopyrronium bromide** (as a 0.05% solution) in the iontophoretic treatment of hyperhidrosis of palms and soles.

Botulinum A toxin-haemagglutinin complex (section 4.9.3) is licensed for use intradermally for severe hyperhidrosis of the axillae unresponsive to topical antiperspirant or other antihidrotic treatment; intradermal treatment is unlikely to be tolerated by most children and should be administered under hospital specialist supervision.

ALUMINIUM SALTS

Cautions avoid contact with eyes or mucous membranes; avoid use on broken or irritated skin; do not shave axillae or use depilatories within 12 hours of application; avoid contact with clothing

Side-effects skin irritation

Licensed use licensed for use in children (age range not specified by manufacturer)

13 Skin

◻ **ALUMINIUM SALTS (continued)**

Indication and dose

> Hyperhidrosis affecting axillae, hands or feet
> Apply liquid formulation at night to dry skin, wash off the following morning, initially apply daily then reduce frequency as condition improves—do not bathe immediately before use

> Hyperhidrosis, bromidrosis, intertrigo, and prevention of tinea pedis and related conditions
> Apply powder to dry skin

Anhydrol® Forte (Dermal)
Solution (= application), aluminium chloride hexahydrate 20% in an alcoholic basis, net price 60-mL bottle with roll-on applicator = £2.62. Label: 15
Excipients none as listed in section 13.1.3

¹**Driclor®** (Stiefel)
Application, aluminium chloride hexahydrate 20% in an alcoholic basis, net price 60-mL bottle with roll-on applicator = £2.82. Label: 15
Excipients none as listed in section 13.1.3
1. A 30-mL pack is on sale to the public

ZeaSORB® (Stiefel)
Dusting powder, aldioxa 0.22%, chloroxylenol 0.5%, net price 50 g = £2.61
Excipients include fragrance

◼ GLYCOPYRRONIUM BROMIDE

Cautions see section 15.1.3 (but poorly absorbed and systemic effects unlikely)

Contra-indications see section 15.1.3 (but poorly absorbed and systemic effects unlikely), infections affecting the treatment site

Side-effects see section 15.1.3 (but poorly absorbed and systemic effects unlikely), tingling at administration site

Licensed use licensed for use in children (age range not specified by manufacturer)

Indication and dose

> Iontophoretic treatment of hyperhidrosis
> consult product literature; only 1 site to be treated at a time, max. 2 sites treated in any 24 hours, treatment not to be repeated within 7 days

> **Other indications** section 15.1.3

Robinul® (Antigen) PoM
Powder, glycopyrronium bromide, net price 3 g = £110.00

13.13 Topical circulatory preparations

These preparations are used to improve circulation in conditions such as bruising and superficial thrombophlebitis but are of little value. First aid measures such as rest, ice, compression, and elevation should be used. Topical preparations containing heparinoids should not be used on large areas of skin, broken or sensitive skin, or mucous membranes. Chilblains are best managed by avoidance of exposure to cold; neither systemic nor topical vasodilator therapy is established as being effective.

Hirudoid® (Genus) ◢
Cream, heparinoid 0.3% in a vanishing-cream basis, net price 50 g = £3.99
Excipients include cetostearyl alcohol, hydroxybenzoates (parabens)

Dose

> Superficial thrombophlebitis, bruising, and haematoma
> Child 5–18 years apply up to 4 times daily

Gel, heparinoid 0.3%, net price 50 g = £3.99
Excipients include propylene glycol, fragrance

Dose

> Superficial thrombophlebitis, bruising, and haematoma
> Child 5–18 years apply up to 4 times daily

13 Skin

14 Immunological products and vaccines

14.1 Active immunity...725

14.2 Passive immunity 729

14.3 Storage and use 729

14.4 Vaccines and antisera..730

14.5 Immunoglobulins...754

14.6 International travel...758

14.1 Active immunity

Active immunity can be acquired by natural disease or by vaccination. **Vaccines** stimulate production of antibodies and other components of the immune mechanism; they consist of either:

1. a *live attenuated* form of a virus (e.g. measles, mumps and rubella vaccine) or bacteria (e.g. BCG vaccine), or
2. *inactivated* preparations of a virus (e.g. influenza vaccine) or bacteria, or
3. *extracts of* or *detoxified* exotoxins produced by a micro-organism (e.g. tetanus vaccine).

Live attenuated vaccines usually produce a durable immunity but not always as long-lasting as that resulting from natural infection.

Inactivated vaccines may require a primary series of injections of vaccine to produce adequate antibody response and in most cases booster (reinforcing) injections are required; the duration of immunity varies from months to many years. Some inactivated vaccines are adsorbed onto an adjuvant (such as aluminium hydroxide) to enhance the antibody response.

> Advice in this chapter reflects that in the handbook *Immunisation against Infectious Disease* (2006), which in turn reflects the guidance of the Joint Committee on Vaccination and Immunisation (JCVI).
>
> Chapters from the handbook are available at www.dh.gov.uk
>
> The advice in this chapter also incorporates changes announced by the Chief Medical Officer and Health Department Updates.

Cautions Most children can safely receive the majority of vaccines. Vaccination may be postponed if the child is suffering from an acute illness, however, it is not necessary to postpone immunisation in children with minor illnesses without fever or systemic upset. See also Predisposition to Neurological Problems, below. For individuals with bleeding disorders, see Route of Administration, below. If alcohol or disinfectant is used for cleansing the skin it should be allowed to evaporate before vaccination to prevent possible inactivation of live vaccines.

When two live virus vaccines are required (and are not available as a combined preparation) they should be given either simultaneously at different sites or separated by an interval of at least 4 weeks. For **interactions** see Appendix 1 (vaccines).

See also Cautions under individual vaccines.

Contra-indications Vaccines are contra-indicated in children who have a confirmed anaphylactic reaction to a preceding dose of a vaccine containing the same antigens or vaccine component (such as antibacterials in viral vaccines). The

14

Immunological products and vaccines

presence of the following excipients in vaccines and immunological products has been noted under the relevant entries:

Gelatin	Neomycin	Streptomycin
Gentamicin	Penicillins	Thiomersal
Kanamycin	Polymyxin B	

Hypersensitivity to egg with evidence of previous anaphylactic reaction, contra-indicates influenza vaccine, tick-borne encephalitis vaccine, and yellow fever vaccine. See also Cautions under MMR vaccine.

See also Vaccines and HIV infection, below.

Live vaccines may be contra-indicated temporarily in children who are:

- immunosuppressed (see Impaired Immune Response, below);
- pregnant (see Pregnancy and Breast-feeding, below).

See also Contra-indications under individual vaccines.

Impaired immune response Immune response to vaccines may be reduced in immunosuppressed children and there is also a risk of generalised infection with live vaccines. Severely immunosuppressed children should not be given live vaccines (including those with severe primary immunodeficiency). Specialist advice should be sought for children being treated with high doses of corticosteroids (dose equivalents of prednisolone: **children**, 2 mg/kg (or more than 40 mg) daily for at least 1 week or 1 mg/kg daily for 1 month), or other immunosuppressive drugs[1], and for children with malignant conditions undergoing chemotherapy or generalised radiotherapy[1,2]. For special reference to *HIV infection*, see below.

The Royal College of Paediatrics and Child Health has produced a statement, *Immunisation of the Immunocompromised Child (2002)* (available at www.rcpch.ac.uk).

Pregnancy and breast-feeding Live vaccines should not be administered routinely during pregnancy because of the theoretical risk of fetal infection but where there is a significant risk of exposure to disease (e.g. to yellow fever), the need for vaccination usually outweighs any possible risk to the fetus. Termination of pregnancy following inadvertent immunisation is not recommended. Although there is a theoretical risk of live vaccine being present in breast milk, vaccination is not contra-indicated for women who are breast-feeding when there is significant risk of exposure to disease. There is no evidence of risk from vaccinating pregnant women, or those who are breast-feeding, with inactivated viral or bacterial vaccines or toxoids. For use of specific vaccines during pregnancy or breast-feeding, see under individual vaccines.

Side-effects Injection of a vaccine may be followed by local reactions such as pain, inflammation, redness, and lymphangitis. An induration or sterile abscess may develop at the injection site. Gastro-intestinal disturbances, fever, headache, irritability, loss of appetite, fatigue, myalgia, and malaise are among the most commonly reported side-effects. Other side-effects include influenza-like symptoms, dizziness, paraesthesia, asthenia, drowsiness, arthralgia, rash, and lymphadenopathy. Hypersensitivity reactions, such as bronchospasm, angioedema, urticaria, and anaphylaxis, are very rare but can be fatal (see section 3.4.3 for management of allergic emergencies).

Oral vaccines such as cholera, live poliomyelitis, rotavirus, and live typhoid can also cause gastro-intestinal disturbances such as nausea, vomiting, abdominal pain and cramps, and diarrhoea.

See also Predisposition to Neurological Problems, below.

Some vaccines (e.g. poliomyelitis) produce very few reactions, while others (e.g. measles, mumps and rubella) may cause a very mild form of the disease. Occasionally more serious adverse reactions can occur—these should always be reported to the CHM (see Adverse Reactions to Drugs, p. 21).

1. Live vaccines should be postponed until at least 3 months after stopping high-dose systemic corticosteroids and at least 6 months after stopping other immunosuppressive drugs or generalised radiotherapy (at least 12 months after discontinuing immunosuppressants following bone-marrow transplantation).
2. Use of normal immunoglobulin should be considered after exposure to measles (see p. 756) and varicella–zoster immunoglobulin considered after exposure to chickenpox or herpes zoster (see p. 757).

There is no evidence that premature babies are at increased risk of adverse reactions from vaccines, see also Prematurity, below.

Predisposition to neurological problems

When there is a personal or family history of *febrile* convulsions, there is an increased risk of these occurring during fever from any cause including immunisation, but this is not a contra-indication to immunisation. In children who have had a seizure associated with fever without neurological deterioration, immunisation is *recommended*; advice on the *prevention of fever* (see Post-immunisation Pyrexia in Infants, below) should be given before immunisation. When a child has had a convulsion not associated with fever, and the neurological condition is not deteriorating, immunisation is *recommended*.

Children with stable neurological disorders (e.g. spina bifida, congenital brain abnormality, and peri-natal hypoxic-ischaemic encephalopathy) should be immunised according to the recommended schedule.

Where there is a *still evolving neurological problem*, including poorly controlled epilepsy, immunisation should be deferred and the child referred to a specialist. Immunisation is recommended if a cause for the neurological disorder is identified. If a cause is not identified, immunisation should be deferred until the condition is stable.

Post-immunisation pyrexia in infants

The parent should be advised that if pyrexia develops after childhood immunisation, the infant can be given a dose of paracetamol and, if necessary, a second dose given 6 hours later; ibuprofen may be used if paracetamol is unsuitable. The parent should be warned to seek medical advice if the pyrexia persists.

For post-immunisation pyrexia in an infant aged 2–3 months, the dose of paracetamol is 60 mg; the dose of ibuprofen is 50 mg (on doctor's advice). An oral syringe can be obtained from any pharmacy to give the small volume required.

Further information on adverse effects associated with specific vaccines can be found under individual vaccines.

Vaccines and HIV infection   HIV-positive children with or without symptoms can receive the following live vaccines:

MMR (but avoid if immunity significantly impaired), varicella-zoster (but avoid if immunity significantly impaired—consult product literature);[1]

and the following inactivated vaccines:

anthrax, cholera (oral), diphtheria, haemophilus influenzae type b, hepatitis A, hepatitis B, human papilloma virus, influenza, meningococcal, pertussis, pneumococcal, poliomyelitis[2], rabies, tetanus, tick-borne encephalitis, typhoid (injection).

HIV-positive children should **not** receive:

BCG, typhoid (oral), yellow fever[3]

Note The above advice differs from that for other immunocompromised children; Immunisation of HIV-infected Children issued by Children's HIV Association (CHIVA) are available at www.chiva.org.uk

Vaccines and asplenia   The following vaccines are recommended for asplenic children or those with splenic dysfunction:

haemophilus influenzae type b, influenza, meningococcal group C, pneumococcal.

For antibiotic prophylaxis in asplenia see p. 305.

1. Use of normal immunoglobulin should be considered after exposure to measles (see p. 756) and varicella–zoster immunoglobulin considered after exposure to chickenpox or herpes zoster (see p. 757).
2. Inactivated poliomyelitis vaccine is now used instead of oral poliomyelitis vaccine for routine immunisation of children.
3. If yellow fever risk is unavoidable, specialist advice should be sought.

14 Immunological products and vaccines

![Immunisation schedule]

Immunisation schedule

Vaccines for the childhood immunisation schedule should be obtained from **local health organisations** or **direct from Movianto**—not to be prescribed on FP10 (HS21 in Northern Ireland; GP10 in Scotland; WP10 in Wales).

> ### Prematurity
> Children born prematurely should receive all routine immunisations based on the actual date of birth. There is no evidence that premature infants are at increased risk of adverse reactions directly related to vaccines. However, for those in neonatal units with cardiorespiratory problems, and those infants who have had more than one apnoeic attack in the 24 hours prior to immunisation, it may be appropriate to monitor for apnoea for 48 hours after immunisation. Seroconversion may be unreliable in babies born earlier than 28 weeks' gestation or in babies treated with corticosteroids for chronic lung disease; consideration should be given to testing for antibodies against *Haemophilus influenzae* (type b), meningococcal C, and hepatitis B after primary immunisation.

When to immunise (for pre-mature infants—see note above)	Vaccine given and dose schedule (for details of dose, see under individual vaccines)
Neonates at risk only	• **BCG Vaccine** See section 14.4, BCG Vaccines • **Hepatitis B Vaccine** See section 14.4, Hepatitis B Vaccine
2 months	• **Diphtheria, Tetanus, Pertussis (Acellular, Component), Poliomyelitis (Inactivated), and Haemophilus Type b Conjugate Vaccine (Adsorbed)** First dose • **Pneumococcal Polysaccharide Conjugate Vaccine (Adsorbed)** First dose
3 months	• **Diphtheria, Tetanus, Pertussis (Acellular, Component), Poliomyelitis (Inactivated), and Haemophilus Type b Conjugate Vaccine (Adsorbed)** Second dose • **Meningococcal Group C Conjugate Vaccine** First dose
4 months	• **Diphtheria, Tetanus, Pertussis (Acellular, Component), Poliomyelitis (Inactivated), and Haemophilus Type b Conjugate Vaccine (Adsorbed)** Third dose • **Meningococcal Group C Conjugate Vaccine** Second dose • **Pneumococcal Polysaccharide Conjugate Vaccine (Adsorbed)** Second dose
12 months	• **Haemophilus Type b Conjugate Vaccine and Meningococcal Group C Conjugate Vaccine** Single booster dose
13 months	• **Measles, Mumps and Rubella Vaccine, Live (MMR)** First dose • **Pneumococcal Polysaccharide Conjugate Vaccine (Adsorbed)** Single booster dose
Between 3 years and 4 months, and 5 years	• **Adsorbed Diphtheria [low dose], Tetanus, Pertussis (Acellular, Component) and Poliomyelitis (Inactivated) Vaccine** *or* **Adsorbed Diphtheria, Tetanus, Pertussis (Acellular, Component) and Poliomyelitis (Inactivated) Vaccine** *or* **Diphtheria, Tetanus, Pertussis (Acellular, Component) Poliomyelitis (Inactivated) and Haemophilus Type b Conjugate Vaccine (Adsorbed)** Single booster dose **Note:** Preferably allow interval of at least 3 years after completing primary course; can be given at same session as MMR Vaccine but use separate syringe and needle, and give in different limb • **Measles, Mumps and Rubella Vaccine, Live (MMR)** Second dose
12–13 years (females only)	• **Human Papilloma Virus Vaccine** 3 doses; second dose 1–2 months, and third dose 6 months after first dose[1,2]
13–18 years	• **Adsorbed Diphtheria [low dose], Tetanus, and Poliomyelitis (Inactivated) Vaccine** Single booster dose
During adult life Women of child-bearing age susceptible to rubella	• **Measles, Mumps and Rubella Vaccine, Live (MMR)** Women of child-bearing age who have not received 2 doses of a rubella-containing vaccine or who do not have a positive antibody test for rubella should be offered rubella immunisation (using the MMR vaccine)—exclude pregnancy before immunisation, but see also section 14.4, Measles, Mumps and Rubella Vaccine
During adult life If not previously immunised	• **Adsorbed Diphtheria [low dose], Tetanus, and Poliomyelitis (inactivated) Vaccine** 3 doses at intervals of 1 month Booster dose at least 1 year after primary course and again 5–10 years later

1. The two human papilloma virus vaccines are not interchangeable and one vaccine product should be used for the entire course; however, Department of Health (November 2008) states for individuals with previous incomplete vaccination with *Gardasil®*, who are eligible for HPV vaccination under the national programme, *Cervarix®* can be used to complete the vaccination course if necessary; the individual must be informed that *Cervarix®* does not protect against genital warts.
2. For females aged 14 to under 18 years, see 'Catch-Up' Programme, p. 740.

14 **Immunological products and vaccines**

Route of administration   Vaccines should not be given intravenously. Most vaccines are given by the intramuscular route; some vaccines are given by other routes—the intradermal route for BCG vaccine, deep subcutaneous route for Japanese encephalitis and varicella vaccines, and the oral route for cholera, live poliomyelitis, rotavirus, and live typhoid vaccines. The intramuscular route should not be used in children with **bleeding disorders** such as haemophilia or thrombocytopenia; vaccines usually given by the intramuscular route should be given by deep subcutaneous injection instead.

Note The Department of Health has advised *against the use of jet guns* for vaccination owing to the risk of transmitting blood-borne infections, such as HIV.

High-risk groups

For information on high-risk groups, see section 14.4 under individual vaccines

BCG Vaccines, p. 730

Hepatitis A Vaccine, p. 736

Hepatitis B Vaccine, p. 737

Influenza Vaccine, p. 741

Pneumococcal Vaccines, p. 746

Tetanus Vaccines, p. 751

Children with unknown or incomplete immunisation history

For children born in the UK who present with an inadequate or unknown immunisation history, investigation into immunisations received should be carried out. Outstanding doses should be administered where the routine childhood immunisation schedule has not been completed.

For advice on the immunisation of children coming to the UK, consult the handbook *Immunisation against Infectious Disease* (2006) (available at www.dh.gov.uk)

14.2 Passive immunity

Immunity with immediate protection against certain infective organisms can be obtained by injecting preparations made from the plasma of immune individuals with adequate levels of antibody to the disease for which protection is sought (see under Immunoglobulins, section 14.5). The duration of this passive immunity varies according to the dose and the type of immunoglobulin. Passive immunity may last only a few weeks; where necessary, passive immunisation can be repeated.

Antibodies of human origin are usually termed *immunoglobulins*. The term *antiserum* is applied to material prepared in animals. Because of serum sickness and other allergic-type reactions that may follow injections of antisera, this therapy has been replaced wherever possible by the use of immunoglobulins. Reactions are theoretically possible after injection of human immunoglobulins but reports of such reactions are very rare.

14.3 Storage and use

Care must be taken to store all vaccines and other immunological products under the conditions recommended in the product literature, otherwise the preparation may become ineffective. **Refrigerated storage** is usually necessary; many vaccines and immunoglobulins need to be stored at 2–8°C and not allowed to freeze. Vaccines and immunoglobulins should be protected from light. Reconstituted vaccines and opened multi-dose vials must be used within the period recommended in the product literature. Unused vaccines should be disposed of by incineration at a registered disposal contractor.

Particular attention must be paid to instructions on the use of diluents. Vaccines which are liquid suspensions or are reconstituted before use should be adequately mixed to ensure uniformity of the material to be injected.

Vaccines and antisera

Availability   Anthrax and yellow fever vaccines, botulism antitoxin, diphtheria antitoxin, and snake and spider venom antitoxins are available from local designated holding centres.

For antivenom, see Emergency Treatment of Poisoning, p. 47.

Enquiries for vaccines not available commercially can also be made to:

Immunisation Policy, Monitoring and Surveillance
Department of Health
Wellington House
133–155 Waterloo Road
London, SE1 8UG.
Tel: (020) 7972 4047

In Scotland information about availability of vaccines can be obtained from a Specialist in Pharmaceutical Public Health. In Wales enquiries for vaccines not commercially available should be directed to:

Welsh Medicines Information Centre
University Hospital of Wales
Cardiff, CF14 4XW.
Tel: (029) 2074 2979

and in Northern Ireland:

Regional Pharmacist (procurement co-ordination)
United Hospitals Trust Pharmacy Dept
Whiteabbey Hospital
Doagh Road
Newtownabbey, BT37 9RH.
Tel: (028) 9086 5181 ext 2386

For further details of availability, see under individual vaccines.

Anthrax vaccine

Anthrax vaccine is rarely required for children. For further information see BNF section 14.4.

BCG vaccines

BCG (Bacillus Calmette-Guérin) is a live attenuated strain derived from *Mycobacterium bovis* which stimulates the development of hypersensitivity to *M. tuberculosis*. BCG vaccine should be given intradermally by operators skilled in the technique (see below).

The expected reaction to successful BCG vaccination is induration at the site of injection followed by a local lesion which starts as a papule 2 or more weeks after vaccination; the lesion may ulcerate then subside over several weeks or months, leaving a small flat scar. A dry dressing may be used if the ulcer discharges, but air should **not** be excluded.

All children of 6 years and over being considered for BCG immunisation must first be given a skin test for hypersensitivity to tuberculoprotein (see under Diagnostic agents, below). A skin test is not necessary for a child under 6 years provided that the child has not stayed for longer than 3 months in a country with an incidence[1] of tuberculosis of greater than 40 per 100 000, the child has not had contact with a person with tuberculosis, and there is no family history of tuberculosis within the last 5 years.

BCG is recommended for the following groups of children if BCG immunisation has not previously been carried out and they are negative for tuberculoprotein hypersensitivity:

- all neonates and infants (0–12 months) born in areas where the incidence[1] of tuberculosis is greater than 40 per 100 000;

14   Immunological products and vaccines

---

1. List of countries or primary care trusts where the incidence of tuberculosis is greater than 40 cases per 100 000 is available at www.hpa.org.uk

- neonates, infants, and children under 16 years with a parent or grandparent born in a country with an incidence[1] of tuberculosis greater than 40 per 100 000;

- new immigrants aged under 16 years who were born in, or lived for more than 3 months in a country with an incidence[1] of tuberculosis greater than 40 per 100 000;

- new immigrants aged 16–18 years from Sub-Saharan Africa or a country[1] with an incidence of tuberculosis greater than 500 per 100 000;

- contacts of those with active respiratory tuberculosis;

- children under 16 years intending to live with local people for more than 3 months in a country with an incidence[1] of tuberculosis greater than 40 per 100 000 (section 14.6).

BCG vaccine can be given simultaneously with another live vaccine (see also section 14.1), but if they are not given at the same time, an interval of 4 weeks should normally be allowed between them. When BCG is given to infants, there is no need to delay routine primary immunisations. No further vaccination should be given in the arm used for BCG vaccination for at least 3 months because of the risk of regional lymphadenitis.

For advice on chemoprophylaxis against tuberculosis, see section 5.1.9; for treatment of infection following vaccination, seek expert advice.

◼ BACILLUS CALMETTE-GUÉRIN VACCINE
BCG vaccine

Cautions see section 14.1; **interactions**: Appendix 1 (vaccines)

Contra-indications see section 14.1; also neonate in household contact with known or suspected case of active tuberculosis; generalised septic skin conditions (for children with eczema, lesion-free site should be used)

Side-effects see section 14.1 and notes above; *also* at the injection-site, subcutaneous abscess, prolonged ulceration; *rarely* disseminated complications such as osteitis or osteomyelitis

Indication and dose

Immunisation against tuberculosis
- **By intradermal injection**

  Neonate 0.05 mL

  Child 1 month–1 year 0.05 mL

  Child 1–18 years 0.1 mL

Intradermal injection technique Skin is stretched between thumb and forefinger and needle (size 25G or 26G) inserted (bevel upwards) for about 3 mm into superficial layers of dermis (almost parallel with surface). Needle should be short with short bevel (can usually be seen through epidermis during insertion). Tense raised blanched bleb showing tips of hair follicles is sign of correct injection; 7 mm bleb ≡ 0.1 mL injection, 3 mm bleb ≡ 0.05 mL injection; if considerable resistance not felt, needle is too deep and should be removed and reinserted before giving more vaccine.
To be injected at insertion of deltoid muscle onto humerus (keloid formation more likely with sites higher on arm); tip of shoulder should be **avoided**.

◀ Intradermal
Bacillus Calmette-Guérin Vaccine ⬚PoM⬚
BCG Vaccine, Dried/Tub/BCG
Injection, (powder for suspension), freeze-dried preparation of live bacteria of a strain derived from the bacillus of Calmette and Guérin
Available from health organisations or direct from Movianto (SSI brand, multidose vial with diluent)

Diagnostic agents

The *Mantoux test* is recommended for tuberculin skin testing, but no licensed preparation is currently available. Guidance for healthcare professionals is available at www.immunisation.nhs.uk.

In the Mantoux test, the diagnostic dose is administered by intradermal injection of Tuberculin Purified Protein Derivative (PPD).

The *Heaf test* (involving the use of multiple-puncture apparatus) is no longer available.

Note Response to tuberculin may be suppressed by live viral vaccines, viral infection, sarcoidosis, corticosteroid therapy, or immunosuppression due to disease or treatment. Tuberculin testing should not be carried out within 4 weeks of receiving a live viral vaccine

1. List of countries or primary care trusts where the incidence of tuberculosis is greater than 40 cases per 100 000 is available at www.hpa.org.uk

14

Immunological products and vaccines

Two interferon gamma release assay (IGRA) tests are also available as an aid in the diagnosis of tuberculosis infection: *QuantiFERON®-TB Gold* and *T-SPOT®.TB*. Both tests measure T-cell mediated immune response to synthetic antigens. For further information on the use of interferon gamma release assay tests for tuberculosis, see www.hpa.org.uk.

Tuberculin Purified Protein Derivative PoM
(Tuberculin PPD)
Injection, heat-treated products of growth and lysis of appropriate *Mycobacterium* spp. 20 units/mL (2 units/0.1-mL dose) (for routine use), 1.5-mL vial; 100 units/mL (10 units/0.1-mL dose), 1.5-mL vial

Dose
Mantoux test
• **By intradermal injection**

2 units (0.1 mL of 20 units/mL strength) for routine Mantoux test; if first test is negative and a further test is considered appropriate 10 units (0.1 mL of 100 units/mL strength)

Available from Movianto (SSI brand)

Important The strength of tuberculin PPD in this product may be different to the strengths of products used previously for the Mantoux test; care is required to select the correct strength

Botulism antitoxin

A polyvalent botulism antitoxin is available for the post-exposure prophylaxis of botulism and for the treatment of children thought to be suffering from botulism. It specifically neutralises the toxins produced by *Clostridium botulinum* types A, B, and E. It is not effective against infantile botulism as the toxin (type A) is seldom, if ever, found in the blood in this type of infection.

Hypersensitivity reactions are a problem. It is essential to read the contra-indications, warnings, and details of sensitivity tests on the package insert. Prior to treatment checks should be made regarding previous administration of any antitoxin and history of any allergic condition, e.g. asthma, hay fever, etc. All children should be tested for sensitivity (diluting the antitoxin if history of allergy).

Botulism Antitoxin PoM
A preparation containing the specific antitoxic globulins that have the power of neutralising the toxins formed by types A, B, and E of *Clostridium botulinum*.

Note The BP title Botulinum Antitoxin is not used because the preparation currently in use may have a different specification

Dose
Prophylaxis
Consult product literature

Available from local designated centres, for details see TOXBASE (requires registration) www.toxbase.org. For supplies outside working hours apply to other designated centres and, as a last resort, to the duty doctor at the Health Protection Agency (Tel (020) 8200 6868). For major incidents, obtain supplies from the local blood bank

Cholera vaccine

Cholera vaccine (oral) contains inactivated Inaba (including El-Tor biotype) and Ogawa strains of *Vibrio cholerae*, serotype O1 together with recombinant B-subunit of the cholera toxin produced in Inaba strains of *V.cholerae*, serotype O1.

Oral cholera vaccine is licensed for travellers to endemic or epidemic areas on the basis of current recommendations (see also section 14.6). Immunisation should be completed at least 1 week before potential exposure. However, there is no requirement for cholera vaccination for international travel.

Immunisation with cholera vaccine does not provide complete protection and all travellers to a country where cholera exists should be warned that scrupulous attention to food, water, and personal hygiene is **essential**.

Injectable cholera vaccine provides unreliable protection and is no longer available in the UK.

CHOLERA VACCINE

Cautions see section 14.1 and notes above
Contra-indications see section 14.1
Side-effects see section 14.1; also *rarely* respiratory symptoms such as rhinitis and cough; *very rarely* sore throat, insomnia

Indication and dose
See notes above
• **By mouth**
Child 2–6 years 3 doses each separated by an interval of 1–6 weeks

Child 6–18 years 2 doses separated by an interval of 1–6 weeks
Note If more than 6 weeks have elapsed between doses, the primary course should be restarted
A single booster dose can be given 2 years after primary course for children 6–18 years, and 6 months after primary course for children 2–6 years. If more than 2 years have elapsed since the last vaccination, the primary course should be repeated

Administration Dissolve effervescent sodium bicarbonate granules in a glassful of

◻ **CHOLERA VACCINE (*continued*)**

water (approximately 150 mL). For child over 6 years, add vaccine suspension to make one dose. For child 2–6 years, discard half (approximately 75 mL) of the solution, then add vaccine suspension to make one dose. Drink within 2 hours. Food, drink and other oral medicines should be avoided for 1 hour before and after vaccination

Dukoral® (Novartis Vaccines) ℙᴏᴹ
Oral suspension, for dilution with solution of effervescent sodium bicarbonate granules, heat- and formaldehyde-inactivated Inaba (including El-Tor biotype) and Ogawa strains of *Vibrio cholerae* bacteria and recombinant cholera toxin B-subunit produced in *V. cholerae*, net price 2-dose pack = £23.42. Counselling, administration

Diphtheria Vaccines

Diphtheria vaccines are prepared from the toxin of *Corynebacterium diphtheriae* and adsorption on aluminium hydroxide or aluminium phosphate improves antigenicity. The vaccine stimulates the production of the protective antitoxin. The quantity of diphtheria toxoid in a preparation determines whether the vaccine is defined as 'high dose' or 'low dose'. Vaccines containing the higher dose of diphtheria toxoid are used for primary immunisation of children under 10 years of age. Vaccines containing the lower dose of diphtheria toxoid are used for primary immunisation in children over 10 years. Single-antigen diphtheria vaccine is not available and adsorbed diphtheria vaccine is given as a combination product containing other vaccines.

For primary immunisation *of children aged between 2 months and 10 years* vaccination is recommended usually in the form of 3 doses (separated by 1-month intervals) of **diphtheria, tetanus, pertussis (acellular, component), poliomyelitis (inactivated) and haemophilus type b conjugate vaccine (adsorbed)** (see Immunisation schedule, section 14.1). In unimmunised children aged *over 10 years* the primary course comprises of 3 doses of **adsorbed diphtheria** [low dose], **tetanus and inactivated poliomyelitis vaccine.**

A booster dose should be given 3 years after the primary course (this interval can be reduced to a minimum of 1 year if the primary course was delayed). Children *under 10 years* should receive *either* **adsorbed diphtheria, tetanus, pertussis (acellular, component) and inactivated poliomyelitis vaccine** *or* **adsorbed diphtheria** [low dose], **tetanus, pertussis (acellular, component) and inactivated poliomyelitis vaccine.** Children aged *over 10 years* should receive **adsorbed diphtheria** [low dose], **tetanus, and inactivated poliomyelitis vaccine.**

A second booster dose, of adsorbed diphtheria [low dose], tetanus and inactivated poliomyelitis vaccine, should be given 10 years after the previous booster dose (this interval can be reduced to a minimum of 5 years if previous doses were delayed). For children who have been vaccinated following a tetanus-prone wound, see Tetanus vaccines, p. 751.

Travel Children travelling to areas with a risk of diphtheria infection should be fully immunised according to the UK schedule (see also section 14.6). If more than 10 years have lapsed since completion of the UK schedule, a dose of **adsorbed diphtheria** [low dose], **tetanus and inactivated poliomyelitis vaccine** should be administered.

Contacts Advice on the management of cases of diphtheria, carriers, contacts and outbreaks must be sought from health protection units. The immunisation history of infected children and their contacts should be determined; those who have been incompletely immunised should complete their immunisation and fully immunised individuals should receive a reinforcing dose. For advice on antibacterial treatment to prevent a secondary case of diphtheria in a non-immune child, see Table 2, section 5.1.

DIPHTHERIA-CONTAINING VACCINES

Cautions see section 14.1; see also individual components of vaccines

Contra-indications see section 14.1; see also individual components of vaccines

Side-effects see section 14.1; also restlessness, sleep disturbances, and unusual crying in infants;

Licensed use *Infanrix-IPV + Hib®* not licensed for use in children over 36 months; *Pediacel®* not licensed in children over 4 years but Department

◻ **DIPHTHERIA-CONTAINING VACCINES (***continued***)**

of Health recommends that these be used for children up to 10 years

Indication and dose

> See notes above and under preparations

◢ Diphtheria-containing vaccines for children under 10 years

Important **Not** recommended for children *aged 10 years or over* (see Diphtheria vaccines for children over 10)

Diphtheria, Tetanus, Pertussis (Acellular, Component), Poliomyelitis (Inactivated) and Haemophilus Type b Conjugate Vaccine (Adsorbed) PoM

Injection, suspension of diphtheria toxoid, tetanus toxoid, acellular pertussis, inactivated poliomyelitis and *Haemophilus influenzae* type b (conjugated to tetanus protein), net price 0.5-mL prefilled syringe = £19.94
Excipients may include neomycin, polymyxin B and streptomycin

Dose

> Primary immunisation
> • **By intramuscular injection**
> > **Child 2 months–10 years** 3 doses each of 0.5 mL separated by intervals of 1 month; *see also* notes on booster doses, above

Available as part of childhood immunisation schedule, from health organisations or Moviano; brands include *Infanrix-IPV+Hib*®, *Pediacel*®

Adsorbed Diphtheria, Tetanus, Pertussis (Acellular, Component) and Inactivated Poliomyelitis Vaccine PoM

Injection, suspension of diphtheria toxoid, tetanus toxoid, acellular pertussis and inactivated poliomyelitis vaccine components adsorbed on a mineral carrier, net price 0.5-mL prefilled syringe = £17.56
Excipients may include neomycin and polymyxin B

Dose

> First booster dose
> • **By intramuscular injection**
> > **Child 3–10 years** 0.5 mL 3 years after primary immunisation; *see also* notes on booster doses, above

Available as part of childhood immunisation schedule, from health organisations or Moviano; brands include *Infanrix-IPV*®

Adsorbed Diphtheria [low dose], Tetanus, Pertussis (Acellular, Component) and Inactivated Poliomyelitis Vaccine PoM

Injection, suspension of diphtheria toxoid [low dose], tetanus toxoid, acellular pertussis and inactivated poliomyelitis vaccine components adsorbed on a mineral carrier, net price 0.5-mL prefilled syringe = £11.98
Excipients may include neomycin, polymyxin B and streptomycin

Dose

> First booster dose
> • **By intramuscular injection**
> > **Child 3–10 years** 0.5 mL 3 years after primary immunisation; *see also* notes on booster doses, above

Available as part of childhood immunisation schedule, from health organisations or Moviano; brands include *Repevax*®

◢ Diphtheria-containing vaccines for children over 10 years

A low dose of diphtheria toxoid is sufficient to recall immunity in older children previously immunised against diphtheria but whose immunity may have diminished with time; it is insufficient to cause serious reactions in a child who is already immune. Preparations containing low dose diphtheria should be used for children *over 10 years*, both for primary immunisation and booster doses.

Adsorbed Diphtheria [low dose], Tetanus and Inactivated Poliomyelitis Vaccine PoM

Injection, suspension of diphtheria toxoid [low dose], tetanus toxoid and inactivated poliomyelitis vaccine components adsorbed on a mineral carrier, net price 0.5-mL prefilled syringe = £6.74
Excipients may include neomycin, polymyxin B and streptomycin

Dose

> Primary immunisation
> • **By intramuscular injection**
> > **Child 10–18 years** 3 doses each of 0.5 mL separated by intervals of 1 month; second booster dose, 0.5 mL given 10 years after first booster dose (may also be used as first booster dose in those over 10 years who have received only 3 previous doses of a diphtheria-containing vaccine); see also notes on booster doses, above

Available as part of childhood schedule, from health organisations or Moviano; brands include *Revaxis*®

◢ Diphtheria antitoxin

Diphtheria antitoxin is used for passive immunisation in suspected cases of diphtheria only (without waiting for bacteriological confirmation); tests for hypersensitivity should be first carried out. It is derived from horse serum, and reactions are common after administration; resuscitation facilities should be available immediately.

It is no longer used for prophylaxis because of the risk of hypersensitivity; unimmunised contacts should be promptly investigated and given antibacterial prophylaxis (Table 2, section 5.1) and vaccine (see Contacts above, p. 733).

Diphtheria Antitoxin PoM
Dip/Ser

Dose

> Prophylaxis not recommended therefore no dose stated (see notes above)

> Treatment
> > Consult product literature

Available from Centre for Infections (Tel (020) 8200 6868) or in Northern Ireland from Public Health Laboratory, Belfast City Hospital (Tel (028) 9032 9241).

Haemophilus type B conjugate vaccine

Haemophilus influenzae type b (Hib) vaccine is made from capsular polysaccharide; it is conjugated with a protein such as tetanus toxoid to increase immunogenicity, especially in young children. Haemophilus influenzae type b vaccine is given in combination with diphtheria, tetanus, pertussis (acellular, component) and inactivated poliomyelitis vaccine, (see under Diphtheria containing Vaccines) as a component of the primary course of childhood immunisation (see Immunisation schedule, section 14.1) For infants under 1 year, the course consists of 3 doses of a vaccine containing haemophilus influenzae type b component, with an interval of 1 month between doses. A booster dose of haemophilus influenzae type b vaccine (combined with meningococcal group C conjugate vaccine) should be given at around 12 months of age.

Children 1–10 years who have not been immunised against *Haemophilus influenzae type b* need to receive only 1 dose of the vaccine (combined with meningococcal group C conjugate vaccine). However, if a primary course of immunisation has not been completed, these children should be given 3 doses of diphtheria, tetanus, pertussis (acellular, component), poliomyelitis (inactivated) and haemophilus type b conjugate vaccine (adsorbed). The risk of infection falls sharply in older children and the vaccine is not normally required for children over 10 years.

Haemophilus influenzae type b vaccine may be given to those over 10 years who are considered to be at increased risk of invasive *H. influenzae* type b disease (such as those with sickle-cell disease and those receiving treatment for malignancy).

For use of rifampicin in the prevention of secondary cases of Haemophilus influenza type b disease, see Table 2, section 5.1

Asplenia or splenic dysfunction Haemophilus influenzae type b vaccine is recommended for children with asplenia or splenic dysfunction. Immunised children over 1 year, who develop splenic dysfunction, should be given 1 additional dose of haemophilus influenzae type b vaccine combined with meningococcal group C conjugate vaccine). For elective splenectomy, the vaccine should ideally be given at least 2 weeks before surgery. Children over 1 year, who are not immunised against *Haemophilus influenzae* type b, should be given 2 doses of haemophilus influenzae type b vaccine (combined with meningococcal group C conjugate vaccine) with an interval of 2 months between doses. However, children under 10 years, who are not immunised against diphtheria, tetanus, pertussis, poliomyelitis, and *Haemophilus influenzae* type b should be given 3 doses (with an interval of 1 month between doses) of combined diphtheria, tetanus, pertussis (acellular component), poliomyelitis (inactivated) and haemophilus type b conjugate vaccine.

HAEMOPHILUS TYPE B CONJUGATE VACCINE

Cautions see section 14.1

Contra-indications see section 14.1

Side-effects see section 14.1; also, atopic dermatitis, hypotonia

Licensed use *Menitorix®* is not licensed for use in children over 2 years

Indication and dose

See notes above and under preparation

   Primary immunisation, see under Diphtheria-containing vaccines

Menitorix® (GSK) PoM

Injection, powder for reconstitution, capsular polysaccharide of *Haemophilus influenzae* type b and capsular polysaccharide of *Neisseria meningitidis* group C (both conjugated to tetanus protein),

net price single dose vial (with syringe containing 0.5 mL diluent) = £39.87

Dose

- **By intramuscular injection**

   CHILD 1 –10 years , 0.5 mL

   CHILD over 1 year , with asplenia or splenic dysfunction (see notes above), 0.5 mL

Available as part of the childhood immunisation schedule from Movianto

◀Combined vaccines

See also Diphtheria-containing vaccines

Hepatitis A vaccine

Hepatitis A vaccine is prepared from formaldehyde-inactivated hepatitis A virus grown in human diploid cells.

Immunisation is recommended for:

- residents of homes for those with severe learning difficulties;
- children with haemophilia treated with plasma-derived clotting factors;
- children with severe liver disease;
- children travelling to high-risk areas (see p. 759);
- adolescents who are at risk due to their sexual behaviour;
- parenteral drug abusers.

Immunisation should be considered for:

- children with chronic liver disease including chronic hepatitis B or chronic hepatitis C;
- prevention of secondary cases in close contacts of confirmed cases of hepatitis A, within 7 days of onset of disease in the primary case.

A booster dose of hepatitis A vaccine is usually given 6–12 months after the initial dose. A second booster dose can be given 20 years after the previous booster dose to those who continue to be at risk. Specialist advice should be sought on re-immunisation of immunocompromised individuals.

In children under 16 years, a single dose of the combined vaccine *Ambirix*® can be used to provide rapid protection against hepatitis A.

◾ HEPATITIS A VACCINE

Cautions section 14.1

Contra-indications section 14.1

Side-effects section 14.1; for combination vaccines, see also Typhoid vaccines, p. 752

Indication and dose

Immunisation against hepatitis A infection

for dose, see under preparations

◢ Single component

Avaxim® (Sanofi Pasteur) (PoM)

Injection, suspension of formaldehyde-inactivated hepatitis A virus (GBM grown in human diploid cells) 320 antigen units/mL adsorbed onto aluminium hydroxide, net price 0.5-mL prefilled syringe = £19.19

Excipients include neomycin

Dose

- **By intramuscular injection**

  (see note below)

  Child 16–18 years 0.5 mL as a single dose; booster dose 0.5 mL 6–12 months after initial dose

  Note Booster dose may be delayed by up to 3 years if not given after recommended interval following primary dose with *Avaxim*®. The deltoid region is the preferred site of injection; not to be injected into the buttock (vaccine efficacy reduced). The subcutaneous route may be used for children with bleeding disorders

Epaxal® (MASTA) (PoM)

Injection, suspension of formaldehyde-inactivated hepatitis A virus (RG-SB grown in human diploid cells) at least 48 units/mL, net price 0.5-mL pre-filled syringe = £23.81

Dose

- **By intramuscular injection**

  (see note below)

  Child 1–18 years 0.5 mL as a single dose; booster dose 0.5 mL 6–12 months after initial dose (1–6 months if splenectomised)

  Note Booster dose may be delayed by up to 4 years if not given after recommended interval following primary dose. The deltoid region is the preferred site of

injection. The subcutaneous route may be used for children with bleeding disorders

Important *Epaxal*® contains influenza virus haemagglutinin grown in the allantoic cavity of chick embryos, therefore contra-indicated in those hypersensitive to eggs or chicken protein.

Havrix Monodose® (GSK) (PoM)

Injection, suspension of formaldehyde-inactivated hepatitis A virus (HM 175 grown in human diploid cells) 1440 ELISA units/mL adsorbed onto aluminium hydroxide, net price 1-mL prefilled syringe = £22.14, 0.5-mL (720 ELISA units) prefilled syringe (*Havrix Junior Monodose*®) = £16.77

Excipients include neomycin

Dose

- **By intramuscular injection**

  (see note below)

  Child 1–15 years 0.5 mL as a single dose; booster dose 0.5 mL 6–12 months after initial dose

  Child 16–18 years 1 mL as a single dose; booster dose 1 mL 6–12 months after initial dose

  Note Booster dose may be delayed by up to 3 years if not given after recommended interval following primary dose with *Havrix Monodose*®. The deltoid region is the preferred site of injection. The subcutaneous route may be used for children with bleeding disorders

Vaqta® **Paediatric** (Sanofi Pasteur) (PoM)

Injection, suspension of formaldehyde-inactivated hepatitis A virus (grown in human diploid cells) 50 antigen units/mL adsorbed onto aluminium hydroxyphosphate sulphate, net price 0.5-mL pre-filled syringe = £15.65

Excipients include neomycin

Dose

- **By intramuscular injection**

  (see note below)

  Child 1–18 years 0.5 mL as a single dose; booster dose 0.5 mL 6–18 months after initial dose

  Note The deltoid region is the preferred site of injection. The subcutaneous route may be used for children with bleeding disorders (but immune response may be reduced)

◁ **HEPATITIS A VACCINE (continued)**

◢**With hepatitis B vaccine**
Ambirix® (GSK) ▼ PoM

Injection, suspension of inactivated hepatitis A virus (grown in human diploid cells) 720 ELISA units/mL absorbed onto aluminium hydroxide, and recombinant (DNA) hepatitis B surface antigen (grown in yeast cells) 20 micrograms/mL adsorbed onto aluminium hydroxide and aluminium phosphate, net price 1-mL prefilled syringe = £31.18
Excipients include neomycin and traces of thiomersal

Dose

- **By intramuscular injection**
  (see note below)

  Child 1–15 years primary course, 2 doses of 1 mL, the second 6–12 months after initial dose

  Note Primary course should be completed with *Ambirix®* (single component vaccines given at appropriate intervals may be used for booster dose); the deltoid region is the preferred site of injection in older children; anterolateral thigh is the preferred site in infants; not to be injected into the buttock (vaccine efficacy reduced); subcutaneous route used for children with bleeding disorders (but immune response may be reduced)

  Important *Ambirix®* not recommended for post-exposure prophylaxis following percutaneous (needle-stick), ocular, or mucous membrane exposure to hepatitis B virus

Twinrix® (GSK) PoM

Injection, inactivated hepatitis A virus (grown in human diploid cells) 720 ELISA units absorbed onto aluminium hydroxide, and recombinant (DNA) hepatitis B surface antigen (grown in yeast cells) 20 micrograms/mL adsorbed onto aluminium hydroxide and aluminium phosphate, net price 1-mL prefilled syringe (*Twinrix® Adult*) = £27.76, 0.5-mL prefilled syringe (*Twinrix® Paediatric*) = £20.79
Excipients include neomycin and traces of thiomersal

Dose

- **By intramuscular injection**
  (see note below)

  Child 1–15 years primary course 3 doses of 0.5 mL, the second 1 month and the third 6 months after first dose

  Child 16–18 years primary course, 3 doses of 1 mL, the second 1 month and the third 6 months after first dose

  Accelerated schedule (e.g. for travellers departing within 1 month) for child over 16 years, second dose given 7 days after first dose, third dose after further 14 days and fourth dose 12 months after the first dose

  Note Primary course should be completed with *Twinrix®* (single component vaccines given at appropriate intervals

may be used for booster dose); the deltoid region is the preferred site of injection in older children; anterolateral thigh is the preferred site in infants; not to be injected into the buttock (vaccine efficacy reduced); subcutaneous route used for children with bleeding disorders (but immune response may be reduced).

Important *Twinrix®* **not** recommended for post-exposure prophylaxis following percutaneous (needle-stick), ocular or mucous membrane exposure to hepatitis B virus.

◢**With typhoid vaccine**
Hepatyrix® (GSK) PoM

Injection, suspension of inactivated hepatitis A virus (grown in human diploid cells) 1440 ELISA units/mL adsorbed onto aluminium hydroxide, combined with typhoid vaccine containing 25 micrograms/mL virulence polysaccharide antigen of *Salmonella typhi*, net price 1-mL prefilled syringe = £32.08
Excipients include neomycin

Dose

- **By intramuscular injection**
  (see note below)

  Child 15-18 years 1 mL as a single dose; booster doses, see under single component hepatitis A vaccine (above) and under polysaccharide typhoid vaccine, p. 752

  Note The deltoid region is the preferred site of injection; not to be injected into the buttock (vaccine efficacy reduced). The subcutaneous route may be used for children with bleeding disorders

ViATIM® (Sanofi Pasteur) PoM

Injection, suspension of inactivated hepatitis A virus (grown in human diploid cells) 160 antigen units/mL adsorbed onto aluminium hydroxide, combined with typhoid vaccine containing 25 micrograms/mL virulence polysaccharide antigen of *Salmonella typhi*, net price 1-mL prefilled syringe = £30.22

Dose

- **By intramuscular injection**
  (see note below)

  Child 16-18 years 1 mL as a single dose; booster doses, see under single component hepatitis A vaccine (above) and under polysaccharide typhoid vaccine, p. 752

  Note The deltoid region is the preferred site of injection; not to be injected into the buttock (vaccine efficacy reduced). The subcutaneous route may be used for children with bleeding disorders

Hepatitis B vaccine

Hepatitis B vaccine contains inactivated hepatitis B virus surface antigen (HBsAg) adsorbed on aluminium hydroxide adjuvant. It is made biosynthetically using recombinant DNA technology. The vaccine is used in individuals at high risk of contracting hepatitis B.

In the UK, high-risk groups include:

- parenteral drug misusers, their sexual partners, and household contacts; other drug misusers who are likely to 'progress' to injecting;

- adolescents who are at risk from their sexual behaviour,

- close family contacts of a case or individual with chronic hepatitis B infection;

- babies whose mothers have had acute hepatitis B during pregnancy *or* are positive for hepatitis B surface antigen (regardless of e-antigen markers); hepatitis B vaccination is started immediately on delivery and *hepatitis B immunoglobulin* (see p. 757) given at the same time (but preferably at a different site). Babies whose mothers are positive for hepatitis B surface antigen and for e-antigen antibody should receive the vaccine only (but babies weighing 1.5 kg or less should receive the immunoglobulin regardless of the mother's e-antigen antibody status);

- children with haemophilia, those receiving regular blood transfusions or blood products, and carers responsible for the administration of such products;
- children with chronic renal failure including those on haemodialysis. Children receiving haemodialysis should be monitored for antibodies annually and re-immunised if necessary. Home carers (of dialysis patients) should be vaccinated;
- children with chronic liver disease;
- patients of day-care or residential accommodation for those with severe learning difficulties;
- children in custodial institutions;
- children travelling to areas of high or intermediate prevalence who are at increased risk or who plan to remain there for lengthy periods (see p. 759);
- families adopting children from countries with a high or intermediate prevalence of hepatitis B;
- foster carers and their families.

Different immunisation schedules for hepatitis B vaccine are recommended for specific circumstances (see under individual preparations); an 'accelerated schedule' is recommended for pre-exposure prophylaxis in high–risk groups where rapid protection is required, and for post-exposure prophylaxis (see below). Generally, three or four doses are required for primary immunisation. Immunisation may take up to 6 months to confer adequate protection; the duration of immunity is not known precisely, but a single booster 5 years after the primary course may be sufficient to maintain immunity for those who continue to be at risk.

Immunisation does not eliminate the need for commonsense precautions for avoiding the risk of infection from known carriers by the routes of infection which have been clearly established, consult *Guidance for Clinical Health Care Workers: Protection against Infection with Blood-borne Viruses* (available at www.dh.gov.uk). Accidental inoculation of hepatitis B virus-infected blood into a wound, incision, needle-prick, or abrasion may lead to infection, whereas it is unlikely that indirect exposure to a carrier will do so.

Following significant exposure to hepatits B, an accelerated schedule, with the second dose given 1 month, and the third dose 2 months after the initial dose, is recommended. For those at continued risk, a fourth dose should be given 12 months after the first dose. More detailed guidance is given in the memorandum *Immunisation against Infectious Disease*.

Specific **hepatitis B immunoglobulin** ('HBIG') is available for use with the vaccine in those accidentally inoculated and in neonates at special risk of infection (section 14.5).

A combined hepatitis A and hepatitis B vaccine is also available.

◢ HEPATITIS B VACCINE

Cautions section 14.1

Contra-indications section 14.1

Side-effects section 14.1

Indication and dose

Immunisation against hepatitis B infection
for dose see under preparations

◢ **Single component**
Engerix B® (GSK) (PoM)
Injection, suspension of hepatitis B surface antigen (prepared from yeast cells by recombinant DNA technique) 20 micrograms/mL adsorbed onto aluminium hydroxide, net price 0.5-mL (paediatric) prefilled syringe = £9.67, 1-mL vial = £12.34, 1-mL prefilled syringe = £12.99
Excipients include traces of thiomersal

Dose
- **By intramuscular injection**
  (see note below)

  Neonate (except if born to hepatitis B surface antigen-positive mother, see below), 3 doses of 10 micrograms, second dose 1 month and third dose 6 months after first dose

◁ **HEPATITIS B VACCINE (continued)**

Child 1 month–16 years 3 doses of 10 micrograms, second dose 1 month and third dose 6 months after first dose

Child 16–18 years 3 doses of 20 micrograms, second dose 1 month and third dose 6 months after first dose
Accelerated schedule (all age groups), second dose 1 month after first dose, third dose 2 months after first dose and fourth dose 12 months after first dose
Alternative schedule for Child 11–15 years, 2 doses of 20 micrograms, the second dose 6 months after the first dose (this schedule not suitable if high risk of infection between doses or if compliance with second dose uncertain)

Infant born to hepatitis B surface antigen-positive mother (see also notes above)
• **By intramuscular injection**
  (see note below)

Neonate 4 doses of 10 micrograms, first dose at birth with hepatitis B immunoglobulin injection (separate site) the second 1 month, the third 2 months and the fourth 12 months after first dose

Renal insufficiency (including haemodialysis) patients)
• **By intramuscular injection**
  (see note below)

Neonate (except if born to hepatitis B surface antigen positive mother, see above), 3 doses of 10 micrograms, second dose 1 month and third dose 6 months after first dose *or* accelerated schedule, 4 doses of 10 micrograms, second dose 1 month, third dose 2 months, and fourth dose 12 months after first dose; immunisation schedule and booster doses may need to be adjusted in those with low antibody concentration

Child 1 month–16 years 3 doses of 10 micrograms, second dose 1 month and third dose 6 months after first dose *or* accelerated schedule, 4 doses of 10 micrograms, second dose 1 month, third dose 2 months, and fourth dose 12 months after first dose; immunisation schedule and booster doses may need to be adjusted in those with low antibody concentration

Child 16–18 years 4 doses of 40 micrograms, the second 1 month, the third 2 months and the fourth 6 months after the first dose; immunisation schedule and booster doses may need to be adjusted in those with low antibody concentration

Note Deltoid muscle is preferred site of injection in older children; anterolateral thigh is preferred site in neonates, infants and young children; not to be injected into the buttock (vaccine efficacy reduced)

Fendrix® (GSK) [PoM]
Injection, suspension of hepatitis B surface antigen (prepared from yeast cells by recombinant DNA technique) 40 micrograms/mL adsorbed onto aluminium phosphate, net price 0.5-mL prefilled syringe = £38.10
Excipients include traces of thiomersal

Dose
Renal insufficiency patients (including pre-haemodialysis and haemodialysis patients)
• **By intramuscular injection**
  (see note below)

Child 15–18 years 4 doses of 20 micrograms, the second 1 month, the third 2 months and the fourth 6 months after the first dose; immunisation schedule and booster doses may need to be adjusted in those with low antibody concentration
Note Deltoid muscle is preferred site of injection; not to be injected into the buttock (vaccine efficacy reduced)

HBvaxPRO® (Sanofi Pasteur) [PoM]
Injection, suspension of hepatitis B surface antigen (prepared from yeast cells by recombinant DNA technique) 10 micrograms/mL adsorbed onto aluminium hydroxyphosphate sulphate, net price 0.5-mL (5-microgram) prefilled syringe = £9.50, 1-mL (10-microgram) prefilled syringe = £12.95; 40 micrograms/mL, 1-mL (40-microgram) vial = £29.30

Dose
• **By intramuscular injection**
  (see note below)

Neonate (except if born to hepatitis B surface antigen-positive mother, see below), 3 doses of 5 micrograms, second dose 1 month and third dose 6 months after first dose

Child 1 month–16 years 3 doses of 5 micrograms, second dose 1 month and third dose 6 months after first dose

Child 16–18 years 3 doses of 10 micrograms, second dose 1 month and third dose 6 months after first dose
Accelerated schedule (all age groups), second dose 1 month after first dose, third dose 2 months after first dose with fourth dose at 12 months
Booster doses may be required in immunocompromised patients with low antibody concentration

Infant born to hepatitis B surface antigen-positive mother (see also notes above)
• **By intramuscular injection**
  (see note below)

Neonate 5 micrograms, first dose at birth with hepatitis B immunoglobulin injection (separate site), the second 1 month, the third 2 months and the fourth 12 months after the first dose

Chronic haemodialysis patients
• **By intramuscular injection**
  (see note below)

Child 16–18 years 3 doses of 40 micrograms, second dose 1 month and third dose 6 months after first dose; booster doses may be required in those with low antibody concentration

Note Deltoid muscle is preferred site of injection in older children; anterolateral thigh is preferred site in neonates and infants; not to be injected into the buttock (vaccine efficacy reduced)

◢**With hepatitis A vaccine**
See Hepatitis A Vaccine

Human papilloma virus vaccines

Human papilloma virus vaccine is available as a bivalent vaccine (*Cervarix®*) or a quadrivalent vaccine (*Gardasil®*). *Cervarix®* is licensed for use in females for the prevention of cervical cancer and other pre-cancerous lesions caused by human papilloma virus types 16 and 18. *Gardasil®* is licensed for use in females for the prevention of cervical cancer, genital warts and pre-cancerous lesions caused by human papilloma virus types 6, 11, 16 and 18. The two vaccines are not interchangeable and one vaccine product should be used for an entire course. However, the Department of Health (November 2008) states for individuals with previous incomplete vaccination with *Gardasil®*, who are eligible for HPV vaccination under the national programme, *Cervarix®* can be used to complete the vaccination course if necessary; the individual must be informed that *Cervarix®* does not protect against genital warts.

Human papilloma virus vaccine will be most effective if given before sexual activity starts. The first dose is given to females aged 12 to 13 years, the second and third doses are given 1–2 and 6 months after the first dose (see Immunisation schedule, section 14.1); all 3 doses should be given within a 12-month period. If the course is interrupted, it should be resumed but not repeated, allowing the appropriate interval between the remaining doses. Where there are significant challenges in scheduling vaccination, or a high likelihood that the third dose will not be given, the third dose of *Cervarix®* can be given 3 months after the second dose. Where appropriate, immunisation with human papillomavirus vaccine should be offered to females coming into the UK as they may not have been offered protection in their country of origin. The duration of protection has not been established, but current studies suggest that protection is maintained for at least 6 years after completion of primary course.

> Human papilloma virus vaccine 'Catch up' programme for England, Wales and Northern Ireland
> A 'catch up' programme will be offered as follows:
> - from September 2008 [January 2009 in Wales] to all females born between 1 September 1990 and 31 August 1991 (aged 17–18 years)
> - from September 2009 to all females born between 1 September 1991 and 31 August 1995 (aged 14–18 years)

> Human papilloma virus vaccine 'Catch up' programme for Scotland
> The 'catch up' programme in Scotland will be offered as follows:
> - from 1 September 2008 to all females aged 16–17 years
> - from September 2009 to all females aged 14–16 years

HUMAN PAPILLOMA VIRUS VACCINES

Cautions see section 14.1

Contra-indications see section 14.1

Side-effects see section 14.1

Indication and dose

> see notes above and under preparations
> Note To avoid confusion, prescribers should specify the brand to be dispensed

Cervarix® (GSK) ▼ [PoM]
Injection, suspension of virus-like particles of human papilloma virus type 16 (40 micrograms/mL), type 18 (40 micrograms/mL) capsid protein (prepared by recombinant DNA technique using a Baculovirus expression system) in monopho-

sphoryl lipid A adjuvant adsorbed onto aluminium hydroxide, net price 0.5-mL prefilled syringe = £80.50

Note To avoid confusion, prescribers should specify the brand to be dispensed

Dose

> Prevention of premalignant genital lesions and cervical cancer (see notes above)
> - By intramuscular injection into deltoid region
>   Child **10–18 years** 3 doses of 0.5 mL, the second 1 month and the third 6 months after the first dose

Gardasil® (Sanofi Pasteur) ▼ [PoM]
Injection, suspension of virus-like particles of human papilloma virus type 6 (40 micrograms/mL), type 11 (80 micrograms/mL), type 16 (80 micrograms/mL), type 18 (40 micrograms/mL) capsid protein (prepared from yeast cells by

◻ **HUMAN PAPILLOMA VIRUS VACCINES (*continued*)**

recombinant DNA technique) adsorbed onto aluminium hydroxyphosphate sulphate, net price 0.5-mL prefilled syringe = £80.50

Note To avoid confusion, prescribers should specify the brand to be dispensed

Dose

Prevention of premalignant genital lesions, cervical cancer and genital warts (see notes above)

• **By intramuscular injection preferably into deltoid region or higher anterolateral thigh**

Child 9–18 years 3 doses of 0.5 mL, the second 2 months and the third 6 months after the first dose

Alternative schedule for Child 9–18 years, 3 doses of 0.5 mL, the second at least 1 month and the third at least 4 months after the first dose; schedule should be completed within 12 months

---

Influenza vaccine

While most viruses are antigenically stable, the influenza viruses A and B (especially A) are constantly altering their antigenic structure as indicated by changes in the haemagglutinins (H) and neuraminidases (N) on the surface of the viruses. It is essential that influenza vaccines in use contain the H and N components of the prevalent strain or strains recommended each year by the World Health Organization.

Influenza vaccines will not control epidemics — immunisation is recommended *only for persons at high risk*. Annual immunisation is strongly recommended for children (including infants that were preterm or low birth-weight) aged over 6 months with the following conditions:

• chronic respiratory disease (includes asthma treated with continuous or repeated use of inhaled or systemic corticosteroids or asthma with previous exacerbations requiring hospital admission);

• chronic heart disease;

• chronic liver disease;

• chronic renal disease;

• chronic neurological disease;

• diabetes mellitus;

• immunosuppression because of disease (including asplenia or splenic dysfunction) or treatment (including chemotherapy and prolonged corticosteroid treatment);

• HIV infection (regardless of immune status).

Influenza immunisation is also recommended for children living in long-stay facilities. Influenza immunisation should also be considered for household contacts of immunocompromised individuals.

Where possible, pregnant women and children should receive a thiomersal-free influenza vaccine; if this is not available, a thiomersal-containing influenza vaccine should be given.

Information on pandemic influenza and avian influenza may be found at www.dh.gov.uk/pandemicflu and www.hpa.org.uk.

◢ INFLUENZA VACCINES

Cautions see section 14.1; **interactions**: Appendix 1 (vaccines)

Contra-indications see section 14.1

Side-effects see section 14.1; also reported, febrile convulsions and trasient thrombocytopenia

Licensed use Inactivated Influenza Vaccine (Surface Antigen) and *Fluvirin*® are not licensed for use in children under 4 years

Indication and dose

Annual immunisation against influenza

• **By intramuscular injection**

Child 6 months–3 years 0.25–0.5 mL (repeated after 4–6 weeks in children not previously vaccinated)

Child 3–13 years 0.5 mL (repeated after 4–6 weeks in children not previously vaccinated)

Child 13–18 years 0.5 mL as a single dose

Inactivated Influenza Vaccine (Split Virion) (PoM)

Flu

Injection, suspension of formaldehyde-inactivated influenza virus (split virion) grown in fertilised hens' eggs, net price 0.25-mL prefilled syringe = £6.29, 0.5-mL prefilled syringe = £6.29

Excipients may include neomycin and polymyxin

Available from Sanofi Pasteur

◻ **INFLUENZA VACCINES** (*continued*)

Inactivated Influenza Vaccine (Surface Antigen) PoM

Flu or Flu(adj)
Injection, suspension of propiolactone-inactivated influenza virus (surface antigen) grown in fertilised hens' eggs, net price 0.5-mL prefilled syringe = £4.40
Excipients may include neomycin, polymyxin B and traces of thiomersal
Available from Novartis Vaccines

Agrippal® (Novartis Vaccines) PoM
Injection, suspension of formaldehyde-inactivated influenza virus (surface antigen) grown in fertilised hens' eggs, net price 0.5-mL prefilled syringe = £5.85
Excipients include kanamycin and neomycin

Begrivac® (Novartis Vaccines) PoM
Injection, suspension of formaldehyde-inactivated influenza virus (split virion) grown in fertilised hens' eggs, net price 0.5-mL prefilled syringe = £5.85
Excipients include polymyxin B

Enzira® (Wyeth) PoM
Injection, suspension of inactivated influenza virus (split virion) grown in fertilised hens' eggs, net price 0.5-mL prefilled syringe = £6.59
Excipients include neomycin and polymyxin B

Fluarix® (GSK) PoM
Injection, suspension of formaldehyde-inactivated influenza virus (split virion) grown in fertilised hens' eggs, net price 0.5-mL prefilled syringe = £4.49
Excipients include gentamicin

Fluvirin® (Novartis Vaccines) PoM
Injection, suspension of formaldehyde-inactivated influenza virus (surface antigen) grown in fertilised hens' eggs, net price 0.5mL prefilled syringe = £5.55
Excipients include neomycin, polymyxin B, and traces of thiomersal

Imuvac® (Solvay) PoM
Injection, suspension of formaldehyde-inactivated influenza virus (surface antigen) grown in fertilised hens' eggs, net price 0.5-mL prefilled syringe = £6.59
Excipients include gentamicin

Influvac Sub-unit® (Solvay) PoM
Injection, suspension of formaldehyde-inactivated influenza virus (surface antigen) grown in fertilised hens' eggs, net price 0.5-mL prefilled syringe = £5.22
Excipients include gentamicin

Mastaflu® (MASTA) PoM
Injection, suspension of formaldehyde-inactivated influenza virus (surface antigen) grown in fertilised hens' eggs, net price 0.5-mL prefilled syringe = £6.50
Excipients include gentamicin

Viroflu® (Sanofi Pasteur) PoM
Injection, suspension of inactivated influenza virus (surface antigen, virosome) grown in fertilised hens' eggs, net price 0.5-mL prefilled syringe = £6.59
Excipients include neomycin and polymyxin B

Measles vaccine

Measles vaccine has been replaced by a combined live measles, mumps and rubella vaccine (MMR vaccine).

MMR vaccine may be used in the control of outbreaks of measles (see under MMR Vaccine).

◢**Single antigen vaccine**
No longer available in the UK

◢**Combined vaccines**
See MMR vaccine, below

Measles, Mumps and Rubella (MMR) vaccine

A combined live **measles, mumps, and rubella vaccine** (MMR vaccine) aims to eliminate measles, mumps and rubella (and congenital rubella syndrome). Every child should receive two doses of MMR vaccine by entry to primary school, unless there is a valid contra-indication (see section 14.1). MMR vaccine should be given irrespective of previous measles, mumps, or rubella infection or vaccination.

The first dose of MMR vaccine is given to children aged 13 months. A second dose is given before starting school at 3–5 years of age (see Immunisation schedule, section 14.1).

When protection against measles is required urgently (e.g. during a measles outbreak), the second dose of MMR vaccine can be given 1 month after the first dose; if the second dose is given before 18 months of age, then children should still receive the routine dose before starting school at 3–5 years of age.

Children presenting for pre-school booster who have not received the first dose of MMR vaccine should be given a dose of MMR vaccine followed 3 months later by a second dose. At school-leaving age or at entry into further education, MMR immunisation should be offered to individuals of both sexes who have not received 2 doses during childhood. In a young adult who has received only a single dose of MMR in childhood, a second dose is recommended to achieve full protection. If 2 doses of MMR vaccine are required, the second dose should be given one month after the initial dose.

MMR vaccine should be used to protect against rubella in *seronegative females of child-bearing age* (see Immunisation schedule, section 14.1). MMR vaccine may also be offered to previously *unimmunised and seronegative post-partum* mothers—vaccination a few days after delivery is important because about 60% of congenital abnormalities from rubella infection occur in babies of mothers who have borne more than one child. Immigrants arriving after the age of school immunisation are particularly likely to require immunisation.

Contacts   MMR vaccine may also be used in the control of outbreaks of measles and should be offered to susceptible children including babies aged over 6 months who are contacts of a case, within 3 days of exposure to infection; these children should still receive routine MMR vaccinations at the recommended ages. Children aged under 9 months for whom avoidance of measles infection is particularly important (such as those with history of recent severe illness) can be given normal immunoglobulin (section 14.5, p. 755) after exposure to measles; routine MMR immunisation should then be given after at least 3 months at the appropriate age.

MMR vaccine is **not suitable** for prophylaxis following exposure to mumps or rubella since the antibody response to the mumps and rubella components is too slow for effective prophylaxis.

Children with impaired immune response should not receive live vaccines (for advice on HIV see section 14.1). If they have been exposed to measles infection they should be given normal immunoglobulin (section 14.5).

Travel   Unimmunised children over 6 months of age travelling to areas where measles is endemic or epidemic should receive MMR vaccine. Children immunised before 12 months of age should still receive two doses of MMR at the recommended ages. If one dose of MMR has already been given to a child, then the second dose should be brought forward to at least one month after the first, to ensure complete protection. If the child is under 18 months of age and the second dose is given within 3 months of the first, then the routine dose, before starting school at 3–5 years, should still be given.

Side-effects   See section 14.1. Also malaise, fever, or a rash may occur after the first dose of MMR vaccine, most commonly about a week after vaccination and lasting about 2 to 3 days. Leaflets are available for parents on advice for reducing fever (including the use of paracetamol). Febrile seizures occur less commonly 6 to 11 days after MMR vaccination; the incidence of febrile seizures is lower than that following measles infection. Parotid swelling occurs occasionally, usually in the third week, and rarely, arthropathy 2 to 3 weeks after immunisation. Adverse reactions are considerably less frequent after the second dose of MMR vaccine than after the first dose.

Idiopathic thrombocytopenic purpura has occurred rarely following MMR vaccination, usually within 6 weeks of the first dose. The risk of developing idiopathic thrombocytopenic purpura after MMR vaccine is much less than the risk of developing it after infection with wild measles or rubella virus. The CSM has recommended that children who develop idiopathic thrombocytopenic purpura within 6 weeks of the first dose of MMR should undergo serological testing before the second dose is due; if the results suggest incomplete immunity against measles, mumps or rubella then a second dose of MMR is recommended. The Specialist and Reference Microbiology Division, Health Protection Agency offers free serological testing for children who develop idiopathic thrombocytopenic purpura *within 6 weeks* of the first dose of MMR.

Post-vaccination aseptic meningitis was reported (rarely and with complete recovery) following vaccination with MMR vaccine containing Urabe mumps vaccine, which has now been discontinued; no cases have been confirmed in association with the currently used Jeryl Lynn mumps vaccine. Children with post-vaccination symptoms are not infectious.

> Reviews undertaken on behalf of the CSM, the Medical Research Council, and the Cochrane Collaboration, have not found any evidence of a link between MMR vaccination and bowel disease or autism. The Chief Medical Officers have advised that the MMR vaccine is the safest and best way to protect children against measles, mumps, and rubella. Information (including fact sheets and a list of references) may be obtained from:
> www.immunisation.nhs.uk and www.immunisation.nhs.uk/Vaccines/MMR

◢ MEASLES, MUMPS AND RUBELLA VACCINE, LIVE

Cautions see section 14.1; also after immuno-globulin administration or blood transfusion, leave an interval of at least 3 months before MMR immunisation as antibody response to measles component may be reduced; **interactions:** Appendix 1 (vaccines)

Hypersensitivity to egg There is increasing evidence that MMR vaccine can be given safely even when the child has had an anaphylactic reaction to food containing egg (dislike of egg or refusal to eat egg is not a contra-indication). For children with a confirmed anaphylactic reaction to egg-containing food, MMR vaccine should be administered in a hospital setting.

Contra-indications see section 14.1

Pregnancy avoid vaccination during pregnancy; avoid pregnancy for at least 1 month after vaccination

Side-effects see section 14.1 and notes above; also *less commonly* sleep disturbance, unusual crying in infants, also reported peripheral and optic neuritis.

Licensed use *Priorix*® not licensed for use in children under 9 months, and *MMRvaxPro*® not licensed for use in children under 1 year

Indication and dose

Immunisation against measles, mumps, and rubella

• **By intramuscular or deep subcutaneous injection**

CHILD **6 months–18 years** primary immunisation, 2 doses each of 0.5 mL, see Immunisation schedule, section 14.1, p. 728; see also notes above for use in outbreaks, for contacts of cases, and for travel

◢ **Combined vaccines**

MMRvaxPro® (Sanofi Pasteur) ▼ [PoM]

Injection, powder for reconstitution, live attenuated, measles virus (Enders' Edmonston strain) and mumps virus (Jeryl Lynn [Level B] strain) prepared in chick embryo cells, and rubella virus (Wistar RA 27/3 strain); single-dose vial (with syringe containing solvent)

Excipients include gelatin and neomycin

Only available as part of childhood immunisation schedule from health organisations or Movianto

Priorix® (GSK) [PoM]

Injection,, powder for reconstitution, live attenuated, measles virus (Schwarz strain) and mumps virus (RIT 4385 strain) prepared in chick embryo cells, and rubella virus (Wistar RA 27/3 strain), net price single-dose vial (with syringe containing solvent) = £6.37

Excipients include neomycin

Also available as part of childhood immunisation schedule from health organisations or Movianto

Meningococcal vaccines

Almost all childhood meningococcal disease in the UK is caused by *Neisseria meningitidis* serogroups B and C. **Meningococcal Group C conjugate vaccine** protects only against infection by serogroup C. The risk of meningococcal disease declines with age—immunisation is not generally recommended after the age of 25 years.

Childhood immunisation Meningococcal Group C conjugate vaccine provides long-term protection against infection by serogroup C of *Neisseria meningitidis*. Immunisation consists of 2 doses given at 3 months and 4 months of age; a booster dose should be given at 12 months of age, usually combined with haemophilus influenzae type b vaccine. This routine booster dose should be given one month before the booster dose of pneumococcal conjugate vaccine (see Immunisation schedule, section 14.1, p. 728). It is recommended that meningococcal group C conjugate vaccine be given to anyone aged under 25 years who has not been vaccinated previously with this vaccine; those over 1 year receive a single dose.

Meningococcal group C conjugate vaccine in patients with asplenia or splenic dysfunction Meningococcal group C conjugate vaccine is recommended for children with asplenia or splenic dysfunction. Children under 1 year should be vaccinated according to the Immunisation Schedule (section 14.1). Unimmunised children over 1 year should be given 2 doses of meningococcal group C conjugate vaccine (usually combined with haemophilus influenzae type b vaccine) with an interval of 2 months between doses. Immunised children who develop splenic dysfunction should be given 1 additional dose of meningococcal group C conjugate vaccine (usually combined with haemophilus influenzae type b vaccine).

Travel Children travelling to countries of risk (see below) should be immunised with a meningococcal polysaccharide vaccine that covers serotypes **A, C, W135 and Y**, even if they have previously received meningitis C conjugate vaccine. If the child has recently received meningococcal group C conjugate vaccine an interval of at least 2 weeks should be allowed before administration of the tetravalent (A, C, W135, and Y) vaccine. The antibody response to serotype C in unconjugated meningococcal polysaccharide vaccines in children under 18 months may be suboptimal.

Vaccination is particularly important for those living with local people or visiting an area of risk during outbreaks.

Immunisation recommendations and requirements for visa entry for individual countries should be checked before travelling, particularly to countries in Sub-Saharan Africa, Asia, and the Indian sub-continent where outbreaks and epidemics of meningococcal infection are reported. Country-by-country information is available from the National Travel Health Network and Centre (www.nathnac.org). Proof of vaccination with the tetravalent (A, C, W135 and Y) meningococcal vaccine is required for those travelling to Saudi Arabia during the Hajj and Umrah pilgrimages (where outbreaks of the W135 strain have occurred).

Contacts For advice on the immunisation of *laboratory workers and close contacts* of cases of meningococcal disease in the UK and on the role of the vaccine in the control of *local outbreaks*, consult Guidelines for Public Health Management of Meningococcal Disease in the UK at www.hpa.org.uk. See Table 2, section 5.1 for antibacterial prophylaxis for prevention of secondary cases of meningococcal meningitis.

◢ MENINGOCOCCAL VACCINES

Cautions see section 14.1

Contra-indications see section 14.1

Side-effects see section 14.1; also *rarely* symptoms of meningitis reported (but no evidence that vaccine causes meningococcal C meningitis)

Licensed use *ACWYVax* not licensed in children under 2 years

Indication and dose

Immunisation against *Neisseria meningitidis*
for dose, see under preparations

◢ Meningococcal Group C conjugate vaccine
Meningitec® (Wyeth) [PoM]
Injection, suspension of capsular polysaccharide antigen of *Neisseria meningitidis* group C (conjugated to *Corynebacterium diphtheriae* protein), adsorbed onto aluminium phosphate, net price 0.5-mL prefilled syringe = £7.50

Dose
• **By intramuscular injection**
  Child 2 months–1 year for routine immunisation, 0.5 mL, see notes above and Immunisation schedule, section 14.1
  Child 1–18 years 0.5 mL as a single dose
  Note Subcutaneous route used for children with bleeding disorders

Available as part of childhood immunisation schedule from Movianto

Menjugate Kit® (Sanofi Pasteur) [PoM]
Injection, powder for reconstitution, capsular polysaccharide antigen of *Neisseria meningitidis* group C (conjugated to *Corynebacterium diphtheriae* protein), adsorbed onto aluminium hydroxide, single-dose vials

Dose
• **By intramuscular injection**
  Child 2 months–1 year for routine immunisation, 0.5 mL, see notes above and Immunisation schedule, section 14.1
  Child 1–18 years 0.5 mL as a single dose
  Note Subcutaneous route used for children with bleeding disorders

NeisVac-C® (Baxter) [PoM]
Injection, suspension of polysaccharide antigen of *Neisseria meningitidis* group C (conjugated to tetanus toxoid protein), adsorbed onto aluminium hydroxide, 0.5-mL prefilled syringe

Dose
• **By intramuscular injection**
  Child 3 months–1 year for routine immunisation, 0.5 mL, see notes above and Immunisation schedule, section 14.1
  Child 1–18 years 0.5 mL as a single dose

Available from Movianto

14

Immunological products and vaccines

◻ **MENINGOCOCCAL VACCINES** (*continued*)

◢Meningococcal Group C conjugate vaccine with Haemophilus Influenzae type B vaccine
See *Haemophilus Influenzae* type B vaccine

◢Meningococcal polysaccharide A, C, W135 and Y vaccine

ACWY Vax® (GSK) ▼ PoM
Injection, powder for reconstitution, capsular polysaccharide antigens of *Neisseria meningitidis*

groups A, C, W135 and Y, net price single-dose vial (with syringe containing diluent) = £16.73

Dose
• **By deep subcutaneous injection**
  Child 3 months–2 years 2 doses (each of 0.5 mL) separated by an interval of 3 months; antibody response may be suboptimal in this age group
  Child 2–18 years 0.5 mL as a single dose; booster dose for those at continued risk, 0.5mL 5 years after initial dose (children under 5 years when first vaccinated, should be given a booster dose after 2–3 years)

Mumps vaccine

◢Single antigen vaccine
No longer available in the UK

◢Combined vaccines
See MMR Vaccine, p. 742

Pertussis vaccine

Pertussis vaccine is given as a combination preparation containing other vaccines (see Diphtheria Vaccines). Acellular vaccines are derived from highly purified components of *Bordetella pertussis*. Primary immunisation against pertussis (whooping cough) requires 3 doses of an acellular pertussis-containing vaccine (see Immunisation schedule, section 14.1, p. 728), given at intervals of 1 month from the age of 2 months.

A booster dose of an acellular pertussis-containing vaccine should be given 3 years after the primary course.

All children up to the age of 10 years should receive primary immunisation with diphtheria, tetanus, pertussis (acellular, component), poliomyelitis (inactivated) and haemophilus type b conjugate vaccine (adsorbed).

Children aged 1–10 years who have not received a *pertussis-containing* vaccine as part of their primary immunisation schedule should be offered 1 dose of a suitable pertussis-containing vaccine; after an interval of at least 1 year, a booster dose of a suitable pertussis-containing vaccine should be given. Immunisation against pertussis is not currently recommended in individuals over 10 years of age.

Cautions   Section 14.1

Contra-indications   Section 14.1

Side effects   See also section 14.1. The incidence of local and systemic effects is generally lower with vaccines containing acellular pertussis components than with the whole-cell pertussis vaccine used. However, compared with primary vaccination, booster doses with vaccines containing acellular pertussis are reported to increase the risk of injection-site reactions (some of which affect the entire limb); local reactions do not contra-indicate further doses (see below).

The vaccine should not be withheld from children with a history to a preceding dose of:

• fever, irrespective of severity;

• persistent crying or screaming for more than 3 hours;

• severe local reaction, irrespective of extent.

These side-effects were associated with whole-cell pertussis vaccine.

◢Combined vaccines
Combined vaccines, see under Diphtheria vaccines

Pneumococcal vaccines

Pneumococcal vaccines protect against infection with *Streptococcus pneumoniae* (pneumococcus); the vaccines contain polysaccharide from capsular pneumococci. **Pneumococcal polysaccharide vaccine** contains purified polysaccharide from 23 capsular types of pneumococci whereas **pneumococcal polysaccharide**

conjugated vaccine (adsorbed) contains polysaccharide from 7 capsular types, the polysaccharide being conjugated to protein.

The conjugate vaccine is used for childhood immunisation. The recommended schedule consists of 3 doses, the first at 2 months of age, the second at 4 months, and the third at 13 months (see Immunisation Schedule, section 14.1).

Pneumococcal vaccination is recommended for individuals at increased risk of pneumococcal infection as follows:

- child under 5 years with a history of invasive pneumococcal disease;
- asplenia or splenic dysfunction (including homozygous sickle cell disease and coeliac disease which could lead to splenic dysfunction);
- chronic respiratory disease (includes asthma treated with continuous or frequent use of a systemic corticosteroid);
- chronic heart disease;
- chronic renal disease;
- chronic liver disease;
- diabetes mellitus;
- immune deficiency because of disease (e.g. HIV infection) or treatment (including prolonged systemic corticosteroid treatment);
- presence of cochlear implant;
- conditions where leakage of cerebrospinal fluid could occur.

Where possible, the vaccine should be given at least 2 weeks before splenectomy, cochlear implant surgery, and chemotherapy; children and carers should be given advice about increased risk of pneumococcal infection. Prophylactic antibacterial therapy against pneumococcal infection (Table 2, section 5.1, p. 305) should not be stopped after immunisation. A patient card and information leaflet for patients with asplenia are available from the Department of Health or in Scotland from the Scottish Executive, Public Health Division 1 (Tel (0131) 244 2501).

Choice of vaccine   Children under 2 years at increased risk of pneumococcal infection (see list above) should receive pneumococcal polysaccharide conjugate vaccine (adsorbed) at the recommended ages, followed by a single dose of the 23-valent pneumococcal polysaccharide vaccine after their second birthday (see below). Children at increased risk of pneumococcal infection presenting late for vaccination should receive 2 doses (separated by at least 1 month) of pneumo-coccal polysaccharide conjugate vaccine (adsorbed) before the age of 12 months, and a third dose at 13 months. Children over 12 months and under 5 years (who have not been vaccinated or not completed the primary course) should receive a single dose of pneumococcal polysaccharide conjugate vaccine (adsorbed) (2 doses separated by an interval of 2 months in the immunocompromised or those with asplenia or splenic dysfunction). All children under 5 years at increased risk of pneumococcal infection should receive a single dose of the 23-valent pneumo-coccal polysaccharide vaccine after their second birthday and at least 2 months after the final dose of the 7-valent pneumococcal polysaccharide conjugate vaccine (adsorbed).

Children over 5 years who are at increased risk of pneumococcal disease should receive a single dose of the 23-valent unconjugated pneumococcal polysaccha-ride vaccine.

Revaccination   In individuals with higher concentrations of antibodies to pneumococcal polysaccharides, revaccination with the 23-valent pneumococcal polysaccharide vaccine more commonly produces adverse reactions. Revaccina-tion is therefore not recommended, except every 5 years in individuals in whom the antibody concentration is likely to decline rapidly (e.g. asplenia, splenic dysfunction and nephrotic syndrome). If there is doubt, the need for revaccination should be discussed with a haematologist, immunologist, or microbiologist.

14 Immunological products and vaccines

▲ PNEUMOCOCCAL VACCINES

Cautions see section 14.1

Contra-indications see section 14.1

Side-effects see section 14.1; *also* Revaccination, above

Indication and dose

> Immunisation against pneumococcal infection
>
> for dose see under preparations

◢Pneumococcal polysaccharide vaccines

Pneumovax® II (Sanofi Pasteur) [PoM]

Injection, polysaccharide from each of 23 capsular types of pneumococcus, net price 0.5-mL vial = £8.83

Dose

> • **By subcutaneous or intramuscular injection**
>
> **Child 2–18 years** 0.5 mL; revaccination, see notes above

◢Pneumococcal polysaccharide conjugate vaccine (adsorbed)

Prevenar® (Wyeth) ▼ [PoM]

Injection, polysaccharide from each of 7 capsular types of pneumococcus (conjugated to diphtheria toxoid) adsorbed onto aluminium phosphate, net price 0.5-mL prefilled syringe = £34.50

Dose

> • **By intramuscular injection**
>
> **Child 2 months–5 years** 0.5 mL (see notes above and Immunisation schedule, section 14.1)
>
> Note Deltoid muscle is preferred site of injection in young children; anterolateral thigh is preferred site in infants
>
> The dose in *BNF for Children* may differ from that in product literature

Poliomyelitis vaccines

There are two types of poliomyelitis vaccine (containing strains of poliovirus types 1, 2, and 3) available, inactivated poliomyelitis vaccine (for injection) and live (oral) poliomyelitis vaccine. **Inactivated poliomyelitis vaccine**, only available in combined preparation (see under Diphtheria vaccines, combined), is recommended for routine immunisation; it is given by injection and contains inactivated strains of human poliovirus types 1, 2 and 3.

A course of primary immunisation consists of 3 doses of a combined preparation containing inactivated poliomyelitis vaccine starting at 2 months of age with intervals of 1 month between doses (see Immunisation schedule, section 14.1). A course of 3 doses should also be given to all unimmunised children; no child should remain unimmunised against poliomyelitis.

Two booster doses of a preparation containing inactivated poliomyelitis vaccine are recommended, the first before school entry and the second before leaving school (see Immunisation schedule, section 14.1). Further booster doses should be given every 10 years only to individuals at special risk.

Preparations containing inactivated poliomyelitis vaccine can be used to complete an immunisation course initiated with the live (oral) poliomyelitis vaccine. **Live (oral) poliomyelitis vaccine** is available only for use during outbreaks. The live (oral) vaccine poses a very rare risk of vaccine-associated paralytic polio because the attenuated strain of the virus can revert to a virulent form. For this reason the live (oral) vaccine must **not** be used for immunosuppressed individuals or their household contacts. The use of inactivated poliomyelitis vaccine removes the risk of vaccine-associated paralytic polio altogether.

Travel Unimmunised travellers to areas with a high incidence of poliomyelitis should receive a full 3–dose course of a preparation containing inactivated poliomyelitis vaccine. Those who have not been vaccinated in the last 10 years should receive a booster dose of **adsorbed diphtheria [low dose], tetanus and inactivated poliomyelitis vaccine**. Information about countries with a high incidence of poliomyelitis can be obtained from www.travax.nhs.uk or from the National Travel Health Network and Centre, p. 760 (www.nathnac.org).

▲ POLIOMYELITIS VACCINES

Cautions see section 14.1; *also for live vaccine,* interactions: Appendix 1 (vaccines)

Contra-indications see notes above and section 14.1

Side-effects see notes above and section 14.1

Indication and dose

> See under preparations

◢Combined vaccines

See under Diphtheria-containing Vaccines

◢Inactivated (Salk) Vaccine

See under Diphtheria-containing Vaccines

◁ **POLIOMYELITIS VACCINES** (*continued*)

▲Live (oral) (Sabin) vaccine
Poliomyelitis Vaccine, Live (Oral) (GSK) [PoM]
OPV
A suspension of suitable live attenuated strains of
poliomyelitis virus, types 1, 2, and 3. Available in
single-dose and 10-dose containers
Excipients include neomycin and polymyxin B

Dose
Control of outbreaks
• By mouth
   Child 1 month–18 years 3 drops; may be given on a
   lump of sugar; not to be given with foods which
   contain preservatives

Note Live poliomyelitis vaccine loses potency once the
container has been opened—any vaccine remaining at the
end of an immunisation session should be discarded;
whenever possible sessions should be arranged to avoid
undue wastage.

Rabies vaccine

Rabies vaccine contains inactivated rabies virus cultivated in either human diploid
cells or purified chick embryo cells; vaccines are used for pre- and post-exposure
prophylaxis.

Pre-exposure prophylaxis   Immunisation should be offered to children at high
risk of exposure to rabies—where there is limited access to prompt medical care
for those living in areas where rabies is enzootic, for those travelling to such areas
for longer than 1 month, and for those on shorter visits who may be exposed to
unusual risk. Transmission of rabies by humans has not been recorded but it is
advised that those caring for children with the disease should be vaccinated.

Immunisation against rabies is indicated during pregnancy if there is substantial
risk of exposure to rabies and rapid access to post-exposure prophylaxis is likely
to be limited.

Up-to-date country-by-country information on the incidence of rabies can be
obtained from the National Travel Health Network and Centre (www.nathnac.org)
and, in Scotland, from Health Protection Scotland (www.hps.scot.nhs.uk).

Immunisation against rabies requires 3 doses of rabies vaccine, with further
booster doses for those who remain at continued risk.

Post-exposure management   Following potential exposure to rabies, the wound
or site of exposure (e.g. mucous membrane) should be cleansed under running
water and washed for several minutes with soapy water as soon as possible after
exposure. Disinfectant and a simple dressing can be applied, but suturing should
be delayed because it may increase the risk of introducing rabies virus into the
nerves.

Post-exposure prophylaxis against rabies depends on the level of risk in the
country, the nature of exposure, and the individual's immunity. In each case,
expert risk assessment and advice on appropriate management should be
obtained from the Health Protection Agency Virus Reference Department, Colin-
dale, London (tel. (020) 8200 4400) or the Centre for Infections (tel. (020) 8200
6868), in Scotland from Health Protection Scotland (tel. (0141) 300 1100), in
Northern Ireland from the Public Health Laboratory, Belfast City Hospital (tel.
(028) 9032 9241).

There are no specific contra-indications to the use of rabies vaccine for post-
exposure prophylaxis and its use should be considered whenever a child has been
attacked by an animal in a country where rabies is enzootic, even if there is no
direct evidence of rabies in the attacking animal. Because of the potential
consequences of untreated rabies exposure and because rabies vaccination has
not been associated with fetal abnormalities, pregnancy is not considered a
contra-indication to post-exposure prophylaxis.

For post-exposure prophylaxis of *fully immunised* individuals (who have previously
received pre-exposure or post-exposure prophylaxis with cell-derived rabies
vaccine), 2 doses of cell-derived vaccine, given on day 0 and day 3, are likely
to be sufficient. Rabies immunoglobulin is not necessary in such cases.

Post-exposure treatment for *unimmunised individuals* (or those whose prophylaxis
is possibly incomplete) comprises 5 doses of rabies vaccine given over 1 month
(on days 0, 3, 7, 14, and 30); also, depending on the level of risk (determined by
factors such as the nature of the bite and the country where it was sustained),
rabies immunoglobulin (section 14.5) is given on day 0. The immunisation course
can be discontinued if it is proved that the child was not at risk.

Immunological products and vaccines

◼ RABIES VACCINE

Cautions see section 14.1

Contra-indications see section 14.1; but see also Post-exposure Management in notes above

Side-effects see section 14.1; also reported paresis

Indication and dose

Pre-exposure immunisation against rabies

• **By intramuscular injection in deltoid region or anterolateral thigh in infants**

Child 1 month–18 years 1 mL on days 0, 7, and 21 or 28; for those at continued risk give a single reinforcing dose 1 year after the primary course is completed and booster doses every 3–5 years; for those at intermittent risk give booster doses every 2–5 years

Post-exposure immunisation against rabies

• **By intramuscular injection in deltoid region or anterolateral thigh in infants**

Child 1 month–18 years 1 mL (see notes above)

Rabies Vaccine (Sanofi Pasteur) (PoM)
Rab
Injection, powder for reconstitution, freeze-dried inactivated Wistar rabies virus strain PM/ WI 38 1503-3M cultivated in human diploid cells, net price single-dose vial with syringe containing diluent = £24.40
Excipients include neomycin

Rabipur® (Novartis Vaccines) (PoM)
Injection, powder for reconstitution, freeze-dried inactivated Flury LEP rabies virus strain cultivated in chick embryo cells, net price single-dose vial = £24.40
Excipients include neomycin

Rotavirus vaccine

Rotavirus vaccine is a live, oral vaccine licensed for immunisation of infants over 6 weeks of age for protection against gastro-enteritis caused by rotavirus infection.

The rotavirus vaccine virus is excreted in the stool and may be transmitted to close contacts; the vaccine should be used with caution in those with immunosuppressed close contacts. Carers of a recently vaccinated baby should be advised of the need to wash their hands after changing the baby's nappies.

◼ ROTAVIRUS VACCINE

Cautions see section 14.1; *also* diarrhoea or vomiting (postpone vaccination); immunosuppressed close contacts (see notes above); **interactions**: Appendix 1 (vaccines)

Contra-indications see section 14.1; also predisposition to, or history of, intussusception

Side-effects see section 14.1

Indication and dose

Immunisation against gastro-enteritis caused by rotavirus infection

• **By mouth**

Child over 6 weeks 2 doses of 1 mL, separated by an interval of at least 4 weeks; course should

be completed before 24 weeks of age (preferably before 16 weeks)

Rotarix® (GSK) ▼ (PoM)
Oral suspension, powder for reconstitution, live attenuated rotavirus RIX4414 strain, net price single-dose vial (with oral syringe containing diluent) = £41.38

Rubella vaccine

A combined measles, mumps and rubella vaccine (MMR vaccine) aims to eliminate rubella (German measles) and congenital rubella syndrome. MMR vaccine is used for childhood vaccination as well as for vaccinating adults (including women of child-bearing age) who do not have immunity against rubella the combined live measles, mumps and rubella vaccine is a suitable alternative.

◀ Single antigen vaccine
No longer available in the UK; see MMR vaccine, p. 742

◀ Combined vaccines
see MMR vaccine

Smallpox vaccine

Limited supplies of **smallpox vaccine** are held at the Specialist and Reference Microbiology Division, Health Protection Agency (Tel. (020) 8200 4400) for the exclusive use of workers in laboratories where pox viruses (such as vaccinia) are handled.

If a wider use of the vaccine is being considered, *Guidelines for smallpox response and management in the post-eradication era* should be consulted at www.dh.gov.uk

Tetanus vaccines

Tetanus vaccine contains a cell-free purified toxin of *Clostridium tetani* adsorbed on aluminium hydroxide or aluminium phosphate to improve antigenicity.

Primary immunisation for children under 10 years consists of 3 doses of a combined preparation containing adsorbed tetanus vaccine (see Diphtheria-containing Vaccines), with an interval of 1 month between doses. Following routine childhood vaccination, 2 booster doses of a preparation containing adsorbed tetanus vaccine are recommended, the first before school entry and the second before leaving school. (see Immunisation schedule, section 14.1).

The recommended schedule of tetanus vaccination not only gives protection against tetanus in childhood but also gives the basic immunity for subsequent booster doses. In most circumstances, a total number of 5 doses of tetanus vaccine is considered sufficient for long-term protection.

For primary immunisation of children over 10 years previously unimmunised against tetanus, 3 doses of **adsorbed diphtheria [low dose], tetanus and inactivated poliomyelitis vaccine** are given with an interval of 1 month between doses (see Diphtheria-containing Vaccines).

Cautions   See also Section 14.1. When a child presents for a booster dose but has been vaccinated following a tetanus-prone wound, the vaccine preparation administered at the time of injury should be determined. If this is not possible, the booster should still be given to ensure adequate protection against all antigens in the booster vaccine.

Very rarely, tetanus has developed after abdominal surgery; carers of children awaiting elective surgery should be asked about the child's tetanus immunisation status and the child should be immunised if necessary.

Parenteral drug abuse is also associated with tetanus; those abusing drugs by injection should be vaccinated if unimmunised—booster doses should be given if there is any doubt about their immunisation status.

Travel recommendations see section 14.6.

Contra-indications   See section 14.1

Side-effects   See section 14.1

Wounds   Wounds are considered to be tetanus-prone if they are sustained more than 6 hours before surgical treatment *or* at any interval after injury and are puncture-type (particularly if contaminated with soil or manure) *or* show much devitalised tissue *or* are septic *or* are compound fractures *or* contain foreign bodies. All wounds should receive thorough cleansing.

- For *clean wounds*: fully immunised individuals (those who have received a total of 5 doses of a tetanus-containing vaccine at appropriate intervals) and those whose primary immunisation is complete (with boosters up to date), do not require tetanus vaccine; individuals whose primary immunisation is incomplete or whose boosters are not up to date require a reinforcing dose of a tetanus-containing vaccine (followed by further doses as required to complete the schedule); non-immunised individuals (or those whose immunisation status is not known or who have been fully immunised but are now immunocompromised) should be given a dose of the appropriate tetanus-containing vaccine immediately (followed by completion of the full course of the vaccine if records confirm the need).

- For *tetanus-prone wounds*: management is as for clean wounds with the addition of a dose of tetanus immunoglobulin (section 14.5) given at a different site; in fully immunised individuals and those whose primary immunisation is complete (with boosters up to date) the immunoglobulin is needed only if the risk of infection is especially high (e.g. contamination with manure). Antibacterial prophylaxis (with benzylpenicillin, co-amoxiclav, or metronidazole) may also be required for tetanus-prone wounds.

◀Combined vaccines
See Diphtheria-containing Vaccines

14 Immunological products and vaccines

Tick-borne encephalitis vaccine

Tick-borne encephalitis vaccine contains inactivated tick-bourne encephalitis virus cultivated in chick embryo cells. It is recommended for immunisation of those living in or visiting high-risk areas (see International Travel, section 14.6). Children walking or camping in warm forested areas of Central and Eastern Europe and Scandinavia, particularly from April to October when ticks are most prevalent, are at greatest risk of tick-borne encephalitis. For full protection, 3 doses of the vaccine are required; booster doses are required every 3–5 years for those still at risk. Ideally, immunisation should be completed at least one month before travel.

TICK-BORNE ENCEPHALITIS VACCINE, INACTIVATED

Cautions see section 14.1

Contra-indications see section 14.1

Side-effects see section 14.1

Indication and dose

Immunisation against tick-borne encephalitis

• **By intramuscular injection in deltoid region or anterolateral thigh in infants**

Child 1–16 years initial immunisation, 3 doses of 0.25 mL, second dose after 1–3 months and third dose after a further 5–12 months

Child 16–18 years 3 doses each of 0.5 mL, second dose after 1–3 months and third dose after further 5–12 months

Immunocompromised (including those receiving immunosuppressants), antibody concentra- tion may be measured 4 weeks after second dose and dose repeated if protective levels not achieved

Note To achieve more rapid protection, second dose may be given 14 days after first dose.

Booster doses, give first dose within 3 years after initial course, then every 3–5 years

TicoVac® (MASTA) [PoM]

Injection, suspension, formaldehyde-inactivated Neudörfl tick-borne encephalitis virus strain, (cultivated in chick embryo cells) adsorbed onto hydrated aluminium hydroxide, net price 0.25-mL prefilled syringe (*TicoVac Junior®*) = £28.00, 0.5-mL prefilled syringe = £32.00

Excipients include gentamicin and neomycin

Typhoid vaccines

Typhoid vaccine is available as Vi capsular polysaccharide injectable vaccine (from *Salmonella typhi*) for injection; and as live attenuated *Salmonella typhi* vaccine for oral use.

Typhoid immunisation is advised for children travelling to:

• areas where typhoid is endemic, especially if staying with or visiting local people

• endemic areas where frequent or prolonged exposure to poor sanitation and poor food hygiene is likely

Typhoid vaccination is not a substitute for scrupulous personal hygiene (see p. 759).

Capsular **polysaccharide typhoid vaccine** is usually given by *intramuscular* injection. Children under 2 years may respond suboptimally to the vaccine, but children aged between 1–2 years should be immunised if the risk of typhoid fever is considered high (immunisation is not recommended for infants under 12 months). Booster doses are needed every 3 years on continued exposure.

Oral typhoid vaccine is a **live attenuated** vaccine contained in an enteric-coated capsule. 3 doses of one capsule taken on alternate days, provides protection 7–10 days after the last dose. Protection may persist for up to 3 years in those constantly (or repeatedly) exposed to *Salmonella typhi*, but occasional travellers require further courses at intervals of 1 year.

Interactions   Oral typhoid vaccine is inactivated by concomitant administration of antibacterials or antimalarials:

• Antibacterials should be avoided for 3 days before and after oral typhoid vaccination;

• Mefloquine should be avoided for at least 12 hours before or after oral typhoid;

• For other antimalarials, vaccination with oral typhoid vaccine should be completed at least 3 days before the first dose of the antimalarial (except proguanil hydrochloride with atovaquone, which may be given concomitantly).

◢ TYPHOID VACCINE

Cautions   section 14.1; **interactions**: see above and Appendix 1 (vaccines)

Contra-indications   section 14.1; also for *oral* vaccine, acute gastro-intestinal illness

Side-effects   section 14.1

Indication and dose

Immunisation against typhoid fever

for dose see under preparations

◢Typhoid polysaccharide vaccine for injection
Typherix® (GSK) ᴘᴏᴹ

Injection, Vi capsular polysaccharide typhoid vaccine, 50 micrograms/mL virulence poly-saccharide antigen of *Salmonella typhi*, net price 0.5-mL prefilled syringe = £9.93

Dose

• **By intramuscular injection**

Child under 2 years [unlicensed use], 0.5 mL, at least 2 weeks before potential exposure to typhoid infection; response may be suboptimal (see notes above)

Child 2–18 years 0.5 mL, at least 2 weeks before potential exposure to typhoid infection

Typhim Vi® (Sanofi Pasteur) ᴘᴏᴹ

Injection, Vi capsular polysaccharide typhoid vaccine, 50 micrograms/mL virulence poly-saccharide antigen of formaldehyde-inactivated *Salmonella typhi*, net price 0.5-mL prefilled syringe = £9.49

Dose

• **By intramuscular injection**

Child under 2 years [unlicensed use], 0.5 mL, at least 2 weeks before potential exposure to typhoid infection; response may be suboptimal (see notes above)

Child 2–18 years 0.5 mL, at least 2 weeks before potential exposure to typhoid infection

◢Polysaccharide vaccine with hepatitis A vaccine
See Hepatitis A Vaccine

◢Typhoid vaccine, live (oral)
Vivotif® (MASTA) ᴘᴏᴹ

Capsules, e/c, live attenuated *Salmonella typhi* (Ty21a), net price 3-cap pack = £14.77. Label: 23, 25, counselling, administration

Dose

• **By mouth**

Child 6–18 years 1 capsule on days 1, 3, and 5

Counselling. Swallow as soon as possible after placing in mouth with a cold or lukewarm drink; it is important to store capsules in a refrigerator

---

Varicella–zoster vaccine

Varicella–zoster vaccine (live) is licensed for immunisation against varicella in seronegative individuals. It is not recommended for routine use in children but can be given to seronegative healthy children over 1 year who come into close contact with individuals at high risk of severe varicella infections.

Rarely, the varicella–zoster vaccine virus has been transmitted from the vaccinated individual to close contacts. Therefore, contact with the following should be avoided if a vaccine-related cutaneous rash develops within 4–6 weeks of the first or second dose:

• varicella-susceptible pregnant females;

• individuals at high risk of severe varicella, including those with immunodeficiency or those receiving immunosuppressive therapy.

Varicella–zoster immunoglobulin is used to protect susceptible children at increased risk of varicella infection, see p. 758

◢ VARICELLA–ZOSTER VACCINES

Cautions   see section 14.1; also post-vaccination close-contact with susceptible individuals (see notes above): **interactions**: Appendix 1 (vaccines)

Contra-indications   see section 14.1

Pregnancy   avoid pregnancy for 3 months after vaccination

Side-effects   see section 14.1; *also* varicella-like rash; *rarely* thrombocytopenia

Indication and dose

Immunisation against varicella infection (see notes above)

For dose, see under preparations

Varilrix® (GSK) ▼ ᴘᴏᴹ

Injection, powder for reconstitution, live attenuated varicella–zoster virus (Oka strain) propagated in human diploid cells, net price 0.5-mL vial (with diluent) = £27.31
Excipients include neomycin

Dose

• **By subcutaneous injection preferably into deltoid region**

Child 1–18 years (see notes above), 2 doses of 0.5 mL separated by an interval of at least 6 weeks (minimum 4 weeks)

14

Immunological products and vaccines

▱ **VARICELLA–ZOSTER VACCINES (continued)**

Varivax® (Sanofi Pasteur) ▼ PoM
Injection powder for reconstitution, live attenuated varicella-zoster virus (Oka/Merck strain) propagated in human diploid cells, net price 0.5-mL vial (with diluent) = £32.14
Excipients include gelatin and neomycin

Dose
- **By intramuscular or subcutaneous injection into deltoid region (or higher anterolateral thigh in young children)**

  Child 1–13 years (see notes above) 2 doses of 0.5 mL separated by an interval of at least 4 weeks (2 doses separated by 12 weeks in children with asymptomatic HIV infection)

  Child 13–18 years 2 doses of 0.5 mL separated by 4–8 weeks

Yellow fever vaccine

Live yellow fever vaccine is indicated for those travelling to or living in areas where infection is endemic (see p. 758). Infants under 6 months of age should not be vaccinated because there is a small risk of encephalitis; infants aged 6–9 months should be vaccinated only if the risk of yellow fever is high and unavoidable (seek expert advice). The immunity which probably lasts for life is officially accepted for 10 years starting from 10 days after primary immunisation and for a further 10 years immediately after revaccination.

Very rarely vaccine-associated adverse effects have been reported, such as viscerotropic disease (yellow fever vaccine-associated viscerotropic disease, YEL-AVD), a syndrome which may include metabolic acidosis, muscle and liver cytolysis, and multi-organ failure. Neurological disorders (yellow fever vaccine-associated neurotropic disease, YEL-AND) such as encephalitis have also been reported. These *very rare* adverse effects have usually occured after the first dose of yellow fever vaccine in those with no previous immunity.

Pregnancy and breast-feeding Live yellow fever vaccine should not be given during pregnancy but if a significant risk of exposure cannot be avoided then vaccination should be delayed to the third trimester if possible (but the need for immunisation usually outweighs risk to the fetus). Vaccination should be considered in breast-feeding women when there is a real risk to the mother from yellow fever disease.

YELLOW FEVER VACCINE

Cautions see section 14.1; pregnancy and breast-feeding, see notes above; also see **interactions**: Appendix 1 (vaccines)

Contra-indications see section 14.1 and notes above; also children under 6 months; history of thymus dysfunction

Side-effects see section 14.1; *also* reported neurotropic disease, and viscerotropic disease (see notes above)

Indication and dose

Immunisation against yellow fever
- **By deep subcutaneous injection**

  Child 9 months–18 years 0.5 mL (see also notes above)

Yellow Fever Vaccine, Live PoM
Yel(live)
Injection, powder for reconstitution, live, attenuated 17D-204 strain of yellow fever virus, cultivated in chick embryos; single dose vial with syringe containing 0.5 mL diluent
Available (only to designated Yellow Fever Vaccination centres) as *Stamaril®*

14.5 Immunoglobulins

Human immunoglobulins have replaced immunoglobulins of animal origin (antisera) which were frequently associated with hypersensitivity. Injection of immunoglobulins produces immediate protection lasting for several weeks.

Immunoglobulins are produced from pooled human plasma or serum, and are tested and found non-reactive for hepatitis B surface antigen and for antibodies against hepatitis C virus and human immunodeficiency virus (types 1 and 2)

The two types of human immunoglobulin preparation are **normal immuno-globulin** and **specific immunoglobulins**.

Further information about immunoglobulins is included in *Immunisation against Infectious Disease* (see section 14.1) and in the Health Protection Agency's *Immunoglobulin Handbook*: www.hpa.org.uk.

Availability **Normal immunoglobulin** is available from Health Protection and microbiology laboratories only for contacts and the control of outbreaks. It is available commercially for other purposes.

Specific immunoglobulins are available from Health Protection and microbiology laboratories with the exception of **tetanus immunoglobulin** which is distributed through BPL to hospital pharmacies or blood transfusion departments and is also available to general medical practitioners. **Rabies immunoglobulin** is available from the Specialist and Reference Microbiology Division, Health Protection Agency. The large amounts of **hepatitis B immunoglobulin** required by transplant centres should be obtained commercially.

In Scotland all immunoglobulins are available from the *Blood Transfusion Service*. **Tetanus immunoglobulin** is distributed by the *Blood Transfusion Service* to hospitals and general medical practitioners on demand.

Normal immunoglobulin

Human **normal immunoglobulin** ('HNIG') is prepared from pools of at least 1000 donations of human plasma; it contains antibody to measles, mumps, varicella, hepatitis A, and other viruses that are currently prevalent in the general population.

Cautions and side-effects Normal immunoglobulin is **contra-indicated** in patients with known class specific antibody to immunoglobulin A (IgA).

> **CHM advice**
> Intravenous normal immunoglobulin may very rarely induce thromboembolic events and should be used with caution in those with risk factors for arterial or venous thrombotic events and in obese individuals.

Normal immunoglobulin may **interfere with the immune response to live virus vaccines** which should therefore only be given **at least 3 weeks before or 3 months after** an injection of normal immunoglobulin (this does not apply to yellow fever vaccine since normal immunoglobulin does not contain antibody to this virus).

Side-effects of immunoglobulins include malaise, chills, fever, and rarely anaphylaxis.

Uses Normal immunoglobulin is administered by intramuscular injection for the protection of susceptible contacts against **hepatitis A** virus (infectious hepatitis), **measles** and, to a lesser extent, **rubella**.

Special formulations of immunoglobulins for intravenous administration are available for *replacement therapy* for children with congenital agammaglobulinaemia and hypogammaglobulinaemia, for the treatment of idiopathic thrombocytopenic purpura and Kawasaki syndrome (see section 2.9), and for the prophylaxis of infection following bone-marrow transplantation and in children with symptomatic HIV infection who have recurrent bacterial infections. Normal immunoglobulin may also be given intramuscularly or subcutaneously for replacement therapy, but intravenous formulations are normally preferred.

Intravenous immunoglobulin is also used in the treatment of Guillain-Barré syndrome in preference to plasma exchange.

Hepatitis A **Hepatitis A vaccine** is preferred for children at risk of infection (see p. 736) including those visiting areas where the disease is highly endemic (all countries excluding Northern and Western Europe, North America, Japan, Australia, and New Zealand). In unimmunised children, transmission of hepatitis A is reduced by good hygiene. Intramuscular normal immunoglobulin is no longer recommended for routine prophylaxis in travellers but it may be indicated for immunocompromised patients if their antibody response to vaccine is unlikely to be adequate.

14 Immunological products and vaccines

Intramuscular normal immunoglobulin is of value in the prevention of infection in close contacts of confirmed cases of hepatitis A where there has been a delay of more than 7 days in identifying contacts, or for close contacts at high risk of severe disease.

Measles   Intramuscular normal immunoglobulin may be given to prevent or attenuate an attack of measles in individuals who do not have adequate immunity. Children with compromised immunity who have come into contact with measles should receive intramuscular normal immunoglobulin as soon as possible after exposure. It is most effective if given within 72 hours but can be effective if given within 6 days. For individuals receiving intravenous immunoglobulin, 100 mg/kg given within 3 weeks before measles exposure should prevent measles. Intramuscular normal immunoglobulin should also be considered for the following individuals if they have been in contact with a confirmed case of measles or with a person associated with a local outbreak:

• non-immune pregnant women

• infants under 9 months

Further advice should be sought from the Centre for Infections, Health Protection Agency (tel. (020) 8200 6868).

Individuals with normal immunity who are not in the above categories and who have not been fully immunised against measles, can be given MMR vaccine (section 14.4) for prophylaxis following exposure to measles.

Rubella   Intramuscular immunoglobulin after exposure to rubella does **not** prevent infection in non-immune contacts and is **not** recommended for protection of pregnant females exposed to rubella. It may, however, reduce the likelihood of a clinical attack which may possibly reduce the risk to the fetus. It should be used only if termination of pregnancy would be unacceptable to the pregnant individual, when it should be given as soon as possible after exposure. Serological follow-up of recipients is essential. For routine prophylaxis, see MMR vaccine (p. 742).

◢For intramuscular use
Normal Immunoglobulin (PoM)

Normal immunoglobulin injection. 250-mg vial; 750-mg vial

Dose

To control outbreaks of hepatitis A (see notes above)
• **By deep intramuscular injection**
  Child under 10 years 250 mg
  Child 10–18 years 500 mg

Measles prophylaxis or to attenuate an attack
• **By deep intramuscular injection**
  Child under 1 year 250 mg
  Child 1–3 years 500 mg
  Child 3–18 years 750 mg

Rubella in pregnancy, prevention of clinical attack
• **By deep intramuscular injection**
  750 mg

Available from the Centre for Infections and other regional Health Protection Agency offices (for contacts and control of outbreaks only, see above)

◢For subcutaneous use
Subcuvia® (Baxter) (PoM)

Normal immunoglobulin injection, net price 5-mL vial = £32.56, 10-mL vial = £65.12

Dose

Antibody deficiency syndromes
• **By subcutaneous injection**

  Consult product literature
  Note May be administered by intramuscular injection (if subcutaneous route not possible) but **not** for patients with bleeding disorders

Subgam® (BPL) (PoM)

Normal immunoglobulin injection, net price 250-mg vial = £11.20, 750-mg vial = £28.50, 1.5-g vial = £57.00

Dose

Antibody deficiency syndromes
• **By subcutaneous injection**

  Consult product literature
  Note May be administered by intramuscular injection (if subcutaneous route not possible) but **not** for patients with bleeding disorders

Vivaglobin® (CSL Behring) (PoM)

Normal immunoglobulin injection, net price 3-mL vial £17.76, 10-mL vial = £59.20, 20-mL vial = £118.40

Dose

Antibody deficiency syndromes
• **By subcutaneous injection**

  Consult product literature

◀ For intravenous use

Normal Immunoglobulin for Intravenous Use PoM

Brands include *Flebogamma®* 5% (0.5 g, 2.5 g, 5 g, 10 g); *Gammagard® S/D* (0.5 g, 2.5 g, 5 g, 10 g); *Octagam®* ▼ (5%—2.5 g, 5 g, 10 g; 10%—5g, 10g); *Privigen®* ▼ (5g, 10g, 20g); *Sandoglobulin NF®* (6 g, 12 g); *Vigam® S* (2.5 g, 5 g); *Vigam® Liquid* (2.5 g, 5 g, 10 g)

Dose

Kawasaki syndrome
• By intravenous infusion
  Child 1 month–12 years 2 g/kg as a single dose within 10 days of onset of symptoms (but children with a delayed diagnosis may also benefit)

Other indications Consult product literature

Specific immunoglobulins

Specific immunoglobulins are prepared by pooling the plasma of selected donors with high levels of the specific antibody required.

Although a hepatitis B vaccine is now available for those at high risk of infection, specific **hepatitis B immunoglobulin** ('HBIG') is available for use in association with hepatitis B vaccine for the prevention of infection in infants born to mothers who have become infected with this virus in pregnancy or who are high-risk carriers (see Hepatitis B Vaccine, p. 737).

Following exposure of an unimmunised individual to an animal in or from a high-risk country, the site of the bite should be washed with soapy water and specific **rabies immunoglobulin** of human origin should be administered; as much of the dose as possible should be injected in and around the cleansed wound. Rabies vaccine should also be given (for details see Rabies Vaccine, BNF section 14.4).

For the management of tetanus-prone wounds, **tetanus immunoglobulin** of human origin ('HTIG') should be used in addition to wound cleansing and, where appropriate, antibacterial prophylaxis and a tetanus-containing vaccine (section 14.4). Tetanus immunoglobulin, together with metronidazole (section 5.1.11) and wound cleansing, should also be used for the treatment of established cases of tetanus.

Varicella–zoster immunoglobulin (VZIG) is recommended for individuals who are at increased risk of severe varicella *and* who have no antibodies to varicella–zoster virus *and* who have significant exposure to chickenpox or herpes zoster. Those at increased risk include:

● neonates whose mothers develop chickenpox in the period 7 days before to 7 days after delivery;

● susceptible neonates exposed in the first 7 days of life;

● susceptible neonates or infants exposed whilst requiring intensive or prolonged special care nursing;

● susceptible women exposed at any stage of pregnancy (but when supplies of VZIG are short, may only be issued to those exposed in the first 20 weeks' gestation or to those near term) providing VZIG is given within 10 days of contact;

● immunosuppressed individuals including those who have received corticosteroids in the previous 3 months at the following dose equivalents of prednisolone: *children* 2 mg/kg daily (or more than 40 mg) for at least 1 week or 1 mg/kg daily for 1 month.

Important: for full details consult *Immunisation against Infectious Disease*. **Varicella–zoster vaccine** is available—see section 14.4.

◀ Hepatitis B

Hepatitis B Immunoglobulin PoM

See notes above

Dose

• By intramuscular injection
  (as soon as possible after exposure; ideally within 12 hours, but no later than 7 days after exposure)

Neonate 200 units as soon as possible after birth; for full details consult *Immunisation against Infectious Disease*

Child 1 month–5 years 200 units

Child 5–10 years 300 units

Child 10–18 years 500 units

Available from selected Health Protection Agency and NHS laboratories (except for Transplant Centres, see p. 755), also available from BPL and SNBTS (as *Liberim HB®*)

Note Hepatitis B immunoglobulin for intravenous use is available from BPL on a named-patient basis.

14

Immunological products and vaccines

◢Rabies

Rabies Immunoglobulin PoM
(Antirabies Immunoglobulin Injection)

See notes above

Dose

20 units/kg, *by infiltration* in and around the cleansed wound; if the wound not visible or healed or if infiltration of whole volume not possible, give remainder *by intramuscular injection* into anterolateral thigh (remote from vaccination site)

Available from Specialist and Reference Microbiology Division, Health Protection Agency (also from BPL)

◢Tetanus

Tetanus Immunoglobulin PoM
(Antitetanus Immunoglobulin Injection)

See notes above

Dose

Prophylaxis
• By intramuscular injection

250 units, increased to 500 units if more than 24 hours have elapsed or there is risk of heavy contamination or following burns

Therapeutic
• By intramuscular injection

150 units/kg (multiple sites)

Available from BPL
Note May be difficult to obtain

◢Varicella–zoster

Varicella–Zoster Immunoglobulin PoM
(Antivaricella–zoster Immunoglobulin)

See notes above

Dose

Prophylaxis (as soon as possible—not later than 10 days after exposure)
• By deep intramuscular injection

Neonate 250 mg

Child 1 month–6 years 250 mg

Child 6–11 years 500 mg

Child 11–15 years 750 mg

Child 15–18 years 1 g

Give second dose if further exposure occurs more than 3 weeks after first dose

Note No evidence that effective in treatment of severe disease. Normal immunoglobulin for intravenous use may be used in those unable to receive intramuscular injection.
Available from selected Health Protection Agency and NHS laboratories (also from BPL)

Anti-D (Rh$_0$) immunoglobulin

This section is not included in *BNF for Children*. See BNF for use of Anti-D (Rh$_0$) immunoglobulin

---

14.6 International travel

Note For advice on **malaria chemoprophylaxis**, see section 5.4.1.

No special immunisation is required for travellers to the United States, Europe, Australia, or New Zealand although all travellers should have immunity to tetanus and poliomyelitis (and childhood immunisations should be up to date). Certain precautions are required in Non-European areas surrounding the Mediterranean, in Africa, the Middle East, Asia, and South America.

Travellers to areas that have a high incidence of **poliomyelitis** or **tuberculosis** should be immunised with the appropriate vaccine; in the case of poliomyelitis previously immunised adults may be given a booster dose of a preparation containing inactivated poliomyelitis vaccine. BCG immunisation is recommended for travellers aged under 16 years proposing to stay for longer than 3 months (or in close contact with the local population) in countries with an incidence[1] of tuberculosis greater than 40 per 100 000; it should preferably be given three months or more before departure.

Yellow fever immunisation is recommended for travel to the endemic zones of Africa and South America. Many countries require an International Certificate of Vaccination from individuals arriving from, or who have been travelling through, endemic areas, whilst other countries require a certificate from all entering travellers (consult the Department of Health handbook, *Health Information for Overseas Travel*, www.dh.gov.uk).

---

1. List of countries where the incidence of tuberculosis is greater than 40 cases per 100 000 is available at www.hpa.org.uk

Immunisation against **meningococcal meningitis** is recommended for a number of areas of the world (for details, see p. 744).

Protection against **hepatitis A** is recommended for travellers to high-risk areas outside Northern and Western Europe, North America, Japan, Australia and New Zealand. Hepatitis A vaccine (see p. 736) is preferred and it is likely to be effective even if given shortly before departure; normal immunoglobulin is no longer given routinely but may be indicated in the immunocompromised (see p. 755). Special care must also be taken with food hygiene (see below).

Hepatitis B vaccine (see p. 737) is recommended for those travelling to areas of high prevalence who plan to remain there for lengthy periods and who may therefore be at increased risk of acquiring infection as the result of medical or dental procedures carried out in those countries. Short-term tourists are not generally at increased risk of infection but may place themselves at risk by their sexual behaviour when abroad.

Prophylactic immunisation against **rabies** (see Rabies Vaccine, BNF section 14.4) is recommended for travellers to enzootic areas on long journeys or to areas out of reach of immediate medical attention.

Travellers who have not had a **tetanus** booster in the last 10 years and are visiting areas where medical attention may not be accessible should receive a booster dose of adsorbed diphtheria [low dose], tetanus and inactivated poliomyelitis vaccine (see p. 733), even if they have received 5 doses of a tetanus-containing vaccine previously.

Typhoid vaccine is indicated for travellers to those countries where typhoid is endemic but the vaccine is no substitute for personal precautions (see below).

There is no requirement for cholera vaccination as a condition for entry into any country, but **oral cholera vaccine** (see p. 732) may be considered for backpackers and those travelling to situations where the risk is greatest (e.g. refugee camps). Regardless of vaccination, travellers to areas where cholera is endemic should take special care with food hygiene (see below).

Advice on **diphtheria**, on **Japanese encephalitis**[1] (vaccine available on named-patient basis from Sanofi Pasteur and MASTA) and on **tick-borne encephalitis** is included in *Health Information for Overseas Travel*, see below.

Food hygiene   In areas where sanitation is poor, good food hygiene is important to help prevent hepatitis A, typhoid, cholera, and other diarrhoeal diseases (including travellers' diarrhoea). Food should be freshly prepared and hot, and uncooked vegetables (including green salads) should be avoided; only fruits which can be peeled should be eaten. Only suitable bottled water, or tap water that has been boiled, or treated with sterilising tablets should be used for drinking.

Information on health advice for travellers
The Department of Health booklet, *Health Advice For Travellers* (code: T7.1) includes information on immunisation requirements (or recommendations) around the world and precautions for avoiding disease, while travelling. The booklet can be obtained from GP surgeries, travel agents, or post-offices, or by telephoning (24-hour service) 0300 123 1002; also available on the Internet at: www.dh.gov.uk or email: dh@prolog.uk.com

The Department of Health handbook, *Health Information for Overseas Travel* (2001), which draws together essential information *for healthcare professionals* regarding health advice for travellers, can be obtained from

The Stationery Office

PO Box 29, Norwich NR3 1GN

Telephone orders, 0870 600 5522

Fax: 0870 600 5533

www.tso.co.uk

14 Immunological products and vaccines

---

1. Japanese encephalitis vaccine not prescribable on the NHS; health authorities may investigate circumstances under which vaccine prescribed

Immunisation requirements change from time to time, and information on the current requirements for any particular country may be obtained from the embassy or legation of the appropriate country or from:

National Travel Health Network and Centre
Hospital for Tropical Diseases
Mortimer Market Centre
Capper Street, off Tottenham Court Road
London, WC1E 6AU.
Tel: 0845 602 6712
(9 a.m.–noon, 2–4.30 p.m. weekdays for healthcare professionals **only**)
www.nathnac.org

Travel Medicine Team
Health Protection Scotland
Clifton House
Clifton Place
Glasgow, G3 7LN.
Tel: (0141) 300 1100
(2 p.m.–4 p.m. weekdays)
www.travax.nhs.uk (registration required. Annual fee may be payable for users outside NHS Scotland)

Welsh Medicines Information Centre
University Hospital of Wales
Cardiff, CF14 4XW.
Tel: (029) 2074 2979
(08.30 a.m.–5 p.m. weekdays for health professionals in Wales **only**)

Department of Health and Social Services
Castle Buildings
Stormont
Belfast, BT4 3PP.
Tel: (028) 9052 0000

15 Anaesthesia

15.1 General anaesthesia **761**
15.1.1 Intravenous anaesthetics 763
15.1.2 Inhalational anaesthetics 766
15.1.3 Antimuscarinic drugs 769
15.1.4 Sedative and analgesic peri-operative drugs 771
15.1.5 Neuromuscular blocking drugs 778
15.1.6 Drugs for reversal of neuromuscular blockade 783
15.1.7 Antagonists for central and respiratory depression 784
15.1.8 Drugs for malignant hyperthermia 786
15.2 Local anaesthesia **786**

15.1 General anaesthesia

15.1.1 Intravenous anaesthetics
15.1.2 Inhalational anaesthetics
15.1.3 Antimuscarinic drugs
15.1.4 Sedative and analgesic peri-operative drugs
15.1.5 Neuromuscular blocking drugs
15.1.6 Drugs for reversal of neuromuscular blockade
15.1.7 Antagonists for central and respiratory depression
15.1.8 Drugs for malignant hyperthermia

> **Note**
> The drugs in section 15.1 should be used only by experienced personnel and where adequate resuscitation equipment is available.

Several different types of drug are given together during general anaesthesia. Anaesthesia is induced with either a volatile drug given by inhalation (section 15.1.2) or with an intravenously administered drug (section 15.1.1); anaesthesia is maintained with an intravenous or inhalational anaesthetic. Analgesics (section 15.1.4), usually short-acting opioids, are also used. The use of neuromuscular blocking drugs (section 15.1.5) necessitates intermittent positive-pressure ventilation. Following surgery, anticholinesterases (section 15.1.6) can be given to reverse the effects of neuromuscular blocking drugs; specific antagonists (section 15.1.7) can be used to reverse central and respiratory depression caused by some drugs used in surgery. A topical local anaesthetic (section 15.2) can be used to reduce pain at the injection site.

Individual requirements vary considerably and the recommended doses are only a guide. Smaller doses are indicated in ill, shocked, or debilitated children and in significant hepatic impairment, while robust individuals may require larger doses. The required dose of induction agent may be less if the patient has been premedicated with a sedative agent (section 15.1.4) or if an opioid analgesic has been used.

Surgery and long-term medication   The risk of losing disease control on stopping long-term medication before surgery is often greater than the risk posed by continuing it during surgery. It is vital that the anaesthetist knows about **all** drugs that a child is (or has been) taking.

Children with adrenal atrophy resulting from long-term corticosteroid use (section 6.3.2) may suffer a precipitous fall in blood pressure unless corticosteroid cover is provided during anaesthesia and in the immediate postoperative period. Anaesthetists must therefore know whether a child is, or has been, receiving corticosteroids (including high-dose inhaled corticosteroids).

15 Anaesthesia

Other drugs that should normally not be stopped before surgery include drugs for epilepsy, asthma, immunosuppression, and metabolic, endocrine and cardiovascular disorders (but see potassium sparing diuretics, below). Expert advice is required for children receiving antivirals for HIV infection. For general advice on surgery in children with diabetes, see section 6.1.1.

Children taking aspirin or an oral anticoagulant present an increased risk for surgery. In these circumstances, the anaesthetist and surgeon should assess the relative risks and decide jointly whether aspirin or the anticoagulant should be stopped or replaced with heparin therapy.

Drugs that should be stopped before surgery include combined oral contraceptives (see Surgery, section 7.3.1 for details). If antidepressants need to be stopped, they should be withdrawn gradually to avoid withdrawal symptoms. Tricyclic antidepressants need not be stopped, but there may be an increased risk of arrhythmias and hypotension (and dangerous interactions with vasopressor drugs); therefore, the anaesthetist should be informed if they are not stopped. Lithium should be stopped 24 hours before major surgery but the normal dose can be continued for minor surgery (with careful monitoring of fluids and electrolytes). Potassium-sparing diuretics may need to be withheld on the morning of surgery because hyperkalaemia may develop if renal perfusion is impaired or if there is tissue damage.

Anaesthesia and skilled tasks   Children and their carers should be very carefully warned about the risk of undertaking skilled tasks after the use of sedatives and analgesics during minor outpatient procedures. For intravenous benzodiazepines and for a short general anaesthetic the risk extends to **at least 24 hours** after administration. Responsible persons should be available to take children home. The dangers of taking **alcohol** should also be emphasised.

Prophylaxis of acid aspiration   Regurgitation and aspiration of gastric contents (Mendelson's syndrome) is an important complication of general anaesthesia, particularly in obstetrics, during emergency surgery and in gastro-oesophageal reflux disease; prophylaxis against acid aspiration may be required in children.

An **H$_2$-receptor antagonist** (section 1.3.1) or a **proton pump inhibitor** (section 1.3.5) such as omeprazole may be used before surgery to increase the pH and reduce the volume of gastric fluid. They do not affect the pH of fluid already in the stomach and this limits their value in emergency procedures; oral H$_2$-receptor antagonists can be given 1–2 hours before the procedure but omeprazole must be given at least 12 hours earlier. Antacids are frequently used to neutralise the acidity of the fluid already in the stomach; 'clear' (non-particulate) antacids such as sodium citrate are preferred. Sodium citrate 300 mmol/litre (88.2 mg/mL) oral solution is licensed for use before general anaesthesia for caesarean section (available from Viridian).

Anaesthesia, sedation and resuscitation in dental practice

For details see *A Conscious Decision: A review of the use of general anaesthesia and conscious sedation in primary dental care*; report by a group chaired by the Chief Medical Officer and Chief Dental Officer, July 2000 and associated documents. Further details can also be found in *Conscious Sedation in the Provision of Dental Care*; report of an Expert Group on Sedation for Dentistry (commissioned by the Department of Health), 2003. Both documents are available at www.dh.gov.uk.

Guidance is also included in *Standards for Dental Professionals*, London, General Dental Council, May 2005 (and as amended subsequently) and *Conscious Sedation in Dentistry: Dental Clinical Guidance*, Scottish Dental Clinical Effectiveness Programme, May 2006.

Gas cylinders

Each gas cylinder bears a label with the name of the gas contained in the cylinder. The name or chemical symbol of the gas appears on the shoulder of the cylinder and is also clearly and indelibly stamped on the cylinder valve.

15 Anaesthesia

The colours on the valve end of the cylinder extend down to the shoulder; in the case of mixed gases the colours for the individual gases are applied in four segments, two for each colour.

Gas cylinders should be stored in a cool well-ventilated room, free from flammable materials.

No lubricant of any description should be used on the cylinder valves.

15.1.1 Intravenous anaesthetics

Intravenous anaesthetics may be used either to induce anaesthesia or for maintenance of anaesthesia throughout surgery. Intravenous anaesthetics nearly all produce their effect in one arm-brain circulation time and can cause apnoea and hypotension, and so adequate resuscitative facilities **must** be available. They are **contra-indicated** if the anaesthetist is not confident of being able to maintain the airway. Extreme care is required in surgery of the mouth, pharynx, or larynx and in children with acute circulatory failure (shock) or fixed cardiac output.

To facilitate tracheal intubation, induction is usually followed by a neuromuscular blocking drug (section 15.1.5) or short-acting opioid (section 15.1.4.3).

Total intravenous anaesthesia   This is a technique in which surgery is carried out with all drugs given intravenously. Respiration can be spontaneous, or controlled with oxygen-enriched air. Neuromuscular blocking drugs can be used to provide relaxation and prevent reflex muscle movements. The main problem to be overcome is the assessment of depth of anaesthesia. Target Controlled Infusion (TCI) systems can be used to titrate intravenous anaesthetic infusions to predicted plasma-drug concentrations; specific models with paediatric pharmacokinetic data should be used for children.

Anaesthesia and skilled tasks   See section 15.1.

Drugs used for intravenous anaesthesia   **Propofol** is associated with rapid recovery without a hangover effect and it is very widely used. There is sometimes pain on intravenous injection which can be reduced by intravenous lidocaine. Significant extraneous muscle movements may occur. Convulsions, anaphylaxis, and delayed recovery from anaesthesia can occur after propofol administration; since the onset of convulsions can be delayed, the CSM has advised special caution after day surgery. Propofol has been associated with bradycardia, occasionally profound; intravenous administration of an antimuscarinic drug may prevent this.

Thiopental sodium (thiopentone sodium) is a barbiturate that is used widely for induction of anaesthesia, but it has no analgesic properties. Induction is generally smooth and rapid, but dose-related cardiorespiratory depression can occur. Awakening from a moderate dose of thiopental is rapid because the drug redistributes into other tissues, particularly fat. However, metabolism is slow and sedative effects can persist for 24 hours. Repeated doses have a cumulative effect particularly in neonates, and recovery is much slower.

Etomidate is an induction agent associated with rapid recovery without a hangover effect. It causes less hypotension than thiopental and propofol during induction. It produces a high incidence of extraneous muscle movement, which can be minimised by an opioid analgesic or a short-acting benzodiazepine given just before induction. Pain on injection can be reduced by injecting into a larger vein or by giving an opioid analgesic just before induction. Etomidate may suppress adrenocortical function, particularly on continuous administration, and it should not be used for maintenance of anaesthesia.

Ketamine has good analgesic properties at sub-anaesthetic dosage and it causes less hypotension than thiopental and propofol during induction. It is often used in children requiring repeat anaesthesia (such as for serial burns dressings), however recovery is relatively slow and there is a high incidence of extraneous muscle movements. The main disadvantage of ketamine is the high incidence of hallucinations, nightmares, and other transient psychotic effects; these can be reduced by a benzodiazepine, such as diazepam or midazolam. Ketamine also has abuse potential and may lead to dependence.

15 Anaesthesia

ETOMIDATE

Cautions see notes above; avoid in acute porphyria (section 9.8.2); **interactions:** Appendix 1 (anaesthetics, general)

Hepatic impairment reduce dose in liver cirrhosis

Pregnancy depresses neonatal respiration in third trimester

Breast-feeding avoid for 24 hours after administration

Contra-indications see notes above

Side-effects see notes above; also coughing, hiccups, shivering, allergic reactions (including bronchospasm and anaphylaxis); respiratory depression, arrhythmias, and convulsions also reported

Indication and dose

See under preparations

Etomidate-Lipuro® (Braun) (PoM)
Injection (emulsion), etomidate 2 mg/mL, net price 10-mL amp = £1.53
Dose

> Induction of anaesthesia
> • By slow intravenous injection
>   Child 1 month–18 years 150–300 micrograms/kg; child under 10 years may need up to 400 micrograms/kg

Hypnomidate® (Janssen-Cilag) (PoM)
Injection, etomidate 2 mg/mL, net price 10-mL amp = £1.47
Excipients include propylene glycol (see Excipients, p. 3)
Dose

> Induction of anaesthesia
> • By slow intravenous injection
>   Child 1 month–18 years 300 micrograms/kg; max. total dose 60 mg

KETAMINE

Cautions see notes above; increased cerebrospinal fluid pressure; predisposition to hallucinations or nightmares; **interactions:** Appendix 1 (anaesthetics, general)

Pregnancy depresses neonatal respiration in third trimester

Contra-indications see notes above; hypertension, pre-eclampsia or eclampsia, severe cardiac disease, stroke; raised intracranial pressure; head trauma; acute porphyria (section 9.8.2)

Side-effects see notes above; also tachycardia, hypertension, arrhythmias, hypotension, bradycardia; increased salivation, laryngospasm; anxiety, insomnia, diplopia, nystagmus, raised intra-ocular pressure; rashes, injection-site reactions; anaphylaxis also reported

Indication and dose

Premedication prior to invasive or painful procedures
• By intravenous injection
  Child 1 month–18 years 1–2 mg/kg as a single dose

Induction and maintenance of anaesthesia (short procedures)
• By intravenous injection over at least 60 seconds

  Neonate 1–2 mg/kg produces 5–10 minutes of surgical anaesthesia, adjusted according to response

  Child 1 month–12 years 1–2 mg/kg produces 5–10 minutes of surgical anaesthesia, adjusted according to response

  Child 12–18 years 1–4.5 mg/kg (usually 2 mg/kg) produces 5–10 minutes of surgical anaesthesia, adjusted according to response

• By intramuscular injection

  Neonate 4 mg/kg usually produces 15 minutes of surgical anaesthesia, adjusted according to response

  Child 1 month–18 years 4–13 mg/kg (4 mg/kg sufficient for some diagnostic procedures), adjusted according to response; 10 mg/kg usually produces 12–25 minutes of surgical anaesthesia

Induction and maintenance of anaesthesia (longer procedures)
• By continuous intravenous infusion

  Neonate initially 0.5–2 mg/kg followed by a continuous intravenous infusion of 500 micrograms/kg/hour adjusted according to response; up to 2 mg/kg/hour may be used to produce deep anaesthesia

  Child 1 month–18 years initially 0.5–2 mg/kg followed by a continuous intravenous infusion of 0.6–2.7 mg/kg/hour adjusted according to response

Administration for *continuous intravenous infusion*, dilute to a concentration of 1 mg/mL with Glucose 5% *or* Sodium Chloride 0.9%; use microdrip infusion for maintenance of anaesthesia

For *intravenous injection*, dilute 100 mg/mL strength to a concentration of not more than 50 mg/mL with Glucose 5% *or* Sodium Chloride 0.9% *or* Water for Injections

Ketalar® (Pfizer) (PoM)
Injection, ketamine (as hydrochloride) 10 mg/mL, net price 20-mL vial = £4.22; 50 mg/mL, 10-mL vial = £8.77; 100 mg/mL, 10-mL vial = £16.10

PROPOFOL

Cautions see notes above; cardiac impairment; respiratory impairment; hypovolaemia; epilepsy; hypotension; raised intracranial pressure; monitor blood-lipid concentration if risk of fat overload or if sedation longer than 3 days; **interactions**: Appendix 1 (anaesthetics, general)

Hepatic impairment use with caution

Renal impairment use with caution

Pregnancy depresses neonatal respiration in third trimester; for maintenance of anaesthesia, doses of propofol should not exceed 6 mg/kg/hour

Breast-feeding present in milk but amount probably too small to be harmful

Contra-indications see notes above; sedation of ventilated children under 17 years in intensive care (risk of potentially fatal effects including metabolic acidosis, cardiac failure, rhabdomyolysis, hyperlipidaemia, and hepatomegaly)

Side-effects see notes above; also hypotension, tachycardia, flushing; transient apnoea, hyperventilation, coughing, and hiccup during induction; headache; *less commonly* thrombosis, phlebitis; *rarely* arrhythmia, headache, vertigo, shivering, euphoria; *very rarely* pancreatitis, pulmonary oedema, sexual disinhibition, and discoloration of urine; serious and sometimes fatal side-effects reported with prolonged infusion of doses exceeding 5 mg/kg/hour, including metabolic acidosis, rhabdomyolysis, hyperkalaemia, and cardiac failure, dystonia and dyskinesia also reported

Licensed use *Diprivan®* 2%, *Propofol-Lipuro®* 2%, and *Propoven®* 2% not licensed for use in children under 3 years; *Diprofusor®* TCI ('target controlled infusion') system not licensed for use in children

Indication and dose

Induction of anaesthesia
- **By intravenous injection or by intravenous infusion**

   Child 1 month–3 years 2.5–4 mg/kg administered slowly until response (using *Diprivan®* 1%, *Propofol-Lipuro®* 1%, and *Propoven®* 1% only)

   Child 3–8 years 2.5–4 mg/kg administered slowly until response

   Child 8–12 years 2.5 mg/kg administered slowly until response

   Child 12–18 years 1.5–2.5 mg/kg at a rate of 20–40 mg every 10 seconds until response

Maintenance of anaesthesia
- **By continuous intravenous infusion**

   Child 1 month–3 years 9–15 mg/kg/hour (using *Diprivan®* 1%, *Propofol-Lipuro®* 1%, and *Propoven®* 1% only), adjusted according to response

   Child 3–12 years 9–15 mg/kg/hour, adjusted according to response

   Child 12–18 years 4–12 mg/kg/hour, adjusted according to response

Sedation of ventilated children in intensive care
- **By continuous intravenous infusion**

   Child 17–18 years 0.3–4 mg/kg/hour, adjusted according to response

Induction of sedation for surgical and diagnostic procedures (1% emulsion only)
- **By intravenous injection over 1–5 minutes**

   Child 17–18 years 0.5–1 mg/kg

Maintenance of sedation for surgical and diagnostic procedures (1% emulsion only)
- **By intravenous infusion**

   Child 17–18 years 1.5–4.5 mg/kg/hour (additionally if rapid increase in sedation required, *by intravenous injection* 10–20 mg)

Administration for *continuous intravenous infusion*; microbiological filter not recommended; **1% emulsion** may be infused undiluted using a suitable infusion pump; may also be administered via a Y-piece close to injection site co-administered with Glucose 5% *or* Sodium Chloride 0.9%; *alternatively* dilute to a concentration not less than 2 mg/mL with Glucose 5% (*or* Sodium Chloride 0.9% for *Propofol-Lipuro®*, *Propoven®*, Braun, and Fresenius Kabi brands); use glass or PVC containers (if PVC bag used, it should be full—withdraw volume of infusion fluid equal to that of propofol to be added); give within 6 hours of preparation

2% emulsion do not dilute; may be administered via a Y-piece close to injection site co-administered with Glucose 5% *or* Sodium Chloride 0.9%

Propofol (Non-proprietary) ⓅⓄⓂ
1% injection (emulsion), propofol 10 mg/mL, net price 20-mL amp = £2.33, 50-mL bottle = £5.82, 100-mL bottle = £11.64

2% injection (emulsion), propofol 20 mg/mL, net price 50-mL vial = £11.64
Brands include *Propofol-Lipuro®*, *Propoven®*

Diprivan® (AstraZeneca) ⓅⓄⓂ
1% injection (emulsion), propofol 10 mg/mL, net price 20-mL amp = £3.88, 50-mL prefilled syringe (for use with *Diprifusor®* TCI system) = £10.67

2% injection (emulsion), propofol 20 mg/mL, net price 50-mL prefilled syringe (for use with *Diprifusor®* TCI system) = £20.37

THIOPENTAL SODIUM
(Thiopentone sodium)

Cautions see notes above; cardiovascular disease; reconstituted solution is highly alkaline—extravasation causes tissue necrosis and severe pain; avoid intra-arterial injection; **interactions**: Appendix 1 (anaesthetics, general)

Hepatic impairment reduce induction dose in severe liver disease

Pregnancy depresses neonatal respiration in the third trimester—dose should not exceed 250 mg

15

Anaesthesia

◻ **THIOPENTAL SODIUM** (*continued*)

Contra-indications see notes above; acute porphyria (section 9.8.2); myotonic dystrophy

Breast-feeding present in milk—manufacturer advises avoid

Side-effects hypotension, arrhythmias, myocardial depression, laryngeal spasm, cough, sneezing; hypersensitivity reactions; rash, injection-site reactions; excessive doses associated with hypothermia and profound reduction in cerebral function

Licensed use not licensed for use in status epilepticus; not licensed for use by intravenous infusion

Indication and dose

Induction of anaesthesia
• **By slow intravenous injection**

Neonate initially up to 2 mg/kg, then 1 mg/kg repeated as necessary (max. total dose 4 mg/kg)

Child 1 month–18 years initially up to 4 mg/kg, then 1 mg/kg repeated as necessary (max. total dose 7 mg/kg)

Prolonged status epilepticus
• **By slow intravenous injection and intravenous infusion**

Neonate initially up to 2 mg/kg by intravenous injection, then up to 8 mg/kg/hour by continuous intravenous infusion, adjusted according to response

Child 1 month–18 years initially up to 4 mg/kg by intravenous injection, then up to 8 mg/kg/hour by continuous intravenous infusion, adjusted according to response

Administration For *intravenous injection*, dilute to a concentration of 25 mg/mL with Water for Injections, and give over at least 10–15 seconds; for *intravenous infusion* dilute to a concentration of 2.5 mg/mL with Sodium Chloride 0.9%

Thiopental (Link) [PoM]
Injection, powder for reconstitution, thiopental sodium, net price 500-mg vial = £3.06

15.1.2 Inhalational anaesthetics

Inhalational anaesthetics may be gases or volatile liquids. They can be used both for induction and maintenance of anaesthesia and can also be used following induction with an intravenous anaesthetic (section 15.1.1).

Gaseous anaesthetics require suitable equipment for storage and administration. They may be supplied via hospital pipelines or from metal cylinders. *Volatile liquid anaesthetics* are administered using calibrated vaporisers, using air, oxygen, or nitrous oxide–oxygen mixtures as the carrier gas; all can trigger malignant hyperthermia (section 15.1.8) and are contra-indicated in those susceptible to malignant hyperthermia. Volatile liquid anaesthetics can increase cerebrospinal pressure and should be used with caution in children with raised intracranial pressure.

In children with neuromuscular disease, inhalational anaesthetics are associated with very rare cases of hyperkalaemia resulting in cardiac arrhythmias and death.

To prevent hypoxia, the inspired gas mixture should contain a minimum of 25% oxygen at all times. Higher concentrations of oxygen (greater than 30%) are usually required during inhalational anaesthesia with nitrous oxide, see Nitrous oxide, p. 768.

Anaesthesia and skilled tasks See section 15.1.

Volatile liquid anaesthetics

Isoflurane is a volatile liquid anaesthetic. Heart rhythm is generally stable during isoflurane anaesthesia, but heart-rate can rise. Systemic arterial pressure can fall and cardiac output can decrease, owing to a decrease in systemic vascular resistance. Respiration is depressed. Muscle relaxation occurs and the effects of muscle relaxant drugs are potentiated. Isoflurane can cause hepatotoxicity in those sensitised to halogenated anaesthetics.

Desflurane is a rapid acting volatile liquid anaesthetic; it is reported to have about one-fifth the potency of isoflurane. Emergence and recovery from anaesthesia are particularly rapid because of its low solubility. Desflurane is not recommended for induction of anaesthesia as it is irritant to the upper respiratory tract; cough, breath-holding, apnoea, laryngospasm, and increased secretions can occur. The risk of hepatotoxicity with desflurane in those sensitised to halogenated anaesthetics appears to be remote.

Sevoflurane is a rapid acting volatile liquid anaesthetic and is more potent than desflurane. Emergence and recovery are particularly rapid but slower than desflurane. Sevoflurane is non-irritant and is therefore used for inhalational induction of anaesthesia. Sevoflurane can interact with carbon dioxide absorbents to form compound A, a potentially nephrotoxic vinyl ether. However, in spite of extensive use, no cases of sevoflurane-induced permanent renal injury have been reported and the carbon dioxide absorbents used in the UK produce very low concentrations of compound A.

Halothane is a volatile liquid anaesthetic. It has largely been superceded by newer agents, but is used by very specialised paediatric anaesthetists to manage difficult airways (with careful monitoring for cardiorespiratory depression and arrhythmias). Its advantages are that it is potent, induction is smooth, and the vapour is non-irritant and seldom induces coughing or breathholding. Despite these advantages, halothane is not widely used because of its association with *severe hepatotoxicity* (**important:** see CSM advice, below).

Halothane causes cardiorespiratory depression. Respiratory depression results in raised arterial carbon dioxide tension and sometimes ventricular arrhythmias. Halothane also depresses the cardiac muscle fibres and can cause bradycardia, resulting in diminished cardiac output and fall of arterial pressure. Adrenaline (epinephrine) infiltrations should be avoided in children anaesthetised with halothane because ventricular arrhythmias can result.

Halothane produces moderate muscle relaxation, but this may be inadequate for major abdominal surgery for which specific muscle relaxants should be used.

> **CSM advice (halothane hepatotoxicity)**
> *Severe hepatotoxicity* can follow halothane anaesthesia. The CSM has reported that this occurs more frequently after repeated exposure to halothane and has a high mortality. The risk of severe hepatotoxicity appears to be increased by repeated exposures within a short time interval, but even after a long interval (sometimes of several years), susceptible patients have been reported to develop jaundice. Since there is no reliable way of identifying susceptible patients, the CSM recommends the following precautions before the use of halothane:
> - a careful anaesthetic history should be taken to determine previous exposure and previous reactions to halothane;
> - repeated exposure to halothane within a period of **at least** 3 months should be **avoided** unless there are **overriding** clinical circumstances;
> - a history of unexplained jaundice or pyrexia in a patient following exposure to halothane is an absolute **contra-indication** to its future use in that patient.

DESFLURANE

Cautions see notes above; **interactions:** Appendix 1 (anaesthetics, general)

    Pregnancy depresses neonatal respiration in third trimester

Contra-indications see notes above

Side-effects see notes above

Indication and dose

  Induction of anaesthesia
- By inhalation through specifically calibrated vaporiser

    Child 12–18 years 4–11%, but **not** recommended (see notes above)

Maintenance of anaesthesia
- By inhalation through specifically calibrated vaporiser

    Neonate 2–6% in nitrous oxide-oxygen; 2.5–8.5% in oxygen or oxygen-enriched air

    Child 1 month–18 years 2–6% in nitrous oxide-oxygen; 2.5–8.5% in oxygen or oxygen-enriched air

Suprane® (Baxter) (PoM)
Desflurane, net price 240 mL = £58.62

HALOTHANE

Cautions see notes above (**important:** CSM advice above); avoid for dental procedures in those under 18 years unless treated in hospital (high risk of arrhythmia); avoid in acute porphyria (section 9.8.2); **interactions:** Appendix 1 (anaesthetics, general)

Hepatic impairment avoid if history of unexplained pyrexia or jaundice following previous exposure to halothane

Pregnancy depresses neonatal respiration in third trimester

◁ **HALOTHANE (continued)**

Breast-feeding excreted in milk

Contra-indications see notes above

Side-effects see notes above

Indication and dose

Induction of anaesthesia
* **By inhalation through specifically calibrated vaporiser**

    Child 1 month–18 years initially 0.5% then increased gradually according to response to 2–4% in oxygen or nitrous oxide–oxygen

Maintenance of anaesthesia
* **By inhalation through specifically calibrated vaporiser**

    Child 1 month–18 years 0.5–2% in oxygen or nitrous oxide–oxygen

Halothane (Non-proprietary) PoM
Available from 'special-order' manufacturers or specialist importing companies, see p. 943

ISOFLURANE

Cautions see notes above; **interactions:** Appendix 1 (anaesthetics, general)

Pregnancy depresses neonatal respiration in third trimester

Contra-indications see notes above

Side-effects see notes above

Indication and dose

Induction of anaesthesia
* **By inhalation through specifically calibrated vaporiser**

    Neonate increased gradually according to response from 0.5–3% in oxygen or nitrous oxide-oxygen

    Child 1 month–18 years increased gradually according to response from 0.5–3% in oxygen or nitrous oxide-oxygen

Maintenance of anaesthesia
* **By inhalation through specifically calibrated vaporiser**

    Neonate 1–2.5% in nitrous oxide-oxygen; additional 0.5–1% may be required if given with oxygen alone

    Child 1 month–18 years 1–2.5% in nitrous oxide-oxygen; additional 0.5–1% may be required if given with oxygen alone; caesarean section, 0.5–0.75% in nitrous oxide-oxygen

Isoflurane (Abbott)
Isoflurane, net price 250 mL = £47.50

AErrane® (Baxter)
Isoflurane, net price 250 mL = £27.00

SEVOFLURANE

Cautions see notes above; **interactions:** Appendix 1 (anaesthetics, general)

Renal impairment manufacturer advises use with caution

Pregnancy depresses neonatal respiration in third trimester

Contra-indications see notes above

Side-effects see notes above; also agitation; hepatitis and seizures also reported

Indication and dose

Induction of anaesthesia
* **By inhalation through specifically calibrated vaporiser**

    Neonate up to 4% in oxygen or nitrous oxide-oxygen, according to response

    Child 1 month–18 years initially 0.5–1% then increased gradually up to 8% in oxygen or nitrous oxide-oxygen, according to response

Maintenance of anaesthesia
* **By inhalation through specifically calibrated vaporiser**

    Neonate 0.5–2% in oxygen or nitrous oxide-oxygen, according to response

    Child 1 month–18 years 0.5–3% in oxygen or nitrous oxide-oxygen, according to response

Sevoflurane (Non-proprietary) PoM
Sevoflurane, net price 250 mL = £123.00

Nitrous oxide

Nitrous oxide is used for maintenance of anaesthesia and, in sub-anaesthetic concentrations, for analgesia. For *anaesthesia* it is commonly used in a concentration of 50 to 66% in oxygen as part of a balanced technique in association with other inhalational or intravenous agents. Nitrous oxide is unsatisfactory as a sole anaesthetic owing to lack of potency, but is useful as part of a combination of drugs since it allows a significant reduction in dosage.

For *analgesia* (without loss of consciousness) a mixture of nitrous oxide and oxygen containing 50% of each gas (*Entonox®*, *Equanox®*) is used. Self-administration using a demand valve may be used in children who are able to self-regulate their intake (usually over 5 years of age) for painful dressing changes, as an aid to postoperative physiotherapy, for wound debridement and in emergency ambulances.

Nitrous oxide may have a deleterious effect if used in children with an air-containing closed space since nitrous oxide diffuses into such a space with a resulting increase in pressure. This effect may be dangerous in the presence of a pneumothorax, which may enlarge to compromise respiration, or in the presence of intracranial air after head injury. Hypoxia can occur immediately following the administration of nitrous oxide; additional oxygen should always be given for several minutes after stopping the flow of nitrous oxide.

Exposure of children to nitrous oxide for prolonged periods, either by continuous or by intermittent administration, may result in megaloblastic anaemia owing to interference with the action of vitamin B_{12}; neurological toxic effects can occur without preceding overt haematological changes. For the same reason, exposure of theatre staff to nitrous oxide should be minimised. Depression of white cell formation may also occur.

Assessment of plasma-vitamin B_{12} concentration should be considered before nitrous oxide anaesthesia in children at risk of deficiency, including children who have a poor or vegetarian diet and children with a history of anaemia. Nitrous oxide should **not** be given continuously for longer than 24 hours or more frequently than every 4 days without close supervision and haematological monitoring.

NITROUS OXIDE

Cautions see notes above; **interactions:** Appendix 1 (anaesthetics, general)

Pregnancy depresses neonatal respiration in third trimester

Side-effects see notes above

Indication and dose

Maintenance of light anaesthesia
• By inhalation using suitable anaesthetic apparatus

Neonate up to 66% in oxygen

Child 1 month–18 years up to 66% in oxygen

Analgesia
• By inhalation using suitable anaesthetic apparatus
(see also notes above)

Neonate up to 50% in oxygen, according to the child's needs

Child 1 month–18 years up to 50% in oxygen, according to the child's needs

15.1.3 Antimuscarinic drugs

Antimuscarinic drugs are used (less commonly nowadays) as premedicants to dry bronchial and salivary secretions which are increased by intubation, upper airway surgery, or some inhalational anaesthetics, but they should not be used for this indication in children with cystic fibrosis. Antimuscarinics are also used before or with neostigmine (section 15.1.6) to prevent bradycardia, excessive salivation, and other muscarinic actions of neostigmine. They also prevent bradycardia and hypotension associated with drugs such as halothane, propofol, and suxamethonium.

Atropine sulphate is now rarely used for premedication but still has an emergency role in the treatment of vagotonic side-effects. For its role in cardiopulmonary resuscitation, see section 2.7.3.

Hyoscine hydrobromide reduces secretions and also provides a degree of amnesia, sedation and anti-emesis. Unlike atropine it may produce bradycardia rather than tachycardia. In some children hyoscine may cause the central anticholinergic syndrome (excitement, ataxia, hallucinations, behavioural abnormalities, and drowsiness).

Glycopyrronium bromide reduces salivary secretions. When given intravenously it produces less tachycardia than atropine. It is widely used with neostigmine for reversal of non-depolarising muscle relaxants (section 15.1.5).

Glycopyrronium or hyoscine hydrobromide are also used to control excessive secretions in upper airways or hypersalivation in palliative care and in children

15 Anaesthesia

unable to control posture or with abnormal swallowing reflex; effective dose varies and tolerance may develop. The intramuscular route should be avoided if possible. Hyoscine transdermal patches may also be used (section 4.6).

◢ ATROPINE SULPHATE

Cautions Down's syndrome; gastro-oesophageal reflux disease, diarrhoea, ulcerative colitis, paralytic ileus, pyloric stenosis, cardiovascular disease, hypertension, conditions characterised by tachycardia (including hyperthyroidism, cardiac insufficiency, cardiac surgery), myasthenia gravis, pyrexia, urinary retention, individuals susceptible to angle-closure glaucoma; **interactions**: Appendix 1 (antimuscarinics)

Pregnancy not known to be harmful; manufacturer advises caution

Breast-feeding small amount present in milk— manufacturer advises caution

Duration of action Since atropine has a shorter duration of action than neostigmine, late unopposed bradycardia may result; close monitoring of the patient is necessary

Side-effects constipation, tachycardia, transient bradycardia (followed by tachycardia, palpitation and arrhythmias), reduced bronchial secretions, urinary urgency and retention, dilatation of the pupils with loss of accommodation, photophobia, dry mouth, flushing, dryness of the skin; *less commonly* nausea, vomiting, giddiness, confusion

Licensed use not licensed for use by oral route; not licensed for use in children under 12 years for intra-operative bradycardia

Indication and dose

Premedication
- **By mouth 1–2 hours before induction**

  Neonate 20–40 micrograms/kg

  Child 1 month–18 years 20–40 micrograms/kg (max. 900 micrograms)

- **By subcutaneous or intramuscular injection 30–60 minutes before induction**

  Neonate 10–15 micrograms/kg (subcutaneous route recommended)

  Child 1 month–12 years 10–30 micrograms/kg (minimum 100 micrograms, max. 600 micrograms)

  Child 12–18 years 300–600 micrograms

Intra-operative bradycardia
- **By intravenous injection**

  Neonate 20 micrograms/kg

  Child 1 month–12 years 10–20 micrograms/kg

  Child 12–18 years 300–600 micrograms (larger doses in emergencies)

Control of muscarinic side-effects of neostigmine in reversal of competitive neuromuscular block
- **By intravenous injection**

  Neonate 20 micrograms/kg

  Child 1 month–12 years 20 micrograms/kg (max. 600 micrograms)

  Child 12–18 years 0.6–1.2 mg

Control of muscarinic side-effects of edrophonium in reversal of competitive neuromuscular block
- **By intravenous injection**

  Child 1 month–18 years 7 micrograms/kg (max. 600 micrograms)

Cycloplegia, anterior uveitis (section 11.5)

Administration for administration *by mouth*, injection solution may be given orally

¹**Atropine** (Non-proprietary) (PoM)
Injection, atropine sulphate 600 micrograms/mL, net price 1-mL amp = 60p
Note Other strengths also available

Injection, prefilled disposable syringe, atropine sulphate 100 micrograms/mL, net price 5 mL = £4.58, 10 mL = £5.39, 30 mL = £8.95

Injection, prefilled disposable syringe, atropine sulphate 200 micrograms/mL, net price 5 mL = £5.37; 300 micrograms/mL, 10 mL = £5.37; 600 micrograms/mL, 1 mL = £4.67

Oral solution, atropine sulphate 100 micrograms/ mL available from 'special-order' manufacturers or specialist importing companies, see p. 943
1. (PoM) restriction does not apply where administration is for saving life in emergency

¹**Minijet® Atropine** (UCB Pharma) (PoM)
Injection, atropine sulphate 100 micrograms/mL, net price 5 mL = £4.58, 10 mL = £5.39, 30 mL = £8.95
1. (PoM) restriction does not apply where administration is for saving life in emergency

◢ GLYCOPYRRONIUM BROMIDE
(Glycopyrrolate)

Cautions see under Atropine Sulphate; **interactions**: Appendix 1 (antimuscarinics)

Side-effects see under Atropine Sulphate

Licensed use not licensed for use in control of upper airways secretion and hypersalivation

Indication and dose

Premedication at induction
- **By intravenous or intramuscular injection**

  Neonate 5 micrograms/kg

  Child 1 month–18 years 4–8 micrograms/kg (max. 200 micrograms)

15 Anaesthesia

◁ **GLYCOPYRRONIUM BROMIDE** (*continued*)

Intra-operative bradycardia
• **By intravenous injection**

Neonate 10 micrograms/kg, repeated if necessary

Child 1 month–18 years 4–8 micrograms/kg (max. 200 micrograms), repeated if necessary

Control of muscarinic side-effects of neostigmine in reversal of competitive neuromuscular block
• **By intravenous injection**

Neonate 10 micrograms/kg

Child 1 month–18 years 10 micrograms/kg (max. 500 micrograms)

Control of upper airways secretion and hypersalivation
• **By mouth**

Child 1 month–18 years 40–100 micrograms/kg 3–4 times daily, adjusted according to response (max. 2 mg)

• **By subcutaneous infusion**

Child 1 month–12 years 12–40 micrograms/kg/24 hours (max. 1.2 mg)

Child 12–18 years 0.6–1.2 mg/24 hours

• **By subcutaneous or intramuscular injection (but see notes above)**

Child 1 month–12 years 4–10 micrograms/kg (max. 200 micrograms) 4 times a day when required

Child 12–18 years 200 micrograms every 4 hours when required

Administration for administration *by mouth*, injection solution may be given or crushed tablets suspended in water

Glycopyrronium bromide (Non-proprietary)
Tablets, glycopyrronium bromide 1 mg and 2 mg
Available on a named-patient basis from specialist importing companies, p. 943

Robinul® (Anpharm) PoM
Injection, glycopyrronium bromide 200 micrograms/mL, net price 1-mL amp = 70p; 3-mL amp = £1.50
Note May be difficult to obtain

◢With neostigmine metilsulphate
Section 15.1.6

◢ **HYOSCINE HYDROBROMIDE**
(Scopolamine hydrobromide)

Cautions see under Hyoscine hydrobromide (section 4.6); also paralytic ileus, myasthenia gravis, epilepsy, susceptibility to angle-closure glaucoma

Side-effects see under Atropine Sulphate; also bradycardia

Indication and dose
Premedication
• **By subcutaneous or intramuscular injection 30–60 minutes before induction**

Child 1–12 years 15 micrograms/kg (max. 600 micrograms)

Child 12–18 years 200–600 micrograms

Note Same dose may be given by intravenous injection immediately before induction

Motion sickness, excessive respiratory secretions see p. 245

Hyoscine (Non-proprietary) PoM
Injection, hyoscine hydrobromide 400 micrograms/mL, net price 1-mL amp = £2.67; 600 micrograms/mL, 1-mL amp = £2.67

◢Preparations
For transdermal and oral preparations see section 4.6

15.1.4 Sedative and analgesic peri-operative drugs

15.1.4.1   Anxiolytics and neuroleptics
15.1.4.2   Non-opioid analgesics
15.1.4.3   Opioid analgesics

Premedication   These drugs are given to allay fear and anxiety in the pre-operative period (including the night before an operation), to relieve pain and discomfort when present, and to augment the action of subsequent anaesthetic agents. A number of the drugs used also provide some degree of pre-operative amnesia. The choice will vary with the individual child, the nature of the operative procedure, the anaesthetic to be used, and other prevailing circumstances such as outpatients, obstetrics, and recovery facilities. The choice also varies between elective and emergency operations. Oral administration is preferred where possible; the rectal route should only be used in exceptional circumstances.

The use of anxiolytic or sedative drugs as premedication in children is declining, but can be useful in selected cases. Sedative premedication should be avoided in

15 Anaesthesia

children with a compromised airway, CNS depression, or a history of sleep apnoea.

Application of a local anaesthetic (section 15.2) to the injection site can help to prevent pain.

Sedation for clinical procedures Anxiety about a clinical procedure can be minimised by using a sedative drug, usually a benzodiazepine, for its anxiolytic and amnesic effect. The child should be **monitored carefully** as soon as the sedative is given until recovery after the procedure; concomitant use of sedatives potentiates the CNS depressant effects of analgesics. For a painful procedure, the sedative may be given with a local anaesthetic (administered topically, by infiltration or as a nerve block as appropriate) and an analgesic such as paracetamol or an NSAID.

Oral **midazolam** is the most common premedicant for children. Midazolam is suitable for sedating a child for a procedure lasting no longer than 20 minutes; it is given by mouth 30–60 minutes before the procedure. Alternatively, **temazepam** may be given by mouth 60–90 minutes before the procedure. If the procedure is likely to last 20–60 minutes, **chloral hydrate** or **triclofos** (section 4.1.1) by mouth are effective, especially in children of pre-school age; secobarbital (quinalbarbitone) can be used in older children but the risk of excessive sedation and cardiorespiratory depression is greater. The antihistamine **alimemazine** (trimeprazine, section 3.4.1) is occasionally used orally as a premedicant, but when given alone it may cause postoperative restlessness in the presence of pain. Alimemazine also has antiemetic properties though it is rarely used for this indication.

If deep sedation is required a general anaesthetic (e.g. propofol or ketamine), or a potent opioid (e.g. fentanyl) can be used, however they should be used only under the supervision of a specialist experienced in the use of these drugs.

Dental procedures Anxiolytics diminish tension, anxiety and panic, and may benefit anxious children, however they should be used under specialist supervision only. Children and their carers should be carefully warned about the risk of undertaking skilled tasks (**important**: for general advice on anaesthesia and skilled tasks, see p. 762). For futher information on hypnotics and anxiolytics, see p. 211. For further information on hypnotics used for dental procedures, see p. 212.

Anaesthesia and skilled tasks See section 15.1.

15.1.4.1 Anxiolytics and neuroleptics

Benzodiazepines

Benzodiazepines possess useful properties for premedication including relief of anxiety, sedation, and amnesia; short-acting benzodiazepines taken by mouth are the most common premedicants. They have no analgesic effect so an opioid analgesic may sometimes be required for pain.

Benzodiazepines can alleviate anxiety at doses that do not necessarily cause excessive sedation and they are of particular value during short procedures or during operations under local anaesthesia (including dentistry). Amnesia reduces the likelihood of any unpleasant memories of the procedure (although benzodiazepines, particularly when used for more profound sedation, can sometimes induce sexual fantasies in adolescents). Benzodiazepines are also used in intensive care units for sedation, particularly in those receiving assisted ventilation.

Benzodiazepines may occasionally cause marked respiratory depression and facilities for its treatment are essential; flumazenil (section 15.1.7) is used to antagonise the effects of benzodiazepines. They are best avoided in myasthenia gravis, especially peri-operatively.

Diazepam is used to produce mild sedation with amnesia. It is a long-acting drug with active metabolites and a second period of drowsiness can occur several hours after its administration. Peri-operative use of diazepam is not generally recommended; its effect and timing of response are unreliable and paradoxical effects may occur.

Diazepam is relatively insoluble in water and preparations formulated in organic solvents are painful on intravenous injection and give rise to a high incidence of venous thrombosis (which may not be noticed for several days after the injection). Intramuscular injection of diazepam is also painful and absorption is erratic; administration by the intramuscular route is not recommended. An emulsion formulated for intravenous injection is less irritant and reduces the risk of venous thrombosis; it is not suitable for intramuscular injection. Diazepam is also available as a rectal solution.

Temazepam is given by mouth in older children and has a shorter duration of action and a more rapid onset than diazepam given by mouth. It has been used as a premedicant in inpatient and day-case surgery; anxiolytic and sedative effects last about 90 minutes although there may be residual drowsiness.

Lorazepam produces more prolonged sedation than temazepam and it has marked amnesic effects. It is used as a premedicant the night before major surgery; a further, smaller dose may be required the following morning if any delay in starting surgery is anticipated. Alternatively the first dose may be given early in the morning on the day of operation.

Midazolam is a water-soluble benzodiazepine which is often used by intravenous injection in preference to intravenous diazepam; it has a quick onset of action and recovery is faster than from diazepam, making it suitable for day cases. Midazolam can be given by mouth but its bitter acidic taste may need to be disguised. It can also be given buccally and intranasally; use of the intranasal route is limited by nasal discomfort and is not recommended. Midazolam is associated with profound sedation when high doses are given or when used with certain other drugs. It can cause severe disinhibition and restlessness in some children. Midazolam is not recommended for prolonged sedation in neonates; drug accumulation is likely to occur.

There have been reports of overdosage in adults when high strength midazolam injection has been used for conscious sedation. The use of high strength midazolam (5 mg/mL in 2 mL and 10 mL ampoules, or 2 mg/mL in 5 mL ampoules) should be restricted to general anaesthesia, intensive care, palliative care, or other situations where the risk has been assessed. It is advised that flumazenil (section 15.1.7) is available where midazolam is used, to reverse the effects if necessary.

DIAZEPAM

Cautions see notes above and section 4.8.2

Contra-indications see section 4.8.2

Side-effects see notes above and section 4.8.2

Indication and dose

Premedication and sedation for clinical procedures (but see notes above)

- **By mouth 45–60 minutes before procedure**

  Child 1 month–12 years 200–300 micrograms/kg (max. 10 mg)

  Child 12–18 years 200–300 micrograms/kg (max. 20 mg)

- **By intravenous injection over 2–4 minutes into large vein (specialist use only); emulsion preparation preferred**

  Child 1 month–12 years 100–200 micrograms/kg (max. 5 mg) immediately before procedure

  Child 12–18 years 100–200 micrograms/kg (max. 20 mg) immediately before procedure

- **By rectum (as rectal solution) approximately 30 minutes before procedure**

  Child 1–3 years 5 mg

  Child 3–12 years 5–10 mg

  Child 12–18 years 10 mg

Status epilepticus section 4.8.2

Febrile convulsions section 4.8.3

Muscle spasm section 10.2.2

Diazepam (Non-proprietary) ⟨PoM⟩
Tablets, diazepam 2 mg, net price 28 = 95p; 5 mg, 28 = 98p; 10 mg, 28 = £1.08. Label: 2 or 19
Brands include *Rimapam*® ⟨JHS⟩, *Tensium*® ⟨JHS⟩

Oral solution, diazepam 2 mg/5 mL, net price 100 mL = £6.75. Label: 2 or 19
Brands include *Dialar*® ⟨JHS⟩

Strong oral solution, diazepam 5 mg/5 mL, net price 100-mL pack = £6.38. Label: 2 or 19 ⟨JHS⟩
Brands include *Dialar*® ⟨JHS⟩

Dental prescribing on NHS Diazepam Tablets or Diazepam Oral Solution 2 mg/5 mL may be prescribed

◀ Parenteral preparations and rectal solution
Section 4.8.2

15

Anaesthesia

LORAZEPAM

Cautions see notes above and section 4.8.2; **interactions**: Appendix 1 (anxiolytics and hypnotics)

Contra-indications see under Diazepam (section 4.8.2)

Side-effects see notes above and under Diazepam (section 4.8.2)

Licensed use not licensed for use in children under 5 years by mouth; not licensed for use in children under 12 years by intravenous injection

Indication and dose

> Status epilepticus section 4.8.2

> **Premedication**
> * **By mouth**
>
>   **Child 1 month–12 years** 50–100 micrograms/kg (max. 4 mg) at least 1 hour before surgery
>
>   **Child 12–18 years** 1–4 mg at least 1 hour before surgery
>   Note Same dose may be given the night before surgery in addition to, or to replace, dose before surgery

* **By intravenous injection**

     Child 1 month–18 years 50–100 micrograms/kg (max. 4 mg)
     Note Give intravenous injection 30–45 minutes before surgery

Administration for *intravenous injection*, dilute injection solution with an equal volume of Sodium Chloride 0.9% *or* Water for Injections; give over 3–5 minutes; max. rate 50 micrograms/kg over 3 minutes

Lorazepam (Non-proprietary) ℗ₒₘ

Tablets, lorazepam 1 mg, net price 28-tab pack = £8.28; 2.5 mg, 28-tab pack = £15.08. Label: 2 or 19

Injection, lorazepam 4 mg/mL, net price 1-mL amp = 37p
Excipients include benzyl alcohol (avoid in neonates see Excipients, p. 3), propylene glycol
Brands include *Ativan*®

◢ Extemporaneous formulations available see Extemporaneous Preparations, p. 8

MIDAZOLAM

Cautions see notes above; cardiac disease; respiratory disease; myasthenia gravis; neonates; history of drug or alcohol abuse; reduce dose if debilitated; risk of severe hypotension in hypovolaemia, vasoconstriction, hypothermia; avoid prolonged use (and abrupt withdrawal thereafter); **interactions**: Appendix 1 (anxiolytics and hypnotics)

Hepatic impairment can precipitate coma

Renal impairment start with small doses in severe renal impairment; increased cerebral sensitivity

Pregnancy use only if clear indication such as seizure control (high doses during late pregnancy or labour may cause neonatal hypothermia, hypotonia, and respiratory depression)

Breast-feeding present in milk—manufacturer advises avoid breast-feeding for 24 hours after administration

Contra-indications marked neuromuscular respiratory weakness including unstable myasthenia gravis; severe respiratory depression; acute pulmonary insufficiency

Side-effects see notes above; gastro-intestinal disturbances, increased appetite, jaundice; hypotension, cardiac arrest, heart rate changes, anaphylaxis, thrombosis; laryngospasm, bronchospasm, respiratory depression and respiratory arrest (particularly with high doses or on rapid injection); drowsiness, confusion, ataxia, amnesia, headache, euphoria, hallucinations, convulsions (more common in neonates), fatigue, dizziness, vertigo, involuntary movements, paradoxical excitement and aggression, dysarthria; urinary retention, incontinence; blood disorders; muscle weakness; visual disturbances; salivation changes; skin reactions; injection-site reactions; with *intranasal administration* burning sensation, lacrimation, and severe irritation of nasal mucosa

Licensed use not licensed for use in children under 6 months for premedication and conscious sedation; not licensed for use by mouth, or by buccal administration

Indication and dose

> Sedation (but see notes above)
> * **By mouth**
>
>   **Child 1 month–18 years** 500 micrograms/kg (max. 20 mg) 30–60 minutes before procedure
>
> * **By buccal administration**
>
>   **Child 6 months–10 years** 200–300 micrograms/kg (max. 5 mg)
>
>   **Child 10–18 years** 6–7 mg (max. 8 mg if 70 kg or over)
>
> * **By rectum**
>
>   **Child 6 months–12 years** 300–500 micrograms/kg 15–30 minutes before procedure
>
> * **By intravenous injection over 2–3 minutes 5–10 minutes before procedure**
>
>   **Child 1 month–6 years** initially 25–50 micrograms/kg, increased if necessary in small steps (max. total dose 6 mg)
>
>   **Child 6–12 years** initially 25–50 micrograms/kg, increased if necessary in small steps (max. total dose 10 mg)
>
>   **Child 12–18 years** initially 25–50 micrograms/kg, increased if necessary in small steps (max. total dose 7.5 mg)

> Premedication (but see notes above)
> * **By mouth**
>
>   **Child 1 month–18 years** 500 micrograms/kg (max. 20 mg) 15–30 minutes before the procedure

15 Anaesthesia

◻ **MIDAZOLAM** *(continued)*

- **By rectum**

  Child 6 months–12 years 300–500 micrograms/kg 15–30 minutes before induction

- **By intravenous injection**

  Child 12–18 years 25–50 micrograms/kg repeated as required (max. total dose 7.5 mg)

Induction of anaesthesia (but rarely used)
- **By slow intravenous injection**

  Child 7–18 years initially 150 micrograms/kg (max. 7.5 mg) given in steps of 50 micrograms/kg (max. 2.5 mg) over 2–5 minutes; wait for 2–5 minutes then give additional doses of 50 micrograms/kg (max. 2.5 mg) every 2 minutes if necessary; max. total dose 500 micrograms/kg (not exceeding 25 mg)

Sedation in intensive care
- **By intravenous injection and continuous intravenous infusion**

  Neonate less than 32 weeks gestational age 30 micrograms/kg/hour *by continuous intravenous infusion* adjusted according to response

  Neonate over 32 weeks gestational age 60 micrograms/kg/hour *by continuous intravenous infusion* adjusted according to response

  Child 1–6 months 60 micrograms/kg/hour *by continuous intravenous infusion* adjusted according to response

  Child 6 months–12 years initially 50–200 micrograms/kg *by slow intravenous injection* over at least 3 minutes followed by 30–120 micrograms/kg/hour *by continuous intravenous infusion* adjusted according to response

  Child 12–18 years initially 30–300 micrograms/kg *by slow intravenous injection* given in steps of 1–2.5 mg every 2 minutes followed by 30–200 micrograms/kg/hour *by continuous intravenous infusion* adjusted according to response
  Note Initial dose may not be required and lower maintenance doses needed if opioid analgesics also used; reduce dose (or reduce or omit initial dose) in hypovolaemia, vasoconstriction, or hypothermia

Status epilepticus section 4.8.2

Administration for administration *by mouth*, injection solution may be diluted with apple or black currant juice, chocolate sauce, or cola

For *buccal administration*, administer half of the dose between the upper lip and gum on each side of the mouth using an oral syringe; retain in the mouth for at least 5 minutes then swallow

For *continuous intravenous infusion*, dilute with Glucose 5% *or* Sodium Chloride 0.9%; for neonates and children under 15 kg body-weight, dilute to a max. concentration of 1 mg/mL

Neonatal intensive care, body-weight under 3.3 kg, dilute 15 mg/kg body-weight to a final volume of 50 mL with infusion fluid; an intravenous infusion rate of 0.1 mL/hour provides a dose of 30 micrograms/kg/hour; body-weight over 3.3kg, dilute 50 mg to final volume of 50 mL with infusion fluid, max. concentration of 1mg/mL; an intravenous infusion rate of 0.05–0.1 mL/kg/hour provides a dose of 50–100micrograms/kg/hour

For *rectal administration* of the injection solution, attach a plastic applicator onto the end of a syringe; if the volume to be given rectally is too small, dilute with Water for Injections

Midazolam (Non-proprietary) ⒸⒹ
Oral liquid, midazolam 2.5 mg/mL, 100 mL
Available from 'special-order' manufacturers or specialist importing companies, see p. 943

Buccal liquid, midazolam 10 mg/mL, 5 mL and 25 mL
Available from 'special-order' manufacturers or specialist importing companies, see p. 943 (*Epistatus*® and *Consed*®)

Injection, midazolam (as hydrochloride) 1 mg/mL, net price 2-mL amp = 50p, 5-mL amp = 60p, 50-mL vial = £7.87; 2 mg/mL, 5-mL amp = 65p; 5 mg/mL, 2-mL amp = 58p, 10-mL amp = £2.50

Hypnovel® (Roche) ⒸⒹ
Injection, midazolam (as hydrochloride) 2 mg/mL, net price 5-mL amp = 75p; 5 mg/mL, 2-mL amp = 90p

---

▰ **TEMAZEPAM**

Cautions see notes above and under Diazepam (section 4.8.2); **interactions:** Appendix 1 (anxiolytics and hypnotics)

Contra-indications see under Diazepam (section 4.8.2)

Side-effects see notes above and under Diazepam (section 4.8.2)

Licensed use tablets not licensed for use in children

Indication and dose

Premedication and sedation for clinical procedures
- **By mouth**

  Child 1–12 years 1 mg/kg (max. 30 mg) 1 hour before surgery

  Child 12–18 years 20–30 mg 1 hour before surgery

Temazepam (Non-proprietary) ⒸⒹ
Tablets, temazepam 10 mg, net price 28-tab pack = £3.89; 20 mg, 28-tab pack = £1.64. Label: 19

Oral solution, temazepam 10 mg/5 mL, net price 300 mL = £18.96. Label: 19

Note Sugar-free versions are available and can be ordered by specifying 'sugar-free' on the prescription
Dental prescribing on NHS Temazepam Tablets or Oral Solution may be prescribed
Note See p. 17 for prescribing requirements of controlled drugs

15

Anaesthesia

15.1.4.2 **Non-opioid analgesics**

Since non-steroidal anti-inflammatory drugs (NSAIDs) do not depress respiration, do not impair gastro-intestinal motility, and do not cause dependence, they may be useful alternatives (or adjuncts) to the use of opioids for the relief of postoperative pain. NSAIDs may be inadequate for the relief of severe pain.

Diclofenac, ibuprofen (section 10.1.1), **paracetamol** (section 4.7.1), and **ketorolac** are used to relieve postoperative pain in children; diclofenac and paracetamol can be given parenterally and rectally as well as by mouth. Intramuscular injections of diclofenac are given deep into the gluteal muscle to minimise pain and tissue damage; diclofenac can also be given by intravenous infusion for the treatment or prevention of postoperative pain.

Ketorolac is less irritant on intramuscular injection but pain has been reported; it can also be given by mouth or by intravenous injection.

KETOROLAC TROMETAMOL

Cautions section 10.1.1; avoid in acute porphyria (section 9.8.2); **interactions**: Appendix 1 (NSAIDs)

Renal impairment reduce dose (max. 60 mg daily by intramuscular or intravenous injection) and monitor renal function; manufacturer advises avoid if serum creatinine greater than 160 mmol/litre

Breast-feeding amount too small to be harmful but manufacturer advises avoid

Contra-indications section 10.1.1; also complete or partial syndrome of nasal polyps; haemorrhagic diatheses (including coagulation disorders) and following operations with high risk of haemorrhage or incomplete haemostasis; confirmed or suspected cerebrovascular bleeding; hypovolaemia or dehydration

Pregnancy contra-indicated during pregnancy, labour and delivery

Side-effects section 10.1.1; also gastro-intestinal disturbances; flushing, bradycardia, palpitation, chest pain; dyspnoea, asthma; malaise, euphoria, psychosis, paraesthesia, convulsions, abnormal dreams, hyperkinesia; infertility, urinary frequency, thirst; hyponatraemia, hyperkalaemia, myalgia; visual disturbances (including optic neuritis); pallor, purpura, pain at injection site

Licensed use not licensed for use in children under 16 years

Indication and dose

Short-term management of moderate to severe acute postoperative pain only
• By mouth
 Child 16–18 years 10 mg every 4–6 hours as required; max. 40 mg daily; max. duration of treatment 7 days

• By intravenous injection over at least 15 seconds
 Child 6 months–16 years initially 0.5–1 mg/kg (max. 15 mg), then 500 micrograms/kg (max. 15 mg) every 6 hours as required; max. 60 mg daily; max. duration of treatment 2 days

• By intramuscular injection *or* by intravenous injection over at least 15 seconds
 Child 16–18 years initially 10 mg, then 10–30 mg every 4–6 hours as required (up to every 2 hours during initial postoperative period); max. 90 mg daily (children weighing less than 50 kg max. 60 mg daily); max. duration of treatment 2 days
 Note When converting from parenteral to oral administration, total combined dose on the day of converting should not exceed 90 mg (60 mg in children weighing less than 50 kg) of which the oral component should not exceed 40 mg

Ketorolac (Non-proprietary) PoM
Injection, ketorolac trometamol 30 mg/mL, net price 1-mL amp = £1.14

Toradol® (Roche) PoM
Tablets, ivory, f/c, ketorolac trometamol 10 mg, net price 20-tab pack = £5.79. Label: 17, 21

Injection, ketorolac trometamol 10 mg/mL, net price 1-mL amp = 94p; 30 mg/mL, 1-mL amp = £1.14

15.1.4.3 **Opioid analgesics**

Opioid analgesics are now rarely used as premedicants; they are more likely to be administered at induction. Pre-operative use of opioid analgesics is generally limited to children who require control of existing pain. The main side-effects of opioid analgesics are respiratory depression, cardiovascular depression, nausea, and vomiting; for general notes on opioid analgesics and their use in postoperative pain, see section 4.7.2.

For the management of opioid-induced respiratory depression, see section 15.1.7.

Intra-operative analgesia Opioid analgesics given in small doses before or with induction reduce the dose requirement of some drugs used during anaesthesia.

Alfentanil, **fentanyl**, and **remifentanil** are particularly useful because they act within 1–2 minutes and have short durations of action. The initial doses of alfentanil or fentanyl are followed either by successive intravenous injections or by an intravenous infusion; prolonged infusions increase the duration of effect. Repeated intra-operative doses of alfentanil or fentanyl should be given with care since the resulting respiratory depression can persist postoperatively and occasionally it may become apparent for the first time postoperatively when monitoring of the child might be less intensive. Alfentanil, fentanyl, and remifentanil can cause muscle rigidity, particularly of the chest wall muscle or jaw muscle, which can be managed by the use of neuromuscular blocking drugs.

In contrast to other opioids which are metabolised in the liver, remifentanil undergoes rapid metabolism by non-specific blood and tissue esterases; its short duration of action allows prolonged administration at high dosage, without accumulation, and with little risk of residual postoperative respiratory depression. Remifentanil should not be given by intravenous injection intra-operatively, but it is well suited to continuous infusion; a supplementary analgesic is given before stopping the infusion of remifentanil.

Neonates   The half-life of fentanyl and alfentanil is prolonged in neonates and accumulation is likely with prolonged use.

ALFENTANIL

Cautions   section 4.7.2 and notes above
Contra-indications   section 4.7.2
Side-effects   section 4.7.2 and notes above; also hypertension, myoclonic movements; *less commonly* arrhythmias, cough, hiccup, laryngospasm; also reported cardiac arrest, convulsions, and pyrexia

Indication and dose

To avoid excessive dosage in obese children, dose may need to be calculated on the basis of ideal weight for height

Analgesia especially during short procedures; enhancement of anaesthesia
- **By intravenous injection over 30 seconds (with assisted ventilation)**

  Neonate initially 5–20 micrograms/kg; supplemental doses up to 10 micrograms/kg

  Child 1 month–18 years initially 10–20 micrograms/kg; supplemental doses up to 10 micrograms/kg

- **By intravenous infusion (with assisted ventilation)**

  Neonate initially 10–50 micrograms/kg over 10 minutes followed by 30–60 micrograms/kg/hour

  Child 1 month–18 years initially 50–100 micrograms/kg over 10 minutes followed by 30–60 micrograms/kg/hour

Administration   for *continuous or intermittent intravenous infusion* dilute in Glucose 5% *or* Sodium Chloride 0.9% *or* Compound Sodium Lactate

Rapifen® (Janssen-Cilag) CD
Injection, alfentanil (as hydrochloride) 500 micrograms/mL, net price 2-mL amp = 67p; 10-mL amp = £3.08

Intensive care injection, alfentanil (as hydrochloride) 5 mg/mL. To be diluted before use, net price 1-mL amp = £2.46

FENTANYL

Cautions   section 4.7.2 and notes above
Contra-indications   section 4.7.2
Side-effects   section 4.7.2 and notes above; also myoclonic movements; *less commonly* laryngospasm; *rarely* asystole, insomnia

Indication and dose

To avoid excessive dosage in obese children, dose may need to be calculated on the basis of ideal weight for height

Analgesia during operation, enhancement of anaesthesia with spontaneous respiration
- **By intravenous injection over at least 30 seconds**

  Child 1 month–12 years initially 1–3 micrograms/kg, then 1 microgram/kg as required

  Child 12–18 years initially 50–200 micrograms, then 50 micrograms as required

Analgesia during operation, enhancement of anaesthesia with assisted ventilation
- **By intravenous injection over at least 30 seconds**

  Neonate initially 1–5 micrograms/kg, then 1–3 micrograms/kg as required

  Child 1 month–12 years initially 1–5 micrograms/kg, then 1–3 micrograms/kg as required

  Child 12–18 years initially 0.3–3.5 mg, then 100–200 micrograms as required

15

Anaesthesia

◁ **FENTANYL (continued)**

Analgesia and respiratory depressant with assisted ventilation in intensive care
• **By intravenous infusion**

Neonate initially 1–5 micrograms/kg, then adjusted according to response

Child 1 month–18 years initially 1–5 micrograms/kg, then adjusted according to response

Analgesia in other situations section 4.7.2

Administration for *intravenous infusion*, injection solution may be diluted in Glucose 5% *or* Sodium Chloride 0.9%

Fentanyl (Non-proprietary) ⒸⒹ
Injection, fentanyl (as citrate) 50 micrograms/mL, net price 2-mL amp = 54p, 10-mL amp = £1.65

Sublimaze® (Janssen-Cilag) ⒸⒹ
Injection, fentanyl (as citrate) 50 micrograms/mL, net price 2-mL amp = 22p, 10-mL amp = £1.11

▌ REMIFENTANIL

Cautions section 4.7.2 (but no dose adjustment necessary in renal impairment) and notes above

Contra-indications section 4.7.2 and notes above; left ventricular dysfunction

Side-effects section 4.7.2 and notes above; also hypertension, hypoxia; *very rarely* asystole and anaphylaxis

Indication and dose

To avoid excessive dosage in obese children, dose should be calculated on the basis of ideal weight for height

Enhancement and maintenance of anaesthesia
• **By intravenous injection and by continuous intravenous infusion**

Neonate by *intravenous infusion* 24–60 micrograms/kg/hour; additional doses of 1 microgram/kg can be given by *intravenous injection* during the intravenous infusion

Child 1–12 years initially by *intravenous injection* 0.1–1 micrograms/kg over at least 30 seconds (omitted if not required) then by *intravenous infusion* 3–80 micrograms/kg/hour according to anaesthetic technique and adjusted according to

response; additional doses can be given by *intravenous injection* during the intravenous infusion

Child 12–18 years initially by *intravenous injection* 0.1–1 micrograms/kg over at least 30 seconds (omitted if not required) then by *intravenous infusion* 3–120 micrograms/kg/hour according to anaesthetic technique and adjusted according to response; additional doses can be given by *intravenous injection* during the intravenous infusion

Administration for *intravenous injection*, reconstitute to a concentration of 1 mg/mL; for *continuous intravenous infusion*, dilute further with Glucose 5% *or* Sodium Chloride 0.9% *or* Water for Injections to a concentration of 20–25 micrograms/mL for Child 1–12 years or 20–250 micrograms/mL (usually 50 micrograms/mL) for Child 12–18 years

Ultiva® (GSK) ⒸⒹ
Injection, powder for reconstitution, remifentanil (as hydrochloride), net price 1-mg vial = £5.12; 2-mg vial = £10.23; 5-mg vial = £25.58

15.1.5 Neuromuscular blocking drugs

Neuromuscular blocking drugs used in anaesthesia are also known as **muscle relaxants**. By specific blockade of the neuromuscular junction they enable light anaesthesia to be used with adequate relaxation of the muscles of the abdomen and diaphragm. They also relax the vocal cords and allow the passage of a tracheal tube. Their action differs from the muscle relaxants used in musculoskeletal disorders (section 10.2.2) that act on the spinal cord or brain.

Children who have received a neuromuscular blocking drug should **always** have their respiration assisted or controlled until the drug has been inactivated or antagonised (section 15.1.6). They should also receive sufficient concomitant inhalational or intravenous anaesthetic or sedative drugs to prevent awareness.

Non-depolarising neuromuscular blocking drugs

Non-depolarising neuromuscular blocking drugs (also known as competitive muscle relaxants) compete with acetylcholine for receptor sites at the neuromuscular junction and their action can be reversed with anticholinesterases, such as neostigmine (section 15.1.6). Non-depolarising neuromuscular blocking drugs can be divided into the **aminosteroid** group, comprising pancuronium, rocuronium, and vecuronium, and the **benzylisoquinolinium** group, which includes atracurium, cisatracurium, and mivacurium.

Non-depolarising neuromuscular blocking drugs have a slower onset of action than suxamethonium. These drugs can be classified by their duration of action as short-acting (15–30 minutes), intermediate-acting (30–40 minutes), and long-acting (60–120 minutes), although duration of action is dose-dependent. Drugs with a shorter or intermediate duration of action, such as atracurium and vecuronium, are more widely used than those with a longer duration of action, such as pancuronium.

Non-depolarising neuromuscular blocking drugs have no sedative or analgesic effects and are not considered to trigger malignant hyperthermia.

For children receiving intensive care and who require tracheal intubation and mechanical ventilation, a non-depolarising neuromuscular blocking drug is chosen according to its onset of effect, duration of action, and side-effects. Rocuronium, with a rapid onset of effect, may facilitate intubation. Atracurium or cisatracurium may be suitable for long-term neuromuscular blockade since their duration of action is not dependent on elimination by the liver or the kidneys.

Cautions   Allergic cross-reactivity between neuromuscular blocking drugs has been reported; caution is advised in cases of hypersensitivity to these drugs. Their activity is prolonged in children with myasthenia gravis and in hypothermia, therefore lower doses are required. Non-depolarising neuromuscular blocking drugs should be used with great care in those with other neuromuscular disorders and those with fluid and electrolyte disturbances, as response in these children is unpredictable. Resistance may develop in children with burns who may require increased doses; low plasma cholinesterase activity in these children requires dose titration for mivacurium. **Interactions:** Appendix 1 (muscle relaxants).

Side-effects   Benzylisoquinolinium non-depolarising neuromuscular blocking drugs (except cisatracurium) are associated with histamine release, which can cause skin flushing, hypotension, tachycardia, bronchospasm, and very rarely, anaphylactoid reactions. Most aminosteroid neuromuscular blocking drugs produce minimal histamine release. Drugs with vagolytic activity can counteract any bradycardia that occurs during surgery. Acute myopathy has also been reported after prolonged use in intensive care.

Atracurium, a mixture of 10 isomers, is a benzylisoquinolinium neuromuscular blocking drug with an intermediate duration of action. It undergoes non-enzymatic metabolism which is independent of liver and kidney function, thus allowing its use in children with hepatic or renal impairment. Cardiovascular effects are associated with significant histamine release. Neonates may be more sensitive to the effects of atracurium and lower doses may be required.

Cisatracurium is a single isomer of atracurium. It is more potent and has a slightly longer duration of action than atracurium and provides greater cardiovascular stability because cisatracurium lacks histamine-releasing effects. In children aged 1 month to 12 years, cisatracurium has a shorter duration of action and produces faster spontaneous recovery.

Mivacurium, a benzylisoquinolinium neuromuscular blocking drug, has a short duration of action. It is metabolised by plasma cholinesterase and muscle paralysis is prolonged in individuals deficient in this enzyme. It is not associated with vagolytic activity or ganglionic blockade although histamine release can occur, particularly with rapid injection. In children under 12 years mivacurium has a faster onset, shorter duration of action, and produces more rapid spontaneous recovery.

Pancuronium, an aminosteroid neuromuscular blocking drug, has a long duration of action and is often used in children receiving long-term mechanical ventilation in intensive care units. It lacks a histamine-releasing effect, but vagolytic and sympathomimetic effects can cause tachycardia and hypertension. The half-life of pancuronium is prolonged in neonates; neonates should receive post-operative intermittent positive pressure ventilation

Rocuronium exerts an effect within 2 minutes and has the most rapid onset of any of the non-depolarising neuromuscular blocking drugs. It is an aminosteroid neuromuscular blocking drug with an intermediate duration of action. It is reported to have minimal cardiovascular effects; high doses produce mild vagolytic activity. In children under 12 years, rocuronium has a faster onset and shorter duration of action.

Vecuronium, an aminosteroid neuromuscular blocking drug, has an intermediate duration of action. It does not generally produce histamine release and lacks

15

Anaesthesia

cardiovascular effects. In neonates and infants, vecuronium has a faster onset and a longer duration of action; recovery is longer in these children. Unexpected sustained neuromuscular blockade may occur in neonates.

ATRACURIUM BESILATE
(Atracurium besylate)

Cautions see notes above

Pregnancy does not cross placenta in significant amounts but manufacturer advises use only if potential benefit outweighs risk

Breast-feeding unlikely to be harmful following recovery from neuromuscular block; some manufacturers advise avoiding breast-feeding for 24 hours after administration

Side-effects see notes above; seizures also reported

Licensed use not licensed for use in neonates

Indication and dose

To avoid excessive dosage in obese children, dose should be calculated on the basis of ideal weight for height

Neuromuscular blockade (short to intermediate duration) for surgery or during intensive care
• By intravenous administration

Neonate initially by *intravenous injection* 300–500 micrograms/kg followed *either* by *intravenous injection*, 100–200 micrograms/kg repeated as necessary *or* by *intravenous infusion*, 300–400 micrograms/kg/hour adjusted according to response

Child 1 month–18 years initially by *intravenous injection* 300–600 micrograms/kg then 100–200 micrograms/kg repeated as necessary *or* initially by *intravenous injection* 200–600 micrograms/kg followed by *intravenous infusion*, 300–600 micrograms/kg/hour adjusted to response; higher doses may be necessary in intensive care

Administration for *continuous intravenous infusion*, dilute to a concentration of 0.5–5 mg/mL with Glucose 5% *or* Sodium Chloride 0.9% *or* Ringer's solution *or* Compound Sodium Lactate; stability varies with diluent.
Neonatal intensive care, dilute 60 mg/kg body-weight to a final volume of 50 mL with Glucose 5% or Sodium Chloride 0.9%; minimum concentration of 500 micrograms/mL, max. concentration of 5 mg/mL; an intravenous infusion rate of 0.1 mL/hour provides a dose of 120 micrograms/kg/hour

Atracurium (Non-proprietary) ▣PoM
Injection, atracurium besilate 10 mg/mL, net price 2.5-mL amp = £1.85; 5-mL amp = £3.37; 25-mL amp = £14.45

Tracrium® (GSK) ▣PoM
Injection, atracurium besilate 10 mg/mL, net price 2.5-mL amp = £1.66; 5-mL amp = £3.00; 25-mL amp = £12.91

CISATRACURIUM

Cautions see notes above

Pregnancy manufacturer advises avoid—no information available

Breast-feeding no information available

Side-effects see notes above

Indication and dose

To avoid excessive dosage in obese children, dose should be calculated on the basis of ideal weight for height

Neuromuscular blockade (intermediate duration) for intubation and during surgery
• By intravenous injection

Child 1 month–2 years initially 150 micrograms/kg, then 30 micrograms/kg repeated approx. every 20 minutes as necessary

Child 2–12 years initially 150 micrograms/kg (80–100 micrograms/kg if not for intubation), then 20 micrograms/kg repeated approx. every 10 minutes as necessary

Child 12–18 years initially 150 micrograms/kg, then 30 micrograms/kg repeated approx. every 20 minutes as necessary

• By intravenous infusion

Child 2–18 years initially 180 micrograms/kg/hour, reduced to 60–120 micrograms/kg/hour when stable; dose reduced by up to 40% if used with isoflurane

Administration for *continuous intravenous infusion*, dilute to a concentration of 0.1–2 mg/mL with Glucose 5% *or* Sodium Chloride 0.9%; solutions of 2 mg/mL and 5 mg/mL may be infused undiluted

Nimbex® (GSK) ▣PoM
Injection, cisatracurium (as besilate) 2 mg/mL, net price 10-mL amp = £7.55

Forte injection, cisatracurium (as besilate) 5 mg/mL, net price 30-mL vial = £31.09

MIVACURIUM

Cautions see notes above; low plasma cholinesterase activity

Hepatic impairment reduce dose in severe impairment

Renal impairment clinical effect prolonged in renal failure—reduce dose according to response

Pregnancy manufacturer advises avoid—no information available

△ **MIVACURIUM** (*continued*)

Side-effects   see notes above

Indication and dose

> To avoid excessive dosage in obese children, dose should be calculated on the basis of ideal weight for height

Neuromuscular blockade (short duration) during surgery

- **By intravenous administration**

 Child 2–6 months by *intravenous injection* initially 150 micrograms/kg, then *either* by *intravenous injection* 100 micrograms/kg repeated every 6–9 minutes as necessary *or* by *intravenous infusion*, 8–10 micrograms/kg/minute, adjusted if necessary every 3 minutes by 1 microgram/kg/minute to usual dose 11–14 micrograms/kg/minute

 Child 6 months–12 years by *intravenous injection* initially 200 micrograms/kg, then *either* by *intravenous injection* 100 micrograms/kg repeated every 6–9 minutes as necessary *or* by *intravenous infusion*, 8–10 micrograms/kg/minute, adjusted if necessary every 3 minutes by 1 microgram/kg/minute to usual dose 11–14 micrograms/kg/minute

 Child 12–18 years by *intravenous injection* initially 70–250 micrograms/kg, then *either* by *intravenous injection* 100 micrograms/kg repeated every 15 minutes as necessary *or* by *intravenous infusion*, 8–10 micrograms/kg/minute, adjusted if necessary every 3 minutes by 1 microgram/kg/minute to usual dose of 6–7 micrograms/kg/minute

Administration   for *intravenous injection*, give undiluted or dilute in Glucose 5% *or* Sodium Chloride 0.9%. Doses up to 150 micrograms/kg may be given over 5–15 seconds, higher doses should be given over 30 seconds. In asthma, cardiovascular disease or in those sensitive to reduced arterial blood pressure, give over 60 seconds.

Mivacron® (GSK) [PoM]
 Injection, mivacurium (as chloride) 2 mg/mL, net price 5-mL amp = £2.79; 10-mL amp = £4.51

▎**PANCURONIUM BROMIDE**

Cautions   see notes above

 Hepatic impairment   possibly slower onset, higher dose requirement, and prolonged recovery time

 Renal impairment   manufacturer advises caution; prolonged duration of block

 Pregnancy   crosses placenta in small amounts—manufacturer advises avoid

 Breast-feeding   no information available—manufacturer advises avoid

Side-effects   see notes above

Indication and dose

> To avoid excessive dosage in obese children, dose should be calculated on the basis of ideal weight for height

Neuromuscular blockade (long duration) during surgery

- **By intravenous injection**

 Neonate initially 100 micrograms/kg, then 50 micrograms/kg repeated as necessary

 Child 1 month–18 years initially 100 micrograms/kg, then 20 micrograms/kg repeated as necessary

Administration   for *intravenous injection*, give undiluted *or* dilute in Glucose 5% *or* Sodium Chloride 0.9%

Pancuronium (Non-proprietary) [PoM]
 Injection, pancuronium bromide 2 mg/mL, net price 2-mL amp = £1.20

▎**ROCURONIUM BROMIDE**

Cautions   see notes above

 Hepatic impairment   reduce dose

 Renal impairment   reduce maintenance dose; prolonged paralysis

 Pregnancy   manufacturer advises caution

 Breast-feeding   present in milk in *animal* studies—manufacturer advises avoid unless potential benefit outweighs risk

Side-effects   see notes above

Indication and dose

> To avoid excessive dosage in obese children, dose should be calculated on the basis of ideal weight for height

Neuromuscular blockade (intermediate duration) during surgery

- **By intravenous administration**

 Child 1 month–18 years initially by *intravenous injection* 600 micrograms/kg, then *either* by *intravenous injection*, 150 micrograms/kg repeated as required *or* by *intravenous infusion*, 300–600 micrograms/kg/hour adjusted according to response

Administration   for *continuous intravenous infusion* or via drip tubing, may be diluted with Glucose 5% *or* Sodium Chloride 0.9%

Esmeron® (Organon) [PoM]
 Injection, rocuronium bromide 10 mg/mL, net price 5-mL vial = £3.01, 10-mL vial = £6.01

15

Anaesthesia

▲ VECURONIUM BROMIDE

Cautions see notes above

Pregnancy manufacturer advises avoid unless
potential benefit outweighs risk—no information
available

Breast-feeding no information available

Side-effects see notes above

Licensed use not licensed for assisted ventilation
in intensive care; not licensed without a test dose
in children under 5 months for neuromuscular
blockade during surgery

Indication and dose

> To avoid excessive dosage in obese children, dose
> should be calculated on the basis of ideal weight for
> height

Neuromuscular blockade (intermediate duration) during surgery
• By intravenous administration

Neonate by *intravenous injection* initially 80–
100 micrograms/kg, then 30–50 micrograms/kg
adjusted according to response

Child 1 month–18 years by *intravenous injection*
initially 80–100 micrograms/kg, then *either* by
intravenous injection, 20–30 micrograms/kg
repeated as required *or* by *intravenous infusion*,
50–80 micrograms/kg/hour, adjusted according to response

Assisted ventilation in intensive care
• By intravenous injection

Neonate initially 80–100 micrograms/kg, then
30–50 micrograms/kg adjusted according to
response usually every 2–4 hours

• By intravenous infusion

Child 1 month–18 years initially 80–100 micrograms/kg then 50–80 micrograms/kg/hour,
adjusted according to response; up to
200 micrograms/kg/hour may be required

Administration reconstitute each vial with 5 mL
Water for Injections to give 2 mg/mL solution;
alternatively reconstitute with up to 10 mL Glucose 5% *or* Sodium Chloride 0.9% *or* Water for
Injections *or* Ringer's solution—unsuitable for
further dilution if not reconstituted with Water for
Injections.

For *continuous intravenous infusion*, dilute reconstituted solution to a concentration up to
40 micrograms/mL with Glucose 5% *or* Sodium
Chloride 0.9% *or* Ringer's solution; reconstituted
solution can also be given via drip tubing

Norcuron® (Organon) [PoM]
Injection, powder for reconstitution, vecuronium
bromide, net price 10-mg vial = £3.95 (with water
for injections)

Depolarising neuromuscular blocking drugs

Suxamethonium has the most rapid onset of action of any of the neuromuscular
blocking drugs and is ideal if fast onset and brief duration of action are required
e.g. with tracheal intubation. Neonates and young children are less sensitive to
suxamethonium and a higher dose may be required.

Suxamethonium acts by mimicking acetylcholine at the neuromuscular junction
but hydrolysis is much slower than for acetylcholine; depolarisation is therefore
prolonged, resulting in neuromuscular blockade. Unlike the non-depolarising
neuromuscular blocking drugs, its action cannot be reversed and recovery is
spontaneous; anticholinesterases such as neostigmine potentiate the neuromuscular block.

Suxamethonium should be given after anaesthetic induction because paralysis is
usually preceded by painful muscle fasciculations. Bradycardia may occur; premedication with atropine (section 15.1.3) reduces bradycardia as well as the
excessive salivation associated with suxamethonium use.

Prolonged paralysis may occur in **dual block**, which occurs with high or repeated
doses of suxamethonium and is caused by the development of a non-depolarising
block following the initial depolarising block; edrophonium (section 15.1.6) may
be used to confirm the diagnosis of dual block. Children with myasthenia gravis
are resistant to suxamethonium but can develop dual block resulting in delayed
recovery. Prolonged paralysis may also occur in those with low or atypical plasma
cholinesterase. Assisted ventilation should be continued until muscle function is
restored.

▲ SUXAMETHONIUM CHLORIDE
(Succinylcholine chloride)

Cautions see notes above; hypersensitivity to
other neuromuscular blocking drugs; patients
with cardiac, respiratory or neuromuscular disease; raised intra-ocular pressure (avoid in

penetrating eye injury); severe sepsis (risk of
hyperkalaemia); **interactions:** Appendix 1
(muscle relaxants)

Pregnancy mildly prolonged maternal paralysis
may occur

◻ **SUXAMETHONIUM CHLORIDE (continued)**

Contra-indications family history of malignant hyperthermia, hyperkalaemia; major trauma, severe burns, neurological disease involving acute wasting of major muscle, prolonged immobilisation—risk of hyperkalaemia, personal or family history of congenital myotonic disease, Duchenne muscular dystrophy, low plasma-cholinesterase activity (including severe liver disease, see below)

Hepatic impairment prolonged apnoea may occur in severe liver disease because of reduced hepatic synthesis of pseudocholinesterase

Side-effects see notes above; also increased gastric pressure; hyperkalaemia; postoperative muscle pain, myoglobinuria, myoglobinaemia; increased intraocular pressure; flushing, rash; *rarely* arrhythmias, cardiac arrest; bronchospasm, apnoea, prolonged respiratory depression; limited jaw mobility; *very rarely* anaphylactic reactions, malignant hyperthermia; *also reported* hypertension, hypotension, rhabdomyolysis

Indication and dose

Neuromuscular blockade during surgery
• **By intravenous injection**

Neonate 2 mg/kg produces 5-10 minutes paralysis; 3mg/kg results in full neuromuscular block

Child 1 month–1 year initially 2 mg/kg, maintenance usually 1–2 mg/kg at 5–10 minute intervals as necessary

Child 1–18 years initially 1 mg/kg, then 0.5–1 mg/kg repeated every 5–10 minutes as necessary

• **By intramuscular injection**

Neonate up to 4–5 mg/kg produces 10–30 minutes paralysis (after 2–3 minute delay)

Child 1 month–1 year up to 4–5 mg/kg (paralysis after 2–3 minute delay)

Child 1–12 years up to 4 mg/kg (paralysis after 2–3 minute delay); max. 150 mg

Administration for *intravenous injection*, give undiluted *or* dilute with Glucose 5% *or* Sodium Chloride 0.9%

Suxamethonium Chloride (Non-proprietary) PoM
Injection, suxamethonium chloride 50 mg/mL, net price 2-mL amp = 64p, 2-mL prefilled syringe = £7.35

Anectine® (GSK) PoM
Injection, suxamethonium chloride 50 mg/mL, net price 2-mL amp = 71p

---

15.1.6 ▌ **Drugs for reversal of neuromuscular blockade**

▌ **Anticholinesterases**

Anticholinesterases reverse the effects of the non-depolarising (competitive) neuromuscular blocking drugs such as pancuronium, but they prolong the action of the depolarising neuromuscular blocking drug suxamethonium.

Edrophonium has a transient action and may be used in the diagnosis of suspected dual block due to suxamethonium. Atropine (section 15.1.3) is given before or with edrophonium to prevent muscarinic effects of edrophonium; it is also used in the diagnosis of myasthenia gravis (section 10.2.1).

Neostigmine has a longer duration of action than edrophonium and is used specifically for reversal of non-depolarising (competitive) blockade. It acts within one minute of intravenous injection and its effects last for 20 to 30 minutes; a second dose may then be necessary. Glycopyrronium or alternatively atropine (section 15.1.3), given before or with neostigmine, prevent bradycardia, excessive salivation, and other muscarinic effects of neostigmine.

▌ **EDROPHONIUM CHLORIDE**

Cautions section 10.2.1; atropine should also be given

Contra-indications section 10.2.1

Side-effects section 10.2.1

Indication and dose

Brief reversal of non-depolarising neuromuscular blockade
• **By intravenous injection over several minutes**

Child 1 month–18 years 500–700 micrograms/kg (after or with atropine)

Myasthenia gravis (section 10.2.1)

Edrophonium (Cambridge) PoM
Injection, edrophonium chloride 10 mg/mL, net price 1-mL amp = £6.55

15 Anaesthesia

NEOSTIGMINE METILSULFATE
(Neostigmine methylsulphate)

Cautions section 10.2.1; glycopyrronium or atropine should also be given

Contra-indications section 10.2.1

Side-effects section 10.2.1

Indication and dose

> Reversal of non-depolarising muscle block
> • By intravenous injection over 1 minute
>
> **Neonate** 50–80 micrograms/kg, after or with glycopyrronium or atropine
>
> **Child 1 month–12 years** 50–80 micrograms/kg (max. 2.5 mg) after or with glycopyrronium or atropine
>
> **Child 12–18 years** 50–80 micrograms/kg (max. 5 mg) after or with glycopyrronium or atropine

> Myasthenia gravis section 10.2.1

Administration for *intravenous injection*, give undiluted *or* dilute with Glucose 5% *or* Sodium Chloride 0.9% *or* Water for Injections

Neostigmine (Non-proprietary) [PoM]
Injection, neostigmine metilsulfate 2.5 mg/mL, net price 1-mL amp = 58p

◢ **With glycopyrronium**

Robinul-Neostigmine® (Anpharm) [PoM]
Injection, neostigmine metilsulfate 2.5 mg, glycopyrronium bromide 500 micrograms/mL, net price 1-mL amp = £1.15

Dose

> Reversal of non-depolarising neuromuscular blockade
> • By intravenous injection over 10–30 seconds
>
> **Child 1 month–18 years** 0.02 mL/kg (*or* 0.2 mL/kg of a 1 in 10 dilution), dose may be repeated if required (total max. 2 mL)

Administration for *intravenous injection*, may be diluted with Sodium Chloride 0.9% *or* Water for Injections
Note May be difficult to obtain

Other drugs for reversal of neuromuscular blockade

Sugammadex is a modified gamma cyclodextrin used for reversal of neuromuscular blockade induced by rocuronium (section 15.1.5).

SUGAMMADEX

Cautions recurrence of neuromuscular blockade—monitor respiratory function until fully recovered; recovery may be delayed in cardiovascular disease; wait 24 hours before re-administering rocuronium; **interactions:** Appendix 1 (sugammadex)

Renal impairment avoid if estimated glomerular filtration rate less then 30 mL/minute/1.73 m^2

Pregnancy manufacturer advises caution—no information available

Side-effects taste disturbances; *less commonly* allergic reactions; bronchospasm also reported

Indication and dose

> Routine reversal of neuromuscular blockade induced by rocuronium
> • By intravenous injection
>
> **Child 2–18 years** 2 mg/kg (consult product literature)

Administration for *intravenous injection* dose may be diluted to a concentration of 10 mg/mL with Sodium Chloride 0.9%

Bridion® (Schering-Plough) ▼ [PoM]
Injection, sugammadex (as sodium salt) 100 mg/mL, net price 2-mL amp = £59.64, 5-mL amp = £149.10
Electrolytes Na$^+$ 0.42 mmol/mL

15.1.7 **Antagonists for central and respiratory depression**

Respiratory depression is a major concern with opioid analgesics and it may be treated by artificial ventilation or be reversed by an opioid antagonist. **Naloxone** given intravenously immediately reverses opioid-induced respiratory depression but the dose may have to be repeated because of its **short duration of action**. Intramuscular injection of naloxone produces a more gradual and prolonged effect but absorption may be erratic. Care is required in children requiring pain relief because naloxone also antagonises the analgesic effect of opioids.

Neonates Naloxone is used in newborn infants to reverse respiratory depression and sedation resulting from the use of opioids by the mother, usually for pain during labour. In neonates the effects of opioids may persist for up to 48 hours and in such cases naloxone is often given by intramuscular injection for its prolonged effect. In severe respiratory depression after birth, breathing should first be established (using artificial means if necessary) and naloxone administered only if use of opioids by the mother is thought to cause the respiratory depression; the infant should be monitored closely and further doses of naloxone administered as necessary.

Flumazenil is a benzodiazepine antagonist for the reversal of the central sedative effects of benzodiazepines after anaesthetic and similar procedures. Flumazenil has a shorter half-life and duration of action than diazepam and midazolam, so children may become resedated.

Doxapram (section 3.5.1) is a central and respiratory stimulant but is of limited value in anaesthesia.

FLUMAZENIL

Cautions short-acting (repeat doses may be necessary—benzodiazepine effects may persist for at least 24 hours); benzodiazepine dependence (may precipitate withdrawal symptoms); prolonged benzodiazepine therapy for epilepsy (risk of convulsions); history of panic disorders (risk of recurrence); ensure neuromuscular blockade cleared before giving; avoid rapid injection in high-risk or anxious children and following major surgery; head injury (rapid reversal of benzodiazepine sedation may cause convulsions)

Hepatic impairment carefully titrate dose

Pregnancy may cross placenta in small amounts—manufacturer advises avoid unless potential benefit outweighs risk

Contra-indications life-threatening condition (e.g. raised intracranial pressure, status epilepticus) controlled by benzodiazepines

Side-effects nausea, vomiting, and flushing; if wakening too rapid, agitation, anxiety, and fear; transient increase in blood pressure and heart-rate in intensive care patients; *very rarely* convulsions (particularly in those with epilepsy), hypersensitivity reactions including anaphylaxis

Licensed use not licensed for use in children

Indication and dose

Reversal of sedative effects of benzodiazepines
• **By intravenous injection over 15 seconds (question aetiology if no response to repeated injection)**

Neonate 10 micrograms/kg, repeat at 1-minute intervals if required

Child 1 month–12 years 10 micrograms/kg (max. single dose 200 micrograms), repeated at 1-minute intervals if required; max. total dose of 40 micrograms/kg (1 mg) (2 mg in intensive care)

Child 12–18 years 200 micrograms, repeated at 1-minute intervals if required; max. total dose 1 mg (2 mg in intensive care)

• **By intravenous infusion, if drowsiness recurs after injection**

Neonate 2–10 micrograms/kg/hour, adjusted according to response

Child 1 month–18 years 2–10 micrograms/kg/hour, adjusted according to response; max. 400 micrograms/hour

Administration for *continuous intravenous infusion*, dilute with Glucose 5% *or* Sodium Chloride 0.9%

Flumazenil (Non-proprietary) (PoM)
Injection, flumazenil 100 micrograms/mL, net price 5-mL amp = £14.49

Anexate® (Roche) (PoM)
Injection, flumazenil 100 micrograms/mL, net price 5-mL amp = £14.49

NALOXONE HYDROCHLORIDE

Cautions cardiovascular disease or those receiving cardiotoxic drugs (serious adverse cardiovascular effects reported); maternal physical dependence on opioids (may precipitate withdrawal in newborn); pain (see also under Titration of Dose, below); has short duration of action (see notes above)

Titration of dose In postoperative use, the dose should be titrated for each child in order to obtain sufficient respiratory response; however, naloxone antagonises analgesia

Pregnancy manufacturer advises use only if potential benefit outweighs risk

Side-effects hypotension, hypertension, ventricular tachycardia and fibrillation, cardiac arrest; hyperventilation, dyspnoea, pulmonary oedema; *less commonly* agitation, excitement, paraesthesia

Indication and dose

Reversal of respiratory and CNS depression in neonate following maternal opioid use during labour
• **By intramuscular injection**

Neonate 200 micrograms (60 micrograms/kg) as a single dose at birth

• **By intravenous or subcutaneous injection**

Neonate 10 micrograms/kg, repeated every 2–3 minutes if required

15

Anaesthesia

◿ **NALOXONE HYDROCHLORIDE** *(continued)*

Reversal of opioid-induced respiratory depression
• By intravenous injection
  Neonate 5–10 micrograms/kg, repeated every 2–3 minutes if required

  Child 1 month–12 years 5–10 micrograms/kg; if response inadequate, give a subsequent dose of 100 micrograms/kg (max. 2 mg)

  Child 12–18 years 1.5–3 micrograms/kg; if response inadequate, give subsequent doses of 100 micrograms every 2 minutes

• By continuous intravenous infusion
  Neonate 5–20 micrograms/kg/hour, adjusted according to response

  Child 1 month–18 years 5–20 micrograms/kg/hour, adjusted according to response

Overdosage with opioids see Emergency Treatment of Poisoning p. 39

Administration for *continuous intravenous infusion*, dilute to a concentration of 4 micrograms/mL (24 micrograms/mL if fluid restricted) with Glucose 5% *or* Sodium Chloride 0.9%

Naloxone PoM
See under Emergency Treatment of Poisoning p. 40

15.1.8 Drugs for malignant hyperthermia

Malignant hyperthermia is a rare but potentially lethal complication of anaesthesia. It is characterised by a rapid rise in temperature, increased muscle rigidity, tachycardia, and acidosis. The most common triggers of malignant hyperthermia are the volatile anaesthetics. Suxamethonium has also been implicated, but malignant hyperthermia is more likely if it is given following a volatile anaesthetic. Volatile anaesthetics and suxamethonium should be avoided during anaesthesia in children at high risk of malignant hyperthermia.

Dantrolene is used in the treatment of malignant hyperthermia. It acts on skeletal muscle cells by interfering with calcium efflux, thereby stopping the contractile process.

▌ DANTROLENE SODIUM

Cautions avoid extravasation (risk of tissue necrosis); **interactions**: Appendix 1 (muscle relaxants)

Pregnancy use only if potential benefit outweighs risk

Breast-feeding present in milk—manufacturer advises use only if potential benefit outweighs the risk

Side-effects hepatotoxicity, pulmonary oedema, dizziness, weakness, and injection-site reactions including erythema, rash, swelling, and thrombophlebitis

Indication and dose
Malignant hyperthermia
• By rapid intravenous injection
  Child 1 month–18 years initially 2–3 mg/kg, then 1 mg/kg repeated as required (total max. dose 10 mg/kg)

Chronic severe spasticity of voluntary muscle see section 10.2.2

Dantrium Intravenous® (Procter & Gamble Pharm.) PoM
Injection, powder for reconstitution, dantrolene sodium, net price 20-mg vial = £15.08 (hosp. only)

15.2 Local anaesthesia

The use of local anaesthetics by injection or by application to mucous membranes to produce local analgesia is discussed in this section.

See also section 1.7 (anus), section 11.7 (eye), section 12.3 (oropharynx), and section 13.3 (skin).

Use of local anaesthetics Local anaesthetic drugs act by causing a reversible block to conduction along nerve fibres. The drugs used vary widely in their potency, toxicity, duration of action, stability, solubility in water, and ability to penetrate mucous membranes. These variations determine their suitability for use by various routes, e.g. topical (surface), infiltration, peripheral nerve block, intravenous regional anaesthesia (Bier's block), plexus, epidural (extradural) or spinal block. Local anaesthetics may also be used for postoperative pain relief, thereby reducing the need for analgesics such as opioids.

15 Anaesthesia

Administration   In estimating the safe dosage of these drugs it is important to take account of the rate at which they are absorbed and excreted as well as their potency. The child's age, weight, physique, and clinical condition, the degree of vascularity of the area to which the drug is to be applied, and the duration of administration are other factors which must be taken into account.

Local anaesthetics do not rely on the circulation to transport them to their sites of action, but uptake into the systemic circulation is important in terminating their action and producing toxicity. Following most regional anaesthetic procedures, maximum arterial plasma concentrations of anaesthetic develop within about 10 to 25 minutes, so **careful surveillance** for toxic effects is necessary during the first 30 minutes after injection. Great care must be taken to avoid accidental intravascular injection. Local anaesthesia around the oral cavity may impair swallowing and therefore increase the risk of aspiration.

Epidural anaesthesia is commonly used during surgery, often combined with general anaesthesia, because of its protective effect against the stress response of surgery. It is often used for major surgery in children, including orthopaedic and abdominal surgery.

Toxicity   Toxic effects associated with local anaesthetics usually result from excessively high plasma concentrations; single application of topical lidocaine preparations does not generally cause systemic side-effects. Effects initially include a feeling of inebriation and lightheadedness followed by sedation, circumoral paraesthesia and twitching; convulsions can occur in severe reactions. On intravenous injection convulsions and cardiovascular collapse may occur very rapidly. Hypersensitivity reactions occur mainly with the ester-type local anaesthetics such as benzocaine, procaine, and tetracaine (amethocaine); reactions are less frequent with the amide types such as lidocaine (lignocaine), bupivacaine, levobupivacaine, prilocaine, and ropivacaine. Local anaesthetics may be associated with methaemoglobinaemia; prilocaine and benzocaine have been implicated.

When prolonged analgesia is required, a long-acting local anaesthetic is preferred to minimise the likelihood of cumulative systemic toxicity. Local anaesthetic injections should be given slowly in order to detect inadvertent intravascular administration. Local anaesthetics should **not** be injected into inflamed or infected tissues nor should they be applied to the traumatised urethra. In such cases absorption into the blood may increase the possibility of systemic side-effects. The local anaesthetic effect may also be reduced by the altered local pH. Local anaesthetics can also be ototoxic and should **not** be applied to the middle ear.

Use of vasoconstrictors   Most local anaesthetics cause dilation of blood vessels. The addition of a vasoconstrictor such as **adrenaline (epinephrine)** diminishes local blood flow, slows the rate of absorption of the local anaesthetic, and prolongs its local effect. Adrenaline must be used in a low concentration (e.g. 1 in 400 000–1 in 200 000) for this purpose and it should **not** be given with a local anaesthetic injection in digits and appendages; it may produce ischaemic necrosis.

When adrenaline is included the final concentration should be no more than 1 in 200 000 (5 micrograms/mL), but see also Dental Anaesthesia, below. The total dose of adrenaline should **not** exceed 5 micrograms/kg (1 mL/kg of a 1 in 200 000 solution). Care must also be taken to calculate a safe maximum dose of local anaesthetic when using combination products. For general cautions associated with the use of adrenaline, see section 2.7.3. For drug interactions, see Appendix 1 (sympathomimetics).

Dental anaesthesia   **Lidocaine** (lignocaine) is widely used in dental procedures; it is most often used in combination with **adrenaline** (epinephrine). Lidocaine 2% combined with adrenaline 1 in 80 000 (12.5 micrograms/mL) is a safe and effective preparation; there is no justification for using higher concentrations of adrenaline.

The local anaesthetics **articaine** (carticaine) and **mepivacaine** are also used in dentistry; they are available in cartridges suitable for dental use. Mepivacaine is available with or without adrenaline (as *Scandonest*®) and articaine is available with adrenaline (as *Septanest*®).

15

Anaesthesia

In children with severe hypertension or unstable cardiac rhythm, the use of adrenaline in a local anaesthetic may be hazardous. For these children **prilocaine** with or without felypressin can be used but there is no evidence that it is any safer.

Great care should be taken to avoid inadvertent intravenous administration of a preparation containing adrenaline.

Lidocaine

Lidocaine (lignocaine) is effectively absorbed from mucous membranes and is a useful surface anaesthetic in concentrations up to 10%. Except for surface anaesthesia and dental anaesthesia, solutions should not usually exceed 1% in strength. The duration of the block (with adrenaline) is about 90 minutes.

Application of a mixture of lidocaine and prilocaine (*EMLA®*) under an occlusive dressing provides surface anaesthesia for 1–2 hours. *EMLA®* does not appear to be effective in providing local anaesthesia for heel lancing in neonates.

LIDOCAINE HYDROCHLORIDE
(Lignocaine hydrochloride)

Cautions see notes above; see section 2.3.2 for effects on heart; also epilepsy, respiratory impairment, impaired cardiac conduction, bradycardia, severe shock; acute porphyria (section 9.8.2); myasthenia gravis; reduce dose in debilitated; resuscitative equipment should be available; **interactions**: Appendix 1 (lidocaine)

Hepatic impairment manufacturer advises caution—increased risk of side-effects

Renal impairment possible accumulation of lidocaine and active metabolite; manufacturers advise caution in severe impairment

Pregnancy with large doses, neonatal respiratory depression, hypotonia and bradycardia after paracervical or epidural block

Breast-feeding amount too small to be harmful

Contra-indications see notes above; also hypovolaemia, complete heart block; do not use solutions containing adrenaline for anaesthesia in appendages

Side-effects see notes above and section 2.3.2; also CNS effects include confusion, respiratory depression and convulsions; hypotension and bradycardia (may lead to cardiac arrest); hypersensitivity reported

Licensed use *EMLA®* cream not licensed for use in children under 1 year

Indication and dose

Local anaesthesia
- By local infiltration
  (see also Administration p. 787 and *Safe Practice* warning below)

  Neonate according to nature of procedure, up to 3 mg/kg (0.3 mL/kg of 1% solution), repeated not more often than every 4 hours

  Child 1 month–12 years according to nature of procedure, up to 3 mg/kg (0.3 mL/kg of 1% solution), repeated not more often than every 4 hours

  Child 12–18 years according to nature of procedure, up to 200 mg, repeated not more often than every 4 hours

Ventricular arrhythmias section 2.3.2

Intravenous regional anaesthesia and nerve blocks seek expert advice

Dental anaesthesia seek expert advice

Safe Practice The licensed doses stated above may not be appropriate in some settings and expert advice should be sought

◢ **Lidocaine hydrochloride injections**
Lidocaine (Non-proprietary) PoM
Injection 0.5%, lidocaine hydrochloride 5 mg/mL, net price 10-mL amp = 35p

Injection 1%, lidocaine hydrochloride 10 mg/mL, net price 2-mL amp = 21p; 5-mL amp = 25p; 10-mL amp = 38p; 10-mL prefilled syringe = £4.53; 20-mL amp = 78p

Injection 2%, lidocaine hydrochloride 20 mg/mL, net price 2-mL amp = 27p; 5-mL amp = 28p

Xylocaine® (AstraZeneca) PoM
Injection 1% with adrenaline 1 in 200 000, anhydrous lidocaine hydrochloride 10 mg/mL, adrenaline 1 in 200 000 (5 micrograms/mL), net price 20-mL vial = 99p

Injection 2% with adrenaline 1 in 200 000, anhydrous lidocaine hydrochloride 20 mg/mL, adrenaline 1 in 200 000 (5 micrograms/mL), net price 20-mL vial = £1.04

◢ **Lidocaine injections for dental use**
Note Consult expert dental sources for specific advice in relation to dose of lidocaine for dental anaesthesia

A variety of lidocaine injections with adrenaline are available in dental cartridges; brand names include *Lignospan Special®*, *Rexocaine®*, *Xylocaine®*, and *Xylotox®*.

◢ **Lidocaine for surface anaesthesia**
Important. Rapid and extensive absorption may result in systemic side-effects

Lidocaine (Non-proprietary)
Ointment, lidocaine hydrochloride 5%, net price 15 g = 88p
Dose
  Dental practice
    Child rub gently into dry gum

◁ **LIDOCAINE HYDROCHLORIDE (continued)**

Pain relief (in anal fissures, haemorrhoids, pruritus ani, pruritus vulvae, herpes zoster)
    Child 1–2 mL applied when necessary; avoid long-term use

Solution, lidocaine hydrochloride 4%, net price 25 mL = £1.35

Dose

Biopsy in mouth
    Child up to 3 mg/kg with suitable spray or swab (with adrenaline if necessary); max. 5 mL

Puncture of maxillary sinus or polypectomy
    Child up to 3 mg/kg; apply with swab for 2–3 minutes (with adrenaline)

Bronchoscopy and bronchography
    Child up to 3 mg/kg; 2–3 mL with suitable spray

EMLA® (AstraZeneca)
Drug Tariff cream, lidocaine 2.5%, prilocaine 2.5%, net price 5-g tube = £1.73

Surgical pack cream, lidocaine 2.5%, prilocaine 2.5%, net price 30-g tube = £10.25

Premedication pack cream, lidocaine 2.5%, prilocaine 2.5%, net price 5 × 5-g tube with 12 occlusive dressings = £9.75

Cautions not for preterm neonates, children under 1 year receiving treatment with methaemoglobin-inducing agents, wounds, mucous membranes, or atopic dermatitis; avoid use near eyes or middle ear; although systemic absorption low, caution in anaemia, in congenital or acquired methaemoglobinaemia or in G6PD deficiency (see also Prilocaine, p. 791)

Side-effects include administration site reactions such as transient paleness, redness, oedema, itching, burning sensation, and localised lesions

Dose

Anaesthesia before minor skin procedures including venepuncture

    Neonate apply max. 1 g under occlusive dressing for max. 1 hour before procedure; max. 1 dose in 24 hours

    Child 1–3 months or body-weight less than 5 kg apply max. 1 g under occlusive dressing for max. 1 hour before procedure; max. 1 dose in 24 hours

    Child 3 months–1 year and body weight over 5 kg apply max. 2 g under occlusive dressing for max. 4 hours before procedure; max. 2 doses in 24 hours

    Child 1–18 years apply thick layer under occlusive dressing 1–5 hours before procedure (2–5 hours before procedures on large areas e.g. split skin grafting); max. 2 doses in 24 hours for child 1–12 years

Note Shorter application time of 15–30 minutes is recommended for children with atopic dermatitis

Instillagel® (CliniMed)
Gel, lidocaine hydrochloride 2%, chlorhexidine gluconate solution 0.25%, in a sterile lubricant basis in disposable syringe, net price 6-mL syringe = £1.41, 11-mL syringe = £1.58
Excipients include hydroxybenzoates (parabens)

Laryngojet® (UCB Pharma) [PoM]
Jet spray 4% (disposable kit for laryngotracheal anaesthesia), lidocaine hydrochloride 40 mg/mL, net price per unit (4-mL vial and disposable sterile cannula with cover and vial injector) = £5.10

Cautions may be rapidly and almost completely absorbed from respiratory tract and systemic side-effects may occur; extreme caution if mucosa has been traumatised or if sepsis present

Dose

Bronchoscopy, laryngoscopy, oesophagoscopy, endotracheal intubation, and biopsy
    Child up to 0.075 mL/kg (3 mg/kg) as a single dose instilled as jet spray or applied with a swab; max. 5 mL (200 mg)

LMX 4® (Ferndale)
Cream lidocaine 4%, net price 5-g tube = £2.98; 5 × 5-g tube with 10 occlusive dressings = £16.90
Excipients include benzyl alcohol and propylene glycol

Cautions not for wounds, mucous membranes or atopic dermatitis, avoid use near eyes or middle ear; although systemic absorption low, caution in severe hepatic impairment, acutely ill or debilitated children

Side-effects irritation and rash

Dose

Anaesthesia before venous cannulation or vene-puncture
    Child 1 month–18 years apply thick layer (1–2.5 g; child under 1 year max 1 g) to small area (2.5 cm × 2.5 cm) of non-irritated skin at least 30 minutes before procedure (max 60 minutes); remove cream with gauze and perform procedure after approximately 5 minutes

Rapydan® (EUSA Pharma) [PoM]
Medicated plasters, lidocaine 70 mg, tetracaine 70 mg, net price 25 = £98.00
Excipients include hydroxybenzoates (parabens)

Dose

Needle puncture
    Child 3–18 years apply 1–2 plasters to intact skin 30 minutes before needle puncture; max. 2 plasters daily

Xylocaine® (AstraZeneca)
Spray (= pump spray), lidocaine 10% (100 mg/g) supplying 10 mg lidocaine/dose; 500 spray doses per container, net price 50-mL bottle = £3.13

Dose

Bronchoscopy, laryngoscopy, oesophagoscopy, endotracheal intubation
    Child up to 18 years up to 3 mg/kg

Note Lidocaine can damage plastic cuffs of endotracheal tubes

◀**Lidocaine for ear, nose, and oropharyngeal use**
For **cautions**, **contra-indications** and **side-effects** of phenylephrine, see section 2.7.2

Lidocaine with Phenylephrine (Non-proprietary)
Topical solution, lidocaine hydrochloride 5%, phenylephrine hydrochloride 0.5%, net price 2.5 mL (with nasal applicator) = £9.60

15 Anaesthesia

Bupivacaine

The advantage of bupivacaine over other local anaesthetics is its longer duration of action (3–7 hours). It has a slow onset of action, taking up to 30 minutes for full effect. It is often used in lumbar epidural blockade and is particularly suitable for continuous epidural analgesia in labour or for postoperative pain relief. It is the principal drug used for spinal anaesthesia.

BUPIVACAINE HYDROCHLORIDE

Cautions see under Lidocaine Hydrochloride and notes above; myocardial depression may be more severe and more resistant to treatment; **interactions**: Appendix 1 (bupivacaine)

Hepatic impairment manufacturer advises caution in severe impairment

Renal impairment manufacturer advises caution

Pregnancy large doses during the third trimester can cause neonatal respiratory depression, hypotonia, and bradycardia after paracervical or epidural block; lower doses for intrathecal use during late pregnancy

Breast-feeding amount too small to be harmful

Contra-indications see under Lidocaine Hydrochloride and notes above; intravenous regional anaesthesia (Bier's block)

Side-effects see under Lidocaine Hydrochloride and notes above

Indication and dose

Adjusted according to child's physical status and nature of procedure, seek expert advice—**important**: see also under Administration, p. 787

Bupivacaine (Non-proprietary) PoM

Injection, anhydrous bupivacaine hydrochloride 2.5 mg/mL (0.25%), net price 10 mL = 82p; 5 mg/mL (0.5%), 10 mL = 94p

Note Bupivacaine hydrochloride injection 0.25% and 0.5% are available in glass or plastic ampoules, and sterile-wrapped glass ampoules

Infusion, anhydrous bupivacaine hydrochloride 1 mg/mL (0.1%), net price 100 mL = £8.41, 250 mL = £10.59; 1.25 mg/mL (0.125%), 250 mL = £10.80

Marcain® (AstraZeneca) PoM

Injection, anhydrous bupivacaine hydrochloride 2.5 mg/mL (*Marcain® 0.25%*), net price 10-mL *Polyamp®* = £1.06; 5 mg/mL (*Marcain® 0.5%*), 10-mL *Polyamp®* = £1.21

Marcain Heavy® (AstraZeneca) PoM

Injection, anhydrous bupivacaine hydrochloride 5 mg, glucose 80 mg/mL, net price 4-mL amp = £1.21

◀ With adrenaline

Bupivacaine and Adrenaline (Non-proprietary) PoM

Injection, anhydrous bupivacaine hydrochloride 2.5 mg/mL (0.25%), adrenaline 1 in 200 000 (5 micrograms/mL), net price 10-mL amp = £1.23

Injection, anhydrous bupivacaine hydrochloride 5 mg/mL (0.5%), adrenaline 1 in 200 000 (5 micrograms/mL), net price 10-mL amp = £1.40

Levobupivacaine

Levobupivacaine, an isomer of bupivacaine, has anaesthetic and analgesic properties similar to bupivacaine but is thought to have fewer adverse effects.

LEVOBUPIVACAINE

Note Levobupivacaine is an isomer of bupivacaine

Cautions see under Lidocaine Hydrochloride and notes above; **interactions**: Appendix 1 (levobupivacaine)

Hepatic impairment manufacturer advises caution

Pregnancy large doses during the third trimester can cause neonatal respiratory depression, hypotonia, and bradycardia after paracervical or epidural block; manufacturer advises avoid if possible—toxicity in *animal* studies

Breast-feeding likely to be present in milk but risk to infant minimal

Contra-indications see under Lidocaine Hydrochloride and notes above; intravenous regional anaesthesia (Bier's block); paracervical block in obstetrics

Side-effects see under Lidocaine Hydrochloride and notes above

Licensed use not licensed for use in children by epidural infusion

Indication and dose

Adjusted according to child's physical status and nature of procedure, seek expert advice—**important**: see also under Administration, p. 787

Chirocaine® (Abbott) PoM

Injection, levobupivacaine (as hydrochloride) 2.5 mg/mL, net price 10-mL amp = £1.66; 5 mg/mL, 10-mL amp = £1.90; 7.5 mg/mL, 10-mL amp = £2.85

Infusion, levobupivacaine (as hydrochloride) 625 micrograms/mL, net price 100 mL = £7.80, 200 mL = £10.40; 1.25 mg/mL, net price 100 mL = £8.54, 200 mL = £12.20

Prilocaine

Prilocaine is a local anaesthetic of low toxicity which is similar to lidocaine (lignocaine). If used in high doses, methaemoglobinaemia may occur which can be treated with intravenous injection of methylthioninium chloride (methylene blue) 1% using a dose of 1 mg/kg. Neonates and infants under 6 months are particularly susceptible to methaemoglobinaemia.

▲ PRILOCAINE HYDROCHLORIDE

Cautions see under Lidocaine Hydrochloride and notes above; severe or untreated hypertension, severe heart disease; concomitant drugs which cause methaemoglobinaemia; hepatic impairment; renal impairment; **interactions**: Appendix 1 (prilocaine)

Hepatic impairment manufacturer advises caution

Renal impairment manufacturer advises caution

Pregnancy large doses during the third trimester can cause neonatal respiratory depression, hypotonia, and bradycardia after paracervical or epidural block; neonatal methaemoglobinaemia reported after paracervical block or pudendal block

Breast-feeding present in milk but not known to be harmful

Contra-indications see under Lidocaine Hydrochloride and notes above; anaemia or congenital or acquired methaemoglobinaemia

Side-effects see under Lidocaine Hydrochloride and notes above; ocular toxicity (including blindness) reported with excessively high strengths used for ophthalmic procedures

Indication and dose

> Infiltration anaesthesia (higher strengths for dental use only), nerve block
> See under preparations below, seek expert advice—**important**: see also under Administration, p. 787

Citanest® (AstraZeneca) ▣PoM
Injection 1%, prilocaine hydrochloride 10 mg/mL, net price 50-mL multidose vial = £2.01

Dose

> **Child 6 months–12 years** up to 5 mg/kg adjusted according to site of administration and response; max. 400 mg
> **Child 12–18 years** 100–200 mg/minute, or in incremental doses, to max. total dose 400 mg (adjusted according to site of administration and response)

◢With lidocaine
EMLA®
See Lidocaine, p. 789

◢For dental use
Note Consult expert dental sources for specific advice in relation to dose of prilocaine for dental anaesthesia

Citanest® (Dentsply) ▣PoM
Injection 4%, prilocaine hydrochloride 40 mg/mL, net price 2.2-mL cartridge = 17p

Citanest with Octapressin® (Dentsply) ▣PoM
Injection 3%, prilocaine hydrochloride 30 mg/mL, felypressin 0.03 unit/mL, net price 1.8-mL cartridge and self-aspirating cartridge (both) = 15p

Ropivacaine

Ropivacaine is an amide-type local anaesthetic agent similar to bupivacaine. It is less cardiotoxic than bupivacaine, but also less potent.

▲ ROPIVACAINE HYDROCHLORIDE

Cautions see under Lidocaine Hydrochloride and notes above; **interactions**: Appendix 1 (ropivacaine)

Hepatic impairment manufacturer advises caution in severe impairment

Renal impairment manufacturer advises caution in severe impairment

Pregnancy safety not established but not known to be harmful

Breast-feeding not known to be harmful

Contra-indications see under Lidocaine Hydrochloride and notes above; intravenous regional anaesthesia (Bier's block); paracervical block in obstetrics

Side-effects see under Lidocaine Hydrochloride and notes above

Licensed use not licensed for use in children by epidural infusion

Indication and dose

> Adjust according to child's physical status and nature of procedure, seek expert advice—**important**: see also under Administration, p. 787

Naropin® (AstraZeneca) ▣PoM
Injection, ropivacaine hydrochloride 2 mg/mL, net price 10-mL *Polyamp®* = £1.78; 7.5 mg/mL, 10-mL *Polyamp®* = £2.65; 10 mg/mL, 10-mL *Polyamp®* = £3.20

Epidural infusion, ropivacaine hydrochloride 2 mg/mL, net price 200-mL *Polybag®* = £14.45

15

Anaesthesia

Tetracaine

Tetracaine (amethocaine) is an effective local anaesthetic for topical application; a 4% gel is indicated for anaesthesia prior to venepuncture or venous cannulation. Tetracaine remains effective for 4–6 hours after a single application in most children. It does not appear to be effective prior to neonatal heel lancing.

Tetracaine is rapidly absorbed from mucous membranes and should **never** be applied to inflamed, traumatised, or highly vascular surfaces. It should **never** be used to provide anaesthesia for bronchoscopy or cystoscopy, as lidocaine (lignocaine) is a safer alternative. It is used in ophthalmology (section 11.7) and in skin preparations (section 13.3). Hypersensitivity to tetracaine has been reported.

TETRACAINE
(Amethocaine)

Cautions see notes above

Contra-indications see notes above

Side-effects see notes above; also erythema, oedema and pruritus; very rarely blistering
Important. Rapid and extensive absorption may result in systemic side-effects (see also notes above)

Licensed use not licensed for use in neonates

Ametop® (S&N Hlth.)
Gel, tetracaine 4%, net price 1.5-g tube = £1.08

Dose

> **Neonate** apply contents of tube (or appropriate proportion) to site of venepuncture or venous cannulation and cover with occlusive dressing; remove gel and dressing after 30 minutes for venepuncture and after 45 minutes for venous cannulation

> **Child 1 month–18 years** apply contents of tube (or appropriate proportion) to site of venepuncture or venous cannulation and cover with occlusive dressing; remove gel and dressing after 30 minutes for venepuncture and after 45 minutes for venous cannulation
> **Note** Child over 5 years, contents of max. 5 tubes applied at separate sites at a single time, child 1 month–5 years, contents of max. 1 tube applied at separate sites at a single time

◢ **With lidocaine**
Rapydan®
see Lidocaine, p. 789

A1 Interactions

Two or more drugs given at the same time may exert their effects independently or may interact. The interaction may be potentiation or antagonism of one drug by another, or occasionally some other effect. Adverse drug interactions should be reported to the CHM as for other adverse drug reactions.

Drug interactions may be **pharmacodynamic** or **pharmacokinetic**.

Pharmacodynamic interactions

These are interactions between drugs which have similar or antagonistic pharmacological effects or side-effects. They may be due to competition at receptor sites, or occur between drugs acting on the same physiological system. They are usually predictable from a knowledge of the pharmacology of the interacting drugs; in general, those demonstrated with one drug are likely to occur with related drugs. They occur to a greater or lesser extent in most patients who receive the interacting drugs.

Pharmacokinetic interactions

These occur when one drug alters the absorption, distribution, metabolism, or excretion of another, thus increasing or reducing the amount of drug available to produce its pharmacological effects. They are not easily predicted and many of them affect only a small proportion of patients taking the combination of drugs. Pharmacokinetic interactions occurring with one drug cannot be assumed to occur with related drugs unless their pharmacokinetic properties are known to be similar.

Pharmacokinetic interactions are of several types:

Affecting absorption   The rate of absorption or the total amount absorbed can both be altered by drug interactions. Delayed absorption is rarely of clinical importance unless high peak plasma concentrations are required (e.g. when giving an analgesic). Reduction in the total amount absorbed, however, may result in ineffective therapy.

Due to changes in protein binding   To a variable extent most drugs are loosely bound to plasma proteins. Protein-binding sites are non-specific and one drug can displace another thereby increasing its proportion free to diffuse from plasma to its site of action. This only produces a detectable increase in effect if it is an extensively bound drug (more than 90%) that is not widely distributed throughout the body. Even so displacement rarely produces more than transient potentiation because this increased concentration of free drug results in an increased rate of elimination.

Displacement from protein binding plays a part in the potentiation of warfarin by sulphonamides, and tolbutamide but the importance of these interactions is due mainly to the fact that warfarin metabolism is also inhibited.

Affecting metabolism   Many drugs are metabolised in the liver. Induction of the hepatic microsomal enzyme system by one drug can gradually increase the rate of metabolism of another, resulting in lower plasma concentrations and a reduced effect. On withdrawal of the inducer plasma concentrations increase and toxicity may occur. Barbiturates, griseofulvin, many antiepileptics, and rifampicin are the most important enzyme inducers. Drugs affected include warfarin and the oral contraceptives.

Conversely when one drug inhibits the metabolism of another higher plasma concentrations are produced, rapidly resulting in an increased effect with risk of toxicity. Some drugs which potentiate warfarin and phenytoin do so by this mechanism.

Appendix 1: Interactions

Isoenzymes of the hepatic cytochrome P450 system interact with a wide range of drugs. Drugs may be substrates, inducers or inhibitors of the different isoenzymes. A great deal of *in-vitro* information is available on the effect of drugs on the isoenzymes; however, since drugs are eliminated by a number of different metabolic routes as well as renal excretion, the clinical effects of interactions cannot be predicted accurately from laboratory data on the cytochrome P450 isoenzymes. Except where a combination of drugs is specifically contra-indicated, the BNF presents only interactions that have been reported in clinical practice. In all cases the possibility of an interaction must be considered if toxic effects occur or if the activity of a drug diminishes.

Affecting renal excretion Drugs are eliminated through the kidney both by glomerular filtration and by active tubular secretion. Competition occurs between those which share active transport mechanisms in the proximal tubule. For example, salicylates and some other NSAIDs delay the excretion of methotrexate; serious methotrexate toxicity is possible.

Relative importance of interactions

Many drug interactions are harmless and many of those which are potentially harmful only occur in a small proportion of patients; moreover, the severity of an interaction varies from one patient to another. Drugs with a small therapeutic ratio (e.g. phenytoin) and those which require careful control of dosage (e.g. anticoagulants, antihypertensives, and antidiabetics) are most often involved.

Patients at increased risk from drug interactions include those with impaired renal or liver function.

Hazardous interactions The symbol • has been placed against interactions that are **potentially hazardous** and where combined administration of the drugs involved should be **avoided** (or only undertaken with caution and appropriate monitoring).

Interactions that have no symbol do not usually have serious consequences.

List of drug interactions

The following is an alphabetical list of drugs and their interactions; to avoid excessive cross-referencing each drug or group is listed twice: in the alphabetical list and also against the drug or group with which it interacts.

For explanation of symbol • see above

Abacavir

Analgesics: abacavir possibly reduces plasma concentration of methadone

Antibacterials: plasma concentration of abacavir possibly reduced by rifampicin

Antiepileptics: plasma concentration of abacavir possibly reduced by phenytoin

• Antivirals: plasma concentration of abacavir reduced by •tipranavir

Barbiturates: plasma concentration of abacavir possibly reduced by phenobarbital

Abatacept

Adalimumab: increased risk of side-effects when abatacept given with adalimumab

Etanercept: increased risk of side-effects when abatacept given with etanercept

Infliximab: increased risk of side-effects when abatacept given with infliximab

• Vaccines: avoid concomitant use of abatacept with live •vaccines (see p. 725)

Acarbose *see* Antidiabetics

ACE Inhibitors

Alcohol: enhanced hypotensive effect when ACE inhibitors given with alcohol

Aldesleukin: enhanced hypotensive effect when ACE inhibitors given with aldesleukin

Allopurinol: increased risk of leucopenia and hypersensitivity reactions when ACE inhibitors given with allopurinol especially in renal impairment

Alpha-blockers: enhanced hypotensive effect when ACE inhibitors given with alpha-blockers

Anaesthetics, General: enhanced hypotensive effect when ACE inhibitors given with general anaesthetics

Analgesics: increased risk of renal impairment when ACE inhibitors given with NSAIDs, also hypotensive effect antagonised

Angiotensin-II Receptor Antagonists: increased risk of hyperkalaemia when ACE inhibitors given with angiotensin-II receptor antagonists

Antacids: absorption of ACE inhibitors possibly reduced by antacids; absorption of captopril, enalapril and fosinopril reduced by antacids

Antibacterials: plasma concentration of active metabolite of imidapril reduced by rifampicin (reduced antihypertensive effect); quinapril tablets reduce absorption of tetracyclines (quinapril tablets contain magnesium carbonate)

Anticoagulants: increased risk of hyperkalaemia when ACE inhibitors given with heparins

Antidepressants: hypotensive effect of ACE inhibitors possibly enhanced by MAOIs

Antidiabetics: ACE inhibitors possibly enhance hypoglycaemic effect of insulin, metformin and sulphonylureas

Antipsychotics: enhanced hypotensive effect when ACE inhibitors given with antipsychotics

ACE Inhibitors (continued)

Anxiolytics and Hypnotics: enhanced hypotensive effect when ACE inhibitors given with anxiolytics and hypnotics

Beta-blockers: enhanced hypotensive effect when ACE inhibitors given with beta-blockers

Calcium-channel Blockers: enhanced hypotensive effect when ACE inhibitors given with calcium-channel blockers

Cardiac Glycosides: captopril possibly increases plasma concentration of digoxin

● Ciclosporin: increased risk of hyperkalaemia when ACE inhibitors given with ●ciclosporin

Clonidine: enhanced hypotensive effect when ACE inhibitors given with clonidine; antihypertensive effect of captopril possibly delayed by previous treatment with clonidine

Corticosteroids: hypotensive effect of ACE inhibitors antagonised by corticosteroids

Cytotoxics: increased risk of anaemia or leucopenia when captopril given with azathioprine especially in renal impairment; increased risk of anaemia when enalapril given with azathioprine especially in renal impairment

Diazoxide: enhanced hypotensive effect when ACE inhibitors given with diazoxide

● Diuretics: enhanced hypotensive effect when ACE inhibitors given with ●diuretics; increased risk of severe hyperkalaemia when ACE inhibitors given with ●potassium-sparing diuretics and aldosterone antagonists (monitor potassium concentration with low-dose spironolactone in heart failure)

Dopaminergics: enhanced hypotensive effect when ACE inhibitors given with levodopa

● Lithium: ACE inhibitors reduce excretion of ●lithium (increased plasma concentration)

Methyldopa: enhanced hypotensive effect when ACE inhibitors given with methyldopa

Moxisylyte (thymoxamine): enhanced hypotensive effect when ACE inhibitors given with moxisylyte

Moxonidine: enhanced hypotensive effect when ACE inhibitors given with moxonidine

Muscle Relaxants: enhanced hypotensive effect when ACE inhibitors given with baclofen or tizanidine

Nitrates: enhanced hypotensive effect when ACE inhibitors given with nitrates

Oestrogens: hypotensive effect of ACE inhibitors antagonised by oestrogens

● Potassium Salts: increased risk of severe hyperkalaemia when ACE inhibitors given with ●potassium salts

Probenecid: excretion of captopril reduced by probenecid

Prostaglandins: enhanced hypotensive effect when ACE inhibitors given with alprostadil

Vasodilator Antihypertensives: enhanced hypotensive effect when ACE inhibitors given with hydralazine, minoxidil or sodium nitroprusside

Acebutolol see Beta-blockers
Aceclofenac see NSAIDs
Acemetacin see NSAIDs
Acenocoumarol (nicoumalone) see Coumarins
Acetazolamide see Diuretics
Aciclovir
Note. Interactions do not apply to topical aciclovir preparations
Note. Valaciclovir interactions as for aciclovir
Ciclosporin: increased risk of nephrotoxicity when aciclovir given with ciclosporin
Cytotoxics: plasma concentration of aciclovir increased by mycophenolate, also plasma concentration of inactive metabolite of mycophenolate increased
Probenecid: excretion of aciclovir reduced by probenecid (increased plasma concentration)
Tacrolimus: possible increased risk of nephrotoxicity when aciclovir given with tacrolimus

Acitretin see Retinoids
Adalimumab
Abatacept: increased risk of side-effects when adalimumab given with abatacept
● Anakinra: avoid concomitant use of adalimumab with ●anakinra
● Vaccines: avoid concomitant use of adalimumab with live ●vaccines (see p. 725)
Adefovir
Antivirals: avoidance of adefovir advised by manufacturer of tenofovir
Adenosine
Note. Possibility of interaction with drugs tending to impair myocardial conduction
Anaesthetics, Local: increased myocardial depression when anti-arrhythmics given with bupivacaine, levobupivacaine, prilocaine or ropivacaine
● Anti-arrhythmics: increased myocardial depression when anti-arrhythmics given with other ●anti-arrhythmics
● Antipsychotics: increased risk of ventricular arrhythmias when anti-arrhythmics that prolong the QT interval given with ●antipsychotics that prolong the QT interval
● Beta-blockers: increased myocardial depression when anti-arrhythmics given with ●beta-blockers
● Dipyridamole: effect of adenosine enhanced and extended by ●dipyridamole (important risk of toxicity)
Theophylline: anti-arrhythmic effect of adenosine antagonised by theophylline
Adrenaline (epinephrine) see Sympathomimetics
Adrenergic Neurone Blockers
Alcohol: enhanced hypotensive effect when adrenergic neurone blockers given with alcohol
Alpha-blockers: enhanced hypotensive effect when adrenergic neurone blockers given with alpha-blockers
● Anaesthetics, General: enhanced hypotensive effect when adrenergic neurone blockers given with ●general anaesthetics
Analgesics: hypotensive effect of adrenergic neurone blockers antagonised by NSAIDs
Angiotensin-II Receptor Antagonists: enhanced hypotensive effect when adrenergic neurone blockers given with angiotensin-II receptor antagonists
Antidepressants: enhanced hypotensive effect when adrenergic neurone blockers given with MAOIs; hypotensive effect of adrenergic neurone blockers antagonised by tricyclics
Antipsychotics: hypotensive effect of adrenergic neurone blockers antagonised by haloperidol; hypotensive effect of adrenergic neurone blockers antagonised by higher doses of chlorpromazine; enhanced hypotensive effect when adrenergic neurone blockers given with phenothiazines
Anxiolytics and Hypnotics: enhanced hypotensive effect when adrenergic neurone blockers given with anxiolytics and hypnotics
Beta-blockers: enhanced hypotensive effect when adrenergic neurone blockers given with beta-blockers
Calcium-channel Blockers: enhanced hypotensive effect when adrenergic neurone blockers given with calcium-channel blockers
Clonidine: enhanced hypotensive effect when adrenergic neurone blockers given with clonidine
Corticosteroids: hypotensive effect of adrenergic neurone blockers antagonised by corticosteroids
Diazoxide: enhanced hypotensive effect when adrenergic neurone blockers given with diazoxide
Diuretics: enhanced hypotensive effect when adrenergic neurone blockers given with diuretics
Dopaminergics: enhanced hypotensive effect when adrenergic neurone blockers given with levodopa

Appendix 1: Interactions

Adrenergic Neurone Blockers *(continued)*

Methyldopa: enhanced hypotensive effect when adrenergic neurone blockers given with methyldopa

Moxisylyte (thymoxamine): enhanced hypotensive effect when adrenergic neurone blockers given with moxisylyte

Moxonidine: enhanced hypotensive effect when adrenergic neurone blockers given with moxonidine

Muscle Relaxants: enhanced hypotensive effect when adrenergic neurone blockers given with baclofen or tizanidine

Nitrates: enhanced hypotensive effect when adrenergic neurone blockers given with nitrates

Oestrogens: hypotensive effect of adrenergic neurone blockers antagonised by oestrogens

Pizotifen: hypotensive effect of adrenergic neurone blockers antagonised by pizotifen

Prostaglandins: enhanced hypotensive effect when adrenergic neurone blockers given with alprostadil

● Sympathomimetics: hypotensive effect of adrenergic neurone blockers antagonised by ●ephedrine, ●isometheptene, ●metaraminol, ●methylphenidate, ●noradrenaline (norepinephrine), ●oxymetazoline, ●phenylephrine, ●pseudoephedrine and ●xylometazoline

Vasodilator Antihypertensives: enhanced hypotensive effect when adrenergic neurone blockers given with hydralazine, minoxidil or sodium nitroprusside

Adsorbents *see* Kaolin

Agalsidase Alfa and Beta

Anti-arrhythmics: effects of agalsidase alfa and beta possibly inhibited by amiodarone (manufacturers of agalsidase alfa and beta advise avoid concomitant use)

Antibacterials: effects of agalsidase alfa and beta possibly inhibited by gentamicin (manufacturers of agalsidase alfa and beta advise avoid concomitant use)

Antimalarials: effects of agalsidase alfa and beta possibly inhibited by chloroquine and hydroxy-chloroquine (manufacturers of agalsidase alfa and beta advise avoid concomitant use)

Alcohol

ACE Inhibitors: enhanced hypotensive effect when alcohol given with ACE inhibitors

Adrenergic Neurone Blockers: enhanced hypotensive effect when alcohol given with adrenergic neurone blockers

Alpha-blockers: increased sedative effect when alcohol given with indoramin; enhanced hypotensive effect when alcohol given with alpha-blockers

Analgesics: enhanced hypotensive and sedative effects when alcohol given with opioid analgesics

Angiotensin-II Receptor Antagonists: enhanced hypotensive effect when alcohol given with angiotensin-II receptor antagonists

● Antibacterials: disulfiram-like reaction when alcohol given with metronidazole; possibility of disulfiram-like reaction when alcohol given with tinidazole; increased risk of convulsions when alcohol given with ●cycloserine

● Anticoagulants: major changes in consumption of alcohol may affect anticoagulant control with ●coumarins or ●phenindione

● Antidepressants: some beverages containing alcohol and some dealcoholised beverages contain tyramine which interacts with ●MAOIs (hypertensive crisis)—if no tyramine, enhanced hypotensive effect; sedative effects possibly increased when alcohol given with SSRIs; increased sedative effect when alcohol given with ●mirtazapine, ●tricyclic-related antidepressants or ●tricyclics

Antidiabetics: alcohol enhances hypoglycaemic effect of antidiabetics; increased risk of lactic acidosis when alcohol given with metformin; flushing, in

Alcohol

Antidiabetics *(continued)*

susceptible subjects, when alcohol given with chlorpropamide

Antiepileptics: alcohol possibly increases CNS side-effects of carbamazepine; increased sedative effect when alcohol given with primidone

Antifungals: effects of alcohol possibly enhanced by griseofulvin

Antihistamines: increased sedative effect when alcohol given with antihistamines (possibly less effect with non-sedating antihistamines)

Antimuscarinics: increased sedative effect when alcohol given with hyoscine

Antipsychotics: increased sedative effect when alcohol given with antipsychotics

Anxiolytics and Hypnotics: increased sedative effect when alcohol given with anxiolytics and hypnotics

Barbiturates: increased sedative effect when alcohol given with barbiturates

Beta-blockers: enhanced hypotensive effect when alcohol given with beta-blockers

Calcium-channel Blockers: enhanced hypotensive effect when alcohol given with calcium-channel blockers; plasma concentration of alcohol possibly increased by verapamil

Clonidine: enhanced hypotensive effect when alcohol given with clonidine

Cytotoxics: disulfiram-like reaction when alcohol given with procarbazine

Diazoxide: enhanced hypotensive effect when alcohol given with diazoxide

Disulfiram: disulfiram reaction when alcohol given with disulfiram (see BNF section 4.10)

Diuretics: enhanced hypotensive effect when alcohol given with diuretics

Dopaminergics: alcohol reduces tolerance to bromocriptine

Levamisole: possibility of disulfiram-like reaction when alcohol given with levamisole

Lofexidine: increased sedative effect when alcohol given with lofexidine

Methyldopa: enhanced hypotensive effect when alcohol given with methyldopa

Moxonidine: enhanced hypotensive effect when alcohol given with moxonidine

Muscle Relaxants: increased sedative effect when alcohol given with baclofen, methocarbamol or tizanidine

Nabilone: increased sedative effect when alcohol given with nabilone

Nicorandil: alcohol possibly enhances hypotensive effect of nicorandil

Nitrates: enhanced hypotensive effect when alcohol given with nitrates

● Paraldehyde: increased sedative effect when alcohol given with ●paraldehyde

● Retinoids: presence of alcohol causes etretinate to be formed from ●acitretin (increased risk of teratogenicity in women of child-bearing potential)

Vasodilator Antihypertensives: enhanced hypotensive effect when alcohol given with hydralazine, minoxidil or sodium nitroprusside

Aldesleukin

ACE Inhibitors: enhanced hypotensive effect when aldesleukin given with ACE inhibitors

Alpha-blockers: enhanced hypotensive effect when aldesleukin given with alpha-blockers

Angiotensin-II Receptor Antagonists: enhanced hypotensive effect when aldesleukin given with angiotensin-II receptor antagonists

Beta-blockers: enhanced hypotensive effect when aldesleukin given with beta-blockers

Calcium-channel Blockers: enhanced hypotensive effect when aldesleukin given with calcium-channel blockers

Aldesleukin *(continued)*

Clonidine: enhanced hypotensive effect when aldesleukin given with clonidine

Diazoxide: enhanced hypotensive effect when aldesleukin given with diazoxide

Diuretics: enhanced hypotensive effect when aldesleukin given with diuretics

Methyldopa: enhanced hypotensive effect when aldesleukin given with methyldopa

Moxonidine: enhanced hypotensive effect when aldesleukin given with moxonidine

Nitrates: enhanced hypotensive effect when aldesleukin given with nitrates

Vasodilator Antihypertensives: enhanced hypotensive effect when aldesleukin given with hydralazine, minoxidil or sodium nitroprusside

Alendronic Acid *see* Bisphosphonates

Alfentanil *see* Opioid Analgesics

Alfuzosin *see* Alpha-blockers

Alimemazine (trimeprazine) *see* Antihistamines

Aliskiren

Angiotensin-II Receptor Antagonists: plasma concentration of aliskiren possibly reduced by irbesartan

Anticoagulants: increased risk of hyperkalaemia when aliskiren given with heparins

Antifungals: plasma concentration of aliskiren increased by ketoconazole

Diuretics: aliskiren reduces plasma concentration of furosemide (frusemide); increased risk of hyperkalaemia when aliskiren given with potassium-sparing diuretics and aldosterone antagonists

Potassium Salts: increased risk of hyperkalaemia when aliskiren given with potassium salts

Alitretinoin *see* Retinoids

Alkylating Drugs *see* Busulfan, Carmustine, Cyclophosphamide, Ifosfamide, Lomustine, Melphalan, and Thiotepa

Allopurinol

ACE Inhibitors: increased risk of leucopenia and hypersensitivity reactions when allopurinol given with ACE inhibitors especially in renal impairment

Antibacterials: increased risk of rash when allopurinol given with amoxicillin or ampicillin

Anticoagulants: allopurinol possibly enhances anticoagulant effect of coumarins

• Antivirals: allopurinol increases plasma concentration of ●didanosine (risk of toxicity)—avoid concomitant use

Ciclosporin: allopurinol possibly increases plasma concentration of ciclosporin (risk of nephrotoxicity)

• Cytotoxics: allopurinol enhances effects and increases toxicity of ●azathioprine and ●mercaptopurine (reduce dose of azathioprine and mercaptopurine to one quarter of usual dose); avoidance of allopurinol advised by manufacturer of ●capecitabine

Diuretics: increased risk of hypersensitivity when allopurinol given with thiazides and related diuretics especially in renal impairment

Theophylline: allopurinol possibly increases plasma concentration of theophylline

Almotriptan *see* 5HT$_1$ Agonists

Alpha$_2$-adrenoceptor Stimulants *see* Apraclonidine, Brimonidine, Clonidine and Methyldopa

Alpha-blockers

ACE Inhibitors: enhanced hypotensive effect when alpha-blockers given with ACE inhibitors

Adrenergic Neurone Blockers: enhanced hypotensive effect when alpha-blockers given with adrenergic neurone blockers

Alcohol: enhanced hypotensive effect when alpha-blockers given with alcohol; increased sedative effect when indoramin given with alcohol

Aldesleukin: enhanced hypotensive effect when alpha-blockers given with aldesleukin

Alpha-blockers *(continued)*

• Anaesthetics, General: enhanced hypotensive effect when alpha-blockers given with ●general anaesthetics

Analgesics: hypotensive effect of alpha-blockers antagonised by NSAIDs

Angiotensin-II Receptor Antagonists: enhanced hypotensive effect when alpha-blockers given with angiotensin-II receptor antagonists

• Antidepressants: enhanced hypotensive effect when alpha-blockers given with MAOIs; manufacturer of indoramin advises avoid concomitant use with ●MAOIs

Antipsychotics: enhanced hypotensive effect when alpha-blockers given with antipsychotics

• Antivirals: plasma concentration of alfuzosin possibly increased by ●ritonavir—avoid concomitant use

Anxiolytics and Hypnotics: enhanced hypotensive and sedative effects when alpha-blockers given with anxiolytics and hypnotics

• Beta-blockers: enhanced hypotensive effect when alpha-blockers given with ●beta-blockers, also increased risk of first-dose hypotension with post-synaptic alpha-blockers such as prazosin

• Calcium-channel Blockers: enhanced hypotensive effect when alpha-blockers given with ●calcium-channel blockers, also increased risk of first-dose hypotension with post-synaptic alpha-blockers such as prazosin

Cardiac Glycosides: prazosin increases plasma concentration of digoxin

Clonidine: enhanced hypotensive effect when alpha-blockers given with clonidine

Corticosteroids: hypotensive effect of alpha-blockers antagonised by corticosteroids

Diazoxide: enhanced hypotensive effect when alpha-blockers given with diazoxide

• Diuretics: enhanced hypotensive effect when alpha-blockers given with ●diuretics, also increased risk of first-dose hypotension with post-synaptic alpha-blockers such as prazosin

Dopaminergics: enhanced hypotensive effect when alpha-blockers given with levodopa

Methyldopa: enhanced hypotensive effect when alpha-blockers given with methyldopa

• Moxisylyte (thymoxamine): possible severe postural hypotension when alpha-blockers given with ●moxisylyte

Moxonidine: enhanced hypotensive effect when alpha-blockers given with moxonidine

Muscle Relaxants: enhanced hypotensive effect when alpha-blockers given with baclofen or tizanidine

Nitrates: enhanced hypotensive effect when alpha-blockers given with nitrates

Oestrogens: hypotensive effect of alpha-blockers antagonised by oestrogens

Prostaglandins: enhanced hypotensive effect when alpha-blockers given with alprostadil

• Sildenafil: enhanced hypotensive effect when alpha-blockers given with ●sildenafil (avoid alpha-blockers for 4 hours after sildenafil)

• Sympathomimetics: avoid concomitant use of tolazoline with ●adrenaline (epinephrine) or ●dopamine

• Tadalafil: enhanced hypotensive effect when alpha-blockers given with ●tadalafil—avoid concomitant use

• Ulcer-healing Drugs: effects of tolazoline antagonised by ●cimetidine and ●ranitidine

• Vardenafil: enhanced hypotensive effect when alpha-blockers (excludes tamsulosin) given with ●vardenafil—avoid vardenafil for 6 hours after alpha-blockers

Vasodilator Antihypertensives: enhanced hypotensive effect when alpha-blockers given with hydralazine, minoxidil or sodium nitroprusside

Alpha-blockers (post-synaptic) *see* Alpha-blockers

Alprazolam *see* Anxiolytics and Hypnotics

Alprostadil *see* Prostaglandins

Aluminium Hydroxide *see* Antacids

Amantadine

Antimuscarinics: increased risk of antimuscarinic side-effects when amantadine given with antimuscarinics

Antipsychotics: increased risk of extrapyramidal side-effects when amantadine given with antipsychotics

Bupropion: increased risk of side-effects when amantadine given with bupropion

Domperidone: increased risk of extrapyramidal side-effects when amantadine given with domperidone

• Memantine: increased risk of CNS toxicity when amantadine given with ●memantine (manufacturer of memantine advises avoid concomitant use); effects of dopaminergics possibly enhanced by memantine

Methyldopa: increased risk of extrapyramidal side-effects when amantadine given with methyldopa; antiparkinsonian effect of dopaminergics antagonised by methyldopa

Metoclopramide: increased risk of extrapyramidal side-effects when amantadine given with metoclopramide

Tetrabenazine: increased risk of extrapyramidal side-effects when amantadine given with tetrabenazine

Amikacin *see* Aminoglycosides

Amiloride *see* Diuretics

Aminoglycosides

Agalsidase Alfa and Beta: gentamicin possibly inhibits effects of agalsidase alfa and beta (manufacturers of agalsidase alfa and beta advise avoid concomitant use)

Analgesics: plasma concentration of amikacin and gentamicin in neonates possibly increased by indometacin

Antibacterials: neomycin reduces absorption of phenoxymethylpenicillin; increased risk of nephrotoxicity when aminoglycosides given with colistin or polymyxins; increased risk of nephrotoxicity and ototoxicity when aminoglycosides given with capreomycin, teicoplanin or vancomycin; possible increased risk of nephrotoxicity when aminoglycosides given with cephalosporins

• Anticoagulants: experience in anticoagulant clinics suggests that INR possibly altered when neomycin (given for local action on gut) is given with ●coumarins or ●phenindione

Antidiabetics: neomycin possibly enhances hypoglycaemic effect of acarbose, also severity of gastrointestinal effects increased

Antifungals: increased risk of nephrotoxicity when aminoglycosides given with amphotericin

Bisphosphonates: increased risk of hypocalcaemia when aminoglycosides given with bisphosphonates

Cardiac Glycosides: neomycin reduces absorption of digoxin; gentamicin possibly increases plasma concentration of digoxin

• Ciclosporin: increased risk of nephrotoxicity when aminoglycosides given with ●ciclosporin

• Cytotoxics: neomycin possibly reduces absorption of methotrexate; increased risk of nephrotoxicity and possibly of ototoxicity when aminoglycosides given with ●platinum compounds

• Diuretics: increased risk of ototoxicity when aminoglycosides given with ●loop diuretics

• Muscle Relaxants: aminoglycosides enhance effects of ●non-depolarising muscle relaxants and ●suxamethonium

Oestrogens: antibacterials that do not induce liver enzymes possibly reduce contraceptive effect of oestrogens (risk probably small, see p. 478)

• Parasympathomimetics: aminoglycosides antagonise effects of ●neostigmine and ●pyridostigmine

• Tacrolimus: increased risk of nephrotoxicity when aminoglycosides given with ●tacrolimus

Aminoglycosides *(continued)*

Vaccines: antibacterials inactivate oral typhoid vaccine–see p. 752

Vitamins: neomycin possibly reduces absorption of vitamin A

Aminophylline *see* Theophylline

Aminosalicylates

Cardiac Glycosides: sulfasalazine possibly reduces absorption of digoxin

Cytotoxics: possible increased risk of leucopenia when aminosalicylates given with azathioprine or mercaptopurine

Folates: sulfasalazine possibly reduces absorption of folic acid

Amiodarone

Note. Amiodarone has a long half-life; there is a potential for drug interactions to occur for several weeks (or even months) after treatment with it has been stopped

Agalsidase Alfa and Beta: amiodarone possibly inhibits effects of agalsidase alfa and beta (manufacturers of agalsidase alfa and beta advise avoid concomitant use)

Anaesthetics, Local: increased myocardial depression when anti-arrhythmics given with bupivacaine, levobupivacaine, prilocaine or ropivacaine

• Anti-arrhythmics: increased myocardial depression when anti-arrhythmics given with other ●anti-arrhythmics; increased risk of ventricular arrhythmias when amiodarone given with ●disopyramide—avoid concomitant use; amiodarone increases plasma concentration of ●flecainide (halve dose of flecainide)

• Antibacterials: increased risk of ventricular arrhythmias when amiodarone given with parenteral ●erythromycin—avoid concomitant use; increased risk of ventricular arrhythmias when amiodarone given with ●levofloxacin or ●moxifloxacin—avoid concomitant use; increased risk of ventricular arrhythmias when amiodarone given with ●sulfamethoxazole and ●trimethoprim (as co-trimoxazole)—avoid concomitant use of co-trimoxazole

• Anticoagulants: amiodarone inhibits metabolism of ●coumarins and ●phenindione (enhanced anticoagulant effect); amiodarone increases plasma concentration of ●dabigatran etexilate (reduce dose of dabigatran etexilate)

• Antidepressants: increased risk of ventricular arrhythmias when amiodarone given with ●tricyclics—avoid concomitant use

• Antiepileptics: amiodarone inhibits metabolism of ●phenytoin (increased plasma concentration)

• Antihistamines: increased risk of ventricular arrhythmias when amiodarone given with ●mizolastine—avoid concomitant use

• Antimalarials: avoidance of amiodarone advised by manufacturer of artemether/lumefantrine (risk of ventricular arrhythmias); increased risk of ventricular arrhythmias when amiodarone given with ●chloroquine and hydroxychloroquine, ●mefloquine or ●quinine—avoid concomitant use

• Antimuscarinics: increased risk of ventricular arrhythmias when amiodarone given with ●tolterodine

• Antipsychotics: increased risk of ventricular arrhythmias when anti-arrhythmics that prolong the QT interval given with ●antipsychotics that prolong the QT interval; increased risk of ventricular arrhythmias when amiodarone given with ●benperidol—manufacturer of benperidol advises avoid concomitant use; increased risk of ventricular arrhythmias when amiodarone given with ●amisulpride, ●haloperidol, ●phenothiazines, ●pimozide, ●sertindole or ●zuclopenthixol—avoid concomitant use; increased risk of ventricular arrhythmias when amiodarone given with ●sulpiride

• Antivirals: plasma concentration of amiodarone possibly increased by ●atazanavir; plasma concentration

Amiodarone
- Antivirals *(continued)*
  of amiodarone possibly increased by •fosamprenavir (increased risk of ventricular arrhythmias—avoid concomitant use); plasma concentration of amiodarone possibly increased by •indinavir—avoid concomitant use; increased risk of ventricular arrhythmias when amiodarone given with •nelfinavir—avoid concomitant use; plasma concentration of amiodarone increased by •ritonavir (increased risk of ventricular arrhythmias—avoid concomitant use)
- Atomoxetine: increased risk of ventricular arrhythmias when amiodarone given with •atomoxetine
- Beta-blockers: increased risk of bradycardia, AV block and myocardial depression when amiodarone given with •beta-blockers; increased myocardial depression when anti-arrhythmics given with •beta-blockers; increased risk of ventricular arrhythmias when amiodarone given with •sotalol—avoid concomitant use
- Calcium-channel Blockers: increased risk of bradycardia, AV block and myocardial depression when amiodarone given with •diltiazem or •verapamil
- Cardiac Glycosides: amiodarone increases plasma concentration of •digoxin (halve dose of digoxin)
  Ciclosporin: amiodarone possibly increases plasma concentration of ciclosporin
  Diuretics: increased cardiac toxicity with amiodarone if hypokalaemia occurs with acetazolamide, loop diuretics or thiazides and related diuretics; amiodarone increases plasma concentration of eplerenone (reduce dose of eplerenone)
  Grapefruit Juice: plasma concentration of amiodarone increased by grapefruit juice
- $5HT_3$ Antagonists: increased risk of ventricular arrhythmias when amiodarone given with •dolasetron—avoid concomitant use
- Ivabradine: increased risk of ventricular arrhythmias when amiodarone given with •ivabradine
- Lipid-regulating Drugs: increased risk of myopathy when amiodarone given with •simvastatin
- Lithium: manufacturer of amiodarone advises avoid concomitant use with •lithium (risk of ventricular arrhythmias)
  Orlistat: plasma concentration of amiodarone possibly reduced by orlistat
- Pentamidine Isetionate: increased risk of ventricular arrhythmias when amiodarone given with •pentamidine isetionate—avoid concomitant use
  Thyroid Hormones: for concomitant use of amiodarone and thyroid hormones see p. 109
  Ulcer-healing Drugs: plasma concentration of amiodarone increased by cimetidine

Amisulpride *see* Antipsychotics
Amitriptyline *see* Antidepressants, Tricyclic
Amlodipine *see* Calcium-channel Blockers
Amobarbital *see* Barbiturates
Amoxicillin *see* Penicillins
Amphotericin
  Note. Close monitoring required with concomitant administration of nephrotoxic drugs or cytotoxics
  Antibacterials: increased risk of nephrotoxicity when amphotericin given with aminoglycosides or polymyxins; possible increased risk of nephrotoxicity when amphotericin given with vancomycin
  Antifungals: amphotericin reduces renal excretion and increases cellular uptake of flucytosine (toxicity possibly increased); effects of amphotericin possibly antagonised by imidazoles and triazoles
- Cardiac Glycosides: hypokalaemia caused by amphotericin increases cardiac toxicity with •cardiac glycosides
- Ciclosporin: increased risk of nephrotoxicity when amphotericin given with •ciclosporin

Amphotericin *(continued)*
- Corticosteroids: increased risk of hypokalaemia when amphotericin given with •corticosteroids—avoid concomitant use unless corticosteroids needed to control reactions
  Diuretics: increased risk of hypokalaemia when amphotericin given with loop diuretics or thiazides and related diuretics
  Pentamidine Isetionate: possible increased risk of nephrotoxicity when amphotericin given with pentamidine isetionate
- Tacrolimus: increased risk of nephrotoxicity when amphotericin given with •tacrolimus

Ampicillin *see* Penicillins
Anabolic Steroids
- Anticoagulants: anabolic steroids enhance anticoagulant effect of •coumarins and •phenindione
  Antidiabetics: anabolic steroids possibly enhance hypoglycaemic effect of antidiabetics

Anaesthetics, General
  Note. See also Surgery and Long-term Medication, p. 761
  ACE Inhibitors: enhanced hypotensive effect when general anaesthetics given with ACE inhibitors
- Adrenergic Neurone Blockers: enhanced hypotensive effect when general anaesthetics given with •adrenergic neurone blockers
- Alpha-blockers: enhanced hypotensive effect when general anaesthetics given with •alpha-blockers
  Angiotensin-II Receptor Antagonists: enhanced hypotensive effect when general anaesthetics given with angiotensin-II receptor antagonists
  Antibacterials: general anaesthetics possibly potentiate hepatotoxicity of isoniazid; effects of thiopental enhanced by sulphonamides; hypersensitivity-like reactions can occur when general anaesthetics given with intravenous vancomycin
- Antidepressants: Because of hazardous interactions between general anaesthetics and •MAOIs, MAOIs should normally be stopped 2 weeks before surgery; increased risk of arrhythmias and hypotension when general anaesthetics given with tricyclics
- Antipsychotics: enhanced hypotensive effect when general anaesthetics given with •antipsychotics
  Anxiolytics and Hypnotics: increased sedative effect when general anaesthetics given with anxiolytics and hypnotics
  Beta-blockers: enhanced hypotensive effect when general anaesthetics given with beta-blockers
- Calcium-channel Blockers: enhanced hypotensive effect when general anaesthetics or isoflurane given with calcium-channel blockers; general anaesthetics enhance hypotensive effect of •verapamil (also AV delay)
  Clonidine: enhanced hypotensive effect when general anaesthetics given with clonidine
- Cytotoxics: nitrous oxide increases antifolate effect of •methotrexate—avoid concomitant use
  Diazoxide: enhanced hypotensive effect when general anaesthetics given with diazoxide
  Diuretics: enhanced hypotensive effect when general anaesthetics given with diuretics
- Dopaminergics: increased risk of arrhythmias when volatile liquid general anaesthetics given with •levodopa
  Ergot Alkaloids: halothane reduces effects of ergometrine on the parturient uterus
- Memantine: increased risk of CNS toxicity when ketamine given with •memantine (manufacturer of memantine advises avoid concomitant use)
  Methyldopa: enhanced hypotensive effect when general anaesthetics given with methyldopa
  Moxonidine: enhanced hypotensive effect when general anaesthetics given with moxonidine
- Muscle Relaxants: increased risk of myocardial depression and bradycardia when propofol given with •suxamethonium; volatile liquid general anaes-

Anaesthetics, General
- Muscle Relaxants *(continued)*
  thetics enhance effects of non-depolarising muscle relaxants and suxamethonium; ketamine enhances effects of atracurium
  Nitrates: enhanced hypotensive effect when general anaesthetics given with nitrates
  Oxytocin: oxytocic effect possibly reduced, also enhanced hypotensive effect and risk of arrhythmias when volatile liquid general anaesthetics given with oxytocin
  Probenecid: effects of thiopental possibly enhanced by probenecid
- Sympathomimetics: increased risk of arrhythmias when volatile liquid general anaesthetics given with ●adrenaline (epinephrine); increased risk of hypertension when volatile liquid general anaesthetics given with ●methylphenidate
  Theophylline: increased risk of convulsions when ketamine given with theophylline; increased risk of arrhythmias when halothane given with theophylline
  Vasodilator Antihypertensives: enhanced hypotensive effect when general anaesthetics given with hydralazine, minoxidil or sodium nitroprusside

Anaesthetics, General (intravenous) *see* Anaesthetics, General

Anaesthetics, General (volatile liquids) *see* Anaesthetics, General

Anaesthetics, Local *see* Bupivacaine, Levobupivacaine, Lidocaine (lignocaine), Prilocaine, Procaine, and Ropivacaine

Anagrelide
- Cilostazol: manufacturer of anagrelide advises avoid concomitant use with ●cilostazol
- Phosphodiesterase Inhibitors: manufacturer of anagrelide advises avoid concomitant use with ●enoximone and ●milrinone

Anakinra
- Adalimumab: avoid concomitant use of anakinra with ●adalimumab
- Etanercept: increased risk of side-effects when anakinra given with ●etanercept—avoid concomitant use
- Infliximab: avoid concomitant use of anakinra with ●infliximab
- Vaccines: avoid concomitant use of anakinra with live ●vaccines (see p. 725)

Analgesics *see* Aspirin, Nefopam, NSAIDs, Opioid Analgesics, and Paracetamol

Angiotensin-II Receptor Antagonists
  ACE Inhibitors: increased risk of hyperkalaemia when angiotensin-II receptor antagonists given with ACE inhibitors
  Adrenergic Neurone Blockers: enhanced hypotensive effect when angiotensin-II receptor antagonists given with adrenergic neurone blockers
  Alcohol: enhanced hypotensive effect when angiotensin-II receptor antagonists given with alcohol
  Aldesleukin: enhanced hypotensive effect when angiotensin-II receptor antagonists given with aldesleukin
  Aliskiren: irbesartan possibly reduces plasma concentration of aliskiren
  Alpha-blockers: enhanced hypotensive effect when angiotensin-II receptor antagonists given with alpha-blockers
  Anaesthetics, General: enhanced hypotensive effect when angiotensin-II receptor antagonists given with general anaesthetics
  Analgesics: increased risk of renal impairment when angiotensin-II receptor antagonists given with NSAIDs, also hypotensive effect antagonised
  Anticoagulants: increased risk of hyperkalaemia when angiotensin-II receptor antagonists given with heparin

Angiotensin-II Receptor Antagonists *(continued)*
  Antidepressants: hypotensive effect of angiotensin-II receptor antagonists possibly enhanced by MAOIs
  Antipsychotics: enhanced hypotensive effect when angiotensin-II receptor antagonists given with antipsychotics
  Anxiolytics and Hypnotics: enhanced hypotensive effect when angiotensin-II receptor antagonists given with anxiolytics and hypnotics
  Beta-blockers: enhanced hypotensive effect when angiotensin-II receptor antagonists given with beta-blockers
  Calcium-channel Blockers: enhanced hypotensive effect when angiotensin-II receptor antagonists given with calcium-channel blockers
- Ciclosporin: increased risk of hyperkalaemia when angiotensin-II receptor antagonists given with ●ciclosporin
  Clonidine: enhanced hypotensive effect when angiotensin-II receptor antagonists given with clonidine
  Corticosteroids: hypotensive effect of angiotensin-II receptor antagonists antagonised by corticosteroids
  Diazoxide: enhanced hypotensive effect when angiotensin-II receptor antagonists given with diazoxide
- Diuretics: enhanced hypotensive effect when angiotensin-II receptor antagonists given with ●diuretics; increased risk of hyperkalaemia when angiotensin-II receptor antagonists given with ●potassium-sparing diuretics and aldosterone antagonists
  Dopaminergics: enhanced hypotensive effect when angiotensin-II receptor antagonists given with levodopa
- Lithium: angiotensin-II receptor antagonists reduce excretion of ●lithium (increased plasma concentration)
  Methyldopa: enhanced hypotensive effect when angiotensin-II receptor antagonists given with methyldopa
  Moxisylyte (thymoxamine): enhanced hypotensive effect when angiotensin-II receptor antagonists given with moxisylyte
  Moxonidine: enhanced hypotensive effect when angiotensin-II receptor antagonists given with moxonidine
  Muscle Relaxants: enhanced hypotensive effect when angiotensin-II receptor antagonists given with baclofen or tizanidine
  Nitrates: enhanced hypotensive effect when angiotensin-II receptor antagonists given with nitrates
  Oestrogens: hypotensive effect of angiotensin-II receptor antagonists antagonised by oestrogens
- Potassium Salts: increased risk of hyperkalaemia when angiotensin-II receptor antagonists given with ●potassium salts
  Prostaglandins: enhanced hypotensive effect when angiotensin-II receptor antagonists given with alprostadil
  Tacrolimus: increased risk of hyperkalaemia when angiotensin-II receptor antagonists given with tacrolimus
  Vasodilator Antihypertensives: enhanced hypotensive effect when angiotensin-II receptor antagonists given with hydralazine, minoxidil or sodium nitroprusside

Antacids
Note. Antacids should preferably not be taken at the same time as other drugs since they may impair absorption
  ACE Inhibitors: antacids possibly reduce absorption of ACE inhibitors; antacids reduce absorption of captopril, enalapril and fosinopril
  Analgesics: alkaline urine due to some antacids increases excretion of aspirin
  Antibacterials: antacids reduce absorption of azithromycin, cefaclor, cefpodoxime, ciprofloxacin, isoniazid, levofloxacin, moxifloxacin, norfloxacin, ofloxacin, rifampicin and tetracyclines; oral

Antacids
Antibacterials *(continued)*
magnesium salts (as magnesium trisilicate) reduce absorption of nitrofurantoin

Antiepileptics: antacids reduce absorption of gabapentin and phenytoin

Antifungals: antacids reduce absorption of itraconazole and ketoconazole

Antihistamines: antacids reduce absorption of fexofenadine

Antimalarials: antacids reduce absorption of chloroquine and hydroxychloroquine; oral magnesium salts (as magnesium trisilicate) reduce absorption of proguanil

Antipsychotics: antacids reduce absorption of phenothiazines and sulpiride

Antivirals: antacids possibly reduce plasma concentration of atazanavir; antacids possibly reduce absorption of fosamprenavir; antacids reduce absorption of tipranavir

Bile Acids: antacids possibly reduce absorption of bile acids

Bisphosphonates: antacids reduce absorption of bisphosphonates

Cardiac Glycosides: antacids possibly reduce absorption of digoxin

Corticosteroids: antacids reduce absorption of deflazacort

Cytotoxics: antacids reduce absorption of mycophenolate

Deferasirox: antacids containing aluminium possibly reduce absorption of deferasirox (manufacturer of deferasirox advises avoid concomitant use)

Dipyridamole: antacids possibly reduce absorption of dipyridamole

Iron: oral magnesium salts (as magnesium trisilicate) reduce absorption of *oral* iron

Lipid-regulating Drugs: antacids reduce absorption of rosuvastatin

Lithium: sodium bicarbonate increases excretion of lithium (reduced plasma concentration)

Penicillamine: antacids reduce absorption of penicillamine

Thyroid Hormones: antacids possibly reduce absorption of levothyroxine (thyroxine)

Ulcer-healing Drugs: antacids possibly reduce absorption of lansoprazole

Antazoline *see* Antihistamines

Anti-arrhythmics *see* Adenosine, Amiodarone, Disopyramide, Flecainide, Lidocaine (lignocaine), and Propafenone

Antibacterials *see* individual drugs

Antibiotics (cytotoxic) *see* Bleomycin, Doxorubicin, Epirubicin, Mitomycin

Anticoagulants *see* Coumarins, Dabigatran etexilate, Heparins, Phenindione, and Rivaroxaban

Antidepressants *see* Antidepressants, SSRI; Antidepressants, Tricyclic; Antidepressants, Tricyclic (related); MAOIs; Mirtazapine; Moclobemide; Reboxetine; St John's Wort; Tryptophan; Venlafaxine

Antidepressants, Noradrenaline Re-uptake Inhibitors *see* Reboxetine

Antidepressants, SSRI
Alcohol: sedative effects possibly increased when SSRIs given with alcohol

Anaesthetics, Local: fluvoxamine inhibits metabolism of ropivacaine—avoid prolonged administration of ropivacaine

● **Analgesics:** increased risk of bleeding when SSRIs given with ●NSAIDs or ●aspirin; fluvoxamine possibly increases plasma concentration of methadone; increased risk of CNS toxicity when SSRIs given with ●tramadol

Anti-arrhythmics: fluoxetine increases plasma concentration of flecainide; paroxetine possibly inhibits

Antidepressants, SSRI
Anti-arrhythmics *(continued)*
metabolism of propafenone (increased risk of toxicity)

● **Anticoagulants:** SSRIs possibly enhance anticoagulant effect of ●coumarins

● **Antidepressants:** avoidance of fluvoxamine advised by manufacturer of ●reboxetine; possible increased serotonergic effects when SSRIs given with duloxetine; fluvoxamine inhibits metabolism of ●duloxetine—avoid concomitant use; citalopram, escitalopram, fluvoxamine or paroxetine should not be started until 2 weeks after stopping ●MAOIs, also MAOIs should not be started until at least 1 week after stopping citalopram, escitalopram, fluvoxamine or paroxetine; CNS effects of SSRIs increased by ●MAOIs (risk of serious toxicity); sertraline should not be started until 2 weeks after stopping ●MAOIs, also MAOIs should not be started until at least 2 weeks after stopping sertraline; fluoxetine should not be started until 2 weeks after stopping ●MAOIs, also MAOIs should not be started until at least 5 weeks after stopping fluoxetine; increased risk of CNS toxicity when escitalopram given with ●moclobemide, preferably avoid concomitant use; after stopping citalopram, fluvoxamine or paroxetine do not start ●moclobemide for at least 1 week; after stopping fluoxetine do not start ●moclobemide for 5 weeks; after stopping sertraline do not start ●moclobemide for 2 weeks; increased serotonergic effects when SSRIs given with ●St John's wort—avoid concomitant use; SSRIs increase plasma concentration of some ●tricyclics; agitation and nausea may occur when SSRIs given with ●tryptophan

● **Antiepileptics:** SSRIs antagonise anticonvulsant effect of ●antiepileptics (convulsive threshold lowered); fluoxetine and fluvoxamine increase plasma concentration of ●carbamazepine; plasma concentration of paroxetine reduced by carbamazepine, phenytoin and primidone; fluoxetine and fluvoxamine increase plasma concentration of ●phenytoin

Antihistamines: antidepressant effect of SSRIs possibly antagonised by cyproheptadine

● **Antimalarials:** avoidance of antidepressants advised by manufacturer of ●artemether/lumefantrine

Antimuscarinics: paroxetine increases plasma concentration of darifenacin and procyclidine

● **Antipsychotics:** fluoxetine increases plasma concentration of ●clozapine, ●haloperidol, risperidone, ●sertindole and ●zotepine; paroxetine inhibits metabolism of perphenazine (reduce dose of perphenazine); fluoxetine and paroxetine possibly inhibit metabolism of ●aripiprazole (reduce dose of aripiprazole); fluvoxamine, paroxetine and sertraline increase plasma concentration of ●clozapine; citalopram possibly increases plasma concentration of clozapine (increased risk of toxicity); fluvoxamine increases plasma concentration of olanzapine; SSRIs possibly increase plasma concentration of ●pimozide (increased risk of ventricular arrhythmias—avoid concomitant use); paroxetine possibly increases plasma concentration of risperidone (increased risk of toxicity); paroxetine increases plasma concentration of ●sertindole

● **Antivirals:** plasma concentration of paroxetine and sertraline possibly reduced by darunavir; plasma concentration of SSRIs possibly increased by ●ritonavir; plasma concentration of paroxetine possibly reduced by ritonavir

● **Anxiolytics and Hypnotics:** fluvoxamine increases plasma concentration of some benzodiazepines; fluvoxamine increases plasma concentration of ●melatonin—avoid concomitant use; sedative effects possibly increased when sertraline given with zolpidem

Antidepressants, SSRI *(continued)*

Atomoxetine: possible increased risk of convulsions when antidepressants given with atomoxetine; fluoxetine and paroxetine possibly inhibit metabolism of atomoxetine

Barbiturates: SSRIs antagonise anticonvulsant effect of barbiturates (convulsive threshold lowered); plasma concentration of paroxetine reduced by phenobarbital

Beta-blockers: paroxetine possibly increases plasma concentration of metoprolol (enhanced effect); citalopram and escitalopram increase plasma concentration of metoprolol; fluvoxamine increases plasma concentration of propranolol

Bupropion: plasma concentration of citalopram possibly increased by bupropion

Calcium-channel Blockers: fluoxetine possibly inhibits metabolism of nifedipine (increased plasma concentration)

• Dopaminergics: caution with paroxetine advised by manufacturer of entacapone; fluoxetine should not be started until 2 weeks after stopping •rasagiline, also rasagiline should not be started until at least 5 weeks after stopping fluoxetine; increased risk of CNS toxicity when SSRIs given with •rasagiline; fluvoxamine should not be started until 2 weeks after stopping •rasagiline; increased risk of hypertension and CNS excitation when paroxetine or sertraline given with •selegiline (selegiline should not be started until 2 weeks after stopping paroxetine or sertraline, avoid paroxetine or sertraline for 2 weeks after stopping selegiline); increased risk of hypertension and CNS excitation when fluvoxamine given with •selegiline (selegiline should not be started until 1 week after stopping fluvoxamine, avoid fluvoxamine for 2 weeks after stopping selegiline); increased risk of hypertension and CNS excitation when fluoxetine given with •selegiline (selegiline should not be started until 5 weeks after stopping fluoxetine, avoid fluoxetine for 2 weeks after stopping selegiline); theoretical risk of serotonin syndrome if citalopram given with selegiline (especially if dose of selegiline exceeds 10 mg daily); manufacturer of escitalopram advises caution with selegiline

• $5HT_1$ Agonists: fluvoxamine inhibits the metabolism of frovatriptan; possible increased serotonergic effects when SSRIs given with frovatriptan; increased risk of CNS toxicity when citalopram, escitalopram, fluoxetine, fluvoxamine or paroxetine given with •sumatriptan; increased risk of CNS toxicity when sertraline given with •sumatriptan (manufacturer of sertraline advises avoid concomitant use); fluvoxamine possibly inhibits metabolism of zolmitriptan (reduce dose of zolmitriptan)

• Lithium: Increased risk of CNS effects when SSRIs given with •lithium (lithium toxicity reported)

• Muscle Relaxants: fluvoxamine increases plasma concentration of •tizanidine (increased risk of toxicity)—avoid concomitant use

Parasympathomimetics: paroxetine increases plasma concentration of galantamine

• Sibutramine: increased risk of CNS toxicity when SSRIs given with •sibutramine (manufacturer of sibutramine advises avoid concomitant use)

Sympathomimetics: metabolism of SSRIs possibly inhibited by methylphenidate

• Theophylline: fluvoxamine increases plasma concentration of •theophylline (concomitant use should usually be avoided, but where not possible halve theophylline dose and monitor plasma-theophylline concentration)

Ulcer-healing Drugs: plasma concentration of citalopram, escitalopram and sertraline increased by cimetidine; fluvoxamine possibly increases plasma

Antidepressants, SSRI

Ulcer-healing Drugs *(continued)*
concentration of lansoprazole; plasma concentration of escitalopram increased by omeprazole

Antidepressants, SSRI (related) *see* Duloxetine and Venlafaxine

Antidepressants, Tricyclic

Adrenergic Neurone Blockers: tricyclics antagonise hypotensive effect of adrenergic neurone blockers

• Alcohol: increased sedative effect when tricyclics given with •alcohol

Alpha$_2$-adrenoceptor Stimulants: avoidance of tricyclics advised by manufacturer of apraclonidine and brimonidine

Anaesthetics, General: increased risk of arrhythmias and hypotension when tricyclics given with general anaesthetics

• Analgesics: increased risk of CNS toxicity when tricyclics given with •tramadol; side-effects possibly increased when tricyclics given with nefopam; sedative effects possibly increased when tricyclics given with opioid analgesics

• Anti-arrhythmics: increased risk of ventricular arrhythmias when tricyclics given with •amiodarone—avoid concomitant use; increased risk of ventricular arrhythmias when tricyclics given with •disopyramide or •flecainide; increased risk of arrhythmias when tricyclics given with •propafenone

• Antibacterials: increased risk of ventricular arrhythmias when tricyclics given with •moxifloxacin—avoid concomitant use; plasma concentration of tricyclics possibly reduced by rifampicin

• Anticoagulants: tricyclics may enhance or reduce anticoagulant effect of •coumarins

• Antidepressants: possible increased serotonergic effects when amitriptyline or clomipramine given with duloxetine; increased risk of hypertension and CNS excitation when tricyclics given with •MAOIs, tricyclics should not be started until 2 weeks after stopping MAOIs (3 weeks if starting clomipramine or imipramine), also MAOIs should not be started for at least 1–2 weeks after stopping tricyclics (3 weeks in the case of clomipramine or imipramine); after stopping tricyclics do not start •moclobemide for at least 1 week; plasma concentration of some tricyclics increased by •SSRIs; plasma concentration of amitriptyline reduced by St John's wort

• Antiepileptics: tricyclics antagonise anticonvulsant effect of •antiepileptics (convulsive threshold lowered); metabolism of tricyclics accelerated by •carbamazepine (reduced plasma concentration and reduced effect); plasma concentration of tricyclics possibly reduced by •phenytoin; tricyclics antagonises anticonvulsant effect of •primidone (convulsive threshold lowered), also metabolism of tricyclics possibly accelerated (reduced plasma concentration)

Antifungals: plasma concentration of imipramine and nortriptyline possibly increased by terbinafine

Antihistamines: increased antimuscarinic and sedative effects when tricyclics given with antihistamines

• Antimalarials: avoidance of antidepressants advised by manufacturer of •artemether/lumefantrine

Antimuscarinics: increased risk of antimuscarinic side-effects when tricyclics given with antimuscarinics

• Antipsychotics: plasma concentration of tricyclics increased by •antipsychotics—possibly increased risk of ventricular arrhythmias; possibly increased antimuscarinic side-effects when tricyclics given with clozapine; increased risk of antimuscarinic side-effects when tricyclics given with phenothiazines; increased risk of ventricular arrhythmias when tricyclics given with •pimozide—avoid concomitant use

• Antivirals: side-effects of tricyclics possibly increased by fosamprenavir; plasma concentration of tricyclics possibly increased by •ritonavir

Antidepressants, Tricyclic *(continued)*

Anxiolytics and Hypnotics: increased sedative effect when tricyclics given with anxiolytics and hypnotics

• Atomoxetine: increased risk of ventricular arrhythmias when tricyclics given with •atomoxetine; possible increased risk of convulsions when antidepressants given with atomoxetine

• Barbiturates: tricyclics antagonise anticonvulsant effect of •barbiturates (convulsive threshold lowered), also metabolism of tricyclics possibly accelerated (reduced plasma concentration)

• Beta-blockers: plasma concentration of imipramine increased by labetalol and propranolol; increased risk of ventricular arrhythmias when tricyclics given with •sotalol

Calcium-channel Blockers: plasma concentration of imipramine increased by diltiazem and verapamil; plasma concentration of tricyclics possibly increased by diltiazem and verapamil

• Clonidine: tricyclics antagonise hypotensive effect of •clonidine, also increased risk of hypertension on clonidine withdrawal

Disulfiram: metabolism of tricyclics inhibited by disulfiram (increased plasma concentration); concomitant amitriptyline reported to increase disulfiram reaction with alcohol

Diuretics: increased risk of postural hypotension when tricyclics given with diuretics

• Dopaminergics: caution with tricyclics advised by manufacturer of entacapone; increased risk of CNS toxicity when tricyclics given with •rasagiline; CNS toxicity reported when tricyclics given with •selegiline

Lithium: risk of toxicity when tricyclics given with lithium

Muscle Relaxants: tricyclics enhance muscle relaxant effect of baclofen

Nicorandil: tricyclics possibly enhance hypotensive effect of nicorandil

Nitrates: tricyclics reduce effects of sublingual tablets of nitrates (failure to dissolve under tongue owing to dry mouth)

Oestrogens: antidepressant effect of tricyclics antagonised by oestrogens (but side-effects of tricyclics possibly increased due to increased plasma concentration)

• Pentamidine Isetionate: increased risk of ventricular arrhythmias when tricyclics given with •pentamidine isetionate

• Sibutramine: increased risk of CNS toxicity when tricyclics given with •sibutramine (manufacturer of sibutramine advises avoid concomitant use)

Sodium Oxybate: increased risk of side-effects when tricyclics given with sodium oxybate

• Sympathomimetics: increased risk of hypertension and arrhythmias when tricyclics given with •adrenaline (epinephrine) (but local anaesthetics with adrenaline appear to be safe); metabolism of tricyclics possibly inhibited by methylphenidate; increased risk of hypertension and arrhythmias when tricyclics given with •noradrenaline (norepinephrine)

Thyroid Hormones: effects of tricyclics possibly enhanced by thyroid hormones; effects of amitriptyline and imipramine enhanced by thyroid hormones

Ulcer-healing Drugs: plasma concentration of tricyclics possibly increased by cimetidine; metabolism of amitriptyline, doxepin, imipramine and nortriptyline inhibited by cimetidine (increased plasma concentration)

Antidepressants, Tricyclic (related)

• Alcohol: increased sedative effect when tricyclic-related antidepressants given with •alcohol

Alpha₂-adrenoceptor Stimulants: avoidance of tricyclic-related antidepressants advised by manufacturer of apraclonidine and brimonidine

Antidepressants, Tricyclic (related) *(continued)*

• Antidepressants: tricyclic-related antidepressants should not be started until 2 weeks after stopping •MAOIs, also MAOIs should not be started until at least 1–2 weeks after stopping tricyclic-related antidepressants; after stopping tricyclic-related antidepressants do not start •moclobemide for at least 1 week

• Antiepileptics: tricyclic-related antidepressants possibly antagonise anticonvulsant effect of •antiepileptics (convulsive threshold lowered); plasma concentration of mianserin reduced by •carbamazepine and •phenytoin; metabolism of mianserin accelerated by •primidone (reduced plasma concentration)

Antihistamines: possible increased antimuscarinic and sedative effects when tricyclic-related antidepressants given with antihistamines

• Antimalarials: avoidance of antidepressants advised by manufacturer of •artemether/lumefantrine

Antimuscarinics: possibly increased antimuscarinic side-effects when tricyclic-related antidepressants given with antimuscarinics

Antivirals: side-effects possibly increased when trazodone given with ritonavir

Anxiolytics and Hypnotics: increased sedative effect when tricyclic-related antidepressants given with anxiolytics and hypnotics

Atomoxetine: possible increased risk of convulsions when antidepressants given with atomoxetine

• Barbiturates: tricyclic-related antidepressants possibly antagonise anticonvulsant effect of •barbiturates (convulsive threshold lowered); metabolism of mianserin accelerated by •phenobarbital (reduced plasma concentration)

Diazoxide: enhanced hypotensive effect when tricyclic-related antidepressants given with diazoxide

Nitrates: tricyclic-related antidepressants possibly reduce effects of sublingual tablets of nitrates (failure to dissolve under tongue owing to dry mouth)

• Sibutramine: increased risk of CNS toxicity when tricyclic-related antidepressants given with •sibutramine (manufacturer of sibutramine advises avoid concomitant use)

Vasodilator Antihypertensives: enhanced hypotensive effect when tricyclic-related antidepressants given with hydralazine or sodium nitroprusside

Antidiabetics

Note. Other oral drugs may be taken at least 1 hour before or 4 hours after exenatide injection, or taken with a meal when exenatide is not administered, to minimise possible interference with absorption

ACE Inhibitors: hypoglycaemic effect of insulin, metformin and sulphonylureas possibly enhanced by ACE inhibitors

Alcohol: hypoglycaemic effect of antidiabetics enhanced by alcohol; increased risk of lactic acidosis when metformin given with alcohol; flushing, in susceptible subjects, when chlorpropamide given with alcohol

Anabolic Steroids: hypoglycaemic effect of antidiabetics possibly enhanced by anabolic steroids

• Analgesics: effects of sulphonylureas possibly enhanced by •NSAIDs; effects of tolbutamide enhanced by •azapropazone (avoid concomitant use)

Anti-arrhythmics: hypoglycaemic effect of gliclazide, insulin and metformin possibly enhanced by disopyramide

• Antibacterials: hypoglycaemic effect of acarbose possibly enhanced by neomycin, also severity of gastrointestinal effects increased; effects of repaglinide enhanced by clarithromycin; effects of glibenclamide possibly enhanced by ciprofloxacin and norfloxacin; plasma concentration of nateglinide reduced by rifampicin; hypoglycaemic effect of repaglinide possibly antagonised by rifampicin; plasma concentration of rosiglitazone reduced by •rifampicin—

Appendix 1: Interactions

Antidiabetics
- Antibacterials (continued)
consider increasing dose of rosiglitazone; effects of sulphonylureas enhanced by ●chloramphenicol; metabolism of sulphonylureas possibly accelerated by ●rifamycins (reduced effect); metabolism of chlorpropamide and tolbutamide accelerated by ●rifamycins (reduced effect); effects of sulphonylureas rarely enhanced by sulphonamides and trimethoprim; hypoglycaemic effect of repaglinide possibly enhanced by trimethoprim—manufacturer advises avoid concomitant use
- Anticoagulants: exenatide possibly enhances anticoagulant effect of warfarin; hypoglycaemic effect of sulphonylureas possibly enhanced by ●coumarins, also possible changes to anticoagulant effect
Antidepressants: hypoglycaemic effect of insulin, metformin and sulphonylureas enhanced by MAOIs; hypoglycaemic effect of antidiabetics possibly enhanced by MAOIs
Antiepileptics: tolbutamide transiently increases plasma concentration of phenytoin (possibility of toxicity); plasma concentration of glibenclamide possibly reduced by topiramate
- Antifungals: plasma concentration of sulphonylureas increased by ●fluconazole and ●miconazole; hypoglycaemic effect of gliclazide and glipizide enhanced by ●miconazole—avoid concomitant use; hypoglycaemic effect of nateglinide possibly enhanced by fluconazole; hypoglycaemic effect of repaglinide possibly enhanced by itraconazole; hypoglycaemic effect of glipizide possibly enhanced by posaconazole; plasma concentration of sulphonylureas possibly increased by voriconazole
Antihistamines: thrombocyte count depressed when metformin given with ketotifen (manufacturer of ketotifen advises avoid concomitant use)
Antipsychotics: hypoglycaemic effect of sulphonylureas possibly antagonised by phenothiazines
Antivirals: plasma concentration of tolbutamide possibly increased by ritonavir
Aprepitant: plasma concentration of tolbutamide reduced by aprepitant
Beta-blockers: warning signs of hypoglycaemia (such as tremor) with antidiabetics may be masked when given with beta-blockers; hypoglycaemic effect of insulin enhanced by beta-blockers
- Bosentan: increased risk of hepatotoxicity when glibenclamide given with ●bosentan—avoid concomitant use
Calcium-channel Blockers: glucose tolerance occasionally impaired when insulin given with nifedipine
Cardiac Glycosides: acarbose possibly reduces plasma concentration of digoxin; sitagliptin increases plasma concentration of digoxin
Ciclosporin: hypoglycaemic effect of repaglinide possibly enhanced by ciclosporin
Corticosteroids: hypoglycaemic effect of antidiabetics antagonised by corticosteroids
- Cytotoxics: avoidance of repaglinide advised by manufacturer of ●lapatinib; metabolism of rosiglitazone possibly inhibited by paclitaxel
Deferasirox: plasma concentration of repaglinide increased by deferasirox
Diazoxide: hypoglycaemic effect of antidiabetics antagonised by diazoxide
Diuretics: hypoglycaemic effect of antidiabetics antagonised by loop diuretics and thiazides and related diuretics; increased risk of hyponatraemia when chlorpropamide given with potassium-sparing diuretics and aldosterone antagonists plus thiazide; increased risk of hyponatraemia when chlorpropamide given with thiazides and related diuretics plus potassium-sparing diuretic
Hormone Antagonists: requirements for insulin, metformin, repaglinide and sulphonylureas possibly

Antidiabetics
Hormone Antagonists (continued)
reduced by lanreotide; requirements for insulin, metformin, repaglinide and sulphonylureas possibly reduced by octreotide
Leflunomide: hypoglycaemic effect of tolbutamide possibly enhanced by leflunomide
- Lipid-regulating Drugs: hypoglycaemic effect of acarbose possibly enhanced by colestyramine; hypoglycaemic effect of nateglinide possibly enhanced by gemfibrozil; increased risk of severe hypoglycaemia when repaglinide given with ●gemfibrozil—avoid concomitant use; plasma concentration of rosiglitazone increased by ●gemfibrozil (consider reducing dose of rosiglitazone); plasma concentration of glibenclamide possibly increased by fluvastatin; may be improved glucose tolerance and an additive effect when insulin or sulphonylureas given with fibrates
Oestrogens: hypoglycaemic effect of antidiabetics antagonised by oestrogens
Orlistat: avoidance of acarbose advised by manufacturer of orlistat
Pancreatin: hypoglycaemic effect of acarbose antagonised by pancreatin
Probenecid: hypoglycaemic effect of chlorpropamide possibly enhanced by probenecid
Progestogens: hypoglycaemic effect of antidiabetics antagonised by progestogens
- Sulfinpyrazone: effects of sulphonylureas enhanced by ●sulfinpyrazone
Testosterone: hypoglycaemic effect of antidiabetics possibly enhanced by testosterone
Ulcer-healing Drugs: excretion of metformin reduced by cimetidine (increased plasma concentration); hypoglycaemic effect of sulphonylureas enhanced by cimetidine

Antiepileptics see Carbamazepine, Ethosuximide, Gabapentin, Lacosamide, Lamotrigine, Levetiracetam, Oxcarbazepine, Phenytoin, Primidone, Rufinamide, Stiripentol, Tiagabine, Topiramate, Valproate, Vigabatrin, and Zonisamide

Antifungals see Amphotericin; Antifungals, Imidazole; Antifungals, Triazole; Caspofungin; Flucytosine; Griseofulvin; Micafungin; Terbinafine

Antifungals, Imidazole
Aliskiren: ketoconazole increases plasma concentration of aliskiren
- Analgesics: ketoconazole inhibits metabolism of ●buprenorphine (reduce dose of buprenorphine)
Antacids: absorption of ketoconazole reduced by antacids
- Anti-arrhythmics: increased risk of ventricular arrhythmias when ketoconazole given with ●disopyramide—avoid concomitant use
- Antibacterials: metabolism of ketoconazole accelerated by ●rifampicin (reduced plasma concentration), also plasma concentration of rifampicin may be reduced by ketoconazole; plasma concentration of ketoconazole possibly reduced by isoniazid; avoidance of concomitant ketoconazole in severe renal and hepatic impairment advised by manufacturer of ●telithromycin
- Anticoagulants: ketoconazole enhances anticoagulant effect of ●coumarins; miconazole enhances anticoagulant effect of ●coumarins (miconazole oral gel and possibly vaginal formulations absorbed); ketoconazole increases plasma concentration of ●rivaroxaban—avoid concomitant use
- Antidepressants: avoidance of imidazoles advised by manufacturer of ●reboxetine; ketoconazole increases plasma concentration of mirtazapine
- Antidiabetics: miconazole enhances hypoglycaemic effect of ●gliclazide and ●glipizide—avoid concomitant use; miconazole increases plasma concentration of ●sulphonylureas

Antifungals, Imidazole *(continued)*
- Antiepileptics: ketoconazole and miconazole possibly increase plasma concentration of carbamazepine; plasma concentration of ketoconazole reduced by ●phenytoin; miconazole enhances anticonvulsant effect of ●phenytoin (plasma concentration of phenytoin increased)

Antifungals: imidazoles possibly antagonise effects of amphotericin

- Antihistamines: manufacturer of loratadine advises ketoconazole possibly increases plasma concentration of loratadine; imidazoles possibly inhibit metabolism of ●mizolastine (avoid concomitant use); ketoconazole inhibits metabolism of ●mizolastine—avoid concomitant use

- Antimalarials: avoidance of imidazoles advised by manufacturer of ●artemether/lumefantrine

Antimuscarinics: absorption of ketoconazole reduced by antimuscarinics; ketoconazole increases plasma concentration of darifenacin—avoid concomitant use; manufacturer of fesoterodine advises dose reduction when ketoconazole given with fesoterodine—consult fesoterodine product literature; ketoconazole increases plasma concentration of solifenacin; avoidance of ketoconazole advised by manufacturer of tolterodine

- Antipsychotics: ketoconazole inhibits metabolism of ●aripiprazole (reduce dose of aripiprazole); increased risk of ventricular arrhythmias when imidazoles given with ●pimozide—avoid concomitant use; imidazoles possibly increase plasma concentration of quetiapine (reduce dose of quetiapine); increased risk of ventricular arrhythmias when ketoconazole given with ●sertindole—avoid concomitant use; possible increased risk of ventricular arrhythmias when imidazoles given with ●sertindole—avoid concomitant use

- Antivirals: plasma concentration of both drugs increased when ketoconazole given with darunavir; plasma concentration of ketoconazole increased by fosamprenavir; ketoconazole increases plasma concentration of ●indinavir and ●maraviroc (consider reducing dose of indinavir and maraviroc); plasma concentration of ketoconazole reduced by ●nevirapine—avoid concomitant use; combination of ketoconazole with ●ritonavir may increase plasma concentration of either drug (or both); ketoconazole increases plasma concentration of saquinavir; imidazoles possibly increase plasma concentration of saquinavir

- Anxiolytics and Hypnotics: ketoconazole increases plasma concentration of alprazolam; ketoconazole increases plasma concentration of ●midazolam (risk of prolonged sedation)

Aprepitant: ketoconazole increases plasma concentration of aprepitant

Bosentan: ketoconazole increases plasma concentration of bosentan

- Calcium-channel Blockers: ketoconazole inhibits metabolism of ●felodipine (increased plasma concentration); avoidance of ketoconazole advised by manufacturer of lercanidipine; ketoconazole possibly inhibits metabolism of dihydropyridines (increased plasma concentration)

- Ciclosporin: ketoconazole inhibits metabolism of ●ciclosporin (increased plasma concentration); miconazole possibly inhibits metabolism of ●ciclosporin (increased plasma concentration)

- Cilostazol: ketoconazole possibly increases plasma concentration of ●cilostazol—avoid concomitant use

Cinacalcet: ketoconazole inhibits metabolism of cinacalcet (increased plasma concentration)

Corticosteroids: ketoconazole possibly inhibits metabolism of corticosteroids; ketoconazole increases plasma concentration of inhaled and oral budesonide; ketoconazole increases plasma concentration

Antifungals, Imidazole
Corticosteroids *(continued)*
of active metabolite of ciclesonide; ketoconazole inhibits the metabolism of methylprednisolone; ketoconazole increases plasma concentration of inhaled mometasone

- Cytotoxics: ketoconazole inhibits metabolism of erlotinib and sunitinib (increased plasma concentration); ketoconazole increases plasma concentration of bortezomib and imatinib; ketoconazole increases plasma concentration of ●lapatinib and ●nilotinib—avoid concomitant use; ketoconazole increases plasma concentration of active metabolite of ●temsirolimus—avoid concomitant use; *in vitro* studies suggest a possible interaction between ketoconazole and docetaxel (consult docetaxel product literature); ketoconazole reduces plasma concentration of ●irinotecan (but concentration of active metabolite of irinotecan increased)—avoid concomitant use

- Diuretics: ketoconazole increases plasma concentration of ●eplerenone—avoid concomitant use

- Domperidone: ketoconazole possibly increases risk of arrhythmias with ●domperidone

- Ergot Alkaloids: increased risk of ergotism when imidazoles given with ●ergotamine and methysergide—avoid concomitant use

- 5HT$_1$ Agonists: ketoconazole increases plasma concentration of almotriptan (increased risk of toxicity); ketoconazole increases plasma concentration of ●eletriptan (risk of toxicity)—avoid concomitant use

- Ivabradine: ketoconazole increases plasma concentration of ●ivabradine—avoid concomitant use

Lanthanum: absorption of ketoconazole possibly reduced by lanthanum (give at least 2 hours apart)

- Lipid-regulating Drugs: possible increased risk of myopathy when imidazoles given with atorvastatin or simvastatin; increased risk of myopathy when ketoconazole given with ●simvastatin (avoid concomitant use); possible increased risk of myopathy when miconazole given with ●simvastatin—avoid concomitant use

Oestrogens: anecdotal reports of contraceptive failure when imidazoles or ketoconazole given with oestrogens

Parasympathomimetics: ketoconazole increases plasma concentration of galantamine

Retinoids: ketoconazole increases plasma concentration of alitretinoin

Rimonabant: ketoconazole increases plasma concentration of rimonabant

Sildenafil: ketoconazole increases plasma concentration of sildenafil—reduce initial dose of sildenafil

- Sirolimus: ketoconazole increases plasma concentration of ●sirolimus—avoid concomitant use; miconazole increases plasma concentration of ●sirolimus

- Tacrolimus: imidazoles possibly increase plasma concentration of ●tacrolimus; ketoconazole increases plasma concentration of ●tacrolimus

Tadalafil: ketoconazole increases plasma concentration of tadalafil

- Theophylline: ketoconazole possibly increases plasma concentration of ●theophylline

Ulcer-healing Drugs: absorption of ketoconazole reduced by histamine H$_2$-antagonists, proton pump inhibitors and sucralfate

- Vardenafil: ketoconazole increases plasma concentration of ●vardenafil—avoid concomitant use

Vitamins: ketoconazole possibly increases plasma concentration of paricalcitol

Antifungals, Polyene *see* Amphotericin
Antifungals, Triazole
Note. In general, fluconazole interactions relate to multiple-dose treatment
- Analgesics: fluconazole increases plasma concentration of celecoxib (halve dose of celecoxib); vorico-

Antifungals, Triazole

- Analgesics *(continued)*

nazole increases plasma concentration of diclofenac and ibuprofen; fluconazole increases plasma concentration of parecoxib (reduce dose of parecoxib); voriconazole increases plasma concentration of ●alfentanil and ●methadone (consider reducing dose of alfentanil and methadone); fluconazole inhibits metabolism of alfentanil (risk of prolonged or delayed respiratory depression); itraconazole possibly inhibits metabolism of alfentanil; fluconazole and itraconazole possibly increase plasma concentration of fentanyl

Antacids: absorption of itraconazole reduced by antacids

- Anti-arrhythmics: manufacturer of itraconazole advises avoid concomitant use with ●disopyramide

- Antibacterials: plasma concentration of itraconazole increased by clarithromycin; triazoles possibly increase plasma concentration of ●rifabutin (increased risk of uveitis—reduce rifabutin dose); posaconazole increases plasma concentration of ●rifabutin (also plasma concentration of posaconazole reduced); voriconazole increases plasma concentration of ●rifabutin, also rifabutin reduces plasma concentration of voriconazole (increase dose of voriconazole and also monitor for rifabutin toxicity); fluconazole increases plasma concentration of ●rifabutin (increased risk of uveitis—reduce rifabutin dose); plasma concentration of itraconazole reduced by ●rifabutin—avoid concomitant use; plasma concentration of posaconazole reduced by ●rifampicin; plasma concentration of voriconazole reduced by ●rifampicin—avoid concomitant use; metabolism of fluconazole and itraconazole accelerated by ●rifampicin (reduced plasma concentration)

- Anticoagulants: fluconazole, itraconazole and voriconazole enhance anticoagulant effect of ●coumarins; avoidance of itraconazole, posaconazole and voriconazole advised by manufacturer of rivaroxaban

- Antidepressants: avoidance of triazoles advised by manufacturer of ●reboxetine; plasma concentration of voriconazole reduced by ●St John's wort—avoid concomitant use

- Antidiabetics: posaconazole possibly enhances hypoglycaemic effect of glipizide; fluconazole possibly enhances hypoglycaemic effect of nateglinide; itraconazole possibly enhances hypoglycaemic effect of repaglinide; voriconazole possibly increases plasma concentration of sulphonylureas; fluconazole increases plasma concentration of ●sulphonylureas

- Antiepileptics: fluconazole possibly increases plasma concentration of carbamazepine; plasma concentration of voriconazole possibly reduced by ●carbamazepine and ●primidone—avoid concomitant use; plasma concentration of itraconazole and posaconazole possibly reduced by ●carbamazepine; fluconazole increases plasma concentration of ●phenytoin (consider reducing dose of phenytoin); voriconazole increases plasma concentration of ●phenytoin, also phenytoin reduces plasma concentration of voriconazole (increase dose of voriconazole and also monitor for phenytoin toxicity); plasma concentration of posaconazole reduced by ●phenytoin; plasma concentration of itraconazole reduced by ●phenytoin—avoid concomitant use; plasma concentration of posaconazole possibly reduced by ●primidone

Antifungals: triazoles possibly antagonise effects of amphotericin; plasma concentration of itraconazole increased by micafungin (consider reducing dose of itraconazole)

- Antihistamines: itraconazole inhibits metabolism of ●mizolastine—avoid concomitant use

Antifungals, Triazole *(continued)*

- Antimalarials: avoidance of triazoles advised by manufacturer of ●artemether/lumefantrine

Antimuscarinics: avoidance of itraconazole advised by manufacturer of darifenacin and tolterodine; manufacturer of fesoterodine advises dose reduction when itraconazole given with fesoterodine—consult fesoterodine product literature; itraconazole increases plasma concentration of solifenacin

- Antipsychotics: itraconazole possibly inhibits metabolism of ●aripiprazole (reduce dose of aripiprazole); increased risk of ventricular arrhythmias when triazoles given with ●pimozide—avoid concomitant use; triazoles possibly increase plasma concentration of quetiapine (reduce dose of quetiapine); increased risk of ventricular arrhythmias when itraconazole given with ●sertindole—avoid concomitant use; possible increased risk of ventricular arrhythmias when triazoles given with ●sertindole—avoid concomitant use

- Antivirals: posaconazole increases plasma concentration of ●atazanavir; plasma concentration of itraconazole and posaconazole reduced by ●efavirenz; plasma concentration of voriconazole reduced by ●efavirenz, also plasma concentration of efavirenz increased (consider increasing voriconazole dose and reducing efavirenz dose); plasma concentration of itraconazole possibly increased by fosamprenavir; itraconazole increases plasma concentration of ●indinavir (consider reducing dose of indinavir); plasma concentration of itraconazole possibly reduced by nevirapine—consider increasing dose of itraconazole; fluconazole increases plasma concentration of ●nevirapine, ritonavir and tipranavir; plasma concentration of voriconazole reduced by ●ritonavir—avoid concomitant use; combination of itraconazole with ●ritonavir may increase plasma concentration of either drug (or both); triazoles possibly increase plasma concentration of saquinavir; fluconazole increases plasma concentration of ●zidovudine (increased risk of toxicity)

- Anxiolytics and Hypnotics: itraconazole increases plasma concentration of alprazolam; posaconazole increases plasma concentration of ●midazolam; fluconazole and itraconazole increase plasma concentration of ●midazolam (risk of prolonged sedation); itraconazole increases plasma concentration of buspirone (reduce dose of buspirone)

- Barbiturates: plasma concentration of voriconazole possibly reduced by ●phenobarbital—avoid concomitant use; plasma concentration of itraconazole and posaconazole possibly reduced by ●phenobarbital

- Bosentan: fluconazole possibly increases plasma concentration of ●bosentan—avoid concomitant use; itraconazole possibly increases plasma concentration of bosentan

- Calcium-channel Blockers: negative inotropic effect possibly increased when itraconazole given with calcium-channel blockers; itraconazole inhibits metabolism of ●felodipine (increased plasma concentration); avoidance of itraconazole advised by manufacturer of lercanidipine; itraconazole possibly inhibits metabolism of dihydropyridines (increased plasma concentration)

- Cardiac Glycosides: itraconazole increases plasma concentration of ●digoxin

- Ciclosporin: fluconazole, itraconazole, posaconazole and voriconazole inhibit metabolism of ●ciclosporin (increased plasma concentration)

Corticosteroids: itraconazole possibly inhibits metabolism of corticosteroids and methylprednisolone; itraconazole increases plasma concentration of inhaled budesonide

- Cytotoxics: itraconazole inhibits metabolism of busulfan (increased risk of toxicity); itraconazole possibly increases side-effects of cyclophosphamide; avoid-

Antifungals, Triazole

- Cytotoxics *(continued)*
ance of itraconazole, posaconazole and voriconazole advised by manufacturer of ●lapatinib; avoidance of itraconazole and voriconazole advised by manufacturer of ●nilotinib; posaconazole possibly inhibits metabolism of ●vinblastine and ●vincristine (increased risk of neurotoxicity); itraconazole possibly inhibits metabolism of ●vincristine (increased risk of neurotoxicity)
- Diuretics: fluconazole increases plasma concentration of eplerenone (reduce dose of eplerenone); itraconazole increases plasma concentration of ●eplerenone—avoid concomitant use; plasma concentration of fluconazole increased by hydrochlorothiazide
- Ergot Alkaloids: increased risk of ergotism when triazoles given with ●ergotamine and methysergide—avoid concomitant use
- 5HT$_1$ Agonists: itraconazole increases plasma concentration of ●eletriptan (risk of toxicity)—avoid concomitant use
- Ivabradine: fluconazole increases plasma concentration of ivabradine—reduce initial dose of ivabradine; itraconazole possibly increases plasma concentration of ●ivabradine—avoid concomitant use
- Lipid-regulating Drugs: possible increased risk of myopathy when triazoles given with atorvastatin or simvastatin; increased risk of myopathy when itraconazole or posaconazole given with ●atorvastatin (avoid concomitant use); fluconazole increases plasma concentration of fluvastatin; increased risk of myopathy when itraconazole or posaconazole given with ●simvastatin (avoid concomitant use)

Oestrogens: anecdotal reports of contraceptive failure when fluconazole or itraconazole given with oestrogens

Sildenafil: itraconazole increases plasma concentration of sildenafil—reduce initial dose of sildenafil

- Sirolimus: posaconazole possibly increases plasma concentration of sirolimus; itraconazole and voriconazole increase plasma concentration of ●sirolimus—avoid concomitant use
- Tacrolimus: triazoles possibly increase plasma concentration of ●tacrolimus; posaconazole increases plasma concentration of ●tacrolimus (reduce dose of tacrolimus); fluconazole, itraconazole and voriconazole increase plasma concentration of ●tacrolimus

Tadalafil: itraconazole possibly increases plasma concentration of tadalafil

- Theophylline: fluconazole possibly increases plasma concentration of ●theophylline
- Ulcer-healing Drugs: plasma concentration of posaconazole reduced by ●cimetidine; voriconazole possibly increases plasma concentration of esomeprazole; voriconazole increases plasma concentration of omeprazole (consider reducing dose of omeprazole); absorption of itraconazole reduced by histamine H$_2$-antagonists and proton pump inhibitors
- Vardenafil: itraconazole possibly increases plasma concentration of ●vardenafil—avoid concomitant use

Antihistamines

Note. Sedative interactions apply to a lesser extent to the non-sedative antihistamines. Interactions do not generally apply to antihistamines used for topical action (including inhalation)

Alcohol: increased sedative effect when antihistamines given with alcohol (possibly less effect with non-sedating antihistamines)

Analgesics: sedative effects possibly increased when sedating antihistamines given with ●opioid analgesics

Antacids: absorption of fexofenadine reduced by antacids

Antihistamines *(continued)*

- Anti-arrhythmics: increased risk of ventricular arrhythmias when mizolastine given with ●amiodarone, ●disopyramide, ●flecainide or ●propafenone—avoid concomitant use
- Antibacterials: manufacturer of loratadine advises plasma concentration possibly increased by erythromycin; metabolism of mizolastine inhibited by ●erythromycin—avoid concomitant use; increased risk of ventricular arrhythmias when mizolastine given with ●moxifloxacin—avoid concomitant use; metabolism of mizolastine possibly inhibited by ●macrolides (avoid concomitant use)

Antidepressants: increased antimuscarinic and sedative effects when antihistamines given with MAOIs or tricyclics; cyproheptadine possibly antagonises antidepressant effect of SSRIs; possible increased antimuscarinic and sedative effects when antihistamines given with tricyclic-related antidepressants

Antidiabetics: thrombocyte count depressed when ketotifen given with metformin (manufacturer of ketotifen advises avoid concomitant use)

- Antifungals: manufacturer of loratadine advises plasma concentration possibly increased by ketoconazole; metabolism of mizolastine inhibited by ●itraconazole or ●ketoconazole—avoid concomitant use; metabolism of mizolastine possibly inhibited by ●imidazoles (avoid concomitant use)

Antimuscarinics: increased risk of antimuscarinic side-effects when antihistamines given with antimuscarinics

Antivirals: plasma concentration of loratadine possibly increased by fosamprenavir; plasma concentration of chlorphenamine (chlorpheniramine) possibly increased by lopinavir; plasma concentration of non-sedating antihistamines possibly increased by ritonavir

Anxiolytics and Hypnotics: increased sedative effect when antihistamines given with anxiolytics and hypnotics

- Beta-blockers: increased risk of ventricular arrhythmias when mizolastine given with ●sotalol—avoid concomitant use

Betahistine: antihistamines theoretically antagonise effect of betahistine

Ulcer-healing Drugs: manufacturer of loratadine advises plasma concentration possibly increased by cimetidine

Antihistamines, Non-sedating *see* Antihistamines

Antihistamines, Sedating *see* Antihistamines

Antimalarials *see* Artemether with Lumefantrine, Chloroquine and Hydroxychloroquine, Mefloquine, Primaquine, Proguanil, and Quinine

Antimetabolites *see* Cytarabine, Fludarabine, Fluorouracil, Mercaptopurine, Methotrexate, and Tioguanine

Antimuscarinics

Note. Many drugs have antimuscarinic effects; concomitant use of two or more such drugs can increase side-effects such as dry mouth, urine retention, and constipation; concomitant use can also lead to confusion in the elderly. Interactions do not generally apply to antimuscarinics used by inhalation

Alcohol: increased sedative effect when hyoscine given with alcohol

Analgesics: increased risk of antimuscarinic side-effects when antimuscarinics given with nefopam

- Anti-arrhythmics: increased risk of ventricular arrhythmias when tolterodine given with ●amiodarone, ●disopyramide or ●flecainide; increased risk of antimuscarinic side-effects when antimuscarinics given with disopyramide

Antibacterials: manufacturer of fesoterodine advises dose reduction when fesoterodine given with clarithromycin and telithromycin—consult fesoterodine product literature; manufacturer of tolterodine advises avoid concomitant use with

Antimuscarinics

Antibacterials *(continued)*

clarithromycin and erythromycin; plasma concentration of darifenacin possibly increased by erythromycin; plasma concentration of active metabolite of fesoterodine reduced by rifampicin

Antidepressants: plasma concentration of darifenacin and procyclidine increased by paroxetine; increased risk of antimuscarinic side-effects when antimuscarinics given with MAOIs or tricyclics; possibly increased antimuscarinic side-effects when antimuscarinics given with tricyclic-related antidepressants

Antifungals: antimuscarinics reduce absorption of ketoconazole; manufacturer of fesoterodine advises dose reduction when fesoterodine given with itraconazole and ketoconazole—consult fesoterodine product literature; plasma concentration of darifenacin increased by ketoconazole—avoid concomitant use; plasma concentration of solifenacin increased by itraconazole and ketoconazole; manufacturer of tolterodine advises avoid concomitant use with itraconazole and ketoconazole; manufacturer of darifenacin advises avoid concomitant use with itraconazole

Antihistamines: increased risk of antimuscarinic side-effects when antimuscarinics given with antihistamines

Antipsychotics: antimuscarinics possibly reduce effects of haloperidol; increased risk of antimuscarinic side-effects when antimuscarinics given with clozapine; antimuscarinics reduce plasma concentration of phenothiazines, but risk of antimuscarinic side-effects increased

Antivirals: manufacturer of darifenacin advises avoid concomitant use with atazanavir, fosamprenavir, indinavir, lopinavir, nelfinavir, ritonavir, saquinavir and tipranavir; manufacturer of fesoterodine advises dose reduction when fesoterodine given with atazanavir, indinavir, nelfinavir, ritonavir and saquinavir—consult fesoterodine product literature; manufacturer of tolterodine advises avoid concomitant use with fosamprenavir, indinavir, lopinavir, nelfinavir, ritonavir and saquinavir; plasma concentration of solifenacin increased by nelfinavir and ritonavir

• Beta-blockers: increased risk of ventricular arrhythmias when tolterodine given with ●sotalol

Calcium-channel Blockers: manufacturer of darifenacin advises avoid concomitant use with verapamil

Cardiac Glycosides: darifenacin possibly increases plasma concentration of digoxin

Ciclosporin: manufacturer of darifenacin advises avoid concomitant use with ciclosporin

Domperidone: antimuscarinics antagonise effects of domperidone on gastro-intestinal activity

Dopaminergics: increased risk of antimuscarinic side-effects when antimuscarinics given with amantadine; antimuscarinics possibly reduce absorption of levodopa

Memantine: effects of antimuscarinics possibly enhanced by memantine

Metoclopramide: antimuscarinics antagonise effects of metoclopramide on gastro-intestinal activity

Nitrates: antimuscarinics possibly reduce effects of sublingual tablets of nitrates (failure to dissolve under tongue owing to dry mouth)

Parasympathomimetics: antimuscarinics antagonise effects of parasympathomimetics

Antipsychotics

Note. Increased risk of toxicity with myelosuppressive drugs

Note. Avoid concomitant use of clozapine with drugs that have a substantial potential for causing agranulocytosis

ACE Inhibitors: enhanced hypotensive effect when antipsychotics given with ACE inhibitors

Antipsychotics *(continued)*

Adrenergic Neurone Blockers: enhanced hypotensive effect when phenothiazines given with adrenergic neurone blockers; higher doses of chlorpromazine antagonise hypotensive effect of adrenergic neurone blockers; haloperidol antagonises hypotensive effect of adrenergic neurone blockers

Adsorbents: absorption of phenothiazines possibly reduced by kaolin

Alcohol: increased sedative effect when antipsychotics given with alcohol

Alpha-blockers: enhanced hypotensive effect when antipsychotics given with alpha-blockers

• Anaesthetics, General: enhanced hypotensive effect when antipsychotics given with ●general anaesthetics

• Analgesics: avoid concomitant use of clozapine with ●azapropazone (increased risk of agranulocytosis); possible severe drowsiness when haloperidol given with indometacin; increased risk of convulsions when antipsychotics given with tramadol; enhanced hypotensive and sedative effects when antipsychotics given with opioid analgesics

Angiotensin-II Receptor Antagonists: enhanced hypotensive effect when antipsychotics given with angiotensin-II receptor antagonists

Antacids: absorption of phenothiazines and sulpiride reduced by antacids

• Anti-arrhythmics: increased risk of ventricular arrhythmias when antipsychotics that prolong the QT interval given with ●anti-arrhythmics that prolong the QT interval; increased risk of ventricular arrhythmias when amisulpride, haloperidol, pimozide, sertindole or zuclopenthixol given with ●amiodarone—avoid concomitant use; increased risk of ventricular arrhythmias when benperidol given with ●amiodarone—manufacturer of benperidol advises avoid concomitant use; increased risk of ventricular arrhythmias when sulpiride given with ●amiodarone or ●disopyramide; increased risk of ventricular arrhythmias when amisulpride, pimozide, sertindole or zuclopenthixol given with ●disopyramide—avoid concomitant use; increased risk of ventricular arrhythmias when phenothiazines given with ●disopyramide; increased risk of arrhythmias when clozapine given with ●flecainide

• Antibacterials: increased risk of ventricular arrhythmias when pimozide given with ●clarithromycin, ●moxifloxacin or ●telithromycin—avoid concomitant use; increased risk of ventricular arrhythmias when sertindole given with ●erythromycin or ●moxifloxacin—avoid concomitant use; increased risk of ventricular arrhythmias when amisulpride or zuclopenthixol given with parenteral ●erythromycin—avoid concomitant use; plasma concentration of clozapine possibly increased by ●erythromycin (possible increased risk of convulsions); possible increased risk of ventricular arrhythmias when pimozide given with ●erythromycin—avoid concomitant use; increased risk of ventricular arrhythmias when sulpiride given with parenteral ●erythromycin; plasma concentration of clozapine increased by ciprofloxacin; plasma concentration of olanzapine possibly increased by ciprofloxacin; increased risk of ventricular arrhythmias when haloperidol, phenothiazines or zuclopenthixol given with ●moxifloxacin—avoid concomitant use; increased risk of ventricular arrhythmias when benperidol given with ●moxifloxacin—manufacturer of benperidol advises avoid concomitant use; plasma concentration of aripiprazole possibly reduced by ●rifabutin and ●rifampicin—increase dose of aripiprazole; plasma concentration of clozapine possibly reduced by rifampicin; metabolism of haloperidol accelerated by ●rifampicin (reduced plasma concentration); avoid

Antipsychotics
- Antibacterials *(continued)*
concomitant use of clozapine with
●chloramphenicol or ●sulphonamides (increased risk
of agranulocytosis); plasma concentration of quetiapine possibly increased by macrolides (reduce dose
of quetiapine); possible increased risk of ventricular
arrhythmias when sertindole given with
●macrolides—avoid concomitant use
- Antidepressants: plasma concentration of clozapine
possibly increased by citalopram (increased risk of
toxicity); metabolism of aripiprazole possibly inhibited by ●fluoxetine and ●paroxetine (reduce dose of
aripiprazole); plasma concentration of clozapine,
haloperidol, risperidone, sertindole and zotepine
increased by ●fluoxetine; plasma concentration of
clozapine and olanzapine increased by
●fluvoxamine; plasma concentration of
clozapine and sertindole increased by ●paroxetine;
plasma concentration of risperidone possibly
increased by paroxetine (increased risk of toxicity);
metabolism of perphenazine inhibited by paroxetine
(reduce dose of perphenazine); plasma concentration
of clozapine increased by ●sertraline and
●venlafaxine; plasma concentration of haloperidol
increased by venlafaxine; clozapine possibly
increases CNS effects of ●MAOIs; plasma concentration of pimozide possibly increased by ●SSRIs
(increased risk of ventricular arrhythmias—avoid
concomitant use); plasma concentration of aripiprazole possibly reduced by ●St John's wort—increase
dose of aripiprazole; antipsychotics increase plasma
concentration of ●tricyclics—possibly increased risk
of ventricular arrhythmias; increased risk of antimuscarinic side-effects when phenothiazines given
with tricyclics; increased risk of ventricular arrhythmias when pimozide given with ●tricyclics—avoid
concomitant use; possibly increased antimuscarinic
side-effects when clozapine given with tricyclics
- Antidiabetics: phenothiazines possibly antagonise
hypoglycaemic effect of sulphonylureas
- Antiepileptics: metabolism of clozapine accelerated by
●carbamazepine (reduced plasma concentration),
also avoid concomitant use of drugs with substantial
potential for causing agranulocytosis; metabolism of
haloperidol, olanzapine, quetiapine, risperidone and
sertindole accelerated by carbamazepine (reduced
plasma concentration); plasma concentration of
aripiprazole reduced by ●carbamazepine—increase
dose of aripiprazole; plasma concentration of paliperidone reduced by carbamazepine; antipsychotics
antagonise anticonvulsant effect of ●carbamazepine,
●ethosuximide, ●oxcarbazepine, ●phenytoin,
●primidone and ●valproate (convulsive threshold
lowered); metabolism of clozapine, quetiapine and
sertindole accelerated by phenytoin (reduced plasma
concentration); plasma concentration of aripiprazole
possibly reduced by ●phenytoin and ●primidone—
increase dose of aripiprazole; metabolism of haloperidol accelerated by primidone (reduced plasma
concentration); increased risk of neutropenia when
olanzapine given with ●valproate
- Antifungals: metabolism of aripiprazole inhibited by
●ketoconazole (reduce dose of aripiprazole);
increased risk of ventricular arrhythmias when
sertindole given with ●itraconazole or
●ketoconazole—avoid concomitant use; metabolism
of aripiprazole possibly inhibited by ●itraconazole
(reduce dose of aripiprazole); possible increased risk
of ventricular arrhythmias when sertindole given
with ●imidazoles or ●triazoles—avoid concomitant
use; plasma concentration of quetiapine possibly
increased by imidazoles and triazoles (reduce dose of
quetiapine); increased risk of ventricular arrhythmias
when pimozide given with ●imidazoles or
●triazoles—avoid concomitant use

Antipsychotics *(continued)*
- Antimalarials: avoidance of antipsychotics advised by
manufacturer of ●artemether/lumefantrine;
increased risk of ventricular arrhythmias when
pimozide given with ●mefloquine or ●quinine—avoid
concomitant use
- Antimuscarinics: increased risk of antimuscarinic side-
effects when clozapine given with antimuscarinics;
plasma concentration of phenothiazines reduced by
antimuscarinics, but risk of antimuscarinic side-
effects increased; effects of haloperidol possibly
reduced by antimuscarinics
- Antipsychotics: avoid concomitant use of clozapine
with depot formulation of ●flupentixol,
●fluphenazine, ●haloperidol, ●pipotiazine,
●risperidone or ●zuclopenthixol as cannot be withdrawn quickly if neutropenia occurs; increased risk
of ventricular arrhythmias when sulpiride given with
●haloperidol; increased risk of ventricular arrhythmias when sertindole given with ●amisulpride—
avoid concomitant use; increased risk of ventricular
arrhythmias when pimozide given with
●phenothiazines—avoid concomitant use; increased
risk of ventricular arrhythmias when pimozide given
with ●sulpiride
- Antivirals: plasma concentration of pimozide possibly
increased by ●atazanavir—avoid concomitant use;
metabolism of aripiprazole possibly inhibited by
●atazanavir, ●fosamprenavir, ●indinavir, ●lopinavir,
●nelfinavir, ●ritonavir and ●saquinavir (reduce dose
of aripiprazole); plasma concentration of pimozide
possibly increased by ●efavirenz, ●indinavir,
●nelfinavir and ●saquinavir (increased risk of ventricular arrhythmias—avoid concomitant use); plasma
concentration of aripiprazole possibly reduced by
●efavirenz and ●nevirapine—increase dose of aripiprazole; plasma concentration of pimozide and
sertindole increased by ●fosamprenavir (increased
risk of ventricular arrhythmias—avoid concomitant
use); plasma concentration of clozapine possibly
increased by fosamprenavir; plasma concentration of
sertindole increased by ●indinavir, ●lopinavir,
●nelfinavir, ●ritonavir and ●saquinavir (increased risk
of ventricular arrhythmias—avoid concomitant use);
plasma concentration of olanzapine reduced by
ritonavir—consider increasing dose of olanzapine;
plasma concentration of clozapine increased by
●ritonavir (increased risk of toxicity)—avoid concomitant use; plasma concentration of antipsychotics possibly increased by ●ritonavir; plasma
concentration of pimozide increased by ●ritonavir
(increased risk of ventricular arrhythmias—avoid
concomitant use)
- Anxiolytics and Hypnotics: increased sedative effect
when antipsychotics given with anxiolytics and
hypnotics; plasma concentration of zotepine
increased by diazepam; increased risk of hypotension, bradycardia and respiratory depression
when intramuscular olanzapine given with parenteral
●benzodiazepines; plasma concentration of haloperidol increased by buspirone
- Aprepitant: avoidance of pimozide advised by manufacturer of ●aprepitant
- Atomoxetine: increased risk of ventricular arrhythmias
when antipsychotics that prolong the QT interval
given with ●atomoxetine
- Barbiturates: antipsychotics antagonise anticonvulsant
effect of ●barbiturates (convulsive threshold
lowered); metabolism of haloperidol accelerated by
phenobarbital (reduced plasma concentration);
plasma concentration of both drugs reduced when
chlorpromazine given with phenobarbital; plasma
concentration of aripiprazole possibly reduced by
●phenobarbital—increase dose of aripiprazole
- Beta-blockers: enhanced hypotensive effect when
phenothiazines given with beta-blockers; plasma

Antipsychotics

- Beta-blockers *(continued)*
concentration of both drugs may increase when chlorpromazine given with ●propranolol; increased risk of ventricular arrhythmias when amisulpride, phenothiazines, pimozide, sertindole or sulpiride given with ●sotalol; increased risk of ventricular arrhythmias when zuclopenthixol given with ●sotalol—avoid concomitant use

Calcium-channel Blockers: enhanced hypotensive effect when antipsychotics given with calcium-channel blockers

Clonidine: enhanced hypotensive effect when phenothiazines given with clonidine

- Cytotoxics: avoid concomitant use of clozapine with ●cytotoxics (increased risk of agranulocytosis); avoidance of pimozide advised by manufacturer of ●lapatinib

Desferrioxamine: manufacturer of levomepromazine (methotrimeprazine) advises avoid concomitant use with desferrioxamine; avoidance of prochlorperazine advised by manufacturer of desferrioxamine

Diazoxide: enhanced hypotensive effect when phenothiazines given with diazoxide

- Diuretics: risk of ventricular arrhythmias with amisulpride or sertindole increased by hypokalaemia caused by ●diuretics; risk of ventricular arrhythmias with pimozide increased by hypokalaemia caused by ●diuretics (avoid concomitant use); enhanced hypotensive effect when phenothiazines given with diuretics

Dopaminergics: increased risk of extrapyramidal side-effects when antipsychotics given with amantadine; antipsychotics antagonise effects of apomorphine, levodopa and pergolide; antipsychotics antagonise hypoprolactinaemic and antiparkinsonian effects of bromocriptine and cabergoline; manufacturer of amisulpride advises avoid concomitant use of levodopa (antagonism of effect); avoidance of antipsychotics advised by manufacturer of pramipexole, ropinirole and rotigotine (antagonism of effect)

- Ivabradine: increased risk of ventricular arrhythmias when pimozide or sertindole given with ●ivabradine

- Lithium: increased risk of ventricular arrhythmias when sertindole given with ●lithium—avoid concomitant use; increased risk of extrapyramidal side-effects and possibly neurotoxicity when clozapine, flupentixol, haloperidol, phenothiazines or zuclopenthixol given with lithium; increased risk of extrapyramidal side-effects when sulpiride given with lithium

Memantine: effects of antipsychotics possibly reduced by memantine

Methyldopa: enhanced hypotensive effect when antipsychotics given with methyldopa (also increased risk of extrapyramidal effects)

Metoclopramide: increased risk of extrapyramidal side-effects when antipsychotics given with metoclopramide

Moxonidine: enhanced hypotensive effect when phenothiazines given with moxonidine

Muscle Relaxants: promazine possibly enhances effects of suxamethonium

Nitrates: enhanced hypotensive effect when phenothiazines given with nitrates

- Penicillamine: avoid concomitant use of clozapine with ●penicillamine (increased risk of agranulocytosis)

- Pentamidine Isetionate: increased risk of ventricular arrhythmias when amisulpride given with ●pentamidine isetionate—avoid concomitant use; increased risk of ventricular arrhythmias when phenothiazines given with ●pentamidine isetionate

- Sibutramine: increased risk of CNS toxicity when antipsychotics given with ●sibutramine (manufacturer of sibutramine advises avoid concomitant use)

Sodium Benzoate: haloperidol possibly reduces effects of sodium benzoate

Antipsychotics *(continued)*

Sodium Oxybate: antipsychotics possibly enhance effects of sodium oxybate

Sodium Phenylbutyrate: haloperidol possibly reduces effects of sodium phenylbutyrate

Sympathomimetics: antipsychotics antagonise hypertensive effect of sympathomimetics

Tetrabenazine: increased risk of extrapyramidal side-effects when antipsychotics given with tetrabenazine

- Ulcer-healing Drugs: effects of antipsychotics, chlorpromazine and clozapine possibly enhanced by cimetidine; increased risk of ventricular arrhythmias when sertindole given with ●cimetidine—avoid concomitant use; plasma concentration of clozapine possibly reduced by omeprazole; absorption of sulpiride reduced by sucralfate

Vasodilator Antihypertensives: enhanced hypotensive effect when phenothiazines given with hydralazine, minoxidil or sodium nitroprusside

Antivirals *see* Abacavir, Aciclovir, Adefovir, Atazanavir, Cidofovir, Darunavir, Didanosine, Efavirenz, Emtricitabine, Etravirine, Famciclovir, Fosamprenavir, Foscarnet, Ganciclovir, Indinavir, Lamivudine, Lopinavir, Maraviroc, Nelfinavir, Nevirapine, Raltegravir, Ribavirin, Ritonavir, Saquinavir, Stavudine, Telbivudine, Tenofovir, Tipranavir, Valaciclovir, and Zidovudine

Anxiolytics and Hypnotics

ACE Inhibitors: enhanced hypotensive effect when anxiolytics and hypnotics given with ACE inhibitors

Adrenergic Neurone Blockers: enhanced hypotensive effect when anxiolytics and hypnotics given with adrenergic neurone blockers

Alcohol: increased sedative effect when anxiolytics and hypnotics given with alcohol

Alpha-blockers: enhanced hypotensive and sedative effects when anxiolytics and hypnotics given with alpha-blockers

Anaesthetics, General: increased sedative effect when anxiolytics and hypnotics given with general anaesthetics

Analgesics: increased sedative effect when anxiolytics and hypnotics given with opioid analgesics

Angiotensin-II Receptor Antagonists: enhanced hypotensive effect when anxiolytics and hypnotics given with angiotensin-II receptor antagonists

- Antibacterials: metabolism of midazolam inhibited by ●clarithromycin, ●erythromycin, ●quinupristin/ dalfopristin and ●telithromycin (increased plasma concentration with increased sedation); plasma concentration of buspirone increased by erythromycin (reduce dose of buspirone); metabolism of zopiclone inhibited by erythromycin and quinupristin/dalfopristin; metabolism of benzodiazepines possibly accelerated by rifampicin (reduced plasma concentration); metabolism of diazepam accelerated by rifampicin (reduced plasma concentration); metabolism of buspirone and zaleplon possibly accelerated by rifampicin; metabolism of zolpidem accelerated by rifampicin (reduced plasma concentration and reduced effect); plasma concentration of zopiclone significantly reduced by rifampicin; metabolism of diazepam inhibited by isoniazid

Anticoagulants: chloral and triclofos may transiently enhance anticoagulant effect of coumarins

- Antidepressants: plasma concentration of melatonin increased by ●fluvoxamine—avoid concomitant use; plasma concentration of some benzodiazepines increased by fluvoxamine; sedative effects possibly increased when zolpidem given with sertraline; manufacturer of buspirone advises avoid concomitant use with MAOIs; plasma concentration of oral midazolam possibly reduced by St John's wort; increased sedative effect when anxiolytics and hypnotics given with mirtazapine, tricyclic-related antidepressants or tricyclics

Anxiolytics and Hypnotics *(continued)*

Antiepileptics: plasma concentration of midazolam reduced by carbamazepine; plasma concentration of clonazepam often reduced by carbamazepine, phenytoin and primidone; benzodiazepines possibly increase or decrease plasma concentration of phenytoin; diazepam increases or decreases plasma concentration of phenytoin; plasma concentration of clobazam increased by stiripentol; plasma concentration of diazepam and lorazepam possibly increased by valproate; increased risk of side-effects when clonazepam given with valproate; clobazam possibly increases plasma concentration of valproate

• Antifungals: plasma concentration of alprazolam increased by itraconazole and ketoconazole; plasma concentration of midazolam increased by •fluconazole, •itraconazole and •ketoconazole (risk of prolonged sedation); plasma concentration of buspirone increased by itraconazole (reduce dose of buspirone); plasma concentration of midazolam increased by •posaconazole

Antihistamines: increased sedative effect when anxiolytics and hypnotics given with antihistamines

• Antipsychotics: increased sedative effect when anxiolytics and hypnotics given with antipsychotics; buspirone increases plasma concentration of haloperidol; increased risk of hypotension, bradycardia and respiratory depression when parenteral benzodiazepines given with intramuscular •olanzapine; diazepam increases plasma concentration of zotepine

• Antivirals: plasma concentration of midazolam possibly increased by •atazanavir—avoid concomitant use of oral midazolam; increased risk of prolonged sedation when midazolam given with •efavirenz—avoid concomitant use; increased risk of prolonged sedation and respiratory depression when alprazolam, clonazepam, diazepam, flurazepam or midazolam given with •fosamprenavir; plasma concentration of midazolam possibly increased by •indinavir, •nelfinavir and •ritonavir (risk of prolonged sedation—avoid concomitant use of oral midazolam); increased risk of prolonged sedation when alprazolam given with •indinavir—avoid concomitant use; plasma concentration of alprazolam, diazepam, flurazepam and zolpidem possibly increased by •ritonavir (risk of extreme sedation and respiratory depression —avoid concomitant use); plasma concentration of anxiolytics and hypnotics possibly increased by •ritonavir; plasma concentration of buspirone increased by ritonavir (increased risk of toxicity); plasma concentration of midazolam increased by •saquinavir (risk of prolonged sedation—avoid concomitant use of oral midazolam)

Aprepitant: plasma concentration of midazolam increased by aprepitant (risk of prolonged sedation)

Barbiturates: plasma concentration of clonazepam often reduced by phenobarbital

Beta-blockers: enhanced hypotensive effect when anxiolytics and hypnotics given with beta-blockers

Calcium-channel Blockers: enhanced hypotensive effect when anxiolytics and hypnotics given with calcium-channel blockers; midazolam increases absorption of lercanidipine; metabolism of midazolam inhibited by diltiazem and verapamil (increased plasma concentration with increased sedation); plasma concentration of buspirone increased by diltiazem and verapamil (reduce dose of buspirone)

Cardiac Glycosides: alprazolam increases plasma concentration of digoxin (increased risk of toxicity)

Clonidine: enhanced hypotensive effect when anxiolytics and hypnotics given with clonidine

Cytotoxics: plasma concentration of midazolam increased by nilotinib

Anxiolytics and Hypnotics *(continued)*

Deferasirox: plasma concentration of midazolam possibly reduced by deferasirox

Diazoxide: enhanced hypotensive effect when anxiolytics and hypnotics given with diazoxide

Disulfiram: metabolism of benzodiazepines inhibited by disulfiram (increased sedative effects); increased risk of temazepam toxicity when given with disulfiram

Diuretics: enhanced hypotensive effect when anxiolytics and hypnotics given with diuretics; administration of chloral or triclofos with parenteral furosemide (frusemide) may displace thyroid hormone from binding sites

Dopaminergics: benzodiazepines possibly antagonise effects of levodopa

Grapefruit Juice: plasma concentration of buspirone increased by grapefruit juice

Lofexidine: increased sedative effect when anxiolytics and hypnotics given with lofexidine

Methyldopa: enhanced hypotensive effect when anxiolytics and hypnotics given with methyldopa

Moxonidine: enhanced hypotensive effect when anxiolytics and hypnotics given with moxonidine; sedative effects possibly increased when benzodiazepines given with moxonidine

Muscle Relaxants: increased sedative effect when anxiolytics and hypnotics given with baclofen or tizanidine

Nabilone: increased sedative effect when anxiolytics and hypnotics given with nabilone

Nitrates: enhanced hypotensive effect when anxiolytics and hypnotics given with nitrates

Oestrogens: plasma concentration of melatonin increased by oestrogens

Probenecid: excretion of lorazepam reduced by probenecid (increased plasma concentration); excretion of nitrazepam possibly reduced by probenecid (increased plasma concentration)

• Sodium Oxybate: benzodiazepines enhance effects of •sodium oxybate (avoid concomitant use)

Theophylline: effects of benzodiazepines possibly reduced by theophylline

Ulcer-healing Drugs: plasma concentration of melatonin increased by cimetidine; metabolism of benzodiazepines, clomethiazole and zaleplon inhibited by cimetidine (increased plasma concentration); metabolism of diazepam possibly inhibited by esomeprazole and omeprazole (increased plasma concentration)

Vasodilator Antihypertensives: enhanced hypotensive effect when anxiolytics and hypnotics given with hydralazine, minoxidil or sodium nitroprusside

Apomorphine

Antipsychotics: effects of apomorphine antagonised by antipsychotics

Dopaminergics: effects of apomorphine possibly enhanced by entacapone

Memantine: effects of dopaminergics possibly enhanced by memantine

Methyldopa: antiparkinsonian effect of dopaminergics antagonised by methyldopa

Apraclonidine

Antidepressants: manufacturer of apraclonidine advises avoid concomitant use with MAOIs, tricyclic-related antidepressants and tricyclics

Aprepitant

Note. Fosaprepitant is a prodrug of aprepitant

Antibacterials: plasma concentration of aprepitant possibly increased by clarithromycin and telithromycin; plasma concentration of aprepitant reduced by rifampicin

Anticoagulants: aprepitant possibly reduces anticoagulant effect of warfarin

• Antidepressants: manufacturer of aprepitant advises avoid concomitant use with •St John's wort

Appendix 1: Interactions

Aprepitant *(continued)*

Antidiabetics: aprepitant reduces plasma concentration of tolbutamide

Antiepileptics: plasma concentration of aprepitant possibly reduced by carbamazepine and phenytoin

Antifungals: plasma concentration of aprepitant increased by ketoconazole

• Antipsychotics: manufacturer of aprepitant advises avoid concomitant use with ●pimozide

Antivirals: plasma concentration of aprepitant possibly increased by ritonavir

Anxiolytics and Hypnotics: aprepitant increases plasma concentration of midazolam (risk of prolonged sedation)

Barbiturates: plasma concentration of aprepitant possibly reduced by phenobarbital

Corticosteroids: aprepitant inhibits metabolism of dexamethasone and methylprednisolone (reduce dose of dexamethasone and methylprednisolone)

• Oestrogens: aprepitant possibly causes contraceptive failure of hormonal contraceptives containing ●oestrogens (alternative contraception recommended)

• Progestogens: aprepitant possibly causes contraceptive failure of hormonal contraceptives containing ●progestogens (alternative contraception recommended)

Aripiprazole *see* Antipsychotics

Artemether with Lumefantrine

• Anti-arrhythmics: manufacturer of artemether/lumefantrine advises avoid concomitant use with ●amiodarone, ●disopyramide or ●flecainide (risk of ventricular arrhythmias)

• Antibacterials: manufacturer of artemether/lumefantrine advises avoid concomitant use with ●macrolides and ●quinolones

• Antidepressants: manufacturer of artemether/lumefantrine advises avoid concomitant use with ●antidepressants

• Antifungals: manufacturer of artemether/lumefantrine advises avoid concomitant use with ●imidazoles and ●triazoles

• Antimalarials: manufacturer of artemether/lumefantrine advises avoid concomitant use with ●antimalarials; increased risk of ventricular arrhythmias when artemether/lumefantrine given with ●quinine

• Antipsychotics: manufacturer of artemether/lumefantrine advises avoid concomitant use with ●antipsychotics

Antivirals: manufacturer of artemether/lumefantrine advises caution with atazanavir, darunavir, fosamprenavir, indinavir, lopinavir, nelfinavir, ritonavir, saquinavir and tipranavir

• Beta-blockers: manufacturer of artemether/lumefantrine advises avoid concomitant use with ●metoprolol and ●sotalol

Grapefruit Juice: plasma concentration of artemether/lumefantrine possibly increased by grapefruit juice

• Ulcer-healing Drugs: manufacturer of artemether/lumefantrine advises avoid concomitant use with ●cimetidine

Vaccines: antimalarials inactivate oral typhoid vaccine—see p. 752

Ascorbic acid *see* Vitamins

Aspirin

Adsorbents: absorption of aspirin possibly reduced by kaolin

• Analgesics: avoid concomitant use of aspirin with ●NSAIDs (increased side-effects); antiplatelet effect of aspirin possibly reduced by ibuprofen

Antacids: excretion of aspirin increased by alkaline urine due to some antacids

• Anticoagulants: increased risk of bleeding when aspirin given with ●coumarins or ●phenindione (due to

Aspirin

• Anticoagulants *(continued)*
antiplatelet effect); aspirin enhances anticoagulant effect of ●heparins

• Antidepressants: increased risk of bleeding when aspirin given with ●SSRIs or ●venlafaxine

Antiepileptics: aspirin enhances effects of phenytoin and valproate

Cilostazol: manufacturer of cilostazol recommends dose of aspirin should not exceed 80 mg daily when given with cilostazol

Clopidogrel: increased risk of bleeding when aspirin given with clopidogrel

Corticosteroids: increased risk of gastro-intestinal bleeding and ulceration when aspirin given with corticosteroids, also corticosteroids reduce plasma concentration of salicylate

• Cytotoxics: aspirin reduces excretion of ●methotrexate (increased risk of toxicity)

Diuretics: aspirin antagonises diuretic effect of spironolactone; increased risk of toxicity when high-dose aspirin given with carbonic anhydrase inhibitors

Iloprost: increased risk of bleeding when aspirin given with iloprost

Leukotriene Receptor Antagonists: aspirin increases plasma concentration of zafirlukast

Metoclopramide: rate of absorption of aspirin increased by metoclopramide (enhanced effect)

Probenecid: aspirin antagonises effects of probenecid

Sibutramine: increased risk of bleeding when aspirin given with sibutramine

Sulfinpyrazone: aspirin antagonises effects of sulfinpyrazone

Atazanavir

Antacids: plasma concentration of atazanavir possibly reduced by antacids

• Anti-arrhythmics: atazanavir possibly increases plasma concentration of ●amiodarone and ●lidocaine (lignocaine)

• Antibacterials: plasma concentration of both drugs increased when atazanavir given with clarithromycin; atazanavir increases plasma concentration of ●rifabutin (reduce dose of rifabutin); plasma concentration of atazanavir reduced by ●rifampicin—avoid concomitant use; avoidance of concomitant atazanavir in severe renal and hepatic impairment advised by manufacturer of ●telithromycin

Anticoagulants: atazanavir may enhance or reduce anticoagulant effect of warfarin; avoidance of atazanavir advised by manufacturer of rivaroxaban

• Antidepressants: plasma concentration of atazanavir reduced by ●St John's wort—avoid concomitant use

• Antifungals: plasma concentration of atazanavir increased by ●posaconazole

Antimalarials: caution with atazanavir advised by manufacturer of artemether/lumefantrine

Antimuscarinics: avoidance of atazanavir advised by manufacturer of darifenacin; manufacturer of fesoterodine advises dose reduction when atazanavir given with fesoterodine—consult fesoterodine product literature

• Antipsychotics: atazanavir possibly inhibits metabolism of ●aripiprazole (reduce dose of aripiprazole); atazanavir possibly increases plasma concentration of ●pimozide—avoid concomitant use

• Antivirals: manufacturer of atazanavir advises avoid concomitant use with ●efavirenz (plasma concentration of atazanavir reduced); avoid concomitant use of atazanavir with ●indinavir; atazanavir increases plasma concentration of ●maraviroc (consider reducing dose of maraviroc); plasma concentration of atazanavir possibly reduced by ●nevirapine—avoid concomitant use; atazanavir increases plasma concentration of saquinavir; plasma concentration of atazanavir reduced by

Atazanavir
- Antivirals *(continued)*
tenofovir, also plasma concentration of tenofovir possibly increased; atazanavir increases plasma concentration of tipranavir (also plasma concentration of atazanavir reduced)
- Anxiolytics and Hypnotics: atazanavir possibly increases plasma concentration of ●midazolam—avoid concomitant use of oral midazolam
- Calcium-channel Blockers: atazanavir increases plasma concentration of ●diltiazem (reduce dose of diltiazem); atazanavir possibly increases plasma concentration of verapamil
- Ciclosporin: atazanavir possibly increases plasma concentration of ●ciclosporin
- Cytotoxics: atazanavir possibly inhibits metabolism of ●irinotecan (increased risk of toxicity)
- Ergot Alkaloids: atazanavir possibly increases plasma concentration of ●ergot alkaloids—avoid concomitant use
- Lipid-regulating Drugs: possible increased risk of myopathy when atazanavir given with atorvastatin; possible increased risk of myopathy when atazanavir given with ●rosuvastatin—avoid concomitant use; increased risk of myopathy when atazanavir given with ●simvastatin (avoid concomitant use)
- Oestrogens: atazanavir increases plasma concentration of ●ethinylestradiol—avoid concomitant use
- Sildenafil: atazanavir possibly increases side-effects of ●sildenafil
- Sirolimus: atazanavir possibly increases plasma concentration of ●sirolimus
- Tacrolimus: atazanavir possibly increases plasma concentration of ●tacrolimus
- Ulcer-healing Drugs: plasma concentration of atazanavir possibly reduced by histamine H$_2$-antagonists; plasma concentration of atazanavir reduced by ●proton pump inhibitors

Atenolol *see* Beta-blockers
Atomoxetine
- Analgesics: increased risk of ventricular arrhythmias when atomoxetine given with ●methadone; possible increased risk of convulsions when atomoxetine given with tramadol
- Anti-arrhythmics: increased risk of ventricular arrhythmias when atomoxetine given with ●amiodarone or ●disopyramide
- Antibacterials: increased risk of ventricular arrhythmias when atomoxetine given with parenteral ●erythromycin; increased risk of ventricular arrhythmias when atomoxetine given with ●moxifloxacin
- Antidepressants: metabolism of atomoxetine possibly inhibited by fluoxetine and paroxetine; possible increased risk of convulsions when atomoxetine given with antidepressants; atomoxetine should not be started until 2 weeks after stopping ●MAOIs, also MAOIs should not be started until at least 2 weeks after stopping atomoxetine; increased risk of ventricular arrhythmias when atomoxetine given with ●tricyclics
- Antimalarials: increased risk of ventricular arrhythmias when atomoxetine given with ●mefloquine
- Antipsychotics: increased risk of ventricular arrhythmias when atomoxetine given with ●antipsychotics that prolong the QT interval
- Beta-blockers: increased risk of ventricular arrhythmias when atomoxetine given with ●sotalol
Bupropion: possible increased risk of convulsions when atomoxetine given with bupropion
- Diuretics: risk of ventricular arrhythmias with atomoxetine increased by hypokalaemia caused by ●diuretics
Sympathomimetics, Beta$_2$: Increased risk of cardiovascular side-effects when atomoxetine given with parenteral salbutamol

Atorvastatin *see* Statins

Atovaquone
- Antibacterials: plasma concentration of atovaquone reduced by ●rifabutin and ●rifampicin (possible therapeutic failure of atovaquone); plasma concentration of atovaquone reduced by tetracycline
Antivirals: atovaquone possibly reduces plasma concentration of indinavir; atovaquone possibly inhibits metabolism of zidovudine (increased plasma concentration)
Metoclopramide: plasma concentration of atovaquone reduced by metoclopramide

Atracurium *see* Muscle Relaxants
Atropine *see* Antimuscarinics
Auranofin *see* Gold
Azapropazone *see* NSAIDs
Azathioprine
ACE Inhibitors: increased risk of anaemia or leucopenia when azathioprine given with captopril especially in renal impairment; increased risk of anaemia when azathioprine given with enalapril especially in renal impairment
- Allopurinol: enhanced effects and increased toxicity of azathioprine when given with ●allopurinol (reduce dose of azathioprine to one quarter of usual dose)
Aminosalicylates: possible increased risk of leucopenia when azathioprine given with aminosalicylates
- Antibacterials: increased risk of haematological toxicity when azathioprine given with ●sulfamethoxazole (as co-trimoxazole); increased risk of haematological toxicity when azathioprine given with ●trimethoprim (also with co-trimoxazole)
- Anticoagulants: azathioprine possibly reduces anticoagulant effect of ●coumarins
Antiepileptics: cytotoxics possibly reduce absorption of phenytoin
- Antipsychotics: avoid concomitant use of cytotoxics with ●clozapine (increased risk of agranulocytosis)
Cardiac Glycosides: cytotoxics reduce absorption of digoxin tablets

Azithromycin *see* Macrolides
Aztreonam
- Anticoagulants: aztreonam possibly enhances anticoagulant effect of ●coumarins
Oestrogens: antibacterials that do not induce liver enzymes possibly reduce contraceptive effect of oestrogens (risk probably small, see p. 478)
Vaccines: antibacterials inactivate oral typhoid vaccine–see p. 752

Baclofen *see* Muscle Relaxants
Balsalazide *see* Aminosalicylates
Bambuterol *see* Sympathomimetics, Beta$_2$
Barbiturates
Alcohol: increased sedative effect when barbiturates given with alcohol
Analgesics: barbiturates possibly increase CNS effects of opioid analgesics
Anti-arrhythmics: barbiturates accelerate metabolism of disopyramide (reduced plasma concentration)
- Antibacterials: barbiturates accelerate metabolism of ●chloramphenicol, doxycycline and metronidazole (reduced plasma concentration); phenobarbital possibly reduces plasma concentration of rifampicin; phenobarbital reduces plasma concentration of ●telithromycin (avoid during and for 2 weeks after phenobarbital)
- Anticoagulants: barbiturates accelerate metabolism of ●coumarins (reduced anticoagulant effect)
- Antidepressants: phenobarbital reduces plasma concentration of paroxetine; phenobarbital accelerates metabolism of ●mianserin (reduced plasma concentration); anticonvulsant effect of barbiturates possibly antagonised by MAOIs and ●tricyclic-related antidepressants (convulsive threshold lowered); anticonvulsant effect of barbiturates antagonised by SSRIs (convulsive threshold lowered); avoid concomitant use of phenobarbital with ●St John's wort; anti-

Barbiturates

- **Antidepressants** *(continued)*
  convulsant effect of barbiturates antagonised by
  ●tricyclics (convulsive threshold lowered), also
  metabolism of tricyclics possibly accelerated
  (reduced plasma concentration)
- **Antiepileptics:** phenobarbital reduces plasma concentration of carbamazepine, lamotrigine, tiagabine and
  zonisamide; phenobarbital possibly reduces plasma
  concentration of ethosuximide; plasma concentration of phenobarbital increased by oxcarbazepine,
  also plasma concentration of an active metabolite of
  oxcarbazepine reduced; plasma concentration of
  phenobarbital often increased by phenytoin, plasma
  concentration of phenytoin often reduced but may
  be increased; increased sedative effect when barbiturates given with primidone; plasma concentration of phenobarbital increased by ●stiripentol;
  plasma concentration of phenobarbital increased by
  valproate (also plasma concentration of valproate
  reduced); plasma concentration of phenobarbital
  possibly reduced by vigabatrin
- **Antifungals:** phenobarbital possibly reduces plasma
  concentration of itraconazole and ●posaconazole;
  phenobarbital possibly reduces plasma concentration of ●voriconazole—avoid concomitant use;
  phenobarbital reduces absorption of griseofulvin
  (reduced effect)
- **Antipsychotics:** anticonvulsant effect of barbiturates
  antagonised by ●antipsychotics (convulsive threshold lowered); phenobarbital accelerates metabolism
  of haloperidol (reduced plasma concentration);
  plasma concentration of both drugs reduced when
  phenobarbital given with chlorpromazine; phenobarbital possibly reduces plasma concentration of
  ●aripiprazole—increase dose of aripiprazole
- **Antivirals:** phenobarbital possibly reduces plasma
  concentration of abacavir, darunavir,
  fosamprenavir and ●lopinavir; avoidance of phenobarbital advised by manufacturer of etravirine; barbiturates possibly reduce plasma concentration of
  ●indinavir, ●nelfinavir and ●saquinavir; phenobarbital
  possibly reduces plasma concentration of ●indinavir,
  also plasma concentration of phenobarbital possibly
  increased
  Anxiolytics and Hypnotics: phenobarbital often
  reduces plasma concentration of clonazepam
  Aprepitant: phenobarbital possibly reduces plasma
  concentration of aprepitant
  Beta-blockers: barbiturates reduce plasma concentration of metoprolol and timolol; barbiturates possibly
  reduce plasma concentration of propranolol
- **Calcium-channel Blockers:** barbiturates reduce effects
  of ●felodipine and ●isradipine; barbiturates probably
  reduce effects of ●dihydropyridines, ●diltiazem and
  ●verapamil
  Cardiac Glycosides: barbiturates accelerate metabolism of digitoxin (reduced effect)
- **Ciclosporin:** barbiturates accelerate metabolism of
  ●ciclosporin (reduced effect)
- **Corticosteroids:** barbiturates accelerate metabolism of
  ●corticosteroids (reduced effect)
  Cytotoxics: phenobarbital possibly reduces plasma
  concentration of etoposide; phenobarbital reduces
  plasma concentration of irinotecan and its active
  metabolite
- **Diuretics:** phenobarbital reduces plasma concentration
  of ●eplerenone—avoid concomitant use; increased
  risk of osteomalacia when phenobarbital given with
  carbonic anhydrase inhibitors
  Folates: plasma concentration of phenobarbital possibly reduced by folates
  Hormone Antagonists: barbiturates accelerate metabolism of gestrinone (reduced plasma concentration);
  barbiturates possibly accelerate metabolism of toremifene (reduced plasma concentration)

Barbiturates *(continued)*
  Leukotriene Receptor Antagonists: phenobarbital
  reduces plasma concentration of montelukast
  Lofexidine: increased sedative effect when barbiturates
  given with lofexidine
  Memantine: effects of barbiturates possibly reduced by
  memantine
- **Oestrogens:** barbiturates accelerate metabolism of
  ●oestrogens (reduced contraceptive effect—see
  p. 478)
- **Progestogens:** barbiturates accelerate metabolism of
  ●progestogens (reduced contraceptive effect—see
  p. 478)
- **Sodium Oxybate:** barbiturates enhance effects of
  ●sodium oxybate (avoid concomitant use)
  Sympathomimetics: plasma concentration of phenobarbital possibly increased by methylphenidate
- **Tacrolimus:** phenobarbital reduces plasma concentration of ●tacrolimus
  Theophylline: barbiturates accelerate metabolism of
  theophylline (reduced effect)
  Thyroid Hormones: barbiturates accelerate metab-
  olism of thyroid hormones (may increase require-
  ments for thyroid hormones in hypothyroidism)
  Tibolone: barbiturates accelerate metabolism of tibol-
  one (reduced plasma concentration)
  Vitamins: barbiturates possibly increase requirements
  for vitamin D
Beclometasone *see* Corticosteroids
Bemiparin *see* Heparins
Bendroflumethiazide (bendrofluazide) *see* Diuretics
Benperidol *see* Antipsychotics
Benzodiazepines *see* Anxiolytics and Hypnotics
Benzthiazide *see* Diuretics
Benzylpenicillin *see* Penicillins
Beta-blockers
  Note. Since systemic absorption may follow topical
  application of beta-blockers to the eye the possibility of
  interactions, in particular, with drugs such as verapamil
  should be borne in mind
  ACE Inhibitors: enhanced hypotensive effect when
  beta-blockers given with ACE inhibitors
  Adrenergic Neurone Blockers: enhanced hypotensive
  effect when beta-blockers given with adrenergic
  neurone blockers
  Alcohol: enhanced hypotensive effect when beta-
  blockers given with alcohol
  Aldesleukin: enhanced hypotensive effect when beta-
  blockers given with aldesleukin
- **Alpha-blockers:** enhanced hypotensive effect when
  beta-blockers given with ●alpha-blockers, also
  increased risk of first-dose hypotension with post-
  synaptic alpha-blockers such as prazosin
  Anaesthetics, General: enhanced hypotensive effect
  when beta-blockers given with general anaesthetics
  Anaesthetics, Local: propranolol increases risk of
  ●bupivacaine toxicity
  Analgesics: hypotensive effect of beta-blockers antagonised by NSAIDs; plasma concentration of esmolol
  possibly increased by morphine
  Angiotensin-II Receptor Antagonists: enhanced hypotensive effect when beta-blockers given with angiotensin-II receptor antagonists
- **Anti-arrhythmics:** increased myocardial depression
  when beta-blockers given with ●anti-arrhythmics;
  increased risk of ventricular arrhythmias when
  sotalol given with ●amiodarone or ●disopyramide—
  avoid concomitant use; increased risk of bradycardia,
  AV block and myocardial depression when beta-
  blockers given with ●amiodarone; increased risk of
  myocardial depression and bradycardia when beta-
  blockers given with ●flecainide; propranolol
  increases risk of ●lidocaine (lignocaine) toxicity;
  plasma concentration of metoprolol and propranolol
  increased by propafenone
- **Antibacterials:** increased risk of ventricular arrhythmias
  when sotalol given with ●moxifloxacin—avoid con-

Beta-blockers

- Antibacterials *(continued)*
  comitant use; metabolism of bisoprolol and
  propranolol accelerated by rifampicin (plasma concentration significantly reduced); plasma concentration of carvedilol, celiprolol and metoprolol reduced
  by rifampicin
- Antidepressants: plasma concentration of metoprolol
  increased by citalopram and escitalopram; plasma
  concentration of propranolol increased by fluvoxamine; plasma concentration of metoprolol possibly
  increased by paroxetine (enhanced effect);
  labetalol and propranolol increase plasma concentration of imipramine; enhanced hypotensive effect
  when beta-blockers given with MAOIs; increased
  risk of ventricular arrhythmias when sotalol given
  with ●tricyclics
  Antidiabetics: beta-blockers may mask warning signs
  of hypoglycaemia (such as tremor) with antidiabetics; beta-blockers enhance hypoglycaemic effect
  of insulin
- Antihistamines: increased risk of ventricular arrhythmias when sotalol given with ●mizolastine—avoid
  concomitant use
- Antimalarials: avoidance of metoprolol and sotalol
  advised by manufacturer of ●artemether/lumefan-
  trine; increased risk of bradycardia when beta-
  blockers given with mefloquine
- Antimuscarinics: increased risk of ventricular arrhythmias when sotalol given with ●tolterodine
- Antipsychotics: plasma concentration of both drugs
  may increase when propranolol given with
  ●chlorpromazine; increased risk of ventricular
  arrhythmias when sotalol given with
  ●zuclopenthixol—avoid concomitant use; increased
  risk of ventricular arrhythmias when sotalol given
  with ●amisulpride, ●phenothiazines, ●pimozide,
  ●sertindole or ●sulpiride; enhanced hypotensive
  effect when beta-blockers given with phenothiazines
- Antivirals: avoidance of metoprolol for heart failure
  advised by manufacturer of ●tipranavir
  Anxiolytics and Hypnotics: enhanced hypotensive
  effect when beta-blockers given with anxiolytics and
  hypnotics
- Atomoxetine: increased risk of ventricular arrhythmias
  when sotalol given with ●atomoxetine
  Barbiturates: plasma concentration of metoprolol and
  timolol reduced by barbiturates; plasma concentration of propranolol possibly reduced by barbiturates
- Calcium-channel Blockers: enhanced hypotensive
  effect when beta-blockers given with calcium-
  channel blockers; possible severe hypotension and
  heart failure when beta-blockers given with
  ●nifedipine; increased risk of AV block and bradycardia when beta-blockers given with ●diltiazem;
  asystole, severe hypotension and heart failure when
  beta-blockers given with ●verapamil (see p. 140)
  Cardiac Glycosides: increased risk of AV block and
  bradycardia when beta-blockers given with cardiac
  glycosides
- Ciclosporin: carvedilol increases plasma concentration
  of ●ciclosporin
- Clonidine: increased risk of withdrawal hypertension
  when beta-blockers given with ●clonidine (withdraw
  beta-blockers several days before slowly withdrawing clonidine)
  Corticosteroids: hypotensive effect of beta-blockers
  antagonised by corticosteroids
  Diazoxide: enhanced hypotensive effect when beta-
  blockers given with diazoxide
- Diuretics: enhanced hypotensive effect when beta-
  blockers given with diuretics; risk of ventricular
  arrhythmias with sotalol increased by hypokalaemia
  caused by ●loop diuretics or ●thiazides and related
  diuretics

Beta-blockers *(continued)*
  Dopaminergics: enhanced hypotensive effect when
  beta-blockers given with levodopa
  Ergot Alkaloids: increased peripheral vasoconstriction
  when beta-blockers given with ergotamine and
  methysergide
  $5HT_1$ Agonists: propranolol increases plasma concentration of rizatriptan (manufacturer of rizatriptan
  advises halve dose and avoid within 2 hours of
  propranolol)
- $5HT_3$ Antagonists: increased risk of ventricular arrhythmias when sotalol given with ●dolasetron—avoid
  concomitant use
- Ivabradine: increased risk of ventricular arrhythmias
  when sotalol given with ●ivabradine
  Methyldopa: enhanced hypotensive effect when beta-
  blockers given with methyldopa
- Moxisylyte (thymoxamine): possible severe postural
  hypotension when beta-blockers given with
  ●moxisylyte
  Moxonidine: enhanced hypotensive effect when beta-
  blockers given with moxonidine
  Muscle Relaxants: propranolol enhances effects of
  muscle relaxants; enhanced hypotensive effect when
  beta-blockers given with baclofen; possible
  enhanced hypotensive effect and bradycardia when
  beta-blockers given with tizanidine
  Nitrates: enhanced hypotensive effect when beta-
  blockers given with nitrates
  Oestrogens: hypotensive effect of beta-blockers
  antagonised by oestrogens
  Parasympathomimetics: propranolol antagonises
  effects of neostigmine and pyridostigmine; increased
  risk of arrhythmias when beta-blockers given with
  pilocarpine
  Prostaglandins: enhanced hypotensive effect when
  beta-blockers given with alprostadil
- Sympathomimetics: increased risk of severe hypertension and bradycardia when non-cardioselective
  beta-blockers given with ●adrenaline (epinephrine),
  also reponse to adrenaline (epinephrine) may be
  reduced; increased risk of severe hypertension and
  bradycardia when non-cardioselective beta-blockers
  given with ●dobutamine; possible increased risk of
  severe hypertension and bradycardia when non-
  cardioselective beta-blockers given with ●noradren-
  aline (norepinephrine)
  Thyroid Hormones: metabolism of propranolol accelerated by levothyroxine (thyroxine)
  Ulcer-healing Drugs: plasma concentration of labetalol,
  metoprolol and propranolol increased by cimetidine
  Vasodilator Antihypertensives: enhanced hypotensive
  effect when beta-blockers given with hydralazine,
  minoxidil or sodium nitroprusside
Betahistine
  Antihistamines: effect of betahistine theoretically
  antagonised by antihistamines
Betamethasone *see* Corticosteroids
Betaxolol *see* Beta-blockers
Bethanechol *see* Parasympathomimetics
Bexarotene
  Antiepileptics: cytotoxics possibly reduce absorption
  of phenytoin
- Antipsychotics: avoid concomitant use of cytotoxics
  with ●clozapine (increased risk of agranulocytosis)
  Cardiac Glycosides: cytotoxics reduce absorption of
  digoxin tablets
- Lipid-regulating Drugs: plasma concentration of bex-
  arotene increased by ●gemfibrozil—avoid concomi-
  tant use
Bezafibrate *see* Fibrates
Bicalutamide
  Anticoagulants: bicalutamide possibly enhances antic-
  oagulant effect of coumarins
Biguanides *see* Antidiabetics

Bile Acid Sequestrants *see* Colesevelam, Colestipol, and Colestyramine
Bile Acids *see* Ursodeoxycholic Acid
Bisoprolol *see* Beta-blockers
Bisphosphonates
  Analgesics: bioavailability of tiludronic acid increased by indometacin
  Antacids: absorption of bisphosphonates reduced by antacids
  Antibacterials: increased risk of hypocalcaemia when bisphosphonates given with aminoglycosides
  Calcium Salts: absorption of bisphosphonates reduced by calcium salts
  Iron: absorption of bisphosphonates reduced by *oral* iron
Bleomycin
  Antiepileptics: cytotoxics possibly reduce absorption of phenytoin
  • Antipsychotics: avoid concomitant use of cytotoxics with •clozapine (increased risk of agranulocytosis)
  Cardiac Glycosides: cytotoxics reduce absorption of digoxin tablets
  • Cytotoxics: increased pulmonary toxicity when bleomycin given with •cisplatin
Bortezomib
  Antiepileptics: cytotoxics possibly reduce absorption of phenytoin
  Antifungals: plasma concentration of bortezomib increased by ketoconazole
  • Antipsychotics: avoid concomitant use of cytotoxics with •clozapine (increased risk of agranulocytosis)
  Cardiac Glycosides: cytotoxics reduce absorption of digoxin tablets
Bosentan
  • Antibacterials: plasma concentration of bosentan reduced by •rifampicin—avoid concomitant use
  Anticoagulants: manufacturer of bosentan recommends monitoring anticoagulant effect of coumarins
  • Antidiabetics: increased risk of hepatotoxicity when bosentan given with •glibenclamide—avoid concomitant use
  • Antifungals: plasma concentration of bosentan increased by ketoconazole; plasma concentration of bosentan possibly increased by •fluconazole—avoid concomitant use; plasma concentration of bosentan possibly increased by itraconazole
  Antivirals: plasma concentration of bosentan possibly increased by ritonavir
  • Ciclosporin: plasma concentration of bosentan increased by •ciclosporin (also plasma concentration of ciclosporin reduced—avoid concomitant use)
  Lipid-regulating Drugs: bosentan reduces plasma concentration of simvastatin
  • Oestrogens: bosentan possibly causes contraceptive failure of hormonal contraceptives containing •oestrogens (alternative contraception recommended)
  • Progestogens: bosentan possibly causes contraceptive failure of hormonal contraceptives containing •progestogens (alternative contraception recommended)
  Sildenafil: bosentan reduces plasma concentration of sildenafil
Brimonidine
  Antidepressants: manufacturer of brimonidine advises avoid concomitant use with MAOIs, tricyclic-related antidepressants and tricyclics
Brinzolamide *see* Diuretics
Bromocriptine
  Alcohol: tolerance of bromocriptine reduced by alcohol
  Antibacterials: plasma concentration of bromocriptine increased by erythromycin (increased risk of toxicity); plasma concentration of bromocriptine possibly increased by macrolides (increased risk of toxicity)

Bromocriptine *(continued)*
  Antipsychotics: hypoprolactinaemic and antiparkinsonian effects of bromocriptine antagonised by antipsychotics
  Domperidone: hypoprolactinaemic effect of bromocriptine possibly antagonised by domperidone
  Hormone Antagonists: plasma concentration of bromocriptine increased by octreotide
  Memantine: effects of dopaminergics possibly enhanced by memantine
  Methyldopa: antiparkinsonian effect of dopaminergics antagonised by methyldopa
  Metoclopramide: hypoprolactinaemic effect of bromocriptine antagonised by metoclopramide
  • Sympathomimetics: risk of toxicity when bromocriptine given with •isometheptene
Buclizine *see* Antihistamines
Budesonide *see* Corticosteroids
Bumetanide *see* Diuretics
Bupivacaine
  Anti-arrhythmics: increased myocardial depression when bupivacaine given with anti-arrhythmics
  • Beta-blockers: increased risk of bupivacaine toxicity when given with •propranolol
Buprenorphine *see* Opioid Analgesics
Bupropion
  Note. Bupropion should be administered with extreme caution to patients receiving other medication known to lower the seizure threshold—see CSM advice BNF section 4.10 and Cautions, Contra-indications and Side-effects of individual drugs
  • Antidepressants: bupropion possibly increases plasma concentration of citalopram; manufacturer of bupropion advises avoid for 2 weeks after stopping •MAOIs; manufacturer of bupropion advises avoid concomitant use with •moclobemide
  Antiepileptics: plasma concentration of bupropion reduced by carbamazepine and phenytoin; metabolism of bupropion inhibited by valproate
  • Antivirals: plasma concentration of bupropion increased or decreased by •ritonavir
  Atomoxetine: possible increased risk of convulsions when bupropion given with atomoxetine
  Dopaminergics: increased risk of side-effects when bupropion given with amantadine or levodopa
Buspirone *see* Anxiolytics and Hypnotics
Busulfan
  Analgesics: metabolism of *intravenous* busulfan possibly inhibited by paracetamol (manufacturer of *intravenous* busulfan advises caution within 72 hours of paracetamol)
  • Antibacterials: plasma concentration of busulfan increased by •metronidazole (increased risk of toxicity)
  Antiepileptics: cytotoxics possibly reduce absorption of phenytoin; plasma concentration of busulfan possibly reduced by phenytoin
  Antifungals: metabolism of busulfan inhibited by itraconazole (increased risk of toxicity)
  • Antipsychotics: avoid concomitant use of cytotoxics with •clozapine (increased risk of agranulocytosis)
  Cardiac Glycosides: cytotoxics reduce absorption of digoxin tablets
  Cytotoxics: increased risk of hepatotoxicity when busulfan given with tioguanine
Butobarbital *see* Barbiturates
Butyrophenones *see* Antipsychotics
Cabergoline
  Antibacterials: plasma concentration of cabergoline increased by erythromycin (increased risk of toxicity); plasma concentration of cabergoline possibly increased by macrolides (increased risk of toxicity)
  Antipsychotics: hypoprolactinaemic and antiparkinsonian effects of cabergoline antagonised by antipsychotics
  Domperidone: hypoprolactinaemic effect of cabergoline possibly antagonised by domperidone

Cabergoline *(continued)*

Memantine: effects of dopaminergics possibly enhanced by memantine

Methyldopa: antiparkinsonian effect of dopaminergics antagonised by methyldopa

Metoclopramide: hypoprolactinaemic effect of cabergoline antagonised by metoclopramide

Calcium Salts

Note. see also Antacids

Antibacterials: calcium salts reduce absorption of ciprofloxacin and tetracycline

Bisphosphonates: calcium salts reduce absorption of bisphosphonates

Cardiac Glycosides: large intravenous doses of calcium salts can precipitate arrhythmias when given with cardiac glycosides

Corticosteroids: absorption of calcium salts reduced by corticosteroids

Diuretics: increased risk of hypercalcaemia when calcium salts given with thiazides and related diuretics

Fluorides: calcium salts reduce absorption of fluorides

Iron: calcium salts reduce absorption of *oral* iron

Thyroid Hormones: calcium salts reduce absorption of levothyroxine (thyroxine)

Zinc: calcium salts reduce absorption of zinc

Calcium-channel Blockers

Note. Dihydropyridine calcium-channel blockers include amlodipine, felodipine, isradipine, lacidipine, lercanidipine, nicardipine, nifedipine, and nimodipine

ACE Inhibitors: enhanced hypotensive effect when calcium-channel blockers given with ACE inhibitors

Adrenergic Neurone Blockers: enhanced hypotensive effect when calcium-channel blockers given with adrenergic neurone blockers

Alcohol: enhanced hypotensive effect when calcium-channel blockers given with alcohol; verapamil possibly increases plasma concentration of alcohol

Aldesleukin: enhanced hypotensive effect when calcium-channel blockers given with aldesleukin

• Alpha-blockers: enhanced hypotensive effect when calcium-channel blockers given with ●alpha-blockers, also increased risk of first-dose hypotension with post-synaptic alpha-blockers such as prazosin

• Anaesthetics, General: enhanced hypotensive effect when calcium-channel blockers given with general anaesthetics or isoflurane; hypotensive effect of verapamil enhanced by ●general anaesthetics (also AV delay)

Analgesics: hypotensive effect of calcium-channel blockers antagonised by NSAIDs; diltiazem inhibits metabolism of alfentanil (risk of prolonged or delayed respiratory depression)

Angiotensin-II Receptor Antagonists: enhanced hypotensive effect when calcium-channel blockers given with angiotensin-II receptor antagonists

• Anti-arrhythmics: increased risk of bradycardia, AV block and myocardial depression when diltiazem or verapamil given with ●amiodarone; increased risk of myocardial depression and asystole when verapamil given with ●disopyramide or ●flecainide

• Antibacterials: metabolism of verapamil possibly inhibited by ●clarithromycin and ●erythromycin (increased risk of toxicity); metabolism of felodipine possibly inhibited by erythromycin (increased plasma concentration); manufacturer of lercanidipine advises avoid concomitant use with erythromycin; metabolism of diltiazem, nifedipine, nimodipine and verapamil accelerated by ●rifampicin (plasma concentration significantly reduced); metabolism of isradipine and nicardipine possibly accelerated by ●rifampicin (possible significantly reduced plasma concentration); plasma concentration of nifedipine increased by ●quinupristin/ dalfopristin

Antidepressants: metabolism of nifedipine possibly inhibited by fluoxetine (increased plasma concen-

Calcium-channel Blockers

Antidepressants *(continued)*

tration); diltiazem and verapamil increase plasma concentration of imipramine; enhanced hypotensive effect when calcium-channel blockers given with MAOIs; plasma concentration of amlodipine possibly reduced by St John's wort; diltiazem and verapamil possibly increase plasma concentration of tricyclics

Antidiabetics: glucose tolerance occasionally impaired when nifedipine given with insulin

• Antiepileptics: effects of dihydropyridines, nicardipine and nifedipine probably reduced by carbamazepine; effects of felodipine and isradipine reduced by carbamazepine; diltiazem and verapamil enhance effects of ●carbamazepine; effects of dihydropyridines, nicardipine and nifedipine probably reduced by ●phenytoin; effects of felodipine, isradipine and verapamil reduced by phenytoin; diltiazem increases plasma concentration of ●phenytoin but also effect of diltiazem reduced; effects of felodipine and isradipine reduced by ●primidone; effects of dihydropyridines, diltiazem and verapamil probably reduced by ●primidone

• Antifungals: metabolism of dihydropyridines possibly inhibited by itraconazole and ketoconazole (increased plasma concentration); metabolism of felodipine inhibited by ●itraconazole and ●ketoconazole (increased plasma concentration); manufacturer of lercanidipine advises avoid concomitant use with itraconazole and ketoconazole; negative inotropic effect possibly increased when calcium-channel blockers given with itraconazole; plasma concentration of nifedipine increased by micafungin

Antimalarials: possible increased risk of bradycardia when calcium-channel blockers given with mefloquine

Antimuscarinics: avoidance of verapamil advised by manufacturer of darifenacin

Antipsychotics: enhanced hypotensive effect when calcium-channel blockers given with antipsychotics

• Antivirals: plasma concentration of verapamil possibly increased by atazanavir; plasma concentration of diltiazem increased by ●atazanavir (reduce dose of diltiazem); plasma concentration of diltiazem reduced by efavirenz; manufacturer of lercanidipine advises avoid concomitant use with ritonavir; plasma concentration of calcium-channel blockers possibly increased by ●ritonavir

Anxiolytics and Hypnotics: enhanced hypotensive effect when calcium-channel blockers given with anxiolytics and hypnotics; diltiazem and verapamil inhibit metabolism of midazolam (increased plasma concentration with increased sedation); absorption of lercanidipine increased by midazolam; diltiazem and verapamil increase plasma concentration of buspirone (reduce dose of buspirone)

• Barbiturates: effects of dihydropyridines, diltiazem and verapamil probably reduced by ●barbiturates; effects of felodipine and isradipine reduced by ●barbiturates

• Beta-blockers: enhanced hypotensive effect when calcium-channel blockers given with beta-blockers; increased risk of AV block and bradycardia when diltiazem given with ●beta-blockers; asystole, severe hypotension and heart failure when verapamil given with ●beta-blockers (see p. 140); possible severe hypotension and heart failure when nifedipine given with ●beta-blockers

Calcium-channel Blockers: plasma concentration of both drugs may increase when diltiazem given with nifedipine

• Cardiac Glycosides: nifedipine possibly increases plasma concentration of ●digoxin; diltiazem, lercanidipine and nicardipine increase plasma concentration of ●digoxin; verapamil increases plasma

Calcium-channel Blockers

- Cardiac Glycosides *(continued)*
concentration of •digoxin, also increased risk of AV block and bradycardia
- Ciclosporin: diltiazem, nicardipine and verapamil increase plasma concentration of •ciclosporin; combination of lercanidipine with •ciclosporin may increase plasma concentration of either drug (or both)—avoid concomitant use; plasma concentration of nifedipine possibly increased by ciclosporin (increased risk of toxicity including gingival hyperplasia)
- Cilostazol: diltiazem increases plasma concentration of •cilostazol—avoid concomitant use

Clonidine: enhanced hypotensive effect when calcium-channel blockers given with clonidine

Corticosteroids: hypotensive effect of calcium-channel blockers antagonised by corticosteroids

Cytotoxics: nifedipine possibly inhibits metabolism of vincristine

Diazoxide: enhanced hypotensive effect when calcium-channel blockers given with diazoxide

Diuretics: enhanced hypotensive effect when calcium-channel blockers given with diuretics; diltiazem and verapamil increase plasma concentration of eplerenone (reduce dose of eplerenone)

Dopaminergics: enhanced hypotensive effect when calcium-channel blockers given with levodopa

Grapefruit Juice: plasma concentration of felodipine, isradipine, lacidipine, lercanidipine, nicardipine, nifedipine, nimodipine and verapamil increased by grapefruit juice

Hormone Antagonists: diltiazem and verapamil increase plasma concentration of dutasteride

- Ivabradine: diltiazem and verapamil increase plasma concentration of •ivabradine—avoid concomitant use
- Lipid-regulating Drugs: diltiazem increases plasma concentration of atorvastatin; possible increased risk of myopathy when diltiazem given with simvastatin; increased risk of myopathy when verapamil given with •simvastatin

Lithium: neurotoxicity may occur when diltiazem or verapamil given with lithium without increased plasma concentration of lithium

- Magnesium (parenteral): profound hypotension reported with concomitant use of nifedipine and •parenteral magnesium in pre-eclampsia

Methyldopa: enhanced hypotensive effect when calcium-channel blockers given with methyldopa

Moxisylyte (thymoxamine): enhanced hypotensive effect when calcium-channel blockers given with moxisylyte

Moxonidine: enhanced hypotensive effect when calcium-channel blockers given with moxonidine

Muscle Relaxants: verapamil enhances effects of non-depolarising muscle relaxants and suxamethonium; enhanced hypotensive effect when calcium-channel blockers given with baclofen or tizanidine; hypotension, myocardial depression, and hyperkalaemia when verapamil given with intravenous dantrolene; risk of arrhythmias when diltiazem given with intravenous dantrolene; nifedipine enhances effects of non-depolarising muscle relaxants

Nitrates: enhanced hypotensive effect when calcium-channel blockers given with nitrates

Oestrogens: hypotensive effect of calcium-channel blockers antagonised by oestrogens

Prostaglandins: enhanced hypotensive effect when calcium-channel blockers given with alprostadil

Sildenafil: enhanced hypotensive effect when amlodipine given with sildenafil

- Sirolimus: diltiazem increases plasma concentration of •sirolimus; plasma concentration of both drugs increased when verapamil given with •sirolimus

Calcium-channel Blockers *(continued)*

- Tacrolimus: diltiazem and nifedipine increase plasma concentration of •tacrolimus; felodipine, nicardipine and verapamil possibly increase plasma concentration of tacrolimus
- Theophylline: calcium-channel blockers possibly increase plasma concentration of •theophylline (enhanced effect); diltiazem increases plasma concentration of theophylline; verapamil increases plasma concentration of •theophylline (enhanced effect)

Ulcer-healing Drugs: metabolism of calcium-channel blockers possibly inhibited by cimetidine (increased plasma concentration); plasma concentration of isradipine increased by cimetidine (halve dose of isradipine)

Vardenafil: enhanced hypotensive effect when nifedipine given with vardenafil

Vasodilator Antihypertensives: enhanced hypotensive effect when calcium-channel blockers given with hydralazine, minoxidil or sodium nitroprusside

Calcium-channel Blockers (dihydropyridines) *see* Calcium-channel Blockers

Candesartan *see* Angiotensin-II Receptor Antagonists

Capecitabine *see* Fluorouracil

Capreomycin

Antibacterials: increased risk of nephrotoxicity when capreomycin given with colistin or polymyxins; increased risk of nephrotoxicity and ototoxicity when capreomycin given with aminoglycosides or vancomycin

Cytotoxics: increased risk of nephrotoxicity and ototoxicity when capreomycin given with platinum compounds

Oestrogens: antibacterials that do not induce liver enzymes possibly reduce contraceptive effect of oestrogens (risk probably small, see p. 478)

Vaccines: antibacterials inactivate oral typhoid vaccine—see p. 752

Captopril *see* ACE Inhibitors

Carbamazepine

Alcohol: CNS side-effects of carbamazepine possibly increased by alcohol

- Analgesics: effects of carbamazepine enhanced by •dextropropoxyphene; carbamazepine reduces plasma concentration of methadone; carbamazepine reduces effects of tramadol; carbamazepine possibly accelerates metabolism of paracetamol
- Antibacterials: plasma concentration of carbamazepine increased by •clarithromycin and •erythromycin; plasma concentration of carbamazepine reduced by •rifabutin; carbamazepine accelerates metabolism of doxycycline (reduced effect); plasma concentration of carbamazepine increased by •isoniazid (also possibly increased isoniazid hepatotoxicity); carbamazepine reduces plasma concentration of •telithromycin (avoid during and for 2 weeks after carbamazepine)
- Anticoagulants: carbamazepine accelerates metabolism of •coumarins (reduced anticoagulant effect)
- Antidepressants: plasma concentration of carbamazepine increased by •fluoxetine and •fluvoxamine; carbamazepine reduces plasma concentration of •mianserin, mirtazapine and paroxetine; manufacturer of carbamazepine advises avoid for 2 weeks after stopping •MAOIs, also antagonism of anticonvulsant effect; anticonvulsant effect of antiepileptics possibly antagonised by MAOIs and •tricyclic-related antidepressants (convulsive threshold lowered); anticonvulsant effect of antiepileptics antagonised by •SSRIs and •tricyclics (convulsive threshold lowered); avoid concomitant use of antiepileptics with •St John's wort; carbamazepine accelerates metabolism of •tricyclics (reduced plasma concentration and reduced effect)

Carbamazepine *(continued)*
- Antiepileptics: carbamazepine possibly reduces plasma concentration of ethosuximide; carbamazepine often reduces plasma concentration of lamotrigine, also plasma concentration of an active metabolite of carbamazepine sometimes raised (but evidence is conflicting); plasma concentration of carbamazepine sometimes reduced by oxcarbazepine (but concentration of an active metabolite of carbamazepine may be increased), also plasma concentration of an active metabolite of oxcarbazepine often reduced; plasma concentration of both drugs often reduced when carbamazepine given with phenytoin, also plasma concentration of phenytoin may be increased; plasma concentration of carbamazepine often reduced by primidone, also plasma concentration of primidone sometimes reduced (but concentration of an active metabolite of primidone often increased); plasma concentration of carbamazepine increased by ●stiripentol; carbamazepine reduces plasma concentration of tiagabine and zonisamide; carbamazepine often reduces plasma concentration of topiramate; carbamazepine reduces plasma concentration of valproate, also plasma concentration of active metabolite of carbamazepine increased
- Antifungals: plasma concentration of carbamazepine possibly increased by fluconazole, ketoconazole and miconazole; carbamazepine possibly reduces plasma concentration of itraconazole and ●posaconazole; carbamazepine possibly reduces plasma concentration of ●voriconazole—avoid concomitant use; carbamazepine possibly reduces plasma concentration of caspofungin—consider increasing dose of caspofungin
- Antimalarials: possible increased risk of convulsions when antiepileptics given with chloroquine and hydroxychloroquine; anticonvulsant effect of antiepileptics antagonised by ●mefloquine
- Antipsychotics: anticonvulsant effect of carbamazepine antagonised by ●antipsychotics (convulsive threshold lowered); carbamazepine accelerates metabolism of haloperidol, olanzapine, quetiapine, risperidone and sertindole (reduced plasma concentration); carbamazepine reduces plasma concentration of ●aripiprazole—increase dose of aripiprazole; carbamazepine accelerates metabolism of ●clozapine (reduced plasma concentration), also avoid concomitant use of drugs with substantial potential for causing agranulocytosis; carbamazepine reduces plasma concentration of paliperidone
- Antivirals: carbamazepine possibly reduces plasma concentration of darunavir, fosamprenavir, lopinavir, nelfinavir, saquinavir and tipranavir; plasma concentration of both drugs reduced when carbamazepine given with efavirenz; avoidance of carbamazepine advised by manufacturer of etravirine; carbamazepine possibly reduces plasma concentration of ●indinavir, also plasma concentration of carbamazepine possibly increased; plasma concentration of carbamazepine possibly increased by ●ritonavir

Anxiolytics and Hypnotics: carbamazepine often reduces plasma concentration of clonazepam; carbamazepine reduces plasma concentration of midazolam

Aprepitant: carbamazepine possibly reduces plasma concentration of aprepitant

Barbiturates: plasma concentration of carbamazepine reduced by phenobarbital

Bupropion: carbamazepine reduces plasma concentration of bupropion
- Calcium-channel Blockers: carbamazepine reduces effects of felodipine and isradipine; carbamazepine probably reduces effects of dihydropyridines, nicardipine and nifedipine; effects of carbamazepine enhanced by ●diltiazem and ●verapamil

Carbamazepine *(continued)*

Cardiac Glycosides: carbamazepine accelerates metabolism of digitoxin (reduced effect)
- Ciclosporin: carbamazepine accelerates metabolism of ●ciclosporin (reduced plasma concentration)
- Corticosteroids: carbamazepine accelerates metabolism of ●corticosteroids (reduced effect)
- Cytotoxics: carbamazepine reduces plasma concentration of ●imatinib and ●lapatinib—avoid concomitant use; carbamazepine reduces plasma concentration of irinotecan and its active metabolite
- Diuretics: increased risk of hyponatraemia when carbamazepine given with diuretics; plasma concentration of carbamazepine increased by ●acetazolamide; carbamazepine reduces plasma concentration of ●eplerenone—avoid concomitant use
- Hormone Antagonists: metabolism of carbamazepine inhibited by ●danazol (increased risk of toxicity); carbamazepine accelerates metabolism of gestrinone (reduced plasma concentration); carbamazepine possibly accelerates metabolism of toremifene (reduced plasma concentration)

5HT$_3$ Antagonists: carbamazepine accelerates metabolism of ondansetron (reduced effect)

Lithium: neurotoxicity may occur when carbamazepine given with lithium without increased plasma concentration of lithium

Muscle Relaxants: carbamazepine antagonises muscle relaxant effect of non-depolarising muscle relaxants (accelerated recovery from neuromuscular blockade)
- Oestrogens: carbamazepine accelerates metabolism of ●oestrogens (reduced contraceptive effect—see p. 478)
- Progestogens: carbamazepine accelerates metabolism of ●progestogens (reduced contraceptive effect—see p. 478)

Retinoids: plasma concentration of carbamazepine possibly reduced by isotretinoin

Theophylline: carbamazepine accelerates metabolism of theophylline (reduced effect)

Thyroid Hormones: carbamazepine accelerates metabolism of thyroid hormones (may increase requirements for thyroid hormones in hypothyroidism)

Tibolone: carbamazepine accelerates metabolism of tibolone (reduced plasma concentration)
- Ulcer-healing Drugs: metabolism of carbamazepine inhibited by ●cimetidine (increased plasma concentration)

Vitamins: carbamazepine possibly increases requirements for vitamin D

Carbapenems *see* Doripenem, Ertapenem, Imipenem with Cilastatin, and Meropenem

Carbonic Anhydrase Inhibitors *see* Diuretics

Carboplatin *see* Platinum Compounds

Carboprost *see* Prostaglandins

Cardiac Glycosides

ACE Inhibitors: plasma concentration of digoxin possibly increased by captopril

Alpha-blockers: plasma concentration of digoxin increased by prazosin

Aminosalicylates: absorption of digoxin possibly reduced by sulfasalazine

Analgesics: plasma concentration of cardiac glycosides possibly increased by NSAIDs, also possible exacerbation of heart failure and reduction of renal function

Antacids: absorption of digoxin possibly reduced by antacids
- Anti-arrhythmics: plasma concentration of digoxin increased by ●amiodarone and ●propafenone (halve dose of digoxin)

Antibacterials: plasma concentration of digoxin possibly increased by gentamicin, telithromycin and trimethoprim; absorption of digoxin reduced by

Cardiac Glycosides

Antibacterials *(continued)*
neomycin; plasma concentration of digoxin possibly reduced by rifampicin; plasma concentration of digoxin increased by macrolides (increased risk of toxicity); metabolism of digitoxin accelerated by rifamycins (reduced effect)

- Antidepressants: plasma concentration of digoxin reduced by ●St John's wort—avoid concomitant use

Antidiabetics: plasma concentration of digoxin possibly reduced by acarbose; plasma concentration of digoxin increased by sitagliptin

Antiepileptics: metabolism of digitoxin accelerated by carbamazepine, phenytoin and primidone (reduced effect); plasma concentration of digoxin possibly reduced by phenytoin

- Antifungals: increased cardiac toxicity with cardiac glycosides if hypokalaemia occurs with ●amphotericin; plasma concentration of digoxin increased by ●itraconazole
- Antimalarials: plasma concentration of digoxin possibly increased by ●chloroquine and hydroxychloroquine; possible increased risk of bradycardia when digoxin given with mefloquine; plasma concentration of digoxin increased by ●quinine

Antimuscarinics: plasma concentration of digoxin possibly increased by darifenacin

Antivirals: plasma concentration of digoxin increased by etravirine; plasma concentration of digoxin possibly increased by ritonavir

Anxiolytics and Hypnotics: plasma concentration of digoxin increased by alprazolam (increased risk of toxicity)

Barbiturates: metabolism of digitoxin accelerated by barbiturates (reduced effect)

Beta-blockers: increased risk of AV block and bradycardia when cardiac glycosides given with beta-blockers

Calcium Salts: arrhythmias can be precipitated when cardiac glycosides given with large intravenous doses of calcium salts

- Calcium-channel Blockers: plasma concentration of digoxin increased by ●diltiazem, ●lercanidipine and ●nicardipine; plasma concentration of digoxin possibly increased by ●nifedipine; plasma concentration of digoxin increased by ●verapamil, also increased risk of AV block and bradycardia
- Ciclosporin: plasma concentration of digoxin increased by ●ciclosporin (increased risk of toxicity)

Corticosteroids: increased risk of hypokalaemia when cardiac glycosides given with corticosteroids

Cytotoxics: absorption of digoxin tablets reduced by cytotoxics

- Diuretics: increased cardiac toxicity with cardiac glycosides if hypokalaemia with ●acetazolamide, ●loop diuretics or ●thiazides and related diuretics; plasma concentration of digoxin possibly increased by potassium canrenoate; plasma concentration of digitoxin possibly affected by spironolactone; plasma concentration of digoxin increased by ●spironolactone

Lenalidomide: plasma concentration of digoxin possibly increased by lenalidomide

Lipid-regulating Drugs: absorption of cardiac glycosides possibly reduced by colestipol and colestyramine; plasma concentration of digoxin possibly increased by atorvastatin

Muscle Relaxants: risk of ventricular arrhythmias when cardiac glycosides given with suxamethonium; possible increased risk of bradycardia when cardiac glycosides given with tizanidine

Penicillamine: plasma concentration of digoxin possibly reduced by penicillamine

Sympathomimetics, Beta$_2$: plasma concentration of digoxin possibly reduced by salbutamol

Cardiac Glycosides *(continued)*

Ulcer-healing Drugs: plasma concentration of digoxin possibly slightly increased by proton pump inhibitors; absorption of cardiac glycosides possibly reduced by sucralfate

Carisoprodol *see* Muscle Relaxants

Carmustine

Antiepileptics: cytotoxics possibly reduce absorption of phenytoin

- Antipsychotics: avoid concomitant use of cytotoxics with ●clozapine (increased risk of agranulocytosis)

Cardiac Glycosides: cytotoxics reduce absorption of digoxin tablets

Ulcer-healing Drugs: myelosuppressive effects of carmustine possibly enhanced by cimetidine

Carteolol *see* Beta-blockers

Carvedilol *see* Beta-blockers

Caspofungin

Antibacterials: plasma concentration of caspofungin initially increased and then reduced by rifampicin (consider increasing dose of caspofungin)

Antiepileptics: plasma concentration of caspofungin possibly reduced by carbamazepine and phenytoin—consider increasing dose of caspofungin

Antivirals: plasma concentration of caspofungin possibly reduced by efavirenz and nevirapine—consider increasing dose of caspofungin

- Ciclosporin: plasma concentration of caspofungin increased by ●ciclosporin (manufacturer of caspofungin recommends monitoring liver enzymes)

Corticosteroids: plasma concentration of caspofungin possibly reduced by dexamethasone—consider increasing dose of caspofungin

- Tacrolimus: caspofungin reduces plasma concentration of ●tacrolimus

Cefaclor *see* Cephalosporins

Cefadroxil *see* Cephalosporins

Cefalexin *see* Cephalosporins

Cefixime *see* Cephalosporins

Cefotaxime *see* Cephalosporins

Cefpodoxime *see* Cephalosporins

Cefradine *see* Cephalosporins

Ceftazidime *see* Cephalosporins

Ceftriaxone *see* Cephalosporins

Cefuroxime *see* Cephalosporins

Celecoxib *see* NSAIDs

Celiprolol *see* Beta-blockers

Cephalosporins

Antacids: absorption of cefaclor and cefpodoxime reduced by antacids

Antibacterials: possible increased risk of nephrotoxicity when cephalosporins given with aminoglycosides

- Anticoagulants: cephalosporins possibly enhance anticoagulant effect of ●coumarins

Oestrogens: antibacterials that do not induce liver enzymes possibly reduce contraceptive effect of oestrogens (risk probably small, see p. 478)

Probenecid: excretion of cephalosporins reduced by probenecid (increased plasma concentration)

Ulcer-healing Drugs: absorption of cefpodoxime reduced by histamine H$_2$-antagonists

Vaccines: antibacterials inactivate oral typhoid vaccine—see p. 752

Cetirizine *see* Antihistamines

Chloral *see* Anxiolytics and Hypnotics

Chloramphenicol

Antibacterials: metabolism of chloramphenicol accelerated by rifampicin (reduced plasma concentration)

- Anticoagulants: chloramphenicol enhances anticoagulant effect of ●coumarins
- Antidiabetics: chloramphenicol enhances effects of ●sulphonylureas
- Antiepileptics: chloramphenicol increases plasma concentration of ●phenytoin (increased risk of toxicity); metabolism of chloramphenicol accelerated by ●primidone (reduced plasma concentration)

Chloramphenicol *(continued)*
- Antipsychotics: avoid concomitant use of chloramphenicol with ●clozapine (increased risk of agranulocytosis)
- Barbiturates: metabolism of chloramphenicol accelerated by ●barbiturates (reduced plasma concentration)
- Ciclosporin: chloramphenicol possibly increases plasma concentration of ●ciclosporin

  Hydroxocobalamin: chloramphenicol reduces response to hydroxocobalamin

  Oestrogens: antibacterials that do not induce liver enzymes possibly reduce contraceptive effect of oestrogens (risk probably small, see p. 478)
- Tacrolimus: chloramphenicol possibly increases plasma concentration of ●tacrolimus

  Vaccines: antibacterials inactivate oral typhoid vaccine–see p. 752

Chlordiazepoxide *see* Anxiolytics and Hypnotics
Chloroquine and Hydroxychloroquine

  Adsorbents: absorption of chloroquine and hydroxychloroquine reduced by kaolin

  Agalsidase Alfa and Beta: chloroquine and hydroxychloroquine possibly inhibit effects of agalsidase alfa and beta (manufacturers of agalsidase alfa and beta advise avoid concomitant use)

  Antacids: absorption of chloroquine and hydroxychloroquine reduced by antacids
- Anti-arrhythmics: increased risk of ventricular arrhythmias when chloroquine and hydroxychloroquine given with ●amiodarone—avoid concomitant use
- Antibacterials: increased risk of ventricular arrhythmias when chloroquine and hydroxychloroquine given with ●moxifloxacin—avoid concomitant use

  Antiepileptics: possible increased risk of convulsions when chloroquine and hydroxychloroquine given with antiepileptics
- Antimalarials: avoidance of antimalarials advised by manufacturer of ●artemether/lumefantrine; increased risk of convulsions when chloroquine and hydroxychloroquine given with ●mefloquine
- Cardiac Glycosides: chloroquine and hydroxychloroquine possibly increase plasma concentration of ●digoxin
- Ciclosporin: chloroquine and hydroxychloroquine increase plasma concentration of ●ciclosporin (increased risk of toxicity)

  Lanthanum: absorption of chloroquine and hydroxychloroquine possibly reduced by lanthanum (give at least 2 hours apart)

  Laronidase: chloroquine and hydroxychloroquine possibly inhibit effects of laronidase (manufacturer of laronidase advises avoid concomitant use)

  Parasympathomimetics: chloroquine and hydroxychloroquine have potential to increase symptoms of myasthenia gravis and thus diminish effect of neostigmine and pyridostigmine

  Ulcer-healing Drugs: metabolism of chloroquine and hydroxychloroquine inhibited by cimetidine (increased plasma concentration)

  Vaccines: antimalarials inactivate oral typhoid vaccine–see p. 752

Chlorothiazide *see* Diuretics
Chlorphenamine (chlorpheniramine) *see* Antihistamines
Chlorpromazine *see* Antipsychotics
Chlorpropamide *see* Antidiabetics
Chlortalidone *see* Diuretics
Ciclesonide *see* Corticosteroids
Ciclosporin
- ACE Inhibitors: increased risk of hyperkalaemia when ciclosporin given with ●ACE inhibitors

  Allopurinol: plasma concentration of ciclosporin possibly increased by allopurinol (risk of nephrotoxicity)
- Analgesics: increased risk of nephrotoxicity when ciclosporin given with ●NSAIDs; ciclosporin

Ciclosporin
- Analgesics *(continued)*

  increases plasma concentration of ●diclofenac (halve dose of diclofenac)
- Angiotensin-II Receptor Antagonists: increased risk of hyperkalaemia when ciclosporin given with ●angiotensin-II receptor antagonists

  Anti-arrhythmics: plasma concentration of ciclosporin possibly increased by amiodarone and propafenone
- Antibacterials: metabolism of ciclosporin inhibited by ●clarithromycin and ●erythromycin (increased plasma concentration); metabolism of ciclosporin accelerated by ●rifampicin (reduced plasma concentration); plasma concentration of ciclosporin possibly reduced by ●sulfadiazine; plasma concentration of ciclosporin possibly increased by ●chloramphenicol, ●doxycycline and ●telithromycin; increased risk of nephrotoxicity when ciclosporin given with ●aminoglycosides, ●polymyxins, ●quinolones, ●sulphonamides or ●vancomycin; increased risk of myopathy when ciclosporin given with ●daptomycin (preferably avoid concomitant use); metabolism of ciclosporin possibly inhibited by ●macrolides (increased plasma concentration); plasma concentration of ciclosporin increased by ●quinupristin/dalfopristin; increased risk of nephrotoxicity when ciclosporin given with ●trimethoprim, also plasma concentration of ciclosporin reduced by intravenous trimethoprim
- Antidepressants: plasma concentration of ciclosporin reduced by ●St John's wort—avoid concomitant use

  Antidiabetics: ciclosporin possibly enhances hypoglycaemic effect of repaglinide
- Antiepileptics: metabolism of ciclosporin accelerated by ●carbamazepine and ●phenytoin (reduced plasma concentration); plasma concentration of ciclosporin possibly reduced by oxcarbazepine; metabolism of ciclosporin accelerated by ●primidone (reduced effect)
- Antifungals: metabolism of ciclosporin inhibited by ●fluconazole, ●itraconazole, ●ketoconazole, ●posaconazole and ●voriconazole (increased plasma concentration); metabolism of ciclosporin possibly inhibited by ●miconazole (increased plasma concentration); increased risk of nephrotoxicity when ciclosporin given with ●amphotericin; ciclosporin increases plasma concentration of ●caspofungin (manufacturer of caspofungin recommends monitoring liver enzymes); plasma concentration of ciclosporin possibly reduced by griseofulvin and terbinafine; plasma concentration of ciclosporin possibly increased by micafungin
- Antimalarials: plasma concentration of ciclosporin increased by ●chloroquine and hydroxychloroquine (increased risk of toxicity)

  Antimuscarinics: avoidance of ciclosporin advised by manufacturer of darifenacin
- Antivirals: increased risk of nephrotoxicity when ciclosporin given with aciclovir; plasma concentration of ciclosporin possibly increased by ●atazanavir, ●nelfinavir and ●ritonavir; plasma concentration of ciclosporin possibly reduced by efavirenz; plasma concentration of ciclosporin increased by ●indinavir; plasma concentration of both drugs increased when ciclosporin given with ●saquinavir
- Barbiturates: metabolism of ciclosporin accelerated by ●barbiturates (reduced effect)
- Beta-blockers: plasma concentration of ciclosporin increased by ●carvedilol
- Bile Acids: absorption of ciclosporin increased by ●ursodeoxycholic acid
- Bosentan: ciclosporin increases plasma concentration of ●bosentan (also plasma concentration of ciclosporin reduced—avoid concomitant use)
- Calcium-channel Blockers: combination of ciclosporin with ●lercanidipine may increase plasma concentra-

Ciclosporin
- Calcium-channel Blockers (continued)
tion of either drug (or both)—avoid concomitant use; plasma concentration of ciclosporin increased by ●diltiazem, ●nicardipine and ●verapamil; ciclosporin possibly increases plasma concentration of nifedipine (increased risk of toxicity including gingival hyperplasia)
- Cardiac Glycosides: ciclosporin increases plasma concentration of ●digoxin (increased risk of toxicity)
- Colchicine: possible increased risk of nephrotoxicity and myotoxicity when ciclosporin given with ●colchicine (increased plasma concentration of ciclosporin)
- Corticosteroids: plasma concentration of ciclosporin increased by high-dose ●methylprednisolone (risk of convulsions); ciclosporin increases plasma concentration of prednisolone
- Cytotoxics: increased risk of nephrotoxicity when ciclosporin given with ●melphalan; increased risk of neurotoxicity when ciclosporin given with ●doxorubicin; risk of toxicity when ciclosporin given with ●methotrexate; plasma concentration of ciclosporin possibly increased by imatinib; in vitro studies suggest a possible interaction between ciclosporin and docetaxel (consult docetaxel product literature); ciclosporin possibly increases plasma concentration of etoposide (increased risk of toxicity)
- Diuretics: increased risk of hyperkalaemia when ciclosporin given with ●potassium-sparing diuretics and aldosterone antagonists; increased risk of nephrotoxicity and possibly hypermagnesaemia when ciclosporin given with thiazides and related diuretics
- Grapefruit Juice: plasma concentration of ciclosporin increased by ●grapefruit juice (increased risk of toxicity)
- Hormone Antagonists: metabolism of ciclosporin inhibited by ●danazol (increased plasma concentration); plasma concentration of ciclosporin reduced by lanreotide and ●octreotide
- Lipid-regulating Drugs: increased risk of renal impairment when ciclosporin given with bezafibrate or fenofibrate; increased risk of myopathy when ciclosporin given with ●rosuvastatin (avoid concomitant use); plasma concentration of both drugs may increase when ciclosporin given with ●ezetimibe; increased risk of myopathy when ciclosporin given with ●statins
Mannitol: possible increased risk of nephrotoxicity when ciclosporin given with mannitol
- Metoclopramide: plasma concentration of ciclosporin increased by ●metoclopramide
- Modafinil: plasma concentration of ciclosporin reduced by ●modafinil
Oestrogens: plasma concentration of ciclosporin possibly increased by oestrogens
- Orlistat: absorption of ciclosporin possibly reduced by ●orlistat
- Potassium Salts: increased risk of hyperkalaemia when ciclosporin given with ●potassium salts
- Progestogens: metabolism of ciclosporin inhibited by ●progestogens (increased plasma concentration)
Sevelamer: plasma concentration of ciclosporin possibly reduced by sevelamer
Sirolimus: ciclosporin increases plasma concentration of sirolimus
- Sitaxentan: ciclosporin increases plasma concentration of ●sitaxentan—avoid concomitant use
- Sulfinpyrazone: plasma concentration of ciclosporin reduced by ●sulfinpyrazone
- Tacrolimus: plasma concentration of ciclosporin increased by ●tacrolimus (increased risk of nephrotoxicity)—avoid concomitant use
- Ulcer-healing Drugs: plasma concentration of ciclosporin possibly increased by ●cimetidine; plasma

Ciclosporin
- Ulcer-healing Drugs (continued)
concentration of ciclosporin possibly affected by omeprazole
Cidofovir
Antivirals: combination of cidofovir with tenofovir may increase plasma concentration of either drug (or both)
Cilazapril see ACE Inhibitors
Cilostazol
- Anagrelide: avoidance of cilostazol advised by manufacturer of ●anagrelide
Analgesics: manufacturer of cilostazol recommends dose of concomitant aspirin should not exceed 80 mg daily
- Antibacterials: plasma concentration of cilostazol increased by ●erythromycin (also plasma concentration of erythromycin reduced)—avoid concomitant use
- Antifungals: plasma concentration of cilostazol possibly increased by ●ketoconazole—avoid concomitant use
- Antivirals: plasma concentration of cilostazol possibly increased by ●fosamprenavir, ●indinavir, ●lopinavir, ●nelfinavir, ●ritonavir and ●saquinavir—avoid concomitant use
- Calcium-channel Blockers: plasma concentration of cilostazol increased by ●diltiazem—avoid concomitant use
- Ulcer-healing Drugs: plasma concentration of cilostazol possibly increased by ●cimetidine and ●lansoprazole—avoid concomitant use; plasma concentration of cilostazol increased by ●omeprazole (risk of toxicity)—avoid concomitant use
Cimetidine see Histamine H₂-antagonists
Cinacalcet
Antifungals: metabolism of cinacalcet inhibited by ketoconazole (increased plasma concentration)
Tobacco: metabolism of cinacalcet increased by tobacco smoking (reduced plasma concentration)
Cinnarizine see Antihistamines
Ciprofibrate see Fibrates
Ciprofloxacin see Quinolones
Cisatracurium see Muscle Relaxants
Cisplatin see Platinum Compounds
Citalopram see Antidepressants, SSRI
Clarithromycin see Macrolides
Clemastine see Antihistamines
Clindamycin
- Muscle Relaxants: clindamycin enhances effects of ●non-depolarising muscle relaxants and ●suxamethonium
Oestrogens: antibacterials that do not induce liver enzymes possibly reduce contraceptive effect of oestrogens (risk probably small, see p. 478)
Parasympathomimetics: clindamycin antagonises effects of neostigmine and pyridostigmine
Vaccines: antibacterials inactivate oral typhoid vaccine—see p. 752
Clobazam see Anxiolytics and Hypnotics
Clomethiazole see Anxiolytics and Hypnotics
Clomipramine see Antidepressants, Tricyclic
Clonazepam see Anxiolytics and Hypnotics
Clonidine
ACE Inhibitors: enhanced hypotensive effect when clonidine given with ACE inhibitors; previous treatment with clonidine possibly delays antihypertensive effect of captopril
Adrenergic Neurone Blockers: enhanced hypotensive effect when clonidine given with adrenergic neurone blockers
Alcohol: enhanced hypotensive effect when clonidine given with alcohol
Aldesleukin: enhanced hypotensive effect when clonidine given with aldesleukin

Clonidine (continued)

Alpha-blockers: enhanced hypotensive effect when clonidine given with alpha-blockers

Anaesthetics, General: enhanced hypotensive effect when clonidine given with general anaesthetics

Analgesics: hypotensive effect of clonidine antagonised by NSAIDs

Angiotensin-II Receptor Antagonists: enhanced hypotensive effect when clonidine given with angiotensin-II receptor antagonists

• Antidepressants: enhanced hypotensive effect when clonidine given with MAOIs; hypotensive effect of clonidine antagonised by ●tricyclics, also increased risk of hypertension on clonidine withdrawal

Antipsychotics: enhanced hypotensive effect when clonidine given with phenothiazines

Anxiolytics and Hypnotics: enhanced hypotensive effect when clonidine given with anxiolytics and hypnotics

• Beta-blockers: increased risk of withdrawal hypertension when clonidine given with ●beta-blockers (withdraw beta-blockers several days before slowly withdrawing clonidine)

Calcium-channel Blockers: enhanced hypotensive effect when clonidine given with calcium-channel blockers

Corticosteroids: hypotensive effect of clonidine antagonised by corticosteroids

Diazoxide: enhanced hypotensive effect when clonidine given with diazoxide

Diuretics: enhanced hypotensive effect when clonidine given with diuretics

Dopaminergics: enhanced hypotensive effect when clonidine given with levodopa

Methyldopa: enhanced hypotensive effect when clonidine given with methyldopa

Moxisylyte (thymoxamine): enhanced hypotensive effect when clonidine given with moxisylyte

Moxonidine: enhanced hypotensive effect when clonidine given with moxonidine

Muscle Relaxants: enhanced hypotensive effect when clonidine given with baclofen or tizanidine

Nitrates: enhanced hypotensive effect when clonidine given with nitrates

Oestrogens: hypotensive effect of clonidine antagonised by oestrogens

Prostaglandins: enhanced hypotensive effect when clonidine given with alprostadil

• Sympathomimetics: possible risk of hypertension when clonidine given with adrenaline (epinephrine) or noradrenaline (norepinephrine); serious adverse events reported with concomitant use of clonidine and ●methylphenidate (causality not established)

Vasodilator Antihypertensives: enhanced hypotensive effect when clonidine given with hydralazine, minoxidil or sodium nitroprusside

Clopamide see Diuretics

Clopidogrel

Analgesics: increased risk of bleeding when clopidogrel given with NSAIDs or aspirin

• Anticoagulants: manufacturer of clopidogrel advises avoid concomitant use with ●warfarin; antiplatelet action of clopidogrel enhances anticoagulant effect of ●coumarins and ●phenindione; increased risk of bleeding when clopidogrel given with heparins

Dipyridamole: increased risk of bleeding when clopidogrel given with dipyridamole

Iloprost: increased risk of bleeding when clopidogrel given with iloprost

Ulcer-healing Drugs: antiplatelet effect of clopidogrel possibly reduced by proton pump inhibitors

Clotrimazole see Antifungals, Imidazole

Clozapine see Antipsychotics

Co-amoxiclav see Penicillins

Co-beneldopa see Levodopa

Co-careldopa see Levodopa

Codeine see Opioid Analgesics

Co-fluampicil see Penicillins

Colchicine

• Antibacterials: increased risk of colchicine toxicity when given with ●clarithromycin or ●erythromycin

• Ciclosporin: possible increased risk of nephrotoxicity and myotoxicity when colchicine given with ●ciclosporin (increased plasma concentration of ciclosporin)

• Lipid-regulating Drugs: possible increased risk of myopathy when colchicine given with ●statins

Colesevelam

Note. Other drugs should be taken at least 1 hour before or 4 hours after colesevelam to reduce possible interference with absorption

Colestipol

Note. Other drugs should be taken at least 1 hour before or 4-6 hours after colestipol to reduce possible interference with absorption

Antibacterials: colestipol possibly reduces absorption of tetracycline

Bile Acids: colestipol possibly reduces absorption of bile acids

Cardiac Glycosides: colestipol possibly reduces absorption of cardiac glycosides

Diuretics: colestipol reduces absorption of thiazides and related diuretics (give at least 2 hours apart)

Thyroid Hormones: colestipol reduces absorption of thyroid hormones

Colestyramine

Note. Other drugs should be taken at least 1 hour before or 4-6 hours after colestyramine to reduce possible interference with absorption

Analgesics: colestyramine increases the excretion of meloxicam; colestyramine reduces absorption of paracetamol

Antibacterials: colestyramine possibly reduces absorption of tetracycline; colestyramine antagonises effects of oral vancomycin

• Anticoagulants: colestyramine may enhance or reduce anticoagulant effect of ●coumarins and ●phenindione

Antidiabetics: colestyramine possibly enhances hypoglycaemic effect of acarbose

Antiepileptics: colestyramine possibly reduces absorption of valproate

Bile Acids: colestyramine possibly reduces absorption of bile acids

Cardiac Glycosides: colestyramine possibly reduces absorption of cardiac glycosides

Cytotoxics: colestyramine reduces absorption of mycophenolate

Diuretics: colestyramine reduces absorption of thiazides and related diuretics (give at least 2 hours apart)

Leflunomide: colestyramine significantly decreases effect of leflunomide (enhanced elimination)—avoid unless drug elimination desired

Raloxifene: colestyramine reduces absorption of raloxifene (manufacturer of raloxifene advises avoid concomitant administration)

Thyroid Hormones: colestyramine reduces absorption of thyroid hormones

Colistin see Polymyxins

Contraceptives, oral see Oestrogens and Progestogens

Corticosteroids

Note. Interactions do not generally apply to corticosteroids used for topical action (including inhalation) unless specified

ACE Inhibitors: corticosteroids antagonise hypotensive effect of ACE inhibitors

Adrenergic Neurone Blockers: corticosteroids antagonise hypotensive effect of adrenergic neurone blockers

Alpha-blockers: corticosteroids antagonise hypotensive effect of alpha-blockers

Corticosteroids *(continued)*

Analgesics: increased risk of gastro-intestinal bleeding and ulceration when corticosteroids given with NSAIDs; increased risk of gastro-intestinal bleeding and ulceration when corticosteroids given with aspirin, also corticosteroids reduce plasma concentration of salicylate

Angiotensin-II Receptor Antagonists: corticosteroids antagonise hypotensive effect of angiotensin-II receptor antagonists

Antacids: absorption of deflazacort reduced by antacids

• Antibacterials: plasma concentration of methylprednisolone possibly increased by clarithromycin; metabolism of corticosteroids possibly inhibited by erythromycin; metabolism of methylprednisolone inhibited by erythromycin; corticosteroids possibly reduce plasma concentration of isoniazid; metabolism of corticosteroids accelerated by •rifamycins (reduced effect)

• Anticoagulants: corticosteroids may enhance or reduce anticoagulant effect of •coumarins (high-dose corticosteroids enhance anticoagulant effect)

Antidiabetics: corticosteroids antagonise hypoglycaemic effect of antidiabetics

• Antiepileptics: metabolism of corticosteroids accelerated by •carbamazepine, •phenytoin and •primidone (reduced effect)

• Antifungals: metabolism of corticosteroids possibly inhibited by itraconazole and ketoconazole; plasma concentration of active metabolite of ciclesonide increased by ketoconazole; plasma concentration of inhaled mometasone increased by ketoconazole; plasma concentration of inhaled and oral budesonide increased by ketoconazole; metabolism of methylprednisolone inhibited by ketoconazole; increased risk of hypokalaemia when corticosteroids given with •amphotericin—avoid concomitant use unless corticosteroids needed to control reactions; plasma concentration of inhaled budesonide increased by itraconazole; metabolism of methylprednisolone possibly inhibited by itraconazole; dexamethasone possibly reduces plasma concentration of caspofungin—consider increasing dose of caspofungin

• Antivirals: dexamethasone possibly reduces plasma concentration of indinavir, lopinavir and saquinavir; plasma concentration of corticosteroids, dexamethasone and prednisolone possibly increased by ritonavir; plasma concentration of inhaled and intranasal budesonide and fluticasone increased by •ritonavir

Aprepitant: metabolism of dexamethasone and methylprednisolone inhibited by aprepitant (reduce dose of dexamethasone and methylprednisolone)

• Barbiturates: metabolism of corticosteroids accelerated by •barbiturates (reduced effect)

Beta-blockers: corticosteroids antagonise hypotensive effect of beta-blockers

Calcium Salts: corticosteroids reduce absorption of calcium salts

Calcium-channel Blockers: corticosteroids antagonise hypotensive effect of calcium-channel blockers

Cardiac Glycosides: increased risk of hypokalaemia when corticosteroids given with cardiac glycosides

• Ciclosporin: high-dose methylprednisolone increases plasma concentration of •ciclosporin (risk of convulsions); plasma concentration of prednisolone increased by ciclosporin

Clonidine: corticosteroids antagonise hypotensive effect of clonidine

• Cytotoxics: increased risk of haematological toxicity when corticosteroids given with •methotrexate

Diazoxide: corticosteroids antagonise hypotensive effect of diazoxide

Diuretics: corticosteroids antagonise diuretic effect of diuretics; increased risk of hypokalaemia when

Corticosteroids

Diuretics *(continued)*
corticosteroids given with acetazolamide, loop diuretics or thiazides and related diuretics

Methyldopa: corticosteroids antagonise hypotensive effect of methyldopa

Mifepristone: effect of corticosteroids (including inhaled corticosteroids) may be reduced for 3–4 days after mifepristone

Moxonidine: corticosteroids antagonise hypotensive effect of moxonidine

Muscle Relaxants: corticosteroids possibly antagonise effects of pancuronium and vecuronium

Nitrates: corticosteroids antagonise hypotensive effect of nitrates

Oestrogens: plasma concentration of corticosteroids increased by oral contraceptives containing oestrogens

Sodium Benzoate: corticosteroids possibly reduce effects of sodium benzoate

Sodium Phenylbutyrate: corticosteroids possibly reduce effects of sodium phenylbutyrate

Somatropin: corticosteroids may inhibit growth-promoting effect of somatropin

Sympathomimetics: metabolism of dexamethasone accelerated by ephedrine

Sympathomimetics, Beta$_2$: increased risk of hypokalaemia when corticosteroids given with high doses of beta$_2$ sympathomimetics—for CSM advice (hypokalaemia) see p. 173

Theophylline: increased risk of hypokalaemia when corticosteroids given with theophylline

• Vaccines: high doses of corticosteroids impair immune response to •vaccines, avoid concomitant use with live vaccines (see p. 725)

Vasodilator Antihypertensives: corticosteroids antagonise hypotensive effect of hydralazine, minoxidil and sodium nitroprusside

Cortisone *see* Corticosteroids

Co-trimoxazole *see* Trimethoprim and Sulfamethoxazole

Coumarins
Note. Change in patient's clinical condition, particularly associated with liver disease, intercurrent illness, or drug administration, necessitates more frequent testing. Major changes in diet (especially involving salads and vegetables) and in alcohol consumption may also affect anticoagulant control

• Alcohol: anticoagulant control with coumarins may be affected by major changes in consumption of •alcohol

Allopurinol: anticoagulant effect of coumarins possibly enhanced by allopurinol

• Anabolic Steroids: anticoagulant effect of coumarins enhanced by •anabolic steroids

• Analgesics: anticoagulant effect of coumarins possibly enhanced by •NSAIDs; anticoagulant effect of coumarins enhanced by •azapropazone (avoid concomitant use); increased risk of haemorrhage when anticoagulants given with intravenous •diclofenac (avoid concomitant use, including low-dose heparin); increased risk of haemorrhage when anticoagulants given with •ketorolac (avoid concomitant use, including low-dose heparin); anticoagulant effect of coumarins enhanced by •tramadol; increased risk of bleeding when coumarins given with •aspirin (due to antiplatelet effect); anticoagulant effect of coumarins possibly enhanced by prolonged regular use of paracetamol

• Anti-arrhythmics: metabolism of coumarins inhibited by •amiodarone (enhanced anticoagulant effect); anticoagulant effect of coumarins enhanced by •propafenone

• Antibacterials: experience in anticoagulant clinics suggests that INR possibly altered when coumarins are given with •neomycin (given for local action on gut); anticoagulant effect of coumarins possibly enhanced by •azithromycin, •aztreonam,

Coumarins

- Antibacterials *(continued)*
  ●cephalosporins, levofloxacin, ●tetracyclines, tigecycline and trimethoprim; anticoagulant effect of coumarins enhanced by ●chloramphenicol, ●ciprofloxacin, ●clarithromycin, ●erythromycin, ●metronidazole, ●nalidixic acid, ●norfloxacin, ●ofloxacin and ●sulphonamides; studies have failed to demonstrate an interaction with coumarins, but common experience in anticoagulant clinics is that INR can be altered by a course of broad-spectrum penicillins such as ampicillin; metabolism of coumarins accelerated by ●rifamycins (reduced anticoagulant effect)
- Antidepressants: anticoagulant effect of warfarin possibly enhanced by ●venlafaxine; anticoagulant effect of coumarins possibly enhanced by ●SSRIs; anticoagulant effect of coumarins reduced by ●St John's wort (avoid concomitant use); anticoagulant effect of warfarin enhanced by mirtazapine; anticoagulant effect of coumarins may be enhanced or reduced by ●tricyclics
- Antidiabetics: anticoagulant effect of warfarin possibly enhanced by exenatide; coumarins possibly enhance hypoglycaemic effect of ●sulphonylureas, also possible changes to anticoagulant effect
- Antiepileptics: metabolism of coumarins accelerated by ●carbamazepine and ●primidone (reduced anticoagulant effect); metabolism of coumarins accelerated by ●phenytoin (possibility of reduced anticoagulant effect, but enhancement also reported); anticoagulant effect of coumarins possibly enhanced by valproate
- Antifungals: anticoagulant effect of coumarins enhanced by ●fluconazole, ●itraconazole, ●ketoconazole and ●voriconazole; anticoagulant effect of coumarins enhanced by ●miconazole (miconazole oral gel and possibly vaginal formulations absorbed); anticoagulant effect of coumarins reduced by ●griseofulvin
  Antimalarials: isolated reports that anticoagulant effect of warfarin may be enhanced by proguanil
- Antivirals: anticoagulant effect of warfarin may be enhanced or reduced by atazanavir, ●nevirapine and ●ritonavir; anticoagulant effect of coumarins may be enhanced or reduced by fosamprenavir; anticoagulant effect of coumarins possibly enhanced by ●ritonavir; anticoagulant effect of warfarin possibly enhanced by saquinavir
  Anxiolytics and Hypnotics: anticoagulant effect of coumarins may transiently be enhanced by chloral and triclofos
  Aprepitant: anticoagulant effect of warfarin possibly reduced by aprepitant
- Barbiturates: metabolism of coumarins accelerated by ●barbiturates (reduced anticoagulant effect)
  Bosentan: monitoring anticoagulant effect of coumarins recommended by manufacturer of bosentan
- Clopidogrel: anticoagulant effect of coumarins enhanced due to antiplatelet action of ●clopidogrel; avoidance of warfarin advised by manufacturer of ●clopidogrel
- Corticosteroids: anticoagulant effect of coumarins may be enhanced or reduced by ●corticosteroids (high-dose corticosteroids enhance anticoagulant effect)
- Cranberry Juice: anticoagulant effect of coumarins possibly enhanced by ●cranberry juice—avoid concomitant use
- Cytotoxics: anticoagulant effect of coumarins possibly enhanced by ●etoposide, ●ifosfamide and ●sorafenib; anticoagulant effect of coumarins enhanced by ●fluorouracil; anticoagulant effect of coumarins possibly reduced by ●azathioprine, ●mercaptopurine and ●mitotane; increased risk of bleeding when coumarins given with ●erlotinib; replacement of warfarin with a heparin advised by

Coumarins

- Cytotoxics *(continued)*
  manufacturer of imatinib (possibility of enhanced warfarin effect)
- Dipyridamole: anticoagulant effect of coumarins enhanced due to antiplatelet action of ●dipyridamole
- Disulfiram: anticoagulant effect of coumarins enhanced by ●disulfiram
- Dopaminergics: anticoagulant effect of warfarin enhanced by ●entacapone
- Enteral Foods: anticoagulant effect of coumarins antagonised by vitamin K (present in some ●enteral feeds)
- Glucosamine: anticoagulant effect of warfarin enhanced by ●glucosamine (avoid concomitant use)
- Hormone Antagonists: anticoagulant effect of coumarins possibly enhanced by bicalutamide and ●toremifene; metabolism of coumarins inhibited by ●danazol (enhanced anticoagulant effect); anticoagulant effect of coumarins enhanced by ●flutamide and ●tamoxifen
  Iloprost: anticoagulant effect of coumarins possibly enhanced by iloprost
  Lactulose: anticoagulant effect of coumarins possibly enhanced by lactulose
  Leflunomide: anticoagulant effect of warfarin possibly enhanced by leflunomide
  Leukotriene Receptor Antagonists: anticoagulant effect of warfarin enhanced by zafirlukast
- Levamisole: anticoagulant effect of warfarin possibly enhanced by ●levamisole
- Lipid-regulating Drugs: anticoagulant effect of coumarins may be enhanced or reduced by ●colestyramine; anticoagulant effect of warfarin may be transiently reduced by atorvastatin; anticoagulant effect of coumarins enhanced by ●fibrates, ●fluvastatin and simvastatin; anticoagulant effect of coumarins possibly enhanced by ezetimibe and ●rosuvastatin
  Memantine: anticoagulant effect of warfarin possibly enhanced by memantine
- Oestrogens: anticoagulant effect of coumarins may be enhanced or reduced by ●oestrogens
  Orlistat: monitoring anticoagulant effect of coumarins recommended by manufacturer of orlistat
- Progestogens: anticoagulant effect of coumarins may be enhanced or reduced by ●progestogens
  Raloxifene: anticoagulant effect of coumarins antagonised by raloxifene
- Retinoids: anticoagulant effect of coumarins possibly reduced by ●acitretin
  Sibutramine: increased risk of bleeding when anticoagulants given with sibutramine
- Sitaxentan: anticoagulant effect of coumarins enhanced by ●sitaxentan
- Sulfinpyrazone: anticoagulant effect of coumarins enhanced by ●sulfinpyrazone
- Sympathomimetics: anticoagulant effect of coumarins possibly enhanced by ●methylphenidate
  Terpene Mixture: anticoagulant effect of coumarins possibly reduced by Rowachol®
- Testolactone: anticoagulant effect of coumarins enhanced by ●testolactone
- Testosterone: anticoagulant effect of coumarins enhanced by ●testosterone
- Thyroid Hormones: anticoagulant effect of coumarins enhanced by ●thyroid hormones
  Ubidecarenone: anticoagulant effect of warfarin may be enhanced or reduced by ubidecarenone
- Ulcer-healing Drugs: metabolism of coumarins inhibited by ●cimetidine (enhanced anticoagulant effect); anticoagulant effect of coumarins possibly enhanced by ●esomeprazole, ●omeprazole and pantoprazole; absorption of coumarins possibly reduced by ●sucralfate (reduced anticoagulant effect)

Coumarins (continued)

Vaccines: anticoagulant effect of warfarin possibly enhanced by influenza vaccine
• Vitamins: anticoagulant effect of coumarins antagonised by •vitamin K

Cranberry Juice

• Anticoagulants: cranberry juice possibly enhances anticoagulant effect of •coumarins—avoid concomitant use

Cyclizine see Antihistamines

Cyclopenthiazide see Diuretics

Cyclopentolate see Antimuscarinics

Cyclophosphamide

Antiepileptics: cytotoxics possibly reduce absorption of phenytoin
Antifungals: side-effects of cyclophosphamide possibly increased by itraconazole
• Antipsychotics: avoid concomitant use of cytotoxics with •clozapine (increased risk of agranulocytosis)
Cardiac Glycosides: cytotoxics reduce absorption of digoxin tablets
• Cytotoxics: increased toxicity when high-dose cyclophosphamide given with •pentostatin—avoid concomitant use
Muscle Relaxants: cyclophosphamide enhances effects of suxamethonium

Cycloserine

• Alcohol: increased risk of convulsions when cycloserine given with •alcohol
Antibacterials: increased risk of CNS toxicity when cycloserine given with isoniazid
Oestrogens: antibacterials that do not induce liver enzymes possibly reduce contraceptive effect of oestrogens (risk probably small, see p. 478)
Vaccines: antibacterials inactivate oral typhoid vaccine—see p. 752

Cyproheptadine see Antihistamines

Cytarabine

Antiepileptics: cytotoxics possibly reduce absorption of phenytoin
Antifungals: cytarabine possibly reduces plasma concentration of flucytosine
• Antipsychotics: avoid concomitant use of cytotoxics with •clozapine (increased risk of agranulocytosis)
Cardiac Glycosides: cytotoxics reduce absorption of digoxin tablets
Cytotoxics: intracellular concentration of cytarabine increased by fludarabine

Cytotoxics see individual drugs

Dabigatran Etexilate

• Analgesics: possible increased risk of bleeding when dabigatran etexilate given with •NSAIDs; increased risk of haemorrhage when anticoagulants given with intravenous •diclofenac (avoid concomitant use, including low-dose heparin); increased risk of haemorrhage when anticoagulants given with •ketorolac (avoid concomitant use, including low-dose heparin)
• Anti-arrhythmics: plasma concentration of dabigatran etexilate increased by •amiodarone (reduce dose of dabigatran etexilate)
Sibutramine: increased risk of bleeding when anticoagulants given with sibutramine

Dairy Products

Antibacterials: dairy products reduces absorption of ciprofloxacin and norfloxacin; dairy products reduces absorption of tetracyclines (except doxycycline and minocycline)

Dalteparin see Heparins

Danazol

• Anticoagulants: danazol inhibits metabolism of •coumarins (enhanced anticoagulant effect)
• Antiepileptics: danazol inhibits metabolism of •carbamazepine (increased risk of toxicity)
• Ciclosporin: danazol inhibits metabolism of •ciclosporin (increased plasma concentration)

Danazol (continued)

• Lipid-regulating Drugs: possible increased risk of myopathy when danazol given with •simvastatin
Tacrolimus: danazol possibly increases plasma concentration of tacrolimus

Dantrolene see Muscle Relaxants

Dapsone

Antibacterials: plasma concentration of dapsone reduced by rifamycins; plasma concentration of both drugs may increase when dapsone given with trimethoprim
Antivirals: plasma concentration of dapsone possibly increased by fosamprenavir
Oestrogens: antibacterials that do not induce liver enzymes possibly reduce contraceptive effect of oestrogens (risk probably small, see p. 478)
Probenecid: excretion of dapsone reduced by probenecid (increased risk of side-effects)
Vaccines: antibacterials inactivate oral typhoid vaccine—see p. 752

Daptomycin

• Ciclosporin: increased risk of myopathy when daptomycin given with •ciclosporin (preferably avoid concomitant use)
• Lipid-regulating Drugs: increased risk of myopathy when daptomycin given with •fibrates or •statins (preferably avoid concomitant use)
Oestrogens: antibacterials that do not induce liver enzymes possibly reduce contraceptive effect of oestrogens (risk probably small, see p. 478)
Vaccines: antibacterials inactivate oral typhoid vaccine—see p. 752

Darifenacin see Antimuscarinics

Darunavir

Anti-arrhythmics: darunavir possibly increases plasma concentration of lidocaine (lignocaine)—avoid concomitant use
• Antibacterials: darunavir increases plasma concentration of •rifabutin (reduce dose of rifabutin); plasma concentration of darunavir significantly reduced by •rifampicin—avoid concomitant use
Anticoagulants: avoidance of darunavir advised by manufacturer of rivaroxaban
• Antidepressants: darunavir possibly reduces plasma concentration of paroxetine and sertraline; plasma concentration of darunavir reduced by •St John's wort—avoid concomitant use
Antiepileptics: plasma concentration of darunavir possibly reduced by carbamazepine and phenytoin
Antifungals: plasma concentration of both drugs increased when darunavir given with ketoconazole
Antimalarials: caution with darunavir advised by manufacturer of artemether/lumefantrine
• Antivirals: plasma concentration of darunavir reduced by efavirenz and saquinavir; plasma concentration of both drugs increased when darunavir given with indinavir; plasma concentration of darunavir reduced by •lopinavir, also plasma concentration of lopinavir increased (avoid concomitant use); darunavir increases plasma concentration of •maraviroc (consider reducing dose of maraviroc)
Barbiturates: plasma concentration of darunavir possibly reduced by phenobarbital
• Lipid-regulating Drugs: darunavir possibly increases plasma concentration of pravastatin; possible increased risk of myopathy when darunavir given with •rosuvastatin—avoid concomitant use

Dasatinib

• Antibacterials: metabolism of dasatinib accelerated by •rifampicin (reduced plasma concentration—avoid concomitant use)
Antiepileptics: cytotoxics possibly reduce absorption of phenytoin
• Antipsychotics: avoid concomitant use of cytotoxics with •clozapine (increased risk of agranulocytosis)

Dasatinib *(continued)*

Cardiac Glycosides: cytotoxics reduce absorption of digoxin tablets

Lipid-regulating Drugs: dasatinib possibly increases plasma concentration of simvastatin

Ulcer-healing Drugs: plasma concentration of dasatinib possibly reduced by famotidine

Deferasirox

Antacids: absorption of deferasirox possibly reduced by antacids containing aluminium (manufacturer of deferasirox advises avoid concomitant use)

Antibacterials: plasma concentration of deferasirox reduced by rifampicin

Antidiabetics: deferasirox increases plasma concentration of repaglinide

Anxiolytics and Hypnotics: deferasirox possibly reduces plasma concentration of midazolam

Deflazacort *see* Corticosteroids

Demeclocycline *see* Tetracyclines

Desferrioxamine

Antipsychotics: avoidance of desferrioxamine advised by manufacturer of levomepromazine (methotrimeprazine); manufacturer of desferrioxamine advises avoid concomitant use with prochlorperazine

Desflurane *see* Anaesthetics, General

Desloratadine *see* Antihistamines

Desmopressin

Analgesics: effects of desmopressin enhanced by indometacin

Loperamide: plasma concentration of *oral* desmopressin increased by loperamide

Desogestrel *see* Progestogens

Dexamethasone *see* Corticosteroids

Dexamfetamine *see* Sympathomimetics

Dexibuprofen *see* NSAIDs

Dexketoprofen *see* NSAIDs

Dextromethorphan *see* Opioid Analgesics

Dextropropoxyphene *see* Opioid Analgesics

Diamorphine *see* Opioid Analgesics

Diazepam *see* Anxiolytics and Hypnotics

Diazoxide

ACE Inhibitors: enhanced hypotensive effect when diazoxide given with ACE inhibitors

Adrenergic Neurone Blockers: enhanced hypotensive effect when diazoxide given with adrenergic neurone blockers

Alcohol: enhanced hypotensive effect when diazoxide given with alcohol

Aldesleukin: enhanced hypotensive effect when diazoxide given with aldesleukin

Alpha-blockers: enhanced hypotensive effect when diazoxide given with alpha-blockers

Anaesthetics, General: enhanced hypotensive effect when diazoxide given with general anaesthetics

Analgesics: hypotensive effect of diazoxide antagonised by NSAIDs

Angiotensin-II Receptor Antagonists: enhanced hypotensive effect when diazoxide given with angiotensin-II receptor antagonists

Antidepressants: enhanced hypotensive effect when diazoxide given with MAOIs or tricyclic-related antidepressants

Antidiabetics: diazoxide antagonises hypoglycaemic effect of antidiabetics

Antiepileptics: diazoxide reduces plasma concentration of phenytoin, also effect of diazoxide may be reduced

Antipsychotics: enhanced hypotensive effect when diazoxide given with phenothiazines

Anxiolytics and Hypnotics: enhanced hypotensive effect when diazoxide given with anxiolytics and hypnotics

Beta-blockers: enhanced hypotensive effect when diazoxide given with beta-blockers

Diazoxide *(continued)*

Calcium-channel Blockers: enhanced hypotensive effect when diazoxide given with calcium-channel blockers

Clonidine: enhanced hypotensive effect when diazoxide given with clonidine

Corticosteroids: hypotensive effect of diazoxide antagonised by corticosteroids

Diuretics: enhanced hypotensive and hyperglycaemic effects when diazoxide given with diuretics

Dopaminergics: enhanced hypotensive effect when diazoxide given with levodopa

Methyldopa: enhanced hypotensive effect when diazoxide given with methyldopa

Moxisylyte (thymoxamine): enhanced hypotensive effect when diazoxide given with moxisylyte

Moxonidine: enhanced hypotensive effect when diazoxide given with moxonidine

Muscle Relaxants: enhanced hypotensive effect when diazoxide given with baclofen or tizanidine

Nitrates: enhanced hypotensive effect when diazoxide given with nitrates

Oestrogens: hypotensive effect of diazoxide antagonised by oestrogens

Prostaglandins: enhanced hypotensive effect when diazoxide given with alprostadil

Vasodilator Antihypertensives: enhanced hypotensive effect when diazoxide given with hydralazine, minoxidil or sodium nitroprusside

Diclofenac *see* NSAIDs

Dicycloverine (dicyclomine) *see* Antimuscarinics

Didanosine

Note. Antacids in tablet formulation may affect absorption of other drugs

● Allopurinol: plasma concentration of didanosine increased by ●allopurinol (risk of toxicity)—avoid concomitant use

● Antivirals: plasma concentration of didanosine possibly increased by ganciclovir; increased risk of side-effects when didanosine given with ●ribavirin—avoid concomitant use; increased risk of side-effects when didanosine given with ●stavudine; plasma concentration of didanosine increased by ●tenofovir (increased risk of toxicity)—avoid concomitant use; plasma concentration of didanosine reduced by ●tipranavir

● Cytotoxics: increased risk of toxicity when didanosine given with ●hydroxycarbamide—avoid concomitant use

Digitoxin *see* Cardiac Glycosides

Digoxin *see* Cardiac Glycosides

Dihydrocodeine *see* Opioid Analgesics

Diltiazem *see* Calcium-channel Blockers

Dimercaprol

● Iron: avoid concomitant use of dimercaprol with ●iron

Dimethyl sulfoxide

● Analgesics: avoid concomitant use of dimethyl sulfoxide with ●sulindac

Dinoprostone *see* Prostaglandins

Diphenoxylate *see* Opioid Analgesics

Dipipanone *see* Opioid Analgesics

Dipivefrine *see* Sympathomimetics

Dipyridamole

Antacids: absorption of dipyridamole possibly reduced by antacids

● Anti-arrhythmics: dipyridamole enhances and extends the effects of ●adenosine (important risk of toxicity)

● Anticoagulants: antiplatelet action of dipyridamole enhances anticoagulant effect of ●coumarins and ●phenindione; dipyridamole enhances anticoagulant effect of heparins

Clopidogrel: increased risk of bleeding when dipyridamole given with clopidogrel

Cytotoxics: dipyridamole possibly reduces effects of fludarabine

Disodium Etidronate *see* Bisphosphonates

Disodium Pamidronate *see* Bisphosphonates

Disopyramide

- Anaesthetics, Local: increased myocardial depression when anti-arrhythmics given with bupivacaine, levobupivacaine, prilocaine or ropivacaine
- Anti-arrhythmics: increased myocardial depression when anti-arrhythmics given with other ●anti-arrhythmics; increased risk of ventricular arrhythmias when disopyramide given with ●amiodarone—avoid concomitant use
- Antibacterials: plasma concentration of disopyramide possibly increased by ●clarithromycin (increased risk of toxicity); plasma concentration of disopyramide increased by ●erythromycin (increased risk of toxicity); increased risk of ventricular arrhythmias when disopyramide given with ●moxifloxacin or ●quinupristin/dalfopristin—avoid concomitant use; metabolism of disopyramide accelerated by ●rifamycins (reduced plasma concentration)
- Antidepressants: increased risk of ventricular arrhythmias when disopyramide given with ●tricyclics
- Antidiabetics: disopyramide possibly enhances hypoglycaemic effect of gliclazide, insulin and metformin
- Antiepileptics: plasma concentration of disopyramide reduced by phenytoin; metabolism of disopyramide accelerated by primidone (reduced plasma concentration)
- Antifungals: increased risk of ventricular arrhythmias when disopyramide given with ●ketoconazole—avoid concomitant use; avoidance of disopyramide advised by manufacturer of ●itraconazole
- Antihistamines: increased risk of ventricular arrhythmias when disopyramide given with ●mizolastine—avoid concomitant use
- Antimalarials: avoidance of disopyramide advised by manufacturer of ●artemether/lumefantrine (risk of ventricular arrhythmias)
- Antimuscarinics: increased risk of antimuscarinic side-effects when disopyramide given with antimuscarinics; increased risk of ventricular arrhythmias when disopyramide given with ●tolterodine
- Antipsychotics: increased risk of ventricular arrhythmias when anti-arrhythmics that prolong the QT interval given with ●antipsychotics that prolong the QT interval; increased risk of ventricular arrhythmias when disopyramide given with ●amisulpride, ●pimozide, ●sertindole or ●zuclopenthixol—avoid concomitant use; increased risk of ventricular arrhythmias when disopyramide given with ●phenothiazines or ●sulpiride
- Antivirals: plasma concentration of disopyramide possibly increased by ●ritonavir (increased risk of toxicity)
- Atomoxetine: increased risk of ventricular arrhythmias when disopyramide given with ●atomoxetine
- Barbiturates: metabolism of disopyramide accelerated by barbiturates (reduced plasma concentration)
- Beta-blockers: increased myocardial depression when anti-arrhythmics given with ●beta-blockers; increased risk of ventricular arrhythmias when disopyramide given with ●sotalol—avoid concomitant use
- Calcium-channel Blockers: increased risk of myocardial depression and asystole when disopyramide given with ●verapamil
- Diuretics: increased cardiac toxicity with disopyramide if hypokalaemia occurs with ●acetazolamide, ●loop diuretics or ●thiazides and related diuretics
- 5HT₃ Antagonists: increased risk of ventricular arrhythmias when disopyramide given with ●dolasetron—avoid concomitant use
- Ivabradine: increased risk of ventricular arrhythmias when disopyramide given with ●ivabradine
- Nitrates: disopyramide reduces effects of sublingual tablets of nitrates (failure to dissolve under tongue owing to dry mouth)

Distigmine *see* Parasympathomimetics

Disulfiram

- Alcohol: disulfiram reaction when disulfiram given with alcohol (see BNF section 4.10)
- Antibacterials: psychotic reaction reported when disulfiram given with metronidazole
- Anticoagulants: disulfiram enhances anticoagulant effect of ●coumarins
- Antidepressants: increased disulfiram reaction with alcohol reported with concomitant amitriptyline; disulfiram inhibits metabolism of tricyclics (increased plasma concentration)
- Antiepileptics: disulfiram inhibits metabolism of ●phenytoin (increased risk of toxicity)
- Anxiolytics and Hypnotics: disulfiram increases risk of temazepam toxicity; disulfiram inhibits metabolism of benzodiazepines (increased sedative effects)
- Paraldehyde: risk of toxicity when disulfiram given with ●paraldehyde
- Theophylline: disulfiram inhibits metabolism of theophylline (increased risk of toxicity)

Diuretics

Note. Since systemic absorption may follow topical application of brinzolamide to the eye, the possibility of interactions should be borne in mind

Note. Since systemic absorption may follow topical application of dorzolamide to the eye, the possibility of interactions should be borne in mind

- ACE Inhibitors: enhanced hypotensive effect when diuretics given with ●ACE inhibitors; increased risk of severe hyperkalaemia when potassium-sparing diuretics and aldosterone antagonists given with ●ACE inhibitors (monitor potassium concentration with low-dose spironolactone in heart failure)
- Adrenergic Neurone Blockers: enhanced hypotensive effect when diuretics given with adrenergic neurone blockers
- Alcohol: enhanced hypotensive effect when diuretics given with alcohol
- Aldesleukin: enhanced hypotensive effect when diuretics given with aldesleukin
- Aliskiren: plasma concentration of furosemide (frusemide) reduced by aliskiren; increased risk of hyperkalaemia when potassium-sparing diuretics and aldosterone antagonists given with aliskiren
- Allopurinol: increased risk of hypersensitivity when thiazides and related diuretics given with allopurinol especially in renal impairment
- Alpha-blockers: enhanced hypotensive effect when diuretics given with ●alpha-blockers, also increased risk of first-dose hypotension with post-synaptic alpha-blockers such as prazosin
- Anaesthetics, General: enhanced hypotensive effect when diuretics given with general anaesthetics
- Analgesics: Diuretic effect of potassium canrenoate possibly antagonised by NSAIDs; possibly increased risk of hyperkalaemia when potassium-sparing diuretics and aldosterone antagonists given with NSAIDs; diuretics increase risk of nephrotoxicity of NSAIDs, also antagonism of diuretic effect; effects of diuretics antagonised by indometacin and ketorolac; increased risk of hyperkalaemia when potassium-sparing diuretics and aldosterone antagonists given with indometacin; occasional reports of reduced renal function when triamterene given with ●indometacin—avoid concomitant use; increased risk of toxicity when carbonic anhydrase inhibitors given with high-dose aspirin; diuretic effect of spironolactone antagonised by aspirin
- Angiotensin-II Receptor Antagonists: enhanced hypotensive effect when diuretics given with ●angiotensin-II receptor antagonists; increased risk of hyperkalaemia when potassium-sparing diuretics and aldosterone antagonists given with ●angiotensin-II receptor antagonists
- Anti-arrhythmics: plasma concentration of eplerenone increased by amiodarone (reduce dose of eplere-

Diuretics

Diuretics

- **Anti-arrhythmics** *(continued)*
none); hypokalaemia caused by acetazolamide, loop
diuretics or thiazides and related diuretics increases
cardiac toxicity with amiodarone; hypokalaemia
caused by acetazolamide, loop diuretics or thiazides
and related diuretics increases cardiac toxicity with
●disopyramide; hypokalaemia caused by acetazolamide, loop diuretics or thiazides and related diuretics increases cardiac toxicity with ●flecainide;
hypokalaemia caused by acetazolamide, loop
diuretics or thiazides and related diuretics antagonises action of ●lidocaine (lignocaine)
- **Antibacterials:** plasma concentration of eplerenone
increased by ●clarithromycin and ●telithromycin—
avoid concomitant use; plasma concentration of
eplerenone increased by erythromycin (reduce dose
of eplerenone); plasma concentration of eplerenone
reduced by ●rifampicin—avoid concomitant use;
avoidance of diuretics advised by manufacturer of
lymecycline; increased risk of ototoxicity when loop
diuretics given with ●aminoglycosides,
●polymyxins or ●vancomycin; acetazolamide antagonises effects of ●methenamine; increased risk of
hyperkalaemia when eplerenone given with trimethoprim
- **Antidepressants:** possible increased risk of hypokalaemia when loop diuretics or thiazides and related
diuretics given with reboxetine; enhanced hypotensive effect when diuretics given with MAOIs; plasma
concentration of eplerenone reduced by ●St John's
wort—avoid concomitant use; increased risk of
postural hypotension when diuretics given with
tricyclics
Antidiabetics: loop diuretics and thiazides and related
diuretics antagonise hypoglycaemic effect of antidiabetics; increased risk of hyponatraemia when
thiazides and related diuretics plus potassium-
sparing diuretic given with chlorpropamide;
increased risk of hyponatraemia when potassium-
sparing diuretics and aldosterone antagonists plus
thiazide given with chlorpropamide
- **Antiepileptics:** plasma concentration of eplerenone
reduced by ●carbamazepine and ●phenytoin—avoid
concomitant use; increased risk of hyponatraemia
when diuretics given with carbamazepine; acetazolamide increases plasma concentration of
●carbamazepine; effects of furosemide (frusemide)
antagonised by phenytoin; increased risk of osteomalacia when carbonic anhydrase inhibitors given
with phenytoin or primidone; acetazolamide possibly
reduces plasma concentration of primidone
- **Antifungals:** plasma concentration of eplerenone
increased by ●itraconazole and ●ketoconazole—
avoid concomitant use; increased risk of hypokalaemia when loop diuretics or thiazides and related
diuretics given with amphotericin; hydrochlorothiazide increases plasma concentration of fluconazole; plasma concentration of eplerenone increased
by fluconazole (reduce dose of eplerenone)
- **Antipsychotics:** hypokalaemia caused by diuretics
increases risk of ventricular arrhythmias with
●amisulpride and ●sertindole; enhanced hypotensive
effect when diuretics given with phenothiazines;
hypokalaemia caused by diuretics increases risk of
ventricular arrhythmias with ●pimozide (avoid concomitant use)
- **Antivirals:** plasma concentration of eplerenone
increased by ●nelfinavir and ●ritonavir—avoid concomitant use; plasma concentration of eplerenone
increased by saquinavir (reduce dose of eplerenone)
Anxiolytics and Hypnotics: enhanced hypotensive
effect when diuretics given with anxiolytics and
hypnotics; administration of parenteral furosemide
(frusemide) with chloral or triclofos may displace
thyroid hormone from binding sites

Diuretics *(continued)*

- **Atomoxetine:** hypokalaemia caused by diuretics
increases risk of ventricular arrhythmias with
●atomoxetine
- **Barbiturates:** increased risk of osteomalacia when
carbonic anhydrase inhibitors given with phenobarbital; plasma concentration of eplerenone reduced
by ●phenobarbital—avoid concomitant use
- **Beta-blockers:** enhanced hypotensive effect when
diuretics given with beta-blockers; hypokalaemia
caused by loop diuretics or thiazides and related
diuretics increases risk of ventricular arrhythmias
with ●sotalol
Calcium Salts: increased risk of hypercalcaemia when
thiazides and related diuretics given with calcium
salts
Calcium-channel Blockers: enhanced hypotensive
effect when diuretics given with calcium-channel
blockers; plasma concentration of eplerenone
increased by diltiazem and verapamil (reduce dose of
eplerenone)
- **Cardiac Glycosides:** hypokalaemia caused by acetazolamide, loop diuretics or thiazides and related
diuretics increases cardiac toxicity with ●cardiac
glycosides; spironolactone possibly affects plasma
concentration of digitoxin; spironolactone increases
plasma concentration of ●digoxin; potassium canrenoate possibly increases plasma concentration of
digoxin
- **Ciclosporin:** increased risk of nephrotoxicity and
possibly hypermagnesaemia when thiazides and
related diuretics given with ciclosporin; increased
risk of hyperkalaemia when potassium-sparing diuretics and aldosterone antagonists given with
●ciclosporin
Clonidine: enhanced hypotensive effect when diuretics
given with clonidine
Corticosteroids: diuretic effect of diuretics antagonised
by corticosteroids; increased risk of hypokalaemia
when acetazolamide, loop diuretics or thiazides and
related diuretics given with corticosteroids
Cytotoxics: avoidance of spironolactone advised by
manufacturer of mitotane (antagonism of effect);
increased risk of nephrotoxicity and ototoxicity when
diuretics given with platinum compounds
Diazoxide: enhanced hypotensive and hyperglycaemic
effects when diuretics given with diazoxide
Diuretics: increased risk of hypokalaemia when loop
diuretics or thiazides and related diuretics given with
acetazolamide; profound diuresis possible when
metolazone given with furosemide (frusemide);
increased risk of hypokalaemia when thiazides and
related diuretics given with loop diuretics
Dopaminergics: enhanced hypotensive effect when
diuretics given with levodopa
Hormone Antagonists: increased risk of hypercalcaemia when thiazides and related diuretics given
with toremifene; increased risk of hyperkalaemia
when potassium-sparing diuretics and aldosterone
antagonists given with trilostane
Lipid-regulating Drugs: absorption of thiazides and
related diuretics reduced by colestipol and colestyramine (give at least 2 hours apart)
- **Lithium:** loop diuretics and thiazides and related
diuretics reduce excretion of ●lithium (increased
plasma concentration and risk of toxicity)—loop
diuretics safer than thiazides; potassium-sparing
diuretics and aldosterone antagonists reduce excretion of ●lithium (increased plasma concentration and
risk of toxicity); acetazolamide increases the excretion of ●lithium
Methyldopa: enhanced hypotensive effect when diuretics given with methyldopa
Moxisylyte (thymoxamine): enhanced hypotensive
effect when diuretics given with moxisylyte

Diuretics *(continued)*

Moxonidine: enhanced hypotensive effect when diuretics given with moxonidine

Muscle Relaxants: enhanced hypotensive effect when diuretics given with baclofen or tizanidine

Nitrates: enhanced hypotensive effect when diuretics given with nitrates

Oestrogens: diuretic effect of diuretics antagonised by oestrogens

• Potassium Salts: increased risk of hyperkalaemia when potassium-sparing diuretics and aldosterone antagonists given with ●potassium salts

Progestogens: risk of hyperkalaemia when potassium-sparing diuretics and aldosterone antagonists given with drospirenone (monitor serum potassium during first cycle)

Prostaglandins: enhanced hypotensive effect when diuretics given with alprostadil

Sympathomimetics, Beta$_2$: increased risk of hypokalaemia when acetazolamide, loop diuretics or thiazides and related diuretics given with high doses of beta$_2$ sympathomimetics—for CSM advice (hypokalaemia) see p. 173

• Tacrolimus: increased risk of hyperkalaemia when potassium-sparing diuretics and aldosterone antagonists given with ●tacrolimus

Theophylline: increased risk of hypokalaemia when acetazolamide, loop diuretics or thiazides and related diuretics given with theophylline

Vasodilator Antihypertensives: enhanced hypotensive effect when diuretics given with hydralazine, minoxidil or sodium nitroprusside

Vitamins: increased risk of hypercalcaemia when thiazides and related diuretics given with vitamin D

Diuretics, Loop *see* Diuretics

Diuretics, Potassium-sparing and Aldosterone Antagonists *see* Diuretics

Diuretics, Thiazide and related *see* Diuretics

Dobutamine *see* Sympathomimetics

Docetaxel

Antibacterials: *in vitro* studies suggest a possible interaction between docetaxel and erythromycin (consult docetaxel product literature)

Antiepileptics: cytotoxics possibly reduce absorption of phenytoin

Antifungals: *in vitro* studies suggest a possible interaction between docetaxel and ketoconazole (consult docetaxel product literature)

• Antipsychotics: avoid concomitant use of cytotoxics with ●clozapine (increased risk of agranulocytosis)

Cardiac Glycosides: cytotoxics reduce absorption of digoxin tablets

Ciclosporin: *in vitro* studies suggest a possible interaction between docetaxel and ciclosporin (consult docetaxel product literature)

Cytotoxics: plasma concentration of docetaxel increased by sorafenib

Dolasetron *see* 5HT$_3$ Antagonists

Domperidone

Analgesics: effects of domperidone on gastro-intestinal activity antagonised by opioid analgesics

• Antifungals: risk of arrhythmias with domperidone possibly increased by ●ketoconazole

Antimuscarinics: effects of domperidone on gastro-intestinal activity antagonised by antimuscarinics

Dopaminergics: increased risk of extrapyramidal side-effects when domperidone given with amantadine; domperidone possibly antagonises hypoprolactinaemic effects of bromocriptine and cabergoline

Donepezil *see* Parasympathomimetics

Dopamine *see* Sympathomimetics

Dopaminergics *see* Amantadine, Apomorphine, Bromocriptine, Cabergoline, Entacapone, Levodopa, Pergolide, Pramipexole, Quinagolide, Rasagiline, Ropinirole, Rotigotine, Selegiline, and Tolcapone

Dopexamine *see* Sympathomimetics

Doripenem

Antiepileptics: doripenem possibly reduces plasma concentration of valproate

Oestrogens: antibacterials that do not induce liver enzymes possibly reduce contraceptive effect of oestrogens (risk probably small, see p. 478)

Probenecid: excretion of doripenem reduced by probenecid (manufacturers of doripenem advise avoid concomitant use)

Vaccines: antibacterials inactivate oral typhoid vaccine—see p. 752

Dorzolamide *see* Diuretics

Dosulepin (dothiepin) *see* Antidepressants, Tricyclic

Doxapram

Antidepressants: effects of doxapram enhanced by MAOIs

Sympathomimetics: increased risk of hypertension when doxapram given with sympathomimetics

Theophylline: increased CNS stimulation when doxapram given with theophylline

Doxazosin *see* Alpha-blockers

Doxepin *see* Antidepressants, Tricyclic

Doxorubicin

Antiepileptics: cytotoxics possibly reduce absorption of phenytoin

• Antipsychotics: avoid concomitant use of cytotoxics with ●clozapine (increased risk of agranulocytosis)

Antivirals: doxorubicin possibly inhibits effects of stavudine

Cardiac Glycosides: cytotoxics reduce absorption of digoxin tablets

• Ciclosporin: increased risk of neurotoxicity when doxorubicin given with ●ciclosporin

Cytotoxics: plasma concentration of doxorubicin possibly increased by sorafenib

Doxycycline *see* Tetracyclines

Drospirenone *see* Progestogens

Drotrecogin Alfa

• Anticoagulants: manufacturer of drotrecogin alfa advises avoid concomitant use with high doses of ●heparin—consult product literature

Duloxetine

Analgesics: possible increased serotonergic effects when duloxetine given with pethidine or tramadol

• Antibacterials: metabolism of duloxetine inhibited by ●ciprofloxacin—avoid concomitant use

• Antidepressants: metabolism of duloxetine inhibited by ●fluvoxamine—avoid concomitant use; possible increased serotonergic effects when duloxetine given with SSRIs, St John's wort, amitriptyline, clomipramine, ●moclobemide, tryptophan or venlafaxine; duloxetine should not be started until 2 weeks after stopping ●MAOIs, also MAOIs should not be started until at least 5 days after stopping duloxetine; after stopping SSRI-related antidepressants do not start ●moclobemide for at least 1 week

• Antimalarials: avoidance of antidepressants advised by manufacturer of ●artemether/lumefantrine

Atomoxetine: possible increased risk of convulsions when antidepressants given with atomoxetine

5HT$_1$ Agonists: possible increased serotonergic effects when duloxetine given with 5HT$_1$ agonists

• Sibutramine: increased risk of CNS toxicity when SSRI-related antidepressants given with ●sibutramine (manufacturer of sibutramine advises avoid concomitant use)

Dutasteride

Calcium-channel Blockers: plasma concentration of dutasteride increased by diltiazem and verapamil

Dydrogesterone *see* Progestogens

Edrophonium *see* Parasympathomimetics

Efalizumab

• Vaccines: discontinue efalizumab 8 weeks before and until 2 weeks after vaccination with live or live-attenuated ●vaccines

Efavirenz

Analgesics: efavirenz reduces plasma concentration of methadone

Antibacterials: increased risk of rash when efavirenz given with clarithromycin; efavirenz reduces plasma concentration of rifabutin—increase dose of rifabutin; plasma concentration of efavirenz reduced by rifampicin—increase dose of efavirenz

• Antidepressants: plasma concentration of efavirenz reduced by •St John's wort—avoid concomitant use

Antiepileptics: plasma concentration of both drugs reduced when efavirenz given with carbamazepine

• Antifungals: efavirenz reduces plasma concentration of itraconazole and •posaconazole; efavirenz reduces plasma concentration of •voriconazole, also plasma concentration of efavirenz increased (consider increasing voriconazole dose and reducing efavirenz dose); efavirenz possibly reduces plasma concentration of caspofungin—consider increasing dose of caspofungin

• Antipsychotics: efavirenz possibly reduces plasma concentration of •aripiprazole—increase dose of aripiprazole; efavirenz possibly increases plasma concentration of •pimozide (increased risk of ventricular arrhythmias—avoid concomitant use)

• Antivirals: avoidance of efavirenz advised by manufacturer of •atazanavir (plasma concentration of atazanavir reduced); efavirenz reduces plasma concentration of darunavir, fosamprenavir and indinavir; efavirenz possibly reduces plasma concentration of •etravirine—avoid concomitant use; efavirenz reduces plasma concentration of •lopinavir—consider increasing dose of lopinavir; efavirenz possibly reduces plasma concentration of •maraviroc—consider increasing dose of maraviroc; plasma concentration of efavirenz reduced by nevirapine; toxicity of efavirenz increased by ritonavir, monitor liver function tests; efavirenz significantly reduces plasma concentration of saquinavir

• Anxiolytics and Hypnotics: increased risk of prolonged sedation when efavirenz given with •midazolam—avoid concomitant use

Calcium-channel Blockers: efavirenz reduces plasma concentration of diltiazem

• Ciclosporin: efavirenz possibly reduces plasma concentration of •ciclosporin

• Ergot Alkaloids: increased risk of ergotism when efavirenz given with •ergot alkaloids—avoid concomitant use

Grapefruit Juice: plasma concentration of efavirenz possibly increased by grapefruit juice

Lipid-regulating Drugs: efavirenz reduces plasma concentration of atorvastatin, pravastatin and simvastatin

Oestrogens: efavirenz possibly reduces contraceptive effect of oestrogens

• Tacrolimus: efavirenz possibly affects plasma concentration of •tacrolimus

Eletriptan see 5HT₁ Agonists

Emtricitabine

Antivirals: manufacturer of emtricitabine advises avoid concomitant use with lamivudine

Enalapril see ACE Inhibitors

Enoxaparin see Heparins

Enoximone see Phosphodiesterase Inhibitors

Entacapone

• Anticoagulants: entacapone enhances anticoagulant effect of •warfarin

• Antidepressants: manufacturer of entacapone advises caution with moclobemide, paroxetine, tricyclics and venlafaxine; avoid concomitant use of entacapone with non-selective •MAOIs

Dopaminergics: entacapone possibly enhances effects of apomorphine; entacapone possibly reduces plasma concentration of rasagiline; manufacturer of

Entacapone

Dopaminergics *(continued)*
entacapone advises max. dose of 10 mg selegiline if used concomitantly

Iron: absorption of entacapone reduced by *oral* iron

Memantine: effects of dopaminergics possibly enhanced by memantine

Methyldopa: entacapone possibly enhances effects of methyldopa; antiparkinsonian effect of dopaminergics antagonised by methyldopa

Sympathomimetics: entacapone possibly enhances effects of adrenaline (epinephrine), dobutamine, dopamine and noradrenaline (norepinephrine)

Enteral Foods

• Anticoagulants: the presence of vitamin K in some enteral feeds can antagonise the anticoagulant effect of •coumarins and •phenindione

Antiepileptics: enteral feeds possibly reduce absorption of phenytoin

Ephedrine see Sympathomimetics

Epinephrine (adrenaline) see Sympathomimetics

Epirubicin

Antiepileptics: cytotoxics possibly reduce absorption of phenytoin

• Antipsychotics: avoid concomitant use of cytotoxics with •clozapine (increased risk of agranulocytosis)

Cardiac Glycosides: cytotoxics reduce absorption of digoxin tablets

• Ulcer-healing Drugs: plasma concentration of epirubicin increased by •cimetidine

Eplerenone see Diuretics

Eprosartan see Angiotensin-II Receptor Antagonists

Eptifibatide

Iloprost: increased risk of bleeding when eptifibatide given with iloprost

Ergometrine see Ergot Alkaloids

Ergot Alkaloids

Anaesthetics, General: effects of ergometrine on the parturient uterus reduced by halothane

• Antibacterials: increased risk of ergotism when ergotamine and methysergide given with •macrolides or •telithromycin—avoid concomitant use; avoidance of ergotamine and methysergide advised by manufacturer of •quinupristin/dalfopristin; increased risk of ergotism when ergotamine and methysergide given with tetracyclines

Antidepressants: possible risk of hypertension when ergotamine and methysergide given with reboxetine

• Antifungals: increased risk of ergotism when ergotamine and methysergide given with •imidazoles or •triazoles—avoid concomitant use

• Antivirals: plasma concentration of ergot alkaloids possibly increased by •atazanavir—avoid concomitant use; increased risk of ergotism when ergot alkaloids given with •efavirenz—avoid concomitant use; increased risk of ergotism when ergotamine and methysergide given with •fosamprenavir, •indinavir, •nelfinavir, •ritonavir or •saquinavir—avoid concomitant use

Beta-blockers: increased peripheral vasoconstriction when ergotamine and methysergide given with beta-blockers

• 5HT₁ Agonists: increased risk of vasospasm when ergotamine and methysergide given with •almotriptan, •rizatriptan, •sumatriptan or •zolmitriptan (avoid ergotamine and methysergide for 6 hours after almotriptan, rizatriptan, sumatriptan or zolmitriptan, avoid almotriptan, rizatriptan, sumatriptan or zolmitriptan for 24 hours after ergotamine and methysergide); increased risk of vasospasm when ergotamine and methysergide given with •eletriptan or •frovatriptan (avoid ergotamine and methysergide for 24 hours after eletriptan or frovatriptan, avoid eletriptan or frovatriptan for 24 hours after ergotamine and methysergide)

Ergot Alkaloids (continued)

Sympathomimetics: increased risk of ergotism when ergotamine and methysergide given with sympathomimetics

- Ulcer-healing Drugs: increased risk of ergotism when ergotamine and methysergide given with ●cimetidine—avoid concomitant use

Ergotamine and Methysergide see Ergot Alkaloids

Erlotinib

- Analgesics: increased risk of bleeding when erlotinib given with ●NSAIDs

Antibacterials: metabolism of erlotinib accelerated by rifampicin (reduced plasma concentration)

- Anticoagulants: increased risk of bleeding when erlotinib given with ●coumarins

Antiepileptics: cytotoxics possibly reduce absorption of phenytoin

Antifungals: metabolism of erlotinib inhibited by ketoconazole (increased plasma concentration)

- Antipsychotics: avoid concomitant use of cytotoxics with ●clozapine (increased risk of agranulocytosis)

Cardiac Glycosides: cytotoxics reduce absorption of digoxin tablets

Cytotoxics: plasma concentration of erlotinib possibly increased by capecitabine

Tobacco: plasma concentration of erlotinib reduced by tobacco smoking

Ertapenem

Antiepileptics: ertapenem possibly reduces plasma concentration of valproate

Oestrogens: antibacterials that do not induce liver enzymes possibly reduce contraceptive effect of oestrogens (risk probably small, see p. 478)

Vaccines: antibacterials inactivate oral typhoid vaccine—see p. 752

Erythromycin see Macrolides

Escitalopram see Antidepressants, SSRI

Esmolol see Beta-blockers

Esomeprazole see Proton Pump Inhibitors

Estradiol see Oestrogens

Estriol see Oestrogens

Estrone see Oestrogens

Estropipate see Oestrogens

Etanercept

Abatacept: increased risk of side-effects when etanercept given with abatacept

- Anakinra: increased risk of side-effects when etanercept given with ●anakinra—avoid concomitant use

- Vaccines: avoid concomitant use of etanercept with live ●vaccines (see p. 725)

Ethinylestradiol see Oestrogens

Ethosuximide

- Antibacterials: metabolism of ethosuximide inhibited by ●isoniazid (increased plasma concentration and risk of toxicity)

- Antidepressants: anticonvulsant effect of antiepileptics possibly antagonised by MAOIs and ●tricyclic-related antidepressants (convulsive threshold lowered); anticonvulsant effect of antiepileptics antagonised by ●SSRIs and ●tricyclics (convulsive threshold lowered); avoid concomitant use of antiepileptics with ●St John's wort

- Antiepileptics: plasma concentration of ethosuximide possibly reduced by carbamazepine and primidone; plasma concentration of ethosuximide possibly reduced by ●phenytoin, also plasma concentration of phenytoin possibly increased; plasma concentration of ethosuximide possibly increased by valproate

- Antimalarials: possible increased risk of convulsions when antiepileptics given with chloroquine and hydroxychloroquine; anticonvulsant effect of antiepileptics antagonised by ●mefloquine

- Antipsychotics: anticonvulsant effect of ethosuximide antagonised by ●antipsychotics (convulsive threshold lowered)

Ethosuximide (continued)

Barbiturates: plasma concentration of ethosuximide possibly reduced by phenobarbital

Etodolac see NSAIDs

Etomidate see Anaesthetics, General

Etonogestrel see Progestogens

Etoposide

- Anticoagulants: etoposide possibly enhances anticoagulant effect of ●coumarins

Antiepileptics: plasma concentration of etoposide possibly reduced by phenytoin; cytotoxics possibly reduce absorption of phenytoin

- Antipsychotics: avoid concomitant use of cytotoxics with ●clozapine (increased risk of agranulocytosis)

Barbiturates: plasma concentration of etoposide possibly reduced by phenobarbital

Cardiac Glycosides: cytotoxics reduce absorption of digoxin tablets

Ciclosporin: plasma concentration of etoposide possibly increased by ciclosporin (increased risk of toxicity)

Etoricoxib see NSAIDs

Etravirine

- Antibacterials: plasma concentration of etravirine increased by ●clarithromycin, also plasma concentration of clarithromycin reduced; plasma concentration of both drugs reduced when etravirine given with ●rifabutin; manufacturer of etravirine advises avoid concomitant use with rifampicin

Antidepressants: manufacturer of etravirine advises avoid concomitant use with St John's wort

Antiepileptics: manufacturer of etravirine advises avoid concomitant use with carbamazepine and phenytoin

- Antivirals: plasma concentration of etravirine possibly reduced by ●efavirenz and ●nevirapine—avoid concomitant use; etravirine increases plasma concentration of ●fosamprenavir (consider reducing dose of fosamprenavir); etravirine possibly reduces plasma concentration of ●indinavir—avoid concomitant use; etravirine possibly reduces plasma concentration of maraviroc; etravirine possibly increases plasma concentration of nelfinavir—avoid concomitant use; plasma concentration of etravirine reduced by ●tipranavir, also plasma concentration of tipranavir increased (avoid concomitant use)

Barbiturates: manufacturer of etravirine advises avoid concomitant use with phenobarbital

Cardiac Glycosides: etravirine increases plasma concentration of digoxin

Lipid-regulating Drugs: etravirine possibly reduces plasma concentration of atorvastatin

Sildenafil: etravirine reduces plasma concentration of sildenafil

Etynodiol see Progestogens

Exemestane

Antibacterials: plasma concentration of exemestane possibly reduced by rifampicin

Ezetimibe

Anticoagulants: ezetimibe possibly enhances anticoagulant effect of coumarins

- Ciclosporin: plasma concentration of both drugs may increase when ezetimibe given with ●ciclosporin

Lipid-regulating Drugs: increased risk of cholelithiasis and gallbladder disease when ezetimibe given with fibrates—discontinue if suspected

Famciclovir

Probenecid: excretion of famciclovir possibly reduced by probenecid (increased plasma concentration)

Famotidine see Histamine H$_2$-antagonists

Felodipine see Calcium-channel Blockers

Fenbufen see NSAIDs

Fenofibrate see Fibrates

Fenoprofen see NSAIDs

Fenoterol see Sympathomimetics, Beta$_2$

Fentanyl see Opioid Analgesics

Ferrous Salts see Iron

Fesoterodine *see* Antimuscarinics
Fexofenadine *see* Antihistamines
Fibrates
- Antibacterials: increased risk of myopathy when fibrates given with •daptomycin (preferably avoid concomitant use)
- Anticoagulants: fibrates enhance anticoagulant effect of •coumarins and •phenindione
- Antidiabetics: gemfibrozil increases plasma concentration of •rosiglitazone (consider reducing dose of rosiglitazone); fibrates may improve glucose tolerance and have an additive effect with insulin or sulphonylureas; gemfibrozil possibly enhances hypoglycaemic effect of nateglinide; increased risk of severe hypoglycaemia when gemfibrozil given with •repaglinide—avoid concomitant use
  Ciclosporin: increased risk of renal impairment when bezafibrate or fenofibrate given with ciclosporin
- Cytotoxics: gemfibrozil increases plasma concentration of •bexarotene—avoid concomitant use
- Lipid-regulating Drugs: increased risk of cholelithiasis and gallbladder disaese when fibrates given with ezetimibe—discontinue if suspected; increased risk of myopathy when fibrates given with •statins; increased risk of myopathy when gemfibrozil given with •statins (preferably avoid concomitant use)
Filgrastim
  Note. Pegfilgrastim interactions as for filgrastim
  Cytotoxics: neutropenia possibly exacerbated when filgrastim given with fluorouracil
Flavoxate *see* Antimuscarinics
Flecainide
  Anaesthetics, Local: increased myocardial depression when anti-arrhythmics given with bupivacaine, levobupivacaine, prilocaine or ropivacaine
- Anti-arrhythmics: increased myocardial depression when anti-arrhythmics given with other •anti-arrhythmics; plasma concentration of flecainide increased by •amiodarone (halve dose of flecainide)
- Antidepressants: plasma concentration of flecainide increased by fluoxetine; increased risk of ventricular arrhythmias when flecainide given with •tricyclics
- Antihistamines: increased risk of ventricular arrhythmias when flecainide given with •mizolastine—avoid concomitant use
- Antimalarials: avoidance of flecainide advised by manufacturer of •artemether/lumefantrine (risk of ventricular arrhythmias); plasma concentration of flecainide increased by •quinine
- Antimuscarinics: increased risk of ventricular arrhythmias when flecainide given with •tolterodine
- Antipsychotics: increased risk of ventricular arrhythmias when anti-arrhythmics that prolong the QT interval given with •antipsychotics that prolong the QT interval; increased risk of arrhythmias when flecainide given with •clozapine
- Antivirals: plasma concentration of flecainide possibly increased by •fosamprenavir, •indinavir, •lopinavir and •ritonavir (increased risk of ventricular arrhythmias—avoid concomitant use)
- Beta-blockers: increased risk of myocardial depression and bradycardia when flecainide given with •beta-blockers; increased myocardial depression when anti-arrhythmics given with •beta-blockers
- Calcium-channel Blockers: increased risk of myocardial depression and asystole when flecainide given with •verapamil
- Diuretics: increased cardiac toxicity with flecainide if hypokalaemia occurs with •acetazolamide, •loop diuretics or •thiazides and related diuretics
- 5HT₃ Antagonists: increased risk of ventricular arrhythmias when flecainide given with •dolasetron—avoid concomitant use
  Ulcer-healing Drugs: metabolism of flecainide inhibited by cimetidine (increased plasma concentration)
Flucloxacillin *see* Penicillins

Fluconazole *see* Antifungals, Triazole
Flucytosine
  Antifungals: renal excretion of flucytosine decreased and cellular uptake increased by amphotericin (toxicity possibly increased)
  Cytotoxics: plasma concentration of flucytosine possibly reduced by cytarabine
Fludarabine
  Antiepileptics: cytotoxics possibly reduce absorption of phenytoin
- Antipsychotics: avoid concomitant use of cytotoxics with •clozapine (increased risk of agranulocytosis)
  Cardiac Glycosides: cytotoxics reduce absorption of digoxin tablets
- Cytotoxics: fludarabine increases intracellular concentration of cytarabine; increased pulmonary toxicity when fludarabine given with •pentostatin (unacceptably high incidence of fatalities)
  Dipyridamole: effects of fludarabine possibly reduced by dipyridamole
Fludrocortisone *see* Corticosteroids
Flunisolide *see* Corticosteroids
Fluorides
  Calcium Salts: absorption of fluorides reduced by calcium salts
Fluorouracil
  Note. Capecitabine is a prodrug of fluorouracil
  Note. Tegafur is a prodrug of fluorouracil
- Allopurinol: manufacturer of capecitabine advises avoid concomitant use with •allopurinol
  Antibacterials: metabolism of fluorouracil inhibited by metronidazole (increased toxicity)
- Anticoagulants: fluorouracil enhances anticoagulant effect of •coumarins
  Antiepileptics: fluorouracil possibly inhibits metabolism of phenytoin (increased risk of toxicity); cytotoxics possibly reduce absorption of phenytoin
- Antipsychotics: avoid concomitant use of cytotoxics with •clozapine (increased risk of agranulocytosis)
  Cardiac Glycosides: cytotoxics reduce absorption of digoxin tablets
  Cytotoxics: capecitabine possibly increases plasma concentration of erlotinib
  Filgrastim: neutropenia possibly exacerbated when fluorouracil given with filgrastim
- Temoporfin: increased skin photosensitivity when topical fluorouracil used with •temoporfin
  Ulcer-healing Drugs: metabolism of fluorouracil inhibited by cimetidine (increased plasma concentration)
Fluoxetine *see* Antidepressants, SSRI
Flupentixol *see* Antipsychotics
Fluphenazine *see* Antipsychotics
Flurazepam *see* Anxiolytics and Hypnotics
Flurbiprofen *see* NSAIDs
Flutamide
- Anticoagulants: flutamide enhances anticoagulant effect of •coumarins
Fluticasone *see* Corticosteroids
Fluvastatin *see* Statins
Fluvoxamine *see* Antidepressants, SSRI
Folates
  Aminosalicylates: absorption of folic acid possibly reduced by sulfasalazine
  Antiepileptics: folates possibly reduce plasma concentration of phenytoin and primidone
  Barbiturates: folates possibly reduce plasma concentration of phenobarbital
Folic Acid *see* Folates
Folinic Acid *see* Folates
Formoterol (eformoterol) *see* Sympathomimetics, Beta₂
Fosamprenavir
  Note. Fosamprenavir is a prodrug of amprenavir
  Analgesics: fosamprenavir reduces plasma concentration of methadone
  Antacids: absorption of fosamprenavir possibly reduced by antacids

Fosamprenavir *(continued)*

- Anti-arrhythmics: fosamprenavir possibly increases plasma concentration of ●amiodarone, ●flecainide and ●propafenone (increased risk of ventricular arrhythmias—avoid concomitant use); fosamprenavir possibly increases plasma concentration of ●lidocaine (lignocaine)—avoid concomitant use

- Antibacterials: plasma concentration of both drugs increased when fosamprenavir given with erythromycin; fosamprenavir increases plasma concentration of ●rifabutin (reduce dose of rifabutin); plasma concentration of fosamprenavir significantly reduced by ●rifampicin—avoid concomitant use; fosamprenavir possibly increases plasma concentration of dapsone; avoidance of concomitant fosamprenavir in severe renal and hepatic impairment advised by manufacturer of ●telithromycin

  Anticoagulants: fosamprenavir may enhance or reduce anticoagulant effect of coumarins; avoidance of fosamprenavir advised by manufacturer of rivaroxaban

- Antidepressants: plasma concentration of fosamprenavir reduced by ●St John's wort—avoid concomitant use; fosamprenavir possibly increases side-effects of tricyclics

  Antiepileptics: plasma concentration of fosamprenavir possibly reduced by carbamazepine and phenytoin

  Antifungals: fosamprenavir increases plasma concentration of ketoconazole; fosamprenavir possibly increases plasma concentration of itraconazole

  Antihistamines: fosamprenavir possibly increases plasma concentration of loratadine

  Antimalarials: caution with fosamprenavir advised by manufacturer of artemether/lumefantrine

  Antimuscarinics: avoidance of fosamprenavir advised by manufacturer of darifenacin and tolterodine

- Antipsychotics: fosamprenavir possibly inhibits metabolism of ●aripiprazole (reduce dose of aripiprazole); fosamprenavir possibly increases plasma concentration of clozapine; fosamprenavir increases plasma concentration of ●pimozide and ●sertindole (increased risk of ventricular arrhythmias—avoid concomitant use)

- Antivirals: plasma concentration of fosamprenavir reduced by efavirenz and ●tipranavir; plasma concentration of fosamprenavir increased by ●etravirine (consider reducing dose of fosamprenavir); plasma concentration of fosamprenavir reduced by lopinavir, effect on lopinavir plasma concentration not predictable—avoid concomitant use; plasma concentration of fosamprenavir possibly reduced by nevirapine

- Anxiolytics and Hypnotics: increased risk of prolonged sedation and respiratory depression when fosamprenavir given with ●alprazolam, clonazepam, ●diazepam, ●flurazepam or ●midazolam

  Barbiturates: plasma concentration of fosamprenavir possibly reduced by phenobarbital

- Cilostazol: fosamprenavir possibly increases plasma concentration of ●cilostazol—avoid concomitant use

- Ergot Alkaloids: increased risk of ergotism when fosamprenavir given with ●ergotamine and methysergide—avoid concomitant use

- Lipid-regulating Drugs: possible increased risk of myopathy when fosamprenavir given with atorvastatin; possible increased risk of myopathy when fosamprenavir given with ●rosuvastatin or ●simvastatin—avoid concomitant use

  Oestrogens: fosamprenavir increases plasma concentration of oestrogens, also plasma concentration of fosamprenavir reduced—alternative contraception recommended

  Progestogens: fosamprenavir increases plasma concentration of progestogens, also plasma concentra-

Fosamprenavir

  Progestogens *(continued)*
  tion of fosamprenavir reduced—alternative contraception recommended

  Sildenafil: fosamprenavir possibly increases plasma concentration of sildenafil—reduce initial dose of sildenafil

  Tadalafil: fosamprenavir possibly increases plasma concentration of tadalafil

  Ulcer-healing Drugs: fosamprenavir possibly increases plasma concentration of cimetidine

  Vardenafil: fosamprenavir possibly increases plasma concentration of vardenafil

Fosaprepitant *see* Aprepitant

Foscarnet

  Antivirals: avoidance of foscarnet advised by manufacturer of lamivudine

Fosinopril *see* ACE Inhibitors

Fosphenytoin *see* Phenytoin

Framycetin *see* Aminoglycosides

Frovatriptan *see* 5HT$_1$ Agonists

Furosemide (frusemide) *see* Diuretics

Fusidic Acid

- Antivirals: plasma concentration of both drugs increased when fusidic acid given with ●ritonavir—avoid concomitant use

- Lipid-regulating Drugs: possible increased risk of myopathy when fusidic acid given with atorvastatin; increased risk of myopathy when fusidic acid given with ●simvastatin

  Oestrogens: antibacterials that do not induce liver enzymes possibly reduce contraceptive effect of oestrogens (risk probably small, see p. 478)

  Sugammadex: fusidic acid possibly reduces response to sugammadex

  Vaccines: antibacterials inactivate oral typhoid vaccine—see p. 752

Gabapentin

  Antacids: absorption of gabapentin reduced by antacids

- Antidepressants: anticonvulsant effect of antiepileptics possibly antagonised by MAOIs and ●tricyclic-related antidepressants (convulsive threshold lowered); anticonvulsant effect of antiepileptics antagonised by ●SSRIs and ●tricyclics (convulsive threshold lowered); avoid concomitant use of antiepileptics with ●St John's wort

- Antimalarials: possible increased risk of convulsions when antiepileptics given with chloroquine and hydroxychloroquine; anticonvulsant effect of antiepileptics antagonised by ●mefloquine

Galantamine *see* Parasympathomimetics

Ganciclovir

  Note. Increased risk of myelosuppression with other myelosuppressive drugs—consult product literature

  Note. Valganciclovir interactions as for ganciclovir

- Antibacterials: increased risk of convulsions when ganciclovir given with ●imipenem with cilastatin

- Antivirals: ganciclovir possibly increases plasma concentration of didanosine; avoidance of intravenous ganciclovir advised by manufacturer of lamivudine; profound myelosuppression when ganciclovir given with ●zidovudine (if possible avoid concomitant administration, particularly during initial ganciclovir therapy)

  Cytotoxics: plasma concentration of ganciclovir possibly increased by mycophenolate, also plasma concentration of inactive metabolite of mycophenolate possibly increased

  Probenecid: excretion of ganciclovir reduced by probenecid (increased plasma concentration and risk of toxicity)

  Tacrolimus: possible increased risk of nephrotoxicity when ganciclovir given with tacrolimus

Gemeprost *see* Prostaglandins

Gemfibrozil *see* Fibrates

Gentamicin *see* Aminoglycosides
Gestodene *see* Progestogens
Gestrinone

  Antibacterials: metabolism of gestrinone accelerated by rifampicin (reduced plasma concentration)
  Antiepileptics: metabolism of gestrinone accelerated by carbamazepine, phenytoin and primidone (reduced plasma concentration)
  Barbiturates: metabolism of gestrinone accelerated by barbiturates (reduced plasma concentration)

Glibenclamide *see* Antidiabetics
Gliclazide *see* Antidiabetics
Glimepiride *see* Antidiabetics
Glipizide *see* Antidiabetics
Glucosamine

• Anticoagulants: glucosamine enhances anticoagulant effect of ●warfarin (avoid concomitant use)

Glyceryl Trinitrate *see* Nitrates
Glycopyrronium *see* Antimuscarinics
Gold

  Penicillamine: avoidance of gold advised by manufacturer of penicillamine (increased risk of toxicity)

Grapefruit Juice

  Anti-arrhythmics: grapefruit juice increases plasma concentration of amiodarone
  Antimalarials: grapefruit juice possibly increases plasma concentration of artemether/lumefantrine
  Antivirals: grapefruit juice possibly increases plasma concentration of efavirenz
  Anxiolytics and Hypnotics: grapefruit juice increases plasma concentration of buspirone
  Calcium-channel Blockers: grapefruit juice increases plasma concentration of felodipine, isradipine, lacidipine, lercanidipine, nicardipine, nifedipine, nimodipine and verapamil

• Ciclosporin: grapefruit juice increases plasma concentration of ●ciclosporin (increased risk of toxicity)
• Cytotoxics: avoidance of grapefruit juice advised by manufacturer of ●lapatinib and ●nilotinib

  Ivabradine: grapefruit juice increases plasma concentration of ivabradine

• Lipid-regulating Drugs: grapefruit juice possibly increases plasma concentration of atorvastatin; grapefruit juice increases plasma concentration of ●simvastatin—avoid concomitant use

  Sildenafil: grapefruit juice possibly increases plasma concentration of sildenafil

• Sirolimus: grapefruit juice increases plasma concentration of ●sirolimus—avoid concomitant use
• Tacrolimus: grapefruit juice increases plasma concentration of ●tacrolimus

  Tadalafil: grapefruit juice possibly increases plasma concentration of tadalafil

• Vardenafil: grapefruit juice possibly increases plasma concentration of ●vardenafil—avoid concomitant use

Griseofulvin

  Alcohol: griseofulvin possibly enhances effects of alcohol

• Anticoagulants: griseofulvin reduces anticoagulant effect of ●coumarins

  Antiepileptics: absorption of griseofulvin reduced by primidone (reduced effect)
  Barbiturates: absorption of griseofulvin reduced by phenobarbital (reduced effect)
  Ciclosporin: griseofulvin possibly reduces plasma concentration of ciclosporin

• Oestrogens: griseofulvin accelerates metabolism of ●oestrogens (reduced contraceptive effect—see p. 478)
• Progestogens: griseofulvin accelerates metabolism of ●progestogens (reduced contraceptive effect—see p. 478)

Guanethidine *see* Adrenergic Neurone Blockers
Haloperidol *see* Antipsychotics
Halothane *see* Anaesthetics, General

Heparin *see* Heparins
Heparins

  ACE Inhibitors: increased risk of hyperkalaemia when heparins given with ACE inhibitors
  Aliskiren: increased risk of hyperkalaemia when heparins given with aliskiren

• Analgesics: possible increased risk of bleeding when heparins given with NSAIDs; increased risk of haemorrhage when anticoagulants given with intravenous ●diclofenac (avoid concomitant use, including low-dose heparin); increased risk of haemorrhage when anticoagulants given with ●ketorolac (avoid concomitant use, including low-dose heparin); anticoagulant effect of heparins enhanced by ●aspirin

  Angiotensin-II Receptor Antagonists: increased risk of hyperkalaemia when heparin given with angiotensin-II receptor antagonists
  Clopidogrel: increased risk of bleeding when heparins given with clopidogrel
  Dipyridamole: anticoagulant effect of heparins enhanced by dipyridamole

• Drotrecogin Alfa: avoidance of concomitant use of high doses of heparin with drotrecogin alfa advised by manufacturer of ●drotrecogin alfa—consult product literature

  Iloprost: anticoagulant effect of heparins possibly enhanced by iloprost

• Nitrates: anticoagulant effect of heparins reduced by infusion of ●glyceryl trinitrate

  Sibutramine: increased risk of bleeding when anticoagulants given with sibutramine

Histamine H$_2$-antagonists

• Alpha-blockers: cimetidine and ranitidine antagonise effects of ●tolazoline

  Analgesics: cimetidine possibly increases plasma concentration of azapropazone; cimetidine inhibits metabolism of opioid analgesics (increased plasma concentration)

• Anti-arrhythmics: cimetidine increases plasma concentration of amiodarone and ●propafenone; cimetidine inhibits metabolism of flecainide (increased plasma concentration); cimetidine increases plasma concentration of ●lidocaine (lignocaine) (increased risk of toxicity)

  Antibacterials: histamine H$_2$-antagonists reduce absorption of cefpodoxime; cimetidine increases plasma concentration of erythromycin (increased risk of toxicity, including deafness); cimetidine inhibits metabolism of metronidazole (increased plasma concentration); metabolism of cimetidine accelerated by rifampicin (reduced plasma concentration)

• Anticoagulants: cimetidine inhibits metabolism of ●coumarins (enhanced anticoagulant effect)

  Antidepressants: cimetidine increases plasma concentration of citalopram, escitalopram, mirtazapine and sertraline; cimetidine inhibits metabolism of amitriptyline, doxepin, imipramine and nortriptyline (increased plasma concentration); cimetidine increases plasma concentration of moclobemide (halve dose of moclobemide); cimetidine possibly increases plasma concentration of tricyclics
  Antidiabetics: cimetidine reduces excretion of metformin (increased plasma concentration); cimetidine enhances hypoglycaemic effect of sulphonylureas

• Antiepileptics: cimetidine inhibits metabolism of ●carbamazepine, ●phenytoin and ●valproate (increased plasma concentration)

• Antifungals: histamine H$_2$-antagonists reduce absorption of itraconazole and ketoconazole; cimetidine reduces plasma concentration of ●posaconazole; cimetidine increases plasma concentration of terbinafine

Histamine H$_2$-antagonists *(continued)*

Antihistamines: manufacturer of loratadine advises cimetidine possibly increases plasma concentration of loratadine

- Antimalarials: avoidance of cimetidine advised by manufacturer of ●artemether/lumefantrine; cimetidine inhibits metabolism of chloroquine and hydroxychloroquine and quinine (increased plasma concentration)

- Antipsychotics: cimetidine possibly enhances effects of antipsychotics, chlorpromazine and clozapine; increased risk of ventricular arrhythmias when cimetidine given with ●sertindole—avoid concomitant use

Antivirals: histamine H$_2$-antagonists possibly reduce plasma concentration of atazanavir; plasma concentration of fosamprenavir possibly increased by fosamprenavir; histamine H$_2$-antagonists possibly increase plasma concentration of raltegravir—manufacturer of raltegravir advises avoid concomitant use

Anxiolytics and Hypnotics: cimetidine inhibits metabolism of benzodiazepines, clomethiazole and zaleplon (increased plasma concentration); cimetidine increases plasma concentration of melatonin

Beta-blockers: cimetidine increases plasma concentration of labetalol, metoprolol and propranolol

Calcium-channel Blockers: cimetidine possibly inhibits metabolism of calcium-channel blockers (increased plasma concentration); cimetidine increases plasma concentration of isradipine (halve dose of isradipine)

- Ciclosporin: cimetidine possibly increases plasma concentration of ●ciclosporin

- Cilostazol: cimetidine possibly increases plasma concentration of ●cilostazol—avoid concomitant use

- Cytotoxics: cimetidine possibly enhances myelosuppressive effects of carmustine and lomustine; cimetidine increases plasma concentration of ●epirubicin; cimetidine inhibits metabolism of fluorouracil (increased plasma concentration); famotidine possibly reduces plasma concentration of dasatinib; histamine H$_2$-antagonists possibly reduce absorption of lapatinib

Dopaminergics: cimetidine reduces excretion of pramipexole (increased plasma concentration)

- Ergot Alkaloids: increased risk of ergotism when cimetidine given with ●ergotamine and methysergide—avoid concomitant use

Hormone Antagonists: absorption of cimetidine possibly delayed by octreotide

5HT$_1$ Agonists: cimetidine inhibits metabolism of zolmitriptan (reduce dose of zolmitriptan)

Mebendazole: cimetidine possibly inhibits metabolism of mebendazole (increased plasma concentration)

Sildenafil: cimetidine increases plasma concentration of sildenafil (reduce initial dose of sildenafil)

- Theophylline: cimetidine inhibits metabolism of ●theophylline (increased plasma concentration)

Thyroid Hormones: cimetidine reduces absorption of levothyroxine (thyroxine)

Homatropine *see* Antimuscarinics

Hormone Antagonists *see* Bicalutamide, Danazol, Dutasteride, Exemestane, Flutamide, Gestrinone, Lanreotide, Octreotide, Tamoxifen, Toremifene, and Trilostane

5HT$_1$ Agonists

- Antibacterials: plasma concentration of eletriptan increased by ●clarithromycin and ●erythromycin (risk of toxicity)—avoid concomitant use; metabolism of zolmitriptan possibly inhibited by quinolones (reduce dose of zolmitriptan)

- Antidepressants: increased risk of CNS toxicity when sumatriptan given with ●citalopram, ●escitalopram, ●fluoxetine, ●fluvoxamine or ●paroxetine; metabolism of frovatriptan inhibited by fluvoxamine; metabolism of zolmitriptan possibly inhibited by fluvoxamine (reduce dose of zolmitriptan); increased

5HT$_1$ Agonists

- Antidepressants *(continued)*
risk of CNS toxicity when sumatriptan given with ●sertraline (manufacturer of sertraline advises avoid concomitant use); possible increased serotonergic effects when 5HT$_1$ agonists given with duloxetine; risk of CNS toxicity when rizatriptan or sumatriptan given with ●MAOIs (avoid rizatriptan or sumatriptan for 2 weeks after MAOIs); increased risk of CNS toxicity when zolmitriptan given with ●MAOIs; risk of CNS toxicity when rizatriptan or sumatriptan given with ●moclobemide (avoid rizatriptan or sumatriptan for 2 weeks after moclobemide); risk of CNS toxicity when zolmitriptan given with ●moclobemide (reduce dose of zolmitriptan); possible increased serotonergic effects when frovatriptan given with SSRIs; increased serotonergic effects when 5HT$_1$ agonists given with ●St John's wort—avoid concomitant use

- Antifungals: plasma concentration of eletriptan increased by ●itraconazole and ●ketoconazole (risk of toxicity)—avoid concomitant use; plasma concentration of almotriptan increased by ketoconazole (increased risk of toxicity)

- Antivirals: plasma concentration of eletriptan increased by ●indinavir, ●nelfinavir and ●ritonavir (risk of toxicity)—avoid concomitant use

Beta-blockers: plasma concentration of rizatriptan increased by propranolol (manufacturer of rizatriptan advises halve dose and avoid within 2 hours of propranolol)

- Ergot Alkaloids: increased risk of vasospasm when eletriptan or frovatriptan given with ●ergotamine and methysergide (avoid ergotamine and methysergide for 24 hours after eletriptan or frovatriptan, avoid eletriptan or frovatriptan for 24 hours after ergotamine and methysergide); increased risk of vasospasm when almotriptan, rizatriptan, sumatriptan or zolmitriptan given with ●ergotamine and methysergide (avoid ergotamine and methysergide for 6 hours after almotriptan, rizatriptan, sumatriptan or zolmitriptan, avoid almotriptan, rizatriptan, sumatriptan or zolmitriptan for 24 hours after ergotamine and methysergide)

Ulcer-healing Drugs: metabolism of zolmitriptan inhibited by cimetidine (reduce dose of zolmitriptan)

5HT$_3$ Antagonists

Analgesics: ondansetron possibly antagonises effects of tramadol

- Anti-arrhythmics: increased risk of ventricular arrhythmias when dolasetron given with ●amiodarone, ●disopyramide, ●flecainide, ●lidocaine (lignocaine) or ●propafenone—avoid concomitant use

Antibacterials: metabolism of ondansetron accelerated by rifampicin (reduced effect)

Antiepileptics: metabolism of ondansetron accelerated by carbamazepine and phenytoin (reduced effect)

- Beta-blockers: increased risk of ventricular arrhythmias when dolasetron given with ●sotalol—avoid concomitant use

Hydralazine *see* Vasodilator Antihypertensives

Hydrochlorothiazide *see* Diuretics

Hydrocortisone *see* Corticosteroids

Hydroflumethiazide *see* Diuretics

Hydromorphone *see* Opioid Analgesics

Hydrotalcite *see* Antacids

Hydroxocobalamin

Antibacterials: response to hydroxocobalamin reduced by chloramphenicol

Hydroxycarbamide

Antiepileptics: cytotoxics possibly reduce absorption of phenytoin

- Antipsychotics: avoid concomitant use of cytotoxics with ●clozapine (increased risk of agranulocytosis)

Hydroxycarbamide *(continued)*
- Antivirals: increased risk of toxicity when hydroxycarbamide given with ●didanosine and ●stavudine—avoid concomitant use

Cardiac Glycosides: cytotoxics reduce absorption of digoxin tablets

Hydroxychloroquine *see* Chloroquine and Hydroxychloroquine

Hydroxyzine *see* Antihistamines

Hyoscine *see* Antimuscarinics

Ibandronic Acid *see* Bisphosphonates

Ibuprofen *see* NSAIDs

Ifosfamide
- Anticoagulants: ifosfamide possibly enhances anticoagulant effect of ●coumarins

Antiepileptics: cytotoxics possibly reduce absorption of phenytoin
- Antipsychotics: avoid concomitant use of cytotoxics with ●clozapine (increased risk of agranulocytosis)

Cardiac Glycosides: cytotoxics reduce absorption of digoxin tablets

Iloprost
Analgesics: increased risk of bleeding when iloprost given with NSAIDs or aspirin

Anticoagulants: iloprost possibly enhances anticoagulant effect of coumarins and heparins; increased risk of bleeding when iloprost given with phenindione

Clopidogrel: increased risk of bleeding when iloprost given with clopidogrel

Eptifibatide: increased risk of bleeding when iloprost given with eptifibatide

Tirofiban: increased risk of bleeding when iloprost given with tirofiban

Imatinib
- Antibacterials: plasma concentration of imatinib reduced by ●rifampicin—avoid concomitant use

Anticoagulants: manufacturer of imatinib advises replacement of warfarin with a heparin (possibility of enhanced warfarin effect)
- Antidepressants: plasma concentration of imatinib reduced by ●St John's wort—avoid concomitant use
- Antiepileptics: plasma concentration of imatinib reduced by ●carbamazepine, ●oxcarbazepine and ●phenytoin—avoid concomitant use; cytotoxics possibly reduce absorption of phenytoin

Antifungals: plasma concentration of imatinib increased by ketoconazole
- Antipsychotics: avoid concomitant use of cytotoxics with ●clozapine (increased risk of agranulocytosis)

Cardiac Glycosides: cytotoxics reduce absorption of digoxin tablets

Ciclosporin: imatinib possibly increases plasma concentration of ciclosporin

Lipid-regulating Drugs: imatinib increases plasma concentration of simvastatin

Thyroid Hormones: imatinib possibly reduces plasma concentration of levothyroxine (thyroxine)

Imidapril *see* ACE Inhibitors

Imipenem with Cilastatin
Antiepileptics: imipenem with cilastatin reduces plasma concentration of valproate
- Antivirals: increased risk of convulsions when imipenem with cilastatin given with ●ganciclovir

Oestrogens: antibacterials that do not induce liver enzymes possibly reduce contraceptive effect of oestrogens (risk probably small, see p. 478)

Vaccines: antibacterials inactivate oral typhoid vaccine—see p. 752

Imipramine *see* Antidepressants, Tricyclic

Immunoglobulins
Note. For advice on immunoglobulins and live virus vaccines, see under Normal Immunoglobulin, p. 755

Immunosuppressants (antiproliferative) *see* Azathioprine and Mycophenolate Mofetil

Indapamide *see* Diuretics

Indinavir
- Anti-arrhythmics: indinavir possibly increases plasma concentration of ●amiodarone—avoid concomitant use; indinavir possibly increases plasma concentration of ●flecainide (increased risk of ventricular arrhythmias—avoid concomitant use)
- Antibacterials: indinavir increases plasma concentration of ●rifabutin—avoid concomitant use; metabolism of indinavir accelerated by ●rifampicin (reduced plasma concentration—avoid concomitant use); avoidance of concomitant indinavir in severe renal and hepatic impairment advised by manufacturer of ●telithromycin

Anticoagulants: avoidance of indinavir advised by manufacturer of rivaroxaban
- Antidepressants: plasma concentration of indinavir reduced by ●St John's wort—avoid concomitant use
- Antiepileptics: plasma concentration of indinavir possibly reduced by ●carbamazepine and ●phenytoin, also plasma concentration of carbamazepine and phenytoin possibly increased; plasma concentration of indinavir possibly reduced by ●primidone
- Antifungals: plasma concentration of indinavir increased by ●itraconazole and ●ketoconazole (consider reducing dose of indinavir)

Antimalarials: caution with indinavir advised by manufacturer of artemether/lumefantrine

Antimuscarinics: avoidance of indinavir advised by manufacturer of darifenacin and tolterodine; manufacturer of fesoterodine advises dose reduction when indinavir given with fesoterodine—consult fesoterodine product literature
- Antipsychotics: indinavir possibly inhibits metabolism of ●aripiprazole (reduce dose of aripiprazole); indinavir possibly increases plasma concentration of ●pimozide (increased risk of ventricular arrhythmias—avoid concomitant use); indinavir increases plasma concentration of ●sertindole (increased risk of ventricular arrhythmias—avoid concomitant use)
- Antivirals: avoid concomitant use of indinavir with ●atazanavir; plasma concentration of both drugs increased when indinavir given with darunavir; plasma concentration of indinavir reduced by efavirenz and nevirapine; plasma concentration of indinavir possibly reduced by ●etravirine—avoid concomitant use; indinavir increases plasma concentration of ●maraviroc (consider reducing dose of maraviroc); combination of indinavir with nelfinavir may increase plasma concentration of either drug (or both); plasma concentration of indinavir increased by ritonavir; indinavir increases plasma concentration of saquinavir
- Anxiolytics and Hypnotics: increased risk of prolonged sedation when indinavir given with ●alprazolam—avoid concomitant use; indinavir possibly increases plasma concentration of ●midazolam (risk of prolonged sedation—avoid concomitant use of oral midazolam)

Atovaquone: plasma concentration of indinavir possibly reduced by atovaquone
- Barbiturates: plasma concentration of indinavir possibly reduced by ●barbiturates; plasma concentration of indinavir possibly reduced by ●phenobarbital, also plasma concentration of phenobarbital possibly increased
- Ciclosporin: indinavir increases plasma concentration of ●ciclosporin
- Cilostazol: indinavir possibly increases plasma concentration of ●cilostazol—avoid concomitant use

Corticosteroids: plasma concentration of indinavir possibly reduced by dexamethasone
- Ergot Alkaloids: increased risk of ergotism when indinavir given with ●ergotamine and methysergide—avoid concomitant use

Indinavir (continued)
- 5HT$_1$ Agonists: indinavir increases plasma concentration of ●eletriptan (risk of toxicity)—avoid concomitant use
- Lipid-regulating Drugs: possible increased risk of myopathy when indinavir given with atorvastatin; possible increased risk of myopathy when indinavir given with ●rosuvastatin—avoid concomitant use; increased risk of myopathy when indinavir given with ●simvastatin (avoid concomitant use)
- Sildenafil: indinavir increases plasma concentration of ●sildenafil—reduce initial dose of sildenafil
  Tadalafil: indinavir possibly increases plasma concentration of tadalafil
- Vardenafil: indinavir increases plasma concentration of ●vardenafil—avoid concomitant use

Indometacin see NSAIDs
Indoramin see Alpha-blockers
Infliximab
  Abatacept: increased risk of side-effects when infliximab given with abatacept
- Anakinra: avoid concomitant use of infliximab with ●anakinra
- Vaccines: avoid concomitant use of infliximab with live ●vaccines (see p. 725)
Influenza Vaccine see Vaccines
Insulin see Antidiabetics
Interferon Alfa see Interferons
Interferon Gamma see Interferons
Interferons
  Note. Peginterferon alfa interactions as for interferon alfa
- Antivirals: increased risk of peripheral neuropathy when interferon alfa given with ●telbivudine
  Theophylline: interferon alfa inhibits metabolism of theophylline (increased plasma concentration)
  Vaccines: manufacturer of interferon gamma advises avoid concomitant use with vaccines
Ipratropium see Antimuscarinics
Irbesartan see Angiotensin-II Receptor Antagonists
Irinotecan
- Antidepressants: metabolism of irinotecan accelerated by ●St John's wort (reduced plasma concentration—avoid concomitant use)
  Antiepileptics: plasma concentration of irinotecan and its active metabolite reduced by carbamazepine and phenytoin; cytotoxics possibly reduce absorption of phenytoin
- Antifungals: plasma concentration of irinotecan reduced by ●ketoconazole (but concentration of active metabolite of irinotecan increased)—avoid concomitant use
- Antipsychotics: avoid concomitant use of cytotoxics with ●clozapine (increased risk of agranulocytosis)
- Antivirals: metabolism of irinotecan possibly inhibited by ●atazanavir (increased risk of toxicity)
  Barbiturates: plasma concentration of irinotecan and its active metabolite reduced by phenobarbital
  Cardiac Glycosides: cytotoxics reduce absorption of digoxin tablets
  Cytotoxics: plasma concentration of irinotecan possibly increased by sorafenib
Iron
  Antacids: absorption of *oral* iron reduced by oral magnesium salts (as magnesium trisilicate)
  Antibacterials: *oral* iron reduces absorption of ciprofloxacin, levofloxacin, moxifloxacin, norfloxacin and ofloxacin; *oral* iron reduces absorption of tetracyclines, also absorption of *oral* iron reduced by tetracyclines
  Bisphosphonates: *oral* iron reduces absorption of bisphosphonates
  Calcium Salts: absorption of *oral* iron reduced by calcium salts
  Cytotoxics: *oral* iron reduces absorption of mycophenolate

Iron (continued)
- Dimercaprol: avoid concomitant use of iron with ●dimercaprol
  Dopaminergics: *oral* iron reduces absorption of entacapone; *oral* iron possibly reduces absorption of levodopa
  Methyldopa: *oral* iron antagonises hypotensive effect of methyldopa
  Penicillamine: *oral* iron reduces absorption of penicillamine
  Thyroid Hormones: *oral* iron reduces absorption of levothyroxine (thyroxine) (give at least 2 hours apart)
  Trientine: absorption of *oral* iron reduced by trientine
  Zinc: *oral* iron reduces absorption of zinc, also absorption of *oral* iron reduced by zinc
Isocarboxazid see MAOIs
Isoflurane see Anaesthetics, General
Isometheptene see Sympathomimetics
Isoniazid
  Anaesthetics, General: hepatotoxicity of isoniazid possibly potentiated by general anaesthetics
  Antacids: absorption of isoniazid reduced by antacids
  Antibacterials: increased risk of CNS toxicity when isoniazid given with cycloserine
- Antiepileptics: isoniazid increases plasma concentration of ●carbamazepine (also possibly increased isoniazid hepatotoxicity); isoniazid inhibits metabolism of ●ethosuximide (increased plasma concentration and risk of toxicity); isoniazid inhibits metabolism of ●phenytoin (increased plasma concentration)
  Antifungals: isoniazid possibly reduces plasma concentration of ketoconazole
  Anxiolytics and Hypnotics: isoniazid inhibits the metabolism of diazepam
  Corticosteroids: plasma concentration of isoniazid possibly reduced by corticosteroids
  Oestrogens: antibacterials that do not induce liver enzymes possibly reduce contraceptive effect of oestrogens (risk probably small, see p. 478)
  Theophylline: isoniazid possibly increases plasma concentration of theophylline
  Vaccines: antibacterials inactivate oral typhoid vaccine—see p. 752
Isosorbide Dinitrate see Nitrates
Isosorbide Mononitrate see Nitrates
Isotretinoin see Retinoids
Isradipine see Calcium-channel Blockers
Itraconazole see Antifungals, Triazole
Ivabradine
- Anti-arrhythmics: increased risk of ventricular arrhythmias when ivabradine given with ●amiodarone or ●disopyramide
- Antibacterials: plasma concentration of ivabradine possibly increased by ●clarithromycin and ●telithromycin—avoid concomitant use; increased risk of ventricular arrhythmias when ivabradine given with ●erythromycin—avoid concomitant use
  Antidepressants: plasma concentration of ivabradine reduced by St John's wort—avoid concomitant use
- Antifungals: plasma concentration of ivabradine increased by ●ketoconazole—avoid concomitant use; plasma concentration of ivabradine increased by fluconazole—reduce initial dose of ivabradine; plasma concentration of ivabradine possibly increased by ●itraconazole—avoid concomitant use
- Antimalarials: increased risk of ventricular arrhythmias when ivabradine given with ●mefloquine
- Antipsychotics: increased risk of ventricular arrhythmias when ivabradine given with ●pimozide or ●sertindole
- Antivirals: plasma concentration of ivabradine possibly increased by ●nelfinavir and ●ritonavir—avoid concomitant use
- Beta-blockers: increased risk of ventricular arrhythmias when ivabradine given with ●sotalol

Ivabradine *(continued)*
- Calcium-channel Blockers: plasma concentration of ivabradine increased by ●diltiazem and ●verapamil—avoid concomitant use

  Grapefruit Juice: plasma concentration of ivabradine increased by grapefruit juice
- Pentamidine Isetionate: increased risk of ventricular arrhythmias when ivabradine given with ●pentamidine isetionate

Kaolin

  Analgesics: kaolin possibly reduces absorption of aspirin

  Antibacterials: kaolin possibly reduces absorption of tetracyclines

  Antimalarials: kaolin reduces absorption of chloroquine and hydroxychloroquine

  Antipsychotics: kaolin possibly reduces absorption of phenothiazines

Ketamine *see* Anaesthetics, General

Ketoconazole *see* Antifungals, Imidazole

Ketoprofen *see* NSAIDs

Ketorolac *see* NSAIDs

Ketotifen *see* Antihistamines

Labetalol *see* Beta-blockers

Lacidipine *see* Calcium-channel Blockers

Lacosamide

- Antidepressants: anticonvulsant effect of antiepileptics possibly antagonised by MAOIs and ●tricyclic-related antidepressants (convulsive threshold lowered); anticonvulsant effect of antiepileptics antagonised by ●SSRIs and ●tricyclics (convulsive threshold lowered); avoid concomitant use of antiepileptics with ●St John's wort
- Antimalarials: possible increased risk of convulsions when antiepileptics given with chloroquine and hydroxychloroquine; anticonvulsant effect of antiepileptics antagonised by ●mefloquine

Lactulose

  Anticoagulants: lactulose possibly enhances anticoagulant effect of coumarins

Lamivudine

  Antibacterials: plasma concentration of lamivudine increased by trimethoprim (as co-trimoxazole)—avoid concomitant use of high-dose co-trimoxazole

  Antivirals: avoidance of lamivudine advised by manufacturer of emtricitabine; manufacturer of lamivudine advises avoid concomitant use with foscarnet; manufacturer of lamivudine advises avoid concomitant use of intravenous ganciclovir

Lamotrigine

- Antibacterials: plasma concentration of lamotrigine reduced by ●rifampicin
- Antidepressants: anticonvulsant effect of antiepileptics possibly antagonised by MAOIs and ●tricyclic-related antidepressants (convulsive threshold lowered); anticonvulsant effect of antiepileptics antagonised by ●SSRIs and ●tricyclics (convulsive threshold lowered); avoid concomitant use of antiepileptics with ●St John's wort

  Antiepileptics: plasma concentration of lamotrigine often reduced by carbamazepine, also plasma concentration of an active metabolite of carbamazepine sometimes raised (but evidence is conflicting); plasma concentration of lamotrigine reduced by phenytoin and primidone; plasma concentration of lamotrigine reduced by valproate
- Antimalarials: possible increased risk of convulsions when antiepileptics given with chloroquine and hydroxychloroquine; anticonvulsant effect of antiepileptics antagonised by ●mefloquine

  Barbiturates: plasma concentration of lamotrigine reduced by phenobarbital
- Oestrogens: plasma concentration of lamotrigine reduced by ●oestrogens
- Progestogens: plasma concentration of lamotrigine reduced by ●progestogens

Lanreotide

  Antidiabetics: lanreotide possibly reduces requirements for insulin, metformin, repaglinide and sulphonylureas

  Ciclosporin: lanreotide reduces plasma concentration of ciclosporin

Lansoprazole *see* Proton Pump Inhibitors

Lanthanum

  Antifungals: lanthanum possibly reduces absorption of ketoconazole (give at least 2 hours apart)

  Antimalarials: lanthanum possibly reduces absorption of chloroquine and hydroxychloroquine (give at least 2 hours apart)

Lapatinib

- Antibacterials: manufacturer of lapatinib advises avoid concomitant use with ●rifabutin, ●rifampicin and ●telithromycin
- Antidepressants: manufacturer of lapatinib advises avoid concomitant use with ●St John's wort
- Antidiabetics: manufacturer of lapatinib advises avoid concomitant use with ●repaglinide
- Antiepileptics: plasma concentration of lapatinib reduced by ●carbamazepine—avoid concomitant use; cytotoxics possibly reduce absorption of phenytoin; manufacturer of lapatinib advises avoid concomitant use with ●phenytoin
- Antifungals: plasma concentration of lapatinib increased by ●ketoconazole—avoid concomitant use; manufacturer of lapatinib advises avoid concomitant use with ●itraconazole, ●posaconazole and ●voriconazole
- Antipsychotics: avoid concomitant use of cytotoxics with ●clozapine (increased risk of agranulocytosis); manufacturer of lapatinib advises avoid concomitant use with ●pimozide
- Antivirals: manufacturer of lapatinib advises avoid concomitant use with ●ritonavir and ●saquinavir

  Cardiac Glycosides: cytotoxics reduce absorption of digoxin tablets
- Grapefruit Juice: manufacturer of lapatinib advises avoid concomitant use with ●grapefruit juice

  Ulcer-healing Drugs: absorption of lapatinib possibly reduced by histamine H_2-antagonists and proton pump inhibitors

Laronidase

  Anaesthetics, Local: effects of laronidase possibly inhibited by procaine (manufacturer of laronidase advises avoid concomitant use)

  Antimalarials: effects of laronidase possibly inhibited by chloroquine and hydroxychloroquine (manufacturer of laronidase advises avoid concomitant use)

Leflunomide

  Note. Increased risk of toxicity with other haematotoxic and hepatotoxic drugs

  Antibacterials: plasma concentration of active metabolite of leflunomide possibly increased by rifampicin

  Anticoagulants: leflunomide possibly enhances anticoagulant effect of warfarin

  Antidiabetics: leflunomide possibly enhances hypoglycaemic effect of tolbutamide

  Antiepileptics: leflunomide possibly increases plasma concentration of phenytoin

  Lipid-regulating Drugs: the effect of leflunomide is significantly decreased by colestyramine (enhanced elimination)—avoid unless drug elimination desired
- Vaccines: avoid concomitant use of leflunomide with live ●vaccines (see p. 725)

Lenalidomide

  Cardiac Glycosides: lenalidomide possibly increases plasma concentration of digoxin

Lercanidipine *see* Calcium-channel Blockers

Leukotriene Receptor Antagonists

  Analgesics: plasma concentration of zafirlukast increased by aspirin

Leukotriene Receptor Antagonists *(continued)*

Antibacterials: plasma concentration of zafirlukast reduced by erythromycin

Anticoagulants: zafirlukast enhances anticoagulant effect of warfarin

Antiepileptics: plasma concentration of montelukast reduced by primidone

Barbiturates: plasma concentration of montelukast reduced by phenobarbital

Theophylline: zafirlukast possibly increases plasma concentration of theophylline, also plasma concentration of zafirlukast reduced

Levamisole

Alcohol: possibility of disulfiram-like reaction when levamisole given with alcohol

• Anticoagulants: levamisole possibly enhances anticoagulant effect of •warfarin

Antiepileptics: levamisole possibly increases plasma concentration of phenytoin

Levetiracetam

• Antidepressants: anticonvulsant effect of antiepileptics possibly antagonised by MAOIs and •tricyclic-related antidepressants (convulsive threshold lowered); anticonvulsant effect of antiepileptics antagonised by •SSRIs and •tricyclics (convulsive threshold lowered); avoid concomitant use of antiepileptics with •St John's wort

• Antimalarials: possible increased risk of convulsions when antiepileptics given with chloroquine and hydroxychloroquine; anticonvulsant effect of antiepileptics antagonised by •mefloquine

Levobunolol *see* Beta-blockers

Levobupivacaine

Anti-arrhythmics: increased myocardial depression when levobupivacaine given with anti-arrhythmics

Levocetirizine *see* Antihistamines

Levodopa

ACE Inhibitors: enhanced hypotensive effect when levodopa given with ACE inhibitors

Adrenergic Neurone Blockers: enhanced hypotensive effect when levodopa given with adrenergic neurone blockers

Alpha-blockers: enhanced hypotensive effect when levodopa given with alpha-blockers

Anaesthetics, General: increased risk of arrhythmias when levodopa given with •volatile liquid general anaesthetics

Angiotensin-II Receptor Antagonists: enhanced hypotensive effect when levodopa given with angiotensin-II receptor antagonists

• Antidepressants: risk of hypertensive crisis when levodopa given with •MAOIs, avoid levodopa for at least 2 weeks after stopping MAOIs; increased risk of side-effects when levodopa given with moclobemide

Antiepileptics: effects of levodopa possibly reduced by phenytoin

Antimuscarinics: absorption of levodopa possibly reduced by antimuscarinics

Antipsychotics: effects of levodopa antagonised by antipsychotics; avoidance of levodopa advised by manufacturer of amisulpride (antagonism of effect)

Anxiolytics and Hypnotics: effects of levodopa possibly antagonised by benzodiazepines

Beta-blockers: enhanced hypotensive effect when levodopa given with beta-blockers

Bupropion: increased risk of side-effects when levodopa given with bupropion

Calcium-channel Blockers: enhanced hypotensive effect when levodopa given with calcium-channel blockers

Clonidine: enhanced hypotensive effect when levodopa given with clonidine

Diazoxide: enhanced hypotensive effect when levodopa given with diazoxide

Diuretics: enhanced hypotensive effect when levodopa given with diuretics

Levodopa *(continued)*

Dopaminergics: enhanced effects and increased toxicity of levodopa when given with selegiline (reduce dose of levodopa)

Iron: absorption of levodopa possibly reduced by *oral* iron

Memantine: effects of dopaminergics possibly enhanced by memantine

Methyldopa: enhanced hypotensive effect when levodopa given with methyldopa; antiparkinsonian effect of dopaminergics antagonised by methyldopa

Moxonidine: enhanced hypotensive effect when levodopa given with moxonidine

Muscle Relaxants: possible agitation, confusion and hallucinations when levodopa given with baclofen

Nitrates: enhanced hypotensive effect when levodopa given with nitrates

Vasodilator Antihypertensives: enhanced hypotensive effect when levodopa given with hydralazine, minoxidil or sodium nitroprusside

Vitamins: effects of levodopa reduced by pyridoxine when given without dopa-decarboxylase inhibitor

Levofloxacin *see* Quinolones

Levomepromazine (methotrimeprazine) *see* Antipsychotics

Levonorgestrel *see* Progestogens

Levothyroxine (thyroxine) *see* Thyroid Hormones

Lidocaine (lignocaine)

Note. Interactions less likely when lidocaine used topically

Anaesthetics, Local: increased myocardial depression when anti-arrhythmics given with bupivacaine, levobupivacaine, prilocaine or ropivacaine

• Anti-arrhythmics: increased myocardial depression when anti-arrhythmics given with other •anti-arrhythmics

• Antibacterials: increased risk of ventricular arrhythmias when lidocaine (lignocaine) given with •quinupristin/dalfopristin—avoid concomitant use

• Antipsychotics: increased risk of ventricular arrhythmias when anti-arrhythmics that prolong the QT interval given with •antipsychotics that prolong the QT interval

• Antivirals: plasma concentration of lidocaine (lignocaine) possibly increased by •atazanavir and lopinavir; plasma concentration of lidocaine (lignocaine) possibly increased by darunavir and •fosamprenavir—avoid concomitant use

• Beta-blockers: increased myocardial depression when anti-arrhythmics given with •beta-blockers; increased risk of lidocaine (lignocaine) toxicity when given with •propranolol

• Diuretics: action of lidocaine (lignocaine) antagonised by hypokalaemia caused by •acetazolamide, •loop diuretics or •thiazides and related diuretics

• 5HT$_3$ Antagonists: increased risk of ventricular arrhythmias when lidocaine (lignocaine) given with •dolasetron—avoid concomitant use

Muscle Relaxants: neuromuscular blockade enhanced and prolonged when lidocaine (lignocaine) given with suxamethonium

• Ulcer-healing Drugs: plasma concentration of lidocaine (lignocaine) increased by •cimetidine (increased risk of toxicity)

Linezolid

Note. Linezolid is a reversible, non-selective MAO inhibitor—see interactions of MAOIs

Oestrogens: antibacterials that do not induce liver enzymes possibly reduce contraceptive effect of oestrogens (risk probably small, see p. 478)

Vaccines: antibacterials inactivate oral typhoid vaccine—see p. 752

Liothyronine *see* Thyroid Hormones

Lipid-regulating Drugs *see* Colestipol, Colestyramine, Ezetimibe, Fibrates, Nicotinic Acid, and Statins

Lisinopril *see* ACE Inhibitors

Lithium
- ACE Inhibitors: excretion of lithium reduced by ●ACE inhibitors (increased plasma concentration)
- Analgesics: excretion of lithium reduced by ●NSAIDs (increased risk of toxicity); excretion of lithium reduced by ●ketorolac (increased risk of toxicity)—avoid concomitant use
- Angiotensin-II Receptor Antagonists: excretion of lithium reduced by ●angiotensin-II receptor antagonists (increased plasma concentration)

  Antacids: excretion of lithium increased by sodium bicarbonate (reduced plasma concentration)
- Anti-arrhythmics: avoidance of lithium advised by manufacturer of ●amiodarone (risk of ventricular arrhythmias)

  Antibacterials: increased risk of lithium toxicity when given with metronidazole
- Antidepressants: possible increased serotonergic effects when lithium given with venlafaxine; increased risk of CNS effects when lithium given with ●SSRIs (lithium toxicity reported); risk of toxicity when lithium given with tricyclics

  Antiepileptics: neurotoxicity may occur when lithium given with carbamazepine or phenytoin without increased plasma concentration of lithium; plasma concentration of lithium possibly affected by topiramate
- Antipsychotics: increased risk of extrapyramidal side-effects and possibly neurotoxicity when lithium given with clozapine, flupentixol, haloperidol, phenothiazines or zuclopenthixol; increased risk of ventricular arrhythmias when lithium given with ●sertindole—avoid concomitant use; increased risk of extrapyramidal side-effects when lithium given with sulpiride

  Calcium-channel Blockers: neurotoxicity may occur when lithium given with diltiazem or verapamil without increased plasma concentration of lithium
- Diuretics: excretion of lithium increased by ●acetazolamide; excretion of lithium reduced by ●loop diuretics and ●thiazides and related diuretics (increased plasma concentration and risk of toxicity)—loop diuretics safer than thiazides; excretion of lithium reduced by ●potassium-sparing diuretics and aldosterone antagonists (increased plasma concentration and risk of toxicity)
- Methyldopa: neurotoxicity may occur when lithium given with ●methyldopa without increased plasma concentration of lithium

  Muscle Relaxants: lithium enhances effects of muscle relaxants; hyperkinesis caused by lithium possibly aggravated by baclofen

  Parasympathomimetics: lithium antagonises effects of neostigmine and pyridostigmine

  Theophylline: excretion of lithium increased by theophylline (reduced plasma concentration)
Lofepramine *see* Antidepressants, Tricyclic
Lofexidine

  Alcohol: increased sedative effect when lofexidine given with alcohol

  Anxiolytics and Hypnotics: increased sedative effect when lofexidine given with anxiolytics and hypnotics

  Barbiturates: increased sedative effect when lofexidine given with barbiturates
Lomustine

  Antiepileptics: cytotoxics possibly reduce absorption of phenytoin
- Antipsychotics: avoid concomitant use of cytotoxics with ●clozapine (increased risk of agranulocytosis)

  Cardiac Glycosides: cytotoxics reduce absorption of digoxin tablets

  Ulcer-healing Drugs: myelosuppressive effects of lomustine possibly enhanced by cimetidine
Loperamide

  Desmopressin: loperamide increases plasma concentration of *oral* desmopressin

Lopinavir
  Note. In combination with ritonavir as *Kaletra®* (ritonavir is present to inhibit lopinavir metabolism and increase plasma-lopinavir concentration)—see also Ritonavir
- Anti-arrhythmics: lopinavir possibly increases plasma concentration of ●flecainide (increased risk of ventricular arrhythmias—avoid concomitant use); lopinavir possibly increases plasma concentration of lidocaine (lignocaine)
- Antibacterials: plasma concentration of lopinavir reduced by ●rifampicin—avoid concomitant use; avoidance of concomitant lopinavir in severe renal and hepatic impairment advised by manufacturer of ●telithromycin

  Anticoagulants: avoidance of lopinavir advised by manufacturer of rivaroxaban
- Antidepressants: plasma concentration of lopinavir reduced by ●St John's wort—avoid concomitant use
- Antiepileptics: plasma concentration of lopinavir possibly reduced by carbamazepine, phenytoin and ●primidone

  Antihistamines: lopinavir possibly increases plasma concentration of chlorphenamine (chlorpheniramine)

  Antimalarials: caution with lopinavir advised by manufacturer of artemether/lumefantrine

  Antimuscarinics: avoidance of lopinavir advised by manufacturer of darifenacin and tolterodine
- Antipsychotics: lopinavir possibly inhibits metabolism of ●aripiprazole (reduce dose of aripiprazole); lopinavir increases plasma concentration of ●sertindole (increased risk of ventricular arrhythmias—avoid concomitant use)
- Antivirals: lopinavir reduces plasma concentration of ●darunavir, also plasma concentration of lopinavir increased (avoid concomitant use); plasma concentration of lopinavir reduced by ●efavirenz—consider increasing dose of lopinavir; lopinavir reduces plasma concentration of fosamprenavir, effect on lopinavir plasma concentration not predictable—avoid concomitant use; lopinavir increases plasma concentration of ●maraviroc (consider reducing dose of maraviroc); plasma concentration of lopinavir reduced by nelfinavir, also plasma concentration of active metabolite of nelfinavir increased; plasma concentration of lopinavir possibly reduced by ●nevirapine—consider increasing dose of lopinavir; lopinavir increases plasma concentration of saquinavir and tenofovir; plasma concentration of lopinavir reduced by ●tipranavir
- Barbiturates: plasma concentration of lopinavir possibly reduced by ●phenobarbital
- Cilostazol: lopinavir possibly increases plasma concentration of ●cilostazol—avoid concomitant use

  Corticosteroids: plasma concentration of lopinavir possibly reduced by dexamethasone
- Lipid-regulating Drugs: possible increased risk of myopathy when lopinavir given with atorvastatin; possible increased risk of myopathy when lopinavir given with ●rosuvastatin or ●simvastatin—avoid concomitant use

  Sirolimus: lopinavir possibly increases plasma concentration of sirolimus
Loprazolam *see* Anxiolytics and Hypnotics
Loratadine *see* Antihistamines
Lorazepam *see* Anxiolytics and Hypnotics
Lormetazepam *see* Anxiolytics and Hypnotics
Losartan *see* Angiotensin-II Receptor Antagonists
Lumefantrine *see* Artemether with Lumefantrine
Lymecycline *see* Tetracyclines
Macrolides
  Note. See also Telithromycin
  Note. Interactions do not apply to small amounts of erythromycin used topically

  Analgesics: erythromycin increases plasma concentration of alfentanil

Appendix 1: Interactions

Macrolides *(continued)*

Antacids: absorption of azithromycin reduced by antacids

- Anti-arrhythmics: increased risk of ventricular arrhythmias when parenteral erythromycin given with ●amiodarone—avoid concomitant use; erythromycin increases plasma concentration of ●disopyramide (increased risk of toxicity); clarithromycin possibly increases plasma concentration of ●disopyramide (increased risk of toxicity)
- Antibacterials: increased risk of ventricular arrhythmias when parenteral erythromycin given with ●moxifloxacin—avoid concomitant use; macrolides possibly increase plasma concentration of ●rifabutin (increased risk of uveitis—reduce rifabutin dose); clarithromycin increases plasma concentration of ●rifabutin (increased risk of uveitis—reduce rifabutin dose); plasma concentration of clarithromycin reduced by rifamycins
- Anticoagulants: azithromycin possibly enhances anticoagulant effect of ●coumarins; clarithromycin and erythromycin enhance anticoagulant effect of ●coumarins
- Antidepressants: avoidance of macrolides advised by manufacturer of ●reboxetine

Antidiabetics: clarithromycin enhances effects of repaglinide

- Antiepileptics: clarithromycin and erythromycin increase plasma concentration of ●carbamazepine; clarithromycin inhibits metabolism of phenytoin (increased plasma concentration); erythromycin possibly inhibits metabolism of valproate (increased plasma concentration)

Antifungals: clarithromycin increases plasma concentration of itraconazole

- Antihistamines: manufacturer of loratadine advises erythromycin possibly increases plasma concentration of loratadine; macrolides possibly inhibit metabolism of ●mizolastine (avoid concomitant use); erythromycin inhibits metabolism of ●mizolastine—avoid concomitant use
- Antimalarials: avoidance of macrolides advised by manufacturer of ●artemether/lumefantrine

Antimuscarinics: erythromycin possibly increases plasma concentration of darifenacin; manufacturer of fesoterodine advises dose reduction when clarithromycin given with fesoterodine—consult fesoterodine product literature; avoidance of clarithromycin and erythromycin advised by manufacturer of tolterodine

- Antipsychotics: increased risk of ventricular arrhythmias when parenteral erythromycin given with ●amisulpride or ●zuclopenthixol—avoid concomitant use; erythromycin possibly increases plasma concentration of ●clozapine (possible increased risk of convulsions); increased risk of ventricular arrhythmias when clarithromycin given with ●pimozide—avoid concomitant use; possible increased risk of ventricular arrhythmias when erythromycin given with ●pimozide—avoid concomitant use; macrolides possibly increase plasma concentration of quetiapine (reduce dose of quetiapine); possible increased risk of ventricular arrhythmias when macrolides given with ●sertindole—avoid concomitant use; increased risk of ventricular arrhythmias when erythromycin given with ●sertindole—avoid concomitant use; increased risk of ventricular arrhythmias when parenteral erythromycin given with ●sulpiride
- Antivirals: plasma concentration of both drugs increased when clarithromycin given with atazanavir; increased risk of rash when clarithromycin given with efavirenz; clarithromycin increases plasma concentration of ●etravirine, also plasma concentration of clarithromycin reduced; plasma concentration of both drugs increased when erythromycin given with fosamprenavir; clarithromycin possibly increases plasma concentration of ●maraviroc (con-

Macrolides

- Antivirals *(continued)* sider reducing dose of maraviroc); plasma concentration of azithromycin and erythromycin possibly increased by ritonavir; plasma concentration of clarithromycin increased by ●ritonavir (reduce dose of clarithromycin in renal impairment); plasma concentration of clarithromycin increased by ●tipranavir (reduce dose of clarithromycin in renal impairment), also clarithromycin increases plasma concentration of tipranavir; clarithromycin tablets reduce absorption of zidovudine (give at least 2 hours apart)
- Anxiolytics and Hypnotics: clarithromycin and erythromycin inhibit metabolism of ●midazolam (increased plasma concentration with increased sedation); erythromycin increases plasma concentration of buspirone (reduce dose of buspirone); erythromycin inhibits the metabolism of zopiclone

Aprepitant: clarithromycin possibly increases plasma concentration of aprepitant

- Atomoxetine: increased risk of ventricular arrhythmias when parenteral erythromycin given with ●atomoxetine
- Calcium-channel Blockers: erythromycin possibly inhibits metabolism of felodipine (increased plasma concentration); avoidance of erythromycin advised by manufacturer of lercanidipine; clarithromycin and erythromycin possibly inhibit metabolism of ●verapamil (increased risk of toxicity)

Cardiac Glycosides: macrolides increase plasma concentration of digoxin (increased risk of toxicity)

- Ciclosporin: macrolides possibly inhibit metabolism of ●ciclosporin (increased plasma concentration); clarithromycin and erythromycin inhibit metabolism of ●ciclosporin (increased plasma concentration)
- Cilostazol: erythromycin increases plasma concentration of ●cilostazol (also plasma concentration of erythromycin reduced)—avoid concomitant use
- Colchicine: clarithromycin or erythromycin increase risk of ●colchicine toxicity

Corticosteroids: erythromycin possibly inhibits metabolism of corticosteroids; clarithromycin possibly increases plasma concentration of methylprednisolone; erythromycin inhibits the metabolism of methylprednisolone

- Cytotoxics: avoidance of clarithromycin advised by manufacturer of ●nilotinib; *in vitro* studies suggest a possible interaction between erythromycin and docetaxel (consult docetaxel product literature); erythromycin increases toxicity of ●vinblastine—avoid concomitant use
- Diuretics: clarithromycin increases plasma concentration of ●eplerenone—avoid concomitant use; erythromycin increases plasma concentration of eplerenone (reduce dose of eplerenone)

Dopaminergics: macrolides possibly increase plasma concentration of bromocriptine and cabergoline (increased risk of toxicity); erythromycin increases plasma concentration of bromocriptine and cabergoline (increased risk of toxicity)

- Ergot Alkaloids: increased risk of ergotism when macrolides given with ●ergotamine and methysergide—avoid concomitant use
- 5HT₁ Agonists: clarithromycin and erythromycin increase plasma concentration of ●eletriptan (risk of toxicity)—avoid concomitant use
- Ivabradine: clarithromycin possibly increases plasma concentration of ●ivabradine—avoid concomitant use; increased risk of ventricular arrhythmias when erythromycin given with ●ivabradine—avoid concomitant use

Leukotriene Receptor Antagonists: erythromycin reduces plasma concentration of zafirlukast

- Lipid-regulating Drugs: clarithromycin increases plasma concentration of ●atorvastatin and prava-

Macrolides

* Lipid-regulating Drugs *(continued)*
  statin; possible increased risk of myopathy when erythromycin given with atorvastatin; erythromycin increases plasma concentration of pravastatin; erythromycin reduces plasma concentration of rosuvastatin; increased risk of myopathy when clarithromycin or erythromycin given with ●simvastatin (avoid concomitant use)

  Oestrogens: antibacterials that do not induce liver enzymes possibly reduce contraceptive effect of oestrogens (risk probably small, see p. 478)

  Parasympathomimetics: erythromycin increases plasma concentration of galantamine

* Pentamidine Isetionate: increased risk of ventricular arrhythmias when parenteral erythromycin given with ●pentamidine isetionate

  Sildenafil: clarithromycin possibly increases plasma concentration of sildenafil—reduce initial dose of sildenafil; erythromycin increases plasma concentration of sildenafil—reduce initial dose of sildenafil

* Sirolimus: clarithromycin increases plasma concentration of ●sirolimus—avoid concomitant use; plasma concentration of both drugs increased when erythromycin given with ●sirolimus

* Tacrolimus: clarithromycin and erythromycin increase plasma concentration of ●tacrolimus

  Tadalafil: clarithromycin and erythromycin possibly increase plasma concentration of tadalafil

* Theophylline: azithromycin possibly increases plasma concentration of theophylline; clarithromycin inhibits metabolism of ●theophylline (increased plasma concentration); erythromycin inhibits metabolism of ●theophylline (increased plasma concentration), if erythromycin given by mouth, also decreased plasma-erythromycin concentration

  Ulcer-healing Drugs: plasma concentration of erythromycin increased by cimetidine (increased risk of toxicity, including deafness); plasma concentration of both drugs increased when clarithromycin given with omeprazole

  Vaccines: antibacterials inactivate oral typhoid vaccine—see p. 752

  Vardenafil: erythromycin increases plasma concentration of vardenafil (reduce dose of vardenafil)

Magnesium (parenteral)

* Calcium-channel Blockers: profound hypotension reported with concomitant use of parenteral magnesium and ●nifedipine in pre-eclampsia

  Muscle Relaxants: parenteral magnesium enhances effects of non-depolarising muscle relaxants and suxamethonium

Magnesium Salts (oral) *see* Antacids

Mannitol

  Ciclosporin: possible increased risk of nephrotoxicity when mannitol given with ciclosporin

MAOIs

  Note. For interactions of reversible MAO-A inhibitors (RIMAs) see Moclobemide, and for interactions of MAO-B inhibitors see Rasagiline and Selegiline; the antibacterial Linezolid is a reversible, non-selective MAO inhibitor

  ACE Inhibitors: MAOIs possibly enhance hypotensive effect of ACE inhibitors

  Adrenergic Neurone Blockers: enhanced hypotensive effect when MAOIs given with adrenergic neurone blockers

* Alcohol: MAOIs interact with tyramine found in some beverages containing ●alcohol and some dealcoholised beverages (hypertensive crisis)—if no tyramine, enhanced hypotensive effect

  Alpha$_2$-adrenoceptor Stimulants: avoidance of MAOIs advised by manufacturer of apraclonidine and brimonidine

* Alpha-blockers: avoidance of MAOIs advised by manufacturer of ●indoramin; enhanced hypotensive effect when MAOIs given with alpha-blockers

MAOIs *(continued)*

* Anaesthetics, General: Because of hazardous interactions between MAOIs and ●general anaesthetics, MAOIs should normally be stopped 2 weeks before surgery

* Analgesics: CNS excitation or depression (hypertension or hypotension) when MAOIs given with ●pethidine—avoid concomitant use and for 2 weeks after stopping MAOIs; avoidance of MAOIs advised by manufacturer of ●nefopam; possible CNS excitation or depression (hypertension or hypotension) when MAOIs given with ●opioid analgesics—avoid concomitant use and for 2 weeks after stopping MAOIs

  Angiotensin-II Receptor Antagonists: MAOIs possibly enhance hypotensive effect of angiotensin-II receptor antagonists

* Antidepressants: increased risk of hypertension and CNS excitation when MAOIs given with ●reboxetine (MAOIs should not be started until 1 week after stopping reboxetine, avoid reboxetine for 2 weeks after stopping MAOIs); after stopping MAOIs do not start ●citalopram, ●escitalopram, ●fluvoxamine or ●paroxetine for 2 weeks, also MAOIs should not be started until at least 1 week after stopping citalopram, escitalopram, fluvoxamine or paroxetine; after stopping MAOIs do not start ●fluoxetine for 2 weeks, also MAOIs should not be started until at least 5 weeks after stopping fluoxetine; after stopping MAOIs do not start ●mirtazapine or ●sertraline for 2 weeks, also MAOIs should not be started until at least 2 weeks after stopping mirtazapine or sertraline; after stopping MAOIs do not start ●duloxetine for 2 weeks, also MAOIs should not be started until at least 5 days after stopping duloxetine; enhanced CNS effects and toxicity when MAOIs given with ●venlafaxine (venlafaxine should not be started until 2 weeks after stopping MAOIs, avoid MAOIs for 1 week after stopping venlafaxine); increased risk of hypertension and CNS excitation when MAOIs given with other ●MAOIs (avoid for at least 2 weeks after stopping previous MAOIs and then start at a reduced dose); after stopping MAOIs do not start ●moclobemide for at least 1 week; MAOIs increase CNS effects of ●SSRIs (risk of serious toxicity); after stopping MAOIs do not start ●tricyclic-related antidepressants for 2 weeks, also MAOIs should not be started until at least 1–2 weeks after stopping tricyclic-related antidepressants; increased risk of hypertension and CNS excitation when MAOIs given with ●tricyclics, tricyclics should not be started until 2 weeks after stopping MAOIs (3 weeks if starting clomipramine or imipramine), also MAOIs should not be started for at least 1–2 weeks after stopping tricyclics (3 weeks in the case of clomipramine or imipramine); CNS excitation and confusion when MAOIs given with ●tryptophan (reduce dose of tryptophan)

  Antidiabetics: MAOIs possibly enhance hypoglycaemic effect of antidiabetics; MAOIs enhance hypoglycaemic effect of insulin, metformin and sulphonylureas

* Antiepileptics: MAOIs possibly antagonise anticonvulsant effect of antiepileptics (convulsive threshold lowered); avoidance for 2 weeks after stopping MAOIs advised by manufacturer of ●carbamazepine, also antagonism of anticonvulsant effect

  Antihistamines: increased antimuscarinic and sedative effects when MAOIs given with antihistamines

* Antimalarials: avoidance of antidepressants advised by manufacturer of ●artemether/lumefantrine

  Antimuscarinics: increased risk of antimuscarinic side-effects when MAOIs given with antimuscarinics

* Antipsychotics: CNS effects of MAOIs possibly increased by ●clozapine

  Anxiolytics and Hypnotics: avoidance of MAOIs advised by manufacturer of buspirone

MAOIs *(continued)*

- Atomoxetine: after stopping MAOIs do not start ●atomoxetine for 2 weeks, also MAOIs should not be started until at least 2 weeks after stopping atomoxetine; possible increased risk of convulsions when antidepressants given with atomoxetine

Barbiturates: MAOIs possibly antagonise anticonvulsant effect of barbiturates (convulsive threshold lowered)

Beta-blockers: enhanced hypotensive effect when MAOIs given with beta-blockers

- Bupropion: avoidance of bupropion for 2 weeks after stopping MAOIs advised by manufacturer of ●bupropion

Calcium-channel Blockers: enhanced hypotensive effect when MAOIs given with calcium-channel blockers

Clonidine: enhanced hypotensive effect when MAOIs given with clonidine

Diazoxide: enhanced hypotensive effect when MAOIs given with diazoxide

Diuretics: enhanced hypotensive effect when MAOIs given with diuretics

- Dopaminergics: avoid concomitant use of non-selective MAOIs with ●entacapone; risk of hypertensive crisis when MAOIs given with ●levodopa, avoid levodopa for at least 2 weeks after stopping MAOIs; risk of hypertensive crisis when MAOIs given with ●rasagiline, avoid MAOIs for at least 2 weeks after stopping rasagiline; enhanced hypotensive effect when MAOIs given with selegiline; avoid concomitant use of MAOIs with tolcapone

Doxapram: MAOIs enhance effects of doxapram

- 5HT₁ Agonists: risk of CNS toxicity when MAOIs given with ●rizatriptan or ●sumatriptan (avoid rizatriptan or sumatriptan for 2 weeks after MAOIs); increased risk of CNS toxicity when MAOIs given with ●zolmitriptan
- Methyldopa: avoidance of MAOIs advised by manufacturer of ●methyldopa

Moxonidine: enhanced hypotensive effect when MAOIs given with moxonidine

Muscle Relaxants: phenelzine enhances effects of suxamethonium

Nicorandil: enhanced hypotensive effect when MAOIs given with nicorandil

Nitrates: enhanced hypotensive effect when MAOIs given with nitrates

- Sibutramine: increased CNS toxicity when MAOIs given with ●sibutramine (manufacturer of sibutramine advises avoid concomitant use), also avoid sibutramine for 2 weeks after stopping MAOIs
- Sympathomimetics: risk of hypertensive crisis when MAOIs given with ●sympathomimetics; risk of hypertensive crisis when MAOIs given with ●methylphenidate, some manufacturers advise avoid methylphenidate for at least 2 weeks after stopping MAOIs
- Tetrabenazine: risk of CNS excitation and hypertension when MAOIs given with ●tetrabenazine

Vasodilator Antihypertensives: enhanced hypotensive effect when MAOIs given with hydralazine, minoxidil or sodium nitroprusside

MAOIs, reversible *see* Moclobemide

Maraviroc

- Antibacterials: plasma concentration of maraviroc possibly increased by ●clarithromycin and ●telithromycin (consider reducing dose of maraviroc); plasma concentration of maraviroc reduced by ●rifampicin—consider increasing dose of maraviroc
- Antidepressants: plasma concentration of maraviroc possibly reduced by ●St John's wort—avoid concomitant use

Maraviroc *(continued)*

- Antifungals: plasma concentration of maraviroc increased by ●ketoconazole (consider reducing dose of maraviroc)
- Antivirals: plasma concentration of maraviroc increased by ●atazanavir, ●darunavir, ●indinavir, ●lopinavir and ●saquinavir (consider reducing dose of maraviroc); plasma concentration of maraviroc possibly reduced by ●efavirenz—consider increasing dose of maraviroc; plasma concentration of maraviroc possibly reduced by etravirine; plasma concentration of maraviroc possibly increased by ●nelfinavir (consider reducing dose of maraviroc)

Mebendazole

Ulcer-healing Drugs: metabolism of mebendazole possibly inhibited by cimetidine (increased plasma concentration)

Medroxyprogesterone *see* Progestogens

Mefenamic Acid *see* NSAIDs

Mefloquine

- Anti-arrhythmics: increased risk of ventricular arrhythmias when mefloquine given with ●amiodarone—avoid concomitant use
- Antibacterials: increased risk of ventricular arrhythmias when mefloquine given with ●moxifloxacin—avoid concomitant use; plasma concentration of mefloquine reduced by ●rifampicin—avoid concomitant use
- Antiepileptics: mefloquine antagonises anticonvulsant effect of ●antiepileptics
- Antimalarials: avoidance of antimalarials advised by manufacturer of ●artemether/lumefantrine; increased risk of convulsions when mefloquine given with ●chloroquine and hydroxychloroquine; increased risk of convulsions when mefloquine given with ●quinine (but should not prevent the use of intravenous quinine in severe cases)
- Antipsychotics: increased risk of ventricular arrhythmias when mefloquine given with ●pimozide—avoid concomitant use
- Atomoxetine: increased risk of ventricular arrhythmias when mefloquine given with ●atomoxetine

Beta-blockers: increased risk of bradycardia when mefloquine given with beta-blockers

Calcium-channel Blockers: possible increased risk of bradycardia when mefloquine given with calcium-channel blockers

Cardiac Glycosides: possible increased risk of bradycardia when mefloquine given with digoxin

- Ivabradine: increased risk of ventricular arrhythmias when mefloquine given with ●ivabradine

Vaccines: antimalarials inactivate oral typhoid vaccine–see p. 752

Megestrol *see* Progestogens

Melatonin *see* Anxiolytics and Hypnotics

Meloxicam *see* NSAIDs

Melphalan

Antibacterials: increased risk of melphalan toxicity when given with nalidixic acid

Antiepileptics: cytotoxics possibly reduce absorption of phenytoin

- Antipsychotics: avoid concomitant use of cytotoxics with ●clozapine (increased risk of agranulocytosis)

Cardiac Glycosides: cytotoxics reduce absorption of digoxin tablets

- Ciclosporin: increased risk of nephrotoxicity when melphalan given with ●ciclosporin

Memantine

- Anaesthetics, General: increased risk of CNS toxicity when memantine given with ●ketamine (manufacturer of memantine advises avoid concomitant use)
- Analgesics: increased risk of CNS toxicity when memantine given with ●dextromethorphan (manufacturer of memantine advises avoid concomitant use)

Memantine *(continued)*

Anticoagulants: memantine possibly enhances anticoagulant effect of warfarin

Antiepileptics: memantine possibly reduces effects of primidone

Antimuscarinics: memantine possibly enhances effects of antimuscarinics

Antipsychotics: memantine possibly reduces effects of antipsychotics

Barbiturates: memantine possibly reduces effects of barbiturates

• Dopaminergics: memantine possibly enhances effects of dopaminergics and selegiline; increased risk of CNS toxicity when memantine given with •amantadine (manufacturer of memantine advises avoid concomitant use)

Muscle Relaxants: memantine possibly modifies effects of baclofen and dantrolene

Mepacrine

Antimalarials: mepacrine increases plasma concentration of primaquine (increased risk of toxicity)

Meprobamate *see* Anxiolytics and Hypnotics

Meptazinol *see* Opioid Analgesics

Mercaptopurine

• Allopurinol: enhanced effects and increased toxicity of mercaptopurine when given with •allopurinol (reduce dose of mercaptopurine to one quarter of usual dose)

Aminosalicylates: possible increased risk of leucopenia when mercaptopurine given with aminosalicylates

• Antibacterials: increased risk of haematological toxicity when mercaptopurine given with •sulfamethoxazole (as co-trimoxazole); increased risk of haematological toxicity when mercaptopurine given with •trimethoprim (also with co-trimoxazole)

• Anticoagulants: mercaptopurine possibly reduces anticoagulant effect of •coumarins

Antiepileptics: cytotoxics possibly reduce absorption of phenytoin

• Antipsychotics: avoid concomitant use of cytotoxics with •clozapine (increased risk of agranulocytosis)

Cardiac Glycosides: cytotoxics reduce absorption of digoxin tablets

Meropenem

Antiepileptics: meropenem reduces plasma concentration of valproate

Oestrogens: antibacterials that do not induce liver enzymes possibly reduce contraceptive effect of oestrogens (risk probably small, see p. 478)

Probenecid: excretion of meropenem reduced by probenecid (manufacturers of meropenem advise avoid concomitant use)

Vaccines: antibacterials inactivate oral typhoid vaccine—see p. 752

Mesalazine *see* Aminosalicylates

Mestranol *see* Oestrogens

Metaraminol *see* Sympathomimetics

Metformin *see* Antidiabetics

Methadone *see* Opioid Analgesics

Methenamine

• Antibacterials: increased risk of crystalluria when methenamine given with •sulphonamides

• Diuretics: effects of methenamine antagonised by •acetazolamide

Oestrogens: antibacterials that do not induce liver enzymes possibly reduce contraceptive effect of oestrogens (risk probably small, see p. 478)

Potassium Salts: avoid concomitant use of methenamine with potassium citrate

Vaccines: antibacterials inactivate oral typhoid vaccine—see p. 752

Methocarbamol *see* Muscle Relaxants

Methotrexate

• Anaesthetics, General: antifolate effect of methotrexate increased by •nitrous oxide—avoid concomitant use

Methotrexate *(continued)*

• Analgesics: excretion of methotrexate probably reduced by •NSAIDs (increased risk of toxicity); excretion of methotrexate reduced by •azapropazone (avoid concomitant use); excretion of methotrexate reduced by •aspirin, •diclofenac, •ibuprofen, •indometacin, •ketoprofen, •meloxicam and •naproxen (increased risk of toxicity)

• Antibacterials: absorption of methotrexate possibly reduced by neomycin; excretion of methotrexate possibly reduced by ciprofloxacin (increased risk of toxicity); increased risk of haematological toxicity when methotrexate given with •sulfamethoxazole (as co-trimoxazole); increased risk of methotrexate toxicity when given with doxycycline, sulphonamides or tetracycline; excretion of methotrexate reduced by penicillins (increased risk of toxicity); increased risk of haematological toxicity when methotrexate given with •trimethoprim (also with co-trimoxazole)

Antiepileptics: antifolate effect of methotrexate increased by phenytoin; cytotoxics possibly reduce absorption of phenytoin

• Antimalarials: antifolate effect of methotrexate increased by •pyrimethamine

• Antipsychotics: avoid concomitant use of cytotoxics with •clozapine (increased risk of agranulocytosis)

Cardiac Glycosides: cytotoxics reduce absorption of digoxin tablets

• Ciclosporin: risk of toxicity when methotrexate given with •ciclosporin

• Corticosteroids: increased risk of haematological toxicity when methotrexate given with •corticosteroids

• Cytotoxics: increased pulmonary toxicity when methotrexate given with •cisplatin

• Probenecid: excretion of methotrexate reduced by •probenecid (increased risk of toxicity)

• Retinoids: plasma concentration of methotrexate increased by •acitretin (also increased risk of hepatotoxicity)—avoid concomitant use

Theophylline: methotrexate possibly increases plasma concentration of theophylline

Ulcer-healing Drugs: excretion of methotrexate possibly reduced by omeprazole (increased risk of toxicity)

Methoxamine *see* Sympathomimetics

Methyldopa

ACE Inhibitors: enhanced hypotensive effect when methyldopa given with ACE inhibitors

Adrenergic Neurone Blockers: enhanced hypotensive effect when methyldopa given with adrenergic neurone blockers

Alcohol: enhanced hypotensive effect when methyldopa given with alcohol

Aldesleukin: enhanced hypotensive effect when methyldopa given with aldesleukin

Alpha-blockers: enhanced hypotensive effect when methyldopa given with alpha-blockers

Anaesthetics, General: enhanced hypotensive effect when methyldopa given with general anaesthetics

Analgesics: hypotensive effect of methyldopa antagonised by NSAIDs

Angiotensin-II Receptor Antagonists: enhanced hypotensive effect when methyldopa given with angiotensin-II receptor antagonists

• Antidepressants: manufacturer of methyldopa advises avoid concomitant use with •MAOIs

Antipsychotics: enhanced hypotensive effect when methyldopa given with antipsychotics (also increased risk of extrapyramidal effects)

Anxiolytics and Hypnotics: enhanced hypotensive effect when methyldopa given with anxiolytics and hypnotics

Beta-blockers: enhanced hypotensive effect when methyldopa given with beta-blockers

Appendix 1: Interactions

Methyldopa *(continued)*

Calcium-channel Blockers: enhanced hypotensive effect when methyldopa given with calcium-channel blockers

Clonidine: enhanced hypotensive effect when methyldopa given with clonidine

Corticosteroids: hypotensive effect of methyldopa antagonised by corticosteroids

Diazoxide: enhanced hypotensive effect when methyldopa given with diazoxide

Diuretics: enhanced hypotensive effect when methyldopa given with diuretics

Dopaminergics: methyldopa antagonises antiparkinsonian effect of dopaminergics; increased risk of extrapyramidal side-effects when methyldopa given with amantadine; effects of methyldopa possibly enhanced by entacapone; enhanced hypotensive effect when methyldopa given with levodopa

Iron: hypotensive effect of methyldopa antagonised by oral iron

• Lithium: neurotoxicity may occur when methyldopa given with •lithium without increased plasma concentration of lithium

Moxisylyte (thymoxamine): enhanced hypotensive effect when methyldopa given with moxisylyte

Moxonidine: enhanced hypotensive effect when methyldopa given with moxonidine

Muscle Relaxants: enhanced hypotensive effect when methyldopa given with baclofen or tizanidine

Nitrates: enhanced hypotensive effect when methyldopa given with nitrates

Oestrogens: hypotensive effect of methyldopa antagonised by oestrogens

Prostaglandins: enhanced hypotensive effect when methyldopa given with alprostadil

• Sympathomimetics, Beta$_2$: acute hypotension reported when methyldopa given with infusion of •salbutamol

Vasodilator Antihypertensives: enhanced hypotensive effect when methyldopa given with hydralazine, minoxidil or sodium nitroprusside

Methylphenidate *see* Sympathomimetics

Methylprednisolone *see* Corticosteroids

Methysergide *see* Ergot Alkaloids

Metipranolol *see* Beta-blockers

Metoclopramide

Analgesics: metoclopramide increases rate of absorption of aspirin (enhanced effect); effects of metoclopramide on gastro-intestinal activity antagonised by opioid analgesics; metoclopramide increases rate of absorption of paracetamol

Antimuscarinics: effects of metoclopramide on gastro-intestinal activity antagonised by antimuscarinics

Antipsychotics: increased risk of extrapyramidal side-effects when metoclopramide given with antipsychotics

Atovaquone: metoclopramide reduces plasma concentration of atovaquone

• Ciclosporin: metoclopramide increases plasma concentration of •ciclosporin

Dopaminergics: increased risk of extrapyramidal side-effects when metoclopramide given with amantadine; metoclopramide antagonises hypoprolactinaemic effects of bromocriptine and cabergoline; metoclopramide antagonises antiparkinsonian effect of pergolide; avoidance of metoclopramide advised by manufacturer of ropinirole and rotigotine (antagonism of effect)

Muscle Relaxants: metoclopramide enhances effects of suxamethonium

Tetrabenazine: increased risk of extrapyramidal side-effects when metoclopramide given with tetrabenazine

Metolazone *see* Diuretics

Metoprolol *see* Beta-blockers

Metronidazole

Note. Interactions do not apply to topical metronidazole preparations

Alcohol: disulfiram-like reaction when metronidazole given with alcohol

• Anticoagulants: metronidazole enhances anticoagulant effect of •coumarins

• Antiepileptics: metronidazole inhibits metabolism of •phenytoin (increased plasma concentration); metabolism of metronidazole accelerated by primidone (reduced plasma concentration)

Barbiturates: metabolism of metronidazole accelerated by barbiturates (reduced plasma concentration)

• Cytotoxics: metronidazole increases plasma concentration of •busulfan (increased risk of toxicity); metronidazole inhibits metabolism of fluorouracil (increased toxicity); metronidazole possibly reduces bioavailability of mycophenolate

Disulfiram: psychotic reaction reported when metronidazole given with disulfiram

Lithium: metronidazole increases risk of lithium toxicity

Oestrogens: antibacterials that do not induce liver enzymes possibly reduce contraceptive effect of oestrogens (risk probably small, see p. 478)

Ulcer-healing Drugs: metabolism of metronidazole inhibited by cimetidine (increased plasma concentration)

Vaccines: antibacterials inactivate oral typhoid vaccine–see p. 752

Mianserin *see* Antidepressants, Tricyclic (related)

Micafungin

Antifungals: micafungin increases plasma concentration of itraconazole (consider reducing dose of itraconazole)

Calcium-channel Blockers: micafungin increases plasma concentration of nifedipine

Ciclosporin: micafungin possibly increases plasma concentration of ciclosporin

Sirolimus: micafungin increases plasma concentration of sirolimus

Miconazole *see* Antifungals, Imidazole

Midazolam *see* Anxiolytics and Hypnotics

Mifepristone

Corticosteroids: mifepristone may reduce effect of corticosteroids (including inhaled corticosteroids) for 3–4 days

Milrinone *see* Phosphodiesterase Inhibitors

Minocycline *see* Tetracyclines

Minoxidil *see* Vasodilator Antihypertensives

Mirtazapine

• Alcohol: increased sedative effect when mirtazapine given with •alcohol

Anticoagulants: mirtazapine enhances anticoagulant effect of warfarin

• Antidepressants: mirtazapine should not be started until 2 weeks after stopping •MAOIs, also MAOIs should not be started until at least 2 weeks after stopping mirtazapine; after stopping mirtazapine do not start •moclobemide for at least 1 week

Antiepileptics: plasma concentration of mirtazapine reduced by carbamazepine and phenytoin

Antifungals: plasma concentration of mirtazapine increased by ketoconazole

• Antimalarials: avoidance of antidepressants advised by manufacturer of •artemether/lumefantrine

Anxiolytics and Hypnotics: increased sedative effect when mirtazapine given with anxiolytics and hypnotics

Atomoxetine: possible increased risk of convulsions when antidepressants given with atomoxetine

• Sibutramine: increased risk of CNS toxicity when mirtazapine given with •sibutramine (manufacturer of sibutramine advises avoid concomitant use)

Ulcer-healing Drugs: plasma concentration of mirtazapine increased by cimetidine

Mitomycin

Antiepileptics: cytotoxics possibly reduce absorption of phenytoin

● Antipsychotics: avoid concomitant use of cytotoxics with ●clozapine (increased risk of agranulocytosis)
Cardiac Glycosides: cytotoxics reduce absorption of digoxin tablets

Mitotane

● Anticoagulants: mitotane possibly reduces anticoagulant effect of ●coumarins
Antiepileptics: cytotoxics possibly reduce absorption of phenytoin

● Antipsychotics: avoid concomitant use of cytotoxics with ●clozapine (increased risk of agranulocytosis)
Cardiac Glycosides: cytotoxics reduce absorption of digoxin tablets
Diuretics: manufacturer of mitotane advises avoid concomitant use of spironolactone (antagonism of effect)

Mivacurium see Muscle Relaxants
Mizolastine see Antihistamines
Moclobemide

● Analgesics: possible CNS excitation or depression (hypertension or hypotension) when moclobemide given with ●dextromethorphan or ●pethidine—avoid concomitant use; possible CNS excitation or depression (hypertension or hypotension) when moclobemide given with ●opioid analgesics

● Antidepressants: moclobemide should not be started for at least 1 week after stopping ●MAOIs, ●SSRI-related antidepressants, ●citalopram, ●fluvoxamine, ●mirtazapine, ●paroxetine, ●tricyclic-related antidepressants or ●tricyclics; increased risk of CNS toxicity when moclobemide given with ●escitalopram, preferably avoid concomitant use; moclobemide should not be started until 5 weeks after stopping ●fluoxetine; moclobemide should not be started until 2 weeks after stopping ●sertraline; possible increased serotonergic effects when moclobemide given with ●duloxetine

● Antimalarials: avoidance of antidepressants advised by manufacturer of ●artemether/lumefantrine
Atomoxetine: possible increased risk of convulsions when antidepressants given with atomoxetine

● Bupropion: avoidance of moclobemide advised by manufacturer of ●bupropion

● Dopaminergics: caution with moclobemide advised by manufacturer of entacapone; increased risk of side-effects when moclobemide given with levodopa; avoid concomitant use of moclobemide with ●selegiline

● 5HT$_1$ Agonists: risk of CNS toxicity when moclobemide given with ●rizatriptan or ●sumatriptan (avoid rizatriptan or sumatriptan for 2 weeks after moclobemide); risk of CNS toxicity when moclobemide given with ●zolmitriptan (reduce dose of zolmitriptan)

● Sibutramine: increased CNS toxicity when moclobemide given with ●sibutramine (manufacturer of sibutramine advises avoid concomitant use, also avoid sibutramine for 2 weeks after stopping moclobemide)

● Sympathomimetics: risk of hypertensive crisis when moclobemide given with ●sympathomimetics
Ulcer-healing Drugs: plasma concentration of moclobemide increased by cimetidine (halve dose of moclobemide)

Modafinil

Antiepileptics: modafinil possibly increases plasma concentration of phenytoin

● Ciclosporin: modafinil reduces plasma concentration of ●ciclosporin

● Oestrogens: modafinil accelerates metabolism of ●oestrogens (reduced contraceptive effect—see p. 478)

Moexipril see ACE Inhibitors

Mometasone see Corticosteroids
Monobactams see Aztreonam
Montelukast see Leukotriene Receptor Antagonists
Morphine see Opioid Analgesics
Moxifloxacin see Quinolones
Moxisylyte (thymoxamine)

ACE Inhibitors: enhanced hypotensive effect when moxisylyte given with ACE inhibitors
Adrenergic Neurone Blockers: enhanced hypotensive effect when moxisylyte given with adrenergic neurone blockers

● Alpha-blockers: possible severe postural hypotension when moxisylyte given with ●alpha-blockers
Angiotensin-II Receptor Antagonists: enhanced hypotensive effect when moxisylyte given with angiotensin-II receptor antagonists

● Beta-blockers: possible severe postural hypotension when moxisylyte given with ●beta-blockers
Calcium-channel Blockers: enhanced hypotensive effect when moxisylyte given with calcium-channel blockers
Clonidine: enhanced hypotensive effect when moxisylyte given with clonidine
Diazoxide: enhanced hypotensive effect when moxisylyte given with diazoxide
Diuretics: enhanced hypotensive effect when moxisylyte given with diuretics
Methyldopa: enhanced hypotensive effect when moxisylyte given with methyldopa
Moxonidine: enhanced hypotensive effect when moxisylyte given with moxonidine
Nitrates: enhanced hypotensive effect when moxisylyte given with nitrates
Vasodilator Antihypertensives: enhanced hypotensive effect when moxisylyte given with hydralazine, minoxidil or sodium nitroprusside

Moxonidine

ACE Inhibitors: enhanced hypotensive effect when moxonidine given with ACE inhibitors
Adrenergic Neurone Blockers: enhanced hypotensive effect when moxonidine given with adrenergic neurone blockers
Alcohol: enhanced hypotensive effect when moxonidine given with alcohol
Aldesleukin: enhanced hypotensive effect when moxonidine given with aldesleukin
Alpha-blockers: enhanced hypotensive effect when moxonidine given with alpha-blockers
Anaesthetics, General: enhanced hypotensive effect when moxonidine given with general anaesthetics
Analgesics: hypotensive effect of moxonidine antagonised by NSAIDs
Angiotensin-II Receptor Antagonists: enhanced hypotensive effect when moxonidine given with angiotensin-II receptor antagonists
Antidepressants: enhanced hypotensive effect when moxonidine given with MAOIs
Antipsychotics: enhanced hypotensive effect when moxonidine given with phenothiazines
Anxiolytics and Hypnotics: enhanced hypotensive effect when moxonidine given with anxiolytics and hypnotics; sedative effects possibly increased when moxonidine given with benzodiazepines
Beta-blockers: enhanced hypotensive effect when moxonidine given with beta-blockers
Calcium-channel Blockers: enhanced hypotensive effect when moxonidine given with calcium-channel blockers
Clonidine: enhanced hypotensive effect when moxonidine given with clonidine
Corticosteroids: hypotensive effect of moxonidine antagonised by corticosteroids
Diazoxide: enhanced hypotensive effect when moxonidine given with diazoxide
Diuretics: enhanced hypotensive effect when moxonidine given with diuretics

Moxonidine *(continued)*

Dopaminergics: enhanced hypotensive effect when moxonidine given with levodopa

Methyldopa: enhanced hypotensive effect when moxonidine given with methyldopa

Moxisylyte (thymoxamine): enhanced hypotensive effect when moxonidine given with moxisylyte

Muscle Relaxants: enhanced hypotensive effect when moxonidine given with baclofen or tizanidine

Nitrates: enhanced hypotensive effect when moxonidine given with nitrates

Oestrogens: hypotensive effect of moxonidine antagonised by oestrogens

Prostaglandins: enhanced hypotensive effect when moxonidine given with alprostadil

Vasodilator Antihypertensives: enhanced hypotensive effect when moxonidine given with hydralazine, minoxidil or sodium nitroprusside

Muscle Relaxants

ACE Inhibitors: enhanced hypotensive effect when baclofen or tizanidine given with ACE inhibitors

Adrenergic Neurone Blockers: enhanced hypotensive effect when baclofen or tizanidine given with adrenergic neurone blockers

Alcohol: increased sedative effect when baclofen, methocarbamol or tizanidine given with alcohol

Alpha-blockers: enhanced hypotensive effect when baclofen or tizanidine given with alpha-blockers

• Anaesthetics, General: effects of atracurium enhanced by ketamine; increased risk of myocardial depression and bradycardia when suxamethonium given with •propofol; effects of non-depolarising muscle relaxants and suxamethonium enhanced by volatile liquid general anaesthetics

Anaesthetics, Local: neuromuscular blockade enhanced and prolonged when suxamethonium given with procaine

Analgesics: excretion of baclofen possibly reduced by NSAIDs (increased risk of toxicity); excretion of baclofen reduced by ibuprofen (increased risk of toxicity)

Angiotensin-II Receptor Antagonists: enhanced hypotensive effect when baclofen or tizanidine given with angiotensin-II receptor antagonists

Anti-arrhythmics: neuromuscular blockade enhanced and prolonged when suxamethonium given with lidocaine (lignocaine)

• Antibacterials: effects of non-depolarising muscle relaxants and suxamethonium enhanced by piperacillin; plasma concentration of tizanidine increased by •ciprofloxacin (increased risk of toxicity)—avoid concomitant use; effects of non-depolarising muscle relaxants and suxamethonium enhanced by •aminoglycosides; effects of non-depolarising muscle relaxants and suxamethonium enhanced by •clindamycin; effects of non-depolarising muscle relaxants and suxamethonium enhanced by •polymyxins; effects of suxamethonium enhanced by •vancomycin

• Antidepressants: plasma concentration of tizanidine increased by •fluvoxamine (increased risk of toxicity)—avoid concomitant use; effects of suxamethonium enhanced by phenelzine; muscle relaxant effect of baclofen enhanced by tricyclics

Antiepileptics: muscle relaxant effect of non-depolarising muscle relaxants antagonised by carbamazepine and phenytoin (accelerated recovery from neuromuscular blockade)

Antimalarials: effects of suxamethonium possibly enhanced by quinine

Antipsychotics: effects of suxamethonium possibly enhanced by promazine

Anxiolytics and Hypnotics: increased sedative effect when baclofen or tizanidine given with anxiolytics and hypnotics

Muscle Relaxants *(continued)*

Beta-blockers: enhanced hypotensive effect when baclofen given with beta-blockers; possible enhanced hypotensive effect and bradycardia when tizanidine given with beta-blockers; effects of muscle relaxants enhanced by propranolol

Calcium-channel Blockers: enhanced hypotensive effect when baclofen or tizanidine given with calcium-channel blockers; effects of non-depolarising muscle relaxants enhanced by nifedipine and verapamil; risk of arrhythmias when intravenous dantrolene given with diltiazem; hypotension, myocardial depression, and hyperkalaemia when intravenous dantrolene given with verapamil; effects of suxamethonium enhanced by verapamil

Cardiac Glycosides: possible increased risk of bradycardia when tizanidine given with cardiac glycosides; risk of ventricular arrhythmias when suxamethonium given with cardiac glycosides

Clonidine: enhanced hypotensive effect when baclofen or tizanidine given with clonidine

Corticosteroids: effects of pancuronium and vecuronium possibly antagonised by corticosteroids

Cytotoxics: effects of suxamethonium enhanced by cyclophosphamide and thiotepa

Diazoxide: enhanced hypotensive effect when baclofen or tizanidine given with diazoxide

Diuretics: enhanced hypotensive effect when baclofen or tizanidine given with diuretics

Dopaminergics: possible agitation, confusion and hallucinations when baclofen given with levodopa

Lithium: effects of muscle relaxants enhanced by lithium; baclofen possibly aggravates hyperkinesis caused by lithium

Magnesium (parenteral): effects of non-depolarising muscle relaxants and suxamethonium enhanced by parenteral magnesium

Memantine: effects of baclofen and dantrolene possibly modified by memantine

Methyldopa: enhanced hypotensive effect when baclofen or tizanidine given with methyldopa

Metoclopramide: effects of suxamethonium enhanced by metoclopramide

Moxonidine: enhanced hypotensive effect when baclofen or tizanidine given with moxonidine

Nitrates: enhanced hypotensive effect when baclofen or tizanidine given with nitrates

Oestrogens: plasma concentration of tizanidine possibly increased by oestrogens (increased risk of toxicity)

Parasympathomimetics: effects of suxamethonium possibly enhanced by donepezil; effects of non-depolarising muscle relaxants possibly antagonised by donepezil; effects of suxamethonium enhanced by edrophonium, galantamine, neostigmine, pyridostigmine and rivastigmine; effects of non-depolarising muscle relaxants antagonised by edrophonium, neostigmine, pyridostigmine and rivastigmine

Progestogens: plasma concentration of tizanidine possibly increased by progestogens (increased risk of toxicity)

Sympathomimetics, Beta$_2$: effects of suxamethonium enhanced by bambuterol

Vasodilator Antihypertensives: enhanced hypotensive effect when baclofen or tizanidine given with hydralazine; enhanced hypotensive effect when baclofen or tizanidine given with minoxidil; enhanced hypotensive effect when baclofen or tizanidine given with sodium nitroprusside

Muscle Relaxants, depolarising *see* Muscle Relaxants
Muscle Relaxants, non-depolarising *see* Muscle Relaxants
Mycophenolate

Antacids: absorption of mycophenolate reduced by antacids

Mycophenolate *(continued)*

- Antibacterials: bioavailability of mycophenolate possibly reduced by metronidazole and norfloxacin; plasma concentration of active metabolite of mycophenolate reduced by ●rifampicin

  Antiepileptics: cytotoxics possibly reduce absorption of phenytoin

- Antipsychotics: avoid concomitant use of cytotoxics with ●clozapine (increased risk of agranulocytosis)

  Antivirals: mycophenolate increases plasma concentration of aciclovir, also plasma concentration of inactive metabolite of mycophenolate increased; mycophenolate possibly increases plasma concentration of ganciclovir, also plasma concentration of inactive metabolite of mycophenolate possibly increased

  Cardiac Glycosides: cytotoxics reduce absorption of digoxin tablets

  Iron: absorption of mycophenolate reduced by *oral* iron

  Lipid-regulating Drugs: absorption of mycophenolate reduced by colestyramine

  Sevelamer: plasma concentration of mycophenolate possibly reduced by sevelamer

Mycophenolate Mofetil *see* Mycophenolate

Mycophenolate Sodium *see* Mycophenolate

Mycophenolic Acid *see* Mycophenolate

Nabilone

  Alcohol: increased sedative effect when nabilone given with alcohol

  Anxiolytics and Hypnotics: increased sedative effect when nabilone given with anxiolytics and hypnotics

Nabumetone *see* NSAIDs

Nadolol *see* Beta-blockers

Nalidixic Acid *see* Quinolones

Nandrolone *see* Anabolic Steroids

Naproxen *see* NSAIDs

Naratriptan *see* 5HT₁ Agonists

Nateglinide *see* Antidiabetics

Nebivolol *see* Beta-blockers

Nefopam

- Antidepressants: manufacturer of nefopam advises avoid concomitant use with ●MAOIs; side-effects possibly increased when nefopam given with tricyclics

  Antimuscarinics: increased risk of antimuscarinic side-effects when nefopam given with antimuscarinics

Nelfinavir

  Analgesics: nelfinavir reduces plasma concentration of methadone

- Anti-arrhythmics: increased risk of ventricular arrhythmias when nelfinavir given with ●amiodarone—avoid concomitant use

- Antibacterials: nelfinavir increases plasma concentration of ●rifabutin (halve dose of rifabutin); plasma concentration of nelfinavir significantly reduced by ●rifampicin—avoid concomitant use; avoidance of concomitant nelfinavir in severe renal and hepatic impairment advised by manufacturer of ●telithromycin

  Anticoagulants: avoidance of nelfinavir advised by manufacturer of rivaroxaban

- Antidepressants: plasma concentration of nelfinavir reduced by ●St John's wort—avoid concomitant use

- Antiepileptics: plasma concentration of nelfinavir possibly reduced by carbamazepine and ●primidone; nelfinavir reduces plasma concentration of phenytoin

  Antimalarials: caution with nelfinavir advised by manufacturer of artemether/lumefantrine

  Antimuscarinics: avoidance of nelfinavir advised by manufacturer of darifenacin and tolterodine; manufacturer of fesoterodine advises dose reduction when nelfinavir given with fesoterodine—consult fesoterodine product literature; nelfinavir increases plasma concentration of solifenacin

Nelfinavir *(continued)*

- Antipsychotics: nelfinavir possibly inhibits metabolism of ●aripiprazole (reduce dose of aripiprazole); nelfinavir possibly increases plasma concentration of ●pimozide (increased risk of ventricular arrhythmias—avoid concomitant use); nelfinavir increases plasma concentration of ●sertindole (increased risk of ventricular arrhythmias—avoid concomitant use)

- Antivirals: plasma concentration of nelfinavir possibly increased by etravirine—avoid concomitant use; combination of nelfinavir with indinavir, ritonavir or saquinavir may increase plasma concentration of either drug (or both); nelfinavir reduces plasma concentration of lopinavir, also plasma concentration of active metabolite of nelfinavir increased; nelfinavir possibly increases plasma concentration of ●maraviroc (consider reducing dose of maraviroc)

- Anxiolytics and Hypnotics: nelfinavir possibly increases plasma concentration of ●midazolam (risk of prolonged sedation—avoid concomitant use of oral midazolam)

- Barbiturates: plasma concentration of nelfinavir possibly reduced by ●barbiturates

- Ciclosporin: nelfinavir possibly increases plasma concentration of ●ciclosporin

- Cilostazol: nelfinavir possibly increases plasma concentration of ●cilostazol—avoid concomitant use

  Cytotoxics: nelfinavir increases plasma concentration of paclitaxel

- Diuretics: nelfinavir increases plasma concentration of ●eplerenone—avoid concomitant use

- Ergot Alkaloids: increased risk of ergotism when nelfinavir given with ●ergotamine and methysergide—avoid concomitant use

- 5HT₁ Agonists: nelfinavir increases plasma concentration of ●eletriptan (risk of toxicity)—avoid concomitant use

- Ivabradine: nelfinavir possibly increases plasma concentration of ●ivabradine—avoid concomitant use

- Lipid-regulating Drugs: possible increased risk of myopathy when nelfinavir given with atorvastatin; possible increased risk of myopathy when nelfinavir given with ●rosuvastatin—avoid concomitant use; increased risk of myopathy when nelfinavir given with ●simvastatin (avoid concomitant use)

- Oestrogens: nelfinavir accelerates metabolism of ●oestrogens (reduced contraceptive effect—see p. 478)

  Progestogens: nelfinavir possibly reduces contraceptive effect of progestogens

  Sildenafil: nelfinavir possibly increases plasma concentration of sildenafil—reduce initial dose of sildenafil

- Tacrolimus: nelfinavir possibly increases plasma concentration of ●tacrolimus

- Ulcer-healing Drugs: plasma concentration of nelfinavir reduced by ●omeprazole—avoid concomitant use

Neomycin *see* Aminoglycosides

Neostigmine *see* Parasympathomimetics

Nevirapine

  Analgesics: nevirapine possibly reduces plasma concentration of methadone

- Antibacterials: nevirapine possibly increases plasma concentration of rifabutin; plasma concentration of nevirapine reduced by ●rifampicin—avoid concomitant use

- Anticoagulants: nevirapine may enhance or reduce anticoagulant effect of ●warfarin

- Antidepressants: plasma concentration of nevirapine reduced by ●St John's wort—avoid concomitant use

- Antifungals: nevirapine reduces plasma concentration of ●ketoconazole—avoid concomitant use; plasma concentration of nevirapine increased by ●fluconazole; nevirapine possibly reduces plasma concentration of caspofungin and itraconazole—

Nevirapine
- Antifungals *(continued)*
    consider increasing dose of caspofungin and itraconazole
- Antipsychotics: nevirapine possibly reduces plasma concentration of ●aripiprazole—increase dose of aripiprazole
- Antivirals: nevirapine possibly reduces plasma concentration of ●atazanavir and ●etravirine—avoid concomitant use; nevirapine reduces plasma concentration of efavirenz and indinavir; nevirapine possibly reduces plasma concentration of fosamprenavir; nevirapine possibly reduces plasma concentration of ●lopinavir—consider increasing dose of lopinavir
- Oestrogens: nevirapine accelerates metabolism of ●oestrogens (reduced contraceptive effect—see p. 478)
- Progestogens: nevirapine accelerates metabolism of ●progestogens (reduced contraceptive effect—see p. 478)

Nicardipine *see* Calcium-channel Blockers

Nicorandil
    Alcohol: hypotensive effect of nicorandil possibly enhanced by alcohol
    Antidepressants: enhanced hypotensive effect when nicorandil given with MAOIs; hypotensive effect of nicorandil possibly enhanced by tricyclics
- Sildenafil: hypotensive effect of nicorandil significantly enhanced by ●sildenafil (avoid concomitant use)
- Tadalafil: hypotensive effect of nicorandil significantly enhanced by ●tadalafil (avoid concomitant use)
- Vardenafil: possible increased hypotensive effect when nicorandil given with ●vardenafil—avoid concomitant use
    Vasodilator Antihypertensives: possible enhanced hypotensive effect when nicorandil given with hydralazine, minoxidil or sodium nitroprusside

Nicotinic Acid
    Note. Interactions apply to lipid-regulating doses of nicotinic acid
- Lipid-regulating Drugs: increased risk of myopathy when nicotinic acid given with ●statins (applies to lipid regulating doses of nicotinic acid)

Nifedipine *see* Calcium-channel Blockers

Nilotinib
- Antibacterials: manufacturer of nilotinib advises avoid concomitant use with ●clarithromycin, ●moxifloxacin and ●telithromycin
    Antiepileptics: cytotoxics possibly reduce absorption of phenytoin
- Antifungals: plasma concentration of nilotinib increased by ●ketoconazole—avoid concomitant use; manufacturer of nilotinib advises avoid concomitant use with ●itraconazole and ●voriconazole
- Antipsychotics: avoid concomitant use of cytotoxics with ●clozapine (increased risk of agranulocytosis)
- Antivirals: manufacturer of nilotinib advises avoid concomitant use with ●ritonavir
    Anxiolytics and Hypnotics: nilotinib increases plasma concentration of midazolam
    Cardiac Glycosides: cytotoxics reduce absorption of digoxin tablets
- Grapefruit Juice: manufacturer of nilotinib advises avoid concomitant use with ●grapefruit juice

Nimodipine *see* Calcium-channel Blockers

Nitrates
    ACE Inhibitors: enhanced hypotensive effect when nitrates given with ACE inhibitors
    Adrenergic Neurone Blockers: enhanced hypotensive effect when nitrates given with adrenergic neurone blockers
    Alcohol: enhanced hypotensive effect when nitrates given with alcohol
    Aldesleukin: enhanced hypotensive effect when nitrates given with aldesleukin

Nitrates *(continued)*
    Alpha-blockers: enhanced hypotensive effect when nitrates given with alpha-blockers
    Anaesthetics, General: enhanced hypotensive effect when nitrates given with general anaesthetics
    Analgesics: hypotensive effect of nitrates antagonised by NSAIDs
    Angiotensin-II Receptor Antagonists: enhanced hypotensive effect when nitrates given with angiotensin-II receptor antagonists
    Anti-arrhythmics: effects of sublingual tablets of nitrates reduced by disopyramide (failure to dissolve under tongue owing to dry mouth)
- Anticoagulants: infusion of glyceryl trinitrate reduces anticoagulant effect of ●heparins
    Antidepressants: enhanced hypotensive effect when nitrates given with MAOIs; effects of sublingual tablets of nitrates possibly reduced by tricyclic-related antidepressants (failure to dissolve under tongue owing to dry mouth); effects of sublingual tablets of nitrates reduced by tricyclics (failure to dissolve under tongue owing to dry mouth)
    Antimuscarinics: effects of sublingual tablets of nitrates possibly reduced by antimuscarinics (failure to dissolve under tongue owing to dry mouth)
    Antipsychotics: enhanced hypotensive effect when nitrates given with phenothiazines
    Anxiolytics and Hypnotics: enhanced hypotensive effect when nitrates given with anxiolytics and hypnotics
    Beta-blockers: enhanced hypotensive effect when nitrates given with beta-blockers
    Calcium-channel Blockers: enhanced hypotensive effect when nitrates given with calcium-channel blockers
    Clonidine: enhanced hypotensive effect when nitrates given with clonidine
    Corticosteroids: hypotensive effect of nitrates antagonised by corticosteroids
    Diazoxide: enhanced hypotensive effect when nitrates given with diazoxide
    Diuretics: enhanced hypotensive effect when nitrates given with diuretics
    Dopaminergics: enhanced hypotensive effect when nitrates given with levodopa
    Methyldopa: enhanced hypotensive effect when nitrates given with methyldopa
    Moxisylyte (thymoxamine): enhanced hypotensive effect when nitrates given with moxisylyte
    Moxonidine: enhanced hypotensive effect when nitrates given with moxonidine
    Muscle Relaxants: enhanced hypotensive effect when nitrates given with baclofen or tizanidine
    Oestrogens: hypotensive effect of nitrates antagonised by oestrogens
    Prostaglandins: enhanced hypotensive effect when nitrates given with alprostadil
- Sildenafil: hypotensive effect of nitrates significantly enhanced by ●sildenafil (avoid concomitant use)
- Tadalafil: hypotensive effect of nitrates significantly enhanced by ●tadalafil (avoid concomitant use)
- Vardenafil: possible increased hypotensive effect when nitrates given with ●vardenafil—avoid concomitant use
    Vasodilator Antihypertensives: enhanced hypotensive effect when nitrates given with hydralazine, minoxidil or sodium nitroprusside

Nitrazepam *see* Anxiolytics and Hypnotics

Nitrofurantoin
    Antacids: absorption of nitrofurantoin reduced by oral magnesium salts (as magnesium trisilicate)
    Oestrogens: antibacterials that do not induce liver enzymes possibly reduce contraceptive effect of oestrogens (risk probably small, see p. 478)
    Probenecid: excretion of nitrofurantoin reduced by probenecid (increased risk of side-effects)

Nitrofurantoin *(continued)*

Sulfinpyrazone: excretion of nitrofurantoin reduced by sulfinpyrazone (increased risk of toxicity)

Vaccines: antibacterials inactivate oral typhoid vaccine–see p. 752

Nitroimidazoles *see* Metronidazole and Tinidazole

Nitrous Oxide *see* Anaesthetics, General

Nizatidine *See* Histamine H$_2$-antagonists

Noradrenaline (norepinephrine) *see* Sympathomimetics

Norelgestromin *see* Progestogens

Norepinephrine (noradrenaline) *see* Sympathomimetics

Norethisterone *see* Progestogens

Norfloxacin *see* Quinolones

Norgestimate *see* Progestogens

Norgestrel *see* Progestogens

Nortriptyline *see* Antidepressants, Tricyclic

NSAIDs

Note. See also Aspirin. Interactions do not generally apply to topical NSAIDs

ACE Inhibitors: increased risk of renal impairment when NSAIDs given with ACE inhibitors, also hypotensive effect antagonised

Adrenergic Neurone Blockers: NSAIDs antagonise hypotensive effect of adrenergic neurone blockers

Alpha-blockers: NSAIDs antagonise hypotensive effect of alpha-blockers

• Analgesics: avoid concomitant use of NSAIDs with •NSAIDs or •aspirin (increased side-effects); avoid concomitant use of NSAIDs with •ketorolac (increased side-effects and haemorrhage); ibuprofen possibly reduces antiplatelet effect of aspirin

Angiotensin-II Receptor Antagonists: increased risk of renal impairment when NSAIDs given with angiotensin-II receptor antagonists, also hypotensive effect antagonised

• Antibacterials: indometacin possibly increases plasma concentration of amikacin and gentamicin in neonates; plasma concentration of etoricoxib reduced by rifampicin; possible increased risk of convulsions when NSAIDs given with •quinolones

• Anticoagulants: increased risk of haemorrhage when intravenous diclofenac given with •anticoagulants (avoid concomitant use, including low-dose heparin); increased risk of haemorrhage when ketorolac given with •anticoagulants (avoid concomitant use, including low-dose heparin); azapropazone enhances anticoagulant effect of •coumarins (avoid concomitant use); NSAIDs possibly enhance anticoagulant effect of •coumarins and •phenindione; possible increased risk of bleeding when NSAIDs given with •dabigatran etexilate or heparins

• Antidepressants: increased risk of bleeding when NSAIDs given with •SSRIs or •venlafaxine

• Antidiabetics: azapropazone enhances effects of •tolbutamide (avoid concomitant use); NSAIDs possibly enhance effects of •sulphonylureas

• Antiepileptics: azapropazone significantly increases plasma concentration of •phenytoin—avoid concomitant use; NSAIDs possibly enhance effects of •phenytoin

Antifungals: plasma concentration of parecoxib increased by fluconazole (reduce dose of parecoxib); plasma concentration of celecoxib increased by fluconazole (halve dose of celecoxib); plasma concentration of diclofenac and ibuprofen increased by voriconazole

• Antipsychotics: possible severe drowsiness when indometacin given with haloperidol; avoid concomitant use of azapropazone with •clozapine (increased risk of agranulocytosis)

• Antivirals: plasma concentration of NSAIDs possibly increased by ritonavir; plasma concentration of piroxicam increased by •ritonavir (risk of toxicity)—avoid concomitant use; increased risk of haematological toxicity when NSAIDs given with zidovudine

NSAIDs *(continued)*

Beta-blockers: NSAIDs antagonise hypotensive effect of beta-blockers

Bisphosphonates: indometacin increases bioavailability of tiludronic acid

Calcium-channel Blockers: NSAIDs antagonise hypotensive effect of calcium-channel blockers

Cardiac Glycosides: NSAIDs possibly increase plasma concentration of cardiac glycosides, also possible exacerbation of heart failure and reduction of renal function

• Ciclosporin: increased risk of nephrotoxicity when NSAIDs given with •ciclosporin; plasma concentration of diclofenac increased by •ciclosporin (halve dose of diclofenac)

Clonidine: NSAIDs antagonise hypotensive effect of clonidine

Clopidogrel: increased risk of bleeding when NSAIDs given with clopidogrel

Corticosteroids: increased risk of gastro-intestinal bleeding and ulceration when NSAIDs given with corticosteroids

• Cytotoxics: NSAIDs probably reduce excretion of •methotrexate (increased risk of toxicity); azapropazone reduces excretion of •methotrexate (avoid concomitant use); diclofenac, ibuprofen, indometacin, ketoprofen, meloxicam and naproxen reduce excretion of •methotrexate (increased risk of toxicity); increased risk of bleeding when NSAIDs given with •erlotinib

Desmopressin: indometacin enhances effects of desmopressin

Diazoxide: NSAIDs antagonise hypotensive effect of diazoxide

• Dimethyl sulfoxide: avoid concomitant use of sulindac with •dimethyl sulfoxide

• Diuretics: risk of nephrotoxicity of NSAIDs increased by diuretics, also antagonism of diuretic effect; indometacin and ketorolac antagonise effects of diuretics; NSAIDs possibly antagonise diuretic effect of potassium canrenoate; occasional reports of reduced renal function when indometacin given with •triamterene—avoid concomitant use; increased risk of hyperkalaemia when indometacin given with potassium-sparing diuretics and aldosterone antagonists; possibly increased risk of hyperkalaemia when NSAIDs given with potassium-sparing diuretics and aldosterone antagonists

Iloprost: increased risk of bleeding when NSAIDs given with iloprost

Lipid-regulating Drugs: excretion of meloxicam increased by colestyramine

• Lithium: NSAIDs reduce excretion of •lithium (increased risk of toxicity); ketorolac reduces excretion of •lithium (increased risk of toxicity)—avoid concomitant use

Methyldopa: NSAIDs antagonise hypotensive effect of methyldopa

Moxonidine: NSAIDs antagonise hypotensive effect of moxonidine

Muscle Relaxants: NSAIDs possibly reduce excretion of baclofen (increased risk of toxicity); ibuprofen reduces excretion of baclofen (increased risk of toxicity)

Nitrates: NSAIDs antagonise hypotensive effect of nitrates

Oestrogens: etoricoxib increases plasma concentration of ethinylestradiol

Penicillamine: possible increased risk of nephrotoxicity when NSAIDs given with penicillamine

• Pentoxifylline (oxpentifylline): possible increased risk of bleeding when NSAIDs given with pentoxifylline (oxpentifylline); increased risk of bleeding when ketorolac given with •pentoxifylline (oxpentifylline) (avoid concomitant use)

Appendix 1: Interactions

NSAIDs *(continued)*

- Probenecid: excretion of dexketoprofen, indometacin, ketoprofen and naproxen reduced by ●probenecid (increased plasma concentration); excretion of ketorolac reduced by ●probenecid (increased plasma concentration)—avoid concomitant use

  Sibutramine: increased risk of bleeding when NSAIDs given with sibutramine

- Tacrolimus: possible increased risk of nephrotoxicity when NSAIDs given with tacrolimus; increased risk of nephrotoxicity when ibuprofen given with ●tacrolimus

  Ulcer-healing Drugs: plasma concentration of azapropazone possibly increased by cimetidine

  Vasodilator Antihypertensives: NSAIDs antagonise hypotensive effect of hydralazine, minoxidil and sodium nitroprusside

Octreotide

  Antidiabetics: octreotide possibly reduces requirements for insulin, metformin, repaglinide and sulphonylureas

- Ciclosporin: octreotide reduces plasma concentration of ●ciclosporin

  Dopaminergics: octreotide increases plasma concentration of bromocriptine

  Ulcer-healing Drugs: octreotide possibly delays absorption of cimetidine

Oestrogens

  Note. Interactions of combined oral contraceptives may also apply to combined contraceptive patches and vaginal rings

  ACE Inhibitors: oestrogens antagonise hypotensive effect of ACE inhibitors

  Adrenergic Neurone Blockers: oestrogens antagonise hypotensive effect of adrenergic neurone blockers

  Alpha-blockers: oestrogens antagonise hypotensive effect of alpha-blockers

  Analgesics: plasma concentration of ethinylestradiol increased by etoricoxib

  Angiotensin-II Receptor Antagonists: oestrogens antagonise hypotensive effect of angiotensin-II receptor antagonists

- Antibacterials: contraceptive effect of oestrogens possibly reduced by antibacterials that do not induce liver enzymes (risk probably small, see p. 478); metabolism of oestrogens accelerated by ●rifamycins (reduced contraceptive effect—see p. 478)

- Anticoagulants: oestrogens may enhance or reduce anticoagulant effect of ●coumarins; oestrogens antagonise anticoagulant effect of ●phenindione

- Antidepressants: contraceptive effect of oestrogens reduced by ●St John's wort (avoid concomitant use); oestrogens antagonise antidepressant effect of tricyclics (but side-effects of tricyclics possibly increased due to increased plasma concentration)

  Antidiabetics: oestrogens antagonise hypoglycaemic effect of antidiabetics

- Antiepileptics: metabolism of oestrogens accelerated by ●carbamazepine, ●oxcarbazepine, ●phenytoin, ●primidone, ●rufinamide and ●topiramate (reduced contraceptive effect—see p. 478); oestrogens reduce plasma concentration of ●lamotrigine

- Antifungals: anecdotal reports of contraceptive failure when oestrogens given with fluconazole, imidazoles, itraconazole or ketoconazole; metabolism of oestrogens accelerated by ●griseofulvin (reduced contraceptive effect—see p. 478); occasional reports of breakthrough bleeding when oestrogens (used for contraception) given with terbinafine

- Antivirals: plasma concentration of ethinylestradiol increased by ●atazanavir—avoid concomitant use; contraceptive effect of oestrogens possibly reduced by efavirenz; plasma concentration of oestrogens increased by fosamprenavir, also plasma concentration of fosamprenavir reduced—alternative contraception recommended; metabolism of oestro-

Oestrogens

- Antivirals *(continued)*
  gens accelerated by ●nelfinavir, ●nevirapine and ●ritonavir (reduced contraceptive effect—see p. 478)

  Anxiolytics and Hypnotics: oestrogens increase plasma concentration of melatonin

- Aprepitant: possible contraceptive failure of hormonal contraceptives containing oestrogens when given with ●aprepitant (alternative contraception recommended)

- Barbiturates: metabolism of oestrogens accelerated by ●barbiturates (reduced contraceptive effect—see p. 478)

  Beta-blockers: oestrogens antagonise hypotensive effect of beta-blockers

  Bile Acids: elimination of cholesterol in bile increased when oestrogens given with bile acids

- Bosentan: possible contraceptive failure of hormonal contraceptives containing oestrogens when given with ●bosentan (alternative contraception recommended)

  Calcium-channel Blockers: oestrogens antagonise hypotensive effect of calcium-channel blockers

  Ciclosporin: oestrogens possibly increase plasma concentration of ciclosporin

  Clonidine: oestrogens antagonise hypotensive effect of clonidine

  Corticosteroids: oral contraceptives containing oestrogens increase plasma concentration of corticosteroids

  Diazoxide: oestrogens antagonise hypotensive effect of diazoxide

  Diuretics: oestrogens antagonise diuretic effect of diuretics

  Dopaminergics: oestrogens increase plasma concentration of ropinirole; oestrogens increase plasma concentration of selegiline (increased risk of toxicity)

  Lipid-regulating Drugs: plasma concentration of ethinylestradiol increased by atorvastatin and rosuvastatin

  Methyldopa: oestrogens antagonise hypotensive effect of methyldopa

- Modafinil: metabolism of oestrogens accelerated by ●modafinil (reduced contraceptive effect—see p. 478)

  Moxonidine: oestrogens antagonise hypotensive effect of moxonidine

  Muscle Relaxants: oestrogens possibly increase plasma concentration of tizanidine (increased risk of toxicity)

  Nitrates: oestrogens antagonise hypotensive effect of nitrates

  Sitaxentan: plasma concentration of oestrogens increased by sitaxentan

  Somatropin: oestrogens (when used as oral replacement therapy) may increase dose requirements of somatropin

  Sugammadex: plasma concentration of oestrogens possibly reduced by sugammadex

  Tacrolimus: metabolism of oestrogens possibly inhibited by tacrolimus; ethinylestradiol possibly increases plasma concentration of tacrolimus

  Theophylline: oestrogens reduce excretion of theophylline (increased plasma concentration)

  Thyroid Hormones: oestrogens may increase requirements for thyroid hormones in hypothyroidism

  Vasodilator Antihypertensives: oestrogens antagonise hypotensive effect of hydralazine, minoxidil and sodium nitroprusside

Oestrogens, conjugated *see* Oestrogens

Ofloxacin *see* Quinolones

Olanzapine *see* Antipsychotics

Olmesartan *see* Angiotensin-II Receptor Antagonists

Olsalazine *see* Aminosalicylates

Omeprazole *see* Proton Pump Inhibitors

Ondansetron *see* 5HT₃ Antagonists

Opioid Analgesics

Alcohol: enhanced hypotensive and sedative effects when opioid analgesics given with alcohol

Antibacterials: plasma concentration of alfentanil increased by erythromycin; avoidance of premedication with opioid analgesics advised by manufacturer of ciprofloxacin (reduced plasma concentration of ciprofloxacin) when ciprofloxacin used for surgical prophylaxis; metabolism of methadone accelerated by rifampicin (reduced effect)

• Anticoagulants: tramadol enhances anticoagulant effect of ●coumarins

• Antidepressants: plasma concentration of methadone possibly increased by fluvoxamine; possible increased serotonergic effects when pethidine or tramadol given with duloxetine; CNS excitation or depression (hypertension or hypotension) when pethidine given with ●MAOIs—avoid concomitant use and for 2 weeks after stopping MAOIs; possible CNS excitation or depression (hypertension or hypotension) when opioid analgesics given with ●MAOIs—avoid concomitant use and for 2 weeks after stopping MAOIs; possible CNS excitation or depression (hypertension or hypotension) when opioid analgesics given with ●moclobemide; possible CNS excitation or depression (hypertension or hypotension) when dextromethorphan or pethidine given with ●moclobemide—avoid concomitant use; increased risk of CNS toxicity when tramadol given with ●SSRIs or ●tricyclics; sedative effects possibly increased when opioid analgesics given with tricyclics

• Antiepileptics: dextropropoxyphene enhances effects of ●carbamazepine; effects of tramadol reduced by carbamazepine; plasma concentration of methadone reduced by carbamazepine; metabolism of methadone accelerated by phenytoin (reduced effect and risk of withdrawal effects)

• Antifungals: metabolism of buprenorphine inhibited by ●ketoconazole (reduce dose of buprenorphine); metabolism of alfentanil inhibited by fluconazole (risk of prolonged or delayed respiratory depression); plasma concentration of fentanyl possibly increased by fluconazole and itraconazole; metabolism of alfentanil possibly inhibited by itraconazole; plasma concentration of alfentanil and methadone increased by ●voriconazole (consider reducing dose of alfentanil and methadone)

• Antihistamines: sedative effects possibly increased when opioid analgesics given with ●sedating antihistamines

Antipsychotics: enhanced hypotensive and sedative effects when opioid analgesics given with antipsychotics; increased risk of convulsions when tramadol given with antipsychotics

• Antivirals: plasma concentration of methadone possibly reduced by abacavir and nevirapine; plasma concentration of methadone reduced by efavirenz, fosamprenavir, nelfinavir and ritonavir; plasma concentration of dextropropoxyphene increased by ●ritonavir (risk of toxicity)—avoid concomitant use; plasma concentration of buprenorphine possibly increased by ritonavir; plasma concentration of alfentanil and fentanyl increased by ●ritonavir; plasma concentration of pethidine reduced by ●ritonavir, but plasma concentration of toxic pethidine metabolite increased (avoid concomitant use); plasma concentration of morphine possibly reduced by ritonavir; methadone possibly increases plasma concentration of zidovudine

Anxiolytics and Hypnotics: increased sedative effect when opioid analgesics given with anxiolytics and hypnotics

• Atomoxetine: increased risk of ventricular arrhythmias when methadone given with ●atomoxetine; possible

Opioid Analgesics

• Atomoxetine *(continued)*
increased risk of convulsions when tramadol given with atomoxetine

Barbiturates: CNS effects of opioid analgesics possibly increased by barbiturates

Beta-blockers: morphine possibly increases plasma concentration of esmolol

Calcium-channel Blockers: metabolism of alfentanil inhibited by diltiazem (risk of prolonged or delayed respiratory depression)

Domperidone: opioid analgesics antagonise effects of domperidone on gastro-intestinal activity

• Dopaminergics: risk of CNS toxicity when pethidine given with ●rasagiline (avoid pethidine for 2 weeks after rasagiline); avoid concomitant use of dextromethorphan with ●rasagiline; caution with tramadol advised by manufacturer of selegiline; hyperpyrexia and CNS toxicity reported when pethidine given with ●selegiline (avoid concomitant use)

5HT$_3$ Antagonists: effects of tramadol possibly antagonised by ondansetron

• Memantine: increased risk of CNS toxicity when dextromethorphan given with ●memantine (manufacturer of memantine advises avoid concomitant use)

Metoclopramide: opioid analgesics antagonise effects of metoclopramide on gastro-intestinal activity

• Sodium Oxybate: opioid analgesics enhance effects of ●sodium oxybate (avoid concomitant use)

Ulcer-healing Drugs: metabolism of opioid analgesics inhibited by cimetidine (increased plasma concentration)

Orciprenaline *see* Sympathomimetics

Orlistat

Anti-arrhythmics: orlistat possibly reduces plasma concentration of amiodarone

Anticoagulants: manufacturer of orlistat recommends monitoring anticoagulant effect of coumarins

Antidiabetics: manufacturer of orlistat advises avoid concomitant use with acarbose

• Ciclosporin: orlistat possibly reduces absorption of ●ciclosporin

Orphenadrine *see* Antimuscarinics

Oxaliplatin *see* Platinum Compounds

Oxandrolone *see* Anabolic Steroids

Oxazepam *see* Anxiolytics and Hypnotics

Oxcarbazepine

• Antidepressants: anticonvulsant effect of antiepileptics possibly antagonised by MAOIs and ●tricyclic-related antidepressants (convulsive threshold lowered); anticonvulsant effect of antiepileptics antagonised by ●SSRIs and ●tricyclics (convulsive threshold lowered); avoid concomitant use of antiepileptics with ●St John's wort

Antiepileptics: oxcarbazepine sometimes reduces plasma concentration of carbamazepine (but concentration of an active metabolite of carbamazepine may be increased), also plasma concentration of an active metabolite of oxcarbazepine often reduced; oxcarbazepine increases plasma concentration of phenytoin, also plasma concentration of an active metabolite of oxcarbazepine reduced; plasma concentration of an active metabolite of oxcarbazepine sometimes reduced by valproate

• Antimalarials: possible increased risk of convulsions when antiepileptics given with chloroquine and hydroxychloroquine; anticonvulsant effect of antiepileptics antagonised by ●mefloquine

• Antipsychotics: anticonvulsant effect of oxcarbazepine antagonised by ●antipsychotics (convulsive threshold lowered)

Barbiturates: oxcarbazepine increases plasma concentration of phenobarbital, also plasma concentration of an active metabolite of oxcarbazepine reduced

Oxcarbazepine (continued)

Ciclosporin: oxcarbazepine possibly reduces plasma concentration of ciclosporin

• Cytotoxics: oxcarbazepine reduces plasma concentration of •imatinib—avoid concomitant use

• Oestrogens: oxcarbazepine accelerates metabolism of •oestrogens (reduced contraceptive effect—see p. 478)

• Progestogens: oxcarbazepine accelerates metabolism of •progestogens (reduced contraceptive effect—see p. 478)

Oxprenolol see Beta-blockers

Oxybutynin see Antimuscarinics

Oxycodone see Opioid Analgesics

Oxymetazoline see Sympathomimetics

Oxytetracycline see Tetracyclines

Oxytocin

Anaesthetics, General: oxytocic effect possibly reduced, also enhanced hypotensive effect and risk of arrhythmias when oxytocin given with volatile liquid general anaesthetics

Prostaglandins: uterotonic effect of oxytocin potentiated by prostaglandins

Sympathomimetics: risk of hypertension when oxytocin given with vasoconstrictor sympathomimetics (due to enhanced vasopressor effect)

Paclitaxel

Antidiabetics: paclitaxel possibly inhibits metabolism of rosiglitazone

Antiepileptics: cytotoxics possibly reduce absorption of phenytoin

• Antipsychotics: avoid concomitant use of cytotoxics with •clozapine (increased risk of agranulocytosis)

Antivirals: plasma concentration of paclitaxel increased by nelfinavir and ritonavir

Cardiac Glycosides: cytotoxics reduce absorption of digoxin tablets

Paliperidone see Antipsychotics

Pancreatin

Antidiabetics: pancreatin antagonises hypoglycaemic effect of acarbose

Pancuronium see Muscle Relaxants

Pantoprazole see Proton Pump Inhibitors

Papaveretum see Opioid Analgesics

Paracetamol

Anticoagulants: prolonged regular use of paracetamol possibly enhances anticoagulant effect of coumarins

Antiepileptics: metabolism of paracetamol possibly accelerated by carbamazepine

Cytotoxics: paracetamol possibly inhibits metabolism of intravenous busulfan (manufacturer of intravenous busulfan advises caution within 72 hours of paracetamol)

Lipid-regulating Drugs: absorption of paracetamol reduced by colestyramine

Metoclopramide: rate of absorption of paracetamol increased by metoclopramide

Paraldehyde

• Alcohol: increased sedative effect when paraldehyde given with •alcohol

• Disulfiram: risk of toxicity when paraldehyde given with •disulfiram

Parasympathomimetics

Anti-arrhythmics: effects of neostigmine and pyridostigmine possibly antagonised by propafenone

• Antibacterials: plasma concentration of galantamine increased by erythromycin; effects of neostigmine and pyridostigmine antagonised by •aminoglycosides; effects of neostigmine and pyridostigmine antagonised by clindamycin; effects of neostigmine and pyridostigmine antagonised by •polymyxins

Antidepressants: plasma concentration of galantamine increased by paroxetine

Antifungals: plasma concentration of galantamine increased by ketoconazole

Parasympathomimetics (continued)

Antimalarials: effects of neostigmine and pyridostigmine may be diminished because of potential for chloroquine and hydroxychloroquine to increase symptoms of myasthenia gravis

Antimuscarinics: effects of parasympathomimetics antagonised by antimuscarinics

Beta-blockers: increased risk of arrhythmias when pilocarpine given with beta-blockers; effects of neostigmine and pyridostigmine antagonised by propranolol

Lithium: effects of neostigmine and pyridostigmine antagonised by lithium

Muscle Relaxants: donepezil possibly enhances effects of suxamethonium; edrophonium, galantamine, neostigmine, pyridostigmine and rivastigmine enhance effects of suxamethonium; donepezil possibly antagonises effects of non-depolarising muscle relaxants; edrophonium, neostigmine, pyridostigmine and rivastigmine antagonise effects of non-depolarising muscle relaxants

Parecoxib see NSAIDs

Paricalcitol see Vitamins

Paroxetine see Antidepressants, SSRI

Pegfilgrastim see Filgrastim

Peginterferon Alfa see Interferons

Penicillamine

Analgesics: possible increased risk of nephrotoxicity when penicillamine given with NSAIDs

Antacids: absorption of penicillamine reduced by antacids

• Antipsychotics: avoid concomitant use of penicillamine with •clozapine (increased risk of agranulocytosis)

Cardiac Glycosides: penicillamine possibly reduces plasma concentration of digoxin

Gold: manufacturer of penicillamine advises avoid concomitant use with gold (increased risk of toxicity)

Iron: absorption of penicillamine reduced by oral iron

Zinc: penicillamine reduces absorption of zinc, also absorption of penicillamine reduced by zinc

Penicillins

Allopurinol: increased risk of rash when amoxicillin or ampicillin given with allopurinol

Antibacterials: absorption of phenoxymethylpenicillin reduced by neomycin

Anticoagulants: common experience in anticoagulant clinics is that INR can be altered by a course of broad-spectrum penicillins such as ampicillin, although studies have failed to demonstrate an interaction with coumarins or phenindione

Cytotoxics: penicillins reduce excretion of methotrexate (increased risk of toxicity)

Muscle Relaxants: piperacillin enhances effects of non-depolarising muscle relaxants and suxamethonium

Oestrogens: antibacterials that do not induce liver enzymes possibly reduce contraceptive effect of oestrogens (risk probably small, see p. 478)

Probenecid: excretion of penicillins reduced by probenecid (increased plasma concentration)

Sugammadex: flucloxacillin possibly reduces response to sugammadex

Sulfinpyrazone: excretion of penicillins reduced by sulfinpyrazone

Vaccines: antibacterials inactivate oral typhoid vaccine–see p. 752

Pentamidine Isetionate

• Anti-arrhythmics: increased risk of ventricular arrhythmias when pentamidine isetionate given with •amiodarone—avoid concomitant use

• Antibacterials: increased risk of ventricular arrhythmias when pentamidine isetionate given with parenteral •erythromycin; increased risk of ventricular arrhythmias when pentamidine isetionate given with •moxifloxacin—avoid concomitant use

Pentamidine Isetionate *(continued)*
- Antidepressants: increased risk of ventricular arrhythmias when pentamidine isetionate given with ●tricyclics

Antifungals: possible increased risk of nephrotoxicity when pentamidine isetionate given with amphotericin
- Antipsychotics: increased risk of ventricular arrhythmias when pentamidine isetionate given with ●amisulpride—avoid concomitant use; increased risk of ventricular arrhythmias when pentamidine isetionate given with ●phenothiazines
- Ivabradine: increased risk of ventricular arrhythmias when pentamidine isetionate given with ●ivabradine

Pentazocine *see* Opioid Analgesics
Pentostatin
Antiepileptics: cytotoxics possibly reduce absorption of phenytoin
- Antipsychotics: avoid concomitant use of cytotoxics with ●clozapine (increased risk of agranulocytosis)

Cardiac Glycosides: cytotoxics reduce absorption of digoxin tablets
- Cytotoxics: increased toxicity when pentostatin given with high-dose ●cyclophosphamide—avoid concomitant use; increased pulmonary toxicity when pentostatin given with ●fludarabine (unacceptably high incidence of fatalities)

Pentoxifylline (oxpentifylline)
- Analgesics: possible increased risk of bleeding when pentoxifylline (oxpentifylline) given with NSAIDs; increased risk of bleeding when pentoxifylline (oxpentifylline) given with ●ketorolac (avoid concomitant use)

Theophylline: pentoxifylline (oxpentifylline) increases plasma concentration of theophylline

Pergolide
Antipsychotics: effects of pergolide antagonised by antipsychotics

Memantine: effects of dopaminergics possibly enhanced by memantine

Methyldopa: antiparkinsonian effect of dopaminergics antagonised by methyldopa

Metoclopramide: antiparkinsonian effect of pergolide antagonised by metoclopramide

Pericyazine *see* Antipsychotics
Perindopril *see* ACE Inhibitors
Perphenazine *see* Antipsychotics
Pethidine *see* Opioid Analgesics
Phenazocine *see* Opioid Analgesics
Phenelzine *see* MAOIs
Phenindione
Note. Change in patient's clinical condition particularly associated with liver disease, intercurrent illness, or drug administration, necessitates more frequent testing. Major changes in diet (especially involving salads and vegetables) and in alcohol consumption may also affect anticoagulant control
- Alcohol: anticoagulant control with phenindione may be affected by major changes in consumption of ●alcohol
- Anabolic Steroids: anticoagulant effect of phenindione enhanced by ●anabolic steroids
- Analgesics: anticoagulant effect of phenindione possibly enhanced by ●NSAIDs; increased risk of haemorrhage when anticoagulants given with intravenous ●diclofenac (avoid concomitant use, including low-dose heparin); increased risk of haemorrhage when anticoagulants given with ●ketorolac (avoid concomitant use, including low-dose heparin); increased risk of bleeding when phenindione given with ●aspirin (due to antiplatelet effect)
- Anti-arrhythmics: metabolism of phenindione inhibited by ●amiodarone (enhanced anticoagulant effect)
- Antibacterials: experience in anticoagulant clinics suggests that INR possibly altered when phenindione is given with ●neomycin (given for local action on gut); anticoagulant effect of phenindione possibly

Phenindione
- Antibacterials *(continued)*
enhanced by levofloxacin and ●tetracyclines; studies have failed to demonstrate an interaction with phenindione, but common experience in anticoagulant clinics is that INR can be altered by a course of broad-spectrum penicillins such as ampicillin
- Antivirals: anticoagulant effect of phenindione possibly enhanced by ●ritonavir
- Clopidogrel: anticoagulant effect of phenindione enhanced due to antiplatelet action of ●clopidogrel
- Dipyridamole: anticoagulant effect of phenindione enhanced due to antiplatelet action of ●dipyridamole
- Enteral Foods: anticoagulant effect of phenindione antagonised by vitamin K (present in some ●enteral feeds)

Iloprost: increased risk of bleeding when phenindione given with iloprost
- Lipid-regulating Drugs: anticoagulant effect of phenindione may be enhanced or reduced by ●colestyramine; anticoagulant effect of phenindione possibly enhanced by ●rosuvastatin; anticoagulant effect of phenindione enhanced by ●fibrates
- Oestrogens: anticoagulant effect of phenindione antagonised by ●oestrogens
- Progestogens: anticoagulant effect of phenindione antagonised by ●progestogens

Sibutramine: increased risk of bleeding when anticoagulants given with sibutramine
- Testolactone: anticoagulant effect of phenindione enhanced by ●testolactone
- Testosterone: anticoagulant effect of phenindione enhanced by ●testosterone
- Thyroid Hormones: anticoagulant effect of phenindione enhanced by ●thyroid hormones
- Vitamins: anticoagulant effect of phenindione antagonised by ●vitamin K

Phenobarbital *see* Barbiturates
Phenothiazines *see* Antipsychotics
Phenoxybenzamine *see* Alpha-blockers
Phenoxymethylpenicillin *see* Penicillins
Phentolamine *see* Alpha-blockers
Phenylephrine *see* Sympathomimetics
Phenytoin
Note. Fosphenytoin interactions as for phenytoin
- Analgesics: effects of phenytoin possibly enhanced by ●NSAIDs; plasma concentration of phenytoin significantly increased by ●azapropazone—avoid concomitant use; phenytoin accelerates metabolism of methadone (reduced effect and risk of withdrawal effects); effects of phenytoin enhanced by aspirin

Antacids: absorption of phenytoin reduced by antacids
- Anti-arrhythmics: metabolism of phenytoin inhibited by ●amiodarone (increased plasma concentration); phenytoin reduces plasma concentration of disopyramide
- Antibacterials: metabolism of phenytoin inhibited by clarithromycin, ●isoniazid and ●metronidazole (increased plasma concentration); plasma concentration of phenytoin increased or decreased by ciprofloxacin; phenytoin accelerates metabolism of doxycycline (reduced plasma concentration); plasma concentration of phenytoin increased by ●chloramphenicol (increased risk of toxicity); metabolism of phenytoin accelerated by ●rifamycins (reduced plasma concentration); plasma concentration of phenytoin possibly increased by sulphonamides; phenytoin reduces plasma concentration of ●telithromycin (avoid during and for 2 weeks after phenytoin); plasma concentration of phenytoin increased by ●trimethoprim (also increased antifolate effect)
- Anticoagulants: phenytoin accelerates metabolism of ●coumarins (possibility of reduced anticoagulant effect, but enhancement also reported)

Phenytoin *(continued)*
- Antidepressants: plasma concentration of phenytoin increased by ●fluoxetine and ●fluvoxamine; phenytoin reduces plasma concentration of ●mianserin, mirtazapine and paroxetine; anticonvulsant effect of antiepileptics possibly antagonised by MAOIs and ●tricyclic-related antidepressants (convulsive threshold lowered); anticonvulsant effect of antiepileptics antagonised by ●SSRIs and ●tricyclics (convulsive threshold lowered); avoid concomitant use of antiepileptics with ●St John's wort; phenytoin possibly reduces plasma concentration of ●tricyclics

Antidiabetics: plasma concentration of phenytoin transiently increased by tolbutamide (possibility of toxicity)

- Antiepileptics: plasma concentration of both drugs often reduced when phenytoin given with carbamazepine, also plasma concentration of phenytoin may be increased; plasma concentration of phenytoin possibly increased by ●ethosuximide, also plasma concentration of ethosuximide possibly reduced; phenytoin reduces plasma concentration of lamotrigine, tiagabine and zonisamide; plasma concentration of phenytoin increased by oxcarbazepine, also plasma concentration of an active metabolite of oxcarbazepine reduced; phenytoin possibly reduces plasma concentration of primidone (but concentration of an active metabolite increased), plasma concentration of phenytoin often reduced but may be increased; plasma concentration of phenytoin possibly increased by rufinamide; plasma concentration of phenytoin increased by ●stiripentol; plasma concentration of phenytoin increased by ●topiramate (also plasma concentration of topiramate reduced); plasma concentration of phenytoin increased or possibly reduced when given with valproate, also plasma concentration of valproate reduced; plasma concentration of phenytoin reduced by vigabatrin

- Antifungals: phenytoin reduces plasma concentration of ●ketoconazole and ●posaconazole; anticonvulsant effect of phenytoin enhanced by ●miconazole (plasma concentration of phenytoin increased); plasma concentration of phenytoin increased by ●fluconazole (consider reducing dose of phenytoin); phenytoin reduces plasma concentration of ●itraconazole—avoid concomitant use; plasma concentration of phenytoin increased by ●voriconazole, also phenytoin reduces plasma concentration of voriconazole (increase dose of voriconazole and also monitor for phenytoin toxicity); phenytoin possibly reduces plasma concentration of caspofungin—consider increasing dose of caspofungin

- Antimalarials: possible increased risk of convulsions when antiepileptics given with chloroquine and hydroxychloroquine; anticonvulsant effect of antiepileptics antagonised by ●mefloquine; anticonvulsant effect of phenytoin antagonised by ●pyrimethamine, also increased antifolate effect

- Antipsychotics: anticonvulsant effect of phenytoin antagonised by ●antipsychotics (convulsive threshold lowered); phenytoin possibly reduces plasma concentration of ●aripiprazole—increase dose of aripiprazole; phenytoin accelerates metabolism of clozapine, quetiapine and sertindole (reduced plasma concentration)

- Antivirals: phenytoin possibly reduces plasma concentration of abacavir, darunavir, fosamprenavir, lopinavir and saquinavir; avoidance of phenytoin advised by manufacturer of etravirine; phenytoin possibly reduces plasma concentration of ●indinavir, also plasma concentration of phenytoin possibly increased; plasma concentration of phenytoin reduced by nelfinavir; phenytoin possibly reduces plasma concentration of ritonavir, also plasma concentration of phenytoin possibly affected; plasma

Phenytoin
- Antivirals *(continued)*
  concentration of phenytoin increased or decreased by zidovudine

Anxiolytics and Hypnotics: phenytoin often reduces plasma concentration of clonazepam; plasma concentration of phenytoin increased or decreased by diazepam; plasma concentration of phenytoin possibly increased or decreased by benzodiazepines

Aprepitant: phenytoin possibly reduces plasma concentration of aprepitant

Barbiturates: phenytoin often increases plasma concentration of phenobarbital, plasma concentration of phenytoin often reduced but may be increased

Bupropion: phenytoin reduces plasma concentration of bupropion

- Calcium-channel Blockers: phenytoin reduces effects of felodipine, isradipine and verapamil; phenytoin probably reduces effects of dihydropyridines, nicardipine and ●nifedipine; plasma concentration of phenytoin increased by ●diltiazem but also effect of diltiazem reduced

Cardiac Glycosides: phenytoin accelerates metabolism of digitoxin (reduced effect); phenytoin possibly reduces plasma concentration of digoxin

- Ciclosporin: phenytoin accelerates metabolism of ●ciclosporin (reduced plasma concentration)

- Corticosteroids: phenytoin accelerates metabolism of ●corticosteroids (reduced effect)

- Cytotoxics: phenytoin possibly reduces plasma concentration of busulfan and etoposide; metabolism of phenytoin possibly inhibited by fluorouracil (increased risk of toxicity); phenytoin increases antifolate effect of methotrexate; absorption of phenytoin possibly reduced by cytotoxics; phenytoin reduces plasma concentration of ●imatinib—avoid concomitant use; avoidance of phenytoin advised by manufacturer of ●lapatinib; phenytoin reduces plasma concentration of irinotecan and its active metabolite

Diazoxide: plasma concentration of phenytoin reduced by diazoxide, also effect of diazoxide may be reduced

- Disulfiram: metabolism of phenytoin inhibited by ●disulfiram (increased risk of toxicity)

- Diuretics: phenytoin antagonises effects of furosemide (frusemide); phenytoin reduces plasma concentration of ●eplerenone—avoid concomitant use; increased risk of osteomalacia when phenytoin given with carbonic anhydrase inhibitors

Dopaminergics: phenytoin possibly reduces effects of levodopa

Enteral Foods: absorption of phenytoin possibly reduced by enteral feeds

Folates: plasma concentration of phenytoin possibly reduced by folates

Hormone Antagonists: phenytoin accelerates metabolism of gestrinone (reduced plasma concentration); phenytoin possibly accelerates metabolism of toremifene

5HT$_3$ Antagonists: phenytoin accelerates metabolism of ondansetron (reduced effect)

Leflunomide: plasma concentration of phenytoin possibly increased by leflunomide

Levamisole: plasma concentration of phenytoin possibly increased by levamisole

Lipid-regulating Drugs: combination of phenytoin with fluvastatin may increase plasma concentration of either drug (or both)

Lithium: neurotoxicity may occur when phenytoin given with lithium without increased plasma concentration of lithium

Modafinil: plasma concentration of phenytoin possibly increased by modafinil

Muscle Relaxants: phenytoin antagonises muscle relaxant effect of non-depolarising muscle relaxants (accelerated recovery from neuromuscular blockade)

Phenytoin *(continued)*
- Oestrogens: phenytoin accelerates metabolism of
  ●oestrogens (reduced contraceptive effect—see
  p. 478)
- Progestogens: phenytoin accelerates metabolism of
  ●progestogens (reduced contraceptive effect—see
  p. 478)
- Sulfinpyrazone: plasma concentration of phenytoin
  increased by ●sulfinpyrazone
  Sympathomimetics: plasma concentration of phenytoin increased by methylphenidate
  Tacrolimus: phenytoin reduces plasma concentration
  of tacrolimus, also plasma concentration of phenytoin possibly increased
- Theophylline: plasma concentration of both drugs
  reduced when phenytoin given with ●theophylline
  Thyroid Hormones: phenytoin accelerates metabolism
  of thyroid hormones (may increase requirements in
  hypothyroidism), also plasma concentration of
  phenytoin possibly increased
  Tibolone: phenytoin accelerates metabolism of tibolone
- Ulcer-healing Drugs: metabolism of phenytoin inhibited by ●cimetidine (increased plasma concentration); effects of phenytoin enhanced by
  ●esomeprazole; effects of phenytoin possibly
  enhanced by omeprazole; absorption of phenytoin
  reduced by ●sucralfate
  Vaccines: effects of phenytoin enhanced by influenza
  vaccine
  Vitamins: phenytoin possibly increases requirements
  for vitamin D
Phosphodiesterase Inhibitors
- Anagrelide: avoidance of enoximone and milrinone
  advised by manufacturer of ●anagrelide
Physostigmine *see* Parasympathomimetics
Pilocarpine *see* Parasympathomimetics
Pimozide *see* Antipsychotics
Pindolol *see* Beta-blockers
Pioglitazone *see* Antidiabetics
Piperacillin *see* Penicillins
Pipotiazine *see* Antipsychotics
Piroxicam *see* NSAIDs
Pivmecillinam *see* Penicillins
Pizotifen
  Adrenergic Neurone Blockers: pizotifen antagonises
  hypotensive effect of adrenergic neurone blockers
Platinum Compounds
- Antibacterials: increased risk of nephrotoxicity and
  possibly of ototoxicity when platinum compounds
  given with ●aminoglycosides or ●polymyxins;
  increased risk of nephrotoxicity and ototoxicity when
  platinum compounds given with capreomycin;
  increased risk of nephrotoxicity and possibly of
  ototoxicity when cisplatin given with vancomycin
  Antiepileptics: cytotoxics possibly reduce absorption
  of phenytoin
- Antipsychotics: avoid concomitant use of cytotoxics
  with ●clozapine (increased risk of agranulocytosis)
  Cardiac Glycosides: cytotoxics reduce absorption of
  digoxin tablets
- Cytotoxics: increased pulmonary toxicity when cisplatin given with ●bleomycin and ●methotrexate
  Diuretics: increased risk of nephrotoxicity and ototoxicity when platinum compounds given with diuretics
Polymyxin B *see* Polymyxins
Polymyxins
  Antibacterials: increased risk of nephrotoxicity when
  colistin or polymyxins given with aminoglycosides;
  increased risk of nephrotoxicity when colistin or
  polymyxins given with capreomycin; increased risk
  of nephrotoxicity and ototoxicity when colistin given
  with teicoplanin or vancomycin; increased risk of
  nephrotoxicity when polymyxins given with vancomycin

Polymyxins *(continued)*
  Antifungals: increased risk of nephrotoxicity when
  polymyxins given with amphotericin
- Ciclosporin: increased risk of nephrotoxicity when
  polymyxins given with ●ciclosporin
- Cytotoxics: increased risk of nephrotoxicity and
  possibly of ototoxicity when polymyxins given with
  ●platinum compounds
- Diuretics: increased risk of otoxicity when polymyxins
  given with ●loop diuretics
- Muscle Relaxants: polymyxins enhance effects of
  ●non-depolarising muscle relaxants and
  ●suxamethonium
  Oestrogens: antibacterials that do not induce liver
  enzymes possibly reduce contraceptive effect of
  oestrogens (risk probably small, see p. 478)
- Parasympathomimetics: polymyxins antagonise effects
  of ●neostigmine and ●pyridostigmine
  Vaccines: antibacterials inactivate oral typhoid
  vaccine—see p. 752
Polystyrene Sulphonate Resins
  Thyroid Hormones: polystyrene sulphonate resins
  reduce absorption of levothyroxine (thyroxine)
Posaconazole *see* Antifungals, Triazole
Potassium Canrenoate *see* Diuretics
Potassium Aminobenzoate
  Antibacterials: potassium aminobenzoate inhibits
  effects of sulphonamides
Potassium Bicarbonate *see* Potassium Salts
Potassium Chloride *see* Potassium Salts
Potassium Citrate *see* Potassium Salts
Potassium Salts
  Note. Includes salt substitutes
- ACE Inhibitors: increased risk of severe hyperkalaemia
  when potassium salts given with ●ACE inhibitors
  Aliskiren: increased risk of hyperkalaemia when
  potassium salts given with aliskiren
- Angiotensin-II Receptor Antagonists: increased risk of
  hyperkalaemia when potassium salts given with
  ●angiotensin-II receptor antagonists
  Antibacterials: avoid concomitant use of potassium
  citrate with methenamine
- Ciclosporin: increased risk of hyperkalaemia when
  potassium salts given with ●ciclosporin
- Diuretics: increased risk of hyperkalaemia when
  potassium salts given with ●potassium-sparing diuretics and aldosterone antagonists
- Tacrolimus: increased risk of hyperkalaemia when
  potassium salts given with ●tacrolimus
Pramipexole
  Antipsychotics: manufacturer of pramipexole advises
  avoid concomitant use of antipsychotics (antagonism
  of effect)
  Memantine: effects of dopaminergics possibly
  enhanced by memantine
  Methyldopa: antiparkinsonian effect of dopaminergics
  antagonised by methyldopa
  Ulcer-healing Drugs: excretion of pramipexole reduced
  by cimetidine (increased plasma concentration)
Pravastatin *see* Statins
Prazosin *see* Alpha-blockers
Prednisolone *see* Corticosteroids
Prilocaine
  Anti-arrhythmics: increased myocardial depression
  when prilocaine given with anti-arrhythmics
  Antibacterials: increased risk of methaemoglobinaemia
  when prilocaine given with sulphonamides
Primaquine
- Antimalarials: avoidance of antimalarials advised by
  manufacturer of ●artemether/lumefantrine
  Mepacrine: plasma concentration of primaquine
  increased by mepacrine (increased risk of toxicity)
  Vaccines: antimalarials inactivate oral typhoid
  vaccine—see p. 752

Primidone

Alcohol: increased sedative effect when primidone given with alcohol

Anti-arrhythmics: primidone accelerates metabolism of disopyramide (reduced plasma concentration)

● Antibacterials: primidone accelerates metabolism of ●chloramphenicol, doxycycline and metronidazole (reduced plasma concentration); primidone reduces plasma concentration of ●telithromycin (avoid during and for 2 weeks after primidone)

● Anticoagulants: primidone accelerates metabolism of ●coumarins (reduced anticoagulant effect)

● Antidepressants: primidone reduces plasma concentration of paroxetine; primidone accelerates metabolism of ●mianserin (reduced plasma concentration); anticonvulsant effect of antiepileptics possibly antagonised by MAOIs and ●tricyclic-related antidepressants (convulsive threshold lowered); anticonvulsant effect of antiepileptics antagonised by ●SSRIs and ●tricyclics (convulsive threshold lowered); avoid concomitant use of antiepileptics with ●St John's wort; anticonvulsant effect of primidone antagonised by ●tricyclics (convulsive threshold lowered), also metabolism of tricyclics possibly accelerated (reduced plasma concentration)

● Antiepileptics: primidone often reduces plasma concentration of carbamazepine, also plasma concentration of primidone sometimes reduced (but concentration of an active metabolite of primidone often increased); primidone possibly reduces plasma concentration of ethosuximide; primidone reduces plasma concentration of lamotrigine and tiagabine; plasma concentration of primidone possibly reduced by phenytoin (but concentration of an active metabolite increased), plasma concentration of phenytoin often reduced but may be increased; plasma concentration of primidone possibly increased by valproate (plasma concentration of active metabolite of primidone increased), also plasma concentration of valproate reduced; plasma concentration of primidone possibly reduced by vigabatrin

● Antifungals: primidone possibly reduces plasma concentration of ●posaconazole; primidone possibly reduces plasma concentration of ●voriconazole—avoid concomitant use; primidone reduces absorption of griseofulvin (reduced effect)

● Antimalarials: possible increased risk of convulsions when antiepileptics given with chloroquine and hydroxychloroquine; anticonvulsant effect of antiepileptics antagonised by ●mefloquine

● Antipsychotics: anticonvulsant effect of primidone antagonised by ●antipsychotics (convulsive threshold lowered); primidone accelerates metabolism of haloperidol (reduced plasma concentration); primidone possibly reduces plasma concentration of ●aripiprazole—increase dose of aripiprazole

● Antivirals: primidone possibly reduces plasma concentration of ●indinavir, ●lopinavir, ●nelfinavir and ●saquinavir

Anxiolytics and Hypnotics: primidone often reduces plasma concentration of clonazepam

Barbiturates: increased sedative effect when primidone given with barbiturates

● Calcium-channel Blockers: primidone reduces effects of ●felodipine and ●isradipine; primidone probably reduces effects of ●dihydropyridines, ●diltiazem and ●verapamil

Cardiac Glycosides: primidone accelerates metabolism of digitoxin (reduced effect)

● Ciclosporin: primidone accelerates metabolism of ●ciclosporin (reduced effect)

● Corticosteroids: primidone accelerates metabolism of ●corticosteroids (reduced effect)

Diuretics: plasma concentration of primidone possibly reduced by acetazolamide; increased risk of osteo-

Primidone *(continued)*

Diuretics: malacia when primidone given with carbonic anhydrase inhibitors

Folates: plasma concentration of primidone possibly reduced by folates

Hormone Antagonists: primidone accelerates metabolism of gestrinone and toremifene (reduced plasma concentration)

Leukotriene Receptor Antagonists: primidone reduces plasma concentration of montelukast

Memantine: effects of primidone possibly reduced by memantine

● Oestrogens: primidone accelerates metabolism of ●oestrogens (reduced contraceptive effect—see p. 478)

● Progestogens: primidone accelerates metabolism of ●progestogens (reduced contraceptive effect—see p. 478)

Sympathomimetics: plasma concentration of primidone possibly increased by methylphenidate

Theophylline: primidone accelerates metabolism of theophylline (reduced effect)

Thyroid Hormones: primidone accelerates metabolism of thyroid hormones (may increase requirements for thyroid hormones in hypothyroidism)

Tibolone: primidone accelerates metabolism of tibolone (reduced plasma concentration)

Vitamins: primidone possibly increases requirements for vitamin D

Probenecid

ACE Inhibitors: probenecid reduces excretion of captopril

Anaesthetics, General: probenecid possibly enhances effects of thiopental

● Analgesics: probenecid reduces excretion of ●dexketoprofen, ●indometacin, ●ketoprofen and ●naproxen (increased plasma concentration); probenecid reduces excretion of ●ketorolac (increased plasma concentration)—avoid concomitant use; effects of probenecid antagonised by aspirin

Antibacterials: probenecid reduces excretion of doripenem and meropenem (manufacturers of doripenem and meropenem advise avoid concomitant use); probenecid reduces excretion of cephalosporins, ciprofloxacin, nalidixic acid, norfloxacin and penicillins (increased plasma concentration); probenecid reduces excretion of dapsone and nitrofurantoin (increased risk of side-effects); effects of probenecid antagonised by pyrazinamide

Antidiabetics: probenecid possibly enhances hypoglycaemic effect of chlorpropamide

● Antivirals: probenecid reduces excretion of aciclovir (increased plasma concentration); probenecid possibly reduces excretion of famciclovir (increased plasma concentration); probenecid reduces excretion of ganciclovir and ●zidovudine (increased plasma concentration and risk of toxicity)

Anxiolytics and Hypnotics: probenecid reduces excretion of lorazepam (increased plasma concentration); probenecid possibly reduces excretion of nitrazepam (increased plasma concentration)

● Cytotoxics: probenecid reduces excretion of ●methotrexate (increased risk of toxicity)

Sodium Benzoate: probenecid possibly reduces excretion of conjugate formed by sodium benzoate

Sodium Phenylbutyrate: probenecid possibly reduces excretion of conjugate formed by sodium phenylbutyrate

Procaine

Laronidase: procaine possibly inhibits effects of laronidase (manufacturer of laronidase advises avoid concomitant use)

Muscle Relaxants: neuromuscular blockade enhanced and prolonged when procaine given with suxamethonium

Procarbazine

    Alcohol: disulfiram-like reaction when procarbazine given with alcohol

    Antiepileptics: cytotoxics possibly reduce absorption of phenytoin

• Antipsychotics: avoid concomitant use of cytotoxics with •clozapine (increased risk of agranulocytosis)

    Cardiac Glycosides: cytotoxics reduce absorption of digoxin tablets

Prochlorperazine *see* Antipsychotics

Procyclidine *see* Antimuscarinics

Progesterone *see* Progestogens

Progestogens

    Note. Interactions of combined oral contraceptives may also apply to combined contraceptive patches and vaginal rings

• Antibacterials: metabolism of progestogens accelerated by •rifamycins (reduced contraceptive effect—see p. 478)

• Anticoagulants: progestogens may enhance or reduce anticoagulant effect of •coumarins; progestogens antagonise anticoagulant effect of •phenindione

• Antidepressants: contraceptive effect of progestogens reduced by •St John's wort (avoid concomitant use)

    Antidiabetics: progestogens antagonise hypoglycaemic effect of antidiabetics

• Antiepileptics: metabolism of progestogens accelerated by •carbamazepine, •oxcarbazepine, •phenytoin, •primidone, •rufinamide and •topiramate (reduced contraceptive effect—see p. 478); progestogens reduce plasma concentration of •lamotrigine

• Antifungals: metabolism of progestogens accelerated by •griseofulvin (reduced contraceptive effect—see p. 478); occasional reports of breakthrough bleeding when progestogens (used for contraception) given with terbinafine

• Antivirals: plasma concentration of progestogens increased by fosamprenavir, also plasma concentration of fosamprenavir reduced—alternative contraception recommended; contraceptive effect of progestogens possibly reduced by nelfinavir; metabolism of progestogens accelerated by •nevirapine (reduced contraceptive effect—see p. 478)

• Aprepitant: possible contraceptive failure of hormonal contraceptives containing progestogens when given with •aprepitant (alternative contraception recommended)

• Barbiturates: metabolism of progestogens accelerated by •barbiturates (reduced contraceptive effect—see p. 478)

• Bosentan: possible contraceptive failure of hormonal contraceptives containing progestogens when given with •bosentan (alternative contraception recommended)

• Ciclosporin: progestogens inhibit metabolism of •ciclosporin (increased plasma concentration)

    Diuretics: risk of hyperkalaemia when drospirenone given with potassium-sparing diuretics and aldosterone antagonists (monitor serum potassium during first cycle)

    Dopaminergics: progestogens increase plasma concentration of selegiline (increased risk of toxicity)

    Lipid-regulating Drugs: plasma concentration of norethisterone increased by atorvastatin; plasma concentration of norgestrel increased by rosuvastatin

    Muscle Relaxants: progestogens possibly increase plasma concentration of tizanidine (increased risk of toxicity)

    Sitaxentan: plasma concentration of progestogens increased by sitaxentan

    Sugammadex: plasma concentration of progestogens possibly reduced by sugammadex

    Tacrolimus: metabolism of progestogens possibly inhibited by tacrolimus

Proguanil

    Antacids: absorption of proguanil reduced by oral magnesium salts (as magnesium trisilicate)

    Anticoagulants: isolated reports that proguanil may enhance anticoagulant effect of warfarin

• Antimalarials: avoidance of antimalarials advised by manufacturer of •artemether/lumefantrine; increased antifolate effect when proguanil given with pyrimethamine

    Vaccines: antimalarials inactivate oral typhoid vaccine—see p. 752

Promazine *see* Antipsychotics

Promethazine *see* Antihistamines

Propafenone

    Anaesthetics, Local: increased myocardial depression when anti-arrhythmics given with bupivacaine, levobupivacaine, prilocaine or ropivacaine

• Anti-arrhythmics: increased myocardial depression when anti-arrhythmics given with other •anti-arrhythmics

• Antibacterials: metabolism of propafenone accelerated by •rifampicin (reduced effect)

• Anticoagulants: propafenone enhances anticoagulant effect of •coumarins

• Antidepressants: metabolism of propafenone possibly inhibited by paroxetine (increased risk of toxicity); increased risk of arrhythmias when propafenone given with •tricyclics

• Antihistamines: increased risk of ventricular arrhythmias when propafenone given with •mizolastine—avoid concomitant use

• Antipsychotics: increased risk of ventricular arrhythmias when anti-arrhythmics that prolong the QT interval given with •antipsychotics that prolong the QT interval

• Antivirals: plasma concentration of propafenone possibly increased by •fosamprenavir (increased risk of ventricular arrhythmias—avoid concomitant use); plasma concentration of propafenone increased by •ritonavir (increased risk of ventricular arrhythmias—avoid concomitant use)

• Beta-blockers: increased myocardial depression when anti-arrhythmics given with •beta-blockers; propafenone increases plasma concentration of metoprolol and propranolol

• Cardiac Glycosides: propafenone increases plasma concentration of •digoxin (halve dose of digoxin)

    Ciclosporin: propafenone possibly increases plasma concentration of ciclosporin

• 5HT$_3$ Antagonists: increased risk of ventricular arrhythmias when propafenone given with •dolasetron—avoid concomitant use

    Parasympathomimetics: propafenone possibly antagonises effects of neostigmine and pyridostigmine

    Theophylline: propafenone increases plasma concentration of theophylline

• Ulcer-healing Drugs: plasma concentration of propafenone increased by •cimetidine

Propantheline *see* Antimuscarinics

Propiverine *see* Antimuscarinics

Propofol *see* Anaesthetics, General

Propranolol *see* Beta-blockers

Prostaglandins

    ACE Inhibitors: enhanced hypotensive effect when alprostadil given with ACE inhibitors

    Adrenergic Neurone Blockers: enhanced hypotensive effect when alprostadil given with adrenergic neurone blockers

    Alpha-blockers: enhanced hypotensive effect when alprostadil given with alpha-blockers

    Angiotensin-II Receptor Antagonists: enhanced hypotensive effect when alprostadil given with angiotensin-II receptor antagonists

    Beta-blockers: enhanced hypotensive effect when alprostadil given with beta-blockers

Prostaglandins *(continued)*

Calcium-channel Blockers: enhanced hypotensive effect when alprostadil given with calcium-channel blockers

Clonidine: enhanced hypotensive effect when alprostadil given with clonidine

Diazoxide: enhanced hypotensive effect when alprostadil given with diazoxide

Diuretics: enhanced hypotensive effect when alprostadil given with diuretics

Methyldopa: enhanced hypotensive effect when alprostadil given with methyldopa

Moxonidine: enhanced hypotensive effect when alprostadil given with moxonidine

Nitrates: enhanced hypotensive effect when alprostadil given with nitrates

Oxytocin: prostaglandins potentiate uterotonic effect of oxytocin

Vasodilator Antihypertensives: enhanced hypotensive effect when alprostadil given with hydralazine, minoxidil or sodium nitroprusside

Protein Kinase Inhibitors *see* Dasatinib, Erlotinib, Imatinib, Lapatinib, Nilotinib, Sorafenib, Sunitinib, and Temsirolimus

Proton Pump Inhibitors

Antacids: absorption of lansoprazole possibly reduced by antacids

Antibacterials: plasma concentration of both drugs increased when omeprazole given with clarithromycin

• Anticoagulants: esomeprazole, omeprazole and pantoprazole possibly enhance anticoagulant effect of •coumarins

Antidepressants: omeprazole increases plasma concentration of escitalopram; plasma concentration of lansoprazole possibly increased by fluvoxamine

• Antiepileptics: omeprazole possibly enhances effects of phenytoin; esomeprazole enhances effects of •phenytoin

Antifungals: proton pump inhibitors reduce absorption of itraconazole and ketoconazole; plasma concentration of esomeprazole possibly increased by voriconazole; plasma concentration of omeprazole increased by voriconazole (consider reducing dose of omeprazole)

Antipsychotics: omeprazole possibly reduces plasma concentration of clozapine

• Antivirals: proton pump inhibitors reduce plasma concentration of •atazanavir; omeprazole reduces plasma concentration of •nelfinavir—avoid concomitant use; omeprazole increases plasma concentration of •raltegravir—avoid concomitant use; proton pump inhibitors possibly increase plasma concentration of raltegravir—manufacturer of raltegravir advises avoid concomitant use; omeprazole increases plasma concentration of saquinavir; plasma concentration of esomeprazole and omeprazole reduced by •tipranavir

Anxiolytics and Hypnotics: esomeprazole and omeprazole possibly inhibit metabolism of diazepam (increased plasma concentration)

Cardiac Glycosides: proton pump inhibitors possibly slightly increase plasma concentration of digoxin

Ciclosporin: omeprazole possibly affects plasma concentration of ciclosporin

• Cilostazol: omeprazole increases plasma concentration of •cilostazol (risk of toxicity)—avoid concomitant use; lansoprazole possibly increases plasma concentration of •cilostazol—avoid concomitant use

Clopidogrel: proton pump inhibitors possibly reduce antiplatelet effect of clopidogrel

Cytotoxics: omeprazole possibly reduces excretion of methotrexate (increased risk of toxicity); proton pump inhibitors possibly reduce absorption of lapatinib

Proton Pump Inhibitors *(continued)*

Tacrolimus: omeprazole possibly increases plasma concentration of tacrolimus

Ulcer-healing Drugs: absorption of lansoprazole possibly reduced by sucralfate

Pseudoephedrine *see* Sympathomimetics

Pyrazinamide

Oestrogens: antibacterials that do not induce liver enzymes possibly reduce contraceptive effect of oestrogens (risk probably small, see p. 478)

Probenecid: pyrazinamide antagonises effects of probenecid

Sulfinpyrazone: pyrazinamide antagonises effects of sulfinpyrazone

Vaccines: antibacterials inactivate oral typhoid vaccine–see p. 752

Pyridostigmine *see* Parasympathomimetics

Pyridoxine *see* Vitamins

Pyrimethamine

• Antibacterials: increased antifolate effect when pyrimethamine given with •sulphonamides or •trimethoprim

• Antiepileptics: pyrimethamine antagonises anticonvulsant effect of •phenytoin, also increased antifolate effect

• Antimalarials: avoidance of antimalarials advised by manufacturer of •artemether/lumefantrine; increased antifolate effect when pyrimethamine given with proguanil

Antivirals: increased antifolate effect when pyrimethamine given with zidovudine

• Cytotoxics: pyrimethamine increases antifolate effect of •methotrexate

Vaccines: antimalarials inactivate oral typhoid vaccine–see p. 752

Quetiapine *see* Antipsychotics

Quinagolide

Memantine: effects of dopaminergics possibly enhanced by memantine

Methyldopa: antiparkinsonian effect of dopaminergics antagonised by methyldopa

Quinapril *see* ACE Inhibitors

Quinine

• Anti-arrhythmics: increased risk of ventricular arrhythmias when quinine given with •amiodarone—avoid concomitant use; quinine increases plasma concentration of •flecainide

• Antibacterials: increased risk of ventricular arrhythmias when quinine given with •moxifloxacin—avoid concomitant use

• Antimalarials: avoidance of antimalarials advised by manufacturer of •artemether/lumefantrine; increased risk of ventricular arrhythmias when quinine given with •artemether/lumefantrine; increased risk of convulsions when quinine given with •mefloquine (but should not prevent the use of intravenous quinine in severe cases)

• Antipsychotics: increased risk of ventricular arrhythmias when quinine given with •pimozide—avoid concomitant use

• Cardiac Glycosides: quinine increases plasma concentration of •digoxin

Muscle Relaxants: quinine possibly enhances effects of suxamethonium

Ulcer-healing Drugs: metabolism of quinine inhibited by cimetidine (increased plasma concentration)

Vaccines: antimalarials inactivate oral typhoid vaccine–see p. 752

Quinolones

• Analgesics: possible increased risk of convulsions when quinolones given with •NSAIDs; manufacturer of ciprofloxacin advises avoid premedication with opioid analgesics (reduced plasma concentration of ciprofloxacin) when ciprofloxacin used for surgical prophylaxis

Quinolones *(continued)*

    Antacids: absorption of ciprofloxacin, levofloxacin, moxifloxacin, norfloxacin and ofloxacin reduced by antacids

- Anti-arrhythmics: increased risk of ventricular arrhythmias when levofloxacin or moxifloxacin given with ●amiodarone—avoid concomitant use; increased risk of ventricular arrhythmias when moxifloxacin given with ●disopyramide—avoid concomitant use
- Antibacterials: increased risk of ventricular arrhythmias when moxifloxacin given with parenteral ●erythromycin—avoid concomitant use
- Anticoagulants: levofloxacin possibly enhances anticoagulant effect of coumarins and phenindione; ciprofloxacin, nalidixic acid, norfloxacin and ofloxacin enhance anticoagulant effect of ●coumarins
- Antidepressants: ciprofloxacin inhibits metabolism of ●duloxetine—avoid concomitant use; increased risk of ventricular arrhythmias when moxifloxacin given with ●tricyclics—avoid concomitant use
    Antidiabetics: ciprofloxacin and norfloxacin possibly enhance effects of glibenclamide
    Antiepileptics: ciprofloxacin increases or decreases plasma concentration of phenytoin
- Antihistamines: increased risk of ventricular arrhythmias when moxifloxacin given with ●mizolastine—avoid concomitant use
- Antimalarials: avoidance of quinolones advised by manufacturer of ●artemether/lumefantrine; increased risk of ventricular arrhythmias when moxifloxacin given with ●chloroquine and hydroxychloroquine, ●mefloquine or ●quinine—avoid concomitant use
- Antipsychotics: increased risk of ventricular arrhythmias when moxifloxacin given with ●benperidol—manufacturer of benperidol advises avoid concomitant use; increased risk of ventricular arrhythmias when moxifloxacin given with ●haloperidol, ●phenothiazines, ●pimozide, ●sertindole or ●zuclopenthixol—avoid concomitant use; ciprofloxacin increases plasma concentration of clozapine; ciprofloxacin possibly increases plasma concentration of olanzapine
- Atomoxetine: increased risk of ventricular arrhythmias when moxifloxacin given with ●atomoxetine
- Beta-blockers: increased risk of ventricular arrhythmias when moxifloxacin given with ●sotalol—avoid concomitant use
    Calcium Salts: absorption of ciprofloxacin reduced by calcium salts
- Ciclosporin: increased risk of nephrotoxicity when quinolones given with ●ciclosporin
- Cytotoxics: nalidixic acid increases risk of melphalan toxicity; ciprofloxacin possibly reduces excretion of methotrexate (increased risk of toxicity); norfloxacin possibly reduces bioavailability of mycophenolate; avoidance of moxifloxacin advised by manufacturer of ●nilotinib
    Dairy Products: absorption of ciprofloxacin and norfloxacin reduced by dairy products
    Dopaminergics: ciprofloxacin inhibits metabolism of ropinirole (increased plasma concentration)
    5HT₁ Agonists: quinolones possibly inhibit metabolism of zolmitriptan (reduce dose of zolmitriptan)
    Iron: absorption of ciprofloxacin, levofloxacin, moxifloxacin, norfloxacin and ofloxacin reduced by *oral* iron
- Muscle Relaxants: ciprofloxacin increases plasma concentration of ●tizanidine (increased risk of toxicity)—avoid concomitant use
    Oestrogens: antibacterials that do not induce liver enzymes possibly reduce contraceptive effect of oestrogens (risk probably small, see p. 478)
- Pentamidine Isetionate: increased risk of ventricular arrhythmias when moxifloxacin given with ●pentamidine isetionate—avoid concomitant use

Quinolones *(continued)*

    Probenecid: excretion of ciprofloxacin, nalidixic acid and norfloxacin reduced by probenecid (increased plasma concentration)
    Sevelamer: bioavailability of ciprofloxacin reduced by sevelamer
    Strontium Ranelate: absorption of quinolones reduced by strontium ranelate (manufacturer of strontium ranelate advises avoid concomitant use)
- Theophylline: possible increased risk of convulsions when quinolones given with ●theophylline; ciprofloxacin and norfloxacin increase plasma concentration of ●theophylline
    Ulcer-healing Drugs: absorption of ciprofloxacin, levofloxacin, moxifloxacin, norfloxacin and ofloxacin reduced by sucralfate
    Vaccines: antibacterials inactivate oral typhoid vaccine–see p. 752
    Zinc: absorption of ciprofloxacin, levofloxacin, moxifloxacin, norfloxacin and ofloxacin reduced by zinc

Quinupristin with Dalfopristin

- Anti-arrhythmics: increased risk of ventricular arrhythmias when quinupristin/dalfopristin given with ●disopyramide or ●lidocaine (lignocaine)—avoid concomitant use
    Antibacterials: manufacturer of quinupristin/dalfopristin recommends monitoring liver function when given with rifampicin
    Antivirals: quinupristin/dalfopristin possibly increases plasma concentration of saquinavir
- Anxiolytics and Hypnotics: quinupristin/dalfopristin inhibits metabolism of ●midazolam (increased plasma concentration with increased sedation); quinupristin/dalfopristin inhibits the metabolism of zopiclone
- Calcium-channel Blockers: quinupristin/dalfopristin increases plasma concentration of ●nifedipine
- Ciclosporin: quinupristin/dalfopristin increases plasma concentration of ●ciclosporin
- Ergot Alkaloids: manufacturer of quinupristin/dalfopristin advises avoid concomitant use with ●ergotamine and methysergide
    Oestrogens: antibacterials that do not induce liver enzymes possibly reduce contraceptive effect of oestrogens (risk probably small, see p. 478)
- Tacrolimus: quinupristin/dalfopristin increases plasma concentration of ●tacrolimus
    Vaccines: antibacterials inactivate oral typhoid vaccine–see p. 752

Rabeprazole *see* Proton Pump Inhibitors

Raloxifene

    Anticoagulants: raloxifene antagonises anticoagulant effect of coumarins
    Lipid-regulating Drugs: absorption of raloxifene reduced by colestyramine (manufacturer of raloxifene advises avoid concomitant administration)

Raltegravir

- Antibacterials: plasma concentration of raltegravir reduced by ●rifampicin—consider increasing dose of raltegravir
- Ulcer-healing Drugs: plasma concentration of raltegravir increased by ●omeprazole—avoid concomitant use; plasma concentration of raltegravir possibly increased by histamine H₂-antagonists and proton pump inhibitors—manufacturer of raltegravir advises avoid concomitant use

Ramipril *see* ACE Inhibitors

Ranitidine *see* Histamine H₂-antagonists

Rasagiline

    Note. Rasagiline is a MAO-B inhibitor

- Analgesics: avoid concomitant use of rasagiline with ●dextromethorphan; risk of CNS toxicity when rasagiline given with ●pethidine (avoid pethidine for 2 weeks after rasagiline)
- Antidepressants: after stopping rasagiline do not start ●fluoxetine for 2 weeks, also rasagiline should not be

Rasagiline

- Antidepressants *(continued)*
  started until at least 5 weeks after stopping fluoxetine; after stopping rasagiline do not start
  ●fluvoxamine for 2 weeks; risk of hypertensive crisis
  when rasagiline given with ●MAOIs, avoid MAOIs
  for at least 2 weeks after stopping rasagiline;
  increased risk of CNS toxicity when rasagiline given
  with ●SSRIs or ●tricyclics
  Dopaminergics: plasma concentration of rasagiline
  possibly reduced by entacapone
  Memantine: effects of dopaminergics possibly
  enhanced by memantine
  Methyldopa: antiparkinsonian effect of dopaminergics
  antagonised by methyldopa
- Sympathomimetics: avoid concomitant use of rasagiline with ●sympathomimetics

Reboxetine

- Antibacterials: manufacturer of reboxetine advises
  avoid concomitant use with ●macrolides
- Antidepressants: manufacturer of reboxetine advises
  avoid concomitant use with ●fluvoxamine; increased
  risk of hypertension and CNS excitation when
  reboxetine given with ●MAOIs (MAOIs should not be
  started until 1 week after stopping reboxetine, avoid
  reboxetine for 2 weeks after stopping MAOIs)
- Antifungals: manufacturer of reboxetine advises avoid
  concomitant use with ●imidazoles and ●triazoles
- Antimalarials: avoidance of antidepressants advised by
  manufacturer of ●artemether/lumefantrine
  Atomoxetine: possible increased risk of convulsions
  when antidepressants given with atomoxetine
  Diuretics: possible increased risk of hypokalaemia
  when reboxetine given with loop diuretics or thiazides and related diuretics
  Ergot Alkaloids: possible risk of hypertension when
  reboxetine given with ergotamine and methysergide
- Sibutramine: increased risk of CNS toxicity when
  noradrenaline re-uptake inhibitors given with
  ●sibutramine (manufacturer of sibutramine advises
  avoid concomitant use)

Remifentanil *see* Opioid Analgesics

Repaglinide *see* Antidiabetics

Retinoids

- Alcohol: etretinate formed from acitretin in presence of
  ●alcohol (increased risk of teratogenecity in women
  of child-bearing potential)
- Antibacterials: possible increased risk of benign intracranial hypertension when retinoids given with
  ●tetracyclines (avoid concomitant use)
- Anticoagulants: acitretin possibly reduces anticoagulant effect of ●coumarins
  Antiepileptics: isotretinoin possibly reduces plasma
  concentration of carbamazepine
  Antifungals: plasma concentration of alitretinoin
  increased by ketoconazole
- Cytotoxics: acitretin increases plasma concentration of
  ●methotrexate (also increased risk of hepatotoxicity)—avoid concomitant use
  Lipid-regulating Drugs: alitretinoin reduces plasma
  concentration of simvastatin
  Vitamins: risk of hypervitaminosis A when retinoids
  given with vitamin A

Ribavirin

- Antivirals: increased risk of side-effects when ribavirin
  given with ●didanosine—avoid concomitant use;
  ribavirin possibly inhibits effects of ●stavudine;
  increased risk of anaemia when ribavirin given with
  ●zidovudine—avoid concomitant use

Rifabutin *see* Rifamycins

Rifampicin *see* Rifamycins

Rifamycins

  ACE Inhibitors: rifampicin reduces plasma concentration of active metabolite of imidapril (reduced
  antihypertensive effect)

Rifamycins *(continued)*

  Analgesics: rifampicin reduces plasma concentration of
  etoricoxib; rifampicin accelerates metabolism of
  methadone (reduced effect)
  Antacids: absorption of rifampicin reduced by antacids
- Anti-arrhythmics: rifamycins accelerate metabolism of
  ●disopyramide (reduced plasma concentration); rifampicin accelerates metabolism of ●propafenone
  (reduced effect)
- Antibacterials: rifamycins reduce plasma concentration
  of clarithromycin and dapsone; plasma concentration of rifabutin increased by ●clarithromycin
  (increased risk of uveitis—reduce rifabutin dose);
  rifampicin accelerates metabolism of chloramphenicol (reduced plasma concentration); plasma concentration of rifabutin possibly increased by
  ●macrolides (increased risk of uveitis—reduce rifabutin dose); monitoring of liver function with rifampicin recommended by manufacturer of
  quinupristin/dalfopristin; rifampicin reduces plasma
  concentration of ●telithromycin (avoid during and for
  2 weeks after rifampicin); rifampicin possibly reduces
  plasma concentration of trimethoprim
- Anticoagulants: rifamycins accelerate metabolism of
  ●coumarins (reduced anticoagulant effect); rifampicin reduces plasma concentration of rivaroxaban
  Antidepressants: rifampicin possibly reduces plasma
  concentration of tricyclics
- Antidiabetics: rifamycins accelerate metabolism of
  ●chlorpropamide and ●tolbutamide (reduced effect);
  rifampicin reduces plasma concentration of
  ●rosiglitazone—consider increasing dose of rosiglitazone; rifampicin reduces plasma concentration of
  nateglinide; rifampicin possibly antagonises hypoglycaemic effect of repaglinide; rifamycins possibly
  accelerate metabolism of ●sulphonylureas (reduced
  effect)
- Antiepileptics: rifabutin reduces plasma concentration
  of ●carbamazepine; rifampicin reduces plasma concentration of ●lamotrigine; rifamycins accelerate
  metabolism of ●phenytoin (reduced plasma concentration)
- Antifungals: rifampicin accelerates metabolism of
  ●ketoconazole (reduced plasma concentration), also
  plasma concentration of rifampicin may be reduced
  by ketoconazole; plasma concentration of rifabutin
  increased by ●fluconazole (increased risk of uveitis—
  reduce rifabutin dose); rifampicin accelerates
  metabolism of ●fluconazole and ●itraconazole
  (reduced plasma concentration); rifabutin reduces
  plasma concentration of ●itraconazole—avoid concomitant use; plasma concentration of rifabutin
  increased by ●posaconazole (also plasma concentration of posaconazole reduced); rifampicin reduces
  plasma concentration of ●posaconazole and
  ●terbinafine; plasma concentration of rifabutin
  increased by ●voriconazole, also rifabutin reduces
  plasma concentration of voriconazole (increase dose
  of voriconazole and also monitor for rifabutin
  toxicity); rifampicin reduces plasma concentration of
  ●voriconazole—avoid concomitant use; rifampicin
  initially increases and then reduces plasma concentration of caspofungin (consider increasing dose of
  caspofungin); plasma concentration of rifabutin
  possibly increased by ●triazoles (increased risk of
  uveitis—reduce rifabutin dose)
- Antimalarials: rifampicin reduces plasma concentration
  of ●mefloquine—avoid concomitant use
  Antimuscarinics: rifampicin reduces plasma concentration of active metabolite of fesoterodine
- Antipsychotics: rifampicin accelerates metabolism of
  ●haloperidol (reduced plasma concentration);
  rifabutin and rifampicin possibly reduce plasma
  concentration of ●aripiprazole—increase dose of

Rifamycins

- Antipsychotics *(continued)*
  aripiprazole; rifampicin possibly reduces plasma concentration of clozapine
- Antivirals: rifampicin possibly reduces plasma concentration of abacavir and ritonavir; plasma concentration of rifabutin increased by ●atazanavir, ●darunavir, ●fosamprenavir and ●tipranavir (reduce dose of rifabutin); rifampicin reduces plasma concentration of ●atazanavir, ●lopinavir and ●nevirapine—avoid concomitant use; rifampicin significantly reduces plasma concentration of ●darunavir, ●fosamprenavir and ●nelfinavir—avoid concomitant use; rifampicin reduces plasma concentration of efavirenz—increase dose of efavirenz; plasma concentration of rifabutin reduced by efavirenz—increase dose of rifabutin; avoidance of rifampicin advised by manufacturer of etravirine and zidovudine; plasma concentration of both drugs reduced when rifampicin given with ●etravirine; rifampicin accelerates metabolism of ●indinavir (reduced plasma concentration—avoid concomitant use); plasma concentration of rifabutin increased by ●indinavir—avoid concomitant use; rifampicin reduces plasma concentration of ●maraviroc and ●raltegravir—consider increasing dose of maraviroc and raltegravir; plasma concentration of rifabutin increased by ●nelfinavir (halve dose of rifabutin); plasma concentration of rifabutin possibly increased by nevirapine; plasma concentration of rifabutin increased by ●ritonavir (increased risk of toxicity); rifampicin significantly reduces plasma concentration of ●saquinavir, also risk of hepatotoxicity—avoid concomitant use; rifabutin reduces plasma concentration of ●saquinavir; rifampicin possibly reduces plasma concentration of ●tipranavir—avoid concomitant use
  Anxiolytics and Hypnotics: rifampicin accelerates metabolism of diazepam (reduced plasma concentration); rifampicin possibly accelerates metabolism of benzodiazepines (reduced plasma concentration); rifampicin possibly accelerates metabolism of buspirone and zaleplon; rifampicin accelerates metabolism of zolpidem (reduced plasma concentration and reduced effect); rifampicin significantly reduces plasma concentration of zopiclone
  Aprepitant: rifampicin reduces plasma concentration of aprepitant
- Atovaquone: rifabutin and rifampicin reduce plasma concentration of ●atovaquone (possible therapeutic failure of atovaquone)
  Barbiturates: plasma concentration of rifampicin possibly reduced by phenobarbital
  Beta-blockers: rifampicin accelerates metabolism of bisoprolol and propranolol (plasma concentration significantly reduced); rifampicin reduces plasma concentration of carvedilol, celiprolol and metoprolol
- Bosentan: rifampicin reduces plasma concentration of ●bosentan—avoid concomitant use
- Calcium-channel Blockers: rifampicin possibly accelerates metabolism of ●isradipine and ●nicardipine (possible significantly reduced plasma concentration); rifampicin accelerates metabolism of ●diltiazem, ●nifedipine, ●nimodipine and ●verapamil (plasma concentration significantly reduced)
  Cardiac Glycosides: rifamycins accelerate metabolism of digitoxin (reduced effect); rifampicin possibly reduces plasma concentration of digoxin
- Ciclosporin: rifampicin accelerates metabolism of ●ciclosporin (reduced plasma concentration)
- Corticosteroids: rifamycins accelerate metabolism of ●corticosteroids (reduced effect)
- Cytotoxics: rifampicin reduces plasma concentration of active metabolite of ●mycophenolate; rifampicin accelerates metabolism of ●dasatinib (reduced

Rifamycins

- Cytotoxics *(continued)*
  plasma concentration—avoid concomitant use); rifampicin accelerates metabolism of erlotinib and sunitinib (reduced plasma concentration); rifampicin reduces plasma concentration of ●imatinib—avoid concomitant use; avoidance of rifabutin and rifampicin advised by manufacturer of ●lapatinib; rifampicin reduces plasma concentration of sorafenib; rifampicin reduces plasma concentration of active metabolite of ●temsirolimus—avoid concomitant use
  Deferasirox: rifampicin reduces plasma concentration of deferasirox
- Diuretics: rifampicin reduces plasma concentration of ●eplerenone—avoid concomitant use
  Hormone Antagonists: rifampicin possibly reduces plasma concentration of exemestane; rifampicin accelerates metabolism of gestrinone (reduced plasma concentration)
  $5HT_3$ Antagonists: rifampicin accelerates metabolism of ondansetron (reduced effect)
  Leflunomide: rifampicin possibly increases plasma concentration of active metabolite of leflunomide
  Lipid-regulating Drugs: rifampicin possibly reduces plasma concentration of atorvastatin and simvastatin; rifampicin accelerates metabolism of fluvastatin (reduced effect)
- Oestrogens: rifamycins accelerate metabolism of ●oestrogens (reduced contraceptive effect—see p. 478); antibacterials that do not induce liver enzymes possibly reduce contraceptive effect of oestrogens (risk probably small, see p. 478)
- Progestogens: rifamycins accelerate metabolism of ●progestogens (reduced contraceptive effect—see p. 478)
- Sirolimus: rifabutin and rifampicin reduce plasma concentration of ●sirolimus—avoid concomitant use
- Tacrolimus: rifampicin reduces plasma concentration of ●tacrolimus
  Tadalafil: rifampicin reduces plasma concentration of tadalafil
  Theophylline: rifampicin accelerates metabolism of theophylline (reduced plasma concentration)
  Thyroid Hormones: rifampicin accelerates metabolism of levothyroxine (thyroxine) (may increase requirements for levothyroxine (thyroxine) in hypothyroidism)
  Tibolone: rifampicin accelerates metabolism of tibolone (reduced plasma concentration)
  Ulcer-healing Drugs: rifampicin accelerates metabolism of cimetidine (reduced plasma concentration)
  Vaccines: antibacterials inactivate oral typhoid vaccine—see p. 752

Rimonabant

  Antifungals: plasma concentration of rimonabant increased by ketoconazole

Risedronate Sodium *see* Bisphosphonates

Risperidone *see* Antipsychotics

Ritodrine *see* Sympathomimetics, Beta$_2$

Ritonavir

- Alpha-blockers: ritonavir possibly increases plasma concentration of ●alfuzosin—avoid concomitant use
- Analgesics: ritonavir possibly increases plasma concentration of NSAIDs and buprenorphine; ritonavir increases plasma concentration of ●dextropropoxyphene and ●piroxicam (risk of toxicity)—avoid concomitant use; ritonavir increases plasma concentration of ●alfentanil and ●fentanyl; ritonavir reduces plasma concentration of methadone; ritonavir possibly reduces plasma concentration of morphine; ritonavir reduces plasma concentration of ●pethidine, but increases plasma concentration of toxic metabolite of pethidine (avoid concomitant use)

Ritonavir *(continued)*
- Anti-arrhythmics: ritonavir increases plasma concentration of •amiodarone and •propafenone (increased risk of ventricular arrhythmias—avoid concomitant use); ritonavir possibly increases plasma concentration of •disopyramide (increased risk of toxicity); ritonavir possibly increases plasma concentration of •flecainide (increased risk of ventricular arrhythmias—avoid concomitant use)
- Antibacterials: ritonavir possibly increases plasma concentration of azithromycin and erythromycin; ritonavir increases plasma concentration of •clarithromycin (reduce dose of clarithromycin in renal impairment); ritonavir increases plasma concentration of •rifabutin (increased risk of toxicity); plasma concentration of ritonavir possibly reduced by rifampicin; plasma concentration of both drugs increased when ritonavir given with •fusidic acid—avoid concomitant use; avoidance of concomitant ritonavir in severe renal and hepatic impairment advised by manufacturer of •telithromycin
- Anticoagulants: ritonavir may enhance or reduce anticoagulant effect of •warfarin; ritonavir possibly enhances anticoagulant effect of •coumarins and •phenindione; ritonavir increases plasma concentration of •rivaroxaban—manufacturer of rivaroxaban advises avoid concomitant use
- Antidepressants: ritonavir possibly reduces plasma concentration of paroxetine; side-effects possibly increased when ritonavir given with trazodone; ritonavir possibly increases plasma concentration of •SSRIs and •tricyclics; plasma concentration of ritonavir reduced by •St John's wort—avoid concomitant use
- Antidiabetics: ritonavir possibly increases plasma concentration of tolbutamide
- Antiepileptics: ritonavir possibly increases plasma concentration of •carbamazepine; plasma concentration of ritonavir possibly reduced by phenytoin, also plasma concentration of phenytoin possibly affected
- Antifungals: combination of ritonavir with •itraconazole or •ketoconazole may increase plasma concentration of either drug (or both); plasma concentration of ritonavir increased by fluconazole; ritonavir reduces plasma concentration of •voriconazole—avoid concomitant use
- Antihistamines: ritonavir possibly increases plasma concentration of non-sedating antihistamines
- Antimalarials: caution with ritonavir advised by manufacturer of artemether/lumefantrine
- Antimuscarinics: avoidance of ritonavir advised by manufacturer of darifenacin and tolterodine; manufacturer of fesoterodine advises dose reduction when ritonavir given with fesoterodine—consult fesoterodine product literature; ritonavir increases plasma concentration of solifenacin
- Antipsychotics: ritonavir possibly increases plasma concentration of •antipsychotics; ritonavir possibly inhibits metabolism of •aripiprazole (reduce dose of aripiprazole); ritonavir increases plasma concentration of •clozapine (increased risk of toxicity)—avoid concomitant use; ritonavir reduces plasma concentration of olanzapine—consider increasing dose of olanzapine; ritonavir increases plasma concentration of •pimozide and •sertindole (increased risk of ventricular arrhythmias—avoid concomitant use)
- Antivirals: ritonavir increases toxicity of efavirenz, monitor liver function tests; ritonavir increases plasma concentration of indinavir and •saquinavir; combination of ritonavir with nelfinavir may increase plasma concentration of either drug (or both)
- Anxiolytics and Hypnotics: ritonavir possibly increases plasma concentration of •anxiolytics and hypnotics; ritonavir possibly increases plasma concentration of •alprazolam, •diazepam, •flurazepam and

Ritonavir
- Anxiolytics and Hypnotics *(continued)*
  •zolpidem (risk of extreme sedation and respiratory depression —avoid concomitant use); ritonavir possibly increases plasma concentration of •midazolam (risk of prolonged sedation—avoid concomitant use of oral midazolam); ritonavir increases plasma concentration of buspirone (increased risk of toxicity)
- Aprepitant: ritonavir possibly increases plasma concentration of aprepitant
- Bosentan: ritonavir possibly increases plasma concentration of bosentan
- Bupropion: ritonavir increases or decreases plasma concentration of •bupropion
- Calcium-channel Blockers: ritonavir possibly increases plasma concentration of •calcium-channel blockers; avoidance of ritonavir advised by manufacturer of lercanidipine
- Cardiac Glycosides: ritonavir possibly increases plasma concentration of digoxin
- Ciclosporin: ritonavir possibly increases plasma concentration of •ciclosporin
- Cilostazol: ritonavir possibly increases plasma concentration of •cilostazol—avoid concomitant use
- Corticosteroids: ritonavir possibly increases plasma concentration of corticosteroids, dexamethasone and prednisolone; ritonavir increases plasma concentration of inhaled and intranasal budesonide and •fluticasone
- Cytotoxics: avoidance of ritonavir advised by manufacturer of •lapatinib and •nilotinib; ritonavir increases plasma concentration of paclitaxel
- Diuretics: ritonavir increases plasma concentration of •eplerenone—avoid concomitant use
- Ergot Alkaloids: increased risk of ergotism when ritonavir given with •ergotamine and methysergide—avoid concomitant use
- 5HT$_1$ Agonists: ritonavir increases plasma concentration of •eletriptan (risk of toxicity)—avoid concomitant use
- Ivabradine: ritonavir possibly increases plasma concentration of •ivabradine—avoid concomitant use
- Lipid-regulating Drugs: possible increased risk of myopathy when ritonavir given with atorvastatin; possible increased risk of myopathy when ritonavir given with •rosuvastatin—avoid concomitant use; increased risk of myopathy when ritonavir given with •simvastatin (avoid concomitant use)
- Oestrogens: ritonavir accelerates metabolism of •oestrogens (reduced contraceptive effect—see p. 478)
- Sildenafil: ritonavir significantly increases plasma concentration of •sildenafil—avoid concomitant use
- Sympathomimetics: ritonavir possibly increases plasma concentration of dexamfetamine
- Tacrolimus: ritonavir possibly increases plasma concentration of •tacrolimus
- Tadalafil: ritonavir increases plasma concentration of tadalafil
- Theophylline: ritonavir accelerates metabolism of •theophylline (reduced plasma concentration)
- Vardenafil: ritonavir possibly increases plasma concentration of •vardenafil—avoid concomitant use

Rivaroxaban
- Analgesics: increased risk of haemorrhage when anticoagulants given with intravenous •diclofenac (avoid concomitant use, including low-dose heparin); increased risk of haemorrhage when anticoagulants given with •ketorolac (avoid concomitant use, including low-dose heparin)
- Antibacterials: plasma concentration of rivaroxaban reduced by rifampicin
- Antifungals: plasma concentration of rivaroxaban increased by •ketoconazole—avoid concomitant use; manufacturer of rivaroxaban advises avoid

Rivaroxaban

- Antifungals *(continued)*
  concomitant use with itraconazole, posaconazole and voriconazole
- Antivirals: manufacturer of rivaroxaban advises avoid concomitant use with atazanavir, darunavir, fosamprenavir, indinavir, lopinavir, nelfinavir, saquinavir and tipranavir; plasma concentration of rivaroxaban increased by ●ritonavir—manufacturer of rivaroxaban advises avoid concomitant use
  Sibutramine: increased risk of bleeding when anticoagulants given with sibutramine

Rivastigmine *see* Parasympathomimetics

Rizatriptan *see* 5HT₁ Agonists

Rocuronium *see* Muscle Relaxants

Ropinirole

  Antibacterials: metabolism of ropinirole inhibited by ciprofloxacin (increased plasma concentration)
  Antipsychotics: manufacturer of ropinirole advises avoid concomitant use of antipsychotics (antagonism of effect)
  Memantine: effects of dopaminergics possibly enhanced by memantine
  Methyldopa: antiparkinsonian effect of dopaminergics antagonised by methyldopa
  Metoclopramide: manufacturer of ropinirole advises avoid concomitant use of metoclopramide (antagonism of effect)
  Oestrogens: plasma concentration of ropinirole increased by oestrogens

Ropivacaine

  Anti-arrhythmics: increased myocardial depression when ropivacaine given with anti-arrhythmics
  Antidepressants: metabolism of ropivacaine inhibited by fluvoxamine—avoid prolonged administration of ropivacaine

Rosiglitazone *see* Antidiabetics

Rosuvastatin *see* Statins

Rotigotine

  Antipsychotics: manufacturer of rotigotine advises avoid concomitant use of antipsychotics (antagonism of effect)
  Memantine: effects of dopaminergics possibly enhanced by memantine
  Methyldopa: antiparkinsonian effect of dopaminergics antagonised by methyldopa
  Metoclopramide: manufacturer of rotigotine advises avoid concomitant use of metoclopramide (antagonism of effect)

Rowachol®

  Anticoagulants: Rowachol® possibly reduces anticoagulant effect of coumarins

Rufinamide

- Antidepressants: anticonvulsant effect of antiepileptics possibly antagonised by MAOIs and ●tricyclic-related antidepressants (convulsive threshold lowered); anticonvulsant effect of antiepileptics antagonised by ●SSRIs and ●tricyclics (convulsive threshold lowered); avoid concomitant use of antiepileptics with ●St John's wort
  Antiepileptics: rufinamide possibly increases plasma concentration of phenytoin; plasma concentration of rufinamide possibly increased by valproate (reduce dose of rufinamide)
- Antimalarials: possible increased risk of convulsions when antiepileptics given with chloroquine and hydroxychloroquine; anticonvulsant effect of antiepileptics antagonised by ●mefloquine
- Oestrogens: rufinamide accelerates metabolism of ●oestrogens (reduced contraceptive effect—see p. 478)
- Progestogens: rufinamide accelerates metabolism of ●progestogens (reduced contraceptive effect—see p. 478)

St John's Wort

- Antibacterials: St John's wort reduces plasma concentration of ●telithromycin (avoid during and for 2 weeks after St John's wort)
- Anticoagulants: St John's wort reduces anticoagulant effect of ●coumarins (avoid concomitant use)
- Antidepressants: possible increased serotonergic effects when St John's wort given with duloxetine; St John's wort reduces plasma concentration of amitriptyline; increased serotonergic effects when St John's wort given with ●SSRIs—avoid concomitant use
- Antiepileptics: avoid concomitant use of St John's wort with ●antiepileptics
- Antifungals: St John's wort reduces plasma concentration of ●voriconazole—avoid concomitant use
- Antimalarials: avoidance of antidepressants advised by manufacturer of ●artemether/lumefantrine
- Antipsychotics: St John's wort possibly reduces plasma concentration of ●aripiprazole—increase dose of aripiprazole
- Antivirals: St John's wort reduces plasma concentration of ●atazanavir, ●darunavir, ●efavirenz, ●fosamprenavir, ●indinavir, ●lopinavir, ●nelfinavir, ●nevirapine, ●ritonavir and ●saquinavir—avoid concomitant use; avoidance of St John's wort advised by manufacturer of etravirine; St John's wort possibly reduces plasma concentration of ●maraviroc and ●tipranavir—avoid concomitant use
  Anxiolytics and Hypnotics: St John's wort possibly reduces plasma concentration of oral midazolam
- Aprepitant: avoidance of St John's wort advised by manufacturer of ●aprepitant
  Atomoxetine: possible increased risk of convulsions when antidepressants given with atomoxetine
- Barbiturates: avoid concomitant use of St John's wort with ●phenobarbital
  Calcium-channel Blockers: St John's wort possibly reduces plasma concentration of amlodipine
- Cardiac Glycosides: St John's wort reduces plasma concentration of ●digoxin—avoid concomitant use
- Ciclosporin: St John's wort reduces plasma concentration of ●ciclosporin—avoid concomitant use
- Cytotoxics: St John's wort reduces plasma concentration of ●imatinib—avoid concomitant use; avoidance of St John's wort advised by manufacturer of ●lapatinib; St John's wort accelerates metabolism of ●irinotecan (reduced plasma concentration—avoid concomitant use)
- Diuretics: St John's wort reduces plasma concentration of ●eplerenone—avoid concomitant use
- 5HT₁ Agonists: increased serotonergic effects when St John's wort given with ●5HT₁ agonists—avoid concomitant use
  Ivabradine: St John's wort reduces plasma concentration of ivabradine—avoid concomitant use
  Lipid-regulating Drugs: St John's wort reduces plasma concentration of simvastatin
- Oestrogens: St John's wort reduces contraceptive effect of ●oestrogens (avoid concomitant use)
- Progestogens: St John's wort reduces contraceptive effect of ●progestogens (avoid concomitant use)
- Tacrolimus: St John's wort reduces plasma concentration of ●tacrolimus—avoid concomitant use
- Theophylline: St John's wort reduces plasma concentration of ●theophylline—avoid concomitant use

Salbutamol *see* Sympathomimetics, Beta₂

Salmeterol *see* Sympathomimetics, Beta₂

Saquinavir

- Antibacterials: plasma concentration of saquinavir reduced by ●rifabutin; plasma concentration of saquinavir significantly reduced by ●rifampicin, also risk of hepatotoxicity—avoid concomitant use; plasma concentration of saquinavir possibly increased by quinupristin/dalfopristin; avoidance of concomitant saquinavir in severe renal and hepatic

Saquinavir
- Antibacterials *(continued)*
  impairment advised by manufacturer of
  •telithromycin
  Anticoagulants: saquinavir possibly enhances anticoagulant effect of warfarin; avoidance of saquinavir
  advised by manufacturer of rivaroxaban
- Antidepressants: plasma concentration of saquinavir
  reduced by •St John's wort—avoid concomitant use
- Antiepileptics: plasma concentration of saquinavir
  possibly reduced by carbamazepine, phenytoin and
  •primidone
  Antifungals: plasma concentration of saquinavir
  increased by ketoconazole; plasma concentration of
  saquinavir possibly increased by imidazoles and
  triazoles
  Antimalarials: caution with saquinavir advised by
  manufacturer of artemether/lumefantrine
  Antimuscarinics: avoidance of saquinavir advised by
  manufacturer of darifenacin and tolterodine; manufacturer of fesoterodine advises dose reduction when
  saquinavir given with fesoterodine—consult fesoterodine product literature
- Antipsychotics: saquinavir possibly inhibits metabolism
  of •aripiprazole (reduce dose of aripiprazole);
  saquinavir possibly increases plasma concentration
  of •pimozide (increased risk of ventricular arrhythmias—avoid concomitant use); saquinavir increases
  plasma concentration of •sertindole (increased risk
  of ventricular arrhythmias—avoid concomitant use)
- Antivirals: plasma concentration of saquinavir
  increased by atazanavir, indinavir, lopinavir and
  •ritonavir; saquinavir reduces plasma concentration
  of darunavir; plasma concentration of saquinavir
  significantly reduced by efavirenz; saquinavir
  increases plasma concentration of •maraviroc (consider reducing dose of maraviroc); combination of
  saquinavir with nelfinavir may increase plasma
  concentration of either drug (or both); plasma
  concentration of saquinavir reduced by •tipranavir
- Anxiolytics and Hypnotics: saquinavir increases
  plasma concentration of •midazolam (risk of prolonged sedation—avoid concomitant use of oral
  midazolam)
- Barbiturates: plasma concentration of saquinavir possibly reduced by •barbiturates
- Ciclosporin: plasma concentration of both drugs
  increased when saquinavir given with •ciclosporin
- Cilostazol: saquinavir possibly increases plasma concentration of •cilostazol—avoid concomitant use
  Corticosteroids: plasma concentration of saquinavir
  possibly reduced by dexamethasone
- Cytotoxics: avoidance of saquinavir advised by manufacturer of •lapatinib
  Diuretics: saquinavir increases plasma concentration of
  eplerenone (reduce dose of eplerenone)
- Ergot Alkaloids: increased risk of ergotism when
  saquinavir given with •ergotamine and methysergide—avoid concomitant use
- Lipid-regulating Drugs: possible increased risk of
  myopathy when saquinavir given with atorvastatin;
  possible increased risk of myopathy when saquinavir
  given with •rosuvastatin—avoid concomitant use;
  increased risk of myopathy when saquinavir given
  with •simvastatin (avoid concomitant use)
  Sildenafil: saquinavir possibly increases plasma concentration of sildenafil—reduce initial dose of
  sildenafil
- Tacrolimus: saquinavir increases plasma concentration
  of •tacrolimus (consider reducing dose of tacrolimus)
  Tadalafil: saquinavir possibly increases plasma concentration of tadalafil—reduce initial dose of tadalafil
  Ulcer-healing Drugs: plasma concentration of saquinavir increased by omeprazole

Saquinavir *(continued)*
  Vardenafil: saquinavir possibly increases plasma concentration of vardenafil—reduce initial dose of
  vardenafil
Secobarbital *see* Barbiturates
Selegiline
Note. Selegiline is a MAO-B inhibitor
- Analgesics: hyperpyrexia and CNS toxicity reported
  when selegiline given with •pethidine (avoid concomitant use); manufacturer of selegiline advises
  caution with tramadol
- Antidepressants: theoretical risk of serotonin syndrome
  if selegiline given with citalopram (especially if dose
  of selegiline exceeds 10 mg daily); caution with
  selegiline advised by manufacturer of escitalopram;
  increased risk of hypertension and CNS excitation
  when selegiline given with •fluoxetine (selegiline
  should not be started until 5 weeks after stopping
  fluoxetine, avoid fluoxetine for 2 weeks after
  stopping selegiline); increased risk of hypertension
  and CNS excitation when selegiline given with
  •fluvoxamine or •venlafaxine (selegiline should not
  be started until 1 week after stopping fluvoxamine or
  venlafaxine, avoid fluvoxamine or venlafaxine for 2
  weeks after stopping selegiline); increased risk of
  hypertension and CNS excitation when selegiline
  given with •paroxetine or •sertraline (selegiline
  should not be started until 2 weeks after stopping
  paroxetine or sertraline, avoid paroxetine or sertraline for 2 weeks after stopping selegiline); enhanced
  hypotensive effect when selegiline given with
  MAOIs; avoid concomitant use of selegiline with
  •moclobemide; CNS toxicity reported when selegiline given with •tricyclics
  Dopaminergics: max. dose of 10 mg selegiline advised
  by manufacturer of entacapone if used concomitantly; selegiline enhances effects and increases
  toxicity of levodopa (reduce dose of levodopa)
  Memantine: effects of dopaminergics and selegiline
  possibly enhanced by memantine
  Methyldopa: antiparkinsonian effect of dopaminergics
  antagonised by methyldopa
  Oestrogens: plasma concentration of selegiline
  increased by oestrogens (increased risk of toxicity)
  Progestogens: plasma concentration of selegiline
  increased by progestogens (increased risk of toxicity)
- Sympathomimetics: risk of hypertensive crisis when
  selegiline given with •dopamine
Selenium
  Vitamins: absorption of selenium possibly reduced by
  ascorbic acid (give at least 4 hours apart)
Sertindole *see* Antipsychotics
Sertraline *see* Antidepressants, SSRI
Sevelamer
  Antibacterials: sevelamer reduces bioavailability of
  ciprofloxacin
  Ciclosporin: sevelamer possibly reduces plasma con-
  centration of ciclosporin
  Cytotoxics: sevelamer possibly reduces plasma con-
  centration of mycophenolate
  Tacrolimus: sevelamer possibly reduces plasma con-
  centration of tacrolimus
Sevoflurane *see* Anaesthetics, General
Sibutramine
  Analgesics: increased risk of bleeding when sibutramine given with NSAIDs or aspirin
  Anticoagulants: increased risk of bleeding when
  sibutramine given with anticoagulants
- Antidepressants: increased CNS toxicity when sibutramine given with •MAOIs or •moclobemide (manufacturer of sibutramine advises avoid concomitant
  use), also avoid sibutramine for 2 weeks after
  stopping MAOIs or moclobemide; increased risk of
  CNS toxicity when sibutramine given with •SSRI-
  related antidepressants, •SSRIs, •mirtazapine,
  •noradrenaline re-uptake inhibitors, •tricyclic-

Sibutramine
- Antidepressants *(continued)*
  related antidepressants, ●tricyclics or ●tryptophan (manufacturer of sibutramine advises avoid concomitant use)
- Antipsychotics: increased risk of CNS toxicity when sibutramine given with ●antipsychotics (manufacturer of sibutramine advises avoid concomitant use)

Sildenafil
- Alpha-blockers: enhanced hypotensive effect when sildenafil given with ●alpha-blockers (avoid alpha-blockers for 4 hours after sildenafil)
  Antibacterials: plasma concentration of sildenafil possibly increased by clarithromycin and telithromycin—reduce initial dose of sildenafil; plasma concentration of sildenafil increased by erythromycin—reduce initial dose of sildenafil
  Antifungals: plasma concentration of sildenafil increased by itraconazole and ketoconazole—reduce initial dose of sildenafil
- Antivirals: side-effects of sildenafil possibly increased by ●atazanavir; plasma concentration of sildenafil reduced by etravirine; plasma concentration of sildenafil possibly increased by fosamprenavir, nelfinavir and saquinavir—reduce initial dose of sildenafil; plasma concentration of sildenafil increased by ●indinavir—reduce initial dose of sildenafil; plasma concentration of sildenafil significantly increased by ●ritonavir—avoid concomitant use
  Bosentan: plasma concentration of sildenafil reduced by bosentan
  Calcium-channel Blockers: enhanced hypotensive effect when sildenafil given with amlodipine
  Grapefruit Juice: plasma concentration of sildenafil possibly increased by grapefruit juice
- Nicorandil: sildenafil significantly enhances hypotensive effect of ●nicorandil (avoid concomitant use)
- Nitrates: sildenafil significantly enhances hypotensive effect of ●nitrates (avoid concomitant use)
  Ulcer-healing Drugs: plasma concentration of sildenafil increased by cimetidine (reduce initial dose of sildenafil)

Simvastatin *see* Statins

Sirolimus
- Antibacterials: plasma concentration of sirolimus increased by ●clarithromycin and ●telithromycin—avoid concomitant use; plasma concentration of both drugs increased when sirolimus given with ●erythromycin; plasma concentration of sirolimus reduced by ●rifabutin and ●rifampicin—avoid concomitant use
- Antifungals: plasma concentration of sirolimus increased by ●itraconazole, ●ketoconazole and ●voriconazole—avoid concomitant use; plasma concentration of sirolimus increased by micafungin and ●miconazole; plasma concentration of sirolimus possibly increased by posaconazole
- Antivirals: plasma concentration of sirolimus possibly increased by ●atazanavir and lopinavir
- Calcium-channel Blockers: plasma concentration of sirolimus increased by ●diltiazem; plasma concentration of both drugs increased when sirolimus given with ●verapamil
  Ciclosporin: plasma concentration of sirolimus increased by ciclosporin
- Grapefruit Juice: plasma concentration of sirolimus increased by ●grapefruit juice—avoid concomitant use

Sitaxentan
- Anticoagulants: sitaxentan enhances anticoagulant effect of ●coumarins
- Ciclosporin: plasma concentration of sitaxentan increased by ●ciclosporin—avoid concomitant use
  Oestrogens: sitaxentan increases plasma concentration of oestrogens

Sitaxentan *(continued)*
  Progestogens: sitaxentan increases plasma concentration of progestogens

Sodium Aurothiomalate *see* Gold

Sodium Benzoate
  Antiepileptics: effects of sodium benzoate possibly reduced by valproate
  Antipsychotics: effects of sodium benzoate possibly reduced by haloperidol
  Corticosteroids: effects of sodium benzoate possibly reduced by corticosteroids
  Probenecid: excretion of conjugate formed by sodium benzoate possibly reduced by probenecid

Sodium Bicarbonate *see* Antacids

Sodium Clodronate *see* Bisphosphonates

Sodium Nitroprusside *see* Vasodilator Antihypertensives

Sodium Oxybate
- Analgesics: effects of sodium oxybate enhanced by ●opioid analgesics (avoid concomitant use)
  Antidepressants: increased risk of side-effects when sodium oxybate given with tricyclics
  Antipsychotics: effects of sodium oxybate possibly enhanced by antipsychotics
- Anxiolytics and Hypnotics: effects of sodium oxybate enhanced by ●benzodiazepines (avoid concomitant use)
- Barbiturates: effects of sodium oxybate enhanced by ●barbiturates (avoid concomitant use)

Sodium Phenylbutyrate
  Antiepileptics: effects of sodium phenylbutyrate possibly reduced by valproate
  Antipsychotics: effects of sodium phenylbutyrate possibly reduced by haloperidol
  Corticosteroids: effects of sodium phenylbutyrate possibly reduced by corticosteroids
  Probenecid: excretion of conjugate formed by sodium phenylbutyrate possibly reduced by probenecid

Sodium Valproate *see* Valproate

Solifenacin *see* Antimuscarinics

Somatropin
  Corticosteroids: growth-promoting effect of somatropin may be inhibited by corticosteroids
  Oestrogens: increased doses of somatropin may be needed when given with oestrogens (when used as oral replacement therapy)

Sorafenib
  Antibacterials: plasma concentration of sorafenib reduced by rifampicin
- Anticoagulants: sorafenib possibly enhances anticoagulant effect of ●coumarins
  Antiepileptics: cytotoxics possibly reduce absorption of phenytoin
- Antipsychotics: avoid concomitant use of cytotoxics with ●clozapine (increased risk of agranulocytosis)
  Cardiac Glycosides: cytotoxics reduce absorption of digoxin tablets
  Cytotoxics: sorafenib possibly increases plasma concentration of doxorubicin and irinotecan; sorafenib increases plasma concentration of docetaxel

Sotalol *see* Beta-blockers

Spironolactone *see* Diuretics

Statins
  Antacids: absorption of rosuvastatin reduced by antacids
- Anti-arrhythmics: increased risk of myopathy when simvastatin given with ●amiodarone
- Antibacterials: plasma concentration of atorvastatin and pravastatin increased by ●clarithromycin; increased risk of myopathy when simvastatin given with ●clarithromycin, ●erythromycin or ●telithromycin (avoid concomitant use); plasma concentration of rosuvastatin reduced by erythromycin; possible increased risk of myopathy when atorvastatin given with erythromycin or fusidic acid; plasma concentration of pravastatin increased by erythromycin; plasma concentration of

Statins
- Antibacterials *(continued)*
atorvastatin and simvastatin possibly reduced by rifampicin; metabolism of fluvastatin accelerated by rifampicin (reduced effect); increased risk of myopathy when statins given with ●daptomycin (preferably avoid concomitant use); increased risk of myopathy when simvastatin given with ●fusidic acid; increased risk of myopathy when atorvastatin given with ●telithromycin (avoid concomitant use)
- Anticoagulants: atorvastatin may transiently reduce anticoagulant effect of warfarin; rosuvastatin possibly enhances anticoagulant effect of ●coumarins and ●phenindione; fluvastatin and simvastatin enhance anticoagulant effect of ●coumarins

Antidepressants: plasma concentration of simvastatin reduced by St John's wort

Antidiabetics: fluvastatin possibly increases plasma concentration of glibenclamide

Antiepileptics: combination of fluvastatin with phenytoin may increase plasma concentration of either drug (or both)
- Antifungals: increased risk of myopathy when simvastatin given with ●itraconazole, ●ketoconazole or ●posaconazole (avoid concomitant use); possible increased risk of myopathy when simvastatin given with ●miconazole—avoid concomitant use; plasma concentration of fluvastatin increased by fluconazole; increased risk of myopathy when atorvastatin given with ●itraconazole or ●posaconazole (avoid concomitant use); possible increased risk of myopathy when atorvastatin or simvastatin given with imidazoles; possible increased risk of myopathy when atorvastatin or simvastatin given with triazoles
- Antivirals: possible increased risk of myopathy when rosuvastatin given with ●atazanavir, ●darunavir, ●fosamprenavir, ●indinavir, ●lopinavir, ●nelfinavir, ●ritonavir, ●saquinavir or ●tipranavir—avoid concomitant use; increased risk of myopathy when simvastatin given with ●atazanavir, ●indinavir, ●nelfinavir, ●ritonavir or ●saquinavir (avoid concomitant use); possible increased risk of myopathy when atorvastatin given with atazanavir, fosamprenavir, indinavir, lopinavir, nelfinavir, ritonavir or saquinavir; plasma concentration of pravastatin possibly increased by darunavir; plasma concentration of atorvastatin, pravastatin and simvastatin reduced by efavirenz; plasma concentration of atorvastatin possibly reduced by etravirine; possible increased risk of myopathy when simvastatin given with ●fosamprenavir or ●lopinavir—avoid concomitant use

Bosentan: plasma concentration of simvastatin reduced by bosentan
- Calcium-channel Blockers: plasma concentration of atorvastatin increased by diltiazem; possible increased risk of myopathy when simvastatin given with diltiazem; increased risk of myopathy when simvastatin given with ●verapamil

Cardiac Glycosides: atorvastatin possibly increases plasma concentration of digoxin
- Ciclosporin: increased risk of myopathy when statins given with ●ciclosporin; increased risk of myopathy when rosuvastatin given with ●ciclosporin (avoid concomitant use)
- Colchicine: possible increased risk of myopathy when statins given with ●colchicine

Cytotoxics: plasma concentration of simvastatin possibly increased by dasatinib; plasma concentration of simvastatin increased by imatinib
- Grapefruit Juice: plasma concentration of atorvastatin possibly increased by grapefruit juice; plasma concentration of simvastatin increased by ●grapefruit juice—avoid concomitant use
- Hormone Antagonists: possible increased risk of myopathy when simvastatin given with ●danazol

Statins *(continued)*
- Lipid-regulating Drugs: increased risk of myopathy when statins given with ●gemfibrozil (preferably avoid concomitant use); increased risk of myopathy when statins given with ●fibrates; increased risk of myopathy when statins given with ●nicotinic acid (applies to lipid regulating doses of nicotinic acid)

Oestrogens: atorvastatin and rosuvastatin increase plasma concentration of ethinylestradiol

Progestogens: atorvastatin increases plasma concentration of norethisterone; rosuvastatin increases plasma concentration of norgestrel

Retinoids: plasma concentration of simvastatin reduced by alitretinoin

Stavudine
- Antivirals: increased risk of side-effects when stavudine given with ●didanosine; effects of stavudine possibly inhibited by ●ribavirin; effects of stavudine possibly inhibited by ●zidovudine (manufacturers advise avoid concomitant use)
- Cytotoxics: effects of stavudine possibly inhibited by doxorubicin; increased risk of toxicity when stavudine given with ●hydroxycarbamide—avoid concomitant use

Stiripentol
- Antidepressants: anticonvulsant effect of antiepileptics possibly antagonised by MAOIs and ●tricyclic-related antidepressants (convulsive threshold lowered); anticonvulsant effect of antiepileptics antagonised by ●SSRIs and ●tricyclics (convulsive threshold lowered); avoid concomitant use of antiepileptics with ●St John's wort
- Antiepileptics: stiripentol increases plasma concentration of ●carbamazepine and ●phenytoin
- Antimalarials: possible increased risk of convulsions when antiepileptics given with chloroquine and hydroxychloroquine; anticonvulsant effect of antiepileptics antagonised by ●mefloquine

Anxiolytics and Hypnotics: stiripentol increases plasma concentration of clobazam
- Barbiturates: stiripentol increases plasma concentration of ●phenobarbital

Streptomycin *see* Aminoglycosides

Strontium Ranelate

Antibacterials: strontium ranelate reduces absorption of quinolones and tetracyclines (manufacturer of strontium ranelate advises avoid concomitant use)

Sucralfate

Antibacterials: sucralfate reduces absorption of ciprofloxacin, levofloxacin, moxifloxacin, norfloxacin, ofloxacin and tetracyclines
- Anticoagulants: sucralfate possibly reduces absorption of ●coumarins (reduced anticoagulant effect)
- Antiepileptics: sucralfate reduces absorption of ●phenytoin

Antifungals: sucralfate reduces absorption of ketoconazole

Antipsychotics: sucralfate reduces absorption of sulpiride

Cardiac Glycosides: sucralfate possibly reduces absorption of cardiac glycosides

Theophylline: sucralfate possibly reduces absorption of theophylline (give at least 2 hours apart)

Thyroid Hormones: sucralfate reduces absorption of levothyroxine (thyroxine)

Ulcer-healing Drugs: sucralfate possibly reduces absorption of lansoprazole

Sugammadex

Antibacterials: response to sugammadex possibly reduced by flucloxacillin and fusidic acid

Hormone Antagonists: response to sugammadex possibly reduced by toremifene

Oestrogens: sugammadex possibly reduces plasma concentration of oestrogens

Progestogens: sugammadex possibly reduces plasma concentration of progestogens

Sulfadiazine *see* Sulphonamides
Sulfadoxine *see* Sulphonamides
Sulfamethoxazole *see* Sulphonamides
Sulfasalazine *see* Aminosalicylates
Sulfinpyrazone
    Analgesics: effects of sulfinpyrazone antagonised by aspirin
    Antibacterials: sulfinpyrazone reduces excretion of nitrofurantoin (increased risk of toxicity); sulfinpyrazone reduces excretion of penicillins; effects of sulfinpyrazone antagonised by pyrazinamide
  • Anticoagulants: sulfinpyrazone enhances anticoagulant effect of •coumarins
  • Antidiabetics: sulfinpyrazone enhances effects of •sulphonylureas
  • Antiepileptics: sulfinpyrazone increases plasma concentration of •phenytoin
  • Ciclosporin: sulfinpyrazone reduces plasma concentration of •ciclosporin
    Theophylline: sulfinpyrazone reduces plasma concentration of theophylline
Sulindac *see* NSAIDs
Sulphonamides
    Anaesthetics, General: sulphonamides enhance effects of thiopental
    Anaesthetics, Local: increased risk of methaemoglobinaemia when sulphonamides given with prilocaine
  • Anti-arrhythmics: increased risk of ventricular arrhythmias when sulfamethoxazole (as co-trimoxazole) given with •amiodarone—avoid concomitant use of co-trimoxazole
  • Antibacterials: increased risk of crystalluria when sulphonamides given with •methenamine
  • Anticoagulants: sulphonamides enhance anticoagulant effect of •coumarins
    Antidiabetics: sulphonamides rarely enhance the effects of sulphonylureas
    Antiepileptics: sulphonamides possibly increase plasma concentration of phenytoin
  • Antimalarials: increased antifolate effect when sulphonamides given with •pyrimethamine
  • Antipsychotics: avoid concomitant use of sulphonamides with •clozapine (increased risk of agranulocytosis)
  • Ciclosporin: increased risk of nephrotoxicity when sulphonamides given with •ciclosporin; sulfadiazine possibly reduces plasma concentration of •ciclosporin
  • Cytotoxics: increased risk of haematological toxicity when sulfamethoxazole (as co-trimoxazole) given with •azathioprine, •mercaptopurine or •methotrexate; sulphonamides increase risk of methotrexate toxicity
    Oestrogens: antibacterials that do not induce liver enzymes possibly reduce contraceptive effect of oestrogens (risk probably small, see p. 478)
    Potassium Aminobenzoate: effects of sulphonamides inhibited by potassium aminobenzoate
    Vaccines: antibacterials inactivate oral typhoid vaccine—see p. 752
Sulphonylureas *see* Antidiabetics
Sulpiride *see* Antipsychotics
Sumatriptan *see* 5HT$_1$ Agonists
Sunitinib
    Antibacterials: metabolism of sunitinib accelerated by rifampicin (reduced plasma concentration)
    Antiepileptics: cytotoxics possibly reduce absorption of phenytoin
    Antifungals: metabolism of sunitinib inhibited by ketoconazole (increased plasma concentration)
  • Antipsychotics: avoid concomitant use of cytotoxics with •clozapine (increased risk of agranulocytosis)
    Cardiac Glycosides: cytotoxics reduce absorption of digoxin tablets
Suxamethonium *see* Muscle Relaxants

Sympathomimetics
  • Adrenergic Neurone Blockers: ephedrine, isometheptene, metaraminol, methylphenidate, noradrenaline (norepinephrine), oxymetazoline, phenylephrine, pseudoephedrine and xylometazoline antagonise hypotensive effect of •adrenergic neurone blockers
  • Alpha-blockers: avoid concomitant use of adrenaline (epinephrine) or dopamine with •tolazoline
  • Anaesthetics, General: increased risk of hypertension when methylphenidate given with •volatile liquid general anaesthetics; increased risk of arrhythmias when adrenaline (epinephrine) given with •volatile liquid general anaesthetics
  • Anticoagulants: methylphenidate possibly enhances anticoagulant effect of •coumarins
  • Antidepressants: risk of hypertensive crisis when sympathomimetics given with •MAOIs or •moclobemide; risk of hypertensive crisis when methylphenidate given with •MAOIs, some manufacturers advise avoid methylphenidate for at least 2 weeks after stopping MAOIs; methylphenidate possibly inhibits metabolism of SSRIs and tricyclics; increased risk of hypertension and arrhythmias when adrenaline (epinephrine) given with •tricyclics (but local anaesthetics with adrenaline appear to be safe); increased risk of hypertension and arrhythmias when noradrenaline (norepinephrine) given with •tricyclics
    Antiepileptics: methylphenidate increases plasma concentration of phenytoin; methylphenidate possibly increases plasma concentration of primidone
    Antipsychotics: hypertensive effect of sympathomimetics antagonised by antipsychotics
    Antivirals: plasma concentration of dexamfetamine possibly increased by ritonavir
    Barbiturates: methylphenidate possibly increases plasma concentration of phenobarbital
  • Beta-blockers: increased risk of severe hypertension and bradycardia when adrenaline (epinephrine) given with non-cardioselective •beta-blockers, also response to adrenaline (epinephrine) may be reduced; increased risk of severe hypertension and bradycardia when dobutamine given with non-cardioselective •beta-blockers; possible increased risk of severe hypertension and bradycardia when noradrenaline (norepinephrine) given with non-cardioselective •beta-blockers
  • Clonidine: possible risk of hypertension when adrenaline (epinephrine) or noradrenaline (norepinephrine) given with clonidine; serious adverse events reported with concomitant use of methylphenidate and •clonidine (causality not established)
    Corticosteroids: ephedrine accelerates metabolism of dexamethasone
  • Dopaminergics: risk of toxicity when isometheptene given with •bromocriptine; effects of adrenaline (epinephrine), dobutamine, dopamine and noradrenaline (norepinephrine) possibly enhanced by entacapone; avoid concomitant use of sympathomimetics with •rasagiline; risk of hypertensive crisis when dopamine given with •selegiline
    Doxapram: increased risk of hypertension when sympathomimetics given with doxapram
    Ergot Alkaloids: increased risk of ergotism when sympathomimetics given with ergotamine and methysergide
    Oxytocin: risk of hypertension when vasoconstrictor sympathomimetics given with oxytocin (due to enhanced vasopressor effect)
  • Sympathomimetics: effects of adrenaline (epinephrine) possibly enhanced by •dopexamine; dopexamine possibly enhances effects of •noradrenaline (norepinephrine)
    Theophylline: avoidance of ephedrine in children advised by manufacturer of theophylline

Sympathomimetics, Beta$_2$

Atomoxetine: Increased risk of cardiovascular side-effects when parenteral salbutamol given with atomoxetine

Cardiac Glycosides: salbutamol possibly reduces plasma concentration of digoxin

Corticosteroids: increased risk of hypokalaemia when high doses of beta$_2$ sympathomimetics given with corticosteroids—for CSM advice (hypokalaemia) see p. 173

Diuretics: increased risk of hypokalaemia when high doses of beta$_2$ sympathomimetics given with acetazolamide, loop diuretics or thiazides and related diuretics—for CSM advice (hypokalaemia) see p. 173

• Methyldopa: acute hypotension reported when infusion of salbutamol given with ●methyldopa

Muscle Relaxants: bambuterol enhances effects of suxamethonium

Theophylline: increased risk of hypokalaemia when high doses of beta$_2$ sympathomimetics given with theophylline—for CSM advice (hypokalaemia) see p. 173

Tacrolimus

Note. Interactions do not generally apply to tacrolimus used topically; risk of facial flushing and skin irritation with alcohol consumption (p. 692) does not apply to tacrolimus taken systemically

• Analgesics: possible increased risk of nephrotoxicity when tacrolimus given with NSAIDs; increased risk of nephrotoxicity when tacrolimus given with ●ibuprofen

Angiotensin-II Receptor Antagonists: increased risk of hyperkalaemia when tacrolimus given with angiotensin-II receptor antagonists

• Antibacterials: plasma concentration of tacrolimus increased by ●clarithromycin, ●erythromycin and ●quinupristin/dalfopristin; plasma concentration of tacrolimus reduced by ●rifampicin; increased risk of nephrotoxicity when tacrolimus given with ●aminoglycosides; plasma concentration of tacrolimus possibly increased by ●chloramphenicol and ●telithromycin; possible increased risk of nephrotoxicity when tacrolimus given with vancomycin

• Antidepressants: plasma concentration of tacrolimus reduced by ●St John's wort—avoid concomitant use

Antiepileptics: plasma concentration of tacrolimus reduced by phenytoin, also plasma concentration of phenytoin possibly increased

• Antifungals: plasma concentration of tacrolimus increased by ●fluconazole, ●itraconazole, ●ketoconazole and ●voriconazole; increased risk of nephrotoxicity when tacrolimus given with ●amphotericin; plasma concentration of tacrolimus increased by ●posaconazole (reduce dose of tacrolimus); plasma concentration of tacrolimus reduced by ●caspofungin; plasma concentration of tacrolimus possibly increased by ●imidazoles and ●triazoles

• Antivirals: possible increased risk of nephrotoxicity when tacrolimus given with aciclovir or ganciclovir; plasma concentration of tacrolimus possibly increased by ●atazanavir, ●nelfinavir and ●ritonavir; plasma concentration of tacrolimus possibly affected by ●efavirenz; plasma concentration of tacrolimus increased by ●saquinavir (consider reducing dose of tacrolimus)

• Barbiturates: plasma concentration of tacrolimus reduced by ●phenobarbital

• Calcium-channel Blockers: plasma concentration of tacrolimus possibly increased by felodipine, nicardipine and verapamil; plasma concentration of tacrolimus increased by ●diltiazem and ●nifedipine

• Ciclosporin: tacrolimus increases plasma concentration of ●ciclosporin (increased risk of nephrotoxicity)—avoid concomitant use

Tacrolimus *(continued)*

• Diuretics: increased risk of hyperkalaemia when tacrolimus given with ●potassium-sparing diuretics and aldosterone antagonists

• Grapefruit Juice: plasma concentration of tacrolimus increased by ●grapefruit juice

Hormone Antagonists: plasma concentration of tacrolimus possibly increased by danazol

Oestrogens: tacrolimus possibly inhibits metabolism of oestrogens; plasma concentration of tacrolimus possibly increased by ethinylestradiol

• Potassium Salts: increased risk of hyperkalaemia when tacrolimus given with ●potassium salts

Progestogens: tacrolimus possibly inhibits metabolism of progestogens

Sevelamer: plasma concentration of tacrolimus possibly reduced by sevelamer

Ulcer-healing Drugs: plasma concentration of tacrolimus possibly increased by omeprazole

Tadalafil

• Alpha-blockers: enhanced hypotensive effect when tadalafil given with ●alpha-blockers—avoid concomitant use

Antibacterials: plasma concentration of tadalafil possibly increased by clarithromycin and erythromycin; plasma concentration of tadalafil reduced by rifampicin

Antifungals: plasma concentration of tadalafil increased by ketoconazole; plasma concentration of tadalafil possibly increased by itraconazole

Antivirals: plasma concentration of tadalafil possibly increased by fosamprenavir and indinavir; plasma concentration of tadalafil increased by ritonavir; plasma concentration of tadalafil possibly increased by saquinavir—reduce initial dose of tadalafil

Grapefruit Juice: plasma concentration of tadalafil possibly increased by grapefruit juice

• Nicorandil: tadalafil significantly enhances hypotensive effect of ●nicorandil (avoid concomitant use)

• Nitrates: tadalafil significantly enhances hypotensive effect of ●nitrates (avoid concomitant use)

Tamoxifen

• Anticoagulants: tamoxifen enhances anticoagulant effect of ●coumarins

Tamsulosin *see* Alpha-blockers

Taxanes *see* Docetaxel and Paclitaxel

Tegafur with uracil *see* Fluorouracil

Teicoplanin

Antibacterials: increased risk of nephrotoxicity and ototoxicity when teicoplanin given with aminoglycosides or colistin

Oestrogens: antibacterials that do not induce liver enzymes possibly reduce contraceptive effect of oestrogens (risk probably small, see p. 478)

Vaccines: antibacterials inactivate oral typhoid vaccine—see p. 752

Telbivudine

• Interferons: increased risk of peripheral neuropathy when telbivudine given with ●interferon alfa

Telithromycin

• Antibacterials: plasma concentration of telithromycin reduced by ●rifampicin (avoid during and for 2 weeks after rifampicin)

• Antidepressants: plasma concentration of telithromycin reduced by ●St John's wort (avoid during and for 2 weeks after St John's wort)

• Antiepileptics: plasma concentration of telithromycin reduced by ●carbamazepine, ●phenytoin and ●primidone (avoid during and for 2 weeks after carbamazepine, phenytoin and primidone)

• Antifungals: manufacturer of telithromycin advises avoid concomitant use with ●ketoconazole in severe renal and hepatic impairment

Antimuscarinics: manufacturer of fesoterodine advises dose reduction when telithromycin given with

Telithromycin

  Antimuscarinics *(continued)*
    fesoterodine—consult fesoterodine product literature

- Antipsychotics: increased risk of ventricular arrhythmias when telithromycin given with ●pimozide—avoid concomitant use

- Antivirals: manufacturer of telithromycin advises avoid concomitant use with ●atazanavir, ●fosamprenavir, ●indinavir, ●lopinavir, ●nelfinavir, ●ritonavir, ●saquinavir and ●tipranavir in severe renal and hepatic impairment; telithromycin possibly increases plasma concentration of ●maraviroc (consider reducing dose of maraviroc)

- Anxiolytics and Hypnotics: telithromycin inhibits metabolism of ●midazolam (increased plasma concentration with increased sedation)

  Aprepitant: telithromycin possibly increases plasma concentration of aprepitant

- Barbiturates: plasma concentration of telithromycin reduced by ●phenobarbital (avoid during and for 2 weeks after phenobarbital)

  Cardiac Glycosides: telithromycin possibly increases plasma concentration of digoxin

- Ciclosporin: telithromycin possibly increases plasma concentration of ●ciclosporin

- Cytotoxics: avoidance of telithromycin advised by manufacturer of ●lapatinib and ●nilotinib

- Diuretics: telithromycin increases plasma concentration of ●eplerenone—avoid concomitant use

- Ergot Alkaloids: increased risk of ergotism when telithromycin given with ●ergotamine and methysergide—avoid concomitant use

- Ivabradine: telithromycin possibly increases plasma concentration of ●ivabradine—avoid concomitant use

- Lipid-regulating Drugs: increased risk of myopathy when telithromycin given with ●atorvastatin or ●simvastatin (avoid concomitant use)

  Oestrogens: antibacterials that do not induce liver enzymes possibly reduce contraceptive effect of oestrogens (risk probably small, see p. 478)

  Sildenafil: telithromycin possibly increases plasma concentration of sildenafil—reduce initial dose of sildenafil

- Sirolimus: telithromycin increases plasma concentration of ●sirolimus—avoid concomitant use

- Tacrolimus: telithromycin possibly increases plasma concentration of ●tacrolimus

  Vaccines: antibacterials inactivate oral typhoid vaccine–see p. 752

Telmisartan *see* Angiotensin-II Receptor Antagonists

Temazepam *see* Anxiolytics and Hypnotics

Temocillin *see* Penicillins

Temoporfin

- Cytotoxics: increased skin photosensitivity when temoporfin given with topical ●fluorouracil

Temozolomide

  Antiepileptics: cytotoxics possibly reduce absorption of phenytoin; plasma concentration of temozolomide increased by valproate

- Antipsychotics: avoid concomitant use of cytotoxics with ●clozapine (increased risk of agranulocytosis)
  Cardiac Glycosides: cytotoxics reduce absorption of digoxin tablets

Temsirolimus

  Note. The main active metabolite of temsirolimus is sirolimus —*see also* interactions of sirolimus and consult product literature

- Antibacterials: plasma concentration of active metabolite of temsirolimus reduced by ●rifampicin—avoid concomitant use

  Antiepileptics: cytotoxics possibly reduce absorption of phenytoin

Temsirolimus *(continued)*

- Antifungals: plasma concentration of active metabolite of temsirolimus increased by ●ketoconazole—avoid concomitant use

- Antipsychotics: avoid concomitant use of cytotoxics with ●clozapine (increased risk of agranulocytosis)
  Cardiac Glycosides: cytotoxics reduce absorption of digoxin tablets

Tenofovir

- Antivirals: manufacturer of tenofovir advises avoid concomitant use with adefovir; tenofovir reduces plasma concentration of atazanavir, also plasma concentration of tenofovir possibly increased; combination of tenofovir with cidofovir may increase plasma concentration of either drug (or both); tenofovir increases plasma concentration of ●didanosine (increased risk of toxicity)—avoid concomitant use; plasma concentration of tenofovir increased by lopinavir

Tenoxicam *see* NSAIDs

Terazosin *see* Alpha-blockers

Terbinafine

- Antibacterials: plasma concentration of terbinafine reduced by ●rifampicin

  Antidepressants: terbinafine possibly increases plasma concentration of imipramine and nortriptyline

  Ciclosporin: terbinafine possibly reduces plasma concentration of ciclosporin

  Oestrogens: occasional reports of breakthrough bleeding when terbinafine given with oestrogens (when used for contraception)

  Progestogens: occasional reports of breakthrough bleeding when terbinafine given with progestogens (when used for contraception)

  Ulcer-healing Drugs: plasma concentration of terbinafine increased by cimetidine

Terbutaline *see* Sympathomimetics, Beta$_2$

Terpene Mixture *see* Rowachol®

Testolactone

- Anticoagulants: testolactone enhances anticoagulant effect of ●coumarins and ●phenindione

Testosterone

- Anticoagulants: testosterone enhances anticoagulant effect of ●coumarins and ●phenindione

  Antidiabetics: testosterone possibly enhances hypoglycaemic effect of antidiabetics

Tetrabenazine

- Antidepressants: risk of CNS excitation and hypertension when tetrabenazine given with ●MAOIs

  Antipsychotics: increased risk of extrapyramidal side-effects when tetrabenazine given with antipsychotics

  Dopaminergics: increased risk of extrapyramidal side-effects when tetrabenazine given with amantadine

  Metoclopramide: increased risk of extrapyramidal side-effects when tetrabenazine given with metoclopramide

Tetracosactide *see* Corticosteroids

Tetracycline *see* Tetracyclines

Tetracyclines

  ACE Inhibitors: absorption of tetracyclines reduced by quinapril tablets (quinapril tablets contain magnesium carbonate)

  Adsorbents: absorption of tetracyclines possibly reduced by kaolin

  Antacids: absorption of tetracyclines reduced by antacids

- Anticoagulants: tetracyclines possibly enhance anticoagulant effect of ●coumarins and ●phenindione

  Antiepileptics: metabolism of doxycycline accelerated by carbamazepine (reduced effect); metabolism of doxycycline accelerated by phenytoin and primidone (reduced plasma concentration)

  Atovaquone: tetracycline reduces plasma concentration of atovaquone

  Barbiturates: metabolism of doxycycline accelerated by barbiturates (reduced plasma concentration)

Tetracyclines *(continued)*

Calcium Salts: absorption of tetracycline reduced by calcium salts

• Ciclosporin: doxycycline possibly increases plasma concentration of •ciclosporin

Cytotoxics: doxycycline or tetracycline increase risk of methotrexate toxicity

Dairy Products: absorption of tetracyclines (except doxycycline and minocycline) reduced by dairy products

Diuretics: manufacturer of lymecycline advises avoid concomitant use with diuretics

Ergot Alkaloids: increased risk of ergotism when tetracyclines given with ergotamine and methysergide

Iron: absorption of tetracyclines reduced by *oral* iron, also absorption of *oral* iron reduced by tetracyclines

Lipid-regulating Drugs: absorption of tetracycline possibly reduced by colestipol and colestyramine

Oestrogens: antibacterials that do not induce liver enzymes possibly reduce contraceptive effect of oestrogens (risk probably small, see p. 478)

• Retinoids: possible increased risk of benign intracranial hypertension when tetracyclines given with •retinoids (avoid concomitant use)

Strontium Ranelate: absorption of tetracyclines reduced by strontium ranelate (manufacturer of strontium ranelate advises avoid concomitant use)

Ulcer-healing Drugs: absorption of tetracyclines reduced by sucralfate and tripotassium dicitratobismuthate

Vaccines: antibacterials inactivate oral typhoid vaccine–see p. 752

Zinc: absorption of tetracyclines reduced by zinc, also absorption of zinc reduced by tetracyclines

Theophylline

Allopurinol: plasma concentration of theophylline possibly increased by allopurinol

Anaesthetics, General: increased risk of convulsions when theophylline given with ketamine; increased risk of arrhythmias when theophylline given with halothane

Anti-arrhythmics: theophylline antagonises anti-arrhythmic effect of adenosine; plasma concentration of theophylline increased by propafenone

• Antibacterials: plasma concentration of theophylline possibly increased by azithromycin and isoniazid; metabolism of theophylline inhibited by •clarithromycin (increased plasma concentration); metabolism of theophylline inhibited by •erythromycin (increased plasma concentration), if erythromycin given by mouth, also decreased plasma-erythromycin concentration; plasma concentration of theophylline increased by •ciprofloxacin and •norfloxacin; metabolism of theophylline accelerated by rifampicin (reduced plasma concentration); possible increased risk of convulsions when theophylline given with •quinolones

• Antidepressants: plasma concentration of theophylline increased by •fluvoxamine (concomitant use should usually be avoided, but where not possible halve theophylline dose and monitor plasma-theophylline concentration); plasma concentration of theophylline reduced by •St John's wort—avoid concomitant use

• Antiepileptics: metabolism of theophylline accelerated by carbamazepine and primidone (reduced effect); plasma concentration of both drugs reduced when theophylline given with •phenytoin

• Antifungals: plasma concentration of theophylline possibly increased by •fluconazole and •ketoconazole

• Antivirals: metabolism of theophylline accelerated by •ritonavir (reduced plasma concentration)

Anxiolytics and Hypnotics: theophylline possibly reduces effects of benzodiazepines

Theophylline *(continued)*

Barbiturates: metabolism of theophylline accelerated by barbiturates (reduced effect)

• Calcium-channel Blockers: plasma concentration of theophylline possibly increased by •calcium-channel blockers (enhanced effect); plasma concentration of theophylline increased by diltiazem; plasma concentration of theophylline increased by •verapamil (enhanced effect)

Corticosteroids: increased risk of hypokalaemia when theophylline given with corticosteroids

Cytotoxics: plasma concentration of theophylline possibly increased by methotrexate

Disulfiram: metabolism of theophylline inhibited by disulfiram (increased risk of toxicity)

Diuretics: increased risk of hypokalaemia when theophylline given with acetazolamide, loop diuretics or thiazides and related diuretics

Doxapram: increased CNS stimulation when theophylline given with doxapram

Interferons: metabolism of theophylline inhibited by interferon alfa (increased plasma concentration)

Leukotriene Receptor Antagonists: plasma concentration of theophylline possibly increased by zafirlukast, also plasma concentration of zafirlukast reduced

Lithium: theophylline increases excretion of lithium (reduced plasma concentration)

Oestrogens: excretion of theophylline reduced by oestrogens (increased plasma concentration)

Pentoxifylline (oxpentifylline): plasma concentration of theophylline increased by pentoxifylline (oxpentifylline)

Sulfinpyrazone: plasma concentration of theophylline reduced by sulfinpyrazone

Sympathomimetics: manufacturer of theophylline advises avoid concomitant use with ephedrine in children

Sympathomimetics, Beta$_2$: increased risk of hypokalaemia when theophylline given with high doses of beta$_2$ sympathomimetics—for CSM advice (hypokalaemia) see p. 173

Tobacco: metabolism of theophylline increased by tobacco smoking (reduced plasma concentration)

• Ulcer-healing Drugs: metabolism of theophylline inhibited by •cimetidine (increased plasma concentration); absorption of theophylline possibly reduced by sucralfate (give at least 2 hours apart)

Vaccines: plasma concentration of theophylline possibly increased by influenza vaccine

Thiazolidinediones *see* Antidiabetics

Thiopental *see* Anaesthetics, General

Thiotepa

Antiepileptics: cytotoxics possibly reduce absorption of phenytoin

• Antipsychotics: avoid concomitant use of cytotoxics with •clozapine (increased risk of agranulocytosis)

Cardiac Glycosides: cytotoxics reduce absorption of digoxin tablets

Muscle Relaxants: thiotepa enhances effects of suxamethonium

Thioxanthenes *see* Antipsychotics

Thyroid Hormones

Antacids: absorption of levothyroxine (thyroxine) possibly reduced by antacids

Anti-arrhythmics: for concomitant use of thyroid hormones and amiodarone see p. 109

Antibacterials: metabolism of levothyroxine (thyroxine) accelerated by rifampicin (may increase requirements for levothyroxine (thyroxine) in hypothyroidism)

• Anticoagulants: thyroid hormones enhance anticoagulant effect of •coumarins and •phenindione

Antidepressants: thyroid hormones enhance effects of amitriptyline and imipramine; thyroid hormones possibly enhance effects of tricyclics

Thyroid Hormones *(continued)*

Antiepileptics: metabolism of thyroid hormones accelerated by carbamazepine and primidone (may increase requirements for thyroid hormones in hypothyroidism); metabolism of thyroid hormones accelerated by phenytoin (may increase requirements in hypothyroidism), also plasma concentration of phenytoin possibly increased

Barbiturates: metabolism of thyroid hormones accelerated by barbiturates (may increase requirements for thyroid hormones in hypothyroidism)

Beta-blockers: levothyroxine (thyroxine) accelerates metabolism of propranolol

Calcium Salts: absorption of levothyroxine (thyroxine) reduced by calcium salts

Cytotoxics: plasma concentration of levothyroxine (thyroxine) possibly reduced by imatinib

Iron: absorption of levothyroxine (thyroxine) reduced by *oral* iron (give at least 2 hours apart)

Lipid-regulating Drugs: absorption of thyroid hormones reduced by colestipol and colestyramine

Oestrogens: requirements for thyroid hormones in hypothyroidism may be increased by oestrogens

Polystyrene Sulphonate Resins: absorption of levothyroxine (thyroxine) reduced by polystyrene sulphonate resins

Ulcer-healing Drugs: absorption of levothyroxine (thyroxine) reduced by cimetidine and sucralfate

Tiagabine

● Antidepressants: anticonvulsant effect of antiepileptics possibly antagonised by MAOIs and ●tricyclic-related antidepressants (convulsive threshold lowered); anticonvulsant effect of antiepileptics antagonised by ●SSRIs and ●tricyclics (convulsive threshold lowered); avoid concomitant use of antiepileptics with ●St John's wort

Antiepileptics: plasma concentration of tiagabine reduced by carbamazepine, phenytoin and primidone

● Antimalarials: possible increased risk of convulsions when antiepileptics given with chloroquine and hydroxychloroquine; anticonvulsant effect of antiepileptics antagonised by ●mefloquine

Barbiturates: plasma concentration of tiagabine reduced by phenobarbital

Tiaprofenic Acid *see* NSAIDs

Tibolone

Antibacterials: metabolism of tibolone accelerated by rifampicin (reduced plasma concentration)

Antiepileptics: metabolism of tibolone accelerated by carbamazepine and primidone (reduced plasma concentration); metabolism of tibolone accelerated by phenytoin

Barbiturates: metabolism of tibolone accelerated by barbiturates (reduced plasma concentration)

Ticarcillin *see* Penicillins

Tigecycline

Anticoagulants: tigecycline possibly enhances anticoagulant effect of coumarins

Oestrogens: antibacterials that do not induce liver enzymes possibly reduce contraceptive effect of oestrogens (risk probably small, see p. 478)

Vaccines: antibacterials inactivate oral typhoid vaccine–see p. 752

Tiludronic Acid *see* Bisphosphonates

Timolol *see* Beta-blockers

Tinidazole

Alcohol: possibility of disulfiram-like reaction when tinidazole given with alcohol

Oestrogens: antibacterials that do not induce liver enzymes possibly reduce contraceptive effect of oestrogens (risk probably small, see p. 478)

Vaccines: antibacterials inactivate oral typhoid vaccine–see p. 752

Tinzaparin *see* Heparins

Tioguanine

Antiepileptics: cytotoxics possibly reduce absorption of phenytoin

● Antipsychotics: avoid concomitant use of cytotoxics with ●clozapine (increased risk of agranulocytosis)

Cardiac Glycosides: cytotoxics reduce absorption of digoxin tablets

Cytotoxics: increased risk of hepatotoxicity when tioguanine given with busulfan

Tiotropium *see* Antimuscarinics

Tipranavir

Antacids: absorption of tipranavir reduced by antacids

● Antibacterials: tipranavir increases plasma concentration of ●clarithromycin (reduce dose of clarithromycin in renal impairment), also plasma concentration of tipranavir increased by clarithromycin; tipranavir increases plasma concentration of ●rifabutin (reduce dose of rifabutin); plasma concentration of tipranavir possibly reduced by ●rifampicin—avoid concomitant use; avoidance of concomitant tipranavir in severe renal and hepatic impairment advised by manufacturer of ●telithromycin

Anticoagulants: avoidance of tipranavir advised by manufacturer of rivaroxaban

● Antidepressants: plasma concentration of tipranavir possibly reduced by ●St John's wort—avoid concomitant use

Antiepileptics: plasma concentration of tipranavir possibly reduced by carbamazepine

Antifungals: plasma concentration of tipranavir increased by fluconazole

Antimalarials: caution with tipranavir advised by manufacturer of artemether/lumefantrine

Antimuscarinics: avoidance of tipranavir advised by manufacturer of darifenacin

● Antivirals: tipranavir reduces plasma concentration of ●abacavir, ●didanosine, ●fosamprenavir, ●lopinavir, ●saquinavir and ●zidovudine; plasma concentration of tipranavir increased by atazanavir (also plasma concentration of atazanavir reduced); tipranavir reduces plasma concentration of ●etravirine, also plasma concentration of tipranavir increased (avoid concomitant use)

● Beta-blockers: manufacturer of tipranavir advises avoid concomitant use with ●metoprolol for heart failure

● Lipid-regulating Drugs: possible increased risk of myopathy when tipranavir given with ●rosuvastatin—avoid concomitant use

● Ulcer-healing Drugs: tipranavir reduces plasma concentration of ●esomeprazole and ●omeprazole

Vitamins: increased risk of bleeding when tipranavir given with high doses of vitamin E

Tirofiban

Iloprost: increased risk of bleeding when tirofiban given with iloprost

Tizanidine *see* Muscle Relaxants

Tobacco

Cinacalcet: tobacco smoking increases cinacalcet metabolism (reduced plasma concentration)

Cytotoxics: tobacco smoking reduces plasma concentration of erlotinib

Theophylline: tobacco smoking increases theophylline metabolism (reduced plasma concentration)

Tobramycin *see* Aminoglycosides

Tolazoline *see* Alpha-blockers

Tolbutamide *see* Antidiabetics

Tolcapone

Antidepressants: avoid concomitant use of tolcapone with MAOIs

Memantine: effects of dopaminergics possibly enhanced by memantine

Methyldopa: antiparkinsonian effect of dopaminergics antagonised by methyldopa

Tolfenamic Acid *see* NSAIDs

Tolterodine *see* Antimuscarinics

Topiramate
- Antidepressants: anticonvulsant effect of antiepileptics possibly antagonised by MAOIs and •tricyclic-related antidepressants (convulsive threshold lowered); anticonvulsant effect of antiepileptics antagonised by •SSRIs and •tricyclics (convulsive threshold lowered); avoid concomitant use of antiepileptics with •St John's wort

  Antidiabetics: topiramate possibly reduces plasma concentration of glibenclamide
- Antiepileptics: plasma concentration of topiramate often reduced by carbamazepine; topiramate increases plasma concentration of •phenytoin (also plasma concentration of topiramate reduced)
- Antimalarials: possible increased risk of convulsions when antiepileptics given with chloroquine and hydroxychloroquine; anticonvulsant effect of antiepileptics antagonised by •mefloquine

  Lithium: topiramate possibly affects plasma concentration of lithium
- Oestrogens: topiramate accelerates metabolism of •oestrogens (reduced contraceptive effect—see p. 478)
- Progestogens: topiramate accelerates metabolism of •progestogens (reduced contraceptive effect—see p. 478)

Torasemide *see* Diuretics

Toremifene
- Anticoagulants: toremifene possibly enhances anticoagulant effect of •coumarins

  Antiepileptics: metabolism of toremifene possibly accelerated by carbamazepine (reduced plasma concentration); metabolism of toremifene possibly accelerated by phenytoin; metabolism of toremifene accelerated by primidone (reduced plasma concentration)

  Barbiturates: metabolism of toremifene possibly accelerated by barbiturates (reduced plasma concentration)

  Diuretics: increased risk of hypercalcaemia when toremifene given with thiazides and related diuretics

  Sugammadex: toremifene possibly reduces response to sugammadex

Trabectedin

  Antiepileptics: cytotoxics possibly reduce absorption of phenytoin
- Antipsychotics: avoid concomitant use of cytotoxics with •clozapine (increased risk of agranulocytosis)

  Cardiac Glycosides: cytotoxics reduce absorption of digoxin tablets

Tramadol *see* Opioid Analgesics

Trandolapril *see* ACE Inhibitors

Tranylcypromine *see* MAOIs

Trazodone *see* Antidepressants, Tricyclic (related)

Tretinoin *see* Retinoids

Triamcinolone *see* Corticosteroids

Triamterene *see* Diuretics

Triclofos *see* Anxiolytics and Hypnotics

Trientine

  Iron: trientine reduces absorption of *oral* iron

  Zinc: trientine reduces absorption of zinc, also absorption of trientine reduced by zinc

Trifluoperazine *see* Antipsychotics

Trihexyphenidyl (benzhexol) *see* Antimuscarinics

Trilostane

  Diuretics: increased risk of hyperkalaemia when trilostane given with potassium-sparing diuretics and aldosterone antagonists

Trimethoprim
- Anti-arrhythmics: increased risk of ventricular arrhythmias when trimethoprim (as co-trimoxazole) given with •amiodarone—avoid concomitant use of co-trimoxazole

  Antibacterials: plasma concentration of trimethoprim possibly reduced by rifampicin; plasma concentra-

Trimethoprim *(continued)*

  tion of both drugs may increase when trimethoprim given with dapsone

  Anticoagulants: trimethoprim possibly enhances anticoagulant effect of coumarins

  Antidiabetics: trimethoprim possibly enhances hypoglycaemic effect of repaglinide—manufacturer advises avoid concomitant use; trimethoprim rarely enhances the effects of sulphonylureas
- Antiepileptics: trimethoprim increases plasma concentration of •phenytoin (also increased antifolate effect)
- Antimalarials: increased antifolate effect when trimethoprim given with •pyrimethamine

  Antivirals: trimethoprim (as co-trimoxazole) increases plasma concentration of lamivudine—avoid concomitant use of high-dose co-trimoxazole

  Cardiac Glycosides: trimethoprim possibly increases plasma concentration of digoxin
- Ciclosporin: increased risk of nephrotoxicity when trimethoprim given with •ciclosporin, also plasma concentration of ciclosporin reduced by intravenous trimethoprim
- Cytotoxics: increased risk of haematological toxicity when trimethoprim (also with co-trimoxazole) given with •azathioprine, •mercaptopurine or •methotrexate

  Diuretics: increased risk of hyperkalaemia when trimethoprim given with eplerenone

  Oestrogens: antibacterials that do not induce liver enzymes possibly reduce contraceptive effect of oestrogens (risk probably small, see p. 478)

  Vaccines: antibacterials inactivate oral typhoid vaccine—see p. 752

Trimipramine *see* Antidepressants, Tricyclic

Tripotassium Dicitratobismuthate

  Antibacterials: tripotassium dicitratobismuthate reduces absorption of tetracyclines

Tropicamide *see* Antimuscarinics

Trospium *see* Antimuscarinics

Tryptophan
- Antidepressants: possible increased serotonergic effects when tryptophan given with duloxetine; CNS excitation and confusion when tryptophan given with •MAOIs (reduce dose of tryptophan); agitation and nausea may occur when tryptophan given with •SSRIs
- Antimalarials: avoidance of antidepressants advised by manufacturer of •artemether/lumefantrine

  Atomoxetine: possible increased risk of convulsions when antidepressants given with atomoxetine
- Sibutramine: increased risk of CNS toxicity when tryptophan given with •sibutramine (manufacturer of sibutramine advises avoid concomitant use)

Typhoid Vaccine (oral) *see* Vaccines

Typhoid Vaccine (parenteral) *see* Vaccines

Ubidecarenone

  Anticoagulants: ubidecarenone may enhance or reduce anticoagulant effect of warfarin

Ulcer-healing Drugs *see* Histamine H_2-antagonists, Proton Pump Inhibitors, Sucralfate, and Tripotassium Dicitratobismuthate

Ursodeoxycholic Acid

  Antacids: absorption of bile acids possibly reduced by antacids
- Ciclosporin: ursodeoxycholic acid increases absorption of •ciclosporin

  Lipid-regulating Drugs: absorption of bile acids possibly reduced by colestipol and colestyramine

  Oestrogens: elimination of cholesterol in bile increased when bile acids given with oestrogens

Vaccines

Note. For a general warning on live vaccines and high doses of corticosteroids or other immunosuppressive drugs, see p. 725; for advice on live vaccines and immunoglobulins, see under Normal Immunoglobulin, p. 755

- Abatacept: avoid concomitant use of live vaccines with •abatacept (see p. 725)
- Adalimumab: avoid concomitant use of live vaccines with •adalimumab (see p. 725)
- Anakinra: avoid concomitant use of live vaccines with •anakinra (see p. 725)

  Antibacterials: oral typhoid vaccine inactivated by antibacterials–see p. 752

  Anticoagulants: influenza vaccine possibly enhances anticoagulant effect of warfarin

  Antiepileptics: influenza vaccine enhances effects of phenytoin

  Antimalarials: oral typhoid vaccine inactivated by antimalarials–see p. 752
- Corticosteroids: immune response to vaccines impaired by high doses of •corticosteroids, avoid concomitant use with live vaccines (see p. 725)
- Efalizumab: live or live-attenuated vaccines should be given 2 weeks before •efalizumab or withheld until 8 weeks after discontinuation
- Etanercept: avoid concomitant use of live vaccines with •etanercept (see p. 725)
- Infliximab: avoid concomitant use of live vaccines with •infliximab (see p. 725)

  Interferons: avoidance of vaccines advised by manufacturer of interferon gamma
- Leflunomide: avoid concomitant use of live vaccines with •leflunomide (see p. 725)

  Theophylline: influenza vaccine possibly increases plasma concentration of theophylline

Valaciclovir *see* Aciclovir

Valganciclovir *see* Ganciclovir

Valproate

Analgesics: effects of valproate enhanced by aspirin

Antibacterials: plasma concentration of valproate possibly reduced by doripenem and ertapenem; plasma concentration of valproate reduced by imipenem with cilastatin and meropenem; metabolism of valproate possibly inhibited by erythromycin (increased plasma concentration)

Anticoagulants: valproate possibly enhances anticoagulant effect of coumarins

- Antidepressants: anticonvulsant effect of antiepileptics possibly antagonised by MAOIs and •tricyclic-related antidepressants (convulsive threshold lowered); anticonvulsant effect of antiepileptics antagonised by •SSRIs and •tricyclics (convulsive threshold lowered); avoid concomitant use of antiepileptics with •St John's wort
- Antiepileptics: plasma concentration of valproate reduced by carbamazepine, also plasma concentration of active metabolite of carbamazepine increased; valproate possibly increases plasma concentration of ethosuximide; valproate increases plasma concentration of lamotrigine; valproate sometimes reduces plasma concentration of an active metabolite of oxcarbazepine; valproate increases or possibly decreases plasma concentration of phenytoin, also plasma concentration of valproate reduced; valproate possibly increases plasma concentration of •primidone (plasma concentration of active metabolite of primidone increased), also plasma concentration of valproate reduced; valproate possibly increases plasma concentration of rufinamide (reduce dose of rufinamide)
- Antimalarials: possible increased risk of convulsions when antiepileptics given with chloroquine and hydroxychloroquine; anticonvulsant effect of antiepileptics antagonised by •mefloquine
- Antipsychotics: anticonvulsant effect of valproate antagonised by •antipsychotics (convulsive thresh-

Valproate

- Antipsychotics *(continued)*
  old lowered); increased risk of neutropenia when valproate given with •olanzapine

  Antivirals: valproate possibly increases plasma concentration of zidovudine (increased risk of toxicity)

  Anxiolytics and Hypnotics: plasma concentration of valproate possibly increased by clobazam; increased risk of side-effects when valproate given with clonazepam; valproate possibly increases plasma concentration of diazepam and lorazepam

  Barbiturates: valproate increases plasma concentration of phenobarbital (also plasma concentration of valproate reduced)

  Bupropion: valproate inhibits the metabolism of bupropion

  Cytotoxics: valproate increases plasma concentration of temozolomide

  Lipid-regulating Drugs: absorption of valproate possibly reduced by colestyramine

  Sodium Benzoate: valproate possibly reduces effects of sodium benzoate

  Sodium Phenylbutyrate: valproate possibly reduces effects of sodium phenylbutyrate
- Ulcer-healing Drugs: metabolism of valproate inhibited by •cimetidine (increased plasma concentration)

Valsartan *see* Angiotensin-II Receptor Antagonists

Vancomycin

Anaesthetics, General: hypersensitivity-like reactions can occur when intravenous vancomycin given with general anaesthetics

Antibacterials: increased risk of nephrotoxicity and ototoxicity when vancomycin given with aminoglycosides, capreomycin or colistin; increased risk of nephrotoxicity when vancomycin given with polymyxins

Antifungals: possible increased risk of nephrotoxicity when vancomycin given with amphotericin
- Ciclosporin: increased risk of nephrotoxicity when vancomycin given with •ciclosporin

  Cytotoxics: increased risk of nephrotoxicity and possibly of ototoxicity when vancomycin given with cisplatin
- Diuretics: increased risk of otoxicity when vancomycin given with •loop diuretics

  Lipid-regulating Drugs: effects of oral vancomycin antagonised by colestyramine
- Muscle Relaxants: vancomycin enhances effects of •suxamethonium

  Oestrogens: antibacterials that do not induce liver enzymes possibly reduce contraceptive effect of oestrogens (risk probably small, see p. 478)

  Tacrolimus: possible increased risk of nephrotoxicity when vancomycin given with tacrolimus

  Vaccines: antibacterials inactivate oral typhoid vaccine–see p. 752

Vardenafil
- Alpha-blockers: enhanced hypotensive effect when vardenafil given with •alpha-blockers (excludes tamsulosin)—avoid vardenafil for 6 hours after alpha-blockers

  Antibacterials: plasma concentration of vardenafil increased by erythromycin (reduce dose of vardenafil)
- Antifungals: plasma concentration of vardenafil increased by •ketoconazole—avoid concomitant use; plasma concentration of vardenafil possibly increased by •itraconazole—avoid concomitant use
- Antivirals: plasma concentration of vardenafil possibly increased by fosamprenavir; plasma concentration of vardenafil increased by •indinavir—avoid concomitant use; plasma concentration of vardenafil possibly increased by •ritonavir—avoid concomitant use; plasma concentration of vardenafil possibly increased by saquinavir—reduce initial dose of vardenafil

Vardenafil *(continued)*

Calcium-channel Blockers: enhanced hypotensive effect when vardenafil given with nifedipine

- Grapefruit Juice: plasma concentration of vardenafil possibly increased by ●grapefruit juice—avoid concomitant use
- Nicorandil: possible increased hypotensive effect when vardenafil given with ●nicorandil—avoid concomitant use
- Nitrates: possible increased hypotensive effect when vardenafil given with ●nitrates—avoid concomitant use

Vasodilator Antihypertensives

ACE Inhibitors: enhanced hypotensive effect when hydralazine, minoxidil or sodium nitroprusside given with ACE inhibitors

Adrenergic Neurone Blockers: enhanced hypotensive effect when hydralazine, minoxidil or sodium nitroprusside given with adrenergic neurone blockers

Alcohol: enhanced hypotensive effect when hydralazine, minoxidil or sodium nitroprusside given with alcohol

Aldesleukin: enhanced hypotensive effect when hydralazine, minoxidil or sodium nitroprusside given with aldesleukin

Alpha-blockers: enhanced hypotensive effect when hydralazine, minoxidil or sodium nitroprusside given with alpha-blockers

Anaesthetics, General: enhanced hypotensive effect when hydralazine, minoxidil or sodium nitroprusside given with general anaesthetics

Analgesics: hypotensive effect of hydralazine, minoxidil and sodium nitroprusside antagonised by NSAIDs

Angiotensin-II Receptor Antagonists: enhanced hypotensive effect when hydralazine, minoxidil or sodium nitroprusside given with angiotensin-II receptor antagonists

Antidepressants: enhanced hypotensive effect when hydralazine, minoxidil or sodium nitroprusside given with MAOIs; enhanced hypotensive effect when hydralazine or sodium nitroprusside given with tricyclic-related antidepressants

Antipsychotics: enhanced hypotensive effect when hydralazine, minoxidil or sodium nitroprusside given with phenothiazines

Anxiolytics and Hypnotics: enhanced hypotensive effect when hydralazine, minoxidil or sodium nitroprusside given with anxiolytics and hypnotics

Beta-blockers: enhanced hypotensive effect when hydralazine, minoxidil or sodium nitroprusside given with beta-blockers

Calcium-channel Blockers: enhanced hypotensive effect when hydralazine, minoxidil or sodium nitroprusside given with calcium-channel blockers

Clonidine: enhanced hypotensive effect when hydralazine, minoxidil or sodium nitroprusside given with clonidine

Corticosteroids: hypotensive effect of hydralazine, minoxidil and sodium nitroprusside antagonised by corticosteroids

Diazoxide: enhanced hypotensive effect when hydralazine, minoxidil or sodium nitroprusside given with diazoxide

Diuretics: enhanced hypotensive effect when hydralazine, minoxidil or sodium nitroprusside given with diuretics

Dopaminergics: enhanced hypotensive effect when hydralazine, minoxidil or sodium nitroprusside given with levodopa

Methyldopa: enhanced hypotensive effect when hydralazine, minoxidil or sodium nitroprusside given with methyldopa

Moxisylyte (thymoxamine): enhanced hypotensive effect when hydralazine, minoxidil or sodium nitroprusside given with moxisylyte

Vasodilator Antihypertensives *(continued)*

Moxonidine: enhanced hypotensive effect when hydralazine, minoxidil or sodium nitroprusside given with moxonidine

Muscle Relaxants: enhanced hypotensive effect when hydralazine, minoxidil or sodium nitroprusside given with baclofen; enhanced hypotensive effect when hydralazine, minoxidil or sodium nitroprusside given with tizanidine

Nicorandil: possible enhanced hypotensive effect when hydralazine, minoxidil or sodium nitroprusside given with nicorandil

Nitrates: enhanced hypotensive effect when hydralazine, minoxidil or sodium nitroprusside given with nitrates

Oestrogens: hypotensive effect of hydralazine, minoxidil and sodium nitroprusside antagonised by oestrogens

Prostaglandins: enhanced hypotensive effect when hydralazine, minoxidil or sodium nitroprusside given with alprostadil

Vasodilator Antihypertensives: enhanced hypotensive effect when hydralazine given with minoxidil or sodium nitroprusside; enhanced hypotensive effect when minoxidil given with sodium nitroprusside

Vecuronium *see* Muscle Relaxants

Venlafaxine

- Analgesics: increased risk of bleeding when venlafaxine given with ●NSAIDs or ●aspirin
- Anticoagulants: venlafaxine possibly enhances anticoagulant effect of ●warfarin
- Antidepressants: possible increased serotonergic effects when venlafaxine given with duloxetine; enhanced CNS effects and toxicity when venlafaxine given with ●MAOIs (venlafaxine should not be started until 2 weeks after stopping MAOIs, avoid MAOIs for 1 week after stopping venlafaxine); after stopping SSRI-related antidepressants do not start ●moclobemide for at least 1 week
- Antimalarials: avoidance of antidepressants advised by manufacturer of ●artemether/lumefantrine
- Antipsychotics: venlafaxine increases plasma concentration of ●clozapine and haloperidol

Atomoxetine: possible increased risk of convulsions when antidepressants given with atomoxetine

- Dopaminergics: caution with venlafaxine advised by manufacturer of entacapone; increased risk of hypertension and CNS excitation when venlafaxine given with ●selegiline (selegiline should not be started until 1 week after stopping venlafaxine, avoid venlafaxine for 2 weeks after stopping selegiline)

Lithium: possible increased serotonergic effects when venlafaxine given with lithium

- Sibutramine: increased risk of CNS toxicity when SSRI-related antidepressants given with ●sibutramine (manufacturer of sibutramine advises avoid concomitant use)

Verapamil *see* Calcium-channel Blockers

Vigabatrin

- Antidepressants: anticonvulsant effect of antiepileptics possibly antagonised by MAOIs and ●tricyclic-related antidepressants (convulsive threshold lowered); anticonvulsant effect of antiepileptics antagonised by ●SSRIs and ●tricyclics (convulsive threshold lowered); avoid concomitant use of antiepileptics with ●St John's wort

Antiepileptics: vigabatrin reduces plasma concentration of phenytoin; vigabatrin possibly reduces plasma concentration of primidone

- Antimalarials: possible increased risk of convulsions when antiepileptics given with chloroquine and hydroxychloroquine; anticonvulsant effect of antiepileptics antagonised by ●mefloquine

Barbiturates: vigabatrin possibly reduces plasma concentration of phenobarbital

Vildagliptin *see* Antidiabetics

Vinblastine
- Antibacterials: toxicity of vinblastine increased by ●erythromycin—avoid concomitant use
  Antiepileptics: cytotoxics possibly reduce absorption of phenytoin
- Antifungals: metabolism of vinblastine possibly inhibited by ●posaconazole (increased risk of neurotoxicity)
- Antipsychotics: avoid concomitant use of cytotoxics with ●clozapine (increased risk of agranulocytosis)
  Cardiac Glycosides: cytotoxics reduce absorption of digoxin tablets

Vincristine
  Antiepileptics: cytotoxics possibly reduce absorption of phenytoin
- Antifungals: metabolism of vincristine possibly inhibited by ●itraconazole and ●posaconazole (increased risk of neurotoxicity)
- Antipsychotics: avoid concomitant use of cytotoxics with ●clozapine (increased risk of agranulocytosis)
  Calcium-channel Blockers: metabolism of vincristine possibly inhibited by nifedipine
  Cardiac Glycosides: cytotoxics reduce absorption of digoxin tablets

Vinorelbine
  Antiepileptics: cytotoxics possibly reduce absorption of phenytoin
- Antipsychotics: avoid concomitant use of cytotoxics with ●clozapine (increased risk of agranulocytosis)
  Cardiac Glycosides: cytotoxics reduce absorption of digoxin tablets

Vitamin A see Vitamins
Vitamin D see Vitamins
Vitamin E see Vitamins
Vitamin K (Phytomenadione) see Vitamins

Vitamins
  Antibacterials: absorption of vitamin A possibly reduced by neomycin
- Anticoagulants: vitamin K antagonises anticoagulant effect of ●coumarins and ●phenindione
  Antiepileptics: vitamin D requirements possibly increased when given with carbamazepine, phenytoin or primidone
  Antifungals: plasma concentration of paricalcitol possibly increased by ketoconazole
  Antivirals: increased risk of bleeding when high doses of vitamin E given with tipranavir
  Barbiturates: vitamin D requirements possibly increased when given with barbiturates
  Diuretics: increased risk of hypercalcaemia when vitamin D given with thiazides and related diuretics
  Dopaminergics: pyridoxine reduces effects of levodopa when given without dopa-decarboxylase inhibitor
  Retinoids: risk of hypervitaminosis A when vitamin A given with retinoids
  Selenium: ascorbic acid possibly reduces absorption of selenium (give at least 4 hours apart)

Voriconazole see Antifungals, Triazole
Warfarin see Coumarins
Xipamide see Diuretics
Xylometazoline see Sympathomimetics
Zafirlukast see Leukotriene Receptor Antagonists
Zaleplon see Anxiolytics and Hypnotics

Zidovudine
  Note. Increased risk of toxicity with nephrotoxic and myelosuppressive drugs—for further details consult product literature
  Analgesics: increased risk of haematological toxicity when zidovudine given with NSAIDs; plasma con-

Zidovudine
  Analgesics *(continued)*
    centration of zidovudine possibly increased by methadone
  Antibacterials: absorption of zidovudine reduced by clarithromycin tablets (give at least 2 hours apart); manufacturer of zidovudine advises avoid concomitant use with rifampicin
  Antiepileptics: zidovudine increases or decreases plasma concentration of phenytoin; plasma concentration of zidovudine possibly increased by valproate (increased risk of toxicity)
- Antifungals: plasma concentration of zidovudine increased by ●fluconazole (increased risk of toxicity)
  Antimalarials: increased antifolate effect when zidovudine given with pyrimethamine
- Antivirals: profound myelosuppression when zidovudine given with ●ganciclovir (if possible avoid concomitant administration, particularly during initial ganciclovir therapy); increased risk of anaemia when zidovudine given with ●ribavirin—avoid concomitant use; zidovudine possibly inhibits effects of ●stavudine (manufacturers advise avoid concomitant use); plasma concentration of zidovudine reduced by ●tipranavir
  Atovaquone: metabolism of zidovudine possibly inhibited by atovaquone (increased plasma concentration)
- Probenecid: excretion of zidovudine reduced by ●probenecid (increased plasma concentration and risk of toxicity)

Zinc
  Antibacterials: zinc reduces absorption of ciprofloxacin, levofloxacin, moxifloxacin, norfloxacin and ofloxacin; zinc reduces absorption of tetracyclines, also absorption of zinc reduced by tetracyclines
  Calcium Salts: absorption of zinc reduced by calcium salts
  Iron: absorption of zinc reduced by *oral* iron, also absorption of *oral* iron reduced by zinc
  Penicillamine: absorption of zinc reduced by penicillamine, also absorption of penicillamine reduced by zinc
  Trientine: absorption of zinc reduced by trientine, also absorption of trientine reduced by zinc

Zoledronic Acid see Bisphosphonates
Zolmitriptan see 5HT$_1$ Agonists
Zolpidem see Anxiolytics and Hypnotics

Zonisamide
- Antidepressants: anticonvulsant effect of antiepileptics possibly antagonised by MAOIs and ●tricyclic-related antidepressants (convulsive threshold lowered); anticonvulsant effect of antiepileptics antagonised by ●SSRIs and ●tricyclics (convulsive threshold lowered); avoid concomitant use of antiepileptics with ●St John's wort
  Antiepileptics: plasma concentration of zonisamide reduced by carbamazepine and phenytoin
- Antimalarials: possible increased risk of convulsions when antiepileptics given with chloroquine and hydroxychloroquine; anticonvulsant effect of antiepileptics antagonised by ●mefloquine
  Barbiturates: plasma concentration of zonisamide reduced by phenobarbital

Zopiclone see Anxiolytics and Hypnotics
Zotepine see Antipsychotics
Zuclopenthixol see Antipsychotics

A2 Borderline substances

A2.1 Enteral feeds (non-disease specific) 879

A2.2 Nutritional supplements (non-disease specific) 890

A2.3 Specialised formulas 896

A2.4 Feed supplements 904

A2.5 Feed additives 909

A2.6 Foods for special diets 910

A2.7 Nutritional supplements for metabolic diseases 912

In certain conditions some foods (and toilet preparations) have characteristics of drugs and the Advisory Committee on Borderline Substances (ACBS) advises as to the circumstances in which such substances may be regarded as drugs. Prescriptions issued in accordance with the Committee's advice and endorsed 'ACBS' will normally not be investigated.

> General Practitioners are reminded that the ACBS recommends products on the basis that they may be regarded as drugs for the management of specified conditions. Doctors should satisfy themselves that the products can safely be prescribed, that patients are adequately monitored and that, where necessary, expert hospital supervision is available.

Foods which may be prescribed on FP10, GP10 (Scotland), or when available WP10 (Wales)

Note All the food products listed in this appendix have ACBS approval. The clinical condition for which the product has been approved is included with each entry.

Foods included in this Appendix may contain cariogenic sugars and appropriate oral hygiene measures should be taken.

Note Feeds containing more than 6 g/100 mL protein or 2 g/100 mL fibre should be avoided in children unless recommended by an appropriate specialist or dietician.

Enteral foods and supplements   For most enteral feeds and nutritional supplements, the main source of **carbohydrate** is either maltodextrin or glucose syrup; other carbohydrate sources are listed in the relevant table, below. Feeds containing residual lactose (less than 1 g lactose/100 mL formula) are described as 'clinically lactose-free' or 'lactose-free' by some manufacturers. The presence of lactose (including residual lactose) in feeds is indicated in the relevant table, below. The primary sources of **protein** or **amino acids** are included with each product entry. The **fat** or **oil** content is derived from a variety of sources such as vegetables, soya bean, corn, palm nuts, and seeds; where the fat content is derived from animal or fish sources, this information is included in the relevant table, below. The presence of medium chain triglycerides (MCT) is also noted where the quantity exceeds 30% of the fat content.

Enteral feeds and nutritional supplements can contain varying amounts of **vitamins**, **minerals**, and **trace elements**—the manufacturer's product literature should be consulted for more detailed information. For further information on enteral nutrition, see section 9.4.2. Feeds containing vitamin K may affect the INR in children receiving warfarin; see **interactions**: Appendix 1 (vitamins).

The suitability of food products for patients requiring a vegan, kosher, halal, or other compliant diet should be confirmed with individual manufacturers.

> **Standard ACBS indications:**
> Disease-related malnutrition, intractable malabsorption, pre-operative preparation of malnourished patients, dysphagia, proven inflammatory bowel disease, following total gastrectomy, short-bowel syndrome, bowel fistula
>
> **Paediatric ACBS indications:**
> Disease-related malnutrition, intractable malabsorption, growth failure, pre-operative preparation of malnourished patients, dysphagia, short-bowel syndrome, bowel fistula

A2.1 Enteral feeds (non-disease specific)

A2.1.1 Enteral feeds (non-disease specific): less than 5 g protein/100 mL

For further information on composition of feeds, see p.878

A2.1.1.1 Enteral feeds: 1 kcal/mL and less than 5 g protein/100 mL

Not suitable for use in child under 1 year; not recommended for child 1–6 years unless otherwise stated

Product	Formulation	Energy	Protein	Carbohydrate	Fat	Fibre	Special Characteristics	ACBS Indications	Presentation & Flavour
Fresubin® Original (Fresenius Kabi)	Liquid (sip or tube feed)	420 kJ (100 kcal) **per 100 mL**	3.8 g cows' milk soya	13.8 g (sugars 3.5 g[1])	3.4 g	Nil	Gluten-free Residual lactose Contains fish gelatin Feed in flexible pack contains fish oil and fish gelatin	Standard, p.878	Bottle: 200 mL = £1.66 Black currant, chocolate, mocha, nut, peach, vanilla Flexible pack: 500 mL = £3.21 1000 mL = £6.33 1500 mL = £9.51
Fresubin® Original Fibre (Fresenius Kabi)	Liquid (tube feed)	420 kJ (100 kcal) **per 100 mL**	3.8 g cows' milk soya	13.8 g (sugars 1 g)	3.4 g	2 g	Gluten-free Residual lactose Contains fish oil and fish gelatin	Standard, p.878 except bowel fistula. Not suitable for child under 2 years	Flexible pack: 500 mL = £3.63 1000 mL = £7.24 1500 mL = £10.20
Isosource® Fibre (Nestlé)	Liquid (tube feed)	422 kJ (100 kcal) **per 100 mL**	3.8 g cows' milk	13.6 g	3.4 g	1.4 g	Gluten-free Residual lactose	Standard, p.878 Not suitable for child under 2 years	Flexible pack: 500 mL = £3.39 1000 mL = £6.77
Isosource® Standard (Nestlé)	Liquid (tube feed)	420 kJ (100 kcal) **per 100 mL**	4 g cows' milk	13.6 g	3.3 g	Nil	Gluten-free Residual lactose	Standard, p.878	Flexible pack: 500 mL = £2.98 1000 mL = £5.95
Jevity® (Abbott)	Liquid (tube feed)	441 kJ (106 kcal) **per 100 mL**	4 g caseinates	14.1 g (sugars 470 mg)	3.47 g	1.76 g	Gluten-free Residual lactose	Standard, p.878 except bowel fistula. Not suitable for child under 2 years	Flexible pack: 500 mL = £3.85 1000 mL = £7.23 1500 mL = £10.86
Modulen IBD® (Nestlé)	Standard dilution (20%) of powder (sip or tube feed)	420 kJ (100 kcal) **per 100mL**	3.6 g casein	11 g (sugars 3.98 g)	4.7 g	Nil	Gluten-free Residual lactose	Crohn's disease active phase, and in remission if malnourished	Can: 400 g = £13.60 Unflavoured[2] (8.3-g measuring scoop provided)

Powder provides: protein 18 g, carbohydrate 54 g, fat 23 g, 2070 kJ (500kcal)/100 g

1. Sugar content varies with flavour
2. Flavouring: see *Flavour Mix*, p. 909

Appendix 2: Borderline substances

Appendix 2: Borderline substances

A2.1.1.1 Enteral feeds: 1 kcal/mL and less than 5 g protein/100 mL *(product list continued)*

Not suitable for use in child under 1 year; not recommended for child 1–6 years unless otherwise stated

Product	Formulation	Energy	Protein	Carbohydrate	Fat	Fibre	Special Characteristics	ACBS Indications	Presentation & Flavour
Novasource® GI Control (Nestlé)	Liquid (tube feed)	444 kJ (106 kcal) **per 100 mL**	4.1 g cows' milk	14.4 g (sugars 500 mg)	3.5 g (MCT 40%)	2.2 g	Gluten-free Residual lactose	Standard, p.878	Flexible pack: 500 mL = £4.52
Nutrison® (Nutricia Clinical)	Liquid (tube feed)	420 kJ (100 kcal) **per 100 mL**	4 g cows' milk	12.3 g (sugars 1 g)	3.9 g	Nil	Gluten-free Residual lactose	Standard, p.878	Bottle: 500 mL = £3.65 Flexible pack: 500 mL = £4.05 1000 mL = £7.11 1500 mL = £10.65
Formerly *Nutrison® Standard*									
Nutrison® Multi Fibre (Nutricia Clinical)	Liquid (tube feed)	420 kJ (100 kcal) **per 100 mL**	4 g cows' milk	12.3 g (sugars 1 g)	3.9 g	1.5 g	Gluten-free Residual lactose	Standard, p.878 except for bowel fistula	Bottle: 500 mL = £3.97 Flexible pack: 500 mL = £4.38 1000 mL = £7.92 1500 mL = £11.89
Osmolite® (Abbott)	Liquid (tube feed)	424 kJ (100 kcal) **per 100 mL**	4 g caseinates soy isolate	13.6 g (sugars 630 mg)	3.4 g	Nil	Gluten-free Residual lactose	Standard, p.878	Can: 250 mL = £1.79 Bottle: 500 mL = £3.39 1000 mL = £6.46 1500 mL = £9.69

■ **Soya protein formula** (see also section A2.3.1)

Product	Formulation	Energy	Protein	Carbohydrate	Fat	Fibre	Special Characteristics	ACBS Indications	Presentation & Flavour
Nutrison® Soya (Nutricia Clinical)	Liquid (tube feed)	420 kJ (100 kcal) **per 100 mL**	4 g soy isolate	12.3 g (sugars 1 g)	3.9 g	Nil	Gluten-free Residual lactose Milk protein-free	Standard, p.878; *also* cows' milk and protein and lactose intolerance	Bottle: 500 mL = £4.12 Flexible pack: 1000 mL = £8.24
Nutrison® Soya Multi Fibre (Nutricia Clinical)	Liquid (tube feed)	420 kJ (100 kcal) **per 100 mL**	4 g soy isolate	12.3 g (sugars 700 mg)	3.9 g	1.5 g	Gluten-free Residual lactose Milk protein-free	Standard, p.878 except for bowel fistula; *also* cows' milk protein and lactose intolerance	Flexible pack: 1500 mL = £13.25

Peptide-based formula

Product	Formulation	Energy	Protein	Carbohydrate	Fat	Fibre	Special Characteristics	ACBS Indications	Presentation & Flavour
Peptamen® (Nestlé)	Liquid (sip or tube feed)	420 kJ (100 kcal) per 100 mL	4 g whey peptides	12.7 g (sugars 480 mg[1])	3.7 g (MCT 70%)	Nil	Gluten-free Residual lactose	Short bowel syndrome, intractable malabsorption, proven inflammatory bowel disease, bowel fistula	Cup (vanilla flavour): 200 mL = £2.68, Can (unflavoured[2]): 375 mL = £4.84, Flexible pack: 500 mL = £5.38, 1000 mL = £10.10
Peptisorb® (Nutricia Clinical)	Liquid (tube feed)	425 kJ (100 kcal) per 100 mL	4 g whey protein hydrolysate	17.6 g (sugars 1.7 g)	1.7 g (MCT 47%)	Nil	Gluten-free Residual lactose	Short bowel syndrome, intractable malabsorption, proven inflammatory bowel disease, bowel fistula	Bottle: 500 mL = £5.50, Flexible pack: 500 mL = £6.04, 1000 mL = £10.92
Survimed® OPD (Fresenius Kabi)	Liquid (tube feed)	420 kJ (100 kcal) per 100 mL	4.5 g lactalbumin hydrolysate	15 g (sugars 300 mg)	2.4 g (MCT 54%)	Nil	Gluten-free Residual lactose Contains fish oil and fish gelatin	Standard, p.878; *also* growth failure	Flexible pack: 500 mL = £5.34

1. Sugar content varies with flavour
2. Flavouring: see *Flavour Mix*, p. 909

A2.1.1.2 Enteral feeds: Less than 1 kcal/mL and less than 5 g protein/100 mL

Not suitable for use in child under 1 year; not recommended for child 1–6 years unless otherwise stated

Product	Formulation	Energy	Protein	Carbohydrate	Fat	Fibre	Special Characteristics	ACBS Indications	Presentation & Flavour

Amino acid formula (essential and non-essential amino acids)

Product	Formulation	Energy	Protein	Carbohydrate	Fat	Fibre	Special Characteristics	ACBS Indications	Presentation & Flavour
Elemental 028® Extra (SHS)	Liquid (sip or tube feed)	360 kJ (86 kcal) per 100 mL	2.5 g (protein equivalent)	11 g (sugars 4.7 g)	3.5 g (MCT 35%)	Nil		Short bowel syndrome, intractable malabsorption, proven inflammatory bowel disease, bowel fistula	Carton: 250 mL = £2.88, Grapefruit, orange and pineapple, orange, summer fruits
	Standard dilution (20%) of powder (sip or tube feed)	374 kJ[1] (89 kcal) per 100 mL	2.5 g (protein equivalent)	11.8 g (sugars 1.8 g)	3.5 g (MCT 35%)	Nil			Sachet: 100 g = £5.60, Banana, citrus, orange, unflavoured[2]

Powder provides protein equivalent 12.5 g, carbohydrate 59 g, fat 17.45 g, energy 1871 kJ (443 kcal)/100 g

1. Nutritional values may vary with flavour—consult product literature
2. Flavouring: see *Modjul® Flavour System*, p. 909

Appendix 2: Borderline substances

Appendix 2: Borderline substances

A2.1.2 Enteral feeds (non-disease specific); 5 g (or more) protein/100 mL
For further information on the composition of feeds, see p. 878

A2.1.2.1 Enteral feeds: 1.5 kcal/mL and 5 g (or more) protein/100 mL
Not suitable for use in child under 1 year; not recommended for child 1–6 years unless otherwise stated

Product	Formulation	Energy	Protein	Carbohydrate	Fat	Fibre	Special Characteristics	ACBS Indications	Presentation & Flavour
Clinutren® 1.5 (Nestlé)	Liquid (sip feed)	630 kJ (150 kcal) **per 100 mL**	5.6 g cows' milk	21 g (sugars 5.2 g[1])	5 g	less than 500 mg	Gluten-free Residual lactose	Standard, p. 878 Not suitable for use in child under 3 years	Plastic cup: 4 × 200 mL = £6.59 Apricot, banana, chocolate, coffee, strawberry-raspberry, vanilla
Clinutren® 1.5 Fibre (Nestlé)	Liquid (sip feed)	630 kJ (150 kcal) **per 100 mL**	5.7 g cows' milk	19 g (sugars 6.1 g)	5.9 g	2.6 g	Gluten-free Residual lactose	Standard, p. 878 except bowel fistula Not suitable for use in child under 3 years	Plastic cup: 4 × 200 mL = £6.59 Plum or vanilla
Fresubin® 2250 Complete (Fresenius Kabi) (Formerly Fresubin® Energy Fibre)	Liquid (tube feed)	630 kJ (150 kcal) **per 100mL**	5.6 g cows' milk	18.8 g (sugars 1.5 g)	5.8 g	2 g	Gluten-free Residual lactose Contains fish oil and fish gelatin	Standard, p. 878	Flexible pack: 1500 mL = £11.39
Fresubin® Energy (Fresenius Kabi)	Liquid (sip feed)	630 kJ (150 kcal) **per 100mL**	5.6 g cows' milk	18.8 g (sugars[1])	5.8 g	Nil	Gluten-free[2] Residual lactose Contains fish gelatin	Standard, p. 878	Bottle: 200 mL = £1.66 Banana, black currant, cappuccino, chocolate, lemon, neutral, strawberry, tropical fruits, vanilla Flexible pack: 500 mL = £3.91 1000 mL = £7.70 1500 mL = £10.32
	Liquid (tube feed)	630 kJ (150 kcal) **per 100mL**	5.6 g cows' milk	18.8 g (sugars 1.4 g)	5.8 g	Nil	Gluten-free Residual lactose Contains fish gelatin	Standard, p. 878	
Fresubin® Energy Fibre (Fresenius Kabi)	Liquid (sip feed)	630 kJ (150 kcal) **per 100mL**	5.6 g cows' milk	18.8 g (sugars[1])	5.8 g	2 g	Gluten-free Residual lactose Contains fish gelatin	Standard, p. 878	Bottle: 200 mL = £1.74 Banana, caramel, cherry, chocolate, strawberry, vanilla
	Liquid (tube feed)	630 kJ (150 kcal) **per 100mL**	5.6 g cows' milk	18.8 g (sugars 1.5 g)	5.8 g	2 g	Gluten-free Residual lactose Contains fish oil and fish gelatin	Standard, p. 878	Flexible pack: 500 mL = £4.30 1000 mL = £8.20

1. Sugar content varies with flavour
2. Strawberry flavour may contain traces of wheat starch and egg

Product	Form	Energy	Protein	Carbohydrate	Fat	Fibre	Characteristics	Indication	Price
Fresubin® HP Energy (Fresenius Kabi)	Liquid (tube feed)	630 kJ (150 kcal) per 100 mL	7.5 g cows' milk	17 g (sugars 1 g)	5.8g (MCT 57%)	Nil	Gluten-free, Residual lactose, Contains fish oil and fish gelatin	Standard, p.878; *also* CAPD and haemodialysis	Flexible pack: 500 mL = £3.99, 1000 mL = £8.00
Isosource® Energy (Nestlé)	Liquid (tube feed)	670 kJ (160 kcal) per 100 mL	5.7 g cows' milk	20 g	6.2 g	Nil	Gluten-free, Residual lactose	Standard, p.878	Flexible pack: 500 mL = £3.66, 1000 mL = £7.31
Isosource® Energy Fibre (Nestlé)	Liquid (tube feed)	630 kJ (150 kcal) per 100 mL	4.9 g cows' milk	20.2 g	5.5 g	1.5 g	Gluten-free, Residual lactose	Standard, p.878 except bowel fistula	Flexible pack: 500 mL = £3.96, 1000 mL = £7.93
Jevity® 1.5 kcal (Abbott)	Liquid (tube feed)	640 kJ (152 kcal) per 100 mL	6.38 g caseinates and soy isolate	20.1 g (sugars 1.47 g)	4.9 g	2.2 g	Gluten-free, Residual lactose	Standard, p.878 Not suitable for child under 2 years; not recommended for child 2–10 years	Flexible pack: 500 mL = £4.69, 1000 mL = £8.70, 1500 mL = £13.58
Novasource® GI Forte (Nestlé)	Liquid (tube feed)	631 kJ (150 kcal) per 100 mL	6 g cows' milk	18.3 g (sugars 1.8 g)	5.9 g	2.2 g	Gluten-free, Residual lactose	Standard, p.878	Flexible pack: 500 mL = £4.49, 1000 mL = £8.98
Nutrison® Energy (Nutricia Clinical)	Liquid (tube feed)	630 kJ (150 kcal) per 100 mL	6 g cows' milk	18.5 g (sugars 1.5 g)	5.8g	Nil	Gluten-free, Residual lactose	Standard, p.878	Bottle: 500 mL = £4.25, Flexible pack: 500 mL = £4.72, 1000 mL = £8.55, 1500 mL = £12.80
Nutrison® Energy Multi Fibre (Nutricia Clinical)	Liquid (tube feed)	630 kJ (150 kcal) per 100 mL	6 g cows' milk	18.5 g (sugars 1.5 g)	5.8 g	1.5 g	Gluten-free, Residual lactose	Standard, p.878	Bottle: 500 mL = £4.76, Flexible pack: 500 mL = £5.23, 1000 mL = £9.49, 1500 mL = £15.20
Osmolite® 1.5 kcal (Abbott) Formerly *Ensure® Plus* (Ready to Hang)	Liquid (tube feed)	632 kJ (150 kcal) per 100 mL	6.25 g cows' milk soya protein isolate	20 g (sugars 4.9 g)	5 g	Nil	Gluten-free, Residual lactose	Standard, p.878	Flexible pack: 500mL = £4.15, 1000mL = £8.10, 1500mL = £12.13

Appendix 2: Borderline substances

Appendix 2: Borderline substances

A2.1.2.2 Enteral feeds: Less than 1.5 kcal/mL and 5 g (or more) protein/100 mL

Not suitable for use in child under 1 year; not recommended for child 1–6 years unless otherwise stated

Product	Formulation	Energy	Protein	Carbohydrate	Fat	Fibre	Special Characteristics	ACBS Indications	Presentation & Flavour
Fresubin® 1000 Complete (Fresenius Kabi)	Liquid (tube feed)	420 kJ (100 kcal) **per 100 mL**	5.5 g cows' milk	12.5 g (sugars 1.1 g)	3.1 g	2 g	Gluten-free Residual lactose Contains fish oil	Standard, p. 878	Flexible pack: 1000 mL = £8.20
Fresubin® 1200 Complete (Fresenius Kabi)	Liquid (tube feed)	500 kJ (120 kcal) **per 100 mL**	6 g cows' milk	15 g (sugars 1.22 g)	4.1 g	2 g	Gluten-free Residual lactose Contains fish oil	Standard, p. 878	Flexible pack: 1000 mL = £10.61
Jevity® Plus (Abbott)	Liquid (tube feed)	504 kJ (120 kcal) **per 100 mL**	5.5 g caseinates soy isolates	15.1 g (sugars 890 mg)	3.93 g	2.2 g	Gluten-free Residual lactose	Standard, p. 878 Not suitable for child under 2 years; not recommended for child 2–10 years	Flexible pack: 500 mL = £4.24 1000 mL = £9.77 1500 mL = £11.57
Jevity® Promote (Abbott)	Liquid (tube feed)	427 kJ (101 kcal) **per 100 mL**	5.55 g caseinates soy isolates	12 g (sugars 670 mg)	3.32 g	1.7 g	Gluten-free Residual lactose	Standard, p. 878 Not suitable for child under 2 years; not recommended for child 2–10 years	Flexible pack: 1000 mL = £8.49
Nutrison® MCT (Nutricia Clinical)	Liquid (tube feed)	420 kJ (100 kcal) **per 100 mL**	5 g cows' milk	12.6 g (sugars 1 g)	3.3 g (MCT 61%)	Nil	Gluten-free Residual lactose	Standard, p. 878	Flexible pack: 1000 mL = £7.73
Nutrison® Protein Plus (Nutricia Clinical)	Liquid (tube feed)	525 kJ (125 kcal) **per 100 mL**	6.3 g cows' milk	14.2 g (sugars 1.1 g)	4.9 g	Nil	Gluten-free Residual lactose	Standard, p. 878	Flexible pack: 1000 mL = £7.95
Nutrison® Protein Plus Multi Fibre (Nutricia Clinical)	Liquid (tube feed)	525 kJ (125 kcal) **per 100 mL**	6.3 g cow's milk	14.1 g (sugars 1.1 g)	4.9 g	1.5 g	Gluten-free Residual lactose	Disease related malnutrition	Flexible pack: 1000 mL = £8.85
Nutrison® 1000 Complete Multi Fibre (Nutricia Clinical)	Liquid (tube feed)	420 kJ (100 kcal) **per 100 mL**	5.5 g cows' milk	11.3 g (sugars 700 mg)	3.7 g	2 g	Gluten-free Residual lactose	Disease related malnutrition in patients with low energy and/or low fluid requirements	Flexible pack: 1000 mL = £8.59
Nutrison® 1200 Complete Multi Fibre (Nutricia Clinical)	Liquid (tube feed)	505 kJ (120 kcal) **per 100 mL**	5.5 g cows' milk	15 g (sugars 1.2 g)	4.3 g	2 g	Gluten-free Residual lactose	Standard, p. 878 except bowel fistula	Bottle: 500 mL = £4.55 Flexible pack: 1000 mL = £9.10 1500 mL = £13.66

Product	Formulation	Energy	Protein	Carbohydrate	Fat	Fibre	Special Characteristics	ACBS Indications	Presentation & Flavour
Osmolite® Plus (Abbott)	Liquid (tube feed)	508 kJ (121 kcal) **per 100 mL**	5.55 g caseinates	15.8 g (sugars 730 mg)	3.93 g	Nil	Gluten-free Residual lactose	Standard, p.878 Not recommended for child 1–10 years	Flexible pack: 500 mL = £3.96 1000 mL = £7.64 1500 mL = £11.44
Peptamen® HN (Nestlé)	Liquid (tube feed)	556 kJ (133 kcal) **per 100 mL**	6.6 g whey protein hydrolysates	15.6 g (sugars 1.4 g)	4.9 g (MCT 70%)	Nil	Gluten-free Residual lactose Hydrolysed with pork trypsin	Short bowel syndrome, intractable malabsorption, proven inflammatory bowel disease, bowel fistula Not suitable for child under 3 years	Flexible pack: 500 mL = £5.97
Perative® (Abbott)	Liquid (sip or tube feed)	552 kJ (131 kcal) **per 100 mL**	6.7 g caseinate whey protein hydrolysates	17.7 g (sugars 660 mg)	3.7 g (MCT 42%)	Nil	Gluten-free Residual lactose	Standard, p.878 Not suitable for child under 5 years	Flexible pack: 500 mL = £5.52 1000 mL = £11.04

A2.1.2.3 Enteral feeds: More than 1.5 kcal/mL and 5 g (or more) protein/100 mL

Not suitable for use in child under 1 year; not recommended for child 1–6 years unless otherwise stated

Product	Formulation	Energy	Protein	Carbohydrate	Fat	Fibre	Special Characteristics	ACBS Indications	Presentation & Flavour
Ensure® Twocal (Abbott)	Liquid (sip or tube feed)	838 kJ (200 kcal) **per 100 mL**	8.4 g cows' milk	21 g (sugars 4.5 g)	8.9 g	1 g	Gluten-free Residual lactose	Standard, p.878; *also* haemodialysis and CAPD	Carton: 200 mL = £2.03 Banana, neutral, strawberry, vanilla

A2.1.3 Enteral feeds (non-disease specific): Child under 12 years

For further information on composition of feeds, see p.878

A2.1.3.1 Enteral feeds, Child: Less than 1 kcal/mL and less than 4 g protein/100 mL

Product	Formulation	Energy	Protein	Carbohydrate	Fat	Fibre	Special Characteristics	ACBS Indications	Presentation & Flavour
Nutrini® Low Energy Multi Fibre (Nutricia Clinical)	Liquid (tube feed)	315 kJ (75 kcal) **per 100 mL**	2.1 g whey protein and caseinate	9.3 g (sugars 600 mg)	3.3 g	800 mg	Gluten-free Residual lactose Contains fish oil	Paediatric, p.878 except bowel fistula, in child 1–6 years, body-weight 8–20 kg	Bottle: 200 mL = £2.05 Flexible pack: 500 mL = £5.18
Nutriprem® 1 (Cow & Gate)	Liquid (sip feed)	335 kJ (80 kcal) **per 100 mL**	2.5 g whey protein and casein	7.6 g (lactose 6.3 g)	4.4 g	800 mg	Contains soya, fish oil and egg lipid	Low birth-weight formula	Bottle: 60 mL Hospital supply only

Appendix 2: Borderline substances

Appendix 2: Borderline substances

A2.1.3.1 Enteral feeds, Child: Less than 1 kcal/mL and less than 4 g protein/100 mL *(product list continued)*

Product	Formulation	Energy	Protein	Carbohydrate	Fat	Fibre	Special Characteristics	ACBS Indications	Presentation & Flavour
Nutriprem® 2 (Cow & Gate)	Liquid (sip feed)	310 kJ (75 kcal) **per 100 mL**	2 g whey protein and casein	7.4 g (lactose 5.8 g)	4.1 g	800 mg	Contains soya, fish oil and egg lipid	Catch-up growth in pre-term infants (less than 35 weeks at birth) and small for gestational-age infants up to 6 months corrected age	Carton: 200 mL = £1.54 (Bottle: 100 mL Hospital supply only) Can: 900 g = £10.28 (5.1-g measuring scoop provided)
	Standard dilution (15.4%) of powder (sip feed)	315 kJ (75 kcal) **per 100 mL**	2 g whey protein and casein	7.4 g (lactose 5.8 g)	4.1 g (including MCT oil)	800 mg			

Powder provides: protein 13 g, carbohydrate 48.3 g, fat 26.7 g, fibre 5.2 g, energy 2030 kJ (485 kcal)/100 g

SMA® High Energy (SMA Nutrition)	Liquid (sip feed)	382 kJ (91 kcal) **per 100 mL**	2 g whey protein and casein	9.8 g lactose	4.9 g	Nil	Contains lactose	Disease related malnutrition and malabsorption, and growth failure in child from birth to 18 months	Carton: 250 mL = £2.07

▪ Amino acid formula (essential and non-essential amino acids)

Emsogen® (SHS)	Standard dilution (20%) of powder (sip or tube feed)	368 kJ[1] (88 kcal) **per 100 mL**	2.5 g protein equivalent (essential and non-essential amino acids)	12 g (sugars 1.6 g)	3.3 g[2] (MCT 83%)	Nil	Lactose-free	Short-bowel syndrome, intractable malabsorption, proven inflammatory bowel disease, bowel fistula Not suitable for child under 1 year or as sole source of nutrition in child 1–5 years	Sachet: 100 g = £5.54 Orange Unflavoured[3]

Powder provides: protein equivalent 12.5 g, carbohydrate 60 g, fat 16.4 g, energy 1839 kJ (438 kcal)/100 g

1. Nutritional values may vary with flavour—consult product literature
2. Additional source of alpha linolenic acid needed if used as sole source of nutrition
3. Flavouring: see *Modjul® Flavour System*, p. 909

A2.1.3.2 Enteral feeds, Child: 1 kcal/mL and less than 4 g protein/100 mL

Not suitable for child under 1 year unless otherwise stated

Product	Formulation	Energy	Protein	Carbohydrate	Fat	Fibre	Special Characteristics	ACBS Indications	Presentation & Flavour
Clinutren® Junior (Nestlé)	Standard dilution (22%) of powder (sip or tube feed)	420 kJ (100 kcal) **per 100 mL**	2.97 g whey protein and caseinate	13.3 g	3.9 g	Nil	Gluten-free Residual lactose	Standard, p.878; *also* growth failure in child 1–10 years	Can: 400 g = £9.72 Vanilla (7.85-g measuring scoop provided)

Powder provides: protein 13.9 g, carbohydrate 62.2 g, fat 18.3 g, energy 1950 kJ (467 kcal)/100 g

Product	Form	Energy	Protein	Carbohydrate	Fat	Sodium	Characteristics	Use	Presentation
Frebini® Original (Fresenius Kabi)	Liquid (tube feed)	420 kJ (100 kcal) **per 100 mL**	2.5 g cows' milk	12.5 g (sugars 700 mg)	4.4 g	Nil	Gluten-free Residual lactose Contains fish oils and fish gelatin	Standard, p.878; *also* growth failure in child 1–10 years, body-weight 8–30 kg	Flexible pack: 500 mL = £4.73
Frebini® Original Fibre (Fresenius Kabi)	Liquid (tube feed)	420 kJ (100 kcal) **per 100 mL**	2.5 g cows' milk	12.5 g (sugars 700 mg)	4.4 g	750 mg	Gluten-free Residual lactose Contains fish oils and fish gelatin	Standard, p.878; *also* growth failure in child 1–10 years, body-weight 8–30 kg	Flexible pack: 500 mL = £5.25
Infatrini® (Nutricia Clinical)	Liquid (sip or tube feed)	415 kJ (100 kcal) **per 100 mL**	2.6 g cows' milk	10.3 g (lactose 5.2 g)	5.4 g	800 mg	Gluten-free Contains fish oil	Failure to thrive, disease-related malnutrition and malabsorption, in child from birth up to body-weight 8 kg	Bottle: 100 mL = £1.05 200 mL = £2.01 500 mL = £5.25
Nutrini® (Nutricia Clinical)	Liquid (tube feed)	420 kJ (100 kcal) **per 100 mL**	2.8 g cows' milk	12.3 g (sugars 1 g)	4.4 g	Nil	Gluten-free Residual lactose	Standard, p.878; *also* growth failure in child 1–6 years, body-weight 8–20 kg	Bottle: 200 mL = £2.11 Flexible pack: 500 mL = £5.28
Nutrini® Multi Fibre (Nutricia Clinical)	Liquid (tube feed)	420 kJ (100 kcal) **per 100 mL**	2.8 g whey protein and caseinate	12.3 g (sugars 800 mg)	4.4 g	800 mg	Gluten-free Residual lactose Contains fish oil	Standard, p.878; *also* growth failure in child 1–6 years, body-weight 8–20 kg	Bottle: 200 mL = £2.35 Flexible pack: 500 mL = £5.87
Paediasure® (Abbott)	Liquid (sip or tube feed)	422 kJ (100 kcal)[1] **per 100 mL**	2.8 g cows' milk	11.2 g (sugars 3.92 g)	4.98 g	Nil	Gluten-free Residual lactose	Paediatric, p.878 in child 1–10 years, body-weight 8–30 kg	Can: 250 mL = £2.54 Vanilla Carton: 200 mL = £2.04 Banana, chocolate, strawberry, vanilla (bottle)[1] Flexible pack: 500 mL = £5.09 Vanilla
Paediasure® Fibre (Abbott)	Liquid (sip or tube feed)	420 kJ (100 kcal) **per 100 mL**	2.8 g caseinates and whey protein	10.9 g (sugars 3.84 g)	4.98 g	730 mg	Gluten-free Residual lactose	Paediatric, p.878 in child 1–10 years, body-weight 8–30 kg	Carton: 200 mL = £2.19 Banana, strawberry, vanilla Flexible pack: 500 mL = £5.52 Vanilla
Tentrini® (Nutricia Clinical)	Liquid (tube feed)	420 kJ (100 kcal) **per 100 mL**	3.3 g whey protein and caseinate	12.3 g (sugars 800 mg)	4.2 g	Nil	Gluten-free Residual lactose Contains fish oil	Standard, p.878; *also* growth failure in child 7–12 years, body-weight 21–45 kg	Bottle or Flexible pack: 500 mL = £4.66

1. Nutritional values may vary with flavour—consult product literature

Appendix 2: Borderline substances

Appendix 2: Borderline substances

A2.1.3.2 Enteral feeds, Child: 1 kcal/mL and less than 4 g protein/100 mL *(product list continued)*

Not suitable for child under 1 year unless otherwise stated

Product	Formulation	Energy	Protein	Carbohydrate	Fat	Fibre	Special Characteristics	ACBS Indications	Presentation & Flavour
Tentrini® Multi Fibre (Nutricia Clinical)	Liquid (tube feed)	420 kJ (100 kcal) per 100 mL	3.3 g whey protein and caseinate	12.3 g (sugars 800 mg)	4.2 g	1.1 g	Gluten-free Residual lactose Contains fish oil	Standard, p. 878 except bowel fistula; *also* growth failure in child 7–12 years body-weight 21–45 kg	Bottle or Flexible pack: 500 mL = £5.12
Nutrini® Peptisorb (Nutricia Clinical) Formerly *Nutrini® Pepti*	Liquid (tube feed)	420 kJ (100 kcal) per 100 mL	2.8 g whey protein hydrolysate	13.7 g (sugars 800 mg)	3.9 g (MCT 46%)	Nil	Gluten-free Residual lactose	Standard, p. 878; *also* growth failure in child 1–6 years, body-weight 8–20 kg	Flexible pack: 500 mL = £8.15
Peptamen® Junior (Nestlé)	Liquid (tube feed)	420 kJ (100 kcal) per 100 mL	3 g whey protein hydrolysate	13.2 g	4 g (MCT 60%)	Nil	Gluten-free Residual lactose Hydrolysed with pork trypsin	Short bowel syndrome, intractable malabsorption, proven inflammatory bowel disease, bowel fistula, in child 1–10 years	Flexible pack: 500 mL = £5.54
	Standard dilution (22% of powder) (sip or tube feed)	420 kJ (100 kcal) per 100 mL	3 g whey protein hydrolysate	13.8 g	3.85 g (MCT 60%)	Nil	Gluten-free Residual lactose Hydrolysed with bacterial trypsin		Can: 400 g = £14.52 Vanilla (7.86-g measuring scoop provided)

Powder provides: protein 13.7 g, carbohydrate 62.9 g, fat 17.5 g, energy 1910 kJ (457 kcal)/100 g

■ **Hydrolysate Formula** See also Infant Formula (Hydrolysate), section 2.3.1

A2.1.3.3 Enteral feeds, Child: More than 1 kcal/mL and less than 4 g protein/100 mL

Not suitable for child under 1 year unless otherwise stated

Product	Formulation	Energy	Protein	Carbohydrate	Fat	Fibre	Special Characteristics	ACBS Indications	Presentation & Flavour
Isosource® Junior (Nestlé)	Liquid (tube feed)	512 kJ (122 kcal) per 100 mL	2.7 g cows' milk	17 g	4.7 g	Nil	Gluten-free Residual lactose	Standard, p. 878; *also* growth failure in child 1–6 years, body-weight 8–20 kg	Flexible pack: 500 mL = £4.84
Fortini® (Nutricia Clinical)	Liquid (sip feed)	630 kJ (150 kcal) per 100 mL	3.4 g cows' milk	18.8 g (sugars 7.4 g)	6.8 g	Nil	Gluten-free Residual lactose	Disease-related malnutrition and growth failure in child 1–6 years, body-weight 8–20 kg	Bottle: 200 mL = £2.52 Strawberry, vanilla
Fortini® Multifibre (Nutricia Clinical)	Liquid (sip feed)	630 kJ (150 kcal) per 100 mL	3.4 g cows' milk	18.8 g (sugars 7.4 g)	6.8 g	1.5 g	Gluten-free Residual lactose	Disease-related malnutrition and growth failure in child 1–6 years, body-weight 8–20 kg	Bottle: 200 mL = £2.65 Banana, chocolate, strawberry, vanilla

Product	Formulation	Energy	Protein	Carbohydrate	Fat	Fibre	Special Characteristics	ACBS Indications	Presentation & Flavour
Frebini® Energy Drink (Fresenius Kabi)	Liquid (sip feed)	630 kJ (150 kcal) **per 100 mL**	3.8 g cows' milk	18.7 g (sugars 4.5 g)	6.7 g	Nil	Gluten-free Residual lactose	Disease-related malnutrition and growth failure in child 1–10 years, body-weight 8–30 kg	Bottle: 200 mL = £2.25 Banana, strawberry
Frebini® Energy (Fresenius Kabi)	Liquid (tube feed)	630 kJ (150 kcal) **per 100 mL**	3.75 g cows' milk	18.75 g (sugars 830 mg)	6.7 g	Nil	Gluten-free Residual lactose Contains fish oil and fish gelatin	Standard, p.878; *also* growth failure in child 1–10 years, body-weight 8–30 kg	Flexible pack: 500 mL = £5.93
Frebini® Energy Fibre Drink (Fresenius Kabi)	Liquid (sip feed)	630 kJ (150 kcal) **per 100 mL**	3.8 g cows' milk	18.75 g (sugars 4.5 g[1])	6.7 g	1.1 g	Gluten-free Residual lactose	Disease-related malnutrition and growth failure in child 1–10 years, body-weight 8–30 kg	Bottle: 200 mL = £2.30 Chocolate, vanilla
Frebini® Energy Fibre (Fresenius Kabi)	Liquid (tube feed)	630 kJ (150 kcal) **per 100 mL**	3.75 g cows' milk	18.75 g (sugars 830 mg)	6.7 g	1.13 g	Gluten-free Residual lactose Contains fish oils and fish gelatin	Standard, p.878; *also* growth failure in child 1–10 years, body-weight 8–30 kg	Flexible pack: 500 mL = £6.34
Resource® Junior (Nestlé)	Liquid (sip feed)	630 kJ (150 kcal)[2] **per 100 mL**	3 g cows' milk	20.6 g (sugars 4.9 g)	6.2 g	Nil	Gluten-free Residual lactose	Standard, p.878 in child 1–10 years	Carton: 200 mL = £1.69 Chocolate, strawberry, vanilla

1. Sugar content varies with flavour

2. Nutritional values may vary with flavour—consult product literature

A2.1.3.4 Enteral feeds, Child: 1.5 kcal/mL and more than 4 g protein/100 mL

Not suitable for child under 1 year unless otherwise stated

Product	Formulation	Energy	Protein	Carbohydrate	Fat	Fibre	Special Characteristics	ACBS Indications	Presentation & Flavour
Nutrini® Energy (Nutricia Clinical)	Liquid (tube feed)	630 kJ (150 kcal) **per 100 mL**	4.1 g caseinate whey protein	18.5 g (sugars 1.1 g)	6.7 g	Nil	Gluten-free Residual lactose Contains fish oil	Standard, p.878; *also* growth failure in child 1–6 years, body-weight 8–20 kg	Bottle: 200 mL = £2.59 Flexible pack: 500 mL £6.62
Nutrini® Energy Multi Fibre (Nutricia Clinical)	Liquid (tube feed)	630 kJ (150 kcal) **per 100 mL**	4.1 g caseinate whey protein	18.5 g (sugars 1.1 g)	6.7 g	800 mg	Gluten-free Residual lactose Contains fish oil	Paediatric, p.878 except bowel fistula; *also* total gastrectomy, in child 1–6 years, body-weight 8–20 kg	Bottle: 200 mL = £2.74 Flexible pack: 500 mL £6.82
Paediasure® Plus (Abbott)	Liquid (sip or tube feed)	632 kJ (151 kcal) **per 100 mL**	4.2 g caseinates whey protein	16.7 g[1]	7.47 g	Nil	Gluten-free Residual lactose	Paediatric, p.878 in child 1–10 years, body-weight 8–30 kg	Carton: 200 mL = £2.43 Banana, strawberry, vanilla Flexible pack: 500 mL = £6.23 Vanilla

1. Sugar content varies with presentation

Appendix 2: Borderline substances

Appendix 2: Borderline substances

A2.1.3.4 Enteral feeds, Child: 1.5 kcal/mL and more than 4 g protein/100 mL *(product list continued)*

Not suitable for child under 1 year unless otherwise stated

Product	Formulation	Energy	Protein	Carbohydrate	Fat	Fibre	Special Characteristics	ACBS Indications	Presentation & Flavour
Paediasure® Plus Fibre (Abbott)	Liquid (sip or tube feed)	626 kJ (150 kcal) **per 100 mL**	4.2 g caseinates whey protein	16.4 g¹	7.47 g	1.1 g	Gluten-free Residual lactose	Paediatric, p.878 in child 1–10 years, body-weight 8–30 kg	Carton: 200 mL = £2.64 Vanilla; Flexible pack: 500 mL = £6.63 Vanilla
Tentrini® Energy (Nutricia Clinical)	Liquid (tube feed)	630 kJ (150 kcal) **per 100 mL**	4.9 g whey protein and caseinate	18.5 g (sugars 1.1 g)	6.3 g	Nil	Gluten-free Residual lactose Contains fish oil	Standard, p. 878; *also growth failure, in child 7–12 years, body-weight 21–45 kg*	Bottle or Flexible pack: 500 mL = £5.76
Tentrini® Energy Multi Fibre (Nutricia Clinical)	Liquid (tube feed)	630 kJ (150 kcal) **per 100 mL**	4.9 g whey protein and caseinate	18.5 g (sugars 1.1 g)	6.3 g	1.1 g	Gluten-free Residual lactose Contains fish oil	Paediatric, p. 878; *also proven inflammatory bowel disease, in child 7–12 years, body-weight 21–45 kg*	Bottle or Flexible pack: 500 mL = £6.35

1. Sugar content varies with presentation

A2.2 Nutritional supplements (non-disease specific)

A2.2.1 Nutritional supplements: less than 5g protein/100mL

For further information on composition of feeds, see p.878

A2.2.1.1 Nutritional supplements: 1kcal/mL and less than 5g protein/100mL

Not suitable for use in child under 1 year; use with caution in child 1–5 years unless otherwise stated

Product	Formulation	Energy	Protein	Carbohydrate	Fat	Fibre	Special Characteristics	ACBS Indications	Presentation & Flavour
Enrich® (Abbott)	Liquid (sip or tube feed)	431 kJ (103 kcal) **per 100 mL**	3.76 g caseinates soy isolate	14 g (sugars 4.96 g)	3.52 g	1.36 g	Gluten-free Residual lactose	Standard, p.878 except bowel fistula	Can: 250 mL = £2.24 Vanilla
Ensure® (Abbott)	Liquid (sip or tube feed)	423 kJ (100 kcal)¹ **per 100 mL**	4 g caseinates soy isolate	13.6 g (sugars 3.93 g)	3.36 g	Nil	Gluten-free Residual lactose	Standard, p.878	Can: 250 mL £1.96 Chocolate, vanilla

1. Nutritional values may vary with flavour—consult product literature

A2.2.1.2 Nutritional supplements: More than 1kcal/mL and less than 5g protein/100mL

Not suitable for use in child under 1 year; use with caution in child 1–5 years unless otherwise stated

Product	Formulation	Energy	Protein	Carbohydrate	Fat	Fibre	Special Characteristics	ACBS Indications	Presentation & Flavour
Clinutren® Fruit (Nestlé)	Liquid (sip feed)	520 kJ (125 kcal) **per 100 mL**	4 g whey protein hydrolysate	27 g (sugars 9.5 g[1])	less than 200 mg	less than 200 mg[2]	Gluten-free Residual lactose Non-milk taste	Standard, p. 878 Not suitable for child under 3 years	Carton: 4×200 mL = £6.63 Apple, grapefruit, orange, pear-cherry, raspberry-black currant
Ensure® Plus Juce (Abbott)	Liquid (sip feed)	638 kJ (150kcal) **per 100 mL**	4.8 g whey protein isolate	32.7 g (sugars 9.4 g[1])	Nil	Nil	Gluten-free Residual lactose Non-milk taste	Standard, p. 878	Bottle: 220 mL = £1.75 Apple, fruit punch, grapefruit, lemon-lime, orange, peach, pineapple, strawberry
Fortijuce® (Nutricia Clinical)	Liquid (sip feed)	640 kJ (150 kcal) **per 100 mL**	4.0 g cows' milk	33.5 g (sugars 13.1 g[1])	Nil	Nil	Gluten-free Residual lactose Non-milk taste	Standard, p. 878 Not suitable for child under 3 years	Bottle: 200 mL = £1.80 Starter pack: 4×200 mL = £7.00 Apple, black currant, forest fruits, lemon, orange, strawberry, tropical Starter pack (mixed) 4×200 mL = £7.00
Provide® Xtra Juice Drink (Fresenius Kabi)	Liquid (sip feed)	525 kJ (125 kcal) **per 100 mL**	3.75 g pea and soya protein hydrolysates	27.5 g[1]	Nil	Nil[2]	Gluten-free Lactose-free Non-milk taste Sweet-flavoured products contain fish gelatin	Standard, p. 878	Carton: 200 mL = £1.63 Apple, black currant, carrot-apple, cherry, citrus-cola, lemon-lime, melon, orange-pineapple, tomato
Resource® Dessert Energy (Nestlé)	Semi-solid	671 kJ (160 kcal) **per 100 g**	4.8 g cows' milk	21.2 g (sugars 9.9 g[1])	6.2 g	Nil	Gluten-free Contains lactose	Standard, p. 878; *also* CAPD, haemodialysis	Cup: 125 g = £1.35 Caramel, chocolate, vanilla
Resource® Fruit Flavour Drink (Nestlé)	Liquid (sip feed)	638 kJ (150 kcal) **per 100 mL**	4.0 g cows' milk	33.5 g (sugars 8 g[1])	Nil	Nil	Gluten-free Residual lactose Non-milk taste	Standard, p. 878 Not suitable for child under 3 years	Carton: 200 mL = £1.53 Apple, orange, pineapple

1. Sugar content varies with flavour
2. Fibre content varies with flavour

Appendix 2: Borderline substances

Appendix 2: Borderline substances

A2.2.2 Nutritional supplements: 5g (or more) protein/100mL
For further information on composition of feeds, see p.878

A2.2.2.1 Nutritional supplements: 1.5 kcal/mL and 5 g (or more) protein/100 mL
Not suitable for use in child under 1 year; use with caution in child 1–5 years unless otherwise stated

Product	Formulation	Energy	Protein	Carbohydrate	Fat	Fibre	Special Characteristics	ACBS Indications	Presentation & Flavour
Ensure® Plus Fibre (Abbott)	Liquid (sip or tube feed)	642 kJ (153 kcal)[1] **per 100 mL**	6.25 g cows' milk soya protein isolate	20.2 g (sugars 5.5 g)	4.92 g	2.5 g	Gluten-free Residual lactose	Standard, p.878; *also* CAPD, haemodialysis	Bottle: 200 mL = £1.74 Banana, chocolate, fruits of the forest, raspberry, strawberry, vanilla
Ensure® Plus Milkshake style (Abbott)	Liquid (sip or tube feed)	632 kJ (150 kcal)[1] **per 100 mL**	6.25 g cows' milk soya protein isolate	20.2 g (sugars 5.6 g)	4.92 g	Nil	Gluten-free Residual lactose	Standard, p.878; *also* CAPD, haemodialysis	Can: 250 mL = £2.22 (vanilla) 250 mL = £2.16 (chicken or mushroom) Bottle: 220 mL = £1.73 Banana, black currant, caramel, chocolate, coffee, fruits of the forest, orange, peach, raspberry, strawberry, vanilla, neutral
Ensure® Plus Yoghurt style (Abbott)	Liquid (sip feed)	632 kJ (150 kcal)[1] **per 100 mL**	6.25 g cows' milk	20.2 g (sugars 11.7 g)	4.92 g	Nil	Gluten-free Residual lactose	Standard, p.878; *also* CAPD, haemodialysis	Bottle: 220 mL = £1.73 Orange, peach, pineapple, strawberry
Ensure® Plus Commence (Abbott)	Starter pack (5–10 day's supply), contains: *Ensure® Plus Milkshake Style* (various flavours), 1 pack (10 × 220-mL) = £18.00.								
Enmix® Plus Commence (Abbott)	Starter pack (5–10 day's supply), contains: *Ensure® Plus* (Milkshake, Yoghurt, & Juce style; various flavours), 1 pack (10 × 220-mL) = £17.80.								
Fortisip® Bottle (Nutricia Clinical)	Liquid (sip feed)	630 kJ (150 kcal) **per 100 mL**	6 g cows' milk	18.4 g[2]	5.8 g	Nil	Gluten-free Residual lactose	Standard, p.878 Not suitable for child under 3 years	Bottle: 200 mL = £1.80 Banana, chocolate, neutral, orange, strawberry, toffee, tropical fruits, vanilla
Fortisip® Multi Fibre (Nutricia Clinical)	Liquid (sip feed)	630 kJ (150 kcal) **per 100 mL**	6 g cows' milk	18.4 g (sugars 7.0 g)	5.8 g	2.3 g	Gluten-free Residual lactose	Standard, p.878 Not suitable for child under 3 years	Bottle: 200 mL = £1.85 Banana, chocolate, orange, strawberry, tomato, vanilla

1. Minor nutritional variations between flavours—consult product literature
2. Sugar content varies with flavour

Fortisip® Yoghurt Style (Nutricia Clinical)	Liquid (sip feed)	630 kJ (150 kcal) per 100 mL	6 g cows' milk	18.7 g (sugars 10.8 g)	5.8 g	200 mg	Gluten-free Contains lactose	Standard, p. 878 Not suitable for child under 3 years	Bottle: 200 mL = £1.80 Peach-orange, raspberry, vanilla-lemon
Fortisip® Range (Nutricia Clinical)	Starter pack contains 4 × Fortisip® Bottle, 4 × Fortijuce®, 2 × Fortisip® Yogurt Style, 1 pack (10 × 200 mL) = £17.46.								
Fresubin® Protein Energy Drink (Fresenius Kabi)	Liquid (sip feed)	630 kJ (150 kcal) per 100 mL	10 g cows' milk	12.4 g (sugars 6.4 g[1])	6.7 g	Nil[2]	Gluten-free Residual lactose Contains fish gelatin	Standard, p. 878; also CAPD, haemodialysis	Bottle: 200 mL = £1.69 Cappuccino, chocolate, strawberry, tropical fruits, vanilla

1. Sugar content varies with flavour
2. Fibre content varies with flavour

A2.2.2.2 Nutritional supplements: Less than 1.5kcal/mL and 5g (or more) protein/100mL

Not suitable for use in child under 1 year; use with caution in child 1–5 years unless otherwise stated

Product	Formulation	Energy	Protein	Carbohydrate	Fat	Fibre	Special Characteristics	ACBS Indications	Presentation & Flavour
Clinutren® Dessert (Nestlé)	Semi-solid	520 kJ (125 kcal) per 100 g	9.5 g cows' milk	15.5 g (sugars 14 g[1])	2.6 g	500 mg[2]	Gluten-free Contains lactose	Standard, p. 878; also CAPD, haemodialysis Not suitable for child under 3 years	Pot: 4 × 125 g = £5.40 Caramel, chocolate, peach, vanilla
Ensure® Plus Crème (Abbott)	Semi-solid	574 kJ (137 kcal)[3] per 100 g	5.68 g milk protein isolate soy protein isolate	18.4 g (sugars 12.4 g)	4.47 g	Nil	Gluten-free Residual lactose Contains soya	Standard, p. 878; also CAPD, haemodialysis Not suitable for child under 3 years	Pot: 125 g = £1.63 Banana, chocolate, neutral, vanilla
Fortimel® Regular (Nutricia Clinical) (Formerly Fortimel®)	Liquid (sip feed)	420 kJ (100 kcal) per 100 mL	10 g cows' milk	10.3 g (sugars 8.1 g[1])	2.1 g	Nil	Gluten-free Contains lactose	Standard, p. 878 Not suitable for child under 3 years	Bottle: 200 mL = £1.52 Chocolate, forest fruits, strawberry, vanilla
Fortisip® Fruit Dessert (Nutricia Clinical)	Semi-Solid	560 kJ (133 kcal) per 100 g	7 g whey isolate	16.7 g (sugars 11.3 g)	4 g	2.6 g	Residual lactose	Standard, p. 878 except bowel fistula; also CAPD, haemodialysis Not suitable for child under 3 years	Pot: 3 × 150 g = £6.09 Apple
Resource® Protein (Nestlé)	Liquid (sip feed)	530 kJ (125 kcal) per 100 mL	9.4 g cows' milk	14 g (sugars 4.5 g[4])	3.5 g	Nil	Gluten-free Contains lactose	Standard, p. 878 Not suitable for child under 3 years	Bottle: 200 mL = £1.33 Apricot, chocolate, forest fruits, strawberry, vanilla

1. Sugar content varies with flavour
2. Fibre content varies with flavour
3. Minor nutritional variations between flavours—consult product literature
4. Nutritional values may vary with flavour—consult product literature

Appendix 2: Borderline substances

Appendix 2: Borderline substances

A2.2.3 Nutritional supplements: More than 1.5kcal/mL and 5g (or more) protein/100mL

Not suitable for use in child under 1 year; use with caution in child 1–5 years unless otherwise stated

Product	Formulation	Energy	Protein	Carbohydrate	Fat	Fibre	Special Characteristics	ACBS Indications	Presentation & Flavour
Complan® Shake (Complan Foods)	Powder	1057 kJ[1] (251 kcal) **per 57 g**	8.8 g cows' milk	35.2 g (sugars 22.7 g)	8.4 g	Trace	Gluten-free Contains lactose	Standard, p. 878	Sachet: 4 × 57 g = £3.26 Banana, chocolate, milk, strawberry, vanilla
							Powder 57 g reconstituted with 200 mL whole milk provides: protein 15.6 g, carbohydrate 44.5 g, fat 16.4 g, energy 1621 kJ (387 kcal)		
Foodlink® Complete (Foodlink)	Powder	1838 kJ[1] (437 kcal) **per 100 g**	21.9 g cows' milk	57.3 g	13.3 g	Nil	Contains lactose	Standard, p. 878	Carton: 450 g = £3.29 Banana, chocolate, neutral, strawberry
							Recommended serving = 3 heaped tablespoonfuls in 250 mL water provides: protein 12.5 g, carbohydrate 32.7 g, fat 7.6 g, energy 1048 kJ (249 kcal)[1]		
Foodlink® Complete with Fibre (Foodlink)	Powder	1804 kJ (428 kcal)[1] **per 100 g**	19.5 g cows' milk	57.1 g (sugars 36.8 g)	12.3 g	8 g	Contains lactose	Standard, p. 878	Sachet: 10 × 63 g = £6.67 Vanilla + fibre
							Recommended serving = 4 heaped tablespoonfuls in 250 mL water provides: protein 12.3 g, carbohydrate 38 g, fat 7.5 g, fibre 5 g, energy 1137 kJ (270 kcal)[1]		
Forticreme® Complete (Nutricia Clinical)	Semi-solid	675 kJ (160 kcal) **per 100 g**	9.5 g cows' milk	19.2 g (sugars 10.6 g)	5 g	100 mg[2]	Gluten-free Residual lactose	Standard, p. 878; *also* CAPD, haemodialysis Not suitable for child under 3 years	Pot: 4 × 125 g = £6.99 Banana, chocolate, forest fruits, vanilla
Fortisip® Extra (Nutricia Clinical)	Liquid (sip feed)	675 kJ (160 kcal) **per 100 mL**	10 g cows' milk	18.1 g (sugars 9 g)	5.3 g	Nil[2]	Gluten-free Contains lactose	Standard, p. 878 Not suitable for child under 3 years	Bottle: 200 mL = £1.80 Chocolate, forest fruits, mocha, strawberry, vanilla
Fresubin® 2kcal (Fresenius Kabi)	Liquid (sip feed)	840 kJ (200 kcal) **per 100 mL**	10 g cows' milk	22.5 g (sugars 5.8 g)	7.8 g	Nil	Gluten-free Contains lactose	Standard, p. 878; *also* CAPD, haemodialysis	Bottle: 200 mL = £1.69 Fruits of the forest, cappuccino, vanilla
Fresubin® 2kcal Fibre (Fresenius Kabi)	Liquid (sip feed)	840 kJ (200 kcal) **per 100 mL**	10 g cows' milk	22.5 g (sugars 5.8 g)	7.8 g	1.6 g	Gluten-free Contains lactose	Standard, p. 878; *also* CAPD, haemodialysis	Bottle: 200 mL = £1.69 Chocolate
Fresubin® Crème (Fresenius Kabi)	Semi-solid	756 kJ (180 kcal) **per 100 g**	10 g cows' milk	19 g (sugars 14.4 g)	7.2 g	2 g	Gluten-free Residual lactose	Standard, p. 878; *also* CAPD, haemodialysis Not suitable for child under 3 years	Pot: 4 × 125 g = £6.92 Cappuccino, strawberry, vanilla
Renilon® 7.5 (Nutricia Clinical)	Liquid (sip feed)	840 kJ (200 kcal) **per 100 mL**	7.5 g cows' milk	20 g (sugars 4.8 g)	10 g	Nil	Gluten-free Residual lactose	Standard, p. 878 Not suitable for child under 3 years	Carton: 125 mL = £1.79 Apricot, caramel

1. Nutritional values may vary with flavour—consult product literature
2. Fibre content varies with flavour

Product	Form	Energy	Protein	Carbohydrate	Fat		Characteristics	Suitable	Presentation / flavour
Resource® 2.0 Fibre (Nestlé)	Liquid (sip feed)	836 kJ (200 kcal)[1] **per 100 mL**	9 g cows' milk	21.4 g (sugars 5.5 g)	8.7 g	2.5 g	Gluten-free Residual lactose	Standard, p.878 Not suitable for child under 6 years; caution in child 6–10 years	Carton: 200 mL = £1.65 Apricot, coffee, neutral, strawberry, summer fruits, vanilla
Resource® Dessert Fruit (Nestlé)	Semi-solid	678 kJ (160 kcal)[1] **per 100 g**	5 g cows' milk	24 g (sugars 16.4 g)	5 g	1.4 g	Gluten-free Residual lactose	Standard, p.878; also CAPD, haemodialysis	Cup: 3 × 125 g = £4.05 Apple, apple-peach, apple-strawberry[2]
Resource® Shake (Nestlé)	Liquid (sip feed)	730 kJ (174 kcal)[1] **per 100 mL**	5.1 g cows' milk	22.6 g (sugars 6.4 g)	7 g	Nil	Gluten-free Residual lactose	Standard, p.878	Carton: 175 mL = £1.50 Banana, chocolate, lemon, strawberry, summer fruits, toffee, vanilla
Vegenat-med® Balanced Protein (Vegenat)	Powder	1924 kJ (458 kcal)[1] **per 110 g serving**	18 g cows' milk	62 g	15.35 g	5.8 g	Gluten-free Residual lactose	Standard, p.878 except bowel fistula Not suitable for child under 14 years	Sachet: 12 × 110 g = £33.89 Apple, chocolate, honey, orange
Vegenat-med® High Protein (Vegenat)	Powder	1940 kJ (463 kcal)[1] **per 110 g serving**	23.3 g cows' milk	57.2 g	15.6 g	6 g	Gluten-free Residual lactose	Standard, p.878 except bowel fistula Not suitable for child under 14 years	Sachet: 12 × 110 g = £47.44 Chicken, chickpea, fish, fish-vegetable, ham, lentil, veal, vegetable, winter vegetable 12 × 110 g = £45.75 Curry chicken 12 × 110 g = £45.07 Lemon, rice with lemon 24 × 55 g = £43.46 Rice with apple

1. Nutritional values may vary with flavour—consult product literature
2. Flavour not suitable for child under 3 years

Appendix 2: Borderline substances

Appendix 2: Borderline substances

A2.3 Specialised formulas

For further information on composition of feeds, see p.878

A2.3.1 Specialised formulas: Infant and child

Specialised formulas are suitable for infants from birth unless otherwise indicated (*see also* A2.1.3.1 Enteral feeds (non-disease specific); Child under 12 years)

■ **Specialised formulas: Infant and child: Amino acid-based formula**

ACBS Indications: Proven whole protein intolerance, short bowel syndrome, intractable malabsorption, or other gastro-intestinal disorders where an elemental diet is indicated

Product	Formulation	Energy	Protein	Carbohydrate	Fat	Fibre	Special Characteristics	ACBS Indications	Presentation & Flavour
Neocate® Active (SHS)	Standard dilution (21%) of powder	1255 kJ (300 kcal) **per 300 mL serving** (63-g sachet made up to 300 mL with water)	8.3 g protein equivalent (essential and non-essential amino acids)	34 g (sugars 3.1 g[1])	14.5 g	Nil	Milk protein-free	See above Nutritional supplement only Not suitable for child under 1 year	Sachet: 14 × 63 g = £49.14 Black currant, unflavoured[2]
Powder provides: protein equivalent 13.1 g, carbohydrate 54 g, fat 23 g, energy 1992 kJ (475 kcal)/100 g									
Neocate® Advance (SHS)	Standard dilution (25%) of powder	420 kJ (100 kcal) **per 100 mL**	2.5 g protein equivalent (essential and non-essential amino acids)	14.6 g (sugars 1.3 g[1])	3.5 g (MCT 35%)	Nil	Milk protein-free	See above Not suitable for child under 1 year	Sachet: 100 g = £4.82 Unflavoured[2] 15 × 50 g = £38.43 Banana-vanilla
Powder provides: protein equivalent 10 g, carbohydrate 58.5 g, fat 14 g, energy 1683 kJ (400 kcal)/100 g									
Neocate® LCP (SHS)	Standard dilution (14.7%) of powder	293 kJ (70 kcal) **per 100 mL**	1.9 g protein equivalent (essential and non-essential amino acids)	7.9 g (sugars 720 mg)	3.4 g	Nil	Milk protein-free	Cows' milk allergy, multiple food protein intolerance, and conditions requiring an elemental diet	Can: 400 g = £22.91 (4.9-g measuring scoop provided)
Powder provides: protein equivalent 13 g, carbohydrate 54 g, fat 23 g, energy 1990 kJ (475 kcal)/100 g									

1. Sugar content varies with flavour

2. Flavouring: see *Modjul® Flavour System*, p.909

Product	Dilution	Energy	Protein	Carbohydrate	Fat		Notes	Indication	Pack
Nutramigen® AA (Mead Johnson)	Standard dilution (13.6%) of powder	286 kJ (68 kcal) per 100 mL	1.89 g essential and non-essential amino acids	7 g	3.6 g	Nil	Gluten-free Lactose-free	Severe cows' milk protein intolerance, or multiple food intolerance, and other gastro-intestinal disorders where an elemental diet is specifically indicated	Can: 400 g = £21.22 (4.5-g measuring scoop provided)

Powder provides: protein 13.9 g, carbohydrate 51 g, fat 26 g, energy 2092 kJ (498 kcal)/100 g

■ Specialised formulas: Infant and child: Hydrolysate formula

Product	Dilution	Energy	Protein	Carbohydrate	Fat		Notes	Indication	Pack
Cow & Gate Pepti® (Cow & Gate)	Standard dilution (13.6%) of powder	275 kJ (66 kcal) per 100 mL	1.6 g whey hydrolysed	7.1 g (sugars 6.4 g)	3.5 g	800 mg	Contains lactose and fish oil	Established cows' milk protein intolerance, with or without secondary lactose intolerance	Can: 900 g = £19.39 (4.5-g measuring scoop provided)

Powder provides: protein 11.6 g, carbohydrate 52 g, fat 25.6 g, energy 2025 kJ (484 kcal)/100 g

| Cow & Gate Pepti-Junior® (Cow & Gate) | Standard dilution (12.8%) of powder | 275 kJ (66 kcal) per 100 mL | 1.8 g whey hydrolysed | 6.8 g (sugars 1.1 g) | 3.5 g | Nil | Residual lactose Contains fish oil | Disaccharide and/or whole protein intolerance, or where amino acids and peptides are indicated in conjunction with medium chain triglycerides | Can: 450 g = £10.68 (4.3-g measuring scoop provided) |

Powder provides: protein 14 g, carbohydrate 53.4 g, fat 27.3 g, energy 2155 kJ (515 kcal)/100 g

| Nutramigen® 1 (Mead Johnson) | Standard dilution (13.5%) of powder | 280 kJ (68 kcal) per 100 mL | 1.9 g casein hydrolysed | 7.5 g | 3.4 g | Nil | Gluten-free Lactose-free | Disaccharide and/or whole protein intolerance where additional medium chain triglycerides are not included | Can: 400 g = £8.61 (4.5-g measuring scoop provided) |

Powder provides: protein 14 g, carbohydrate 55 g, fat 25 g, energy 2100 kJ (500 kcal)/100 g

| Nutramigen® 2 (Mead Johnson) | Standard dilution (14.6%) of powder | 285 kJ (68 kcal) per 100 mL | 1.7 g casein hydrolysed | 8.6 g | 2.9 g | Nil | Gluten-free Lactose-free | Established disaccharide and/or whole protein intolerance (where additional chain triglycerides are not indicated) Not suitable for child under 6 months | Can: 400 g = £8.61 (4.9-g measuring scoop provided) |

Powder provides: protein 11.6 g, carbohydrate 59 g, fat 20 g, energy 1950 kJ (466 kcal)/100 g

| Pepdite® (SHS) | Standard dilution (15%) of powder | 297 kJ (71 kcal) per 100 mL | 2.1 g protein equivalent (non-milk hydrolysate) | 7.8 g (sugars 700 mg) | 3.5 g | Nil | Lactose-free Contains meat (pork) and soya derivatives | Disaccharide and/or whole protein intolerance | Can: 400 g = £14.70 (5-g measuring scoop provided) |

Powder provides: protein equivalent 13.8 g, carbohydrate 52 g, fat 23.2 g, energy 1977 kJ (472 kcal)/100 g

Appendix 2: Borderline substances

Appendix 2: Borderline substances

A2.3.1 Specialised formulas: Infant and child: Hydrolysate formula (product list continued)

Product	Formulation	Energy	Protein	Carbohydrate	Fat	Fibre	Special Characteristics	ACBS Indications	Presentation & Flavour
Pepdite® 1+ (SHS)	Standard dilution (22.8%) of powder	423 kJ (100 kcal) per 100 mL	3.1 g protein equivalent (non-milk hydrolysate, essential amino acids)	13 g (sugars 1.2 g)	3.9 g (MCT 35%)	Nil	Lactose-free Contains meat (pork) and soya derivatives	Disaccharide and/or whole protein intolerance, or where amino acids or peptides are indicated in conjunction with medium chain triglycerides. Not suitable for child under 1 year	Can: 400 g = £15.44 Unflavoured[1]
	Powder provides: protein equivalent 13.8 g, carbohydrate 57 g, fat 17.3 g, energy 1844 kJ (439 kcal)/100 g								
Pregestimil® (Mead Johnson)	Standard dilution (13.5%) of powder	280 kJ (68 kcal) per 100 mL	1.89 g casein hydrolysed	6.9 g	3.8 g (MCT 54%)	Nil	Gluten-free Lactose-free	Disaccharide and/or whole protein intolerance, or where amino acids or peptides are indicated in conjunction with medium chain triglycerides	Can: 400 g = £9.44 (4.5-g measuring scoop provided)
	Powder provides: protein 14 g, carbohydrate 51 g, fat 28 g, energy 2100 kJ (500 kcal)/100 g								
Prejomin® (Milupa)	Standard dilution (15%) of powder	315 kJ (75 kcal) per 100 mL	2 g soya, collagen (porcine) hydrolysate	8.6 g (sugars 400 mg)	3.6 g	Nil	Gluten-free Lactose-free Contains meat (pork) derivatives	Disaccharide and/or whole protein intolerance, where additional medium chain triglycerides are not indicated	Can: 400 g = £10.12 (5-g measuring scoop provided)
	Powder provides: protein 13.5 g, carbohydrate 57.1 g, fat 24 g, energy 2085 kJ (497 kcal)/100 g								

◼ Specialised formulas: Infant and child: Residual lactose formula

Product	Formulation	Energy	Protein	Carbohydrate	Fat	Fibre	Special Characteristics	ACBS Indications	Presentation & Flavour
Enfamil® O-Lac (Mead Johnson)	Standard dilution (13%) of powder	280 kJ (68 kcal) per 100 mL	1.42 g cows' milk	7.2 g	3.7 g	Nil	Gluten-free Residual lactose	Proven lactose intolerance	Can: 400 g = £3.86 (4.3-g measuring scoop provided)
	Powder provides: protein 10.9 g, carbohydrate 55 g, fat 28 g, energy 2200 kJ (520 kcal)/100 g								
Galactomin 17® (SHS)	Standard dilution (13.6%) of powder	295 kJ (70 kcal) per 100 mL	1.7 g protein equivalent (cows' milk)	7.5 g (sugars 1.4 g)	3.7 g	Nil	Residual lactose	Proven lactose intolerance in preschool children, galactosaemia, and galactokinase deficiency	Can: 400 g = £13.16 Unflavoured[1] (4.3-g measuring scoop provided)
	Powder provides: protein equivalent 12.3 g, carbohydrate 55.3 g, fat 27.2 g, energy 2155 kJ (515 kcal)/100 g								
SMA® LF (SMA Nutrition)	Standard dilution (13%) of powder	281 kJ (67 kcal) per 100 mL	1.5 g casein, whey	7.2 g (sugars 2.6 g)	3.6 g	Nil	Residual lactose	Proven lactose intolerance	Can: 430 g = £4.57
	Powder provides: protein 12 g, carbohydrate 55.6 g, fat 28 g, energy 2185 kJ (522 kcal)/100 g								

1. Flavouring: see Modjul® Flavour System, p. 909

Specialised formulas: Infant and child: MCT-enhanced formula

	Standard dilution	Energy	Protein	Carbohydrate	Fat	Fibre	Special characteristics	Indications	Presentation
Caprilon® (SHS)	Standard dilution (12.7%) of powder	277 kJ (66 kcal) **per 100 mL**	1.5 g cows' milk	7 g (sugars 1.3 g)	3.6 g (MCT 75%)	Nil	Contains lactose	Disorders in which a high intake of MCT is beneficial	Can: 420 g = £14.28 (4.2-g measuring scoop provided)

Powder provides: protein equivalent 11.8 g, carbohydrate 55.1 g, fat 28.3 g, energy 2184 kJ (522 kcal)/100 g

	Standard dilution	Energy	Protein	Carbohydrate	Fat	Fibre	Special characteristics	Indications	Presentation
MCT Pepdite® (SHS)	Standard dilution (15%) of powder	286 kJ (68 kcal) **per 100 mL**	2 g protein equivalent (non-milk peptides, essential amino acids)	8.8 g (sugars 1.2 g)	2.7 g (MCT 75%)	Nil	Gluten-free Lactose-free Contains meat (pork) and soya derivatives	Disorders in which a high intake of MCT is beneficial	Can: 400 g = £16.01 (5-g measuring scoop provided)

Powder provides: protein equivalent 13.8 g, carbohydrate 59 g, fat 18 g, energy 1903 kJ (453 kcal)/100 g

	Standard dilution	Energy	Protein	Carbohydrate	Fat	Fibre	Special characteristics	Indications	Presentation
MCT Pepdite® +1 (SHS)	Standard dilution (20%) of powder	381 kJ (91 kcal) **per 100 mL**	2.8 g protein equivalent (non-milk peptides, essential amino acids)	11.8 g (sugars 1.6 g)	3.6 g (MCT 75%)	Nil	Gluten-free Lactose-free Contains meat (pork) and soya derivatives	Disorders in which a high intake of MCT is beneficial Not suitable for child under 1 year	Can: 400 g = £16.01 Unflavoured[1]

Powder provides: protein equivalent 13.8 g, carbohydrate 59 g, fat 18 g, energy 1903 kJ (453 kcal)/100 g

	Standard dilution	Energy	Protein	Carbohydrate	Fat	Fibre	Special characteristics	Indications	Presentation
Monogen® (SHS)	Standard dilution (17.5%) of powder	313 kJ (74 kcal) **per 100 mL**	2 g protein equivalent (whey)	12 g (sugars 1.2 g)	2.1 g (MCT 90%)	Nil	Residual lactose Supplementation with essential fatty acids may be needed	Long-chain acyl-CoA dehydrogenase deficiency (LCAD), carnitine palmitoyl transferase deficiency (CPTD), primary and secondary lipoprotein lipase deficiency	Can: 400 g = £15.91 Unflavoured[1] (5-g measuring scoop provided)

Powder provides: protein equivalent 11.4 g, carbohydrate 68 g, fat 11.8 g, energy 1786 kJ (424 kcal)/100 g

Specialised formulas: Infant and child: Soya-based formula

	Standard dilution	Energy	Protein	Carbohydrate	Fat	Fibre	Special characteristics	Indications	Presentation
InfaSoy® (Cow & Gate)	Standard dilution (12.7%) of powder	275 kJ (66 kcal) **per 100 mL**	1.8 g soya	6.6 g (sugars 1 g)	3.6 g	Nil	Lactose-free	Proven lactose and associated sucrose intolerance in pre-school children, galactokinase deficiency, galactosaemia, and proven whole cows' milk sensitivity	Can: 900 g = £7.47 (4.2-g measuring scoop provided)

Powder provides: protein equivalent 14.2 g, carbohydrate 52 g, fat 28.3 g, energy 2170 kJ (519 kcal)/100 g

	Standard dilution	Energy	Protein	Carbohydrate	Fat	Fibre	Special characteristics	Indications	Presentation
Isomil® (Abbott)	Standard dilution (13.2%) of powder	284 kJ (68 kcal) **per 100 mL**	1.8 g soya protein isolate	6.9 g (sugars 2.4 g)	3.7 g	Nil	Gluten-free Lactose-free	Proven lactose intolerance in pre-school children, galactokinase deficiency, galactosaemia, and proven whole cows' milk sensitivity	Can: 400 g = £3.38 4.4 g (measuring scoop provided)

Powder provides: protein 13.7 g, carbohydrate 52.4 g, fat 28.1 g, energy 2163 kJ (517 kcal)/100 g

1. Flavouring: see *Modjul® Flavour System*, p.909

Appendix 2: Borderline substances

Appendix 2: Borderline substances

A2.3.1 Specialised formulas: Infant and child: Soya-based formula (product list continued)

Product	Formulation	Energy	Protein	Carbohydrate	Fat	Fibre	Special Characteristics	ACBS Indications	Presentation & Flavour
Wysoy® (Wyeth)	Standard dilution (13.2%) of powder	280 kJ (67 kcal) **per 100 mL**	1.8 g soya protein isolate	6.9 g (sugars 2.5 g)	3.6 g	Nil	Lactose-free	Proven lactose and associated sucrose intolerance in pre-school children, galactokinase deficiency, galactosaemia, and proven whole cows' milk sensitivity	Can: 430 g = £4.44 860 g = £8.41

Powder provides: protein 14 g, carbohydrate 54 g, fat 27 g, energy 2155 kJ (515 kcal)/100 g

■ Specialised formulas: Infant and child: Low calcium formula

Product	Formulation	Energy	Protein	Carbohydrate	Fat	Fibre	Special Characteristics	ACBS Indications	Presentation & Flavour
Locasol® (SHS)	Standard dilution (13.1%) of powder	278 kJ (66 kcal) **per 100 mL**	1.9 g cows' milk	7 g (sugars 6.9 g)	3.4 g	Nil	Contains lactose Calcium less than 7 mg/100 mL No added vitamin D	Conditions of calcium intolerance requiring restriction of calcium and vitamin D intake	Can: 400 g = £18.29 (4.4-g measuring scoop provided)

Powder provides: protein 14.6 g, carbohydrate 53.7 g, fat 26.1 g, energy 2125 kJ (508 kcal)/100 g

■ Specialised formulas: Infant and child: Fructose-based formula

Product	Formulation	Energy	Protein	Carbohydrate	Fat	Fibre	Special Characteristics	ACBS Indications	Presentation & Flavour
Galactomin 19® (SHS)	Standard dilution (12.9%) of powder	288 kJ (69 kcal) **per 100 mL**	1.9 g protein equivalent (cows' milk)	6.4 g (fructose 6.3 g)	4 g	Nil	Residual lactose, galactose and glucose	Conditions of glucose plus galactose intolerance	Can: 400 g = £34.65

Powder provides: protein equivalent 14.6 g, carbohydrate 49.7 g, fat 30.8 g, energy 2233 kJ (534 kcal)/100 g

■ Specialised formulas: Infant and child: Pre-thickened infant feeds

Not to be used for a period of more than 6 months; not to be used in conjunction with any other feed thickener or antacid products

Product	Formulation	Energy	Protein	Carbohydrate	Fat	Fibre	Special Characteristics	ACBS Indications	Presentation & Flavour
Enfamil® AR (Mead Johnson)	Standard dilution (13.5%) of powder	285 kJ (68 kcal) **per 100 mL**	1.7 g cows' milk	7.6 g (lactose 4.6 g)	3.5 g	Nil	Contains lactose, pregelatinised rice starch	Significant gastro-oesophageal reflux	Can: 400 g = £2.90 (4.5-g measuring scoop provided)

Powder provides: protein 12.5 g, carbohydrate 56 g, fat 26 g, energy 2093 kJ (500 kcal)/100 g

Product	Formulation	Energy	Protein	Carbohydrate	Fat	Fibre	Special Characteristics	ACBS Indications	Presentation & Flavour
SMA® Staydown (SMA Nutrition)	Standard dilution (12.9%) of powder	279 kJ (67 kcal) **per 100 mL**	1.6 g casein, whey	7 g (lactose 5 g)	3.6 g	Nil	Contains lactose, precooked corn starch	Significant gastro-oesophageal reflux	Can: 900 g = £6.49

Powder provides: protein 12.4 g, carbohydrate 54.3 g, fat 28 g, energy 2166 kJ (518 kcal)/100 g

A2.3.2 Modular feeds for specific clinical conditions

For further information on composition of feeds, see p.878

Product	Formulation	Energy	Protein	Carbohydrate	Fat	Fibre	Special Characteristics	ACBS Indications	Presentation & Flavour
Alicalm® (SHS)	Standard dilution (30%) of powder	567 kJ (135 kcal) **per 100 mL**	4.5 g caseinate whey	17.4 g (sugars 3.2 g)	5.3 g	Nil	Residual lactose	Crohn's disease Not suitable for child under 1 year; use as nutritional supplement only in children 1–6 years	Powder: 400 g = £16.20 Vanilla
Powder provides: protein 15 g, carbohydrate 58 g, fat 17.5 g, energy 1889 kJ (450 kcal)/100 g									
Casilan 90® (Heinz)	Powder	1572 kJ (370 kcal) **per 100 g**	90 g cows' milk	300 mg	1 g	Nil	Gluten-free Electrolytes/100 g: Na⁺ 1.3 mmol K⁺ 8.7 mmol Ca²⁺ 35 mmol P⁺ 22.6 mmol	Nutritional supplement for use in biochemically proven hypoproteinaemia	Can: 250 g = £5.90
Forticare® (Nutricia Clinical)	Liquid (sip feed)	675 kJ (160 kcal) **per 100 mL**	9 g cows' milk	19.1 g (sugars 13.6 g)	5.3 g	2.1 g	Gluten-free Residual lactose Contains fish oil	Nutritional supplement in patients with lung cancer undergoing chemotherapy, or with pancreatic cancer Not suitable for child under 3 years	Carton: 125 mL = £1.92 Cappuccino, orange-lemon, peach-ginger
Generaid® (SHS)	Powder	1586 kJ (374 kcal) **per 100 g**	76 g protein equivalent (whey protein, plus branched chain amino acids)	5 g (sugars 5 g)	5.5 g	Nil	Electrolytes/100 g: Na⁺ 6.1 mmol K⁺ 10.8 mmol Ca²⁺ 6.5 mmol P⁺ 6.45 mmol	Nutritional supplement for use in chronic liver disease and/or porto-hepatic encephalopathy	Tub: 200 g = £23.97 Unflavoured[1]
Generaid® Plus (SHS)	Standard dilution (22%) of powder	428 kJ (102 kcal) **per 100 mL**	2.4 g protein equivalent (whey protein, branched chain amino acids)	13.6 g (sugars 1.4 g)	4.2 g (MCT 32%)	Nil	Electrolytes/100 mL: Na⁺ 0.7 mmol K⁺ 2.7 mmol Ca²⁺ 1.72 mmol P⁺ 1.67 mmol	A sole source of nutrition or nutritional supplement in children over 1 year with hepatic disorders	Can: 400 g = £17.15 Unflavoured[1] (5-g measuring scoop provided)
Powder provides: protein equivalent 11 g, carbohydrate 62 g, fat 19 g, energy 1944 kJ (463 kcal)/100 g									

1. Flavouring: see *Modjul® Flavour System*, p.909

Appendix 2: Borderline substances

Appendix 2: Borderline substances

A2.3.2 Modular feeds for specific clinical conditions (product list continued)

Product	Formulation	Energy	Protein	Carbohydrate	Fat	Fibre	Special Characteristics	ACBS Indications	Presentation & Flavour
KetoCal® (SHS)	Standard dilution (20%) of powder	602 kJ (146 kcal) **per 100 mL**	3.1 g cows' milk with additional amino acids	600 mg (sugars 120 mg)	14.6 g (LCT 100%)	Nil	Electrolytes/100 mL: Na+ 4.3 mmol K+ 4.1 mmol Ca2+ 2.15 mmol P+ 2.77 mmol	Sole source of nutrition or nutritional supplement as part of ketogenic diet in management of epilepsy resistant to drug therapy, in children over 1 year, only on the advice of secondary care physician with experience of ketogenic diet	Can: 300 g = £23.87 Vanilla, Unflavoured
Powder provides: protein 15.25 g, carbohydrate 3 g, fat 73 g, energy 3011 kJ (730 kcal)/100 g										
Kindergen® (SHS)	Standard dilution (20%) of powder	421 kJ (101 kcal) **per 100 mL**	1.5 g whey protein	11.8 mg (sugars 1.2 g)	5.3 g (LCT 93%)	Nil	Electrolytes/100 mL: Na+ 2 mmol K+ 0.6 mmol Ca2+ 2.8 mmol P+ 3 mmol Low Vitamin A	Sole source of nutrition or nutritional supplement for infants and children with chronic renal failure receiving peritoneal rapid overnight dialysis	Tub: 400 g = £15.18 (5-g measuring scoop provided)
Powder provides: protein 7.5 g, carbohydrate 59 g, fat 26.3 g, energy 2104 kJ (504 kcal)/100 g										
Medium-chain Triglyceride (MCT) Oil (SHS)	Liquid	3515 kJ (855 kcal) **per 100 mL**	Nil	Nil	MCT 100%	Nil		Nutritional supplement for steatorrhoea associated with cystic fibrosis of the pancreas, intestinal lymphangiectasia, intestinal surgery, chronic liver disease and liver cirrhosis, other proven malabsorption syndromes, ketogenic diet in management of epilepsy, type 1 hyperlipoproteinaemia	Bottle: 500 mL = £11.50
Nepro® (Abbott)	Liquid (sip or tube feed)	838 kJ (200 kcal) **per 100 mL**	7 g cows' milk	20.6 g (sugars 3.26 g)	9.6 g	1.56 g	Gluten-free Residual lactose Electrolytes/100 mL: Na+ 3.67 mmol K+ 2.72 mmol Ca2+ 3.43 mmol P+ 2.23 mmol	Sole source of nutrition or nutritional supplement in patients with chronic renal failure who are on haemodialysis or CAPD, or with cirrhosis, or other conditions requiring a high energy, low fluid, low electrolyte diet. Not suitable for child under 1 year; use with caution in child 1–5 years	Carton: 200 mL = £2.28 Strawberry, vanilla[1] Flexible pack: 500 mL = £4.95 Vanilla

1. Minor nutritional variations between flavours—consult product literature

| ProSure® (Abbott) | Liquid (sip or tube feed) | 529 kJ (125 kcal) **per 100 mL** | 6.65 g cows' milk | 18.3 g (sugars 2.95 g) | 2.56 g | 2.07 g | Gluten-free Residual lactose Contains fish oil | Nutritional supplement for patients with pancreatic cancer Not suitable for child under 1 year; use with caution in child 1–4 years | Carton: 240 mL = £2.70 Banana, vanilla[1] |
| Protifar® (Nutricia Clinical) | Powder | 1580 kJ (373 kcal) **per 100 g** | 88.5 g cows' milk | less than 1.5 g | 1.6 g | Nil | Gluten-free Residual lactose Electrolytes/100 mL: Na$^+$ 1.3 mmol K$^+$ 1.28 mmol Ca^{2+} 33.75 mmol P$^+$ 22.58 mmol | Nutritional supplement for use in biochemically proven hypoproteinaemia | Can: 225 g = £7.22 Unflavoured (2.5-g measuring scoop provided) |

Powder provides: protein 2.2 g per 2.5 g

| Renamil® (KoRa) | Powder (sip or tube feed when reconstituted) | 2003 kJ (477 kcal) **per 100 g** | 4.6 g cows' milk | 70.8 g | 19.3 g | Nil | Contains lactose Gluten-free Electrolytes/100 g: Na$^+$ 1.04 mmol K$^+$ 0.13 mmol Ca^{2+} 10.22 mmol P$^+$ 1.06 mmol Contains no vitamin A or vitamin D | Sole source of nutrition or nutritional supplement for adults and children over 1 year with chronic renal failure | Sachet: 10 × 100 g = £25.40 |
| Renapro® (KoRa) | Powder | 1580 kJ (372 kcal) **per 100 g** | 90 g whey protein | 800 mg | 1 g | Nil | Gluten-free Residual lactose Electrolytes/100 g: Na$^+$ 23 mmol K$^+$ 2 mmol Ca^{2+} 4.99 mmol P$^+$ 4.84 mmol | Nutritional supplement for biochemically proven hypoproteinaemia and patients undergoing dialysis Not suitable for child under 1 year | Sachet: 30 × 20 g = £69.60 |

Powder provides: protein 18 g, energy 316 kJ (74 kcal)/20-g sachet

| Suplena® (Abbott) | Liquid (sip or tube feed) | 840 kJ (200 kcal) **per 100 mL** | 3 g caseinates | 25.5 g (sugars 2.7 g) | 9.6 g | Nil | Gluten-free Residual lactose Electrolytes/100 mL: Na$^+$ 3.39 mmol K$^+$ 2.87 mmol Ca^{2+} 3.48 mmol P$^+$ 2.39 mmol | A sole source of nutrition or nutritional supplement in patients with chronic or acute renal failure who are not undergoing dialysis, or with chronic or acute liver disease with fluid restriction; other conditions requiring high energy, low protein, low electrolyte, low volume enteral feed Not suitable for child under 1 year; use with caution in child 1–5 years | Can: 237 mL = £2.34 Vanilla |

1. Minor nutritional variations between flavours—consult product literature

Appendix 2: Borderline substances

Appendix 2: Borderline substances

A2.4 Feed supplements

A2.4.1 High-energy supplements

For further information on composition of feeds, see p. 878

A2.4.1.1 High-energy supplements: carbohydrate

Flavoured carbohydrate supplements are not suitable for child under 1 year; liquid supplements should be diluted before use in child under 5 years

ACBS Indications: disease-related malnutrition, malabsorption states, or other conditions requiring fortification with a high or readily available carbohydrate supplement

Product	Formulation	Energy	Protein	Carbohydrate	Fat	Fibre	Special Characteristics	ACBS Indications	Presentation & Flavour
Caloreen® (Nestlé)	Powder	1640 kJ (390 kcal) **per 100 g**	Nil	96 g Maltodextrin	Nil	Nil	Gluten-free Lactose-free	See above Not suitable for child under 3 years	Powder: 500 g = £3.42 Unflavoured (10-g measuring scoop provided)
Maxijul® Super Soluble (SHS)	Powder	1615 kJ (380 kcal) **per 100g**	Nil	95 g Glucose polymer (sugars 8.6 g)	Nil	Nil	Gluten-free Lactose-free	See above	Sachets: 4 × 132 g = £5.04 Can: 200 g = £1.96 2.5 kg = £17.94 25 kg = £121.85 Unflavoured
Maxijul® Liquid (SHS)	Liquid	850 kJ (200 kcal) **per 100 mL**	Nil	50 g Glucose polymer (sugars 4.5 g[1])	Nil	Nil	Gluten-free Lactose-free	See above	Carton: 200 mL = £1.28 Orange, unflavoured
Polycal® (Nutricia Clinical)	Powder	1630 kJ (384 kcal) **per 100g**	Nil	96 g Maltodextrin (sugars 6 g)	Nil	Nil	Gluten-free Lactose-free	See above	Can: 400 g = £3.55 Neutral (5-g measuring scoop provided)
	Liquid	1050 kJ (247 kcal) **per 100mL**	Nil	61.9 g Maltodextrin (sugars 12.2 g)	Nil	Nil	Gluten-free Lactose-free	Liquid not suitable for child under 3 years	Bottle: 200 mL = £1.42 Neutral, orange
Vitajoule® (Vitaflo)	Powder	1610 kJ (380 kcal) **per 100g**	Nil	96 g Dried glucose syrup	Nil	Nil	Gluten-free Lactose-free	See above	Can: 500 g = £3.48 2.5 kg = £17.14 25 kg = £101.97 (10-g measuring scoop provided)

1. Sugar content varies with flavour

A2.4.1.2 High-energy supplements: fat

Liquid supplements should be diluted before use in child under 5 years

ACBS indications: disease-related malnutrition, malabsorption states, or other conditions requiring fortification with a high fat (or fat and carbohydrate) supplement

Product	Formulation	Energy	Protein	Carbohydrate	Fat	Fibre	Special Characteristics	ACBS Indications	Presentation & Flavour
Calogen® (Nutricia Clinical)	Liquid (emulsion)	1850 kJ (450 kcal)[1] **per 100 mL**	Nil	100 mg	50 g (LCT 100%)	Nil	Gluten-free Lactose-free	See above.	Bottle: 200mL = £3.80 500mL = £9.32 Banana[2], neutral, strawberry[2]
Liquigen® (SHS)	Liquid (emulsion)	1850 kJ (450 kcal) **per 100mL**	Nil	Nil	50 g (MCT 97%) Fractionated coconut oil	Nil	Gluten-free Lactose-free Not suitable for child under 1 year	Steatorrhoea associated with cystic fibrosis of the pancreas, intestinal lymphangiectasia, intestinal surgery, chronic liver disease, liver cirrhosis, other proven malabsorption syndromes, ketogenic diet in epilepsy, and in type 1 lipoproteinaemia	Bottle: 250 mL = £7.26
◼ Fat and Carbohydrate									
Duobar® (SHS)	Bar	1211 kJ (292 kcal) **per 45g**	Less than 20 mg	22.5 g (sucrose)	22.5 g	Nil	Contains phenylalanine 180 micrograms/45-g bar Gluten-free Lactose-free	See above	Bar: 45 g = £1.54 Neutral, strawberry, toffee
Duocal® (SHS)	Liquid	695 kJ (166 kcal) **per 100 mL**	Nil	23.7 g (sugars 2.1 g)	7.9 g (MCT 30%)	Nil	Contains vitamin E	See above	Bottle: 250 mL = £3.14
Duocal® Super Soluble (SHS)	Powder	2061 kJ (492 kcal) **per 100 g**	Nil	72.7 g (sugars 6.5 g)	22.3 g (MCT 35%)	Nil	Gluten-free Lactose-free	See above	Can: 400 g = £14.16 (5-g measuring scoop provided)
Energivit® (SHS)	Standard dilution (15%) of powder	309 kJ (74 kcal) **per 100 mL**	Nil	10 g (sugars 900 mg)/100 g	3.75 g	Nil	Lactose-free With vitamins, minerals, and trace elements	For children requiring additional energy, vitamins, minerals, and trace elements following a protein-restricted diet	Can: 400 g = £17.23 (5-g measuring scoop provided)
Powder provides: carbohydrate 66.7 g, fat 25 g, energy 2059 kJ (492 kcal)/100 g									
MCT Duocal (SHS)	Powder	2082 kJ (497 kcal) **per 100 g**	Nil	72 g (sugars 10.1g)	23.2 g (MCT 83%)	Nil		See above	Can: 400 g = £16.84

1. Nutritional values may vary with flavour—consult product literature
2. Flavour not suitable for child under 3 years

Appendix 2: Borderline substances

Appendix 2: Borderline substances

A2.4.1.3 High-energy supplements: protein

ACBS indications: disease-related malnutrition, malabsorption states, or other conditions requiring fortification with a high fat or carbohydrate (with protein) supplement

Product	Formulation	Energy	Protein	Carbohydrate	Fat	Fibre	Special Characteristics	ACBS Indications	Presentation & Flavour
Vitapro® (Vitaflo)	Powder	1506 kJ (360 kcal) **per 100 g**	75 g whey protein isolate	9 g	6 g	Nil	Contains lactose	Biochemically proven hypoproteinaemia	Tub: 250 g = £7.10, 2kg = £55.73 (5-g measuring scoop provided)

■ Protein and carbohydrate

Dialamine® (SHS)	Standard dilution (20%) of powder	264 kJ (62 kcal) **per 100 mL**	4.3 g protein equivalent (essential and non-essential amino acids)	11.2 g (sugars 10.2 g)	Nil	Nil	Contains vitamin C	Hypoproteinaemia, chronic renal failure, wound fistula leakage with excessive protein loss, conditions requiring a controlled nitrogen intake, and haemodialysis. Not suitable for child under 6 months	Can: 400 g = £57.53, Orange

Powder provides: protein equivalent 25 g, carbohydrate 65 g, vitamin C 125 mg, energy 1530 kJ (360 kcal)/100 g

■ Protein, fat, and carbohydrate

Calshake® (Fresenius Kabi)	Powder	1841 kJ (439 kcal) **per 87 g**[1]	4.1 g cows' milk	56.4 g (sugars 20 g)	22 g	Nil	Contains lactose, Gluten-free	See above. Not suitable for child under 1 year	Sachet: 87 g = £1.87 Banana, neutral, strawberry, vanilla; 90 g = £1.87 Chocolate

Powder: one sachet reconstituted with 240 mL whole milk provides approx. 2 kcal/mL and protein 12 g

Enshake® (Abbott)	Powder	1893 kJ (450 kcal) **per 100 g**[1]	8.4 g cows' milk, soy protein isolate	69 g (sugars 14.5 g)	15.6 g	Nil	Residual lactose, With vitamins and minerals	See above. Not suitable for child under 1 year; use with caution in child 1–6 years	Sachet: 96.5 g = £1.87 Banana, chocolate, strawberry, vanilla

Powder: 96.5 g reconstituted with 240 mL whole milk provides approx. 2 kcal/mL and protein 16 g

Pro-Cal® (Vitaflo)	Powder	2788 kJ (667 kcal) **per 100 g**	13.5 g cows' milk	27 g	56 g	Nil	Contains lactose	See above. Not suitable for child under 1 year	Sachets: 25 × 15 g = £12.83; Tub: 510 g = £11.88, 1.5 kg = £24.21, 12.5 kg = £172.13, 25 kg = £265.25 (15-g measuring scoop provided)

Powder 15 g provides: protein 2 g, carbohydrate 4 g, fat 8.4 g, energy 418 kJ (100 kcal)

1. Nutritional values may vary with flavour—consult product literature

Product	Formulation	Energy	Protein	Carbohydrate	Fat	Fibre	Special Characteristics	ACBS Indications	Presentation & Flavour
Pro-Cal® Shot (Vitaflo)	Liquid	1393 kJ (334 kcal) per 100 mL	6.7 g cows' milk	13.4 g	28.2 g	Nil	Contains lactose	See above. Not suitable for child under 1 year	Bottle: 6 × 250 mL = £25.80 Banana, neutral, strawberry[1]
QuickCal® (Vitaflo)	Powder	3263 kJ (780 kcal) per 100 g	4.6 g cows' milk	17 g	77 g	Nil	Contains lactose	See above. Not suitable for child under 1 year	Sachets: 25 × 13 g = £11.54

Powder 13 g provides: protein 600 mg, carbohydrate 2.2 g, fat 10 g, energy 418 kJ (100 kcal)

Product	Formulation	Energy	Protein	Carbohydrate	Fat	Fibre	Special Characteristics	ACBS Indications	Presentation & Flavour
Scandishake® Mix (Nutricia Clinical)	Powder	2099 kJ (500 kcal) per 100 g[2]	4.7 g cows' milk	65 g (sugars 14.3 g)	24.7 g	Nil	Gluten-free. Contains lactose	See above. Not suitable for child under 3 years	Sachet: 85 g = £2.02 Banana, caramel, chocolate, strawberry, vanilla, unflavoured

Powder: 85 g reconstituted with 240 mL whole milk provides: protein 11.7 g, carbohydrate 66.8 g, fat 30.4 g, energy 2457 kJ (588 kcal)

Product	Formulation	Energy	Protein	Carbohydrate	Fat	Fibre	Special Characteristics	ACBS Indications	Presentation & Flavour
Vitasavoury® (Vitaflo)	Powder	2590 kJ (619 kcal) per 100 g[2]	12.7 g cows' milk	23.5 g (sugars 1.5 g)	52.3 g	6.2 g	Contains lactose	See above. Not suitable for child under 3 years	Cup (200 kcal): 24 × 33 g = £25.76 Sachet (300 kcal): 10 × 50 g = £15.52 Chicken, leek and potato, mushroom, vegetable

1. Flavour not suitable for child under 3 years
2. Nutritional values may vary with flavour—consult product literature

A2.4.2 Fibre, vitamin, and mineral supplements

Product	Formulation	Energy	Protein	Carbohydrate	Fat	Fibre	Special Characteristics	ACBS Indications	Presentation & Flavour
High-fibre supplements									
Resource® Benefiber® (Nestlé)	Powder	323 kJ (76 kcal) per 100 g	Nil	19 g guar gum, partially hydrolysed	Nil	78 g	Gluten-free. Lactose-free	Standard, p. 878 except dysphagia. Not suitable for child under 5 years	Sachets 16 × 8 g = £5.72 Can: 250 g = £8.76 (5-g measuring scoop provided)

Appendix 2: Borderline substances

Appendix 2: Borderline substances

A2.4.2 Fibre, vitamin, and mineral supplements *(product list continued)*

Product	Formulation	Energy	Protein	Carbohydrate	Fat	Fibre	Special Characteristics	ACBS Indications	Presentation & Flavour
■ Vitamin and Mineral supplements									
Metabolic Mineral Mixture® (SHS)	Powder	729 kJ (175 kcal) **per 100 g**	Nil	Nil	Nil	Nil	Contains trace elements Electrolytes/100 g: Na⁺ 172 mmol K⁺ 212 mmol Ca²⁺ 205 mmol P⁺ 192 mmol Energy source: Calcium lactate	Mineral supplement for synthetic diets Suitable for infants (but may require further dilution)	Tub: 100 g = £9.94
Paediatric Seravit® (SHS)	Powder	1275 kJ (300 kcal) **per 100 g**	Nil	75 g¹ (sugars 6.75 g)	Nil	Nil		Vitamin and mineral supplement in infants and children with restrictive therapeutic diets	Tub: 200 g = £14.03 Unflavoured² 200 g = £14.94 Pineapple³ (5-g measuring scoop provided)

1. Sugar content varies with flavour
2. Flavouring: see *Modjul® Flavour System*, p.909
3. Flavour not suitable for child under 6 months

A2.5 Feed additives

A2.5.1 Special foods for conditions of intolerance

Colief® (Britannia)
Liquid, lactase 50 000 units/g, net price 7-mL dropper bottle = £7.00
For the relief of symptoms associated with lactose intolerance in infants, provided that lactose intolerance is confirmed by the presence of reducing substances and/or excessive acid in stools, a low concentration of the corresponding disaccharide enzyme on intestinal biopsy or

by breath hydrogen test or lactose intolerance test. For dosage and administration details, consult product literature

Fructose
(Laevulose)
For proven glucose/galactose intolerance

A2.5.2 Feed thickeners and pre-thickened foods

Carobel, Instant® (Cow & Gate)
Powder, carob seed flour. Net price 135 g = £2.81.
For thickening feeds in the treatment of vomiting

Nutilis® (Nutricia Clinical)
Powder, modified maize starch, gluten- and lactose-free, net price 20 × 9-g sachets = £5.71, 225 g = £4.38.
For thickening of foods in dysphagia. Not to be prescribed for children under 3 years

Resource® Thickened Drink (Nestlé)
Liquid, carbohydrate 22 g, energy: orange 375 kJ (89 kcal); apple 375 kJ (89 kcal)/100 mL. Syrup and custard consistencies. Gluten-free; clinically lactose free, net price 12 × 114-mL cups = £7.08.
For dysphagia. Not suitable for children under 1 year

Resource® ThickenUp® (Nestlé)
Powder, modified maize starch. Gluten- and lactose-free, net price 227 g = £4.11; 75 × 6.4-g sachet = £15.75.
For thickening of foods in dysphagia. Not to be prescribed for children under 1 year

SLO Drinks® (SLO Drinks)
Powder, carbohydrate content varies with flavour and chosen consistency (3 consistencies available), see pro-

duct literature. Flavours: black currant, lemon, orange, or peach, net price 25 × 115 mL = £7.50
Nutritional supplement for patient hydration in the dietary management of dysphagia. Not to be used in children under 3 years

Thick and Easy® (Fresenius Kabi)
Powder. Modified maize starch, net price 225-g can = £4.15; 100 × 9-g sachets = £26.35; 4.54 kg = £70.53.
Thickened Juices, liquid, modified food starch. Flavours: apple, orange, net price 118-mL pot = 54p; apple, black currant, cranberry, kiwi-strawberry, and orange, 1.42-litre bottle = £3.61.
For thickening of foods in dysphagia. Not suitable for children under 1 year except in cases of failure to thrive

Thixo-D® (Sutherland)
Powder, modified maize starch, gluten-free. Net price 375-g tub = £6.75.
For thickening of foods in dysphagia. Not to be prescribed for children under 1 year except in cases of failure to thrive

Vitaquick® (Vitaflo)
Powder. Modified maize starch. Net price 300 g = £6.40; 2 kg = £32.59; 6 kg = £83.40.
For thickening of foods in dysphagia. Not to be prescribed for children under 1 year except in cases of failure to thrive

A2.5.3 Flavouring preparations

Flavour Mix® (Nestlé)
Powder. Flavours: banana, chocolate, coffee, lemon-lime, strawberry. Net price 60 g = £5.62

FlavourPac® (Vitaflo)
Powder, flavours: black currant, lemon, orange, tropical or raspberry, net price 30 × 4-g sachets = £11.29
For use with Vitaflo's range of unflavoured protein substitutes for metabolic diseases

Modjul® Flavour System (SHS)
Powder, carbohydrate-based flavours, black currant, orange, pineapple, 100 g = £9.54; cherry-vanilla, grapefruit, lemon-lime, 20 × 5-g sachets = £9.54
For use with unflavoured SHS products based on peptides or amino acids; not suitable for child under 6 months

Appendix 2: Borderline substances

A2.6 Foods for special diets

A2.6.1 Gluten-free foods

> **ACBS indications:** gluten-sensitive enteropathies including steatorrhoea due to gluten sensitivity, coeliac disease, and dermatitis herpetiformis.

Aproten® (Ultrapharm)
Gluten-free. Flour. Net price 500 g = £4.99.

Barkat® (Gluten Free Foods Ltd)
Gluten-free. Baguettes (par-baked), net price 200 g = £2.99. Bread (white, par-baked, sliced), 300 g = £2.40; country loaf (par-baked, sliced), 250 g = £2.99; rolls (par-baked), 300 g = 2.99. Bread mix, 500 g = £5.10. Multi grain bread, 500 g = £3.95. Rice bread (sliced), brown or white, 450 g = £3.95. Crackers (matzo), 200 g = £2.24. Biscuits (coffee) 200 g = £1.49. Pasta (animal shapes, macaroni, spaghetti, spirals, tagliatelle), 500 g = £4.40, buckwheat (penne or spirals) 250 g = £1.79. Rice pizza crust, brown or white, 150 g = £3.40. Flour mix, 750 g = £4.75.

Bi-Aglut® (Ultrapharm)
Gluten-free. Bread flour mix or plain flour, net price 500 g = £4.75. Bread rolls, 150 g = £1.77. Bread sticks, 150 g = £1.95. Biscuits, 180 g = £2.89. Crackers, 150 g = £2.36. Cracker toast, 240 g = £4.18. Pasta (fusilli, macaroni, penne, spaghetti), 500 g = £5.23.

Dietary Specials (Nutrition Point)
Gluten-free. Bread, loaf, sliced (brown, white or multi-grain), net price 400 g = £2.80; bread rolls, long (white) 3 = £1.75. Bread mix, 500 g = £4.95; cracker bread, 150 g = £1.80; cake mix (white), 750 g = £4.95; white mix, 500 g = £4.95. Tea biscuits, 220 g = £2.00. Pasta (spaghetti, penne, fusilli), 500 g = £3.20. Pizza base 2 × 150 g = £4.90.

Ener-G® (General Dietary)
Gluten-free. Cookies (vanilla flavour), net price 435 g = £5.00. Rolls, dinner, 6 = £2.97, long, white 220 g = £2.39, round, white 220 g = £2.39; Rice bread (sliced), brown, 474 g = £4.39; white, 456 g = £4.39. Rice loaf (sliced), 612 g = £4.39. Seattle brown loaf, 600 g = £5.05. Tapioca bread (sliced), 480 g = £4.39. Rice pasta (macaroni, shells, small shells, and lasagne), 454 g = £4.08; spaghetti, 447 g = £3.98; tagliatelle, 400 g = £3.98; vermicelli, 300 g = £4.08; cannelloni, 335 g = £3.98. Brown rice pasta: lasagne, 454 g = £3.98; macaroni, 454 g = £3.98; spaghetti, 447 g = £3.98. Xanthan gum, 170 g = £6.93.

Freebake® (Freebake)
Gluten-free. Bread mix, net price 2.4 kg = £12.15, cake mix, 2.4 kg = £11.90, pizza base mix, 2.4 kg = £12.00. Flour (plain), 2.4 kg = £11.50.

Gadsby's
Gluten-free. White bread flour, net price 1 kg = £4.99. Bread, white (sliced or unsliced), 400 g = £2.50. Bread rolls, white, 4 × 75 g = £2.00

Glutafin® (Nutricia Dietary)
Gluten-free. Bread loaf, fibre or white (sliced), 400 g = £3.25; rolls, fibre or white, 4 = £3.25. Pasta, savoury, 125 g = £1.80, savoury shorts 150 g = £2.47. Biscuits, digestive, sweet or tea, 150 g = £1.80. Biscuits, 200 g = £3.51. Biscuits, shortbread, 100 g = £1.49. Mixes, bread, fibre or white, 500 g = 5.63, cake, 500 g = £5.63. Crackers, 200 g = £2.93. High fibre crackers, 200 g = £2.46. Pasta (penne, shells, spirals, spaghetti), 500 g = £5.69; (lasagne, tagliatelle), 250 g = £2.98. Pizza bases, 2 × 150 g = £7.40.

Select Gluten-free. Bread, fibre loaf (sliced), 400 g = £2.89; part-baked, 400 g = £3.25, fresh, white or brown, (sliced), 400 g = £3.02. Seeded loaf, 400 g = £3.15. White loaf (sliced), 400 g = £2.89; part-baked, 400 g = £3.25. Fibre rolls, 4 = £3.25, White rolls, 4 = £3.25; part-baked, 4 = £3.25; long, part-baked, 2 = £3.25. Mixes (bread, cake, fibre, fibre bread, pastry, and white), 500 g = £5.63

Heron Foods® (Gluten Free Foods Ltd)
Gluten-free. Bread mix, organic (standard or fibre), net price 500 g = £4.12

Il Pane di Anna® (Gluten Free Foods Ltd)
Gluten-free. Bread mix, white, net price 500 g = £5.25, cake mix, white, 500 g = £5.25, pizza base mix, 500 g = £5.25

Juvela® (SHS)
Gluten-free. Harvest mix, fibre mix, and flour mix, net price 500 g = £6.06. Bread (whole or sliced), 400-g loaf = £2.92; part-baked loaf (with or without fibre), 400 g = £3.13; fresh sliced loaf (white) 400 g = £3.17, (fibre) 400 g = £2.92. Fibre bread (sliced and unsliced), 400 g = £2.92. Bread rolls, white, 5 × 85 g = £3.94, fibre bread rolls, 5 × 85 g = £3.94, part-baked rolls (with or without fibre), 5 × 75 g = £4.07. Crispbread, 210 g = £3.82. Pasta (fibre linguine, fibre penne, fusilli, macaroni, spaghetti), 500 g = £5.94; lasagne, 250 g = £3.03; tagliatelle, 250 g = £2.86. Pizza bases, 2 × 180 g = £7.24. Digestive biscuits, 150 g = £2.51. Savoury biscuits, 150 g = £3.15. Sweet biscuits, 150 g = £2.38. Tea biscuits, 160 g = £2.51.

Lifestyle® (Ultrapharm)
Gluten-free. Brown bread (sliced and unsliced), net price 400 g = £2.82. White bread (sliced and unsliced), 400 g = £2.82. High fibre bread (sliced or unsliced), 400 g = £2.82. Bread rolls (brown, white, or high-fibre) 400 g = £2.82.

Livwell® (Livwell)
Gluten-free. Bread, sliced (brown) net price 225 g = £2.25, (white), 200 g = £2.25; baguette (white) 250 g = £2.50; rolls (white) 4 = £2.50

Orgran® (Community)
Gluten-free. Pasta: lasagne (corn, rice and maize), 150 g = £2.89; macaroni (rice and maize), 250 g = £2.25; shells (split pea and soya), 200 g = £2.25; spaghetti (corn, rice, rice and maize), 250 g = £2.25; spirals (buckwheat, corn, rice, rice and millet, rice and maize), 250 g = £2.25, spirals (organic brown rice), 250 g = £2.60. Crispbread (corn or rice), 200 g = £2.56. Pizza and pastry mix, 375 g = £3.33. Flour, self-raising, 500 g = £2.89. Bread mix, 450 g = £3.10

Proceli® (Generpharm)
Gluten-free. Bread (white, sliced), net price 165 g = £2.24; sandwich bread, 155 g = £2.18; baguettes (part-baked), 2 × 125 g = £2.96. Bread buns, 4 × 50 g = £3.25. Dinner rolls (white, part-baked), 4 × 35 g = £1.91. Flat bread (part-baked), 3 × 40 g = £3.99. Hotdog rolls (white, part-baked), 3 × 35 g = £1.95. Long rolls (white, part-baked), 3 × 83 g = £2.81. Lunch rolls (white), 6 × 45 g = £3.22. Flour (white), 1 kg = £6.88. Pasta (macaroni, small macaroni, puntini, short spaghetti, spirals), 250 g = £2.99. Pizza bases, 3 × 12 g = £5.99. Rice bread (sandwich loaf), 200 g = £2.32, rice bread (brown), 220 g = £2.32.

Pure® (Innovative)
Gluten-free. Blended flour, net price 1 kg = £3.75; potato starch flour, 500 g = £1.49; rice flour, (brown), 500 g = £1.40, (white), 500 g = £1.50; tapioca starch flour, 500 g = £1.99; teff flour, (brown or white), 1 kg = £4.20; xanthan gum, 100 g = £5.75

Rite-Diet® (Nutricia Dietary)
Gluten-free. Flour mix (white or fibre), 500 g = £5.22.

Rizopia® (PGR Health Foods)
Gluten-free. Brown rice pasta (fusilli, penne, spaghetti), 500 g = £2.50, (lasagne), 375 g = £2.50

Schar® (Nutrition Point)
Gluten-free. Bread.(white, sliced), net price 2 x 200 g = £2.90. Baguette (french bread), 400 g = £3.05. Bread rolls, 150 g = £1.82. Lunch rolls, 150 g = £1.85. Bread mix, 1 kg = £4.75. Ertha brown bread, 2 × 250 g = £3.10. Cake mix, 500 g = £4.50. Flour mix, 1 kg = £4.75. Breadsticks (Grissini), 150 g = £1.95. Cracker toast, 150 g = £2.10. Crackers, 200 g = £2.55. Crispbread, 250 g = £3.50. Pasta (fusilli, penne), 500 g = £3.30; lasagne, 250 g = £3.30; macaroni pipette, 500 g = £3.30; spaghetti, 500 g = £3.30. Biscuits (frollini tea), 200 g = £2.00. Savoy biscuits, 200 g = £2.45.

Sunnyvale® (Everfresh)
Gluten-free. Mixed grain bread (sour dough), net price 400 g = £1.91.

Tritamyl® (Gluten Free Foods Ltd)
Gluten-free. Flour, net price 1 kg = £5.60. Brown bread mix, 1 kg = £5.60. White bread mix, 1 kg = £5.60.

Ultra® (Ultrapharm)
Gluten-free. Baguette, net price 400 g = £2.46. Bread, 400 g = £2.46. High-fibre bread, 500 g = £3.35. Bread rolls, 400 g = £2.46. Crackerbread, 100 g = £1.77. Sweet biscuits, 250 g = £2.93. Pasta (fusilli, penne, spaghetti, tagliatelle), 250 g = £2.93. Pizza base, 400 g = £2.65.

Valpiform® (Ultrapharm)
Gluten-free. Bread mix, 2 × 500 g = £6.73. Bread, country loaf (sliced), 400 g = £3.75. Crac'form toast, 2 × 125 g = £3.52. Crisp rolls, 220 g = £3.60; Baguettes, maxi, 2 × 200 g = £4.49, petites, 2 × 160 g = £2.99. Pastry mix, 2 × 500 g = £6.73.

Wellfoods® (Wellfoods)
Gluten-free. Bread, loaf (unsliced), net price 600 g = £4.85, (sliced) 600 g = £4.95; burger buns, 4 = £3.95; rolls, 4 = £3.65. Flour alternative, 1 kg = £7.65. Pizza base, 2 = £8.95

A2.6.1.1 Gluten- and wheat-free foods

ACBS indications: established gluten enteropathy with coexisting established wheat sensitivity only.

Ener-G® (General Dietary)
Gluten-free, wheat-free. Pizza bases, 372 g = £3.75. Six flour bread loaf, 576 g = £3.60. Seattle brown rolls (round or long), 4 × 119 g = £3.00

Glutafin® (Nutricia Dietary)
Gluten-free, wheat-free. Crisp bread, 2 × 125 g = £3.82. Mixes (fibre bread, bread), 500 g = £5.63; cake or pastry mix, 500 g = £5.63.

Heron Foods® (Gluten Free Foods Ltd)
Gluten-free, wheat-free. Bread mix, organic (fibre), net price 500 g = £4.12; bread and cake mix, organic, 500 g = £4.12

A2.6.2 Low-protein foods

ACBS indications: inherited metabolic disorders, renal or liver failure, requiring a low-protein diet

Aproten® (Ultrapharm)
Low protein. Low Na^+ and K^+. Biscuits, net price 180 g (36) = £2.88. Bread mix, 250 g = £2.17. Crispbread, 260 g = £4.06. Pasta (anellini, ditalini, rigatini, spaghetti) 500 g = £4.06, (tagliatelle), 250 g = £2.16.

Ener-G (General Dietary)
Low protein. Egg replacer, net price 454 g = £4.05. Rice bread, 600 g = £4.39

Fate® (Fate)
Low protein. Mix (all-purpose), net price 500 g = £6.35. Cake mix, 2 × 250 g = £6.35, (chocolate-flavour), 2 × 250 g = £6.35.

Harifen® (Ultrapharm)
Low protein. Cracker toast, net price 200 g = £2.75. Cookies, white chip, 200 g = £2.25

Juvela® (SHS)
Low protein. Mix, net price 500 g = £6.66. Bread (sliced), 400-g loaf = £3.12. Bread rolls, 5 × 70 g = £3.87. Biscuits, orange and cinnamon flavour, 125 g = £6.51; chocolate chip, 130 g = £6.51. Pizza base, 2 = £7.37

Loprofin® (SHS)
Low protein. Sweet biscuits, net price 150 g = £2.08; chocolate cream-filled biscuits, 125 g = £2.08; cookies (chocolate chip or cinnamon), 100 g = £5.51; crunch bar, 8 × 41 g = £11.09; wafers (orange, vanilla, or chocolate), 100 g = £2.02. Breakfast cereal, (loops) 375 g = £6.23, (flakes) 375 g = £6.24. Egg replacer, 500 g = £12.14. Egg-white replacer, 100 g = £7.81. Bread (sliced), 400-g loaf = £3.12. Bread rolls, (white), 4 = £2.91, (part-baked) 4 × 65 g = £3.28. Mix, 500 g = £6.61. Cake mix (chocolate or

lemon), 500 g = £6.99. Dessert mix (chocolate, strawberry, vanilla), 150 g = £3.82. Crackers, 150 g = £2.84. Herb crackers, 150 g = £2.84. Pasta (fusilli, penne, spaghetti), 500 g = £6.91, (macaroni, puntoni, tagliatelle), 250 g = £3.32, (conchigle, gnoccetti sardi), 500 g = £6.66, (lasagne), 250 g = £3.36, (animal shapes), 500 g = £6.64, (vermicelli), 250 g = £3.44. Snack Pot (curry, or tomato and basil), 47 g = £3.67. Rice, 500 g = £6.71.

Low protein drink (Milupa)
Powder, protein (whey) 450 mg, carbohydrate 6 g, fat 3 g, energy 220 kJ (53 kcal)/10 g, with vitamins, minerals, and trace elements. Net price 400 g = £7.23.
For inherited disorders of amino acid metabolism in childhood
Note Termed *Milupa® lp-drink* by manufacturer

PK Foods (Gluten Free Foods Ltd)
Low protein. Bread, white (sliced), 550 g = £4.00. Crispbread, 75 g = £2.00. Pasta (spirals), 250 g = £2.00. *Aminex®* biscuits, 200 g = £3.75, cookies, 150 g = £3.75, rusks, 200 g = £4.25
For phenylketonuria and similar amino acid abnormalities
Cookies (chocolate chip, orange, or cinnamon), 150 g = £3.75. Egg replacer, 350 g = £3.75. Flour mix, 750 g = £6.99. Jelly (orange or cherry flavour), 4 × 80 g = £5.76.
For phenylketonuria only

Promin® (Firstplay Dietary)
Low protein. Burger mix, 2 × 62 g = £5.60, (lamb and mint), 4 × 72 g = £5.60. Sausage mix (apple and sage, tomato and basil, or original), 4 × 30 g = £6.30. Cous Cous, 500 g = £6.35. Pasta (alphabets, macaroni, shells, shortcut spaghetti, spirals) and pasta tricolour (alphabets, shells, spirals), 500 g = £6.35; Lasagne sheets, 200 g =

£2.70. Pasta shells in tomato, pepper and herb sauce, 4 x 72-g sachets = £7.32; Pasta elbows in cheese and broccoli sauce, 4 x 66- g sachets = £7.32. Pasta spirals in Moroccan sauce, 4 × 72 g = £7.32. Pasta meal, 500 g = £6.35. Pasta imitation rice, 500 g = £6.35. Rice pudding imitation (apple, banana, strawberry, and original flavours), 4 × 69-g sachets = £5.60. Dessert, (chocolate and banana, strawberry and vanilla, custard, or caramel), 6 × 36.5-g sachets = £5.60. Hot breakfast (apple and cinnamon, banana, chocolate, original), 6 × 57-g sachets = £7.14. Spread, chocolate and hazelnut, 230 g = £6.80

Rite-Diet® Low-protein (SHS)
Low protein. Baking mix. Net price 500 g = £6.36.

Sno-Pro® (SHS)
Low protein. Drink, protein 220 mg (phenylalanine 12.5 mg), carbohydrate 8 g, fat 3.8 g, energy 280 kJ (67 kcal)/100 mL. Net price 200 mL = 98p.

Taranis® (Firstplay Dietary)
Low protein. Cake bars (lemon), net price 6 × 40 g = £5.25

Ultra® (Ultrapharm)
Low protein. PKU bread, 400 g = £2.25. PKU flour, 500 g = £3.07. PKU biscuits, 200 g = £2.21. PKU pizza base, 400 g = £2.35. PKU savoy biscuits, 150 g = £2.06.

Valpiform® (Ultrapharm)
Low protein. Biscuits, shortbread, net price 120 g = £4.06

Vita Bite® (Vitaflo)
Low protein. Bar, protein 30 mg (less than 2.5 mg phenylalanine), carbohydrate 15.35 g, fat 8.4 g, energy 572 kJ (137 kcal)/25 g. Chocolate flavoured, net price 25 g = 96p.
Not recommended for any child under 1 year

A2.7 Nutritional supplements for metabolic diseases

Glutaric aciduria (type 1)

GA Gel® (Vitaflo)
Gel, protein equivalent (essential and non-essential amino acids except lysine, and low tryptophan) 8.4 g, carbohydrate 8.6 g. fat trace, energy 286 kJ (68 kcal)/20 g, with vitamins, minerals, and trace elements. Unflavoured (flavouring: see *FlavourPac®*, p. 909), net price 30 × 20-g sachets = £141.51
Nutritional supplement for dietary management of type 1 glutaric aciduria in children 6 months–10 years

[1]XLYS, Low TRY, Analog (SHS)
Powder, protein equivalent (essential and non-essential amino acids except lysine and low tryptophan) 13 g, carbohydrate 54 g, fat 23 g, energy 1990 kJ (475 kcal)/100 g, with vitamins, minerals, and trace elements; *standard dilution* (15%) provides protein equivalent 1.95 g, carbohydrate 8.1 g, fat 3.5 g, energy 300 kJ (72kcal)/100 mL. Unflavoured, net price 400 g = £28.22 (5-g measuring scoop provided).
Nutritional supplement for dietary management of type 1 glutaric aciduria

[2]XLYS, Low TRY, Maxamaid (SHS)
Powder, protein equivalent (essential and non-essential amino acids except lysine, and low tryptophan) 25 g, carbohydrate 51 g, fat less than 500 mg, energy 1311 kJ (309 kcal)/100 g, with vitamins, minerals, and trace elements. Unflavoured, (flavouring: see *Modjul* Flavour System, p. 909), net price 500 g = £76.94.
Nutritional supplement for dietary management of type 1 glutaric aciduria

XLYS, TRY, Glutaridon (SHS)
Powder, protein equivalent (essential and non-essential amino acids except lysine and tryptophan) 79 g, carbohydrate 4 g, energy 1411 kJ (332 kcal)/100 g, Lactose-free. Unflavoured, (flavouring: see *Modjul* Flavour System, p. 909), net price 2 × 500 g = £291.46
Nutritional supplement for type 1 glutaric aciduria in children and adults; requires additional source of vitamins, minerals and trace elements

Glucogen storage disease

Corn flour and corn starch
For hypoglycaemia associated with glycogen-storage disease

Glucose
(Dextrose monohydrate)
Net price 100 g = 39p.
For glycogen storage disease and sucrose/isomaltose intolerance

Glycosade® (Vitaflo)
Powder, protein 200 mg, carbohydrate (maize starch) 47.6 g, fat 100 mg, fibre less than 600 mg, energy 803 kJ (192 kcal)/60 g, net price 30 × 60-g sachets = £90.00
A nutritional supplement for use in the dietary management of glycogen storage disease and other metabolic conditions where a constant supply of glucose is essential. Not suitable for use in children under 2 years

Homocystinuria or hypermethionimaemia

HCU cooler® (Vitaflo)
Liquid, protein (essential and non-essential amino acids except methionine) 15 g, carbohydrate 7.8 g, fat trace, energy 386 kJ (92 kcal)/130 mL, with vitamins, minerals and trace elements. Orange flavour, net price 30 × 130-mL pouch = £258.30
A methionine-free protein substitute for use as a nutritional supplement in children over 3 years with homocystinuria

HCU Express® (Vitaflo)
Powder, protein (essential and non-essential amino acids except methionine) 15 g, carbohydrate 3.8 g, fat 30 mg,

energy 315 kJ (75.3 kcal)/25 g with vitamins, minerals and trace elements. Unflavoured, (flavouring: see *Flavour Pac®*, p. 909), net price 30 × 25- g sachets = £253.24
A methionine-free protein substitute for use as a nutritional supplement in children over 8 years with homocystinuria

HCU gel® (Vitaflo)
Powder, protein (essential and non-essential amino acids except methionine) 8.4 g, carbohydrate 8.6 g, fat 30 mg, energy 286 kJ (68 kcal)/20 g with vitamins, minerals and

---

1. Analog products are generally intended for use in children up to 1 year
2. Maxamaid products are generally intended for use in children 1–8 years

trace elements. Unflavoured, (flavouring: see *Flavour Pac®*, p. 909), net price 30 × 20- g sachets = £141.51

A methionine-free protein substitute for use as a nutritional supplement for the dietary management of children 1–10 years with homocystinuria

HCU LV® (SHS)

Powder, protein (essential and non-essential amino acids except methionine) 20 g, carbohydrate 2.5 g, fat 190 mg, energy 390 kJ (92 kcal)/27.8-g sachet, with vitamins, minerals and trace elements. Unflavoured (flavouring: see *Modjul®* Flavour System, p. 909),or tropical flavour (formulation varies slightly), net price 30 × 27.8-g sachets = £386.17

A nutritional supplement for the dietary management of hypermethioninaemia or vitamin B₆ non-responsive homocystinuria in children over 8 years

¹XMET Analog (SHS)

Powder, protein equivalent (essential and non-essential amino acids except methionine) 13 g, carbohydrate 54 g, fat 23 g, energy 1990 kJ (475 kcal)/100 g, with vitamins, minerals, and trace elements; *standard dilution* (15%) provides protein equivalent 1.95 g, carbohydrate 8.1 g, fat 3.5 g, energy 300 kJ (72 kcal)/100 mL. Unflavoured, net price 400 g = £28.22 (5-g measuring scoop provided)

Nutritional supplement for the dietary management of hypermethioninaemia or homocystinuria

Hyperlysinaemia

¹XLYS Analog (SHS)

Powder, protein equivalent (essential and non-essential amino acids except lysine) 13 g, carbohydrate 54 g, fat 23 g, energy 1990 kJ (475 kcal)/100 g with vitamins, minerals, and trace elements; *standard dilution* (15%) provides protein equivalent 1.95 g, carbohydrate 8.1 g, fat 3.5 g, energy 300 kJ(72 kcal)/100 mL. Unflavoured, net price 400 g = £28.22 (5-g measuring scoop provided).

Nutritional supplement for the dietary management of hyperlysinaemia

Isovaleric acidaemia

¹XLEU Analog (SHS)

Powder, protein equivalent (essential and non-essential amino acids except leucine) 13 g, carbohydrate 54 g, fat 23 g, energy 1990 kJ (475 kcal)/100 g, with vitamins, minerals, and trace elements; *standard dilution* (15%) provides protein equivalent 1.95 g, carbohydrate 8.1 g, fat 3.5 g, energy 300 kJ (72 kcal)/100 mL. Unflavoured, net price 400 g = £28.22 (5-g measuring scoop provided)

Nutritional supplement for the dietary management of isovaleric acidaemia

XLEU Faladon (SHS)

Powder, protein equivalent (essential and non-essential amino acids except leucine) 77 g, carbohydrate 4.5 g, fat nil, energy 1386 kJ (326 kcal)/100 g with vitamins, minerals, and trace elements. Unflavoured, (flavouring:

Maple syrup urine disease

Isoleucine Amino Acid Supplement (Vitaflo)

Powder, isoleucine 50 mg, carbohydrate 4 g, fat nil, energy 64 kJ (15 kcal)/4-g, net price 30 × 4-g sachets = £42.23

Nutritional supplement for use in the dietary management of maple syrup urine disease and other inborn errors of amino acid metabolism in children over 1 year and adults

Mapleflex® (SHS)

Powder, protein equivalent (essential and non-essential amino acids except isoleucine, leucine, and valine) 8.4 g,

XMET Homidon (SHS)

Powder, protein equivalent (essential and non-essential amino acids, except methionine) 77 g, carbohydrate 4.5 g, fat nil, energy 1386 kJ (326 kcal)/100 g, with vitamins, minerals, and trace elements. Unflavoured, (flavouring: see *Modjul®* Flavour System, p. 909), net price 500 g = £145.76.

Nutritional supplement for the dietary management of hypermethioninaemia or homocystinuria in children

²XMET Maxamaid (SHS)

Powder, protein equivalent (essential and non-essential amino acids except methionine) 25 g, carbohydrate 51 g, fat less than 500 mg, energy 1311 kJ (309 kcal)/100 g, with vitamins, minerals, and trace elements. Unflavoured (flavouring: see *Modjul®* Flavour System, p. 909), net price 500 g = £76.94

Nutritional supplement for the dietary management of hypermethioninaemia or homocystinuria

³XMET Maxamum® (SHS)

Powder, protein equivalent (essential and non-essential amino acids except methionine) 39 g, carbohydrate 34 g, fat less than 500 mg, energy 1260 kJ (297 kcal)/100 g, with vitamins, minerals, and trace elements. Unflavoured, (flavouring: see *Modjul®* Flavour System, p. 909), net price 500 g = £123.34.

Nutritional supplement for the dietary management of hypermethioninaemia or homocystinuria

²XLYS Maxamaid (SHS)

Powder, protein equivalent (essential and non-essential amino acids except lysine) 25 g, carbohydrate 51 g, fat less than 500 mg, energy 1311 kJ (309 kcal)/100 g with vitamins, minerals, and trace elements. Unflavoured, (flavouring: see *Modjul®* Flavour System, p. 909), net price 500 g = £76.94.

Nutritional supplement for the dietary management of hyperlysinaemia

see *Modjul®* Flavour System, p. 909), net price 200 g = £58.29.

Nutritional supplement for the dietary management of isovaleric acidaemia in children

²XLEU Maxamaid (SHS)

Powder, protein equivalent (essential and non-essential amino acids except leucine) 25 g, carbohydrate 51 g, fat less than 500 mg, energy 1311 kJ (309 kcal)/100 g with vitamins, minerals, and trace elements. Unflavoured, (flavouring: see *Modjul®* Flavour System, p. 909), net price 500 g = £76.94.

Nutritional supplement for the dietary management of isovaleric acidaemia

carbohydrate 11 g, fat 3.9 g, energy 474 kJ (113 kcal)/29-g sachet, with vitamins, minerals, and trace elements. Unflavoured, (flavouring: see *Modjul®* Flavour System, p. 909), net price 30 × 29-g sachets = £162.82.

Nutritional supplement for the dietary management of maple syrup urine disease in children 1–10 years

MSUD Aid III® (SHS)

Powder, protein equivalent (essential and non-essential amino acids except isoleucine, leucine, and valine) 77 g, carbohydrate 4.5 g, fat nil, energy 1386 kJ (326 kcal)/

Appendix 2: Borderline substances

1. Analog products are generally intended for use in children up to 1 year
2. Maxamaid products are generally intended for use in children 1–8 years
3. Maxamum products are generally intended for use in children over 8 years

100 g with vitamins, minerals, and trace elements. Unflavoured, (flavouring: see *Modjul*® Flavour System, p. 909),
net price 500 g = £145.76.

Nutritional supplement for the dietary management of
maple syrup urine disease and related conditions in children and adults where it is necessary to limit the intake of
branched chain amino acids

¹**MSUD Analog** (SHS)
Powder, protein equivalent (essential and non-essential
amino acids except isoleucine, leucine, and valine) 13 g,
carbohydrate 54 g, fat 23 g, energy 1990 kJ (475 kcal)/
100 g, with vitamins, minerals, and trace elements; *standard dilution* (15%) provides protein equivalent 1.95g,
carbohydrate 8.1 g, fat 3.5 g, energy 300 kJ (72 kcal)/
100 mL. Unflavoured, net price 400 g = £28.22 (5-g measuring scoop provided).

Nutritional supplement for the dietary management of
maple syrup urine disease

MSUD express® (Vitaflo)
Powder, protein equivalent (essential and non-essential
amino acids except leucine, isoleucine, and valine) 15 g,
carbohydrate 3.8 g, fat less than 100 mg, energy 315 kJ
(75 kcal)/25 g, with vitamins, minerals, and trace elements. Unflavoured, (flavouring: see *Flavour Pac*®, p. 909),
net price 30 × 25-g sachets = £253.24.

Nutritional supplement for the dietary management of
maple syrup urine disease in children over 8 years and
adults

MSUD express cooler® (Vitaflo)
Liquid, protein equivalent (essential and non-essential
amino acids except leucine, isoleucine, and valine) 15 g,
carbohydrate 7.8 g, fat trace, energy 386 kJ (92 kcal)/130-
mL pouch, with vitamins, minerals, and trace elements.
Orange flavour, net price 30 × 130-mL = £258.30.

Nutritional supplement for the dietary management of
maple syrup urine disease in children over 3 years and
adults

MSUD Gel® (Vitaflo)
Powder, protein equivalent (essential and non-essential
amino acids except leucine, isoleucine, and valine) 8.4 g,
carbohydrate 8.6 g, fat less than 100 mg, energy 286 kJ
(68 kcal)/20 g, with vitamins, minerals, and trace elements. Unflavoured, (flavouring: see *Flavour Pac*®, p. 909),
net price 30 × 20-g sachets = £141.51.

Nutritional supplement for the dietary management of
maple syrup urine disease in children 1–10 years

²**MSUD Maxamaid**® (SHS)
Powder, protein equivalent (essential and non-essential
amino acids except isoleucine, leucine, and valine) 25 g,
carbohydrate 51 g, fat less than 500 mg, energy 1311 kJ
(309 kcal)/100 g, with vitamins, minerals, and trace elements. Unflavoured, (flavouring: see *Modjul*® Flavour
System, p. 909), net price 500 g = £76.94.

Nutritional supplement for the dietary management of
maple syrup urine disease

³**MSUD Maxamum**® (SHS)
Powder, protein equivalent (essential and non-essential
amino acids except isoleucine, leucine, and valine) 39 g,
carbohydrate 34 g, fat less than 500 mg, energy 1260 kJ
(297 kcal)/100 g, with vitamins, minerals, and trace elements. Orange flavour or unflavoured, (flavouring: see
Modjul® Flavour System, p. 909), net price 500 g =
£123.34.

Nutritional supplement for the dietary management of
maple syrup urine disease

Valine Amino Acid Supplement (Vitaflo)
Powder, valine 50 mg, carbohydrate 4 g, fat nil, energy
64 kJ (15 kcal)/4 g, net price 30 × 4-g sachets = £42.23

Nutritional supplement for the dietary management of
maple syrup urine disease and other inborn errors of
amino acid metabolism in children over 1 year

Methylmalonic propionic acidaemia

¹**XMTVI Analog** (SHS)
Powder, protein equivalent (essential and non-essential
amino acids except methionine, threonine, and valine, and
low isoleucine) 13 g, carbohydrate 54 g, fat 23 g, energy
1990 kJ (475 kcal)/100 g, with vitamins, minerals, and
trace elements; *standard dilution* (15%) provides protein
equivalent 1.95 g, carbohydrate 8.1 g, fat 3.5 g, energy
300 kJ (72 kcal)/100 mL. Unflavoured, net price 400 g =
£28.22 (5-g measuring scoop provided).

Nutritional supplement for the dietary management of
methylmalonic acidaemia or propionic acidaemia

XMTVI Asadon (SHS)
Powder, protein equivalent (essential and non-essential
amino acids except methionine, threonine, and valine, and
low isoleucine) 77 g, carbohydrate 4.5 g, fat nil, energy
1386 kJ (326 kcal)/100 g, with vitamins, minerals, and
trace elements. Unflavoured, (flavouring: see *Modjul*®
Flavour System, p. 909), net price 200 g = £58.29.

Nutritional supplement for the dietary management of
methylmalonic acidaemia or propionic acidaemia in
children and adults

²**XMTVI Maxamaid** (SHS)
Powder, protein equivalent (essential and non-essential
amino acids except methionine, threonine, and valine, and
low isoleucine) 25 g, carbohydrate 51 g, fat less than
500 mg, energy 1311 kJ (309 kcal)/100 g, with vitamins,
minerals, and trace elements. Unflavoured, (flavouring:
see *Modjul*® Flavour System, p. 909), net price 500 g =
£76.94.

Nutritional supplement for the dietary management of
methylmalonic acidaemia or propionic acidaemia

³**XMTVI Maxamum** (SHS)
Powder, protein equivalent (essential and non-essential
amino acids except methionine, threonine, and valine, and
low isoleucine) 39 g, carbohydrate 34 g, fat less than
500 mg, energy 1260 kJ (297 kcal)/100 g, with vitamins,
minerals, and trace elements. Unflavoured, (flavouring:
see *Modjul*® Flavour System, p. 909), net price 500 g =
£123.34.

Nutritional supplement for the dietary management of
methylmalonic acidaemia or propionic acidaemia

Other inborn errors of metabolism

Cystine Amino Acid Supplement (Vitaflo)
Powder, cystine 500 mg, carbohydrate 3.4 g, fat nil, energy
63 kJ (15 kcal)/4 g, net price 30 × 4-g sachets = £42.23

Nutritional supplement for the dietary management of
inborn errors of amino acid metabolism in children over 1
year

EAA® **Supplement** (Vitaflo)
Powder, protein equivalent (essential amino acids) 5 g,
carbohydrate 4 g, fat nil, energy 151 kJ (36 kcal)/12.5 g,
with vitamins, minerals, and trace elements. Tropical
flavour, net price 50 × 12.5-g sachets = £165.67

Nutritional supplement for the dietary management of
disorders of protein metabolism including urea cycle
disorders in children over 3 years

---

1. Analog products are generally intended for use in children up to 1 year
2. Maxamaid products are generally intended for use in children 1–8 years
3. Maxamum products are generally intended for use in children over 8 years

Key Omega® (Vitaflo)
Powder, protein (cows' milk, soya) 170 mg, carbohydrate 2.8 g, fat 800 mg (of which arachidonic acid 200 mg, docosahexaenoic acid 100 mg), energy 80 kJ (19 kcal)/4 g, net price 30 × 4-g sachet = £32.30
Nutritional supplement for the dietary management of inborn errors of metabolism

Leucine Amino Acid Supplement (Vitaflo)
Powder, leucine 100 mg, carbohydrate 4 g, fat nil, energy 64 kJ (15 kcal)/4 g, net price 30 × 4-g sachets = £42.23
Nutritional supplement for the dietary management of inborn errors of amino acid metabolism in children over 1 year

Phenylketonuria

Add-Ins® (SHS)
Powder, protein equivalent (containing essential and nonessential amino acids except phenylalanine) 10 g, carbohydrate nil, fat 5.1 g, energy 359 kJ (86 kcal)/18.2-g sachet, with vitamins, minerals, and trace elements. Unflavoured, net price 60 × 18.2-g sachets = £294.00.
Nutritional supplement for the dietary management of proven phenylketonuria in children over 4 years

Easiphen® (SHS)
Liquid, protein equivalent (containing essential and nonessential amino acids except phenylalanine) 6.7 g, carbohydrate 5.1 g, fat 2 g, energy 275 kJ (65 kcal)/100 mL with vitamins, minerals, and trace elements. Forest berries, orange, or tropical flavour, net price 250-mL carton = £7.56.
Nutritional supplement for the dietary management of proven phenylketonuria in children over 8 years

Lophlex® (SHS)
Powder, protein equivalent (essential and non-essential amino acids except phenylalanine) 20 g, carbohydrate 2.5 g, fat 60 mg, fibre 220 mg, energy 385 kJ (91 kcal)/27.8-g sachet, with vitamins, minerals, and trace elements. Flavours: berry, orange, or unflavoured, net price 30 x 27.8-g sachets = £226.87.
Nutritional supplement for the dietary management of proven phenylketonuria in children over 8 years and adults including pregnant women

Lophlex LQ® (SHS)
Liquid, protein equivalent (essential and non-essential amino acids except phenylalanine) 20 g, carbohydrate 8.8 g, fibre 340 mg, energy 490 kJ (115 kcal)/125 mL, with vitamins, minerals, and trace elements. Flavours: berry, citrus, or orange, net price 3 × 125 mL = £24.27.
Nutritional supplement for the dietary management of phenylketonuria in children over 8 years and adults including pregnant women

Lophlex® LQ 10 (SHS)
Liquid, protein equivalent (essential and non-essential amino acids except phenylalanine) 10 g, carbohydrate 4.4 g, fibre 170 mg, energy 245 kJ (58 kcal)/62.5 mL, with vitamins, minerals, and trace elements. Berry flavour, net price 60 × 62.5 mL = £243.00.
Nutritional supplement for the dietary management of phenylketonuria in children over 4 years and adults including pregnant women

Loprofin® PKU Drink (SHS)
Liquid, protein (cows' milk) 400 mg (phenylalanine 10 mg), lactose 9.4 g, fat 2 g, energy 165 kJ (40 kcal)/100 mL. Net price 200-mL carton = 60p.
Nutritional supplement for the dietary management of phenylketonuria in children over 1 year

Milupa PKU 2-prima® (Milupa)
Powder, protein equivalent (essential and non-essential amino acids except phenylalanine) 60 g, carbohydrate 10 g, fat nil, energy 1190 kJ (280 kcal)/100 g, with vitamins, minerals, and trace elements. Vanilla flavour, net price 500 g = £122.70
Nutritional supplement for the dietary management of phenylketonuria in children 1–8 years

Milupa PKU 2-secunda® (Milupa)
Powder, protein equivalent (essential and non-essential amino acids except phenylalanine) 70 g, carbohydrate 6.8 g, fat nil, energy 1306 kJ (307 kcal)/100 g, with vitamins, minerals, and trace elements. Vanilla flavour, net price 500 g = £143.15
Nutritional supplement for the dietary management of phenylketonuria in children 9–15 years

Milupa PKU 3-advanta® (Milupa)
Powder, protein equivalent (essential and non-essential amino acids except phenylalanine) 70 g, carbohydrate 4.7 g, fat nil, energy 1270 kJ (299 kcal)/100 g, with vitamins, minerals, and trace elements. Vanilla flavour, net price 500 g = £143.15
Nutritional supplement for the dietary management of phenylketonuria in children over 15 years

Minaphlex® (SHS)
Liquid, protein equivalent (essential and non-essential amino acids except phenylalanine) 8.4 g, carbohydrate 9.9 g, fat 3.9 g, energy 455 kJ (108 kcal)/29-g sachet, with vitamins, minerals, and trace elements. Chocolate, pineapple-vanilla. Unflavoured (carbohydrate 11 g, energy 474 kJ (113 kcal)/29-g sachet), net price 30 × 29-g sachets = £98.92.
Nutritional supplement for the dietary management of phenylketonuria in children 1–10 years

Phlexy-10® Exchange System (SHS)
Bar, protein equivalent (essential and non-essential amino acids except phenylalanine) 8.33 g, carbohydrate 20.5 g, fat 3.7 g, fibre 1.7 g/42-g bar. Citrus fruit flavour. Net price per bar = £4.76

Capsules, protein equivalent (essential and non-essential amino acids except phenylalanine) 416.5 mg/capsule. Net price 200-cap pack = £33.33

Tablets, protein equivalent (essential and non-essential amino acids except phenylalanine) 833 mg tablet. Net price 75-tab pack = £21.59

Drink Mix, powder, (essential and non-essential amino acids except phenylalanine) 8.33 g, carbohydrate 8.8 g/20-g sachet. Apple-black currant, citrus, or tropical flavour. Net price 30 × 20-g sachet = £100.51
Nutritional supplement for the dietary management of phenylketonuria

Phlexy-Vits® (SHS)
Powder, vitamins, minerals, and trace elements, net price 30 × 7-g sachets = £56.08.

Tablets, vitamins, minerals, and trace elements, net price 180-tab pack = £68.69.
For use as a vitamin and mineral component of restricted therapeutic diets in children over 11 years and adults with phenylketonuria and similar amino acid abnormalities

PK Aid 4® (SHS)
Powder, protein equivalent (essential and non-essential amino acids except phenylalanine) 79 g, carbohydrate 4.5 g, fat nil, energy 1420 kJ (334 kcal)/100 g. Unflavoured, (flavouring: see *Modjul®* Flavour System, p. 909), net price 500 g = £112.04 (5-g measuring scoop provided).
Nutritional supplement for the dietary management of phenylketonuria in children and adults

PKU Anamix Junior LQ® (SHS)
Liquid, protein equivalent (essential and non-essential amino acids except phenylalanine) 10 g, carbohydrate 8.8 g, fat 4.8 g, fibre 310 mg, energy 497 kJ (118 kcal)/125 mL, with vitamins, minerals, and trace elements. Lactose-free. Flavours: Berry or orange, net price 125-mL

carton = £4.50
Nutritional supplement for the dietary supplement of
phenyketonuria in children 1–10 years

PKU cooler10® (Vitaflo)
Liquid, protein equivalent (essential and non-essential
amino acids except phenylalanine) 10 g, carbohydrate
5.1 g, energy 258 kJ (62 kcal)/87-mL pouch, with vitamins, minerals, and trace elements. Orange or purple
option, net price 30 × 87-mL = £105.00.
Nutritional supplement for the dietary management of
phenylketonuria in children over 3 years

PKU cooler15® (Vitaflo)
Liquid, protein equivalent (essential and non-essential
amino acids except phenylalanine) 15 g, carbohydrate
7.8 g, energy 386 kJ (92 kcal)/130-mL pouch, with vitamins, minerals, and trace elements. Orange or purple
option, net price 30 x 130 mL = £156.60.
Nutritional supplement for the dietary management of
phenylketonuria in children over 3 years

PKU cooler20® (Vitaflo)
Liquid, protein equivalent (essential and non-essential
amino acids except phenylalanine) 20 g, carbohydrate
10.2 g, energy 517 kJ (124 kcal)/174 mL pouch, with
vitamins, minerals, and trace elements. Orange or purple
option, net price 30 × 174 mL = £210.00.
Nutritional supplement for the dietary management of
phenylketonuria in children over 3 years

PKU express® (Vitaflo)
Powder, protein equivalent (essential and non-essential
amino acids except phenylalanine) 15 g, carbohydrate
3.8 g, energy 315 kJ (76 kcal)/25 g, with vitamins, minerals, and trace elements. Lemon, orange, tropical, or
unflavoured, net price 30 x 25-g sachets = £153.53.
Nutritional supplement for the dietary management of
phenylketonuria in children over 8 years

PKU gel® (Vitaflo)
Powder, protein equivalent (essential and non-essential
amino acids except phenylalanine) 8.4 g, carbohydrate
8.6 g, fat less than 100 mg, energy 286 kJ (68 kcal)/20 g,
with vitamins, minerals and trace elements. Orange,
raspberry, or unflavoured (flavouring: see *Flavour Pac®*,
p. 909), net price 30 × 20-g sachets = £88.51.
For use as part of the low-protein dietary management of
phenylketonuria in children 1–10 years

PKU Start® (Vitaflo)
Liquid, protein equivalent (essential and non-essential
amino acids except phenylalanine) 2 g, carbohydrate
8.3 g, fat 2.9 g, energy 286 kJ (68 kcal)/100 mL with vita-

mins, minerals, and trace elements. Contains lactose and
fish oil. Net price 500-mL bottle = £5.30
For the dietary management of phenylketonuria in children under 12 months

L-Tyrosine (SHS)
Powder, net price 100 g = £12.53.
For use as a supplement in maternal phenylketonurics
who have low plasma tyrosine concentrations

[1]XP Analog (SHS)
Powder, protein equivalent (essential and non-essential
amino acids except phenylalanine) 13 g, carbohydrate
54 g, fat 23 g (of which LCT 95%), energy 1990 kJ
(475 kcal)/100 g, with vitamins, minerals, and trace elements; *standard dilution* (15%) provides protein equivalent
1.95 g, carbohydrate 8.1 g, fat 3.5 g, energy 300 kJ
(72 kcal)/100 mL. Net price 400 g = £22.54 (5-g measuring
scoop provided).
Nutritional supplement for the dietary management of
phenylketonuria in children under 1 year

XP Analog LCP (SHS)
Powder, protein equivalent (essential and non-essential
amino acids except phenylalanine) 13 g, carbohydrate
54 g, fat 23 g (of which LCT 98.7%), energy 1990 kJ
(475 kcal)/100 g, with vitamins, minerals, and trace elements; *standard dilution* (15%) provides protein equivalent
1.95 g, carbohydrate 8.1 g, fat 3.5 g, energy 300 kJ
(72 kcal)/100 mL Net price 400 g = £25.64 (5-g measuring
scoop provided).
Nutritional supplement for the dietary management of
phenylketonuria in children under 1 year

[2]XP Maxamaid (SHS)
Powder, protein equivalent (essential and non-essential
amino acids except phenylalanine) 25 g, carbohydrate
51 g, fat less than 500 mg, energy 1311 kJ (309 kcal)/
100 g, with vitamins, minerals, and trace elements.
Orange flavour, or unflavoured, net price 500 g = £45.52.
Nutritional supplement for the dietary management of
phenylketonuria in children 1– 8 years

[3]XP Maxamum® (SHS)
Powder, protein equivalent (essential and non-essential
amino acids except phenylalanine) 39 g, carbohydrate
34 g, fat less than 500 mg, energy 1260 kJ (297 kcal)/
100 g, with vitamins, minerals, and trace elements.
Orange, or unflavoured, net price 30 × 50-g sachets =
£211.14, 500 g = £70.39.
Nutritional supplement for the dietary management of
phenylketonuria in children over 8 years

Tyrosinaemia

TYR cooler® (Vitaflo)
Liquid, protein equivalent (essential and non-essential
amino acids except tyrosine and phenylalanine) 15 g,
carbohydrate 7.8 g, fat nil, energy 386 kJ (92 kcal)/
130 mL, with vitamins, minerals, and trace elements.
Orange flavour, net price 30 × 130-mL pouch = £258.30.
Nutritional supplement for the dietary management of
tyrosinaemia in children over 8 years

TYR express® (Vitaflo)
Powder, protein equivalent (essential and non-essential
amino acids except tyrosine and phenylalanine) 15 g,
carbohydrate 3.8 g, fat less than 100 mg, energy 315 kJ
(76 kcal)/25 g, with vitamins, minerals, and trace elements. Unflavoured (flavouring: see *Flavour Pac®*, p. 909),
net price 30 × 25-g sachets = £253.24
Nutritional supplement for the dietary management of
tyrosinaemia in children over 8 years

TYR Gel® (Vitaflo)
Gel, protein equivalent (essential and non-essential amino
acids except tyrosine and phenylalanine) 8.4 g, carbohydrate 8.6 g, fat less than 100 mg, energy 286 kJ (68 kcal)/
20 g, with vitamins, minerals, and trace elements. Unflavoured (flavouring: see *Flavour Pac®*, p. 909), net price 30
× 20-g sachets = £141.51
Nutritional supplement for the dietary management of
tyrosinaemia in children 1–10 years

Tyrosine Amino Acid Supplement (Vitaflo)
Powder, tyrosine 1 g, carbohydrate 2.9 g, energy 62 kJ
(15 kcal)/4-g sachet, net price 30 × 4-g sachet = £37.80.
Nutritional supplement for the dietary management of
tyrosinaemia and other inborn errors of amino acid
metabolism

1. Analog products are generally intended for use in children up to 1 year
2. Maxamaid products are generally intended for use in children 1–8 years
3. Maxamum products are generally intended for use in children over 8 years

¹**XPHEN TYR Analog** (SHS)
Powder, protein equivalent (essential and non-essential amino acids except phenylalanine and tyrosine) 13 g, carbohydrate 54 g, fat 23 g (of which LCT 95%), energy 1990 kJ (475 kcal)/100 g, with vitamins, minerals, and trace elements; *standard dilution* (15%) provides protein equivalent 1.95 g, carbohydrate 8.1 g, fat 3.5 g, energy 300 kJ (72 kcal)/100 mL. Unflavoured, net price 400 g = £28.22.
Nutritional supplement for dietary management of tyrosinaemia in children under 1 year

²**XPHEN TYR Maxamaid** (SHS)
Powder, protein equivalent (essential and non-essential amino acids except phenylalanine and tyrosine) 25 g, carbohydrate 51 g, fat less than 500 mg, energy 1311 kJ (309 kcal)/100 g, with vitamins, minerals, and trace elements. Unflavoured (flavouring: see *Modjul®* Flavour System, p. 909), net price 500 g = £76.94.
Nutritional supplement for the dietary management of tyrosinaemia in children 1–8 years

XPHEN TYR Tyrosidon (SHS)
Powder, protein equivalent (essential and non-essential amino acids except phenylalanine and tyrosine) 77 g, carbohydrate 4.5 g, fat nil, energy 1386 kJ (326 kcal)/

100 g. Unflavoured (flavouring: see *Modjul®* Flavour System, p. 909), net price 500 g = £145.76
Nutritional supplement for the management of tyrosinaemia in children and adults where plasma-methionine concentrations are normal

¹**XPTM Analog** (SHS)
Powder, protein equivalent (essential and non-essential amino acids except methionine, phenylalanine, and tyrosine) 13 g, carbohydrate 54 g, fat 23 g (of which LCT 95%), energy 1990 kJ (475 kcal)/100 g, with vitamins, minerals, and trace elements, *standard dilution* (15%) provides protein equivalent 1.95 g, carbohydrate 8.1 g, fat 3.5 g, energy 300 kJ (72 kcal)/100 mL. Unflavoured, net price 400 g = £28.22
Nutritional supplement for the dietary management of tyrosinaemia type 1 in children under 1 year

XPTM Tyrosidon (SHS)
Powder, protein equivalent (essential and non-essential amino acids except methionine, phenylalanine, and tyrosine) 77 g, carbohydrate 4.5 g, fat nil, energy 1386 kJ (326 kcal)/100 g. Unflavoured (flavouring: see *Modjul®* Flavour System, p. 909), net price 500 g = £145.76.
Nutritional supplement for the dietary management of tyrosinaemia type I in children and adults where plasma-methionine concentrations are above normal

Urea cycle disorders (other than arginase deficiency)

L-Arginine (SHS)
Powder, net price 100 g = £10.64.
For use as a supplement in urea cycle disorders other than arginase deficiency, such as hyperammonaemia types I and II, citrullaemia, arginosuccinic aciduria, and deficiency of N-acetyl glutamate synthetase

Conditions for which ACBS products can be prescribed

Note This is a list of clinical conditions for which the ACBS has approved toilet preparations. For details of the preparations see Chapter 13.

Birthmarks
See Disfiguring skin lesions, below

Dermatitis
Aveeno Bath Oil; Aveeno Cream; Aveeno Colloidal; E45 Emollient Bath Oil; E45 Emollient Wash Cream; E45 Lotion

Dermatitis herpetiformis
See also Gluten-sensitive enteropathies, p. 910

Disfiguring skin lesions (birthmarks, mutilating lesions, scars, vitiligo)
Covermark classic foundation and finishing powder; Dermacolor Camouflage cream and fixing powder; Keromask masking cream and finishing powder; Veil Cover cream and Finishing Powder. (Cleansing Creams, Cleansing Milks, and Cleansing Lotions are excluded)

Disinfectants (antiseptics)
May be prescribed on an FP10 only when ordered in such quantities and with such directions as are appropriate for the treatment of patients, but not for general hygenic purposes.

Eczema
See Dermatitis, above

Photodermatoses (skin protection in)
Delph Sun Lotion SPF 30; E45 Sun SPF 50; Spectraban Ultra; Sunsense Ultra; Uvistat Lipscreen SPF 50, Uvistat Suncream SPF 30 and 50.

Pruritus
See Dermatitis, above

1. Analog products are generally intended for use in children up to 1 year
2. Maxamaid products are generally intended for use in children 1–8 years

A3 Cautionary and advisory labels for dispensed medicines

Preparations in the *BNF for Children* include code numbers of the cautionary labels that pharmacists are recommended to add when dispensing. It is also expected that, when necessary, pharmacists will counsel children or their carers.

Counselling needs to be related to the age, experience, background, and understanding of the child or carer. The pharmacist should ensure understanding of how to take or use the medicine and how to follow the correct dosage schedule. Any effects of the medicine on co-ordination, performance of skilled tasks, any foods or medicines to be avoided, and what to do if a dose is missed should also be explained. Other matters, such as the possibility of staining of the clothes or skin, or discoloration of urine or stools by a medicine should also be mentioned.

For some preparations there is a special need for counselling, such as an unusual method or time of administration or a potential interaction with a common food or domestic remedy, and this should be mentioned where necessary.

Original packs   Most preparations are now dispensed in unbroken original packs (see Patient Packs, p. xii) that include further advice for the patient in the form of patient information leaflets. The advice in patient information leaflets may be less appropriate when the medicine is for a child, particularly for unlicensed medicines or indications. Pharmacists should explain discrepancies to carers, if necessary. The patient information leaflet should only be withheld in exceptional circumstances because it contains other information that should be provided. Label 10 may be of value where appropriate. More general leaflets advising on the administration of preparations such as eye drops, eye ointments, inhalers, and suppositories are also available.

Scope of labels   In general, no label recommendations are provided for injections on the assumption that they will be administered by a healthcare professional or a well-instructed child or carer. The labelling is not exhaustive and pharmacists are recommended to use their professional discretion in labelling new preparations and those for which no labels are shown.

Individual labelling advice is not given on the administration of the large variety of antacids. In the absence of instructions from the prescriber, and if on enquiry the patient has had no verbal instructions, the directions given under 'Dose' should be used on the label.

It is recognised that there may be occasions when pharmacists will use their knowledge and professional discretion and decide to omit one or more of the recommended labels for a particular child. In this case counselling is of the utmost importance. There may also be an occasion when a prescriber does not wish additional cautionary labels to be used, in which case the prescription should be endorsed 'NCL' (no cautionary labels). The exact wording that is required instead should then be specified on the prescription.

Pharmacists label medicines with various wordings in addition to those directions specified on the prescription. Such labels include 'Shake the bottle', 'For external use only', and 'Store in a cool place', as well as 'Discard . . . . days after opening' and 'Do not use after . . . .', which apply particularly to antibiotic mixtures, diluted liquid and topical preparations, and to eye-drops. Although not listed in the *BNF for Children* these labels should continue to be used when appropriate; indeed, 'For external use only' is a legal requirement on external liquid preparations, while 'Keep out of the reach of children' is a legal requirement on all dispensed medicines. Care should be taken not to obscure other relevant information with adhesive labelling.

It is the usual practice for patients to take standard tablets with water or other liquid and for this reason no separate label has been recommended.

The label wordings recommended by the *BNF for Children* apply to medicines dispensed against a prescription. Children and carers should be made aware that a dispensed medicine should never be taken by, or shared with, anyone other than for whom the prescriber intended it. Therefore, the *BNF for Children* does not include warnings against the use of a dispensed medicine by persons other than for whom it was specifically prescribed.

The label or labels for each preparation are recommended after careful consideration of the information available. However, it is recognised that in some cases this information may be either incomplete or open to a different interpretation. The BNF will therefore be grateful to receive any constructive comments on the labelling suggested for any preparation.

Recommended label wordings

Wordings which can be given as separate warnings are labels 1–19 and labels 29–33. Wordings which can be incorporated in an appropriate position in the directions for dosage or administration are labels 21–28. A label has been omitted for number 20.

If separate labels are used it is recommended that the wordings be used without modification. If changes are made to suit computer requirements, care should be taken to retain the sense of the original.

1   Warning. May cause drowsiness

To be used on *preparations for children* containing antihistamines, or other preparations given to children where the warnings of label 2 on driving or alcohol would not be appropriate.

2   Warning. May cause drowsiness. If affected do not drive or operate machinery. Avoid alcoholic drink

To be used on *preparations for adults that can cause drowsiness*, thereby affecting coordination and the ability to drive and operate hazardous machinery; label 1 is more appropriate for children. *It is an offence to drive while under the influence of drink or drugs.* It should be remembered that children and adolescents do, on occasion, consume alcohol and should be made aware of potential problems.

Some of these preparations only cause drowsiness in the first few days of treatment and some only cause drowsiness in higher doses.

In such cases the patient should be told that the advice applies until the effects have worn off. However many of these preparations can produce a slowing of reaction time and a loss of mental concentration that can have the same effects as drowsiness.

Avoidance of alcoholic drink is recommended because the effects of CNS depressants are enhanced by alcohol. Strict prohibition however could lead to some patients not taking the medicine. Pharmacists should therefore explain the risk and encourage compliance, particularly in patients who may think they already tolerate the effects of alcohol (see also label 3). Queries from patients with epilepsy regarding fitness to drive should be referred back to the patient's doctor.

Side-effects unrelated to drowsiness that may affect a patient's ability to drive or operate machinery safely include *blurred vision, dizziness, or nausea*. In general, no label has been recommended to cover these cases, but the patient should be suitably counselled.

3   Warning. May cause drowsiness. If affected do not drive or operate machinery

To be used on *preparations containing monoamine-oxidase inhibitors*; the warning to avoid alcohol and dealcoholised (low alcohol) drink is covered by the patient information leaflet.

Also to be used as for label 2 but where alcohol is not an issue.

4   Warning. Avoid alcoholic drink

To be used on *preparations where a reaction such as flushing may occur if alcohol is taken* (e.g. metronidazole and chlorpropamide). Alcohol may also enhance the hypoglycaemia produced by some oral antidiabetic drugs but routine application of a warning label is not considered necessary.

5   Do not take indigestion remedies at the same time of day as this medicine

To be used with label 25 on *preparations coated to resist gastric acid* (e.g. enteric-coated tablets). This is to avoid the possibility of premature dissolution of the coating in the presence of an alkaline pH.

Label 5 also applies to drugs such as ketoconazole *where the absorption is significantly affected by antacids*; the usual period of avoidance recommended is 2 to 4 hours.

6   Do not take indigestion remedies or medicines containing iron or zinc at the same time of day as this medicine

To be used on *preparations containing ofloxacin and some other quinolones, doxycycline, lymecycline, minocycline, and penicillamine*. These drugs chelate calcium, iron and zinc and are less well absorbed when taken with calcium-containing antacids or preparations containing iron or zinc. These incompatible preparations should be taken 2-3 hours apart.

7   Do not take milk, indigestion remedies, or medicines containing iron or zinc at the same time of day as this medicine

To be used on *preparations containing ciprofloxacin, norfloxacin or tetracyclines that chelate calcium, iron, magnesium, and zinc*, and are thus less available for absorption; these incompatible preparations should be taken 2-3 hours apart. Doxycycline, lymecycline and minocycline are less liable to form chelates and therefore only require label 6 (see above).

8   Do not stop taking this medicine except on your doctor's advice

To be used on *preparations that contain a drug which is required to be taken over long periods without the patient necessarily perceiving any benefit* (e.g. antituberculous drugs).

Also to be used on *preparations that contain a drug whose withdrawal is likely to be a particular hazard* (e.g. clonidine for hypertension). Label 10 (see below) is more appropriate for corticosteroids.

9 **Take at regular intervals. Complete the prescribed course unless otherwise directed**

To be used on *preparations where a course of treatment should be completed* to reduce the incidence of relapse or failure of treatment.

The preparations are antimicrobial drugs given by mouth. Very occasionally, some may have severe side-effects (e.g. diarrhoea in patients receiving clindamycin) and in such cases the patient may need to be advised of reasons for stopping treatment quickly and returning to the doctor.

10 **Warning. Follow the printed instructions you have been given with this medicine**

To be used particularly on *preparations containing anticoagulants, lithium and oral corticosteroids.* The appropriate treatment card should be given to the patient and any necessary explanations given.

This label may also be used on other preparations to remind the patient of the instructions that have been given.

11 **Avoid exposure of skin to direct sunlight or sun lamps**

To be used on *preparations that may cause phototoxic or photoallergic reactions* if the patient is exposed to ultraviolet radiation. Many drugs other than those listed (e.g. phenothiazines and sulphonamides) may, on rare occasions, cause reactions in susceptible patients. Exposure to high intensity ultraviolet radiation from sunray lamps and sunbeds is particularly likely to cause reactions.

12 **Do not take anything containing aspirin while taking this medicine**

To be used on *preparations containing probenecid and sulfinpyrazone* whose activity is reduced by aspirin.

Label 12 should not be used for anticoagulants since label 10 is more appropriate.

13 **Dissolve or *mix with water* before taking**

To be used on *preparations that are intended to be dissolved in water* (e.g. soluble tablets) or *mixed with water* (e.g. powders, granules) before use. In a few cases other liquids such as fruit juice or milk may be used.

14 **This medicine may colour the urine**

To be used on *preparations that may cause the patient's urine to turn an unusual colour.* These include phenolphthalein (alkaline urine pink), triamterene (blue under some lights), levodopa (dark reddish), and rifampicin (red).

15 **Caution flammable: keep away from fire or flames**

To be used on *preparations containing sufficient flammable solvent to render them flammable if exposed to a naked flame.*

16 **Allow to dissolve under the tongue. Do not transfer from this container. Keep tightly closed. Discard eight weeks after opening**

To be used on *glyceryl trinitrate tablets* to remind the patient not to transfer them to plastic or less suitable containers.

17 **Do not take more than . . . in 24 hours**

To be used on *preparations for the treatment of acute migraine* except those containing ergotamine, for which label 18 is used. The dose form should be specified, e.g. tablets or capsules.

It may also be used on preparations for which no dose has been specified by the prescriber.

18 **Do not take more than . . . in 24 hours or . . . in any one week**

To be used on preparations containing ergotamine. The dose form should be specified, e.g. tablets or suppositories.

19 **Warning. Causes drowsiness which may continue the next day. If affected do not drive or operate machinery. Avoid alcoholic drink**

To be used on *preparations containing hypnotics (or some other drugs with sedative effects) prescribed to be taken at night.* On the rare occasions (e.g.

nitrazepam in epilepsy) when hypnotics are prescribed for daytime administration this label would clearly not be appropriate. Also to be used as an *alternative to the label 2 wording* (the choice being at the discretion of the pharmacist) *for anxiolytics prescribed to be taken at night.*

It is hoped that this wording will convey adequately the problem of residual morning sedation after taking 'sleeping tablets'.

21 **. . . with or after food**

To be used on *preparations that are liable to cause gastric irritation, or those that are better absorbed with food.*

Patients should be advised that a *small amount of food is sufficient.*

22 **. . . half to one hour before food**

To be used on some preparations *whose absorption is thereby improved.*

Most oral antibacterials require label 23 instead (see below).

23 **. . . an hour before food or on an empty stomach**

To be used on *oral preparations whose absorption may be reduced by the presence of food and acid in the stomach.*

24 **. . . sucked or chewed**

To be used on *preparations that should be sucked or chewed.*

The pharmacist should use discretion as to which of these words is appropriate.

25 **. . . swallowed whole, not chewed**

To be used on *preparations that are enteric-coated or designed for modified-release.*

Also to be used on *preparations that taste very unpleasant or may damage the mouth* if not swallowed whole.

26 **. . . dissolved under the tongue**

To be used on *preparations designed for sublingual use.* Patients should be advised to hold under the tongue and avoid swallowing until dissolved. The buccal mucosa between the gum and cheek is occasionally specified by the prescriber.

27 **. . . with plenty of water**

To be used on *preparations that should be well diluted* (e.g. chloral hydrate), *where a high fluid intake is required* (e.g. sulphonamides), or *where water is required to aid the action* (e.g. methylcellulose). The patient should be advised that 'plenty' means at least 150 mL (about a tumblerful). In most cases fruit juice, tea, or coffee may be used.

28 **To be spread thinly . . .**

To be used on *external preparations* that should be applied sparingly (e.g. corticosteroids, dithranol).

29 **Do not take more than 2 at any one time. Do not take more than 8 in 24 hours**

To be used on containers of dispensed *solid dose preparations containing paracetamol for adults when the instruction on the label indicates that the dose can be taken on an 'as required' basis.* The dose form should be specified, e.g. tablets or capsules.

This label has been introduced because of the serious consequences of overdosage with paracetamol.

30 **Do not take with any other paracetamol products**

To be used on all containers of dispensed *preparations containing paracetamol.*

31 **Contains aspirin and paracetamol. Do not take with any other paracetamol products**

To be used on all containers of dispensed *preparations containing aspirin and paracetamol.*

32 **Contains aspirin**

To be used on containers of dispensed *preparations containing aspirin when the name on the label does not include the word 'aspirin'.*

33 **Contains an aspirin-like medicine**

To be used on containers of dispensed *preparations containing aspirin derivatives.*

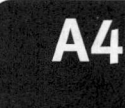Intravenous infusions for neonatal intensive care

Intravenous policy A local policy on the dilution of drugs with intravenous fluids should be drawn up by a multi-disciplinary team and issued as a document to the members of staff concerned.

Centralised additive services are provided in a number of hospital pharmacy departments and should be used in preference to making additions on wards.

The information that follows should be read in conjunction with local policy documents.

Guidelines

1. Drugs should only be diluted with infusion fluid when constant plasma concentrations are needed or when the administration of a more concentrated solution would be harmful.
2. In general, only one drug should be mixed with an infusion fluid in a syringe and the components should be compatible. Ready-prepared solutions should be used whenever possible. Drugs should not normally be added to blood products, mannitol, or sodium bicarbonate. Only specially formulated additives should be used with fat emulsions or amino-acid solutions (section 9.3).
3. Solutions should be thoroughly mixed by shaking and checked for absence of particulate matter before use.
4. Strict asepsis should be maintained throughout and in general the giving set should not be used for more than 24 hours (for drug admixtures).
5. The infusion syringe should be labelled with the neonate's name and hospital number, the name and quantity of drug, the infusion fluid, and the expiry date and time. If a problem occurs during administration, containers should be retained for a period after use in case they are needed for investigation.
6. Administration using a suitable motorised syringe driver is advocated for preparations where strict control over administration is required.
7. It is good practice to examine intravenous infusions from time to time while they are running. If cloudiness, crystallisation, change of colour, or any other sign of interaction or contamination is observed the infusion should be discontinued.

Problems

Microbial contamination The accidental entry and subsequent growth of micro-organisms converts the infusion fluid pathway into a potential vehicle for infection with micro-organisms, particularly species of Candida, Enterobacter, and Klebsiella. Ready-prepared infusions containing the additional drugs, or infusions prepared by an additive service (when available) should therefore be used in preference to making extemporaneous additions to infusion containers on wards etc. However, when this is necessary strict aseptic procedure should be followed.

Incompatibility Physical and chemical incompatibilities may occur with loss of potency, increase in toxicity, or other adverse effect. The solutions may become opalescent or precipitation may occur, but in many instances there is no visual indication of incompatibility. Interaction may take place at any point in the infusion fluid pathway, and the potential for incompatibility is increased when more than one substance is added to the infusion fluid.

Common incompatibilities Precipitation reactions are numerous and varied and may occur as a result of pH, concentration changes, 'salting-out' effects, complexation or other chemical changes. Precipitation or other particle formation must be avoided since, apart from lack of control of dosage on administration, it may initiate or exacerbate adverse effects. This is particularly important in the case of drugs which have been implicated in either thrombophlebitis (e.g. diazepam) or in skin sloughing or necrosis caused by extravasation (e.g. sodium bicarbonate and parenteral nutrition). It is also especially important to effect solution of colloidal drugs and to prevent their subsequent precipitation in order to avoid a pyrogenic reaction (e.g. amphotericin).

It is considered undesirable to mix beta-lactam antibiotics, such as semi-synthetic penicillins and cephalosporins, with proteinaceous materials on the grounds that immunogenic and allergenic conjugates could be formed.

A number of preparations undergo significant loss of potency when added singly or in combination to large volume infusions. Examples include ampicillin in infusions that contain glucose or lactates.

Blood Because of the large number of incompatibilities, drugs should not be added to blood and blood products for infusion purposes. Examples of incompatibility with blood include hypertonic mannitol solutions (irreversible crenation of red cells), dextrans (rouleaux formation and interference with cross-matching), glucose (clumping of red cells), and oxytocin (inactivated).

If the giving set is not changed after the administration of blood, but used for other infusion fluids, a fibrin clot may form which, apart from blocking the set, increases the likelihood of microbial growth.

Intravenous fat emulsions These may break down with coalescence of fat globules and separation of phases when additions such as antibacterials or electrolytes are made, thus increasing the possibility of embolism. Only specially formulated products such as *Vitlipid N*® (section 9.3) may be added to appropriate intravenous fat emulsions.

Other infusions Infusions that frequently give rise to incompatibility include amino acids, mannitol, and sodium bicarbonate.

Method

Ready-prepared infusions should be used whenever available. When addition is required to be made extemporaneously, any product reconstitution instructions such as those relating to concentration, vehicle, mixing, and handling precautions should be strictly followed using an aseptic technique throughout. Once the product has been reconstituted, further dilution with the infusion fluid should be made immediately in order to minimise microbial contamination and, with certain products, to prevent degradation or other formulation change which may occur; e.g. reconstituted ampicillin injection degrades rapidly on standing, and also may form polymers which could cause sensitivity reactions.

It is also important in certain instances that an infusion fluid of specific pH be used (e.g. **furosemide** injection requires dilution in infusions of pH greater than 5.5).

When drug dilutions are made it is important to mix thoroughly; additions should not be made to an infusion container that has been connected to a giving set, as mixing is hampered. If the solutions are not thoroughly mixed, a concentrated layer of the drug may form owing to differences in density. **Potassium chloride** is particularly prone to this 'layering' effect when added without adequate mixing to infusions; if such a mixture is administered it may have a serious effect on the heart.

A time limit between dilution and completion of administration must be imposed for certain admixtures to guarantee satisfactory drug potency and compatibility. For admixtures in which degradation occurs without the formation of toxic substances, an acceptable limit is the time taken for 10% decomposition of the drug. When toxic substances are produced stricter limits may be imposed. Because of the risk of microbial contamination a maximum time limit of 24 hours may be appropriate for additions made elsewhere than in hospital pharmacies offering central additive service.

Certain injections must be protected from light during continuous infusion to minimise oxidation, e.g. amphotericin and sodium nitroprusside.

![ ] **Table of drugs given by continuous intravenous infusion to neonates**
The table lists key drugs given by continuous intravenous infusion to neonates.

> Covers addition to *Glucose intravenous infusion* 5% and 10% and *Sodium chloride intravenous infusion* 0.9%. Compatibility with glucose 5% and with sodium chloride 0.9% indicates compatibility with *Sodium chloride and glucose intravenous infusion*. Infusion of a large volume of hypotonic solution should be avoided, therefore care should be taken if water for injections is used.

Adrenaline/Epinephrine (p. 146)

Dilute 3 mg/kg body-weight to a final volume of 50 mL with Glucose 5% *or* Sodium Chloride 0.9%; an intravenous infusion rate of 0.1 mL/hour provides a dose of 100 nanograms/kg/minute; infuse through a central venous catheter. Incompatible with bicarbonate and alkaline solutions.
Note Usually made up with adrenaline 1 in 1000 (1 mg/mL) solution; this concentration of adrenaline is not licensed for intravenous administration

Alprostadil (*Prostin VR®*) (p. 166)

Dilute 150 micrograms/kg body-weight to a final volume of 50 mL with Glucose 5% *or* Sodium Chloride 0.9%; an intravenous infusion rate of 0.1 mL/hour provides a dose of 5 nanograms/kg/minute. Undiluted solution must not come into contact with the barrel of the plastic syringe; add the required volume of alprostadil to a volume of infusion fluid in the syringe, and then make up to final volume

Atracurium besilate (p. 780)

Dilute 60 mg/kg body-weight to a final volume of 50 mL with Glucose 5% *or* Sodium Chloride 0.9%; an intravenous infusion rate of 0.1 mL/hour provides a dose of 120 micrograms/kg/hour; minimum concentration of 500 micrograms/mL, max. concentration of 5 mg/mL.

Dobutamine (as hydrochloride) (p. 143)

Dilute 30 mg/kg body-weight to a final volume of 50 mL with Glucose 5% *or* Sodium Chloride 0.9%; an intravenous infusion rate of 0.5 mL/hour provides a dose of 5 micrograms/kg/minute; max. concentration of 5 mg/mL; infuse higher concentration solutions through central venous catheter only. Incompatible with bicarbonate and other strong alkaline solutions

Dopamine hydrochloride (p. 143)

Dilute 30 mg/kg body-weight to a final volume of 50 mL with Glucose 5% *or* Sodium Chloride 0.9%; an intravenous infusion rate of 0.3 mL/hour provides a dose of 3 micrograms/kg/minute; max. concentration of 3.2 mg/mL; infuse higher concentration solutions through central venous catheter. Incompatible with bicarbonate and other alkaline solutions

Glyceryl trinitrate (p. 135)

Dilute 3 mg/kg body-weight to a final volume of 50 mL with Glucose 5% *or* Sodium Chloride 0.9%; an intravenous infusion rate of 1 mL/hour provides a dose of 1 microgram/kg/minute; max. concentration of 400 micrograms/mL (but concentration of 1 mg/mL has been used via a central venous catheter).
Note Glass or polyethylene apparatus is preferable; loss of potency will occur if PVC is used

Heparin (as sodium) (p. 148)

Maintenance of umbilical arterial catheter, dilute 50 units to a final volume of 50 mL with Sodium Chloride 0.45% *or* use ready-made bag containing 500 units in 500 mL Sodium Chloride 0.9%; infuse at 0.5 mL/hour

Treatment of thrombosis, dilute 1250 units/kg body-weight to a final volume of 50 mL with Glucose 5% *or* Sodium Chloride 0.9%; an intravenous infusion rate of 1 mL/hour provides a dose of 25 units/kg/hour

Insulin (soluble) (p. 423)

Dilute 5 units to a final volume of 50 mL with Sodium Chloride 0.9% and mix thoroughly; an intravenous infusion rate of 0.1 mL/kg/hour provides a dose of 0.01 units/kg/hour
Note Insulin may be absorbed by plastics, flush giving set with 5 mL of infusion fluid containing insulin

> Intravenous infusion information for neonatal intensive care *only*; for information in other children, see individual drug monographs

Midazolam (p. 774)

Neonate body-weight under 3.3 kg, dilute 15 mg/kg body-weight to a final volume of 50 mL with Glucose 5% *or* Sodium Chloride 0.9%; an intravenous infusion rate of 0.1 mL/hour provides a dose of 30 micrograms/kg/hour

Neonate body-weight over 3.3 kg, dilute 50 mg to a final volume of 50 mL with Glucose 5% *or* Sodium Chloride 0.9%; an intravenous infusion rate of 0.05–0.1 mL/kg/hour provides a dose of 50–100 micrograms/kg/hour

Morphine sulphate (p. 255)

Dilute 2.5 mg/kg body-weight to a final volume of 50 mL with Glucose 5% *or* 10% *or* Sodium Chloride 0.9%; an intravenous infusion rate of 0.1 mL/hour provides a dose of 5 micrograms/kg/hour

Noradrenaline/Norepinephrine (p. 145)

Dilute 600 micrograms (base)/kg body-weight to a final volume of 50 mL with Glucose 5% *or* Sodium Chloride and Glucose; an intravenous infusion rate of 0.1 mL/hour provides a dose of 20 nanograms (base)/kg/minute; infuse through central venous catheter; max. concentration of noradrenaline (base) 40 micrograms/mL (higher concentrations can be used if fluid restricted). Discard if discoloured. Incompatible with bicarbonate or alkaline solutions
Note 1 mg of noradrenaline acid tartrate is equivalent to 500 micrograms of the base. Dose expressed as the base

Dental Practitioners' Formulary

List of Dental Preparations

The following list has been approved by the appropriate Secretaries of State, and the preparations therein may be prescribed by dental practitioners on form FP10D (GP14 in Scotland, WP10D in Wales).

Sugar-free versions, where available, are preferred.

Aciclovir Cream, BP
Aciclovir Oral Suspension, BP, 200 mg/5 mL
Aciclovir Tablets, BP, 200 mg
Aciclovir Tablets, BP, 800 mg
Amoxicillin Capsules, BP
Amoxicillin Oral Powder, DPF[1]
Amoxicillin Oral Suspension, BP
Amphotericin Lozenges, BP
Ampicillin Capsules, BP
Ampicillin Oral Suspension, BP
Artificial Saliva, DPF[2]
Artificial Saliva Substitutes as listed below (to be prescribed only for indications approved by ACBS[3]):
    AS Saliva Orthana®
    Glandosane®
    Biotene Oralbalance®
    BioXtra®
    Saliveze®
    Salivix®
Aspirin Tablets, Dispersible, BP[4]
Azithromycin Oral Suspension, 200 mg/5 mL, DPF
Beclomethasone Pressurised Inhalation, BP, 50 micrograms/metered inhalation, CFC-free, as:
    Clenil Modulite®
Benzydamine Mouthwash, BP 0.15%
Benzydamine Oromucosal Spray, BP 0.15%
Betamethasone Soluble Tablets, 500 micrograms, DPF
Carbamazepine Tablets, BP
Carmellose Gelatin Paste, DPF
Cefalexin Capsules, BP
Cefalexin Oral Suspension, BP
Cefalexin Tablets, BP
Cefradine Capsules, BP
Cefradine Oral Solution, DPF
Cetirizine Hydrochloride Tablets, 10 mg, DPF
Chlorhexidine Gluconate 1% Gel, DPF
Chlorhexidine Mouthwash, BP
Chlorhexidine Oral Spray, DPF
Chlorphenamine Oral Solution, BP
Chlorphenamine Tablets, BP
Choline Salicylate Dental Gel, BP
Clindamycin Capsules, BP
Co-amoxiclav Tablets, BP, 250/125 (amoxicillin 250 mg as trihydrate, clavulanic acid 125 mg as potassium salt)
Diazepam Oral Solution, BP, 2 mg/5 mL
Diazepam Tablets, BP
Diclofenac Sodium Tablets, BP

Dihydrocodeine Tablets, BP, 30 mg
Doxycycline Capsules, BP, 100 mg
Doxycycline Tablets, 20 mg, DPF
Ephedrine Nasal Drops, BP
Erythromycin Ethyl Succinate Oral Suspension, BP
Erythromycin Ethyl Succinate Tablets, BP
Erythromycin Stearate Tablets, BP
Erythromycin Tablets, BP
Fluconazole Capsules, 50 mg, DPF
Fluconazole Oral Suspension, 50 mg/5 mL, DPF
Hydrocortisone Cream, BP, 1%
Hydrocortisone Oromucosal Tablets, BP
Hydrogen Peroxide Mouthwash, BP
Ibuprofen Oral Suspension, BP, sugar-free
Ibuprofen Tablets, BP
Lansoprazole Capsules, DPF
Lidocaine 5% Ointment, DPF
Lidocaine Spray 10%, DPF
Loratadine Tablets, 10 mg, DPF
Menthol and Eucalyptus Inhalation, BP 1980[5]
Metronidazole Oral Suspension, BP
Metronidazole Tablets, BP
Miconazole Cream, BP
Miconazole Oromucosal Gel, BP
Miconazole and Hydrocortisone Cream, BP
Miconazole and Hydrocortisone Ointment, BP
Mouthwash Solution-tablets, DPF
Nitrazepam Tablets, BP
Nystatin Oral Suspension, BP
Gastro-resistant Omeprazole Capsules, BP
Oxytetracycline Tablets, BP
Paracetamol Oral Suspension, BP[6]
Paracetamol Tablets, BP
Paracetamol Tablets, Soluble, BP
Penciclovir Cream, DPF
Phenoxymethylpenicillin Oral Solution, BP
Phenoxymethylpenicillin Tablets, BP
Promethazine Hydrochloride Tablets, BP
Promethazine Oral Solution, BP
Saliva Stimulating Tablets, DPF
Sodium Chloride Mouthwash, Compound, BP
Sodium Fluoride Mouthwash, BP
Sodium Fluoride Oral Drops, BP
Sodium Fluoride Tablets, BP
Sodium Fluoride Toothpaste 0.619%, DPF
Sodium Fluoride Toothpaste 1.1%, DPF
Sodium Fusidate Ointment, BP
Temazepam Oral Solution, BP
Temazepam Tablets, BP
Tetracycline Tablets, BP
Triamcinolone Dental Paste, BP

---

1. Amoxicillin Dispersible Tablets are no longer available
2. Supplies may be difficult to obtain
3. Indications approved by the ACBS are: patients suffering from dry mouth as a result of having (or having undergone) radiotherapy or sicca syndrome
4. The BP directs that when soluble aspirin tablets are prescribed, dispersible aspirin tablets should be dispensed
5. This preparation does not appear in subsequent editions of the BP
6. The BP directs that when Paediatric Paracetamol Oral Suspension or Paediatric Paracetamol Mixture is prescribed and no strength stated Paracetamol Oral Suspension 120 mg/5 mL should be dispensed

Nurse Prescribers' Formulary

Nurse Prescribers' Formulary for Community Practitioners

Nurse Prescribers' Formulary Appendix (Appendix NPF). List of preparations approved by the Secretary of State which may be prescribed on form FP10P (form HS21(N) in Northern Ireland, form GP10(N) in Scotland, forms FP10(CN) and FP10(PN) in Wales or, when available, WP10CN and WP10PN in Wales) by Nurses for National Health Service patients.

Community practitioners who have completed the necessary training may only prescribe items appearing in the nurse prescribers' list set out below. Community Practitioner Nurse Prescribers are recommended to prescribe generically, except where this would not be clinically appropriate or where there is no approved generic name.

Medicinal Preparations

Almond Oil Ear Drops, BP
Arachis Oil Enema, NPF
[1]Aspirin Tablets, Dispersible, 300 mg, BP
Bisacodyl Suppositories, BP (includes 5-mg and 10-mg strengths)
Bisacodyl Tablets, BP
Catheter Maintenance Solution, Chlorhexidine, NPF
Catheter Maintenance Solution, Sodium Chloride, NPF
Catheter Maintenance Solution, 'Solution G', NPF
Catheter Maintenance Solution, 'Solution R', NPF
Chlorhexidine Gluconate Alcoholic Solutions containing at least 0.05%
Chlorhexidine Gluconate Aqueous Solutions containing at least 0.05%
Choline Salicylate Dental Gel, BP
Clotrimazole Cream 1%, BP
Co-danthramer Capsules, NPF
Co-danthramer Capsules, Strong, NPF
Co-danthramer Oral Suspension, NPF
Co-danthramer Oral Suspension, Strong, NPF
Co-danthrusate Capsules, BP
Co-danthrusate Oral Suspension, NPF
Crotamiton Cream, BP
Crotamiton Lotion, BP
Dimeticone barrier creams containing at least 10%
Dimeticone Lotion, NPF
Docusate Capsules, BP
Docusate Enema, NPF
Docusate Oral Solution, BP
Docusate Oral Solution, Paediatric, BP
Econazole Cream 1%, BP
Emollients as listed below:
    Aqueous Cream, BP
    Arachis Oil, BP
    Cetraben® Emollient Cream

Decubal® Clinic
Dermamist®
Diprobase® Cream
Diprobase® Ointment
Doublebase®
E45® Cream
Emulsifying Ointment, BP
[2]Epaderm®
Hydromol® Cream
Hydromol® Ointment
Hydrous Ointment, BP
Linola® Gamma Cream
Lipobase®
Liquid and White Soft Paraffin Ointment, NPF
Neutrogena® Dermatological Cream
Oilatum® Cream
Oilatum® Junior Cream
Paraffin, White Soft, BP
Paraffin, Yellow Soft, BP
QV® Cream
QV® Lotion
QV® Wash
Ultrabase®
Unguentum M®
Zerobase® Cream
Emollient Bath Additives as listed below:
    Alpha Keri® Bath Oil
    [3]Balneum®
    Cetraben® Emollient Bath Additive
    Dermalo® Bath Emollient
    Diprobath®
    Doublebase® Emollient Bath Additive
    Doublebase® Emollient Shower Gel
    Hydromol® Emollient
    Imuderm® Bath Oil
    Oilatum® Emollient
    Oilatum® Junior Emollient Bath Additive
    Oilatum® Gel
    QV® Bath Oil

Nurse Prescribers' Formulary

1. Max. 96 tablets; max. pack size 32 tablets
2. Included in the Drug Tariff, Scottish Drug Tariff, and Northern Ireland Drug Tariff
3. Except pack sizes that are not to be prescribed under the NHS (see Part XVIIIA of the Drug Tariff, Part XI of the Northern Ireland Drug Tariff)

Folic Acid 400 micrograms/5 mL Oral Solution, NPF
Folic Acid Tablets 400 micrograms, BP
Glycerol Suppositories, BP
[1]Ibuprofen Oral Suspension, BP
[1]Ibuprofen Tablets, BP
Ispaghula Husk Granules, BP
Ispaghula Husk Granules, Effervescent, BP
Ispaghula Husk Oral Powder, BP
Lactulose Solution, BP
Lidocaine Ointment, BP
Lidocaine and Chlorhexidine Gel, BP
Macrogol Oral Powder, NPF
Macrogol Oral Powder, Compound, NPF
Macrogol Oral Powder, Compound, Half-strength, NPF
Magnesium Hydroxide Mixture, BP
Magnesium Sulphate Paste, BP
Malathion alcoholic lotions containing at least 0.5%
Malathion aqueous lotions containing at least 0.5%
Mebendazole Oral Suspension, NPF
Mebendazole Tablets, NPF
Methylcellulose Tablets, BP
Miconazole Cream 2%, BP
Miconazole Oromucosal Gel, BP
Mouthwash Solution-tablets, NPF
Nicotine Inhalation Cartridge for Oromucosal Use, NPF
Nicotine Lozenge, NPF
Nicotine Medicated Chewing Gum, NPF
Nicotine Nasal Spray, NPF
Nicotine Sublingual Tablets, NPF
Nicotine Transdermal Patches, NPF
Nystatin Oral Suspension, BP
Olive Oil Ear Drops, BP

Paracetamol Oral Suspension, BP (includes 120 mg/5 mL and 250 mg/5 mL strengths—both of which are available as sugar-free formulations)
[2]Paracetamol Tablets, BP
[2]Paracetamol Tablets, Soluble, BP (includes 120-mg and 500-mg tablets)
Permethrin Cream, NPF
Phenothrin Alcoholic Lotion, NPF
Phenothrin Aqueous Lotion, NPF
Phosphates Enema, BP
Phosphate suppositories, NPF
Piperazine and Senna Powder, NPF
Povidone–Iodine Solution, BP
Senna Granules, Standardised, BP
Senna Oral Solution, NPF
Senna Tablets, BP
Senna and Ispaghula Granules, NPF
Sodium Chloride Solution, Sterile, BP
Sodium Citrate Compound Enema, NPF
Sodium Picosulfate Capsules, NPF
Sodium Picosulfate Elixir, NPF
Spermicidal contraceptives as listed below:
  Gygel® Contraceptive Jelly
Sterculia Granules, NPF
Sterculia and Frangula Granules, NPF
Titanium Ointment, BP
Water for Injections, BP
Zinc and Castor Oil Ointment, BP
Zinc Cream, BP
Zinc Ointment, BP
Zinc Oxide and Dimeticone Spray, NPF
Zinc Oxide Impregnated Medicated Bandage, NPF
Zinc Oxide Impregnated Medicated Stocking, NPF
Zinc Paste Bandage, BP 1993
Zinc Paste and Calamine Bandage
Zinc Paste and Ichthammol Bandage, BP 1993

Appliances and Reagents (including Wound Management Products)

Community Practitioner Nurse Prescribers in England, Wales and Northern Ireland can prescribe any appliance or reagent in the relevant Drug Tariff. In the Scottish Drug Tariff, Appliances and Reagents which may **not** be prescribed by Nurses are annotated **Nx**.

The Drug Tariffs can be accessed online at:

National Health Service Drug Tariff for England and Wales: www.ppa.org.uk/ppa/edt_intro.htm

Health and Personal Social Services for Northern Ireland Drug Tariff: www.centralservicesagency.com/display/ni_drug_tariff

Scottish Drug Tariff: www.isdscotland.org/isd/2245.html

Appliances (including Contraceptive Devices[3]) as listed in Part IXA of the Drug Tariff (Part III of the Northern Ireland Drug Tariff, Part 3 (Appliances) and Part 2 (Dressings) of the Scottish Drug Tariff)

Incontinence Appliances as listed in Part IXB of the Drug Tariff (Part III of the Northern Ireland Drug Tariff, Part 5 of the Scottish Drug Tariff)

1. Except for indications and doses that are [PoM]
2. Max. 96 tablets; max. pack size 32 tablets
3. Nurse Prescribers in Family Planning Clinics—where it is not appropriate for nurse prescribers in family planning clinics to prescribe contraceptive devices using form FP10(P) (forms FP10(CN) and FP10(PN), or when available WP10CN and WP10PN, in Wales), they may prescribe using the same system as doctors in the clinic

Stoma Appliances and Associated Products as listed in Part IXC of the Drug Tariff (Part III of the Northern Ireland Drug Tariff, Part 6 of the Scottish Drug Tariff)

Chemical Reagents as listed in Part IXR of the Drug Tariff (Part II of the Northern Ireland Drug Tariff, Part 9 of the Scottish Drug Tariff)

Nurse Independent Prescribing

Nurse Independent Prescribers (formerly known as Extended Formulary Nurse Prescribers) are able to prescribe any licensed medicine for any medical condition, including some Controlled Drugs (see BNF).

Nurse Independent Prescribers must work within their own level of professional competence and expertise. They are recommended to prescribe generically, except where this would not be clinically appropriate or where there is no approved non-proprietary name.

Up-to-date information and guidance on nurse independent prescribing is available on the Department of Health website at
www.dh.gov.uk/nonmedicalprescribing

Non-medical prescribing

A range of non-medical healthcare professionals are able to prescribe medicines for patients as either Independent or Supplementary Prescribers.

Independent prescribers are practitioners responsible and accountable for the assessment of patients with previously undiagnosed or diagnosed conditions and for decisions about the clinical management required, including prescribing. They are recommended to prescribe generically, except where this would not be clinically appropriate or where there is no approved non-proprietary name.

Supplementary prescribing is a partnership between an independent prescriber (a doctor or a dentist) and a supplementary prescriber to implement an agreed individual Clinical Management Plan with the patient's agreement.

Independent and Supplementary Prescribers are identified by an annotation next to their name in the relevant professional register.

Up-to-date information and guidance on non-medical prescribing is available on the Department of Health website at www.dh.gov.uk/nonmedicalprescribing.

Nurses

For further information on Nurse Independent Prescribing, see Nurse Prescribers' Formulary, p. 927.

Optometrists

Optometrist Independent Prescribers are able to prescribe any licensed medicine for ocular conditions affecting the eye and the tissues surrounding the eye, except Controlled Drugs or medicines for parenteral administration. Optometrist Independent Prescribers must work within their own level of professional competence and expertise.

Pharmacists

Pharmacist Independent Prescribers are able to prescribe any licensed medicine, except Controlled Drugs, for any medical condition. Pharmacist Independent Prescribers must work within their own level of professional competence and expertise.

 # Index of manufacturers

3M
3M Health Care Ltd
3M House
Morley St
Loughborough
Leics, LE11 1EP.
tel: (01509) 611611
fax: (01509) 237288

A&H
Allen & Hanburys Ltd
See GSK

A1 Pharmaceuticals
A1 Pharmaceuticals Plc
Units 20+21 Easter Park
Site 8A Beam Reach
Ferry Lane South, Rainham
Essex, RM13 9BP.
tel: (01708) 528 900
fax: (01708) 528 928
sales@a1plc.co.uk

Abbott
Abbott Laboratories Ltd
Abbott House
Norden Rd, Maidenhead
Berks, SL6 4XE.
tel: (01628) 773 355
fax: (01628) 644 185
ukmedinfo@abbott.com

ABT Healthcare
ABT Healthcare UK Ltd
Springwood Booths Hall
Booths Park
Chelford Rd
Knutsford, WA16 8QZ.
tel: (01565) 757783

Acorus
Acorus Therapeutics Ltd
Office Village
Chester Business Park
Chester, CH4 9QZ.
tel: (01244) 625 152
fax: (01244) 625 151
enquiries@acorus-therapeutics.com

Actavis
Actavis UK Ltd
Whiddon Valley
Barnstaple
Devon, EX32 8NS.
tel: (01271) 311 257
fax: (01271) 346 106
medinfo@actavis.co.uk

Actelion
Actelion Pharmaceuticals UK Ltd
BSi Building, 13th Floor
389 Chiswick High Rd, London, W4
4AL.
tel: (020) 8987 3333
fax: (020) 8987 3322

Activa
Activa Healthcare
1 Lancaster Park
Newborough Rd, Needwood
Burton-upon-Trent, Staffs, DE13 9PD.
tel: (0845) 060 6707
fax: (01283) 576 808
advice@activahealthcare.co.uk

Advancis
Advancis Medical Ltd
Lowmoor Business Park
Kirkby-in-Ashfield, Nottingham,
NG17 7JZ.
tel: (01623) 751 500
fax: (0871) 264 8238
info@advancis.co.uk

Agepha
Agepha GmbH
9 High St
Woburn Sands, MK17 8RF.
tel: (0203) 239 6241
uk@agepha.com

Aguettant
Aguettant Ltd
The Barn
41a Main Rd, Cleeve
Somerset, BS49 4NZ.
tel: (01934) 835 694
fax: (01934) 876 790
info@aguettant.co.uk

Air Products
Air Products plc
Medical Group
2 Millennium Gate
Westmere Drive, Crewe
Cheshire, CW1 6AP.
tel: (0800) 373 580
fax: (0800) 214 709

Alan Pharmaceuticals
Alan Pharmaceuticals
2 Kingsgate Ave
London, N3 3BH.
tel: (020) 8346 4311
fax: (020) 8346 5218

Alcon
Alcon Laboratories (UK) Ltd
Pentagon Park
Boundary Way
Hemel Hempstead, Herts, HP2 7UD.
tel: (01442) 341 234
fax: (01442) 341 200

Alembic Products
Alembic Products Ltd
River Lane
Saltney, Chester, Cheshire, CH4 8RQ.
tel: (01244) 680 147
fax: (01244) 680 155

Alexion
Alexion Pharma UK Ltd
3000 Cathedral Hill
Guildford
Surrey, GU2 7YB.
tel: (01483) 246 641
fax: (01483) 245 130
alexion.uk@alxn.com

ALK-Abelló
ALK-Abelló (UK) Ltd
1 Tealgate
Hungerford, Berks, RG17 0YT.
tel: (01488) 686 016
fax: (01488) 685 423
info@uk.alk-abello.com

Allergan
Allergan Ltd
1st Floor Marlow International
The Parkway
Marlow
Bucks, SL7 1YL.
tel: (01628) 494 026
fax: (01628) 494 449

Allergy
Allergy Therapeutics Ltd
Dominion Way
Worthing, West Sussex, BN14 8SA.
tel: (01903) 844 702
fax: (01903) 844 744
infoservices@allergytherapeutics.
com

Alliance
Alliance Pharmaceuticals Ltd
Avonbridge House
2 Bath Rd
Chippenham, Wilts, SN15 2BB.
tel: (01249) 466 966
fax: (01249) 466 977
medinfo@alliancepharma.co.uk

Almirall
Almirall Ltd
4 The Square
Stockley Park
Uxbridge, UB11 1ET.
tel: (0800) 0087399
almirall@professionalinformation.co.
uk

Alpharma
See Actavis

Alphashow
Alphashow Ltd
10 South Rd
Amersham
Bucks, HP6 5LX.
tel: (0870) 240 2775
fax: (01672) 515 614
info@alphashow.co.uk

Altacor
Altacor Ltd
St. John's Innovation Centre
Cowley Road
Cambridge, CB4 0WS.
tel: (01223) 421 411
fax: (01223) 420 844
info@altacor-pharma.com

Amdipharm
Amdipharm plc
Regency House
Miles Gray Rd
Basildon, Essex, SS14 3AF.
tel: (0870) 777 7675
fax: (0870) 777 7875
medinfo@amdipharm.com

Amgen
Amgen Ltd
240 Cambridge Science Park
Milton Rd, Cambridge, CB4 0WD.
tel: (01223) 420 305
fax: (01223) 426 314
infoline@uk.amgen.com

Anglian
Anglian Pharma Sales & Marketing
Titmore Court
Titmore Green
Little Wymondley, Hitchin
Herts, SG4 7XJ.
tel: (01438) 743 070
fax: (01438) 743 080
mail@anglianpharma.com

Anpharm
See Goldshield

Antigen
See Goldshield

Archimedes
Archimedes Pharma UK Ltd
250 South Oak Way
Green Park
Reading
Berks, RG2 6UG.
tel: (0118) 931 5060
fax: (0118) 931 5065
medicalinformation@
archimedespharma.com

Ardana
Ardana Bioscience Ltd
58 Queen St
Edinburgh, EH2 3NS.
tel: (0131) 226 8550
fax: (0131) 226 8551
info@ardana.co.uk

Ardern
Ardern Healthcare Ltd
Pipers Brook Farm
Eastham
Tenbury Wells, Worcs, WR15 8NP.
tel: (01584) 781 777
fax: (01584) 781 788
info@ardernhealthcare.com

Ark Therapeutics
Ark Therapeutics Group Plc
79 New Cavendish St
London, W1W 6XB.
tel: (020) 7388 7722
fax: (020) 7388 7805
info@arktherapeutics.com

AS Pharma
AS Pharma Ltd
PO Box 181
Polegate, East Sussex, BN26 6WD.
tel: (08700) 664 117
fax: (08700) 664 118
info@aspharma.co.uk

Astellas
Astellas Pharma Ltd
Lovett House, Lovett Rd
Staines, TW18 3AZ.
tel: (01784) 419 615
fax: (01784) 419 401

AstraZeneca
AstraZeneca UK Ltd
Horizon Place
600 Capability Green
Luton, Beds, LU1 3LU.
tel: 0800 7830 033
fax: (01582) 838 003
medical.informationuk@astrazeneca.
com

Auden Mckenzie
Auden Mckenzie (Pharma Division)
Ltd
30 Stadium Business Centre
North End Rd
Wembley, Middx, HA9 0AT.
tel: (020) 8900 2122
fax: (020) 8903 9620

Aurum
Aurum Pharmaceuticals Ltd
Hubert Rd
Brentwood
Essex, CM14 4LZ.
tel: (01277) 266600
fax: (01277) 848 976
info@martindalepharma.co.uk

Aventis Pharma
See Sanofi-Aventis

Ayrton Saunders
Ayrton Saunders Ltd
Ayrton House
Commerce Way
Parliament Business Park
Liverpool, Merseyside, L8 7BA.
tel: (0151) 709 2074
fax: (0151) 709 7336
info@ayrtons.com

Bard
Bard Ltd
Forest House
Brighton Rd
Crawley, West Sussex, RH11 9BP.
tel: (01293) 527 888
fax: (01293) 552 428

Basilea
Basilea Pharmaceuticals Ltd
14/16 Frederick Sanger Road
The Surrey Research Park
Guildford
Surrey, GU2 7YD.
tel: (01483) 790 023
fax: (01483) 505 345
ukmedinfo@basilea.com

Bausch & Lomb
Bausch & Lomb UK Ltd
106 London Rd
Kingston-upon-Thames
Surrey, KT2 6TN.
tel: (020) 8781 2900
fax: (020) 8781 2901

Baxter
Baxter Healthcare Ltd
Wallingford Rd
Compton
Newbury
Berks, RG20 7QW.
tel: (01635) 206 345
fax: (01635) 206 071
surecall@baxter.com

Bayer
Bayer plc
Bayer Schering Pharma
Bayer House, Strawberry Hill
Newbury, Berks, RG14 1JA.
tel: (01635) 563 000
fax: (01635) 563 393
medical.science@bayer.co.uk

Bayer Consumer Care
See Bayer

Bayer Diabetes Care
See Bayer

Bayer Diagnostics
See Bayer

BBI Healthcare
BBI Healthcare
Unit A
Kestrel Way
Garngoch Industrial Estate
Gorseinon, Swansea, SA4 9WN.
tel: (01792) 229 333
fax: (01792) 897 311
info@bbihealthcare.com

Beacon
Beacon Pharmaceuticals Ltd
85 High St
Tunbridge Wells, TN1 1YG.
tel: (01892) 600 930
fax: (01892) 600 937
info@beaconpharma.co.uk

Beiersdorf
Beiersdorf UK Ltd
2010 Solihull Parkway
Birmingham Business Park
Birmingham, B37 7YS.
tel: (0121) 329 8800
fax: (0121) 329 8801

Bell and Croyden
John Bell and Croyden
50-54 Wigmore St
London, W1U 2AU.
tel: (020) 7935 5555
fax: (020) 7935 9605
jbc@johnbellcroyden.co.uk

BHR
BHR Pharmaceuticals Ltd
41 Centenary Business Centre
Hammond Close
Attleborough Fields, Nuneaton
Warwickshire, CV11 6RY.
tel: (024) 7635 3742
fax: (024) 7632 7812
info@bhr.co.uk

Bioenvision
Bioenvision Ltd
10 Lockside Place
Edinburgh Park
Edinburgh, EH12 9RG.
tel: (0131) 248 3555
fax: (0131) 2483300
info@bioenvision.com

Biogen
Biogen Idec Ltd
Innovation House
70 Norden Rd
Maidenhead
Berks, SL6 4AY.
tel: (0800) 008 7401
fax: (01628) 501 010

Biolitec
Biolitec Pharma Ltd
Unit 2, Broomhill Business Park
Broomhill Rd
Tallaght
Dublin 24, Ireland.
tel: (00353) 14637415
fax: (00353) 14637411
medical.info@biolitec.com

BioMarin
BioMarin Europe Ltd
3rd Floor
164 Shaftsbury Ave
London, WC2H 8HL.
tel: (020) 7420 0800
fax: (020) 7420 0829

Biotest UK
Biotest (UK) Ltd
28 Monkspath Business Park
Highlands Road
Shirley
Solihull, B90 4NZ.
tel: (0121) 733 3393
fax: (0121) 733 3066
MedicinesInformation@biotestuk.
com

Blackwell
Blackwell Supplies Ltd
Medcare House
Centurion Close
Gillingham Business Park, Gillingham
Kent, ME8 0SB.
tel: (01634) 877 620
fax: (01634) 877 621

Blake
Thomas Blake & Co
The Byre House
Fearby
Nr. Masham
North Yorks, HG4 4NF.
tel: (01765) 689 042
fax: (01765) 689 042
sales@veilcover.com

BOC
BOC Medical
The Priestley Centre,
10 Priestley Rd
Surrey Research Park
Guildford, Surrey, GU2 7XY.
tel: 0800 111 333
fax: 0800 111 555

Boehringer Ingelheim
Boehringer Ingelheim Ltd
Ellesfield Ave
Bracknell
Berks, RG12 8YS.
tel: (01344) 424 600
fax: (01344) 741 444
medinfo@bra.boehringer-ingelheim.
com

Boots
Boots The Chemists
Medical Services
Thane Rd
D90 East S10
Nottingham, NG90 1BS.
tel: (0115) 959 5165
fax: (0115) 959 2565

BPC 100
The Bolton Pharmaceutical 100 Ltd
2 Chapel Drive
Ambrosden
Oxfordshire, OX25 2RS.
tel: (0845) 602 3907
fax: (0845) 602 3908
info@bpc100.com

BPL
Bio Products Laboratory
Dagger Lane
Elstree, Herts, WD6 3BX.
tel: (020) 8258 2200
fax: (020) 8258 2601

Braun
B Braun (Medical) Ltd
Brookdale Rd
Thorncliffe Park Estate
Chapeltown, Sheffield, S35 2PW.
tel: (0114) 225 9000
fax: (0114) 225 9111
info.bbmuk@bbraun.com

Bray
Bray Health & Leisure
1 Regal Way
Faringdon
Oxon, SN7 7BX.
tel: (01367) 240 736
fax: (01367) 242 625
info@bray.co.uk

Bristol-Myers Squibb
Bristol-Myers Squibb
Pharmaceuticals Ltd
Uxbridge Business Park
Sanderson Rd
Uxbridge
Middx, UB8 1DH.
tel: (01895) 523 000
fax: (01895) 523 010
medical.information@bms.com

Britannia
Britannia Pharmaceuticals Ltd
41-51 Brighton Rd
Redhill
Surrey, RH1 6YS.
tel: (01737) 773 741
fax: (01737) 762 672
medicalservices@britannia-pharm.
com

BSN Medical
BSN Medical Ltd
PO Box 258
Willerby
Hull, HU10 6WT.
tel: (0845) 1223 600
fax: (0845) 1223 666

Cambridge
Cambridge Laboratories
Deltic House, Kingfisher Way
Silverlink Business Park, Wallsend
Tyne & Wear, NE28 9NX.
tel: (0191) 296 9300
fax: (0191) 296 9368
customer.services@camb-labs.com

Cardinal
Cardinal Health Martindale Products
Hubert Rd
Brentwood
Essex, CM14 4JY.
tel: (01277) 266 600
fax: (01277) 848 976
info@martindalepharma.co.uk

Castlemead
See Sanofi-Aventis

C D Medical
C D Medical Ltd
Aston Grange
Oker, Matlock, DE4 2JJ.
tel: (01629) 733 860
fax: (01629) 733 414

Celgene
Celgene Ltd
Morgan House
Madeira Walk
Windsor
Berks, SL4 1EP.
tel: (08448) 010 045
fax: (08448) 010 046
medinfo.uk.ire@celgene.com

Centrapharm
See Derma UK

Cephalon
Cephalon Ltd
1 Albany Place
Hyde Way
Welwyn Garden City
Herts, AL7 3BT.
tel: 0800 783 4869
fax: (01483) 765 008
ukmedinfo@cephalon.com

Chattem UK
Chattem UK Ltd
Guerry House
Ringway Centre
Edison Rd
Basingstoke, RG24 6YH.
tel: (01256) 844 144
fax: (01256) 844 145

Chauvin
See Bausch & Lomb

Chefaro UK
Chefaro UK Ltd
Unit 1, Tower Close
St. Peter's Industrial Park
Huntingdon
Cambs, PE29 7DH.
tel: (01480) 421 800
fax: (01480) 434 861

Chemical Search
Chemical Search International Ltd
29th floor
1 Canada Square
Canary Wharf
London, E14 5DY.
tel: (020) 7712 1758
fax: (020) 7712 1759
info@chemicalsearch.co.uk

Chemidex
Chemidex Pharma Ltd
Chemidex House
Egham Business Village
Crabtree Rd, Egham
Surrey, TW20 8RB.
tel: (01784) 477 167
fax: (01784) 471 776
info@chemidex.co.uk

Chiesi
Chiesi Ltd
Cheadle Royal Business Park
Highfield
Cheadle, SK8 3GY.
tel: (0161) 488 5555
fax: (0161) 488 5565

Chiron
See Novartis

CHS
Cambridge Healthcare Supplies Ltd
14D Wendover Rd
Rackheath Industrial Estate
Rackheath
Norwich, NR13 6LH.
tel: (01603) 735 200
fax: (01603) 735 217
customerservices@typharm.com

Chugai
Chugai Pharma UK Ltd
Mulliner House, Flanders Rd
Turnham Green
London, W4 1NN.
tel: (020) 8987 5680
fax: (020) 8987 5661

Clement Clarke
Clement Clarke International Ltd
Edinburgh Way
Harlow
Essex, CM20 2TT.
tel: (01279) 414 969
fax: (01279) 456 304
resp@clement-clarke.com

CliniMed
CliniMed Ltd
Cavell House, Knaves Beech Way
Loudwater
High Wycombe
Bucks, HP10 9QY.
tel: (01628) 850 100
fax: (01628) 850 331
enquires@clinimed.co.uk

Clinisupplies
Clinisupplies Ltd
9 Crystal Way
Elmgrove Rd
Harrow
Middx, HA1 2HP.
tel: (020) 8863 4168
fax: (020) 8426 0768
info@clinisupplies.co.uk

Colgate-Palmolive
Colgate-Palmolive Ltd
Guildford Business Park
Middleton Rd
Guildford
Surrey, GU2 5LZ.
tel: (01483) 302 222
fax: (01483) 303 003

Coloplast
Coloplast Ltd
Peterborough Business Park
Peterborough, PE2 6FX.
tel: (01733) 392 000
fax: (01733) 233 348
gbcareteam@coloplast.com

Community
Community Foods Ltd
Micross, Brent Terrace
London, NW2 1LT.
tel: (020) 8450 9411
fax: (020) 8208 1803
email@communityfoods.co.uk

Complan Foods
Complan Foods Ltd
Imperial House
15–19 Kingsway
London, WC2B 6UN.
tel: (020) 7395 7565
fax: (08704) 434 018

Concord
See Archimedes

ConvaTec
ConvaTec Ltd
Harrington House, Milton Rd
Ickenham
Uxbridge
Middx, UB10 8PU.
tel: (01895) 628 400
fax: (01895) 628 456

Covidien
Covidien UK Commercial Ltd
154 Fareham Rd
Gosport
Hants, PO13 0AS.
tel: (01329) 224 226
fax: (01329) 224 334
medicalcustomerservices@covidien.com

Cow & Gate
See Nutricia Clinical

CP
See Wockhardt

Crawford
Crawford Pharmaceuticals
Cheshire House
164 Main Rd
Goostrey
Cheshire, CW4 8NP.
tel: (01477) 537 596
fax: (01477) 534 262

Crookes
See Reckitt Benckiser

CSL Behring
CSL Behring UK Ltd
Hayworth House
Market Place
Haywards Heath
West Sussex, RH16 1DB.
tel: (01444) 447 400
fax: (01444) 447 403
medinfo@cslbehring.com

Daiichi Sankyo
Daiichi Sankyo UK Ltd
Chiltern Place
Chalfont Park
Gerrards Cross, SL9 0BG.
tel: (01753) 893 600
fax: (01753) 893 894
med.info@daiichi-sankyo.co.uk

Danetre
Danetre Health Products Ltd
Office 4, Broad March
Long March Industrial Estate
Daventry
Northants, NN11 4HE.
tel: (01327) 310 909
fax: (01327) 310 311
enquiries@danetrehealthproducts.com

DDD
DDD Ltd
94 Rickmansworth Rd
Watford
Herts, WD18 7JJ.
tel: (01923) 229 251
fax: (01923) 220 728

Dental Health
Dental Health Products Ltd
60 Boughton Lane
Maidstone
Kent, ME15 9QS.
tel: (01622) 749 222
fax: (01622) 744 672

Dentsply
Dentsply Ltd
Hamm Moor Lane
Addlestone
Weybridge
Surrey, KT15 2SE.
tel: (01932) 837 279
fax: (01932) 858 970

Dermal
Dermal Laboratories Ltd
Tatmore Place
Gosmore
Hitchin
Herts, SG4 7QR.
tel: (01462) 458 866
fax: (01462) 420 565

Derma UK
Derma UK Ltd
ARC Progress
Mill Lane
Stotfold
Beds, SG5 4NY.
tel: (01462) 733 500
fax: (01462) 733 600
info@dermauk.co.uk

De Vilbiss
De Vilbiss Health Care UK Ltd
High Street
Wollaston
West Midlands, DY8 4PS.
tel: (01384) 446 688
fax: (01384) 446 699

De Witt
E C De Witt & Co Ltd
Aegon House
Daresbury Park
Daresbury
Warrington, Cheshire, WA4 4HS.
tel: (01928) 756 800
fax: (01928) 756 818
info@ecdewitt.com

Dexcel
Dexcel-Pharma Ltd
1 Cottesbrooke Park
Heartlands Business Park
Daventry
Northamptonshire, NN11 8YL.
tel: (01327) 312 266
fax: (01327) 312 262
office@dexcelpharma.co.uk

DHP Healthcare
DHP Healthcare Ltd
60 Boughton Lane
Maidstone
Kent, ME15 9QS.
tel: (01622) 749 222
fax: (01622) 743 816
sales@dhphealthcare.co.uk

Diatos
Diatos SA
Immeuble Paris BioPark - 2 etage
11 Rue Watt
75013
Paris, France
tel: (00800) 3286 6966

Dimethaid
Dimethaid International
c/o Benoliel Partners
Linden House, Ewelme
Oxfordshire, OX10 6HQ.
tel: (01491) 825 016
fax: (01491) 834 592
medinfo@dimethaid.com

Dr Falk
Dr Falk Pharma UK Ltd
Bourne End Business, Cores End Rd
Bourne End, Bucks, SL8 5AS.
tel: (01628) 536 600

Durbin
Durbin plc
180 Northolt Rd
South Harrow
Middx, HA2 0LT.
tel: (020) 8869 6500
fax: (020) 8869 6565
info@durbin.co.uk

Easigrip
Easigrip Ltd
Unit 13, Scar Bank
Millers Rd
Warwick
Warwickshire, CV34 5DB.
tel: (01926) 497 108
fax: (01926) 497 109
enquiry@easigrip.co.uk

Ecolab
Ecolab UK
Lotherton Way
Garforth
Leeds, LS25 2JY.
tel: (0113) 232 0066
fax: (0113) 287 1317
info.healthcare@ecolab.co.uk

Egis
Egis Pharmaceuticals UK Ltd
127 Shirland Rd
London, W9 2EP.
tel: (020) 7266 2669
fax: (020) 7266 2702
enquiries@medimpexuk.com

Eisai
Eisai Ltd
European Knowledge Centre
Mosquito Way
Hatfield
Herts, AL10 9SN.
tel: (020) 8600 1400
fax: (020) 8600 1401
Lmedinfo@eisai.net

Elida Fabergé
Elida Fabergé Ltd
Coal Rd
Seacroft
Leeds, LS14 2AR.
tel: (0113) 222 5000
fax: (0113) 222 5362

Encysive
Encysive (UK) Ltd
Regus House
Highbridge, Oxford Rd
Uxbridge
Middlesex, UB8 1HR.
tel: (01895) 876 168
fax: (01895) 876 320
enquiries@encysive.co.uk

Enturia
Enturia Ltd
Reigate Place
43 London Road
Reigate
Surrey, RH2 9PW.
tel: (0800) 043 7546
fax: (01737) 237 950
enquiries@enturia.co.uk

Espere
Espere Healthcare Ltd
Suite G8, Bedford i-Lab
Priory Business Park
Bedford
Beds, MK44 3RZ.
tel: (01234) 834 614
fax: (01234) 834 615
info@esperehealth.co.uk

Ethicon
Ethicon Ltd
P.O. Box 1988
Simpson Parkway
Kirkton Campus
Livingston, EH54 0AB.
tel: (01506) 594 500
fax: (01506) 460 714

Eumedica
Eumedica S.A.
Winston Churchill Avenue 67
1180 Brussels
Belgium
tel: (0208) 444 3377
fax: (0208) 444 6866
enquiries@eumedica.com

EUSA Pharma
EUSA Pharma (Europe) Ltd
Building 3, Arlington Business Park
Whittle Way
Stevenage
Herts, SG1 2FP.
tel: (01438) 740 720
fax: (01438) 735 740
medinfo-uk@eusapharma.com

Everfresh
Everfresh Natural Foods
Gatehouse Close
Aylesbury
Bucks, HP19 3DE.
tel: (01296) 425 333
fax: (01296) 422 545

Exelgyn
Exelgyn Laboratories
PO Box 4511
Henley-on-Thames
Oxon, RG9 5ZQ.
tel: (01491) 642 137
fax: (0800) 731 6120

Fabre
Pierre Fabre Ltd
Hyde Abbey House
23 Hyde St
Winchester
Hampshire, SO23 7DR.
tel: (01962) 874 400
fax: (01962) 874 413
contactus@pierre-fabre.co.uk

Fate
Fate Special Foods
Unit E2
Brook Street Business Centre
Brook St, Tipton
West Midlands, DY4 9DD.
tel: (01215) 224 433
fax: (01215) 224 433

Fenton
Fenton Pharmaceuticals Ltd
4J Portman Mansions
Chiltern St
London, W1U 6NS.
tel: (020) 7224 1388
fax: (020) 7486 7258
mail@Fent-Pharm.co.uk

Ferndale
Ferndale Pharmaceuticals Ltd
Unit 605, Thorp Arch Estate
Wetherby
West Yorks, LS23 7BJ.
tel: (01937) 541 122
fax: (01937) 849 682
info@ferndalepharma.co.uk

Ferring
Ferring Pharmaceuticals (UK)
The Courtyard
Waterside Drive
Langley
Berks, SL3 6EZ.
tel: (01753) 214 800
fax: (01753) 214 801

Firstplay Dietary
Firstplay Dietary Foods Ltd
338 Turncroft Lane
Offerton
Stockport
Cheshire, SK1 4BP.
tel: (0161) 474 7576
fax: (0161) 474 7576

Flynn
Flynn Pharma Ltd
2nd Floor, The Maltings
Bridge St
Hitchin
Herts, SG5 2DE.
tel: (01462) 458 974
fax: (01462) 450 755

Foodlink
Foodlink (UK) Ltd
2B Plymouth Rd
Plympton
Plymouth, PL7 4JR.
tel: (01752) 344 544
fax: (01752) 342 412
info@foodlinkltd.co.uk

Ford
Ford Medical Associates Ltd
8 Wyndham Way
Orchard Heights
Ashford
Kent, TN25 4PZ.
tel: (01233) 633 224
fax: (01223) 646 595
enquiries@fordmedical.co.uk

Forest
Forest Laboratories UK Ltd
Bourne Rd
Bexley
Kent, DA5 1NX.
tel: (01322) 550 550
fax: (01322) 555 469
medinfo@forest-labs.co.uk

Fox
C. H. Fox Ltd
22 Tavistock St
London, WC2E 7PY.
tel: (020) 7240 3111
fax: (020) 7379 3410

FP
Family Planning Sales Ltd
Maerdy Industrial Estate
Rhymney
Gwent, NP22 5PY.
tel: (0870) 4444 620
fax: (0870) 4444 621

Freebake
Freebake Ltd
Unit E3 Blackpole East
Worcs, WR3 8SG.
tel: (0845) 603 9230
info@freebake.co.uk

Fresenius Kabi
Fresenius Kabi Ltd
Cestrian Court
Eastgate Way
Manor Park, Runcorn
Cheshire, WA7 INT.
tel: (01928) 533 533
fax: (01928) 533 534
med.info-uk@fresenius-kabi.com

Frontier
Frontier Multigate
Newbridge Rd Industrial Estate
Blackwood
South Wales, NP12 2YL.
tel: (01495) 233 050
fax: (01495) 233 055
multigate@frontier-group.co.uk

Galderma
Galderma (UK) Ltd
Meridien House
69-71 Clarendon Rd
Watford
Herts, WD17 1DS.
tel: (01923) 208 950
fax: (01923) 208 998

Galen
Galen Ltd
Seagoe Industrial Estate
Craigavon
Northern Ireland, BT63 5UA.
tel: (028) 3833 4974
fax: (028) 3835 0206
customer.services@galen.co.uk

GE Healthcare
GE Healthcare
The Grove Centre, White Lion Rd
Amersham, Bucks, HP7 9LL.
tel: (01494) 544 000

Geistlich
Geistlich Pharma
Newton Bank
Long Lane
Chester, CH2 2PF.
tel: (01244) 347 534
fax: (01244) 319 327

General Dietary
General Dietary Ltd
PO Box 38
Kingston upon Thames
Surrey, KT2 7YP.
tel: (020) 8336 2323
fax: (020) 8942 8274

Generics
Generics (UK) Ltd
Albany Gate
Darkes Lane
Potters Bar
Herts, EN6 1AG.
tel: (01707) 853 000
fax: (01707) 643 148

Generpharm
Generpharm Ltd
See Sigma

Genus
Genus Pharmaceuticals
Park View House
65 London Rd
Newbury
Berks, RG14 1JN.
tel: (01635) 568 400
fax: (01635) 568 401
enquiries@genuspharma.com

Genzyme
Genzyme Therapeutics
4620 Kingsgate
Cascade Way
Oxford Business Park South
Oxford, OX4 2SU.
tel: (01865) 405 200
fax: (01865) 774 172

Gilead
Gilead Sciences
The Flowers Building
Granta Park
Great Abington
Cambs, CB1 6GT.
tel: (01223) 897 300
fax: (01223) 897 291
ukmedinfo@gilead.com

GlaxoSmithKline
See GSK

Glenwood
Glenwood Laboratories Ltd
Jenkins Dale
Chatham
Kent, ME4 5RD.
tel: (01634) 830 535
fax: (01634) 831 345
g.wooduk@virgin.net

Gluten Free Foods Ltd
Gluten Free Foods Ltd
Unit 270 Centennial Park
Centennial Ave
Elstree, Borehamwood
Herts, WD6 3SS.
tel: (020) 8953 4444
fax: (020) 8953 8285
info@glutenfree-foods.co.uk

Goldshield
Goldshield Pharmaceuticals Ltd
NLA Tower
12-16 Addiscombe Rd
Croydon, CR0 0XT.
tel: (020) 8649 8500
fax: (020) 8686 0807

GP Pharma
See Derma UK

Grifols
Grifols UK Ltd
Byron House
Cambridge Business Park
Cowley Road
Cambridge , CB4 0WZ.
tel: (01223) 395 700
fax: (01223) 395 766
reception.uk@grifols.com

Grünenthal
Grünenthal Ltd
2 Beacon Heights Business Park
Ibstone Rd
Stokenchurch
Bucks, HP14 3XR.
tel: (0870) 351 8960
fax: (01494) 486 298
medicalinformationuk@grunenthal.com

GSK
GlaxoSmithKline
Stockley Park West
Uxbridge
Middx, UB11 1BT.
tel: 0800 221 441
fax: (020) 8990 4328
customercontactuk@gsk.com

GSK Consumer Healthcare
GlaxoSmithKline Consumer
Healthcare
GSK House
980 Great West Rd
Brentford
Middx, TW8 9GS.
tel: (020) 8047 2500
fax: (020) 8047 6860
customer.relations@gsk.com

H&R
H&R Healthcare Ltd
Melton Court, Gibson Lane
Melton
East Yorkshire, HU14 3HH.
tel: (01482) 638 491
fax: (01482) 638 485

Hartmann
Paul Hartmann Ltd
Unit P2, Parklands
Heywood Distribution Park
Pilsworth Rd, Heywood
Lancs, OL10 2TT.
tel: (01706) 363 200
fax: (01706) 363 201
info@uk.hartmann.info

Healthcare Logistics
See Movianto

Heinz
H. J. Heinz Company Ltd
South Building
Hayes Park
Hayes, UB4 8AL.
tel: (020) 8573 7757
fax: (020) 8848 2325
Farleys_Heinz@Heinz.co.uk

Henleys
Henleys Medical Supplies Ltd
Brownfields
Welwyn Garden City
Herts, AL7 1AN.
tel: (01707) 333 164
fax: (01707) 334 795

HK Pharma
HK Pharma Ltd
PO Box 105
Hitchin
Herts, SG5 2GG.
tel: (01462) 433 993
fax: (01462) 450 755

Hoechst Marion Roussel
See Sanofi-Aventis

Home Diagnostics
Home Diagnostics (UK) Ltd
25 Barnes Wallis Road
Segensworth East
Fareham
Hants, PO15 5TT.
tel: (01489) 569 469
fax: (01489) 569 424
info@homediagnostics-uk.com

Hospira
Hospira UK Ltd
Queensway
Royal Leamington Spa
Warwickshire, CV31 3RW.
tel: (01926) 820 820
fax: (01926) 821 041
medinfouk@hospira.com

HRA Pharma
Laboratoire HRA Pharma
15 rue Beranger
75003
Paris
France
tel: (0033) 1 40 33 11 30
fax: (0033) 1 40 33 12 31
info@lysodren-europe.com

Huntleigh
Huntleigh Healthcare Ltd
310 - 312 Dallow Rd
Luton, LU1 1TD.
tel: (01582) 413 104

Hypoguard
Hypoguard Ltd
Dock Lane
Melton
Woodbridge
Suffolk, IP12 1PE.
tel: (01394) 387 333
fax: (01394) 380 152
enquiries@hypoguard.com

IDIS
IDIS World Medicines
IDIS House
Churchfield Rd
Weybridge
Surrey, KT13 8DB.
tel: (01932) 824 000
fax: (01932) 824 200
idis@idispharma.com

INCA-Pharm
INCA-Pharm UK
PO Box 122
Richmond, DL10 5HX.
tel: (01748) 828 812
fax: (01748) 828 801
info@inca-pharm.com

Infai
Infai UK Ltd
Innovation Centre
University of York Science Park
University Rd
Heslington, York, YO10 5DG.
tel: (01904) 435 228
fax: (01904) 435 229
paul@infai.co.uk

Innovative
Innovative Solutions UK Ltd
Unit 28
Transpennine Industrial Estate
Gorrels Way, Queensway
Rochdale, Lancs, OL11 2QR.
tel: (01706) 746713
enquiries@innovative-solutions.org.uk

Insense
Insense Ltd
Colworth Science Park
Sharnbrook
Bedford, MK44 1LQ.
tel: (01234) 782 870
fax: (01234) 783 444
enquiries@insense.co.uk

Insight
Insight Medical Products Ltd
Units 1-4 Silk Mill Studios
2 Charlton Rd
Tetbury
Glos, GL8 8DY.
tel: (01666) 500 055
fax: (01666) 500 115
info@insightmedical.net

Intrapharm
Intrapharm Laboratories Ltd
60 Boughton Lane
Maidstone
Kent, ME15 9QS.
tel: (01622) 749 222
fax: (01622) 744 672
sales@intraphamlabs.com

Ipsen
Ipsen Ltd
190 Bath Rd
Slough
Berks, SL1 3XE.
tel: (01753) 627 777
fax: (01753) 627 778
medical.information.uk@ipsen.com

IS Pharmaceuticals
IS Pharmaceuticals Ltd
Office Village
Chester Business Park
Chester, CH4 9QZ.
tel: (01244) 625 152
fax: (01244) 625 151
enquiries@ispharma.plc.uk

IVAX
See TEVA UK

J&J
Johnson & Johnson Ltd
Foundation Park
Roxborough Way
Maidenhead
Berks, SL6 3UG.
tel: (01628) 822 222
fax: (01628) 821 222

J&J Medical
Johnson & Johnson Medical
Coronation Rd
Ascot
Berks, SL5 9EY.
tel: (01344) 871 000
fax: (01344) 872 599

Janssen-Cilag
Janssen-Cilag Ltd
50-100 Holmers Farm Way
High Wycombe
Bucks, HP12 4EG.
tel: (01494) 567 444
fax: (01494) 567 568

Javelin
Javelin Pharmaceuticals UK Ltd
Compass House, Vision Park
Chivers Way
Histon
Cambs, CB4 9AD..
tel: (0800) 066 5446
fax: (01223) 527 800

Jerini
Jerini AG
Invalidenstrasse 130
10115 Berlin
Germany
tel: (00800) 7020 7020

JLB
B. Braun JLB Ltd
Unit 2A
St Columb Industrial Estate
St Columb Major
Cornwall, TR9 6SF.
tel: (01637) 880 065
fax: (01637) 881 549

Jobskin
Jobskin Ltd
Unit 13 Harrington Mill
Leopold St
Long Eaton
Nottingham, NG10 4QG.
tel: (0115) 973 4300
fax: (0115) 973 3902
dw@jobskin.co.uk

Juvela
Juvela (Hero UK) Ltd
19 De-Havilland Drive
Liverpool, L24 8RN.
tel: (0151) 432 5300
fax: (0151) 432 5335
info@juvela.co.uk

K/L
K/L Pharmaceuticals Ltd
21 Macadam Place
South Newmoor
Irvine
Ayrshire, KA11 4HP.
tel: (01294) 215 951
fax: (01294) 221 600

KCI Medical
KCI Medical Ltd
Langford Business Park
Langford Locks
Kidlington
Oxon, OX5 1GF..
tel: (01865) 840 600
fax: (01865) 840 626

Kestrel
Kestrel Ltd
Ashfield House
Resolution Rd
Ashby de la Zouch
Leics, LE65 1HW.
tel: (01530) 562 301
fax: (01530) 562 430
kestrel@ventiv.co.uk

Kestrel Ophthalmics
Kestrel Ophthalmics Ltd
Kestrel House
7 Moor Rd
Broadstone
Dorset, BH18 8AZ.
tel: (01202) 658 444
fax: (01202) 659 599
info@kestrelophthalmics.co.uk

King
King Pharmaceuticals Ltd
2nd Floor, The Maltings
Bridge St
Hitchin
Herts, SG5 2DE.
tel: (01462) 434 366
fax: (01462) 450 755

KoGEN
KoGEN Ltd
Seagoe Industrial Estate
Craigavon, BT63 5UA.
tel: (028) 383 33933
fax: (028) 383 33665
info@kogen.co.uk

KoRa
KoRa Healthcare Ltd
First Floor, Unit 2
Swords Business Park, Swords
Co. Dublin
Ireland
tel: (01142) 994 979
fax: (01142) 994 979
info@kora.ie

Kyowa Hakko
Kyowa Hakko UK Ltd
258 Bath Rd
Slough
Berks, SL1 4DX.
tel: (01753) 566 020
fax: (01753) 566 030

Labopharm
Labopharm Europe Ltd
Unit 5, The Seapoint Building
44-45 Clontarf Road
Dublin 3
Ireland
tel: (0800) 678 3765 (UK only) or
(01908) 542 374
labopharm.uk@canreginc.com

Lantor
Lantor UK Ltd
73 St Helens Rd
Bolton
Lancs, BL3 3PR.
tel: (01204) 855 000
help@lantor.co.uk

Lederle
See Wyeth

LEO
LEO Pharma
Longwick Rd
Princes Risborough
Bucks, HP27 9RR.
tel: (01844) 347 333
fax: (01844) 342 278
medical-info.uk@leo-pharma.com

LifeScan
LifeScan
50-100 Holmers Farm Way
High Wycombe
Bucks, HP12 4DP.
tel: (01494) 658 750
fax: (01494) 658 751

Lilly
Eli Lilly & Co Ltd
Lilly House
Priestley Rd
Basingstoke
Hampshire, RG24 9NL.
tel: (01256) 315 999
ukmedinfo@lilly.com

Lincoln Medical
Lincoln Medical Ltd
13 Boathouse Meadow Business Park
Cherry Orchard Lane
Salisbury
Wilts, SP2 7LD.
tel: (01722) 410 443

Linderma
Linderma Ltd
Allenby Laboratories
Wigan Rd
West Houghton
Bolton, BL5 2AL.
tel: (01942) 816 184
fax: (01942) 813 937
linderma@virgin.net

Link
See Archimedes

Lipomed
Lipomed GmbH
Schonaugasse 11
D-79713
Bad Sackingen
tel: (0049) 776 155 9222
fax: (0049) 776 155 9223
lipomed@lipomed.com

Livwell
Livwell Ltd
PO Box 22
Hull, HU2 0YX.
tel: (0845) 120 0038
info@livwell.eu

Lornamead
Lornamead UK Ltd
Sabre House
377-399 London Road
Camberley
Surrey, GU15 3HL.
tel: (01276) 674000
fax: (01276) 674098
lornamead@dhl.com

LPC
LPC Medical (UK) Ltd
30 Chaul End Lane
Luton, Beds, LU4 8EZ.
tel: (01582) 560 393
fax: (01582) 560 395
info@lpcpharma.com

Lundbeck
Lundbeck Ltd
Lundbeck House
Caldecotte Lake Business Park
Caldecotte, Milton Keynes
Bucks, MK7 8LF.
tel: (01908) 649 966
fax: (01908) 647 888
ukmedicalinformation@lundbeck.com

Manx
Manx Healthcare
Taylor Group House
Wedgnock Lane
Warwick, CV34 5YA.
tel: (01926) 482 511
fax: (01926) 498 711
info@manxhealthcare.com

Marlborough
Marlborough Pharmaceuticals
PO Box 2957
Marlborough
Wilts, SN8 1WS.
tel: (01672) 514 187
fax: (01672) 515 614
info@marlborough-pharma.co.uk

Martindale
See Cardinal

MASTA
MASTA
Moorfield Rd
Yeadon
Leeds, LS19 7BN.
tel: (0113) 238 7500
fax: (0113) 238 7501
medical@masta.org

McNeil
McNeil Products Ltd
Foundation Park
Roxborough Way
Maidenhead
Berks, SL6 3UG.
tel: (01628) 822 222

MDE
MDE Diagnostics Europe Ltd
The Surrey Technology Centre
40 Occam Rd
Surrey Research Park, Guildford
Surrey, GU2 7YG.
tel: (01483) 688 400
info@mdediagnostic.co.uk

Mead Johnson
Mead Johnson Nutritionals
Uxbridge Business Park
Sanderson Rd
Uxbridge
Middx, UB8 1DH.
tel: (01895) 523 764
fax: (01895) 523 103

Meadow
Meadow Laboratories Ltd
18 Avenue Rd
Chadwell Heath
Romford
Essex, RM6 4JF.
tel: (020) 8597 1203
enquiries@meadowlabs.fsnet.co.uk

Meda
Meda Pharmaceuticals Ltd
Skyway House
Parsonage Rd
Takeley
Bishop's Stortford, CM22 6PU.
tel: (01748) 828 810
fax: (0845) 460 0002
meda@professionalinformation.co.uk

Medac
Medac (UK)
Scion House, Stirling University
Stirling, FK9 4NF.
tel: (01786) 458 086
fax: (01786) 458 032
info@medac-uk.co.uk

Medical House
The Medical House plc
199 Newhall Rd
Sheffield, S9 2QJ.
tel: (0114) 261 9011
fax: (0114) 243 1597
info@themedicalhouse.com

Medihoney
Medihoney (Europe) Ltd
200 Brook Drive
Green Park
Reading, RG2 6UB.
tel: (0800) 071 3912

Medix
See Clement Clarke

Medlock
Medlock Medical Ltd
Tubiton House
Medlock St.
Oldham, OL1 3HS.
tel: (0161) 621 2100
fax: (0161) 627 0932
medical.information@
medlockmedical.com

MedLogic
MedLogic Global Ltd
Western Wood Way
Langage Science Park
Plympton
Plymouth, Devon, PL7 5BG.
tel: (01752) 209 955
fax: (01752) 209 956
enquiries@mlgl.co.uk

Menarini
A. Menarini Pharma UK SRL
Menarini House
Mercury Park
Wycombe Lane, Wooburn Green
Bucks, HP10 0HH.
tel: (01628) 856 400
fax: (01628) 856 402

Menarini Diagnostics
A. Menarini Diagnostics
Wharfedale Rd
Winnersh
Wokingham
Berks, RG41 5RA.
tel: (0118) 944 4100
fax: (0118) 944 4111

Merck
See Merck Serono

Merck Serono
Merck Serono Ltd
Bedfont Cross
Stanwell Rd
Feltham
Middx, TW14 8NX.
tel: (020) 8818 7373
fax: (020) 8818 7274
medinfo.uk@merckserono.net

Merck Sharp & Dohme
See MSD

Merz
Merz Pharma UK Ltd
260 Centennial Park
Elstree Hill South
Herts, WD6 3SR.
tel: (020) 8236 0000
fax: (020) 8236 3501
info@merzpharma.co.uk

Micro Medical
Micro Medical Ltd
Quayside
Chatham Maritime
Chatham
Kent, ME4 4QY.
tel: (01634) 893 500
fax: (01634) 893 600
sales@micromedical.co.uk

Milupa
Milupa Ltd
White Horse Business Park
Trowbridge
Wilts, BA14 0XQ.
tel: (01225) 711 511
fax: (01225) 711 970

Mölnlycke
Mölnlycke Health Care Ltd
The Arenson Centre
Arenson Way
Dunstable
Beds, LU5 5UL.
tel: (0161) 777 2628
fax: (0161) 777 2601
info.uk@molnlycke.net

Morningside
Morningside Healthcare Ltd
115 Narborough Rd
Leicester, LE3 0PA.
tel: (0116) 204 5950
fax: (0116) 247 0756

Movianto
Movianto UK
1 Progress Park
Bedford, MK42 9XE.
tel: (01234) 248 500
fax: (01234) 248 700
movianto.uk@movianto.com

MSD
Merck Sharp & Dohme Ltd
Hertford Rd
Hoddesdon
Herts, EN11 9BU.
tel: (01992) 467 272
fax: (01992) 451 066

Nagor
Nagor Ltd
PO Box 21, Global House
Isle of Man Business Park
Douglas
Isle of Man, IM99 1AX.
tel: (01624) 625 556
fax: (01624) 661 656
enquiries@nagor.com

Napp
Napp Pharmaceuticals Ltd
Cambridge Science Park
Milton Rd
Cambs, CB4 0GW.
tel: (01223) 424 444
fax: (01223) 424 441

Neolab
Neolab Ltd
57 High St
Odiham, Hampshire, RG29 1LF.
tel: (01256) 704 110
fax: (01256) 701 144
info@neolab.co.uk

Neomedic
Neomedic Ltd
2a Crofters Rd
Northwood
Middx, HA6 3ED.
tel: (01923) 836 379
fax: (01923) 840 160
marketing@neomedic.co.uk

Nestlé
Nestlé Nutrition
St George's House
Park Lane
Croydon
Surrey, CR9 1NR.
tel: (020) 8667 5130
fax: (020) 8667 5616
nutrition@uk.nestle.com

Nordic
Nordic Pharma UK Ltd
Abbey House
1650 Arlington Business Park
Theale
Reading, RG7 4SA.
tel: (0118) 929 8233
fax: (0118) 929 8234
info@nordicpharma.co.uk

Norgine
Norgine Pharmaceuticals Ltd
Chaplin House
Moorhall Rd
Harefield
Middx, UB9 6NS.
tel: (01895) 826 600
fax: (01895) 825 865

Novartis
Novartis Pharmaceuticals UK Ltd
Frimley Business Park
Frimley
Camberley
Surrey, GU16 7SR.
tel: (01276) 692 255
fax: (01276) 692 508

Novartis Consumer Health
Novartis Consumer Health
Wimblehurst Rd
Horsham
West Sussex, RH12 5AB.
tel: (01403) 210 211
fax: (01403) 323 939
medicalaffairs.uk@novartis.com

Novartis Vaccines
Novartis Vaccines Ltd
Gaskill Rd
Speke
Liverpool, L24 9GR.
tel: (08457) 451 500
fax: (0151) 7055 669
serviceuk@chiron.com

Novo Nordisk
Novo Nordisk Ltd
Broadfield Park
Brighton Rd
Crawley
West Sussex, RH11 9RT.
tel: (01293) 613 555
fax: (01293) 613 535
customercareuk@novonordisk.com

nSPIRE Health
nSPIRE Health Ltd
Unit 10, Harforde Court
John Tate Rd
Hertford
Herts, SG13 7NW.
tel: (01992) 526 300
fax: (01992) 526 320
info@nspirehealth.com

Nutricia Clinical
Nutricia Clinical Care
Nutricia Ltd
White Horse Business Park
Trowbridge
Wilts, BA14 0XQ.
tel: (01225) 711 688
fax: (01225) 711 798
cndirect@nutricia.co.uk

Nutricia Dietary
Nutricia Dietary Care
see Nutricia Clinical

Nutrition Point
Nutrition Point Ltd
13 Taurus Park
Westbrook
Warrington
Cheshire, WA5 7ZT.
tel: (07041) 544 044
fax: (07041) 544 055
info@nutritionpoint.co.uk

Nycomed
Nycomed UK Ltd
3 Globeside Business Park
Fieldhouse Lane
Marlow
Bucks, SL7 1HZ.
tel: (01628) 646 400
fax: (01628) 646 401
medinfo@nycomed.com

Octapharma
Octapharma Ltd
The Zenith Building
26 Spring Gardens
Manchester, M2 1AB.
tel: (0161) 837 3770
octapharma@octapharma.co.uk

Omron
Omron Healthcare (UK) Ltd
Opal Drive
Fox Milne
Milton Keynes, MK15 0DG.
tel: (0870) 750 2771
fax: (0870) 750 2772
info.omronhealthcare.uk@eu.omron.
com

Organon
Organon Laboratories Ltd
Cambridge Science Park
Milton Rd
Cambs, CB4 0FL.
tel: (01223) 432 700
fax: (01223) 424 368
medrequest@organon.co.uk

Orion
Orion Pharma (UK) Ltd
Oaklea Court
22 Park Street
Newbury
Berks, RG14 1EA.
tel: (01635) 520 300
fax: (01635) 520 319
medicalinformation@orionpharma.
com

Orphan Europe
Orphan Europe (UK) Ltd
Isis House
43 Station Rd
Henley-on-Thames
Oxon, RG9 1AT.
tel: (01491) 414 333
fax: (01491) 414 443
info.uk@orphan-europe.com

Otsuka
Otsuka Pharmaceutical (UK) Ltd
BSi Tower
389 Chiswick High Rd, London, W4
4AJ.
tel: (020) 8742 4300
fax: (020) 8994 8548
medinfo@otsuka.co.uk

Ovation
Ovation Healthcare International Ltd
1 Setanta Place
Dublin 2
Ireland
tel: (00353) 161 39 707
fax: (00353) 161 39 708

Owen Mumford
Owen Mumford Ltd
Brook Hill
Woodstock
Oxford, OX20 1TU.
tel: (01993) 812 021
fax: (01993) 813 466
customerservices@owenmumford.
co.uk

Oxford Nutrition
Oxford Nutrition Ltd
Unit 5 Western Units
Pottery Rd
Bovey Tracey, TQ13 9JJ.
tel: (01626) 832 067
fax: (01626) 836 841
info@nutrinox.com

Paines & Byrne
Paines & Byrne Ltd
Lovett House
Lovett Rd
Staines
Middx, TW18 3AZ.
tel: (01784) 419 620
fax: (01784) 419 401

Pari
PARI Medical Ltd
The Old Sorting Office
Rosemount Ave
West Byfleet
Surrey, KT14 6LB.
tel: (01932) 341 122
fax: (01932) 341 134
infouk@pari.de

Parkside
Parkside Healthcare
12 Parkside Ave
Salford, M7 4HB.
tel: (0161) 795 2792
fax: (0161) 795 4076

Peckforton
Peckforton Pharmaceuticals Ltd
Crewe Hall
Crewe
Cheshire, CW1 6UL.
tel: (01270) 582 255
fax: (01270) 582 299
info@peckforton.com

Penn
Penn Pharmaceuticals Services Ltd
Unit 23 & 24, Tafarnaubach Industrial
Estate
Tredegar
Gwent, NP22 3AA.
tel: (01495) 711 222
fax: (01495) 711 225
penn@pennpharm.co.uk

Pfizer
Pfizer Ltd
Walton Oaks
Dorking Rd
Walton-on-the-Hill
Surrey, KT20 7NS.
tel: (01304) 616 161
fax: (01304) 656 221

PGR Health Foods
PGR Health Foods Ltd
PO Box 214
Hertford, SG14 2ZX.
tel: (01992) 581715
fax: (01992) 536594
info@pgrhealthfoods.co.uk

Pharmacia
See Pfizer

Pharma-Global
Pharma-Global Ltd
Hudson Rd
Sandycove
Co. Dublin
Ireland
tel: (0800) 0436 580
fax: (00353) 1280 2419
eyecare@pharmaglobal.ie

Pharma Mar
See IDIS

Pharma Nord
Pharma Nord (UK) Ltd
Telford Court
Morpeth
Northumberland, NE61 2DB.
tel: (01670) 519989
fax: (01670) 534903
info@pharmanord.co.uk

Pharmasure
Pharmasure Ltd
28 Watford Metro Centre
Dwight Rd
Watford, WD18 9SB.
tel: (01923) 233 466
fax: (01923) 233 113
info@pharmasure.co.uk

Pharmexx UK
Pharmexx UK Ltd
98 Crowmarsh Battle Barns
Preston Crowmarsh
Wallingford
Oxon, OX10 6SL.
tel: (01748) 828 888
pharmexx@professionalinformation.
co.uk

Pinewood
Pinewood Healthcare
Ballymacabry
Clonmel, Co Tipperary, Eire
tel: (00353) 523 6253
fax: (00353) 523 6311
info@pinewood.ie

PLIVA
PLIVA Pharma Ltd
Vision House
Bedford Rd
Petersfield
Hampshire, GU32 3QB.
tel: (01730) 710900
fax: (01730) 710901
medinfo@pliva-pharma.co.uk

Potters
Potters Herbal Medicines
1 Botanic Court
Martland Park
Wigan, WN5 0JZ.
tel: (01942) 219 960
fax: (01942) 219 966
info@pottersherbals.co.uk

Procter & Gamble
Procter & Gamble UK
The Heights
Brooklands
Weybridge
Surrey, KT13 0XP.
tel: (01932) 896 000
fax: (01932) 896 200

Procter & Gamble Pharm.
Procter & Gamble Technical Centres
Medical Dept
Rusham Park
Whitehall Lane
Egham, Surrey, TW20 9NW.
tel: (01784) 474 900
fax: (01784) 474 705

Profile
Profile Pharma Ltd
Chichester Business Park
City Fields Way
Chichester
West Sussex, PO20 2FT.
tel: (0800) 1300 855
fax: (0800) 1300 856
info@profilepharma.com

Profile Respiratory
See Respironics

ProStrakan
ProStrakan Ltd
Galabank Business Park
Galashiels, TD1 1QH.
tel: (01896) 664 000
fax: (01896) 664 001
medinfo@prostrakan.com

Protex
Protex Healthcare (UK) Ltd
Unit 5, Molly Millars Lane
Wokingham
Berks, RG41 2Q2.
tel: (08700) 114 112
orders@protexhealthcare.co.uk

Provalis
See KoGEN

R&C
See Reckitt Benckiser

Ranbaxy
Ranbaxy Ltd
CP House
97-107 Uxbridge Rd
Ealing
London, W5 5TL.
tel: (020) 8280 1600
fax: (020) 8280 1996
medinfoeurope@ranbaxy.com

Ransom
Ransom Consumer Healthcare
Alexander House
40A Wilbury Way
Hitchin
Herts, SG5 1LY.
tel: (01462) 437 615
fax: (01462) 420 528
info@williamransom.com

Ratiopharm UK
Ratiopharm UK Ltd
5 Jackson Close
Grove Rd
Cosham
Portsmouth, Hants, PO6 1UP.
tel: (02392) 313 587
fax: (02392) 386 208
info@ratiopharmdirect.co.uk

Reckitt Benckiser
Reckitt Benckiser Healthcare
Dansom Lane
Hull, HU8 7DS.
tel: (01482) 326 151
fax: (01482) 582 526
miu@reckittbenckiser.com

Recordati
Recordati Pharmaceuticals Ltd
Knyvett House
The Causeway
Staines
Middx, TW18 3BA.
tel: (01784) 898 300
fax: (01784) 895 103

Regent Medical
See Mölnlycke

ReSource Medical
ReSource Medical UK Ltd
2 Thorne Rd
Thornton Lodge
Huddersfield, HD1 3JJ.
tel: (01484) 531 489
fax: (01484) 531 584
info@resource-medical.co.uk

Respironics
Respironics (UK) Ltd
Chichester Business Park
City Fields Way
Tangmere, Chichester
West Sussex, PO20 2FT.
tel: (0800) 1300 840
fax: (0800) 1300 841
rukmarketing@respironics.com

Rhône-Poulenc Rorer
See Sanofi-Aventis

Richardson
Richardson Healthcare Ltd
Devonshire House
Manor Way
Borehamwood
Herts, WD6 1QQ.
tel: (08700) 111 126
fax: (08700) 111 127
info@richardsonhealthcare.com

Riemser
Riemser Arzneimittel AG
An der Wiek 7
17493 Greifswald - Insel Riems
Germany
tel: (0049) 38351 76 679
fax: (0049) 38351 76 778
info@RIEMSER.de

RIS Products
RIS Products Ltd
10 Prospect Place
Welwyn
Herts, AL6 9EW.
tel: (01438) 840 135
fax: (01438) 716 067
info@risproducts.co.uk

Robinsons
Robinson Healthcare Ltd
Lawn Rd
Carlton-in-Lindrick Industrial Estate
Worksop
Notts, S81 9LB.
tel: (01909) 735 001
fax: (01909) 731 103
enquiries@robinsoncare.com

Roche
Roche Products Ltd
Hexagon Place
6 Falcon Way, Shire Park
Welwyn Garden City
Herts, AL7 1TW.
tel: (0800) 328 1629
fax: (01707) 384 555
medinfo.uk@roche.com

Roche Consumer Health
See Bayer

Roche Diagnostics
Roche Diagnostics Ltd
Charles Avenue
Burgess Hill
West Sussex, RH15 9RY.
tel: (01444) 256 000
fax: (01444) 256 239
burgesshill.accu-chek@roche.com

Rosemont
Rosemont Pharmaceuticals Ltd
Rosemont House
Yorkdale Industrial Park
Braithwaite St
Leeds, LS11 9XE.
tel: (0113) 244 1999
fax: (0113) 246 0738
infodesk@rosemontpharma.com

Rowa
Rowa Pharmaceuticals Ltd
Bantry
Co Cork
Ireland
tel: (00 353 27) 50077
fax: (00 353 27) 50417
rowa@rowa-pharma.ie

S&N Hlth.
Smith & Nephew Healthcare Ltd
Healthcare House
Goulton St
Hull, HU3 4DJ.
tel: (01482) 222 200
fax: (01482) 222 211
advice@smith-nephew.com

Sagani
Sagani Ltd
Unit 9 Park House
15-19 Greenhill Crescent
Watford Business Park
Watford, WD18 8PH.
tel: (01923) 251 777
fax: (01923) 251 999
sales@sagani.co.uk

Sallis
Sallis Healthcare Ltd
Vernon Works
Waterford St
Basford
Nottingham, NG6 0DH.
tel: (0115) 978 7841
fax: (0115) 942 2272

Sandoz
Sandoz Ltd
Unit 37
Woolmer Way
Bordon
Hants, GU35 9QE.
tel: (01420) 478 301
fax: (01420) 474 427

Sankyo
See Daiichi Sankyo

Sanochemia
Sanochemia Diagnostics UK Ltd
Argentum
510 Bristol Business Park
Coldharbour Lane
Bristol, BS16 1EJ.
tel: (0117) 906 3562
fax: (0117) 906 3709

Sanofi-Aventis
Sanofi-Aventis Ltd
1 Onslow St
Guildford
Surrey, GU1 4YS.
tel: (01483) 505 515
fax: (01483) 535 432
uk-medicalinformation@
sanofi-aventis.com

Sanofi Pasteur
Sanofi Pasteur MSD Ltd
Mallards Reach
Bridge Avenue
Maidenhead
Berks, SL6 1QP.
tel: (01628) 785 291
fax: (01628) 671 722

Sanofi-Synthelabo
See Sanofi-Aventis

Schering Health
See Bayer

Schering-Plough
Schering-Plough Ltd
Shire Park
Welwyn Garden City
Herts, AL7 1TW.
tel: (01707) 363 636
fax: (01707) 363 763
medical.info@spcorp.com

Schuco
Schuco International Ltd
Challenge House
1 Lyndhurst Ave
London, N12 0NE.
tel: (020) 8368 1642
fax: (020) 8361 3761
sales@schuco.co.uk

Serono
See Merck Serono

Servier
Servier Laboratories Ltd
Gallions
Wexham Springs
Framewood Rd
Wexham, SL3 6RJ.
tel: (01753) 666 409
fax: (01753) 666 204
medical.information@uk.netgrs.com

Seven Seas
Seven Seas Ltd
Hedon Rd
Marfleet
Hull, HU9 5NJ.
tel: (01482) 375 234
fax: (01482) 374 345

Shermond
Shermond
Castle House
Sea View Way
Woodingdean
Brighton, East Sussex, BN2 6NT.
tel: (0870) 242 7701
fax: (01273) 391 028
sales@shermond.com

Shire
Shire Pharmaceuticals Ltd
Hampshire International Business
Park
Chineham
Basingstoke
Hants, RG24 8EP.
tel: (0800) 055 6614
fax: (01256) 894 708
medinfoglobal@shire.com

SHS
SHS International Ltd
100 Wavertree Boulevard
Wavertree Technology Park
Liverpool, L7 9PT.
tel: (0151) 228 8161
fax: (0151) 230 5365
nutrition@shsint.co.uk

Sigma
Sigma Pharmaceuticals plc
PO Box 233
Unit 1-7 Colonial Way
Watford
Herts, WD24 4YR.
tel: (01923) 444 999
fax: (01923) 444 998
info@sigpharm.co.uk

Sigma-Tau
Sigma-Tau Pharma Ltd (UK)
Abbey House
1650 Arlington Business Park
Reading
Berks, RG7 4SA.
tel: (0118) 929 8075
fax: (0118) 929 8076
medical.information@sigma-tau.co.
uk

Sinclair
Sinclair Pharmaceuticals Ltd
4 Godalming Business Centre
Woolsack Way
Godalming
Surrey, GU7 1XW.
tel: (01483) 410 600
fax: (01483) 410 620
info@sinclairpharma.com

Skin Camouflage Co.
The Skin Camouflage Company Ltd
Moor Lane
Sotby
Market Rasen, LN8 5LR.
tel: (01507) 343 091
fax: (01507) 343 092
smjcovermark@aol.com

SLO Drinks
SLO Drinks Ltd
Unit 1
Torr Top St
New Mills
High Peak, SK22 4BS.
tel: (08452) 22 22 05
fax: (08452) 22 22 06
info@slodrinks.com

SMA Nutrition
See Wyeth

SNBTS
Scottish National Blood Transfusion
Service
Protein Fractionation Centre
Ellen's Glen Rd
Edinburgh, EH17 7QT.
tel: (0131) 536 5700
fax: (0131) 536 5781
Contact.pfc@snbts.csa.scot.nhs.uk

Solvay
Solvay Healthcare Ltd
Mansbridge Rd
West End
Southampton, SO18 3JD.
tel: (023) 8046 7000
fax: (023) 8046 5350
medinfo.shl@solvay.com

Sovereign
See Amdipharm

SpePharm
SpePharm UK Ltd
2B Bankside
Hanborough Business Park
Long Hanborough
Witney, Oxon, OX29 8LJ.
tel: (0844) 800 7335
fax: (0844) 800 7336
medinfo.uk@spepharm.com

Squibb
See Bristol-Myers Squibb

SSL
SSL International plc
Venus, 1 Old Park Lane
Trafford Park
Urmston
Manchester, M41 7HA.
tel: (08701) 222 690
fax: (08701) 222 692
medical.information@
ssl-international.com

STD Pharmaceutical
STD Pharmaceutical Products Ltd
Plough Lane
Hereford, HR4 0EL.
tel: (01432) 373 555
fax: (01432) 373 556
enquiries@stdpharm.co.uk

Steraid
Steraid (Gainsborough) Ltd
Unit 42
Corringham Road Industrial Estate
Gainsborough , DN21 1QB.
tel: (01427) 677 659
fax: (01427) 677 654

Stiefel
Stiefel Laboratories (UK) Ltd
Holtspur Lane
Wooburn Green
High Wycombe
Bucks, HP10 0AU.
tel: (01628) 524 966
fax: (01628) 810 021
general@stiefel.co.uk

Stragen
Stragen UK Ltd
Castle Court
41 London Rd
Reigate
Surrey, RH2 9RJ.
tel: (0870) 351 8744
fax: (0870) 351 8745
info@stragenuk.com

Strakan
See ProStrakan

Su-Med
Su-Med International UK Ltd
Integrity House
Units 1-2 Graphite Way
Hadfield
Glossop, Derbyshire, SK13 1QH.
tel: (01457) 890 980
fax: (01457) 890 990
sales@sumed.co.uk

Sutherland
Sutherland Health Ltd
Unit 1, Rivermead
Pipers Way
Thatcham
Berks, RG19 4EP.
tel: (01635) 874 488
fax: (01635) 877 622

Swedish Orphan
Swedish Orphan International Ltd
1 Fordham House Court
Fordham House Estate
Newmarket Rd
Fordham, Cambs, CB7 5LL.
tel: (01638) 722 380
fax: (01638) 723 167

Synergy Healthcare
Synergy Healthcare (UK) Ltd
Lion Mill
Fitton St
Royton
Oldham, OL2 5JX.
tel: (0161) 624 5641
fax: (0161) 627 0902
healthcaresolutions@
synergyhealthplc.com

Syner-Med
Syner-Med (Pharmaceutical
Products) Ltd
Beech House
840 Brighton Rd
Purley, CR8 2BH.
tel: (0845) 634 2100
fax: (0845) 634 2101
mail@syner-med.com

Takeda
Takeda UK Ltd
Takeda House, Mercury Park
Wycombe Lane
Wooburn Green
High Wycombe, Bucks, HP10 0HH.
tel: (01628) 537 900
fax: (01628) 526 615

Talley
Talley Group Ltd
Abbey Park Industrial Estate
Premier Way
Romsey
Hants, SO51 9DQ.
tel: (01794) 503 500
fax: (01794) 503 555

Taro
Taro Pharmaceuticals (UK) Ltd
Lakeside
1 Furzeground Way
Stockley Park East
Uxbridge, Middx, UB11 1BD.
tel: (08707) 369 544
fax: (08707) 369 545
customerservice@taropharma.co.uk

Teofarma
Teofarma S.r.l.
c/o Professional Information Ltd
Olliver
Richmond
North Yorkshire, DL10 5HX.
tel: (01748) 828 857
teofarma@professionalinformation.
co.uk

Teva
Teva Pharmaceuticals Ltd
The Gate House
Gatehouse Way
Aylesbury
Bucks, HP19 8DB.
med.info@tevapharma.co.uk

TEVA UK
TEVA UK Ltd
Building V
The London Road Campus
London Rd
Harlow, Essex, CM17 9LP.
tel: (08705) 020 304
fax: (08705) 323 334
medinfo@tevauk.com

Thornton & Ross
Thornton & Ross Ltd
Linthwaite Laboratories
Huddersfield, HD7 5QH.
tel: (01484) 842 217
fax: (01484) 847 301
mail@thorntonross.com

Tillomed
Tillomed Laboratories Ltd
3 Howard Rd
Eaton Socon, St Neots
Cambs, PE19 3ET.
tel: (01480) 402 400
fax: (01480) 402 402
info@tillomed.co.uk

TOL
Tree of Life
Coaldale Rd
Lymedale Business Park
Newcastle Under Lyme
Staff, ST5 9QX.
tel: (01782) 567 100
fax: (01782) 567 199
health@tol-europe.com

TopoTarget
TopoTarget A/S
Symbion Science Park
Fruebjergvej 3
DK-2100
Copenhagen, Denmark
tel: (00 45 39) 178 392
fax: (00 45 39) 179 492

Torbet
Torbet Laboratories Ltd
14D Wendover Rd
Rackheath Industrial Estate
Rackheath
Norwich, NR13 6LH.
tel: (01603) 735 200
fax: (01603) 735 217
torbet@typharm.com

Transdermal
Transdermal Ltd
35 Grimwade Ave
Croydon
Surrey, CR0 5DJ.
tel: (020) 8654 2251
fax: (020) 8654 2252
transdermal@transdermal.co.uk

TRB Chemedica
TRB Chemedica (UK) Ltd
MED IC3
Keele University Science Park
Keele
Staffordshire, ST5 5NP.
tel: (0845) 330 7556
fax: (0845) 330 7557
phunt@trbchemedica.co.uk

Typharm
Typharm Ltd
14D Wendover Rd
Rackheath Industrial Estate
Rackheath
Norwich, NR13 6LH.
tel: (01603) 735 200
fax: (01603) 735 217
customerservices@typharm.com

UCB Pharma
UCB Pharma Ltd
208 Bath Rd
Slough, SL1 3WE.
tel: (01753) 534 655
fax: (01753) 447 647
medicalinformationuk@ucb-group.
com

Ultrapharm
Ultrapharm Ltd
Centenary Business Park
Henley-on-Thames
Oxon, RG9 1DS.
tel: (01491) 578 016
fax: (01491) 570 001
orders@glutenfree.co.uk

Univar
Univar Ltd
International House
Zenith, Paycocke Rd
Basildon
Essex, SS14 3DW.
tel: (01268) 594 400
fax: (01268) 594 481
trientine@univareurope.com

Unomedical
Unomedical Ltd
Thornhill Rd
Redditch, B98 7NL.
tel: (01527) 587 700
fax: (01527) 592 111

Urgo
Urgo Ltd
Sullington Rd
Shepshed
Loughborough
Leics, LE12 9JJ.
tel: (01509) 502 051
fax: (01509) 650 898
medical@parema.com

Valeant
Valeant Pharmaceuticals Ltd
Cedarwood
Chineham Business Park
Crockford Lane, Basingstoke
Hants, RG24 8WD.
tel: (01256) 707 744
fax: (01256) 707 334
valeantuk@valeant.com

Vegenat
c/o Archaelis Ltd
23 Pembridge Gardens
London, W2 4EB.
tel: (0870) 803 2484
info@vegenat.co.uk

Viatris
See Meda

Viridian
Viridian Pharma Ltd
Yew Tree House
Hendrew Lane
Llandevaud
Newport, Gwent, NP18 2AB.
tel: (01633) 400 335
info@viridianpharma.co.uk

Vitaflo
Vitaflo Ltd
11 Century Building
Brunswick Business Park
Liverpool, L3 4BL.
tel: (0151) 709 9020
fax: (0151) 709 9727
vitaflo@vitaflo.co.uk

Vitaline
Vitaline Pharmaceuticals UK Ltd
Chiltern House, Unit P
Howland Rd
Thame
Oxon, OX9 3GQ.
tel: (01844) 269 007
fax: (01844) 269 005
vitalineinfo@aol.com

Vitalograph
Vitalograph Ltd
Maids Moreton
Buckingham, MK18 1SW.
tel: (01280) 827 110
fax: (01280) 823 302
sales@vitalograph.co.uk

Wallace Cameron
Wallace Cameron Ltd
26 Netherhall Rd
Netherton Industrial Estate
Wishaw, ML2 0JG.
tel: (01698) 354 600
fax: (01698) 354 700
sales@wallacecameron.com

Wallace Mfg
Wallace Manufacturing Chemists Ltd
Wallace House
New Abbey Court
51-53 Stert St, Abingdon
Oxon, OX14 3JF.
tel: (01235) 538 700
fax: (01235) 538 800
info@alinter.co.uk

WaveSense
WaveSense Europe Ltd
Harwell Innovation Centre
173 Curie Ave
Harwell Science & Innovation
Campus
Didcot, Oxon, OX11 0QG.
tel: (01235) 838 639
fax: (01235) 838 648
enquiries@wavesense.co.uk

Wellfoods
Wellfoods Ltd
Towngate
Mapplewell
Barnsley
South Yorks, S75 6AS.
tel: (01226) 381 712
fax: (01226) 390 087
wellfoods@talk21.com

Winthrop
Winthrop Pharmaceuticals UK Ltd
PO Box 611
Guildford, Surrey, GU1 4YS.
tel: (01483) 554 101
fax: (01483) 554 810
winthropsales@sanofi-aventis.com

Wockhardt
Wockhardt UK Ltd
Ash Rd North
Wrexham Industrial Estate
Wrexham, LL13 9UF.
tel: (01978) 661 261
fax: (01978) 660 130

Wyeth
Wyeth Pharmaceuticals
Huntercombe Lane South
Taplow
Maidenhead
Berks, SL6 0PH.
tel: (01628) 604 377
fax: (01628) 666 368
ukmedinfo@wyeth.com

Wynlit
Wynlit Laboratories
153 Furzehill Rd
Borehamwood
Herts, WD6 2DR.
tel: (07903) 370 130
fax: (020) 8292 6117

Wyvern
Wyvern Medical Ltd
PO Box 17
Ledbury
Herefordshire, HR8 2ES.
tel: (01531) 631 105
fax: (01531) 634 844

Zeal
G. H. Zeal Ltd
Deer Park Rd
London, SW19 3UU.
tel: (020) 8542 2283
fax: (020) 8543 7840
scientific@zeal.co.uk

Zeneus
See Cephalon

Zeroderma
Zeroderma Ltd
The Manor House
Victor Barns
Northampton Rd, Brixworth
Northampton, NN6 9DQ.
tel: (01604) 889 855
fax: (01604) 883 199
info@ixlpharma.com

ZooBiotic
ZooBiotic Ltd
Biosurgical Research Unit
Surgical Materials Testing Laboratory
Princess of Wales Hospital, Coity Rd
Brigend, Mid Glamorgan, South
Wales, CF31 1RQ.
tel: (0845) 230 1810
fax: (01656) 752 830
maggots@smtl.co.uk

Special-order Manufacturers

Unlicensed medicines are available from 'special-order' manufacturers and specialist-importing companies; the MHRA maintains a register of these companies at www.mhra.gov.uk.

Licensed **hospital manufacturing units** also manufacture 'special-order' products as unlicensed medicines, the principal NHS units are listed below. A database (*Pro-File*; www.pro-file.nhs.uk) provides information on all medicines manufactured in the NHS; access is restricted to NHS pharmacy staff.

The characteristics of unlicensed formulations may vary, see also Unlicensed Medicines (p. 7) and Extemporaneous Preparations (p. 8).

> The MHRA recommends that an unlicensed medicine should only be used when a patient has special requirements that cannot be met by use of a licensed medicine

England

London

Mr P. Forsey
Production Manager
Guy's and St. Thomas' NHS Foundation Trust
Pharmacy Department
St. Thomas' Hospital
Lambeth Palace Rd
London, SE1 7EH.
tel: (020) 7188 5003
fax: (020) 7188 5013
paul.forsey@gstt.nhs.uk

Mr A. Krol
Managing Director
Moorfields Pharmaceuticals
Moorfields Eye Hospital NHS Trust
25 Provost St
London, N1 7NH.
tel: (020) 7684 8555
fax: (020) 7502 2332
alan.krol@moorfields.nhs.uk

Mr V. Kumar
Assistant Chief Pharmacist
Pharmacy Technical Services Department
St George's Healthcare NHS Trust
Lanesborough Wing
Blackshaw Rd
London, SW17 0QT.
tel: (020) 8725 1193
fax: (020) 8725 3947
vinodh.kumar@stgeorges.nhs.uk

Mr M. Lillywhite
Director of Technical Services
Barts and the London NHS Trust
Pathology and Pharmacy Building
80 Newark St
Whitechapel
London, E1 2ES.
tel: (020) 3246 0273
fax: (020) 3246 0268
mike.lillywhite@bartsandthelondon.nhs.uk

Dr K. Middleton
Principal Pharmacist, Technical Services
Department of Pharmacy
Northwick Park and St Mark's Hospital
Watford Rd
Harrow
Middx, HA1 3UJ.
tel: (020) 8869 2204/2223
keith.middleton@nwlh.nhs.uk

Ms C. Trehane
Production Manager
Royal Free Hospital
Pond Street
London, NW3 2QG.
tel: (020) 7830 2282 / orders: 2424
christine.trehane@royalfree.nhs.uk

Midlands and Eastern

Mr C. Hanson
Production Manager
Pharmacy Manufacturing Unit
The Ipswich Hospital NHS Trust
Heath Rd
Ipswich, IP4 5PD.
tel: (01473) 703 603
fax: (01473) 703 609
con.hanson@ipswichhospital.nhs.uk

Ms J. Kendall
Assistant Chief Pharmacist
Pharmacy Production Units
Nottingham University Hospitals NHS Trust
Queens Medical Centre Campus
Nottingham, NG7 2UH.
tel: (0115) 875 4521
fax: (0115) 970 9744
jeanette.kendall@nuh.nhs.uk

Dr S. Langford
Principal Pharmacist, Technical Services
Pharmacy Manufacturing Unit
University Hospital of North Staffs
City General Site
Stoke-on-Trent, ST4 6QG.
tel: (01782) 552 292
stephen.langford@uhns.nhs.uk

Mr B. McElroy
Associate Director of Pharmacy
UHB Medicines (SFMU)
32–34 Melchett Rd, Kings Norton
Business Centre, Kings Norton
Birmingham, B30 3HS.
tel: (0121) 627 2145
fax: (0121) 627 2168
bruce.mcelroy@uhb.nhs.uk

Dr R. Needle
Chief Pharmacist
Essex Rivers Healthcare NHS Trust
Colchester General Hospital
Turner Rd
Colchester, C04 5JL.
tel: (01206) 742 433
fax: (01206) 742 319
richard.needle@essexrivers.nhs.uk

Mr P.G. Williams
Technical and Support Services Manager
Pharmacy Manufacturing Unit
Queens Hospital
Burton Hospitals NHS Trust
Belvedere Rd
Burton-on-Trent, DE13 0RB.
tel: (01283) 511 511 Extn 5138
fax: (01283) 593 036
paul.williams@burtonh-tr.wmids.nhs.uk

North East

Ms S. Klein
Production Manager
Pharmacy Production Unit
Royal Victoria Infirmary
Queen Victoria Rd
Newcastle-upon-Tyne, NE1 4LP.
tel: (0191) 282 0377
fax: (0191) 282 0376
stephanie.klein@nuth.nhs.uk

North West

Mr M.D. Booth
Principal Pharmacist
Production & Aseptic Services
Manager
Stockport Pharmaceuticals
Stepping Hill Hospital
Stockport
Cheshire, SK2 7JE.
tel: (0161) 419 5657
fax: (0161) 419 5664
mike.booth@stockport.nhs.uk

Mr N. Fletcher
Deputy Director of Pharmacy, Technical Services
Preston Pharmaceuticals
Royal Preston Hospital
Fulwood
Preston, PR2 9HT.
tel: (01772) 522 505
fax: (01772) 522 602
neil.fletcher@lthtr.nhs.uk

South East

Mr F. Brown
Head of Production
Pharmacy Department
St Peter's Hospital
Guildford Rd
Chertsey
Surrey, KT16 OPZ.
tel: (01932) 722 886
fax: (01932) 723 209
fraser.brown@asph.nhs.uk

Ms G. Middlehurst
Quality Assurance and Business
Manager
Pharmacy Manufacturing Unit
Queen Alexandra Hospital
Southwick Hill Rd
Cosham
Portsmouth
Hants, PO6 3LY.
tel: (02392) 286 335
fax: (02392) 378 288
gillian.middlehurst@porthosp.nhs.uk

Mr M. Sherwood
Principal Pharmacist (Production)
Eastbourne DGH Pharmaceuticals
Eastbourne DGH Hospital
East Sussex Hospitals NHS Trust
Kings Drive, Eastbourne
East Sussex, BN21 2UD.
tel: (01323) 414 906
fax: (01323) 414 931
mike.sherwood@esht.nhs.uk

South West

Mr P. S. Bendell
Pharmacy Manufacturing Services
Manager
Torbay PMU
South Devon Healthcare
Kemmings Close
Long Rd
Paignton
Devon, TQ4 7TW.
tel: (01803) 664 707
fax: (01803) 664 354
phil.bendell@nhs.net

Yorkshire

Mr R.W. Brookes
Technical Services Manager
Pharmacy Department
Royal Hallamshire Hospital
Glossop Rd
Sheffield, S10 2JF.
tel: (0114) 271 3104
fax: (0114) 271 2783
roger.brookes@sth.nhs.uk

Dr J. Harwood
Production Manager
Pharmacy Manufacturing Unit
Calderdale and Huddersfield NHS
Foundation Trust
Gate 2, School St
Lindley
Huddersfield
West Yorks, HD3 3ET.
tel: (01484) 355 371
fax: (01484) 355 377
john.harwood@cht.nhs.uk

Northern Ireland

Ms C. McBride
Assistant Director of Pharmaceutical
Services
Manufacturing and Royal Group of
Hospitals Belfast
77 Boucher Crescent
Belfast, BT12 6HU.
tel: (028) 9063 3310 or (028) 9055
3407
fax: (028) 9055 3498
colette.mcbride@royalhospitals.n-i.nhs.uk

Scotland

Mr G. Conkie
Manager, Pharmacy Production Unit
Western Infirmary
Dumbarton Road
Glasgow, G11 6NT.
tel: (0141) 211 2882
fax: (0141) 211 1967
graham.conkie@northglasgow.scot.nhs.uk

Mr B. W. Millar
General Manager
Tayside Pharmaceuticals
Ninewells Hospital
Dundee, DD1 9SY.
tel: (01382) 632 183
fax: (01382) 632 060
baxter.w.millar@tuht.scot.nhs.uk

Wales

Mr P. Spark
Principal Pharmacist (Production)
Cardiff and Vale NHS Trust
University Hospital of Wales
Heath Park, Cardiff, CF14 4XW.
tel: (029) 2074 4828
fax: (029) 2074 3114
paul.spark@cardiffandvale.wales.nhs.uk

Index

Principal page references are printed in **bold** type. Proprietary (trade) names are printed in *italic* type; where the BNF for children does not include a full entry for a branded product, the non-proprietary name is shown in brackets. Names of organisms are also shown in *italic* type.

A

Abacavir, 373, **375**
  lamivudine and zidovudine with, 375
  lamivudine with, 375
Abbreviations, *inside back cover*
  Latin, *inside back cover*
  of units, 5
  Symbols, *inside back cover*
Abcare, 429
Abdominal surgery, antibacterial prophylaxis, 306
Abelcet, 363, 364
Abetalipoproteinaemia, 582
Abidec, 584
Able Spacer, 182
Abscess, dental, 302
Absence seizures, 266
Acanthamoeba keratitis, 622
  contact lenses, 640
Acarbose, 432
Acaricides, 715
ACBS
  foods, 878
  toilet preparations, 917
Accolate, 191
Accu-Chek preparations, 437
Accuhaler
  Flixotide, 188
  Seretide, 188
  Serevent, 177
  Ventolin, 176
ACE inhibitors, **130**
  diuretics with, 131
  heart failure, 130
  renal function, 131
Acea, 710
Acepril (captopril), 133
Acetaminophen *see* Paracetamol
Acetazolamide
  diuretic, 107
  epilepsy, 283, **633**
  glaucoma, 631, **633**, 634
  intracranial pressure, raised, **633**
Acetic acid, otitis externa, 643
Acetylcholine chloride, **639**
Acetylcysteine
  cystic fibrosis, 206
  eye, 637
  meconium ileus, 206
  mucolytic, **207**
  paracetamol poisoning, 36, **38**, 39
Acetylsalicylic acid *see* Aspirin
Aciclovir, **386**, 387
  herpes simplex, 386
    eye, 386, **625**
    genital, 386, 475, 715
    labialis, 715
  herpes zoster, 386
  mouth, 657
  skin, **715**
  varicella zoster, 386
Acid aspiration, prophylaxis, 762

Acidex, 53
Acidosis
  lactic, 374
  metabolic, 550, 555
Acitretin, 685, **689**, 690
Acnamino MR, 331
Acne, 692
  infantile, 693, 699
  systemic treatment, 697
  topical treatment, 693
Acnecide, 694
Acnisal, 697
Acnocin (co-cyprindiol), 698
Acrodermatitis enteropathica, 573
ACTH *see* Corticotropin, 459
Actidose-Aqua Advance, 36
Actilyse, 157
Actinic keratoses, 704
Actinomycin D *see* Dactinomycin, **505**
Actiq, 254
Activated charcoal, **35**
Active, 436
Actonel, 470
  Once a Week, 470
Actrapid, 423
Acular, 640
ACWY Vax, 746
Acyclovir *see* Aciclovir
Adalat preparations, 139
Adalimumab, 611, **612**
Adapalene, 693, 695, **696**
Adcal, 566
Adcal-D₃ preparations, 581
Adcortyl
  in *Orabase*, 655
  Intra-articular/Intradermal, 608
Add-Ins, 915
Addiphos, 560
Addison's disease, 442
Additives *see* Excipients
Additrace, 560
Adefovir, 390
Adenocor, 110
Adenoscan (adenosine), 110
Adenosine, 108, **110**
Adenovirus, 392
ADH *see* Antidiuretic hormone, 464
ADHD *see* Attention deficit hyperactivity disorder
Adhesive, tissue, 719
Adipine preparations, 139
Adrenal function test, 459
Adrenal insufficiency, 442
Adrenal suppression
  metyrapone, 470
  surgery, 445
  systemic corticosteroids, 445
  topical corticosteroids, 672
Adrenaline
  anaphylaxis, 198, 199, **200**, 201
  bradycardia, 107
  capillary bleeding, 26
  croup, 169
  eye, 632
  hypotension, 146
  infusion table (neonatal), 923
  local anaesthesia with, 787, 790
  palliative care, 26
  self administration, 200
Adrenergic neurone blocking drugs, 128
Adrenoceptor agonists, 172
Adriamycin (doxorubicin), 506
Adsorbents
  gastro-intestinal, 65
  poisoning, 35
Advagraf, 524

Advantage Plus, 436
Adverse reactions
  prevention of, 23
  reporting, 21
Advisory Committee on Borderline Substances *see* ACBS
Advisory labels *see* Cautionary and advisory labels
Aerobec—discontinued
AeroChamber, 182
Aerrane, 768
Agalsidase
  alfa, **588**
  beta, **588**
Agammaglobulinaemia, congenital, replacement therapy, 755
Agenerase—discontinued
Agrippal, 742
AIDS, 372
  vaccines and, 727
Airomir preparations, 176
Akathisia, 216
Aknemin (minocycline), 331
Aknemycin Plus, 696
Albendazole
  hookworms, 415
  hydatid disease, 415
  larva migrans, 416
  strongyloidiasis, 416
Albumin solution, **556**
Albustix, 437
Albuterol *see* Salbutamol
Alclometasone dipropionate, 677
Alcohol
  poisoning by, 36
  presence of, 3
  skin, 720
Aldactone, 106
Aldara, 702
Aldioxa, 724
Aldomet, 128
Aldosterone antagonists, 105, 106
Aldurazyme, 590
Alemtuzumab, **525**
Alendronate sodium *see* Alendronic acid, 468, 469
Alendronic acid, 468, 469
Alfacalcidol, **580**
Alfentanil, **777**
Alginate-containing antacids, 53
Alglucosidase alfa, 590, **591**
Alicalm, 901
Alimemazine
  allergic disorders, 192, **194**
  premedication, 194, 771
Alkalinisation of urine, 494
Alkeran, 504
Alkylating drugs, 502
Allegron, 231
Allergy, 191
  allergen immunotherapy, 196
  anaphylaxis, 198
  conjunctivitis, 627
  corticosteroids, 444
  food, 76
  rhinitis, 191, 647
Allopurinol, 499, **500**
Almond oil, ear, 647
Alomide, 628
Alpha Keri Bath Oil, 668
Alpha tocopheryl acetate, **582**
Alpha₂-adrenoceptor stimulants
  cardiovascular, 127
  eye, 632, 639
Alpha-adrenoceptor blocking drugs, 128
  urinary tract, 491

Alpha-blockers *see* Alpha-adreno-
ceptor blocking drugs
Alphaderm, 676
Alphosyl 2 in 1, 706
Alphosyl HC, 688
Alprostadil, 165, **166**
infusion table (neonatal), 923
Altacite Plus, 52
Altargo, 708
Alteplase, **156**, 157
Alternative medicine, 2
Alu-Cap, 570
Aluminium acetate, ear, 642, **643**
Aluminium chloride, **723**
Aluminium hydroxide
antacid, 51, 52, 53
simeticone with, 53
hyperphosphataemia,
570
Alvedon (paracetamol), 248
Alverine, **56**, 57
Alvesco, 188
Amantadine, 390
Ambirix, 737
AmBisome, 363, 365
leishmaniasis, 409
Amethocaine *see* Tetracaine
Ametop, 792
Amfetamine *see* Amphetamines
Amidotrizoates, 87
Amikacin, 333, **334**, 335
tuberculosis, 352
Amikin, 335
Amilamont (amiloride), 105
Amiloride, **105**
furosemide with, 106
heart failure, 100
hydrochlorothiazide with, 106
Aminex products, 911
Amino acids
ACBS, 913, 917
intravenous nutrition, 559
Aminobenzoic acid, 575
Aminoglycosides
ear, 643, 647
eye, 622
systemic, 331
Aminophylline, 100, 178, **180**
see also Theophylline
Aminosalicylates, 66, 68
Amiodarone, 108, 109, **110**, 111
Amisulpride, 221, **222**
Amitriptyline
depression, **229**, 230
neuropathic pain, 261
nocturnal enuresis, 494
Amix (amoxicillin), 314
Amlodipine, 136, **137**
see also Calcium-channel block-
ers
Amlostin (amlodipine), 137
Ammonaps, 593
Ammonia, poisoning by, 46
Amoebiasis, 407
Amoebic
abscess, 407
dysentery, 407
Amoebicides, 407
Amoram (amoxicillin), 314
Amorolfine, **711**
Amoxicillin, **313**, 314
Helicobacter pylori eradication,
59
pneumococcal infection prophy-
laxis, 305
Amoxident (amoxicillin), 314
Amoxil preparations, 314
Amoxycillin *see* Amoxicillin

Amphetamines
abuse, 18
poisoning by, 43
Amphocil, 363, 365
Amphotericin, 361, 362, 363, **364**
eye, 636
leishmaniasis, 409
liposomal, 361, 363
mouth, 657, **658**
Ampicillin, 312, **314**, 315
flucloxacillin with [co-
fluampicil], 312
Amsacrine, **513**
Amsidine, 513
Amyben (amiodarone), 111
Anabact, 710
Anabolic steroids, 459
anaemias, 535
Anaemias, 528
aplastic, 535
chronic renal failure, 536
haemolytic, 535
hypoplastic, 535
iron-deficiency, 529
megaloblastic, 533
sideroblastic, 535
Anaesthesia
analgesics, 776
anticholinesterases, 783
anticoagulants, oral and,
761
antidepressants and, 761
antimuscarinics, 769
antiviral drugs and, 761
corticosteroids, 445, 761
dental practice, 762
diuretics, 761
general, 761
inhalational, 766
intravenous, 763
local, 786
adrenaline with, 787
dental practice, 787
eye, 635
mouth, 654
rectal, 88
vasoconstrictors with,
787
muscle relaxants, 778
Anagrelide, **542**
Anal fissure, 89
Analeptics, 202
Analgesics
compound, 247
non-opioid, 245, 246
postoperative, 776
NSAIDs, 245, 246, 600
anaesthesia, 776
poisoning by, 36
rheumatic diseases, 600
opioid, 249
anaesthesia, 776
cough suppressants,
208
dependence on, 18
neuropathic pain, 261
palliative care, 24, 28
poisoning by, 39
Analog preparations, 912, 913, 914,
916, 917
Anapen, 200, 201
Anaphylaxis, 198, 199
Ancotil, 367
Ancylostomiasis, 415
Androcur, 457
Androgens, 455
Andropatch, 457

Anectine, 783
Anexate, 785
Angettes-75, 155
Angilol (propranolol), 116
Angioedema, 201
Angiotensin-converting enzyme
inhibitors *see* ACE inhibitors
Angiotensin-II receptor antagonists,
134
Angular cheilitis, 657, 673
Anhydrol Forte, 724
Anogenital warts, 701
Anorectics, 237
Anorexia, palliative care, 26
Antacids, 51
sodium content, 51
surgery, 762
Antazoline, **627**
Antepsin, 62
Anterior uveitis, 629
Anthelmintics, 413
Anthracyclines, 505
Anthralin *see* Dithranol
Anthraquinones, 79
Anthrax, 357
vaccine, 730
Anti-androgens, 457
Anti-arrhythmic drugs, 107, 108
Antibacterial policies, 296
Antibacterials, **296**
acne, 695, 697
diarrhoea, 64
ear, 642
eye, 622
oral infections, 297
prophylaxis (table), 303
prophylaxis, surgery, 306
skin, 707
therapy, initial (table), 298
vaginal, 473
Antibiotic-associated colitis *see*
Clostridium difficile
Antibiotics *see* Antibacterials
Anticholinergic drugs *see* Antimuscarinics
Anticholinergic syndrome, 769
Anticholinesterases, 614
anaesthesia, 783
Anticoagulant treatment booklets,
153
Anticoagulants
oral, 151
anaesthesia, 761
reversal, 152
surgery, 761
parenteral, 147
Anticonvulsants *see* Antiepileptics
Antidepressants
anaesthesia, 761
choice, 228
hyponatraemia and, 228
monoamine-oxidase inhibitors,
231
poisoning by, 40
serotonin re-uptake inhibitors,
228, 231
surgery, 761
tricyclic, 229
enuresis, 494
withdrawal, 228
Antidiabetic drugs, 418
insulin, 418
oral, 429
Antidiarrhoeal drugs *see* Diarrhoea
Antidiuretic hormone, 464
Antiemetics, 237
cytotoxic therapy and, 497
migraine, 261, 263

Index

Antiepileptic drugs, 264, 266
  breast-feeding and, 266
  pregnancy and, 266
  surgery, 761
Antifibrinolytic drugs, 158
Antifungal drugs, 361
  anogenital, 473
  oropharyngeal, 657
  skin, 710
Antigiardial drugs, 408
Antihepatitis B immunoglobulin, 757
Antihistamines, 191
  breast-feeding, 192
  cough preparations, 208
  eczema, 682
  eye, 627
  hypnotic, 213
  insomnia, 192
  migraine, 263
  nasal allergy, 648
  nausea and vertigo, **239**
  nausea and vomiting, 237, 238
  pregnancy, 192
  skilled tasks and, 192, 194
  skin, 671
Antihypertensives
  ACE inhibitors, 130
  adrenergic neurone blockers, 128
  alpha-blockers, 128
  angiotensin-II receptor antagonists, 134
  beta-blockers, 114
  calcium-channel blockers, 136
  centrally-acting, 127
  vasodilator, 121
Anti-inflammatory analgesics *see* Analgesics, NSAIDs
Antilymphocyte globulin, 535
Antimalarials, 395, 609
Antimanic drugs, 225
Antimetabolites, 507
Antimigraine drugs, 261
Antimotility drugs, 64, 65
Antimuscarinics
  antipsychotics and, 216
  bronchodilator, 178
  dystonias, 289
  eye, 629
  gastro-intestinal, 54
  premedication, 769
  quaternary ammonium, 55
  urinary tract, 492
Antineoplastic drugs, 496
  see also Cytotoxic drugs
Antiperspirants, 723
Antiplatelet drugs, 154
Antiprotozoal drugs, 394
Antipsychotics, 215
  atypical, 221
  depot injections, 225
  equivalent doses, oral, 218
  high doses (caution), 215
  mania, 225
  withdrawal, 216
    atypical, 222
Antirabies immunoglobulin, 758
Antiretrovirals, **372**, 373, 384
  non-nucleoside reverse transcriptase inhibitors, 382
  nucleoside reverse transcriptase inhibitors, 374
  protease inhibitors, 378

Antiseptics
  ACBS, 917
  lozenges, 659
  mouthwashes, 659
  skin, 719
  sprays, oropharynx, 659
Antiserum, 729, 730, 754
Antispasmodics, 54
Antitetanus immunoglobulin, 758
Antithymocyte immunoglobulin, 520, **521**
Antithyroid drugs, 439
Antituberculous drugs, 348
Antitussives, 208
Antivaricella-zoster immunoglobulin, 758
Antivenoms, 47
Antiviral drugs, 372
  anaesthesia, 761
  eye, 625
  mouth, 657
  skin, 715
  surgery, 761
Anugesic-HC, 88
Anusol preparations, 88
Anxiety, 214, 228
  antipsychotics, 215
  palliative care, 26
Anxiolytics, 211, 214
APD *see* Disodium pamidronate, 469
Aphthous ulcers, 654
Apidra, 424
Aplastic anaemia, 535
Apnoea neonatal
  aminophylline, 180
  caffeine, 202
  doxapram, 202
  theophylline, 179
Appetite suppressants, 237
Applications, definition, 664
Apraclonidine, 632, **639**, 640
Apresoline, 122
Aprinox (bendroflumethiazide), 102
Aproten, 910, 911
Aptivus, 382
Aquadrate, 668
Aquasept—discontinued
Aquasol-A, 575
Aqueous cream, 666
Arachis oil
  enema, 82
  presence of, 3
Aranesp preparations, 537
Arcoxia, 603
Aredia Dry Powder, 469
Arginine
  supplement, 917
  urea cycle disorders, **591**, 592
Argipressin *(Pitressin)*, 464
Arovit, 575
Arpicolin, 290
Arrhythmias, **107**
  anti-arrhythmics, 108
  poisoning and, 34
  supraventricular, 97, 108
  ventricular, 108
Artelac (hypromellose), 638
Artelac SDU, 638
Artemether
  lumefantrine with, **401**, 402
Artesunate, 395
Arthritis
  juvenile idiopathic, 608
  rheumatic, 599
  septic, 302
Arthrofen (ibuprofen), 604
Arthroxen (naproxen), 606
Articaine, 787

Artificial saliva, 661
Artificial tears, 636
AS Saliva Orthana, 661
5-ASA, 68
Asacol preparations, 69, 70
Asadon, 914
Ascalix—discontinued
Ascaricides, 414
Ascaris, 414
Ascensia products, 428, 436
Ascites, 104
Ascorbic acid, **578**
  iron excretion, 540
Asilone preparations, 53
Asmabec preparations, 186
Asmanex, 189
Asmasal preparations, 176
Asparaginase, 513
Aspartame, 561
  presence of, 3
Aspergillosis, 361
Aspiration, acid, prophylaxis, 762
Aspirin
  antiplatelet, **154**, 155
  Kawasaki syndrome, 154
Asplenia
  Haemophilus influenzae type b (Hib)
    prophylaxis, 305
    vaccine, 735
  influenza vaccine, 741
  malaria, 397
  meningococcal vaccine, 744
  pneumococcal
    infection, 305
    vaccine, 746
  vaccines and, 727
Asthma, 168
  acute (table), 171
    management, 168
  allergen immunotherapy, 196
  beta$_2$ agonists, 172
  breast-feeding, 168
  chronic (table), 170
  exercise-induced, 172
  pregnancy, 168
  prophylaxis, 184, 189
  sympathomimetics, 172
Astringents
  ear, 642
  skin, 719
Atarax, 195
Atazanavir, 373, **379**
Atenix (atenolol) preparations, 116
Atenolol, 113, **116**
  see also Beta-adrenoceptor blocking drugs
  supraventricular tachycardia, 108
  thyrotoxicosis, 440
Athlete's foot, 710
Atimos Modulite, 174
Ativan (lorazepam), 774
Atomoxetine, **234**
Atonic seizures, 267
Atorvastatin, 159, **160**, 161
Atovaquone
  malaria, 404, 405
  proguanil with, 405
Atracurium, 779, **780**
  infusion table (neonatal), 923
Atrial fibrillation, 97, 108, 151
Atrial flutter, 108
Atriance, 510
Atripla, 378

Atropine sulphate
  anaesthesia, 769, 770
    bradycardia, 770
  anticholinesterases and, 783
  beta-blocker poisoning, 41
  eye, **629**
  organophosphorus poisoning, 47
Atrovent preparations, 178
Attention deficit hyperactivity disorder, 234
Atypical antipsychotics, 221
  poisoning by, 43
Augmentin preparations, 316
Aureocort, 681
Autopen, 428
Avamys, 650
Avaxim, 736
Aveeno preparations, 666, 669
Aviva products, 436
Avloclor, 402
Avoca, 701
Avomine, 240
Azactam, 328
Azamune (azathioprine), 519
Azathioprine, 519
  arthritis, 610
  auto-immune conditions, 610
  Crohn's disease, **74**
  eczema, 690
  inflammatory bowel disease, 66, 67
  rheumatic disease, 610
  transplant rejection, 518, **519**
  ulcerative colitis, **74**
  vasculitis, 610
Azelaic acid, 693, **694**
Azelastine
  eye, **627**
  nose, **648**
Azidothymidine, 378
Azithromycin, 336, **337**, 338
  eye, 622
Azopt, 634
AZT, 378
Aztreonam, **328**

B

Babyhaler, 182
Bacillus Calmette-Guérin
  vaccines, 730, **731**
Bacitracin
  eye, 624
  skin
    polymyxin with, 708
Baclofen, **616**, 617
Bacteroides fragilis infections
  antipseudomonal penicillins in, 317
  clindamycin in, 339
  metronidazole in, 355
Bactroban, 708
  Nasal, 653
BAL, 45
Balanced Salt Solution, 638, 639
Balneum preparations, 668, 669
Balsalazide, 66, 68, **69**
Bandages medicated, 683
Barbiturates, anaesthesia, 763
Barkat, 910
Barrier preparations, 670

Bartter's syndrome, 104
Basiliximab, 520, **522**
Bath additives
  antimicrobial with, 670
  coal tar, 687
  emollient, 668–70
Baxan, 321
Bazetham MR (tamsulosin), 492
BCG vaccines, 730, **731**
BD Micro-Fine products, 428, 429
BD Safe-clip, 429
Becaplermin, **723**
Beclazone (beclometasone) preparations, 185, 186
Beclometasone dipropionate
  asthma, 184, **185**, 186
  mouth ulceration, 654
  nasal allergy, 649
Beclomethasone *see* Beclometasone, 654
Becodisks, 186
Beconase preparations, 649
Bedranol SR (propranolol), 116
Bee sting allergy preparations, 196, 197
Begrivac, 742
Bendrofluazide *see* Bendroflumethiazide, **101**, 102
Bendroflumethiazide, **101**, 102
Benerva, 577
Benoxinate *see* Oxybuprocaine, 635, **636**
Benzalkonium, 706
  cetrimide with, 671
  chlorhexidine with, 668
  dimeticone with, 671
Benzathine benzylpenicillin, 301, 309
Benzatropine—discontinued
Benzhexol *see* Trihexyphenidyl, 289, **290**
Benzodiazepines
  anaesthesia, 771, 772
  antagonist, 785
  anxiolytics, 212
  epilepsy, 281
  mania, 225
  muscle spasm, 616
  neonatal seizures, 267
  poisoning by, 41
Benzoic acid ointment, compound, 711, 712
Benzoin tincture, compound, 208
Benzoyl peroxide, 693
  acne, 694
    clindamycin with, 694
    hydroxyquinoline with, 694
Benzydamine, 654, **655**
Benzyl alcohol, presence of, 3
Benzyl benzoate, 715
Benzylpenicillin sodium, 308, **309**, 310
  gas-gangrene prophylaxis, 306
Beractant, **203**
Beta Prograne (propranolol), 116
Beta$_2$ agonists, 172
  asthma acute, 169
  asthma chronic, 170
Beta-adrenoceptor blocking drugs
  arrhythmias, 108, 109, 114
  atrial fibrillation, 108
  diuretics with, 114
  eye, 631
  heart failure, 114
  hypertension, 114
  poisoning by, 41
  thyrotoxicosis, 114, 440
  verapamil and, 140

Beta-adrenoceptor stimulants
  asthma, 172
Beta-blockers *see* Beta-adrenoceptor blocking drugs
Betacap, 677
Beta-Cardone, 119
Betacarotene, 704
Betadine
  skin, 722
Betagan, 632
Betaine, **594**, 595
Beta-lactamases, 308
Betamethasone, 443, **450**
  mouth, 655
  skin, 677
Betamethasone dipropionate, 677
  calcipotriol with, 686
  clotrimazole with, 678
  salicylic acid with, 678
Betamethasone sodium phosphate
  ear, 644
  eye, 626
  inflammatory and allergic disorders, 450
  mouth, 654
  nose, 649, 653
    neomycin with, 653
Betamethasone valerate
  skin, 677, 678
    clioquinol with, 678
    fusidic acid with, 678
    neomycin with, 678
Betaxolol, 631
Betnesol
  ear, 644
  eye, 626
  inflammatory and allergic disorders, 450
  mouth, 655
  nose, 649
Betnesol-N
  ear, 644
  eye, 626
  nose, 653
Betnovate preparations, 677, 678
Betoptic, 631
Bettamousse, 677
Bezafibrate, **163**, 164
Bezalip preparations, 164
Bi-Aglut, 910
Bicarbonate
  intravenous, 555
  oral, 550
  see also Sodium bicarbonate
Biguanides, 431
Bile acid sequestrants, 92, 161
Bilharziasis, 416
Bimatoprost, 632
Binocrit, 537
BiNovum, 482
Biosimilar medicines, 2
Biotène Oralbalance, 661
Biotin, 575, **595**
BioXtra, 662
Biphosphonates *see* Bisphosphonates
Bipolar disorder, 225, 226
Birthmarks, ACBS, 917
Bisacodyl, 79, 80
Bismuth subgallate, 88
Bisphosphonates
  hypercalcaemia, 567
  osteoporosis, 468

Index

Bites
    animal, 303
    human, 303
    snake, 47
Black triangle symbol, 21
Bladder
    blood clot dissolution,
        495
    irrigations, 494
Bleeding
    mucosal (palliative care),
        27
    variceal, 464
Bleo-Kyowa (bleomycin), 505
Bleomycin, **505**
Blepharitis, 621
BM-Accutest, 436
Body surface area charts, *inside back
    cover*
Bone metabolism, drugs affecting,
    467
Bone tumours, analgesia,
    246
Bonefos, 470
Bone-marrow suppression, cyto-
    toxic drugs, 497
Bonjela preparations (choline salicy-
    late), 656
Borderline substances *see* ACBS
Bosentan, **124**, 125
Botox, 291
Botulinum A toxin-haemagglutinin
    complex
        hyperhidrosis, 723
Botulinum antitoxin, 732
Botulinum toxin type A, **290**, 291
Botulism antitoxin, 732
Bowel
    cleansing solutions, 85
    irrigation, 35
    sterilisation, 333
Bradycardia, 107
    anaesthesia, 769
Bramitob, 335
Bran, 78
Breast-feeding
    corticosteroids and,
        447
    epilepsy and, 266
    prescribing in, 16
Breeze products, 436, 437
Brevibloc, 117
Brevinor, 482
Brevoxyl, 694
Brexidol, 607
Bricanyl preparations, 177
Bridion, 784
Brimonidine, 632
Brinzolamide, 633, **634**
Broflex, 290
Brolene, 624
Bronchodilators
    adrenoceptor agonist,
        172
    antimuscarinic, 178
    compound, 180
    sympathomimetic, 172
    theophylline, 179
Bronchopulmonary dysplasia, 100,
    103
Bronchospasm, 172
Brucellosis, 328, 354
Brufen preparations, 604
Brugia malayi, 416
Buccastem, 241
Buclizine, codeine and paracetamol
    with, 261
Budenofalk, 73

Budesonide
    asthma, 184, **186**, 187
        formoterol with, 187
    bronchopulmonary dysplasia,
        186
    croup, 169, 186
    inflammatory bowel disease, 66
        Crohn's disease, 72, 73
        ulcerative colitis, 72, 73
    nasal
        allergy, 649, 650
        polyps, 649, 650
Bumetanide, 103, **104**
Bupivacaine, 789, **790**
    adrenaline with, 790
Buprenorphine
    intra-operative analgesia, 251
    pain, 249, **251**
    premedication, 251
Burinex, 104
Buscopan, 56
Busilvex, 503
Buspirone, 215
Busulfan, **502**, 503
Busulphan *see* Busulfan, **502**, 503
Butylcyanoacrylate, 719
Butyrophenones, 216

C

C₁ esterase inhibitor, 201
Cacit, 566
Cacit D3, 581
Caffeine, **202**
    citrate, 202
Calaband, 683
Calamine, 671, 672
Calceos, 581
Calchan MR (nifedipine), 139
Calcichew, 566
Calcichew D3, 581
Calcichew D3 Forte, 581
Calciferol, 578
Calciferol *see* Ergocalciferol, 578,
    579, 580
Calcijex, 581
Calcipotriol, 683, 685, **686**
    betamethasone dipropionate
        with, 686
Calcitonin, **467**, 468, 567
Calcitriol
    psoriasis, 683, 685, **686**
    vitamin D deficiency, 579, **581**
Calcium
    colecalciferol with, 581, 582
    ergocalciferol with, 579, 580
    supplements, 565–7
Calcium acetate, 571
Calcium and vitamin D tablets, 580
Calcium balance, maintenance, 467
Calcium carbonate
    colecalciferol with, 581
    hyperphosphataemia, **571**
Calcium chloride, 567
Calcium folinate, 500, 501, 533
Calcium gluconate, 565, 566, 567
Calcium lactate, 566
Calcium leucovorin *see* Calcium
    folinate, 500, 501, 533
Calcium levofolinate, 500, 501

Calcium levoleucovorin *see* Calcium
    levofolinate, 500, 501
Calcium phosphate, 581
Calcium polystyrene sulphonate,
    548
Calcium Resonium, 548
Calcium salts, 571
Calcium-500, 567
Calcium-channel blockers, 136
    angina, 136
    hypertension, 136
    poisoning by, 41
    pulmonary hypertension, 123
Calcium-Sandoz, 567
Calcort, 450
Calfovit D3, 581
Calluses, 700
Calmurid, 668
Calmurid HC, 676
Calogen, 905
Caloreen, 904
Calpol (paracetamol) preparations,
    248
Calprofen (ibuprofen), 604
Calshake, 906
Camcolit, 227
Camouflaging preparations, 704
Campylobacter enteritis, 298, 335
Cancidas, 365
Candidiasis
    intestinal, 363
    oropharyngeal, 657
    perianal, 87
    skin, 711
    systemic, 361
    vaginal, **473**
    vulval, 473
    vulvovaginal, recurrent, 473
Candidosis see Candidiasis
Canesten
    anogenital, 473, 474
    ear, 645
    HC, 676
    Once (clotrimazole), 474
    skin, 712
Cannabinoid, 244
Cannabis, regulations, 19
Capasal, 706
Caplenal (allopurinol), 500
Capoten, 133
Capreomycin, 352
Caprilon, 899
Caprin, 155
Caps, contraceptive, 490
Captopril, **132**, 133
    see also ACE inhibitors
Carace preparations, 134
Carbagen SR, 268
Carbaglu, 592
Carbalax, 85
Carbamazepine
    attention deficit hyperactivity
        disorder, 267
    bipolar disorder, 225
    epilepsy, 266, **267**, 268, 269
    neuropathic pain, 261
    poisoning, elimination, 35
Carbimazole, 440, **441**
Carbocisteine, **207**
    cystic fibrosis, 206
Carbo-Dome, 687
Carbomers, 637
Carbomix, 36
Carbon monoxide poisoning, 46
Carbonic anhydrase inhibitors
    diuresis, 107
    glaucoma, 633
Carboplatin, 515, **516**

Carboxylase defects, 594
Cardene preparations, 138
Cardiac arrest, 146, 555
Cardiac glycosides, 97
Cardiac *see also* Heart
Cardilate MR—discontinued
Cardiopulmonary
    arrest, 146
    resuscitation, 146
        charts, *inside back cover*
Cardioxane, 499
Cardura preparations,
    129
Carglumic acid, 591, 592
Carmellose
    eye, **637**
    mouth, 654, **655**
Carnitine, 587, 588
Carnitor, 588
Carobel, Instant, 909
Carteolol, **631**
Carticaine *see* Articaine, 787
Carvedilol, 100, 113, 114, **117**
    see also Beta-adrenoceptor
    blocking drugs
Carylderm—discontinued
Cascara, 79
Casilan-90, 901
Caspofungin, 361, 363, **365**
Castor oil, 79
Catapres, 127
Catarrh, vernal, 627
Catheter maintenance, 495
Catheter patency solutions
    chlorhexidine, 495
    sodium chloride, 495
    solution G, 495
    solution R, 495
Cautionary and advisory labels,
    918
    see also inside back cover
    counselling, 918
    NCL, 918
    original packs, 918
Ceanel Concentrate, 706
Cefaclor, 319, **320**
Cefadroxil, 319, **320**, 321
Cefalexin, 319, **321**
Cefixime, 319, **321**, 322
Cefotaxime, 319, **322**
Cefpodoxime, 319, **322**, 323
Cefradine, 319, **323**
Ceftazidime, 319, **323**, 324
    eye drops, 636
Ceftriaxone, 319, **324**, 325
    meningococcal meningitis pro-
    phylaxis, 304
Cefuroxime, 319, **325**
    eye drops, 636
Celevac, 79
CellCept, 520
Cellulitis, 303
Celluvisc, 637
Celsentri, 384
Central nervous system stimulants,
    234
Ceph... *see also* Cef...
Cephalosporins, 319
Ceporex, 321
Cepton, 721
Cerazette, 485
Cerebral oedema, 107, 444
Cerezyme, 589
Cernevit, 561
Cerumol, 647
Cervarix, 740
Cetirizine, 192, **193**
Cetraben, 666, 669

Cetrimide
    benzalkonium with, 671
    chlorhexidine with, 721
    dimeticone with, 671
    scalp, 705
    skin, 671, 719, **721**
CFCs, 172, 184
Charcoal, activated, **35**, 36
Charcodote, 36
Cheilitis, angular, 657, 673
Chenodeoxycholic acid, 91, **92**
Chenofalk, 92
Chickenpox, 385, 757
    corticosteroids, 446
Chilblains, 141, 724
Children, prescribing for,
    11
Chirocaine, 790
Chlamydia
    eye, 302, 622
    genital, 301
Chloractil (chlorpromazine),
    218
Chloral betaine *see* Cloral betaine,
    213
Chloral hydrate, **212**, 213
    anaesthesia, 771
Chlorambucil, **503**
Chloramphenicol, 341
    ear, 642, **645**
    eye, 622, **623**
    systemic, **340**
ChloraPrep, 721
Chlorhexidine
    bladder infections, 494
    mouth, 654, 657, **659**, 660
        chlorobutanol with,
        660
    nose, neomycin with, 653
    skin, 719, 721
        benzalkonium with,
        668
        hydrocortisone and nystatin
        with, 676
    skin disinfection, **720**, 721
        cetrimide with, 721
        dusting powder, 721
Chlorine poisoning, 46
Chlorobutanol, 660
Chlorofluorocarbon propellants,
    172, 184
Chlorohex, 660
Chloromycetin, 623
Chloroquine, 402, 403
    malaria
        prophylaxis, 397–9, 400, **402**
        treatment, 396, **402**
    proguanil with, 403
Chlorothiazide
    chronic hypoglycaemia,
    434
    diabetes insipidus, 464
    hypertension, **102**
Chloroxylenol, 724
Chlorphenamine, 192, **194**, 195
    allergic emergencies, 198
Chlorpheniramine *see* Chlorphena-
    mine
Chlorpromazine
    hypothermia induction,
    218
    nausea and vomiting, 237, **241**
    neonatal abstinence syndrome,
    218
    psychosis, 216, **218**
Chlorpropamide, 430
Chlortalidone, **102**
Cholecalciferol *see* Colecalciferol

Cholera vaccine, **732**, 733
    travel, 759
Cholestasis, 91, 92
Cholestatic conditions, 91
Cholesterol, 92
    Smith-Lemli-Opitz syndrome, 92
Cholestyramine *see* Colestyramine
Cholic acid, 91
Choline, 575
Choline salicylate
    dental gel, 654, **656**
Cholinergic crises, 614
Cholinesterase inhibitors, 614, 783
Choragon, 461
Choreas, 290
Chorionic gonadotrophin, 456, **460**,
    461
Chronic myeloid leukaemia,
    514
Churg-Strauss syndrome,
    190
Cicafem (co-cyprindiol), 698
Ciclesonide, **188**
Ciclosporin
    aplastic anaemia,
    535
    eczema, 690, **691**
    immunosuppression, 517, 520,
    522, 523
    nephrotic syndrome, 522
    psoriasis, 690, **691**
    rheumatic disease, 610
    ulcerative colitis, 66, **74**
Cidofovir, 388
Cidomycin, 334
Cigarette smoking, 291
Cilastatin, 325
    imipenem with, 325, 326
Cilest, 483
Ciloxan, 623
Cimetidine, xvi
Cinchocaine
    rectal, 88
    [ingredient], 89
Cinnarizine, **239**
    motion sickness, 239
    nausea and vertigo,
    239
Cipramil, 232
Ciprofloxacin, 357, **358**, 359
    Crohn's disease, 66
    ear, 643, 647
    eye, 622, **623**
    meningococcal meningitis pro-
    phylaxis, 304
Ciproxin, 359
Circadin, 214
Cisatracurium, 779, **780**
Cisplatin, **516**
Citalopram, 231, **232**
Citanest, 791
Citanest with Octapressin,
    791
Citramag, 86
Citrulline, 591, **592**
Claforan—discontinued
Clairette, 698
Clarithromycin, 336, **338**, 339
    Helicobacter pylori eradication,
    59
Clarosip, 338
Clasteon, 470
Clavulanic acid, 312
    amoxicillin with, 312, 315
    ticarcillin with, 317, 318
Cleanlet Fine, 428
Cleansers, skin, 719
Clenil Modulite, 186

Index

Clexane preparations, 150
Clindamycin, **339**, 340
  acne, 695
  bacterial vaginosis, 475
  benzoyl peroxide with, 694
  malaria, 395, 396
  oral infections, 339
  pneumocystis pneumonia,
    411
  vaginal infections, 475
Clinipak syringe, 429
Clinistix, 437
Clinitar, 687
  shampoo, 706
Clinitas, 639
Clinitek Microalbumin, 437
Clinitest, 437
ClinOleic, 559
Clinutren preparations
  enteral feed, 882, 886
  nutritional supplement, 891, 893
Clioquinol
  betamethasone with, 678
  ear, 642, 644
  fluocinolone with, 678
Clobazam, 282
  epilepsy, 266, 267, **281**
Clobetasol propionate, 678
Clobetasone butyrate, 678, 679
  tetracycline with, 679
Clodronate sodium *see* Sodium
  clodronate, 470
Clofarabine, 507, **508**
Clonazepam
  epilepsy, 267, 281, **282**, 284
    status epilepticus, **283**
  neonatal seizures, 267
Clonidine, **127**
Cloral betaine, 213
Clostridium botulinum, 732
Clostridium difficile, 68
  antibacterial therapy, 298
    metronidazole in, 355
    vancomycin in, 342
Clotrimazole
  anogenital, 473
  ear, 645
  skin, 711, **712**
    betamethasone with, 678
    hydrocortisone with, 676
  vulvovaginal candidiasis, recur-
    rent, 473
Clozapine, 216, 221, **222**, 223
  hypersalivation, 222
Clozaril, 223
Cluster headache, 264
CMV, 388
Coal tar, 682, 683, 687, 688
  dithranol and salicylic acid with,
    688
  hydrocortisone with, 688
  scalp, 687, 705, 706
  zinc with, 687
Co-amilofruse, 106
Co-amilozide, 106
Co-amoxiclav, 312, **315**, 316
Cobalin-H (hydroxocobalamin), 535
COC *see* Contraception, oral, com-
  bined, 475
Cocaine, poisoning by, 43
Co-careldopa, **288**, 289
Co-codamol preparations,
  248
Cocois, 687
Co-cyprindiol, **698**
Cod liver oil
  zinc oxide with, 671
Codalax preparations, 80

Co-danthramer preparations,
  80
Co-danthrusate preparations,
  80
Codeine
  cough suppressant, 208
  diarrhoea, 65
  pain, 249, **252**
    buclizine and paracetamol
      with, 261
    paracetamol with, 248
Coeliac disease, 561
  ACBS, 910
Co-enzyme Q10 *see* Ubidecarenone,
  596
Co-fluampicil, 312, 315
Colazide, 69
Cold sores, 715
Colecalciferol, 578, **581**, 582
  calcium with, 581
Colestid, 163
Colestipol, 161, **162**, 163
Colestyramine
  diarrhoea, 64, 92, **93**
  familial hypercholesterolaemia,
    92
  hypercholesterolaemia, 161, **162**
  pruritus, 92, 93
Colief, 909
Colifoam, 73
Colistin, 345, **346**
  eye drops, 636
Colitis
  Clostridium difficile infection,
    68
  ulcerative, 66
Collodion
  definition, 664
  flexible, 714
Colloidal oatmeal, 666, 669
Colofac preparations, 57
Colomycin, 346
Colophony, 700, 719
Colpermin, 57
Coma
  hyperglycaemic, 432
  hyperosmolar nonketotic,
    432
  hypoglycaemic, 433
  hypothyroid, 438
  insulin, 432
  ketoacidotic, 432
Co-magaldrox, 52
Combined hormonal contraceptives,
  479
  see also Contraception
Combivir, 378
Combur-3 Test, 437
Comfort Point, 429
Compact, 436
Complan Shake, 894
Complementary medicine, 2
Compliance, 1
Concerta XL, 236
Condyline, 702
Condylomata acuminata, 701, 702
Congenital agammaglobulinaemia,
  replacement therapy, 755
Conjunctivitis, 302, 621
  allergic, 627
Conotrane, 671
Consed (midazolam), 775
Constipation, 77
  palliative care, 26
Contact lenses, 640
Contiflo XL (tamsulosin), 492
Continuous infusion devices, pallia-
  tive care, 28

Contour products, 436, 437
Contraception, 475
  devices, 488–90
    contraceptive caps, 490
    contraceptive diaphragms,
      490
  implants, 486
  intra-uterine system, 487
  oral, 475
    combined hormonal, 475
    emergency, 490
    missed pill, 477, 484
    progestogen-only, 484
    starting routines, 479, 484
    surgery, **479**, 484
    travel, 476
  parenteral, 485, **486**
  spermicidal, 488
  transdermal, 475, 483
    detached patch, 477
    starting routines, 479
Controlled drugs, 17
  see also preparations identified by
    [CD] throughout *BNF for Children*
  travel abroad, 19
Conversion tables, *inside back cover*
Convulex, 280
Convulsions
  febrile, 287
  palliative care, 26
  poisoning and, 34
  see also Epilepsy
Convulsive status epilepticus, 283
Co-phenotrope, 65
Co-proxamol, poisoning by, 39
Coracten preparations, 139
Cordarone X, 111
Cordilox preparations, 141
Corlan, 656
Corn flour, ACBS, 912
Corn starch, ACBS, 912
Corneal ulcers, 622, 625
Coronary heart disease
  prevention
    antiplatelet therapy, 154
    diabetes, 119
    dyslipidaemia, 160
    hypertension, 119
    non-drug treatment, 119
    obesity, 119
  risk assessment, 160
Corsodyl preparations, 660
Corticorelin, **460**
Corticosteroids, **442**
  administration, 445
  adrenal suppression, 445
  allergic emergencies, 198
  allergy, 444
    nasal, 648, 649
  anaesthesia, 445, 761
  anaphylactic shock, 444
  angioedema, 444
  aphthous ulcers, 654, **655**
  asthma, 184
    acute, severe, 169
    chronic, 170
  blood disorders, 535
  breast-feeding, 447
  cancer, 520
  chickenpox, 446
  croup, 169
  ear, 642
  equivalent doses, 443
  eye, 622, 625
  haemorrhoids, 88
  hypercalcaemia, 567
  immunosuppression, 520

Index

Corticosteroids (*continued*)—
 infantile spasms, 267
 infections, 446
 inflammatory bowel disease, 66, 72
 inhaled, 184
 measles, 446
 mouth, **655**
 myasthenia gravis, 614, 616
 nasal polyps, 648
 neuropathic pain, 261
 pregnancy, 447
 proctitis, 73
 proctosigmoiditis, 73
 psychiatric reactions, 446
 replacement therapy, 442
 rheumatic disease, 607
 septic shock, 444
 side-effects, 448
 skin
  acne, 697
  choice, 672
  eczema, 672, 682
  nappy rash, 670
  potency, 675
  psoriasis, 674, 683
 steroid treatment card, 448
 surgery, 445, 761
 tuberculosis, 349
 ulcerative colitis, 72, 73
 withdrawal of, 446
Corticotrophin *see* Corticotropin, 459
Corticotrophin-releasing hormone *see* Corticorelin, **460**
Corticotropin, 459
Cortisol, 442
Co-simalcite [ingredient], 52
Cosmegen Lyovac, 505
CosmoFer, 532
Cosopt, 634
Cosuric (allopurinol), 500
Co-trimoxazole, 346, **347**, 348
 pneumocystis pneumonia, 346, 347, 411
Cough
 palliative care, 27
 suppressants, 208
Coumarins, 151
Covering creams, 704
Covermark preparations, 705
Cow & Gate Pepti preparations, 897
Cozaar preparations, 134
Crab lice, 716
Cradle cap, 683, 705
Creams
 definition, 664
 suitable quantities, 665
Creatinine clearance *see* Glomerular filtration rate, 13
Creeping eruption *see* Cutaneous larva migrans, 416
Creon preparations, 94, 95
Cretinism *see* Hypothyroidism, neo-natal, 438
CRH Ferring, 460
CRH *see* Corticorelin, **460**
Crisantaspase, **513**
Crixivan, 380
Crohn's disease, 66
 fistulating, 66
Cromoglicate (*or* cromoglycate) *see* Sodium cromoglicate
Crotamiton, 671, 672
 hydrocortisone with, 676
 scabies, 715
Croup, 169
Cryptococcosis, 362

Crystacide, 722
Crystapen, 310
CS gas *see* CS spray, 46
CS spray, 46
Cuplex, 700
Curatoderm, 686
Curosurf, 203
Cushing's syndrome, 453, 470
 corticosteroid-induced, 448
Cutaneous larva migrans, 416
Cutivate, 681
CX Antiseptic Dusting Powder, 721
Cyanides, poisoning by, 44
Cyanocobalamin, 533
Cyanokit, 44
Cyclimorph, 257
Cyclizine, **239**, 240
 motion sickness, 239
Cyclocaps
 beclometasone, 185
 budesonide, 187
 salbutamol, 175
Cyclohaler
 beclometasone, 185
 budesonide, 187
 salbutamol, 175
Cyclopentolate, **629**, 630
Cyclophosphamide, **503**, 504, 518
Cycloplegics, 629
Cycloserine, **352**
Cyclosporin *see* Ciclosporin
Cyklokapron, 158
Cymevene, 389
Cyproterone
 acne, 698
 precocious puberty, **457**
Cystadane, 595
Cystagon, 594
Cysteamine *see* Mercaptamine, 593, **594**
Cysteine amino acid supplement, 914
Cystic fibrosis
 delayed puberty, 453
 fat malabsorption, 93
 respiratory-tract infections, 300, 305, 317
Cysticide, 415, 416
Cystinosis, nephropathic, 593
Cystitis, 494
 haemorrhagic, 502
Cystrin, 493
Cytarabine, 507, **508**
Cytochrome oxidase deficiency, 576
Cytokine modulators
 Crohn's disease, 75
 juvenile idiopathic arthritis, 611
Cytomegalovirus
 infections, 386, 388, 625
Cytotoxic drugs, **496**
 alopecia, 497
 antibiotic, 505
 bone-marrow suppression, 497
 delayed toxicity, 499
 extravasation, 497
 handling guidelines, 496
 hyperuricaemia, 499
 nausea and vomiting, 497
 pregnancy, 498
 urothelial toxicity, 502

D

d4T *see* Stavudine, 373, **377**
Dacarbazine, 513, **514**
Daclizumab—discontinued

Dactinomycin, **505**
Daktacort, 676
Daktarin
 oral gel, 658
 skin, 713
Dalacin preparations, 340
 acne, 695
 vaginal, 475
Dalfopristin, **345**
Dalivit, 585
Dalteparin, **149**
Danaparoid, 150, 151
Dandrazol preparations, 705
Dandruff, 705
Danlax, 80
Danthron *see* Dantron, 79, 80
Dantrium, 618
 Intravenous, 786
Dantrolene
 malignant hyperthermia, **786**
 muscle spasm, 616, **617**, 618
Dantron, 79, 80
Daonil—discontinued
Dapsone
 pneumocystis pneumonia, 411, **412**
 poisoning, elimination, 35
Daraprim, 410
Darbepoetin, **536**, 537
Darier's disease, 685
Darunavir, 373, **379**
Daunorubicin, **505**, 506
DaunoXome, 506
DDAVP, 466
DDI *see* Didanosine, **375**, 376
Decan, 561
Decapeptyl SR, 459
Decongestants
 nasal, 652
 systemic, 210
DEET *see* Diethyltoluamide, 397
Defective medicines, 23
Defenac (diclofenac), 602, 603
Deferasirox, **540**
Deferiprone, **540**, 541
Deferoxamine *see* Desferrioxamine
Deflazacort, 443, **450**
Delph, 703
Deltacortril Enteric (prednisolone), 453
Deltaprim, 399
Demeclocycline, **330**
Demulcent cough preparations, 209
Dendritic ulcer, 625
Dental Practitioners' Formulary, 924
Dental prescribing
 abscess, 302
 anaesthesia
  general, 762
  local, 787
  vasoconstrictors, 787
 angular cheilitis, 657
 endocarditis prophylaxis, 307
 fluoride, 571
 herpes labialis, 385
 herpetic gingivostomatitis, 385
 infections
  bacterial, 297, 302
  fungal, 657
  viral, 385, 657
 joint prosthesis prophylaxis, 307
 oral hygiene, 659
 pain, 246, 251, 600
  postoperative, 246
 sinusitis, 652
Dentinox, colic drops, 53
Denzapine, 223

Dependence *see* Drug dependence
DepoCyte, 508
Depolarising muscle relaxants *see*
  Muscle relaxants
Depo-Medrone, 452, 608
  with Lidocaine, 608
Depo-Provera, 485, 486
Depression, 228
  antipsychotics, 215
  manic, 225, 226
Derbac-M, 717
Dermabond ProPen, 719
Dermacolor preparations, 705
Dermal, 706
Dermalo, 669
Dermamist, 667
Dermatitis
  ACBS, 917
  herpetiformis, 910
  seborrhoeic, 683
  see also Eczema
Dermatophyte infections, 363, 710
Dermol preparations, 668, 670
Dermovate preparations, 678
Desferal, 541
Desferrioxamine
  aluminium overload, **541**
  eye, 636
  iron overload, 539, **541**
  iron poisoning, **42**
Desflurane, 766, **767**
Desloratadine, 192, **193**
Desloughing agents, 723
Desmomelt, 466
Desmopressin, 466, 467
  assessment tests, **464**
  diabetes insipidus, **464**
  haemophilia, 158, **464**
  nocturnal enuresis, **464**, 494
Desmospray, 466, 467
Desmotabs, 466
Desogestrel, 485
  ethinylestradiol with, 481, 483
Destolit, 92
Detrusitol preparations, 493
Dexamethasone, 443, **450**, 451
  bacterial meningitis,
    451
  cerebral oedema, 450
  corticosteroid replacement ther-
    apy, 451
  croup, 169
  inflammatory and allergic disor-
    ders, 450
      ear, 644
      eye, 626
  malignant disease, 520
  nausea and vomiting,
    238
  palliative care, 26
  suppression test, 444
Dexamfetamine, 234, **235**
Dexamphetamine *see* Dexamfeta-
  mine, 234, **235**
Dexedrine, 235
Dexomon (diclofenac), 603
Dexrazoxane, **499**
Dexsol (dexamethasone),
  451
Dextran
  eye, 638
Dextromethorphan, 208
Dextropropoxyphene
  poisoning by, 39
Dextrose monohydrate *see* Glucose
DF-118 Forte, 253
DHC Continus, 253
Diabetes insipidus, 464

Diabetes mellitus, 418
  diagnosis, 438
  management with insulin, 418
  maturity-onset diabetes of the
    young, 418
  monitoring, 420
      glucose, 435
      ketone, 435, 436, 437
      meters, 436, 437
      test strips, 436, 437
  neonatal, 422
  surgery, 421
Diabetic
  ketoacidosis, 432, 554
  nephropathy, 435
  neuropathy, 435
      skin ulcers, 723
Diabur Test-5000, 437
Diacomit, 277
DIAGLYK (gliclazide), 431
Dialamine, 906
Dialar (diazepam), 773
Diamicron, 431
Diamorphine
  morphine equivalence, 29
  pain, 249, **252**, 253
    chronic, 25, 249
Diamox preparations, 634
Dianette, 698
Diaphragms, contraceptive, 490
Diarrhoea, 64
  oral rehydration, 549
Diastix, 437
Diazemuls (diazepam), 285
Diazepam, 773
  anaesthesia, 772, **773**
  convulsions, 34
  epilepsy
      status epilepticus, 283, **284**,
        285
  febrile convulsions, 287
  muscle spasm, 616, 618
  neonatal seizures, 267
  palliative care, 26
  tetanus, 618
Diazepam Rectubes, 285
Diazoxide
  chronic hypoglycaemia, 434
  hypertension, **121**, 122
  hypoglycaemia, **434**
Dibenyline, 130
Dibucaine *see* Cinchocaine
Diclofenac
  actinic keratoses, 704
  eye, 640
  juvenile idiopathic arthritis, 602
  pain and inflammation, **602**, 603
  postoperative pain, 776
  pyrexia, 602
  rheumatic disease, 600, **602**
Dicloflex (diclofenac), 602, 603
Diclomax (diclofenac), 603
Diclozip (diclofenac), 602
Dicobalt edetate, 44
Dicyclomine *see* Dicycloverine, **55**
Dicycloverine, **55**
Didanosine, **375**, 376
Dietary Specialities, 910
Diethylcarbamazine, 416
Diethyltoluamide, 397
Differin, 696
Difflam
  oral rinse, 655
  spray, 655
Diffundox XL (tamsulosin), 492
Diflucan preparations, 367
Diflucortolone valerate, 679
Digibind, 99

Digoxin, **97**, 98
  arrhythmias, 110
  poisoning, 97
Digoxin-specific antibody
  fragments, 97, **98**, 99
Dihydrocodeine, 250, **253**
Dihydropyridine calcium-channel
  blockers, 136
Dihydrotachysterol, 578
Dihydroxycholecalciferol, 578
Diloxanide furoate, **407**
Diltiazem, 136, **137**
  anal fissure, 89
  poisoning by, 41
  see also Calcium-channel block-
    ers
Dimercaprol, 45
Dimeticone
  head lice, 716, **717**
  skin
      benzalkonium with, 671
      cetrimide with, 671
      zinc oxide with, 671
Dinoprostone, 165, **166**
Dioctyl, 81
Dioctyl sodium sulphosuccinate *see*
  Docusate sodium
Dioderm, 675
Dioralyte preparations, 550
Dip/Ser, 734
Dipentum, 71
Dipeptiven, 561
Diphenoxylate, 65
Diphenylbutylpiperidines, 216
Diphosphonates *see* Bisphosphon-
  ates
Diphtheria
  antibacterial prophylaxis, 304
  antitoxin, 734
  benzylpenicillin in, 309
  immunisation
      travel, 733
      vaccines, combined, 733,
        734
Dipivefrine, 632, **633**
Dipotassium hydrogen phosphate,
  570
Diprivan, 765
Diprobase, 667
Diprobath, 669
Diprosalic, 678
Diprosone, 677
Dipyridamole, **155**
Disfiguring skin lesions, ACBS, 917
Disinfectants, 719
  ACBS, 917
Diskhaler
  Becodisks, 186
  Flixotide, 188
  Relenza, 392
  Serevent, 177
Disodium clodronate *see* Sodium
  clodronate, 470
Disodium cromoglicate *see* Sodium
  cromoglicate
Disodium hydrogen phosphate, 570
Disodium pamidronate, 469
Disprol (paracetamol) preparations,
  248
Distaclor preparations, 320
Distal intestinal obstruction
  syndrome
      acetylcysteine, 206
      amidotrizoates, 87
Distamine, 587
Dithranol, 683, **688**
  coal tar and salicylic acid with,
    688

Dithrocream, 688
Ditropan, 493
Diuretics, 100
  anaesthesia and, 761
  beta-blockers with, 114
  carbonic anhydrase inhibitors, 107
  loop, 100, 103
  osmotic, 107
  potassium and, 547
  potassium with, 107
  potassium-sparing, 101, 105
    with other diuretics, 106
  thiazides, 100, 101
Diva (co-cyprindiol), 698
DMPS see Unithiol, 45
DMSA see Succimer, 45
Dobutamine, 142, **143**
  infusion table (neonatal), 923
Docusate sodium
  ear, 647
  laxative, 79, **81**
Docusol, 81
Dolmatil, 221
Domperidone
  gastro-intestinal stasis, 58
  gastro-oesophageal reflux, 58
  migraine, 263
  nausea and vomiting, 238, **242**, 497
  palliative care, 25
Dopamine, 142, **143**, 144
  infusion table (neonatal), 923
Dopram, 203
Dornase alfa, 206, 207
Dorzolamide, 633, **634**
DOT, 349
Doublebase preparations, 667, 669
Dovobet, 686
Dovonex preparations, 686
Doxadura (doxazosin) preparations, 129
Doxapram, **202**, 203, 785
Doxazosin, 128, 129, 491
  cardiovascular, **128**
  urinary tract, **491**
Doxepin, 229, **230**, 672
  topical, 671, 672
Doxorubicin, 505, **506**
Doxycycline, **330**
  acne, 697
  aphthous ulcers, **656**
  malaria prophylaxis, 397, 398, 399, 400, 406, **407**
  malaria treatment, 395, 406
  mouth, 657
  oral infections, 329
  periodontitis, 302, 655, **656**
Doxylar (doxycycline), 330
Dozic, 219
Drapolene, 671
Dressings
  pain on changing, 769
Driclor, 724
Driving and skilled tasks, 3
Dromadol, 259
Drospirenone, ethinylestradiol with, 483
Drug dependence, 251
  management, 291
  prescribing in, 17
Drug interactions, 793
Dry mouth, 661
  palliative care, 26
Duac, 694
Dual block, 782
Ductus arteriosus, 164, 165
Dukoral, 733

Dulcolax (bisacodyl), 80
Dulcolax (sodium picosulfate), 82
Duobar, 905
Duocal preparations, 905
Duofilm, 700
Duphalac (lactulose), 83
Duraphat preparations, 572, 573
Durogesic DTrans, 254
Dusting powders, 664
Dysentery
  amoebic, 407
  bacillary see Shigellosis, 298
Dysfunctional voiding, 491
Dysmenorrhoea, 246
Dyspepsia, 50
Dysphagia, palliative care, 26
Dyspnoea, palliative care, 26
Dysport, 291
Dystonias, 288
  drug-induced, 216, 289

E

E numbers, *inside back cover*
E45 preparations, 667, 669
  Itch Relief, 668
  Sun, 703
EAA supplement, 914
Ear
  infections, 642
  wax removal, 647
EarCalm, 643
Easi-Breathe
  Beclazone, 186
  Salamol, 176
Easiphen, 915
Easyhaler
  beclometasone, 185
  budesonide, 187
  formoterol, 174
  salbutamol, 175
Ebufac (ibuprofen), 604
Echinocandin antifungal drugs, 363
Echinococcosis, 415
Econac (diclofenac), 602
Econacort, 676
Econazole
  anogenital, 473, 474
  skin, 711, **712**
    hydrocortisone with, 676
  vaginal, 474
Ecopace (captopril), 132
Ecostatin
  anogenital, 474
  skin, 712
Ecstacy, liquid (sodium oxybate), 43
Ecstasy
  controlled drug, 17
  poisoning by, 43
Ectopic tachycardia, 108
Eczema, 681
  ACBS, 917
  ear, 643
  scalp, 705
Ednyt (enalapril), 133
Edrophonium
  anaesthesia, **783**
  myasthenia gravis, 614, **615**

Efavirenz, 373, **382**
  emtricitabine and tenofovir with, 378
Efcortelan—discontinued
Efcortesol, 452
Eformoterol see Formoterol
Elaprase, 590
Electrolade, 550
Electrolyte and water replacement
  intravenous, 551
  oral, 546
Electrolyte concentrations, 546
  intravenous fluids, 546
Electrolytes
  intravenous nutrition, 559
Elemental-028 Extra, 881
Elidel, 692
Elocon, 681
Elspar, 513
Eltroxin (levothyroxine), 439
Eludril preparations, 660
Emadine, 627
Emedastine, **627**
Emergencies in the community,
  medical, *inside back cover*
Emergency
  contraception, 490
  supply, medication, 9
Emeside, 270
EMLA, 789
Emollients, 666
  eczema, 681
  pruritus, 671
  psoriasis, 683
Emollin, 667
Emsogen, 886
Emtricitabine, 373, **376**
  efavirenz and tenofovir with, 378
  tenofovir with, 378
Emtriva, 376
Emulsiderm, 670
Emulsifying ointment, 666, 667
Enalapril, **133**
  see also ACE inhibitors
Enbrel, 613
Enbucrilate, 719
Encephalopathy, hepatic, 83
En-De-Kay preparations, 572
Endocarditis, 299, 332
  antibacterial prophylaxis, 307
Endophthalmitis, 622
Ener-G products
  gluten- and wheat-free, 911
  gluten free, 910
  low protein, 911
Energivit, 905
Energy, intravenous nutrition, 559
Enfamil preparations, 898
  thickened, 900
Enfuvirtide, 373, **384**
Engerix B, 738
Enmix Plus Commence, 892
Enoxaparin, **149**, 150
Enoximone, **99**
Enrich, 890
Enshake, 906
Ensure Plus preparations, 891, 892, 893
Ensure preparations, 885, 890
Entamoeba histolytica, 407
Enteral
  feeding tubes
    administering drugs via, 90
    clearing blockages, 91
  nutrition, 562
    Crohn's disease, 66
    foods, ACBS, 878
Enteric infections, 298

Enterobiasis, 413
Enterocolitis, necrotising, 298
Entocort preparations, 73
Entonox, 768
Enuresis, nocturnal, 493
Enzira, 742
Enzyme induction, 793
Enzymes
  fibrinolytic, 156
Epaderm, 667
Epanutin preparations, 275
  Ready Mixed Parenteral, 287
Epaxal, 736
Ephedrine
  hypotension, **144**
  nasal congestion, 651, **652**
Epiglottitis, 299
Epiglu, 719
Epilepsy, 264, 266
  breast-feeding and, 266
  driving, 266
  neonatal seizures, 267
  pregnancy and, 266
  status epilepticus, 283
    non-convulsive, 283
  syndromes, 267
Epilim preparations, 279, 280
Epimaz (carbamazepine), 268
Epinastine, 627, **628**
Epinephrine *see* Adrenaline
Epipen, 200, 201
Epirubicin, 505, **506**
Episenta preparations, 280
Epistatus (midazolam), 775
Epivir, 377
Epoetin
  alfa, **537**, 538
  beta, **537**, 538
  zeta, **537**, 538
Epoprostenol, 123, 124, **125**, 151
Eposin, 512
Eprex, 538
Eptadone (methadone), 255
Equanox, 768
Equasym (methylphenidate), 236
Equasym XL, 236
Ergocalciferol, 578, **579**, 580
Ergot alkaloids, 261
Ertapenem, **326**
Erwinase, 513
Erymax, 337
Erysipelas, 303
Erythema, perianal, 87
Erythrocin, 337
Erythromycin, 335, **336**, 337
  acne, 695, 696, 697
    tretinoin with, 696
  diphtheria prophylaxis, 304
  eye infections, 622
  gastro-intestinal stasis, 58
  pertussis prophylaxis, 305
  rheumatic fever prophylaxis, 303
Erythroped preparations, 337
Erythropoietins, 536
Escitalopram, 231
Esmeron, 781
Esmolol, 108, 114, **117**
  see also Beta-adrenoceptor blocking drugs
Essential amino acids supplement, 914
Estriol, labial adhesions, 472

Etanercept
  juvenile idiopathic arthritis, 611, **612**, 613
  psoriasis, **692**
Ethambutol, 348, 351, **352**
  tuberculosis treatment, 348, 349
Ethinylestradiol
  acne *see* Co-cyprindiol, **698**
  contraception, 475
    desogestrel with, 481, 483
    drospirenone with, 483
    etonogestrel with, 481
    gestodene with, 481, 483
    levonorgestrel with, 481, 482
    norelgestromin with, 483
    norethisterone with, 481, 482
    norgestimate with, 483
  hormone therapy, **454**
Ethinyloestradiol *see* Ethinylestradiol
Ethosuximide, 266, 267, **269**, 270
Ethyl-2-cyanoacrylate, 719
Ethylene glycol, poisoning by, 45
Ethynodiol *see* Etynodiol, 485
Etomidate, 763, **764**
Etomidate-Lipuro, 764
Etonogestrel
  ethinylestradiol with, 481
  implant, 486
Etopophos, 512
Etoposide, **511**, 512
Etoricoxib, 600, **603**
Etravirine, 373, **383**
Etretinate, 685
Etynodiol, 485
Eucalyptus oil, 208
Eucardic, 117
Eucerin, 668
Eudemine
  hypertension, 122
  hypoglycaemia, 434
Euglucon—discontinued
Eumovate, 679
Eurax preparations, 672, 676
European viper venom antiserum, 47
Evening primrose oil, 667
Evohaler
  Flixotide, 188
  Seretide, 189
  Ventolin, 176
Evoltra, 508
Evotrox (levothyroxine), 439
Evra, 483
Excipients
  details provided, 3
  skin preparations and, 665
Exelderm, 714
Exfoliative dermatitis, 444
Exjade, 540
Exocin, 624
Exorex, 687
Expectorants, 209
Extemporaneous preparations, 8
Exterol, 647
Extrapyramidal symptoms
  antipsychotics and, 216
  treatment, 289
Extravasation, 618

Eye
  anaesthesia, local, 635
  antibacterials, 622
    frequency of administration, 622
  antifungals, 624
  antivirals, 625
  contact lenses, 640
  corticosteroids, 625
  cycloplegics, 629
  drops, administration, 620
  glaucoma, 630
  inflammation, 625
  lotions, administration, 620
  microbial contamination, 621
  miotics, 635
  mydriatics, 629
  ointments, administration, 620
  prostaglandins, 631, 632
Ezetimibe, 163
Ezetrol, 163

F

Fabrazyme, 588
Fabry's Disease, 588
Faecal softeners, 82
Falciparum malaria, 395
Fallot's tetralogy *see* Tetralogy of Fallot, 114
Famciclovir, 386, 475
Fansidar, 406
Fasigyn, 408
Fasturtec, 500
Fat emulsions, intravenous, 559
Fate, 911
Faverin, 233
Favism, 542
Febrile convulsions, 287
Fectrim (co-trimoxazole), 348
Feed thickeners, 564, 909
Feeds *see* Foods
Feldene preparations, 607
Felypressin, 788, 791
FemCap, 490
Femidom, 475
Femodene preparations, 483
Femodette, 481
Femulen, 485
Fenactol (diclofenac), 602, 603
Fenbid (ibuprofen), 604
Fendrix, 739
Fenofibrate, 163, **164**
Fenpaed (ibuprofen), 604
Fentanyl, **777**
  analgesia, **253**, 254
    perioperative, 777, 778
  palliative care, 25
    morphine equivalence, 25
Fentazin, 220
Ferinject, 532
Ferric carboxymaltose, **532**
Ferriprox preparations, 541
Ferrous fumarate, 529, **530**, 531
Ferrous gluconate, 529, 531
Ferrous sulphate, 529, **530**
Fersaday, 530
Fersamal, 530
Feverfen (ibuprofen), 604
Fexofenadine, 192, **193**
Fibrates, 163

Fibrelief, 78
Fibrinolytic drugs, 156
Filariasis, 416
Filaricides, 416
Filgrastim, 543, **544**, 545
Finacea, 694
Finepoint, 428
Fingertip unit, 674
Fits *see* Epilepsy
Flagyl preparations, 356, 357
Flamatak (diclofenac), 603
Flamazine, 709
Flamrase (diclofenac), 602, 603
Flavour Mix, 909
Flavouring preparations, 909
FlavourPac, 909
Flebogamma, 757
Flecainide, 108, 110, **111**, 112
Fleet
    Phospho-soda, 86
    Ready-to-use enema, 85
Fletchers' Enemas—discontinued
Flexbumin preparations (albumin),
  557
Flexible collodion, 719
Flexi-T intra-uterine devices, 489
Flexotard MR (diclofenac), 603
Flixonase preparations, 650
Flixotide preparations, 188
Flolan, 125
Flomaxtra XL, 492
Florinef, 443
Flowfusor, 720
Floxapen, 312
Floxapen (flucloxacillin), 312
Flu-Amp (co-fluampicil), 315
Fluarix, 742
Fluclomix (flucloxacillin), 312
Flucloxacillin, 310, **311**, 312
  ampicillin with [co-fluampicil],
    312
  ear infection, 643
Fluconazole, 361, 362, 363, **366**,
  367
    oropharyngeal candidiasis, 657
    vulvovaginal candidiasis, recur-
      rent, 473
Flucytosine, 361, 362, 363, **367**
Fludara, 509
Fludarabine, 507, **509**
Fludrocortisone, 442, **443**
Fludroxycortide, **679**
Fluid and electrolyte replacement,
  546
    neonate, 551
    oral, 546
    parenteral, 551
Flumazenil, 41, **785**
Flumetasone, **644**
Flumethasone *see* Flumetasone, **644**
Flunisolide, **650**
Fluocinolone acetonide, 679, 680
  clioquinol with, 680
  neomycin with, 680
Fluocinonide, 680
Fluocortolone, 680
  [ingredient], 89
Fluor-a-day, 572
Fluorescein, **639**
  lidocaine with, 636
  proxymetacaine with, 636
Fluoride, 571, **572**
FluoriGard preparations, 572, 573
Fluorometholone, 626
Fluorouracil, 704
Fluoxetine, 231, **232**, 233
Flurandrenolone *see* Fludroxycor-
  tide, **679**

Flurbiprofen
  eye, 640
  sore throat, 654, 656
Fluticasone furoate, 650
Fluticasone propionate
  asthma, 184, **188**
  nasal allergy, 650
  nasal polyps, 650
  salmeterol with, 188
  skin, 680, 681
Fluvirin, 742
Fluvoxamine, 231, **233**
FML, 626
Folate deficiency, 533
Folate rescue, 500
Folic acid, 533, **535**
  methotrexate, following, 610
  pregnancy, 533, 534
Folicare, 535
Folinic acid
  rescue, 500
  see also Calcium levofolinate
Folliculitis, 707
Fomepizole, 45
Food allergy, 76
Foodlink preparations, 894
Foods
  ACBS, 878
  enteral, 562, 564
  feed thickeners, 564
  gluten-free, 910
  intolerance, 564, 909
  low-protein, 911
  special diets, 561, 564, 910
    vitamin supplements, 585
  thickened, 909
Foradil, 174
Forceval, 585
Formaldehyde, 700, 701
Formoterol, **174**
  budesonide with, 187
Formulary
  Dental, 924
  Nurse, 925
Forticare, 901
Forticreme, 894
Fortijuce, 891
Fortimel Regular, 893
Fortini preparations, 888
Fortipine LA 40, 139
Fortisip preparations, 892, 893, 894
Fortum, 324
Fosamax preparations, 469
Fosamprenavir, 373, **380**
Foscarnet, 388, **389**
Foscavir, 389
Fosphenytoin, 275, 283, 285
Fragmin, 149
Framycetin
  ear, 644, 645
Frangula, sterculia with, 79
Frebini preparations, 887, 889
Freebake products, 910
FreeStyle products, 428, 436, 437
Fresubin preparations
    enteral feed, 879, 882, 883, 884
    nutritional supplement, 893, 894
Friars' Balsam, 208
Frisium (clobazam), 282
Froop (furosemide), 104
Fructose
  ACBS, 909
  presence of, 3
Frumil preparations (co-amilofruse),
  106
Frusemide *see* Furosemide
Frusol (furosemide), 104
FTU *see* Fingertip unit, 674

Fucibet, 678
Fucidin, 341
  skin, 709
Fucidin H, 676
Fucithalmic, 623
Full Marks, 718
Fungal infections, 361
  anogenital, 473
  eye, 624
  oropharyngeal, 657
  skin, 362, 710
Fungilin lozenges, 658
Fungizone, 364
Furadantin, 361
Furosemide, **103**, 104
  amiloride with, 106
Fusidic acid
  angular cheilitis, 657
  eye, 622, 623
  skin, **709**
    betamethasone with, 678
    hydrocortisone with, 676
  systemic, 341
Fuzeon, 384
Fybogel, 78
Fybogel Mebeverine, 57

G

G6PD deficiency
  drugs to be avoided in, 542
GA gel, 912
Gabapentin, 266, **270**, 271
Gabitril, 277
Gadsby's, 910
Galactomin preparations, 898, 900
Galenamox (amoxicillin), 314
Galenphol, 209
Galfer, 531
Galpseud, 210
Galsulfase, **589**, 590
Gammagard S/D, 757
Gamma-hydroxybutyrate (sodium
  oxybate), 43
Ganciclovir, **388**, 389
Gardasil, 740
Gas cylinders, 762
Gas-gangrene, 309
  prophylaxis, 306
Gastric emptying, poisoning and, 35
Gastrocote, 54
Gastro-enteritis, 64, 298
Gastrografin, 87
Gastro-intestinal procedures, anti-
  bacterial prophylaxis, 306
Gastro-intestinal secretions
  electrolyte content, 546
Gastro-oesophageal reflux disease,
  50
Gaucher's disease, 589
Gaviscon preparations, 54
G-CSF, 544, 545
Gelatin
  infusion, **557**
  succinylated, 557
Gelofusine, 557
Geloplasma, 557
Gels, definition, 664
GelTears, 637

Generaid preparations, 901
General anaesthesia *see* Anaesthesia, general
Generpharm see Proceli products, 910
Genital warts, 701
Genotropin preparations, 462
Gentamicin, 332, **333**, 334
  ear, 645, 646
  eye, 622, 623, 636
Genticin, 334
  ear, 646
  eye, 623
Gentisone HC, 645
German measles *see* Rubella, 267, **276**
Gestodene, ethinylestradiol with, 481, 483
GHB (sodium oxybate), 43
Giardia lamblia, 408
Giardiasis, 408
Gilles de la Tourette syndrome *see* Tourette syndrome, 290
Gingivitis
  antibacterial treatment, 302, 355
  mouthwashes, 659
Glamin, 559
Glandosane, 662
Glaucoma, 630
  steroid, 625
Glibenclamide, **430**
Gliclazide, **430**, 431
Glivec, 515
Glomerular filtration rate, dosage and, 13
GlucaGen HypoKit, 434
Glucagon, **433**, 434
  beta-blocker poisoning, 41
Glucocorticoids
  equivalent doses, 443
  replacement therapy, 442
Glucogel, 433
GlucoMen products, 428, 436, 437
Glucophage, 432
Glucose
  ACBS, 912
  cyanosis, 115
  hypoglycaemia, 433
  infusion, 553, 554
    potassium and, 555
    sodium and, 553
  intravenous nutrition, 559
  oral rehydration, 549
  presence of, 3
  syrup, hydrogenated, presence of, 3
  tests
    blood, 435
    tolerance, 438
    urine, 437
Glucose 6-phosphate dehydrogenase deficiency
  drugs to be avoided in, 542
Glue ear, 646
Glutafin products, 910, 911
Glutaraldehyde, 700, 701
Glutaric
  acidaemias, 576
  aciduria, 912
Glutarol, 701
Gluten, presence of, 3
Gluten-sensitive enteropathies, 910
Glycerin suppositories, 81
Glycerol
  constipation, 79, 81
  glaucoma, 633

Glyceryl trinitrate
  anal fissure, 89
  extravasation, 618
  infusion table (neonatal), 923
  shock, 142
  vasodilation, **135**, 136
Glycogen storage disease
  dietary supplement, 912
  granulocyte-colony stimulating factor, in, 544
  hypoglycaemia, 433
Glycopeptide antibiotics, 341
Glycophos, 561
Glycopyrrolate *see* Glycopyrronium bromide
Glycopyrronium bromide
  airway secretions, 770
  hyperhidrosis, 723, 724
  hypersalivation, **770**
  neostigmine with, 784
  palliative care, 28
  premedication, 769, **770**, 771
Glycosade, 912
Glypressin, 467
GnRH *see* Gonadorelin, **463**
Goitre, lymphadenoid, 438
Gold, 608
Golden Eye Drops (propamidine), 624
Golden Eye Ointment (dibromopropamidine), 624
Gonadorelin, **463**
Gonadorelin analogues, 457
Gonadotrophin deficiency, 453
Gonadotrophin-releasing hormone *see* Gonadorelin, **463**
Gonadotrophins, 460
Gonapeptyl, 459
Gonorrhoea
  eye, 302
  genital, 301
  pharyngeal, 301
GORD *see* Gastro-oesophageal reflux disease, **50**
Goserelin, **458**
Gout, 613
Gramicidin [ingredient]
  ear drops, 644
  eye drops, 624
Graneodin—discontinued
Granisetron, 238, **243**
Granocyte, 545
Granulocyte-colony stimulating factor, 543–5
Grass pollen extracts, 197
Graves' disease, 440
Grazax, 197
Griseofulvin, 362, 363, **367**, 368
Ground-nut oil *see* Arachis oil
Growth factor, platelet derived, 723
Growth hormone, 461
Guillain-Barré syndrome, 755
Gygel, 488
Gynaecological surgery, antibacterial prophylaxis, 306
Gyne T, 488
GyneFix, 488, 489
Gyno-Daktarin Ovule, 474
Gyno-Pevaryl preparations, 474

H

Haelan preparations, 679
Haem arginate, **597**
Haemaccel, 557
Haemodialysis, 35

Haemolytic anaemia, 535
  G6PD deficiency, 542
Haemophilia, 464
Haemophilus influenzae type b (Hib)
  immunisation, **735**
  prophylaxis, 304
  vaccines
    diphtheria with, 734
    meningococcal with, 735
Haemorrhage, 158
  gastro-intestinal, 60
Haemorrhagic disease of newborn, 583
Haemorrhoids, 88
Haemostatics, 158
HAES-steril, 558
Haldol, 219
Haleraid, 182
Half-Beta-Prograne (propranolol), 116
Half-Inderal LA, 116
Half-Securon SR, 141
Haloperidol
  movement disorders, 290
  nausea and vomiting, 237
  palliative care, 28
  psychoses, 217, **219**
  tics, 219
Halothane, **767**, 768
Halycitrol—discontinued
Harifen products, 911
Harlequin ichthyosis, 689
Hartmann's solution *see* Sodium lactate, intravenous infusion, compound, 553
Hashimoto's thyroiditis, 438
Havrix preparations, 736
Hay fever, 191, 648
Hay-Crom preparations (sodium cromoglicate), 628
HBIG *see* Hepatitis B immunoglobulin
HBvaxPRO, 739
HCG *see* Chorionic gonadotrophin, 456, **460**, 461
HCU preparations, 912, 913
Head lice, 716
Headache
  cluster, 264
  migraine, 261
Heaf test, 731
Healthy Start vitamins, 575
Heart failure, 100
  ACE inhibitors, 100
  beta-blockers, 100, 114
  diuretics, 100, 103
  enoximone, 100
  spironolactone, 100
Heart *see also* Cardiac
Hedrin, 717
Helicobacter pylori
  dyspepsia, 50
  eradication, **59**
  test, 60
Helminth infections, 413
Hemohes, 558
Heparin, 147, **148**
  flushes, 151
  infusion table (neonatal), 923
  injection
    calcium, 148
    sodium, 148
Heparinoids, topical, 724
Hepatic
  encephalopathy, 83
  impairment, prescribing in, 12

Index

Hepatitis A
  immunisation, 746
  immunoglobulin, normal, 755
  travel, 759
  vaccine, **736**
    hepatitis B with, 737
    typhoid with, 737
Hepatitis B
  auto immune, 444
  chronic, 377, 390
  chronic active, 526
  immunisation, 748
  immunoglobulin, **757**
  travel, 759
  vaccine, 737, **738**, 739
Hepatitis C
  chronic, 390
  chronic active, 526
Hepatolenticular degeneration *see*
  Wilson's disease, 586
Hepatyrix, 737
Herbal medicines, 2
Hereditary angiodema *see* Angiodema
Heroin *see* Diamorphine
Heron products
  gluten- and wheat-free, 911
  gluten-free, 910
Herpes infections, 385
  eye, 625
  genital, 386, 475
  immunoglobulin, 758
  mouth, 657
  skin, 715
Hewletts, 667
Hexetidine, 660
HFAs, 172, 184
HGH *see* Somatotrophin, 461
Hib see Haemophilus influenzae
  type b
Hibiscrub, 721
Hibisol, 721
Hibitane preparations, 721
Hiccup, 217
  palliative care, 27
Hirsutism, 698
Hirudoid, 724
Histamine H$_1$-antagonists, 191
Histamine H$_2$-antagonists, 60
Histoacryl, 719
Histoplasmosis, 362
HIV infection, 372
  pregnancy, 373
HNIG *see* Immunoglobulins, normal
Hodgkin's disease, 513
Homatropine, **630**
Homocystinuria, 594, 912
Hookworm infections, 415
Hormone replacement, 453
  androgens, 455
  oestrogens, 454
  progestogens, 454
HRF, 463
5HT$_1$ agonists, 261, **262**
5HT$_3$ antagonists, 238, 243, 244,
  497
HTIG *see* Immunoglobulins, tetanus,
  757, 758
Humalog preparations, 424, 427
Human chorionic gonadotrophin *see*
  Chorionic gonadotrophin, 456,
  460, 461
Human normal immunoglobulin *see*
  Immunoglobulins, normal
Human papilloma virus, vaccine,
  740
HumaPen Luxura products, 428
Humatrope, 462

Humira, 612
Humulin I, 426
Humulin M3, 428
Humulin S, 423
Hyaline membrane disease, 203
Hydatid disease, 415
Hydralazine, 121, **122**
Hydrex, 721
Hydrochlorothiazide
  amiloride with, 106
Hydrocortisone, 443, 444, **451**, 452
  asthma, acute, 169
  colitis, 73
  ear, 644, 645
  eye, 626
  haemorrhoids, 88
  intra-articular, 607
  mouth, 654, 656
  pneumocystis pneumonia, 411
  rectal, 88, 89
  replacement therapy, 442
  rheumatic disease, 608
  septic shock, 142
  skin, 675, 676, 677
    chlorhexidine and nystatin
      with, 676
    clotrimazole with, 676
    coal tar with, 688
    crotamiton with, 676
    econazole with, 676
    fusidic acid with, 676
    miconazole with, 676
    nystatin with, 676
    urea with, 676
Hydrocortistab, 608
Hydrocortone—discontinued
Hydrofluoroalkane propellants, 172,
  184
Hydrogen peroxide
  mouthwash, 659, **660**
  skin, **722**
Hydromol preparations, 667, 669
Hydromorphone, **254**, 255
  morphine equivalence, 24
Hydrotalcite, **52**
  simeticone with, 52
Hydrous ointment, 666
Hydroxocobalamin, 533, **534**, 535
  cyanide poisoning, 44
Hydroxycarbamide, **539**
  sickle-cell disease, 539
Hydroxychloroquine, **609**, 610
Hydroxycholecalciferol, 578
Hydroxyethyl starch *see* Starch,
  etherified, 557, 558
Hydroxyethylcellulose, 637
Hydroxyquinoline
  benzoyl peroxide with, 694
Hydroxyurea *see* Hydroxycarbamide
Hydroxyzine, **195**
Hygroton, 102
Hyoscine butylbromide, **55**, 56
  palliative care, 55
Hyoscine hydrobromide, 245
  excessive respiratory secretions,
    26, 245
  hypersalivation, 245
  motion sickness, 239
  nausea and vomiting, **245**
  palliative care, 28
    gastro-intestinal pain, 25
  premedication, 769, **771**
Hyperactivity, attention deficit, 234
Hyperammonaemia, 591
Hypercalcaemia, 467, 567
Hypercalciuria, 567
Hypercholesterolaemia, 159–61,
  163

Hyperemesis gravidarum, 238
Hyperglycaemia, 418
  coma, 432
  neonatal, 422
HyperHAES, 558
Hyperhidrosis, 723
Hypericum perforatum, 228
Hyperinsulinaemic hypoglycaemia,
  434
Hyperinsulinism, 433
Hyperkalaemia, **547**
  see also Salbutamol
Hyperlipidaemia, 159
Hyperlysinaemia, 913
Hypermethioninaemia, 912
Hypernatraemia, 553
Hyperphosphataemia, 570
Hyperprolactinaemia, 453
Hypersalivation, 769
Hypersecretion, airways, 769
Hypersensitivity *see* Allergic disor-
  ders
Hypertension, 101, **119**
  ACE inhibitors, 130
  beta-blockers, 114
  crisis, 120
  diabetes, 119
  diuretics, 100, 103
  malignant, 120
  nephritis, 121
  poisoning and, 34
  portal, variceal bleeding in,
    464
  pregnancy, 119
  pulmonary, 123, 151
  renal disease, 119
Hyperthermia
  malignant, 786
  poisoning and, 34
Hyperthyroidism *see* Thyrotoxicosis
Hypertonic sodium chloride,
  208
Hyperuricaemia, 499
Hypnomidate, 764
Hypnotics, 211, 212
Hypnovel, 775
Hypocalcaemia, 565
Hypodermic equipment, insulin,
  428
Hypodermoclysis, 551
Hypogammaglobulinaemia, 755
Hypoglycaemia, 420
  acute, 433
  chronic, 434
  hyperinsulinaemia, 434
  neonatal, 433
Hypoglycaemic drugs, oral *see* Anti-
  diabetic drugs, oral, 429
Hypogonadism, 453, 455, 460
Hypoguard products, 428, 436, 437
Hypokalaemia
  diuretics and, 100
  intravenous potassium, 554
  potassium, oral, 546, 547
Hypolar Retard 20, 139
Hypomagnesaemia, 568
Hyponatraemia
  neonate, 553
  sodium replacement
    oral, 548
    parenteral, 552
Hypophosphataemia, 569
Hypopituitarism, 442, 455
Hyposensitisation, 196
Hypostop Gel, 433
Hypotension, poisoning and,
  34
Hypothalamic hormones, 463

Index

Hypothermia
  antipsychotics and, 216
  poisoning and, 34
Hypothyroidism, 438
  neonatal, 438
Hypovase, 129
Hypovolaemia, 556
Hypoxaemia, 204
Hypromellose, 638
Hypurin Isophane, 426
  biphasic, 427
Hypurin Lente, 426
Hypurin Neutral, 423
Hypurin Protamine Zinc, 426

I

Ibuprofen
  ductus arteriosus, **164**, 165
  juvenile idiopathic arthritis, 604
  migraine, 261
  pain, 600, **604**
    postoperative, 776
  pyrexia, 604
    post-immunisation, 727
  rheumatic disease, 600, 604
Ichthammol, 682, **683**
  zinc with, 683
Ichthopaste, 683
Ichthyosis, 666, 685, 689
Icthaband—discontinued
Idiopathic thrombocytopenic
  purpura *see* Thrombocytopenic
  purpura
Idrolax—discontinued
Idursulfase, 589, **590**
Ifosfamide, **504**
Il Pane di Anna products, 910
Iloprost
  pulmonary hypertension, 124,
    125
  Raynaud's syndrome, **141**, 142
Ilube, 637
Imatinib, **514**, 515
Imidazole antifungal drugs, 362, 363
Imiglucerase, **589**
Imigran preparations, 262, 263
Imipenem, 325, **326**, 327
Imipramine
  attention deficit hyperactivity
    disorder, 230
  depression, 229
  nocturnal enuresis, **230**, 231,
    494
Imiquimod, **702**
Immukin, 527
Immune interferon *see* Interferons,
  gamma-1b, 527
Immunisation
  immunity
    active, 725
    passive, 729
  international travel, 758
  schedule, 728
Immunodeficiency, 755, 757
  syndrome, acquired, 372
Immunoglobulins, 729, **754**
  aplastic anaemia, 535
  hepatitis B, 757
  Kawasaki syndrome, 757
  myasthenia gravis, 614
  normal, 755–7
  rabies, 757, 758
  tetanus, 757, 758
  thrombocytopenic purpura, 541
  varicella-zoster, 757, 758

Immunostimulants, 525
Immunosuppressants, 517
  malignant disease, 520
  myasthenia gravis, 616
  skin disease, 690
  transplant rejection, 517
Imodium preparations, 66
Impetigo, 303, 707
Implanon, 486
Imuderm, 669
Imuran, 519
Imuvac, 742
Increlex, 471
Independent prescribing, 928
Inderal preparations, 116
Indian hemp *see* Cannabis, 19
Indinavir, 373, **380**
Indocid PDA, 165
Indolar SR (indometacin m/r), 605
Indometacin
  ductus arteriosus, 164, **165**
  juvenile idiopathic arthritis, 604
  pain and inflammation, 604, 605
  rheumatic disease, 600, **604**
Infacol, 53
Infanrix-IPV, 734
Infanrix-IPV+Hib, 734
Infantile
  acne, 693, 699
  spasms, 267
InfaSoy, 899
Infatrini preparations, 887
Infections
  amoebic, 407
  antisera, 730, 754
  ear, 642
  eye, 621
  fungal, 361
  helminth, 413
  immunoglobulins, 754
  nail, fungal, 362
  notifiable diseases, 296
  oropharyngeal, 657
    bacterial, 297, 302
  protozoal, 394
  skin, 707
  trichomonal, 408
  vaccines, 725
  vaginal, 473
  viral, 372
  vulval, 473
Inflammatory bowel disease, 66
Infliximab
  Crohn's disease, 66, **75**, 76
  inflammatory bowel disease, 67
  rheumatic diseases, 611
Influenza
  immunisation
    vaccines, **741**, 742
  prophylaxis, 390
  treatment, 390
Influvac Sub-unit, 742
Information services, poisons, 33
Infusions, intravenous (neonatal),
  921
Inhalations
  aromatic, 208
  Benzoin tincture, compound,
    208
  menthol and eucalyptus, 208
  steam, 651
Inhaler devices, 181
Innohep, 150
Innovace, 133
Innovative products *see* Pure pro-
  ducts, 910
Inositol, 575
Inotropic drugs, positive, 97, 142

Inovelon, 276
Insect stings, 48, 192
Insecticides, poisoning by, 46
Insomnia, 212
  antihistamines, 192
  palliative care, 27
Instillagel, 789
Insulatard preparations, 426
Insulin, 418
  aspart, 422, **423**, 424
    biphasic, 425, **427**
  detemir, **425**
  glargine, **425**
  glulisine, 422, **424**
  human, 418
  infusion
    intravenous, 420, 422
    subcutaneous, 420
  infusion table (neonatal), 923
  injection equipment, 428
  isophane, 425, **426**
    biphasic, 425, **427**, 428
  lispro, 422, **424**
    biphasic, 425, **427**
  protamine zinc, 425, **426**
  soluble, 422, **423**
  zinc suspension, 425, **426**
    crystalline, 425
    mixed, 426
Insulin-like growth factor, 471
Insuman
  Basal, 426
  Comb preparations, 428
  Rapid, 423
Insupak, 429
Intal, 190
  Spincaps—discontinued
Intelence, 383
Interactions, 793
Interferon gamma release assay,
  732
Interferons
  alfa, 526
    chronic hepatitis B, 390
    chronic hepatitis C, 390
    peginterferon, 390
  gamma-1b, 527
International travel, immunisation
  for, 758
Intracranial pressure, raised
  corticosteroids, 444
  osmotic diuretics, 107
  palliative care, 28
Intralipid preparations, 559
Intra-uterine devices
  copper-bearing, 488–90
  progestogen-releasing, 487
Intravenous
  infusion table (neonatal), 923
  infusions, 551
  nutrition, 558
IntronA, 526
Invanz, 326
Invirase, 382
Iocare, 638
Iodide, 441
Iodine
  radioactive, 440
  skin disinfection, **722**
  thyrotoxicosis, 440, 441
    oral solution, 441
Iopidine, 640
Ipocol, 70
Ipratropium
  asthma, **178**
    acute, 169
  rhinorrhoea, 652, **653**
  Steri-Neb, 178

IPV *see* Poliomyelitis, immunisation
Iron
    deficiency, 529
        neonatal, 529
    oral, 529–31
    overload, 539
    parenteral, 532, 533
    poisoning by, 42
Iron dextran, **532**
Iron sucrose, 532, **533**
Ironorm, 530
Irriclens, 720
Irripod, 720
Irritable bowel syndrome, 54, **68**
Isentress, 385
Isoflurane, 766, **768**
Isogel, 78
Isoleucine Amino Acid Supplement, 913
Isomil, 899
Isoniazid, 351, **352**, 353
    tuberculosis prophylaxis, 305
    tuberculosis treatment, 348, 349
Isophane protamine insulin *see* Insulin, isophane
Isoplex, 557
Isoprenaline, 142
Isopto
    Alkaline, 638
    Atropine, 629
    Plain, 638
Isosource preparations, 879, 883, 888
Isotretinoin, 693
    acne
        erythromycin with, 697
        oral, **699**, 700
        topical, 695, **696**, 697
Isotrex, 697
Isotrexin, 697
Isovaleric acidaemia, 913
Isovorin, 501
Ispagel Orange, 78
Ispaghula
    constipation, **78**
    diarrhoea, 65
    mebeverine with, 57
Istin, 137
Itraconazole, 361, 362, 363, **368**, 369
    oropharyngeal candidiasis, 657
IUDs *see* Intra-uterine devices, 487
Ivermectin
    larva migrans, 416
    onchocerciasis, 416
    scabies, 715
    strongyloidiasis, 416
IZS *see* Insulin, zinc suspension

J

Japanese encephalitis, 759
Jet nebulisers, 182
Jevity preparations, 879, 883, 884
Joy-Rides, 245
Juvela preparations, 910, 911

K

Kala-azar, 409
Kaletra, 381
Kaolin, 65
Kaplon (captopril), 132

Karvol preparations, 208
Katya 30/75, 483
Kawasaki syndrome
    aspirin, 154
    immunoglobulin, 154
    immunoglobulin, normal, **757**
Kay-Cee-L, 547
Kefadim, 324
Keflex, 321
Keftid (cefaclor), 320
Kemadrin preparations, 290
Kemicetine, 341
Kenalog Intra-articular/Intramuscular, 608
Keppra, 273
Keratitis, 622
Keratolytics, warts and calluses, 700
Keratosis follicularis, 685
Keromask preparations, 705
Ketalar, 764
Ketamine, 763, **764**
Ketoacidosis, diabetic, 432
KetoCal, 902
Ketoconazole, 362, 363, **369**, 370
    anogenital, 474
    Cushing's syndrome, 471
    scalp, 705
    skin, 711, 712, 713
Ketodiastix, 437
Ketones, tests
    blood, 435
    urine, 437
Ketorolac
    eye, 640
    pain, postoperative, **776**
Ketostix, 437
Ketotifen, **195**
    eye, 627, **628**
Ketovite, 585
Ketur Test, 437
Key Omega, 915
Kindergen, 902
Kivexa, 375
Klaricid preparations, 338, 339
Klean-Prep, 86
Klinefelter's syndrome, 453
Kloref—discontinued
Kolanticon, 55
Konakion preparations, 584
Kuvan, 562
Kwells, 245
Kytril, 243

L

Labelling, cautionary and advisory *see* Cautionary and advisory labels
Labetalol, 113, 114, **117**, 118
    see also Beta-adrenoceptor blocking drugs
Labial adhesions, 472
Labour, analgesia, 250
Labyrinthine disorders, 239
Lacosamide, **271**
Lacri-Lube, 638
Lactase, ACBS, 909
Lactate *see* Sodium lactate, compound
Lactic acid
    hydrocortisone with, 676
    salicylic acid with, 700, 701
Lactic acidosis, 374
    congenital, 576
Lactugal (lactulose), 83
Lactulose, **83**
Ladropen (flucloxacillin), 312

Laevulose *see* Fructose
Lamictal, 272
Lamisil
    oral, 371
    topical, 714
Lamivudine, **376**, 377
    abacavir and zidovudine with, 375
    abacavir with, 375
    chronic hepatitis B, 377, 390
    HIV infection, 373
    zidovudine with, 378
Lamotrigine, 266, 267, 271, **272**
Lancets, sterile, 428
Landau-Kleffner syndrome, 267
Lanolin, excipient, 667
Lanoxin preparations, 98
Lansoprazole, 62, **63**
Lantus preparations, 425
Lanvis, 511
Larapam SR, 259
Largactil, 218
Lariam, 404
Laronidase, 589, **590**
LarvE, 723
Laryng-O-Jet, 789
Lasix, 104
Lassa fever, 392
Lassar's paste, 689
Latanoprost, 632
Latin abbreviations, *inside back cover*
Laxatives, 77
    bulk-forming, 78
    faecal softeners, 82
    osmotic, 83
    stimulant, 79
Laxido, 83
Ledclair, 45
Ledermycin, 330
Legionnaires' disease, 336
Leishmaniasis, 409
Lennox-Gastaut syndrome, 267
Lenograstim, 543, **545**
Leptospirosis, 309, 328
Leucine amino acid supplement, 915
Leukeran, 503
Leukotriene receptor antagonists, 170, 190
Leuprorelin, **458**
Levamisole, **414**, 415
Levemir preparations, 425
Levetiracetam, 266, 267, **273**
Levobunolol, **632**
Levobupivacaine, **790**
Levocetirizine, 192, **193**, 194
Levodopa
    dopa-decarboxylase inhibitor with, 288
    dystonias, 288
    metabolic disorders, 288
Levofloxacin
    eye, 622, **623**
Levofolinic acid *see* Calcium levofolinate, 500, 501
Levomenthol, 208
Levomepromazine, **219**
    nausea and vomiting, 237
    palliative care, 27, 28
Levonelle 1500, 491
Levonelle One Step, 491
Levonorgestrel, 487
    contraception, 485
        emergency, **490**, 491
        ethinylestradiol with, 481, 482
        intra-uterine, 487
    menstrual disorders, 455

Levothyroxine, **438**, 439
Lexpec (folic acid), 535
LH-RH *see* Gonadorelin, **463**
Liberim HB, 757
Lice, 716
Licensed medicines, 3, 7
Lidocaine
    arrhythmias, 110, **113**
    dental, 787, 788
    eye, 635, **636**
        fluorescein with, 636
    local anaesthesia, 787, **788**, 789
        catheterisation, 494
        phenylephrine with, 789
        prilocaine with, 788, 789
        tetracaine with, 789
        urethral pain, 494
    rectal, 88, 89
    ventricular fibrillation, 108
    ventricular tachycardia,
        108
Life support
    newborn, 146
    paediatric, 146
Lifestyle preparations, 910
Lignocaine *see* Lidocaine
Lignospan Special, 788
Li-Liquid, 228
Linezolid, **344**
Linola Gamma, 667
Lioresal, 617
Liothyronine, 438, **439**
Lipantil preparations, 164
Lipid-regulating drugs, 159
Lipitor, 161
Lipobase, 667
Lipodystrophy syndrome,
    374
Lipofundin preparations, 559
Liposic, 637
Lipostat, 161
LiquiBand, 719
Liquid and White Soft Paraffin
    Ointment, 666
Liquid paraffin, xvi
    eye ointment, 638
Liquifilm Tears, 638
Liquigen, 905
Lisinopril, **133**, 134
    see also ACE inhibitors
Liskonum, 227
Lithium
    bipolar disorder, 226
    mania, 226
    poisoning by, 42
    recurrent depression,
        226
    surgery, 761
Lithium carbonate, **226**, 227
Lithium citrate, **227**, 228
Liver *see* Hepatic
Livwell products, 910
LMX 4, 789
Loa loa, 416
Load 375, 489
Local anaesthetics *see* Anaesthesia,
    local
Locasol, 900
Loceryl, 711
Locoid preparations, 676, 677
    Locoid–C—discontinued
Locorten-Vioform, 644
Lodoxamide, 627, **628**
Loestrin-20, 481
Loestrin-30, 482
Logynon preparations, 481, 482
Lomotil (co-phenotrope), 65
Loniten, 123

Loperamide
    diarrhoea, **65**, 66
        simeticone with, 66
    palliative care, 25
Lophlex preparations, 915
Lopinavir, 373, **380**
    ritonavir with, 381
Lopresor preparations, 118
Loprofin
    low protein products, 911
    PKU preparations, 915
Loratadine, 192, **194**
Lorazepam
    anaesthesia, 772, **774**
    convulsions, 34
    epilepsy
        status epilepticus, 283, **285**
    neonatal seizures, 267
Loron, 470
Losartan, **134**
Losec, 64
Lotions
    definition, 664
    eye, 620
    suitable quantities, 665
Lotriderm, 678
Low-protein foods, 911
LSD *see* Lysergide, 19
Luborant, 662
Lubri-Tears, 638
Lugol's solution, 441
Lumefantrine
    artemether with, **401**, 402
Lupus erythematosus
    systemic, 445, 610
Lustral, 233
Lyclear, 718
Lyflex (baclofen), 617
Lyme disease, 312
Lymecycline, **330**, 331
    acne, 697
Lymphogranuloma venereum, 328
Lyrinel XL, 493
Lysergic acid diethylamide *see*
    Lysergide, 19
Lysergide, regulations, 19
Lysodren, 515
Lysosomal storage disorder, 588,
    589

M

Maalox preparations, 52, 53
MabCampath, 525
Mabron, 260
MabThera, 526
Macrobid, 361
Macrodantin, 361
Macrogols, 83, 84
    [ingredient], 86
Macrolides, 335
Magnapen, 315
Magnaspartate, 569
Magnesium citrate, 86
Magnesium glycerophosphate,
    569
Magnesium hydroxide, 84
    antacid, 52, 53
    preparations, 84
Magnesium salts
    constipation, 84

Magnesium sulphate
    arrhythmias, 568
    asthma, 169
    hypocalcaemia neonatal, **568**
    hypomagnesaemia, **568**
    pulmonary hypertension, 123,
        126
    torsade de pointes, **568**
Magnesium trisilicate, **52**
Magnesium-ʟ-aspartate, **569**
Malabsorption syndromes, 68
    electrolytes, 546
    vitamin K, 583
Malaria
    falciparum, 395
    prophylaxis, 397
    treatment, 395, 396
Malarivon, 403
Malarone, **405**
    malaria prophylaxis, 397, 398,
        399, 400, 404
    malaria treatment, 395, 404
        Paediatric, 405
Malathion, 715, 716, **717**, 718
Malignant disease, 496
    pain, 249
        bone, 246
Malignant hyperthermia, 786
Manevac, 82
Mania, 215, 225
Manic depression *see* Bipolar disor-
    der, 225, 226
Mannitol, 107
    diuresis, **107**
    glaucoma, 631
    presence of, 3
Mantoux test, 731
Manufacturers, special order, 943
Maple syrup urine disease, 576, 913
Mapleflex, 913
Maraviroc, 373, **384**
Marcain preparations, 790
Marevan (warfarin), 153
Marine stings, 48
Marketing authorisation, 3
Marvelon, 483
Mastaflu, 742
Matrifen (fentanyl), 254
Maturity-onset diabetes of the
    young, 418
Maxamaid preparations, 912, 913,
    914, 916, 917
Maxamum preparations, 913, 914,
    916
Maxidex, 626
Maxijul preparations, 904
Maxitram SR, 260
Maxitrol, 626
Maxolon preparations, 243
Maxtrex (methotrexate), 611
McCune-Albright syndrome,
    457
MCT Oil, 902
MCT Pepdite preparations, 899
MDMA *see* Methylenedioxy-
    methamphetamine
Measles
    corticosteroids, 446
    immunisation, 742
    immunoglobulin, normal, 756
    vaccines, combined, 742, 744
Measles, mumps and rubella
    vaccine, **744**
Mebendazole, **414**
    hookworm infections, 415
    roundworm infections, 414
    threadworm infections, 413
    whipworm infections, 414

Mebeverine, 56, **57**
  ispaghula with, 57
Mecasermin, **471**
Mecillinam, 318
Meconium
  aspiration syndrome, 203
  ileus, uncomplicated
    amidotrizoates, 87
Mecysteine, 207, 208
Medac, 513
Medicaid, 671
Medical emergencies in the community, *inside back cover*
Medicines information services, *inside front cover*
Medicated bandages, 683
Medicines, unlicensed, 3, 7
Medikinet preparations, 236
Medinol (paracetamol) preparations, 248
MediSense products, 436
Medi-Test products, 437
Medrone, 452
Medroxyprogesterone, 485, 486
Mefenamic acid, **605**
  dysmenorrhoea, 605
  menorrhagia, 605
  pain, 600
  rheumatic disease, 600
Mefloquine, **403**, 404
  malaria prophylaxis, 397, 399, 400
  malaria treatment, 395
Megaloblastic anaemia, 533
Meglumine amidotrizoate, 87
Melatonin, **214**
Meloxicam, 600, **605**, 606
Melphalan, **504**
Menadiol sodium phosphate, **583**
Mendelson's syndrome, 61, 762
Meningitec, 745
Meningitis
  antibacterial therapy, initial, 300
  bacterial
    dexamethasone in, 451
  cryptococcal, 362
  fungal, 362
  haemophilus, 300
  listerial, 300
  meningococcal, 300
    prophylaxis, 304
    travel, 745, 758
    vaccine, 744, **745**, 746
    vaccine, Hib with, 735
  pneumococcal, 300
  streptococcal, 300
Meningococcal *see* Meningitis
Menitorix, 735
Menjugate, 745
Menorrhagia, 487
  antifibrinolytics, 158
Menstruation
  postponement of, 455
Menthol and eucalyptus inhalation, 208
Mepacrine, 609
Mepivacaine, 787
Mepradec (omeprazole), 64
Merbentyl preparations, 55
Mercaptamine (cysteamine), 593, **594**
Mercaptopurine
  Crohn's disease, 74, **75**
  inflammatory bowel disease, 66, 67
  malignant disease, 508, **509**
  ulcerative colitis, 74, **75**
Mercilon, 481

Meronem, 328
Meropenem, 325, **327**, 328
Mesalazine, 66, 68, **69**, 70
Mesna
  cystic fibrosis, 206
  urothelial toxicity, **502**
Mesren MR, 70
Mestinon, 616
Mestranol, norethisterone with, 483
Metabolic acidosis, 555
Metabolic Mineral Mixture, 908
Metals, poisoning by, 45
Metanium, 671
Metaraminol, **145**
Meted, 706
Metenix-5, 103
Metformin, **431**, 432
Methadone
  neonatal abstinence syndrome, 291
  oral solution (1 mg/mL), 255
  pain, 250, **255**
  poisoning by, 39
Methaemoglobinaemia, 791
Methanol, poisoning by, 45
Metharose (methadone), 255
Methicillin-resistant *Staphylococcus aureus see* MRSA
Methionine, 36, 39
Methotrexate
  Crohn's disease, 66, 74, **75**
  folic acid with, 610
  malignant disease, 507, **509**, 510
  psoriasis, 690, **691**
  rheumatic disease, 608, **610**, 611
Methotrimeprazine *see* Levomepromazine
Methyl alcohol *see* Methanol, 45
Methyl cysteine *see* Mecysteine, 207, 208
Methyl salicylate, 720
  dithranol and salicylic acid with, 688
Methyl salicylate [ingredient], 688
Methylated spirit, industrial, 720
Methylcellulose, **78**, 79
  diarrhoea, 65
Methylcysteine *see* Mecysteine, 207, 208
Methyldopa, **127**, 128
Methylene blue *see* Methylthioninium chloride
Methylenedioxymethamphetamine
  controlled drug, 17
  poisoning by, 43
Methylmalonic acidaemia, 914
Methylphenidate, 234, **235**, 236
Methylprednisolone, **452**
  intra-articular, 607
  lidocaine with, 608
  rheumatic disease, 607, 608
Methylthioninium chloride, 791
Meticillin-resistant *Staphylococcus aureus see* MRSA
Metoclopramide
  migraine, 263
  nausea and vomiting, 237, 238, **242**, 243
  paracetamol with, 262
Metoject, 611
Metolazone, 100, 101, **102**, 103
Metopirone, 471
Metoprolol, 113, **118**
  see also Beta-adrenoceptor blocking drugs
Metosyn, 680
Metrogel, 710

Metrolyl, 357
Metronidazole, 355, **356**, 357
  amoebiasis, 407, 408
  bacterial vaginosis, 475
  Crohn's disease, 66
  gas-gangrene prophylaxis, 306
  giardiasis, 408
  Helicobacter pylori eradication, 59
  oral infections, 355
  protozoal infections, 408
  rosacea, 693
  skin infections, 707, **709**, 710
  trichomoniasis, 408
  vaginal, 475
Metrosa, 710
Metrotop, 710
Metsol (metronidazole), 432
Metyrapone, 470, **471**
Miacalcic, 468
Micafungin, 363, **370**
Micanol, 688
Micolette Micro-enema, 85
Miconazole
  anogenital, 473
  mouth, 657, **658**
  skin, 711, **713**
    hydrocortisone with, 676
  vaginal, 474
Micralax Micro-enema, 85
Micral-Test II, 437
Microalbustik, 437
Microbumintest, 437
Microgynon preparations, 482
Microlance, 428
Micronor, 485
MicroPeak, 181
Microphallus, 456
Micropirin (aspirin), 155
Midazolam
  anaesthesia, 771, 772, **774**, 775
  convulsions, 34
  infusion table (neonatal), 923
  neonatal seizures, 267
  palliative care, 28
  status epilepticus, 283, **286**
Miglustat, 589, **595**
Migraine
  acute attack, 261
  beta-blockers, 115
  prophylaxis, 263
Migraleve, 261
Mildison, 675
Milex diaphragms, 490
Milrinone, **99**, 100
Milupa
  Low Protein Drink, 911
  PKU preparations, 915
Milward Steri-Let, 428
Minaphlex, 915
Mineralocorticoids, 442
  replacement therapy, 442
Mini TT 380 Slimline, 489
Minijet
  Adrenaline, 200, 201
  Aminophylline, 180
  Atropine Sulphate, 770
  Furosemide, 104
  Glucose , 554
  Lignocaine, 113
  Magnesium Sulphate, 568
  Morphine Sulphate, 257
  Naloxone, 40
  Sodium Bicarbonate, 556

Index

Minims
  Amethocaine, 636
  Artificial Tears, 637
  Atropine Sulphate, 629
  Benoxinate (Oxybuprocaine),
    636
  Chloramphenicol, 623
  Cyclopentolate, 630
  Dexamethasone, 626
  Fluorescein Sodium, 639
  Lignocaine and Fluorescein, 636
  Phenylephrine, 630
  Pilocarpine Nitrate, 635
  Prednisolone, 627
  Proxymetacaine, 636
  Proxymetacaine and
    Fluorescein, 636
  Saline, 638
  Tropicamide, 630
MiniQuick, 462
Miniversol, 720
Mini-Wright, 181
Minocin preparations, 331
Minocycline, 328, **331**
  acne, 697
Minoxidil, 121, **122**, 123
Miochol-E, 639
Mirena, 487
Mistabron, 206
Misuse of drugs
  Act, 17
  Regulations 2001, 17
Mitochondrial disorders, 594
Mitotane, **515**
Mitoxantrone, 505, **507**
Mitozantrone *see* Mitoxantrone,
  505, **507**
Mivacron, 781
Mivacurium, 779, **780**, 781
Mixtard 30, 428
Mizolastine, 192, **194**
Mizollen, 194
MMR vaccine, 742, 744
MMRvaxPRO, 744
Mobic, 606
Modafinil, 234, **236**
Modjul Flavour System, 909
Modrasone, 677
Modulen IBD, 879
Moduret-25 (co-amilozide), 106
MODY *see* Maturity-onset diabetes
  of the young, 418
Molcer, 647
Mometasone
  asthma, 184, **189**
  nasal allergy, 651
  skin, 681
Monoamine-oxidase inhibitors, 231
Monofluorophosphate, 571
Monogen, 899
Monoject products, 428, 429
Monolet, 428
Montelukast, **190**, 191
Morhulin, 671
Morphine, **255**, 257
  cyclizine with, 257
  diamorphine equivalence, 29
  infusion table (neonatal), 923
  neonatal abstinence syndrome,
    291
  oral solutions, 256
  pain, 249
    chronic, 249
    palliative care, 24
    postoperative, 250
Motifene (diclofenac), 603
Motilium, 242
Motion sickness, 239

Mouth ulceration, 654
Mouthwash solution-tablets, 661
Mouthwashes, 659
Movicol preparations, 84
MPD Ultra Thin, 428
MRSA, 310
  linezolid in, 344
  nasal, 653
  quinupristin and dalfopristin in,
    345
MST Continus, 257
MSUD preparations, 913, 914
MucoClear, 208
Mucodyne, 207
Mucogel, 52
Mucolytics, 206
  eye, 636
Mucopolysaccharidosis, 589
Mucosal bleeding
  palliative care, 27
Mucositis
  methotrexate-induced, 500
  oral, 497
Multiclix, 428
Multiload IUDs, 489
Multiple myeloma, 535
Multivitamins, **584**, 585
Mumps
  vaccines, **746**
    combined, 742, 744
Mupirocin
  nose, 653
  skin, 707, **708**
Muscle relaxants
  anaesthesia, 778
    depolarising, 782
    non-depolarising, 778
  skeletal, 616
Muscle spasm, 616
Musculoskeletal disorders, rheuma-
  tic, 599
Myasthenia gravis
  anticholinesterases, 614
  corticosteroids, 616
  diagnosis, 614
  diagnostic test, 615
  immunosuppressants, 616
Mycamine, 370
Mycobacterium avium complex
  infections, 349, 353
Mycobutin, 354
Mycophenolate mofetil, 518, **519**,
  520
  eczema, 690
Mycoplasma infections, 328
Mycota, 714
Mydriacyl, 630
Mydriatics, 629
Mydrilate, 630
Myleran, 503
Myoclonic seizures, 267
Myozyme, 591
Mysoline, 274
Myxoedema, juvenile, 438

N

Nabilone, 238, **244**
Naglazyme, 590
Nalcrom, 76
Nalidixic acid, 357, **359**
Naloxone
  anaesthesia, 784, **785**
  opioid poisoning, 39, 40
Name changes, xvii

Nappy rash, 670
Naprosyn preparations, 606
Naproxen
  dysmenorrhoea, 606
  juvenile idiopathic arthritis, 606
  pain and inflammation, 600, **606**
  rheumatic disease, 600, 606
Narcolepsy, 234
Narcotic analgesics *see* Analgesics,
  opioid
Narcotic antagonists *see* Opioid
  antagonists
Naropin, 791
Nasacort, 651
Nasal
  allergy, 648
  congestion, 648
  decongestants
    systemic, 210
    topical, 651
  MRSA, 653
  polyps, 648
Naseptin, 653
Nasobec preparations, 649
Nasofan, 650
Nasogastric feeding tubes *see* Ent-
  eral feeding tubes
Nasonex, 651
Natecal D3, 581
Nateglinide, 432
National Institute for Health and
  Clinical Excellence, 4
Nausea, 239
  cytotoxic drugs, 497
  motion sickness, 239
  opioid-induced, 238
  palliative care, 27
  postoperative, 238
  pregnancy, 238
  vomiting and, 237
Navoban—discontinued
NebuChamber, 182
Nebuhaler, 182
Nebulisers, 182
Necatoriasis, 415
Necrotising enterocolitis, 298
Nedocromil
  asthma, 189, 190
  eye, 627, **628**
Needles, insulin, 428, 429
  clipping device, 429
Neimann-Pick type C disease,
  594
NeisVac-C, 745
Nelarabine, 507, **510**
Nelfinavir, 373, **381**
Neocate preparations, 896
Neoclarityn, 193
Neo-Cortef—discontinued
Neo-Cytamen (hydroxocobalamin),
  535
Neo-Mercazole, 441
Neomycin, 333
  ear, 642, 644, 645, **646**
    betamethasone with, 644
    dexamethasone with, 644
    prednisolone with, 645
  eye, 622, 624, 626
    betamethasone with, 626
    prednisolone with, 627
  nose, 653
    chlorhexidine with, 653
  skin, 707, **708**
    betamethasone valerate
      with, 678
    fluocinolone acetonide with,
      680
Neo-NaClex preparations, 102

Neonatal
    abstinence syndrome, 291
    apnoea *see* Apnoea, neonatal
    seizures, 267
Neoral, 523
NeoRecormon, 538
Neosporin, 624
Neostigmine
    anaesthesia, 783, **784**
    glycopyrronium bromide with, 784
    myasthenia gravis, 614, **615**
Neotigason, 690
Nephrocalcinosis, 103
Nephropathic cystinosis, 593
Nephrotic syndrome
    chlortalidone, **102**
    corticosteroids, 445
Nepro, 902
Nerisone preparations, 679
Nerve agent, poisoning by, 46
Nesidioblastosis, 434
Neulactil, 220
Neupogen, 545
Neural tube defects, prevention, 534
Neuralgia, 229
    postherpetic, 261
Neuroleptic malignant syndrome, 216
Neuroleptics *see* Antipsychotics
Neuromuscular
    blocking drugs, 778
    disorders, 614
Neurontin, 271
Neuropathic pain, 261
Neuropathy
    compression, 608
    diabetic, 435
Neutral insulin *see* Insulin, soluble, 422, **423**
Neutropenias, 535, 543
Nevirapine, 373, **383**, 384
NHS Direct, *inside front cover*
Nicam, 697
Nicardipine, 136, **137**, 138
    see also Calcium-channel blockers
NICE *see* National Institute for Health and Clinical Excellence, 4
Nicef (cefradine), 323
Niclosamide, 415
Nicorette preparations, 292
Nicotinamide
    topical, 697
    vitamin supplement, 575, **577**
Nicotine
    replacement therapy, 291
    smoking cessation products, 292–4
Nicotinell preparations, 293
Nifedipine, **138**, 139, 141
    angina, 136
    chronic hypoglycaemia, 434
    pulmonary hypertension, 123
    Raynaud's syndrome, 136
    see also Calcium-channel blockers
Nifedipress MR, 139
Niferex, 531
Nifopress Retard—discontinued
Nimbex, 780
Nimodipine, 136, **140**
Nimotop, 140
Niquitin preparations, 294
Nitisinone, **596**
Nitrates, 135
Nitrazepam, **282**, 283
Nitric oxide, 123, 124

Nitrocine, 136
Nitrofurantoin, **360**, 361
Nitronal, 136
Nitroprusside *see* Sodium nitroprusside, 121, **123**
Nitrous oxide, 768, **769**
Nitrous oxide-oxygen, 768
Nizoral, 370
    anogenital, 474
    scalp, 705
    skin, 713
Nocturnal enuresis, 493
Non-convulsive status epilepticus, 283
Non-depolarising muscle relaxants *see* Muscle relaxants
Non-medical prescribing, 928
Non-nucleoside reverse transcriptase inhibitors, 372, 373, 382
Nonoxinol, 488
Noonan syndrome, 461
Noradrenaline, **145**
    infusion table (neonatal), 923
Norcuron, 782
Norditropin, 462
Norelgestromin, ethinylestradiol with, 483
Norepinephrine *see* Noradrenaline
Norethisterone
    contraception, 485
        ethinylestradiol with, 482
        mestranol with, 483
        parenteral, 486
    delayed puberty, **455**
    menstrual disorders, 455
Norethisterone acetate
    ethinylestradiol with, 481, 482
Norethisterone enantate, 486
Norgalax Micro-enema, 81
Norgestimate, ethinylestradiol with, 483
Norgeston, 485
Norgestrel *see* Levonorgestrel
Noriday, 485
Norimin, 482
Norimode (loperamide), 66
Norinyl-1, 483
Noristerat, 486
Normacol preparations, 79
Normal immunoglobulin *see* Immunoglobulins, normal
Normal saline *see* Sodium chloride
Normasol, 720
Normax, 80
Normosang, 597
Norphyllin SR (aminophylline), 180
Nortriptyline, 229, **231**
    nocturnal enuresis, 494
Norvir, 381
Norzol (metronidazole), 356
Nose *see* Nasal
Notifiable diseases, 296
Novasource preparations, 879, 883
Nova-T, 489
NovoFine products, 429
Novolizer, 187
NovoMix 30, 427
NovoPen, 428
NovoRapid, 424
Nozinan, 219
NPH *see* Insulin, isophane
NSAIDs (non-steroidal anti-inflammatory drugs) *see* Analgesics
NTBC *see* Nitisinone, **596**
Nucleoside analogues *see* Nucleoside reverse transcriptase inhibitors, 372

Nucleoside reverse transcriptase inhibitors, 372, 373, 374
Nuelin SA, 179
Nurofen (ibuprofen) preparations, 604
Nurse independent prescribing, 927
Nurse Prescribers' Formulary, 925,
Nu-Seals Aspirin, 155
Nutilis, 909
Nutramigen preparations, 897
Nutraplus, 668
Nutrini preparations, 885, 887, 888, 889
Nutriprem preparations, 885
Nutrison preparations, 880, 883, 884
Nutrition
    ACBS, foods, 878
    enteral, 561, 562, 878
    intravenous, 558
    oral, 561, 562
    total parenteral, 558
Nutrizym preparations, 95
NutropinAq, 462
NuvaRing, 481
Nyogel, 632
Nystaform, 713
Nystaform-HC, 676
Nystan, 371
    cream and ointment—discontinued
    mouth, 659
Nystatin, 363, **370**, 371
    mouth, 657, 658, 659
    skin, 711, **713**
        chlorhexidine and hydrocortisone with, 676
        hydrocortisone with, 676
        tolnaftate with, 713

O

Obesity, 237
Obstetric surgery, antibacterial prophylaxis, 306
Occlusal, 700
Octagam, 757
Octalbin preparations (albumin), 556, 557
Octim, 467
Octreotide, **435**
    chronic hypoglycaemia, 434
    hyperinsulinaemic hypoglycaemia, 435
    varices, bleeding from, 435, 464
Octylcyanoacrylate, 719
Ocufen, 640
Ocusan, 639
Oedema
    cerebral, 107, 450
    pulmonary, 100
Oesophageal varices, 464
Oesophagitis *see* Gastro-oesophageal reflux disease, **50**
Oestrogens
    hormone therapy, 454
    labial adhesions, 472
    oral contraceptives, 475
Ofloxacin
    ear, 647
    eye, 624

Oftaquix, 623
Oilatum
   cream, 667
   Emollient, 670
   Fragrance Free, 670
   Plus, 670
   shower emollient, 667
Oily cream, 666
Ointments
   definition, 664
   eye, 620
   suitable quantities, 665
Olanzapine, **223**, 224
   mania, 225
   psychoses, 221
Oligospermia, 460
Olive oil, ear, 647
Olopatadine, 627, **628**
Olsalazine, 66, 68, **71**
Omalizumab, 197, **198**
Omeprazole, 62, **63**, 64
Omnic MR (tamsulosin), 492
Omnikan, 429
Omnitrope, 462
Oncaspar, 513
Onchocerciasis, 416
Oncovin, 512
Ondansetron, 238, **244**
Ondemet (ondansetron), 244
One Touch products, 428, 436, 437
One-Alpha, 580
Onkotrone, 507
Onychomycosis *see* Fungal infections, skin, 362, 710
Opatanol, 628
Opioid analgesics *see* Analgesics, opioid
Opioid antagonists, 784
   poisoning by, 39
Optichamber, 182
OptiClik, 428
Opticrom preparations, 628
OptiFlo preparations, 495
Optil (diltiazem), 137
Optilast, 627
OptiPen Pro 1, 428
Optium products, 436, 437
Optive, 637
Optometrist independent prescribing, 928
OPV *see* Poliomyelitis, immunisation
Orabase, 655
Oral balance see *Biotène Oralbalance*
Oral contraceptives *see* Contraception, oral
Oral rehydration
   salts, 549, 550
      WHO formula, 550
Oral syringes, 3
Oraldene, 660
Oramorph preparations, 256
Orap, 220
Orbifen (ibuprofen), 604
Orelox, 323
Orfadin, 596
Organophosphorus insecticides, poisoning by, 46
Orgaran, 151
Orgran, 910
Orlept (sodium valproate), 279
Orlistat, 237
Oropharynx
   infections, 657
   ulceration and inflammation, 654
ORS, 549
ORT, 549
Ortho-Gynest, 472

Orthopaedic surgery
   antibacterial prophylaxis, 306
Oseltamivir, 390, **391**, 392
Osmanil (fentanyl), 254
Osmolite preparations, 880, 883, 885
Osteoarthritis, 599
Osteomyelitis, 302, 339, 341
Osteoporosis, 467
   calcitriol, 579
   corticosteroid-induced, 467
Otex, 647
Otitis externa, 642
   antibacterial choice, 303
Otitis media, 646
   antibacterial choice, 303
Otomize, 644
Otosporin, 645
Otradrops (xylometazoline), 652
Otraspray (xylometazoline), 652
Otrivine (xylometazoline), 652
Otrivine-Antistin, 627
Ovranette, 482
Ovysmen, 482
Oxactin (fluoxetine), 233
Oxandrolone, 455, **459**
Oxazolidinone antibacterials, 344
Oxcarbazepine, 266, 267, **269**
Oxis, 174
Oxyal, 639
Oxybuprocaine, 635, **636**
Oxybutynin, **492**, 493
Oxycodone, **257**, 258
   morphine equivalence, 24
   palliative care, 25
OxyContin, 258
Oxygen, 204
   ambulatory therapy, 205
   arrangements for supply, 205
   asthma acute, 204
   cluster headache, 264
   nitrous oxide and, 768
Oxymetazoline, 651
Oxymetholone, 535
Oxymycin (oxytetracycline), 331
OxyNorm, 258
Oxytetracycline, **331**
   acne, 697
   oral infections, 329

P

PACT, xiii
Paediasure preparations, 887, 889, 890
Paediatric Life Support algorithms, *inside back cover*
Paediatric Seravit, 908
Pain, 245
   bone, 246
   dental, 246, 251, 600
   dressing changes, 769
   ear, 643, 646
   musculoskeletal, 246
   neuropathic, 261
   orofacial, 246, 251, 261, 600
   palliative care, 24
   perioperative, 250, 776
   rheumatic, 599
   sickle-cell disease, 245
   urethral, 494
   visceral, 249
Paldesic (paracetamol) preparations, 248
Palivizumab, 392, **393**
Palladone preparations, 255

Palliative care
   continuous infusion devices, 28
   prescribing, 24
Paludrine, 405
Paludrine/Avloclor, 403
Pamidronate disodium *see* Disodium pamidronate, 469
Panadeine (co-codamol 8/500), 248
Panadol (paracetamol) preparations, 248
Pancrease HL, 95
Pancreatin, 93, **94**, 95
Pancreatitis, chronic, 93
Pancrex preparations, 95
Pancuronium, 779, **781**
Panoxyl preparations, 694
Panthenol, 575
Pantothenic acid, 575
Papaveretum, **258**
Paracetamol, 246, **247**, 248
   buclizine and codeine with, 261
   codeine with, 248
   febrile convulsions, 287
   metoclopramide with, 262
   migraine, 261
   poisoning by, 36
   post-immunisation pyrexia, 727
   tramadol with, 260
Paracodol (co-codamol 8/500), 248
Paraffin
   eye ointment, 638
   liquid and white soft, 666
   white soft, 666
   yellow soft, 666
Parainfluenza virus, 392
Paraldehyde, 267, **286**
Paraldehyde injection—discontinued
Paramax, 262
Paraplatin, 516
Paraproteinaemias, 535
Parasiticidal preparations, 715
Parasympathomimetics
   anaesthesia, 783
   eye conditions, 635
   myasthenia gravis, 614
Pardelprin (indometacin m/r), 605
Parenteral nutrition, 558
   supplements, 560, 561
PARI Vortex Spacer, 182
Parkinsonism
   drug-induced, 216
Parkinsonism, drug-induced, 216
Paromomycin, 409
Paronychia, 303, 711
Paroxetine, 231
Partial seizures, 266
Parvolex, 39
Pastes, definition, 664
Patient group direction, 3
Patient information leaflets, 1
Patient packs, xii
Pavacol-D (pholcodine), 209
Peak flow meters, 181
Peanut oil *see* Arachis oil
Pedea, 165
Pediacel, 734
Pediculosis, 716
Peditrace, 561
Pelvic inflammatory disease, 301
Pemphigus, 444
Penbritin, 315
Penciclovir, 386, **715**
Penfine, 429
Penicillamine, **586**, 587
   cystinuria, 587
   rheumatic disease, 608
   Wilson's disease, 586

Penicillin G see Benzylpenicillin sodium
Penicillin V see Phenoxymethylpenicillin
Penicillin VK see Phenoxymethylpenicillin
Penicillinases, 310
Penicillins, 308
  antipseudomonal, 317
  broad spectrum, 312
  hypersensitivity, 308
  penicillinase-resistant, 310
  penicillinase-sensitive, 308
Pentacarinat, 413
Pentamidine isetionate, **412**, 413
  leishmaniasis, 409, 412
  pneumocystis pneumonia, 411, 412
  trypanosomiasis, 412
Pentasa, 70
Pentastarch, 557, 558
Pentostam, 409
Pentrax, 706
Pepdite preparations, 897, 898, 899
Peppermint oil, 56, **57**
Peptac, 53
Peptamen preparations, 881, 885, 888
Peptisorb preparations, 881
Perative, 885
Perfalgan, 248
Perfan, 99
Periapical abscess, 302
Periciazine see Pericyazine, **219**, 220
Pericoronitis, 302
Pericyazine, **219**, 220
Perinal, 88
Periodontal abscess, 302
Periodontitis, 655
  antibacterial treatment, 302
Periostat, 655, 656
Peritonitis, 298
Permethrin, 715, 716, **717**, **718**
Permitabs, 723
Peroxyl, 660
Perphenazine
  nausea and vomiting, 237, **241**
  psychoses, **220**
Persantin preparations, 155
Pertussis
  immunisation, 746
  prophylaxis, 305
  vaccines, combined, 734, **746**
Pethidine, **258**, 259
  analgesia, 250
    postoperative, 250
Petroleum jelly, 666
Pevaryl, 712
PGD see Patient group direction, 3
PGI$_2$ see Epoprostenol, 123, 124, **125**, 151
Phaeochromocytoma, 114, **129**
Pharmacist independent prescribing, 928
Pharma-Ject Morphine Sulphate, 251
Pharmalgen, 197
Pharmorubicin preparations, 506
Pharyngitis see Throat infections
Pharynx see Oropharynx
Phenergan preparations, 196, 214
Phenobarbital
  epilepsy, 266, **273**, 274
    status epilepticus, 286, 287
  neonatal abstinence syndrome, 291
  neonatal seizures, 267
  poisoning, elimination, 35
Phenobarbitone see Phenobarbital

Phenothiazines
  classification, 216
  nausea and vertigo, 239
  nausea and vomiting, 237, 238
  poisoning by, 43
  psychoses, 216
Phenothrin, 716, **717**, **718**
Phenoxybenzamine, 129, **130**
Phenoxymethylpenicillin, 309, **310**
  pneumococcal infection prophylaxis, 305
  rheumatic fever prophylaxis, 303
Phentolamine, xvi
Phenylephrine
  eye, **630**
  hypotension, **145**, 146
  lidocaine with, 789
Phenylketonuria, 561, 915
Phenytoin
  epilepsy, 274, **275**
    status epilepticus, 283, **287**
  neonatal seizures, 267
Phlexy-10, 915
Phlexy-Vits preparations, 915
Pholcodine, 208, **209**
Phosex, 571
Phosgene, poisoning by, 46
Phosphate supplements, 569
Phosphate-binding agents, 570
Phosphates
  bowel cleansing, 86
  constipation, 83, 85
  hypophosphataemia, 569, **570**
Phosphate-Sandoz, 570
Phosphocysteamine, 593
Phosphodiesterase inhibitors
  cardiovascular, 99
  pulmonary hypertension, 124, 126
Phosphorus, 569
Photochemotherapy, psoriasis, 685
Photodamage, skin, 704
Photodermatoses, 703
  ACBS, 917
Phototherapy, psoriasis, 685
Phyllocontin Continus, 180
Physeptone (methadone), 255
Physiological saline see Sodium chloride
Phytex, 713
Phytomenadione, 153, 583, 584
Picolax, 86
Piko-1, 181
Pilocarpine, **635**
Pimecrolimus, 690, **691**, 692
Pimozide
  psychoses, 216, **220**
  Tourette syndrome, **220**, 290
Pinetarsol, 687
Pinworm infections, 413
Piperacillin, **317**
  tazobactam with, 317
Piperazine, 414
  roundworm infections, 414
  threadworm infections, 413, **414**
Piracetam, 283
Piriton, 195
Piroxicam
  juvenile idiopathic arthritis, 606
  pain and inflammation, 606
  preparations, 606, 607
  rheumatic disease, 600
Pitressin, 464

Pituitary
  function test, 460
    metyrapone, 470
  hormones, 459
    anterior, 459
    posterior, 464
Pityriasis versicolor, 362, 711
Pivmecillinam, **318**
Pizotifen, **263**
PK Aid 4, 915
PK Foods preparations, 911
PKU preparations, 915, 916
Plaque, 659
Plaquenil, 610
Plasma
  concentrations, electrolytes, 546
  substitutes, 556, 557
Plasmapheresis, myasthenia gravis, 614
Plastipak, 429
Platinex (cisplatin), 516
Pneumococcal infection
  antibacterial prophylaxis, 305
  immunisation
    vaccines, 746, **748**
Pneumocystis pneumonia, 411
  prophylaxis, 411
Pneumonia, 299
  hospital-acquired, 299
  pneumococcal, 746
Pneumovax II, 748
Pocket Chamber, 182
Pocketpeak, 181
PocketScan products, 436
Podophyllum resin, salicylic acid with, 700
Podophyllotoxin, 701, **702**
Poisoning, 33
  active elimination, 35
  adsorbents, 35
  hospital admission, 33
Poisons information services, see inside front cover
Polihexanide, 640
Poliomyelitis
  immunisation, 758
  travel, 748
  vaccines, **748**, 749
    combined, 734
Pollen extracts, 197
Pollinex, 197
Polyacrylic acid see Carbomers, 637
Polyarteritis nodosa, 445
Polycal, 904
  glucose tolerance test, 438
Polyene antifungal drugs, 363
Polyethoxylated castor oil see Polyoxyl castor oil, 3
Polyethylene glycols, 83, 86
Polyfax, 708
  eye, 624
Polygeline, 557
Polyhexamethylene biguanide see Polihexanide, 640
Polyhexanide see Polihexanide, 640
Polymethylmethacrylate, 719
Polymyositis, 610
Polymyxin B
  eye, 626
Polymyxins
  ear, 645, 647
  eye, 622, **624**
  inhalation, **346**
  skin, 707, **708**
  systemic, 345, **346**
Polyoxyl castor oil, presence of, 3
Polysaccharide-iron complex, 531

Index

Polystyrene sulphonate resins, 548
Polytar
  AF, 706
  Emollient, 688
  Liquid, 706
  Plus, 706
Polytrim, 624
Polyvinyl alcohol, 638
Pompe disease, 590
Ponstan preparations, 605
POP *see* Progestogens, contra-ceptives, oral, 475, **484**
Poractant alfa, 203
Porphyrias, acute, 597
  drugs to be avoided in, 597
Posalfilin, 701
Posiject, 143
Potassium acid phosphate, 570
Potassium bicarbonate, 550, **551**
  tablets, effervescent, 551
Potassium canrenoate, 105, **106**
Potassium chloride
  infusion
    glucose and, 555
    sodium chloride and, 555
    sodium chloride, glucose and, 555
  oral, **547**
  parenteral, **554**, 555
Potassium citrate, 494
Potassium iodide, 441
Potassium permanganate, 682, 719, **722**, 723
Potassium supplements, 546
Povidone-iodine
  skin, 719, **722**
    shampoo, 705
Prader-Willi syndrome, 461
Pralidoxime chloride, 46, **47**
Pramocaine [ingredient], 88
Pramoxine *see* Pramocaine, 88
Pravastatin, 159, **161**
Praziquantel
  schistosoma, 416
  tapeworm, 415
Prazosin, 128, **129**
Precocious puberty, 457
Pred Forte, 627
Predenema, 73
Predfoam, 74
Prednisolone, 443, **452**, 453
  asthma, acute, 169
  Crohn's disease, 73
  ear, 645
  eye, 626, 627
  haemorrhoids, 89
  hepatitis, 453
  infantile spasms, 267, 453
  inflammatory and allergic disor-ders, 453
  malignant disease, 520
  nephrotic syndrome, 453
  palliative care, 26
  pneumocystis pneumonia, 411
  rectal, 73, 74, 89
  ulcerative colitis, 73
  withdrawal of, 446
Predsol
  ear, 645
  eye, 627
  rectal, 74
Predsol-N
  ear, 645
  eye, 627
Pre-eclampsia, 119
Pregestimil, 898

Pregnancy
  anticoagulants, 152
  antihistamines, 192
  asthma, 168
  corticosteroids, 447
  cytotoxic drugs, 498
  epilepsy and, 266
  folate supplements, 534
  HIV infection, 373
  hypertension in, 119
  immunosuppressants, 518
  iron, 529
  malaria, 397
    prophylaxis, 398
    treatment, 396
  nausea and vomiting, 238
  prescribing in, 15
  tuberculosis and, 349
  urinary infections, 360
Pregnyl, 461
Prejomin, 898
Premedication, 769, 771
Prescribing, xiii
  ACBS, 878
  analyses and cost, xiii
  breast-feeding, 16
  children, 11
  controlled drugs, 17
  hepatic impairment, 12
  independent, 928
  instalments, 17
  palliative care, 24
  patient packs, xii
  pregnancy, 15
  renal impairment, 13
  repeat prescriptions, 17
  supplementary, 928
Prescription forms
  controlled drugs, 17
  nurses, 925
  security, 3
Prescription only medicines *see* pre-parations identified by [PoM] throughout *BNF for Children*
Presinex (desmopressin), 466
Prestige products, 436, 437
Prevenar, 748
Prezista, 379
Priadel, 228
Prices, xiii
Prilocaine, **791**
  dental, 791
  felypressin with, 788, 791
  lidocaine with, 788, 789
Primacine (erythromycin), 337
Primacor, 100
Primaquine
  malaria treatment, 396, **404**
  pneumocystis pneumonia, 411
Primaxin, 327
Primene, 559
Primidone, 273, **274**
Primolut N, 455
Prioderm, 718
Priorix, 744
Pripsen, 414
Privigen, 757
Pro-Banthine, 56
Pro-Cal preparations, 906, 907
Procarbazine, **517**
Proceli products, 910
Prochlorperazine
  nausea and vertigo, 239
  nausea and vomiting, 237, 238, **241**
Proctofoam HC, 88
Proctosedyl, 89

Procyclidine, **289**, 290
Product licence, 3
Pro-Epanutin, 285
Proflavine cream, 719
Progesterone
  hormone therapy, 454
Progestogen-only pill *see* Progesto-gens, contraceptives, oral, 475, **484**
Progestogens
  contraceptives
    emergency, 490
    intra-uterine, **487**
    oral, 475, **484**
    parenteral, 485, **486**
  hormone therapy, 454
Prograf, 524
Proguanil, **404**, 405
  atovaquone with, 405
  chloroquine with, 403
  malaria prophylaxis, 397, 398, 399, 400, 404
Promethazine
  allergic disorders, 192, **196**
  hypnotic, **214**
  motion sickness, 239
  nausea and vomiting, 238, **240**
  sedation, **214**
Promethazine teoclate, **240**
Promin, 911
Promixin, 346
Propamidine isetionate, eye, 622, **624**
Propantheline, 55, **56**
Prophylaxis, antibacterial, 303
Propine, 633
Propionibacterium acnes, 695
Propionic acidaemia, 914
Propofol, 763, **765**
Propofol-Lipuro, 765
Propoven (propofol), 765
Propranolol, **115**, 116
  cardiovascular, 115
  hyperthyroidism, 442
  migraine prophylaxis, **115**, 263
  see also Beta-adrenoceptor blocking drugs
  tetralogy of Fallot, 114, 115
  thyrotoxicosis, 440, 442
  tremor, 290
Propylene glycol
  presence of, 3
Propylthiouracil, 440, **441**, 442
Prostacyclin *see* Epoprostenol, 123, 124, **125**, 151
Prostaglandins
  anticoagulant, 151
  ductus arteriosus, 165
  eye, 631, 632
Prostap preparations, 458
Prostin E2, 166
Prostin VR, 166
Prosulf, 154
ProSure, 903
Protamine sulphate, 147, 153, **154**
Protease inhibitors, 372, 373, 378
Protein
  intravenous nutrition, 559
  urinalysis, 437
Proteus spp infections, 317
Prothionamide *see* Protionamide, 352
Protifar, 903
Protionamide, 352
Protirelin, **463**
Proton pump inhibitors, 62
Protopam, 47

Index

Protopic, 692
Protozoal infections, 394
Provide, 891
Provigil, 236
Proxymetacaine, 635, **636**
  fluorescein with, 636
Prozac, 233
Prozep (fluoxetine), 233
Pruritus, 192
  ACBS, 917
  cholestasis, 92
  palliative care, 27
  perianal, 87
  skin, 671
Pseudoephedrine, **210**
Pseudomembranous colitis
  antibacterial therapy
    metronidazole in, 355
    vancomycin in, 342
Pseudomonas aeruginosa infections,
  317, 319, 328, 331, 345
  eye, 622
Psittacosis, 328
Psoralen, 685
Psoriasis, 683
  corticosteroids, 674
  photochemotherapy, 685
Psoriderm preparations, 687, 688
  scalp, 706
Psorin preparations, 688
Psychiatric reactions
  corticosteroids, 446
Psychoses, 215
Puberty
  delayed, 453, 455, 456, 460
  precocious, 457, 459
Pubic lice, 716
Pulmicort LS—discontinued
Pulmicort preparations, 187
Pulmonary
  hypertension, 123, 151
  oedema, 100, 103, 105
  surfactants, 203
Pulmozyme, 207
Pulvinal
  beclometasone, 185
  salbutamol, 175
Pure products, 910
Puri-Nethol, 509
Purpura, thrombocytopenic,
  541
PUVA, 685
Pyelonephritis, 360
Pyralvex, 656
Pyrazinamide, **353**
  tuberculosis treatment, 348, 349,
    351
Pyrexia
  post immunisation, 727
Pyridostigmine, 614, **615**, 616
Pyridoxine
  anaemias, 535
  isoniazid-induced neuropathy,
    577
  metabolic disorders, 576, **577**
  seizures, 267, 576, 577
  status epilepticus, 283
Pyrimethamine
  malaria, 405
    sulfadoxine with, 395, 405,
      406
  toxoplasmosis, 409, **410**
Pyrithione zinc shampoos,
  705
Pyruvate dehydrogenase defects,
  594

Q

Q-fever, 328
QuantiFERON-TB Gold, 732
Quaternary ammonium compounds,
  55
Quellada M, 718
Questran preparations, 162
Quetiapine, 221, **224**
QuickCal, 907
Quinaband, 683
Quinalbarbitone *see* Secobarbital,
  771
Quinine, **406**
  malaria, 395, 406
  poisoning
    elimination, 35
Quinoderm, 694
Quinolones, 357
  ear, 647
  eye, 622
Quinupristin, **345**
QV preparations, 667, 670
Qvar preparations, 186

R

Rabies
  immunisation, 749
  immunoglobulin, 757, **758**
  travel, 759
  vaccine, **750**
Rabipur, 750
Raltegravir, 373, **384**, 385
Ranitic (ranitidine), 61
Ranitidine, **61**
Rapamune, 523
Rapifen, 777
Rapitil, 628
Rapolyte—discontinued
Rapydan, 789
Rasburicase, 499, **500**
Ratiograstim, 545
Raynaud's syndrome, 136, 141
Rebetol, 394
Red eye, 622, 625
Redoxon, 578
Reflexions diaphragm, 490
Reflux oesophagitis *see* Gastro-
  oesophageal reflux disease, **50**
Refolinon (calcium folinate), 501
Regranex, 723
Regulan, 78
Regulose (lactulose), 83
Rehydration
  oral, 549
  parenteral, 552
Relaxit, 85
Relenza, 392
Relestat, 628
Remicade, 76
Remifentanil, 777, **778**
Renagel, 571
Renal
  excretion, interactions affecting,
    794
  impairment, prescribing in, 13
Renamil, 903
Renapro, 903
Renilon, 894
Rennie Duo, 54
Repevax, 734
Replagal, 588

Resonium A, 548
Resource preparations,
  enteral feed, 889
  fibre supplement, 907
  nutritional supplement, 891,
    893, 895
  thickened, 909
Respiratory
  depression
    poisoning, 33
    postoperative, 784
  distress syndrome, 100, 103
    pulmonary surfactants, 203
  failure, 202
  secretions, excessive (palliative
    care), 26
  stimulants, 202
  syncytial virus infections, 392
Respontin, 178
Restandol, 456
Resuscitation
  cardiopulmonary, 146
  dental practice, 762
Retacrit, 538
Retapamulin, 707, **708**
Retin-A, 696
Retinoids
  acne
    oral, 699
    topical, 695
  leukaemia, 517
  psoriasis, 685, **689**
Retinol *see* Vitamin A
Retrovir, 378
Revatio, 126
Revaxis, 734
Rexocaine, 788
Reyataz, 379
Rheumatac Retard (diclofenac), 603
Rheumatic diseases, 599
  corticosteroid injections, 607
Rheumatic fever
  prophylaxis, 303
Rhinitis, allergic, 647
Rhinocort Aqua, 650
Rhinolast preparations, 648
Rhumalgan (diclofenac), 603
Riamet, 395, 402
Ribavirin, **393**, 394
  chronic hepatitis C, 390, 392
  Lassa fever, 392
  respiratory syncytial virus, 392
Riboflavin, 575, 576
Rickets, 579
  hypophosphataemic, 569, 579
Rickettsia, 328
Rifabutin, 351, **353**, 354
Rifadin, 354
Rifampicin, **354**, 355
  Haemophilus influenzae prophy-
    laxis, 304
  isoniazid and pyrazinamide with,
    355
  isoniazid with, 355
  meningococcal meningitis pro-
    phylaxis, 304
  tuberculosis, 348, 349, 351
    prophylaxis, 305
    treatment, 348, 349
Rifamycins, 348, 349, 351, 353, 354
Rifater, 355
Rifinah preparations, 355
Rimacid (indometacin), 605
Rimacillin (ampicillin), 315
Rimactane, 355
Rimafen (ibuprofen), 604
Rimapam (diazepam), 773
Rimapurinol (allopurinol), 500

Rimoxallin (amoxicillin), 314
Rinatec, 653
Ringer's solution, 553
Ringer-Lactate solution, 553
Ringworm infection *see* Dermato-
    phyte infection, 363, 710
Risedronate sodium, **469**, 470
Risperdal preparations, 225
Risperidone, 221, **224**, 225
Ritalin, 236
Rite-Diet preparations, 910, 912
Ritonavir, 373, **381**
    lopinavir with, 381
    see also Kaletra
Rituximab, 525, 526
Rivotril, 282, 284
Rizopia, 911
Roaccutane, 700
Robinul, 724, 771
Robinul-Neostigmine, 784
Rocaltrol, 581
Rocephin, 325
Rocuronium, 779, **781**
Roferon-A, 526
Ropivacaine, **791**
Rosacea, 693
Rosiced, 710
Rotarix, 750
Rotavirus vaccine, **750**
Roundworm infections, 414
Rozex, 710
Rubella
    immunisation, 750
    immunoglobulin, 756
    vaccines, combined, 742, 744
Rufinamide, 267, **276**
Rusyde (furosemide), 104
Rynacrom preparations, 651

S

Sabril, 281
Saizen preparations, 462
Salactol, 701
Salamol (salbutamol) preparations,
    175, 176
Salapin (salbutamol), 175
Salatac, 701
Salazopyrin, 72
Salbulin Novolizer, 176
Salbutamol, 172, **174**, 175, 176
    asthma, acute, 169
    hyperkalaemia, 174
Salcatonin *see* Calcitonin, **467**, 468,
    567
Salicylates
    aphthous ulcers, 656
Salicylic acid, 689
    acne, 697
    betamethasone with, 678
    fungal infections, 713
    hyperkeratoses, 700
    psoriasis, 683
        coal tar and dithranol with,
            688
        coal tar with, 706
        dithranol with, 688
        sulphur with, 706
        zinc with, 689
    scalp, 705
    warts and calluses, 700, 701
        podophyllum with, 701
Saline *see* Sodium chloride
Salinum, 662
Saliva, artificial, 661
Saliveze, 662

Salivix, 662
Salmeterol, **176**, 177
    fluticasone with, 188
Salmonellosis, 298
Salofalk preparations, 70
Salpingitis, 328
Salt substitutes, 547
Sandimmun, 523
Sandocal preparations, 567
    colecalciferol with, 582
Sandoglobulin NF, 757
Sando-K, 547
Sandostatin, 435
Sanomigran, 263
Sapropterin, **562**
Saquinavir, 373, **381**, 382
Savlon Dry powder, 722
Scabies, 715
Scandishake, 907
Scandonest, 787
Schar, 911
Scheriproct, 89
Schistosoma, 416
Schistosomicides, 416
Schizophrenia, 215
School, managing medicines at, 1
Scopoderm preparations, 245
Scopolamine *see* Hyoscine
Scottish Medicines Consortium, 4
Scottish Prescribing Analysis, xiii
Scurvy, 578
Sebco, 687
Sebomin, 331
Seborrhoeic
    dermatitis, 683
    eczema, 683
Secobarbital, anaesthesia, 771
Securon preparations, 141
Sedation, anaesthesia, 771
Sedatives, 211
    see also Anxiolytics
Segawa syndrome, 288
Seizures
    absence, 266
    neonatal, 267
    see also Epilepsy
Select-A-Jet Dopamine, 144
Selenium sulphide, 705, 706, 711
Selexid, 318
Selsun, 706
Semisodium valproate, 226
Senna, **81**, 82
Senokot, 81, 82
    granules—discontinued
Septanest, 787
Septic arthritis, 302
Septic shock, 444
Septic spots *see* Paronychia, 303,
    711
Septicaemia
    catheter-related, 301
    hospital-acquired, 301
    initial therapy, 301
    meningococcal, 301
Septrin, 348
Serenace, 219
Seretide, 188
Serevent, 177
Seroquel, 224
Serotonin re-uptake inhibitor anti-
    depressants *see* Antidepressants,
    serotonin re-uptake inhibitors, 228,
    231
Sertraline, 231, **233**
Sesame oil, presence of, 3
Sevelamer, 570, **571**
Sevoflurane, 766, **768**
Sevredol, 257

Sex hormones
    androgens, 455
    oestrogens, 454
    progestogens, 454
Shampoos, 705
Shared care, 5
Sharpsguard, 429
Shigellosis, 298
Shingles, 386
Shock, 142
    anaphylactic, 198
    blood-volume expansion, 557
    cardiogenic, 143
    hypovolaemic, 143
    metabolic acidosis, 555
    septic, 142, 444
        neonatal, 142
Sibutramine, 237
Sickle-cell disease, 539
    delayed puberty, 453
    pain, 245
    pneumococcal infection prophy-
        laxis, 305
Siklos, 539
Sildenafil, 124, **126**
Silkis, 686
Silver nitrate, 700, **701**
Silver sulfadiazine, **709**
    skin, 707
Silver sulphadiazine *see* Silver sulfa-
    diazine
Simeticone, **53**
    aluminium hydroxide with, 53
    hydrotalcite with, 52
Simple eye ointment, 638
Simple linctus, 210
    paediatric, 209
SimpleXx, 462
Simulect, 522
Simvador (simvastatin), 161
Simvastatin, 159, **161**
Sinemet preparations, 289
Sinepin, 230
Singulair, 191
Sinusitis, 652
    antibacterial treatment, 303
Siopel, 671
Sirolimus, 520, **523**
Skin preparations
    ACBS, 917
    antibacterials, 707
    antiviral, 715
    barrier, 670
    camouflagers, 704
    cleansing, 719
    corticosteroids, 672
    dilution, 664
    emollient, 666
    excipients, 665
    ulcers, 723
Skinoren, 694
SLO Drinks, 909
Slocinx XL (doxazosin), 129
Slofenac (diclofenac), 603
Slo-Indo (indometacin m/r), 605
Slo-Phyllin, 179
Slo-Pro (propranolol), 116
Slow-K, 547
Slow-Sodium, 549
SMA preparations, 886, 898, 900
Smallpox vaccine, 750
SMC *see* Scottish Medicines Con-
    sortium, 4
Smith-Lemli-Opitz syndrome, 91
Smoking cessation, 291
Snake bites, 47
    antivenom, 47
Sno Tears, 638

Sno-Pro, 912
Soap substitutes, 666
Sodium acid phosphate, 570
Sodium alendronate *see* Alendronic
   acid, 468, 469
Sodium amidotrizoate, 87
Sodium benzoate, 591, **592**, 593
Sodium bicarbonate
   cyanosis, 114
   ear drops, 647
   intravenous, 555, 556
   oral, 550
Sodium calcium edetate, **45**
Sodium calciumedetate *see* Sodium
   calcium edetate, **45**
Sodium carboxymethylcellulose *see*
   Carmellose
Sodium chloride
   bladder irrigation, 495, 720
   electrolyte replacement
      oral, 548, 549
      parenteral, 552, 553
   eye irrigation, 620, **638**, 639
   hypercalcaemia, 567
   hypertonic inhalation, 206
   infusion, 553
      glucose and, 552, 553
      potassium chloride and, 555
      potassium chloride, glucose
         and, 555
   mouthwash, 659, 661
      compound, **661**
   nasal
      congestion, 651
      postoperative douche, 647
   nebuliser solution, 183
      hypertonic, 208
   skin cleansing, 719, **720**
Sodium citrate
   acid aspiration prophylaxis, 762
   bladder irrigation, 495
   rectal, 85
Sodium clodronate, 470
Sodium content, antacids, 51
Sodium cromoglicate
   asthma, 189, **190**
   eye, 627, **628**
   food allergy, **76**
   nose, 648, **651**
Sodium cromoglycate *see* Sodium
   cromoglicate
Sodium dichloroacetate, **596**
Sodium docusate *see* Docusate sod-
   ium
Sodium feredetate, 529, 531
Sodium fluoride, 571, **572**, 573
Sodium fusidate, **341**
   angular cheilitis, 657
   mouth, 657
Sodium hyaluronate, **639**
Sodium iodine, radioactive, 440
Sodium ironedetate *see* Sodium fer-
   edetate, 529, 531
Sodium lactate
   intravenous infusion
      compound, 553
Sodium nitrite, 44
Sodium nitroprusside, 121, **123**
Sodium oxybate, 43
Sodium phenylbutyrate, 591, 593
Sodium picosulfate, **82**, 86
Sodium picosulphate *see* Sodium
   picosulfate, **82**, 86
Sodium pidolate, 667
Sodium polystyrene sulphonate, 548
Sodium stibogluconate, **409**
Sodium thiosulphate, 44, 45
Sodium valproate *see* Valproate

Sofradex
   ear, 644
   eye, 626
Soft tissue disorders, 599
Softclix products, 428
Solaraze, 704
Solian, 222
Solivito N, 561
Solu-Cortef, 452
Solu-Medrone, 452
Solvazinc, 573
Solvents, ear wax removal, 647
Somatomedins, 471
Somatotrophin, 461
Somatropin, **461**, 462, 463
Somnite (nitrazepam), 283
Sorbitol, presence of, 3
Sotacor, 119
Sotalol, 108, 113, 114, **118**, 119
   see also Beta-adrenoceptor
      blocking drugs
      supraventricular tachycardia,
         108
Soya oil, 669
Soya-based infant formula, 899, 900
SPA, xiii
Spacer devices, 182
Spasm
   muscle, 616
   vascular, 136, **140**
Spasmonal preparations, 57
Spasticity, 616
SpectraBan, 704
Spermicides, 488
SPF, 703
Spiramycin, 336, 410
Spirit
   industrial methylated, 720
   surgical, 720
Spironolactone, 104, **105**, 106
   heart failure, 100
   precocious puberty, 457
Splenectomy *see* Asplenia
Sporanox, 369
Sporanox-Pulse, 369
Sport, drugs and, 32
Sprilon, 671
SQ-PEN, 428
SSRIs *see* Antidepressants, serotonin
   re-uptake inhibitors, 228, 231
SST, 662
St John's Wort, 228
Stamaril, 754
Stannous fluoride, 573
Starch, etherified, 557, 558
Statins, 159
Status epilepticus, 283
Stavudine, 373, **377**
Steam inhalations, 651
Stelazine, 221
Stemetil, 241
Sterculia
   constipation, 79
      frangula with, 79
   diarrhoea, 65
Stericlens (sodium chloride), 720
Steri-Neb
   ipratropium, 178
   Salamol (salbutamol), 176
   sodium chloride, 183
Steripaste, 683
Steripod (sodium chloride), 720
Steripoule (sodium chloride), 183
Steroid treatment card, 448
   suppliers, 447
Steroids *see* Anabolic steroids; Cor-
   ticosteroids; Glucocorticoids; or
   Mineralocorticosteroids

Ster-Zac Bath Concentrate—disconti-
   nued
Stesolid (diazepam), 285
Stiemycin, 695
Still's disease *see* Arthritis, juvenile
   idiopathic, 608
Stimulants
   central nervous system, 202
   respiratory, 202
Stings, 48
Stiripentol, 276, **277**
Stoma, drugs and, 90
Stomatitis
   angular, 657
   herpetic, 657
Strattera, 234
Strefen, 656
Streptase, 157
Streptococcal infection
   antibacterial prophylaxis, 304
Streptogramin antibiotics, 345
Streptokinase, **157**
Streptomycin
   brucellosis, 355
   endocarditis, 332
   tuberculosis, 348, 352, **355**
Stronazon MR (tamsulosin), 492
Strongyloidiasis, 416
Stugeron, 239
Subcuvia, 756
Subgam, 756
Sublimaze, 778
Succimer, 45
Succinylcholine *see* Suxamethon-
   ium, **782**, 783
Sucralfate, **62**
Sucrose, presence of, 3
Sudafed, 210
Sudocrem, 671
Sugammadex, **784**
Sugar-free liquid medicines *see* pre-
   parations identified by 'sugar-free'
   throughout *BNF for Children*
Sugar-free, definition, 3
Sulazine EC (sulfasalazine), 72
Sulconazole, 711, **714**
Sulfa... *see also* Sulpha...
Sulfadiazine
   toxoplasmosis, 409, 411
Sulfadiazine, silver, 707, 709
Sulfadoxine
   malaria, 405
      pyrimethamine with, 395,
         406
Sulfamethoxazole, trimethoprim
   with, *see* Co-trimoxazole
Sulfasalazine
   inflammatory bowel disease, 66,
      68, **71**, 72
   rheumatic disease, 608, **613**
Sulpha... *see also* Sulfa...
Sulphasalazine *see* Sulfasalazine
Sulphites, presence of, 3
Sulphonamides, 346
Sulphonylureas, 429
Sulphur, 683, 697
   salicylic acid with, 706
Sulphur dioxide, poisoning,
   46
Sulpiride
   psychoses, 216, **220**, 221
   Tourette syndrome, **220**, 290
Sulpor, 221
Sumatriptan
   cluster headache, 264
   migraine, **262**, 263
Sun protection factor, 703
Sunnyvale, 911

Sunscreens, 703
    ACBS, 917
Sunsense Ultra, 704
Sunya 20/75, 481
Superinfection, 297
Suplena, 903
Supplementary prescribing, 928
Suprane, 767
Suprax, 322
Suramin, 416
Surfactants, pulmonary, 203
Surgery
    antibacterial prophylaxis, 306,
      307
    diabetes and, 421
    long-term medication and, 761
    tetanus vaccine, 751
    wound infection, 303
Surgical spirit, 720
Survanta, 203
Survimed preparations, 881
Sustanon preparations, 456
Sustiva, 382
Suxamethonium, **782**, 783
Symbicort, 187
Symbols, *inside back cover*
Sympathomimetics
    asthma, 172
    eye, 630, 632
    inotropic, 142
    vasoconstrictor, 144
Synacthen, 460
Synacthen Depot, 460
Synagis, 393
Synalar preparations, 680
Synercid, 345
Syner-KINASE, 158
Synflex, 606
Synphase, 482
Syntaris, 650
Synthamin preparations, 559
Syphilis, 301
Syprol (propranolol), 116
Syringe drivers, palliative care, 28
Syringes
    insulin, 429
      blind patients, 429
    oral, 3
Sytron, 531

T

Tabphyn MR (tamsulosin), 492
Tacalcitol, 683, 685, **686**
Tachycardias *see* Arrhythmias
Tacrolimus
    eczema, 690, **692**
    immunosuppression, 517, 520,
      523, 524
Taenicides, 415
Tambocor, 112
Tambocor XL, 112
Tamiflu, 392
Tamsulosin, 491, **492**
Tapeworm infections, 415
Tar, **687**
    see also Coal tar
Taranis products, 912
Tardive dyskinesia, 216

Targocid, 343
Tartrazine, presence of, 3
Tazarotene, 683
Tazobactam, 317
    piperacillin with, 317
Tazocin, 317
3TC *see* Lamivudine
Tear deficiency, 636
Tear gas, 46
Tears Naturale, 638
Tears, artificial, 636
Tegretol preparations, 268, 269
Teicoplanin, 342, **343**
Telangiectasia, hereditary haemor-
    rhagic, 454
Telfast, 193
Telzir, 380
Temazepam, **775**
    premedication, 772
    sedation, 771
Temgesic, 251
Temodal, 514
Temozolomide, 513, **514**
Tendinitis, 608
Tennis elbow, 608
Tenofovir, 373, **377**, 378
    efavirenz and emtricitabine with,
      378
    emtricitabine with, 378
Tenormin preparations, 116
TENS, 25
Tensipine MR, 139
Tensium (diazepam), 773
Tensopril (captopril), 132
Tentrini preparations, 887, 890
Teoptic, 631
Terbinafine, 714
    dermatophyte infections, 362,
      364
        systemic treatment, **371**
        topical treatment, 711, **714**
Terbutaline, **177**
    asthma, 172
      acute, 169
Terlipressin, 464, 467
Terminal care *see* Palliative care
Testolactone, 457, **458**
Testosterone, **456**, 457
    enantate, 455, 456
    esters, 456
    propionate, 455, 456
    undecanoate, 455, 456
Testotoxicosis *see* Puberty, preco-
    cious, 457, 459
Tetanus
    antibacterial treatment,
      309
    immunisation, **751**
    immunoglobulin, 757, **758**
    vaccines, combined, 734, 751
    travel, 759
    wounds, 751
Tetracaine
    eye, 635, **636**
    local anaesthetic, **792**
      lidocaine with, 789
    rectal, 88
Tetracosactide, 459, **460**
Tetracosactrin *see* Tetracosactide,
    459, **460**
Tetracycline, 328, **329**, 330
    acne, 697
    oral infections, 329
    pregnancy, 329
    skin, clobetasone butyrate with,
      679
Tetrahydrobiopterin, **562**

Tetrahydrofolate reductase deficien-
    cy, 594
Tetralogy of Fallot, 114
Tetralysal-300, 331
Tetraspan, 558
Tetrastarch, 557, 558
T-Gel, 706
Thalassaemia, 539
THAM *see* Trometamol, 555, **556**
Theophylline, **179**, 180
    asthma, chronic, 170
    poisoning by, 43
    poisoning, elimination, 35
    see also Aminophylline
Thiabendazole *see* Tiabendazole
Thiamine, 575, **576**, 577
Thiazides, 100, 101
    diabetes insipidus, 464
    see also Diuretics
Thick and Easy, 909
Thickened foods, 909
Thioguanine *see* Tioguanine, 508,
    511
Thiopental
    anaesthesia, 763, **765**, 766
    status epilepticus, 283, **765**
Thiopentone *see* Thiopental
Thiopurine methyltransferase, 518
Thioxanthenes, 216
Thixo-D, 909
Threadworm infections, 413
Throat infections
    antibacterial treatment, 302
    fungal, 657
    gonorrhoea, 301
    viral, 657
Thrombocytopenias, 535
Thrombocytopenic purpura, 541
    immunoglobulins, 755
    prednisolone, 453
Thrombo-embolism, 151
Thrombolytics, 156
Thrombosis
    antiplatelet drugs, 154
    deep-vein, 147, 151
    prophylaxis, 147
Thrush *see* Candidiasis
Thymoglobuline, 521
Thymol, 661
Thyroid
    antagonists, 439
    function test, 463
    hormones, 438
    storm, 440
Thyroidectomy, 439
Thyroiditis, Hashimoto's, 438
Thyrotoxic crisis, 440
Thyrotoxicosis, 439
    beta-blockers, 114, 440
Thyrotoxicosis, neonatal, 440
Thyrotrophin-releasing hormone *see*
    Protirelin, 463
Thyroxine *see* Levothyroxine, **438**,
    439
Tiabendazole
    larva migrans, 416
Tiagabine, 266, **277**
Ticarcillin, 317, **318**
    clavulanic acid with, 317, 318
Tick-borne encephalitis, 759
    immunisation
      vaccine, 752
    immunisation, vaccine, **752**
TicoVac, 752
Tics, 290
Tilade, 190
Tildiem preparations, 137
Tilofyl (fentanyl), 254

Tiloryth (erythromycin), 337
Timentin, 317, 318
Timodine, 676
Timolol, eye, **632**, 634
Timoptol preparations, 632
Tinaderm-M, 713
Tinea infections, 362, 710
Tinidazole, 408
  amoebiasis, 407, 408
  giardiasis, 408
  protozoal infections,
    408
  trichomoniasis, 408
Tinzaparin, 149, **150**
Tioconazole, 711, **714**
Tioguanine, 508, **511**
Tipranavir, 373, **382**
Tisept, 721
Tissue adhesive, 719
Titanium dioxide, 671, 703
Tixycolds preparations, 652
Tobi, 335
Tobramycin, 333, **335**
Tocopherols, 582
Tocopheryl, 582
Toilet preparations, ACBS, 917
Tolazoline, 123, 124, **126**, 127
Tolbutamide, 430, **431**
Tolnaftate, 713
Tolterodine, 492, **493**
Tonic seizures, 266, 267
Tonic-clonic seizures, 266
Tonsillitis *see* Throat infections
Topal, 54
Topamax, 278
Topiramate, 266, 267, 277, **278**
  migraine, 263
Toradol, 776
Torsade de pointes, 108
  magnesium sulphate, 568
Total parenteral nutrition, 558
Tourette syndrome, 290
TOXBASE, 33
Toxoplasma choroidoretinitis, 409
Toxoplasmosis, 409
TPN, 558
Trachoma, 328, 622
Tracleer, 125
Tracrium, 780
Tradorec XL, 260
Tramacet, 260
Tramadol, 250, **259**, 260
  paracetamol with, 260
Tramake preparations, 259
Tramquel SR, 260
Trandate, 118
Tranexamic acid, **158**
  palliative care, 26
Tranquillisers, 211
Transcutaneous electrical nerve sti-
  mulation, 25
Transfusion reactions, 535
Transplant rejection, 517, 518, 520
Travasept-100, 721
Travel, vaccination for, 758
Travellers' diarrhoea, 759
Travoprost, 632
Treatment cards, anticoagulant,
  153
Tree pollen extracts, 197
Tremors, 290
Tretinoin
  acne, 695, 696
    erythromycin with,
      696
  leukaemia, 517
TRH *see* Protirelin, **463**

Tri-Adcortyl preparations—discontinued
Triadene, 483
Triamcinolone
  intra-articular, 607, 608
    rheumatic disease, 608
  mouth, 654, 655
  nasal allergy, 651
  skin, 681
Triazole antifungal drugs, 362, 363
Tribavirin *see* Ribavirin
Trichomonacides, 408
Trichomonal infections, 408
Triclofos, 213
  anaesthesia, 771
  hypnotic, 212, **213**
Tricyclic antidepressants *see* Anti-
  depressants, tricyclic
Trientine, 586, **587**
Trifluoperazine
  anxiety, **221**
  nausea and vomiting, 237, **242**
  psychoses, 217, **221**
Trihexyphenidyl, 289, **290**
Tri-iodothyronine *see* Liothyronine,
  438, **439**
Trileptal, 269
Trimeprazine *see* Alimemazine
Trimethoprim, 347, **348**
  eye infection, 624
  pneumocystis pneumonia, 411
  sulfamethoxazole with, *see* Co-
    trimoxazole
Trimopan (trimethoprim), 348
Trimovate, 679
TriNovum, 482
Triptans *see* 5HT$_1$ agonists, 261, **262**
Triptorelin, **458**, 459
Tris-hydroxymethyl aminomethane
  see Trometamol, 555, **556**
Tritamyl, 911
Trizivir, 375
Trometamol, 555, **556**
Tropical diseases, advice, 394
Tropicamide, 629, **630**
Tropisetron—discontinued
Trosyl, 714
TRUE products, 436, 437
Trusopt, 634
Truvada, 378
Trypanocides, 409
Trypanosomiasis, 409
T-Safe CU 380 A, 489
T-SPOT.TB, 732
TT 380 Slimline, 489
Tub/BCG, Dried, 731
Tuberculin, 731, 732
Tuberculosis, 348
  antibacterial prophylaxis, 349
  diagnosis, 731
  immunisation
    vaccines, 730
  prophylaxis, 305
  travel, 758
Tumour lysis syndrome, 499
Turbohaler
  Bricanyl, 177
  Oxis, 174
  Symbicort, 187
Turner's syndrome, 453, 459, 461
Twinrix preparations, 737
Typherix, 753
Typhim Vi, 753
Typhoid
  fever, treatment, 298
  immunisation
    vaccines, 752, **753**
  travel, 759

TYR preparations, 916
Tyrosinaemia, 594, 916
Tyrosine
  amino acid supplement, 916
  supplement in phenylketonuria,
    916

U

Ubidecarenone, **596**
Ubiquinone *see* Ubidecarenone, **596**
Ucerax, 195
Ulcerative colitis, 66
Ulcerative gingivitis
  antibacterial treatment, 302, 355
  mouthwashes, 659
Ulcer-healing drugs, 58
Ulcers
  aphthous, 654
  corneal, 622, 625
  duodenal, 58, 60
  gastric, 58, 60
  mouth, 654
  NSAID-associated,
    60
  skin, 723
Ultiva, 778
Ultra foods, 911, 912
Ultrabase, 667
Ultralanum Plain, 680
Ultraproct, 89
Ultraviolet radiation,
  703
Umbilical granulomas,
  701
Undecenoates, **714**
Unguentum M, 667
Unifine products, 429
Unilet products, 428
Uniphyllin Continus, 180
Uniroid-HC, 89
Unisept, 721
Unistik products, 428
Unithiol, 45
Univer, 141
Universal, 428
Unlicensed medicines, 3, 7
Urdox, 92
Urea, 666, 668
  hydrocortisone with, 676
Urea cycle disorders, 591, 917
  arginine supplement, 917
  essential amino acids supple-
    ment, 914
Urethritis, non-gonococcal, 301,
  328
Uriben, 359
Uriflex preparations, 495
Urinary
  alkalinisation, 494
  frequency, 492
  incontinence, 492
  infections, 360
    genital, 474
  retention, 491
Urinary-tract
  infections, 301
Urine tests, 437
Uristix, 437
Urokinase, **157**, 158
Uro-Tainer preparations,
  495
Ursodeoxycholic acid, **91**, 92
Ursofalk, 92
Ursogal, 92
Urticaria, 192

UT 380 Short, 490
UT 380 Standard, 490
Utovlan, 455
UVB, psoriasis, 685
Uvistat preparations, 704

V

Vaccination
  HIV-positive subjects, 727
  schedule, 728
  travel, 758
Vaccines
  active immunity, 725
  allergen extract, 196
  breast-feeding, 725
  cautions, 725
  contra-indications, 725
  post-immunisation pyrexia, 727
  pregnancy, 725
  side-effects, 726
  storage and use, 729
Vaginal infection
  oral treatment, 473
Vaginitis
  candidal, 473
Vaginosis, bacterial, 474
Vaginyl (metronidazole), 356
Valaciclovir, 386, **387**, 388
  genito-urinary infection,
    475
  herpetic stomatitis, 657
Valine Amino Acid Supplement, 914
Vallergan, 194
Valni XL, 139
Valoid, 240
Valpiform products, 911, 912
Valproate
  bipolar disorder, 226
  epilepsy, 266, 267, **278**, 279,
    280
Valproic acid *see* Valproate
Valtrex, 388
Vamin, 559
Vaminolact, 559
Vancocin, 343
Vancomycin, 341, **342**, 343
  eye, 636
Vancomycin-resistant enterococci,
  344
Vaqta, 736
Variceal bleeding, 464
Varicella-zoster, 385, 386
  corticosteroids, 446
  immunisation
    vaccine, **753**, 754, 757
    immunoglobulin, 757, **758**
Varilrix, 753
Varivax, 754
Vascular spasm, 136, **140**
Vascular surgery
  antibacterial prophylaxis, 306
Vaseline Dermacare—discontinued
Vasoconstrictors
  local anaesthesia, 787
    dental practice, 787
  sympathomimetic, 144
Vasodilators
  antihypertensive, 121
  peripheral, 141
Vasogen, 671
Vasopressin
  shock, 142
  variceal bleeding, **464**
Vectavir, 715
Vecuronium, 779, **782**

Vegenat-med preparations,
  895
Veil preparations, 705
Velbe, 512
Velosef, 323
Venofer, 533
Ventavis, 125
Ventmax SR, 175
Ventolin preparations, 175, 176
Vepesid, 512
  infusion—discontinued
Veracur, 701
Verapamil, **140**, 141
  arrhythmias, 108, 110, 136
  beta-blockers and, 140
  hypertension, 136
  poisoning by, 41
  see also Calcium-channel block-
    ers
Verapress MR, 141
Vermox, 414
Verrucas, 700
Verrugon, 701
Vertab SR 240, 141
Vertigo, 239
Vesanoid, 517
Vestibular disorders, 239
Vfend, 372
Viagra, 126
ViATIM, 737
Vibramycin-D, 330
Victanyl (fentanyl), 254
Videne, 722
Videx preparations, 376
Vigabatrin, **280**, 281
  infantile spasms, 267, 280
Vigam preparations, 757
Vigranon-B, 578
Vimpat, 271
Vinblastine, 511, **512**
Vinca alkaloids, 511
Vincent's infection
  antibacterial treatment, 302, 355
  mouthwashes, 659
Vincristine, 511, **512**
Vioform-Hydrocortisone—disconti-
  nued
Viper venom antiserum, European,
  47
Viracept, 381
  powder—discontinued
Viraferon—discontinued
Viramune, 384
Virazole, 394
Viread, 378
Viroflu, 742
Virormone injection, 456
Virovir (aciclovir), 387
Virus infections, 372
Visclair, 208
Viscopaste PB7, 683
Viscotears, 637
Vismed preparations, 639
Vistamethasone
  ear, 644
  eye, 626
  nose, 649
Vistamethasone N
  ear, 644
  eye, 626
  nose, 653
Vita-Bite, 912
Vitajoule, 904
Vitalograph, 181
Vitamin A, **574**, 575
  vitamin D and, **575**
Vitamin B group, 575
  preparations, 577, 578

Vitamin B$_{12}$, 533, 535
Vitamin C *see* Ascorbic acid
Vitamin D, 578, 580
  psoriasis, 683, 685
Vitamin D$_2$ *see* Ergocalciferol, 578,
  579, 580
Vitamin D$_3$ *see* Colecalciferol
Vitamin deficiency, 574
Vitamin E, 582
Vitamin K, 583, 584
  deficiency bleeding, 583
Vitamins, 574
  children's drops, 575
  multivitamins, **584**, 585
  parenteral, 560
Vitapro, 906
Vitaquick, 909
Vitasavoury, 907
Vitiligo, 704
  ACBS, 917
Vitlipid N, 561
Vitrex products, 428
Vivaglobin, 756
Vividrin (sodium cromoglicate), 628,
  651
Vivotif, 753
Volmax—discontinued
Volplex, 557
Volsaid (diclofenac), 603
Voltarol preparations, 603
  eye, 640
  Ophtha, 640
  Rapid, 603
Volulyte, 558
Volumatic, 182
Volume expansion, 556
Voluven, 558
Vomiting
  cytotoxic drugs, 497
  motion sickness, 239
  nausea and, 237
  opioid-induced, 238
  palliative care, 27
  postoperative, 238
  pregnancy, 238
Voriconazole, 361, 363, **371**, 372
Vulvitis, candidal, 473
Vulvovaginal candidiasis, recurrent,
  473
VZIG *see* Immunoglobulins, vari-
  cella-zoster, 757, 758

W

Warfarin, **153**
Warticon preparations, 702
Warts, 700
  anogenital, 701
Wasp sting allergy preparations,
  196, 197
Water for injections, 556
WaveSense products, 428, 437
Waxsol, 647
Welldorm, 213
Wellfoods products, 911
West's syndrome, 280
Whitfield's ointment, 711
Whooping cough *see* Pertussis
Wilson's disease, 586
Wilzin, 587
Withdrawal
  antipsychotics
    atypical, 222
  nicotine, 291
  opioids, 251

Wolff-Parkinson-White syndrome, 108
Wool fat, hydrous, 667
Worm infestation, 413
Wuchereria bancrofti, 416
Wysoy, 900

Y

Yasmin, 483
Yeasts, 363
Yellow cards, *inside back cover*, 21
Yellow fever
    immunisation
        vaccine, **754**
    travel, 758

X

Xagrid, 542
Xanthine bronchodilators *see* Theophylline
Xepin, 672
Xerostomia, 661
    palliative care, 26
XLEU preparations, 913
XLYS Low TRY preparations, 912
XLYS preparations, 913
XLYS TRY preparations, 912
XMET preparations, 913
XMTVI preparations, 914
Xolair, 198
XP preparations, 916
XPHEN TYR preparations, 917
XPTM preparations, 917
Xylitol, presence of, 3
Xylocaine, 788, 789
Xylometazoline
    eye, 627
    nose, 651, **652**
Xyloproct, 89
Xylotox, 788
Xyzal, 194

Z

Zaditen, 195, 628
Zafirlukast, 190, **191**
Zamadol preparations, 259, 260
Zanamivir, 390, **392**
Zantac, 61
Zaponex, 223
Zarontin, 270
Zavesca, 595
ZeaSORB, 724
Zeffix, 377
Zenalb preparations (albumin), 556, 557
Zenapax—discontinued
Zeridame SR, 260
Zerit, 377
Zerobase, 667
Zestril, 134
Ziagen, 375
Zidoval, 475
Zidovudine, 373, **378**
    abacavir and lamivudine with, 375
    lamivudine with, 378
Zinacef, 325

Zinc
    bandages
        stocking, 683
    deficiency, **573**
    skin
        bandages, 682, 683
        calamine and, 683
        calamine, clioquinol and, 683
        castor oil and, 671
        coal tar with, 687
        cod liver oil with, 671
        cream, 671
        dimeticone with, 671
        ichthammol with, 682, 683
        ointment, 671
        salicylic acid with, 689
    Wilson's disease (zinc acetate), **587**
Zincaband, 683
Zindaclin, 695
Zineryt, 695
Zinnat, 325
Zipzoc, 683
Zithromax, 338
Zocor, 161
Zofran, 244
Zoladex preparations, 458
Zollinger–Ellison syndrome, 60, 62
Zolvera (verapamil), 141
Zomacton, 463
Zoster *see* Herpes infections
Zoton FasTab, 63
Zovirax preparations, 387
    cold sore cream, 715
    cream, 715
    eye ointment, 625
Zuvogen, 715
Zydol preparations, 259, 260
Zyloric, 500
Zyomet, 710
Zyprexa, 224
Zyvox, 344

Index

NEWBORN LIFE SUPPORT

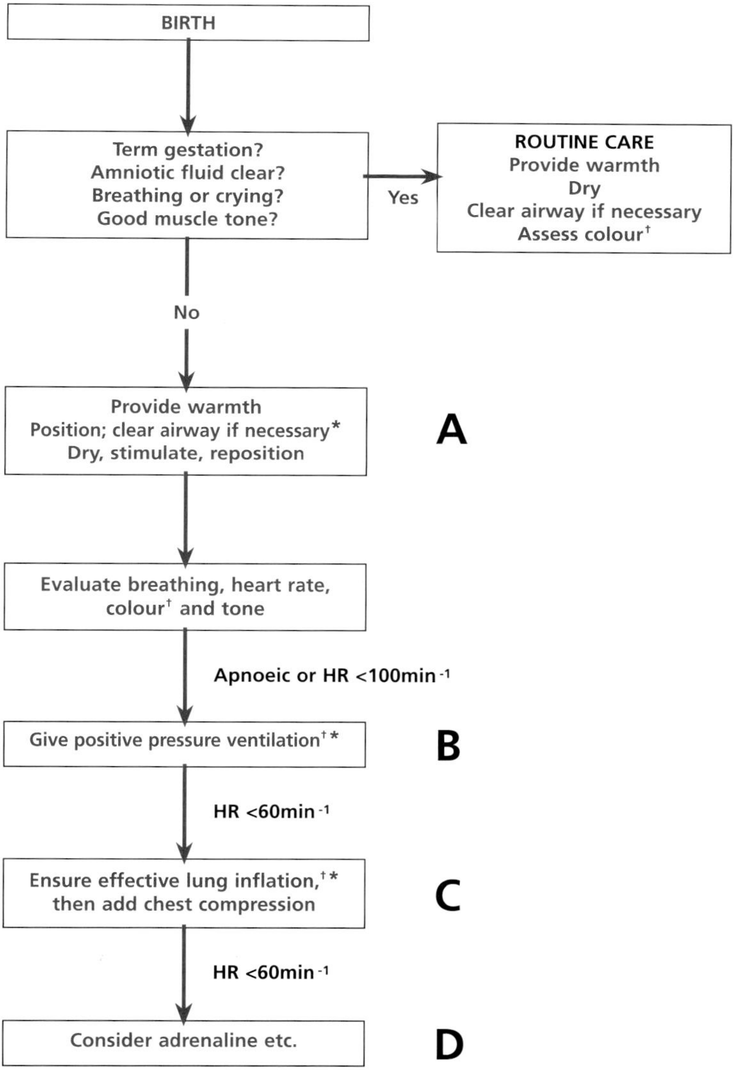

```
                    ┌─────────────────────┐
                    │        BIRTH        │
                    └─────────────────────┘
                              │
                              ▼
        ┌─────────────────────┐           ┌─────────────────────────┐
        │  Term gestation?    │           │      ROUTINE CARE       │
        │  Amniotic fluid clear?│   Yes   │    Provide warmth       │
        │  Breathing or crying?├────────▶ │        Dry              │
        │  Good muscle tone?   │          │  Clear airway if necessary│
        └─────────────────────┘          │    Assess colour†       │
                              │           └─────────────────────────┘
                             No
                              ▼
        ┌─────────────────────────────────┐
        │        Provide warmth           │
        │  Position; clear airway if necessary* │    A
        │    Dry, stimulate, reposition   │
        └─────────────────────────────────┘
                              │
                              ▼
        ┌─────────────────────────────────┐
        │  Evaluate breathing, heart rate,│
        │        colour† and tone         │
        └─────────────────────────────────┘
                              │
              Apnoeic or HR <100min⁻¹
                              ▼
        ┌─────────────────────────────────┐
        │ Give positive pressure ventilation†* │   B
        └─────────────────────────────────┘
                              │
                  HR <60min⁻¹
                              ▼
        ┌─────────────────────────────────┐
        │  Ensure effective lung inflation,†* │   C
        │   then add chest compression    │
        └─────────────────────────────────┘
                              │
                  HR <60min⁻¹
                              ▼
        ┌─────────────────────────────────┐
        │    Consider adrenaline etc.     │    D
        └─────────────────────────────────┘
```

Term gestation?
Amniotic fluid clear?
Breathing or crying?
Good muscle tone?

ROUTINE CARE
Provide warmth
Dry
Clear airway if necessary
Assess colour†

Yes

No

Provide warmth
Position; clear airway if necessary*
Dry, stimulate, reposition

A

Evaluate breathing, heart rate, colour† and tone

Apnoeic or HR <100min⁻¹

Give positive pressure ventilation†*

B

HR <60min⁻¹

Ensure effective lung inflation,†*
then add chest compression

C

HR <60min⁻¹

Consider adrenaline etc.

D

---

*Tracheal intubation may be considered at several steps
†Consider supplemental oxygen at any stage if cyanosis persists

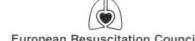

European Resuscitation Council

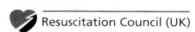

Resuscitation Council (UK)

PAEDIATRIC BASIC LIFE SUPPORT
(Healthcare professionals with a duty to respond)

UNRESPONSIVE?

↓

Shout for help

↓

Open airway

↓

NOT BREATHING NORMALLY?

↓

5 rescue breaths

↓

STILL UNRESPONSIVE?
(no signs of a circulation)

↓

15 chest compressions
2 rescue breaths

After 1 minute call resuscitation team then continue CPR

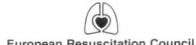

European Resuscitation Council

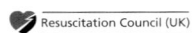

Resuscitation Council (UK)

PAEDIATRIC ADVANCED LIFE SUPPORT

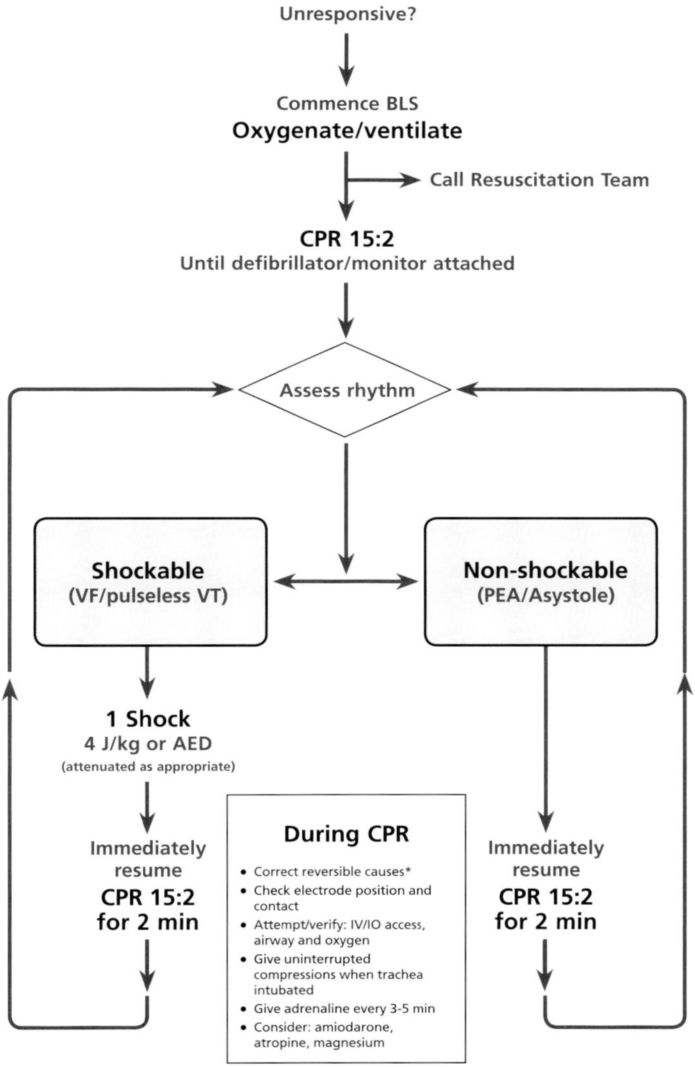

Unresponsive?

↓

Commence BLS
Oxygenate/ventilate

→ **Call Resuscitation Team**

CPR 15:2
Until defibrillator/monitor attached

↓

Assess rhythm

Shockable
(VF/pulseless VT)

←→

Non-shockable
(PEA/Asystole)

1 Shock
4 J/kg or AED
(attenuated as appropriate)

↓

Immediately
resume
CPR 15:2
for 2 min

During CPR

- Correct reversible causes*
- Check electrode position and contact
- Attempt/verify: IV/IO access, airway and oxygen
- Give uninterrupted compressions when trachea intubated
- Give adrenaline every 3-5 min
- Consider: amiodarone, atropine, magnesium

Immediately
resume
CPR 15:2
for 2 min

---

*Reversible causes

Hypoxia	Tension pneumothorax
Hypovolaemia	Tamponade, cardiac
Hypo/hyperkalaemia/metabolic	Toxins
Hypothermia	Thromboembolism

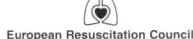

European Resuscitation Council

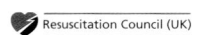

Resuscitation Council (UK)

BODY SURFACE AREA IN CHILDREN

Body-weight under 40kg

Body-weight (kg)	Surface area (m²)
1	0.10
1.5	0.13
2	0.16
2.5	0.19
3	0.21
3.5	0.24
4	0.26
4.5	0.28
5	0.30
5.5	0.32
6	0.34
6.5	0.36
7	0.38
7.5	0.40
8	0.42
8.5	0.44
9	0.46
9.5	0.47
10	0.49
11	0.53
12	0.56
13	0.59
14	0.62
15	0.65
16	0.68
17	0.71
18	0.74
19	0.77
20	0.79
21	0.82
22	0.85
23	0.87
24	0.90
25	0.92
26	0.95
27	0.97
28	1.0
29	1.0
30	1.1
31	1.1
32	1.1
33	1.1
34	1.1
35	1.2
36	1.2
37	1.2
38	1.2
39	1.3
40	1.3

Values are calculated using the Boyd equation

Note Height is not required to estimate body surface area using these tables

Adapted by permission from Macmillan Publishers Ltd: Sharkey I et al, *British Journal of Cancer* 2001; **85** (1): 23–28, © 2001

BODY SURFACE AREA IN CHILDREN
Body-weight over 40kg

Body-weight (kg)	Surface area (m^2)	Body-weight (kg)	Surface area (m^2)
41	1.3	66	1.8
42	1.3	67	1.8
43	1.3	68	1.8
44	1.4	69	1.8
45	1.4	70	1.9
46	1.4	71	1.9
47	1.4	72	1.9
48	1.4	73	1.9
49	1.5	74	1.9
50	1.5	75	1.9
51	1.5	76	2.0
52	1.5	77	2.0
53	1.5	78	2.0
54	1.6	79	2.0
55	1.6	80	2.0
56	1.6	81	2.0
57	1.6	82	2.1
58	1.6	83	2.1
59	1.7	84	2.1
60	1.7	85	2.1
61	1.7	86	2.1
62	1.7	87	2.1
63	1.7	88	2.2
64	1.7	89	2.2
65	1.8	90	2.2

Values are calculated using the Boyd equation

Note Height is not required to estimate body surface area using these tables

Adapted by permission from Macmillan Publishers Ltd: Sharkey I et al, *British Journal of Cancer* 2001; **85** (1): 23–28, © 2001

Medical emergencies in the community

Drug treatment outlined below is intended for use by community healthcare professionals. Only drugs that are used for immediate relief are shown; advice on supporting care is not given. Where the child's condition requires investigation and further treatment, the child should be transferred to hospital promptly.

Anaphylaxis

(section 3.4.3)

Adrenaline injection 1 mg/mL (1 in 1000)

- By intramuscular injection
  Child under 6 years 150 micrograms (0.15 mL), repeated every 5 minutes if necessary
  Child 6–12 years 300 micrograms (0.3 mL), repeated every 5 minutes if necessary
  Child 12–18 years 500 micrograms (0.5 mL), repeated every 5 minutes if necessary; 300 micrograms (0.3 mL) should be given if child is small or prepubertal

Chlorphenamine injection 10 mg/mL

- By intravenous injection over 1 minute or by intramuscular injection
  Child under 6 months 250 micrograms/kg (max. 2.5 mg), repeated if required up to 4 times in 24 hours
  Child 6 months–6 years 2.5 mg, repeated if required up to 4 times in 24 hours
  Child 6–12 years 5mg, repeated if required up to 4 times in 24 hours
  Child 12–18 years 10 mg, repeated if required up to 4 times in 24 hours

High-flow **oxygen** (section 3.6) and **intravenous fluids** should be given if required.

Hydrocortisone (preferably as sodium succinate) by intravenous injection (section 6.3.2) has delayed action but it should be given to severely affected children to prevent further deterioration.

Asthma: acute

(section 3.1)

Regard each emergency consultation as being for **severe acute asthma** until shown otherwise; failure to respond adequately **at any time** requires immediate referral to hospital

Either **salbutamol** aerosol inhaler 100 micrograms/metered inhalation

- By aerosol inhalation via large-volume spacer (and a close-fitting face mask if child under 3 years)
  Child under 18 years 4–10 puffs each inhaled separately, repeated at 10–20 minute intervals or as necessary

or **salbutamol** nebuliser solution 1 mg/mL, 2 mg/mL

- By inhalation of nebulised solution (via oxygen-driven nebuliser if available)
  Child under 5 years 2.5 mg every 10–20 minutes or as necessary
  Child 5–12 years 2.5–5 mg every 10–20 minutes or as necessary
  Child 12–18 years 5 mg every 10–20 minutes or as necessary

or **terbutaline** nebulised solution 2.5 mg/mL

- By inhalation of nebulised solution (via oxygen-driven nebuliser if available)
  Child under 5 years 5 mg every 10–20 minutes or as necessary
  Child 5–12 years 5–10 mg every 10–20 minutes or as necessary
  Child 12–18 years 10 mg every 10–20 minutes or as necessary

If response to beta₂ agonist is poor (while awaiting transfer to hospital) **ipratropium nebuliser solution 250 micrograms/mL**

- By inhalation of nebulised solution (via oxygen-driven nebuliser if available)
  Child under 12 years 250 micrograms every 20–30 minutes if necessary
  Child 12–18 years 500 micrograms every 20–30 minutes if necessary

Plus (in all cases)

Either **prednisolone** soluble tablets 5 mg

- By mouth
  Child under 12 years 1–2 mg/kg (max. 40 mg) daily for 3–5 days; if the child is already taking oral corticosteroids, give prednisolone 2 mg/kg (max. 60 mg)
  Child 12–18 years 40–50 mg daily for at least 5 days

or **hydrocortisone** (preferably as sodium succinate)

- By intravenous injection
  Child under 2 years 4 mg/kg (max. 25 mg) 3–4 times daily, until conversion to oral prednisolone is possible
  Child 2–5 years 4 mg/kg (max. 50 mg) 3–4 times daily, until conversion to oral prednisolone is possible
  Child 5–18 years 4 mg/kg (max. 100 mg) 3–4 times daily, until conversion to oral prednisolone is possible

High-flow **oxygen** (section 3.6) should be given if available

Croup

(section 3.1)

Dexamethasone oral solution 2 mg/5mL

- By mouth
  Child 1 month–2 years 150 micrograms/kg as a single dose

Convulsions

(section 4.8.2)

Either **midazolam** buccal solution 10 mg/mL or injection solution given by buccal route

- By buccal administration, repeated once after 10 minutes if necessary
  Neonate 300 micrograms/kg
  Child 1–6 months 300 micrograms/kg (max. 2.5 mg)
  Child 6 months–1 year 2.5 mg
  Child 1–5 years 5 mg
  Child 5–10 years 7.5 mg
  Child 10–18 years 10 mg

or **diazepam** rectal solution 2 mg/mL, 4 mg/mL

- By rectum, repeated once after 10 minutes if necessary
  Neonate 1.25–2.5 mg
  Child 1 month–2 years 5 mg
  Child 2–12 years 5–10 mg
  Child 12–18 years 10 mg

Febrile convulsions lasting longer than 15 minutes

(section 4.8.3)

Diazepam rectal solution 2 mg/mL, 4 mg/mL

- By rectum, repeated once after 10 minutes if necessary
  Neonate 1.25–2.5 mg
  Child 1 month–2 years 5 mg
  Child 2–12 years 5–10 mg
  Child 12–18 years 10 mg

Diabetic hypoglycaemia

(section 6.1.4)

Glucose or **sucrose**

- By mouth
  Child 2–18 years approx. 10–20 g (2–4 teaspoonfuls of sugar or 3–6 sugar lumps or 55–110 mL *Lucozade® Energy Original* or 100–200 mL *Coca-Cola®*—both non-diet versions or *Glucogel®* one or two 25-g tubes (containing glucose 10 g/25–g tube), repeated after 10–15 minutes if necessary

or if **hypoglycaemia unresponsive** *or* if oral route cannot be used

Glucagon injection 1 mg/mL

- By subcutaneous, intramuscular or intravenous injection
  Child body-weight under 25 kg 500 micrograms (0.5 mL)
  Child body-weight over 25 kg 1 mg (1 mL)

or if **hypoglycaemia prolonged** *or* unresponsive to glucagon after 10 minutes

Glucose intravenous infusion 10%

- By intravenous injection into large vein
  Child 1 month–18 years 5 mL/kg (glucose 500 mg/kg)

Meningococcal disease

(Table 1, section 5.1)

Benzylpenicillin sodium injection 600 mg, 1.2 g

- By intravenous injection (or by intramuscular injection if venous access not available)
  Neonate 300 mg
  Child 1 month–1 year 300 mg
  Child 1–10 years 600 mg
  Child 10–18 years 1.2 g
  Note Give single dose and transfer urgently to hospital

or if history of allergy to penicillin

Cefotaxime injection 1 g

- By intravenous injection (or by intramuscular injection if venous access not available)
  Neonate 50 mg/kg
  Child 1 month–12 years 50 mg/kg (max. 1 g)
  Child 12–18 years 1 g
  Note Give single dose and transfer urgently to hospital

or if history of immediate hypersensitivity reaction (including anaphylaxis, angioedema or urticarial reaction) to penicillin or to cephalosporins

Chloramphenicol injection 1 g

- By intravenous injection
  Child 1 month–18 years 12.5–25 mg/kg
  Note Give single dose and transfer urgently to hospital

Pneumonia: uncomplicated

(Table 1, section 5.1)

Amoxicillin oral suspension 125 mg/5 mL, 250 mg/5 mL; capsules 250 mg

- By mouth
  Child 6 months–1 year 125 mg 3 times daily
  Child 1–5 years 250 mg 3 times daily
  Child 5–18 years 500 mg 3 times daily

or if allergic to penicillin *or* atypical organism suspected

Erythromycin oral suspension 125 mg/5 mL, 250 mg/5 mL; tablets 250 mg

- By mouth
  Child 6 months–2 years 125 mg 4 times daily
  Child 2–8 years 250 mg 4 times daily
  Child 8–18 years 250–500 mg 4 times daily

Prescribing for children

Weight, height, and gender

The table below shows the **mean values** for weight, height and gender by age; these values have been derived from the UK-WHO growth charts 2009 and UK1990 standard centile charts, by extrapolating the 50th centile, and may be used to calculate doses in the absence of actual measurements. However, the child's actual weight and height might vary considerably from the values in the table and it is important to see the child to ensure that the value chosen is appropriate. In most cases the child's actual measurement should be obtained as soon as possible and the dose re-calculated.

Age	Weight kg	Height cm
Full term neonate	3.5	51
1 month	4.3	55
2 months	5.4	58
3 months	6.1	61
4 months	6.7	63
6 months	7.6	67
1 year	9	75
3 years	14	96
5 years	18	109
7 years	23	122
10 years	32	138
12 years	39	149
14 year-old boy	49	163
14 year-old girl	50	159
Adult male	68	176
Adult female	58	164

Approximate conversions and units

lb	kg	stones	kg	mL	fl oz
1	0.45	1	6.35	50	1.8
2	0.91	2	12.70	100	3.5
3	1.36	3	19.05	150	5.3
4	1.81	4	25.40	200	7.0
5	2.27	5	31.75	500	17.6
6	2.72	6	38.10	1000	35.2
7	3.18	7	44.45		
8	3.63	8	50.80		
9	4.08	9	57.15		
10	4.54	10	63.50		
11	4.99	11	69.85		
12	5.44	12	76.20		
13	5.90	13	82.55		
14	6.35	14	88.90		
		15	95.25		

Length

1 metre (m)		= 1000 millimetres (mm)
1 centimetre (cm)		= 10 mm
1 inch (in)		= 25.4 mm
1 foot (ft)	=12 inches	= 304.8 mm

Mass

1 kilogram (kg)	= 1000 grams (g)
1 gram (g)	= 1000 milligrams (mg)
1 milligram (mg)	= 1000 micrograms
1 microgram	= 1000 nanograms
1 nanogram	= 1000 picograms

Volume

1 litre	= 1000 millilitres (mL)
1 millilitre (1 mL)	= 1000 microlitres
1 pint	≈ 568 mL

Other units

1 kilocalorie (kcal)	= 4186.8 joules (J)
1000 kilocalories (kcal)	= 4.1868 megajoules (MJ)
1 megajoule (MJ)	= 238.8 kilocalories (kcal)
1 millimetre of mercury (mmHg)	= 133.3 pascals (Pa)
1 kilopascal (kPa)	= 7.5 mmHg (pressure)

Plasma-drug concentrations in *BNF for Children* are expressed in mass units per litre (e.g. mg/litre). The approximate equivalent in terms of amount of substance units (e.g. micromol/litre) is given in brackets.

Recommended wording of cautionary and advisory labels

For details see Appendix 3

1 Warning. May cause drowsiness

2 Warning. May cause drowsiness. If affected do not drive or operate machinery. Avoid alcoholic drink

3 Warning. May cause drowsiness. If affected do not drive or operate machinery

4 Warning. Avoid alcoholic drink

5 Do not take indigestion remedies at the same time of day as this medicine

6 Do not take indigestion remedies or medicines containing iron or zinc at the same time of day as this medicine

7 Do not take milk, indigestion remedies, or medicines containing iron or zinc at the same time of day as this medicine

8 Do not stop taking this medicine except on your doctor's advice

9 Take at regular intervals. Complete the prescribed course unless otherwise directed

10 Warning. Follow the printed instructions you have been given with this medicine

11 Avoid exposure of skin to direct sunlight or sun lamps

12 Do not take anything containing aspirin while taking this medicine

13 Dissolve or mix with water before taking

14 This medicine may colour the urine

15 Caution flammable: keep away from fire or flames

16 Allow to dissolve under the tongue. Do not transfer from this container. Keep tightly closed. Discard 8 weeks after opening

17 Do not take more than ... in 24 hours

18 Do not take more than ... in 24 hours or ... in any one week

19 Warning. Causes drowsiness which may continue the next day. If affected do not drive or operate machinery. Avoid alcoholic drink

21 ... with or after food

22 ... half to one hour before food

23 ... an hour before food or on an empty stomach

24 ... sucked or chewed

25 ... swallowed whole, not chewed

26 ... dissolved under the tongue

27 ... with plenty of water

28 To be spread thinly ...

29 Do not take more than 2 at any one time. Do not take more than 8 in 24 hours

30 Do not take with any other paracetamol products

31 Contains aspirin and paracetamol. Do not take with any other paracetamol products

32 Contains aspirin

33 Contains an aspirin-like medicine